Oxford Textbook of

Medicine

Project Administrator	Anna McNeil
Project Editor	Dr Irene Butcher
Indexer	Caroline Sheard
Production Manager	Kate Martin
Production Editor	Anna Campbell
Design Manager	Andrew Meaden
Typographer	Jonathan Coleclough
Illustrations	Touch Media, Abingdon
Publisher	Alison Langton

volume **1**

Oxford Textbook of
Medicine
Fourth Edition
Volume 1: Sections 1–10

Edited by

David A. Warrell

Professor of Tropical Medicine and Infectious Diseases and Head, Nuffield Department of Clinical Medicine, University of Oxford; Honorary Consultant Physician, Oxford Radcliffe NHS Trust, UK

Timothy M. Cox

Professor of Medicine, University of Cambridge; Honorary Consultant Physician, Addenbrooke's Hospital, Cambridge, UK

and

John D. Firth

Consultant Physician and Nephrologist Addenbrooke's Hospital, Cambridge, UK

with

Edward J. Benz Jr

President and CEO, Dana Farber Cancer Institute; Richard and Susan Smith, Professor of Medicine, Professor of Pediatrics and Professor of Pathology, Harvard Medical School, Boston, USA

OXFORD
UNIVERSITY PRESS

OXFORD

UNIVERSITY PRESS

Great Clarendon Street, Oxford OX2 6DP

Oxford University Press is a department of the University of Oxford.
It furthers the University's objective of excellence in research, scholarship,
and education by publishing worldwide in

Oxford New York

Auckland Cape Town Dar es Salaam Hong Kong Karachi
Kuala Lumpur Madrid Melbourne Mexico City Nairobi
New Delhi Shanghai Taipei Toronto

With offices in

Argentina Austria Brazil Chile Czech Republic France Greece
Guatemala Hungary Italy Japan Poland Portugal Singapore
South Korea Switzerland Thailand Turkey Ukraine Vietnam

Oxford is a registered trade mark of Oxford University Press
in the UK and in certain other countries

Published in the United States
by Oxford University Press Inc., New York

First published 1983
Second edition published 1987
Third edition published 1996
Fourth edition published 2003
Fourth edition (paperback) published 2005

British Library Cataloguing in Publication Data
Data available

Library of Congress Cataloging in Publication Data
Data available

Typeset by Interactive Sciences Ltd., Gloucester, England
Printed in Italy
on acid-free paper by LegoPrint

ISBN 0–19–856978–5   978–0–19–856978–7 (3 volume set)
Volume 1: 0–19–857014–7 978–0–19–857014–1
Volume 2: 0–19–857015–5 978–0–19–857015–8
Volume 3: 0–19–857013–9 978–0–19–857013–4
Available as 3 volume set only

10 9 8 7 6 5 4 3 2 1

The title page of the 1492 edition of *Rosa Anglica* by John of Gaddesden (1280–1361), which was probably written in 1314. The author was a well known physician attached to Merton College, Oxford in the early part of the 14th century. His famous book was probably the first 'Oxford Textbook of Medicine'. The author was the model for the unsavoury Doctor of Physick in Chaucer's *Canterbury Tales*.

Foreword

by Professor Sir David Weatherall, FRS

It is now 20 years since the first edition of the *Oxford Textbook of Medicine* appeared on the scene, a time when the concept of the all-encompassing textbook of medicine was being questioned. Its predecessor, *Price's Textbook of the Practice of Medicine*, first published in 1922 and by then in its twelfth edition, had come under considerable criticism. One of its most voluble critics, the late J.R.A. Mitchell, had even gone to the trouble of weighing the book, after which he suggested that, because dinosaurs became extinct because of their sheer bulk, medical textbooks would suffer the same fate. In addition, he and many other reviewers suggested that large textbooks are out of date before they are published and hence are of extremely limited value. Notwithstanding Professor Mitchell's outdated views on the extinction of dinosaurs, we thought that he had a point.

After considering these arguments carefully we came to the conclusion that there was still a place for at least one major British work of reference which attempted to cover the whole field of internal medicine. This decision was based largely on the view that, because of the enormous breadth of the subject and the increasing tendency to overspecialization, very few students and practitioners could have immediate access to smaller monographs on every branch of the field; even when they are available they are not always written by those who evaluate their patients in a general medical setting. And if this is true of clinicians in the richer countries, it must apply even more to those in the developing world, where access to libraries and review articles may be limited. Furthermore, although we were well aware that textbooks rapidly become out of date, few advances in medicine lead to major changes in patient care, and those that do often require many years of critical evaluation before they become an integral part of routine clinical practice. For this reason we decided to try to produce a wide-ranging medical textbook which would have a particular emphasis on the global aspects of disease, rather than focus simply on the day-to-day medical problems of the developed world.

Since the *Oxford Textbook of Medicine* first appeared there have been profound changes, both in the practice of medicine and in the problems of the provision of medical care. None of the richer countries has been able to solve the problem of the spiralling costs of health care, which have resulted in part from the introduction of new technology but, even more importantly, from the remarkable increase in the age of their patient populations. If anything, the gap between the quality of the provision of health care between the richer and poorer countries has widened, and although some of the poorer countries have made the epidemiological transition from high death rates due to infection and malnutrition towards a more westernized pattern of illness, particularly in sub-Saharan Africa infectious disease, notably respiratory infection, AIDS, tuberculosis, and malaria, remain the major causes of death; a review of over 11 million childhood deaths in 1998 disclosed, disgracefully, that over 4 million were due to diseases for which adequate vaccines or other forms of prevention already exist. The phenomena of 'globalization', and increasing corporate dominance, are also tending to exacerbate the divide between the rich and poor nations.

Another profound change which has occurred over the last 20 years is the emphasis on the study of disease at the molecular and cellular levels and the increasing role of what is still rather optimistically called 'molecular medicine'. But while this remarkable field promises much for the health of mankind for the future, so far it has had little place in day-to-day clinical practice. Thus, while the fruits of the human genome project offer enormous potential for the better understanding, prevention, and management of the common killers of middle life and old age in richer societies, and the pathogen genome projects offer equal hope for controlling the infectious killers of the developing countries, it is still far from clear when the rich promises of these fields will come to fruition for preventative medicine and clinical care. And there is the danger that when they do, because many of them are likely to be expensive, the gap between the provision of health care in the poorer and richer countries will become even wider. Although many of the solutions to these problems depend on a complete change of attitude of governments and industry in the richer countries, there is no doubt that there will be a rapidly increasing role for their medical schools and doctors to develop collaborative programmes with those of the developing countries and, in general, to take a much more global view of disease, both in medical education and research.

The other major change in the medical field over the last 20 years has been the increasing disquiet about the pattern of medical practice. In many countries doctors have come under increasing criticism for their lack of ability to communicate adequately with patients, for their quality of patient care and, overall, for their lack of humanity. The patient community has become much more sophisticated and demanding, and in most countries there has been a rapid increase in the number of medico-legal actions taken against doctors. This trend has already had wide-ranging repercussions. There has been a major rethink about the pattern of medical education, placing less emphasis on its scientific basis and more on communication skills, ethics, and the social aspects of medicine. The remarkable revolution in the basic biological sciences that underlie medical practice, particularly in the field of genomics, is also raising new ethical issues which would have been undreamed of at the time of the first edition of this book.

In short, medical practice has entered the new millennium in a state of considerable uncertainty. The whole ethos of clinical practice is being questioned, none of the richer countries has got to grips with how to finance the increasing demands of medical care, and many of the poorer countries still have completely dysfunctional health care systems. It is very pleasing therefore to see that the new edition of the *Oxford Textbook of Medicine* reflects so many of these changing issues, as they affect internal medicine. In particular, the textbook has maintained and expanded the aspirations of its original editors towards providing a genuinely global picture of disease, not just as it affects the populations of the richer countries but as it involves the lives of all of those in the poorer countries of the world. As well as continuing to describe the major causes of ill-health and death in the populations of the poorer countries, it includes new sections on screening and the costs of health care, and has greatly increased its coverage of some of the major infectious killers, particularly HIV/AIDS. At the other end of the spectrum it has expanded its sections on the molecular mechanisms of disease and tried to put molecular medicine into perspective by defining its limits. And it has not ignored the remarkable advances in medicine which relate to the richer countries, particularly in its coverage of the problems of the aged. In doing so it has focused on the major killers of Western society, notably cancer, heart disease, and stroke, and has greatly increased the coverage of critical care and emergency medicine. This extensive revision has required the recruitment of many new authors, reflecting a change of over one-third of those from the last edition.

After the publication of the last edition of the *Oxford Textbook of Medicine* my colleague John Ledingham and I decided that it was time to stand aside and pass on our editorial roles to a younger team of editors who are still very active in the fields of medical research and practice. We are delighted to see that our younger colleagues have maintained the tradition of producing a broad-ranging medical textbook which emphasizes the pastoral, scientific, and global aspects of medical care. Despite all its problems medical practice is entering the most exciting and challenging period of its development, and we believe that it still offers the most exciting and enriching of careers for its practitioners. We trust that the 'OTM' will remain their guide and friend for many years to come.

Preface

Textbooks of medicine: *raison d'etre*

Now, in the third millennium, is there any need for a textbook of medicine? Never before has so much information on medical matters been so readily available to so many: physicians are inundated, as are their patients and everyone else. The media seem to carry more and more medical stories in more and more detail every day. The genome has been sequenced. Articulate teenagers speak of stem cells. The internet brings widespread and virtually unlimited access to biomedical information (and misinformation) of a sort: one click of a mouse, and it's all anyone's. A plethora of organizations besieges physicians with guidelines and protocols on every aspect of the practice of medicine. Traditional values are being challenged in all facets of life, including medicine, and there is an unprecedented and entirely appropriate demand for supportive evidence, not just weight of experience, to justify medical interventions.

In these circumstances, some might argue that textbooks of medicine were irrelevant, inappropriate, or even redundant. We strongly refute this. Amidst the maelstrom of 'information' in which physicians now work there is, more than ever, a need for a fixed point of reference, something by which the new, the exciting, and the fashionable can be judged. We make the bold claim that the *Oxford Textbook of Medicine* is just such a fixed point. We argue, unashamedly, that a clinical textbook in the Oslerian tradition is not only required but is essential, to provide expert review, evaluation, and recommendation.

Clinical medicine: changes, challenges, and reconsiderations

This fourth edition of the *Oxford Textbook of Medicine* emerges at a time when discoveries in molecular sciences and advances in technology provide an unprecedented range of diagnostic reagents, drugs, and bioinformatics. Yet, at the same time, there is a widespread recognition that the outcome of treatment for many patients falls short of ideal standards. Microbial resistance to antibiotics, adverse consequences of drugs, and the fallibility of doctors all contribute to failures; and we now realize how dangerous hospitals and clinics can be. Besides this, many contemporary high-tech procedures cannot cure chronic illnesses, and we lack effective weapons to influence the powerful social and behavioural factors that underlie so much illness. The advent of predictive DNA testing also poses complex ethical questions for practitioners, for which few answers are available.

Advances in biomedical science crucially drive innovation and improvement in medical practice. These are not neglected in this book, but the practice of medicine (except in dire emergency) is initiated by a patient talking with a physician and proceeds (as appropriate) through physical examination and investigation to discussion of diagnosis, prognosis, and treatment. These are the core issues of clinical medicine which form the bulk of this textbook.

A culture of public mistrust: the physician–patient relationship

Our political masters in much of the developed world, long tired of being marginalized by old-established networks within the professions, have introduced a new accountability distilled from the concept of audit. This has been exported from the world of finance to embrace the scrutiny of non-financial processes in health care and has created a political climate obsessed with cost effectiveness. The degree of central control often leads to impossible conflicts in the expectations of the public and those entrusted with provision of health care. Baroness O'Neil in her BBC Reith Lectures of 2002* has pointed out that there is often an inconsistency in the demands raised by such control, providing, as it does, perverse incentives for the specious goals and 'output measures' determined by central bodies. While it is true that much better standards of health care delivery are required and careful surveillance of clinical activities is desirable, the *Oxford Textbook of Medicine* presents an affirmation of the physician–patient relationship in the fight against illness, debility, and suffering: for this relationship should remain sacrosanct, based on professional integrity, knowledge, and human feeling.

Aims and emphases: Sir Archibald Garrod's legacy

Garrod first understood the unique interactions between heredity and environment in the genesis of human disease and asked the question: 'Why did this particular person develop this particular illness in this particular environment?' – a question that we are only just beginning to answer in an era of almost naïve enthusiasm for genetics. While the study of the invariant factors in human genetics is almost intoxicating in its simplicity, we now face the formidable challenge of identifying the contribution of the environment, with all its attendant variables, to the generation of the clinical phenotype we define as illness.

This is the background to this edition of the *Oxford Textbook of Medicine*: its remit stretches from disease as it presents to physicians at the bedside, to the attendant disturbances of cellular, tissue, and organ function, all occurring within an individual, inevitably a part of the turmoil of society. To have a complete description of all these aspects of any medical complaint would not be possible, but we recognize that many readers will not have ready access to the latest sources of scientific information. The book is therefore designed to be a proper reference point for both scientific and clinical aspects of medical practice and bears the fingerprints of Osler, Garrod, Doll, and Weatherall, all Regius Professors of Medicine in Oxford.

Limitations and strengths

The bitter practicalities of writing, editing, and producing any book, especially a work of this size, prevent its referring to the last edition of *The*

---

* *A Question of Trust.* Cambridge University Press 2002.

Lancet, Quarterly Journal of Medicine, New England Journal of Medicine, or any other periodical. But this book can and does provide the medical background against which new information should be assessed and understood. Grounded in the principles that have made the first three editions standard reference textbooks, the new edition has, like medicine itself, evolved to bring all contemporary resources to focus on the teaching and interpretation of medicine. Many new approaches and topics are included and we have incorporated the skill, experience, and perspectives of a truly international complement of highly distinguished authors, including the recently honoured Nobel Laureate in Medicine, Dr Sydney Brenner.

This fourth edition includes, for the first time, an editorial adviser based in the United States (EJB) and a greatly increased and broadened representation of North American authors. By adopting this approach, we hope we have been able to integrate and synthesize in this edition the perspectives on shared medical issues as they confront physicians and medical scientists in different countries.

At a time when there is a tendency for physicians in some parts of the world to be more and more proficient about less and less, this book is a means of their grasping what is happening and what is important in all areas of medical practice. When the movement of people, diseases, and doctors around the world is greater than ever, there is a need for a truly global perspective, which this book provides.

Acknowledgements

This edition contains much that is entirely new, but we wish here to acknowledge that it is built on the firm foundations established by the distinguished co-editors of the previous editions, Professor Sir David Weath-

erall and Professor John Ledingham. No work of this kind can be produced without the engagement of dedicated professionals who believe in publishing and commit themselves way beyond healthy expectations to see the task through. Mrs Alison Langton has provided guidance and discipline throughout the production and we are enormously grateful to her and her staff at Oxford University Press for their confidence, commitment, and friendship. We are particularly indebted to Dr Irene Butcher who has worked indefatigably to help us realize our aims and at every level has contributed to the organization of the final text and its complex illustrative material. Her experience, knowledge, and uncompromising attention to detail must surely be unique; her forbearance with the editors and, on rare occasions, errant contributors, has been nothing short of miraculous. We thank our contributors for their patience in delivering their sections and review of proofs for which they are responsible. Ultimately, however, the book and any errors it might contain remain the responsibility of the editors.

Finally we thank Mary, Sue, Helen, and Peggy, our constant, supportive, and forgiving wives; Professor Sir David Weatherall, Professor Alastair Compston, Dr Graham Neale, Professor Michael de Swiet, and Dr Michael Sharpe our section advisers; Professor David Lomas, Professor Julian Hopkin, Professor Michael Doherty, Professor David Isenberg, and Dr Christopher Winearls who gave advice and comment for which the editors are very grateful; and our personal secretaries, Eunice Berry (a veteran of four editions), Joan Grantham, Janet Cameron, Naoe Suzuki, and Beverly Comegys for their exceptional dedication.

Oxford, Cambridge, and Boston   DAW, TMC, JDF, EJB
January 2003

Contents

15 Cardiovascular medicine

17 Respiratory medicine

Volume 3

18 Rheumatology

19 Diseases of the skeleton

20 Nephrology

        D. J. S. Carmichael

21 Sexually-transmitted diseases and sexual health

21.1 Epidemiology 479
       M. W. Adler and A. Meheus

21.2 Sexual behaviour 484
       Anne M. Johnson

21.3 Vaginal discharge 486
       J. Schwebke and S. L. Hillier

21.4 Pelvic inflammatory disease 489
       David Eschenbach

21.5 Infections and other medical problems in homosexual men 491
       A. McMillan

21.6 Cervical cancer and other cancers caused by sexually tramsmitted infections 496
       V. Beral

22 Disorders of the blood

22.1 Introduction 501
       D. J. Weatherall

22.2 Haematopoietic stem cells 508

       22.2.1 Stem cells and haemopoiesis 508
                C. A. Sieff and D. G. Nathan

       22.2.2 Stem-cell disorders 515
                D. C. Linch

22.3 The leukaemias and other disorders of haematopoietic stem cells 520

       22.3.1 Cell and molecular biology of human leukaemias 520
                Thomas Look

       22.3.2 The classification of leukaemia 525
                D. Catovsky

       22.3.3 Acute lymphoblastic leukaemia 529
                Philip J. Burke

       22.3.4 Acute myeloblastic leukaemia 533
                Philip J. Burke

       22.3.5 Chronic lymphocytic leukaemia and other leukaemias of mature B and T cells 539
                D. Catovsky

       22.3.6 Chronic myeloid leukaemia 546
                Tariq I. Mughal and John M. Goldman

       22.3.7 Myelodysplasia 552
                Lawrence B. Gardner and Chi V. Dang

       22.3.8 The polycythaemias 557
                David M. Gustin and Ronald Hoffman

       22.3.9 Idiopathic myelofibrosis 564
                Jerry L. Spivak

       22.3.10 Thrombocytosis 568
                 David M. Gustin and Ronald Hoffman

       22.3.11 Aplastic anaemia and other causes of bone marrow failure 573
                 E. C. Gordon-Smith

       22.3.12 Paroxysmal nocturnal haemoglobinuria 581
                 Lucio Luzzatto

22.4 The white cells and lymphoproliferative disorders 585

       22.4.1 Leucocytes in health and disease 585
                Joseph Sinning and Nancy Berliner

       22.4.2 Introduction to the lymphoproliferative disorders 591
                Barbara A. Degar and Nancy Berliner

       22.4.3 Lymphoma 595
                James O. Armitage

       22.4.4 The spleen and its disorders 609
                D. Swirsky

       22.4.5 Myeloma and paraproteinaemias 616
                Robert A. Kyle

       22.4.6 Eosinophilia 624
                Peter F. Weller

       22.4.7 Histiocytoses 629
                D. K. H. Webb

22.5 The red cell 634

       22.5.1 Erythropoiesis and the normal red cell 634
                Anna Rita Migliaccio and Thalia Papayannopoulou

       22.5.2 Anaemia: pathophysiology, classification, and clinical features 639
                D. J. Weatherall

       22.5.3 Anaemia as a world health problem 644
                D. J. Weatherall

       22.5.4 Iron metabolism and its disorders 648
                T. M. Cox

       22.5.5 Normochromic, normocytic anaemia 657
                D. J. Weatherall

       22.5.6 Megaloblastic anaemia and miscellaneous deficiency anaemias 659
                A. V. Hoffbrand

       22.5.7 Disorders of the synthesis or function of haemoglobin 676
                D. J. Weatherall

       22.5.8 Anaemias resulting from defective red cell maturation 696
                James S. Wiley

25 The eye

26 Psychiatry and drug related problems

Contributors

P. Aaby Research Professor (Novo Nordisk Foundation), Bandim Health Project, Bissau, Guinea-Bissau.
7.10.6 Measles

J. P. Ackers Professor of Postgraduate Education in Public Health, London School of Hygiene and Tropical Medicine, UK.
7.13.13 Trichomoniasis

M. W. Adler Professor of Genitourinary Medicine, Department of Sexually Transmitted Diseases, Royal Free and University College Medical School, London, UK.
21.1 Epidemiology

D. Adu Consultant Nephrologist, Queen Elizabeth Hospital, Birmingham, UK.
20.7.4 Minimal-change nephropathy, focal segmental glomerulosclerosis, and membranous nephtopathy. 20.10.4 The kidney in rheumatological disorders

Graeme J. M. Alexander University Lecturer in Medicine and Honorary Consultant Physician/Hepatologist, University of Cambridge School of Clinical Medicine, Addenbrooke's Hospital, Cambridge, UK.
14.21.4 Liver transplantation

M. Allison Consultant Hepatologist, Hepatobiliary and Transplant Unit, Addenbrooke's Hospital, Cambridge, UK.
5.5 Innate immune system. 14.21.4 Liver transplantation

Chris Andrews Registrar in Anaesthesia, Mater Misericordiae Hospitals, South Brisbane, Queensland, Australia.
8.5.7 Lightning and electrical injuries

Philip Anslow Consultant Neuroradiologist, Radcliffe Infirmary, Oxford, UK.
24.5 Imaging in neurological diseases

Mark J. Arends Senior Lecturer and Honorary Consultant, Pathology Department, University of Cambridge, UK.
4.6 Apoptosis in health and disease

James O. Armitage Dean, College of Medicine, University of Nebraska Medical Center, Omaha, Nebraska, USA.
22.4.3 Lymphoma

J. K. Aronson Reader in Clinical Pharmacology, Radcliffe Infirmary, Oxford, UK.
15.5.1 Pharmacological management of heart failure

Frances M. Ashcroft Royal Society GlaxoSmithKline Research Professor, University Laboratory of Physiology, Oxford, UK.
4.5 Ion channels and disease

T. C. Aw Professor and Head of Division of Occupational Health, Kent Institute of Medicine and Health Sciences, University of Kent at Canterbury, UK.
8.4.1 Occupational and environmental health and safety. 8.5.10 Noise. 8.5.11 Vibration

M. Bagshaw Head of Occupational and Aviation Medicine, British Airways, Harmondsworth, UK.
8.5.5 Aerospace medicine

E. L. Baker Decatur, Georgia, UK.
8.4.1 Occupational and environmental health and safety

L. R. I. Baker Consultant Physician and Nephrologist, London Clinic, London, UK.
20.14 Urinary tract obstruction

C. R. M. Bangham Professor of Immunology, Imperial College Faculty of Medicine, London, UK.
7.10.23 HTLV-I and II and associated diseases

A. P. Banning Consultant Cardiologist, John Radcliffe Hospital, Oxford, UK.
15.3.3 Echocardiography. 15.14.1 Thoracic aortic dissection

D. J. P. Barker Director, MRC Environmental Epidemiology Unit, University of Southampton, UK.
15.4.1.1 Influences acting in utero and early childhood

Roger Barker University Lecturer and Honorary Consultant in Neurology, Department of Neurology, Addenbrooke's Hospital, Cambridge, UK.
24.13.11 Disorders of movement (excluding Parkinson's disease)

D. Barlow Consultant Physician, Department of Genitourinary Medicine, St Thomas's Hospital, London, UK.
7.11.6 Neisseria gonorrhoeae

M. P. Barnes Professor of Neurological Rehabilitation, Hunters Moor Regional Rehabilitation Centre, Newcastle upon Tyne, UK.
24.13.17 Spinal cord injury and its management

John G. Bartlett Chief, Division of Infectious Diseases, Johns Hopkins University School of Medicine, Baltimore, Maryland, USA.
17.5.2.1 Pneumonia—normal host. 17.5.2.2 Nosocomial pneumonia

Christopher Bass Consultant in Liaison Psychiatry, Department of Psychological Medicine, John Radcliffe Hospital, Oxford, UK.
26.5.3 Medically unexplained symptoms in patients attending medical clinics

M. F. Bassendine Professor of Hepatology, Centre for Liver Research, The Medical School, University of Newcastle upon Tyne, UK.
14.20.2.2 Primary biliary cirrhosis

David Bates Professor of Clinical Neurology, Department of Neurology, University of Newcastle upon Tyne, UK.
24.9 Brainstem syndromes. 24.13.1 The unconscious patient

Robert P. Baughman University of Cincinnati Medical Centre, Ohio, USA.
17.11.6 Sarcoidosis

Peter J. Baxter Consultant Physician, Occupational and Environmental Medicine, University of Cambridge, UK.
8.5.12 Disasters: earthquakes, volcanic eruptions, hurricanes, and floods

Peter H. Baylis Provost and Dean of Faculty of Medical Sciences, University of Newcastle upon Tyne, UK.
20.2.1 Water and sodium homeostasis and their disorders

D. Gareth Beevers Professor of Medicine, City Hospital, Birmingham, UK.
15.16.3 Hypertensive emergencies and urgencies

Michael L. Bennish Director, Africa Centre for Health and Population Studies, Mtubatuba, South Africa.
7.11.11 Cholera

M. K. Benson Consultant Physician, Oxford Centre for Respiratory Medicine, Churchill Hospital, Oxford, UK.
17.12 Pleural disease. 17.14.2 Pleural tumours. 17.14.3 Mediastinal tumours and cysts

V. Beral Head, Cancer Research UK Epidemiology Unit, Radcliffe Infirmary, Oxford, UK.
21.6 Cervical cancer and other cancers caused by sexually tramsmitted infections

Anthony R. Berendt Consultant Physician-in-Charge, Bone Infection Unit, Nuffield Orthopaedic Centre, Oxford, UK.
18.7.1 Pyogenic arthritis. 19.3 Osteomyelitis

Nancy Berliner Professor of Medicine and Genetics, Yale School of Medicine, New Haven, Connecticut, USA.
22.4.1 Leucocytes in health and disease. 22.4.2 Introduction to the lymphoproliferative disorders

Michael Besser Professor of Medicine Emeritus, Bart's and The London School of Medicine and Dentistry, Queen Mary College, London, UK.
12.2 Disorders of the anterior pituitary. 12.3 Disorders of the posterior pituitary

Delia B. Bethell Specialist Registrar in Paediatrics, Department of Paediatrics, John Radcliffe Hospital, Oxford, UK.
7.11.1 Diphtheria

Ernest Beutler Chairman, Department of Molecular and Experimental Medicine, The Scripps Research Institute, La Jolla, California, USA.
22.5.11 Erythrocyte enzymopathies

P. C. L. Beverley Professor and Scientific Head, Edward Jenner Institute for Vaccine Research, Compton, Berkshire, UK.
6.5 Tumour immunology

R. W. Bilous Professor of Clinical Medicine, James Cook University Hospital, Middlesbrough, Cleveland, UK.
20.10.1 Diabetes mellitus and the kidney

D. Bilton Consultant in Respiratory Medicine, Papworth Hospital, Cambridge, UK.
17.9 Bronchiectasis

A. E. Bishop Senior Lecturer, Tissue Engineering and Regenerative Medicine Centre, Chelsea and Westminster Hospital, London, UK.
14.8 Hormones and the gastrointestinal tract

Carol M. Black President of the Royal College of Physicians of London and Professor of Rheumatology, Royal Free and University College Medical School, Royal Free Campus, London, UK.
18.10.3 Systemic sclerosis

S. R. Bloom Professor of Medicine and Head, Division of Investigative Science, Imperial College Faculty of Medicine, Hammersmith Campus, London, UK.
12.10 Non-diabetic pancreatic endocrine disorders and multiple endocrine neoplasia. 14.8 Hormones and the gastrointestinal tract

L. D. Blumhardt Emeritus Professor of Clinical Neurology, University of Nottingham, UK.
24.13.5 Syncope. 24.13.16 Diseases of the spinal cord

N. Boon Consultant Cardiologist, Royal Infirmary of Edinburgh, UK.
15.10.4 Cardiac disease in HIV infection

D. R. Booth Senior Hospital Scientist, Institute for Immunology and Allergy Research, Westmead Millennium Institute, Sydney, New South Wales, Australia.
11.12.3 Familial Mediterranean fever and other inherited periodic fever syndromes

Richard T. Booth Professor, Health and Safety Unit, Aston University, Birmingham, UK.
8.4.2 Occupational safety

Leszek K. Borysiewicz Professor and Principal of the Faculty of Medicine, University of Wales, Cardiff, UK.
7.4 The host response to infection

I. C. J. W. Bowler Consultant Microbiologist, Department of Microbiology, John Radcliffe Hospital, Oxford, UK.
7.9 Nosocomial infections

D. J. Bradley Ross Professor of Tropical Hygiene, London School of Hygiene and Tropical Medicine, UK.
7.13.2 Malaria

Thomas Brandt Klinikum Grosshadern, Munich, Germany.
24.12.1 Eye movements and balance

P. Brandtzaeg Professor of Paediatrics, Ullevål University Hospital, University of Oslo, Norway.
7.11.5 Meningococcal infections

P. Brasseur Professor and Head of Department of Parasitology, Faculty of Medicine, Rouen, France.
7.13.3 Babesia

J. Braun Professor and Medical Director, Rheumazentrum Ruhrgebiet, Herne, Germany.
18.6 Spondyloarthritides and related arthritides

Sydney Brenner Research Professor, Salk Institute, La Jolla, California, USA, and Honorary Professor of Genetic Medicine, University of Cambridge, UK.
4.2 The human genome sequence

D. P. Brenton Sub Dean (Curriculum), Royal Free and University College Medical School, London, UK.
11.2 Inborn errors of amino acid and organic acid metabolism

Paul H. Brion Rheumatologist in Private Practice, Vista, California, USA.
18.8 Osteoarthritis

Julian Britton Consultant Surgeon, John Radcliffe Hospital, Oxford, UK.
14.3.1 The acute abdomen. 14.18.3.3 Tumours of the pancreas

Anthony F. T. Brown Associate Professor and Senior Staff Specialist, Department of Emergency Medicine, Royal Brisbane Hospital, Queensland, Australia.
16.4 Anaphylaxis

M. J. Brown Professor of Clinical Pharmacology, University of Cambridge and Honorary Consultant Physician, Addenbrooke's Hospital NHS Trust, Cambridge, UK.
15.16.2.3 Primary hyperaldosteronism (Conn's syndrome). 15.16.2.4 Phaeochromocytoma

A. D. M. Bryceson Emeritus Professor of Tropical Medicine, London School of Hygiene and Tropical Medicine, UK.
7.13.12 Leishmaniasis

Philip J. Burke Johns Hopkins Oncology Center, Baltimore, Maryland, USA.
22.3.3 Acute lymphoblastic leukaemia. 22.3.4 Acute myeloblastic leukaemia

G. M. Burnham Associate Professor of International Health, Johns Hopkins Bloomberg School of Public Health, Baltimore, Maryland, USA.
7.14.1 Cutaneous filariasis

Jacky Burrin Professor of Experimental Endocrinology, Bart's and The London School of Medicine and Dentistry, St Bartholomew's Hospital, London, UK.
12.1 Principles of hormone action

Andy Bush Reader in Paediatric Respirology, London, UK.
17.10 Cystic fibrosis

K. Bushby Professor of Neuromuscular Genetics, Institute of Human Genetics, Newcastle upon Tyne, UK.
24.22.2 Muscular dystrophy

Anthony Busuttil Regius Professor of Forensic Medicine, Forensic Medicine Section, Edinburgh University Medical School, UK.
27 Forensic medicine and the practising doctor

T. Butler Professor of Internal Medicine and Chief of Infectious Diseases, Texas Technical University Health Sciences Center, Lubbock, Texas, USA.
7.11.16 Plague

W. F. Bynum Professor of History of Medicine, Wellcome Trust Centre for the History of Medicine at University College London, UK.
2.1 Science in medicine: when, how, and what

I. Byren Consultant in Infectious Diseases and Genito-Urinary Medicine, John Radcliffe Hospital, Oxford, UK.
15.10.3 Cardiovascular syphilis

John Calam* Professor of Medicine, Imperial College London, UK.
14.7 Peptic ulcer diseases

Donald B. Calne Professor Emeritus, University of British Columbia, Vancouver, Canada.
24.13.10 Parkinsonism and other extrapyramidal diseases

P. M. A. Calverley Professor of Medicine (Pulmonary and Rehabilitation), Clinical Science Centre, University Hospital Aintree, Liverpool, UK.
17.7 Chronic respiratory failure

Giovambattista Capasso Professor of Nephrology, Second University of Naples, Italy.
20.13 Urinary stones, nephrocalcinosis, and renal tubular acidosis

---

* It is with regret that we report the death of Professor John Calam during the preparation of this edition of the textbook.

Jonathan R. Carapetis Senior Lecturer, Research Fellow, and Consultant in Infectious Diseases, Centre for International Child Health, University of Melbourne Department of Paediatrics, Royal Children's Hospital, Melbourne, Australia.
15.10.1 Acute rheumatic fever

Simon Carette Head, Division of Rheumatology, Toronto Western Hospital, Ontario, Canada.
18.4 Back pain and regional disorders

D. J. S. Carmichael Consultant Renal Physician, Southend Hospital, Westcliffe-on-Sea, Essex, UK.
20.16 Drugs and the kidney

D. P. Casemore Senior Research Fellow, CREH, University of Wales, St Asaph, Denbighshire, UK.
7.13.5 Cryptosporidium and cryptosporidiosis. 7.13.6 Cyclospora

D. Catovsky Professor of Haematology, Royal Marsden Hospital and Institute of Cancer Research, London, UK.
22.3.2 The classification of leukaemia. 22.3.5 Chronic lymphocytic leukaemia and other leukaemias of mature B and T cells

Bruce A. Chabner Professor of Medicine, Harvard Medical School and Massachusetts General Hospital, Boston, USA.
6.7 Cancer chemotherapy and radiation therapy

Richard E. Chaisson Professor of Medicine, Epidemiology and International Health, Johns Hopkins University Schools of Medicine and Public Health, Baltimore, Maryland, USA.
7.11.22 Tuberculosis

R. W. Chapman Consultant Gastroenterologist/Hepatologist, John Radcliffe Hospital, Oxford, UK.
14.20.2.3 Primary sclerosing cholangitis

V. Krishna K. Chatterjee Professor of Endocrinology, University of Cambridge, Addenbrooke's Hospital, Cambridge, UK.
12.1 Principles of hormone action

Dominique Chauveau Consultant Nephrologist, Department of Nephrology, Hôpital Necker, Paris, France.
20.9.1 Acute interstitial nephritis

P. F. Chinnery Senior Lecturer in Neurogenetics and Honorary Consultant Neurologist, University of Newcastle upon Tyne and Newcastle upon Tyne Hospitals NHS Trust, UK.
24.22.5 Mitochondrial encephalomyopathies

Seung-Yull Cho Professor, Section of Molecular Parasitology, Sungkyunkwan University School of Medicine, Suwon, Korea.
7.15.4 Pseudophyllidean tapeworms: diphyllobothriasis and sparganosis

Kirpal S. Chugh Professor Emeritus, Department of Nephrology, Postgraduate Institute of Medical Education and Research, Chandigarh, India.
20.7.10 Glomerular disease in the tropics

L. Chwastiak Acting Assistant Professor, Department of Psychiatry, University of Washington, Seattle, USA.
26.5.4 Anxiety and depression

C. M. Clothier Queen's Counsel (retired), London, UK.
1 On being a patient

Andrew J. S. Coats Viscount Royston Professor of Cardiology, Imperial College London and Honorary Consultant Cardiologist, Royal Brompton Hospital, London, UK.
15.2.2 The syndrome of heart failure. 15.5.3 Cardiac rehabilitation

S. M. Cobbe Walton Professor of Medical Cardiology, University of Glasgow, Glasgow Royal Infirmary, UK.
15.2.3 Syncope and palpitation. 15.6 Cardiac arrhythmias

B. J. Cohen Clinical Scientist, Central Public Health Laboratory, London, UK.
7.10.18 Parvovirus B19

J. Cohen Dean and Professor of Infectious Diseases, Brighton and Sussex Medical School, UK.
7.20 Infection in the immunocompromised host

R. D. Cohen Emeritus Professor of Medicine, Bart's and The London School of Medicine and Dentistry, Queen Mary College, University of London, UK.
11.11 Disturbances of acid-base homeostasis

Francis S. Collins Director, National Human Genome Research Institute, Bethesda, Maryland, USA.
4.1 The genomic basis of medicine

R. Collins British Heart Foundation Professor of Medicine and Epidemiology, Clinical Trial Service Unit and Epidemiological Studies Unit, University of Oxford, UK.
2.4.3 Large-scale randomized evidence: trials and overviews

Alastair Compston Professor of Neurology, University of Cambridge, UK.
24.1 Introduction and approach to the patient with neurological disease.
24.16 Demyelinating disorders of the central nervous system

Juliet Compston Reader in Metabolic Bone Diseases and Honorary Consultant Physician, Addenbrooke's Hospital, Cambridge, UK.
19.4 Osteoporosis

C. P. Conlon Consultant Physician in Infectious Diseases, Nuffield Department of Medicine, John Radcliffe Hospital, Oxford, UK.
7.8 Travel and expedition medicine. 7.10.21 HIV and AIDS

Andrew Coop Duke University Medical Center, Durham, North Carolina, USA.
6.2 The nature and development of cancer. 6.3 The genetics of inherited cancers

M. R. Cooper Freelance Science Writer, CAB International, Wallingford, Oxfordshire, UK.
8.3 Poisonous plants and fungi

Susan Copley Consultant Radiologist, Hammersmith Hospital, London, UK.
17.3.1 Thoracic imaging

Fernando F. Costa Professor of Haematology, School of Medical Sciences, Unicamp, Campinas, Brazil.
22.5.10 Disorders of the red cell membrane

J. Couvreur Professeur Associé, Laboratoire de la Toxoplasmose, Institut de Puericulture, Paris, France.
7.13.4 Toxoplasmosis

P. J. Cowen Professor of Psychopharmacology, Warneford Hospital, Oxford, UK.
26.6.1 Psychopharmacology in medical practice

T. M. Cox Professor of Medicine, University of Cambridge, and Honorary Consultant Physician, Addenbrooke's Hospital, Cambridge, UK.
11.3.1 Glycogen storage diseases. 11.3.2 Inborn errors of fructose metabolism. 11.3.3 Disorders of galactose, pentose, and pyruvate metabolism. 11.5 The porphyrias. 11.7.1 Hereditary haemochromatosis. 11.8 Lysosomal storage diseases. 12.13 The pineal gland and melatonin. 14.9.5 Disaccharidase deficiency. 22.5.4 Iron metabolism and its disorders. 33 Emergency medicine

Dorothy H. Crawford Professor of Medical Microbiology, Centre for Infectious Diseases, University of Edinburgh, UK.
7.10.3 The Epstein–Barr virus

Robin A. F. Crawford Consultant Gynaecological Oncologist, Addenbrooke's Hospital, Cambridge, UK.
13.17 Malignant disease in pregnancy

A. J. Crisp Consultant Rheumatologist, Addenbrooke's Hospital, Cambridge, UK.
19.5 Avascular necrosis and related topics

D. W. M. Crook Consultant Microbiologist/Infectious Diseases, John Radcliffe Hospital, Oxford, UK.
24.14.1 Bacterial meningitis

J. Cunningham Professor of Renal and Metabolic Medicine, The Royal London Hospital and Queen Mary's School of Medicine and Dentistry, London, UK.
20.8 Renal tubular disorders

Patrick C. D'Haese Associate Professor, Department of Nephrology and Hypertension, University of Antwerp, Belgium.
20.9.2 Chronic tubulointerstitial nephritis

Tim Dalgleish Research Scientist, MRC Cognitions and Brain Sciences Unit, Cambridge, UK.
26.5.1 Grief, stress, and post-traumatic stress disorder

D. A. B. Dance Director/Consultant Microbiologist, Public Health Laboratory, Derriford Hospital, Plymouth, UK.
7.11.15 Melioidosis and glanders

Chi V. Dang Professor of Medicine and Chief, Hematology Division, Johns Hopkins University School of Medicine, Baltimore, Maryland, USA.
22.3.7 Myelodysplasia

C. J. **Danpure** Professor of Molecular Cell Biology, Department of Biology, University College London, UK.
11.10 Disorders of oxalate metabolism

John H. **Dark** Professor of Cardiothoracic Surgery, Freeman Hospital, Newcastle upon Tyne, UK.
15.5.4 Cardiac transplantation and mechanical circulatory support

A. **Davenport** Consultant Renal Physician/Honorary Senior Lecturer, Centre for Nephrology, Royal Free Hospital, London, UK.
20.3.2 Clinical investigation of renal disease

G. **Davey Smith** Professor of Clinical Epidemiology, University of Bristol, UK.
15.4.1.2 The epidemiology of ischaemic heart disease

Alun **Davies** Reader and Honorary Consultant Surgeon, Department of Vascular Surgery, Faculty of Medicine, Imperial College School of Medicine, Charing Cross Hospital, London, UK.
15.14.2 Peripheral arterial disease

P. D. O. **Davies** Consultant Physician, Fazakerley Hospital, Liverpool, UK.
7.11.23 Disease caused by environmental mycobacteria

Alex M. **Davison** Professor and Consultant Renal Physician, St James's University Hospital, Leeds, UK.
20.3.1 The clinical presentation of renal disease

Marc E. **De Broe** Professor in Medicine, Department of Nephrology, University of Antwerp, Belgium.
20.9.2 Chronic tubulointerstitial nephritis

P. **de la Motte Hall** Professor, Division of Anatomical Pathology, Faculty of Health Sciences, University of Cape Town, South Africa.
14.21.6 Hepatic granulomas

M. **de Swiet** Professor of Obstetric Medicine, Queen Charlotte's and Chelsea Hospital, London, UK.
13.7 Thromboembolism in pregnancy. 13.8 Chest diseases in pregnancy

Barbara A. **Degar** Yale School of Medicine, New Haven, Connecticut, USA.
22.4.2 Introduction to the lymphoproliferative disorders

Eric **Demoncheaux** Research Associate, Medical School, University of Sheffield, UK.
15.15.1 The pulmonary circulation and its influence on gas exchange

D. M. **Denison** Emeritus Professor of Clinical Physiology, Royal Brompton Hospital, London, UK.
8.5.5 Aerospace medicine. 8.5.6 Diving medicine

John **Dent** Director, Department of Gastroenterology, Hepatology and General Medicine and Clinical Professor of Medicine, Royal Adelaide Hospital/ Adelaide University, Australia.
14.6 Diseases of the oesophagus

Christopher P. **Denton** Senior Lecturer/Consultant Rheumatologist, Centre for Rheumatology, Royal Free Hospital, London, UK.
18.10.3 Systemic sclerosis

Ulrich **Desselberger** Consultant Virologist and Director, Clinical Microbiology and Public Health Laboratory, Addenbrooke's Hospital, Cambridge, UK.
7.10.7 Enterovirus infections. 7.10.8 Virus infections causing diarrhoea and vomiting

Charles A. **Dinarello** Professor of Medicine, University of Colorado, Denver, Colorado, USA.
4.4 Cytokines: interleukin-1 and tumour necrosis factor in inflammation

A. K. **Dixon** Professor of Radiology and Honorary Consultant Radiologist, University of Cambridge and Addenbrooke's Hospital, Cambridge, UK.
14.18.2 Computed tomography and magnetic resonance imaging of the liver and pancreas

Michael **Doherty** Professor of Rheumatology, University of Nottingham Medical School, UK.
18.3 Clinical investigation. 18.9 Crystal-related arthropathies

R. **Doll** Emeritus Professor of Medicine and Honorary Member, Cancer Studies Unit, Nuffield Department of Medicine, Radcliffe Infirmary, Oxford, UK.
6.1 Epidemiology of cancer

Michael **Donaghy** Reader in Clinical Neurology, University of Oxford, Honorary Consultant Neurologist, Radcliffe Infirmary, and Honorary Civilian Consultant in Neurology to the Army, Oxford, UK.
24.13.13 The motor neurone diseases

Dominique **Droz** Unite de Pathologie Renale, Hôpital Necker, Paris, France.
20.9.1 Acute interstitial nephritis

R. M. **du Bois** Professor of Respiratory Medicine, National Heart and Lung Institute, University College London and Consultant Physician, Royal Brompton Hospital, London, UK.
17.11.1 Diffuse parenchymal lung disease: an introduction. 17.11.2 Cryptogenic fibrosing alveolitis. 17.11.3 Bronchiolitis obliterans and organizing pneumonia. 17.11.4 The lungs and rheumatological diseases. 17.11.5 The lung in vasculitis

C. R. K. **Dudley** Consultant Renal Physician, The Richard Bright Renal Unit Southmead Hospital, North Bristol NHS Trust, Bristol, UK.
15.14.3 Cholesterol embolism

D. W. **Dunne** Reader in Immunoparasitology, Department of Pathology, University of Cambridge, UK.
7.16.1 Schistosomiasis

David T. **Durack** Consulting Professor of Medicine, Duke University, Durham, North Carolina and Vice-President, Corporate Medical Affairs, Becton Dickinson & Co., Franklin Lakes, New Jersey, USA.
7.2 Fever of unknown origin

S. R. **Durham** Professor of Allergy and Respiratory Medicine, Imperial College Faculty of Medicine, National Heart and Lung Hospital, and Royal Brompton Hospital, London, UK.
17.4.2 Allergic rhinitis ('hay fever')

P. N. **Durrington** Professor of Medicine, University of Manchester Department of Medicine, Manchester Royal Infirmary, UK.
11.6 Lipid and lipoprotein disorders

M. **Eastwood** Post-Retirement Honorary Fellow, Department of Medical Sciences, Western General Hospital, Edinburgh, UK.
10.3 Vitamins and trace elements

Jonathan C. W. **Edwards** Professor in Connective Tissue Medicine, University College London, UK.
18.1 Joints and connective tissue: introduction

Richard **Edwards** Emeritus Professor of Medicine, University of Liverpool, UK.
24.22.4 Metabolic and endocrine disorders

M. **Elia** Professor of Clinical Nutrition and Metabolism, Institute of Human Nutrition, University of Southampton, UK.
10.6 Special nutritional problems and the use of enteral and parenteral nutrition

Matthew J. **Ellis** Associate Professor of Medicine and Director, Breast Cancer Program, Duke University Medical Center, Durham, North Carolina, USA.
6.2 The nature and development of cancer. 6.3 The genetics of inherited cancers

Monique M. **Elseviers** Department of Nephrology-Hypertension, University Hospital Antwerp, Belgium.
20.9.2 Chronic tubulointerstitial nephritis

M. A. **Epstein** Emeritus Professor of Pathology, University of Bristol, UK.
7.10.3 The Epstein–Barr virus

E. **Ernst** Professor and Director, Department of Complementary Medicine, University of Exeter, UK.
2.5 Complementary and alternative medicine

David **Eschenbach** Professor, Department of Obstetrics and Gynecology, University of Washington, Seattle, USA.
21.4 Pelvic inflammatory disease

S. M. **Evans** Specialist Registrar in Gastroenterology, Royal Sussex County Hospital, Brighton, UK.
8.5.8 Podoconiosis

S. J. **Eykyn** Professor (and Honorary Consultant) in Clinical Microbiology, St Thomas' Hospital, London, UK.
7.11.2 Streptococci and enterococci. 7.11.4 Staphylococci. 7.11.10 Anaerobic bacteria. 15.10.2 Infective endocarditis

C. A. **Eynon** Director of Neurosciences Intensive Care, Southampton University Hospital NHS Trust, UK.
16.3 Cardiac arrest. 33 Emergency medicine

Christopher G. **Fairburn** Wellcome Principal Research Fellow and Professor of Psychiatry, Oxford University Department of Psychiatry, Warneford Hospital, Oxford, UK.
26.5.5 Eating disorders

J. J. Farrar Senior Fellow, Wellcome Trust, University of Oxford Clinical Research Unit, The Hospital for Tropical Diseases, Ho Chi Minh, Vietnam.
24.14.1 Bacterial meningitis. 24.14.2 Viral infections of the central nervous system

Ken Farrington Consultant Nephrologist, Lister Hospital, Stevenage, Hertfordshire, UK.
20.6.1 Haemodialysis

D. T. Fearon Wellcome Trust Professor of Medicine, University of Cambridge, UK.
5.5 Innate immune system

John Feehally Professor of Renal Medicine, Leicester General Hospital, UK.
20.7.2 IgA nephropathy and Henoch-Schönlein purpura. 20.7.3 Thin membrane nephropathy

Alvan R. Feinstein* Professor, Yale University School of Medicine, New Haven, Connecticut, USA.
2.4.2 Evidence-based medicine

Eleanor Feldman Consultant Liaison Psychiatrist and Honorary Senior Lecturer, University of Oxford, John Radcliffe Hospital, Oxford, UK.
26.2 Taking a psychiatric history from a medical patient. 26.4 Acute behavioural emergencies

Peter J. Fenner Associate Professor, Schools of Medicine and Health Sciences, James Cook University and National Medical Officer, Surf Life Saving Association of Australia, Mackay, North Queensland, Australia.
8.5.3 Drowning

Robert Ferrari Clinical Assistant Professor, University of Alberta Hospital, Edmonton, Canada.
18.2 Clinical presentation and diagnosis of rheumatic disease

C. ffrench-Constant Professor of Neurological Genetics, University of Cambridge, UK.
24.21 Developmental abnormalities of the central nervous system

R. G. Finch Professor of Infectious Diseases, City Hospital and University of Nottingham, UK.
7.6 Antimicrobial chemotherapy

H. Firth Consultant in Medical Genetics, Department of Medical Genetics, Addenbrooke's Hospital, Cambridge, UK.
24.21 Developmental abnormalities of the central nervous system

J. Firth Consultant Physician and Nephrologist, Addenbrooke's Hospital, Cambridge, UK.
13.5 Renal disease in pregnancy. 15.15.2.2 Pulmonary oedema. 15.15.3.1 Deep venous thrombosis and pulmonary embolism. 15.18 Idiopathic oedema of women. 16.1 The clinical approach to the patient who is very ill. 20.2.2 Disorders of potassium homeostasis. 20.4 Acute renal failure. 33 Emergency medicine

Susan Fisher-Hoch Professor, University of Texas School of Public Health at Brownsville, USA.
7.10.15 Arenaviruses. 7.10.16 Filoviruses

Robert A. Fishman Professor of Neurology Emeritus, University of California San Francisco School of Medicine, USA.
24.7 Lumbar puncture

Edward D. Folland Associate Director of Cardiology and Professor of Medicine, UMass Memorial Medical Center/University of Massachusetts Medical School, Worcester, Maryland, USA.
15.3.6 Cardiac catheterization and angiography. 15.4.2.4 Percutaneous interventional cardiac procedures

J. C. Forfar Consultant Cardiologist, John Radcliffe Hospital, Oxford and Honorary Senior Lecturer, University of Oxford, UK.
13.6 Heart disease in pregnancy

I. S. Foulds Consultant Dermatologist, City Hospital, Birmingham, UK.
8.4.1 Occupational and environmental health and safety

Keith A. A. Fox Professor of Cardiology, Royal Infirmary and University of Edinburgh, UK.
15.4.2.3 Management of acute coronary syndromes: unstable angina and myocardial infarction

Richard Frackowiak Vice Provost (Biomedicine), University College London, Institute of Neurology, London, UK.
24.3 Brain and mind: functional neuroimaging

T. J. R. Francis Consultant in Diving Medicine, Tintagel, Cornwall, UK.
8.5.6 Diving medicine

Keith N. Frayn Professor of Human Metabolism, Oxford Centre for Diabetes, Endocrinology and Metabolism, University of Oxford, UK.
10.2 Nutrition: biochemical background

Alan Freeman Consultant Radiologist, Addenbrooke's Hospital, Cambridge, UK.
14.2.3 Radiology of the gastrointestinal tract

Peggy Frith Consultant Ophthalmic Physician, The Eye Hospital, Radcliffe Infirmary, Oxford and University College London Hospital, UK.
25 The eye in general medicine

Patrick G. Gallagher Associate Professor, Department of Pediatrics, Yale University School of Medicine, New Haven, Connecticut, USA.
22.5.10 Disorders of the red cell membrane

Clare J. Galton Specialist Registrar in Neurology, Neurology Department, Addenbrooke's Hospital, Cambridge, UK.
24.13.8 Alzheimer's disease and other dementias

Hector H. Garcia Associate Professor, Department of Microbiology, Universidad Peruana Cayetano Heredia and Head, Cysticercosis Unit, Department of Transmissible Diseases, Instituto de Ciencias Neurologicas, Lima, Peru.
7.15.1 Cystic hydatid disease (Echinococcus granulosus). 7.15.3 Cysticercosis

K. Gardiner Professor and Managing Director, International Occupational Health Ltd., Birmingham, UK.
8.4.1 Occupational and environmental health and safety

Lawrence B. Gardner Assistant Professor of Medicine, Johns Hopkins University school of Medicine, Baltimore, Maryland, USA.
22.3.7 Myelodysplasia

Christopher S. Garrard Consultant Physician in Intensive Care, John Radcliffe Hospital, Oxford, UK.
16.5.2 The management of respiratory failure

J. S. H. Gaston Professor of Rheumatology, University of Cambridge School of Medicine, Addenbrooke's Hospital, Cambridge, UK.
18.7.2 Reactive arthritis

Duncan Geddes Professor of Respiratory Medicine, Royal Brompton Hospital, London, UK.
17.10 Cystic fibrosis

D. G. Gibson Consultant Cardiologist, Royal Brompton Hospital, London, UK.
15.7 Valve disease. 15.9 Pericardial disease

G. J. Gibson Professor of Respiratory Medicine/Consultant Physician, Freeman Hospital, Newcastle upon Tyne, UK.
17.3.2 Respiratory function tests

A. M. Giles Scientific Officer, Health Systems, Oxford, UK.
32 Reference intervals for biochemical data

I. P. Giles ARC Research Fellow, Bloomsbury Rheumatology Unit, London, UK.
18.10.1 Autoimmune rheumatic disorders and vasculitis

Charles F. Gilks Professor of Tropical Medicine and Senior Adviser on Care, HIV/AIDS Department, World Health Organization, Geneva, Switzerland.
7.10.22 HIV in the developing world

Michael D. J. Gillmer Consultant Obstetrician and Gynaecologist, Women's Centre, John Radcliffe Hospital, Oxford, UK.
13.10 Diabetes in pregnancy

Robert H. Gilman Professor, Department of International Health, Johns Hopkins School of Public Health, Baltimore, Maryland, USA and Research Professor, Universidad Peruana Cayetano Heredia, Lima, Peru.
7.15.3 Cysticercosis

A. E. S. Gimson Consultant Physician and Hepatologist, Cambridge Liver Transplantation Unit, Addenbrooke's Hospital, Cambridge, UK.
13.9 Liver and gastrointestinal diseases during pregnancy. 14.18.1 The structure and function of the liver, biliary tract, and pancreas

P. Glasziou Huntington Centre for Risk Analysis, Boston, Massachusetts, USA.
2.4.1 Bringing the best evidence to the point of care

* It is with regret that we report the death of Professor Alvan R. Feinstein during the preparation of this edition of the textbook.

Peter J. Goadsby Professor of Clinical Neurology, Institute of Neurology, University College and The National Hospital for Neurology and Neurosurgery, London, UK.
24.13.2 Headache

D. Goldblatt Reader in Immunology and Consultant Paediatric Immunologist, Institute of Child Health, Great Ormond Hospital for Children NHS Trust, London, UK.
7.7 Immunization

John M. Goldman Professor of Leukaemia Biology and Chairman, Department of Haematology, Imperial College School of Medicine, London, UK.
22.3.6 Chronic myeloid leukaemia

Irwin Goldstein Director, Institute for Sexual Medicine and Professor of Urology and Gynecology, Boston University School of Medicine, Massachusetts, USA.
12.8.4 Sexual dysfunction

Armando E. Gonzalez Department of Public Health, School of Veterinary Medicine, Universidad Nacional Mayor de San Marcos, Lima, Peru.
7.15.1 Cystic hydatid disease (Echinococcus granulosus)

Timothy H. J. Goodship Reader in Nephrology, University of Newcastle upon Tyne and Consultant Nephrologist, Royal Victoria Infirmary, Newcastle upon Tyne, UK.
20.10.6 Haemolytic uraemic syndrome

Sherwood L. Gorbach Department of Community Health and Medicine, TUFTS University School of Medicine, Boston, Massachusetts, USA.
14.17 Gastrointestinal infections

E. C. Gordon-Smith Professor of Haematology, St George's Hospital Medical School, London, UK.
22.3.11 Aplastic anaemia and other causes of bone marrow failure. 22.8.2 Haemopoietic stem cell transplantation

J. M. Grange Visiting Professor, University College London, Centre for Infectious Diseases and International Health, Royal Free and University College Medical School, London, UK.
7.11.23 Disease caused by environmental mycobacteria

R. Gray Professor of Medical Statistics and Director, University of Birmingham Clinical Trials Unit, UK.
2.4.3 Large-scale randomized evidence: trials and overviews

John R. Graybill Professor, University of Texas Health Science Center, San Antonio, Texas, USA.
7.12.3 Coccidioidomycosis

Jackie Green Director, Centre for Health Promotion Research, Leeds Metropolitan University, Leeds, UK.
3.5 Health promotion

Brian M. Greenwood Professor of Clinical Tropical Medicine, London School of Hygiene and Tropical Medicine, London, UK.
7.11.3 Pneumococcal diseases

Roger Greenwood Consultant Nephrologist and Lead Clinician, Lister Hospital, Stevenage, Hertfordshire, UK.
20.6.1 Haemodialysis

B. Gribbin Honorary Consultant Cardiologist, John Radcliffe Hospital, Oxford, UK.
15.10.3 Cardiovascular syphilis. 15.14.1 Thoracic aortic dissection

John Grimley Evans Professor Emeritus of Clinical Geratology, Green College, Oxford, UK.
30.1 Medicine in old age

Michael L. Grossbard Chief, Hematology/Oncology, St Luke's-Roosevelt Hospital and Beth Israel Medical Center, New York, USA.
6.7 Cancer chemotherapy and radiation therapy

David I. Grove Professor and Director, Clinical Microbiology and Infectious Diseases, The Queen Elizabeth Hospital, Adelaide, Australia.
7.14.5 Nematode infections of lesser importance. 7.16.2 Liver fluke infections. 7.16.4 Intestinal trematode infections

J. P. Grünfeld Professor of Nephrology, Université Paris V - René Descartes and Head of Nephrology, Hôpital Necker, Paris, France.
20.11 Renal involvement in genetic disease

D. J. Gubler Director, Division of Vector-Borne Infectious Diseases, Centers for Disease Control and Prevention, Fort Collins, Colorado, USA.
7.10.11 Alphaviruses. 7.10.13 Flaviviruses

Mark Gurnell Specialist Registrar and Research Fellow, Department of Medicine, Division of Endocrinology and Metabolism, Addenbrooke's Hospital, Cambridge, UK.
12.1 Principles of hormone action

David M. Gustin Section of Hematology–Oncology, University of Chicago, Illinois, USA.
22.3.8 The polycythaemias. 22.3.10 Thrombocytosis

M. R. Haeney Consultant Immunologist, Salford Royal Hospitals NHS Trust, Salford, Manchester, UK.
14.4 Immune disorders of the gastrointestinal tract

Davidson H. Hamer Director, Traveler's Health Service, Tufts-New England Medical Center and Assistant Professor of Medicine and Nutrition, Tufts University, Boston, Massachusetts, USA.
14.17 Gastrointestinal infections

P. J. Hammond Consultant Physician and Endocrinologist, Harrogate District Hospital, Yorkshire, UK.
12.10 Non-diabetic pancreatic endocrine disorders and multiple endocrine neoplasia. 14.8 Hormones and the gastrointestinal tract

J. R. Hampton Professor of Cardiology, Queen's Medical Centre, Nottingham, UK.
15.2.1 Chest pain. 15.2.4 Physical examination of the cardiovascular system

M. Hanna Consultant Neurologist and Reader in Clinical Neurology, National Hospital for Neurology and Neurosurgery and Institute of Neurology, University College London, UK.
24.22.1 Introduction: structure and function

David M. Hansell Professor of Thoracic Imaging, Royal Brompton Hospital, London, UK.
17.3.1 Thoracic imaging

P. Harnden Consultant Urological Pathologist, Cancer Research UK Clinical Centre, St James's University Hospital, Leeds, UK.
20.15 Tumours of the urinary tract

J. M. Harrington Emeritus Professor of Occupational Health, University of Birmingham, UK.
8.4.1 Occupational and environmental health and safety

Anthony Harrison Fellow in Health Systems, King's Fund, London, UK.
3.3 The pattern of care: hospital and community

J. R. Harrison Force Medical Adviser, Sussex Police Authority, Lewes, UK.
8.5.9 Radiation

C. Haslett Professor of Respiratory Medicine, Royal Infirmary, Edinburgh, UK.
16.5.1 Pathophysiology and pathogenesis of acute respiratory distress syndrome. 17.1.3 'First line' defence mechanisms of the lung

Adrian R. W. Hatfield Consultant Gastroenterologist, The Middlesex Hospital, London, UK.
14.2.2 Upper gastrointestinal endoscopy

P. N. Hawkins Professor of Medicine, Royal Free and University College Medical School, London, UK.
11.12.3 Familial Mediterranean fever and other inherited periodic fever syndromes. 11.12.4 Amyloidosis

Keith Hawton Professor of Psychiatry, University Department of Psychiatry and Director and Consultant Psychiatrist, Centre for Suicide Research, Warneford Hospital, Oxford, UK.
26.5.2 The patient who has attempted suicide

R. J. Hay Professor and Dean, Faculty of Medicine and Health Sciences, Queens University, Belfast, UK.
7.11.27 Nocardiosis. 7.12.1 Fungal infections

B. Hazleman Consultant Rheumatologist, Rheumatology Department, Addenbrooke's Hospital, Cambridge, UK.
18.11 Miscellaneous conditions presenting to the rheumatologist

Nick Heather Consultant Clinical Psychologist and Director, Centre for Alcohol and Drug Studies, Newcastle, North Tyneside, and Northumberland Mental Health NHS Trust, Newcastle upon Tyne, UK.
26.7.2 Brief interventions against excessive alcohol consumption

David B. Hellmann Professor, Johns Hopkins University School of Medicine, Baltimore, Maryland, USA.
18.10.7 Polymyositis and dermatomyositis

D. J. Hendrick Consultant Physician and Professor of Occupational Respiratory Medicine, Royal Victoria Infirmary, University of Newcastle upon Tyne, UK.
17.11.8 Pulmonary haemorrhagic disorders. 17.11.9 Eosinophilic pneumonia. 17.11.10 Lymphocytic infiltrations of the lung. 17.11.11 Extrinsic allergic alveolitis. 17.11.12 Eosinophilic granuloma of the lung and pulmonary lymphangiomyomatosis. 17.11.13 Pulmonary alveolar proteinosis. 17.11.14 Pulmonary amyloidosis. 17.11.15 Lipoid (lipid) pneumonia. 17.11.16 Pulmonary alveolar microlithiasis. 17.11.17 Toxic gases and fumes. 17.11.18 Radiation pneumonitis. 17.11.19 Drug-induced lung disease

Mark Herbert Clinical Lecturer in Neonatal Paediatrics, Department of Paediatrics, University of Oxford, UK.
13.15 Infections in pregnancy

Andrew Herxheimer Emeritus Fellow, UK Cochrane Centre, London, UK.
9 Principles of clinical pharmacology and drug therapy

Martin F. Heyworth Chief of Staff and Clinical Professor of Medicine, VA Medical Center and University of Pennsylvania, Philadelphia, USA.
7.13.8 Giardiasis, balantidiasis, isosporiasis, and microsporidiosis

Tim Higenbottam Global Clinical Expert, Astra-Zeneca, Charnwood, Leicestershire and Visiting Professor of Medicine, University of Sheffield, UK.
15.15.1 The pulmonary circulation and its influence on gas exchange. 15.15.2.1 Primary pulmonary hypertension

Katherine A. High William H. Bennett Professor of Pediatrics, University of Pennsylvania School of Medicine and The Children's Hospital of Philadelphia, Pennsylvania, USA.
22.6.4 Genetic disorders of coagulation

S. L. Hillier Research Associate Professor of Obstetrics and Gynecology, University of Washington, Seattle, USA.
21.3 Vaginal discharge

David Hilton-Jones Clinical Director, Oxford MDC Muscle and Nerve Centre, Radcliffe Infirmary, Oxford, UK.
24.17 Disorders of the neuromuscular junction. 24.22.3 Myotonia. 24.22.4 Metabolic and endocrine disorders

John R. Hodges Professor of Behavioural Neurology, MRC Cognition and Brain Sciences Unit and Department of Neurology, Addenbrooke's Hospital, Cambridge, UK.
24.8 Disturbances of higher cerebral function. 24.13.8 Alzheimer's disease and other dementias

H. J. F. Hodgson Sheila Sherlock Professor of Medicine and Director, Centre for Hepatology, Royal Free and University College Medical School, London, UK.
14.9.6 Whipple's disease. 14.20.1 Viral hepatitis—clinical aspects. 14.20.2.1 Autoimmune hepatitis

A. V. Hoffbrand Emeritus Professor of Haematology, Royal Free and University College School of Medicine, London, UK.
22.5.6 Megaloblastic anaemia and miscellaneous deficiency anaemias

Ronald Hoffman Professor, Hematology-Oncology Section University of Illinois College of Medicine, Chicago, USA.
22.3.8 The polycythaemias. 22.3.10 Thrombocytosis

P. A. H. Holloway Consultant Chemical Pathologist in Intensive Care and Honorary Reader in Medicine, John Radcliffe Hospital, Oxford, UK.
32 Reference intervals for biochemical data

Richard H. Holloway Associate Professor of Medicine and Senior Consultant Gastroenterologist, Department of Gastroenterology, Hepatology and General Medicine, Royal Adelaide Hospital, Australia.
14.6 Diseases of the oesophagus

J. M. Hopkin Professor, Experimental Medicine Unit, Swansea Clinical School, University of Wales, Swansea, UK.
17.4.1 Asthma: genetic effects. 17.15 The genetics of lung diseases

Carol Ann Huff Assistant Professor of Oncology, Sidney Kimmel Comprehensive Cancer Care at Johns Hopkins, Baltimore, Maryland, USA.
26.7.3 Problems of alcohol and drug users in the hospital

I. A. Hughes Professor of Paediatrics and Honorary Consultant Paediatric Enterologist, Department of Paediatrics, University of Cambridge, UK.
12.7.2 Congenital adrenal hyperplasia

Lawrence Impey Consultant in Fetal Medicine, The Women's Centre, John Radcliffe Hospital, Oxford, UK.
13.15 Infections in pregnancy

C. W. Imrie Consultant Surgeon and Honorary Professor, Lister Department of Surgery, Royal Infirmary, Glasgow, UK.
14.18.3.1 Acute pancreatitis

H. Irving Consultant Radiologist, St James's University Hospital, Leeds, UK.
20.15 Tumours of the urinary tract

P. G. Isaacson Professor of Histopathology, Royal Free and University College Medical School, London, UK.
14.9.4 Gastrointestinal lymphoma

D. A. Isenberg The Arthritis Research Campaign Professor of Rheumatology at University College London, Centre for Rheumatology, London, UK.
18.10.1 Autoimmune rheumatic disorders and vasculitis. 18.10.2 Systemic lupus erythematosus and related disorders

C. G. Isles Consultant Physician, Medical Unit, Dumfries and Galloway Royal Infirmary, Dumfries, UK.
15.16.1.1 Prevalence, epidemiology, and pathophysiology of hypertension

C. Ison Reader in Medical Microbiology, Department of Infectious Diseases and Microbiology, Faculty of Medicine, Imperial College, St Mary's Campus, London, UK.
7.11.6 Neisseria gonorrhoeae

Alan A. Jackson Professor and Director, Institute of Human Nutrition, University of Southampton, UK.
10.4 Severe malnutrition

H. S. Jacobs Emeritus Professor of Reproductive Endocrinology, University College London Medical School, UK.
12.8.1 Ovarian disorders. 12.8.3 The breast

Robin Jacoby Professor of Old Age Psychiatry, University of Oxford Department of Psychiatry, Warneford Hospital, Oxford, UK.
30.2 Mental disorders of old age

O. F. W. James Head of Clinical Medical Sciences, Medical School, University of Newcastle upon Tyne, UK.
14.21.1 Alcoholic liver disease and non-alcoholic steatosis hepatitis

Paul J. Jenkins Senior Lecturer in Endocrinology, St Bartholomew's Hospital, London, UK.
12.2 Disorders of the anterior pituitary

B. Jennett Emeritus Professor of Neurosurgery, Institute of Neurological Sciences, University of Glasgow, UK.
24.13.6 Brain death and the vegetative state

D. P. Jewell Professor of Gastroenterology, John Radcliffe Hospital, Oxford, UK.
14.9.3 Coeliac disease. 14.10 Crohn's disease. 14.11 Ulcerative colitis. 14.22 Miscellaneous disorders of the gastrointestinal tract and liver

Vivekanand Jha Associate Professor of Nephrology, Postgraduate Institute of Medical Education and Research, Chandigarh, India.
20.7.10 Glomerular disease in the tropics

Anne M. Johnson Professor of Infectious Disease Epidemiology and Head, Department of Primary Care and Population Sciences, University College London, UK.
21.2 Sexual behaviour

A. W. Johnson CAB International, Wallingford, Oxfordshire, UK.
8.3 Poisonous plants and fungi

E. Anthony Jones Chief of Hepatology, Academic Medical Centre, Amsterdam, The Netherlands.
14.21.3 Hepatocellular failure

N. Jones Department of Virology, John Radcliffe Hospital, Oxford, UK.
7.10.25 Orf. 7.10.26 Molluscum contagiosum

S. E. Jones Research Associate, Department of Biology, Imperial College of Science, Technology and Medicine, London, UK.
7.11.33 Syphilis

Kenneth C. Kalunian Professor of Medicine, UCLA School of Medicine, Los Angeles, California, USA.
18.8 Osteoarthritis

Eileen Kaner NHS Primary Care Career Scientist, School of Population and Health Sciences, University of Newcastle upon Tyne, UK.
26.7.2 Brief interventions against excessive alcohol consumption

W. Katon Professor and Vice Chair, Director of Division of Health Services and Psychiatric Epidemiology, University of Washington, Seattle, Washington, USA.
26.5.4 Anxiety and depression

Tomisaku Kawasaki Professor and Director, Japan Kawasaki Disease Research Center, Tokyo, Japan.
18.10.8 Kawasaki syndrome

David Keeling Consultant Haematologist and Director, Oxford Haemophilia Centre and Thrombosis Unit, Churchill Hospital, Oxford, UK.
15.5.2 Therapeutic anticoagulation in atrial fibrillation and heart failure.
15.15.3.2 Therapeutic anticoagulation in deep venous thrombosis and pulmonary embolism

David P. Kelsell Non-Clinical Senior Lecturer, Centre for Cutaneous Research, Barts and The London, Queen Mary's School of Medicine and Dentistry, London, UK.
23.2 Molecular basis of inherited skin disease

John G. Kelton Dean and Vice-President, Faculty of Health Sciences, McMaster University, Hamilton, Ontario, Canada.
22.6.3 Disorders of platelet number and function

Christopher Kennard Professor and Head, Division of Neuroscience and Psychological Medicine, Imperial College London, Charing Cross Campus, London, UK.
24.11 Visual pathways

Rose Anne Kenny Professor of Cardiovascular Research, Institute of Ageing and Health, University of Newcastle upon Tyne, UK.
24.13.5.1 Head-up tilt-table testing in the diagnosis of vasovagal syncope and related disorders

M. G. W. Kettlewell Consultant Surgeon, Oxford Radcliffe Trust, UK.
14.13 Colonic diverticular disease

G. T. Keusch Associate Director for International Research, National Institutes of Health, Bethesda, Maryland, and Professor of Medicine, Tufts-New England Medical Center, Boston, Massachusetts, USA.
7.11.7 Enterobacteria, campylobacter, and miscellaneous food-poisoning bacteria

Munther A. Khamashta Senior Lecturer and Consultant Physician, Lupus Research Unit, The Rayne Institute, St Thomas' Hospital, London, UK.
13.14 Autoimmune rheumatic disorders and vasculitis in pregnancy

Maurice King Honorary Research Fellow, University of Leeds, UK.
3.7.2 Health in a fragile future

Keith P. Klugman Professor of International Health, Rollins School of Public Health and Division of Infectious Diseases, School of Medicine, Emory University, Atlanta, Georgia, USA.
7.11.3 Pneumococcal diseases

R. Knight Associate Specialist in General Medicine, Royal Sussex County Hospital, Brighton, UK.
7.13.1 Amoebic infections. 7.13.9 Blastocystis hominis infection. 7.14.2 Lymphatic filariasis. 7.14.3 Guinea-worm disease: dracunculiasis. 7.14.4 Strongyloidiasis, hookworm, and other gut strongyloid nematodes. 7.14.8 Angiostrongyliasis. 7.15.2 Gut cestodes

Michael D. Kopelman Professor of Clinical Medicine and Deputy Warden, Bart's and The London, Queen Mary's School of Medicine and Dentistry, University of London, UK.
26.3 Neuropsychiatric disorders

Peter G. Kopelman Professor of Clinical Medicine, Bart's and The London Queen Mary's School of Medicine and Dentistry, London, UK.
10.5 Obesity

Christian Krarup Professor, Department of Clinical Neurophysiology, Rigshospitalet, Copenhagen, Denmark.
24.2 Electrophysiology of the central and peripheral nervous systems

J. B. Kurtz Consultant Virologist (retired), Public Health Laboratory, Birmingham Heartlands Hospital, UK.
7.11.35 Legionellosis and legionnaires' disease

Robert A. Kyle Professor of Medicine and Laboratory Medicine, Mayo Clinic, Rochester, Minnesota, USA.
22.4.5 Myeloma and paraproteinaemias

David Lalloo Senior Lecturer in Tropical Medicine, Liverpool School of Tropical Medicine, UK.
7.11.17 Yersinia, Pasteurella, and Francisella

D. J. Lane Consultant Chest Physician (Retired), Oxford Radcliffe Hospital, UK.
17.2 The clinical presentation of chest diseases

Peter Lanyon Consultant Rheumatologist, University Hospital, Queen's Medical Centre, Nottingham, UK.
18.3 Clinical investigation

H. E. Larson Private Practice in Infectious Diseases, Marlborough, Massachusetts, USA.
7.11.21 Botulism, gas gangrene, and clostridial gastrointestinal infections

S. Lawrie Senior Clinical Research Fellow, University Department of Psychiatry, Royal Edinburgh Hospital, UK.
26.5.6 Schizophrenia, bipolar disorder, obsessive–compulsive disorder, and personality disorder

N. F. Lawton Consultant Neurologist, Wessex Neurological Centre, Southampton General Hospital and Honorary Senior Lecturer, University of Southampton, UK.
24.13.19 Benign intracranial hypertension

John H, Lazarus Professor of Clinical Endocrinology, University of Wales College of Medicine, Cardiff, UK.
13.11 Endocrine disease in pregnancy

J. W. LeDuc Director, Division of Viral and Rickettsial Diseases, Centers for Disease Control and Prevention, Atlanta, Georgia, USA.
7.10.14 Bunyaviridae

P. J. Lee Consultant in Metabolic Medicine, Metabolic Unit, National Hospital for Neurology and Neurosurgery, London, UK.
11.2 Inborn errors of amino acid and organic acid metabolism

Tak H. Lee Professor of Allergy and Respiratory Medicine, Guy's, King's and St Thomas' School of Medicine, Guy's Hospital, London, UK.
17.4.3 Basic mechanisms and pathophysiology of asthma

William M. F. Lee Department of Medicine, School of Medicine, University of Pennsylvania, Philadelphia, USA.
4.3 Molecular cell biology

T. Lehner Professor of Basic and Applied Immunology, Department of Immunobiology, Guy's, King's and St Thomas' School of Medicine, London, UK.
14.5 The mouth and salivary glands. 18.10.5 Behçet's disease

Irene M. Leigh Professor of Cellular and Molecular Medicine, Bart's and The London Queen Mary's School of Medicine and Dentistry, University of London, UK.
23.2 Molecular basis of inherited skin disease

G. G. Lennox Consultant Neurologist, Addenbrooke's Hospital, Cambridge, UK.
13.12 Neurological disease in pregnancy

E. A. Letsky Consultant Perinatal Haematologist, Queen Charlotte's and Chelsea Hospital, London, UK.
13.16 Blood disorders in pregnancy

Jeremy Levy Consultant Nephrologist, Imperial College, Hammersmith Hospital, London, UK.
20.7.7 Antiglomerular basement membrane disease

L. M. Lichtenstein Professor of Medicine and Director, Asthma and Allergy Center, Johns Hopkins University School of Medicine, Baltimore, Maryland, USA.
5.2 Allergy

D. C. Linch Professor and Head of Haematology, University College London, UK.
22.2.2 Stem-cell disorders

M. J. Lindop Consultant, Anaesthesia/Intensive Care, Addenbrooke's Hospital, Cambridge, UK.
16.6.3 Brainstem death and organ donation. 16.6.4 The patient without hope

Calvin C. Linnemann, Jr Professor and Director, Infectious Diseases Division, University of Cincinnati Medical Center, Ohio, USA.
7.11.14 Bordetella

Gregory Y. H. Lip Professor of Cardiovascular Medicine, University Department of Medicine, City Hospital, Birmingham, UK.
15.16.3 Hypertensive emergencies and urgencies

P. Little Professor of Primary Care Research, Community Clinical Sciences Division, University of Southampton, UK.
17.5.1 Upper respiratory tract infections

Roderick A. Little Honorary Professor of Surgical Science, University of Manchester, UK.
11.12.2 Metabolic responses to accidental and surgical injury

W. Littler Medical Director, University Hospital NHS Trust, Birmingham, UK.
15.10.2 Infective endocarditis

A. Llanos Cuentas Principal Professor, Facultad de Salud Publica y Administracion, Universidad Peruana Cayetano Heredia, Lima, Peru.
7.11.39.1 Bartonella bacilliformis infection

Diana N. J. Lockwood Consultant Leprologist and Senior Lecturer, Hospital for Tropical Diseases and London School of Hygiene and Tropical Medicine, UK.
7.11.24 Leprosy (Hansen's disease)

S. Logan Senior Lecturer in Paediatric Epidemiology, Institute of Child Health, London, UK.
7.10.12 Rubella

D. J. Lomas Professor of Clinical MRI, University Department of Radiology, Addenbrooke's Hospital, Cambridge, UK.
14.18.2 Computed tomography and magnetic resonance imaging of the liver and pancreas

David A. Lomas Professor of Respiratory Biology and Honorary Consultant Physician, Department of Medicine, University of Cambridge Institute for Medical Research, UK.
11.13 α_1-Antitrypsin deficiency and the serpinopathies

Thomas Look Professor of Pediatrics, Harvard Medical School and Vice-Chair for Research, Pediatric Oncology Department, Dana-Farber Institute, Boston, Massachusetts, USA.
22.3.1 Cell and molecular biology of human leukaemias

A. D. Lopez Senior Science Adviser, World Health Organization, Geneva, Switzerland.
3.1 The Global Burden of Disease Study

Elyse E. Lower Professor of Medicine, University of Cincinnati, Ohio, USA.
17.11.6 Sarcoidosis

Linda M. Luxon Professor of Audiological Medicine, University of London, Institute of Child Health, London, UK and Director, National Institute for Cancer Research, Genova, Italy.
24.12.2 Disorders of hearing

Lucio Luzzatto Professor, Department of Human Genetics, Memorial Sloan-Kettering Cancer Center, New York, USA.
22.3.12 Paroxysmal nocturnal haemoglobinuria. 22.5.12 Glucose-6-phosphate dehydrogenase (G6PD) deficiency

G. A. Luzzi Consultant in Genitourinary/HIV Medicine, South Buckinghamshire NHS Trust, Wycombe Hospital, High Wycombe, Buckinghamshire, UK.
7.10.10 HIV and AIDS

D. C. W. Mabey Professor of Communicable Diseases, London School of Hygiene and Tropical Medicine, London, UK.
7.11.40 Chlamydial infections including lymphogranuloma venerum

P. K. MacCallum Senior Lecturer in Haematology, Barts and The London, Queen Mary's School of Medicine and Dentistry, London, UK.
15.1.2.2 The haemostatic system in arterial disease

J. T. Macfarlane Consultant Physician, Nottingham City Hospital, UK.
7.11.35 Legionellosis and legionnaires' disease

K. T. MacLeod Reader in Cardiac Physiology, Cardiac Medicine, NHLI, Faculty of Medicine, Imperial College London, UK.
15.1.3.1 Physical considerations: biochemistry and cellular physiology of heart muscle

William MacNee Professor of Respiratory and Environmental Medicine, University of Edinburgh, and Honorary Consultant Physician, Lothian University NHS Trust, Edinburgh, UK.
17.6 Chronic obstructive pulmonary disease

M. Monir Madkour Consultant Physician, Military Hospital, Riyadh, Saudi Arabia.
7.11.19 Brucellosis

R. N. Maini Professor of Rheumatology in the University of London, Head of the Kennedy Institute of Rheumatology Division, Faculty of Medicine, Imperial College London, and Honorary Consultant Physician, Charing Cross Hospital, London, UK.
18.5 Rheumatoid arthritis

Hadi Manji Consultant Neurologist, National Hospital for Neurology, London and Ipswich Hospital, Suffolk, UK.
24.14.4 Neurosyphilis and neuroAIDS

J. I. Mann Professor in Human Nutrition and Medicine, University of Otago, Dunedin, New Zealand.
10.1 Diseases of overnourished societies and the need for dietary change

D. Mant Professor of General Practice, Department of Primary Health Care, University of Oxford, UK.
3.4 Preventive medicine

Victor J. Marder Orthopedic Hospital/UCLA Vascular Medicine Program, Los Angeles, California, USA.
22.6.2 Evaluation of the patient with a bleeding diathesis

A. F. Markham Professor of Medicine, St James's University Hospital, Leeds, UK.
14.15 Tumours of the gastrointestinal tract

V. Marks Professor of Clinical Biochemistry Emeritus, Post-Graduate Medical School, University of Surrey, Guildford, UK.
12.11.3 Hypoglycaemia

T. J. Marrie Professor and Chair, Department of Medicine, University of Alberta, Edmonton, Canada.
7.11.38 Coxiella burnetii infections (Q fever)

Helen Marriott Research Associate, Department of Respiratory Medicine, University of Shefffield, UK.
15.15.2.1 Primary pulmonary hypertension

C. D. Marsden* Professor of Neurology, National Hospital for Neurology and Neurosurgery, London, UK.
24.15 Metabolic disorders and the nervous system

Jay W. Mason Professor and Chair, Department of Medicine, University of Kentucky College of Medicine, Lexington, USA.
15.8.1 Myocarditis

V. I. Mathan Professor, ICDDR, Dhaka, Bangladesh.
14.9.8 Malabsorption syndromes in the tropics

Christopher J. Mathias Professor of Neurovascular Medicine and Consultant Physician, Imperial College of Science, Technology and Medicine at St Mary's and National Hospital for Neurology and Neurosurgery, Institute of Neurology, University College London, UK.
24.13.14 Diseases of the autonomic nervous system

Peter W. Mathiesen Professor of Renal Medicine, Academic Renal Unit, University of Bristol, Southmead Hospital, Bristol, UK.
20.7.5 Proliferative glomerulonephritis. 20.7.6 Mesangiocapillary glomerulonephritis

R. McCaig Head, Human Factors Unit, Health Directorate, Health and Safety Executive, Bootle, UK.
8.5.10 Noise. 8.5.11 Vibration

Mary E. McCaul Professor, Department of Psychiatry and Behavioral Sciences, Johns Hopkins University School of Medicine, Baltimore, Maryland, USA.
26.7.1 Alcohol and drug dependence

Joseph McCormick Regional Dean, University of Texas School of Public Health at Brownsville, USA.
7.10.15 Arenaviruses. 7.10.16 Filoviruses

William J. McKenna BHF Professor of Molecular Cardiovascular Sciences, Department of Cardiological Sciences, St George's Hospital Medical School, London, UK.
15.8.2 The cardiomyopathies: hypertrophic, dilated, restrictive, and right ventricular. 15.8.3 Specific heart muscle disorders

* It is with regret that we report the death of Professor C. D. Marsden.

A. J. McMichael Professor and Director, Weatherall Institute of Molecular Medicine, John Radcliffe Hospital, Oxford, UK.
5.1 Principles of immunology.

A. J. McMichael Professor and Director, National Centre for Epidemiology and Population Health, Australian National University, Canberra, Australia.
3.2 Human population size, environment, and health

A. McMillan Consultant Physician, Department of Genito-urinary Medicine, Edinburgh Royal Infirmary, UK.
21.5 Infections and other medical problems in homosexual men

Martin McNally Consultant in Limb Reconstruction and Honorary Senior Lecturer in Orthopaedic Surgery, Bone Infection Unit, Nuffield Orthopaedic Centre, Oxford, UK.
19.3 Osteomyelitis

K. McNeil Director of Transplant Services, The Prince Charles Hospital, Brisbane, Australia.
17.16 Lung and heart–lung transplantation

T. W. Meade Emeritus Professor of Epidemiology, London School of Hygiene and Tropical Medicine, UK.
15.1.2.2 The haemostatic system in arterial disease

A. Meheus Professor, University of Antwerp, Belgium.
21.1 Epidemiology

David K. Menon Professor of Anaesthesia, University of Cambridge, Addenbrooke's Hospital, Cambridge, UK.
16.6.2 Management of raised intracranial pressure

Wayne M. Meyers Chief, Mycobacteriology, Armed Forces Institute of Pathology, Washington DC, USA.
7.11.25 Buruli ulcer: Mycobacterium ulcerans infection

Anna Rita Migliaccio Dirigente de Ricerca in Transfusion Medicine, Laboratory of Clinical Biochemistry, Istituto Superiore dei Sanità, Rome, Italy.
22.5.1 Erythropoiesis and the normal red cell

M. A. Miles Professor, London School of Hygiene and Tropical Medicine, UK.
7.13.11 Chagas' disease

G. J. Miller Professor of Epidemiology, Barts and The London, Queen Mary's School of Medicine and Dentistry, London, UK.
15.1.2.2 The haemostatic system in arterial disease

Mary Miller Consultant in Palliative Medicine, Sir Michael Sobell House, Churchill Hospital, Oxford, UK.
31 Palliative care

Robert F. Miller Reader in Clinical Infection and Consultant Physician, Royal Free and University College Medical School, London, UK.
7.12.5 Pneumocystis carinii

K. R. Mills Professor of Clinical Neurophysiology, King's College Hospital, London, UK.
24.4 Investigation of central motor pathways: magnetic brain stimulation

Philip Minor Public Health and Clinical Microbiology Laboratory, Addenbrooke's Hospital, Cambridge, UK.
7.10.7 Enterovirus infections

Raad H. Mohiaddin Consultant and Honorary Senior Lecturer, Royal Brompton and Harefield NHS Trust, London, JK.
15.3.5 Cardiovascular magnetic resonance and computed X-ray tomography

Andrew J. Molyneux Consultant Neuroradiologist, Radcliffe Infirmary, Oxford, UK.
24.5 Imaging in neurological diseases

Kevin Moore Senior Lecturer, Centre for Hepatology, Royal Free Hospital and University College Medical School, London, UK.
14.21.2 Cirrhosis, portal hypertension, and ascites

Pedro L. Moro Fellow, Vaccine Safety Division, National Immunization Program, Centers for Disease Control and Prevention, Baltimore, Maryland, USA.
7.15.1 Cystic hydatid disease (Echinococcus granulosus)

N. J. McC. Mortensen Professor of Colorectal Surgery, Department of Colorectal Surgery, John Radcliffe Hospital, Oxford, UK.
14.13 Colonic diverticular disease

Peter S. Mortimer Professor of Dermatological Medicine and Consultant Skin Physician, St George's Hospital Medical School, Division of Physiological Medicine, London, UK.
15.17 Lymphoedema

Alastair G. Mowat Clinical Lecturer in Rheumatology, Department of Rheumatology, Nuffield Orthopaedic Centre, Oxford, UK.
18.10.4 Polymyalgia rheumatica and giant-cell arteritis

E. R. Moxon Head, Oxford University Department of Paediatrics, John Radcliffe Hospital, Oxford, UK.
7.11.12 Haemophilus influenzae

M. F. Muers Consultant Physician, Respiratory Medicine, The General Infirmary at Leeds, UK.
17.3.4 Diagnostic bronchoscopy, thoracoscopy, and tissue biopsy

Tariq I. Mughal Consultant Haematologist and Medical Oncologist and Senior Lecturer in Oncology, Lancashire Teaching Hospitals NHS Trust and Preston and Christie Hospital NHS Trust, Manchester, UK.
22.3.6 Chronic myeloid leukaemia

J. A. Muir Gray Director of the UK National Screening Committee, Institute of Health Sciences, Oxford, UK.
3.6 Screening

P. A. Murphy Professor of Medicine and Microbiology, Johns Hopkins University and Chief, Infectious Diseases Division, Johns Hopkins Bayview Hospital, Baltimore, Maryland, USA.
7.5 Physiological changes in infected patients

C. J. L. Murray Global Programme on Evidence for Health Policy, World Health Organization, Geneva, Switzerland.
3.1 The Global Burden of Disease Study

Iain M. Murray-Lyon Consultant Physician and Gastroenterologist, Charing Cross Hospital and Chelsea and Westminster Hospital, London, UK.
14.21.5 Primary and secondary liver tumours

Jean Nachega Assistant Scientist, Johns Hopkins University, Baltimore, Maryland, USA.
7.11.22 Tuberculosis

Robert B. Nadelman Professor of Medicine, Division of Infectious Diseases, New York Medical College, USA.
7.11.29 Lyme borreliosis

N. V. Naoumov Reader in Hepatology/Honorary Consultant Physician, Institute of Hepatology, University College London, UK.
7.10.19 Hepatitis viruses (including TTV)

R. P. Naoumova MRC Senior Clinical Scientist/Honorary Consultant Physician, MRC Clinical Sciences Centre, Hammersmith Hospital, London, UK.
15.1.2.1 The pathogenesis of atherosclerosis

D. G. Nathan President, Dana-Farber Cancer Institute, Boston, Massachusetts, USA.
22.2.1 Stem cells and haemopoiesis

Graham Neale Research Fellow, Clinical Risk Unit, University College London, UK.
14.1 Introduction to gastroenterology. 14.1.1.2 Symptomatology of gastrointestinal disease. 14.16 Vascular and collagen disorders

Catherine Nelson-Piercy Consultant Obstetric Physician, Guy's and St Thomas' Hospitals Trust, London, UK.
13.14 Autoimmune rheumatic disorders and vasculitis in pregnancy

A. R. Ness Senior Lecturer in Epidemiology, Department of Social Medicine, University of Bristol, UK.
15.4.1.2 The epidemiology of ischaemic heart disease

Peter Nestor Neurologist, University of Cambridge Neurology Unit, UK.
24.8 Disturbances of higher cerebral function

J. Neuberger Professor of Hepatology and Consultant Physician, Queen Elizabeth Hospital, Birmingham, UK.
14.21.7 Drugs and liver damage. 14.21.8 The liver in systemic disease

John Newell-Price Senior Lecturer in Endocrinology, Division of Clinical Sciences, Sheffield University, Northern General Hospital, Sheffield, UK.
12.3 Disorders of the posterior pituitary

A. J. Newman Taylor Consultant Physician and Head, Department of Occupational and Environmental Medicine, Royal Brompton Harefield NHS Trust, Faculty of Medicine, Imperial College London, UK.
17.4.4 Asthma. 17.4.5 Occupational asthma

C. S. Ng Assistant Professor, Department of Radiology, University of Texas M. D. Anderson Cancer Center, Houston, USA.
14.18.2 Computed tomography and magnetic resonance imaging of the liver and pancreas

S. Nightingale Consultant Neurologist and Honorary Senior Clinical Lecturer, Royal Shrewsbury Hospital and Birmingham University, Shrewsbury, UK.
7.10.23 HTLV-I and II and associated diseases

T. Northfield Professor Emeritus, Department of Biochemical Medicine, St George's Hospital, London, UK.
14.3.2 Gastrointestinal bleeding

John Nowakowski Assistant Professor of Medicine, Department of Medicine, Division of Infectious Diseases, Westchester Medical Center, Valhalla, New York, USA.
7.11.29 Lyme borreliosis

Fujio Numano Director, Tokyo Vascular Disease Institute, Tokyo, Japan.
15.14.4 Takayasu arteritis

D. O'Gradaigh Research Registrar, Department of Medicine, Addenbrooke's Hospital, Cambridge, UK.
18.11 Miscellaneous conditions presenting to the rheumatologist. 19.5 Avascular necrosis and related topics

Stephen O'Rahilly Professor of Clinical Biochemistry, University of Cambridge, and Honorary Consultant Physician, UK.
10.5 Obesity

S. C. O'Reilly Consultant Rheumatologist, Rheumatology Department, Derbyshire Royal Infirmary, Derby, UK.
18.9 Crystal-related arthropathies

P. J. Oldershaw Consultant Cardiologist, Royal Brompton Hospital, London, UK.
15.13 Congenital heart disease in adolescents and adults

James G. Olson Head, Department of Virology, U. S. Navy Medical Research Center Detachment, Lima, Peru.
7.10.6.1 Nipah and Hendra viruses. 7.11.39 Bartonelloses, excluding Bartonella bacilliformis infections

M. Osame Professor, Third Department of Internal Medicine, Faculty of Medicine, Kagoshima University, Japan.
7.10.23 HTLV-I and II and associated diseases

Jackie Palace Consultant Neurologist, Radcliffe Infirmary, Oxford, UK.
24.17 Disorders of the neuromuscular junction

Thalia Papayannopoulou Professor of Medicine (Hematology), University of Washington, Division of Hematology, Seattle, USA.
22.5.1 Erythropoiesis and the normal red cell

S. Parish Senior Research Fellow, Clinical Trial Service Unit, Nuffield Department of Clinical Medicine, University of Oxford, UK.
2.4.3 Large-scale randomized evidence: trials and overviews

G. R. Park Director of Intensive Care Research, John Farman Intensive Care Unit, Addenbrooke's Hospital, Cambridge, UK.
16.6.1 Sedation and analgesia in the critically ill

David Parkes Professor of Clinical Neurology, King's College Hospital, London, UK.
24.13.4 Narcolepsy

C. Parry University of Oxford–Wellcome Trust Clinical Research Unit, Centre for Tropical Diseases, Ho Chi Minh City, Vietnam.
7.11.8 Typhoid and paratyphoid fevers

Steve W. Parry Consultant Physician and Honorary Senior Lecturer, Freeman Hospital and University of Newcastle upon Tyne, UK.
24.13.5.1 Head-up tilt-table testing in the diagnosis of vasovagal syncope and related disorders

J. Paul Consultant Microbiologist and Director, Brighton Public Health Laboratory, Royal Sussex County Hospital, Brighton, UK.
7.11.42 Newly identified and lesser-known bacteria. 7.17 Non-venomous arthropods

Malik Peiris Professor, Department of Microbiology, University of Hong Kong.
7.10.1 Respiratory tract viruses

Edmund D. Pellegrino Emeritus Professor of Medicine and Medical Ethics, Georgetown University Medical Center, Washington DC, USA.
2.3 Medical ethics

T. H. Pennington Professor of Bacteriology, University of Aberdeen Medical School, UK.
7.3 Biology of pathogenic micro-organisms

M. B. Pepys Professor and Head of Medicine, Department of Medicine, Royal Free Campus, Royal Free and University College Medical School, London, UK.
11.12.1 The acute phase response and C reactive protein. 11.12.4 Amyloidosis

P. L. Perine Professor of Epidemiology, School of Public and Community Medicine, University of Washington, Seattle, USA.
7.11.32 Non-venereal treponematoses: yaws, endemic syphilis (bejel), and pinta

G. D. Perkin Consultant Neurologist, Department of Neurology, Charing Cross Hospital, London, UK.
24.13.3 Epilepsy in later childhood and adults

P. L. Perrotta Assistant Professor, Pathology, Stony Brook University Hospital, New York, USA.
22.8.1 Blood transfusion

H. Persson Medical Director and Consultant Physician, Swedish Poisons Information Centre, Stockholm, Sweden.
8.3 Poisonous plants and fungi

M. C. Petch Consultant Cardiologist, Papworth Hospital, Cambridge, UK.
15.4.2.6 The impact of coronary heart disease on life and work

L. R. Petersen Deputy Director for Science, Centers for Disease Control, Division of Vector-borne Infectious Diseases, Fort Collins, Colorado, USA.
7.10.11 Alphaviruses. 7.10.13 Flaviviruses

R. Peto Professor of Epidemiology and Medical Statistics, University of Oxford, UK.
2.4.3 Large-scale randomized evidence: trials and overviews. 6.1 Epidemiology of cancer

T. E. A. Peto Consultant Physician in Infectious Diseases, Nuffield Department of Medicine, John Radcliffe Hospital, Oxford, UK.
7.10.21 HIV and AIDS

A. Phillips Senior Lecturer, Institute of Nephrology, University of Wales College of Medicine, Cardiff, UK.
20.1 Structure and function of the kidney

R. J. Playford Professor, Imperial College School of Medicine, Hammersmith Hospital, London, UK.
14.9.7 Effects of massive small bowel resection

J. M. Polak Professor and Director, Tissue Engineering and Regenerative Medicine Centre, Imperial College School of Medicine, London, UK.
14.8 Hormones and the gastrointestinal tract

Eleanor S. Pollak Associate Director, Clinical Coagulation Laboratory, Hospital of the University of Pennsylvania, University of Pennsylvania Medical Center, Philadelphia, USA.
22.6.4 Genetic disorders of coagulation

P. A. Poole-Wilson Professor of Cardiology and Cardiac Medicine, National Heart and Lung Institute, Faculty of Medicine, Imperial College London, UK.
15.1.3.1 Physical considerations: biochemistry and cellular physiology of heart muscle

F. M. Pope Consultant Dermatologist, West Middlesex University Hospital, London, UK.
19.2 Inherited defects of connective tissue: Ehlers–Danlos syndrome, Marfan's syndrome, and pseudoxanthoma elasticum

Françoise Portaels Professor and Head, Mycobacteriology Unit, Institute of Tropical Medicine, Antwerp, Belgium.
7.11.25 Buruli ulcer: Mycobacterium ulcerans infection

J. S. Porterfield Formerly Reader in Bacteriology, Sir William Dunn School of Pathology, University of Oxford, UK.
7.10.14 Bunyaviridae

Jerome B. Posner Attending Neurologist, Memorial Sloan-Kettering Cancer Center, New York, USA.
24.18 Paraneoplastic syndromes

William G. Powderly Professor of Medicine, Washington University School of Medicine, St Louis, Missouri, USA.
7.12.2 Cryptococcosis

J. J. Powell Senior Lecturer - Nutrition and Medicine, GI Laboratory, Rayne Institute, St Thomas' Hospital, London, UK.
8.5.8 Podoconiosis

Janet Powell Medical Director, University Hospitals, Coventry and Warwickshire NHS Trust, Coventry, Warwickshire, UK.
15.14.2 Peripheral arterial disease

J. W. Powles University Lecturer in Public Health Medicine, Institute of Public Health, Cambridge, UK.
3.2 Human population size, environment, and health

M. A. Preece Professor of Child Health and Growth, Institute of Child Health, University College London, UK.
12.9.2 Normal growth and its disorders

J. S. Prichard* Professor of Medicine, St James's Hospital, Dublin, Eire.
15.15.2.2 Pulmonary oedema

A. T. Proudfoot Consulting Clinical Toxicologist, National Poisons Information Service, City Hospital, Birmingham, UK.
8.1 Poisoning by drugs and chemicals

Charles Pusey Professor of Renal Medicine, Faculty of Medicine, Imperial College, Hammersmith Hospital, London, UK.
20.7.7 Antiglomerular basement membrane disease

N. P. Quinn Professor of Clinical Neurology, Institute of Neurology and Honorary Consultant Neurologist, The National Hospital for Neurology and Neurosurgery, London, UK.
24.10 Subcortical structures—the cerebellum, thalamus, and basal ganglia

Anisur Rahman Senior Lecturer in Rheumatology, Centre for Rheumatology, Department of Medicine, University College London, UK.
18.10.2 Systemic lupus erythematosus and related disorders

Lawrence E. Ramsay Professor of Clinical Pharmacology and Therapeutics, University of Sheffield and Consultant Physician, Royal Hallamshire Hospital, Sheffield, UK.
15.16.2.1 Hypertension—indications for investigation. 15.16.2.2 Renal and renovascular hypertension. 15.16.2.5 Aortic coarctation. 15.16.2.6 Other rare causes of hypertension. 20.10.2 Hypertension and the kidney

M. Ramsay Consultant Epidemiologist, Immunisation Division, PHLS Communicable Disease Surveillance Centre, London, UK.
7.7 Immunization

A. C. Rankin Reader in Cardiology, Glasgow Royal Infirmary, UK.
15.2.3 Syncope and palpitation. 15.6 Cardiac arrhythmias

C. W. G. Redman Professor of Obstetric Medicine, John Radcliffe Hospital, Oxford, UK.
13.4 Hypertension in pregnancy

Laurence John Reed Academic Unit of Psychiatry, St Thomas' Hospital, London, UK.
26.3 Neuropsychiatric disorders

A. J. Rees Regius Professor of Medicine, Institute of Medical Sciences, University of Aberdeen, UK.
20.10.3 Vasculitis and the kidney

Jeremy Rees Clinical Senior Lecturer in Neuro-oncology, National Hospital for Neurology and Neurosurgery, London, UK.
24.13.18.1 Intracranial tumours

D. Rennie Adjunct Professor of Medicine, Institute for Health Policy Studies, University of California, San Francisco, USA.
8.5.4 Diseases of high terrestrial altitudes

J. Richens Clinical Lecturer, Department of Sexually Transmitted Diseases, Royal Free and University College Medical School, London, UK.
7.11.8 Typhoid and paratyphoid fevers. 7.11.9 Intracellular Klebsiella infections

B. K. Rima Professor of Molecular Biology, Medical Biology Centre, Queen's University of Belfast, UK.
7.10.5 Mumps: epidemic parotitis

A. J. Ritchie Consultant Cardiothoracic Surgeon, Papworth NHS Trust, Cambridge, UK.
15.4.2.5 Coronary artery bypass grafting

Eberhard Ritz Professor and Head, Department of Nephrology, University of Heidelberg, Germany.
20.5.2 Bone disease in chronic renal failure

Harold R. Roberts Sarah Graham Kenan Professor of Medicine and Attending Physician, UNC Hospitals, Chapel Hill, North Carolina, USA.
22.6.1 The biology of haemostasis and thrombosis. 22.6.2 Evaluation of the patient with a bleeding diathesis

William G. Robertson Clinical Scientist, Institute of Urology and Nephrology, University College London, UK.
20.13 Urinary stones, nephrocalcinosis, and renal tubular acidosis

T. A. Rockall Senior Lecturer/Honorary Consultant, St Mary's Hospital, London, UK.
14.3.2 Gastrointestinal bleeding

Allan R. Ronald Professor Emeritus, University of Manitoba, Winnipeg, Canada.
7.11.13 Haemophilus ducreyi and chancroid

P. Ronco Professor of Renal Medicine, Université Pierre et Marie Curie (Paris 6) and Director, Renal Division and INSERM Unit 489, Tenon Hospital (Assistance Publique-Hôpitaux de Paris), Paris, France.
20.10.5 Renal involvement in plasma cell dyscrasias, immunoglobulin-based amyloidoses, and fibrillary glomerulopathies, lymphomas, and leukaemias

Antony Rosen Professor and Director, Division of Rheumatology, Johns Hopkins University School of Medicine, Baltimore, Maryland, USA.
5.3 Autoimmunity

Mark J. Rosen Chief, Division of Pulmonary and Critical Care Medicine, Beth Israel Medical Center, New York, USA.
17.5.2.3 Pulmonary complications of HIV infection

Raymond C. Rosen Professor of Psychiatry, UMDNJ-Robert Wood Johnson Medical School, Department of Psychiatry, Piscataway, New Jersey, USA.
12.8.4 Sexual dysfunction

R. J. M. Ross Professor of Endocrinology, Northern General Hospital, University of Sheffield, UK.
12.9.3 Puberty

D. J. Rowlands Honorary Consultant Cardiologist, Manchester Heart Centre, Manchester Royal Infirmary, UK.
15.3.2 Electrocardiography. 15.3.4 Nuclear techniques

M. B. Rubens Director of Imaging and Consultant Radiologist, Royal Brompton and Harefield NHS Trust, London, UK.
15.3.1 Chest radiography in heart disease. 15.3.5 Cardiovascular magnetic resonance and computed X-ray tomography

David Rubenstein Consultant Physician, Addenbrooke's Hospital, Cambridge, UK.
7.1 The clinical approach to the patient with suspected infection

P. C. Rubin Professor and Dean of Medicine, University of Nottingham, UK.
13.18 Prescribing in pregnancy

Anthony S. Russell Professor of Medicine, University of Alberta, Edmonton, Canada.
18.2 Clinical presentation and diagnosis of rheumatic disease

T. J. Ryan Emeritus Professor of Dermatology, University of Oxford, UK.
23.1 Diseases of the skin

Sara S. T. O. Saad Professor and Haematologist, Department of Internal Medicine, Hematology-Hemotherapy Division, Medical Science Faculty, State University of Campinas, Brazil.
22.5.10 Disorders of the red cell membrane

N. J. Samani Professor of Cardiology, Division of Cardiology, Department of Medicine, University of Leicester, UK.
15.16.1.2 Genetics of hypertension

Brian P. Saunders Senior Lecturer in Endoscopy, St Mark's Hospital, Northwick Park, Harrow, Middlesex, UK.
14.2.1 Colonoscopy and flexible sigmoidoscopy

S. J. Saunders Emeritus Professor, Liver Clinic, Groote Schuur Hospital and Medical Research Council/University of Cape Town Liver Research Centre, Cape Town, South Africa.
14.21.6 Hepatic granulomas

M. O. Savage Professor of Paediatric Endocrinology, St Bartholomew's and The Royal London School of Medicine and Dentistry, London, UK.
12.9.1 Normal and abnormal sexual differentiation. 12.9.3 Puberty

John Savill Professor of Medicine, Royal Infirmary, Edinburgh, UK.
20.7.1 The glomerulus and glomerular injury

* It is with regret that we report the death of Professor J. S. Prichard.

K. P. Schaal Professor and Director, Institute for Medical Microbiology and Immunology, Faculty of Medicine, Rheinische Friedrich-Wilhelms-Universität, Bonn, Germany.
7.11.26 Actinomycosis

Michael Schömig Physician in Charge, Division of Nephrology, Ruperto-Carola-University of Heidelberg, Germany.
20.5.2 Bone disease in chronic renal failure

Ruud B. H. Schutgens Head of Department of Clinical Chemistry, Vrije Universiteit Medical Centre (VUMC), Amsterdam, The Netherlands.
11.9 Peroxisomal diseases

J. Schwebke Associate Professor of Medicine, University of Alabama at Birmingham, USA.
21.3 Vaginal discharge

Neil Scolding Burden Professor of Clinical Neurosciences, University of Bristol Institute of Clinical Neurosciences, Frenchay Hospital, Bristol, UK.
24.15 Metabolic disorders and the nervous system. 24.20 Neurological complications of systemic autoimmune and inflammatory diseases

J. Scott Professor of Medicine, Imperial College Faculty of Medicine, Hammersmith Campus, London, UK.
15.1.2.1 The pathogenesis of atherosclerosis

A. Seaton Professor and Head of Department of Environmental and Occupational Medicine, University of Aberdeen, UK.
17.11.7 Pneumoconioses

G. R. Serjeant Professor Emeritus and Chairman, Sickle Cell Trust, Kingston, Jamaica, West Indies.
20.10.7 Sickle-cell disease and the kidney

N. J. Severs Professor of Cell Biology, National Heart and Lung Institute, Faculty of Medicine, Imperial College London, UK.
15.1.3.1 Physical considerations: biochemistry and cellular physiology of heart muscle

C. A. Seymour Professor of Clinical Biochemistry and Metabolic Medicine and Director for Clinical Advice to The Health Service Ombudsman, St George's Hospital Medical School and Office of Health Service Commissioner, London, UK.
11.7.2 Wilson's disease, Menke's disease: inherited disorders of copper metabolism

K. V. Shah Professor, Johns Hopkins Bloomberg School of Public Health, Baltimore, Maryland, USA.
7.10.17 Papovaviruses

L. M. Shapiro Consultant Cardiologist, Papworth Hospital, Cambridge, UK.
15.4.2.2 Management of stable angina. 15.4.2.5 Coronary artery bypass grafting

Michael Sharpe Reader in Psychological Medicine, University of Edinburgh, Royal Edinburgh Hospital, UK.
7.19 Chronic fatigue syndrome (postviral fatigue syndrome,neurasthenia, and myalgic encephalomyelitis). 26.1 General introduction. 26.5.3 Medically unexplained symptoms in patients attending medical clinics. 26.6.2 Psychological treatment in medical practice

J. M. Shneerson Director, Respiratory Support and Sleep Centre, Papworth Hospital, Cambridge, UK.
17.13 Disorders of the thoracic cage and diaphragm

Tom Siddons Clinical Research Assistant, Pfizer Research and Development (UK), Maidstone, Kent, UK.
15.15.1 The pulmonary circulation and its influence on gas exchange

C. A. Sieff Associate Professor in Pediatrics, Dana Farber Cancer Institute, Boston, Massachusetts, USA.
22.2.1 Stem cells and haemopoiesis

J. Sieper Head of Rheumatology, Department of Medicine, University Hospital Benjamin Franklin, Berlin, Germany.
18.6 Spondyloarthritides and related arthritides

Leslie Silberstein Professor, University of Pennsylvania School of Medicine, Philadelphia, Pennsylvania, USA.
22.5.9 Haemolytic anaemia—congenital and acquired

R. Sinclair Senior Lecturer, Department of Dermatology, University of Melbourne, St Vincent's Hospital, Fitzroy, Victoria, Australia.
23.1 Diseases of the skin

Joseph Sinning Yale School of Medicine, New Haven, Connecticut, USA.
22.4.1 Leucocytes in health and disease

Thira Sirisanthana Professor of Medicine and Director, Research Institute for Health Sciences, Chiang Mai University, Thailand.
7.11.18 Anthrax. 7.12.6 Infection due to Penicillium marneffei

J. G. P. Sissons Professor of Medicine, University of Cambridge and Honorary Consultant Physician, Addenbrooke's Hospital, Cambridge, UK.
7.10.2 Herpesviruses (excluding Epstein–Barr virus)

M. B. Skirrow Honorary Emeritus Consultant Microbiologist, Public Health Laboratory, Gloucester Royal Hospital, UK.
7.11.7 Enterobacteria, campylobacter, and miscellaneous food-poisoning bacteria

Geoffrey L. Smith Professor of Virology and Wellcome Trust Principal Research Fellow, The Wright–Fleming Institute, Faculty of Medicine, Imperial College of Science, Technology and Medicine, St Mary's Campus, London, UK.
7.10.4 Poxviruses

P. H. Smith Department of Urology, St James' University Hospital, Leeds, UK.
20.15 Tumours of the urinary tract

R. Smith Consultant Physician, Nuffield Orthopaedic Centre, Oxford, UK.
19.1 Disorders of the skeleton

E. L. Snyder Professor of Laboratory Medicine, Yale University School of Medicine, New Haven, Connecticut, USA.
22.8.1 Blood transfusion

R. L. Souhami Director of Clinical Research, Cancer Research UK and Emeritus Professor of Medicine, University College London, London, UK.
6.6 Cancer: clinical features and management

C. W. N. Spearman Senior Specialist and Co-Head of Liver Clinic, Groote Schuur Hospital, Cape Town, South Africa.
14.21.6 Hepatic granulomas

C. A. Speed Honorary Consultant Rheumatologist, Addenbrooke's Hospital, Cambridge, UK.
19.5 Avascular necrosis and related topics

G. P. Spickett Consultant Clinical Immunologist, Regional Department of Immunology, Royal Victoria Infirmary, Newcastle upon Tyne, UK.
17.11.8 Pulmonary haemorrhagic disorders. 17.11.9 Eosinophilic pneumonia. 17.11.11 Extrinsic allergic alveolitis. 17.11.19 Drug-induced lung disease

S. G. Spiro Professor of Respiratory Medicine and Medical Director, Medicine, University College London Hospitals NHS Trust, Middlesex Hospital, London, UK.
17.14.1.1 Lung cancer. 17.14.1.2 Pulmonary metastases

Jerry L. Spivak Professor of Medicine and Oncology, Johns Hopkins School of Medicine, Baltimore, Maryland, USA.
22.3.9 Idiopathic myelofibrosis

A. Spurgeon Senior Lecturer, Institute of Occupational Health, University of Birmingham, UK.
8.4.1 Occupational and environmental health and safety

Paul D. Stein Director of Research, St Joseph Mercy-Oakland, Pontiac, Michigan, USA.
15.15.3.1 Deep venous thrombosis and pulmonary embolism

Tom Stevens Consultant Psychiatrist, St Thomas' Hospital and Maudsley NHS Trust, London, UK.
26.3 Neuropsychiatric disorders

J. C. Stevenson Reader and Consultant Physician, Endocrinology and Metabolic Medicine, Faculty of Medicine, Imperial College London, UK.
13.20 Benefits and risks of hormone replacement therapy

P. M. Stewart Professor of Medicine, University of Birmingham and Consultant Physician, Queen Elizabeth Hospital, Birmingham, UK.
12.7.1 Disorders of the adrenal cortex

August Stich Consultant in Tropical Medicine, Medical Mission Institute, Unit of Tropical Medicine and Epidemic Control, Wurzburg, Germany.
7.13.10 Human African trypanosomiasis

John H. Stone Associate Professor of Medicine, Johns Hopkins University, Baltimore, Maryland, USA.
18.10.7 Polymyositis and dermatomyositis

J. R. Stradling Consultant Physician and Professor of Respiratory Medicine, Churchill Hospital, Oxford, UK.
17.1.1 The upper respiratory tract. 17.8.1 Upper airways obstruction. 17.8.2 Sleep-related disorders of breathing

Frank J. Strobl Director, Scientific Affairs, Therakos Inc., Exton, Pennsylvania, USA.
22.5.9 Haemolytic anaemia—congenital and acquired

M. A. Stroud Senior Lecturer in Medicine, Southampton University Hospitals Trust, UK.
8.5.1 Environmental extremes—heat. 8.5.2 Environmental extremes—cold

Michael Strupp Associate Professor of Neurology, Department of Neurology, Klinikum Grosshadern, University of Munich, Germany.
24.12.1 Eye movements and balance

P. H. Sugden Professor of Cellular Biochemistry, Imperial College of Science, Technology and Medicine, London, UK.
15.1.3.1 Physical considerations: biochemistry and cellular physiology of heart muscle

Daniel P. Sulmasy Sisters of Charity Chair in Ethics, St Vincent's Manhattan and New York Medical College, New York, USA.
2.3 Medical ethics

J. A. Summerfield Professor of Experimental Medicine, Faculty of Medicine, Imperial College London, UK.
14.19.1 Congenital disorders of the liver, biliary tract, and pancreas. 14.19.2 Diseases of the gallbladder and biliary tree

Pravan Suntharasamai Emeritus Professor of Tropical Medicine, Faculty of Tropical Medicine, Mahidol University, Bangkok, Thailand.
7.14.9 Gnathostomiasis

J. Swales* Professor of Medicine, University of Leicester, UK.
15.16.1.3 Essential hypertension

P. Sweny Consultant Nephrologist, Royal Free Hospital, London, UK.
20.6.3 Renal transplantation

D. Swirsky Consultant Haematologist, Leeds General Infirmary, UK.
22.4.4 The spleen and its disorders

I. C. Talbot Professor of Histopathology, St Mark's Hospital for Colorectal Disorders, London, UK.
14.15 Tumours of the gastrointestinal tract

D. Tarin Director, UCSD Cancer Center, University of California at San Diego, La Jolla, USA.
6.4 Tumour metastasis

D. Taylor-Robinson Emeritus Professor of Genitourinary Microbiology and Medicine, Division of Medicine, Imperial College of Science, Technology and Medicine, St Mary's Hospital, London, UK.
7.11.40 Chlamydial infections including lymphogranuloma venerum. 7.11.41 Mycoplasmas

P. J. Teddy Consultant Neurosurgeon/Clinical Director, Department of Neurological Surgery, Radcliffe Infirmary, Oxford, UK.
24.14.3 Intracranial abscess

H. J. Testa Professor and Consultant (retired), Royal Infirmary, Manchester, UK.
15.3.4 Nuclear techniques

R. V. Thakker May Professor of Medicine, Nuffield Department of Medicine, University of Oxford, UK.
12.6 Parathyroid disorders and diseases altering calcium metabolism

David G. T. Thomas Professor of Neurological Surgery, National Hospital for Neurology and Neurosurgery, London, UK.
24.13.18.2 Traumatic injuries of the head

D. L. Thomas Associate Professor of Medicine, Johns Hopkins School of Medicine, Baltimore, Maryland, USA.
7.10.20 Hepatitis C virus

P. K. Thomas Emeritus Professor of Neurology, Royal Free Hospital School of Medicine and Institute of Neurology, London, UK.
24.6.1 Inherited disorders. 24.13.15 Disorders of cranial nerves. 24.19 Diseases of the peripheral nerves

D. G. Thompson Professor of Gastroenterology, University of Manchester, UK.
14.1.1.1 Structure and function of the gut. 14.12 Functional bowel disorders and irritable bowel syndrome

R. P. H. Thompson Consultant Physician, St Thomas' Hospital, London, UK.
8.5.8 Podoconiosis. 14.19.3 Jaundice

S. A. Thorne Royal Brompton and Harefield NHS Trust, London, UK.
15.13 Congenital heart disease in adolescents and adults

Ph. Thulliez Head, Laboratoire de la Toxoplasmose, Institut de Puericulture, Paris, France.
7.13.4 Toxoplasmosis

Tran Tin Hien Vice Director, Centre for Tropical Diseases (Cho Quan Hospital), Ho Chi Minh City, Vietnam.
7.11.1 Diphtheria

J. A. Todd Professor of Medical Genetics, University of Cambridge, UK.
12.11.2 The genetics of diabetes melllitus

C. Tomson Consultant Nephrologist, Southmead Hospital, Bristol, UK.
20.12 Urinary tract infection

Keith Tones Professor of Health Education (Emeritus), Leeds Metropolitan University, UK.
3.5 Health promotion

P. A. Tookey Lecturer, Centre for Epidemiology and Biostatistics, Institute of Child Health, London, UK.
7.10.12 Rubella

P. P. Toskes Professor of Medicine, Division of Gastroenterology, Hepatology, and Nutrition, Department of Medicine, University of Florida College of Medicine, Gainsville, USA.
14.9.2 Small bowel bacterial overgrowth. 14.18.3.2 Chronic pancreatitis

Thomas A. Traill Professor of Medicine, Johns Hopkins Hospital, Baltimore, Maryland, USA.
15.11.1 Cardiac myxoma. 15.11.2 Other tumours of the heart. 15.12 Cardiac involvement in genetic disease

David F. Treacher Consultant Physician in Intensive Care, St Thomas' Hospital, Guy's and St Thomas' NHS Trust, London, UK.
16.2 The circulation and circulatory support of the critically ill

A. S. Truswell Emeritus Professor of Human Nutrition, University of Sydney, New South Wales, Australia.
10.1 Diseases of overnourished societies and the need for dietary change

D. M. Turnbull Professor of Neurology, The Medical School, University of Newcastle upon Tyne, UK.
24.22.5 Mitochondrial encephalomyopathies

H. E. Turner Consultant Physician, Radcliffe Infirmary, Oxford, UK.
12.12 Hormonal manifestations of non-endocrine disease

A. Neil Turner Professor of Nephrology, Royal Infirmary, Edinburgh, UK.
20.7.8 Infection-associated nephropathies. 20.7.9 Malignancy-associated renal disease

Robert Twycross Emeritus Clinical Reader in Palliative Medicine, Oxford University, Sir Michael Sobell House, Churchill Hospital, Oxford, UK.
31 Palliative care

F. E. Udwadia Emeritus Professor of Medicine, Grant Medical College and J. J. Hospital, Bombay; Consultant Physician and Director-in-charge of ICU, Breach Candy Hospital; Consultant Physician, Parsee General hospital, Bombay, India.
7.11.20 Tetanus

S. Richard Underwood Professor of Cardiac Imaging, Imperial College of Science, Technology and Medicine, National Heart and Lung Institute, and Royal Brompton Hospital, London, UK.
15.3.5 Cardiovascular magnetic resonance and computed X-ray tomography

Robert J. Unwin Professor of Nephrology and Physiology, Centre for Nephrology, The Middlesex Hospital, London, UK.
20.13 Urinary stones, nephrocalcinosis, and renal tubular acidosis

V. Urquidi Assistant Professor, University of California San Diego Cancer Center and Department of Pathology, La Jolla, California, USA.
6.4 Tumour metastasis

J. A. Vale Director, National Poisons Information Service and West Midlands Poisons Unit, City Hospital, Birmingham, UK.
8.1 Poisoning by drugs and chemicals

---

* It is with regret that we report the death of Professor J. Swales during the preparation of this edition of the textbook.

P. Vallance Professor of Clinical Pharmacology and Therapeutics, Centre for Clinical Pharmacology, University College London, UK.
15.1.1.2 Vascular endothelium, its physiology and pathophysiology

J. van Gijn Professor and Chairman, Department of Neurology, University Medical Centre, Utrecht, The Netherlands.
24.13.7 Stroke: cerebrovascular disease

Sirivan Vanijanonta Emeritus Professor of Tropical Medicine, Faculty of Tropical Medicine, Mahidol University, Bangkok, Thailand.
7.16.3 Lung flukes (paragonimiasis)

Patrick J. W. Venables Professor and Honorary Consultant, Kennedy Institute Division, Imperial College London, UK.
18.10.6 Sjögren's syndrome

B. J. Vennervald Senior Research Scientist, Danish Bilharziasis Laboratory, Charlottenlund, Denmark.
7.16.1 Schistosomiasis

C. M. Verity Consultant Paediatric Neurologist and Associate Lecturer, Faculty of Medicine, University of Cambridge, Addenbrooke's Hospital, Cambridge, UK.
24.21 Developmental abnormalities of the central nervous system

M. P. Vessey Emeritus Professor of Public Health, Unit of Health Care Epidemiology, Department of Public Health, Oxford University, UK.
13.19 Benefits and risks of oral contraceptives

R. Viner Consultant in Adolescent Medicine and Endocrinology, University College London Hospitals and Great Ormond Street Hospital, UK.
29 Adolescent medicine

Peter D. Wagner Professor of Medicine and Bioengineering, University of California, San Diego, USA.
17.1.2 Structure and function of the airways and alveoli

Ann E. Wakefield* Professor of Paediatric Infectious Diseases, Department of Paediatrics, Institute of Molecular Medicine, University of Oxford, UK.
7.12.5 Pneumocystis carinii

D. H. Walker The Carmage and Martha Walls Distinguished Chair in Tropical Diseases, Professor and Chairman, Department of Pathology, and Director, WHO Collaborating Center for Tropical Diseases, Galveston, Texas, USA.
7.11.36 Rickettsial diseases including ehrlichiosis

J. A. Walker-Smith Emeritus Professor of Paediatric Gastroenterology, Royal Free and University College Medical School, London, UK.
14.14 Congenital abnormalities of the gastrointestinal tract

Mark J. Walport Professor of Medicine and Head, Division of Medicine, Faculty of Medicine, Imperial College London, Hammersmith Hospital, London, UK.
5.4 Complement

Julian R. F. Walters Reader in Gastroenterology, Imperial College of Science, Technology and Medicine, Hammersmith Campus, London, UK.
14.2.4 Investigation of gastrointestinal function. 14.9.1 Differential diagnosis and investigation of malabsorption

Gary S. Wand Professor of Medicine, Johns Hopkins University School of Medicine, Baltimore, Maryland, USA.
26.7.1 Alcohol and drug dependence

Ronald J. A. Wanders Professor of Inborn Errors and Metabolism and Deputy Head of the Laboratory for Metabolic Diseases, Academic Medical Centre, Amsterdam, The Netherlands.
11.9 Peroxisomal diseases

B. Ward Anaesthetic Registrar, Coventry School of Anaesthetics, UK.
16.6.1 Sedation and analgesia in the critically ill

T. E. Warkentin Professor, Department of Pathology and Molcular Medicine and Department of Medicine, McMaster University, Hamilton, Ontario, Canada.
22.6.5 Acquired coagulation disorders

D. A. Warrell Professor of Tropical Medicine and Infectious Diseases and Head, Nuffield Department of Clinical Medicine, University of Oxford, UK.
7.8 Travel and expedition medicine. 7.10.9 Rhabdoviruses: rabies and rabies-related viruses. 7.10.10 Colorado tick fever and other arthropod-borne reoviruses. 7.11.28 Rat-bite fevers. 7.11.30 Other borrelia infections. 7.11.32 Non-venereal treponematoses: yaws, endemic syphilis (bejel), and pinta. 7.13.2 Malaria. 7.13.5 Cryptosporidium and cryptosporidiosis. 7.18 Pentostomiasis (porocephalosis). 8.2 Injuries, envenoming, poisoning, and allergic reactions caused by animals. 24.14.1 Bacterial meningitis. 24.14.2 Viral infections of the central nervous system. 24.22.6 Tropical pyomyositis (tropical myositis). 33 Emergency medicine

M. J. Warrell Clinical Virologist, Centre for Tropical Medicine, John Radcliffe Hospital, Oxford, UK.
7.10.9 Rhabdoviruses: rabies and rabies-related viruses. 7.10.10 Colorado tick fever and other arthropod-borne reoviruses

Paul Warwicker Consultant Nephrologist, Renal Unit, Lister Hospital, Stevenage, Hertfordshire, UK.
20.10.6 Haemolytic uraemic syndrome

J. A. H. Wass Professor of Endocrinology and Consultant Physician, Radcliffe Infirmary, Oxford, UK.
12.12 Hormonal manifestations of non-endocrine disease

Laurence Watkins Consultant Neurosurgeon and Senior Lecturer, Institute of Neurology, London, UK.
24.13.18.2 Traumatic injuries of the head

George Watt Department of Medicine, AFRIMS, Bangkok, Thailand.
7.11.31 Leptospirosis. 7.11.37 Scrub typhus

Richard W. E. Watts Visiting Professor and Honorary Consultant Physician, Imperial College School of Medicine, Hammersmith Hospital, London, UK.
11.1 The inborn errors of metabolism: general aspects. 11.4 Disorders of purine and pyrimidine metabolism. 11.10 Disorders of oxalate metabolism

D. J. Weatherall Regius Professor of Medicine Emeritus, University of Oxford, Weatherall Institute of Molecular Medicine, John Radcliffe Hospital, Oxford, UK.
2.2 Scientific method and the art of healing. 22.1 Introduction. 22.5.2 Anaemia: pathophysiology, classification, and clinical features. 22.5.3 Anaemia as a world health problem. 22.5.5 Normochromic, normocytic anaemia. 22.5.7 Disorders of the synthesis or function of haemoglobin. 22.7 The blood in systemic disease

D. K. H. Webb Consultant Paediatric Haematologist, Great Ormond Street Hospital for Children, London, UK.
22.4.7 Histiocytoses

Kathryn E. Webert Clinical Scholar, Hematology and Fellow in Transfusion Medicine, Canadian Blood Services, McMaster University, Hamilton, Ontario, Canada.
22.6.3 Disorders of platelet number and function

A. D. B. Webster Consultant Immunologist, Department of Immunology, Royal Free Hospital, London, UK.
5.6 Immunodeficiency

Anthony P. Weetman Professor of Medicine and Dean, University of Sheffield Medical School, UK.
12.4 The thyroid gland and disorders of thyroid function. 12.5 Thyroid cancer

R. A. Weiss Professor, University College London, UK.
7.10.21 HIV and AIDS. 7.10.24 Viruses and cancer

Peter L. Weissberg BHF Professor of Cardiovascular Medicine, University of Cambridge, UK.
15.1.1.1 Introduction. 15.1.1.3 Vascular smooth muscle cells. 15.4.2.1 The pathophysiology of acute coronary syndromes

Peter F. Weller Professor of Medicine, Harvard Medical School; Chief of Allergy and Inflammation and Co-Chief, Infectious Diseases Division, Beth Israel Deaconess Medical Center, Boston, Massachusetts, USA.
22.4.6 Eosinophilia

A. K. Wells Consultant Respiratory Physician, Royal Brompton Hospital, London, UK.
17.11.4 The lungs and rheumatological diseases

Simon Wessely Professor of Epidemiological Psychiatry, Guy's, King's and St Thomas' School of Medicine and Institute of Psychiatry, London, UK.
26.6.2 Psychological treatment in medical practice

---

* It is with regret that we report the death of Professor Ann E. Wakefield during the preparation of this edition of the textbook.

Gilbert C. White, II John C. Parker Professor of Medicine and Pharmacology and Director, Center for Thrombosis and Hemostasis, University of North Carolina School of Medicine, Chapel Hill, North Carolina, USA.
22.6.1 The biology of haemostasis and thrombosis. 22.6.2 Evaluation of the patient with a bleeding diathesis

Joseph White SPHTM at TUMC, New Orleans, Louisiana, USA.
3.7.1 The cost of health care in Western countries

H. C. Whittle Visiting Professor, London School of Hygiene and Tropical Medicine and Deputy Director, MRC Laboratories, Banjul, The Gambia.
7.10.6 Measles

D. E. L. Wilcken Professor Emeritus of Medicine and Head, Cardiovascular Research Laboratory, University of New South Wales and Prince of Wales Hospital, Sydney, Australia.
15.1.3.2 Clinical physiology of the normal heart

James S. Wiley Professor and Head of Haematology, Nepean Hospital, Penrith, New South Wales, Australia.
22.5.8 Anaemias resulting from defective red cell maturation

P. J. Wilkinson Consultant Medical Microbiologist, University Hospital, Queen's Medical Centre, Nottingham, UK.
7.11.34 Listeriosis

R. G. Will Professor of Clinical Neurology, Western General Hospital, Edinburgh, UK.
24.13.9 Human prion disease

C. B. Williams Consultant Physician in Endoscopy, St Mark's Hospital for Colorectal Disorders, UK.
14.2.1 Colonoscopy and flexible sigmoidoscopy. 14.15 Tumours of the gastrointestinal tract

D. J. Williams Senior Lecturer/Honorary Consultant in Obstetric Medicine, Division of Paediatrics, Obstetrics and Gynaecology, Imperial College of Science, Technology and Medicine, Chelsea and Westminster Hospital, London, UK.
13.1 Physiological changes of normal pregnancy. 13.2 Nutrition in pregnancy. 13.3 Medical management of normal pregnancy

Gareth Williams Professor of Medicine, Department of Medicine, Clinical Sciences Centre, University Hospital Aintree, Liverpool, UK.
12.11.1 Diabetes

J. D. Williams Professor of Nephrology and Consultant Physician, Institute of Nephrology, University of Wales College of Medicine, Cardiff, UK.
20.1 Structure and function of the kidney

Paul F. Williams Consultant Nephrologist, The Ipswich Hospital NHS Trust, UK.
20.6.2 The treatment of endstage renal disease by peritoneal dialysis

Robert Wilson Consultant Physician and Reader, Royal Brompton Hospital and National Heart and Lung Institute, Imperial College of Science, Technology and Medicine, London, UK.
17.3.3 Microbiological methods in the diagnosis of respiratory infections

C. G. Winearls Consultant Nephrologist, Oxford Kidney Unit, Churchill Hospital, Oxford, UK.
20.5.1 Chronic renal failure

F. Wojnarowska Professor of Dermatology and Consultant Dermatologist, Oxford Radcliffe Hospital, Oxford, UK.
13.13 The skin in pregnancy

R. Wolman Consultant in Rheumatology and Sports Medicine, Royal National Orthopaedic Hospital, Stanmore, Middlesex, UK.
28 Sports and exercise medicine

Kathryn J. Wood Professor of Immunology, Nuffield Department of Surgery, University of Oxford, UK.
5.7 Principles of transplantation immunology

Nicholas Wood Professor of Clinical Neurology, Institute of Neurology, London, UK.
24.6.2 Neurogenetics. 24.13.12 Ataxic disorders

Trevor Woodage Clinical Investigator, Celera Genomics, Rockville, Maryland, USA.
4.1 The genomic basis of medicine

H. F. Woods Professor of Medicine, University of Sheffield, UK.
11.11 Disturbances of acid-base homeostasis

Gary P. Wormser Vice Chairman, Department of Medicine, and Chief, Division of Infectious Diseases, New York Medical College, Valhalla, New York, USA.
7.11.29 Lyme borreliosis

D. J. M. Wright Emeritus Reader in Medical Microbiology, Cell and Molecular Biology Section, Imperial College School of Medicine, London, UK.
7.11.33 Syphilis

V. M. Wright Consultant Paediatric Surgeon, Barts and The London NHS Trust, London, UK.
14.14 Congenital abnormalities of the gastrointestinal tract

F. C. W. Wu Senior Lecturer (Endocrinology), Royal Infirmary and University of Manchester, UK.
12.8.2 Disorders of male reproduction

Andrew H. Wyllie Professor and Head of Department of Pathology, University of Cambridge, UK.
4.6 Apoptosis in health and disease

M. A. S. Yasuda Professor, Department of Infectious and Parasitic Diseases, University of São Paulo Medical School, Brazil.
7.12.4 Paracoccidioidomycosis

Newman M. Yeilding Assistant Professor, University of Pennsylvania, Philadelphia, USA.
4.3 Molecular cell biology

Jenny Yiend Postdoctoral Research Assistant, MRC Cognition and Brain Science Unit, Cambridge, UK.
26.5.1 Grief, stress, and post-traumatic stress disorder

V. Zaman Professor, Department of Microbiology, The Aga Khan University, Karachi, Pakistan.
7.13.7 Sarcocystosis. 7.14.6 Other gut nematodes. 7.14.7 Toxocariasis and visceral larva migrans

1

On being a patient

1 On being a patient

C. M. Clothier

'Patior'—'I am suffering'—one recalls being taught at school. Every student knows that a patient is generally, but not always, one who is suffering, and perhaps not very patiently. Only by derivation has the word become associated with the bearing without complaint, of pain, sorrow, or simple irritation with others. Yet this secondary meaning is important in medicine because it reminds us that the great majority of patients do in fact suffer their illnesses with remarkable fortitude and endurance. Might this be another facet of the urge to survive and to minimize disability in the essentially competitive struggle of life? Is it this instinct, perhaps, which leads the average healthy person who stumbles and falls in the street to declare: 'It's nothing really' or 'I'll be all right in a minute', as they try to rise quickly from the fallen position of the vanquished? For falling to the ground in combat is usually fatal, and voluntary prostration of the body usually signifies submission and defeat.

So when otherwise healthy persons seek help from a doctor, or are admitted to hospital, it may be assumed that they are in some perturbation of mind as well as of body. It is this suffering in the mind that makes every patient different, even when their condition is familiar and well recognized, because the mental element in any illness varies enormously with circumstance and temperament.

Visiting the family doctor is usually less of an ordeal for the patient than admission to hospital. The patient often retains the dignity of an upright position *vis-à-vis* the doctor. However, the element of personal distress may still be there and may mask or distort the objective signs and symptoms for which the doctor is trained to look. The 'dependent well' may only be seeking a listening post for the torments of family dissension, personal tragedy, or just old age. Other patients enjoy being examined, manipulated, or injected because of the personal contact and attention involved, which they otherwise lack. How much time to give to each of the greatly diverse patients of a practice or a hospital is a matter of delicate judgement: most will deserve a sympathetic response, but some will seem to merit a rather positive rejection. Yet one must be careful; for there have been recorded instances of patients who complained of bizarre symptoms, signifying no identifiable illness, who were rejected as malingerers but subsequently were shown to have suffered greatly from insidious disease or poison. Those who are truly ill may be brave, or craven, or something in between, depending upon age, circumstance, or personal quality. However, one thing is certain, each patient will think himself or herself to be reacting normally to the predicament of illness, real or imaginary, and will be expecting the same degree of medical attention. If they do not get it they will be offended and angry: whether that reaction should provoke from the doctor sympathy or dismissal may be as crucial a judgement as writing a prescription.

On the other hand, admission to hospital is a fundamentally different experience both for patients and those caring for them. Here the dominant factors are the concession of defeat and the abandonment of the safe haven of home. To lie down in the presence of others in a strange place, to get undressed in the middle of the day, to give specimens of urine or blood, all on the orders of those who remain upright, are acts of submission. The arrival in hospital is accompanied by feelings of anxious apprehension, fear, isolation, and general mental turmoil which caused Osbert Sitwell to speak of 'First depressions on arrival'. Mingled with these feelings may also be some sense of relief in having finally admitted defeat and agreed to surrender one's body into other hands. When one adds to these varied emotions anxiety about work, about the home, or about the patient's spouse or children, it is a wonder that the admitting doctor gets any sensible or accurate answer out of a patient for the first 24 hours after admission. When histories are taken, these widely variable responses to stress, for the most part concealed, should be in the doctor's mind. Even the lay patient is likely to be aware that blood pressure and heart rate are raised when first they are measured in hospital. Symptoms may be minimized, exaggerated consciously or unconsciously, invented, or simply forgotten. Dates and times of episodes or onsets may be so wide of the mark as to be of little use in diagnosis, if not positively dangerous.

The risk, then, is that the patient in hospital becomes merely an interesting focus of medical attention rather than a person with all those confusions of mind that make him or her an individual. This is a very real danger in modern hospital practice, the more so as we are now equipped with the most sophisticated apparatus for diagnosis, facilities that may be seen by some as reducing the need for any contribution from the patient. The feeling of personal unimportance is a marked cause of unhappiness among patients in hospital and a frequent source of complaint against doctors and nurses. Doctors can and sometimes do speak and look as if the patient was no more than an interesting clinical object and nurses can exacerbate the grievance by discussing their private affairs across the bed of the patient to whom they are attending.

In teaching hospitals, the patient's sense of unimportance may be increased by the ordeal of the professional ward round. It has to be stated that even now, at the start of the twenty-second century, there are consultants who persistently treat patients as the fortunate recipients of their attentions, whose views and feelings are of little relevance in the pursuit of a learned profession. Besides being a technical breach of obligation under the terms of a consultant's National Health Service contract, such conduct is rude. A good doctor, who engages the patients' attention and participation in a discussion of their case, may learn a great deal, besides giving the patient immense satisfaction and inspiring confidence. 'Encourage the patient to talk', said a wise old practitioner, 'and he will eventually tell you what is the matter with him'. It is regrettable that those who practise an excessive clinical detachment are not only the old and authoritarian, but include those who have grown up in a world where medical omniscience is no longer taken for granted. Doctors who cannot naturally feel a surge of sympathy for the body prostrated before them should perhaps consider a career in research.

The patients of today are very different from those of half a century ago. Until the advent of the mass media, the relationship between patient and doctor resembled that between parishioner and pastor, schoolmaster and pupil, or lawyer and client. It was impious to question the wisdom or judgement of the learned professional adviser. The remarkable expression 'sapiential authority' sought to encapsulate this ascendancy of doctor over patient. Such a relationship was often quite a happy one for both parties, and perhaps more conducive to treatment and cure than a less trusting one.

However, the mass media, and supremely, television, have changed all that. We have all penetrated behind the camera into the operating theatre and other private places and there seen what doctors and their assistants actually do in the attempt to cure illness or repair damage. However skilful and ingenious, it is obviously not miraculous, and some of it is rather pedestrian. The curtains have been parted and the magic revealed. The magicians themselves have often admitted their humanity and confessed to their failures. When mystery is dispelled, the questions come thick and fast.

It is of no use to resist the tide of doubt and curiosity that now threatens to overwhelm not just medicine but all the learned professions. Family doctors must now expect patients to ask quite penetrating questions about the treatment proposed for them and the drugs it is intended to use. These questions must be answered with some candour if mutual trust is to be maintained. Nothing more disturbs a patient, who may be very intelligent even though not learned in medicine, than hearing their doctor seeking to disguise his own ignorance or doubt by prevarication or deviousness, often easily detected. Besides all of which, it sometimes does professionals in any discipline a great deal of good to be closely questioned about beliefs and practices that they have long held to be unassailably correct; and they should listen to their own explanations and audit them for intelligibility and rationality.

For almost every patient, the general anaesthetic and surgical operation engender particular anxieties which must be recognized and accommodated. It is no small thing to surrender one's consciousness into the hands of others, with all the vulnerability which unconsciousness brings. The intrusion of hands and instruments into the previously intact body equally induces dark fears in many minds. Doctors may not fully appreciate these anxieties, familiar as they are with the procedures used and their general safety and success. Most patients of reasonably resolute temperament face up to these prospects with good enough courage: but having done so, find a postponement of the day especially demoralizing. It is important that surgeons try to arrange lists so that patients do not wait many hours in a state of some tension, only to be told that they must face it all again on another day.

Modern practice and health economics combine nowadays to reduce the patient's stay in hospital to a minimum. Perhaps doctors do not sufficiently realize how much dependence may develop between patients who have been really ill and those who have rescued them from suffering, or even from death, and subsequently cared for them. The cheerful words 'Well, you can go home tomorrow' are not invariably greeted with joy. It is not merely that for some, the attention they receive in hospital is better than anything they get elsewhere: those who have been really ill are often haunted by the prospect of relapse or recurrence and feel a security in hospital, amplified by care and kindness, which they cannot feel at home.

Some introductory words of sympathy for the patient's anxiety and reassurance for their ability to survive outside the hospital are often necessary.

An essay entitled 'On being a patient' ought to contain not merely adjurations for doctors but at least some directions for patients. The foremost of these could be to remember the meaning of the newly acquired status and title. Many patients are irritable and demanding, even when those attributes are not produced or justified by some disease process. They are very unattractive qualities in those who have, after all, been obliged to submit themselves to the care and skill of their fellow beings, sometimes through their own fault or neglect. A little humility and gratitude seem called for and no less because the patient is paying for some part of the services rendered, or believes that he has already done so. It is perhaps one of the least likeable of human attitudes to believe that money buys everything and that plenty of it entitles one to special care and attention. Doctors and nurses do not for the most part do what they do in the expectation of great worldly reward. Patients likewise should recognize and appreciate human kindness when they see it and be grateful for it whether or not they are paying for their treatment.

Finally it is necessary to reflect that, as man is a social animal, the illness of any member of a family affects most of the others. Obviously enough, the spouse of a sick person is liable to be deeply affected by sorrow and by anxiety about the future. Such feelings spring not merely from love and affection but from fear of a future either robbed of economic support or burdened by care for an invalid or disabled person. So a good doctor has more than just the patient to consider and should try to speak to the relatives and to offer them proper and helpful explanations of present treatment and future prospects. It may seem unreasonable to suggest that doctors should treat the relatives of their patients as well as the patients themselves, but human beings are highly interactive and sick people are sensitive to the sorrows and anxieties of their families. If a patient's relatives are much cast down and obviously anxious, this is perceived by the patient and greatly affects morale and the peace of mind that is conducive to recovery.

It is only too tempting to avoid the patient's relatives. Besides being upright and healthy, in contradistinction to the patient, their sorrows and anxieties may make them noisy and demanding. They are apt to ask questions which seem absurd to the doctor and impossible to answer in simple lay terms. However, the effort must be made, not only for humanitarian reasons but because it may rightly be regarded as part of the treatment.

In sum, the patient views those who care for him or her as being in a relationship every bit as confidential and trusting as that which exists within the patient's family, probably more so. The patient has no hesitation in imposing this burdensome connection on one who has hitherto been a total stranger. That is the enormous measure of a doctor's voluntarily assumed responsibilities to the human race.

2

Modern medicine: foundations, achievements, and limitations

2.1 Science in medicine: when, how, and what

W. F. Bynum

Introduction

At least since the Hippocratics, medicine has always aspired to be scientific. What has changed is not so much the aspirations but what it has meant to be 'scientific'.

'Science is the father of knowledge, but opinion breeds ignorance', opined the Hippocratic treatise *The Canon*, and Hippocratic practitioners developed an approach to health, disease, and its treatment based on systematic observation and cumulative experience. Even the word physic, the root of physician as well as physicist, derives from the Greek for 'nature'. Further, Hippocratic medicine was experimental, that word stemming from the same classical roots which gave us 'experience'.

Words, however, can be slippery, as philosophers as divergent as Francis Bacon and Ludwig Wittgenstein have stressed. The science and experiment of the Hippocratics can still inspire, but they are not our science and experiment. During the past two or three centuries, an armoury of sciences and technologies has come to underpin medical practice. This essay attempts briefly to describe these, within the context of distinctive and perennial features of medical practice, that is, suffering individuals whose problems and diseases demand attention.

A typology of historical medicine

The late Erwin Ackerknecht always taught that the history of Western medicine revealed five kinds of medicine: bedside, library, hospital, social, and laboratory. Bedside medicine he equated with Hippocratic, with its emphasis on the individual patient, its tendency towards holism, and a concern with the patient within his or her environment. These are some of the reasons why the Hippocratics are still claimed by both orthodox and alternative practitioners. For Ackerknecht, 'library' medicine dominated in the Middle Ages, when learned medicine retreated into the universities and scholars sometimes assumed that everything worth discovering had been discovered by the ancients, and everything worth being revealed could be found in the Bible. The millennium between the sacking of Rome and the discovery of the New World is often dismissed as a sterile period scientifically, but the physicians of the period, linguistically erudite and philosophically inclined, would have been surprised to be described as unscientific. They simply believed that the road to knowledge was through the book.

They also sometimes engaged with nature, although it is undeniable that nature rather than words became an increasing source of truth and knowledge during the Scientific Revolution, a period stretching roughly from just before Andreas Vesalius (1514–1564) to Isaac Newton (1642–1727). Around 1600, it was becoming apparent to many that the Greeks had not left behind a complete and accurate account of the nature of the world, and that scientific knowledge was cumulative. This 'Battle of the Books', the debate over whether the ancients or the moderns knew more, was decided in favour of the moderns. Many of the outstanding scientific achievements of the era were in astronomy and physics, but medicine, both in its theory and its practice, was also affected. Theory has always been easier to change than practice, of course, and it was famously remarked that William Har-

vey's discovery of the circulation of the blood had no impact on therapeutics. Harvey (1578–1657) also notoriously lamented that his practice actually fell off following the discovery, his patients fearing that he was 'crack-brained'. The fear that too close an identification with science was detrimental to patient confidence recurs in medical history, and is still part of the delicate negotiations between the profession and its public.

Within the discipline of medicine itself there have always been individuals, some of them, like Thomas Sydenham (1624–1689), eminently successful, who believed that experimental science had little to offer to patient care. But these 'artists' of medicine could still invoke the authority of Hippocrates, with its older connotations of knowledge and experience, and during the early modern period, the whole spectrum of the sciences —mathematics, physics, chemistry, the life sciences (not yet called biology)—made their ways into formulations of health and disease. Iatrophysics, iatromathematics, and iatrochemistry all had their advocates in the seventeenth and eighteenth centuries.

That these systems tended to encourage speculation to run ahead of evidence was recognized at the time, and this was part of the reason why 'hospital medicine' had little recourse to those disciplines we now call 'basic medical sciences'. The founders of French hospital medicine, Xavier Bichat (1771–1802), J. N. Corvisart (1755–1821), and R. T. H. Laennec (1781–1826), often referred to chemistry, physiology, and the like as sciences 'accessory' to medicine. The medicine that developed in the Paris hospitals, after the reopening in 1794 of the medical schools closed by the Revolution a couple of years earlier, emphasized above all the study of disease in the sick patient. In a sense, this was Hippocratic medicine writ large, but with some significant differences. First, the hospital offered the curious doctor a vast arena for observing disease. The equivalent of a lifetime's experience of a lone practitioner in the community could be experienced in a few months of hospital work. Hospitals offered the possibility of defining disease based on hundreds of cases. Second, Hippocratic humoralism gradually disappeared as the dominant explanatory framework of health and disease, replaced by the primacy of the lesion, located in the solids—the organs, tissues and, by mid-century, cells. In this new orientation, disease was literally palpable, its lesions to be discovered in life by the systematic use of physical examination—Corvisart rediscovered percussion, Laennec invented the stethoscope—and these findings to be correlated after death by routine autopsy. French high priests of hospital medicine brought diagnosis to a new stage and replaced the older symptom-based nosologies with a more objective, demonstrable one of lesions. The third feature of hospital medicine was what Pierre Louis called the numerical method, the use of numbers to guide both disease classification and therapeutic evaluation.

The philosophy underlying early nineteenth-century French medicine was most systematically expounded by one of the many American students who studied in Paris, Elisha Bartlett, in his *Philosophy of medical science* (1844). The medical science whose philosophy he chronicled was one of facts. All systems of medicine, past and present, were speculative, vague, and useless. Cullen, Brown, Broussais, and Hahnemann were all consigned to the historical dustbin. The new medicine was one of systematic observation and collection of facts, which, properly compared and organized, could provide an objective understanding of disease and a rational basis for its treatment. Bartlett's philosophy was essentially undiluted Baconian inductivism applied to medicine. Unsurprisingly, he counted Hippocrates as well as Pierre Louis among his heroes.

One consequence of the lesion-based medicine was the recognition that not much of what doctors did actually altered the natural history of disease. Therapeutic scepticism, or even nihilism, flourished among doctors whose lives were spent, as Laennec put it, 'among the dead and dying'. It was less likely to be expressed among doctors concerned with earning a living treating private patients, but the concern with medicine's therapeutic impotency also fuelled the movement to prevent disease. Ackerknecht's fourth kind of medicine, social, also flourished in the nineteenth century. Just as hospitals existed long before 'hospital medicine', so epidemics and preventive measures were not invented by the public health movement of the 1830s. Nevertheless, the preventive infrastructures developed partly in response to the cholera pandemics still exist, *mutatis mutandis*. The chief architect of the British public health movement, Edwin Chadwick (1800–1890), was a lawyer who thought that, on the whole, doctors were overrated. (He was neither the first nor the last lawyer to hold that opinion.) He held that epidemic diseases were caused by filth and spread via the foul smells (miasma) of rotting organic matter. His solutions were engineering ones, clean water and efficient waste disposal, which he argued would leave the world an altogether more pleasant and healthier place. His ideas were formed during the 1830s and early 1840s, and they remained more or less fixed for the rest of his long life, which extended well into the bacteriological age. Nevertheless, Chadwick also invoked science in his public health reform programme, above all the science of statistical investigation. His use of statistics can easily be shown to have been naïve, but it was ardent. In his own sphere of enquiry, Chadwick was as much in awe of the unadorned 'fact' as was his contemporary Bartlett. A later generation of Medical Officers of Health and others concerned with disease prevention (or containment) would develop new investigative techniques, more sophisticated statistics, and especially, new theories of disease causation and transmission. But the early public health movement was firmly based on the science of its time.

The final locus of medicine, the laboratory, was also largely a product of the nineteenth century, though of course laboratories (a place where one worked, especially to mutate gold from lead) had existed for much longer. A leading exponent of the laboratory, and one of its most thoughtful philosophers, had experienced Paris hospital medicine as a medical student. Claude Bernard's *Introduction to the study of experimental medicine* (1865) is both an intriguing account of his own brilliant career and a sophisticated analysis of the philosophy of experimentation within the life sciences. Hospitals, he argued, are merely the gateways to medical knowledge, and bedside clinicians can be no more than natural historians of disease. To understand the causes and mechanisms of disease, it is necessary to go into the sanctuary of the laboratory, where experimental conditions can be better controlled. There are in nature no uncaused causes: determinism is the iron law of the universe, extending equally to living systems and inorganic ones. However, organisms present special experimental problems, and it is only through isolating particular features, and holding other parameters as constant as possible, that reliability and reproducibility can be achieved.

Bernard identified three primary branches of experimental medicine: physiology, pathology, and therapeutics. His own research programme touched all three pillars: his research on the roles of the liver and pancreas in sugar metabolism contributed to understanding normal physiology as well as diseases such as diabetes; his investigations of the sites of action of agents such as curare and carbon monoxide foreshadowed structural pharmacology and drug receptor theory; his work on the functions of the sympathetic nerves buttressed his own more general notion of the constancy of *milieu interieur* as the precondition to vital action (and freedom), a precursor of Walter Cannon's concept of homeostasis. Bernard stands supreme as the quintessential advocate of the laboratory.

Who was the first modern medical experimentalist?

When Bernard wrote, experimental medical science was still a fledgling activity, best developed in the universities of the German States and Principalities. The German university ideal of medical education was to be extolled by the American educational reformer Abraham Flexner in the early twentieth century. It was in the reformed and newly created German universities that the forms of modern scientific research were established. Research careers were created; copublication in specialist journals became common; scientific societies flourished. The microscope became the symbol of the medical scientist even as the stethoscope was becoming the hallmark of the forward-looking clinician. In the hands of scientists like Schwann, Virchow, and Weismann, the modern cell theory was developed and applied to medicine and biology more generally. These researchers established the drive to push units of analysis further and further. Eduard Buchner's identification of cell-free ferments in 1897 firmly established the importance of subcellular functions. Pasteur, Koch, Ehrlich, von Behring, and others advanced new notions of the causes of disease, the body's response to infection, and the possibilities of new drugs to combat disease. Any of these scientists might arguably be the answer to the parlour-game question: who was the first modern medical scientist?

The German-speaking lands perfected the modern forms of scientific research, but a good case can be made for a Frenchman to be crowned the first thoroughly modern experimentalist within medicine. François Magendie (1783–1855) (Fig. 1) was a child of the Enlightenment and product of the French Revolution. One of several eminent individuals (Thomas Malthus was another) raised according to the anarchic principles espoused by Jean Jacques Rousseau, Magendie did not learn to read or write till he was 10. His subsequent precocity was such that he was ready for medical studies by the age of 16, learned anatomy and surgery as an apprentice, and made his way through the Paris hospital system. Although he never lost interest in practical medical issues, his reputation was established primarily within the laboratory. His monographs on physiology and pharmacology

Fig. 1 François Magendie. Lithograph by N.E. Maurin. (From Burgess R. Portraits of doctors and scientists in the Wellcome Institute, London, 1973, no.1870.2, by courtesy of the Wellcome Library, London.)

marked new beginnings, and his life manifests three emblematic qualities which make him one of us.

First, he valued facts above theories, evidence above rhetoric. But he went beyond Bartlett and the high priests of hospital medicine in insisting that in experiment, and not simply observation, lay the real future of medical knowledge. Like his pupil Claude Bernard, Magendie was a deft experimentalist. He used animals (and occasionally patients) to probe into a whole range of problems in physiology, pathology, and pharmacology: the functions of the spinal nerves; the physiology of vomiting; important facets of absorption, digestion, circulation, and nutrition; and the actions of drugs and poisons. He described anaphylaxis a century before it was named. He was as philosophically naïve as Bernard was sophisticated: of course he had theories, but his image of himself as a ragpicker with a spiked stick, gathering isolated experimental facts where he found them, is a telling one.

Second, he was modern in sometimes backing the wrong horses. He judged cholera and yellow fever to be non-contagious, was suspicious of anaesthesia, and sometimes claimed more than we might for his newly introduced therapeutic substances, such as strychnine and veratrine.

Finally, Magendie was the scientist who first expunged the double-faced Janus from the medical mentality. William Harvey worshipped Aristotle, Albrecht von Haller was steeped in history, and Isaac Newton popularized the pious conceit of pygmies standing on the shoulders of giants. Magendie looked only in one direction: the future. He had no sense of history and no use for it. He meant what he said when he insisted that most physiological 'facts' had to be verified by new experiments, and he undertook to provide a beginning. He made the laboratory the bedrock of medicine.

What happened next?

Like everyone, Magendie was of his time. Nevertheless, his values were symptomatic of important themes within nineteenth-century medicine and medical science. By the beginning of the First World War, most of the structures and the fundamental concepts of 'our' medicine were in place. Of course, both medical science and medical practice have been utterly transformed since. But the impulse of experimentation and its variable translation into practice were there. We have gone far beyond the cell in our analytical procedures, and our medical, surgical, and therapeutic armamentaria are vastly more sophisticated and powerful.

Our medicine is fundamentally different in one important respect, even if the trend was already evident in the nineteenth century: the fusion of science and technology. Science and technology have become so intertwined that the older distinctions between them are blurred. Technology made a real but minimal impact on nineteenth-century medicine. Some instruments, such as Helmholtz's ophthalmoscope, came into clinical medicine through the laboratory; and German experimental scientists were eager to exploit the latest equipment such as kymographs, sphygmographs, and the profusion of artefacts (Petri dishes, autoclaves, etc.) that Koch and his colleagues devised for the bacteriological laboratory.

Most important of all was probably the X-ray, discovered by Roentgen in late 1895. It made an immediate impact on medical diagnosis, and the associated science of radioactivity soon was felt within therapeutics. Significantly, perhaps, the pioneers of the radioactive phenomena—Roentgen, Becquerel, the Curies—received their Nobel Prizes in physics or chemistry. Hounsfield and Cormack gained theirs for computer-assisted tomography in medicine or physiology. More recently, Kary Mullis's Nobel Prize was for a technological development within molecular biology.

Both medical science and medical practice are now inseparably rooted in technology. So is modern life, another reflection of a perennial historical truth: medical knowledge and medical practice are products of wider social forces with unique historical individualities.

Further reading

Ackerknecht EH (1967). *Medicine at the Paris Hospital, 1784–1848.* Baltimore: Johns Hopkins University Press.

Bynum WF (1994). *Science and the practice of medicine in the nineteenth century.* Cambridge University Press.

Bynum WF, Porter R, eds (1993). *Companion encyclopedia of the history of medicine.* London: Routledge.

Cooter R, Pickstone J, eds (2000). *Medicine in the 20th century.* Amsterdam: Harwood Academic Publishers.

King LS (1982). *Medical thinking: a historical preface.* Princeton University Press, 1982.

Reiser SJ (1978). *Medicine and the reign of technology.* Cambridge University Press.

Weatherall DJ (1995). *Science and the quiet art: medical research and patient care.* Oxford University Press.

2.2 Scientific method and the art of healing

D. J. Weatherall

When Henry Dale, the distinguished British physiologist and pharmacologist, arrived at St Bartholomew's Hospital as a medical student in 1900 he was told by his first clinical teacher, Samuel Gee, that, as medicine was not a science but merely an empirical art, he must forget all the physiology that he had learnt at Cambridge. This advice reflects a deep-rooted tension between the art and science of clinical practice, which still permeates the medical profession.

Patient care, from its earliest beginnings to the present day, has always been a mixture of sympathy and kindness backed up with a well-meaning but often empirical effort to alter the natural course of events. In this sense it has been, and still is, an art, practised against a background of incomplete scientific knowledge about the nature of disease processes. Human beings, like all living things, are immensely complex biological systems. Even today, with all our knowledge of their chemistry and physiology, we have a very limited understanding of the mechanisms that underlie most of the diseases that we encounter in day-to-day practice. Caring for sick people involves making considered judgements based on limited evidence and information. At best, we are slowly reaching the stage at which we are aware of how little we know.

In view of the remarkable progress in the biological sciences over the last few hundred years, today's doctors must try to establish the extent to which the balance of medical practice has shifted from 'craft' to 'science'. How far do the contents of a modern textbook of medicine reflect genuine scientific knowledge as compared with received wisdom and experience? And, of particular relevance to current medical practice and its future development, to what extent have advances in patient care in the twentieth century depended on progress in the basic sciences rather than improvements in our environment and lifestyles? In short, how much of our day-to-day clinical practice depends on a scientifically based understanding of the diseases that we encounter? It is important that we address these questions at a time when there is growing public and governmental disillusion with high-technology scientific medicine, and when many believe that the medical profession has lost its way and become more interested in diseases than in those who suffer from them. Before we tackle these difficult questions it may be helpful to define what we mean by 'scientific medicine' and to outline the way in which it has developed over the years.

Philosophers and historians of science and medicine always seem unhappy when it comes to deciding what is meant by 'scientific medicine'; this is dangerous country for the unwary! Here we shall take a pragmatic (if circular) approach, and use the term simply to describe the prevention and management of illness using methods that have been subjected to the same kinds of rigorous experimental, statistical, and observational scrutiny that are applied in other branches of science.

The earliest documentary evidence to survive from the ancient civilizations of Babylonia, Egypt, China, and India suggests, not surprisingly, that longevity, disease, and death are among our oldest preoccupations. From ancient times to the Renaissance, knowledge of the living world changed very little and the distinction between animate and inanimate objects was blurred. The Babylonians and Egyptions believed that water, air, and earth were the primary constituents of the world; a fourth, fire, was added later.

This notion of the all-pervading influence of the four elements was extended to form a theory about how the human body is constituted. In short, it was thought to consist of four humours, blood, phlegm, yellow bile, and black bile. The notion that disease results from an imbalance of the humours permeated Graeco-Roman medicine and persisted until the seventeenth century. Health was viewed as a harmonious balance of the humours, while disease was thought to reflect an imbalance, or dyscrasia, leading to an abnormal mixture of the humours. This view of pathology, which provided an explanation for both mental and physical illness, formed the basis for what, at the time, was a rational approach to treatment by bleeding, purging, and dietary modification.

The extraordinary developments in natural philosophy in the seventeenth century created an environment that led to the birth of scientific medicine as we now understand it. Modern physics was founded by Isaac Newton, and the work of Boyle and Hooke finally disposed of the Aristotelean elements of earth, fire, and water. The shape of medical and biological thinking was moulded by the French mathematician, philosopher, and biologist René Descartes, who held that material things, whether animals, plants, or inorganic objects, are ruled by the same mechanical laws. All living things, he held, can be looked on as machines. A sick man is like an ill-made clock; a healthy man a well-made clock. And it was during this time that William Harvey published an almost complete description of the circulation of the blood, work that involved many years of animal experimentation and the application of simple statistical methods to determine the output of blood from the heart, and which, in effect, formed the foundation for modern investigative physiology and, later, medicine.

During the eighteenth and nineteenth centuries, the sciences that underpin medicine were further developed. In particular, the concept of the cell became the centrepiece of biology. As perceived by the French Nobel laureate, Francois Jacob, 'with the cell biology discovered its atom'. In 1858 Rudolph Virchow published his celebrated *Die Cellular Pathologie*, in which cell theory was applied to the study of pathology. All diseases, he held, are diseases of cells. This was the dawning of modern cellular pathology and the study of disease at the microscopic, and later submicroscopic, levels. The nineteenth century also saw the gradual decline of vague theories about life forces and a growing belief, helped by the emergence of organic chemistry, that living processes can be understood in terms of chemistry and physics working through complex interactions between the many different types of cells that constitute all living things, a movement that was to culminate in the extraordinary achievements in biochemistry and molecular biology in the twentieth century.

This was also the time when a start was made at assessing the value of therapeutic practices that had gone on largely unchanged for centuries. For despite these rapid advances in the biological sciences, very little could be done for the majority of the disorders that doctors faced in everyday practice. Blood letting and the administration of a variety of useless and potentially harmful treatments were still rife, and although a few drugs of genuine value had been found, foxglove extract and quinine for example, much of the doctors' armamentarium was of unproven value. In the mid-nineteenth century a French clinician, Pierre Charles Alexandre Louis, pioneered the application of statistical analysis to medical practice. One of his earliest ventures was to compile sufficient data to prove that blood letting, which had been practised for centuries, was not only useless but positively harmful in the management of many diseases. During the latter half of the nineteenth century the focus of medical science moved from France to Germany. It was here that, during the late nineteenth and early twentieth centuries, laboratories were set up where men and women could devote their time to research in the blossoming basic sciences, anatomy, physiology, and, later, biochemistry. In this atmosphere a new generation of clinical scientists evolved who became interested in physiological medicine, that is in understanding the fundamental mechanisms of disease.

These developments led to the establishment of university medical schools in the United States and parts of Europe, based on the German tradition. In 1910 the American educationalist Abraham Flexner, after visiting several German medical schools, wrote a withering critique of medical education and science in North America. This attack stimulated the development of specialist clinical departments in many American and European medical schools. Flexner's revolutionary study advocated that medical education should begin with a strong foundation in the basic sciences followed by the study of clinical medicine in an atmosphere of critical thinking and with adequate time and facilities for research. His philosophy was widely accepted, not only in North America but in many European medical schools.

The development of university clinical academic departments in the period between the two world wars, and particularly after the second, led to the emergence of 'clinical science', experimentation on patients or laboratory animals on problems that stemmed directly from observations made at the bedside. Ultimately, this led to a remarkable improvement in our understanding of disease mechanisms. Together with the expanding pharmaceutical industry, it set the scene for the development of modern, high-technology medical practice. Not surprisingly, it also had a profound effect on medical education. Indeed, those who criticize modern methods of teaching doctors, in particular the Cartesian approach to the study of human biology and disease, believe that the organization of university clinical academic departments along Flexner's lines may have done much to concentrate the minds of doctors on diseases rather than those who suffer from them.

The twentieth century has seen a revolution in the basic sciences, which started in physics, spread to chemistry, and, ultimately, completely changed the face of biology. Remarkable developments in physics at the end of the nineteenth century paved the way to an understanding of how atoms are joined together to form molecules and for the development of a new kind of chemistry, which would start to explain the structure of the molecules that make up living things. The amalgamation of physics and chemistry spawned a new discipline, molecular biology, which was to unravel the way in which genetic information is passed from generation to generation and how individual cells function, both as self-contained units and as part of the complex communication network which is the basis of life itself. In the last 20 years there has been a slow shift of emphasis in medical research from the study of disease at the level of patients or their diseased organs to their cells and molecules. Although major scientific achievements do not always have practical benefits for many years, it is already apparent that molecular and cell biology have enormous potential for the future of medical research and practice.

There is no doubt that a combination of improvements in the environment combined with the fruits of scientific medicine have greatly improved the health of Western industrialized societies. In England a century ago, four out of ten babies did not survive to adult life, the life expectancy at birth was only 44 years for boys and 47 for girls, and even as recently as the 1930s 2500 women died each year during pregnancy or childbirth. Today, life expectancy at birth is about 73 years for boys and 78 years for girls. The major triumph for scientific medicine and public health has undoubtedly been the control of many infectious diseases. Consequently, the proportion of deaths due to infection and respiratory diseases has declined dramatically and the major causes of mortality in the West are now vascular disease

and cancer. Although relatively little progress has been made towards their prevention, their management has been transformed by the ingenuity of the pharmaceutical industry combined with development of high-technology medical practice based on a better understanding of disease mechanisms.

Modern scientific medicine is not without its detractors however. Early this century George Bernard Shaw, in his brilliant Preface to *The doctor's dilemma*, derided medical research of his time. His cry 'stimulate the phagocytes' came straight from the laboratory of Almroth Wright at St Mary's Hospital Medical School. But this work was written with style and humour and was concerned mainly with debunking the pomposity of the medical profession. This was not the case in the book, *Medical nemesis*, written by the philosopher and theologian Ivan Illich, which first appeared in 1975. Using a mass of statistics, Illich set out to show that modern medical practice in general, and scientific medicine in particular, has had no effect whatever on the health of society. His thesis holds that common infections such as tuberculosis and poliomyelitis were disappearing long before the advent of antibiotics and vaccines, and, even worse, that modern medicine is a threat to society as well as to individual patients. It is, he believes, more harmful than good because it generates demands for its services and encourages aspects of behaviour that lead to more ill health and reduce our ability to cope with illness and to face suffering and death. Illich concludes that the medical profession, at least in its present form, should be disbanded.

A series of much more thoughtful critiques of modern medicine were published in the late 1970s by Thomas McKeown and others. McKeown extended Illich's thesis that the advent of vaccination, immunization, and antibiotics has had little effect on the control of infectious disease. He argued that the dominance of the mechanistic approach to the problems of disease, which started in the seventeenth century, had caused doctors to overlook important messages that the patterns of disease origins in the past had left for them, and that it had led them to underestimate their potential value for the organization of health care in the future. McKeown believed that the vast majority of diseases are environmental in origin and that if we had been thinking of disease origins rather than mechanisms it would not have taken us so long to suspect the importance of environmental agents or lifestyles in the genesis of our current killers, smoking or lack of exercise as the cause of heart disease for example. In short, writers like Illich and McKeown believe that, because practically all disease stems from the environment, modern scientific medicine, with its accent on disease mechanisms rather than origins, has had little effect on the health of society. While flawed in many ways, particularly with respect to their lack of appreciation of the relative roles of nature and nurture in the genesis of disease, arguments of this kind have had an important influence on current perceptions of the role of science in medicine.

These criticisms of modern scientific medicine have been mirrored by increasing disenchantment with modern medical practice on the part of the public, media, politicians, and even some doctors themselves. Paradoxically, the origins of this mood of disillusionment can be traced to some of the extraordinary successes of scientific medicine earlier this century. In the period after the Second World War, which saw the emergence of vaccines and antibiotics and the control of many infectious diseases, it appeared that medical science was capable of almost anything. The virtual disappearance overnight of scourges like smallpox, diphtheria, and poliomyelitis led to the expectation that similar successes would soon follow. In effect, society came to expect a state of constant rude health as its right. But this did not happen. The diseases that replaced infection, heart attacks, strokes, cancer, rheumatism, and psychiatric disorders, turned out to be much more intractable. Granted there were some remarkable advances in their symptomatic control, but these new killers could not be prevented or cured. As this became clear there was a move on the part of society to alternative medicine; if medical science could not cope with chronic backache or lung cancer why not turn for help to those who claimed they had the answers? Dietary manipulation, food allergy, herbal remedies, and a variety of other approaches to chronic illness were taken up with enthusiasm.

Yet coincident with this disillusionment with modern medicine and the search for better alternatives, it became apparent that the revolution in the biological sciences, stemming from applications of molecular and cell biology, promised to change completely the face of health care in the future. Today, hardly a week goes by without a new breakthrough being splashed all over our television screens and newspapers; another human gene has been isolated and the cause of a disease of which we have never heard is announced. New cures for heart disease or cancer appear to be just round the corner. Whenever these new remarkable discoveries are announced, excited scientists or journalists tell us that they will have a major impact on health care 'within the near future'. Yet time goes by and this doesn't seem to happen. There is a growing feeling that much which goes on in modern science is motivated more by scientists' wish for self-glorification rather than by any practical goals. Furthermore, many believe that modern science, whether it involves the manipulation of human genes or enquires into the origins of the universe, is a debasing activity that is damaging our environment and moving into areas of knowledge that are best left alone. There is a growing fear about the increasing reductionist approach to medical research. This, combined with concerns about the dehumanizing effect of modern hospitals and the feeling that doctors must return to a more holistic approach to their patients, that is to treat them as individuals rather than diseases, is causing increasing concern to our medical educationalists.

Clearly, younger readers of this book are learning their trade at a time when the whole ethos of scientific medicine is being questioned, and when thoughts are turning more to preventive medicine by modification of our environment and lifestyles, with less emphasis on understanding the basic mechanisms of disease. What are they to make of this confusing scene?

In effect, the doctors of today find themselves in a similar position to their predecessors at the beginning of this century. It was already apparent that many of the infectious diseases that were killing their patients could be partly controlled by better housing, hygiene, and other improvements in the environment; a few could be prevented by vaccination. Yet it was far from clear how far measures of this kind would be successful in controlling these diseases. In the meantime there was little that they could do for their patients with tuberculosis, meningitis, poliomyelitis, or puerperal sepsis, except improve their general well-being and manage their symptoms. They knew that there were some exciting developments in the basic biological sciences, microbiology, and, in particular, immunology, which promised to provide the solution to their problems. Yet these fields had been on the move for over half a century and still appeared to be of limited practical value. Hopes for the development of a cure for tuberculosis, following Koch's discovery of the tubercle bacillus in the 1880s, had still come to nothing. In the event it was to be another 60 years before the discovery of streptomycin provided a definitive cure for tuberculosis.

The situation is more or less the same today. We know that we can reduce the frequency of heart disease and cancer by changes in our environment and lifestyles, stopping cigarette smoking for example. But we have no idea of the extent to which we can control our major killers. For this reason it is essential that we continue to support the basic sciences and to provide the doctors of the future with sufficient understanding of them so that, as practical applications come along, as they certainly will, they are in a position to take advantage of them. If the story of the development of scientific medicine from the seventeenth century onwards has anything to tell us, it is simply this. The bulk of our major advances in health care have stemmed from advances in both public health and scientific research, the latter quite often stemming from fields that were driven by curiosity rather than any practical end in view. Harvey's discovery of the circulation of the blood had no practical value for patients with heart disease at the time; it was to be several hundred years before advances stemming from the disparate sciences of physiology, anatomy, pharmacology, and biochemistry, together with the discovery of anaesthesia and remarkable developments in surgical technology, laid the ground for modern cardiological practice. We must not neglect the role of the basic sciences in medical education and practice simply because they do not appear to have any immediate benefits.

As scientifically trained clinicians we try and analyse our patients' illnesses as far as we can with the tools of modern medical science, but frequently we find ourselves in a situation in which knowledge is incomplete and some form of therapy, even if it is of unproven value, has to be tried. The further scientific knowledge increases, the more difficult it is for caring clinicians to dissociate their scientific training from the practical necessity of doing something to relieve suffering, even though they are aware that they are rarely sure about what they are doing. Medicine has remained an art, but one that has become increasingly difficult to practise as knowledge of the scientific ignorance that underlies it has increased. The central problem for those who educate doctors of today is, on the one hand, how to encourage a lifelong attitude of critical, scientific thinking to the management of illness, yet, at the same time, recognize that moment when the scientific approach, because of ignorance, has reached its limits and must be replaced by sympathetic empiricism. Doctors have to learn to live with uncertainty. For many, this can be one of the most difficult and disturbing aspects of their work.

Textbook descriptions of disease are, of necessity, misleading. Even in the case of the most straightforward of illnesses, for which we know the cause down to the last building-block of DNA, the presentation, course, and management is never the same in any two patients. Not only are they modified by the protean physiological adaptations that occur in response to disease, but also by an individual's reaction to illness, depending on their personality, degree of family support, and many other factors that we do not understand. If, as is frequently done in our better teaching hospitals, we attempt to analyse all the features of a patient's illness and explain them in terms of current scientific knowledge, we always fail. And because we know so little about the mechanisms that underlie most of the illnesses that we encounter, a great deal of what we do must still remain empirical. It is the sheer complexity of the manifestations of illness that is responsible for the notion that medicine is still an art. And if this is the case for the relatively well-defined diseases that we see in hospital, the situation is even more complex in the community. The bulk of a family doctor's work involves non-specific complaints that seem totally foreign to anything that they learnt in the laboratory or lecture theatre as a student, often reflecting an individual patient's reactions to stresses of work, family, and environment rather than clearly defined organic disease.

Thus, apart from pastoral qualities, good doctoring requires an ability to cut through many of the unexplained manifestations of disease, to appreciate what is important and what can be disregarded, and hence to get to the core of the problem, knowing when scientific explanation has failed and empiricism must take over. This is the real art of clinical practice. It comes naturally to some doctors, but for others the difficult transition from theory to practice, from the relative certainty of the preclinical sciences to complexities of sick people, is never quite accomplished. This may be the reason for the notion that good medical practice depends more on the acquisition of experience based on long years of practice, rather than on methods of prevention, diagnosis, and treatment based on sound scientific principles. Unfortunately, this view, which may partly reflect doctors' defence mechanisms against continued ignorance, has been responsible for a great deal of poor practice, often based on fashion and anecdote rather than anything more substantive. An overexaggerated perception of the importance of medicine as a craft may also have been responsible for the dogmatism, unhealthy respect for received wisdom of the past, and extreme pomposity that has characterized many aspects of medical practice over the years. Like most human endeavours, the art of medicine has both its good and bad aspects.

In 1941 Sir Arthur Hall wrote:

> Medicine—however much it develops—must always remain an 'applied science' and one differing from all the rest in its applications to man himself. Were there no sick persons there would be no need for Medicine, either the Science or the Art. So long as there are both, both will be necessary. The application of its Science, to be of value, must be made in such a way that it will produce the maximum relief

to the sick man. This calls for certain qualities in the practising physician which differ entirely from anything required in the practice of the other applied sciences. Herein lies the Art of Medicine. The need for it is as great today as it ever was, or ever will be, so long as human sickness continues.

As we have seen, our greatest difficulty is to recognize that moment in caring for a sick patient when the scientific approach, because of ignorance, has reached its limits and has to be replaced by sympathetic empiricism. It is the ability to choose that moment, partly by instinct and partly by experience gained by caring for sick people, that is the main characteristic of a good doctor. Undoubtedly, modern medical science, with its increasingly reductionist approach to the study of disease, has tended to focus our attention more on disease mechanisms than on those who are suffering from the diseases that fascinate us so much. We must redress this balance, and return to a more holistic approach to medical care, without, at the same time, allowing ourselves to develop those uncritical attitudes and reliance on received wisdom which permeated the medical profession for so many centuries. For genuine advances in medicine have stemmed from science, as defined at the beginning of this chapter, regardless of whether it involved cells and molecules, or people and populations.

Further reading

Booth C (1993). History of science in medicine. In: Teeling-Smith G, ed. *Science in medicine: how far has it advanced?*, pp. 11–22. Office of Health Economics, London.

Illich I (1977). *Limits to medicine. Medical nemesis: the expropriation of health.* Penguin Books, Middlesex.

McKeown T (1988). *The origins of human disease.* Blackwell, Oxford.

Weatherall DJ (1995). *Science and the quiet art. The role of research medicine.* Norton, New York.

Weatherall DJ (1999). The conflict between the science and the art of clinical practice in the new Millennium. *Annals of the New York Academy of Sciences* **882**, 240–6.

2.3 Medical ethics

Edmund D. Pellegrino and Daniel P. Sulmasy

Introduction

Clinical ethics, like all ethics, is a practical discipline. Whatever theory it employs, its ultimate aim is a morally defensible decision that is in the patient's best interests. This was the central moral precept of the Hippocratic oath:

> I will follow that system of regimen which, according to my ability and judgement, I consider for the benefit of my patient and I will refrain from whatever is deleterious and mischievous.

Today, this is known as the principle of beneficence, which derives its moral force from the special nature of the relationships between sick persons and health professionals. When patients seek help they are anxious, often in pain, fearful, dependent, and therefore vulnerable and exploitable. In that state, physicians ask then, 'How can I help you?' By that act physicians invite the patient's confidence and trust that they are competent and will use that competence primarily in the patient's interests.

The relationship is therefore not a contract but a covenant of trust, to which physicians must be faithful even if it means some suppression of their own self-interest. The good of the patient is thus a moral compass with four directional guide marks for the physician: medical good (competence), the patient's good expressed in his own preferences (respect for autonomy), the patient's inherent good as a human being (respect for dignity), and the patient's ultimate good (respect for spirituality). To act for the patient's good requires integration of these four elements on behalf of this person who presents as my patient now.

This chapter concentrates on the questions that must be asked, and the conditions that must prevail at the bedside to assure that each of the four levels of the patient's good is attained. Two moral algorithms are provided: one to assess the moral validity of the decision-maker, and the second, to provide a clinical framework or 'work-up' by which to analyse the ethical issues.

Who decides?

Since the good of the patient is far broader than the patient's biomedical good, clinical ethics requires the patient's participation in decision-making. Figure 1 presents an algorithm for determining the morally valid decision-maker. If the patient has sufficient decision-making capacity, the patient is the ultimate decision-maker. If the patient's decision-making capacity is variable, the physician should be guided by the last decision made when the patient was capable. If the patient has never had decision-making capacity (for example an infant or patient with mental retardation), the physician must turn to a morally valid surrogate. If the patient has lost decision-making capacity in a reversible manner (for example through depression) and it can be restored through medical treatment in a timely manner, the decision should be postponed until the patient is treated and capacity restored. If the loss of capacity is irreversible or the decision too urgent, the physician turns to any anticipatory declarations by the patient such as a living will, or the designation of a surrogate decision-maker through a legal document such as a durable power of attorney for health care. Lacking these expressions of the patient's prior wishes, the physician must engage a morally valid surrogate, that is, someone who can responsibly and knowledgeably represent the patient's wishes, and who has intact decision-making capacity and is free of significant conflicts of interest.

Decision-making capacity

Accurate determination of a patient's decision-making capacity is an essential clinical skill. In North American jurisprudence, the term 'incompetence' refers to a judge's decision that an individual has lost all capacity to make decisions. The physician, however, is concerned with a narrower question: is this patient capable of making a decision about *this* clinical option in these particular clinical circumstances? The threshold of capacity will vary according to the gravity of the decision. For example, a patient suffering from suicidal depression might be allowed to refuse venepuncture, but not be allowed to sign out of the hospital against medical advice. Psychiatric consultation is often important, but the determination of decision-making capacity is generally the responsibility of the attending physician. The criteria for decision-making capacity are as follows.

1. What is the patient's neurological status? If the patient is profoundly delirious, demented, obtunded, or aphasic, the patient will not have the capacity to participate in medical decision-making.

2. Does the patient have intact judgement? That is, is the patient free of impulsiveness, able correctly to assess the seriousness of situations, to plan, and to appreciate the connections between acts and consequences?

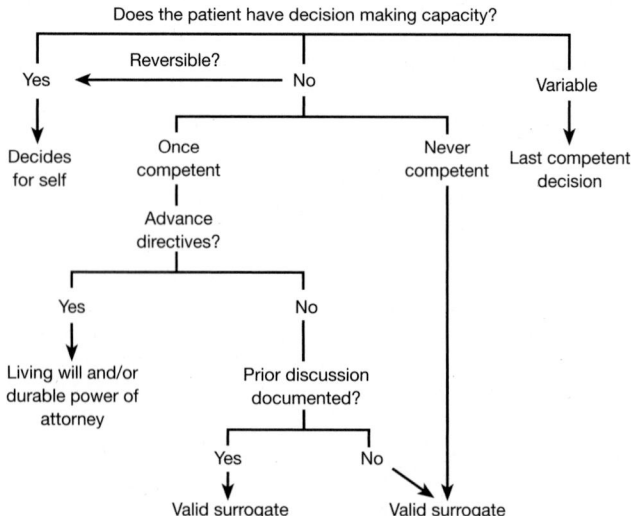

Fig. 1 Who decides?

3. Does the patient understand the nature of the procedure, its risks, benefits, and the consequences of deciding either to accept or to forgo the procedure?

4. Can the patient explain the reasons for a decision in a way that is logical and also consistent with his or her life history and previously held values?

5. Does the patient's decision remain relatively stable over time? Patients must certainly be free to change their minds, but a patient whose decision vacillates minute to minute or who refuses to make any decision may not have intact decision-making capacity.

Informed consent

Every physician must be able to obtain a morally adequate informed consent. This is not synonymous with obtaining a signature on a piece of paper. Informed consent is a process. It is one of the fundamental ways in which the physician shows respect for the good of patients as whole persons.

There are four basic elements in informed consent. The first is that the patient must have decision-making capacity. The rudiments of how to assess decision-making capacity were described above.

Second, the decision by the patient must represent an autonomous authorization, that is, it must be free from coercion, or even subtle manipulation by the physician or by others. Information must be presented in a fair and balanced fashion. This does not imply absolute neutrality nor does it imply that the physician cannot make a recommendation or even try to persuade a patient if the physician thinks the patient is making a mistake. But a physician ought not, for instance, purposefully distort the facts or threaten to sever the physician–patient relationship if the patient does not follow the physician's advice.

Third, all relevant information must be disclosed to the patient. The content to be disclosed should generally include the indications and the nature of the procedure, its potential benefits and risks, and the alternatives, including not having any procedure.

The final element of informed consent, but certainly not the least, is comprehension. The patient must not merely have been told; the patient must understand. The common clinical practice of asking, 'Do you have any questions?' is probably inadequate. If one is seriously interested in being sure that the patient has understood, it is better to ask the patient to explain back in his own words the information just disclosed.

Limits to autonomy

While the good of patients as autonomous agents must be respected, patient autonomy is not absolute. Autonomy is limited, for instance, when there is a probable threat of serious injury to an identifiable third party or parties. An example would be a demand for confidentiality by a patient testing positive for HIV who refuses to tell a sexual partner. Autonomy is further limited by the intellectual integrity of medicine as a practice. For instance, a patient cannot demand a treatment that has been proved ineffective, such as laetrile for cancer. Autonomy can also be limited to protect public health, such as in mandatory vaccination in an epidemic of a lethal infection. Finally, autonomy is limited when it violates the moral integrity of health care professionals as individual moral agents whose freedom of conscience must not be violated; for instance, a physician opposed to euthanasia ought not be forced to comply with a patient request even in settings where this is legal.

The ethics work-up

Once the appropriate decision-maker has been identified, and the conditions for autonomy assured, the physician must turn to analysis of the ethical dilemma and its substantive resolution. Ethics committees and consultations sometimes help, but ultimately clinicians are accountable for what they do or agree to. Every clinician is obliged to master the 'work-up' of the ethical problems just as surely as that of a clinical problem like coma, jaundice, or oedema.

The analytical approach we use consists of the following seven steps.

1. Secure the facts

Good ethics begins with reliable clinical and social data, with as accurate an assessment as possible of factors such as diagnosis, prognosis, effectiveness, benefits, burdens of treatments, brain function, patient preferences, and life situations. Each and all may be ethically relevant.

2. Define the ethical issue

The specifically ethical issue must be identified among the communication, interpersonal, and interprofessional problems, which usually intermingle, especially when conflicts arise. The first step in resolving conflict is clarity in the statement of the issues.

3. Frame the issue

By applying generally accepted ethical principles, one can better understand the important moral dimensions of the issue. These principles are: (i) preservation of the good of the patient as a whole person (the principle of beneficence), and (ii) respecting the good and interests of others (the principle of justice). Beneficence for persons, as noted above, demands an examination of all four aspects of the patient's good—the biomedical good, the good of the patient's autonomous choices, the patient's good as a person, and the patient's own beliefs about the ultimate good. So, for example, a severely anaemic Jehovah's Witness might refuse blood transfusion. Transfusion would serve the biomedical good of the patient, but it would violate the patient's autonomy and idea of the higher or ultimate spiritual good. Or a patient's family might demand continued treatment in the intensive care unit when such care was futile or unnecessary. This might impede other patients' access to intensive care and thus violate the principle of justice.

4. Situate the issue

It is helpful to place the case in relation to one's personal experience and that of the profession. This method of moral analysis is called 'casuistry' and asks whether the case at hand is analogous to any paradigmatic case for which a broad moral consensus has been reached. If so, one could reason by analogy to that case. For example, consider a novel case, such as whether one ought to allow a prisoner who has donated one kidney to his daughter to donate his remaining kidney to her after she has rejected the first kidney. It is useful to ask how this case compares with a more familiar case in which there is a broad moral consensus. For example, this case might be likened to the case of a man who jumps in front of a car to save his daughter's life. Such a man would be considered a hero. Casuistic analysis would ask how analogous these cases really are. What is the same about these two cases? What is different? What is the moral relevance of any similarities or differences?

5. Identify the options

In almost every case, a variety of clinical options are possible. Ethics involves selection of the morally correct choice. It is therefore necessary that all the available clinical options be identified and considered from a clinical as well as a moral point of view. This is where the technically correct and the morally good should intersect for the patient's good.

6. Reason

It is important is to weigh all the facts of the case critically and rigorously in light of one's ethical framework and clinical experience. One must interrelate the facts, the relevant principles, and any paradigm cases. Physicians should also play 'devil's advocate' and examine possible objections to their own positions. They should seek colleagues' input if time permits. An ethics committee or an ethics consultation service may be useful at this juncture. Once resolved, a retrospective critique of the reasoning employed in the case is helpful in preparing for the next time such a situation arises.

7. Decide

In clinical ethics, as in all other aspects of medicine, a decision must be made. Taking all of the aforesaid into account, a choice must be made even in the throes of uncertainty. There is no formula that guarantees the right choices. The answer will require a judicious combination of clinical judgement, practical wisdom, and common sense. In the final analysis, the decision rests with the physician's character and commitment to the good of the patient.

The ethics of end-of-life care

The most common ethical issues faced by clinicians arise at the end of life. Here the good of the patient might include decisions to withhold and withdraw life-sustaining treatments, decisions not to resuscitate, and the use of potent opioid analgesics that may hasten death.

The moral propriety of withholding or withdrawing life-sustaining treatment may be analysed systematically by examining the proposed treatment for its effectiveness, benefit, and burdens. Effective treatments are those that alter the natural history of an illness or alleviate an important symptom. Hippocrates counselled that physicians should 'refuse to treat those who are overmastered by their diseases, recognizing that in such cases medicine is powerless'. When, to a reasonable degree of medical certainty, it can be determined that a treatment will not be effective in securing the goals of treatment mutually determined by the medical team and the patient or the patient's surrogates, that treatment can be called clinically ineffective or 'futile'. In general, there is no moral obligation to provide futile treatment, although allowances must often be made for the psychological unpreparedness of the patient or family to accept the idea of futility.

If it is determined that a medical treatment is biomedically effective, the next question is whether it is beneficial. Beneficial treatments are those that bring some good to the patient beyond the biomedical good. Beneficial treatments serve not only the body, but the good as the patient chooses it, the good of the patient as a human person, or the patient's ultimate sense of the spiritual good. For instance, antibiotic treatment of pneumonia in a patient dying of malignancy might be effective, but it might not be beneficial if it merely postpones dying when the patient sees no benefit in it.

Both the effectiveness and benefits of a treatment must be weighed against their burdens—physical, financial, or emotional. When the burdens are disproportionate to effectiveness and benefits, treatment can be withheld or withdrawn. Planned re-examination of the three variables at previously agreed time intervals will avoid much of the confusion that surrounds do-not-resuscitate orders. Cardiopulmonary resuscitation is a treatment which is ineffective, burdensome, and without benefit in many terminally ill patients. When this is the case, a do-not-resuscitate order is morally licit.

It is incontrovertible that there is a moral mandate to treat pain. None the less, some physicians might hesitate to do so adequately because there is a risk that this might unintentionally hasten the death of the patient. The centuries old Rule of Double Effect may be invoked in such cases. According to this rule, a physician completely opposed to euthanasia can act with clear conscience in administering a drug like morphine to a dying patient if several conditions are met. First, the physician must sincerely intend pain relief, not the death of the patient. Second, the dose must be consistent with a plan to relieve pain through the analgesic effects of morphine, not through causing respiratory arrest and death as the means of relieving pain. Finally, the need for pain relief must be great compared with the risk of respiratory arrest and death in that patient. For example, if a patient is

dying of metastatic breast cancer and is in severe pain, the potential benefit of intravenous morphine would seem overwhelming compared with the small risk that morphine might contribute to hastening an already imminent death. If these conditions are fulfilled, a physician should be able to control pain with a clear conscience, even knowing that death may unintentionally be hastened as a side-effect.

At present, these is significant controversy about whether physicians should be authorized to hasten the death of the patient intentionally through euthanasia or assisted suicide, actions not permitted by Western medicine since the Hippocratic ethic became dominant many centuries ago. Legal bans on these practices are being challenged through legislative initiatives and civil suits. Almost all professional organizations remain opposed.

Conclusion

This chapter has focused on the heart of clinical ethics, that is, acting for the good of the patient. This is the physician's central moral obligation, from which he cannot be relieved since he is bound in a covenant of trust to respond to the sick person who is in need of his medical knowledge.

We have illustrated this moral theme by analysing the four levels of the good of the patient at the bedside in several ways: first, through defining the appropriate decision-maker, the assessment of capacity, and the elements of informed consent; second, through the explication of an ethical work-up for specific cases; and third, by analysing several important ethical decisions in caring for patients at the end of life.

We acknowledge the great importance of many emerging ethical issues such as those raised by genetics, preventive medicine, and information technology. We also recognize that many ethical issues now arise in the context of team care, cost containment, managed care, and in organizational settings in which the physician is simultaneously an employee, a manager, and perhaps even an investor. These issues are too important for superficial treatment. We would only point out that in these instances too the physician's primary responsibility is the good of the sick person. If physicians default on this commitment, the last moral safeguard of the sick will have been compromised to the peril of us all.

Further reading

Beauchamp TL, Childress JF (2001). *The principles of biomedical ethics*, 5th edn. Oxford University Press, New York.

Faden RR, Beauchamp TL (1986). *A history and theory of informed consent*. Oxford University Press, New York.

Gillon R, ed. (1994). *Principles of health care ethics*. John Wiley & Sons, Chichester, UK.

Hippocrates (1939). *Hippocrates, vols I–IV*. Jones WHS, trans. Harvard University Press, Cambridge, Massachusetts.

Jonsen AR (1991). Casuistry as methodology in clinical ethics. *Theoretical Medicine* **12**, 295–307.

Pellegrino ED (1997). Managed care at the bedside: how do we look in the moral mirror? *Kennedy Institute of Ethics Journal* **7**, 321–30.

Pellegrino ED (1989). Withholding and withdrawing treatments: ethics at the bedside. *Clinical Neurosurgery* **35**, 164–84.

Pellegrino ED, Thomasma DC (1988). *For the patient's good: the restoration of beneficence in health care*. Oxford University Press, New York.

Randall F, Downie RS (1996). *Palliative care ethics: a good companion*. Oxford University Press, Oxford.

Reich WT, ed. (1995). *Encyclopedia of bioethics*, 2nd edn. Macmillan, New York.

Sulmasy DP (1992). Physicians, cost-control, and ethics. *Annals of Internal Medicine* **116**, 920–6.

Sulmasy DP (1997). Futility and the varieties of medical judgment. *Theoretical Medicine* **18**, 63–78.

Sulmasy DP, Pellegrino ED (1999). The rule of double effect: clearing up the double talk. *Archives of Internal Medicine* **159**, 545–50.

2.4 The evidence base of modern medicine

2.4.1 Bringing the best evidence to the point of care

P. Glasziou

'You must always be students, learning and unlearning till your life's end'.

Joseph Lister

Imagine you, rather than your patient, have just been diagnosed with a serious cancer outside your field of specialty. Wouldn't you prefer that your oncologist colleague had ready access to all the relevant clinical evidence, such as the results of the relevant randomized trials? But we know this is difficult. Our textbooks are often out of date, and the relevant trials scattered across the vast ocean of medical literature. This inaccessibility of the best research data at the point of clinical decision-making has consequences for patient care, and has given rise to the discipline of evidence-based medicine.

Definition

'Evidence-based medicine is the conscientious, explicit and judicious use of current best evidence in making decisions about the care of individual patients. This practice means integrating individual clinical experience with the best external clinical evidence from systematic research'.

DL Sackett, *et al*. 1996.

History

With basic research continually developing new diagnostic and treatment modalities, we would like to know: what options have been demonstrated to be effective and which is best? These are not new questions. Ambroise Paré faced them in 1536 as surgeon to French soldiers on campaign in Italy. He followed the advice of the most authoritative texts and treated their battle wounds with cautery using 'the oyle the hottest that was possible into the wounds'. However, he eventually ran short of oil and was 'constrained instead to apply a digestive'. After a troubled night, he awoke to find those he had cauterized in great pain, whereas those he had not were doing well. This accidental experiment changed Paré's and French treatment. In 1747, James Lind more deliberately set out to examine alternative treatments for scurvy: he 'took 12 cases of scurvy on board the Salisbury at sea. The cases were as similar as I could have them'. Housing and diet were standardized. Of the six pairs of sailors, the two assigned oranges and lemons recovered within 3 weeks. Unlike Paré's results, Lind's took several decades to be implemented.

The methods for conducting, and the criteria for assessing, research have been considerably strengthened in the twentieth century. Bradford Hill introduced the randomized trial to medicine: the Medical Research Council

trial of streptomycin for pulmonary tuberculosis in 1948. Since then more than a quarter of a million such trials have been conducted. Almost simultaneously, Yerushalmy introduced greater rigour into the evaluation of diagnostic tests by quantifying the accuracy—the sensitivity and specificity—of chest radiograph screening for pulmonary tuberculosis.

Interest in improving clinical evaluation has grown, giving rise to disciplines such as clinical epidemiology and evidence-based medicine, and a flood of clinical research. This is welcome, but has also hampered the dissemination of research results. Medline started in 1966 and currently adds to its 9 million references over 1000 new articles per day (www.nlm.nih.gov/pubs/factsheets/medline.html). Though these are culled from about 4300 journals in 30 languages and 70 countries, it is only a modest portion of the estimated 13 000 to 14 000 biomedical journals currently being published. No clinician's reading time is sufficient to keep up with this flow directly.

Keeping up to date: two strategies

So how can we cope with our information overload? Fortunately, most of the published information is not sufficient to alter clinical practice: much is 'scientist-to-scientist' communication directed at unravelling mechanisms; and many of the clinically relevant studies are not of adequate quality. Thus filtering for quality and clinical relevance reduces the flow to a manageable trickle as illustrated in Fig. 1.

There are two complementary ways of obtaining this filtered information. First we need to keep abreast of major new studies that should alter our clinical practice. However, rather than trying to scan hundreds of journals ourselves, it is wiser to enlist a group of our peers to do this. For example, journals such as the *ACP Journal Club*, *Evidence-Based Medicine*, and *Evidence Based Mental Health* review over 100 journals and appraise the articles for the quality of the research methods (less than 1 in 20 pass), relevance, and interest in order to identify new studies that could change the way we practise. The best systematic reviews and studies are reabstracted and an expert commentary helps place the new data in their current context.

The second, and more radical, process is to formulate and answer clinical questions as they arise with our patients. This is a 'just-in-time'

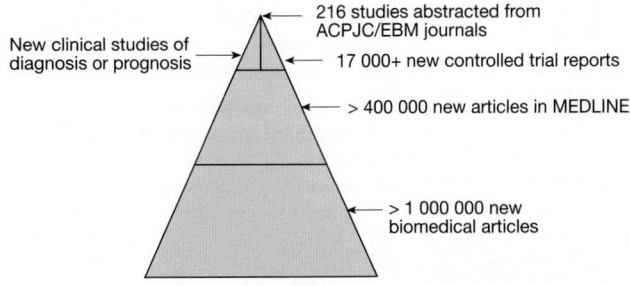

Fig. 1 The yearly flow of new biomedical publications.

approach: instead of trying to keep up to date with all areas of clinical practice, hoping that we have read and remembered the correct articles when we need to apply them, we shift focus to answering questions as they arise. This implies being able to say 'I don't know' and adding 'but I will find out!' When a problem appears, we formulate an answerable question, devise an information-gathering strategy, appraise the information achieved, and take it into account when deciding treatment with our patient. Learning becomes an active, integral, and daily part of clinical practice.

Asking clinical questions

Answering patient-stimulated questions is unlikely to be done unless we can do it rapidly: finding the information in about 30 s and assimilating it within a couple of minutes. This sounds formidable, but has been shown to be feasible. In many ways it is similar to looking up drug doses: the information must be available in our consulting room, it must be well indexed, and the presentation must be readily usable. Currently none of the continually updated evidence-based resources is as comprehensive and rapid as a pharmacopoeia, and we need some skills to navigate those available.

The steps in answering clinical questions are: (i) formulating an answerable question; (ii) formulating an information-gathering strategy; (iii) assessing the quality and relevance of the information retrieved; and (iv) applying the results to our patient. To illustrate these steps consider the following patient:

Case study Case 1. A 74-year-old man presents with his second episode of trigeminal neuralgia. As with the previous episode, he is is managing to control the pain with carbamazepine, but is requiring such large doses that he is drowsy throughout the day. He presents asking about alternatives.

In answering questions, it is helpful to classify questions into the types presented in Table 1: differential diagnosis, diagnostic accuracy, prediction/prognosis, and therapeutic effectiveness. For case 1, the issue is therapy, and a useful breakdown of such questions is: the patient, the intervention, the comparison, and the outcome. So with our patient this might be: 'In patients with trigeminal neuralgia is there a single or combined therapy which is as effective as carbamazepine at controlling pain but with less drowsiness?'

Finding answers

For treatment, we would generally first seek the results of randomized controlled trials; if there were several then we should seek existing systematic reviews. If we had answered this question previously, then the stored result would provide the fastest answer. However, since we hadn't, the first try might be *Best Evidence*: the electronic accumulation of the abstracted articles in the *ACP Journal Club* (since 1991) and *Evidence-Based Medicine* (since 1995), with over 1300 studies reviewed. Searching on the term 'trigeminal' within Therapeutics and Prevention yields one abstract (within 20 s). This was a systematic review of anticonvulsants, including carbamazepine: three placebo controlled trials showed that at 5 to 14 days follow-up 56 per cent of patients had improved with carbamazepine compared with 18 per cent with placebo ($p < 0.001$). The absolute response difference is 38 per cent, and hence for every three patients we treat there will be one additional responder (the number-needed-to-treat). This confirms carbamazepine's efficacy, but does not give us an alternative.

The next possibility is the Cochrane Library which contains Cochrane systematic reviews (the Cochrane Database Systematic Reviews, CDSR), other systematic reviews (the Database of Abstracts of Reviews of Effectiveness, DARE), and a compendium of randomized trials (the Cochrane Controlled Trials Register, CCTR) identified in Medline, EMBASE, and the handsearching by contributors to the Cochrane Collaboration. Starting the Cochrane Library CD and searching on 'trigeminal neuralgia' identifies (within 50 s) one Cochrane review (an update of the McQuay article we found in Best Evidence), and 54 controlled trials. Among these are several trials studying alternatives to carbamazepine. First, a 1988 double-blind crossover study showed baclofen significantly decreased pain in 7 of 10 patients, and in an open label study was useful in combination with carbamazepine. Second, a tantalizing but single-arm study suggested that topical capsaicin was quite effective (a Zhang's systematic review of randomized trials demonstrated clear efficacy in diabetic neuropathy and postherpetic neuralgia). Having discussed these options the patient chose to add baclofen and decrease his carbamazepine. This controlled his symptoms without drowsiness, but he later switched to the topical capsaicin which, applied to two trigger points, appeared effective.

The application of results in Case 1 was straightforward, but this is not always so. The process varies depending on the type of question (Table 1) but there are some overall similarities across these. First, is the study's illness group sufficiently similar (it need not be identical) to our patient to justify a judgement that the biological behaviour of the test or treatment

---

Table 1 Summary of types of clinical questions and the searching and appraising methods for each

Clinical question	Major appraisal issues	Possible sources	Best single Medline search term*
Pretest probabilities	1. Random or consecutive sample 2. Adequate ascertainment (> 80%) 3. Adequate diagnostic work-up	Medline	–
Diagnostic accuracy	1. Random or consecutive sample 2. Independent reading of test and reference standard 3. Adequate verification (> 80% or adjustment for sampling) 4. Adequate reference standard	Best Evidence, Medline	Diagnosis& (pe)
Treatment effects	1. Randomized (concealed) allocation to groups 2. Adequate follow-up (> 80%) 3. Blind and/or objective assessment of outcomes	Cochrane Library, Best Evidence, Clinical Evidence	Clinical-trial (pt)
Prognosis	1. Random or consecutive sample 2. Patients at first presentation (or other defined time-point) in disease 3. Adequate (> 80%) follow-up 4. Adequate measurement of outcomes	Best Evidence, Medline	Exp cohort studies
Multivariate prediction rules (prognostic or diagnostic)	As per diagnostic or prognostic question	Medline, Best Evidence	–

*See Sackett *et al.* for a more complete listing of search strategies.

would not be importantly different? Second, can we implement the test, measure, or treatment in a sufficiently similar manner? If these are fulfilled, then we need to consider how the individual features of our patient might influence the results. The next two sections look at the application of studies of diagnostic tests and of treatments.

Using the results of diagnostic test studies

Most clinical information is imperfect. This includes the history, signs, and laboratory tests. The simplest demonstration of this problem is the extensive data on the lack of agreement among experienced clinicians about the presence or absence of a clinical sign, and even between histopathologists looking at the same image. The sources of this variation and error may be in the patients, in the instruments, or in the observers. For example, true blood pressure varies considerably, but the measured blood pressure varies even more because of different calibration of instruments, cuff sizes, and clinical skill. While it is important to find ways to reduce this variation by standardization and training, some residual error is inevitable.

With experience we learn, implicitly or explicitly, some simple rules to minimize the problems of error. For example, we learn to repeat unexpected abnormal test results: the majority will have disappeared on a second reading, saving us and our patients much anxiety. Experience also teaches us that test results must be interpreted in the light of the clinical picture, or equivalently that we must combine our estimate of the chance a patient has a disease (the pretest probability) with imperfect information from the test. A test's imperfection can be quantified by two measures: (i) the sensitivity, the probability of a positive test result in someone with the target disease, and (ii) the specificity, the probability of a negative test result in someone without the target disease.

Case study Case 2. A 70-year-old man being investigated for fatigue is found to have an iron-deficiency anaemia. As part of the physical examination you do a HemeSelect (a faecal occult blood test) which is negative. Does this obviate the need for a colonoscopy?

Colorectal cancer is clearly high in the differential diagnosis; investigations of consecutive cases of iron-deficiency anaemia suggest a frequency of between 10 and 20 per cent. Let us say our estimate is 16 per cent for our case. To interpret the HemeSelect result we need to know its accuracy, that is, its sensitivity and specificity. A check of the *Best Evidence* CD provides the necessary information (in less than 30 s)—Allison *et al.* followed over 8000 consecutive people screened with three different faecal occult blood tests, with the gold standard being screen-detected cancers or cancers within 2 years of follow-up (which was 96 per cent complete). This study, which is acceptable according to the criteria in Table 1, tells us that the sensitivity is 69 per cent, that is 69 per cent of patients with cancer will have a positive HemeSelect, and the specificity is 94 per cent, that is 94 per cent of patients without cancer will have a negative HemeSelect.

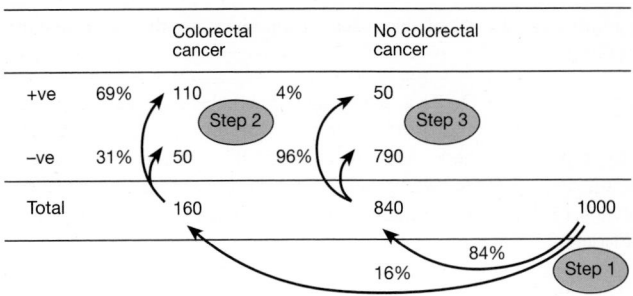

Fig. 2 Breakdown of HemeSelect results for a hypothetical 1000 patients.

To apply this to our patient with iron deficiency we need to work backwards from his chance of cancer before the test—see Fig. 2.

Using a hypothetical 1000 patients similar to our Case 2, Fig. 2 works through this probability in three steps.

1. Of the 1000 similar patients, we would expect 160 to have a colorectal cancer and 840 not (bottom row of Table 1).

2. Of the 160 with cancer 69 per cent (the sensitivity) will have a positive result, that is, $0.69 \times 160 = 110$ and the remaining 50 will have a negative result (column 1),

3. Of the 840 without cancer 94 per cent (the specificity) will have a negative result, that is, $0.94 \times 840 = 790$ and the remaining 50 will have a positive result (column 2).

Thus our patient with the negative HemeSelect is among the 50 (false) + 790 (true) negatives, that is, his chance of cancer is $50/(840) = 6$ per cent (the post-test probability after a negative test).

We clearly cannot repeat such calculations with every patient, but methods have been developed to simplify the process (see Sackett). However, the important principle illustrated here is the need to use both the clinical picture—quantified as the pretest probability—and the test accuracy. Harold Sox has expressed this succinctly: 'What you believe after the test depends on what you believed before the test'. In particular, it is important not to be misled by false positives when screening; nor to be misled by false negatives when attempting to confirm the most likely diagnosis. Figure 3(a) illustrates this geometrically for our case 2, where even after a negative HemeSelect there is still substantial chance of colorectal cancer, whereas in the screening situation of (b) the positive HemeSelect is more likely to be a false than a true positive.

Using the results of treatment studies

The overall results of treatment trials apply to the 'average' patient and need to be individualized. If our patient is at a higher or lower risk, then we need

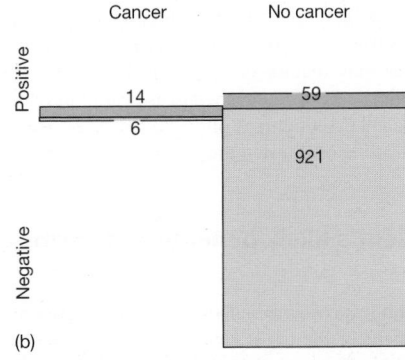

Fig. 3 Interpreting faecal occult blood results in different groups: 2 × 2 tables for (a) patient with iron-deficiency anaemia (16 per cent chance of cancer), and (b) an asymptomatic 70-year-old patient being screened (2 per cent chance of cancer).

to adjust our estimate of the effects of treatment for this. Consider the following case.

Case study Case 3. During a routine check of his blood pressure, a 58-year-old male with stable angina and a history of hypertension was noted to have atrial fibrillation. A check of his chart showed this had been noted several months earlier. Routine investigations revealed no cause, and because of the duration, cardioversion was not warranted. But should he be taking aspirin or warfarin?

The Cochrane Library contains both Cochrane and other systematic reviews of the five relevant randomized trials: warfarin is extremely effective therapy, with a 68 per cent reduction in the risks of ischaemic stroke. However, we must also be concerned about the dangers of anticoagulation— specifically the risks of bleeding, and most crucially the risks of intracranial haemorrhage. Should he be treated? Guidelines seem unhelpful here: a recent review by Thomson showed that the proportion of patients with atrial fibrillation recommended for anticoagulation by the 20 different guidelines ranged from 13 up to 100 per cent!

So how do we apply the systematic review results? The following four questions have been suggested.

1. Is my patient so different from those in the study that the results cannot be applied?

The inclusion and exclusion criteria of clinical trials tell us about the broad category of patients tested in the trials, but are not necessarily a good guide to the applicability of the trials to individuals. A better approach is, first, to think about the potential modifiers of the therapeutic effect, and second, the benefits and harms in the individuals.

The biological effect of an intervention may be modified by several factors: patient characteristics, comorbidities, compliance, or cointerventions. To predict these may require pathophysiological knowledge and empirical data. For example, would a patient with Parkinson's disease having problems with dental hygiene be helped by an electric toothbrush? The randomized trials suggest that certain types of electric brush are clearly better than manual brushing, but did not include patients with Parkinson's disease. However, our knowledge of Parkinson's disease does not suggest there would be any reduction in benefit, and it may be even greater given the effect of bradykinesia on manual brushing.

Treatment decisions must usually balance positive and negative effects of the intervention. For our patient on warfarin the 68 per cent relative reduction in the ischaemic stroke risk must be weighed against the inconvenience of therapeutic monitoring, and more seriously, the risks of major bleeding, particularly the risks of intracranial haemorrhage: an excess of about 1 per cent per year.

2. Is the treatment feasible in my setting?

Barriers to usage include local organization of services, costs, and skills. Patients in remote settings may have difficulty with regular monitoring; service costs and hence access will vary across countries and settings; many new therapies or procedures may require skills or technology that are unavailable, for instance cognitive behavioural therapy is helpful in many conditions but access to a skilled practitioner is often limited. These issues may make the treatment infeasible or threaten the balance of benefits and harms.

3. What are my patient's likely benefits and harms from the treatment?

Low-risk patients usually gain less absolute benefit and high-risk patients more than the 'average' patient in the trials. Hence we need to predict, based on the individual's clinical characteristics, their expected risk. By applying the relative risk reduction seen across the trials, this individualized prognosis can then be used to predict the gains of therapy. Figure 4 summarizes this process. The horizontal axis is the stroke rate per year; the vertical axis is the stroke equivalents prevented by anticoagulation using warfarin. This represents the 68 per cent relative reduction seen across the trials.

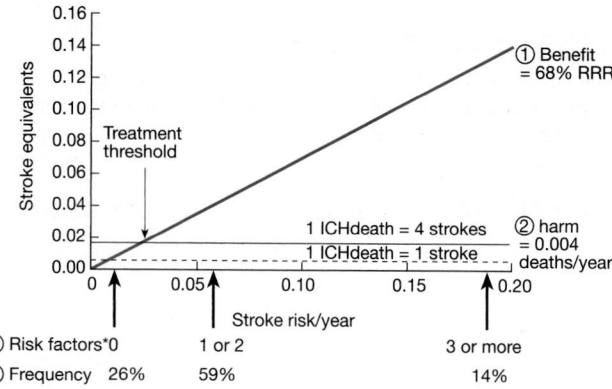

Fig. 4 Warfarin for atrial fibrillation plotting how benefits and harms vary with stroke risk (horizontal axis): (1) Expected benefit from a 68 per cent relative reduction in risk of ischaemic stroke. (2) Expected harms from intracranial haemorrhage: deaths (dashed line) or if one death is considered equal to four strokes (solid line). (3) Predicted risk based on three clinical and two echocardiographic risk factors. (4) The frequency of these risk categories in the Stroke Prevention in Atrial Fibrillation trial.

Where does our patient lie in this spectrum? On the bottom and top axis are marked the clinical risk factors. Our 58-year-old male patient had a normal echocardiogram but ischaemic heart disease and a history of hypertension, and so fitted into the one to two risk-factor category.

4. How will my patient's values influence the decision?

The essence of making wise clinical management is to follow the aphorism of Hippocrates 'Firstly do no (net) harm'. We should now compare the absolute benefits and the absolute harms of therapy, then use the strength of the individual's preferences to weigh these. In large cohort studies of the use of warfarin in the community, the rates of excess intracranial haemorrhage deaths have been about 4 per 1000 per year. This rate is shown as the bottom line in Fig. 4. This line, however, would assume that one death was equivalent to one ischaemic stroke; the line above this values one death equivalent to four ischaemic strokes. The relative value is an individual judgement, but measurements of quality of life in patients after stroke show an average quality of life of roughly 0.75 (on a scale of 0 for death to 1 for normal well health). Where the lines of benefit and harm cross one another, the expected benefit and harms are equal. It is only above this line that we begin to avoid our Hippocratic net harm, and hence the treatment that could be considered worthwhile to the patient, as with case 3.

Conclusions

If we are to advance the use of the best clinical research evidence in patient decision-making then at least two things are required. First, the compilation of the necessary information so that it is quickly accessible by practitioners in the clinic and at the bedside. Answers are needed in minutes not months. The Cochrane Collaboration has gone a long way to achieve this for questions of therapeutic interventions, but similar efforts will be needed for prognosis, diagnosis, and other types of clinical questions. Second, more serious efforts are needed in looking at the applicability and presentation of the results of studies and systematic reviews of studies to allow rapid interpretation and individual application of the results.

Further reading

Allison JE *et al.*(1996). A comparison of fecal occult-blood tests for colorectal-cancer screening. *New England Journal of Medicine* **334**, 155–9.

Anonymous (1996). Anticonvulsant drugs reduce pain in trigeminal neuralgia and diabetic neuropathy and are effective for migraine prophylaxis. *ACP Journal Club* **1124**, 35. *Evidence-Based Medicine* **1**, 89.

Antman EM *et al.* (1992). A comparison of results of meta-analyses of randomized control trials and recommendations of clinical experts. Treatments for myocardial infarction. *Journal of the American Medical Association* **268**, 240–8.

Epstein JB, Marcoe JH (1994). Topical application of capsaicin for treatment of oral neuropathic pain and trigeminal neuralgia. *Oral Surgery, Oral Medicine, and Oral Pathology* **77**, 135–40.

Fromm GH, Terrence CF, Chatta AS (1984). Baclofen in the treatment of trigeminal neuralgia: double-blind study and long-term follow-up. *Annals of Neurology* **15**, 240–4.

Glasziou P *et al.* (1998). Applying the results of trials and systematic reviews to individual patients. *ACP Journal Club* **129**, A-15–16. *Evidence-Based Medicine* **3**, 165–6.

Lind J (1753). *A treatise of the scurvy. In three parts. Containing an inquiry into the nature, causes and cure, of that disease.* Printed by Sands, Murray, & Cochran for A.Kincaid and A Donaldson, Edinburgh. (http://www.rcpe.ac.uk/cochrane/frame.html)

McQuay H *et al.* (1995). Anticonvulsant drugs for management of pain: a systematic review. *British Medical Journal* **311**, 1047–52.

Medical Research Council (1948). Streptomycin treatment of pulmonary tuberculosis: a Medical Research Council investigation. *British Medical Journal* ii, 769–82.

Sackett DL, Haynes RB (1997). Thirteen steps, 100 people, and 1 000 000 thanks. *ACP Journal Club* **127**, A-14. *Evidence-Based Medicine* **2**, 101.

Sackett DL *et al.* (1995). Evidence-based medicine: what it is and what it isn't. *British Medical Journal* **312**, 71–2.

Sackett DL *et al.* (1997). *Evidence-based medicine: how to practice and teach EBM.* Churchill Livingstone, New York.

The Stroke Prevention in Atrial Fibrillation Investigators (1996). Bleeding during antithrombotic therapy in patients with atrial fibrillation. *Archives of Internal Medicine* **156**, 409–16.

The Stroke Prevention in Atrial Fibrillation (SPAF) Investigators (1999). Factors associated with ischemic stroke during aspirin therapy in atrial fibrillation: analysis of 2012 participants in the SPAF I-III clinical trials. *Stroke* **30**, 1223–9.

Thomson R (1998). Guidelines on anticoagulant treatment in atrial fibrillation in Great Britain: variation in content and implications for treatment. *British Medical Journal* **316**, 509–13.

Zhang WY, Li Wan Po A (1994). The effectiveness of topically applied capsaicin: a meta-analysis. *European Journal of Clinical Pharmacology* **46**, 517–22.

2.4.2 Evidence-based medicine

*Alvan R. Feinstein**

Evidence-based medicine can be viewed as a novel form of clinical practice, as a special compendium of approved information, or as a revolutionary change in medical education. After all three views are discussed, the rest of this chapter will describe the advantages and disadvantages of the new approach.

Basic views

Each of the three cited views of evidence-based medicine has been often discussed.

'Novel' form of practice

Despite the apparent novelty of the phrase itself, many practising clinicians believe that evidence-based medicine is 'nothing new'. Almost all thoughtful practitioners have regularly assembled evidence when they reviewed their own experience, developed clinical judgement, read medical literature, attended medical meetings, and talked with one another. This activity seems entirely compatible with statements by evidence-based medicine advocates that the information used to practice evidence-based medicine contains 'clinically relevant research, often from the basic sciences of medicine', including studies of diagnostic tests, prognostic markers, and 'the efficacy and safety of therapeutic, rehabilitative, and preventive regimens'. The traditional mode of clinical practice easily seems to fit not only the foregoing description, but also another statement that the practice of evidence-based medicine consists of 'integrating individual clinical expertise with the best available external clinical evidence from systematic research'.

For these reasons, clinicians may not regard the practice of evidence-based medicine as a novelty, and may wonder why it has received so much exhortation and attention. The source of novelty becomes more apparent, however, in the phrase that evidence-based medicine contains 'the best… evidence from systematic research'. Regardless of what might be offered as criteria for what is best or even good evidence, the evidence-based medicine advocates have a clear, unambiguous requirement. The 'gold standard' is 'the randomized trial, and especially the systematic review of several randomized trials'. This constraint on the acceptable 'best evidence' produces the special compendium of information that is the distinctively novel feature of evidence-based medicine.

Special compendium of information

The new journals and books devoted to evidence-based medicine concentrate on data from randomized trials and their meta-analyses (which are sometimes called 'overviews' or 'systematic reviews'). The volume of work and the scope of topics have been prolific. The first pertinent textbook, in 1996, was followed by a series of additional books, all titled as evidence-based topics in clinical practice, general practice, primary care, health care, family medicine, nursing, cardiology, and consultations. The 'evidence-based' prefix has also been applied in titles for individual articles addressing medical education, prescription guidelines, humanitarian relief intervention, organ allocation, budgeting, and health-care reform.

The intellectual centre of evidence-based medicine is the Cochrane Collaboration, based at Oxford and named after the late Archie Cochrane, a pioneering epidemiologist in urging careful evaluation of health-care interventions. The Collaboration, which co-ordinates the activities of acquiring and maintaining the special compendium, comprises an international consortium of research workers who construct an ever-enlarging data base by contributing results of their own randomized trials, by adding discoveries of previously unpublished trials, and by performing the summary aggregations that constitute the meta-analyses. The collected information, which extends through all branches of medicine, becomes the 'best evidence'. It can be published as reports in conventional literary formats or accessed via electronic media, such as the Internet. Coming mainly from activities in clinical epidemiology, the information has sometimes been called 'epidense' evidence.

*It is with regret that we must report the death of Professor A.R. Feinstein during the preparation of this edition of the textbook.

Revolutionary change in learning

A revolutionary change in medical education is produced by the evidence-based medicine demand that clinical decisions be derived from, or sanctioned by, the contents of the new compendium. The new approach drastically alters the traditional pedagogic system in which medicine was learned from presumably knowledgeable personal authorities. They would express their knowledge either in publications or in the direct supervisory instruction given in the distant past to apprentices, and in modern medicine to students, house officers, and fellows. In the education proposed by evidence-based medicine, however, the wisdom and appraisals of a personal expert are no longer encouraged. They are replaced by the meta-analyses and printouts of the evidence-based medicine computer.

A movement that overthrows academic authorities is not a surprising modern development. The urge to purge leaders of the educational 'establishment' began in universities about 30 years ago, provoked by various national and international political discontents, often arising from the war in Viet Nam. Initiated at a time when many current leaders of evidence-based medicine were undergraduates, this drive was later enhanced by four types of new medical events.

One event, at many academic medical institutions, was the exchanging of part-time teaching faculty, who were clinical practitioners in the neighbouring community, for the increasing numbers of full-time faculty, who were clinical investigators. A second event was the reduced clinical expertise of the clinical investigators. Having been chosen mainly for achievements in laboratory research, the new pedagogic leaders were often more knowledgeable about pathophysiology than therapy and patient care. Both of these events tended to remove expert clinical authorities from being readily available in teaching activities.

A third event was the increasing development and use of randomized trials, which were usually applied to demonstrate the efficacy of new therapeutic agents. When older regimens were occasionally tested, however, the trials sometimes produced dramatic contradictions, showing that firmly-held establishment beliefs were either wrong or harmful. Perhaps the most memorable of these refutations occurred in the randomized trial of high concentration oxygen therapy for newborn premature babies. This treatment had been vigorously endorsed by renowned professors of paediatrics, and it was used for more than a decade, particularly at academic medical centres in the United States, for the goal of preventing respiratory distress. About 10 000 infants were permanently blinded with retrolental fibroplasia before the randomized trial ended the 'academic epidemic' by demonstrating that the oxygen, while avoiding respiratory distress, often produced blindness. The results greatly elevated the reputation of randomized trials for resolving controversies about therapy, but sharply diminished respect for academic authorities as sources of wise clinical advice.

A fourth problem was produced by the enormous expansion of technological tests and treatments. A generalist who could formerly keep track of almost all important changes in the field could no longer do so, and became supplanted by an array of specialists in different organ–system domains, such as cardiology. As new information continued to proliferate, the scope of the specialists also became limited. They often could no longer encompass an entire organ system, and became subspecialized in such subdomains as coronary, congenital, rheumatic, or hypertensive heart disease. The expansion and diffusion of domains of expertise would require a large array of individual authorities, not just a few; and all of them would not be readily available for personal consultation at each teaching institution.

In an atmosphere in which personal authorities were often generally viewed with suspicion, sometimes specifically impugned, and seldom always available, the time was ripe for an entirely new system to replace what was derisively called 'eminence-based' medicine. In the new system, the evidence-based medicine compendium would be the source of 'established wisdom'; and the new authorities would be persons with evidence-based medicine credentials. In medicine, as often in politics, the leaders of the new order would be those who had fomented the overthrow of the old.

Advantages and disadvantages of the new approach

To produce the revolution that would alter long-entrenched patterns of education, the proponents often used extreme vigour and sometimes evangelical fervour in advocating evidence-based medicine and responding to adverse criticism. The zeal itself could evoke either additional admiration or further denunciation. In commenting on complaints, one of the prominent leaders said that 'most of the criticisms have to do with our hubris, style, and conviction'. The value of evidence-based medicine should be judged, however, not by the behaviour of its advocates, but by what it actually does and does not do.

Perhaps the most obvious positive accomplishment of the evidence-based medicine movement is the emphasis on citing explicit data and reasons for clinical decisions. Although this approach had previously been urged for several decades, the renewed demand for citing 'evidence' has helped end the old tradition in which decisions were justified only by non-specific explanations such as 'intuition' or 'judgement'.

A second positive accomplishment has been the demonstration that active clinicians, in an era of extensive and rapid technologic changes, can no longer rely on their previous medical education to provide a permanent basis for clinical practice. Conventional lectures and courses in 'continuing medical education', however, have not offered a satisfactory method to 'keep up' with what is happening. The evidence-based medicine movement has demonstrated a way for clinicians to 'stay alive' by doing computerized searches of accruing literature.

Several other claims of achievement have always been part of good clinical practice, and are not unique to the evidence-based medicine style. Among such claims are the contentions that evidence-based medicine integrates medical education with clinical practice, and that it helps clinicians resist unwarranted pressures.

In the original proposal for evidence-based medicine, a clinical analysis was divided into four main steps. Each step, as discussed in the next four sections, has its own distinctive advantages and disadvantages when conducted with the current evidence-based medicine compendium.

Formulating a question to be answered

The obvious first step in any process of clinical reasoning is to choose a 'prime topic' as the question to be answered. This topic is the doctor's counterpart of the patient's chief complaint. Nevertheless, just as the chief complaint may not always indicate what a patient really wants and expects, the prime topic may not always represent, and may sometimes misrepresent, what is needed for the care of the patient. To be answerable, the chosen question may have to be altered to suit the available data. Thus, the desire to learn about post-therapeutic outcomes, such as relief of symptoms and quality of life, may be diverted to an answer that indicates outcomes such as survival duration and changes in laboratory tests.

A greater, but less apparent, problem is the occasional or frequent mismatch between the available evidence and the nuances of the individual clinical situation. Most published reports of treatment, whether observational studies or randomized trials, will contain results for a stipulated therapy given to patients with a stipulated baseline clinical condition. The stipulations, however, may not include important details—such as concomitant therapy, comorbidity, severity of illness, and functional status—that distinguish the particular patient for whom the question is being asked. The general answer, reflecting results for the larger total group of patients who were treated for the condition, may not be pertinent for the patient's individual distinctions.

This problem is heightened when the evidence comes solely from randomized trials. Designed to answer questions of general efficacy rather than to guide individual treatment, the trials often contain a highly selected group of patients, treated with a relatively rigid therapeutic protocol. Furthermore, with the currently popular intention-to-treat analytic principle, the results of the trials are appraised without regard to whether or how well the patients actually maintained (or even received) the randomly assigned treatment. The results of each trial thus indicate what happens to an 'average' patient assigned to the treatment; and the meta-analyses produce an average of the averages. The average results may be satisfactory for the decisions made by economists, health-plan managers, regulatory agencies, and pharmaceutical companies; but averages are often grossly unsatisfactory for individual decisions about specific patients.

Searching the literature

An important past role of medical textbooks and published 'review articles' was to produce an authoritative summary of pertinent comments and evaluations for each prime topic. The summary may sometimes have been out-of-date, and the authority incorrect, but the search was relatively easy to do and the authority was clearly identified.

With this traditional approach rejected, clinicians are now urged to do their own computerized search of 'the literature'. For only a single topic, among the many others that may be cogent, the computer will regularly produce a large display of multiple reports that can take considerable time to obtain and read. This time can be greatly shortened, however, if clinicians forgo their own full search, and use the approved but highly truncated selection contained in the evidence-based medicine compendium. The clinician thus relies on the evidence-based medicine authorities, who may be relatively anonymous or cited in a multitude of names, instead of the individually identified expert who wrote the section in a chosen textbook or review article.

Relying on the evidence-based medicine compendium, however, can be a frustrating activity in two types of situations. One of them occurs in the 'grey zones of clinical practice' for which gold-standard randomized-trial evidence is available, but inconclusive. In the other situation, the selected prime topic has not been included in the evidence-based medicine collection. Because most randomized trials and their concomitant meta-analyses have been devoted to specific individual therapeutic regimens, very few or no trials have been done for most of the common topics of clinical practice. They include decisions about 'risk factors' and aetiological agents (such as cigarette smoking), pathophysiological challenges (such as restoring electrolyte balance), appraising the relative merits of diagnostic tests, choosing prognostic indicators, or evaluating the 'polypharmacy effects' that occur when several different treatments are used concomitantly. The published literature contains many reports on these topics, but the results come from non-randomized observational studies rather than trials.

Randomized trials (as well as observational studies) are also sparse or non-existent for many interpersonal clinical decisions, such as how to communicate with difficult patients, and how to offer useful reassurance. All of these topics will be omitted from the evidence-based medicine compendium.

Evaluating the literature

The third step in the process is to evaluate what has been found in the literature. The evaluation is relatively quick and easy for topics supplied in the evidence-based medicine compendium, since they have already been assessed and deemed worthwhile. Nevertheless, thoughtful readers may have both qualitative and quantitative difficulties in using the results. Qualitatively, as noted earlier, the evidence-based medicine information may not be suitably pertinent for the individual patient who inspired the search. Quantitatively, the actual magnitude of the cited effects may be difficult to discern and understand when reported in the statistical jargon of proportionate increments, odds ratios, relative risks, and attributable risks.

For example suppose the mortality rates are 24 per cent with treatment A and 18 per cent with the control treatment. This contrast may accurately, but alternatively, be reported as favouring the treatment by a proportional increment of 33 per cent, an odds ratio of 1.44, a relative risk of 1.33, or an attributable risk of 6 per cent.

Aware of the difficulties in interpreting these numbers, the proponents of evidence-based medicine have begun to urge that results be expressed as the inverse of the attributable risk. It is called NNT—the number of patients needed to be treated to produce one extra effect. Its calculation in this example would be $1/0.06 = 16.7$, thus indicating that about 17 patients must be treated to save one more life than would occur with treatment in the 'control' group.

For the same set of data, the realization that 17 patients must be treated to get a single extra 'success' is much easier for clinicians and patients to understand than the possibly misleading improvement proportion of 33 per cent, or the often incomprehensible odds ratio of 1.44. The simple, desirable NNT expressions have not yet become ubiquitous in the evidence-based medicine compendium, however, and many results are still summarized, for statistical convenience, as odds ratios or (even worse) as logarithms of odds ratios.

A separate problem is produced when the quantitative magnitude of the difference is obscured by an evidence-based medicine headline such as 'Treatment A is better than Treatment B for Condition C'. As long as the results have acquired the probabilistic accolade of 'statistical significance', a difference of 0.4 per cent between two treatments may be impressively hailed as 'better', even though 250 patients must receive the 'better' treatment for one to be benefited.

In an era of excessive attention to 'statistical significance', the problem of discerning and interpreting quantitative magnitudes occurs for any type of report, and is not unique to evidence-based medicine. The problem is accentuated, however, when an evidence-based medicine claim of 'better' is accepted uncritically, and particularly when the claim is used to construct guidelines for clinical practice, or criteria for policy recommendations and fiscal reimbursements.

A different type of problem occurs if the desired evidence is not contained in the evidence-based medicine compendium. The clinician must then appraise other sources of information, ranging from published literature to direct discussion with respected colleagues. The evidence-based medicine proponents have offered a hierarchy of rankings for the appraisal of published literature. Randomized trials rank at the top, followed by analyses of non-randomized observational studies, such as the groups appraised in cohort and case–control research. The lowest rank is given to uncontrolled case series, case reports, or the 'anecdotal recommendations' offered by an individual expert.

Although a reasonable generalization, this hierarchy can resemble a ranking of methods for achieving sterile precautions before entering a surgical operating room. Regardless of what is done and how well the precautions are carried out, the most important events occur during the operation, not beforehand. A well conducted observational study that answers the right question can often be more helpful than a randomized trial that is inadequately aimed; and a single case report or small series of cases can sometimes be extraordinarily enlightening. Unfortunately, a concentration on learning the methods of randomized trials and meta-analyses offers no guidance for evaluating non-randomized research, and may lead to underdeveloped critical skills with which 'young physicians who are educated only in evidence-based medicine become completely lost when they have to think about instances in which randomization is impossible'. Evaluating observational research requires special scientific principles for identifying subtle sources of bias that do not occur in randomized trials, but the principles are seldom carefully considered or discussed during an emphasis on randomized trials and meta-analyses.

A separate challenge is to appraise the quality of 'gold' in the 'gold-standard' evidence itself. Diverse 'check-lists' have been proposed for this purpose, but the lists often contain different components; and higher counts of positive components may not always indicate better quality. A major flaw in a crucial single component can invalidate the main results, despite positive counts for all other components.

Implement useful findings

The last step in the recommended process calls for the clinician to implement useful findings. Before beginning the implementation, however, the clinician must first be confident that the findings are indeed useful.

In the old 'eminence-based' system, the authoritative opinions may sometimes have been contradictory, out-of-date, or wrong, but the same phenomena can occur in the evidence-based medicine system. Randomized trials of the same topic have sometimes produced opposing results; different meta-analyses have reached different conclusions for the same set of data; meta-analyses in the evidence-based medicine compendium will often become out-of-date if not promptly revised whenever each pertinent new randomized trial appears; and a later large randomized trial may sometimes contradict results of an existing meta-analysis for smaller previous trials.

A separate problem in usefulness, as discussed earlier, is that the necessary information for an individual patient may be incomplete, inadequate, or wholly absent in the evidence-based medicine compendium. By emphasizing and averaging the 'hard data' of randomized trials, the evidence-based medicine movement can augment the 'statistical reductionism' that tends to dehumanize modern medicine, particularly when evidence-based medicine advocates refer to the care of patients as 'disease management'.

Yet another difficulty in appraising usefulness can arise from the pedagogic revolution that rejects not only the writings of individual authorities, but also their supervisory role in rounds and other teaching activities. When the probing questions of an instructor are replaced by 'evidence carts' or other electronic devices for acquiring evidence-based medicine information, students and house staff are deprived of stimuli that can lead to contemplative thought, and to the learning that comes from justifying decisions and recognizing errors. Without this type of supervisory probing to develop mental agility, young physicians may learn to seek, receive, and excrete the 'best evidence' without simultaneously being challenged to digest, absorb, and evaluate it.

Conclusions

The foregoing comments are not intended to detract from the remarkable accomplishments of the evidence-based medicine movement. Like the Internet itself, evidence-based medicine has had extraordinary growth—developing with unparalleled speed and spreading rapidly throughout the world. The movement has brought a valuable emphasis on the need for using explicit evidence to justify clinical decisions and for maintaining a constant awareness of new and changing evidence. The special evidence-based medicine compendium may contain flaws analogous to those of the old system, but the compendium itself is also a remarkable achievement. It has demonstrated a method to summarize and synthesize a vast plethora of information. The process and the results may be imperfect, but they can serve as a useful basis for future improvements.

The compendium itself, however, can never become fully satisfactory if it continues to rely solely on a 'best evidence' that may sometimes be neither good nor complete, and if the vast bulk of medical evidence, which does not come from randomized trials, continues to be excluded. The methods needed to improve the quality of non-randomized evidence, however, will be delayed or diverted, if talented young clinical investigators, who might construct those methods, are preoccupied with doing meta-analyses for contributions to the evidence-based medicine compendium.

The evidence-based medicine movement can be admired and applauded for its obvious success at inaugurating an exciting new approach to clinical reasoning. The ultimate success of the movement will depend on its ability to escape from self-imposed constraints, and to incorporate all of the contributions, in mind and data, that constitute 'medicine-based evidence'.

Further reading

Cochrane AL, M Blythe (1989). *One man's medicine. An autobiography of Professor Archie Cochrane.* The Memoir Club (British Medical Journal), London.

Ellrodt G, Cook DJ, Lee J, Cho M, Hunt D, Weingarten S (1997). Evidence-based disease management. *Journal of the American Medical Association* **278**, 1687–92.

Evidence-Based Medicine Working Group (1992). Evidence-based medicine: a new approach to teaching the practice of medicine. *Journal of the American Medical Association* **268**, 2420–5.

Feinstein AR (1967). *Clinical judgment.* Williams and Wilkins, Baltimore.

Feinstein AR (1999). Statistical reductionism and clinicians' delinquencies in humanistic research. *Clinical Pharmacology and Therapeutics* **66**, 211–17.

Haynes RB (quoted in Levin A) (1998). Evidence-based medicine gaining supporters. *Annals of Internal Medicine* **128**, 334–6.

Jacobson RM, Feinstein AR (1992). Oxygen as a cause of blindness in premature infants: 'Autopsy' of a decade of errors in clinical epidemiologic research. *Journal of Clinical Epidemiology* **45**, l265–87.

Knottnerus JA, Dinant GJ (1997). Medicine based evidence, a prerequisite for evidence based medicine. *British Medical Journal* **315**, 1109–10.

Laupacis A, Sackett DL, Roberts RS (1988). An assessment of clinically useful measures of the consequences of treatment. *New England Journal of Medicine* **318**, 1728–33.

Naylor CD (1995). Grey zones of clinical practice: some limits to evidence-based medicine. *Lancet* **345**, 840–2.

Sackett DL, Richardson WS, Rosenberg W, Haynes RB (1996). *Evidence-based medicine. How to practice and teach EBM.* Churchill Livingstone, London.

Sackett DL, Rosenberg WMC, Muir Gray JS, et al (1996). Evidence based medicine: what it is and what it isn't. *British Medical Journal* **312**, 71–2.

Vandenbroucke JP (1998). Observational research and evidence-based medicine: What should we teach young physicians? *Journal of Clinical Epidemiology* **51**, 467–72.

Wulff HR, Gøtzsche PC (2000). *Rational diagnosis and treatment. Evidence based clinical decision making,* 3rd edition. Blackwell Science Ltd., Oxford.

2.4.3 Large-scale randomized evidence: trials and overviews

R. Collins, R. Peto, R. Gray, and S. Parish

Introduction and summary

This chapter is intended principally for practising clinicians who need to use the results of clinical trials in their routine practice, and who want to know why some types of evidence are much more reliable than others. It is concerned with treatments that might improve survival (or some other major aspect of long-term disease outcome), and its chief point is that, as long as doctors start with a healthy scepticism about the many apparently striking claims that appear in the medical literature, trials do make sense. The main enemy of common sense is over-optimism: there are a few striking exceptions where treatments for serious disease really do turn out to work extremely well, but in general most of the claims of vast improvements from new therapies turn out to be evanescent. Hence, clinical trials need to be able to detect or to refute more moderate differences in long-term outcome. Once this common-sense idea is explicitly recognized the rest follows naturally, and it becomes obvious what types of evidence can and cannot be trusted. Although the chapter may also be of some interest or encouragement to doctors who are considering participating in (or even planning) large trials, its main intended readers are practising clinicians. For, even the most definite results from large-scale randomized evidence cannot save lives unless such practitioners accept and apply them. This chapter does not include large amounts of statistical detail: instead, it tries to communicate the spirit that underlies the increasing emphasis on large-scale randomized evidence that has developed since the 1980s.

Unrealistic hopes about the chances of discovering large treatment effects can be a serious obstacle not only to appropriate patient care but also to good clinical research. For, such hopes may misleadingly suggest to some research workers or funding agencies that small or even non-randomized studies may suffice. In contrast, realistically moderate expectations of what a treatment might achieve (or, if one treatment is to be compared with another, realistically moderate expectations of how large any difference between these treatments is likely to be) should tend to foster the design of studies that aim to discriminate reliably between: (1) differences in outcome that are realistically moderate but still worthwhile; and (2) differences in outcome that are too small to be of any material importance. Studies having this particular aim must guarantee strict control of bias (which, in general, requires proper randomization and appropriate statistical analysis, with no unduly 'data-dependent' emphasis on specific parts of the overall evidence) and strict control of the play of chance (which, in general, requires large numbers rather than much detail). The conclusion is obvious: moderate biases and moderate random errors must both be avoided if moderate benefits are to be assessed or refuted reliably. This leads to the need for large numbers of properly randomized patients, which in turn leads to both large but simple randomized trials (or 'mega-trials') and large systematic overviews (or 'meta-analyses') of related randomized trials.

Non-randomized evidence, unduly small randomized trials, or unduly small overviews of trials are all much inferior as sources of evidence about current patient management or as foundations for future research strategies. They cannot discriminate reliably between moderate (but worthwhile) differences and negligible differences in outcome, and the mistaken clinical conclusions that they engender could well result in the undertreatment, overtreatment, or other mismanagement of millions of future patients worldwide. In contrast, hundreds of thousands of premature deaths each year could be avoided by seeking appropriately large-scale randomized evidence about various widely practicable treatments for the common causes of death, and by disseminating such evidence appropriately. Likewise, appropriately large-scale randomized evidence could substantially improve the management of many important, but non-fatal, medical problems.

The value of large-scale randomized evidence is illustrated in this chapter by the trials of fibrinolytic therapy for acute myocardial infarction, antiplatelet therapy for a wide range of vascular conditions, hormonal therapy for early breast cancer, and drug therapy for lowering blood pressure. In these examples proof of benefit, that could not have been achieved by either small-scale randomized evidence or non-randomized evidence, has led to widespread changes in practice that are now preventing tens of thousands of premature deaths each year.

Moderate (but worthwhile) effects on major outcomes are generally more plausible than large effects

Some treatments have large, and hence obvious, effects on survival: for example, it is clear without randomized trials that prompt treatment of diabetic coma or cardiac arrest saves lives (and, indeed, a plaque at the entrance to our own hospital records the first clinical use of penicillin). However, perhaps in part because of these striking successes, for the past few decades the hopes of large treatment effects on mortality and major morbidity in other serious diseases have been unrealistically high. Of course, treatments do quite commonly have large effects on various less fundamental measures: drugs readily reduce blood pressure, blood lipids, or blood glucose; many tumours or leukaemias can be controlled temporarily by radiotherapy or chemotherapy; in acute myocardial infarction,

lidocaine (lignocaine) can prevent many arrhythmias and streptokinase can dissolve most coronary thrombi; in early HIV infection, antiretroviral drugs substantially reduce viraemia. However, although all these effects are large, any effects on mortality are much more modest; indeed, there is still dispute as to whether any net improvement in survival is provided by the routine use of radiotherapy for common cancers, lidocaine for acute myocardial infarction, or antiretroviral agents for early HIV infection.

In general, if substantial uncertainty remains about the efficacy of a practicable treatment, its effects on major endpoints are probably either negligibly small, or only moderate, rather than large. Indirect support for this rather pessimistic conclusion comes from many sources, including: the previous few decades of disappointingly slow progress in the curative treatment of the common chronic diseases of middle age; the heterogeneity of each single disease, as evidenced by the unpredictability of survival duration even when apparently similar patients are compared with each other; the variety of different mechanisms in certain diseases that can lead to death, only one of which may be appreciably influenced by any one particular therapy; the modest effects often suggested by systematic overviews (see later) of various therapies; and, in certain special cases, observational epidemiological studies of the strength of the relationship between some disease and the factor that the treatment will modify (for example, blood pressure, blood cholesterol, or blood glucose: see later).

Having accepted that only moderate reductions in mortality are likely with many currently available interventions, how worthwhile might such effects be if they could be detected reliably? To some clinicians, reducing the risk of early death in patients with myocardial infarction from 10 per 100 patients down to 9 or 8 per 100 patients treated may not seem particularly worthwhile, and if such a reduction was only transient, or involved an extremely expensive or toxic treatment, this might well be an appropriate view. Worldwide, however, several million patients a year suffer an acute myocardial infarction, and if just one million were to be given a simple, non-toxic, and widely practicable treatment that reduced the risk of early death from 10 per cent down to 9 or 8 per cent (that is, a proportional reduction of 10 or 20 per cent), this would avoid 10 000 to 20 000 deaths. (For example, about half a million patients a year now receive fibrinolytic therapy for acute myocardial infarction, avoiding about 10 000 early deaths, and large trials have shown that this difference in early mortality persists for several years afterwards.) Such absolute gains are substantial, and might considerably exceed the numbers of lives that could be saved by a much more effective treatment of a much less common disease.

Reliable detection or refutation of moderate differences requires avoidance of both moderate biases and moderate random errors

If realistically moderate differences in outcome are to be reliably detected or reliably refuted, then errors in comparative assessments of the effects of treatment need to be much smaller than the difference between a moderate, but worthwhile, effect and an effect that is too small to be of any material importance. This in turn implies that moderate biases and moderate random errors cannot be tolerated. The only way to guarantee very small random errors is to study really large numbers, and this can be achieved in two main ways: make individual studies large, and combine information from as many relevant studies as possible in systematic overviews (Table 1). However, it is not much use to have very small random errors if there may well be moderate biases, so even the large sizes of some non-randomized analyses of computerized hospital records cannot guarantee medically reliable comparisons between the effects of different treatments.

Avoiding moderate biases

Proper randomization avoids systematic differences between the types of patient in different treatment groups.

Table 1 Requirements for reliable assessment of moderate effects: negligible biases and small random errors

NEGLIGIBLE BIASES
(i.e. guaranteed avoidance of moderate biases)
•**Proper randomization**
(non-randomized methods might suffer moderate biases)
•**Analysis by allocated treatment**
(including all randomized patients: 'intention-to-treat' analysis)
•**Chief emphasis on overall results**
(no unduly data-dependent emphasis on particular subgroups)
•**Systematic overview of all relevant randomized trials**
(no unduly data-dependent emphasis on particular studies)
SMALL RANDOM ERRORS
(i.e. guaranteed avoidance of moderate random errors)
•**Large numbers in any new trials**
(to be really large, trials should be 'streamlined')
•**Systematic overviews of all relevant randomized trials**
(which yield the largest possible total numbers)

The fundamental reason for randomization is to avoid moderate bias, by ensuring that each type of patient can be expected to have been allocated in similar proportions to the different treatment strategies that are to be compared, so that only random differences should affect the final comparisons of outcome. Non-randomized methods, in contrast, cannot generally guarantee that the types of patient given the study treatment do not differ systematically in any important ways from the types of patient given any other treatment(s) with which the study treatment is to be compared. For example, moderate biases might arise if the study treatment was novel and doctors were afraid to use it for the most seriously ill patients, or, conversely, if they were more ready to use it for those who were desperately ill. There may also be other ways in which the severity of the condition differentially affects the likelihood of being assigned to different treatments by the doctor's choice (or by any other non-random procedure).

It might appear at first sight that by collecting enough information about various prognostic features it would be possible to make some mathematical adjustments to correct for any such differences between the types of patients who, in a non-randomized study, receive the different treatments that are to be compared. The hope is that such methods (which are sometimes called 'outcomes analyses') might achieve comparability between those entering the different treatment groups, but they cannot be guaranteed to do so. For, some important prognostic factors may be unrecorded, while others may be difficult to assess exactly and hence difficult to adjust for. There are two reasons for this difficulty. First, it is often not realized that even if there are no systematic differences between one treatment group and another in the accuracy with which prognostic factors are recorded, purely random errors in assessing prognostic factors can introduce systematic biases into the statistically adjusted comparison between treatments in a non-randomized study. Second, in a non-randomized comparison the care with which prognostic factors are recorded may differ between one treatment group and another. Doctors studying a novel treatment may investigate their patients particularly carefully, and, perhaps surprisingly, this extra accuracy can introduce a moderate bias. For example, an unusually careful search of the axilla among women with early breast cancer will sometimes result in the discovery of tiny deposits of cancer cells that would normally have been overlooked, and hence some women who would have been classified as stage I will be reclassified as stage II. The prognosis of these 'down-staged' women is worse than that of those who remain as stage I, but better than that of those already classified as stage II by less intensive investigation. Paradoxically, therefore, such down-staging improves not only the average prognosis of stage I breast cancer but also the average prognosis of stage II breast cancer, biasing any non-randomized comparison with other average women with stage I or stage II disease for whom the staging was less careful.

The machinery of a properly randomized trial: no foreknowledge of treatment allocation, no bias in patient management, unbiased outcome assessment, and no postrandomization exclusions

No foreknowledge of what the next treatment will be

In a properly randomized trial, the decision to enter a patient is made irreversibly and in ignorance of which of the trial treatments he or she will be allocated. The treatment allocation is made after trial entry has been decided upon. (The purpose of this sequence is to ensure that foreknowledge of what the next treatment is going to be cannot affect the decision to enter the patient; if it did, those allocated one treatment might differ systematically from those allocated another.) Ideally, any major prognostic features should also be irreversibly recorded before the treatment is revealed, particularly if these are to be used in any treatment analyses. For, if the recorded value of some prognostic factor might be affected by knowledge of the trial treatment allocation, then treatment comparisons within subgroups defined by that factor might be moderately biased. In particular, treatment comparisons just among 'responders' or just among 'non-responders' can be extremely misleading unless the response is assessed before treatment allocation.

No bias in patient management or in outcome assessment

An additional difficulty, in both randomized and non-randomized comparisons of various treatments, is that there might be systematic differences in the use of other treatments (including general supportive care) or in the assessment of major outcomes. A non-randomized comparison may well suffer from moderate biases due to such systematic differences in ancillary care or assessment, particularly if it merely involves the retrospective review of medical records. In the context of a randomized comparison, however, it is generally possible to devise ways to keep any such biases small. For example, placebo tablets may be given to control-allocated patients and certain subjective assessments may be 'blinded' (although this is less important in studies assessing mortality).

'Intention-to-treat' analyses with no postrandomization exclusions

Even in a properly randomized trial, unnecessary biases may be introduced by inappropriate statistical analysis. One of the most important sources of bias in the analysis is undue concentration on just one part of the evidence, that is to say on 'data-derived subgroup analyses' (see below). Another easily avoided bias is caused by the postrandomization exclusion of patients, particularly if the type (and prognosis) of those excluded from one treatment group differs from that of those excluded from another. Therefore the fundamental statistical analysis of a trial should compare all those originally allocated one treatment (even though some of them may not have actually received it) with all those allocated the other treatment (in other words it should be an 'intention-to-treat' analysis). Additional analyses can also be reported: for example, in describing the frequency of some very specific side-effect it may be preferable to record its incidence only among those who actually received the treatment. (This is because strictly randomized comparisons may not be needed to assess extreme relative risks.) However, in assessing the overall outcome, such 'on-treatment' analyses can be misleading, and 'intention-to-treat' analyses are generally a more trustworthy guide as to whether there is any real difference between the trial treatments in their effects on long-term outcome.

Problems produced by data-dependent emphasis on particular results

Treatment that is appropriate for one patient may be inappropriate for another. Ideally, therefore, what is wanted is not only an answer to the question 'Is this treatment helpful on average for a wide range of patients?', but also an answer to the question 'For which recognizable categories of patient is this treatment helpful?'. However, this ideal is difficult to attain directly because the direct use of clinical trial results in particular subgroups of patients is surprisingly unreliable. Even if the real sizes of the effects of treatment in specific subgroups are importantly different, standard subgroup analyses are so statistically insensitive that they may well fail to demonstrate these differences. Conversely, even if there is a highly significant 'interaction' (that is to say, an apparent difference between the sizes of the therapeutic effects in different subgroups) and the results seem to suggest that the treatment works in some subgroups but not in others (thereby giving the appearance of a 'qualitative interaction'), this may still not be good evidence for subgroup-specific treatment preferences.

Questions about such interactions between patient characteristics and the effects of treatment are easy to ask, but are surprisingly difficult to answer reliably. Apparent interactions can often be produced by the play of chance and, in particular subgroups, can mimic or obscure some of the moderate treatment effects that might realistically be expected. To demonstrate this, a subgroup analysis was performed based on the astrological birth signs of patients randomized in the very large Second International Study of Infarct Survival (**ISIS-2**) trial of the treatment of acute myocardial infarction. Overall in this trial, the 1-month survival advantage produced by aspirin was particularly clearly demonstrated (804 vascular deaths among 8587 patients allocated aspirin, versus 1016 among 8600 allocated as controls; 23 per cent reduction, two-sided p value <0.000001). However, when these analyses were subdivided by the patients' astrological birth signs, to illustrate the unreliability of subgroup analyses, aspirin appeared totally ineffective for those born under Libra or Gemini (Table 2). It would obviously be unwise to conclude from such a result that patients born under the sign of Libra or Gemini should not be given this particular treatment. However, similar conclusions based on 'exploratory' data-derived subgroup analyses, which, from a purely statistical viewpoint, are no more reliable than these, are often reported and believed, with inappropriate effects on practice.

There are three main remedies for this unavoidable conflict between the reliable subgroup-specific conclusions that doctors want and the unreliable findings that direct subgroup analyses can usually offer. However, the extent to which these remedies are helpful in particular instances is one on which informed judgements differ.

First, where there are good *a priori* reasons for anticipating that the effects of treatment might be different in different circumstances then a limited number of subgroup analyses may be **pre**specified in the study protocol, along with a prediction of the direction of such proposed interactions. (For example, it was expected that the benefits of fibrinolytic therapy for acute myocardial infarction would be greater the earlier patients were treated, and so some studies prespecified analyses subdivided by the time from the onset of symptoms to treatment: see later.) These prespecified subgroup-specific analyses are then to be taken much more seriously than other subgroup analyses.

The second approach is to emphasize chiefly the overall results of a trial (or, better still, of all such trials) for particular outcomes, as a guide to—or at least a context for speculation about—the qualitative results in various specific subgroups of patients, and to give less weight to the actual results in each separate subgroup. This is clearly the right way to interpret the findings in Table 2, but it is also likely in many other circumstances to provide the best assessment of whether one treatment is better than another in particular subgroups. Of course, the extrapolation needs to be performed in a sensible way. For example, if one treatment has substantial side-effects, it may be inappropriate for low-risk patients. (In this case, the side-effects in a particular subgroup and the proportional benefit in that subgroup should be estimated separately, but the estimation for both might be more reliable if based on an appropriate extrapolation from the overall results rather than on the results in that one subgroup alone.)

The third approach is to be influenced, in discussing the likely effects on mortality in specific subgroups, not only by the mortality analyses in these subgroups but also by the analyses of recurrence-free survival or some other major 'surrogate' outcome. For, if the overall results are similar but much more highly significant for recurrence-free survival than for mortality, subgroup analyses with respect to the former may be more stable and may provide a better guide as to whether there are any major differences between subgroups in the effects of treatment (particularly if such subgroup analyses were specified before results were available).

Avoiding moderate random errors

The need for large-scale randomization

To distinguish reliably between the two alternatives that there is no worthwhile difference in survival or that treatment confers a moderate, but worthwhile, benefit (for example, 10 or 20 per cent fewer deaths), not only must systematic errors be guaranteed to be small (see above) compared with such a moderate risk reduction, but so too must any of the purely random errors that are produced just by chance. Random errors can be reliably avoided only by studying large enough numbers of patients. However, it is not sufficiently widely appreciated just how large clinical trials need to be in order to detect moderate differences reliably. This can be illustrated by a hypothetical trial that is actually quite inadequate—even though by previous standards it is moderately large—in which a 20 per cent reduction in mortality (from 10 to 8 per cent) is supposed to be detected among 2000 heart attack patients (1000 treated and 1000 controls). In this case, one might predict about 100 deaths (10 per cent) in the control group and 80 deaths (8 per cent) in the treated group. However, even if this difference were observed it would not be conventionally significant ($p = 0.1$); indicating that even if there is no real difference between the effects of the trial treatments, it would still be relatively easy for a result at least as extreme as this to arise by chance alone. Although the play of chance might well increase the difference enough to make it conventionally significant (for example, 110 deaths versus 70 deaths, $2p < 0.001$), it might equally well dilute, obliterate (for example, 90 deaths versus 90 deaths), or even reverse it. The situation in real life is often even worse, as the average trial size may be only a few hundred patients rather than the several thousand that would ideally be needed.

Mega-trials: how to randomize large numbers

One of the chief techniques for obtaining appropriately large-scale randomized evidence is to make trials extremely simple, and then to invite hundreds of hospitals to collaborate. The first of these large simple trials (or mega-trials) were the ISIS and GISSI studies of heart attack treatment, and a few other mega-trials have now been undertaken. However, in terms of medically significant findings, what has been achieved so far is only a fraction of what could quite readily be achieved by the assiduous pursuit of such research strategies. Any obstacle to simplicity is an obstacle to large size, and so it is worth making enormous efforts at the design stage to simplify and streamline the process of entering, treating, and assessing patients. Many trials would be of much greater scientific value if they collected 10 times less data, both at entry and during follow-up, on 10 times more patients. It is particularly important to simplify the entry of patients, otherwise rapid recruitment may be difficult. The current fashions for unduly complicated eligibility criteria, overly detailed 'informed' consent,

Table 2 False-negative mortality effect in a subgroup defined only by the astrological birth sign: the ISIS-2 (1988) trial of aspirin among over 17 000 patients with acute myocardial infarction

Astrological birth sign	No. of 1-month deaths (aspirin versus placebo)	Statistical significance
Libra or Gemini	150 vs. 147	NS
All other signs	654 vs. 869	$2p < 0.000001$
Any birth sign*	804 vs. 1016 (9.4%) (11.8%)	$2p < 0.000001$

* Appropriate overall analysis for assessing the true effect in all subgroups.

excessive 'quality-of-life' assessments, extensive auditing of data, and measurements of the economic costs of treatment are often inappropriate.

Inappropriate inclusion of cost and of 'quality-of-life' indices

Eventually, the cost-effectiveness of various treatments needs to be assessed. However, this does not necessarily imply that costs should be assessed in the same studies in which effectiveness is to be assessed. This is particularly so if attempts to assess costs seriously damage attempts to assess the effects on mortality and major morbidity reliably. Moreover, what really matters is the cost of a treatment in routine practice, not its cost when given in the particular circumstances of a randomized trial.

Likewise, of course, any important ways in which treatments affect the quality of life need to be understood; but again this does not necessarily imply that quality-of-life indices should be assessed in the same trials that assess the main effects of treatment. For, although 20 000 patients may be required for reliable assessment of the effects of treatment on mortality and major morbidity, only a few hundred are likely to be needed for sufficiently reliable assessment of the effects of treatment on various proposed quality-of-life measures (or on costs of treatment). It may be possible to incorporate such assessments within a large mortality study as small sub-studies. But, this may be difficult in practice, and there are many instances where what should be a large simple trial of clinical efficacy should not be jeopardized by the measurement of such factors. Moreover, the effects of a treatment on quality of life in a trial, when both the doctors and the patients are uncertain about any clinical benefits of the treatment, may differ substantially from its effects on quality of life after the treatment has been shown to improve survival. Hence, it may be better to assess these other outcome measures only after having determined whether the treatment has any worthwhile effects on mortality and major morbidity, and if (as is often the case) it does not then any costs and adverse effects on quality of life may be largely irrelevant.

Simplification of entry procedures for trials: the 'uncertainty principle'

For ethical reasons, patients cannot have their treatment chosen at random if either they or their doctor are already reasonably certain what treatment is preferred. Hence, randomization can be offered only if both doctor and patient feel substantially uncertain as to which of the trial treatments is best. The question then arises: 'Which categories of patients about whose treatment there is such uncertainty should be offered randomization?' The obvious answer is all of them, welcoming the heterogeneity that this will produce. (For example, either the treatment of choice will turn out to be the same for men and women, in which case the trial might as well include both, or it will be different, in which case it is particularly important to study both sexes.) In large trials, patient homogeneity is generally a defect, while heterogeneity is generally a strength. Consider, for example, the trials of fibrinolytic therapy for acute myocardial infarction. Some had restrictive entry criteria that allowed inclusion of only those patients who presented between 0 and 6 h after the onset of pain, and so those trials contributed almost nothing to the key question of how late such treatment can still be useful. In contrast, trials with wider and more heterogeneous entry criteria that included some patients with longer delays between pain onset and randomization assessed this question prospectively, and were able to show that fibrinolytic therapy can have definite protective effects when given not only 0 to 6 but also 7 to 12 h after the onset of pain (see later).

This approach of randomizing a wide range of patients in whom there is substantial uncertainty as to which treatment option is best, was used in the Medical Research Council's European Carotid Surgery Trial (**ECST**). This trial compared a policy of immediate carotid endarterectomy with a policy of 'watchful waiting' in patients with partial carotid artery stenosis and a recent minor stroke in that part of the brain supplied by the carotid artery. If a patient was prepared at least to consider surgery, then the neurologist and surgeon responsible for that individual's care considered in their own way whatever medical, personal, or other factors seemed to them to be

relevant (Fig. 1), including, of course, the patient's own preferences and values.

1. If they were then reasonably certain, for any reason, that they **did wish** to recommend immediate surgery for that particular patient, the patient was ineligible for entry into the ECST.

2. Conversely, if they were reasonably certain, for any reason, that they **did not wish** to recommend immediate surgery, the patient was likewise ineligible.

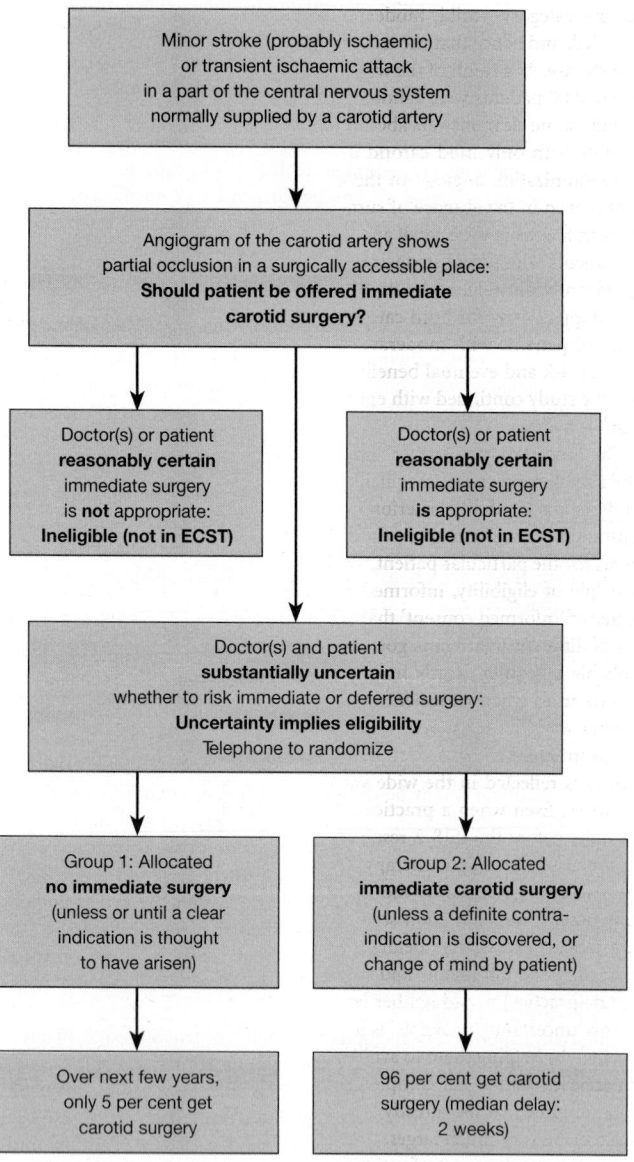

Fig. 1 Example of the 'uncertainty principle' for trial entry: the chief eligibility criterion for the European Carotid Surgery Trial (ECST) was that the doctors and patients should be substantially uncertain whether to risk immediate or deferred surgery. (Partly because this criterion was appropriately flexible, ECST became the largest ever trial of vascular surgery.)

3. If, but only if, they were **substantially uncertain** what to recommend, the patient was automatically eligible for randomization between immediate versus no immediate surgery (with all patients receiving whatever their doctors judged to be the best available medical care, which generally included advice to stop smoking, treatment of hypertension, and the use of aspirin as an antithrombotic drug).

There were substantial differences between individual doctors in the types of patients about whom they were uncertain (in terms of the severity of carotid stenosis, as well as various other characteristics). This guaranteed that no category—mild, moderate, or severe stenosis—would be wholly excluded, and hence that the trial would yield at least some direct evidence in each case. As a result of the wide and simple entry criteria adopted by the ECST, 3000 patients were randomized, and therefore the study was able to provide some clear answers about who needed carotid endarterectomy. For patients with only mild carotid artery stenosis (0–29 per cent) on their prerandomization angiogram there was little risk of ipsilateral ischaemic stroke, even in the absence of surgery, so that any benefits of surgery over the next few years were small and outweighed by its early risks. Conversely, for patients with severe stenosis (70–99 per cent), the risks of surgery were significantly outweighed by its later benefits over the next few years. The trial stopped early for both categories. However, for the intermediate category of patients with moderate stenosis (30–69 per cent) the balance of surgical risk and eventual benefit remained uncertain, and so recruitment into the study continued with entry still governed by the 'uncertainty principle' as before.

The 'uncertainty principle' simultaneously meets the requirements of ethicality, heterogeneity, simplicity, and maximal trial size. It states that the fundamental eligibility criterion is that both patient and doctor should be substantially uncertain about the appropriateness of each of the trial treatments for the particular patient. With such uncertainty as the fundamental principle of eligibility, informed consent can also be simplified. For, the degree of 'informed consent' that is appropriate in a randomized comparison of different treatments governed by the 'uncertainty principle' should probably not differ greatly from that which is applied in routine practice outside trials when treatment is being chosen haphazardly—or, to put it another way, 'double standards' between trial and non-trial situations are inappropriate. The haphazard nature of many non-randomized treatment choices is reflected in the wide variations in practice between and within countries. Even when a practice is similar it may be similarly wrong: for example, before the ISIS-2 results became available (see later), almost no doctors used fibrinolytic therapy for acute myocardial infarction. Provided that trials are governed by the 'uncertainty principle', there is an approximate parallel between good science and good ethics. Indeed, in such circumstances excessively detailed consent procedures (which can be distressing and inhumane, and so would not be considered appropriate in routine practice) would neither be scientifically nor ethically appropriate.

This 'uncertainty principle' is just one of many ways of simplifying trials and thereby helping them to avoid becoming enmeshed in a mass of wholly unnecessary traditional complexity. If randomized trials can be substantially simplified, as has already been achieved for a few major diseases, and hence made very much larger, then they will play an appropriately central role in the development of rational criteria for the planning of healthcare throughout the world.

Minimizing both bias and random error: systematic overviews (meta-analyses) of randomized trials

Cochrane was one of the first people to emphasize the need to bring together, by specialty, the results from all relevant randomized trials, and the Cochrane Collaboration is now attempting to do this systematically. When several trials have all addressed much the same therapeutic question, the traditional procedure of choosing only a few of them as the basis for practice may be a source of serious bias, since chance fluctuations for or against treatment may affect which trials are chosen. To avoid this, it is

appropriate to base inference chiefly on a systematic overview (or meta-analysis) of all the results from all the trials that have addressed a particular type of question (or on an unbiased subset of such trials), and not on some potentially biased subset of the trials. Such overviews will also minimize random errors in the assessment of treatment since, in general, far more patients are involved in an overview than in any contributory individual trial.

The separate trials may well be heterogeneous in their entry criteria, their treatment schedules, their follow-up procedures, their methods of treating relapse, etc. In view of this heterogeneity, at one extreme each trial might be considered in virtual isolation from all others, while at the opposite extreme all might be considered together. Both these extreme views have some merit, and the pursuit of each by different people may prove more illuminating than too definite an insistence on any one particular approach. However, the heterogeneity of the different trials merely argues for careful interpretation of any overviews of different trial results, rather than arguing against any such overviews. For, whatever the difficulties in interpreting overviews may be, without them moderate biases and random errors, which may obscure any moderate treatment effects (or, conversely, may imply effects where none exists), cannot reliably be avoided.

Which overviews are trustworthy?

Since the 1970s, a large (and rapidly increasing) number of meta-analyses of the results of randomized trials have been reported, not all of which are trustworthy. The two fundamental questions are how carefully the overview has been performed and how large it is. The simplest approach is merely to have collected and tabulated the published data from whatever randomized trial reports are easily accessible in the literature, and sometimes this may suffice. At the opposite extreme, extensive efforts may have been made by those organizing the overview to locate every potentially relevant randomized trial, to collaborate closely with the trialists to seek individual data on each patient ever randomized into those trials, and then (after extensive checks and corrections of such data) to produce, in collaboration with those trialists, agreed analyses and publications. The results of some of the largest such collaborations will be described later: the Antiplatelet Trialists' (**APT**) Collaborative Group, the Fibrinolytic Therapy Trialists' (**FTT**) Collaborative Group, and the Early Breast Cancer Trialists' Collaborative Group (**EBCTCG**). Collaboration of the original trialists in the overview process, with collection of individual patient data, can help to avoid or minimize the biases that could be produced by missing trials (for example, owing to the greater likelihood of extremely good, or extremely bad, results being particularly widely known and published), by inappropriate postrandomization withdrawals, or by the failure to allocate treatment properly at random. If randomization was performed properly in the first place, then postrandomization withdrawals can often be followed up and restored to the study for an appropriate 'intention-to-treat' analysis. Knowledge of the exact methods of treatment allocation (backed up by checks on whether the main prognostic factors recorded are non-randomly distributed between the treatment groups in a particular trial) may help to identify trials that were not properly randomized and hence should be excluded from an overview of randomized trials. Overviews based on individual patient data may also provide more information about treatment effects than the more usual overviews of grouped data, for they allow more detailed analyses—indeed, if they are really large then they may actually yield statistically reliable subgroup analyses of the effects of treatment in particular types of patient.

Conversely, even a perfectly conducted overview may not be large enough to be reliable. An overview that brings together complete data from every trial of a certain treatment but which still (because the trials were all small) includes a total of only 100 deaths will have random errors that are no smaller than those for a single trial with 100 deaths among such patients. Small-scale evidence, whether from an overview or from one trial, is often unreliable and will often be found in retrospect to have yielded wrong answers. What is needed is large-scale randomized evidence; it does not matter much whether that evidence comes from a properly conducted overview or a properly conducted trial. The practical medical value of such evidence will now be illustrated by a few recent examples.

Some examples of important results in the treatment of vascular and neoplastic disease that could have been reliably established only by large-scale randomized evidence

Definite result from a single very large trial: benefit from medium-dose aspirin for patients with suspected acute myocardial infarction (and benefits among other groups of patients indicated by overviews of trials)

In the ISIS-2 trial, half of 17 000 patients with suspected acute myocardial infarction were allocated aspirin tablets (162 mg/day for 1 month, which virtually completely inhibits cyclo-oxygenase-dependent platelet activation) and half were allocated placebo tablets. Before 1988, when the ISIS-2 results were published, aspirin was not routinely used in the treatment of acute myocardial infarction, and no other major trial had (or has subsequently) assessed the use of aspirin in cases of suspected acute myocardial infarction. However, the effects of 1 month of aspirin were so definite in ISIS-2 (804/8587 vascular deaths among those who were allocated aspirin versus 1016/8600 among those who were not) that even the lower 99 per cent confidence limit would have represented a worthwhile benefit from such a simple and inexpensive treatment (Fig. 2).

As a result, worldwide treatment patterns changed sharply when the ISIS-2 results emerged, and aspirin is now routinely used in many different countries for the majority of emergency hospital admissions with suspected acute myocardial infarction. In the United Kingdom, for example, two British Heart Foundation surveys found cardiologists reporting that routine aspirin use in acute coronary care had increased from under 10 per cent in 1987 to over 90 per cent in 1989. Worldwide, the annual number of patients with suspected myocardial infarction who would nowadays be given such treatment must be well over a million a year, suggesting that in this clinical context alone aspirin is already preventing tens of thousands of premature deaths each year. However, if the ISIS-2 trial had been a factor of 10 smaller (that is, 1700 instead of 17 000 patients), then exactly the same proportional reduction in mortality as shown in Fig. 2 would not have been conventionally significant and therefore would have been much less likely to influence medical practice—indeed, the result might by chance have appeared exactly flat, greatly damaging future research on aspirin in this

context. Likewise, if the ISIS-2 trial had been non-randomized, then it might well have produced the wrong answer (since in a non-randomized study doctors might tend to give active treatment to patients who are particularly ill, or who are rather different in various other ways from those not given active treatment). In addition, even if a non-randomized study did happen to produce an unbiasedly correct answer, it would be impossible to be sure that it had actually done so, and hence again a non-randomized study might have had much less influence on medical practice than did ISIS-2.

In the ISIS-2 trial aspirin significantly reduced the 1-month mortality figure, but it also significantly reduced the number of non-fatal strokes and non-fatal reinfarctions that were recorded in hospital. Combining all these three outcomes into 'vascular events' (stroke, death, or reinfarction), 13 per cent of those who were allocated aspirin versus 17 per cent of the controls were known to have suffered a vascular event in the month after randomization (Table 3)—an absolute difference of 40 events per 1000 treated (or, perhaps more relevantly, of 40 000 per million). The randomized trials of aspirin, or of other antiplatelet regimens, in other types of high-risk patients (for example, a few years of aspirin for those who have survived a myocardial infarction or stroke) have not been as large as ISIS-2, and so, taken separately, most have yielded false-negative results. However, when the results from many such trials are combined, statistically definite reductions in 'vascular events' are seen (Table 3). Since such treatments do not appear to increase non-vascular mortality, all-cause mortality is also significantly reduced.

In principle, these findings could, if appropriately widely exploited, prevent about 100 000 premature vascular deaths a year in developed countries alone, and there are probably at least as many vascular deaths in less-developed as in developed countries. Hence, with realistically achievable levels of the use of 'medium dose' aspirin (75–325 mg/day) for the secondary prevention of vascular disease, it might well be possible in practice to ensure that aspirin is used in enough high-risk patients to prevent, or substantially delay, at least 100 000 vascular deaths per year worldwide, and such use of aspirin would, in addition, prevent a comparable number of non-fatal strokes or heart attacks. (Medium-dose aspirin was the least expensive and most widely tested antiplatelet regimen: it is of proven efficacy, and on review of all the antiplatelet trials no other antiplatelet regimen has been shown to be of greater efficacy in preventing vascular events; see notes to Table 3.) This large-scale randomized evidence regarding medium-dose aspirin is now changing worldwide clinical practice in ways that will, at low cost, prevent much death and disability in high-risk patients. However, small trials, small overviews, or non-randomized studies (however large) could not possibly have provided appropriately reliable evidence about such moderate risk reductions.

Definite result from a very large overview of trials: benefit from 'adjuvant' therapy with tamoxifen for patients with 'early' breast cancer (and possible benefit suggested with ovarian ablation in younger women)

By definition, in 'early' breast cancer all detectable deposits of disease are limited to the breast and the locoregional lymph nodes, and can be removed surgically. However, experience shows that undetectably small deposits may remain elsewhere that eventually cause clinical recurrence at a distant site, perhaps after a delay of several years, which is then usually followed by death from the disease. These micrometastatic deposits may have been stimulated by the body's own hormones during the years before recurrence became detectable. Therefore, among women who have had the detectable deposits of breast cancer removed by surgery (or by surgery and radiotherapy), there have been many trials of 'adjuvant' treatments that either reduce the production of endogenous oestrogens (for example, various forms of ovarian ablation) or block the access of those oestrogens to the tumour cells (for example, tamoxifen, which blocks the oestrogen receptor protein in some breast cancer cells).

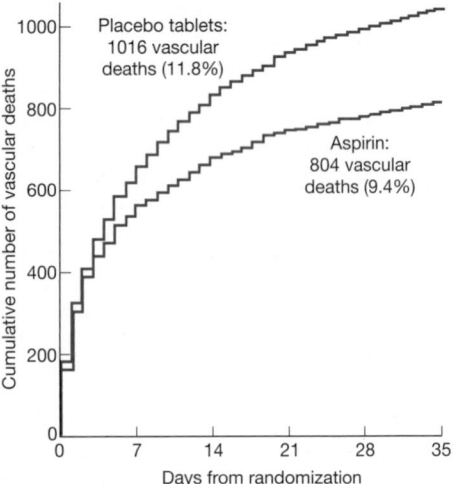

Fig. 2 Effect of administration of aspirin for 1 month on 35-day mortality in the 1988 ISIS-2 trial among over 17 000 patients with acute myocardial infarction. (Absolute survival advantage: 24 SD5 lives saved per 1000 patients allocated aspirin, 2p <0.00001.)

Taken separately, most of these adjuvant trials have been too small to provide reliable evidence about long-term survival. However, if the results of all of them are combined, some very definite differences in 10-year survival rates emerge (Fig. 3). Among women with stage II disease who are less than 50-years old (and therefore generally pre- or perimenopausal), ovarian ablation appears to produce about a 10 per cent absolute difference in the 10-year survival figure (for example, 50 per cent versus 40 per cent). This finding is based on the analysis of only a few hundred deaths so it is still not as reliable as might ideally be wished and, because substantial uncertainty remains, much larger trials are now in progress. Among older women with stage II disease, ovarian ablation is unlikely to be of much relevance (since most of the endogenous oestrogen at older ages comes from sources other than the ovaries), but, in aggregate, the randomized trials among such women have shown very definitely that a few years of tamoxifen therapy also produces about a 10 per cent absolute difference in the 10-year survival rate. A smaller, but still highly significant, reduction in mortality by tamoxifen is also seen among the 10 000 randomized women with stage I disease. Taken separately, however, 37 of the 42 tamoxifen trials were too small to have yielded statistically reliable evidence on their own ($2p > 0.01$), and the five other trials were significant only because, by chance, they had results that were too good to be true.

These tamoxifen overview results have already changed clinical practice substantially, and have redirected research towards large randomized trials of the effects of different durations of tamoxifen treatment: should tamoxifen in asymptomatic women be continued for 2 years, for 5 years, or indefinitely? Large randomized studies of tamoxifen in the primary prevention of breast cancer among high-risk women are only just beginning. However, they have been encouraged by the results from the tamoxifen trials' overview in 30 000 patients with established cancer (stage II or stage I) in one breast, among whom there has been a highly significant reduction of one-third in the likelihood of developing contralateral breast cancer (but a small absolute increase in endometrial cancer). Again, this degree of trustworthy detail would not have been attainable without large-scale randomized evidence.

Promising overview of small trials confirmed by a large trial: benefit from fibrinolytic therapy as emergency treatment for a wide range of patients with acute myocardial infarction

Fibrinolytic drugs that dissolve a thrombus which may be blocking a coronary artery, thereby causing an acute myocardial infarction, were introduced into clinical research in the late 1950s. However, the trials of fibrinolytic drugs in the 1960s and 1970s were too small to be statistically reliable (none involved even 1000 patients). So, by the early 1980s the haemorrhagic side-effects were obvious, the benefits had not been convincingly demonstrated, and these agents were generally considered to be dangerous, ineffective, and hence inappropriate for routine coronary care. Although overviews published in the mid-1980s of the previous small trials (involving a total of only about 6000 patients in 24 trials) indicated a statistically definite benefit, they were not really believed by cardiologists and so such treatments were still not widely used. The situation has been saved by

Table 3 Summary of the overall results of trials of aspirin (or other antiplatelet drugs)* for the prevention of vascular events: the Antiplatelet Trialists' Collaboration (1994), involving a total of about 100 000 randomized patients in over 100 trials

Type of patient	Average scheduled treatment duration (approximate no. of patients randomized)	Proportion who suffered a non-fatal stroke, non-fatal heart attack, or vascular death during the trials		
		Anti-platelet	Control	Events avoided in these trials
High risk:				
Suspected acute heart attack	1 month (20 000)	10%	14%	40 per 1000 ($2p < 0.00001$)
Previous history of heart attack	2 years (20 000)	13%	17%	40 per 1000 ($2p < 0.00001$)
Previous history of stroke or TIA	3 years (10 000)	18%	22%	40 per 1000 ($2p < 0.00001$)
Other vascular disease**	1 year (20 000)	7%	9%	20 per 1000 ($2p < 0.00001$)
Low risk:				
Primary prevention in low-risk people	5 years (30 000)	4.4%	4.8%	4 per 1000 ($2p > 0.05$)

* The most widely tested regimen was medium-dose aspirin, involving an average daily dose of 75–325 mg, and no other antiplatelet regimen appeared to be significantly more or less effective than this in preventing such vascular events. (For comparison, in the United Kingdom or United States, a low-dose aspirin tablet contains about 75–80 mg of aspirin, while a normal-dose tablet contains 300–325 mg.) Pharmacological evidence suggests that, after the first few days, all daily doses of aspirin in the range 75 to 325 mg are likely to be approximately equivalent in their effects on platelets and on the vascular endothelium. Hence, to limit any gastric discomfort with long-term use, a daily dose at the lower end of this range, such as 75, 80, or 100 mg (depending on what is conveniently available), might be slightly preferable. However, in acute emergencies such as suspected myocardial infarction or unstable angina, at least the initial dose should perhaps be at the upper end of the range, such as 250, 300, or 325 mg, so as to achieve a virtually complete antiplatelet effect within less than 1 h (which could then be maintained by a lower daily dose).

** For example, angina, peripheral vascular disease, arterial surgery, or angioplasty, etc.

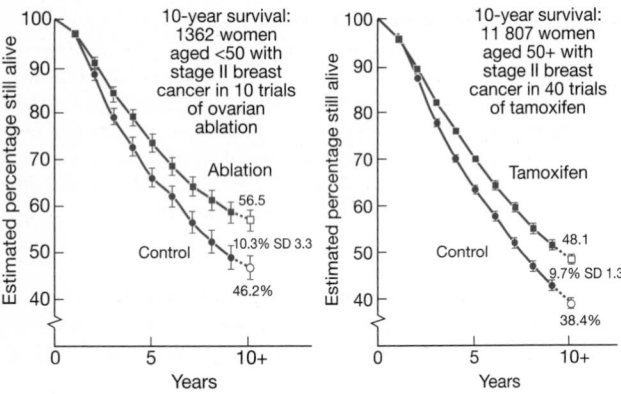

Fig. 3 Effects of hormonal adjuvant treatments for early breast cancer on the 10-year survival rate in a worldwide overview of randomized trials. (Early Breast Cancer Trialists' Collaborative Group, 1992.)

two large randomized trials, ISIS-2 and GISSI-1, both of which involved more than 10 000 patients (and by their aggregation with the seven other randomized trials that involved more than 1000 patients; see below). In ISIS-2, not only were patients randomly allocated to receive aspirin or placebo tablets as described earlier (Fig. 2), but they were also separately allocated to receive intravenous streptokinase (1.5 million units infused over about 60 min) or a placebo infusion. In this 'factorial' design (which allows the separate assessment of more than one treatment without any material loss in the statistical reliability of each comparison), one-quarter of the patients were allocated aspirin alone, one-quarter were allocated streptokinase alone, one-quarter were allocated both streptokinase and aspirin, and one-quarter were allocated neither (that is, they were given placebo tablets and placebo infusion). Streptokinase, like aspirin, produced a highly significant reduction in mortality, and the combination of streptokinase and aspirin was highly significantly better than either aspirin or streptokinase alone (Fig. 4).

The results shown in Fig. 4 might suggest that there was no need to collect any more randomized evidence about fibrinolytic therapy, but this

ignores the potential hazards of such treatment and the heterogeneity of patients. Taken separately, even ISIS-2, the largest of these trials, was not large enough for statistically reliable subgroup analyses, but when the nine largest trials were all taken together they included a total of about 60 000 patients, half of whom were randomly allocated fibrinolytic therapy. Those entering a coronary care unit with a diagnosis of suspected or definite acute myocardial infarction range from patients who are already in cardiogenic shock with low blood pressure and a fast pulse (half of whom will die rapidly) to those who have merely had a history of chest pain and no very definite changes on their ECG (of whom 'only' a small percentage will die before discharge). Fibrinolytic therapy often causes a frightening blood pressure drop: should it be used in patients who are already dangerously hypotensive? It occasionally causes serious strokes: should it be used in patients who are elderly or hypertensive, and therefore already have an above-average risk of stroke (or who have only slight changes on their ECG, and therefore have only a low risk of cardiac death)? Finally, if the coronary artery has been occluded for long enough, the heart muscle that it supplies will have been irreversibly destroyed: how long after the heart attack starts is fibrinolytic treatment still worth risking—3 h? 6 h? 12 h? 24 h?

These questions needed to be answered reliably before appropriate and generally accepted indications for and against such an immediately hazardous, but potentially effective, therapy could be devised. To address them, all fibrinolytic therapy trialists collaborated in a systematic overview of the randomized evidence. On review of the 60 000 patients randomized between fibrinolytic therapy and control in trials of more than 1000 patients, some of the therapeutic questions were relatively easy to answer satisfactorily. For example, it appears that most of those whose ECG is still normal (or shows a pattern that indicates only a low risk of death) can be left untreated, leaving open the option of starting fibrinolytic treatment urgently if their ECG changes suddenly for the worse in the following few hours. Conversely, among those who already had 'high risk' ECG changes when they were randomized, the absolute benefit of immediate fibrinolytic therapy was, if anything, slightly greater than is indicated by Fig. 4. Age, sex, blood pressure, heart rate, diabetes, and a previous history of myocardial infarction could not identify reliably any group that would not, on average, have their chances of survival appreciably increased by treatment.

The longer that fibrinolytic treatment for such patients was delayed, the less benefit it seemed to produce. Among those whose ECG showed a definite ST-segment elevation or bundle-branch block, the benefit was greatest (about 30 lives saved per 1000) among those randomized between 0 and 6 h after the onset of pain (Fig. 5). However, the mortality reduction was still

Fig. 4 Effects of a 1-hour streptokinase infusion (and of aspirin for 1 month) on 35-day mortality in ISIS-2 (1988) among 17 187 patients with acute myocardial infarction who would not normally have received streptokinase or aspirin, divided at random into four similar groups to receive aspirin only, streptokinase only, both, or neither. (Any doctor who believed that a particular patient should be given either treatment gave it, but did not include that patient in ISIS-2.)

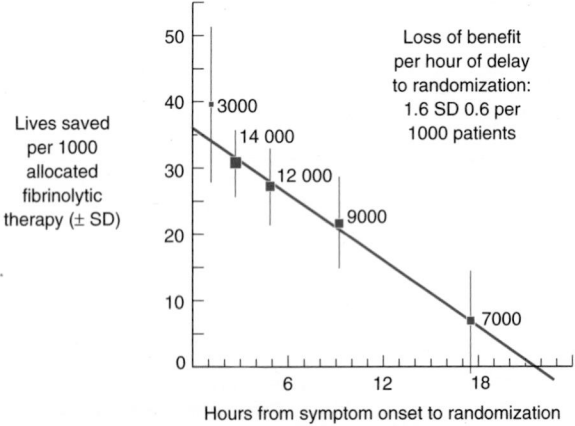

Fig. 5 Benefit versus delay (0–1, 2–3, 4–6, 7–12, or 13–24 h) in the nine largest randomized trials of fibrinolytic therapy versus control in patients with acute myocardial infarction. One-month mortality results for 45 000 patients with ST elevation or bundle-branch block when randomized, showing the definite net benefit even for the 9000 randomized 7–12 h after the onset of pain. (Fibrinolytic Therapy Trialists' Collaboration, 1994.)

Table 4 Magnesium in acute myocardial infarction: contrast between the results of the smaller and the larger randomized trials

	No. of patients randomized	1-month mortality (%)			
		Allocated magnesium		Allocated control	
9 small trials	1500	42/754	(5.6)	86/740	(11.6)
LIMIT-2 trial	2300	90/1159	(7.8)	118/1157	(10.2)
ISIS-4 trial	58000	2216/29011	(7.6)	2103/29039	(7.2)
All trials	62000	2348/30924	(7.59)	2307/30936	(7.46)

There is highly significant heterogeneity (p <0.001) between the group of small trials whose 'hypothesis-generating' results led to the testing of magnesium in ISIS-4 and the pair of larger trials (ISIS-4 and LIMIT-2) whose results tested that hypothesis.

substantial and significant (about 20 per 1000, $2p$ <0.003) when such patients were randomized 7 to 12 h after the onset of pain. Indeed, if they were randomized between 13 and 18 h after the onset of pain there still appeared to be some net reduction in mortality (about 10 per 1000, but not statistically definite). The regression line in Fig. 5 reinforces these separate subgroup analyses in a more reliable way. Yet, before these large trials it was forcefully, but mistakenly, argued that such treatments could not possibly be of any worthwhile benefit if given more than a few hours after the onset of symptoms.

Such detailed inferences are difficult enough with large-scale properly randomized evidence, and would be impossible without it; because of their unknowable biases (see above), non-randomized database analyses are simply not a viable alternative to large-scale randomized evidence. Nor would randomization of 'only' several thousand patients have been sufficient. Indeed, in several important respects what is still needed is more, rather than less, randomized evidence about the effects of fibrinolytic therapy in various particular types of patient. First, it is still unclear whether patients who have definite ECG changes such as ST elevation or bundle-branch block, but who present between 12 and 18 h, or even 18 to 24 h, after the onset of pain should be treated; more randomized evidence is still needed (Fig. 5). Second, for one particular poor-prognosis ECG category (ST depression) the 1-month mortality rates still appear unpromising even when all currently available trials are combined (15 per cent dead among those allocated fibrinolytic therapy versus 14 per cent dead among controls, but based on only 4000 patients). Analogy with the results in other high-risk categories suggests that this result for patients with ST depression may well be a false-negative. Perhaps it has arisen from an unduly data-dependent emphasis on what may, in retrospect, prove to have been a random irregularity in the results in this particular subgroup of only a few thousand individuals. Again, more randomized evidence is needed. Nevertheless, substantial progress has been made in the past decade of mega-trials of fibrinolytic agents. Worldwide, in the mid-1990s, about half a million patients per year were given fibrinolytic therapy, avoiding about 10 000 early deaths each year.

Small trials refuted by a mega-trial: lack of significant benefit from magnesium infusion in suspected acute myocardial infarction

It had been suggested that an infusion of a magnesium salt might reduce early mortality in patients with suspected acute myocardial infarction. Several small trials, involving between them a total of only about 1500 patients, had addressed this question, and their aggregated results indicated a statistically significant, but implausibly large, benefit (42/754 deaths among those allocated magnesium versus 86/740 among the controls, $2p$ <0.001). Some argued that such results constituted proof beyond reasonable doubt that magnesium was of sufficient value to justify its widespread usage without seeking further randomized evidence, but others remained sceptical, arguing that the apparent results were far too good to be true.

Therefore two trials, one (LIMIT-2) involving 2000 patients and one (ISIS-4) involving 58 000 patients, were set up to test the possible effects of magnesium more reliably. The former yielded a moderately promising result (Table 4), indicating avoidance of about one-quarter of the early deaths. However, because of its small size this result was statistically compatible with a true benefit that ranged from no effect to about a halving of early mortality. The much larger ISIS-4 trial yielded a completely unpromising result, and so the overall evidence, based on about 60 000 randomized patients, is now non-significantly adverse.

In view of the striking disparity between the apparent effects of magnesium before and after ISIS-4 had provided large-scale randomized evidence, it is of interest to recall some of the expert views that were expressed while ISIS-4 was in progress. Some felt so strongly that magnesium was already of proven benefit (and hence that further randomization was unethical) that the data-monitoring committee of ISIS-4 was lobbied to try to have the study stopped early and all future patients given magnesium. In contrast, the ISIS-4 steering committee was sufficiently sceptical to want large-scale randomized evidence. They believed that the available evidence was consistent with a negligible benefit, or even a small net hazard, although they all thought it more likely that at least some net benefit would be seen. Even after the LIMIT-2 result was available they continued to hold these opinions, and thought that if there was any real benefit then this was likely to be less than LIMIT-2 had suggested (and hence very much less than the other small trials had suggested).

Those who had trusted the implausibly extreme results from the previous small trials may well have been disappointed by the results of the ISIS-4 mega-trial, which now provide strong evidence that the routine use of magnesium has little or no effect on mortality in acute myocardial infarction. However, in a world where moderate benefits are much more plausible than large benefits, striking results in small-scale trials, in small-scale overviews, or in small subgroups will frequently prove evanescent. The medical assumption that both a moderate mortality difference and a zero mortality difference may be plausible, but that an extreme mortality difference is much less so, has surprisingly strong consequences for the interpretation of randomized evidence. In particular, it implies that even quite highly significant (for example, $2p = 0.001$) mortality differences that are based on only relatively small numbers of deaths may provide untrustworthy evidence of the existence of any real difference.

Trials in their epidemiological context: effects of lower, and of lowering, blood pressure on the risk of stroke and coronary heart disease

Quantitative epidemiological evidence about the effects of long-term differences in risk factors (such as blood pressure or blood cholesterol level) can help in interpreting the results from trials of the effects of reducing these risk factors for only a few years. This may help not only in interpreting previous trials but also in planning the size and duration of any future risk-factor modification trials. For, epidemiological evidence provides approximate upper limits to the risk reductions that could plausibly be expected in the trials, and may also help to identify populations that are particularly likely to benefit from risk-factor modification.

For example, appropriate analyses of prospective, observational epidemiological studies of diastolic blood pressure and disease indicate that, throughout the range of usual diastolic blood pressure in the populations

Fig. 6 Relative risks of stroke and coronary heart disease for five categories of diastolic blood pressure from the combined results of prospective observational studies. Solid squares represent the relative risks of disease in each category relative to the risk in the whole study population, and 95 per cent confidence intervals are denoted by vertical lines (MacMahon, 1994).

studied (that is, about 70–110 mmHg), a lower value was associated with a lower risk of suffering a first stroke or episode of coronary heart disease (that is, there seemed to be neither a 'threshold' value nor a 'J-shape' relationship, Fig. 6). The steepness of this continuous relationship suggests that the eventual risk reductions produced by practicable blood pressure lowering measures (for example, with antihypertensive treatment) may well be worthwhile. Not only may this be the case for certain 'hypertensive' individuals, but also for certain individuals who, although considered 'normotensive', are at high risk for some other reason (for example, as a result of a previous stroke or myocardial infarction).

After making due allowance for the substantial and systematic extent to which the true relationship is diluted by purely random fluctuations in the baseline measurements of blood pressure (that is, the 'regression dilution' bias), the prospective studies suggest that a **prolonged** difference of only 5 mmHg in usual diastolic blood pressure is associated with avoidance of at least one-third of the risk of stroke and at least one-fifth of the risk of coronary heart disease in late middle age. However, although non-randomized, prospective observational studies may be more relevant to the eventual effects of prolonged differences in blood pressure, despite the possibility of confounding by other factors, randomized trials of blood pressure reductions that last for only a few years may be more relevant to assessing the speed with which the epidemiologically expected reductions in stroke or coronary heart disease risk are produced by reducing blood pressure. By comparing the results of a systematic overview of all randomized trials of antihypertensive therapy with the observational epidemiological evidence, it may be possible to estimate the extent to which the eventual effects of a lower blood pressure on disease incidence rates can be achieved within just a few years of treatment in middle or old age. (Ideally, these age ranges should be considered separately, as the fractional avoidance of risk may well be substantially different in middle and in old age.)

Over the past few decades, numerous trials of the treatment of hypertension have been conducted to determine whether blood pressure reduction in middle age reduces the risk of stroke and coronary heart disease. However, although it was fairly rapidly accepted that the treatment of severe hypertension could at least prevent stroke, until recently there has been controversy as to whether the treatment of even severe hypotension could also prevent coronary heart disease. Moreover, questions have also persisted about the effects of the treatment of mild to moderate hypertension on stroke. This continuing uncertainty about the benefits of lowering blood pressure may chiefly have reflected the inability of individual trials (even those with several hundred coronary heart disease events) to detect moderate coronary heart disease reductions reliably, rather than from any important heterogeneity of the real effects of treatment. The mean difference in diastolic blood pressure between treatment and control

groups in the trials was only about 5 to 6 mmHg, and the epidemiological evidence suggests that a long-term difference of this magnitude is associated with only about 20 to 25 per cent less coronary heart disease (and about 35–40 per cent less stroke). Even if such trial treatments would eventually produce between 20 and 25 per cent less coronary heart disease after many years, the effects seen within the 2 or 3 years that are available on average between randomization and death in a 5-year trial might well be somewhat smaller (for example, 15 per cent). Considered separately, however, none of the trials recorded enough coronary heart disease events (or enough vascular deaths) for a statistically reliable assessment of 15 per cent risk reductions.

For stroke, the overview of randomized trials provides direct and highly significant evidence that most, or all, of the stroke avoidance associated with a prolonged difference in usual diastolic blood pressure appears soon after the blood pressure is lowered (Fig. 7). In contrast, the significant reduction in coronary heart disease seen in the trials (16 per cent, SD 4; 95 per cent confidence interval of 8–23 per cent; 2p = 0.0001) falls somewhat short of the difference of about 20 to 25 per cent suggested by the observational epidemiological evidence for a prolonged 5- to 6-mmHg difference in usual diastolic blood pressure. However, this coronary heart disease reduction is substantial and real (2p = 0.0001). Therefore it is

Fig. 7 Reduction in the odds of stroke and coronary heart disease in all unconfounded randomized trials of antihypertensive drug treatment (mean diastolic blood pressure differences of 5–6 mmHg for 5 years). Solid squares represent the odds ratios (treatment:control) for the four larger trials and the properly stratified odds ratio for the combination of the 13 smaller trials. 95 per cent confidence intervals are denoted by horizontal lines (for individual large trials or the combined small trials) and by diamonds (for overviews of all trials) (Collins and Peto, 1994).

reasonable to hope that trials of antihypertensive regimens that can reduce blood pressure to a greater extent than the 5 to 6-mmHg diastolic blood pressure reduction seen in these trials will demonstrate even greater reductions in stroke and coronary heart disease.

The proportional reduction in vascular disease risk observed in the trials appeared to be similar in high- and low-risk individuals, so that the absolute size of the reduction that is produced by treatment may be largely dependent upon the absolute risk. Therefore, for high-risk individuals, the absolute risk reduction produced by antihypertensive treatment might be substantial even among those who are only moderately 'hypertensive'. Indeed, in view of the epidemiological evidence that, for stroke and coronary heart disease risk, there is no 'threshold' level of diastolic blood pressure within the normal range, large randomized trials might even show that blood pressure reduction is of substantial value among many 'normotensive' individuals at high risk of stroke (such as those with a history of cerebral vascular disease) or of coronary heart disease (such as patients with a history of myocardial infarction, angina, peripheral vascular disease, diabetes, or chronic renal failure).

Results from large anonymous trials are relevant to real clinical practice

A clinician is used to dealing with individual patients, and may feel that the results of large trials somehow deny their individuality. This is almost the opposite of the truth, for one of the main reasons why trials have to be large is just because patients are so different from one another. Two apparently similar patients may run entirely different clinical courses, one remaining stable and the other progressing rapidly to severe disability or early death. Consequently, it is only when really large groups of patients are compared that the proportion of patients with a truly good and bad prognosis in each can be relied on to be reasonably similar. One commonly hears statements such as: 'If a treatment effect isn't obvious in a couple of hundred patients then it isn't worth knowing about'. As the previous examples demonstrate, such statements may reveal not clinical wisdom but statistical naïvety.

It is also said that what is really wanted is not a blanket recommendation for everybody, but rather some means of identifying those few individuals who really stand to benefit from therapy. If any criteria (for example, a short-term response to a non-placebo-controlled course of some disease-modifying agent) can be proposed that are likely to discriminate between people who will and will not benefit, then these can be recorded prospectively at entry and the eventual trial results subdivided with respect to them. However, there is a danger in too detailed an analysis of the apparent response of small subgroups chosen for separate emphasis, because of the apparently remarkable effects of treatment in these subgroups. Even if an agent brought no benefit, it would have to be acutely poisonous for it not to appear beneficial in one or two such subgroups! Conversely, if an intervention really avoids an approximately similar proportion of the risk in each category of patient, it will, by chance alone, appear not to do so in some category. The surprising extent to which this happens is evident from the example in Table 2. A large anonymous trial will at least still help to answer the practical question of whether, on average, a policy of widespread treatment (except where clearly contraindicated) is preferable to a general policy of no immediate use of the treatment (except where clearly indicated). Moreover, without a few really large trials it is difficult to see how else many such questions could be resolved over the next few years. For example, digitalis has already been in use for over two centuries, and there is still no reliable consensus as to its net long-term effects on mortality. Trials are at least a practical way of making some solid progress, and it would be unfortunate if desire for the perfect (that is, knowledge of exactly who will benefit from treatment) were to become the enemy of the possible (that is to say, knowledge of the direction and approximate size of the effects of the treatment of many large categories of patient).

Further reading

Antiplatelet Trialists' Collaboration (1994). Collaborative overview of randomised trials of antiplatelet therapy. I: Prevention of death, myocardial infarction, and stroke by prolonged antiplatelet therapy in various categories of patients. *British Medical Journal* **308**, 81–106.

Antithrombotic Trialists' (ATT) Collaboration (writing committee: C Baigent, C Sudlow, R Collins, R Peto) (2002). Collaborative meta-analysis of randomised trials of antiplatelet therapy for prevention of death, myocardial infarction, and stroke in high-risk patients. *British Medical Journal* **324**, 71–86.

Armitage P, Berry G (1994). *Statistical methods in medical research*, 3rd edn. Blackwell Science, Oxford.

Chalmers I (1994). The Cochrane Collaboration: preparing, maintaining and disseminating systematic reviews of the effects of health care. *Annals of the New York Academy of Sciences* **703**, 156–63.

Chalmers TC, Lau J (1993). Meta-analytic stimulus for changes in clinical trials. *Statistical Methods in Medical Research* **2**, 161–72.

Cochrane AL (1979). 1931–1971: a critical review, with particular reference to the medical profession. *Medicines for the year 2000*, pp 1–11. Office of Health Economics, London.

Collins R, Peto R (1994). Antihypertensive drug therapy: effects on stroke and coronary heart disease. *Textbook of hypertension*, p 1156. Blackwell Science, Oxford.

Collins R, MacMahon S (2001). Reliable assessment of the effects of treatment on mortality and major morbidity, I: clinical trials, *Lancet* **357**, 373–80.

Collins R, et al. (1987). Avoidance of large biases and large random errors in the assessment of moderate treatment effects: the need for systematic overviews. *Statistics in Medicine* **6**, 245–50.

Collins R, Doll R, Peto R (1992). Ethics of clinical trials. *Introducing new treatments for cancer: practical, ethical and legal problems*, p 49. Wiley, New York.

Early Breast Cancer Trialists' Collaborative Group (1992). Systemic treatment of early breast cancer by hormonal, cytotoxic, or immune therapy: 133 randomised trials involving 31,000 recurrences and 24,000 deaths among 75,000 women. *Lancet* **339**, 1–15, 71–85.

Early Breast Cancer Trialists' Collaborative Group writing committee (Clarke M, Collins R, Davies C, Godwin J, Gray R, Peto R) (1998). Tamoxifen for early breast cancer: an overview of the randomised trials. *Lancet* **351**, 1451–67.

Early Breast Cancer Trialists' Collaborative Group (writing committee: Clarke M, Collins R, Davies C, Godwin J, Gray R, Peto R) (1998). Polychemotherapy for early breast cancer: an overview of the randomised trials. *Lancet* **352**, 930–42.

European Carotid Surgery Trialists' Collaborative Group (1991). MRC European Carotid Surgery Trial: interim results for symptomatic patients with severe (70–99 per cent) or with mild (0–29 per cent) carotid stenosis. *Lancet* **337**, 1235–43.

Fibrinolytic Therapy Trialists' Collaborative Group (1994). Indications for fibrinolytic therapy in suspected acute myocardial infarction: collaborative overview of early mortality and major morbidity results from all randomised trials of more than 1000 patients. *Lancet* **343**, 311–22.

Heart Protection Study Collaborative Group (writing committee: Collins R, Armitage J, Parish S, Sleight P, Peto R) (2002). MRC/BHF Heart Protection Study of cholesterol lowering with simvastatin in 20,536 high-risk individuals: a randomised placebo-controlled trial. *Lancet* **360**, 7–22.

ISIS-2 (Second International Study of Infarct Survival) Collaborative Group (1988). Randomised trial of intravenous streptokinase, oral aspirin, both, or neither among 17,187 cases of suspected acute myocardial infarction: ISIS-2. *Lancet* **ii**, 349–60.

ISIS-4 (Fourth International Study of Infarct Survival) Collaborative Group (1995). ISIS-4: a randomised factorial trial assessing early oral captopril, oral mononitrate, and intravenous magnesium sulphate in 58050 patients with suspected acute myocardial infarction. *Lancet*.

MacMahon S (1994). Blood pressure and the risks of cardiovascular disease. *Textbook of hypertension*, p 46. Blackwell Science, Oxford.

MacMahon S, Collins R (2001). Reliable assessment of the effects of treatment on mortality and major morbidity, II: observational studies. *Lancet* **357**, 455–62.

Peto R, *et al.* (1976). Design and analysis of randomized clinical trials requiring prolonged observation of each patient. Part I: Introduction and design. *British Journal of Cancer* **34**, 585–612.

Peto R, *et al.* (1977). Design and analysis of randomized clinical trials requiring prolonged observation of each patient. Part II: Analysis and examples. *British Journal of Cancer* **35**, 1–39.

Yusuf S, Collins R, Peto R (1984). Why do we need some large, simple randomized trials? *Statistics in Medicine* **3**, 409–20.

2.5 Complementary and alternative medicine

*E. Ernst**

Definition

Most doctors feel they know intuitively what is meant by complementary and alternative medicine (**CAM**). Yet an adequate definition is hard to find. Often CAM is described by characteristics that exclude it from mainstream medicine, for example:

- not taught in medical school
- not scientifically proven
- not based on a scientific rationale
- not used in routine health care

CAM can be positively defined as 'diagnosis, treatment, and/or prevention which complements mainstream medicine by contributing to a common whole, by satisfying a demand not met by orthodoxy or by diversifying the conceptual frameworks of medicine'.

CAM encompasses a large variety of techniques which have little in common except that they are excluded from mainstream medicine, claim to offer help for every condition, and pride themselves on a holistic approach to patient care (Table 1). Some relate to therapeutic modalities (e.g. herbalism), some to diagnostic techniques (e.g. iridology), and some include both diagnostic and therapeutic modalities (e.g. acupuncture).

There are considerable local differences in what is regarded as CAM or mainstream medicine. In Germany, massage therapy and herbalism are orthodox whereas in English-speaking countries they are usually regarded as CAM. Acupuncture is CAM in the West, while in China it is a widespread, traditional, and accepted form of treatment.

Since most CAM therapies are used as adjuncts to conventional treatments, 'complementary' is a more appropriate term than 'alternative'. When used as a true alternative to mainstream medicine, CAM almost invariably becomes a hazard to patients.

Prevalence

In the United States the prevalence of CAM increased from 33 to 42 per cent in the general population between 1990 and 1997, involving an annual expenditure exceeding US$20 billion. In the United Kingdom, the figures are 20 per cent and £1.6 billion, respectively.

In industrialized countries, typical users of CAM are:

- middle aged
- female
- well educated
- high socio-economic class

Indications for CAM range from chronic benign conditions where mainstream medicine is unable to offer a cure (e.g. back pain) to life-threatening diseases like cancer and AIDS. Most patients try CAM in paral-

lel with conventional treatment, yet 30 to 50 per cent do not tell their doctor. A comprehensive medical history should therefore include questions about CAM.

Reasons for CAM's popularity

The following motivations may be important:

- to leave no option untried
- to take control over one's own health
- to accord one's health care with one's (slightly alternative) world views
- to be given time, understanding, and empathy by a practitioner
- to avoid adverse effects of conventional treatments

Disenchantment with orthodox medicine is a reason for trying CAM that should be taken seriously.

Examples of CAM methods

Acupuncture

Description

The Chinese believed that the life energy flowing in particular channels (meridians) govern the human body; the energy is a balance of opposite characteristics: yin and yang. Illness was understood as an expression of an imbalance between yin and yang. One way of re-establishing the proper equilibrium would be to insert needles in acupuncture points located along the meridians. Instead of needles one can also use pressure (acupressure), laser light (laser acupuncture), electrical currents (electroacupuncture), or heat (moxibustion). Neither the meridians nor the acupuncture points have a morphological basis and the philosophy of yin and yang is unscientific.

Mode of action

Nevertheless, modern neurophysiological research has created a (hypothetical) rationale for acupuncture: activation of brainstem nuclei and the release of neural transmitters and endorphins in the brain and descending inhibitory control systems.

There are considerable differences between traditional Chinese and Western acupuncture. With the former, no conventional diagnoses are sought, treatment is highly individualized according to each patient's particular yin/yang imbalance and is considered as a 'cure all'. Western acupuncturists tailor the treatment to the conventional diagnosis established beforehand and normally strive to identify those diagnoses for which acupuncture is helpful.

Efficacy

Rigorous trials are possible but fraught with methodological problems, for example:

* The constructive comments of Ted Kaptchuk, Harvard School of Medicine, Boston, United States and Adrian White, University of Exeter, United Kingdom are thankfully appreciated.

- What is an adequate sham procedure?
- How can the patient be blinded?
- How can the therapist be blinded?

Several systematic reviews and meta-analyses of clinical trials of acupuncture for defined conditions have been published suggesting that acupuncture is effective for the following conditions:

- back pain
- nausea and vomiting
- dental pain
- migraine

In the following conditions, results are inconclusive:

- addictions (other than nicotine)
- asthma

- headache
- inflammatory rheumatic conditions
- neck pain
- osteoarthritis
- stroke

Acupuncture is no more effective than sham acupuncture or other control interventions for smoking cessation and weight reduction.

Safety

Serious complications include:

- trauma (e.g. cardiac tamponade, pneumothorax)
- infections (e.g. viral hepatitis)

Table 1 Various other forms of therapeutic and diagnostic methods

Name	Principle	Main indications	Efficacy	Safety
Alexander technique	Training process of ideal body posture and movement; developed by F.M. Alexander	Musculoskeletal problems	Very few clinical trials	No serious adverse effects
Applied kinesiology	Diagnostic technique using muscle strength as an indicator; developed by G. Goodheart	Not applicable	Shown to be not valid	Can delay reliable diagnoses
Aromatherapy	Application of essential oils usually through gentle massage techniques; developed by R.M. Gattefossé	Relaxation	Systematic review was inconclusive	Allergic reactions to oils
Autogenic training	Form of self-hypnosis for relaxation and stress reduction; developed by J. Schultz	Stress management	Some evidence for effectiveness	No serious adverse effects
Chelation therapy	Intravenous infusion of EDTA used for 'deblocking' arteries from arteriosclerotic lesions	Circulatory disorders	Shown to be ineffective	Serious adverse effects reported
Chiropractic	Popular manual therapy based on the assumption that most health problems are due to malalignment of the spine and treatable through spinal manipulation; developed by D.D. Palmer; seen as mainstream by many proponents	Back pain	Recent systematic reviews of chiropractic for back pain are inconclusive	Serious adverse effects have been reported, their exact incidence is not known
Colonic irrigation (or colon therapy)	Cleansing of the colon through water enemas to 'free the system of toxins'	Various	No sound evidence for effectiveness	Serious adverse effects reported
Hypnotherapy	Induction of trance-like state to influence the unconscious mind	Various	Some evidence for effectiveness	Adverse effects probably infrequent
Iridology	Diagnostic technique using signs and impurities on the iris	Not applicable	Shown to be not valid	Can delay reliable diagnoses
Macrobiotic diet	Diet based on the ying/yang principle using whole grains and vegetables	Disease prevention	Positive effects on cardiovascular risk factors	Serious adverse effects reported
Massage	Various techniques of manual stimulation of cutaneous, subcutaneous, or muscular structures (deemed mainstream on the European continent)	Musculoskeletal problems	Some evidence for effectiveness in musculoskeletal and psychological problems	No serious adverse effects
Osteopathy	Health problems are thought to be due to malalignment of the spine and corrected through spinal mobilization; developed by T. Still; seen as mainstream by many proponents	Back pain	Systematic reviews of osteopathy for back pain are inconclusive	Adverse effects less than with chiropractic
Reflexology	Internal organs correspond to areas on the sole of the feet and can be influenced through massaging these	Relaxation	Systematic review was inconclusive	No serious adverse effects
Spiritual healing	Channelling of 'healing energy' through a healer into a patient	Re-establishing a wholesome balance	Clinical studies highly contradictory	No serious adverse effects
Yoga	Meditative, postural, and breathing techniques from ancient India	Various	Some evidence for effectiveness in asthma, for instance	No serious adverse effects

EDTA, ethylenediamine tetra-acetic acid.

Phytotherapy

Description

Medical herbalism (phytotherapy) is treatment with whole plants, parts of plants, or plant extracts. The term does not cover treatment with single active constituents such as acetylsalicylic acid, originally from willow bark.

Since all plants contain a multitude of chemicals, phytotherapy involves treatment with a mixture of potentially active compounds. In many cases there is uncertainty about the active ingredients and their pharmacological actions. Herbalists claim that the whole plant (extract) will yield more beneficial effects than any single isolated ingredient.

Most medical cultures have their version of traditional herbalism. Traditional Chinese medicine has a long history of employing mixtures of herbs to prevent and treat disease. This tradition was modified by the Japanese and resulted in Kampo medicine. The Indian tradition has generated Ayurvedic medicine, which relies heavily on plant-based remedies. Likewise, European herbalism has a tradition which is as old as European medicine itself. The scientific investigation of medicinal herbs is, however, a relatively recent innovation.

Mode of action

There are few differences in principle between pharmacotherapy and phytotherapy except that herbal remedies are multicomponent systems which render them pharmacologically more complex. There is no reason why the rules of pharmacokinetics and pharmacodynamics do not apply. For every plant-based medicine discernible modes of action exist. In some cases these have been elucidated; in many other cases they are still hypothetical.

Efficacy

Based on authoritative systematic reviews and meta-analysis, good evidence exists for the efficacy of the following herbal remedies:

- garlic for hypercholesterolaemia
- ginger for nausea and vomiting
- *Ginkgo biloba* for intermittent claudication
- *Ginkgo biloba* to delay the clinical deterioration in dementias
- horse chestnut seed extract for primary venous insufficiency
- kava as an anxiolytic drug
- peppermint oil for irritable bowel syndrome
- saw palmetto for benign prostatic hyperplasia
- St John's Wort for mild to moderate depression

For many other popular medicinal herbs, too few clinical trials have been carried out, or the studies are methodologically flawed, or their results are contradictory. The efficacy of such popular herbal remedies as valerian, aloe vera ,and ginseng is undetermined.

Safety

Many medicinal herbs have serious adverse effects, for example:

- aconite (cardiotoxic)
- aristolochia (nephrotoxic)
- broom (cardiotoxic)
- chaparal (nephrotoxic)
- comfrey (hepatotoxic)
- liquorice root (hypokalaemia)
- pennyroyal (hepatotoxic)
- skullcap (hepatotoxic)

Herbal remedies can also interact with synthetic drugs (Table 2), and Asian herbal medicines have been shown repeatedly to be adulterated with synthetic drugs or heavy metals. In many countries (e.g. the United Kingdom and the United States) herbal medicines are marketed as food supplements with no stringent quality control.

Homoeopathy

Description

Samuel Hahnemann, a German physician, believed in two major principles which formed the basis of an entirely new school of medicine, homoeopathy. The first is known as the 'like cures like' principle. Put simply, it postulates that if a given drug induces symptoms (e.g. a headache) in healthy individuals, this very drug can be employed to treat headaches in patients who suffer from this symptom. The second is that 'potentizing' (i.e. shaking and stepwise diluting) drugs makes them more potent for the treatment of illness. Homoeopathic dilutions prepared thus are believed to be clinically more effective than placebo even if not a single molecule of the original medicine is contained in the potentized remedy. Scientists have for 200 years pointed out that homoeopathy cannot possibly work beyond a placebo effect, but homoeopaths insist that homoeopathic remedies work via 'energy' transfer from the original substance to the diluent (the theory of a 'memory of water').

Homoeopaths do not treat diseases but claim to treat the whole individual. A homoeopath would take a detailed history at each patient's first visit. The aim is to match the totality of the symptoms and characteristics of that patient with a 'drug picture' according to the 'like cures like' principle. This homoeopathic remedy given in the correct potency should then be the optimal treatment for that patient. Clinical improvement may, however, take weeks or months, and in about 20 per cent of all cases symptoms may deteriorate before they become better, a phenomenon termed 'homoeopathic aggravation'.

Homoeopathy has to be seen in its historical context. At the time of Hahnemann it was an important discovery—there were very few effective treatments and many that were overtly harmful. At the very least homoeopathic remedies had virtually no adverse effects. And, if nothing else, Hahnemann can be credited with clinically exploiting the placebo effect to the best benefit of his patients. It is therefore hardly surprising that homoeopathy conquered many countries (e.g. France, the United States, India, and South America) by storm. The advent of more effective and less harmful synthetic drugs eventually led to the decline of homoeopathy. The recent boom of CAM has been associated with a strong revival in homoeopathy.

Mode of action

Even though several hypotheses have been developed to explain the transfer of 'energy' from the mother tincture to the diluent, none have so far withstood the scrutiny of independent assessment. Neither has the 'energy' ever been defined in physical terms, nor are there rational explanations as to how this 'energy' (if it exists) might induce a healing process in a diseased body or organ. Homoeopathy is, therefore, among the least plausible forms of CAM.

Efficacy

A meta-analysis of all 89 randomized or placebo-controlled clinical trials published by 1995 calculated an overall odds ratio of 2.45 in favour of homoeopathy. When only the 26 most rigorous studies were meta-analysed the odds ratio fell to 1.66 but remained statistically significant. However, this publication was criticized for pooling data for all medical conditions and all homoeopathic remedies and for including trials that were not randomized nor placebo-controlled and studies of material (low dilution) remedies where efficacy is not disputed.

The results of further systematic reviews are as follows.

1. The most frequently tested homoeopathic remedy (arnica) has not been conclusively shown to be efficacious beyond a placebo effect by two independent research groups.

Table 2 Possible interactions between some popular herbal remedies and synthetic drugs

Herbal remedy[a]	Usage or pharmacological effect[b]	Possible interaction
Aloe vera (Aloe barbadensis)	Various	With chronic use potentiation of cardiac glycosides or antiarrhythmic drugs due to loss of potassium
Arnica (Arnica montana)	Wound healing	Decreased effects of antihypertensives and anticoagulants
Black cohosh (Cimicifuga racemosa)	Oestrogenic	Increased effects of antihypertensives
Borage (Borago officinalis)	Anti-inflammatory	Interaction with antiepileptics, may increase risk of seizure
Broom (Cystisus scoparius)	Anti-arrhythmic, diuretic	Increased effects of antidepressants, β-blockers, and cardiac glycosides
Cascara (Rhamnus purshiana)	Laxative, cathartic	Loss of potassium with chronic use; potentiation of cardiac glycosides or antiarrhythmic drugs
Camomile (M. chamomilla)	Spasmolytic, anti-inflammatory	May potentiate effects of anticoagulants through its coumarin content
Cranberry (Vaccinum macrocarpon)	Urinary tract infections	May enhance elimination of drugs normally excreted in urine
Ephedra (Ephedra sinica)	CNS stimulant, sympathomimetic	Cardiac glycosides/halothane: arrhythmias; guanethidine: enhanced sympathomimetic effect; MAO inhibitors: enhanced sympathomimetic effect; secale alkaloids/oxytocin: hypertension
Garlic (Allium sativum)	Hypocholesterolaemic	Increased effects of anticoagulants and antiplatelet drugs
Ginger (Zingiber officinalis)	Anti-emetic	Increased effects of anticoagulants
Ginkgo (Ginkgo biloba)	Circulatory diseases	Increased effect of anticoagulants
Ginseng (Panax quinquefolrus)	Various	Interaction with MAO inhibitors; interaction with stimulants and phenelzine; increased effect of hypoglycaemics
Hawthorne (Crataegus)	Digitalis-like	Can increase hypotensive effects of nitrates, antihypotensives, cardiac glycosides, and CNS depressants
Hops (Humulus lupulus)	Hypnotic	Antagonism with antidepressants; can increase effects of CNS depressants and hypnotics; interference with hormonal drugs
Horse chestnut (Aesculus hippocastanum)	Anti-inflammatory	Increased effects of anticoagulants
Kava (Piper methysticum)	Anxiolytic	Potentiation with other axiolytics; can increase Parkinson symptoms with levodopa
Kelp (Laminaria digitata)	Antitumour effects, antiobesity	Increased effects of anticoagulants and antihypertensives
Lavender (Lavandula officinalis)	Sedative	Increased effects of CNS depressants
Liquorice (Glycrrhiza glaba)	Corticosteroid activity for gastric irritation	Potassium loss, e.g. with thiazide diuretics; water and sodium retention with corticosteroids; increased effects of digoxin; decreased effects of antihypertensives
Lily of the valley (Convallaria majalis)	Congestive heart failure	Increased (side-)effects of quinodine, calcium, saluretics, laxatives, glucosteroids, β-blockers, calcium channel blockers, and digitalis
Mistletoe (Visum album)	Anticancer drug	Increased effects of CNS depressants, antihypertensives, and cardiac drugs
Nettle (Urtica dioica)	Diuretic	May potentiate effects of other diuretics
Pumpkin seed (Curcubita)	Anthelmintic, diuretic	Can increase effect of diuretics
Sage (Salvia officinalis)	Antispasmodic	Interaction with antiepileptics, may increase risk of seizure; decreased effect with antiglycaemics
St John's Wort (Hypericum perforatum)	Antidepressant	Increased effects of digoxin MAO inhibitors or serotonin-uptake inhibitors; decreased effect of anticonvulsants and antidiabetic drugs; increased photosensitivity with other such drugs
Valerian (Valerina officinalis)	Hypnotic	Increased effects of CNS depressants and hypnotics
Vitex (Agnus castus)	Hormonal effects	Increased effects of other hormonal drugs
Yew (Taxus brevifolia)	Antirheumatic, anticancer	Chemotherapeutic agents may potentiate its effects

[a]Plant source in brackets; [b]Not comprehensive.

CNS, central nervous system; MAO, monoamine oxidase.

2. The clinical condition which has been tested more than any other (delayed-onset muscle soreness) does not respond to homoeopathic remedies better than it responds to placebo; neither do clinical conditions that are common in everyday homoeopathic practice (e.g. migraine or headaches).

Safety

Highly diluted homoeopathic remedies are probably safe. Whether 'homoeopathic aggravations' represent a safety issue is unclear at present. One 'indirect' safety problem deserves to be mentioned: homoeopaths who are not medically qualified tend to advise their clients against immunization. If this happens on a large scale, we are in danger of losing herd immunity against important infectious diseases.

Other forms of CAM

CAM is a highly diverse field comprising more than 150 different forms of therapeutic and diagnostic methods (Table 1).

Further reading

Ernst E, ed. (2000). *Herbal medicine—a concise overview for healthcare professionals.* Butterworth Heinemann, Oxford.

Ernst E, Hahn EG, eds (1998). *Homoeopathy. A critical appraisal.* Butterworth Heinemann, Oxford.

Ernst E, Pittler MH, Stevinson C, White A, Eisenberg D. (2001). *The desktop guide to complementary and alternative medicine.* Mosby, Edinburgh.

Ernst E, White A, ed. (1999). *Acupuncture a scientific appraisal.* Butterworth Heinemann, Oxford .

Fetow CW, Avila JR (1999*). Professional's handbook of complementary and alternative medicine.* Springhouse, Pennsylvania.

Jonas WB, Levin JS (1999). *Essentials of complementary and alternative medicine.* Lippincott, Williams, Wilkins, Philadelphia.

Schulz V, Häusel R, Tyler VE (1998). *Rational phytotherapy.* Springer Verlag, Berlin.

3

Global patterns of disease and medical practice

3.1 The Global Burden of Disease Study

C. J. L Murray and A. D. Lopez*

Introduction

Reliable, up-to-date epidemiological information is required so that health authorities can assess priorities and evaluate their health systems. National and subnational mortality and morbidity statistics have been published by many countries for several decades. However, before the Global Burden of Disease (**GBD**) Study began in 1992, there had been no attempt to estimate and project the burden of disease and injury globally and regionally, using the same methods and expressing results in a common unit of measurement.

One goal of the GBD Study was to include measures of morbidity in debates about international health policy, which had largely drawn on the available mortality data, much of it referring to children. There was a need to separate epidemiological assessment from advocacy so that estimates of the mortality or disability from a condition were developed as objectively as possible. There was also a need to quantitate the burden of disease using a measure suitable for cost-effectiveness analysis of intervention packages. The GBD method quantifies the impact of premature death and disability on a population, combining these measures into a single unit of measurement of the overall burden of disease in that population. The Study presented the first global and regional estimates of disease and injury burden attributable to 10 important risk factors such as tobacco, alcohol, poor water and sanitation, and unsafe sex. Quantifiable estimates and projections of disease and injury burden from various exposures, measured in a similar fashion, are a key input into priority setting and for policy debates.

In the original GBD Study, 1990 was chosen as the base year for estimating disease burden. A revised Study is now underway to estimate the Global Burden of Disease in 2000, using more extensive and recent data sources, and improved methods, with a broader range of diseases and risk factors. Results of the GBD 2000 Study will be published in 2003; preliminary findings are given in this chapter.

Measuring disease burden

To combine the burden of premature mortality and disability into one summary measure requires a common unit of measurement. Since the late 1940s, it has been generally agreed that time is an appropriate measure: time (in years) lost through premature death, and time (in years) lived with a disability. A range of these time-based measures has been used in different countries, many of them variants of the so-called Quality-Adjusted Life Year or **QALY**. For the GBD, an internationally standardized form of the QALY was developed, called the Disability-Adjusted Life Year (**DALY**). This expresses years of life lost to premature death and years lived with a disability of specified severity. One DALY is one lost year of healthy life. Premature death is defined as occurring before the age to which a person could have expected to survive if he or she were a member of a model population whose life expectancy at birth was approximately equal to that of the world's longest-surviving population, the Japanese.

To calculate total DALYs for a given condition in a population, years of life lost (**YLLs**) and years lived with disability (**YLDs**) for that condition are estimated, and added together. For example, to calculate DALYs incurred through road traffic accidents in India in 1990, the total years of life lost in fatal road accidents must be added to the total years of life lived with disabilities by survivors of such accidents, weighted by the severity of the disability.

To assess premature mortality, the Study used standard life tables for all populations, with life expectancies at birth fixed at 82.5 years for women and 80 years for men. A standard life expectancy allows deaths at the same age to contribute equally to the burden of disease, irrespective of where the death occurs. Other methods, such as using different life expectancies for different populations that more closely match their actual life expectancies, violate this egalitarian principle. As life expectancy is rarely equal for men and women, the GBD assigned men a lower reference life expectancy than women, the magnitude of the difference (2.5 years) being an estimate of the biological advantage of females.

If people are forced to choose between saving a year of life for a 2-year-old and a 22-year-old, most prefer to save the 22 year-old. A range of studies confirm this broad social preference to value a year lived by a young adult more than one lived by a very young child or an older adult. Adults are widely perceived to play a critical role in the family, community, and society. This is why the GBD Study incorporated age-weighting into the DALY. It was assumed that the relative value of a year of life rises rapidly from birth to a peak in the early twenties, after which it steadily declines.

People commonly discount future benefits in the same way that they may discount future against current wealth. Whether a year of healthy life, like money, is also preferred now rather than later, is a matter of debate among economists, medical ethicists, and public health planners, since discounting future health affects both measurements of disease burden and estimates of the cost-effectiveness of an intervention. There are arguments for and against discounting. In the GBD Study, future life years were discounted by 3 per cent per year. This means that a year of healthy life bought for 10 years in the future is worth around 24 per cent less than one bought for now, as discounting is represented as an exponential decay function. Since the impact of discounting is significant, the findings of the GBD Study were published based on DALYs with and without discounting. Discounting future health reduces the relative impact of a child death compared to an adult death. It also reduces the value of interventions that provide benefits largely in the future, such as vaccinating against hepatitis B, which may prevent liver cancer, but some decades later.

In order to measure time lived with a non-fatal disease and assess disabilities in a way that will help to guide health policy, disability must be defined, measured, and valued in a clear framework that inevitably involves simplifying reality. There is surprisingly wide agreement between cultures about what constitutes a severe or a mild disability. For example, a year lived with blindness appears to most people to be a more severe disability than a year lived with watery diarrhoea, while quadriplegia is regarded as

* The authors are extremely grateful to Brodie Ferguson for his assistance in preparing this chapter.

more severe than blindness. These judgements must be made formal and explicit if they are to be incorporated into measurements of disease burden.

To formalize social preferences for different states of health, the GBD Study developed a protocol based on the person trade-off method. In a formal exercise involving health workers from all regions of the world, the severity of a set of 22 indicator disabling conditions—such as blindness, depression, and conditions that cause pain—was weighted between 0 (perfect health) and 1 (equivalent to death). These weights were then grouped into seven classes, where class I has a weight between 0.00 and 0.02 and class VII a weight between 0.7 and 1. Subsequent valuations carried out in various cultures have closely matched the results of the original GBD exercise. For the GBD 2000 Study, disability weights are being determined from an extensive household survey programme to obtain valuations based on a visual analogue scale, with required valuations to be determined on the basis of a more intensive valuation exercise among health professionals to correct for interval-scale biases among respondents.

Sensitivity analyses

To gauge the impact of changing these social choices on the final measures of disease burden, the GBD assessments were recalculated with alternative age-weighting and discount rates, and with alternative methods for weighting the severity of disabilities. Overall, the rankings of diseases and the distribution of burden by broad cause group are largely unaffected by age-weighting, and only slightly affected by changing the method for weighting disability. Changes in the discount rate, by contrast, may have a more significant effect on the overall results. A higher discount rate results in an increased burden in older age groups, while a lower discount rate results in an increased burden in younger age groups. Changes which affect the age distribution of burden, in turn, affect the distribution by cause, as communicable and perinatal conditions are most common in children while non-communicable diseases are most common in adults. The most significant effect of changing the discount and age weights is a reduction in the importance of several psychiatric conditions.

Ultimately, however, the accuracy of the underlying basic epidemiological data from which disease burden is calculated will influence the final results much more than the discount rate, the age weight, or the disability weighting method. If, for example, estimates of the incidence of

blindness are incorrect by a factor of two, the results, whatever the social values used in the unit of measurement, will be substantially incorrect. We conclude that much more effort needs to be invested in improving the basic epidemiological data than in analysing the effects of what are ultimately minor adjustments to the particular summary measure of population health employed.

Estimating mortality and disability

Classification

As most developing countries still have only limited information about the distribution of causes of death in their populations, a primary objective of the GBD has been to develop comprehensive, internally consistent, mortality estimates worldwide for each major cause in 1990. Deaths were classified using a tree structure, in which the first level of disaggregation comprises three broad cause groups:

- *group I*—communicable, maternal, perinatal, and nutritional conditions (ICD-10 codes A00–B99, G00, N70–N73, J00–J06, J10–J18, J20–J22, H65–H66, O00–O99, P00–P96, E00–E02, E40–E46, E50, D50);

- *group II*—non-communicable diseases (ICD-10 codes C00–C97, D00–D48, D51–D89, E03–E07, E10–E16, E20–E34, E51–E89, F00–F99, G03–G99, H00–H61, H68–H95, I00–I99, J30–J99, K00–K92, N00–N64, N75–N99, L00–L99, M00–M99, Q00–Q99); and

- *group III*—injuries (ICD-10 codes V01–Y89).

Each group was then subdivided into categories: for example, cardiovascular diseases and malignant neoplasm are two subcategories of group II. Beyond this level, there are two further disaggregation levels such that 107 individual causes from the International Classification of Diseases (ICD) can be listed separately.

Consistent with the goal of providing disaggregated estimates of disease burden to help set priorities in the health sector, estimates for 1990 were prepared by age and sex and for eight broad geographical regions of the world (Fig. 1)

For the GBD 2000 Study, the regional composition has been adapted to the six WHO regions. However, since these groups can be epidemiologically heterogeneous (for instance, the region of the Americas includes the

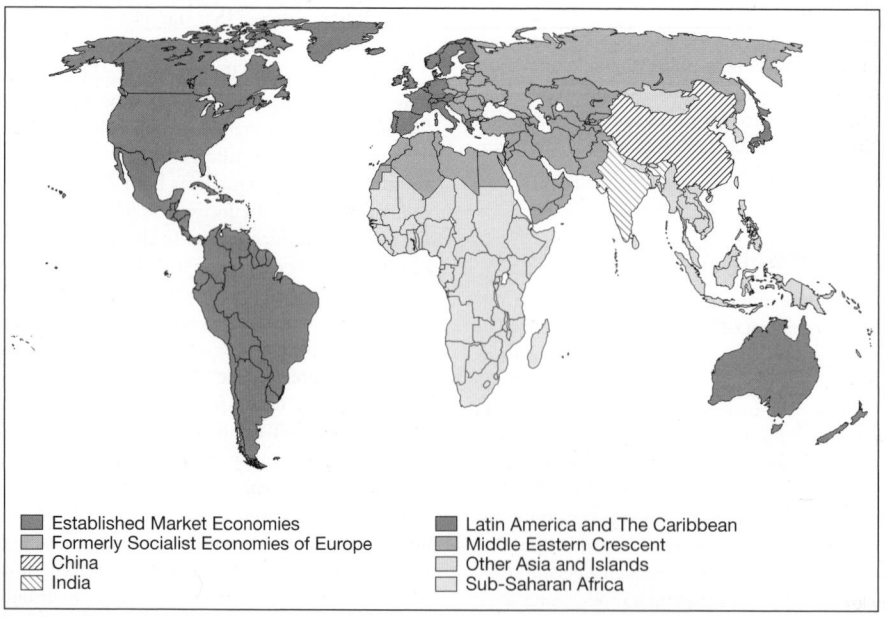

Established Market Economies
Formerly Socialist Economies of Europe
China
India

Latin America and The Caribbean
Middle Eastern Crescent
Other Asia and Islands
Sub-Saharan Africa

Fig. 1 Regions used for the GBD Study, 1990. EME, Established Market Economies; FSE, Former Socialist Economies of Europe; CHN, China; IND, India; LAC, Latin America and the Caribbean; MEC, Middle Eastern Crescent; OAI, other Asia [countries] and Islands; SSA, Sub-Saharan Africa.

United States, Canada, as well as Peru, Bolivia, and Haiti), each region has been subdivided into five categories of countries (labelled A, B, C, D, E) depending on the relationship between child and adult mortality in each country (Fig. 2).

Estimating regional mortality patterns

The Study derived cause-related mortality estimates by using the following four types of data:

1. *Vital registration systems.* Cause-of-death data certified by a physician have been assembled through vital registration systems for over 100 years in some European countries. Data for some 70 countries were available for the 1990s.

2. *Sample death registration systems.* In China, a set of 145 disease surveillance points, representative of both urban and rural areas, and covering about 10 000 000 people, provides useful mortality data. In India, Maharashtra state provides full medical certification for at least 80 per cent of urban deaths, while a rural surveillance system including more than 1300 primary healthcare centres nationwide was used to assess broad rural patterns of mortality. Reliable estimates of age-specific mortality rates in India can be derived, with appropriate adjustment, from the Sample Registration System covering a population of about 6 million but which is representative of all India.

3. *Epidemiological assessments.* Epidemiological estimates exist for specific causes in different regions. These estimates combine information from surveys on the incidence or prevalence of the disease with data on case-fatality rates for both treated and untreated cases.

4. *Cause-of-death models.* These are based on the fact that the broad cause structure of mortality is closely related to the level of mortality in a population. Such models estimate the distribution of deaths by cause in a population from historical studies of mortality patterns in countries with vital registration. The models developed for the initial GBD Study drew on a dataset of 103 observations from 67 countries between 1950 and 1991, and were used primarily to provide plausibility bounds on estimates derived from epidemiological assessments. For the GBD 2000 study, cause-of-death models have been used to ensure that the relative importance of groups I, II, and III as causes of death are consistent with historical observations about the cause structure of mortality, overall mortality, and economic development.

Vital registration data, corrected where necessary for under-registration, were used to construct cause-specific mortality patterns for those regions where registration was complete or virtually complete. For other regions, sex-age-specific mortality rates were estimated from survey and census data on child mortality. Adult mortality levels were inferred from the new WHO model life tables.

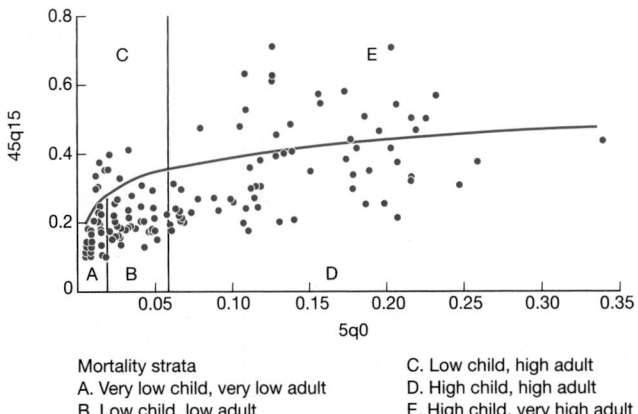

Fig. 2 Child and adult mortality, 1990.

Mortality strata
A. Very low child, very low adult
B. Low child, low adult
C. Low child, high adult
D. High child, high adult
E. High child, very high adult

Assessing disability

A disease or injury may have multiple disabling effects, or sequelae. To estimate the total burden of disability, the Study measured the amount of time lived with each of the various disabling sequelae of diseases and injuries, in both treated and untreated states, and weighted for their severity, in each population. In all, 483 disabling sequelae of disease and injuries were analysed for the Study, for all regions and age groups, and for both sexes.

Calculating the number of years lived with a disabling condition requires information about its incidence, the average age of onset, the average duration of the disability, and the severity weighting of the condition. Epidemiological experts were asked to estimate each variable for each condition based on a thorough review of published and unpublished studies. For each sequela; prevalence, case fatality, remission, and mortality were estimated. This information allowed correction of the preliminary estimates for internal consistency, ensuring that estimated prevalence and estimated incidence were consistent with one another. Consistency was validated using DisMod software specifically developed for the Study (Fig. 3). When inconsistencies were detected, epidemiological experts were asked to revise their initial estimates. The final disability estimates were the result of several rounds of revision over nearly 5 years.

The number of years that each person had lived with a particular disability was calculated from the incidence of the disability, with the 'stream' of disability arising from it measured from the age of onset, the estimated duration of the disability, multiplied by the condition's severity weight. To calculate the YLDs due to a condition in any given population, the number of YLDs lost per incident case must be multiplied by the number of incident cases. A case of asthma, for example, carries a disability weight of 0.1 if untreated and 0.06 if treated. If the annual incidence of asthma in males aged between 15 and 44 years is 1 million cases, the untreated proportion is 35 per cent, and the average duration is 7 years, then this sequela alone is estimated to cause 664 000 YLDs for that demographic group. Unlike the estimates of years of life lost, not all sequelae of all conditions could be explicitly assessed for YLDs. Estimates for conditions not explicitly considered were made on the basis of information about the ratio of total premature mortality to disability (YLDs) for each broad cause group.

The global burden of disease in 1990 and 2000: main findings

The results demonstrate clearly that disability plays a central role in determining the overall health status of a population. Yet that role has until now been almost invisible to public health. The leading causes of disability are shown to be substantially different from the leading causes of death, which has considerable implications for the practice of judging a population's health from its mortality statistics alone.

A key aim of the GBD was to measure the burden of fatal and non-fatal health outcomes in a single measure, the disability-adjusted life year (DALY). This section presents the main results of the assessments of overall

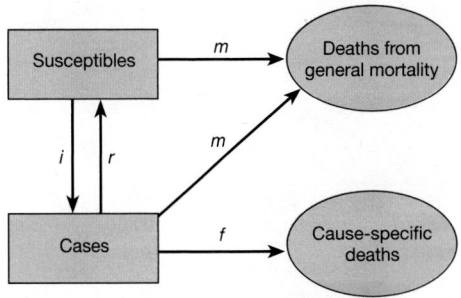

Fig. 3 Basic relationships between susceptibles, cases, and deaths used in developing DisMod.

burden for each region. To calculate DALYs due to each disease or injury in a given year and population, the years of life lost through all deaths in that year were added to the years of life expected to be lived with a disability for all new cases of disease or injury occurring in that year, weighted for the severity of the condition.

Regional imbalances in the burden of disease

Sub-Saharan Africa and India together accounted for more than 40 per cent of the total global burden of disease in 1990, although they make up only 26 per cent of the world's population. By contrast, the Established Market Economies and the Formerly Socialist Economies of Europe, with about one-fifth of the world's population between them, together bore less than 12 per cent of the total disease burden. China emerged as substantially the most 'healthy' of the developing regions, with 15 per cent of the global disease burden and one-fifth of the world's population. This means that about 579 years of healthy life were lost for every 1000 people living in Sub-Saharan Africa, compared with just 124 for every 1000 people in the Established Market Economies (Fig. 4).

The Study found a sevenfold higher risk of a child dying (that is, a newborn dying before the age of 15) in Sub-Saharan Africa compared to a newborn in the Established Market Economies (Fig. 5). This extraordinary excess mortality in many developing regions must remain a priority for global health programmes. Somewhat surprisingly, the risk of adult death in the FSE region, at least for males, was higher than any other region of the world, except Africa (see Fig. 5). This reflects the rapid increase in adult male death rates in the Russian Federation and neighbouring countries since 1987. In 1990, mortality at these ages (15–59 years) was still rising rapidly in Russia, reaching a peak in 1994. Since then, the probability of death between the ages of 15 and 59 has declined as rapidly as it rose, although evidence for 1999 suggests that death rates may be rising again; the trends for females are qualitatively similar, though less extreme.

The leading causes of death for 2000 were similar to those estimated for 1990, with two notable exceptions. HIV/AIDS, which killed an estimated 300 000 people in 1990, claimed 10 times that number in 2000 and the annual mortality toll continues to rise. Conversely, interventions to control measles and diarrhoea have had a marked impact on mortality from the two conditions, with measles deaths falling from 2 million in 1990 to less than 800 000 in 2000. Diarrhoeal deaths had fallen to 2.1 million in 2000, 1.3 million of them in children under 5-years-old.

The GBD Study has provided support for the theory that people in high-income, low-mortality populations not only live longer, but also remain healthier for longer. In recent years, opinion has been divided between the view that ill health is compressed into the last few years of life in these populations, and the view that longer life merely exposes people to a longer

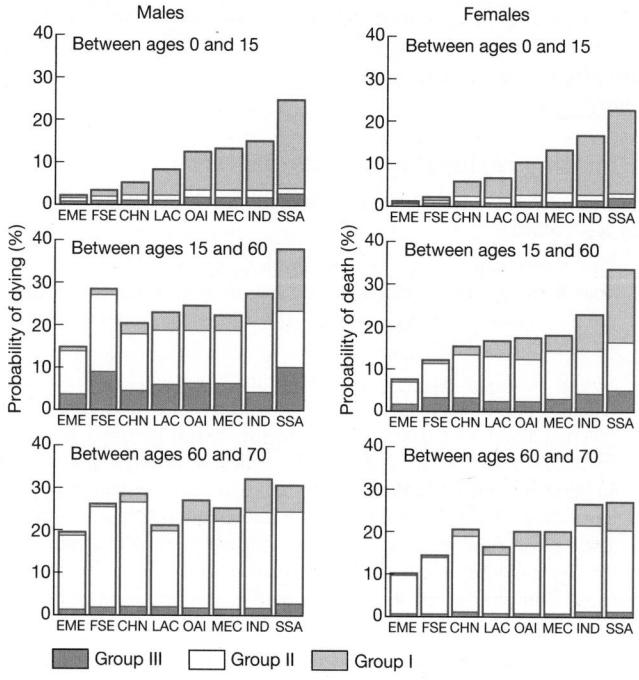

Fig. 5 Regional probabilities of death for males and females by age and group, 1990.

period of poor health. The results suggest that older people in the developed world are healthier than their counterparts in developing countries. It was also found that babies born in Sub-Saharan Africa could expect to spend about 15 per cent of their lifespan disabled, compared to 8 per cent for babies born in the Established Market Economies. The 60-year-olds in Sub-Saharan Africa can expect to spend about half their remaining years with a disability, whereas 60-year-olds in the Established Market Economies are likely to spend one-fifth of those years disabled. The results suggest that the proportion of the lifespan lived with a disability falls as life expectancy rises.

Major causes of disease burden

The leading causes of disease burden in 1990, were lower respiratory infections, diarrhoeal diseases, perinatal causes, and, perhaps unexpectedly, depression (Table 1). The Study showed that the burden of psychiatric disease had been heavily underestimated. Of the ten leading causes of disability worldwide (in YLDs) in 1990, five were psychiatric conditions: unipolar depression, alcohol abuse, bipolar affective disorder, schizophrenia, and obsessive–compulsive disorder. Unipolar depression alone was responsible for more than 1 in every 10 years of life lived with a disability worldwide. Together, psychiatric and neurological conditions accounted for 28 per cent of all YLDs, compared with 1.4 per cent of all deaths and 1.1 per cent of years of life lost. The predominance of these conditions is not restricted to wealthy countries, although their burden is highest there. They were the most important contributors to YLDs in all regions except Sub-Saharan Africa, where they still accounted for 16 per cent of the total.

Alcohol abuse was the leading cause of male disability, and the tenth largest in women, in developed regions and, perhaps surprisingly, the fourth largest cause in men in developing regions. Other important causes of YLDs were anaemia, falls, road traffic accidents, chronic obstructive pulmonary diseases, and osteoarthritis.

Traditional disease burdens in developing societies—communicable, maternal, perinatal conditions, and nutritional deficiencies—remained of major importance in the 1990s. Even though these group I conditions

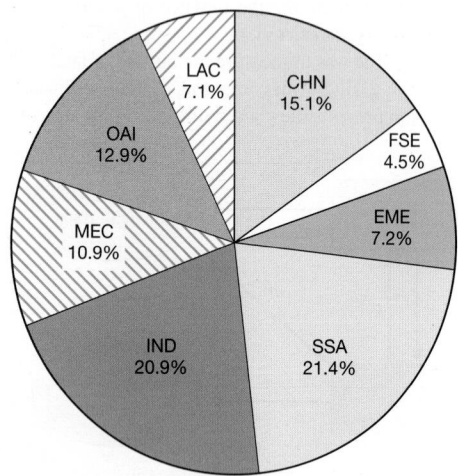

Fig. 4 Distribution of DALYs by region, 1990.

Table 1 Ten leading causes of DALYs 1990 and 2000

1990 Rank	Disease or injury	Cum %	2000 Rank	Disease or injury	Cum %
1	LRI	8.2	1	LRI	6.4
2	Diarrhoeal disease	15.4	2	Perinatal conditions	6.2
3	Perinatal conditions	22.1	3	HIV/AIDS	6.1
4	Depression	25.8	4	Unipolar depressive disorders	4.4
5	IHD	29.2	5	Diarrhoeal disease	4.2
6	Stroke	32.0	6	IHD	3.9
7	Tuberculosis	34.8	7	Cerebrovascular disease	3.2
8	Measles	37.4	8	Road traffic accidents	2.8
9	Road traffic accidents	39.9	9	Malaria	2.7
10	Congenital anomalies	42.3	10	Tuberculosis	2.4

Cum, cumulative; LRI, lower respiratory tract infections; IHD, ischaemic heart disease.

accounted for only 7 per cent of the burden in the Established Market Economies and less than 9 per cent in the Former Socialist Economies, they accounted for more than 40 per cent of the total global burden of disease in 1990, and for 49 per cent in developing regions. In Sub-Saharan Africa, 2 out of every 3 years of healthy life were lost because of group I conditions. Even in China, where the epidemiological transition is far advanced, a quarter of years of healthy life lost were due to this group. Worldwide, five out of ten leading causes of disease burden (as measured by DALYs) are group I conditions: lower respiratory infections (pneumonia); diarrhoeal disease; perinatal conditions; tuberculosis; and measles.

The burden of injury in 1990 was highest (19%) in the FSE region. China had the second largest injury burden, followed by Latin America and the Caribbean. Even in the Established Market Economies the burden of injuries—dominated by road traffic accidents—was almost 12 per cent of the total. In most regions, unintentional injuries were a greater source of ill health in 1990 than intentional injuries such as interpersonal violence and war. The only exception was the Middle Eastern Crescent, where unintentional and intentional injuries took an approximately equal toll because of a particularly high burden of war in the region at the time.

Preliminary estimates of GBD for 2000 suggest that the leading causes are similar to those in 1990, exception for HIV. In 2000, HIV is estimated to have killed 2.95 million people (2.4 million in Africa). HIV/AIDS is the third leading cause of disease burden, accounting for 6.1 per cent of all DALYs lost in 2000, only marginally behind lower respiratory infections (6.4 per cent) and perinatal conditions (6.2 per cent) (Table 1).

Global burden of disease: risk factors

Exposure to particular hazards, such as tobacco, alcohol, unsafe sex, or poor sanitation, can significantly increase people's risks of developing disease. Health policy makers need accurate information on their impact in order to devise effective prevention strategies. The GBD Study assessed, for the first time, the mortality and loss of healthy life that can be attributed to each of 10 major risk factors in each region: malnutrition; poor water supply, sanitation and personal/domestic hygiene; unsafe sex; tobacco abuse; alcohol abuse; occupation; hypertension; physical inactivity; illicit drug use; and air pollution.

The contributions of risk factors to global burden

Malnutrition, poor water, sanitation, and hygiene, unsafe sex, alcohol, tobacco, and occupation proved the most important, accounting together for more than one-third of the total disease burden worldwide in 1990 (see Table 2). Malnutrition and poor sanitation were the dominant hazards, responsible together for almost a quarter of the global burden. Unsafe sex and alcohol each contributed approximately 3.5 per cent, tobacco and occupation hazards just under 3 per cent each. These are similar to the disease burden due to tuberculosis or measles. Major inequalities exist between regions and between men and women in the burdens of most risk

factors. The consequences of unsafe sex, including infections and complications of unwanted pregnancy, are borne disproportionately by women in all regions. In young adult women in Sub-Saharan Africa, unsafe sex accounts for almost one-third of the total disease burden. Tobacco, due to longer exposure, and alcohol caused their heaviest burdens in men in the developed regions, where they accounted together for more than one-fifth of the total burden in 1990. In Asia and other developing regions, the rapid increase in tobacco use over the past few decades is expected to kill many more people in the coming decades than have so far died of this cause in the developed regions.

For the GBD 2000 Study, more than 20 risk factors are being analysed, using a more comparable framework for assessing risk factors. Preliminary results for 2000 suggest little change in the importance of these various risk factors, except for tobacco and unsafe sex, for which disease burdens are rising rapidly, particularly in the developing world. More refined methods have suggested that the blood pressure burden is about twice what was estimated for 1990, although this increase is largely a methodological artefact. Elevated cholesterol is also a major cause of disease burden, about two-thirds that of blood pressure.

Projections of the global burden of disease

To plan health services effectively, policy makers need to know how health needs might change in the future. To meet this need, projections of mortality and disability have been developed for each 5-year period from 1990 to 2020.

Table 2 Contribution of 10 risk factors to the global burden of disease and injury in 1990

Risk factor	Deaths (1000s)	As % of total deaths	DALYs (1000s)	As % of total DALYs
Malnutrition	5881	11.7	219 575	15.9
Poor water supply, sanitation, and personal and domestic hygiene	2668	5.3	93 392	6.8
Unsafe sex	1095	2.2	48 702	3.5
Alcohol	774	1.5	47 687	3.5
Tobacco	3038	6.0	36 182	2.6
Occupation	1129	2.2	37 887	2.7
Hypertension	2918	5.8	19 076	1.4
Physical inactivity	1991	3.9	13 653	1.0
Illicit drugs	100	0.2	8 467	0.6
Air pollution	568	1.1	7 254	0.5

Projection methods

Rather than attempt to model the effects of the many different determinants of disease from the limited data available, mortality change has been modelled as a function of a few socioeconomic variables: (1) income per capita; (2) the average number of years of schooling in adults, termed 'human capital'; and (3) time, a proxy measure for the secular improvement in health this century that results in part from accumulating knowledge and technological development. Historically, these variables have been related to mortality rates: for example, income growth was closely related to the improvement in life expectancy that many countries achieved in the twentieth century. Because of their relationships to death rates, these variables may be regarded as indirect, or distal, determinants of health. A fourth variable, tobacco use, was included, because of its overwhelming impact on the occurrence of chronic diseases, using information from more than four decades of research on the time lag between persistent tobacco use (measured as 'smoking intensity') and its effects on health.

Death rates for all major causes based on historical data for 47 countries from 1950 to 1991 were related to these four variables to generate the projections. A separate model was used for HIV, with modifications for the interaction between HIV and tuberculosis.

Mortality projections

In all regions, life expectancy at birth is expected to increase for women. By 2020, infant girls born in the Established Market Economies may expect to survive to almost 88 years. For men, life expectancy will grow much more slowly, mainly because of the impact of the tobacco epidemic. Nevertheless, by 2020, males born in Sub-Saharan Africa, whose life expectancy at birth was below 50 in 1990, may expect to reach 58 years. Males born in Latin America and the Caribbean, who in 1990 could have expected to live to 65, may expect to reach 71 years. However, for men in the Formerly Socialist Economies of Europe, life expectancy is not expected to increase at all between 1990 and 2020. This is partly due to the fact that life expectancy was falling in 1990, so that any positive change is likely to be merely recovering to the 1990 position.

In young children and adolescents under the age of 15, the risk of death is projected to decline dramatically in all regions, falling by about two-thirds in Sub-Saharan Africa and India. In adult women, too, the risk of death is expected to fall in all regions. Men in the Formerly Socialist Economies of Europe and China, because of the tobacco epidemic, may expect a higher risk of dying between the ages of 15 and 60 than they do today. In other regions, the risk of death for men in this age group is expected to fall, but more modestly than in women. Remarkably, by 2020, men of this age group in the Formerly Socialist Economies of Europe could face a higher risk of death even than men in Sub-Saharan Africa.

Deaths from communicable, maternal and perinatal conditions, and nutritional deficiencies (group I) are expected to fall from 17.3 million in 1990 to 10.3 million in 2020. As a percentage of the total burden, group I conditions are expected to drop by more than half, from 34 per cent to 15 per cent. This projected reduction overall, despite increased burdens due to HIV and possibly tuberculosis, runs counter to the now widely accepted belief that infectious diseases are making a comeback worldwide. It reflects, in part, the relative contraction of the world's 'young' population: the under-15 age group is expected to grow by only 22 per cent between 1990 and 2020, whereas the cohort of adults aged between 15 and 60 is expected to grow by more than 55 per cent. In addition, the projection reflects the observed overall decline in group I conditions over the past four decades, due to increased income, education, and technological progress in the development of antimicrobials and vaccines. Even under the pessimistic scenario, in which both income growth and technological progress are expected to be minimal, deaths from these conditions are still expected to fall slightly to 16.9 million.

It should not be taken for granted that the progress against infectious diseases during the past four decades will be maintained. Antibiotic devel-opment and other control technologies may not keep pace with the emergence of drug-resistant strains of important microbes such as *Mycobacterium tuberculosis*. If such a scenario were to prove correct, and if, in addition, case-fatality rates were to rise because of such drug-resistant strains, the gains of the twentieth century could be halted or even reversed. None the less, the evidence to date, suggests that, as long as current efforts are maintained, group I causes are likely to continue to decline.

While overall, group I conditions are expected to decline, deaths from non-communicable diseases are expected to climb from 28.1 million deaths in 1990 to 49.7 million in 2020, an increase of 77 per cent in absolute numbers. In proportionate terms, group II deaths are expected to increase their share of the total from 55 per cent in 1990 to 73 per cent in 2020. These global figures do not reveal the extreme nature of the change that is projected in some developing regions because they incorporate the projections for the rich nations, which show little change. In India, deaths from non-communicable diseases are projected almost to double, from about 4 million to about 8 million a year, while group I deaths are expected to fall from almost 5 million to below 3 million a year. In the developing world as a whole, deaths from non-communicable diseases are expected to rise from 47 per cent of the total to almost 70 per cent.

The steep projected increase in the burden of non-communicable diseases worldwide is largely driven by population ageing, augmented by the large numbers of people in developing regions who are now exposed to tobacco. Ageing will result in a rise in the absolute numbers of cases of non-communicable diseases and in their increased share of the total disease burden for the population as a whole, but not in any change in the rates of those diseases in any given age group. As studies in the Established Market Economics show, the age-specific rates of some important non-communicable diseases, such as ischaemic heart disease and stroke, have been falling steadily for at least two decades. Whether these rates are also falling in other regions is much less clear. However, any age-specific decrease in the rates of these diseases that may also emerge in low-income countries is likely to be outweighed by the large and demographically driven increase in the absolute numbers of adults at risk from these diseases, augmented by the tobacco epidemic. As with non-communicable diseases, deaths from injury are also expected to rise for mainly demographic reasons. Young adults are generally exposed to greater risks of injury.

Recent health trends in the 1990s: implications for the GBD projections

The original GBD projections were based on data and information about health conditions worldwide during the late 1980s/early 1990s. At that time, two major epidemics were affecting the health of large population groups: the HIV epidemic, particularly in Africa, which killed an estimated 300 000 people worldwide in 1990 but had, by that time, infected millions more; and the explosive increase in the adult mortality rates in Russia and neighbouring countries, particularly from cardiovascular diseases and injuries, and particularly among men. Making projections at a time of such dramatic epidemiological trends is extremely hazardous.

The 1990 GBD Study's HIV/AIDS projections have severely underestimated the spread of the epidemic in Sub-Saharan Africa, particularly in Southern Africa. By 2000, HIV/AIDS was estimated to have killed 2.4 million Africans, several times more than projected on the basis of what was known in 1990. Whether the disease burden will continue to rise, and how far, is uncertain and new projection methods are being developed to forecast the epidemic better, particularly in Africa.

The other large uncertainty in the projections, namely adult mortality in the FSE region, has confounded epidemiologists with the dramatic change in mortality risks during the 1990s. Death rates had been falling markedly in most large countries in this region, and, if they were to continue to do so, the 1990 forecasts will prove to be unduly pessimistic. It is too early to decide whether the recent declines in mortality are the beginning of a long-term secular trend in mortality. Recent evidence for 1999 and 2000 indicates that death rates, particularly in males, have begun to rise again.

Progress in refining the GBD approach

Measuring and evaluating health

An innovation of the GBD Study was the attempt to measure and evaluate states of ill health in a similar way in different societies. This presupposes a common conceptual framework and measurement strategy. In particular, what are the key domains of health that need to be assessed and what is the minimum number of items and response categories needed to measure them? Self-report instruments currently in use lack cross-cultural comparability, with the result that the measurement of health in various populations cannot be compared. The development and implementation of a conceptual framework to measure and describe health in a way that improves comparability across populations is a key challenge for research on burden of disease.

In the GBD Study, comorbid conditions were evaluated separately, and the time spent with these combined states was measured as the sum of the two. This additive model may not be appropriate. More data are required on the prevalence of major comorbidities to avoid multiple attribution in valuing health states.

Conclusions

The GBD Study has provided a picture of current and projected health needs. It has shown that non-communicable diseases are rapidly becoming the dominant causes of ill health in all developing regions except Sub-Saharan Africa; that mental health problems have been underestimated worldwide; and that injuries are important problems in all regions. The findings pose new and immediate challenges to policy makers.

Further reading

Barendregt JJ, Bonneux L, van der Maas, PJ (1998). Health expectancy: from a population health indicator to a tool for policy making. *Journal of Aging and Health* **10**, 242–58.

Murray CJL, Lopez AD, eds (1996). *The global burden of disease: a comprehensive assessment of mortality and disability from diseases, injuries, and risk factors in 1990 and projected to 2020.* Global burden of disease and injury series, Vol. 1. Harvard University Press, Cambridge, MA.

Murray CJL, Lopez AD (1996). *Global health statistics: a compendium of incidence, prevalence and mortality estimates for over 200 conditions.* Global burden of disease and injury series, Vol. 2. Harvard University Press, Cambridge, MA.

Murray CJL, Lopez AD (1999). On the comparable quantification of health risks: lessons from the Global Burden of Disease Study. *Epidemiology* **10**, 594–605.

Murray CJL, Lopez AD (2000). Progress and directions in refining the global burden of disease approach: a response to Williams. *Health Economics* **9**, 69–82.

Murray CJL, Salomon JA, Mathers C (1999). *A critical examination of summary measures of population health.* GPE Working Paper Series, WHO, Geneva.

Peto R, *et al.* (1992). Mortality from tobacco in developed countries: indirect estimation from national vital statistics. *Lancet* **339**, 1268–78.

Sullivan DF (1971). A single index of mortality and morbidity. *Health Reports* **86**, 347–54.

Van de Water HP, Perenboom RJ, Boshuizen HC (1996). Policy relevance of the health expectancy indicator: an inventory of European Union countries. *Health Policy* **36**, 117–29.

Wilkins R, Adams O (1983). Health expectancy in Canada, late 1970's: demographic, regional and social dimensions. *American Journal of Public Health* **73**, 1073–80.

3.2 Human population size, environment, and health

A. J. McMichael and J. W. Powles

Introduction

Homo sapiens originated approximately two hundred thousand years ago. Since then it has undergone three population growth surges: (i) an estimated 50-fold increase as hunter–gatherer humans drifted out of north-eastern Africa and dispersed around the world; (ii) a further 100-fold increase following the advent of agriculture, beginning ten thousand years ago; and then (iii) from just before the industrial revolution, another 10-fold increase from half a billion to six billion.

This third, incomplete, increase has occurred much faster than the two previous increases. Absolute additions to human numbers have been biggest in the past quarter-century, capping an almost-fourfold increase from 1.6 to 6 billion during the twentieth century. However, the annual increase expressed in percentage terms has slowed in the last couple of decades. Demographers expect that by the time the demographic transition is completed worldwide, and birth rates equilibrate with death rates (at historically low levels), world population will have reached between 8 and 11 billion. The medium variant projection for 2050 is approximately 9 billion.

Relationship between environment and population

The relationship between the environment and population size is multifaceted. The main components of that relationships are these: (i) the environment sets limits on the size of the supportable population; (ii) human societies find ways of extending that limit; and (iii) that extension process in turn often leads to the depletion and deterioration of the natural environment.

Carrying capacity

In the natural world, the composition and assets of a species' environment determine the maximum number of individuals of the species that can be supported. For that species, this number is the 'carrying capacity' of its local habitat. There are fluctuations of population size around that number as conditions vary over time. Populations of the human species, uniquely, are not fully constrained by given environmental conditions. Through culture and technology, humans can increase the carrying capacity of their local environments—at least temporarily.

The early domestication of plant species increased food yields and hence population carrying capacity. The subsequent domestication of wild animal species further increased carrying capacity. The advent of agriculture led to a substantial increase in fertility—from an average of 4 to 5 births per completed reproductive lifetime (as reported for traditional hunter–gatherers and, coincidentally, for great apes) to 5 to 7 births per reproductive lifetime in agrarian populations. This greater fecundity meant that the approximate equivalence of birth and death rates in slowly enlarging agrarian populations was attained at very high levels of both. This is well illustrated by India a century ago, when fertility was high (7 to 8 births per

woman) and life expectancy was 20 to 25 years (reflecting especially the high death rates in infancy and childhood).

Overloading the environment

Human communities exploit local natural resource stocks: soil, water, and plants and animals for food and materials. This exploitation, in time, tends to deplete and ultimately degrade environments. Often, the local consequences have been the restriction or decline in human numbers, and impairment of nutritional status and health.

The extent to which humans are disrupting their environment has increased rapidly over the past two centuries, as numbers have expanded and as the material and energy intensities of productive activity have increased. Over the past century or so, adverse environmental effects have mostly been of a localized kind, such as urban-industrial air pollution, chemical pollution of waterways, and urban squalor. Today, human effects on the environment are being played out on a much larger scale—and the longer-term consequences for health could be commensurately more serious. Recent global assessments point to a significant and increasing 'ecological deficit', with manifest decline in natural environmental and ecological resource stocks.

Further, some of these environmental stresses are likely to cause tensions between human communities, leading to armed conflict—another potential source of damage to health. For example, Ethiopia and the Sudan, upstream of Nile-dependent Egypt, increasingly need the Nile's water for their own crop irrigation.

The central issue in all of this is that the ecological underpinnings of human health are being perturbed or depleted. The sustained good health of any population, over time, requires a stable and productive natural environment that: (i) yields assured supplies of food and fresh water, (ii) has a relatively constant climate in which climate-sensitive physical and biological systems do not change for the worse, and (iii) retains biodiversity (a fundamental source of both present and future value). For the human species, as a 'social animal' in the extreme, the richness, texture, and stability of the social environment (i.e. 'social capital') is also important to population health.

A Malthusian perspective on sustainability

Two hundred years ago, Thomas Malthus, responding to the utopian views of William Godwin, de Condorcet, and others about the perfectibility of human institutions, foresaw a potential crisis arising from excessive human numbers within a food-limited environment. The exponential power of population growth would, he concluded, tend always to outstrip the (arithmetic) power of growth in food production. He grimly predicted that population excess in Europe would lead to starvation and die-off—that is, to nature's 'positive checks' that would bring human numbers back in line with food supplies.

In fact, the crisis did not materialize in Europe. Malthus could not have foreseen the remarkable increase in food-producing capacity that the second agricultural revolution, underwritten by mechanization and fossil-fuel energy, would bring during the nineteenth century—or the bonanza of imported grain and meat that Europe's newly-established colonies would provide. Nor could he have foreseen the marked decline in fertility rates that emerged in European populations during the nineteenth century as social modernization occurred and as contraceptive possibilities became widely understood.

Today, nevertheless, a 'Malthusian' perspective is relevant at another level of analysis. In the past quarter-century we have begun to see the evidence that there are limits to the carrying capacity of the globe as a whole. There is mounting evidence, for example, of a damaged stratosphere and of human-induced climate change. These are signs that we are exceeding the carrying capacity of the world as a whole. What might lie in store?

In the natural world, the tendency of plant and animal species to exponential growth is generally constrained by predation, by limits to food supplies, by infectious disease, and, in many animals, by density-dependent changes in reproductive behaviour. As numbers increase, one of the following patterns operates:

(1) logistic (asymptotic) growth, responding to immediate negative feedback, as carrying capacity is approached;

(2) domed or capped growth, responding to deferred negative feedback, necessitating compensatory die-off; or

(3) irruptive growth, with a chaotic post-crash pattern.

Our recognition, today, of the risk of overshoot and collapse (patterns 2 and 3) underlies the increasing attention being paid to the need for 'environmentally sustainable development'. Simplifying, there are two main adverse outcomes to which an excess of human numbers might contribute: (i) recurrent subsistence crises on a subnational or national level, or (ii) 'planetary overload'.

Local subsistence crises

The focus of concern with 'overpopulation' in much of the latter half of the twentieth century was the likelihood that the growth of many local populations would overload local carrying capacities. Chronic food shortages would ensue and undernutrition would force mortality rates up towards equilibrium with fertility, both at unfavourably high levels. The emiserating effects of population pressure would prevent economic development, prolong population growth, and leave such populations 'demographically entrapped'.

So far, however, there appear to have been few developments in this direction. The famines that have occurred in recent decades, the most serious being the Chinese famine of 1959 to 1961 with around 15 to 20 million deaths, have not been attributable primarily to the progressive reduction of food-producing resources per person. Rather, they appear to have arisen from either economic mismanagement (as in the case of the Chinese 'great leap forward') or warfare (as in parts of Africa)—although the contributory causes of some of that strife may include local population pressures on dwindling natural resources. The recent generally favourable trends in per-person food supplies may not be sustainable as populations double (or more) in size in poor countries such as Bangladesh that already have less than one-tenth of a hectare of cropland per person.

Planetary overload

While local subsistence pressures persist or increase in many parts of the world, there is a newer form of pressure arising at the global level. Human population size and the material intensity of our economies are now so great that, at that global level, we are beginning to disrupt some of the biosphere's life-support systems. The clearest evidence of the occurrence of 'global environmental change' is the documented destruction of stratospheric ozone, particularly in polar and subpolar regions, over the past quarter-century and the apparent incipient changes in world climate due to greenhouse-gas accumulation in the lower atmosphere. There is a net ongoing loss of productive soils on all continents; we have overfished most of the ocean fisheries; we have severely depleted many of the great aquifers

upon which irrigated agriculture depends; we are extinguishing at an unprecedented overall rate whole species and many local population;, and, increasingly, persistent human-made organic (especially chlorinated) chemicals are pervading the biosphere.

These various changes are perturbing or weakening systems in the biosphere that provide the stabilization, replenishment, organic production, cleansing, and recycling that our predecessors were able to take for granted in a less populated, less degraded, world. Manifestly we no longer live in such a world. This weakening of Earth's basic life-supporting processes poses a spectrum of long-term risks to human population health. The currently foreseeable risks from these environmental changes include: (i) an anticipated increase in skin cancer rates (and perhaps in ocular disorders and immune system suppression) due to the approximately 10 per cent increase in ultraviolet radiation levels that has now accrued at middle latitudes; (ii) a likely increase in geographical range and seasonality of vector-borne infectious diseases such as malaria and dengue fever under conditions of climate change; (iii) increased exposure, in some parts of the world, to weather extremes and disasters, consequent upon climate change; and (iv) malnutrition and hunger in local populations whose agricultural productivity is adversely affected by changes in climate, soil fertility, freshwater supplies, and the ecology of pests and pathogens.

Contribution of population increase to environmental disruption

The World Wildlife Fund for Nature has analysed in detail the trends over the past three decades in the vitality and function of major categories of ecological systems, including freshwater, marine, and forest ecosystems. Overall, the 'Living Planet Index' has declined by 30 per cent since 1970. Assessments by other international agencies approximately concur.

The three main determinants of human disruption of the environment are population size, the level of material wealth and consumption, and the types of technology. The ongoing climate change debate illustrates well the relativities between the environmental effects of increases in population and consumption. Historically, during the twentieth century, as population increased by just under fourfold the annual fossil fuel emissions of carbon dioxide increased 12-fold. In 1995, the 20 per cent of world population living in high-emission countries accounted for 63 per cent of carbon dioxide emissions, while the lowest-emitting 20 per cent of population contributed just 2 per cent. Over the coming century the projected world population growth will contribute an estimated 35 per cent of growth in carbon dioxide emissions, whereas economic growth would account for the remaining 65 per cent.

If the world were to limit carbon dioxide build-up to a doubling of its preindustrial concentration (i.e. from 275 to 550 p.p.m.)—a level which climatologists think would be tolerable to most ecosystems—then the United Nations medium population projection of 10 to 11 billion by 2100 would allow per-person carbon dioxide emissions similar to those of the 1920 to 1930s. That is approximately two-thirds less than today's level of emissions (see Fig. 1). While that looms as a very demanding task, we actually already have much of the necessary technology to reduce emissions greatly without forfeiture of material standards of living. The real challenge is political—to transform current technologies and economic practice.

Overall, then, the larger potential threat is not from the increase in human numbers *per se* but from mildly environmentally disruptive humans becoming highly disruptive humans—in other words, from a 'development' process that would generalize the patterns of production and consumption typical of today's rich countries. Current practices in rich countries cannot be applied to a human population likely to exceed 10 billion and demanding a higher average standard of living. The Netherlands requires an estimated area 15 times greater than its national size to support its population's way of life. It has been estimated that citizens of high-income countries today each require approximately 4 to 9 ha of the

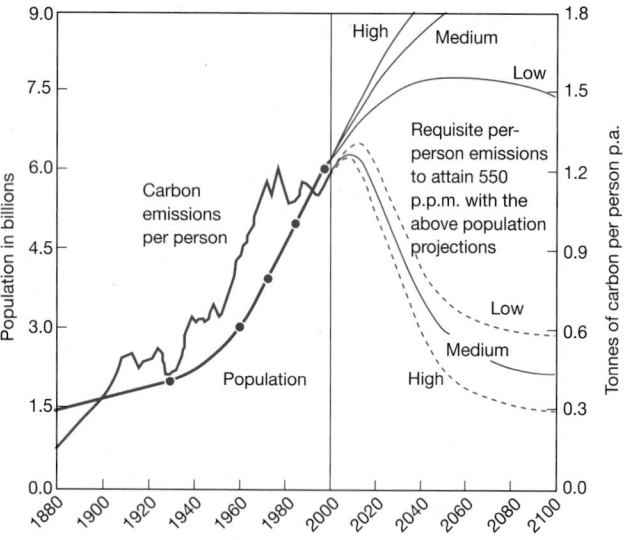

Fig. 1 This shows the configuration of relationships between economic activity, wealth distribution (especially poverty), population size, environmental conditions, and human health. Note that poverty and the material (natural and social) environment are major determinants of health.

Earth's surface to provide the materials for their lifestyle and to absorb their wastes—while India's population gets by on 1 ha per person. There is not enough Earth to allow more than 1 ha of 'ecological footprint' per average-person when the world population reaches 10 billion during the coming century—and yet that future world population will presumably wish to live like Californians, not Calcuttans.

Serious investment in the development and deployment of less environmentally disruptive technologies, and a much greater commitment to international equity, will be required if a smooth and timely transition to an ecologically sustainable world is to be achieved. Because rich countries remain the main source of new knowledge and new technologies, responsibility for finding paths to sustainability rests mainly with them. Minimizing the probabilities of long-term harm to health will be a major consideration. Indeed, this is now becoming the most important health-related aspect of the 'population debate'.

'Green accounting'

We cannot predict, with certainty, how the adverse health effects of ecological disruption will unfold. It therefore makes sense to concentrate, in the short term, on our society's direction of travel, on whether we are moving closer to, or further away from, sustainable paths of economic development. To this end we need to devise and implement new indicators of material progress.

Sustainability has recently been defined by the Environment Department of the World Bank as leaving to future generations 'as many opportunities as we ourselves have had, if not more'. Sustainability can be more readily expressed in operational terms using measures of economic 'stock' (i.e. capital, including natural capital and human resources) than using measures of 'flow' (income). In this context, conventional national income accounts are both biased (they treat living off natural capital as income) and insensitive (they provide little indication of legacies for the future). A broad measure of wealth would combine the estimated values of natural and human resources with those of produced assets (capital as traditionally

considered). Human resources include the 'human capital' embodied in individuals (augmented by health and education levels) and 'social capital' embodied in institutions, customs, and knowledge.

Employing these categories, a pattern of economically sustainable development can be envisaged as one that conserves natural capital while rebuilding (with 'green' technology) the stock of produced assets, and augmenting human and social capital. This shift of emphasis from flows to stocks accords with recent analyses of health trends. For example, in low- and middle-income countries, indicators such as school attendance rates for girls and literacy among adult women are correlated more strongly with the level of child mortality than is income. Countries at similar levels of income may have several-fold differences in child mortality, with the 'better performers' typically showing higher levels of relevant aspects of social capital.

For rich countries, this approach recognizes that health depends less on the consumption opportunities provided by income than on personal and social capacities to protect and enhance health— reflecting, at the individual level, determinants such as schooling and, at the social level, determinants such as food cultures (for example the protection against vascular mortality in Mediterranean populations) and elements of the built environment such as sewers, water supplies, and safe roads. Given that life expectancy differences among high-income countries are, at most, very weakly related to income, it makes little sense to see increasing national income as an important path to sustainable improvements in health.

Conclusion

Over the last two centuries new knowledge of disease and its control, improvements in material conditions, and the enhancement of individual capabilities through education and of social capacities through development of new institutional forms have yielded previously unimaginable improvements in health and longevity. During the historical gap between the fall in the death rates and the fall in birth rates, populations increased rapidly—and are still doing so in many poorer countries. Meanwhile, in high-income countries, attention should be substantially redirected from achieving yet higher local levels of health to developing the conditions necessary to both generalize and sustain good health worldwide.

A first essential is birth control, for without it death control is unsustainable. A second task is to revise our expectations of 'progress' and to reconstruct the milestones by which we measure it, so that the interests of future generations are safeguarded. Physicians are well placed to foster greater public understanding of why large-scale environmental disruption is likely to jeopardize the health of our grandchildren.

Further reading

Intergovernmental Panel on Climate Change (1996). *Second assessment report. Climate change 1995*, Vol. I, II, and III. Cambridge University Press, New York.

Loh J *et al.* (1998). *Living planet report.* World Wildlife Fund International, Gland, Switzerland.

McMichael AJ (1993). *Planetary overload. Global environmental change and the health of the human species.* Cambridge University Press, Cambridge.

UN Department of Economic and Social Affairs (Population Division) (1999). *World population prospects. The 1998 revision*, Document ST/ESA/SER.A/ 177. United Nations, New York.

World Resources Institute, United Nations Environment Programme, United Nations Development Programme, World Bank (1998). *World resources 1998–99.* Oxford University Press, New York.

3.3 The pattern of care: hospital and community

Anthony Harrison

Introduction

Changes in the treatments available over the last 100 years have transformed the care of individuals. Conditions once untreatable, can now be successfully dealt with, while advances in public health have transformed the pattern of disease confronting the health care system, eliminating or virtually eliminating some diseases. These developments have had a strong influence on the pattern of health care delivery. For much of the twentieth century they led to an expansion of the role of hospitals, but towards the end of the century the scope for moving care to other settings was increasingly recognized.

In 1920, a committee chaired by Lord Dawson set out a blueprint for the way that health care services should be delivered in England. The pattern it proposed consisted of primary and secondary care centres, the first located as near as possible to the local population, and the second in any sizeable urban area. If that area was not large enough to support a teaching hospital, the secondary centre and the teaching hospital should be linked professionally. The primary care centres would provide for a wide range of services including general practice and dentistry and, despite their modest size, inpatient beds. Their location in a single facility would, it was hoped, encourage professional interchange and collaboration. This early attempt to set out a vision for the pattern of health care delivery across all services forming a defined geographical area was not implemented even in the country for which it was devised. However, two central issues were presented that continued to preoccupy policymakers ever since.

1. Exactly which clinical services should be provided locally and which regionally or even nationally?

2. How should the various elements be persuaded to work together?

These questions face any health system but the way they are approached varies according to the way that health care is organized and financed. To outside observers, the British National Health Service (**NHS**), funded almost entirely from a single source and under the control of a single central body, in contrast for example to the pluralist systems obtaining in the United States or Germany, has seemed ideally placed to resolve these issues in a systematic way. In practice, however, solutions have remained elusive in all health care systems.

Since Lord Dawson put forward his proposals, the expansion of clinical knowledge, the specialization that goes with it, and the introduction of expensive diagnostic hardware created pressures for larger concentrations of clinical skills within hospitals. That trend was further strengthened by the growth of clinical research in close association with the patient care and teaching functions of the large acute hospital. Hospital development and clinical progress appeared almost synonymous.

Towards the end of the twentieth century, however, that perception began to change. Although the acute hospital has retained a central role in the health care system, its relative importance has begun to decline. Table 1 sums up some of the key changes within England: similar trends are apparent and indeed are in some cases more advanced in other countries.

The growth in activity as measured by the number of patients treated reflects the massive increase in the scope of hospital work brought about by developments in medical technology such as imaging and endoscopy and the vast new range of surgical procedures such as joint replacement, from which a wide range of the population can benefit.

The large acute hospital has been the physical expression of modern medicine through most of the twentieth century, but it became obvious, towards the end of the century, that technological development was allowing effective care to be provided off the hospital site for conditions once treated within it. Consequently, the scale of some elements of hospital care could be reduced.

A combination of developments in clinical technology, particularly in anaesthesia and surgical techniques, and financial pressures imposed by those paying for care, whether government or private insurers attempting to control health care spending, has resulted in continuing losses of bed capacity even while the numbers of treated patients have gone up. Loss of beds was particularly noticeable in surgical specialties as, from the early 1990s onwards, the proportion of patients treated as day (ambulatory) cases rose rapidly. Medical specialties also lost beds, as lengths of stay fell. Thus the acute hospital sector has continued to expand throughout the twentieth century, but its physical capacity, as defined by its bed-stock, has begun to decline. Turnover has become increasingly rapid. This in turn has meant that its efficient operation is increasingly dependent on effective links with community-based services offering aftercare and other forms of support.

These changes in the acute hospital in themselves implied some degree of shift of care to community settings. Rapid discharge schemes and hospital at home schemes have been developed, often administered by community-based nurses. They complemented the hospital's drive to reduce length of stay and use its remaining bed-stock more intensively. Similarly, other parts of what was once the hospital's role, such as check-ups following an inpatient admission, have tended to become the responsibility of general practice.

These changes were part of a wider and more fundamental development—the dispersal of a wide range of hospital activities to other settings, inspired by developments in technology, changes in clinical practice, and the search for lower costs of provision. The rapid introduction of new drugs from the 1950s onwards allowed general practitioners to deal with a large number of conditions which at one time would have been part of the hospital's workload. In some cases, such as diabetes, technological developments—in this case simple self-monitoring devices—allowed some

Table 1 Key changes in the hospital sector since the 1960s

More patients being treated
Much shorter hospital stays
Many more people treated as outpatients
Few long-stay patients
Chronic conditions largely managed in the community
Fewer hospitals

care to be effectively transferred to the patient's own home. Hospitals were needed only for emergencies.

Lord Dawson's proposal for primary care centres was not widely adopted in its country of origin, but the idea that general practice should be the universal front-line of the health service was, in England and many other countries, seen as the foundation of a properly organized health service. General practice offers ready access and continuity of care, but also some control via the gatekeeping function, to the high-cost services of the hospital. This restriction of patient choice has not been universally accepted. Germany for example continues to allow patients to consult specialists directly. The United States has not had the same tradition of general practice and has, until recently, offered freedom of choice. However, financial pressures have led to the creation of managed care organizations aimed at restricting access to specialist, hospital-based care.

The general practitioner or community-based physician has assumed a co-ordinating role. The range of professional services, closely connected to the practice, has grown and with it the concept of an integrated primary care team emerged, reflecting the range of services, such as nursing, physiotherapy, and counselling, that come within the ambit of general practice or work in close association with it.

While the pattern of acute care was changing, an even more dramatic change was taking place in long-stay hospitals housing the elderly, the mentally ill, and those with learning disabilities. Clinical developments, particularly new drugs for the control of severe mental illness, played their part. However, the main explanation for this switch from hospital to community was the perception, which became widespread in the 1980s and 1990s, that most people housed in these institutions did not need to be there. With appropriate support from housing and social services as well as clinical staff, they could perhaps live reasonably normal lives in the community.

However, problems remain. The switch of some care to the community has not been wholly successful. The transfer of care for the mentally ill away from large isolated institutions to smaller local units supported by a network of health care and other community-based services has led to the emergence of a different pattern. Many patients reach specialist care by self-referral or other routes, and for many, the main point of contact is a community nurse and/or social worker rather than a general practitioner. Their roles are central to the creation of community support networks which provide access to housing, and recreational and other facilities essential to everyday life. Such networks have proved hard to manage and, in practice, the necessary liaison between their various elements has not always been possible, particularly in times of crisis.

The switch of care for long-stay groups into the community has led to closures of the large hospital institutions that once housed them. These trends have led to the closure of smaller acute hospitals—or a drastic reduction in the scope of their activity through, for example, the transfer of inpatient admission facilities to other sites. This has been bitterly resisted by local communities, but the combination of cost pressures and clinically based arguments in favour of concentration of services has often proved decisive.

Such rationalizations have been based on the presumption that larger hospitals are better, both economically and clinically. The evidence on both is limited. What exists is often of poor quality since confounding factors make it hard to disentangle the effects of size on the outcomes of care. Overall the available evidence does suggest that specialization of clinical roles with concentration of hospital work in fewer sites produces better results. How far this process should go remains unclear and in some areas of care it may already have gone too far.

Working together

Although most episodes of care are 'singletons' consisting of a visit to one health care professional such as a general practitioner or dentist in the community or the accident and emergency department of a hospital, many are complex, involving many different professionals even within a single hospital institution and extending for long periods. Modern medicine has virtually eradicated some diseases and has contributed, with the social and economic trends associated with the growth of personal incomes, to prolonging life. This has meant that a large part of clinical practice is taken up with chronic conditions and with treating frail elderly people who often need continuing support after, for example, an episode of acute hospital care.

An effective health care system requires that these various contributions are made by the most appropriate professionals and are co-ordinated to prevent the patient falling through gaps between different organizations or professionals. These requirements have proved difficult to fulfil. Even within the British National Health Service funded from a single central source and under unified management, there are frequent failures of the various elements to mesh together properly. Failures often occur at the interface between different organizations. A persistent area of difficulty has been hospital discharge, particularly for those requiring postoperative support. Delays have given rise to the notion of the 'blocked bed'. Blocks can sometimes be attributed to poor internal communications within the hospital. They also reflect failure to co-ordinate the hospital discharge process with provision of community health and social care services. This failure reflects differences in source of funding, which create a division—artificial from the viewpoint of the patient—of responsibility for closely related care functions.

Research has revealed important gaps in the care system, particularly in rehabilitation after stroke or heart attack. As a result, too many people may be prematurely admitted to community long-stay institutions. Again the difficulties can in part be attributed to the failure of the financial mechanism to match clinical and patient requirements.

The search for better service integration has stimulated a number of initiatives. In hospitals, these range from large-scale re-engineering of the hospital as a whole to more modest attempts to improve the care pathways for specific groups of patient such as those receiving new joints or other procedures where some degree of care after discharge is required. In some cases, such pathways extend across care providers. The British government has recently introduced the concept of a national service framework. This is intended to define both the elements required from all forms of provision—hospital and community—and the way they should work together to form a clinically integrated system of care. In principle, this should ensure a correct balance between preventive and curative means and should enable patients needing care to be correctly and promptly routed to an appropriately equipped and trained clinical team. In the United States and elsewhere, disease management programmes have been developed with similar objectives.

Cost pressures have meant that the orchestration of the various contributions of complex episodes of care has been combined with a search for the best combination of professional contributions, where necessary across the boundaries of existing disciplines. It is increasingly accepted that different professional roles are to some extent interchangeable. Many health care systems are experimenting with mixtures of different skills, allowing nurses and in some cases technicians to take over roles which were once exclusively medical.

The emphasis on clinical integration has led to the creation of new professional roles such as liaison nurses. They are intended to co-ordinate contributions by different organizations, for instance that hospital and community professionals co-operate at the point of discharge and that the various elements required for post-discharge support are put in place.

The search for the effective integration of care across the boundary of the hospital and the community continues. In the United Kingdom, the Labour Government's first white paper on health policy, *The new NHS*, suggested ways in which health and social care providers might work together harmoniously.

Conclusions

The pattern of health care services will continue to change, as a result of continuing technical developments within medical and information technology and as a result of social and financial pressures for new forms of service delivery. The balance between hospital and community and between hospitals of different sizes and structure will vary according to the relative advantages in access, cost, and clinical effectiveness of treatment in different locations.

For clinicians, the most important development is the move towards the definition of care pathways and whole systems of care for broad disease groups running across the boundaries of individual hospitals and those of community- and hospital-based organizations. While the bulk of medical training and practice will remain focused on the individual intervention and the patient encounter, the vision of health care delivery is of a series of integrated pathways or networks. Clinicians must start to take responsibility for system management as well as patient care.

Critical future developments may lie as much with the user as the professional. Many health systems have been introducing a new front line—the telephone. In England, after a series of experiments in different parts of the country, the first steps were taken in 1998 towards the introduction of a national network of nurse-provided advice lines. Information technology is making it easier to gain access to knowledge that was once the preserve of the professional. Many large health care institutions in the United States now have websites which are accessible worldwide. The NHS has recently opened a site of its own: NHS Online. Patients are becoming better informed. If these developments succeed in changing the balance between professional and user, new patterns of care will emerge that suit the user rather than the professional. In some areas, such as maternity care and mental health, this is already happening.

Further reading

Ferguson B, Sheldon T, Posnett J, eds (1997). *Concentration and choice in healthcare*. FT Healthcare, London.

Grumbach K, Bodenheimer T (1995). The organization of health care. *Journal of the American Medical Association* **273**, 160–67.

Harrison A (2001). *Making the right connections*. King's Fund Publishing, London.

Johnson S, ed. (1997). *Pathways of care*. Blackwell Science, Oxford.

Leutz WN (1999). Five laws for integrating medical and social services: lessons from the United States and the United Kingdom. *The Milbank Quarterly* **77**, 77–110.

Robinson JC (1994). The changing boundaries of the American hospital. *The Milbank Quarterly* **72**, 259–75.

Shortell SM (1995). Reinventing the American hospital. *The Milbank Quarterly* **73**, 131–59.

Shortell SM *et al.* (1996). *Remaking health care in America: building organized delivery systems*. Jossey-Bass Inc., San Francisco.

Starfield B (1994). Is primary care essential? *The Lancet* **344**, 1129–33.

Starfield B (1998). *Primary care: balancing health needs, services, and technology*. Oxford University Press, New York.

Stevens R (1989). *In sickness and in wealth: American hospitals in the twentieth century*. Basic Books Inc., USA.

Stoeckle JD (1995). The citadel cannot hold: technologies go outside the hospital, patients and doctors too. *The Milbank Quarterly* **73**, 3–17.

Wilson J (1997). *Integrated care management: the path to success*. Butterworth-Heinemann, Oxford.

3.4 Preventive medicine

D. Mant

In his millennium address, Nelson Mandela reminded the world that 'we close the century with most people still languishing in poverty, subjected to hunger, preventable disease, illiteracy and insufficient shelter'. The health gap between rich and poor nations is shameful. For example, life expectancy in Malawi is 34 years compared with 79 years in Sweden. But even in the economically developed world many people still die prematurely. In England and Wales almost 1.4 million years of working life are lost each year due to death before age 65 years. Again, there is a marked gap between rich and poor—the death rate from lung cancer in males aged 20 to 64 years is almost three times as great in social classes IV/V (SMR 151) as in I/II (SMR 58). It is naïve to think that medicine will remedy this situation. The fundamental step in achieving good health remains the elimination of poverty, with consequent access to food, sanitation, education, and shelter. But the power of medicine lies in the scientific understanding it provides of the disease process. Preventive medicine uses this understanding both to try to reduce the risk of disease and to detect and treat appropriately emergent disease before it does damage.

What is the scope for prevention? Figure 1 shows the number of women expected to die at different ages if 10 000 were subject to the age-specific death rates in England and Wales of today compared with the1870s (the pattern is similar for men). The dramatic fall in deaths during childhood and early adulthood has meant that the modal age of death is now over 80 years. However, what medicine cannot offer is immortality. The proportion of women surviving to age 65 who live on to age 100 is still very low, about 0.5 per cent. So there seems to be a reasonable expectation that effective preventive medicine might make death before age 70 or 80 years

uncommon—but the objective is delay of death, and hopefully better quality of life before death, rather than absolute prevention of death.

Preventive strategies

The prevention paradox

The main difference between preventive and curative medicine is the focus on risk. Preventive medicine aims to reduce the risk of disease and the risk of further morbidity and mortality in those who develop disease. It offers hope for the future rather than immediate benefit. The benefit from preventive medicine is the absence of future disease. This is a difficult benefit to champion, particularly to the individual. As Geoffrey Rose pointed out many years ago, not only is the benefit intangible but many people must take precautions in order to prevent illness in only a few. Even in a country where diphtheria is common, several hundred children must be immunized to prevent one death. Rose called this the prevention paradox—a preventive measure which brings large benefits to the community may offer little to each participating individual.

The risk paradox

Epidemiological studies define risk factors for disease—the personal or environmental characteristics which increase the likelihood of developing the disease. One of the risk factors for cardiovascular disease is a high level of cholesterol in the blood. Figure 2 shows the prevalence of high cholesterol in the United Kingdom population, the death rate associated with each cholesterol level, and the proportion of all deaths attributable to cholesterol occurring at each level. The risk paradox is that although those with

Fig. 1 Numbers of women dying at different ages if 10 000 were subject from birth to the mortality rate current in 1871 to 1880 compared with that in 1977–9. (Figure originally drawn by Doll R. *British Medical Journal*, 1982; **286**: 445–53.)

Fig. 2 Proportion of coronary heart disease deaths attributable to raised serum cholesterol occurring at each level (figures above columns). Columns show the prevalence of different levels of cholesterol in the population. The broken line shows coronary heart disease mortality at each level. (Reproduced from Rose G. *Strategy for prevention.* Oxford University Press, 1992: 23.)

a blood cholesterol of 7.5 mmol/l or greater are at highest individual risk of disease, the population at highest risk is that associated with a cholesterol level of 5.5 to 6.0 mmol/l. This is simply because of the number of people at risk—there are far fewer people in the high than in the moderate risk group. Targeting just the high-risk group will have relatively little impact on the total number of deaths.

Defining the at-risk population

As preventive medicine seeks to reduce future disease, its patients are usually identified by characteristics which predict risk of developing the disease. It is usual to define this risk in one of three ways—demographic, phenotypic, or familial. Within each category, further subpopulations may be identified as at particularly high risk.

Demographic risk

This is the most common way to define the target group for preventive medicine. Both the United States and Canadian task forces on prevention (see further reading) classify preventive interventions by the age of the target population. Screening programmes, which often target gender-specific diseases (e.g. breast and cervical cancer), may also specify the target population by sex. Geographical specification of risk tends to reflect health-care system boundaries but some preventive programmes target specific ethnic or socially disadvantaged groups.

Phenotypic risk

A phenotype is a set of observable characteristics of an individual or group. Most epidemiological risk factors for disease (e.g. smoking, obesity, hyperlipidaemia) are phenotypic. Other phenotypic categories used to define at-risk populations are behaviours (e.g. smoking, driving), disease states (e.g. diabetes, angina), and physical characteristics (e.g. obesity, cholesterol level). As phenotypic risks are sometimes interactive (i.e. more than one risk factor influences a specific disease risk), multiple risk assessment is an increasingly common practice.

Familial risk

Recent advances in genetic technology have increased our ability to characterize familial risk accurately, and further advance is likely in the next few years. At present, most preventive medicine programmes in this area use genetic assessment to refine assessment of individual risk in phenotypically identified high-risk families (e.g. cystic fibrosis, neurofibromatosis) or populations (e.g. Down's syndrome). However, the characterization of risk based on population-based genetic screening is already technically feasible in the economically developed world.

Identifying the at-risk population

Some public health interventions can be applied without identifying the at-risk population—you can pass seat belt legislation and increase the tax on tobacco without identifying either drivers or smokers. However, most interventions in clinical preventive medicine are delivered to individuals. It is therefore necessary not only to define the at-risk population but also to identify the individuals within it. You don't just need to know that smokers are at risk, you need to know who smokes. Again, this is usually done in one of three ways—registration, screening, and case-finding.

Registration

Most socialized health systems keep registers. These may be simply demographic (e.g. age, sex, and address) or contain phenotypic or genetic details of individuals. Effective preventive medicine is much easier where registration exists and its accuracy is systematically maintained.

Screening

This topic is covered in Chapter 3.6. The objective is to identify early disease or high risk of disease (e.g. neoplastic dysplasia) before significant morbidity occurs. Its most important feature is that it can do harm as well

as good (it may generate 'false alarms' and detect disease which would not otherwise present during the patient's lifetime) and benefit needs to be carefully assessed, normally in a randomized trial. Population screening is most efficient when based on an accurate population register.

Case-finding

This involves identifying at-risk individuals during routine clinical work (normally in clinical consultations, but sometimes through contact or family tracing). It is less efficient than systematic population screening, but sometimes provides better access to socially disadvantaged groups who may respond poorly to screening invitations or have no registered address. It also allows some interventions to be given at a particularly appropriate moment (e.g. smoking cessation advice at a consultation for cough or contraceptive advice after termination of pregnancy).

Interventions to modify risk

The marked improvements in health which have been achieved in economically developed countries over the past 200 years are not attributable to medicine. Life expectancy has doubled mainly because of environmental control of infectious pathogens (through sanitation and control of insect vectors) and a lifestyle which reduces individual susceptibility to infectious disease (better food, shelter, and education). So although medical science can play an important role in guiding public health policy by improving understanding of the mechanisms of disease, and specific medical interventions allow us to treat disease when it occurs, the role of preventive medicine should not be overestimated. In particular, the medical profession should not take upon itself responsibilities for public health which are more appropriately assumed by governments and other social and environmental agencies.

However, preventive medicine is an important and integral part of good curative medicine. All doctors have a responsibility to think about why someone is ill. Whatever cause is identified (physiological, social, or psychological) the question of whether the cause can be prevented (and the risk of future disease reduced) should be addressed. Doctors who work in a primary care role (particularly those with a registered population) have the added responsibility to ask themselves whether the risk should be addressed at a population rather than just an individual patient level.

Primary and secondary prevention

Preventive interventions have traditionally been categorized as primary, secondary, and tertiary depending on their objectives. However, the term secondary prevention is now commonly used to cover both secondary and tertiary categories. According to this common usage, primary and secondary prevention can be defined as follows.

1. Primary prevention—interventions to reduce the risk of disease in healthy people (e.g. use of seat belts to prevent injury in car accidents; tobacco control to prevent the occurrence of smoking-related disease; immunization against infectious disease).

2. Secondary prevention—interventions to prevent avoidable morbidity in people with disease (e.g. treatment of vascular disease with aspirin; screening for early cancer).

It is immediately obvious that the distinction between primary and secondary is sometimes difficult. Some interventions can fall into more than one category (e.g. stopping smoking reduces the progression as well as onset of many smoking-related diseases) and the definition of disease is not absolute (e.g. many apparently healthy people will have undetected disease). Nevertheless, the pragmatic categorization of preventive interventions into primary and secondary is often useful in practice.

Immunization

Immunity can be induced against many pathogenic bacteria and viruses. Active immunity is usually achieved by stimulating antibody production by

Fig. 3 Laboratory reports of *Haemophilus influenzae* type b before and after introduction of the Hib vaccine (England and Wales 1989 to 1995). (Reproduced by permission of the Controller, Her Majesty's Stationery Office.)

vaccination with an inactivated organism (pertussis, hepatitis A/B), an attenuated live organism (measles, rubella), an antigenic component of the organism (influenza, pneumococcus) or an inactivated toxin (tetanus, diphtheria). Long-lasting immunity can be induced with a single dose of live vaccine. At least two and sometimes three doses are needed for other vaccines, although once an IgG antibody response has been induced, antibody levels are likely to remain high for months or years and can usually be reinforced by a single booster dose. Passive immunity is achieved by injection of human immunoglobulin and therefore protection lasts only a few weeks.

Vaccination can be a very effective preventive strategy. Vaccination against smallpox has led to global eradication of the disease; eradication of polio seems a feasible global objective in the next decade. Vaccination against many other diseases, particularly diseases of childhood such as measles, diphtheria, and polio, has led to rapid and dramatic falls in disease incidence. Figure 3 shows the impact of introduction of the Hib vaccine in 1992 on the incidence of *Haemophilus influenzae* infection in England and Wales.

A number of new and important vaccines are on the horizon—for example, a malaria vaccine. But the existence of an effective vaccine does not guarantee the success of an immunization programme. This depends on the effective delivery of the vaccine to the at-risk population. Vaccination programmes are often limited in their effect by affordability (many vaccines are too expensive for developing countries), acceptability (parental anxiety about the adverse effects of pertussis vaccine has limited its uptake in many countries), and deliverability (vaccines may lose potency if stored outside a refrigerator). There are also potential problems with the antigenic variability of organisms (e.g. influenza) and the difficulty of immunizing at an age young enough to prevent morbidity but old enough to stimulate an immune response (e.g. measles). Nevertheless, immunization is probably the most important medical contribution to primary disease prevention.

Prophylactic treatment

Although most people think of medicines as cures for current illness, many medicines are prescribed with a view to preventing future illness. Antibiotics are given before surgery to prevent postoperative infection, antimalarials to prevent malaria in travellers, anticoagulants to prevent stroke in people with atrial fibrillation, and lipid-lowering agents to prevent heart attacks in people at high risk of cardiovascular disease. The duration of treatment may also be extended beyond the initial treatment phase to achieve a preventive effect. Antidepressants are continued after cure to prevent relapse, ACE inhibitors to prevent worsening of ventricular dysfunction, and uricosuric agents to prevent further episodes of gout.

It must be clear from these examples that many, perhaps most, drugs have the potential to be used for prevention as well as cure. In some cases (e.g. treatment of diabetes) the distinction between prevention and cure is unhelpful—treatment aims to prevent morbidity in both the short and

long term. However, in all the examples given, prescribing is limited to a defined high-risk group. Prophylactic treatment with drugs is less helpful when a high-risk population cannot be easily defined. It is almost always inappropriate to use prophylactic treatment to reduce population risk for three reasons: the strategy is seldom cost-effective, increasing the reliance of the population on medicine is an adverse social outcome, and uncommon adverse effects can easily outweigh any clinical benefit. The last point has been repeatedly demonstrated in clinical trials, including the use of lipid-lowering agents to prevent heart disease and antioxidants to prevent the development of cancer.

Changing behaviour

Environmental factors contribute substantially to differences in premature morbidity and mortality. Many of these environmental factors reflect individual behaviour. Eating more healthily, taking more exercise, and avoiding riding on a motorcycle are all effective ways of preventing disease. People do listen to doctors, and a number of clinical trials have shown advice on behaviour modification to be cost-effective, even though the effect size may be small (e.g. in most studies only about 1 in 20 to 30 smokers given brief advice to stop smoking actually quit). Brief advice is most effective if practical in nature (giving guidance on how change can be achieved) and if backed up by written advice to take home. More intensive interventions tend to be less cost-effective. Time spent on alternative preventive activities (e.g. effective management of chronic disease) may reap greater rewards.

Environmental change

Many environmental causes of disease are best modified on a public health rather than an individual basis. Such factors include the safety of the workplace, environmental pollution, transport safety, food hygiene, and provision of clean water. However, a number of diseases have environmental causes which need to be recognized and avoided by the individual patient. On a global scale, avoidance of insect and other disease vectors (e.g. by netting) and attention to nutritional hygiene (e.g. by filtering water) are probably the most important. In economically developed countries the most common diseases amenable to individual environmental intervention are those associated with atopy—such as asthma and eczema. Not all patients have an identifiable allergenic cause for their symptoms and, even if one is identified, avoidance (e.g. of house dust mite in asthma) may not be easy. But dramatic improvement can occur, and treating contact dermatitis without giving advice on contact avoidance, or treating louse bites without giving advice on how to rid clothes of lice, is bad medical practice.

What interventions work?

It is impossible in a single chapter to cover every possible preventive intervention. It is also undesirable, because many preventive interventions are better seen as part of good routine clinical care (and are included in the relevant chapters on specific diseases). Nevertheless, it is worth listing the preventive interventions which may not be included elsewhere, and for which there is very good evidence of effectiveness from clinical trials. The best sources of evidence are the task force reports from Canada and the United States (see further reading). The evidence cited below is based on the last (1997) update of the Canadian report on clinical preventive health care. It focuses on issues of importance in economically developed countries in which most of the research has been done.

Table 1 lists the preventive interventions shown to be effective for mothers and babies. The target for all but one intervention (screening for haemoglobinopathies) is the whole population. Many of the interventions are usually delivered by midwifery or nursing staff (health visitors in the United Kingdom), but medical staff may be involved in child development and antenatal examinations and it is very important that they reinforce the advice and guidance given by other staff.

Table 1 Preventive interventions with good evidence of effectiveness in mothers and babies

Preventable condition	Preventive intervention	Target population
Neural tube defects	Folic acid supplementation	Women capable of becoming pregnant
Low birth weight	Smoking cessation interventions	Pregnant women
Low cognitive ability of child		
Bacteriuria in pregnancy	Urine culture	Pregnant women
D (Rh) sensitization	D (Rh) antibody screening and immunoglobulin (D Ig) administration after delivery	Pregnant women
Gastrointestinal and respiratory infection in the newborn baby	Counselling on breast feeding; peripartum interventions to increase breast feeding	Pregnant women (or peripartum period)
Phenylketonuria	Serum phenylalanine screening	Neonates
Ophthalmia neonatorum	Ocular prophylaxis	Neonates
Congenital hypothyroidism	Thyroid-stimulating hormone (TSH) test	Neonates
Haemoglobinopathies	Haemoglobin electrophoresis	High-risk neonates
Congenital hip dislocation	Physical examination of hips	Infants
Amblyopia	Eye examination	Infants
Hearing impairment	Hearing examination	Infants
Immunization-preventable disease	Immunizations	Infants and children
Unintentional injury	Counselling on home risk factors, poison control	Parents of infants
Night-time crying	Anticipatory guidance	Parents of infants

Source: Canadian Task Force on Preventive Health Care—last update 1997.

Table 2 deals with children and adolescents. Immunization, dental care, and protection of hearing are interventions which should be offered to all children. All other interventions are targeted at specific high-risk groups, particularly children living in conditions of social disadvantage or with families identified as being at 'high risk' of providing unacceptable levels of child care. Chemoprophylaxis is effective for child contacts of open tuberculosis and for immunocompromised children exposed to influenza. Screening for sexually transmitted disease has been shown to be effective in at-risk adolescents and children.

Table 3 deals with interventions for adults, including the elderly. Only two (hearing impairment and dental care) are targeted at the whole population, although post-fall assessment is targeted at all elderly patients and mammography at all women in the relevant age group. The effectiveness of mammography has again been questioned recently, but the balance of evidence remains in its favour. All other interventions are aimed at high-risk groups. It must be stressed that the omission of many secondary preventive interventions (e.g. management of high blood pressure; rehabilitation after myocardial infarction) reflect their inclusion in other chapters rather than lack of evidence of effectiveness.

What is achievable?

Programme effectiveness

The interventions cited above are known to work because they have been tested in clinical trials. However, clinical trials are often done in settings far removed from everyday life—participants are compliant, those delivering the intervention are highly trained, the technology is of high specification, and quality control is rigorous. These conditions will not hold on a wet Tuesday morning in the boondocks. When preventive interventions fail, the most common reason is lack of effective implementation of the implementation programme, rather than lack of effectiveness of the intervention itself.

The importance of considering programme effectiveness is seen most vividly in relation to immunization and screening programmes. The three most important issues which determine programme effectiveness are the following.

1. Coverage—What proportion of the population at risk receives the intervention?

2. Delivery—Are factors which effect the delivery of the intervention (like the maintenance of equipment, the training of staff, and the storage of biological materials) up to scratch?

3. Quality control—Are standards set and monitored for key indicators of the intervention process (e.g. immune response or predictive value of screening)?

The effect on programme effectiveness of failure in just one of these areas is well documented in the United Kingdom in relation both to immunization (e.g. the resurgence of pertussis after media publicity about potential adverse effects of the vaccine led to a fall in uptake) and to cervical screening (e.g. lack of quality control in cervical sampling and cytological assessment led to false-negative results and avoidable mortality).

Table 2 Preventive interventions with good evidence of effectiveness in children and adolescents

Preventable condition	Preventive intervention	Target population
Dental caries, periodontal disease	Fluoride, toothpaste or supplement, brushing teeth	Children
Hearing impairment	Noise control and hearing protection	Children
Immunization-preventable disease	Immunization	Children and adolescents
Influenza	Chemoprophylaxis	High-risk cases
Tuberculosis	Chemoprophylaxis	High-risk cases
HIV/AIDS, gonorrhoea, chlamydia	Screening for disease	High-risk populations
All-cause morbidity	Day care or preschool programmes	Disadvantaged children
Child maltreatment	Home visits	High-risk families
Tobacco-caused disease	Counselling on smoking cessation	Children and adolescents who smoke

Source: Canadian Task Force on Preventive Health Care—last update 1997.

Table 3 Preventive interventions with good evidence of effectiveness in adults

Preventable condition	Preventive intervention	Target population
Hearing impairment	Noise control and hearing protection	General population
Dental caries, periodontal disease	Fluoride, toothpaste or supplement, brushing and flossing teeth	General population
Tobacco-caused disease	Counselling and offer of nicotine replacement therapy	Smokers
Breast cancer	Mammography and clinical examination	Women aged 50 to 69
Progressive renal disease	Urine dipstick	Adults with insulin-dependent diabetes mellitus
Falls/injury	Multidisciplinary post-fall assessment	Elderly
HIV/AIDS	Voluntary HIV antibody screening	High-risk populations
Gonorrhoea	Cervical or urethral smear	High-risk groups
Influenza	Outreach strategies	High-risk groups; elderly
	Chemoprophylaxis	Contacts
Tuberculosis	Mantoux tuberculin skin test	High-risk groups
	Chemoprophylaxis	Contacts and converters
Pneumococcal pneumonia	Immunization	High-risk elderly

Source: Canadian Task Force on Preventive Health Care—last update 1997.

Cultural constraints

Many preventive interventions aim to change behaviour. Most behaviour has a strong sociocultural component and reflects prevalent attitudes and norms in society. Preventive interventions are severely constrained by this social context—convincing individuals to stop smoking, eat less salt, drink less beer, or drive more slowly is difficult if everyone else is doing the opposite. For example, the mean blood cholesterol level in Finland is almost twice that in Japan (Fig. 4). Migrant studies suggest that this difference is dietary rather than genetic in origin and so medical advice to reduce fat consumption should have the potential to reduce substantially blood cholesterol level. However, even in the context of a clinical trial, dietary advice from health professionals in a community setting seldom achieves a reduction in blood cholesterol of more than 3 to 5 per cent. Studies of salt restriction (to lower blood pressure) show a similar result—intensive intervention and support is needed for an individual patient to achieve a physiologically significant reduction in intake, with many finding such a diet unpalatable. Countercultural change is difficult to achieve.

Time effects

Things change over time. The North Karelia project was a large-scale long-term programme to reduce mortality from cardiovascular disease in northern Finland started in 1972 which involved both public health and individual intervention. Figure 5 compares mortality from cardiovascular disease in North Karelia with that in 10 other provinces in Finland before and during the intervention by plotting two regression lines. The difference in slope of these two lines shows that the intervention was to some extent effective. However, far more impressive in magnitude is the absolute fall in mortality over time in both North Karelia and the other provinces. The lessons for preventive medicine are twofold: the effect of medical intervention may be small in relation to the effect of other economic and social influences; and the change in baseline risk and social context over time may be so rapid that it will substantially influence the absolute benefit of any preventive intervention.

Conclusion

Preventive medicine is an integral part of clinical practice for all doctors. It is our responsibility as clinicians not only to cure the presenting illness but also to take action where possible to prevent future morbidity. However, we must display both humility and assertiveness in our approach. We need to be humble in our approach to patients and to recognize that medicine is not the main determinant of health. At the same time we must display assertiveness in our advocacy of prevention. In the United Kingdom, the

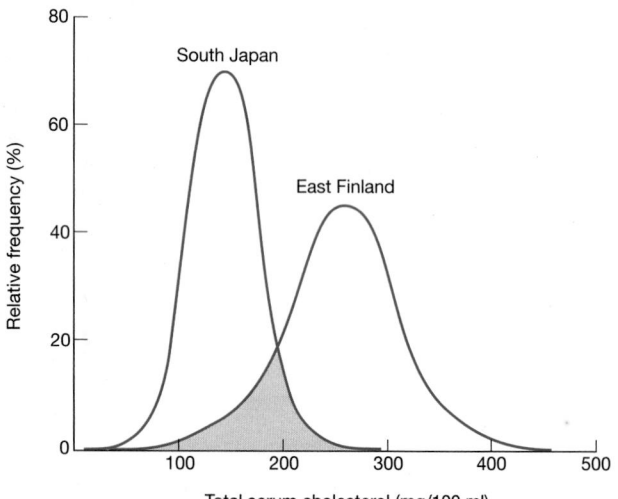

Fig. 4 Distribution of serum cholesterol in southern Japan and eastern Finland. (Reproduced from Rose C. *Strategy of prevention.* Oxford University Press, 1992: 57.)

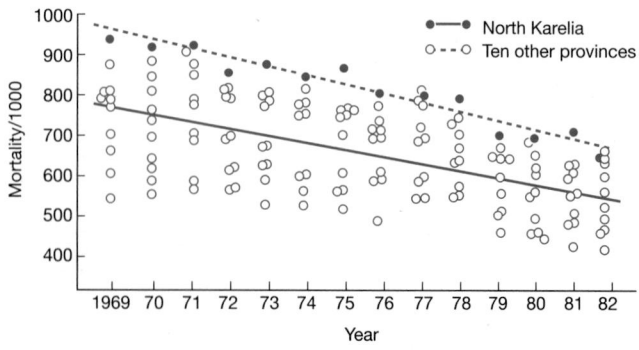

Fig. 5 The North Karelia project. Age-standardized annual mortality from cardiovascular disease in men aged 35 to 64 in Finland, 1969 to 1982. (Redrawn from original data published by Tuomilehto J *et al. British Medical Journal,*1986: **293**: 1068–71.)

Royal College of Physicians' reports, the campaigning of medical charities, and the decision of virtually all doctors to stop smoking have played a major role in influencing both public and political opinion against tobacco use. As a profession, we can make a unique and powerful contribution to prevention by identifying the existence and causes of ill health. We also have a unique and powerful responsibility to act as advocates for our patients in seeking to ensure that these causes are addressed and the risk to their health is minimized. Good clinical practice entails preventive medicine, but good preventive medicine is more than just good clinical practice.

Further reading

Canadian Government (1994, reprinted 1998). *The Canadian guide to preventive health care.* Canadian Government Publishing, Ottawa. [Encyclopaedic (more than 1000 page) summary of current evidence on the effectiveness of preventive health care—updated electronic version at www.fedpubs.com/subject/health/clinpre.htm.]

Goldbloom R, Lawrence R (1990). *Preventing disease—beyond the rhetoric.* Springer Verlag, New York. [Published 10 years ago but a landmark text (based on early work done for the Canadian and US Task Forces on prevention) which made the case for evidence-based prevention.]

Rose G (1992). *The strategy of preventive medicine.* Oxford University Press. [The definitive text on the theory of preventive medicine—short, readable, brilliant.]

UK Joint Committee on Vaccination and Immunisation (1999). *Immunisation against infectious disease. Report of UK Joint Committee on Vaccination and Immunisation.* HMSO, London. [Annually updated short publication which provides a practical, but evidence based, summary of immunization recommendations in the United Kingdom.]

US Preventive Services Task Force (1995). *Guide to clinical preventive services—Report of the US Preventive Services Task Force,* 2nd edn. US Department of Health and Human Services, Washington, DC. [Similarly encyclopaedic (more than 900 page) summary of current evidence on the effectiveness of preventive health care—updated electronic version at www.odphp.osophs.dhhs.gov/pubs/guidecps.]

World Health Organization (1999). *Removing obstacles to healthy development.* World Health Organization, Geneva. [Report focusing on the potential for global prevention of infectious disease—electronic version at www.who.org/infectious-disease-report.]

World Health Organization (2000). *World Health Report 1999. Making a difference.* World Health Organization, Geneva. [Short (121 page) report focusing on what are seen as the two main preventable threats to global health at the millennium—tobacco and malaria.]

3.5 Health promotion

Keith Tones and Jackie Green

Health promotion

Health: meaning and aetiology

Health: the positive dimension

Health promotion is a controversial concept—it means different things to different people. This is not surprising since the notion of health itself is open to many interpretations. The definition of health embodied in the Constitution of the World Health Organization (1946) confirmed that health is not just the absence of disease and infirmity. It is also concerned with positive well being and has mental and social as well as physical dimensions. Although there is a temptation for medical practitioners to dismiss such preoccupations with well being as vague philosophizing, medicine cannot, and should not, discard these broader concerns. For instance, the notion of tertiary prevention has traditionally acknowledged that medicine should aim to maximize the quality of life of those it cannot cure. There is also increasing evidence that life expectancy, in addition to well being, can be influenced by a number of 'positive' individual and social attributes. For instance, the notion of 'social capital' is currently very popular with health policy-makers—it is argued that a high level of social capital supports health through giving access to a range of social networks which provide support and foster a sense of social connectedness. People will be healthier if they feel they are in control of their lives and that their lives are meaningful and make sense emotionally—in other words, they have a 'sense of coherence'. The central concern of health promotion should be not only to add years to life but life to years!

Determinants of health

Whether health is defined as the absence of disease or as a broader more holistic state, it is widely agreed that four major factors determine the extent to which people are or are not healthy. These are shown in Fig.1.

Traditionally, the individual's lifestyle has been the main target of health education—together with exhortations to make proper use of medical services. The current view is that the environment in which we live, work, and play has the most powerful influence, either directly or through the mediation of individuals' behaviour. Accordingly, the most effective health pro-

motion strategies are those that modify the environment to make it safer and more health-enhancing and, most important of all, those which tackle the social and economic factors that cause health inequalities. Environmental circumstances may make it more or less easy for individuals to adopt healthy behaviours. For this reason a central concern for health promotion is to go beyond merely providing education about healthy choices. It should provide a supportive environment such that the 'healthy choice becomes the easy choice'. Of course, changing the environment often requires substantial changes in public policy and associated political action. Health promotion is therefore considered to include both health education and 'healthy public policy'.

Human behaviour in health and illness

Although some medical practitioners have been involved in a wide range of different health promotion activities—including community development and creative arts projects—the face-to-face encounter between doctor and patient is the most common focus of interaction. Every such encounter offers an opportunity for one-to-one health promotion. However, quite often this face-to-face interaction fails to capitalize on the potential offered.

Lessons from failure

Promoting healthy lifestyles is not an easy task and requires a thorough understanding of human behaviour at the social and individual level. The interaction between health professionals and their clients has been subjected to extensive research. This research confirms that, on average, as many as 50 per cent of people fail to co-operate with health advice of any kind, and changes in lifestyle are particularly challenging. A variety of reasons accounts for this failure, for example:

- recipients of, or participants in, health promotion often misinterpret the information provided and a smaller proportion forget key points;

- many people do not believe the information provided because it conflicts with their own ideas and beliefs;

- people may want to change lifestyle but do not believe they can change—because of real or perceived obstacles to action;

- environmental circumstances may be such that there is an absolute barrier to change.

We can and must draw lessons from examples of failure. Typically they are due to inadequate and naïve attempts at health promotion and lack a sound theoretical foundation. There is, however, considerable evidence that allows us to state categorically that health promotion can be effective—provided that appropriate and sufficiently sophisticated interventions are employed. Such interventions should be derived from analysis of the determinants of health and health behaviour, and must be based on a thorough understanding of the psychological, social, and environmental factors that influence people's behaviour in health and illness.

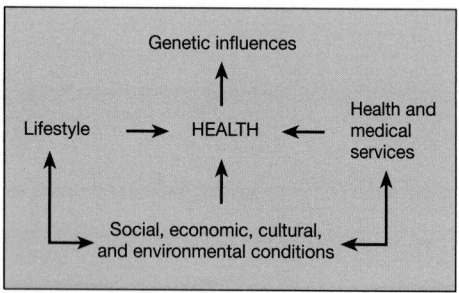

Fig. 1 Determinants of health

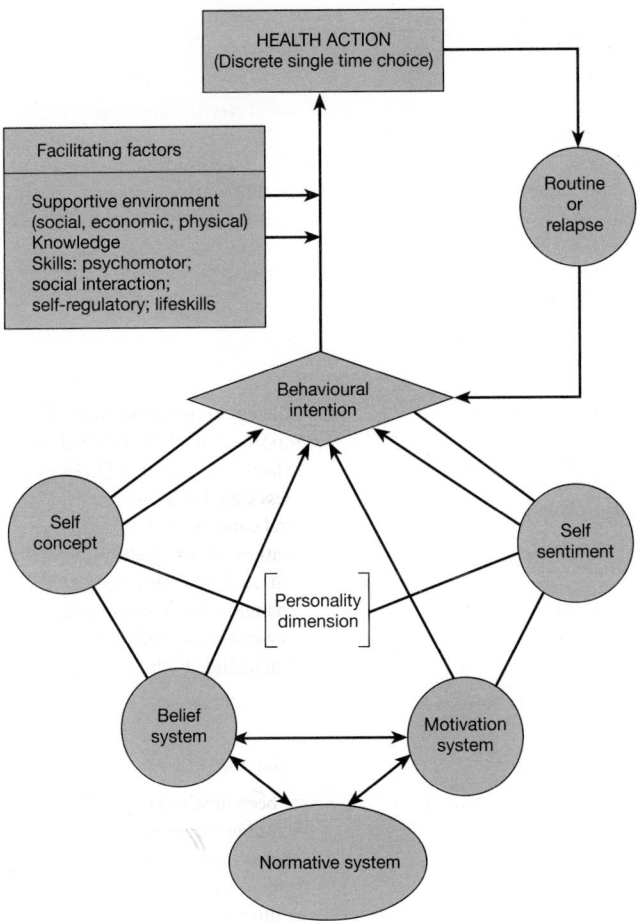

Fig. 2 Determinants of health actions.

The psychosocial and environmental determinants of health actions

Figure 2 summarizes the important factors that determine whether or not individuals will adopt a new and healthier course of action.

Three major systems influence individuals' intention to act, that is the strength of their determination to adopt new types of behaviour or change old habits. These comprise the sum total of their beliefs about carrying out the action, together with their level of motivation to take action. This, in turn, will be the product of all their values and attitudes relating to the action and other emotional states. Finally, their intentions will also be determined by the cumulative influence of social pressures. These pressures will range from the relatively unimportant effect of general norms, conveyed by mass media, through the more powerful community norms, to the much greater influence of close friends, peers, and family.

Even quite firm intentions to adopt a healthy course of action will only be translated into practice if the environment and social circumstances are supportive and there is adequate provision to overcome the various barriers that often stifle action. In other words, it is essential to identify those circumstances that 'make the healthy choice the easy choice' and help avoid relapse into earlier unhealthy habits. The psychosocial and environmental prerequisites for adopting and routinely using condoms as part of a package of safer sex practices provide an illustration of what is required.

Beliefs and motivation

Certain key beliefs will contribute to the intention to use condoms with a sexual partner. First of all, individuals must believe they are susceptible to infection. Furthermore, they must accept that using a condom really will prevent HIV infection (and other sexually transmitted diseases). This belief

will, in turn, depend on their having sufficient understanding about the nature of the virus and its mode of transmission—and by accepting that a condom's thin membrane is an effective barrier to the virus. More importantly, they must be persuaded that using a condom will neither be expensive nor inconvenient. Unfortunately, there is a common belief that condoms reduce sensitivity and gratification, interrupt lovemaking, and generate embarrassment!

A number of key motivational factors may militate against safer sex. Most people value health and are worried about the risk of disease—especially fatal disease. However, many women have been conditioned to believe that casual sex is immoral, a powerful disincentive to taking anticipatory action. This may well create a situation in which a powerful moral value may rule out precautionary action, but be insufficiently powerful to resist sexual passion and their partner's preference.

Social pressure

It is widely recognized that intentions are influenced not only by personal beliefs and values but also by various pressures, real or imagined, from other people. These pressures will include the general influence of social norms in defining 'normal' sexual behaviour, peer expectations and pressures, and also the particularly powerful influence of the partner or potential partner.

Skills and the environment

Good intentions will rarely be implemented unless barriers to action have been minimized and appropriate support has been provided. Three kinds of supportive strategy may be necessary. The first and simplest of these involves access to the information needed to adopt the health action. In this specific example—where to obtain and how to use condoms.

The second prerequisite for making healthy choices is to acquire essential skills:

- assertiveness to negotiate condom use with a partner;
- interpersonal skills and associated confidence needed to obtain condoms;
- psychomotor skills needed for safe and efficient use of the condom.

Third, the provision of a supportive environment is essential. A range of environmental measures will be relevant, including physical measures such as access to condoms and social measures that will create a climate in which condom use is acceptable.

However, the most difficult environmental barriers of all are the socioeconomic circumstances associated with poverty and its accompanying feelings of hopelessness and helplessness. It is no coincidence that the prevalence of preventable disease worldwide—including AIDS—is highest in the lowest socioeconomic groups.

The principle of reciprocal determinism

The principle of reciprocal determinism—drawn from social psychology—has proved to have great explanatory value for understanding efficient health promotion interventions. It asserts that there is typically a continuing interplay between the environment and individual action. On the one hand, social, material, and economic circumstances can facilitate or inhibit individual choice and action; on the other hand, individuals are capable of taking action to change their environment thus effecting change in those circumstances. Health promotion, therefore, is concerned both to reduce environmental barriers to action and, at the same time, strengthen individuals' capacity to challenge and modify their environmental circumstances. For these reasons, empowerment occupies a central place in the philosophy and practice of contemporary health promotion.

Health promotion as 'empowerment'

The World Health Organization has defined the main purpose of health promotion as helping people to take control of their lives and their health by:

- providing individuals with those 'empowerment' skills that generate competence and confidence; and

- removing at least some of the environmental barriers to action.

We noted earlier that health promotion involves a close relationship between health education and 'healthy public policy'. Health education should not be concerned primarily with persuading and cajoling to gain compliance, but rather with reassuring and supporting people to gain their co-operation. A supportive environment will be dependent on healthy public policy, including fiscal and economic measures, environmental engineering, and legislation. The pursuit of healthy public policy itself requires education and lobbying of key figures and activists in the policy arena.

However, it is clear that although lobbying and advocacy are essential to successful health promotion, they will have little impact on entrenched power structures—especially if there are major financial implications—unless they are supported by public pressure. Accordingly, one of the main functions of health education is to create 'critical consciousness'—a process that involves:

- building a sense of community;

- raising people's awareness of, and indignation about, major social and health problems, and developing the skills they need to exert political pressure on government or organizations.

In some instances, this dual process may be sufficient in itself to bring about change but frequently the public's efforts must be supplemented by advocacy on their behalf—and the powerful voice of the medical profession can be especially important in this context.

Furthermore, medical services can contribute in a more general way to both individual and community empowerment and provide a model of good practice for other agencies. The service offered should be 'user-friendly' and responsive to the felt needs of communities.

Settings for health promotion

The 'health career'

The 'health career' is one of the most useful devices for identifying the cumulative influences on health behaviour—and for devising appropriate intervention strategies. In short, it plots key influences that operate over a lifetime. Figure 3 describes its main features. It identifies key agencies, such as the family, and more general influences, such as the community or mass media, that shape beliefs and motivations about health, exert social pressure, and erect barriers to action or, alternatively, provide support for healthy choices.

Settings, alliances, and mass media

The 'health career' analysis makes it possible not only to identify negative influences on health, but also, more positively, to identify agencies, organizations, and settings that can be used to 'deliver' health promotion. For instance, particular interest has been shown recently in the Health Promoting School, the Health Promoting Workplace, and the Health Promoting Hospital; three points merit emphasis:

- the whole ethos of an organization should be health promoting and empowering;

- the impact of any one organization will be maximized by intersectoral working and the creation of healthy alliances;

- mass media can support community health programmes but cannot act as a substitute for interpersonal working.

The doctor's role

It should by now be self-evident that health promotion is a multidisciplinary endeavour. What is the doctor's role? It is clear that the medical profession enjoys a high level of credibility with public and politicians. They

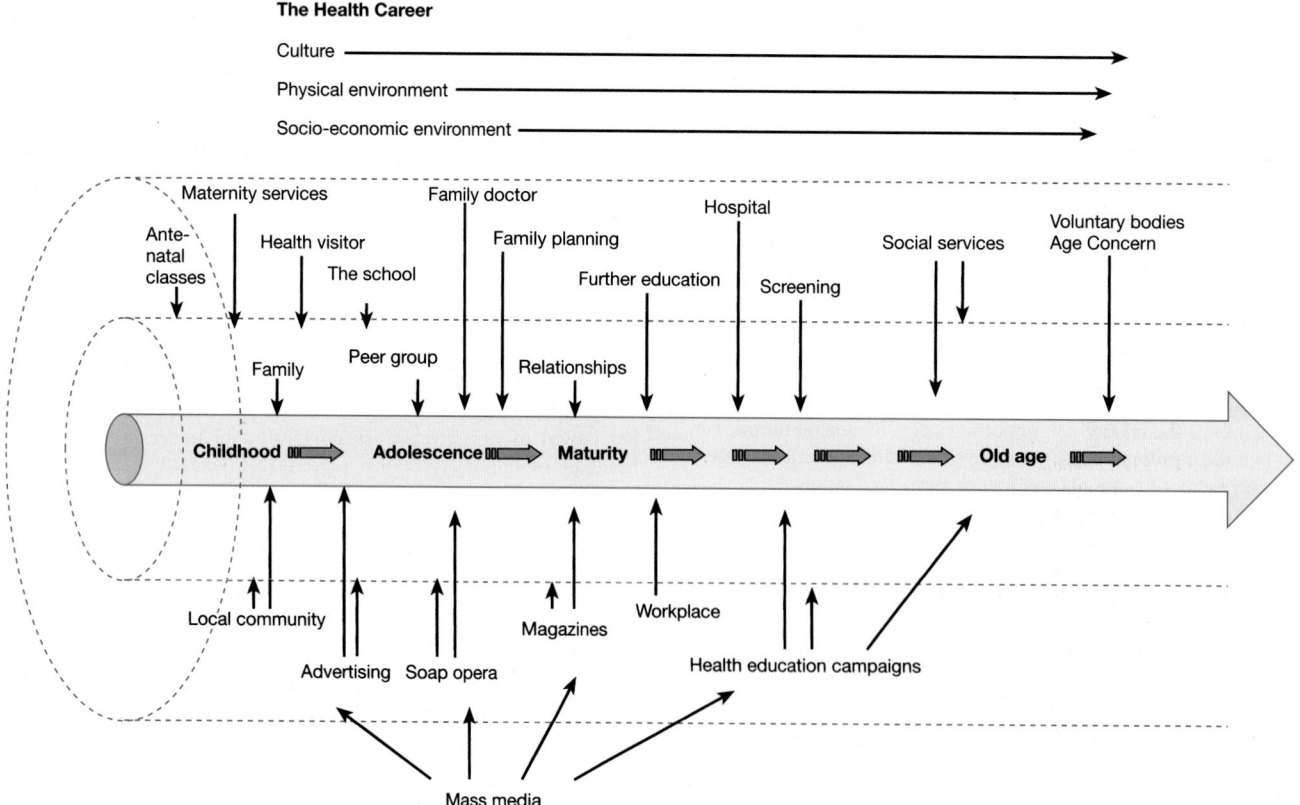

Fig. 3 The Health Career.

are also uniquely placed to have awareness of the broad range of psycho-social and environmental factors influencing the health and well being of patients. Their major contribution may be summarized as follows:

- providing advice on lifestyle;
- delivering medical services in ways that are empowering and contribute to a sense of control;
- acting as advocates for social change—by lobbying and by using creative epidemiology (presenting health data in a dramatic, readily understandable, and compelling way) to create public concern and pressure for political action.

Health promotion methods: the consultation

Ultimately, the effectiveness of health promotion will be directly related to the quality of the specific methods used by health workers. It is clear that the achievement of certain important goals—such as remedying health inequalities—depends on the strength in unity that results from the kinds of alliance and political action mentioned above. However, individual practitioners and organizations such as hospitals can make a substantial impact—if the right techniques and strategies are employed. Box 1 provides guidelines for a health promoting consultation that helps clients take charge of their lives and their health. This approach should avoid the kinds of failure mentioned earlier in this chapter and maximize the chances of achieving real change.

Where consultation time is limited, the task outlined above may appear daunting. However, the following points should be noted:

- The full procedure would be necessary in only a few cases.
- Many interactions with health professionals are continuing and cumulative. A series of meetings may be needed to cover the full 'recipe' for a successful outcome.
- Careful assessment of the stages of readiness to change will allow selection of only those strategies which are pertinent.
- It is frequently possible and desirable to delegate some or all of the task to other staff who may have more time.
- Different methods may be combined to achieve the various subtasks described above, e.g. a support group may use lay 'peer leaders' as health educators.
- Although the consultation offers only limited opportunities for addressing major socioeconomic problems, some action is possible. For instance, a number of health centres have offered 'welfare benefits clinics' in collaboration with a social worker to ensure that patients claim their full entitlement to financial help. Furthermore, by acting as advocates for patients, health workers as a professional group can and should seek to influence local and national policy.

Further reading

Ewles L, Simnett I (1999). *Promoting health: a practical guide.* Baillière Tindall/RCN, London. [A practitioner's guide.]

Jones L, Sidell M, eds. (1997). *The challenge of promoting health: exploration and action.* Macmillan/Open University, London. [Useful on features of health policy, intersectoral working, and the community.]

Tones BK, Tilford S (2001). *Health promotion: effectiveness, efficiency and equity,* 3rd edn. Thornes/Nelson, London. [Standard reference on contribution of health education to health promotion with a slant on evaluation and effectiveness.]

Tones BK (2001). Health promotion, health education and the public health. In: Detels R, McEwen J, Beaglehole R, Tanaka H, eds. *Oxford textbook of public health,* 4th edn, Vol. 2, Ch. 24. Oxford University Press, Oxford. [An overview of the contribution of health promotion to public health, incorporating discussion of philosophy, ethics, programme planning and evaluation.]

Box 1 The health promoting consultation

Needs assessment

- Establish and maintain rapport using appropriate counselling skills.
- Check patients' state of readiness. Have they given any thought to changing their behaviour? Do they think they have a problem? Do they feel it is important for them to change? Are they committed to change but just need some support?

Communication phase

- Provide information at a level appropriate to the patient.
- Ensure that patients pay attention to the message.
- Check that patients have correctly interpreted the message—and fully understood key points. Take account of non-verbal communication.
- Try to ensure that patients remember important points—and provide a written aide-memoire.
- Ensure that any written material has been checked for 'readability'.

Motivation phase: helping patients to change

- Explore patients' existing beliefs and attitudes and those skills necessary for the proposed behaviour change.
- Analyse patients' environmental and social circumstances.
- Seek to modify beliefs and attitudes where appropriate and provide skills training.
- Negotiate and agree a 'contract'.
- Check that the relevant changes in beliefs, attitude, and skills have taken place. Are patients now committed to action?

Support phase

- Provide opportunities for patients to acquire any extra knowledge and skills necessary for translating good intentions into actual practice.
- Help mobilize social and environmental support.
- Consider particularly any skills or support needed to minimize the chance of relapse.
- Keep a check on patients' progress.

Websites

http://www.who.ch [World Health Organization website with search facility. Useful access to health documents, e.g. *Health For All, Ottawa Charter, Jakarta Declaration.*]

http://www.hda-online.org.uk [Health Development Agency. Access to research and information on good practice.]

http://www.healthpromis.had-online.org.uk [Access to 'Healthpromis' the health promotion database for England.]

3.6 Screening

J. A. Muir Gray

All screening programmes do harm; some also have the potential for doing good. In this respect screening is no different from the rest of clinical practice, but there are important differences between screening and clinical practice.

First, the contract, implicit or explicit, between the person being screened and the screener is qualitatively and ethically different from the contract that exists between clinician and patient. A patient who presents with a problem is seeking help and is usually aware of the facts about the limitations of medicine, and does not expect a guaranteed cure or risk-free treatment. This is part of the deal that they make with the clinician when entering the process of care. When, however, a professional or health service, or indeed the government through one of its agencies, writes to a healthy member of the population and asks them to come along for screening, the responsibility on the person issuing the invitation is much heavier. The traditional principle and the first priority to do no harm is even more strongly reinforced when dealing with people who perceive themselves as being healthy. In addition, the limitations and risks of screening must be explicitly and clearly spelt out.

The second way in which screening differs from clinical practice is that screening focuses on populations or on subgroups of the population, although it is often delivered by an individual clinician to an individual member of the public.

Screening is defined by the National Screening Committee in the United Kingdom as 'The systematic application of a test or inquiry, to identify individuals at sufficient risk of a specific disorder to warrant further investigation or direct preventive action, among persons who have not sought medical attention on account of symptoms of that disorder'.

This definition emphasizes that a subgroup of the whole population is selected on the basis of gender, age, or other characteristics, and then offered a test or asked a question. The results of the test may be either positive or negative and both positive and negative results occur in people with the disease or risk factor, and in those without. The relationship between positive and negative test results and those who are positive and negative for the disease is most easily set out in a figure (Fig. 1).

On the basis of these results, it is possible to define certain characteristics of a screening test of which the most important are its sensitivity and specificity.

The sensitivity of a screening test is measured by the proportion of people who actually have the disease or the risk factors sought and who are detected by a positive test.

The specificity of a screening test is measured by the proportion of the people who do not have the disease who are classified as negative by the test result (Fig. 2)

These are the true traditional epidemiological parameters for a screening test, but one of the principles of screening is that screening consists not simply of tests but of a whole set of activities ranging from the identification of the population at risk right through to the diagnosis and treatment of affected individuals.

Appraising the balance of good and harm

The first step in deciding whether or not to introduce a screening programme is to appraise the balance of good and harm.

Screening is delivered as a programme and not as a single test. The sensitivity and specificity of the test, or tests, used in the screening programme are important but criteria have to be used to assess the programme as a whole.

The criteria proposed by the World Health Organization in 1968 have been widely used since then. However, the National Screening Committee in the United Kingdom considered that these criteria, sometimes called the Wilson–Jungner criteria, were not sufficiently robust for the twenty-first century because:

(1) they did not emphasize the need to take into account the adverse effects of screening; and

Fig. 1 The relationship between test results and the presence of disease.

Fig. 2 The calculation of sensitivity and specificity.

(2) they paid insufficient attention to the strength of the evidence on which decisions about screening were to be made.

Accordingly a new set of criteria, set out in Box 1 have been developed.

Measuring the benefits of screening

The first step in appraising a proposed screening programme is to try to measure or estimate the benefits that will result from that programme. But there are two traps that lie in the way of anyone wishing to assess the effectiveness of screening—lead-time bias and length time bias.

Lead-time bias

Proponents of the introduction of any screening programme sometimes base their argument on cohort studies, which are designed to follow a series of people who have had a screening test and compare their survival with that of the general population. However, this is a poor method of evaluating screening, principally because of what is called lead-time bias.

Imagine a disease that has a natural history of 10 years from its beginning to its fatal end, and that causes symptoms after 5 years, which usually prompt the sufferer to visit a doctor; the survival time from the point of symptomatic diagnosis is 5 years (Fig. 3(a)). A test that enables a diagnosis of the disease to be made at an earlier, presymptomatic, stage—for example, at 3 years—will apparently increase survival time (Fig. 3(b)). This apparent increase in survival time does not necessarily mean that screening is effective; it may simply mean that the person with the presymptomatic disease found by screening is aware of the condition for 7 years as opposed to 5—this is referred to as lead-time bias. It is essential that any screening programme is evaluated within a randomized controlled trial which has been designed with death as the outcome in order to control for lead-time bias.

Length-time bias

Imagine a disease that consists of a number of subtypes; almost every disease has been shown to consist of subtypes when more sophisticated methods of diagnosis and classification have been developed. Imagine those subtypes are of two sorts, those that kill very quickly and those that kill very slowly. A screening programme based on regularly repeated tests is inevitably going to identify more of the slow-growing diseases. Thus it might be possible to describe an improvement in survival following the introduction of a screening programme, but if the only people whose survival has been estimated are those with slowly progressing disease, this does not warrant the conclusion that screening is effective.

This problem, sometimes called length-time bias, is classically demonstrated in the case of prostatic cancer. At the age of 80, about one-third of men have evidence of prostate cancer, but only about 8 per cent of men develop symptoms of prostate cancer. It is now thought that there are at least two types of prostate cancer, sometimes called the tigers and the pussycats, with the pussycats being very slow growing and the tigers very rapidly growing. One interpretation of the results of prostate cancer screening is that it is very good at diagnosing the pussycats but has little or no impact on the tigers.

For these reasons it is important to conduct randomized controlled trials of proposed screening programmes and to prepare a systematic review of the evidence from several trials if more than one has been done.

The harm from screening

No screening test is 100 per cent sensitive and specific; furthermore, initiatives to increase sensitivity almost always decrease specificity and, vice versa, initiatives to increase specificity decrease sensitivity.

People who are true positives, who have both the test and the disease, suffer least harm from a screening programme. However, not all the people identified with the disease will benefit from screening; for example, for a proportion of women whose breast cancer is detected by screening the out-

Box 1 Criteria for appraising the viability, effectiveness, and appropriateness of a screening programme

Ideally all the following criteria should be met before screening for a condition is initiated.

The condition

1. The condition should be an important health problem.
2. The epidemiology and natural history of the condition, including development from latent to declared disease, should be adequately understood and there should be a detectable risk factor, disease marker, latent period, or early symptomatic stage.
3. All the cost-effective primary prevention interventions should have been implemented as far as practicable.

The test

4. There should be a simple, safe, precise, and validated screening test.
5. The distribution of test values in the target population should be known and a suitable cut-off level defined and agreed.
6. The test should be acceptable to the population.
7. There should be an agreed policy on the further diagnostic investigation of individuals with a positive test result and on the choices available to those individuals.

The treatment

8. There should be an effective treatment or intervention for patients identified through early detection, with evidence of early treatment leading to better outcomes than late treatment.
9. There should be agreed evidence-based policies covering which individuals should be offered treatment and the appropriate treatment to be offered.
10. Clinical management of the condition and patient outcomes should be optimized in all health care providers prior to participation in a screening programme.

The screening programme

11. There should be evidence from high-quality randomized controlled trials that the screening programme is effective in reducing mortality or morbidity.
12. There should be evidence that the complete screening programme (test, diagnostic procedures, and treatment/ intervention) is clinically, socially, and ethically acceptable to health professionals and the public.
13. The benefit from the screening programme should outweigh the physical and psychological harm (caused by the test, diagnostic procedures, and treatment).
14. The opportunity cost of the screening programme (including testing, diagnosis, and treatment) should be economically balanced in relation to expenditure on medical care as a whole.
15. There should be a plan for managing and monitoring the screening programme and an agreed set of quality assurance standards.
16. Adequate staffing and facilities for testing, diagnosis, treatment, and programme management should be available prior to the commencement of the screening programme.
17. All other options for managing the condition should have been considered (e.g. improving treatment, providing other services).

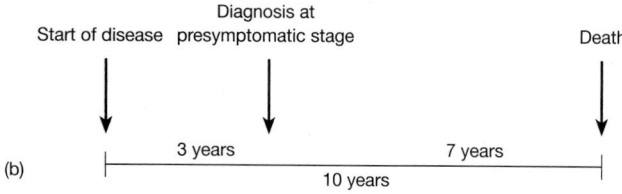

Fig. 3 Lead-time bias.

come remains unchanged—they still die of breast cancer. The effect of screening on the whole population has been to increase the probability of survival but has also meant that when they die this subgroup will have known that they have had cancer for a longer period of time.

People who are false negatives can be said to be harmed by screening if they are falsely reassured, but that harm is minimal. The main harm from screening affects those who have false positive tests. People with false positive tests suffer psychological harm, usually short term, but some may also suffer physical harm from the additional tests or treatments that they undergo. In colorectal cancer screening, for example, it is inevitable that someone who does not have colonic cancer will die from colorectal cancer screening as a result of a complication of colonoscopy.

The special ethical issues of screening

All health care involves risk and many people suffer side-effects from treatment. The ethical difference in screening is, however, that screening tests and programmes are offered to people invited to come for screening by the health service, and the ethical contract between the screening programme and those who are screened is different from that which exists between a clinician doing the best that they can for a patient who has sought help.

The problems that might result from prostate cancer screening illustrate the ethical dilemma. Prostate cancer screening leads to the diagnosis of cancers that would not appear in the lifetime of the individual. In a country the size of the United Kingdom, more than 10 000 people would be identified each year whose cancer would never have become clinically evident in their lifetime. If those people were offered radiotherapy or radical prostatectomy, there would be a mortality of about 1.5 per cent from the effects of treatment alone, and about 30 per cent of those treated would suffer significant side-effects such as incontinence and impotence. Thus the screening programme will harm a large number of people with significant numbers dying as a direct result of screening. These harms must be clearly assessed before screening is started.

Special issues in antenatal screening

For antenatal screening, in which the ethical issues are heightened because the 'outcome' is often abortion, the randomized controlled trial is not necessarily the most appropriate design and for some screening this type of trial is impossible. Of crucial importance in appraising antenatal screening is the sensitivity and specificity of the diagnostic test. With this information it is possible to model the effects of a screening programme. The model for Down's syndrome screening is shown in Fig. 4.

However, even the most elegant research study does not actually make a policy decision; policy-makers in public health have to take the best evidence available and then decide whether or not to introduce the screening programme.

Policy-making: assessing the costs

Once the benefits and harms that might result from screening have been assessed, it is necessary to consider whether or not the introduction of a screening programme that has been shown to do more good than harm is a reasonable use of resources for the population concerned, and policy-makers need to take into account a number of issues, as shown in Fig. 5.

Research produces the evidence of benefit and harm but other factors are equally or more important.

The needs of the population

The needs of the population and the many other demands made on resources need to be taken into account. The decision about whether or not to screen antenatally for HIV infection should be influenced by the prevalence of HIV infection in the population. Similarly, the decision about whether or not to screen for haemoglobinopathies will be influenced by the prevalence of those disorders in the population.

Resources

The cost of the potential screening programme has to be taken into account. One way to think of screening is to think of opportunity costs, namely what else could be done for people with that disease with the money that is being invested in screening. For this reason it is sometimes useful not to think of the proposed screening programme in isolation—for example, not to ask 'shall we screen or not screen?', but to pose the question 'would the resources invested in screening obtain better results if they were put into primary prevention or treatment services for this health problem?'.

The values of the population

Like any other public health service, the values associated with screening are important. Society places a high value on prevention but, for example, if the values of the population are against abortion then many antenatal screening programmes will not even be considered.

Capacity

The results of screening done in research settings are helpful but have their limitation. For example, in considering the results from the Swedish Two Counties study of breast cancer screening, the Department of Health in the United Kingdom had to take into account not only the results of the research but also the facts that:

(1) the research was being done by people who were among the best in the world at mammography and the management of early breast cancer; and

(2) 100 screening teams of the same size as the research team would have to be recruited, trained, and supported for the results obtained in research to be reproduced in practice.

In considering the relevance of research to everyday practice, it is sometimes useful to pilot the proposed screening in an ordinary service setting, principally to see if a sufficient level of quality can be obtained, for without good quality management screening should not be introduced.

Quality management

The quality of a service, as defined by the guru of quality management, Avedis Donabedian, is that quality is measured by the degree to which the service conforms to preset standards of goodness.

The importance of quality assurance

The balance between the good and the harm of a clinician or a service is a function of the quality of the service. If the quality improves, the benefit increases and the harm decreases, and there comes a certain point, as shown in Fig. 6, where a service can do more harm than good.

The challenge for the person responsible for a public health service such as screening is that they are presented with evidence from a research setting which usually has a very high level of quality and they have to ensure that they can achieve the quality standards at point B on Fig. 6, even if they cannot, immediately, achieve the quality standards at point A. Standards are arbitrarily chosen and different levels of standards can be set. The standard set by the research team working to a very tight protocol with highly committed and expert staff is a standard of excellence. The pursuit of excellence is obviously an objective of quality assurance but it is not realistic to expect every service to achieve the level achieved by the best in the world, and a second level, indicated at point B in Fig. 6, is usually defined as the achievable standard. It is also important to identify the minimal acceptable standard below which no service should fall, point C in Fig. 6, for it is important to ensure that of the hundred or so programmes covering an entire population not one of the programmes should fall below the minimal acceptable standard and do more harm than good.

Running screening programmes as systems

A system is a set of activities with a common set of objectives and once the objectives of the programme have been chosen it is possible to identify criteria that can be used to measure progress towards those objectives. Standards can also be set on the basis of the criteria with targets for annual quality improvement being selected.

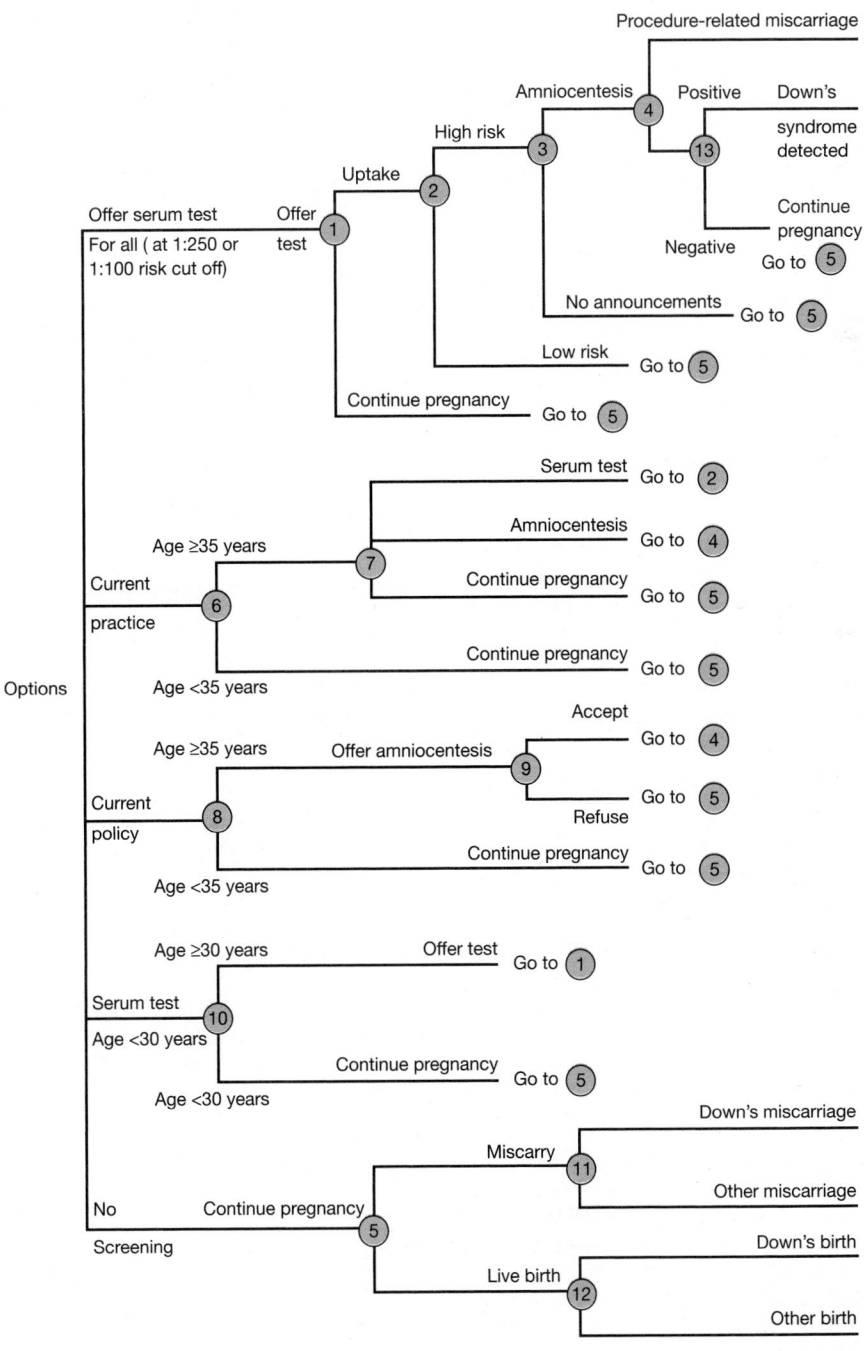

Fig. 4 Decision analysis to show implications of offering screening for Down's syndrome.

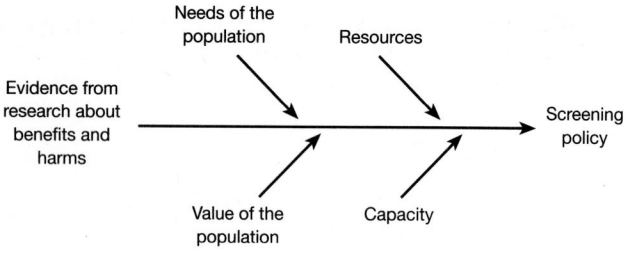

Fig. 5 The ingredients of a screening policy decision.

Fig. 6 The relationship between programme extremes and quality, showing the balance between good and bad effects at different levels of quality.

This approach to systems thinking in screening programme management is shown in Table 1.

The objectives of quality management

Quality management of screening programmes has four objectives.

1. The prevention of quality failures, e.g. by good training and the appropriate choice of equipment.
2. To identify and resolve speedily quality failures that occur; failures in screening programmes are often the focus of intense press and media interest with public alarm being generated by the discovery that one screening programme has a higher number of false negatives than is acceptable.

3. To help all those involved in screening continually to improve their performance; screening is essentially a boring repetitive activity and a high level of commitment is needed to ensure that staff remain motivated; this is particularly important in those screening programmes that depend on the perception of an observer, for example visual perception of cervical smears or mammograms, or the auditory perception of Koratkow sounds.

4. To reset standards regularly; it is not possible to stand still in screening programmes—unless one is constantly striving for improvement there is a risk that the programme will fail because boredom and loss of motivation may reduce quality. The resetting of standards provides new targets at which clinicians and managers can aim.

Achieving continuous quality improvement

Continuous improvement in quality is the objective of screening quality assurance and it requires:

(1) an evidence-based screening system with objectives, criteria, and standards;

(2) an information system that allows performance to be measured and compared with the standards; and

(3) authority to drive quality improvement in all aspects of the programme and to take action if necessary if any part of the programme falls below minimal acceptable standards.

A screening programme requires careful management. The main responsibility for assuring quality rests with the clinicians and managers who are actually responsible for delivering the screening programme, but it is also important for management to invest in quality assurance, activities that are not directly under control of clinicians and managers but which play a part in helping the two groups assess their performance, compare it with the performance of others, and take action either to solve problems or improve performance.

The future of screening

Much has been written about 'genetic screening' but it is in fact hard to generalize about genetic screening for the term is not particularly useful. Certainly new knowledge about genetic risk is raising new opportunities for screening, either in hunting for a particular gene that increases risk or in considering the use of family history as a means of identifying subsets of the population that might be offered screening earlier than the general population, for example breast cancer screening before the age of 50; or offered more intensive screening, for example referral to a cancer genetic clinic. However, the same criteria as outlined above in the section on the good and harm of screening are as relevant to screening based on genetic risk factors as for any other risk factor.

Perhaps more important implications for the future are the changing social attitudes towards technology and risk. Certainly it appears to be much more important to inform people being offered a screening test about the possibility of risk and harm associated with screening. In the past, for example, people have simply been offered blood pressure screening or sometimes been given an antenatal screening test without the implications being fully explained to them. In the twenty-first century this will be unacceptable and all choice will need to be informed. The choice has

Table 1 A systems approach to screening quality assurance

Objectives	Criteria	Standards		Present position	Targets
		Minimal	Achievable		
To cover the population who would benefit from cervical screening	Percentage of women who have not had a hysterectomy who have had a readable smear in the last 5 years	50%	80%	1 out of 70 general practices less than 50%	By the end of year: 70 general practices over 50%
				17 practices more than 80%	35 general practices over 80%

hitherto been based on statistics defined for populations so people can be told, for example, that the benefits of screening for hypertension outweigh the risks. However, in the twenty-first century, with members of the public much better informed and the World Wide Web providing unprecedented access to knowledge, of both good and poor quality, people will increasingly want to know about how the risks relate to them as individuals. Screening is a public health service that focuses on individuals and which brings clinicians in contact with individuals in a manner analogous to traditional clinical practice. In the twenty-first century screening will be based on even sounder epidemiological evidence, derived from studies of whole populations, than has been the case in the twentieth century. Individuals offered screening will need help and advice in deciding whether or not to accept the clinician's proposal and will have an increasingly important part to play in helping them decide whether or not the screening programme offered is appropriate for them as individuals.

Further reading

Donabedian A (1980). The definition of quality: a conceptual exploration. In: *Explorations in quality assessment and monitoring: Vol. I: The definition of quality and approaches to its assessment.* Health Administration Press, Ann Arbor.

Gray JAM (2001). *Evidence-based healthcare*, 2nd edn Churchill Livingstone, Edinburgh.

Wilson JMG, Jungner G. *Principles and practice of screening for disease.* Public Health Paper No. 34. World Health Organization, Geneva.

3.7 The cost of health care

3.7.1 The cost of health care in Western countries

Joseph White

Reasons for interest

The countries conventionally called 'Western' (a term that refers to level of economic development, not geography) have the physical and financial resources needed to provide a high standard of health care to all citizens. Yet doing so at a socially acceptable cost is difficult. Efforts to limit cost may affect the quality of care, access to it, and the work and incomes of medical providers.

Defining the issues

One view of costs emphasizes health care's share of a national economy, and thus the economic 'burden' of care. Another view emphasizes costs relative to service or outcome, and therefore value for money. Those who object most to spending levels, such as employers who contribute to insurance, or government budget-makers, often claim they are concerned with value for money, to show that they are not trying to reduce needed care.

Cost control should be distinguished from 'cost-shifting'. If tight budgets for the British National Health Service cause many patients to 'go private', that is cost control from the government's perspective. From the patients' and providers' vantage point, some costs have been shifted, not reduced.

Why is cost a policy issue?

The cost of health care is more of a public issue than that of most other commodities or services because all Western countries remove much health care from the market's allocation processes. Markets allocate resources by price. A person who cannot afford an item then may save for it, borrow for it, do without, or buy a lower-quality alternative. All of these options can be impracticable or socially unacceptable for a large number of medical needs, so some other method of allocation is needed.

All advanced industrial countries free sick people from worrying (too much) about cost by combining individual contributions into pooled funds. Whether those pools are private or public, and cover all or part of the population of an area, their effect and intent is to protect members from the price constraints that otherwise would limit spending. Some other method of controlling spending on individuals' care is therefore needed, in order to limit contributions to the pool.

Spending trends

Table 1 shows health care spending as a percentage of national economies for 11 countries with constant borders from 1975 to 1995 (Germany is therefore excluded). Generally the 'burden' of health care spending has risen, but much more quickly in some countries than others, and at different rates over time within the same country.

One common explanation of spending increases emphasizes the ageing populations in Western countries. Yet careful analyses suggest that longer life expectancies explain only a small part of the trend, because greater life expectancy implies that mortality, and its attendant costs, are lower at each particular age.

Table 1 Health care spending as a share of gross domestic product: levels and trends, 1975 to 1995

	Spending percentage of GDP			Growth rate of spending share	
	1975	1985	1995	1975–85	1985–95
Australia	7.5	7.7	8.6	0.35	1.12
Canada	7.2	8.4	9.7	1.60	1.43
France	7.0	8.5	9.9	1.98	1.57
Italy	6.2	7.1	7.7	1.31	0.91
Japan	5.5	6.7	7.2	1.95	0.79
The Netherlands	7.5	7.9	8.8	0.52	1.07
Norway	6.1	6.6	8.0	0.79	1.90
Spain	4.9	5.7	7.6	1.50	3.01
Sweden	7.9	9.0	7.2	1.32	−2.14
United Kingdom	5.5	5.9	6.9	0.67	1.73
United States	8.2	10.7	14.2	2.62	2.92

These figures are taken from Organization for Economic Cooperation and Development (OECD) Health Data (1997). Differences in definitions and reliability of data sources across countries mean that different sources may provide different figures.

Some analysts believe that individuals simply prefer health care to other goods so that, once other basic needs are met, higher income will lead to disproportionately higher consumption of health care services. The methods of payment, however, make it hard to determine to what extent spending represents individual preferences.

Rapid innovation in treatments and diffusion of knowledge about them usually interacts with pooled financing to encourage increases in cost. Particularly when policies promise a high standard of care, knowledge of a new, supposedly useful treatment creates pressures to make it available to everyone, as opposed to the norm with market goods, which can be rationed legitimately by price.

In spite of this generally upward trend, Table 1 shows that both spending levels and rates of increase vary greatly. A nation's cost level reflects its history: for instance, the development of national medical capacity, provider income expectations, and practice norms. Spending can also vary due to differences in underlying causes of illness, such as poverty, diet, smoking, alcoholism, violence, and genetic endowments. Yet these factors are unlikely to explain the different rates of growth.

Cost control policies

The main reason why trends in medical costs differ is that nations have made different efforts to restrain them. We can distinguish cost control efforts in terms of the targets of control and the systems of health care finance.

Targets

National policies vary in both the emphasis on and success of targeting different types of services, such as inpatient care or pharmaceuticals. Until recently, national medical norms and the economic and political power of different providers favoured, for example, surgery in the United States and pharmaceutical treatment in Japan. Sometimes advocates argue that higher spending on one service would reduce expenses for others: for instance, that expanded insurance for ambulatory care or pharmaceuticals would reduce hospital costs. Whether such expansions of insurance ever reduce total costs (as opposed to providing better value) is doubtful.

Policies may target different factors that influence spending for a given type of service. For example, they may focus on restraining prices per service or numbers of services or, somehow, both. Another common approach is to limit physical capacity to provide care, and so both volume and prices. For instance, fewer MRI machines per person will probably mean fewer scans and, since each machine is used more often, lower costs per scan.

Research showing that many procedures lack scientific support, and demonstrating wide, medically unexplained variations in practice among communities, encourages another type of policy: measures to make care more 'appropriate', such as treatment guidelines. Sometimes termed 'evidence-based medicine', these measures are promoted as offering savings without harm to patients.

Systems

Cost control is affected by the systems used to pool funds and pay for services.

The extent to which individuals pool their resources may range, in theory, from not at all (individuals pay all costs out of pocket) to total (all care is paid from a single pooled fund). In Western countries, the range is from most people being insured for most services, with some cost-sharing (as in the United States); to virtually everyone insured, for most services, in a single pool (as in Canadian provinces, and the British National Health Service, **NHS**). Both the low and high ends of this continuum are likely to control costs better than some position in the middle. If people pay substantial amounts from personal funds they will face considerable price constraints. But extensive pooling can limit costs, because payment through a

'single pipe' provides a single point of control: limit the total flow, and you can limit spending.

A similar pattern of effectiveness can be seen in choices about how individual caregivers are paid. At one end of this payment continuum, virtually all providers of a given service are paid on the same terms, even if there are multiple payers. Such co-ordination gives the payer(s) dominant market power, which can be used to enforce (relatively) low prices. At the other extreme, payers contract selectively with providers. Then hospitals or doctors may agree to reduce their fees, or accept some outside management of their practices, so as to preserve access to patients. Co-ordinated payment is usual in most Western countries. Selective contracting is the basis of much of American 'managed care', and of 'internal market' reforms such as fundholding by British general practitioners (**GPs**). Unselective contracting by uncoordinated payers, as in the United States around 1990, seems to be the most costly possible approach.

Highly pooled funds tend to be associated with co-ordinated payment. Yet selective contracting may be implemented within a large pool, as in NHS GP fundholding, while high cost-sharing could be combined with standard fees. Thus distinguishing the two dimensions allows more careful analysis than a simple division into more 'market-like' or 'regulatory' approaches.

Choices about targets and systems affect only potential for cost control; performance depends on the specific measures chosen and the commitment of payers to control costs. Extreme positions on these two dimensions none the less have very different risks, both for other health care variables and interests. For example, higher cost-sharing is probably a more direct threat to equity of care, but a lesser threat to the incomes of providers, than some other cost control measures. The much-vaunted 'marketization' of Western systems has generally involved moves towards selective contracting rather than lesser socialization. The evidence does not yet show that highly selective contracting controls costs more effectively than highly co-ordinated payment.

Paying doctors

Cost control choices have many implications for doctors in particular. They tend to prefer higher cost-sharing to alternative cost control measures. But cost-sharing is particularly unpopular with voters, so policies tend to focus instead on the structure of doctors' compensation.

Economists worry that doctors may respond to fee restraints by encouraging patients to consume more services. Capitation or salary would not be vulnerable to that response, but may create incentives to provide fewer services than are necessary. Both private and public policy-makers therefore seek mixed compensation schemes that might limit either failure. In most countries doctors have much preferred fee-for-service payment. Yet methods that reduce fees automatically in response to increased services, as prevailed in Germany from 1985 to 1997, seem to counter the effect of any volume increases, leaving doctors as a group working more for the same money. In many countries, therefore, doctors' organizations are rethinking their preferences about payment methods.

Policy-makers virtually everywhere would like to get the medical profession to 'manage care', making it more appropriate, and to manage the balance among price, volume, and quality within a budget. Unfortunately, even German physicians, with a supportive tradition and institutions, find corporate self-management difficult.

As an alternative, some schemes make individual doctors or groups of doctors responsible for the cost of pharmaceutical, hospital, or other services. Unless these responsibilities are limited and spread across a large payment base, they can create dangerous incentives to deny necessary care.

Fairy tales and the future

Policy-makers and critics dream of more 'rational' measures than those discussed above. One is that policies to keep people healthy would save lots of money on acute care. There is little or no confirming evidence. Another is that societies could prioritize medical services within budgets, excluding those that science shows to be least cost-effective. But such general rules would not be appropriate for many individual cases. The state of Oregon's well-publicized prioritization of treatments in its insurance for the poor has contributed little to cost control, both because the covered list was quite extensive, and capitated providers found that distinguishing covered from uncovered treatments was not worth the trouble. Instead, each Western country must choose its own imperfect policy, with attendant consequences. The trend towards relatively increased spending on health is likely to continue, because longer, less painful lives seem desirable to most people, and modern medicine is believed capable of providing that. But systems will vary in both total costs and cost-effectiveness.

Further reading

Barros PP (1998). The black box of health care expenditure growth determinants. *Health Economics* **7**, 533–44.

Dudley RA *et al.* (1998). The impact of financial incentives on quality of health care. *The Milbank Quarterly* **76**, 649–86.

Jacobs L, Marmor T, Oberlander J (1999). The Oregon health plan and the political paradox of rationing: what advocates and critics have claimed and what Oregon did. *Journal of Health Politics, Policy and Law* **24**, 161–80.

Reinhardt U (1996). Our obsessive campaign to 'gut' the hospital. *Health Affairs* **15**, 145–54.

Rice T, Morrison KR (1994). Patient cost-sharing for medical services: a review of the literature and implications for health care reform. *Medical Care Review* **51**, 235–87.

White J (1999). Targets and systems of health care cost control. *Journal of Health Politics, Policy and Law* **24**, 653–96.

3.7.2 Health in a fragile future

Maurice King

Politics is health. Health is also politics—the operation of power in society—to the grave disadvantage of today's poor and tomorrow's everybody. The traditional enemies of public health—infection, etc.—have been reinforced by those three serpents: the world, the flesh, and the devil, newly armed and globalized for the coming millennium. For 'the world' read 'Mammon'—the overarching quest for wealth, and the power that it brings. For the devil and the flesh read on.

This is written at the start of the new millennium. The human population of the earth has just exceeded 6 billion (12 October 1999), having tripled during the writer's lifetime. Mankind has already passed the high-point in per capita oil consumption (1979) and in grain consumption (1985). The average human is unlikely ever to have so much energy at his disposal again, or to be so well fed.

Wealth

One superpower with 4.6 per cent of the world's population now dominates the earth. Half the world's health expenditure is spent there, and a quarter of its fossil fuel is burnt there. Most serious, that superpower dominates what the world thinks, and it dominates the United Nations system. Within it, money dominates. With a public 'dumbed down' by the media, power is increasingly concentrated, not in Congress and Senate, but in the Department of State, in lobbyists, in think tanks, and in the boardrooms of transnational corporations, especially those which control the media. Domestically, the proper functions of government are being increasingly abrogated to lucrative struggles between lawyers.

The market economy reigns supreme, with no credible alternative on the horizon. The market is now advertisement-driven to produce ever more luxurious resource consumption, and ever less sustainable lifestyles, to the point that tourism has now become the largest industry on earth. The rich become ever richer, and the gap between rich and poor ever wider. More and more wealth is in fewer and fewer hands. For the fortunate, wealth effortlessly creates more wealth as never before. Meanwhile, during the last 20 years, 60 countries have been getting steadily poorer.

With the coming of the new millennium, and the stock markets buoyant, the mood (for the fortunate) is bullish. Unfortunately, the prosperity bubble is fragile. Besides the technical problems of the stability of the global economic system, the bubble can only continue to swell if certain major problems are overlooked—population, global warming, global food, the rising energy costs of fossil fuel exhaustion, and the effects of the media on the stability of the family. One or more of these could prick the bubble and all have the gravest implications for health. In the United States, the market economy requires a per capita carbon dioxide production of 20 tonnes annually, and in the United Kingdom 10 tonnes. Globally, the sustainable fair share is probably about 1.4 tonnes. I argue for radical adaptations in lifestyle, North and South, for equity, frugality, ecology, economy, and for the intense dialogue that must accompany the solution of our major problems. Susan George reminds us that the fossil fuel based economic activity of the present 2 billion 'haves' who burn that fossil fuel, is destroying the world, and that the 9 billion, who by 2050 will want that economic activity, will destroy the world even more disastrously — with no adequate means of either controlling or sharing such economic activity as the world might support sustainably. Meanwhile, the 'have nots' who will not enjoy such benefits are likely to become increasingly violent, North and South. The market economy is therefore destroyed either way. She concludes that we cannot both sustain the liberal free-market economy and continue to tolerate 'the superfluous billions'. This was published in 1999. September 11 2001 has proved how right she is. Before discussing the difficulties of opening this dialogue on a sufficient scale, there is a more immediate problem for physicians.

Health as a free market commodity

Now that the service sector of the economy is growing faster than manufacturing, it has become a tempting source of profit, with the result that the unfettered free market is becoming increasingly perilous for those who cannot afford private health care. Traditionally, most governments have sought to provide some form of insurance-based and tax-supported 'national health service' which was available to everyone, and which strove to 'generalize the adequate' in health care. Of these, the British National Health Service was much admired.

High on the agenda of the World Trade Organization (WTO) is the privatization of education, health, welfare, and social housing. The race is on to capture that share of gross domestic product (GDP) which governments spend on public services, and to open the European public market to transnational competition to the disadvantage of universal coverage, of solidarity through risk pooling, of equity, of comprehensive care, and to the European tradition of democratic accountability—largely in the pursuit of profit.

Opposition to all this is disorganized and inchoate. Over a thousand non-governmental organizations (NGOs) opposed the WTO's 1999 meeting in Seattle. Out of this soup of opposition a coherent, high profile, alternative has yet to crystallize. The problem is that, whereas the WTO's objective is simple—profit—that of the 'the global new green left', if such it can be called, is complex, and lacks a tangible manifesto. It is part green, part animal rights, part local autonomy, part antitransnational, and part much else. It is also divided North/South. Since it is commonly at variance with itself, there is no single voice to articulate the opposition to the free market status quo, and to debate the many problems connected with it. The greatest of these is population.

Demographic disentrapment

Demographic disentrapment is the crux—communities exceeding the carrying capacities of their ecosystems with nowhere to go, and with economies that do not enable them to compete for food on the world market. The Belgian administration had long considered Rwanda trapped. The classic case of as yet peaceable entrapment is Malawi, which has outgrown the carrying capacity of its fragile ecosystem, and where chronic malnutrition is endemic. Half its children are stunted. Expert opinion considers (privately) that much of Africa is trapped. There are also grave doubts about the ability of India to feed a population which is expected to increase by 50 per cent and exceed that of China. Its per capita grain is already falling gently, and water is an even greater constraint than land.

Starvation permitting, Malawi's population, without AIDS, was set to have tripled by 2050, and eventually to have quadrupled. With AIDS it is expected to increase by only 50 per cent. Without AIDS, immediate one-child families would have been essential. Now that AIDS has removed Malawi's demographic momentum, two-child families may be sufficient. The tragedy of AIDS has made the disentrapment of Malawi possible. This opportunity has to be grasped courageously on a continental scale.

Demographic entrapment is tightly taboo to demographers, to development economists, and particularly to the United Nations system. It also taboo to most NGOs. There amounts to what the United States demographer Jason Finkle has termed a 'population policy lockstep', in which demography, the great foundations, and the United Nations agencies support the same policies, and in particular deny (publicly) that demographic entrapment exists. The Cairo population conference in 1994 avoided all population targets, and by 1999 at 'Cairo plus five', population control was even further out of fashion.

There are many reasons for this lockstep. The most politically sensitive one is that that the United States Department of State appears to be actively interested in maintaining it—presumably, since if the South is to restrict its fertility, the North will be expected to restrain its resource consumption, with the serious implications that this has for the market economy, and for United States resource consumption in particular (see http://www.leeds.ac.uk/demographic.disentrapment).

In effect, there appear to be many more 'Chinas' and 'Malawis' in urgent need of one-or-two-child families, if they are to avoid starvation and slaughter, but no demographer dare say so publicly. China's triumph is that one-child families have become the socially-responsible norm. Equity requires that if any community is to be counselled to reduce its fertility drastically, we all should. If therefore the United Nations is to suggest that any country should do so, it will have to be in the context of a United Nations programme for 'a one-or-two-child world'—we are all in it together. This cannot be a tight directive, but has rather to be a 'general political direction' in which the world needs to go. In the uproar over population that would result, Italy for example, with a total fertility of 1.2, and which is afraid that it might disappear, might try to raise its fertility.

Demographic entrapment is only one of many problems in which population plays a part, often a large part. Others include poverty, hunger, malnutrition, increasing global inequality, deforestation, street children, and, indirectly, global warming. To make demographic entrapment taboo is also to hinder gravely the resolution of these other problems —in effect to obstruct the solution of all the major human problems. The consequences of doing this, particularly if the desire to preserve Northern levels of resource consumption, is ultimately the major factor, are diabolical— 'overpowering evil' which, incidentally, the *British Medical Journal* saw fit to list as a technical term.

A common fear underlies all this—that of an anarchic, overcrowded world. '*Quand viennent les Africains?*', a Swiss acquaintance asked, not 'if they come' but 'when are they actually coming?' Many have already come. Equity demands that more should come. Reason argues that all cannot come, say a billion from Africa which is having increasing difficulty feeding itself, and where the fertility of the land is falling widely, and perhaps another half a billion from Asia. The future of the world is brown. How brown? What does seem clear is that for the majority of the trapped, disentrapment will have to take place *in situ*, if they are not to starve or slaughter themselves on the spot. But there is another threat to the family, besides that to its size.

The flesh and the family

The most important institution for human welfare is the family—that cradle of the virtues, 'in sickness and in health', 'for richer for poorer'. The fact that the family is falling apart so widely is thus of the gravest consequences for health and human well being. Why is the family in such decline? Taboos, it seems, are important for maintaining the structure of society. The taboo on entrapment helps to preserve the current North/South power structure. It may well be that the many kinds of taboo with which all societies have surrounded sex—'who may say, or show what, when, where, and to whom', play an important part in maintaining the structure of the family, and that the weakening of the taboos, under the persistent attrition of the media, to which we are all increasingly exposed, from the age of three onwards—in effect 'anything goes'—bears a large part of the blame. We are each the recipients of many years of nurturing in the bosoms of our families. When we die we take these blessings with us. A society which fails to replace the 'social capital' generated by the family, does so at its peril. The consequences of this loss are all around us.

So where is the devil?

Any serious writer or *mediaste* hopes to influence what other people think. The devil lies in what he wants them to think—and not to think—and why, and on the scale and the means by which he does it. Even modest deviance from 'political correctness' becomes ever more difficult in an increasingly 'one-think', one-language, one-superpower, CNN world, with its ever more narrowly focused centres of wealth and power. Frances Stonor Saunders has documented the multifarious ways in which the United States Department of State manipulated the intelligentsia, both left and right, during the Cold War. There is no reason to think that this manipulation has ceased. The policing of the population policy lockstep is a particularly clear example. A really free unlockstepped press capable of debating anything, however alarming, and whatever implications it has for northern lifestyles, is critical.

The idea that, in a world of supposed free speech, the media need to be controlled in order to protect the family, and to prevent our behaviour being too gravely manipulated by scientifically crafted advertisement, and if so how, and by whom, is a thought so outrageous as to defy credulity. But so was the *contagium vivum,* and a spinning earth. We are just starting to think about tempering the free market, the proposed Tobin tax on financial transfers being the outstanding example. But this must be only the beginning.

So as we pore in triumph over the atoms in our chromosomes, let us not forget that we have no clue as to how those atoms bring us conscious minds, and that the devil is as busy as ever in influencing what those minds think, and in narcotizing our consciences so us to prevent our getting to grips with the terrifying problems that beset us—and those who come after us. The first millennium started with a command to care for all men. The important difference now is that we have 30 times as many to care for, and that for 'our fellow men' we should now read 'all terrestrial creation'. Such, then, is the fragile future of public health in a new millennium.

Further reading

Campbell CJ and Lacherrère JH (1998). The end of cheap oil. *Scientific American*, **278**, 78–83.

George S (1999). *The Lugano Report on preserving capitalism in the 21st Century.* Pluto Press, London.

King MH (1999). Commentary: bread for the world—another view. *British Medical Journal* **319**, 991.

King MH (1999). The US Department of State is policing the population policy lockstep. *British Medical Journal* **319**, 998–1001.

King MH and Elliott CM (1997). To the point of farce: A Martian view of the Hardinian taboo—the silence that surrounds population control. *British Medical Journal* **315**, 1441–3.

Saunders FS (1999). *Who paid the piper?* Granta Books, London.

Willey D (1997). Population control: a necessity for the preservation of individual liberty. *Politics and the Life Sciences,* **16**, 228–30.

4

Molecular mechanisms of disease

4.1 The genomic basis of medicine

Trevor Woodage and Francis S. Collins

Introduction

Much of the progress made in biomedical science in the past century has been due to an increasingly sophisticated understanding of the cellular and molecular mechanisms underlying disease processes. Deciphering the nucleotide sequence of the DNA molecules that make up the 46 chromosomes found within each human diploid cell will represent a major milestone in our ability to understand these processes. In particular, knowledge of the sequence of the human genome will help us understand the structure and function of the proteins and RNA molecules that control the developmental programmes and functions of human cells in health and disease. The Human Genome Project is a large, multinational effort that has among its goals determining the complete human genetic sequence by the year 2003, although most of the sequence was already available in 2000, and two groups published draft sequences in 2001. Along with its technical goals, the Human Genome Project has brought dramatic changes in the ways in which biological and medical processes are viewed. This chapter will discuss some of these influences on modern medical theory and practice.

The terms genetics and genomics are often incorrectly used interchangeably. Genetics refers to the study of inherited traits or characteristics, while genomics describes the study of the large-scale structure and composition of the material encoding these genetic instructions. Applying a genomic approach to medicine involves an appreciation of the complex set of interactions that govern the repertoire of genes that are expressed in different tissues under conditions of health and disease.

Scope of the Human Genome Project

Although initially met with widespread scepticism, proposals to determine the complete DNA sequence of the human genome began to circulate in the mid 1980s. This objective was ambitious both in its scientific scope and in its technological requirements. The suggestion that efforts to discover the sequence of individual genes, answering specific biological questions, were to be supplanted by industrial-scale programmes to analyse large numbers of genes or chromosome regions using novel methods and equipment was not well received in all quarters. Debates about the relative merits of gene-based (cDNA) versus whole genome sequencing projects eventually moved to a consensus (but not unanimous) position that both approaches were worth pursuing.

The development of several generations of semiautomated DNA sequencing apparatus that helped to drive down costs gave impetus to arguments that large-scale sequencing efforts were feasible. Even so, the international Human Genome Project was expected to require funding of 3 billion dollars over 15 years to sequence the estimated 3×10^9 base pairs (bp) making up the haploid genome. A substantial proportion of that expense was not directly attributable to DNA sequencing, but rather to providing infrastructure in the form of genetic and physical maps of the human genome, and work on the genomes of model organisms. Construction of these maps, in turn, depended upon the development of new DNA cloning and analytical methods, especially large-insert cloning vehicles such as yeast artificial chromosomes (YACs) and bacterial artificial chromosomes (BACs). YACs and BACs allow the propagation of extended regions of genomic DNA (100 000 to more than 1 million bp) in multiple copies in cultured yeast and bacterial cells respectively. Availability of these cloned DNA molecules allows analysis of large, but manageable, chromosomal fragments that encompass complete genes.

Exceeding expectations, and with the entry of private sector efforts to spur progress, it appears that the complete sequence of the human genome will be available substantially before the initial target date, 2005. In fact, in June 2000 announcements of the completion of the first draft of the human genome sequence were made, and in February 2001 publications appeared describing the draft sequence and its initial analysis. Both public and private sector sequencing efforts arrived at similar estimates of human genome size, at approximately 3.1×10^9 bp, remarkably close to earlier estimates based upon measurements of the amount of DNA contained in an average cell's nucleus. Continuing attempts to provide an essentially complete, ordered representation of the sequence of the human genome are now planned to be finished by 2003.

Generation of these huge amounts of DNA sequence is of little benefit if there is no effective way of interpreting what it means. The creation of large databases containing different kinds of genomic information together with sophisticated software algorithms that can detect protein coding regions, compare related sequences to each other and identify biologically relevant patterns or sequence motifs have given rise to the rapidly expanding discipline of bioinformatics. Although most public attention paid to the Human Genome Project has, naturally enough, been given to sequencing the human genome, early realizations that one of the most effective ways of interpreting sequence data was by cross-species comparison led to the establishment of parallel efforts to sequence a series of model organisms. The complete, or near complete, genomic sequence has been determined for over 20 bacterial species including *E. coli* (5 million bp); *Saccharomyces cerevisae* (12 Mb), a simple, unicellular eukaryote, the common baker's yeast; *Caenorhabditis elegans* (97 Mb), a simple multicellular nematode used in many types of basic research; and *Drosophila melanogaster* (120 Mb), the fruit fly used by biologists for almost 100 years as a model for studying genetics and development. Major efforts to sequence the genomes of the mouse, rat, and zebrafish are underway. These efforts are providing a solid foundation for understanding the genomic basis of many aspects of molecular and cellular physiology.

Implications of genomics for medical practice

Disease gene identification

Initial successes (prior to 1985) in cloning genes that were mutated in human genetic diseases required a detailed understanding of the pathophysiology of the disorder being investigated and the nature of the proteins whose sequences were altered (such as the roles of the α-globin and β-globin genes in the thalassaemias). Unfortunately, such approaches could not be applied in most cases. For example in cystic fibrosis, the most common serious autosomal recessive disease to affect Caucasians, little was known about the molecular causes of the respiratory and gastrointestinal problems that occurred in patients with this uniformly fatal disease. The lack of any detailed knowledge about the protein whose function was disrupted in cystic fibrosis meant that it was impossible to use standard methods to proceed from phenotype to protein to gene. In order to discover the gene that was mutated in cystic fibrosis, it was necessary to follow a novel strategy, which has become known as positional cloning.

Because of its pattern of inheritance, the gene that was mutated in cystic fibrosis was known to lie on one of the autosomes (chromosomes 1–22) rather than on a sex chromosome (the X or Y chromosomes). Cystic fibrosis carriers would have one abnormal copy of the gene and affected individuals would have mutations in both copies of the gene. By examining the pattern of inheritance of a panel of variable DNA markers, it was possible to identify genetic markers lying on the long arm of chromosome 7 whose inheritance patterns correlated with carrier or disease status more often than expected by chance alone. These markers were thus said to show genetic linkage to the cystic fibrosis gene. The cystic fibrosis gene candidate interval was narrowed by identifying additional polymorphic DNA markers that were more finely distributed throughout this part of chromosome 7. Even when this process, linkage analysis, is successful, the chromosomal region containing the disease gene usually consists of several hundred thousand to several million base pairs, typically containing 10 to 100 genes. Clearly, this is a considerable improvement over individually investigating the 30 000 to 40 000 genes that the human genome is estimated to contain, but it is still a daunting target.

The DNA sequences that make up the protein-coding regions of genes occupy only 1.5 per cent of chromosomal DNA (the rest is largely repetitive DNA and spacer elements of unknown function). Thus, it is not a trivial matter to identify all of the genes in a candidate interval of a million or more base pairs. A number of techniques have been developed to identify the genes within a defined interval of chromosomal DNA, most requiring large cloned DNA molecules covering the chromosomal interval under investigation. Recent improvements in the ability to identify and obtain these cloned molecules using BACs and YACs have greatly facilitated gene identification, but all will soon be superceded by the availability of the complete, ordered, human DNA sequence, together with ever-improving annotations of gene location and structure.

Once the genes within the chromosomal segment containing the disease gene have been discovered, the laborious task of finding which of these genes contains the pathogenic mutation is undertaken. In some instances, easily recognized abnormalities such as large deletions or chromosomal translocations disrupt the genes, but in most cases subtle changes in DNA sequence produce disease. The most definitive subtle alterations are mutations that result in the premature termination of a growing peptide chain during the translation of an mRNA coding sequence into protein. Thus, the simple alteration C to A, changing the codon TAC (encoding tyrosine) to TAA (a stop signal) will prematurely terminate protein manufacture. Similarly, the deletion or insertion of a small number of bases (not divisible by three) will cause a frame-shift in which interpretation of codons downstream of the mutation site will be scrambled, and a premature stop codon is usually formed by chance. Simple sequence changes that do not produce premature termination signals may be harder to recognize as being responsible for disease. For example changing a TCG codon to TCA would be unlikely to result in a disease state because both of these nucleotide triplets code for the amino acid serine. Substituting ACG for TCG produces threonine instead of serine. These two amino acids are chemically closely related and substituting one for the other may or may not result in a significant functional alteration. A TCG to CCG change, however, produces proline instead of serine. This amino acid change is non-conservative and more likely to produce a protein that functions differently from the wild-type form. Other subtle mutations that may be difficult to recognize can involve alterations in the DNA sequences that direct the occurrence of normal messenger RNA splicing, or regulatory elements such as promoters, or enhancers which control gene expression.

There are several ways to distinguish between mutations that cause inherited disease and harmless genetic polymorphisms that do not significantly change protein function or patterns of gene expression. A mutation may segregate in families with the presence of disease but not be found in unaffected controls. Cases of highly penetrant autosomal dominant disease that arise spontaneously in pedigrees where the illness has not previously been noted should manifest mutations in the affected proband that are not present in germline DNA from either biological parent. Comparing amino acid sequences of homologous proteins from different species can also help to distinguish between disease-causing mutations and harmless polymorphisms. If the amino acid in question is conserved across a range of species then it is more likely that this specific amino acid residue performs an important role and that altering it would have a significant effect on protein function. Finding pedigree-specific mutations involving different amino acids in the same gene can also add confidence to the search. A more direct test of the significance of a particular sequence change is to examine its effect directly in a functional assay. It may be possible to introduce a copy of a gene containing the sequence change into an appropriate cell line and measure whether protein function has been altered. To perform this type of experiment meaningfully, the protein being studied must be sufficiently understood to develop an assay.

In the case of cystic fibrosis, one of the genes in the candidate interval of chromosome 7 being investigated was found to have a three base pair deletion that segregated with disease status in many affected pedigrees. This results in the absence of a phenylalanine residue at position 508 of the protein, named the cystic fibrosis transmembrane conductance regulator because of its potential effects on ion flow across cell membranes. Loss of the phenylalanine from the protein disturbs intracellular processing, preventing the mature protein from reaching the cell membrane.

In 1989, the feat of identifying the specific 3-bp sequence alteration represented by the mutation known as ΔF508, amidst a genome 3×10^9 bp in size, was a testament to the potential power of positional cloning. However, when practised without a pre-existing framework of polymorphic DNA markers and large-insert DNA clones spanning the genome, this process proved very laborious, time-consuming, and expensive. Fortunately, as a consequence of the Human Genome Project, high-resolution genetic maps now exist for all of the chromosomes. Thus, it is usually no longer necessary to identify novel polymorphic DNA markers when trying to narrow the chromosomal intervals containing disease genes. Further, once a candidate chromosomal interval has been identified, it is now a straightforward matter to obtain DNA clones and most of the sequence covering the region containing the disease gene. The identification of genes lying within a specific genomic interval was previously greatly facilitated by the mapping of a large number of genes to well-defined chromosomal intervals, and is now even more enhanced by the availability of richly annotated genomic sequence databases. Significant technical advances have also been made in the field of identifying sequence variants that represent disease-causing mutations although, in many ways, this area remains the rate-limiting step in positional cloning projects.

Common diseases as complex traits

While great advances have been made in the realm of identification of the causes of single-gene disorders, genetic factors contributing to the development of more common diseases are, on the whole, much less well understood. It is generally accepted that a hereditary component contributes to the aetiology of almost all types of disease. Evidence in support of this contention is provided by observations that family members of affected individuals have the same disease more often than do members of the general population. Of course, a portion of disease familiality may also be due to shared environmental exposures, and care must be taken to consider this when examining such statistics. Nevertheless, careful study designs have allowed the identification of substantial genetic contributions to such common diseases as diabetes mellitus (both types I and II), asthma, essential hypertension, atherosclerosis, degenerative neurological disorders such as senile dementia and Parkinson's disease, the major mental illnesses, and many forms of cancer. Unlike single-gene disorders, common diseases tend not to segregate in families in easily recognized mendelian patterns. For example first-degree relatives of someone with an autosomal dominant disease such as familial hypercholesterolaemia have a 50 per cent chance of carrying the same mutation in the LDL receptor and second-degree relatives have a 25 per cent chance of carrying the mutation. Risk of developing the disease falls with this predictable pattern, depending directly upon the degree of relatedness to the index case. In common polygenic diseases, however, disease risk declines much more rapidly with the genetic distance from the index case. For this reason, familial clusters tend to be fairly small, making them difficult to recognize and study. Such clusters can also be the result of chance, when the disease is common. It is at least partly for these reasons that intensive genetic analyses of many common diseases remain in relatively early stages.

Common diseases are often known as complex traits because they are thought to be due to complex interactions between multiple genetic and environmental factors. Thus, genetic factors that might contribute to type I diabetes mellitus include a locus within the HLA complex, a polymorphic region just upstream of the coding region of the insulin gene and over a dozen other as yet, uncloned genetic loci in addition to presumed environmental exposures such as Coxsackie virus infection. While the presence of HLA-DQw8 has been associated with type I diabetes, possessing this allele does not guarantee that an individual will develop diabetes. In fact, most people with HLA-DQw8 will not become diabetic unless they also carry other predisposing genetic variants and are exposed to certain, largely undefined, environmental factors. In the absence of a complete understanding of these interactions, it is not yet possible, in most instances, to develop models capable of describing precise risk patterns for complex trait inheritance. Nevertheless, a variety of parameters have been used to quantify the relative contribution of various genetic and environmental factors that play a role in the development of disease. One of these quantitative measures is denoted λ, and represents the ratio between the risk of a relative of a patient developing disease compared with the risk of an individual selected at random from the general population. λ_s refers to the λ value for siblings of index cases. Thus, λ_s for type I diabetes is approximately 20, representing the relative risk of a sibling of a diabetic patient developing the disease (6 per cent) compared to the population risk of developing type I diabetes (0.3 per cent). This compares with much higher values for genetic disorders displaying simple mendelian patterns of inheritance. For example the λ_s for cystic fibrosis is approximately 750 in Caucasians (λ_s will tend to be large for rare disorders with low population prevalence). It should be remembered that λ measures the effect of combined genetic and shared environmental factors. Each individual component necessarily must confer a smaller relative risk than the total λ. The manner in which distinct risk factors combine to yield the overall value of λ for a condition can be additive or multiplicative depending upon whether they are independent of each other or synergistic. Values of λ_s for a number of disorders are shown in Table 1. In any case, individual genes that play a role in the development of common diseases may only cause comparatively small increases in the relative risk of developing disease. Assessing the clinical importance of each of these effects may pose substantial challenges in individual patients and they will need to be interpreted in the context of the presence of other genetic variants, exposure to environmental risk factors, and the overall clinical setting. When considered in large populations, however, even sequence variants that are responsible for modest increases in disease risk can be associated with a major public health burden.

While the distinction between 'simple' and 'complex' diseases is a useful one in helping to understand their genetic underpinnings, it is an artificial division. For example approximately 1 in 10 000 individuals possess frameshift mutations that produce truncated and non-functional versions of one copy of their APC genes, causing familial adenomatous polyposis. This

Table 1 Relative risk to siblings (λ_s) of developing particular clinical conditions

Disorder	λ_s
Haemophilia A (males)	3750
Cystic fibrosis	750
Autism	55
Type I diabetes mellitus	20
Multiple sclerosis	15
Schizophrenia	11
Inflammatory bowel disease	10
Grave's disease	5.9
Cholelithiasis	4.5
Type II diabetes mellitus	3.2
Duodenal ulcer	3.0
Migraine	3.0
Lung cancer (adjusted for tobacco exposure)	1.3

condition is characterized by the development of hundreds to thousands of intestinal polyps. Without prophylactic colectomy or other preventive measures, there is a high likelihood that one or more of these polyps will undergo malignant transformation. Untreated, most patients will develop cancer of the colon by 40 years of age. Approximately 7 per cent of Ashkenazi Jews carry a non-truncating T→A sequence variant in APC, rendering the gene unstable and prone to further mutation in dividing cells of the colonic epithelium. This APC mutation appears to be associated with a 1.5 to 2-fold increased risk of developing colorectal carcinoma. This contrast between levels of cancer risk for low-frequency, high-penetrance and high-frequency, low-penetrance alleles of the same gene is an important one, and helps to demonstrate the spectrum of risk associated with different disease-associated alleles. Moreover, it helps to remind us that, strictly speaking, genes do not cause genetic disease, specific alleles of genes confer risk.

The challenge of identifying sequence variants contributing to complex disease

Several of the factors that make it difficult to find DNA sequence changes associated with complex disease have already been alluded to above. They include the absence of large numbers of affected family members sharing identical mutations, the fact that many of the sequence variants found in chronic disease are likely to be subtle changes that are difficult to recognize, and the expectation that the predictive power of particular sequence changes will generally be quite low. Patients with the sequence variant may not have the disease (low penetrance) and some patients with the disease will not carry the sequence variant (phenocopies). In contrast to the situation for simple mendelian disorders in which it may be possible to identify pathogenic mutations by analysing DNA samples from only a small number of cases, for complex disease samples will be needed from hundreds or perhaps thousands of cases. Rather than being able to make simple decisions about whether or not a sequence variant is the causative allele, sophisticated statistical analyses will generally be necessary.

Several approaches are being used to search for disease-associated sequence variants. Instead of relying on collecting large pedigrees, one type of study analyses pairs of affected siblings looking for evidence of excess allele sharing at loci that might be linked to disease. Two siblings can have none, one, or two alleles in common at a particular polymorphic genetic marker, with an expected frequency distribution of 25 per cent, 50 per cent, and 25 per cent respectively. If a particular allele were associated with disease risk, then both siblings with the disease would be expected to carry this allele more often than by chance alone. In large sets of sibling pairs, this would be manifested by statistically significant deviation from the expected distribution of shared alleles.

It is believed that many DNA variants that predispose to common disease traits will be ancient, derived from a common ancestor at some time in the past. More recent examples of shared ancestral alleles causing disease have come from studies of monogenic disorders. For instance in the case of porphyria variegata, two apparently unrelated Afrikaaners with the disease are highly likely to have the same underlying mutation and be descended from a pair of Dutch immigrants who arrived in South Africa in the early seventeenth century. In more outbred populations, the sources of such founder mutations will generally lie in the more distant past. Individuals who carry disease gene variants with common origins will also carry the same alleles at nearby polymorphic markers that were present on the ancestral chromosome on which the mutation first occurred. The distance over which these shared polymorphisms will be observed depends, in part, on the age of the variant. The greater the number of generations that have passed, the greater the chance that meiotic chromosomal recombination will have occurred, creating new patterns of associated markers.

The concept of association between disease status and specific alleles at nearby polymorphic markers in apparently unrelated subjects is known as linkage disequilibrium. Although there remains some uncertainty relating to these estimates, it is likely that, in groups that have not gone through recent population bottlenecks, linkage disequilibrium will extend for regions estimated to be 25 to 30 kb, on average. This means that in order to perform genome-wide scans for disease-associated alleles, roughly 200 000 to 300 000 polymorphic markers will need to be examined (in contrast to the 300–400 markers that are often used to search for monogenic disease genes by linkage analysis in affected families).

Even though characterizing common variants in human DNA was not part of the original goals of the Human Genome Project, that goal has been added. The need for very large numbers of polymorphic markers has meant that a great deal of energy is now being devoted to identifying and cataloguing human genetic variation, and within the next 1 to 2 years it is expected that more than 1 000 000 variants will be found. On average, any two randomly selected chromosomes differ from each other in about one base pair in every thousand. Several efforts have been undertaken to establish databases containing very large numbers of single nucleotide polymorphisms (SNPs). Some methods identify SNPs that are randomly scattered throughout the genome while other approaches target SNP discovery to particular parts of the genome, such as protein coding regions. All of these SNPs may be useful for genetic mapping and linkage disequilibrium studies, though some would argue that focusing on coding region SNPs (cSNPs) will give a higher yield of sequence changes that are more likely to be associated with alterations in gene function. A number of issues relating to the technical and statistical challenges associated with SNP analysis, high through-put genotyping, and the mathematics underlying linkage disequilibrium analysis remain to be resolved. These issues are the subjects of active research.

Changes to medical practice in the age of genomics

Given the great effort needed to define allelic variants contributing to complex disease, it is reasonable to ask whether such a large investment of resources is warranted. To be able to answer in the affirmative, it is necessary to demonstrate that benefits will accrue to everyday medical practice and patient health. Understanding genetic factors that contribute to disease could help establish a more rational basis for many aspects of patient care by providing deep insights into molecular pathogenesis and through improved molecular diagnostic tools that allow individually tailored preventive and/or therapeutic regimens.

Better understanding of molecular mechanisms of disease

Despite the extraordinary advances in our understanding of the functions of cells and organ systems in states of health and disease, it is somewhat humbling that fewer than 5000 human genes have been functionally characterized—many in only a cursory fashion. Clearly, it is difficult to

provide full descriptions of the ways in which disease processes perturb cellular function in the absence of a comprehensive catalogue of genes that are either affected by these disease processes or are involved in the response to disease. The Human Genome Project will provide such a catalogue, giving a complete description of the DNA and protein sequences of all of these genes.

The genome project is providing important tools that will help researchers discover functions of novel proteins. About half of the new genes identified by large-scale DNA sequencing bear some resemblance to other genes that have previously been studied, either in humans or in model organisms. Sequence similarity to previously characterized genes can provide important clues to protein function. In addition to comparisons of primary DNA and protein sequences, computerized approaches to predicting three-dimensional protein structures are becoming increasingly feasible, and may also allow generation of testable predictions about gene function.

Of course, many novel genes do not have any (or enough) similarity to known genes for useful predictions to be made, and direct experimental investigation may be required to determine their function. To deal with the large number of new genes that are being identified by the Human Genome Project, an innovative set of methods has emerged, known collectively as functional genomics, which explore the roles of many genes in parallel. Functional genomics experiments will obtain a great deal of information about patterns of gene expression, protein interactions, and metabolic pathways.

Diagnostic tests

One advance in genomics that is already finding its way into clinical practice is the use of diagnostic tests based on DNA sequence changes. Such tests can be used for several purposes. As with more conventional tests, genetic tests can confirm a specific diagnosis or contribute to the evaluation of problematic differential diagnoses. Presymptomatic diagnostic testing can also be performed in subjects without disease. However, even in the case of high penetrance mutations, such as those found in Huntington's disease, it may be difficult to predict the time at which clinical signs or symptoms will develop. In some cases, measures may be available that will prevent or ameliorate the onset or course of illness. Examples of such conditions include haemochromatosis, in which regular venesection can prevent the sequelae of iron overload, or hereditary non-polyposis colon cancer, in which case colonoscopic removal of premalignant lesions can help to prevent the development of cancer. In the absence of such effective interventions, especially careful consideration must be given to the circumstances in which predictive genetic testing is performed. Some patients find presymptomatic genetic diagnosis helpful because it gives them the opportunity to make long-term plans which include the likelihood (or not) of developing illness. Others prefer 'not to know' and would rather forego testing unless an intervention is available. In many centres, teams that include qualified genetic counsellors are in place to ensure that patients receive appropriate education and non-directive counselling before and after making decisions about whether to undergo testing for serious illnesses.

An important way that DNA testing can differ from conventional diagnostic investigations is in its implications for relatives of the tested proband. A positive (or negative) result may allow one to infer the genotype of individuals other than the proband. For example if a subject had a paternal grandparent with Huntington's disease and was found to have an expanded glutamine-encoding triplet repeat in the Huntington gene herself, then it is virtually certain that her father is also at risk of developing Huntington's disease. Even without his consent to be tested, the father's genotype could be inferred with a high degree of certainty. Such situations can complicate issues relating to informed consent. It is not unusual for several members of a family with a history of a genetic disorder to present for presymptomatic evaluation. Genetic counsellors can help to explore complex issues related to the needs and expectations of different family members while respecting individual autonomy.

To date, most conditions being investigated with DNA-based tests are relatively uncommon, single-gene disorders, and the tests are usually carried out in specialized centres with considerable experience in their execution and interpretation. As the technologies needed to perform these tests become more widely available and the sequence changes being evaluated more frequent, attention will be needed to ensure that procedures relating to DNA-based diagnostics continue to be carefully executed. Such concerns include issues related to quality control, skills in the interpretation of complex test results, provision of adequate genetic counselling, and other matters such as control of record-keeping systems to ensure genetic privacy. As the use of predictive genetic testing becomes more widespread, the associated obligations will fall to an increasingly diverse range of health-care professionals and it is important that they receive adequate training in this area.

Pharmacogenomics

Although not generally thought of in the same way as DNA variations that predispose to complex disease, germ-line sequence changes can also be important determinants of response to pharmacological treatment. The study of DNA sequence polymorphisms affecting metabolism of, and response to, drugs has become known as pharmacogenomics. It has long been recognized that individuals metabolize pharmacological agents at different rates. A substantial proportion of this variation can be due to genetic effects. A classic example of this phenomenon was described well before the modern era of molecular genetics and genomics, with the division of the population into slow and rapid acetylator groups. Approximately 60 per cent of Caucasians, but only 5 to 10 per cent of Asians, show reduced rates of N-acetylation and elimination of a number of drugs, including isoniazid, hydralazine, and caffeine, compared with the remainder of the population who exhibit comparatively rapid N-acetylation. Although initially characterized by standard biochemical tests, the genotypic bases for these metabolic differences in drug metabolism are now known to be several polymorphic variants in the gene N-acetyl-transferase-2 or $NAT2$.

In addition to showing different rates of metabolism and clearance of drugs from the system, subjects are often found to show variable therapeutic responses to these agents. In some cases, this may be due to subtle changes in the structure of drug targets between subjects. For instance several studies have found that schizophrenics with the amino acid histidine at residue 452 of the 5-HT$_{2A}$ serotonin receptor have a poorer antipsychotic response to clozapine than do patients with a tyrosine at this position. In diseases such as essential hypertension that are treated symptomatically, rather than with specific measures, some patients respond better to certain interventions than to others. If the genetic factors that are responsible for different forms of hypertension could be identified, then it might prove possible to tailor treatment regimens specifically directed towards generating responses in the physiological pathways that are perturbed in particular patients. For instance we might be able to predict that a particular patient would be more likely to respond to the antihypertensive effects of β-blockers than ACE inhibitors. We may then be able to use relatively inexpensive, one-time DNA tests, to determine which drugs can be used safely and efficaciously in patients with chronic illness. Such approaches promise to be more effective than the trial and error processes that are now often needed to discover optimal drug treatment regimens.

Development of therapeutic agents

In parallel with the government-funded human genome project, much effort has been expended in the private sector to identify and sequence novel genes. A large part of the motivation behind these efforts is the expectation that new therapeutic agents and targets will be discovered. The distinction between therapeutic agents and targets is one that has important implications for the development strategies that must be used. Therapeutic agents developed from genomic sequence information are usually secreted proteins or hormones that can be made for direct *in vivo* administration. A prime example is the use of recombinant erythropoietin for the treatment of anaemia in chronic renal failure. On the other hand, therapeutic targets can potentially be any proteins that are involved in a disease process or a compensatory response to disease. Once such a target is identified, further effort is needed to develop agents (usually small molecules) that can affect function of the target. Although it remains difficult to predict the three dimensional structure of novel proteins based on amino acid sequence alone, improvements in computational analysis, X-ray crystallography, and nuclear magnetic resonance studies are making it possible to produce increasingly sophisticated models of the active sites of target proteins. Using principles of rational drug design, it will become a more straightforward and less expensive matter to develop new drugs for particular diseases than using the trial-and-error methods that were relied upon in the past. The use of genomic sequence information in identifying targets for drug development is also advancing rapidly in the field of new antibiotic discovery. The genomes of several important microbial pathogens including *H. influenzae*, *S. aureus*, *M. tuberculosis*, and *T. pallidum* have been completely sequenced. Newly identified proteins that are important for bacterial replication or virulence but that do not have close relatives in mammalian cells may provide excellent drug or vaccine targets.

Another exciting possibility that arises from an understanding of the genomic sequence of disease genes is the possibility that the expression of particular proteins might be able to be modulated by developing small molecules that interact specifically with promoter and enhancer elements of the genes coding for these proteins. Considerable advances have been made in both the understanding of factors that influence sequence-specific DNA-binding and the ways in which gene expression are controlled, and it is likely that this knowledge will be used to help develop drugs that can up- or down-regulate gene expression in useful ways for disease treatment or prevention.

Gene therapy

Though they have been slow to come to fruition, the concepts underlying somatic cell gene therapy predate the inception of the Human Genome Project. Initial plans to induce expression of normal proteins in patients with rare genetic defects, such as adenosine deaminase deficiency, have been broadened to include a range of more common diseases such as cancer, atherosclerosis, and AIDS. Achieving clinical benefits from gene therapy has proven to be problematic because of technical difficulties preventing sufficiently high-level expression of recombinant proteins in appropriate tissues. Substantial effort is now being directed to the development of viral and other vectors that will allow more effective delivery of introduced genes to the desired sites. The recent death of a patient involved in a clinical trial using adenovirus as the delivery system has underlined the risks of triggering an overwhelming immune response with such vectors. A full discussion of gene therapies is beyond the scope of this chapter; but clearly, as our understanding of the human and other genomes increases, the range of conditions that are amenable to treatment by various forms of somatic genetic manipulation will also increase.

Public policy implications

With the advances in medical and scientific knowledge that come from the recent, rapid developments in the field of genomics come a host of issues that require consideration by the broader community. Some of these issues have been faced before in other contexts, and some are peculiar to the fields of genetics and genomics.

Genetic privacy

In addition to issues relating to control of access to medical records that are shared with other forms of medical data, there are several privacy concerns that are particular to genetic and DNA sequence-based information. Most people would agree that individuals should have a high degree of control over who has access to information concerning the makeup of their genome. Because relatives share genetic markers, it may be possible to determine a person's genetic constitution without the knowledge or consent of that individual. This can lead to a conflict between one person's desire to be aware of their genetic makeup with another's desire that other people not know his or hers. Deciding 'ownership' of genetic information is not a simple matter and may be difficult to resolve if disputes occur within families. Such disputes also have the potential inadvertently to reveal previously known or unknown instances of non-paternity, with unsettling consequences for those involved.

The use of combinations of polymorphic markers for the purpose of uniquely identifying subjects has found increasing application in non-medical settings, especially forensic science. Privacy concerns have been raised about databases established by government agencies that record DNA profiles of large numbers of individuals. It is important that appropriate safeguards be instituted to ensure that databases that might be used for socially justifiable purposes, such as criminal forensic analysis or identification of deceased military personnel, are not abused.

Health insurance and employment discrimination

Especially in countries such as the United States that do not have universal health insurance programmes, there is concern that people will be denied access to affordable health care because of their genetic makeup. There have been occasional, but well documented, examples of denial of health insurance because patients are at risk of developing genetic illnesses. As the factors underlying genetic contributions to complex disease are elucidated, eventually the majority of people could be found to be at an increased risk of developing one serious medical condition or another. It would be most unfortunate if the possession of an allele that predisposes to cancer of the colon put someone in the position of losing health insurance coverage, rather than the institution of a regular colonoscopy programme that could prevent them from dying of cancer. Legislative solutions are needed to ensure that the availability of health care does not depend upon genetic constitution.

Fears have also been expressed that potential employers could screen applicants for the presence of 'undesirable' genetic traits and use the results of these tests to decide who should be offered positions. Should someone be denied the chance to become an air traffic controller because they were more likely than average to abuse alcohol? Should a person possessing a neurotransmitter receptor variant that makes them prone to depression be prevented from carrying a firearm as a police officer? In general, however, predictions based on such correlations will be rather weak—and thus the strong consensus is that employment decisions should be made solely on the basis of ability to do the job. Here again, legislative protections are needed to prevent discriminatory practices from becoming widespread.

Regulation of novel genetic tests and therapies

Novel diagnostic tests and therapies arising from rapid progress in the field of genomics can pose substantial challenges to statutory regulatory agencies such as the Food and Drug Administration in the United States or the Committee on the Safety of Medicines in the United Kingdom. These authorities may need to acquire quickly the expertise to assess innovative modalities and ensure that they are used appropriately and safely. Many of these issues will best be considered within frameworks similar to those that have been used in other areas of medical practice. The establishment of the Secretary's Advisory Committee on Genetic Testing (SACGT) signals an era of increased scrutiny of predictive genetic tests in the United States.

Many aspects of the traditional drug approval process are being adapted to assess the safety of somatic cell gene therapy and recombinant biotherapeutic agents. Nevertheless, certain of these processes will need to be refined to cope with changes brought about by advances in genomics. Authorities responsible for the governance of genetic testing procedures must address issues relating to informed consent and genetic privacy. Tech-niques with potential to alter the makeup of the human genome, such as germ-line gene therapy and cloning, have already raised thorny moral and philosophical questions.

Education of medical and lay communities

Several factors appear to be responsible for the relatively little attention given by many medical schools to clinical aspects of genetics and genomics. In part because of the relatively large cost of establishing comprehensive research programmes in this area there, has been a tendency for cutting-edge genomics research to be carried out in only a few centres. This, together with the fact that most of the physicians and scientists with experience in genomics tend to be relatively young, has meant that few medical school curricula have received input from senior academics who appreciate the importance of the subject. Clinical genetics has often been taught under the auspices of paediatrics, and has focused on rare diseases. Given the cross-disciplinary nature of the topics that need to be covered to understand genomic aspects of human disease (including clinical medicine, pathology, biochemistry, epidemiology, and biostatistics) and its application to many common diseases of adult onset, it may be that the study of genomics should be considered within a broader context.

With the extensive amount of coverage that has been given to recent advances in genetics and genomics by the print and electronic media, it is not unusual for patients to ask their doctors questions on topics about which the physicians have little information. To meet their patients' needs, and to allow them to be more proactive in addressing preventive medicine and other health concerns, it is important that established medical practitioners and physicians in training have access to continuing medical education resources informing them about genomic aspects of human disease. In the United States, the recent formation of the National Coalition for Health Care Professional Education in Genetics (by the National Human Genome Research Institute, American Medical Association, and American Nursing Association) promises to fuel this effort. Several databases and other resources are already accessible on the world wide web. As a useful starting point, the National Center for Biotechnology Information site (www.ncbi.nlm.nih.gov) provides access to On-line Mendelian Inheritance in Man (OMIM), a comprehensive collection of information related to inherited disease phenotypes. Other highly useful sites include Gene-Clinics (www.geneclinics.org), which provides authoritative reviews on the diagnosis and management of specific genetic disorders, and GeneTests (www.genetests.org), which provides a guide to availability of genetic testing services.

At the same time, members of the lay public will benefit from an increased understanding of how genetic factors might be important in managing their health. Challenges that have to be met in this arena include the sometimes technically complex types of information that need to be understood, as well as the probabilistic nature of many of the clinically relevant associations between genotype and phenotype under consideration. While many patients will take the initiative to try to learn about medical aspects of genomics for themselves, most will benefit from education from a number of sources, especially their physicians and other health-care providers.

Conclusion

It is not an exaggeration to assert that the field of genomics has revolutionized biomedical research in recent years. The process of transition from the laboratory to the clinic is still in its early phases but holds great promise. Insights into the pathological processes underlying many illnesses will expand the range of diagnostic and therapeutic options available to the clinician. Perhaps the most exciting near-term advance that the fruits of the Human Genome Project offers is the opportunity to develop personalized risk profiles based on the particular patterns of DNA sequence variation that individual patients exhibit. These profiles will give us many chances to ameliorate the effects of disease by instituting appropriate preventive health measures and tailoring treatment regimens to specific patients based on their genotypes.

We must be cautious, however, not to overestimate the power of genomics to explain clinical outcomes and other biological phenomena. A comprehensive understanding of the importance of genetic factors in human disease should only serve to highlight the significance of environmental factors as modifiers of genetically coded molecular processes. The effects of genes or DNA sequence variation should not be treated in too deterministic a manner but only regarded as one facet contributing to our understanding of the processes involved in human health and disease.

Further reading

Baxevanis AD, Ouellette BFF, eds (1998). *Bioinformatics: A practical guide to the analysis of genes and proteins*. John Wiley and Sons, New York.

Collins FS (1997). Sequencing the human genome. *Hospital Practice* **15**, 35–43.

Collins FS (1999). Shattuck lecture—medical and societal consequences of the Human Genome Project. *New England Journal of Medicine* **34**, 28–37.

Collins FS, Guyer MS, Chakravarti A (1997). Variations on a theme: cataloging human DNA sequence variation. *Science* **278**, 1580–1.

Evans WE, Relling MV (1999). Pharmacogenomics: translating functional genomics into rational therapeutics. *Science* **286**, 487–91.

Holtzman NA, Murphy PD, Watson MS, Barr PA (1997). Predictive genetic testing: from basic research to clinical practice. *Science* **278**, 602–5.

International Human Genome Sequencing Consortium (2001). Initial sequencing and analysis of the human genome. *Nature* **409**, 860–921.

McCarthy JJ, Hilfiker R (2000). The use of single-nucleotide polymorphism maps in pharmacogenomics. *Nature Biotechnology* **18**, 505–8.

Miklos GL, Rubin GM (1996). The role of the genome project in determining gene function: insights from model organisms. *Cell* **86**, 521–9.

Risch N, Merikangas K (1996). The future of genetic studies of complex human diseases. *Science* **273**, 1516–7.

Venter JC *et al.* (2001). The sequence of the human genome. *Science* **291**, 1304–51.

4.2 The human genome sequence

Sydney Brenner

The modern period in biological research began in 1953 when JD Watson and FHC Crick discovered the double helical structure of DNA. Within the very short period of time of about a decade, the new science of molecular biology uncovered the basic mechanisms of information transfer from genes to proteins in living cells. The nucleotide sequence of a gene was shown to be colinear with the amino acid sequence of the protein that it specified, the genetic code was found to be a triplet code and the correspondences of the three-base codons to each of the 20 amino acids was established. Although there were chemical methods for determining the amino acid sequences of proteins, the structure of the gene was accessible only through mutational changes as recorded by phenotypes. Such mutations defined genes, and these could be mapped by recombination. Research in molecular genetics proceeded most rapidly with bacteria and their viruses which could be handled easily in the laboratory. A beginning was also made to study more complex systems, such as *Drosophila* which had been long established as a laboratory organism for experimental genetics, and *Caenohabditis elegans*, a small, free-living nematode worm.

In the mid 1970s there were two revolutionary, technical innovations which changed the entire course of genetics. The first was a method of cloning and propagating fragments of DNA in bacteria and yeasts and the second was the invention of methods for sequencing DNA. Thus the genome of any organism could be obtained as a library of fragments and the sequences of these fragments could be determined. In principle, therefore, the complete sequence of the genome could be obtained, and since it was possible to clone and sequence cDNA copies of messenger RNA, the expressed genes could be identified and the amino acid sequences of their proteins inferred from the nucleotide sequences. cDNA characterization became important when it was quickly discovered, by the new techniques, that the genes of higher organism were interrupted by intervening sequences called introns which were removed by splicing leaving the coding exons to form a coherent sequence.

For some time the only complete genomes that were sequenced were small, of the order of 100 kb. In 1985, when it was suggested that the complete sequences of the human genome might be obtained, it was realized that not only would there have to be considerable technical improvements, but also the project would have to be on a large scale and require international co-operation. The technical improvements were the automation of many of the laborious steps of the sequencing process, and the availability of sequencing machines and their progressive enhancement in throughput. Larger genomes were tackled and an early accomplishment was the 14-Mb sequence of yeast. This was followed by the sequences of *C. elegans* and *Drosophila*, each of around 100 Mb. In 2001, two groups announced that they had more or less completed the first draft of the human genome sequence, and no doubt this will be subjected to much improvement in future years.

The human genome sequence was seen by many to provide new approaches to human biology and, in particular, to medicine. For example it was claimed that once all the genes were found, all the proteins specified by those genes would be known, and this would allow the uncovering of an enormous number of new targets for the development of new therapeutic agents. In the long run this may prove correct, but before we can use a protein as a drug target we have to know how it functions in the body, and whether any alteration of its activity will have the desired effects. Although the molecular function of a protein can often be specified by comparison of its sequence with proteins of known function, this is insufficient to decide how this activity is translated into a particular cellular process and how this is, in turn, integrated into the physiology of the whole human organism. Thus, for example, while we can readily identify domains with resemblances to proteases, we require additional information to decide what the proteolysis is doing; it may be involved in digestion, in gene regulation, in cell death, in blood coagulation, or the complement pathway. For any protein to be a target we must have something much more than the protein sequence, we must have a therapeutic hypothesis and this will be made possible only by the continuation of conventional biological and clinical research.

There can be no doubt, however, that knowing all or nearly all of the proteins made by cells will spur research on the biochemistry of cells. In particular, this has already had a profound effect on the development of knowledge about cell signalling pathways, DNA repair, protein traffic within cells, and ion channels, to name only a few. In addition, because many of these processes are common to other organisms such as *Drosophila*, the nematode, and even yeast and bacteria, we can draw on research in these organisms to illuminate function in mammalian cells. A whole area of research, called functional genomics by some, relies extensively on this comparative approach. Since mutations in genes are easily obtained in these model organisms, such mutant homologues can inform us about the cellular function of the gene, which can be carried over to the mammalian systems. The main experimental organism for functional analysis is the mouse, a mammalian model organism amenable to a special form of gene manipulation. A line of embryonic cells, ES cells, can be propagated in tissue culture, and when these are injected into a mouse blastula they become incorporated into the embryo and populate both the germline and somatic ells. In this way, transgenic mice can be constructed in which genes have been added or removed from the mouse genome. Mice in which genes have been deleted are called knockout transgenics and can reveal the contribution of the gene to the total phenotype. These methods were used to prove that prions cause the endogenous prion protein to adopt an incorrect form and so cause the neurological disease. Complete removal of the prion gene has no effect of its own but the animals become resistant to infection.

The most significant contribution made by the new genetics has been the identification of the genes involved in single gene mutations in humans. More than 1000 such monogenic, inherited disorders have been identified; some rare, others, such as cystic fibrosis, quite common. These provide the direct test of function and they throw light on the pathogenesis of disease and the underlying molecular causes. In certain areas, such as cholesterol metabolism, the analysis of the changes in certain monogenic diseases has revealed the connections between cholesterol and the ensuing cardiovascular pathology. In addition, even very rare monogenic diseases which resemble the much more common diseases, such as the cases of breast cancer or

Alzheimer's disease, can lead us to understand the pathogenic pathways involved.

There are, however, several very common diseases which can be shown to have a genetic component but are not due to single gene mutations. Schizophrenia, diabetes, and Crohn's disease are common and are about 50 per cent correlated in identical twins. There is, therefore, a large environmental component and the fact that they are polygenic makes it difficult to discover the genes involved. However, the possibility that one might identify the genes with polymorphisms correlating with the disease state has led to the development of what is called predictive medicine or probabilistic medicine. We only have a few of these disease susceptibility marks, but the fact that genetic analysis may be predictive has raised many questions about the ethical, social, and legal consequences of genetic testing. There is very little established work in this field but already there are problems, mostly created by health insurance.

It is clear that in the rush to obtain the sequence, the understanding of the connections between genotype and phenotype has remained superficial. There is a tendency to talk about genes for homosexuality, alcoholism, criminality, and so on. The unravelling of the complex skein of connections between the genes and the final phenotype has only just begun and it will occupy biomedical scientists for the next few decades, at least. DNA sequencing is a unique technology; one can feed a machine with DNA derived from anything—plants, bacteria, humans—and the linear sequence of bases which is the essential information in the DNA can be extracted. There has been an explosion in the amount of data available and there will be much more to come. However, data are not knowledge and only knowledge can lead to understanding the meaning of the sequence and allow us to diagnose and treat human disease.

4.3 Molecular cell biology

William M. F. Lee and Newman M. Yeilding

The molecular mechanisms underlying many cellular and biological functions have been unravelled in recent years and, with this, has come an understanding of the molecular basis of many pathological conditions. This progress promises to provide improved insights into disease pathogenesis, suggest novel opportunities for therapeutic intervention, and launch efforts to make these interventions a part of medical practice. In this chapter, we provide a synopsis of salient features of cell function at the molecular level. Important decisions and events that all cells undergo, such as proliferation, differentiation, and death, are then discussed in molecular terms. Finally, to provide a medical context for this information and illustrate the potential clinical relevance of the knowledge gained, we discuss emerging concepts of the molecular pathogenesis of two important human diseases, cancer and cardiomyopathy. Clearly, none of these sections can hope to be comprehensive given the mass of accumulated knowledge and relatively scant number of pages allotted to this chapter. Accordingly, emphasis has been placed on concepts and principles, with details and examples presented only to better illustrate these paradigms. A further reading list is provided for those seeking more in-depth discussions of the various topics. These are in the nature of review articles and books in order to limit the size of the bibliography. For those with greater interest in the science and who wish to know the details and read the primary articles, the bibliographies of the reviews and book chapters will provide the appropriate references.

Genetic information and information retrieval

No biological process is more universal or fundamental than the way cells store, access, and use the information that is needed for the all the processes involved in creating and sustaining life. Deoxyribonucleic acids (DNA) in the genes of the cell are the repository of this information. DNA is an unbranched, linear polymer constructed of deoxyribonucleotide monomers that are directionally, covalently linked by phosphate bonds between the 5′ hydroxyl group of the deoxyribose sugar moiety of one deoxyribonucleotide and the 3′ hydroxyl group of the deoxyribose moiety of the next deoxyribonucleotide (Fig. 1). Four different deoxyribonucleotides (adenine, A; guanine, G; cytosine, C; and thymine, T) comprise the genetic 'alphabet' with which genetic information is written. Cellular DNA usually exists in a double-stranded (duplex) helical configuration in which one strand is 'zippered' by hydrogen bonds to a second, fully complementary DNA strand. This bonding between complementary strands is established by the nucleotide on one strand interacting with the paired nucleotide on the opposite strand with which it forms the most stable hydrogen bonds: G bonds best with C, C with G, A with T, and T with A. The two strands in duplex DNA maintain full complementarity because, during DNA replication, the DNA polymerase enzymes responsible for synthesis use one strand as template while synthesizing the other through covalent addition of complementary nucleotides to the nascent strand. This type of replication is termed 'semiconservative' because each of the two new daughter DNA strands contains one newly synthesized strand and one previously synthesized strand derived from the original duplex.

In eukaryotic cells, the library of genetic information is stored in chromosomes which consist of exceedingly long strands of DNA with associated proteins that help organize and compact the DNA. The most prominent proteins in chromatin, as chromosomal DNA with associated proteins is called, are the various types of histones. Certain histones form a core around which the DNA is more or less tightly wound, forming a structure called a 'nucleosome'. Nucleosomes are stacked, and stacks of nucleosomes are further organized to allow the very long DNA in chromatin both to fit in chromosomes and, importantly, to be accessible for information

Fig. 1 Chemical structure of DNA and RNA. The chemical structures of the bases that comprise DNA and RNA are depicted in (a). In the nucleotides comprising DNA and RNA, the nitrogen atom at position 9 of purines or position 1 of pyrimidines is covalently bonded to the 1′ carbon atom of a ribose or deoxyribose sugar. DNA and RNA polymers are directionally linked via a phophodiester bond of the 5′ carbon of the sugar moiety of one ribonucleotide or deoxyribonucleotide and the 3′ carbon of another (b). While RNA is most commonly single stranded, DNA primarily exists as a hydrogen-bonded antiparallel duplex between complementary DNA strands (c).

retrieval and replication. Arrayed on each chromosome are a multitude of genes, each of which contains the information necessary to synthesize a functional protein or RNA molecule. Normal somatic cells are diploid, meaning that they possess a pair of every non-sex chromosome (autosomes) and two sex chromosomes, which are either a pair of X chromosomes in cells from females or one X and one Y chromosome in cells from males. This means that two copies of every autosomal gene exist in each cell (one derived from each parent), two copies of X chromosome genes exist in female cells but only one copy in male cells, and one copy of Y chromosome genes exists in male cells and none in female cells. Human cells have 22 pairs of autosomes and two sex chromosomes, so they have 46XX chromosomes if they are female, and 46XY chromosomes if they are male.

An organism's genome contains a complete catalogue of the information required for its development, growth, and function. Proteins are the primary effector molecules responsible for carrying out the instructions written in the genome, and the properties, structure, and function of each protein is largely determined by its amino acid sequence. The principal information carried in the genome is the amino acid sequence of all the proteins produced by that organism. To create these proteins, genomic information is first accessed by transcribing DNA into ribonucleic acid (RNA) format, after which the information in RNA is translated into proteins. The process of gene transcription is carried out by complexes of proteins collectively termed transcription factors and involves the synthesis of RNA copies from DNA templates. RNA differs from DNA structurally in that the sugar moiety is ribose instead of deoxyribose, uracil (U) is incorporated where thymidine (T) is present in DNA, and RNA is usually single-stranded. The absence of a complementary strand means that nucleotides in RNA are free to form hydrogen bonds with other nucleotides in the same RNA (intrachain hydrogen bonding), a property that allows RNA to become highly folded and adopt secondary structures that are functionally important. The three major types of RNA present in cells are:

(1) messenger or mRNA which encode the amino acid sequence of proteins;

(2) ribosomal or rRNA which are components of ribosomes that translate mRNA into proteins; and

(3) transfer or tRNA which actually decode the codons in mRNA transcripts into their respective amino acids during protein synthesis.

Information contained in mRNA for constructing proteins is deciphered through the process of translation. Proteins are polymers composed of 20 different amino acids covalently linked together by peptide bonds. Instructions for the sequence of amino acids in a protein are contained in sequential groups of three consecutive nucleotides, or codons, in mRNA (and the DNA from which it was transcribed), with each codon designating a specific amino acid. Thus, the sequence of specific codons defines the sequence of amino acids that are to be polymerized to create the encoded protein. Since each position in a given codon contains one of four possible nucleotides from which RNA and DNA are made, there are 4^3 or 64 possible nucleotide sequence combinations in a codon triplet. Of these 64 codons, 61 code for 20 different amino acids and 3 (TAA, TAG, and TGA) signal termination of translation. These numbers indicate redundancy in the genetic code, and, in fact, most amino acids are encoded by more than one codon.

The flow of information from DNA to RNA to protein just outlined is the fundamental basis upon which all life on earth is built. However, while this principle is relatively straightforward, the actual process of retrieving information from the genome is much more complicated. Consider that some proteins are needed in large quantities, others are needed in small quantities, and many are needed only some of the time. Yet, two copies of most genes exist in each diploid cell, regardless of the demand or lack of demand for the information they bear. To provide for this requirement that gene expression varies independently of gene copy number, cells have devised elaborate mechanisms for regulating the expression of genes and the activity of their products. That expression of genes is a highly regulated process is hinted at by the fact that the sequences that actually encode pro-

Fig. 2 Transcription and post-transcriptional processing of mRNA. Features of a gene transcriptional unit are shown. Following transcription and generation of a primary mRNA transcript, post-transcriptional processing converts this to a mature mRNA that is ready for export to the cytoplasm and translation. Landmarks in the mature mRNA relevant to translation are shown (UT, untranslated region).

tein occupy only part of the DNA of most genes and only a small proportion of the human genome. Many non-coding regions of the genome have been shown to have important regulatory functions, such as regulating the transcription of genes.

The process of making mRNA transcripts suitable for translation into protein involves the initial synthesis of a primary mRNA copy of the gene and subsequent maturation of this primary transcript to ready it for translation (Fig. 2). Non-coding regions of genes near the start site of transcription or further upstream, termed promoters, initiators, and enhancers, regulate transcription. These elements act only on genes to which they are covalently linked (i.e. they act 'in cis') and function by interacting with proteins that regulate transcription, so-called transcription factors. These proteins non-covalently bind to specific DNA sequence motifs in gene regulatory elements and act 'in trans' to modulate expression of genes by assembling multiprotein complexes that start and control the process of transcription. The abundance and activity of many of these transcription factors are regulated by specific stimuli and environmental factors. Together, these cis- and trans-acting factors regulate mRNA production and determine which genes are expressed, when, and to what extent in different types of cells.

After transcription, mRNAs must undergo additional processing to ready them for translation. The protein coding sequences of many eukaryotic genes are discontinuous and separated by intervening non-coding sequences (introns) which are transcribed and are part of the primary mRNA transcript. Introns must be removed by the process of splicing before the mRNA can be translated, resulting in a spliced mRNA that contains only exon sequences. While their origins are unclear, introns effectively divide protein coding regions of the gene into distinct segments. This gives rise to a form of modularity that can be envisaged as facilitating the modification of existing genes and proteins and the evolution of new ones if exons are moved, mixed, shuffled, duplicated, or deleted. Besides splicing out introns, mRNA maturation involves other events, such as the addition of a special nucleotide 'cap' (7-methyl G) at the proximal or 5' end, cleavage of the distal or 3' end and the addition there of an untemplated string of A residues (polyadenylation). These post-transcriptional modifications of mRNA protect it from degradation by nucleases and make it more translatable once it reaches the cytoplasm.

Mature mRNAs are transported from the nucleus to the cytoplasm where they are translated into the specified amino acid sequence. Ribosomes, which are macromolecular assemblages of multiple RNA and protein components, are the engines of translation and protein synthesis, while multiple species of tRNAs, each charged with its specific amino acid, 'read' the appropriate codons using complementary sequences in their structure. Mature mRNAs contain non-coding sequences preceding and following their coding sequences, and these have been shown to regulate both the efficiency of translation and longevity of the mRNA. During translation, ribosomes must exclude these 5′ and 3′ non-coding sequences from translation or, put another way, they must know where translation should begin and end. Current models of translation suggest that ribosomes attach to the mRNA via its 5′ cap structure and 'scan' down the mRNA until they find the first AUG trinucleotide that is located in a nucleotide sequence context appropriate for translation initiation. This prevents false translation initiation by distinguishing the authentic translation initiation AUG from other AUG trinucleotides that are frequently present upstream. Translation is initiated at the authentic initiation AUG, which encodes methionine, then proceeds down the mRNA in the nucleotide triplet 'reading frame' established by the initiation AUG. Amino acids encoded by each subsequent trinucleotide are covalently added to the elongating polypeptide strand until an 'in-frame' termination codon (UAA, UGA, or UGA) is encountered, at which point translation stops. The reading frame is all important for correctly interpreting the message in mRNA nucleotide sequence and synthesizing the correct protein, since translation of the same sequence in either of the two alternate reading frames will produce totally different, incorrect proteins.

Mutations

Many systems have been built into cells to insure the fidelity of the genetic information transmitted from cell to progeny cell. If DNA errors arise, mechanisms exist to correct them, and if this is not possible, mechanisms exist to cull out the damaged cells. Despite these protective mechanisms, genetic changes and mutations do arise. This is not necessarily bad, for heritable changes drive diversity and the evolution of species. The prejudice against genetic mutations derives, justifiably, from a focus on the individual and the medical problems they may cause. In truth, however, most genetic changes probably have no detectable phenotypic consequences and give rise to so-called DNA sequence or genetic 'polymorphisms' that distinguish the genome of different individuals and have been used for a variety of purposes (e.g. forensics analysis, determining parentage, tracing inheritance of genes, etc.). Because they cause no problems, their occurrence goes unnoticed. On the other hand, mutations that cause disease soon come to medical attention and tend not to remain undetected, especially with the rapid pace of modern genetic analysis. These mutations can cause organ malfunction and developmental abnormalities, particularly those that arise in the germline and are inherited, because all cells in the organism are affected. More frequently, however, genetic mutations arise in somatic cells during a person's life. These may be spontaneous or induced by DNA damaging agents (e.g. gamma or UV radiation or chemical mutagens). Most somatic mutations probably have few if any consequences, because they affect only individual cells, and the vast majority are unaffected. However, when somatic mutations involve important regulatory genes, this may lead to aberrant cell behaviour which, if it involves loss of normal control over cell proliferation, can eventually cause disease, such as cancer.

The nature of genetic errors and their potential consequences are diverse. The complement of chromosomes in somatic cells may deviate from the normal diploid. Aneuploidy may involve either fewer (hypodiploid) or greater (hyperdiploid) numbers of chromosomes, and an aberrant complement of even a single chromosome can be pathogenic (e.g. trisomy 21 causes Down's syndrome). Segments of chromosomes rather than entire chromosomes may be amplified, which can give rise to visible cytogenetic abnormalities, such as chromosomes with 'homogeneously staining regions' (HSR). 'Double minutes' are amplified chromosomal segments that exist free in the nucleus, separated from their chromosome of origin. These cytogenetic abnormalities indicate the presence of genes that are present in many copies in the cell and whose expression may be deregulated. More common than gene amplification are gene deletions, which may or may not be detectable cytogenetically. Chromosomal translocations are yet another aberration and are frequently associated with lymphoid malignancies, probably because gene breakage and rejoining naturally occurs during certain stages of T and B cell development. Translocations juxtapose genetic elements that are normally separate and may cause aberrant regulation of gene expression or fusion of two different genes resulting in the production of a chimeric protein.

The genetic anomalies described so far are detectable cytogenetically, but most mutations are on a much smaller scale. Deletion of whole or portions of genes, which are usually not detectable cytogenetically, cause total loss of the protein product or creation of a truncated protein. Loss (or addition) on a much smaller scale (e.g. of one or two nucleotides), particularly if they occur in protein coding regions of genes, may produce equally devastating effects by shifting the reading frame during translation. Sequences downstream of the nucleotide loss or addition are normal but will be read by ribosomes in an alternate reading frame, resulting in incorporation of totally different amino acids from those intended. Needless to say, unless the frameshift mutation is near the end of the protein coding domain, functionality of the whole protein will be lost. Nucleotide substitutions or 'point' mutation can cause more or less profound disruptions of gene expression and protein function. At one extreme, substitutions may convert a codon for an amino acid into a termination codon ('nonsense' mutation) leading to premature termination of translation. Point mutations outside protein coding regions may also have profound effects if they occur in sequences important for exon–intron splicing or for binding of critical transcription factors. At the other extreme, nucleotide substitutions may be 'silent' when they occur in a nucleotide position that causes no change in the encoded amino acid (due to redundancy in the genetic code). Between these extremes, nucleotide substitutions may alter a codon so that it encodes a different amino acid. These 'missense' mutations may have little effect on the properties of the encoded protein (essentially becoming an amino acid sequence polymorphism) or may critically alter its function. The spectrum of genetic mutations briefly described here will assume greater relevance when the genetic aetiology of cancer is discussed.

Post-translational protein regulation

Cells are highly ordered structures and properly function only when their molecular assemblages and organelles function and interact appropriately. This organization requires that newly synthesized proteins are targeted to the areas of the cell where they are designed to function. For example haemoglobin must be retained within the cytosol of erythrocytes for optimal function, while insulin is secreted and carried via the vasculature to sites distant from the cell that produced it. The molecular beacons that designate the cellular location of proteins are contained in their amino acid sequence. Proteins that integrate in the cell membrane or that are destined for secretion contain a signal peptide, typically an amino-terminal peptide sequence containing one or more positively charged amino acids followed by six to 12 hydrophobic residues. The signal peptide targets proteins for translocation across the endoplasmic reticulum membrane into the lumen as they are being synthesized, after which the peptide is cleaved off, giving the mature protein a different amino terminus from the one initially produced by translation. Endoplasmic reticulum channels are lined by membrane that is contiguous with the plasma membrane, and their lumen is contiguous with the extracellular milieu, so that proteins translocated across the endoplasmic reticulum membrane have access to the cell surface and beyond. Transmembrane proteins are distinguished from secreted proteins by the presence of a transmembrane domain which is comprised of a linear stretch of about 22 hydrophobic amino acids that fixes the protein in the lipid bilayer of cell membranes as it transits into the endoplasmic reticulum during translation. Secreted proteins, in contrast, have no such domain and fail to arrest in the lipid bilayer during membrane transit. The orientation and topography of transmembrane proteins may vary and can be complex, such as in the case of proteins with multiple membrane spanning domains that weave in and out of the cell. Cytosolic and nuclear proteins do not have a signal peptide and are deposited during translation in the cytosol. Nuclear proteins are characterized by the presence of nuclear localization signals which consist of peptides with a preponderance of basic amino acids (lysine or arginines) that target the protein for transport to the nucleus.

Appropriate protein localization within cells and cellular subcompartments is critically important for function. During signal transduction, for example, signals received at the cell surface frequently need to reach the nucleus in order to transcriptionally reprogramme the cell to generate a response. The proper localization of proteins in these signal transduction pathways is crucial so that they are correctly positioned to receive and pass on these signal. As examples Ras and Src proteins function proximally in signal transduction pathways and are kept at the plasma membrane by covalently linked lipid moieties added after translation. Here, they are positioned to interact with upstream signalling molecules, such as transmembrane receptors. The functional importance of this localization is shown by the fact that loss of membrane attachment resulting in cytosolic localization renders Ras and Src inactive. Protein location may be used to regulate their biological activity. Transcription factors obviously have to be in the nucleus to modulate gene expression, and one such factor, NFκB, is kept inactive in the cytoplasm through binding to its inhibitor, IκB. When a signal for NFκB activation is received, IκB is phosphorylated, the complex dissociates, and free NFκB enters the nucleus where it can function. Keeping proteins out of the nuclear compartment until they are needed is a mechanism of regulation for several transcription factors.

Even after appropriate localization, many proteins must have their activity carefully regulated. This is frequently achieved by modifying proteins in one of a number of ways to alter their behaviour and function. Such posttranslational modifications enable the cell to regulate protein activity without having to alter gene expression, resulting in faster, more responsive, and often reversible control. A variety of mechanisms have evolved to regulate protein activity. They may be proteolytically cleaved to generate fragments that have more or different activity from the uncleaved, parent protein. Many secreted enzymes are initially secreted in inactive, proenzyme form and require proteolytic modification for activation. Prime examples include blood coagulation factors which are widely distributed in inactive form and capable of being rapidly activated by proteolysis where and when clot formation is needed. Hormones provide additional examples, some being initially secreted in 'pre' or 'pro' form that require proteolytic processing to become active hormones. Protein function can be altered by covalently modifying the parent protein. For example phosphorylation (attachment of phosphate groups) of the hydroxyl groups of specific serine, threonine, and tyrosine amino acids modifies the activity of many proteins. The enzymes that catalyse such reactions are termed kinases; serine/threonine kinases catalyse phosphorylation of serine and threonine residues, and tyrosine kinases perform the same function for tyrosine residues. Phosphorylation confers a negative charge to these otherwise uncharged amino acids and can change the functional properties of the proteins in which they reside. For example many kinases are themselves substrates for phosphorylation which, in turn, activates their kinase activity. Phosphorylation can also confer upon proteins the ability to interact specifically with other proteins; phosphorylation of certain tyrosine residues allows proteins to bind proteins that have so-called SH2 domains, which are phosphotyrosine binding elements. Modification of proteins by phosphorylation can be reversed through dephosphorylation catalysed by protein phosphatases. The opposing activities of protein kinases and phosphatases and their antagonistic effects on substrate function clearly sets up a highly regulable system for controlling the activity of target proteins. Other examples of post-translational protein modifications with functional consequences include glycosylation, acetylation/deacetylation, ADP ribosylation, sulfa-

tion, and attachment of lipid groups (myristoylation, farnesylation, geranylation, etc.).

Signal transduction

Described above are the basic materials and processes important for the normal function of cells, but normal function of the body as a whole requires more highly co-ordinated, integrated, and orderly function of all of its constituent cells. Significant progress has been achieved in recent decades towards defining the molecular mechanisms involved in the complex and multifaceted inter- and intracellular signalling pathways through which cells and tissues communicate with each other. When functioning normally, these signalling networks allow us to perceive, integrate, and respond to local, environmental, and behavioural stimuli. Deregulated or dysfunctional signalling pathways, on the other hand, are pathogenically associated with many disease states. Cell-to-cell communication occurs through a variety of mechanisms, and the proximity of interacting cells dictates how such communications occur. Cells that are in direct contact with each other can establish direct lines of communication through plasma membrane junctions or pores that allow exchange of small molecules or the propagation of electrical signals to help co-ordinate metabolic, mechanical, or behavioural response. In the absence of direct contact, however, cell-to-cell communication occurs primarily via signalling molecules that are synthesized and released by a signalling cell and elicit a specific response in a target cell. Signalling may be paracrine, with the signalling and responding cells adjacent or nearby, as in the case of signalling at a neuromuscular junction where release of acetylcholine from a neurone elicits a contractile response from its target myocyte. Endocrine signals, on the other hand, use the circulatory system to target more distant cells and may elicit a tissue-specific or tissue non-specific response. For example release of follicle stimulating hormone from the anterior pituitary gland stimulates maturation of an ovarian follicle in a tissue-specific manner, while release of insulin from pancreatic islet cells elicits a more general physiological response from cells throughout the body resulting in their increased uptake of glucose. Cells can also respond to stimuli that they themselves elaborate through autocrine signalling pathways. For example interleukin-2 (IL-2) produced by activated T lymphocytes can stimulate their own IL-2 receptors, leading to autocrine stimulation of proliferation and clonal expansion. This section will address how cells perceive and respond to these signals.

Identification of many of the molecules mediating cell-to-cell communication has facilitated the use of molecular approaches to defining the mechanisms by which target cells respond to signals and modify their behaviour accordingly. Signals are perceived when signalling molecules or ligands bind their cognate receptors. The chemical characteristics of the signalling molecule dictate how and where this interaction occurs. Hydrophilic signalling molecules, for example peptide hormones and small charged molecules, such as epinephrine and histamine, that cannot freely diffuse across the plasma membrane bind receptors located on the cell surface. Some lipophilic signalling molecules, such as prostaglandins, also interact with cell-surface receptors. Others, for example steroid hormones, thyroxine, and retinoids, diffuse across the plasma membrane and interact with receptors located within the cell. Interaction of signalling molecules with their receptors initiates a cascade of chemical reactions that culminates in the modification of the cell's behaviour. These modifications may be rapid and transient, such as the contraction of a muscle cell, or they may be more prolonged, such as the metabolic response initiated by insulin. Some signals initiate a complete and irreversible reprogramming of the cell, as is seen when haematopoietic progenitor cells are induced to terminally differentiate into myeloid or erythroid cells.

The stimulus initiated when a ligand binds to its receptor is usually transduced by a variety of intermediary molecular mechanisms before it affects cell behaviour or produces its response. Conceptually, the most straightforward of these mechanisms is exemplified by the activities of receptors for most steroid hormones, thyroxine, and retinoids. Upon binding, the hormone–receptor complexes are induced to bind specific DNA sequences, called hormone response elements, and regulate the transcription of associated genes (Fig. 3). Up- or down-modulation of the transcription of specific genes reprogrammes the cells toward a defined biological end. For example oestrogens stimulate endometrial growth in preparation for embryonic implantation and growth of the mammary ductal system in preparation for future lactation.

Signalling molecules that cannot diffuse across the plasma membrane are limited to interactions with cell-surface molecules. Therefore, the signals transmitted by hydrophilic ligands or by lipophilic ligands that interact with cell-surface receptors must be transduced by intracellular messengers. Cell-surface receptors transduce signals through three primary mechanisms: activation of ion transport channels; generation of small molecular intermediates ('second messengers') that modulate the activity of specific cellular proteins; or induction of covalent modifications of proteins, thereby modulating their enzymatic activity. The first mechanism, activation of ion transport channels, can alter the electrical potential across the cell membrane as seen when the nicotinic acetylcholine receptor is stimulated by acetylcholine resulting in activation of its Na^+/K^+ ligand-gated ion channel, membrane depolarization, and muscle contraction. This will not be discussed further, and attention will focus on the other two mechanisms by which cell-surface receptors transduce their signals.

Second messengers

Cell surface receptors modulate cell behaviour by activating intracellular signalling networks. Many of these signalling networks involve second messengers, intracellular signalling molecules whose concentration increases or decreases in response to activation of a cell-surface receptor. Second messengers transmit the signal by binding to and altering the activity of specific proteins that modulate cell behaviour. Ionized calcium, Ca^{2+}, serves as a second messenger, as do many small molecular weight intermediates, for example cyclic AMP (cAMP), cyclic GMP (cGMP), 1,2-diacylglycerol, and phosphatidylinositides, produced by enzymes activated directly or indirectly by cell surface receptors. An overview of the mechanisms by which second messengers transmit signals provides insight into the complexities of intracellular signalling networks.

Cyclic AMP

Cytosolic cAMP levels regulate many cellular metabolic responses. Increases in cAMP levels cause an increase in contraction rate in cardiac myocytes, increased gluconeogenesis in hepatocytes, increased thyroxine

Fig. 3 Activation of gene transcription by hormones. After diffusing across the cell membrane, the lipophilic hormone (H) binds to its cytoplasmic or nuclear hormone receptor (R). This induces binding of the receptor to specific DNA sequences, called hormone response elements (HRE), which modulates transcription of associated genes and results in altered gene expression.

Fig. 4 Activation of cyclic AMP-dependent protein kinases by G-protein-coupled receptors. Ligand-induced activation of the G-protein-coupled receptor activates the heterotrimeric G-protein leading to dissociation of the Gα subunit from the Gβ–Gγ complex. Gα activates adenylate cyclase leading to the synthesis of cAMP from ATP. Two cAMP molecules bind to each of the two regulatory subunits of the heterotetrameric cyclic AMP-dependent protein kinase, causing dissociation and activation of the catalytic subunits.

synthesis in thyroid cell, and many other cell type-specific metabolic responses. Levels of cytosolic cAMP are regulated by the enzyme adenylate cyclase, which is located on the inner surface of the plasma membrane and which, when activated, converts ATP to cAMP. Adenylate cyclase activity is regulated by members of a family of cell surface receptors, called G-protein-coupled receptors. These receptors are characterized by a primary amino acid sequence containing seven transmembrane domains that thread the receptor back and forth seven times through the plasma membrane (hence, they are sometimes called seven transmembrane-spanning proteins). These receptors regulate the activity of a family of GTP-dependent regulatory proteins (G-proteins) located at the plasma membrane, which, in turn, regulate adenylate cyclase activity (Fig. 4). Both stimulatory (G_s) and inhibitory (G_i) G-proteins exist which induce or inhibit the activity of adenylate cyclase, respectively, thus providing a mechanism for either increasing or decreasing cAMP levels.

Cytosolic levels of cAMP regulate the activity of a family of cAMP-dependent protein kinases, referred to as protein kinase A. These enzymes are composed of two regulatory (R) and two catalytic (C) subunits that form R_2C_2 tetramers. When cAMP binds to the R subunits, the C subunits dissociate and become catalytically active serine/threonine protein kinases. Phosphorylation of target proteins by protein kinase A modulates their enzymatic activity and leads to the downstream physiological consequences of receptor activation (Fig. 4). These effects of increased levels of cAMP persist until cAMP is hydrolysed to AMP by cAMP phosphodiesterase. The C and R subunits of protein kinase A then reassociate into a catalytically inactive R_2C_2 tetramer, and signalling is terminated.

The cascade of reactions initiated by the signalling network, from hormone to receptor to G-protein to adenylate cyclase to cAMP to protein kinase A activity to biological effect, permits amplification of the hormone signal, comparable to the amplification of chemical reactions initiated by activation of the blood coagulation cascade. One G-protein-coupled hormone receptor can activate as many as 100 G_s-proteins, and activated adenylate cyclase catalyses the production of many cAMP molecules. Such amplification can lead to dramatic augmentation of an initially small signal, and explains why epinephrine levels as low as 10^{-10} M can lead to the generation of as much as 10^{-6} M cAMP, an amplification of 10^4.

Adenylate cyclase is activated by a variety of hormone receptors, yet it leads to different metabolic responses depending on the cell type. For example activation of adenylate cyclase in adipocytes by epinephrine, ACTH, or glucagon results in decreased amino acid uptake and increases lipolysis. In contrast, its activation in hepatocytes increases amino acid uptake, as well as activating pathways that lead to increased gluconeogenesis, ketogenesis, and glycogenolysis. This observation leads to the question:

How do an apparent limited number of signalling proteins generate such diverse cellular responses? While the mechanism of the diversity of biological responses is only partially understood, it is clear that cell context is a major determinant of the biological effect of second messengers. Different cell types express different repertoires of proteins, enzymes, and transcription factors. Second messengers can have diverse biological readouts depending on which factors they interact with, and furthermore, the same signal can have different effects depending on the strength with which it is delivered. Thus, subtle differences in gene expression, signal strength, and amplification can have important biological and physiological consequences.

The clinical relevance of cAMP-mediated signalling pathways is highlighted by the mechanism by which *Vibrio cholerae* induces massive diarrhoea. These bacteria produce cholera toxin, a peptide that irreversibly activates G_s by covalently adding an ADP-ribose moiety to a specific arginine residue. This leads to continuous activation of adenylate cyclase and dramatic increases in cAMP levels in intestinal epithelial cells. Increased cAMP levels alter the activity of ion transport proteins and potentiate the flow of water through intestinal epithelial cells into the intestinal lumen leading to massive diarrhoea.

Other second messengers

The principles outlined above in which receptor activation leads to changes in second messenger concentrations which, in turn, alters the activity of specific effector proteins hold true for other second messengers, including cGMP, Ca^{2+}, and phosphatidylinositides. cGMP levels are regulated by soluble and membrane-bound forms of the enzyme guanylate cyclase. Guanylate cyclase is regulated by a broad spectrum of factors, including atriopeptins (e.g. atial natriuretic peptide, brain natriuretic peptide, and some enterotoxins) which regulate the membrane-bound form, and nitric oxide, nitroglycerine, nitroprusside, and sodium nitrite which diffuse across the plasma membrane to regulate the soluble form. cGMP levels and cGMP-regulated protein kinases play important roles in the regulation of vascular smooth muscle tone, endothelial cell permeability, cardiac contractility, platelet aggregation, intestinal motility and ion transport channel function, bone growth, and neuronal function.

The inositol-lipid signalling pathways are regulated by second messengers derived from two phospholipids located mainly in the inner layer of the plasma membrane lipid bilayer, PIP (phosphatidylinositol 4-phosphate) and PIP_2 (phosphatidylinositol 4,5-bisphosphate). This signalling pathway is activated when G-proteins, G_0 and G_q, activate the enzyme phospholipase C (PLC), which catalyses hydrolysis of PIP_2 to two second messengers, IP_3 (inositol 1,4,5-trisphosphate) and diacylglycerol (Fig. 5). IP_3 diffuses into the cytosol and stimulates Ca^{2+} release from the endoplasmic reticulum by activating IP_3-gated Ca^{2+}-release channels. Ca^{2+}, itself a second messenger, mediates many of its cellular effects through a calcium-dependent regulatory protein, calmodulin. The Ca^{2+}/calmodulin complex is an important regulator of ion transport channels, and structural elements of the cell, for example actin–myosin complexes in smooth muscle cells and microfilaments that mediate many processes such as cell motility, conformation changes, and mitosis. It also regulates a group of enzymes known as Ca^{2+}/calmodulin-dependent protein kinases (CaM-kinases) which affect glycogen breakdown and synthesis of catecholamine neurotransmitters.

In addition to its effects on CaM kinases, increases in intracellular Ca^{2+} mediated by IP_3 stimulates the migration of a cytosolic protein, protein kinase C, to the plasma membrane where it is activated by diacylglycerol, the other product of PIP_2 hydrolysis. Protein kinase C regulates the activity of a number of enzymes complementary to those regulated by CaM-kinases in mediating glycogen breakdown. It also regulates various transcription factors, such as NFκB, to alter the transcriptional programme of the cell. Thus second messengers transduce signals that are important in regulating numerous cell functions, including metabolism, structure, function, proliferation, and differentiation.

Fig. 5 Inositol–phospholipid signalling pathways. Activation of phospholipase C catalyses the hydrolysis of phosphatidylinositol 4,5-bisphosphate to inositol 1,4,5-trisphosphate (IP_3) and diacylglycerol (DAG). IP_3 induces calcium release from the endoplasmic reticulum which acts as a second messenger binding to calmodulin and modulating the activity of CaM kinases. DAG activates protein kinase C which transduces the signal by modulating the activity of a number of downstream enzymes.

Signalling via covalent modifications of proteins

Many recently identified signalling pathways are initiated and conducted by proteins with latent enzyme or functional activity. Stimulation of these pathways by ligand binding to cell surface receptors induces the activity of these signalling proteins. These signalling pathways are initiated by one of four classes of receptors: (1) receptor tyrosine kinases; (2) tyrosine kinase-associated receptors; (3) receptor tyrosine phosphatases; and (4) receptor serine/threonine kinases. Once activated, these receptors induce either phosphorylation or dephosphorylation of target proteins on specific tyrosine, serine, or threonine residues, thereby altering target protein structure and/or function, and initiating a cascade of downstream events.

Receptor tyrosine kinases

Receptor tyrosine kinases (RTKs) make up a family of cell-surface proteins with several common structural features: an extracellular domain that interacts with a specific ligand; a transmembrane domain; and a cytoplasmic domain with regulated tyrosine kinase enzymatic activity. When ligand binds to the extracellular domain, the kinase activity of its cytoplasmic domain is induced through a process involving dimerization or multimerization of the receptor. The kinase domains of the dimerized receptors phosphorylates specific tyrosine residues in the cytoplasmic domain of its dimerization partner, a process termed 'autophosphorylation'. These phosphorylated tyrosine residues serve as high-affinity binding sites for intracellular proteins that transduce the receptor signal.

Once activated, the RTK signal is transduced through two classes of proteins that bind to the receptor: adapter proteins that have no intrinsic enzymatic or signalling properties and enzymes involved in activating downstream events. These two classes of proteins share SH2 domains which are known to mediate binding to phosphotyrosine residues. Through their SH2 domains, adapter proteins and other signalling proteins bind the newly phosphorylated tyrosine residues on the RTK cytoplasmic domain (Fig. 6). The specific residue that each protein binds is determined by the distinct sequence of amino acids surrounding the phosphotyrosine residue. For example Src binds the amino acid sequences phosphotyrosine–glutamate–glutamate–isoleucine through its SH2 domain. By binding adapter proteins and other enzymatically active proteins, the RTK transduces its signal into the cell.

Intracellular signalling pathways activated by receptor tyrosine kinases
Many of the signals initiated by RTKs are transduced by Ras proteins, which are members of a family of low molecular weight proteins that bind guanine nucleotides and possess GTPase activity. They, in turn, regulate a

cascade of serine/threonine kinases that control cell proliferation and differentiation. Ras proteins were initially identified through the role of mutant Ras proteins in carcinogenesis. Ras mutations are estimated to be present in about 30 per cent of human cancers and are among the most common molecular abnormalities found. Ras proteins cycle between an active 'on' state when GTP is bound and an inactive 'off' state when GDP is bound. Cycling between the on and off states is regulated by two classes of signalling molecules: GTPase-activating proteins (GAPs) which increase Ras hydrolysis of bound GTP to GDP, thereby inactivating Ras, and guanine-nucleotide exchange factors which facilitate dissociation of GDP from Ras (Fig. 7). Since the cytosolic concentration of GTP is approximately 10-fold higher than GDP, Ras will tend to bind GTP after dissociation from GDP, resulting in its activation. Many RTKs activate Ras through the actions of two cytosolic proteins, Grb2 and Sos. Grb2 is an adapter protein that contains an SH2 domain through which it bind the tyrosine-phosphorylated RTK, and two Src homology 3 (SH3) domains through which it binds Sos. Sos functions as a guanine-nucleotide exchange factor and activates Ras by facilitating GDP–GTP exchange. In many human cancers, Ras has been mutated so that it no longer hydrolyses GTP to GDP normally, resulting in a Ras protein that is continuously bound to GTP and a signalling pathway that remains turned on.

Many of the cellular changes induced by Ras are mediated by a family of proteins called mitogen-activated protein (MAP) kinases. These kinases are unusual in that they require phosphorylation of both threonine and tyrosine residues to stimulate their full activity, while most kinases catalyse phosphorylation of either tyrosine residues or serine and threonine residues, but not both. The dual function kinase that activates MAP kinase is called MAP-kinase-kinase (MKK, also known as MAPKK or MEK). MKK is activated by a serine/threonine kinase called Raf (also known as MAP-kinase-kinase-kinase or MKKK) which, in turn, is activated by Ras. Once activated by this linear cascade of reactions (Fig. 6), MAP kinases modulate cell behavior by phosphorylating other cellular proteins, including cytosolic proteins and other kinases. They also translocate to the nucleus where they phosphorylate and activate transcription factors, e.g. Elk-1 and serum response factor (SRF).

Fig. 6 Activation of intracellular signalling pathways by receptor tyrosine kinases. Ligand-induced dimerization of receptor tyrosine kinases leads to activation of latent kinase activity and *trans*-phosphorylation of the receptor's cytoplasmic domain. The adapter protein, Grb2, binds specific phosphotyrosine residues in the receptor via its SH2 domain, and it binds Sos via its SH3 domains. Sos functions as a guanine exchange factor, activating Ras by facilitating GDP–GTP exchange. The activated Ras signal is transduced in a linear fashion through Raf to MEK, to MAP kinase. MAP kinases translocate to the nucleus and modulate cell behaviour by regulating the activity of transcription factors, for example Elk-1, and hence gene expression.

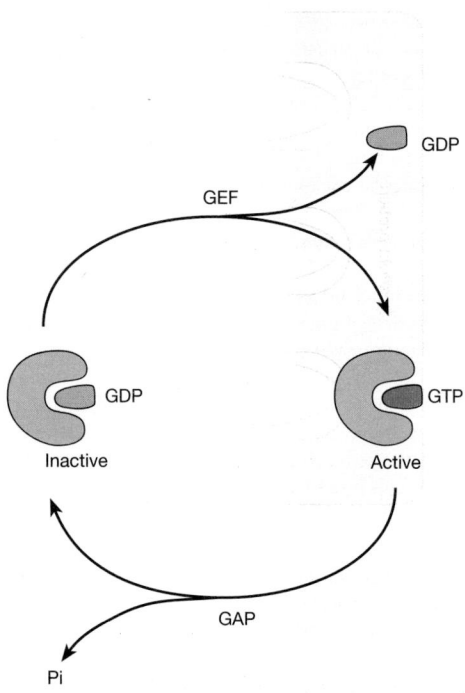

Fig. 7 Activation of Ras proteins. Ras proteins cycle between active and inactive forms. Ras becomes activated when guanine nucleotide exchange factor (GEF) facilitates its dissociation from GDP, enabling it to bind GTP, thus resulting in Ras activation. Ras binding to GTPase-activating proteins (GAP) induces hydrolysis of GTP to GDP resulting in Ras inactivation.

Transcription factors are final participants in afferent signal transduction pathways and initiators of cellular responses to these signals. In general, they are proteins that bind specific DNA sequences and modulate the expression of genes to which they bind. Most bind DNA as dimers, and different transcription factors use specific peptide motifs to dimerize with their partner(s), e.g. 'leucine zippers' and helix-loop-helix domains. Upon binding to DNA, they interact with the basal transcription machinery either directly or via intermediary proteins ('coactivators' and 'corepressors') to initiate, enhance, or inhibit transcription. Transcriptional gene regulation is highly complex, not only due to the multitude of transcription factors present in cells but also due to the ability of many factors to heterodimerize and form combinatorial pairs that have different DNA-binding, transactivation and/or regulatory properties. By transcriptionally reprogramming the cell, these factors regulate cell proliferation or differentiation, survival or apoptosis, and cell structure and function.

Organization of MAP kinase signalling pathways

The RTK–MKKK–MKK–MAP kinase cascade transduces many different signals from the cell surface to the nucleus. To date, 14 MKKKs, five MKKs, and 12 MAP kinases have been identified. Different signal transduction pathways are created by combining different components of each of these kinase families, thus generating diversity in cellular responses. However, some limitations exist in the different components that can be combined. For example MKKs show a fair amount of specificity for the MAP kinases that they activate and are generally coupled to a specific MAP kinase. The MKKs, MEK1 and MEK2, activate MAP kinases involved in cell growth and differentiation, for example ERK1 and ERK2, but they do not activate the MAP kinases involved in response to stress, for example JNK/SAPK kinases or p38 kinases. In contrast, MKKKs are quite promiscuous and can activate multiple MKKs. This promiscuity raises the question of how specificity in signal transduction pathways is generated. This mystery was recently solved by the discovery that scaffold proteins bring together specific components

Fig. 8 Organization of MAP kinase signalling pathways by scaffold proteins. Scaffold proteins can bind multiple members of a signalling pathway, restricting their access to substrates and providing specificity in the signalling response.

of the signalling cascade so that they are sequestered into a signalling unit. Scaffold proteins assure that when a MKKK is activated by a specific signal, only those MKKs and MAP kinases bound to the same scaffold protein are activated (Fig. 8). Thus scaffold proteins bring specificity to signalling pathways so that only the intended cellular responses are generated.

Tyrosine kinase-associated receptors

While RTKs have latent enzymatic activity that is activated by ligand binding, receptors of the tyrosine kinase-associated receptor family lack intrinsic kinase activity, but associate via their cytoplasmic domains with tyrosine kinases located in the cytosol and/or the plasma membrane. Ligand binding induces activity of the associated kinase to transduce the receptor signal. This family includes antigen-specific receptors on T and B lymphocytes and receptors for many of the cytokines that regulate the proliferation and differentiation of haematopoietic cells. These non-catalytic receptors primarily associate with members of the Src family or the Janus family of cytosolic tyrosine kinases (JAK) to transduce their signals. Members of the Src family of tyrosine kinases play important roles in regulating the cell cycle, regulating activation of immune effector cells induced by antigen and Fc receptors, and modulating osteoclast behaviour in bone remodelling.

The more recently described JAKs are involved in signalling pathways initiated by many cytokines, and mediate their effects by activating transcription factors from the STAT (signal transducers and activators of transcription) family. Binding of cytokines such as interferon α, β, or γ or many interleukins to their cognate receptors activates the latent kinase activity of their associated JAKs which, in turn, phosphorylates specific members of the STAT family. Phosphorylation induces the STATs to dimerize and translocate to the nucleus where they activate transcription of specific cytokine-regulated genes.

Receptor tyrosine phosphatases

The currency of signal transduction initiated by RTKs and tyrosine kinase-associated receptors is phosphorylation of specific tyrosine residues. These signalling pathways illustrate the dramatic effect that an apparently simple modification, tyrosine phosphorylation, has on protein function. Receptor tyrosine phosphatases, in contrast, transduce signals by removing phosphate residues from, or dephosphorylating, specific proteins. The CD45 protein is a transmembrane protein expressed on the surface of leucocytes and plays an important role in lymphocyte activation. Upon activation,

CD45 acts as a phosphatase to dephosphorylate target proteins. One such target is Lck, a member of the Src family of tyrosine kinases, whose kinase activity is induced when it is dephosphorylated.

Receptor serine/threonine kinases

The final class of receptors that transduce signals by inducing covalent modifications of target proteins is the serine/threonine kinase receptor family, which, upon activation, catalyses the phosphorylation of target proteins on specific serine and/or threonine residues. Receptors for the transforming growth factor-β (TGF-β) superfamily of ligands, including TGF-β proteins, activins, and bone morphogen proteins (BMP), contain serine/threonine kinase domains through which they modulate signalling pathways. These receptors activate members of the Smad family of proteins by inducing phosphorylation of target serine residues. Activated Smads form heteromeric complexes with other Smad family members, and translocate to the nucleus where they act as transcription factors.

Signalling networks

The events involved in transducing signals from cell surface receptors have been presented as simplified linear pathways leading to predictable cellular responses. However, biological systems are in actuality much more complex with numerous interconnections between the different signalling pathways. These interconnections enable a single signalling event to activate a network of signalling cascades and, thus, to orchestrate complex metabolic, structural, or functional cellular changes. For example activated RTKs typically phosphorylate several tyrosine residues in the RTK cytoplasmic domain which enables the docking of multiple proteins containing SH2 domains. Such proteins, in addition to Grb2, include the γ isoform of phospholipase C (PLC), phosphatidylinositol-3 (PI-3) kinase, tyrosine phosphatases (e.g. Shp2 and Syp), RasGAP (a negative regulator of the Ras GTPase), Src family tyrosine kinases, and multiple adapters (including Shc, Grb7, Nck, etc.). Thus, in addition to activating the MKKK–MKK–MAP kinase pathway, RTKs can also activate numerous accessory signalling pathways (Fig. 9). Moreover, interconnections between signalling pathways exist distal to cell surface receptors. For example, protein kinase C can activate the Ras signalling pathway, and Ras can activate PI-3 kinase to activate the inositol–lipid signalling pathways. Thus complex interconnections exist between different signalling cascades that enable signalling proteins to build a multifaceted signalling network to marshal a cellular response.

Fig. 9 Signalling networks. Signals from activated RTKs can be transduced via multiple signalling pathways, and numerous interconnections exist between different signalling pathways. Thus a single stimulus can orchestrate a complex biological response.

Fates of a cell: proliferation, differentiation, death

Somatic cells undergo one of three general fates: they (a) proliferate by mitotic cell division; (b) differentiate and acquire specialized functions; or (c) die and are eliminated from the body. Cell proliferation is necessary for growth of the organism and insures repletion of cells lost to terminal differentiation, death, or cell loss. In the immune system, lymphocyte proliferation serves the important function of amplifying responses to antigens. Differentiation provides the organism with cells that execute specific and specialized functions. Differentiation tends to be an incremental process, going through stages, but at the end may be 'terminal' so that further cell proliferation is precluded. Cell death as an active process, initiated by the cell itself, is apoptosis. Perhaps not obvious is the fact that this cell fate is as important physiologically as cell proliferation and differentiation. It allows tissue renewal and changes in cellular composition without undesirable or harmful cell accumulation. In the event of exposure to toxic agents, apoptosis eliminates the damaged cells, preventing them from being a burden or harmful to the organism. In complex multicellular organisms, when any of these three cellular processes becomes deregulated and unbalanced, the consequences are usually dire and result in either functional insufficiency or neoplasia. In recent years, some of their mechanisms and regulation have been defined at a molecular level.

Cell proliferation

The cell cycle

Somatic cells proliferate by mitosis, a process that produces two identical progeny from one parental cell. Mitotic cells pass through an ordered series of states collectively termed the 'cell cycle' (Fig. 10). This cycle has four sequential phases, labelled G_1, S, G_2, and M, which are defined biochemically, morphologically, and on the basis of cellular DNA content. S phase is the period of wholesale DNA synthesis during which the parental diploid cell with a '2N' complement of DNA replicates its entire genetic content and becomes a cell with 4N DNA content. M phase or mitosis is the period of nuclear and cell division during which the duplicated DNA complement of the 4N parental cell is divided equally between the two progeny cells which are consequently 2N. M phase is morphologically obvious as the period during which chromosomes condense into their familiar, microscopically visible forms, the nuclear envelope breaks down, the chromosomes segregate into two identical sets, the nuclear envelopes reforms (which completes nuclear division or 'karyokinesis'), and the two progeny cells separate (which completes cell division or 'cytokinesis'). G_1 and G_2 phases were originally conceived as 'gaps' between the distinctive M and S phases of the cell cycle. G_2 is the period between S and M, when cells have finished replicating their DNA, have 4N DNA, and are preparing to divide. G_1 is the period between M and S when cells are 2N, have finished one round of cell division, and have not yet initiated the next.

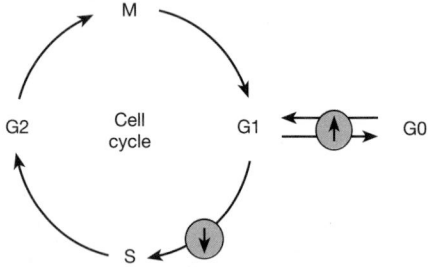

Fig. 10 Cell cycle. The sequential phases of the cell cycle, G_1, S, G_2, and M, are depicted, as well as the resting G_0 phase. Common regulatory points near the end of G_1 and between G_1 and G_0 are shown by circles with arrows within.

The durations of S, G_2, and M tend to be relatively constant, in contrast to that of G_1 which can be highly variable depending on the cell type and is subject to regulation by environmental factors, such as the availability of mitogens and nutrients. It is the period of cell growth, and a certain increase in mass may be required before the cell can enter the next S phase. When conditions are unsuitable for cell proliferation, they arrest in G_1, and those that are already in S, G_2, or M usually complete the round they have entered and arrest only when they reach G_1 again. A point in late G_1 called the 'restriction point' or 'R' has special significance and is the point past which cells become committed to enter S, even if mitogens are withdrawn. Cells may withdraw from the cell cycle and remain for prolonged periods in a metabolically active but non-proliferative state. These cells have 2N DNA content and are described as being in G_0. Terminally differentiated cells are examples of cells in G_0. However, other cells reversibly enter G_0 and may be induced to return to G_1 and begin cycling again under certain conditions (distinction between cells in G_0 and prolonged G_1, admittedly, may be difficult). Hepatocytes are in G_0 unless partial hepatectomy or hepatotoxic insults induce them to proliferate to reconstitute functional liver mass. Resting, antigen-specific lymphocytes remain in G_0 until antigen and cytokine stimulation induces them to proliferate.

Adherence to the G_1–S–G_2–M sequence during normal progression through the cell cycle means that a cell must duplicate its DNA before dividing and that it must divide before duplicating its DNA again. This insures a normal genetic complement in the progeny cells and maintains genetic constancy. The dependence of later events in the cell cycle upon normal completion of earlier events is insured by 'checkpoint' control mechanisms that prevent a cell that has not successfully completed one phase of the cycle from entering the next. Checkpoint activity is seen after cell exposure to DNA-damaging agents, such as ionizing radiation, and is manifest as delayed cell entry into S and M by inducing temporary arrest in G_1 or G_2. This delay allows cells time either to repair its damaged DNA or, if the damage is irreparable, to execute a programme of self-destruction or apoptosis.

Cell cycle regulation: cyclins and cyclin-dependent kinases

Notable progress has been made in understanding the regulation of cell entry and progression through the cell cycle. In brief, cell cycling is regulated by serine/threonine kinases of the Cdk (cyclin-dependent kinase) family. As implied by their name, the catalytic activities of these kinases are dependent on associated regulatory proteins called cyclins. Cyclins were so named because levels of the first to be described were seen to fluctuate periodically with the cell cycle. Numerous Cdks and cyclins exist in the cell and form various combinatorial pairs with distinct activities. Control of cyclin/Cdk activity exists at many levels and occurs by the appearance and disappearance of the cyclins at specific phases of the cell cycle, by post-translational modification of Cdks, and by association with Cdk inhibitors. Cyclin/Cdks, in turn, regulate cell cycling by modulating the activity and behaviour of other proteins, such as transcription factors and structural proteins.

The function of cyclins and Cdks is best exemplified by their regulation of cell entry into M phase. Studies of mutant fission yeast called cdc2 (cell division cycle 2) that tended to arrest in G_1 or G_2 led to the cloning of a 34 kDa serine/threonine kinase ($p34^{cdc2}$) that is required for yeast to enter S or M phase. This protein is evolutionarily conserved, being present in a structurally and functionally similar form in humans. Another line of study showed that cytoplasmic extracts from mature frog eggs, when injected into immature oocytes, induced the oocytes to mature and undergo typical M phase changes. The 'maturation promoting factor' (MPF) activity in these extracts was found to reside in two proteins, frog $p34^{cdc2}$ and a B-type cyclin (Fig. 11). Cyclin B has no intrinsic enzymatic function and plays a regulatory role by associating with $p34^{cdc2}$ which then exhibits kinase/MPF activity. Cyclin B levels increase during S and G_2, and levels of the cyclin B/$p34^{cdc2}$ complex sufficient for the G_2/M transition are reached well before the onset of M. Mitosis is not prematurely triggered, however, because the complex accumulates in an inactive form. During S and G_2, the $p34^{cdc2}$

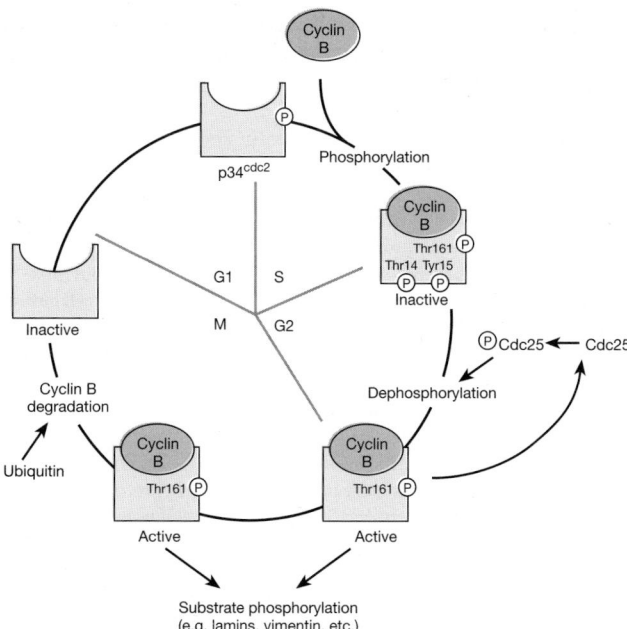

Fig. 11 Activation of mitosis. The G2–M transition activated by cyclin B/p34^{cdc2} is depicted, as well as the phosphorylation and dephosphorylation events leading up to cyclin B/p34^{cdc2} activation and cyclin B degradation during M phase.

complexed with cyclin B accumulates as a multiply phosphorylated protein. In human p34^{cdc2}, phosphorylation of a specific threonine (thr161) stabilizes its association with cyclin B and is essential for activity. On the other hand, phosphorylation of another threonine (thr14) and a tyrosine (tyr15) in p34^{cdc2} suppresses its kinase activity and keeps the cyclin B/p34^{cdc2} complex inactive. Activation of this complex just prior to entry into M requires dephosphorylation of both thr14 and tyr15 which is accomplished by a dual-specificity phosphatase, Cdc25. The kinase and phosphatase that regulate p34^{cdc2} activity and time cell entry into M are themselves regulated by phosphorylation (which inhibits the kinase responsible for tyr15 phosphorylation and enhances the phosphatase function of Cdc25). Once activated, cyclin B/p34^{cdc2} can phosphorylate Cdc25 and create a self-amplifying feedback loop that generates more oocyte MPF activity from a small initial amount of active MPF and the large pre-existing stock of inactive MPF. What starts this sequence of events by initially phosphorylating Cdc25 is unclear, although cyclin A/Cdks are candidates because they are active prior to cyclin B/p34^{cdc2} activation and have MPF activity; also inhibition of cyclin A during S prevents entry into M.

As its name indicates, activated cyclin B/p34^{cdc2} phosphorylates serine and threonine residues in cellular proteins. Discerning its physiological substrates is difficult, however, because there are many potential substrates and other cyclin/Cdk complexes and kinases are active at the same time. Candidates include the lamins and vimentin which are proteins important for the structural organization of cells. They are substrates for cyclin B/p34^{cdc2} kinase activity *in vitro* and undergo M phase phosphorylation *in vivo*. Phosphorylation of lamins is important for nuclear lamina disassembly and envelope breakdown, and phosphorylation of vimentin may cause depolymerization of intermediate filaments in the cytoplasm. If these are physiological substrates, cyclin B/p34^{cdc2} activity may initiate the structural reorganization that is part of mitosis. As M phase progresses, cyclin B/p34^{cdc2} is inactivated by degradation of the cyclin B component. Mutant cyclin B that is resistant to proteolysis induces cell arrest in M, demonstrating that cyclin B degradation is important for cells to exit M.

Cyclins other than cyclin B and Cdks other than p34^{cdc2} regulate other parts of the cell cycle. The behaviour and activity of these others resemble those of cyclin B and p34^{cdc2}, so that the activity of Cdks are regulated by the cyclins with which they pair, and the permitted partnerships determine

where and how in the cell cycle the individual cyclin/Cdk complexes function. The portion of the cell cycle that has received particular attention is G$_1$ and the G$_1$/S boundary, because events here determine commitment to and rates of cell proliferation and have a bearing on neoplastic transformation of cells. Among cyclins, cyclin A and B are unlikely to be important in G$_1$ and the G$_1$/S boundary because they disappear during M and reappear only in S; cyclins D and E are better candidates from a timing standpoint, and D cyclins (there are three types, Dl, D2, and D3) may be especially significant because abnormalities in these have been implicated in the pathogenesis of parathyroid adenomas and certain B cell lymphomas. Cdks that associate with these cyclins are probably important in G$_1$/S regulation: Cdk4 and 6 associate only with cyclin D, and Cdk2 associates with cyclins A, D, and E. These cyclins and Cdks are thought to regulate the G$_1$/S transition through phosphorylation of Rb, the protein product of the retinoblastoma susceptibility gene (Fig. 12). In its hypophosphorylated state, Rb inhibits cell entry into S phase probably by binding to certain members of the E2F family of transcription factors. However, during passage through G$_1$, Rb is phosphorylated on many serine and threonine residues, and hyperphosphorylated Rb releases E2F. E2F, in turn, activates transcription of genes needed for S phase activity and other aspects of cell proliferation (dihydrofolate reductase, thymidine kinase, myc, myb, etc.). Thus, Rb's ability to bind E2F is determined by its phosphorylation state and, in turn, regulates E2F transcriptional activity and cell cycling. Cyclin D/Cdk4 and 6 are among the kinases that can phosphorylate Rb with substrate specificity being conferred, at least in part, by the ability of cyclin D to bind Rb. Others cyclin/Cdk complexes may play important roles in cell cycle regulation as well. For example cyclin E associates primarily with Cdk2, and in G$_1$ cells is found in a quaternary complex with Rb-related p107 protein, E2F, and Cdk2. This complex disappears as cells enter S, just as a similar complex containing cyclin A instead of E makes its appearance. Cyclin E can also phosphorylate Rb and reverse the G$_1$ growth arrest induced by hypophosphorylated Rb. The appearance of cyclin A at the beginning of S, its decline in G$_2$ and M, and its presence in S phase in a quarternary complex with Cdk2, E2F, and p107 suggest that cyclin A plays a role in driving S phase events. Cyclin A in complex with p32^{cdc2} may trigger the G$_2$/M transition by phosphorylating Cdc25 and initiating cyclin B/p32^{cdc2} activation.

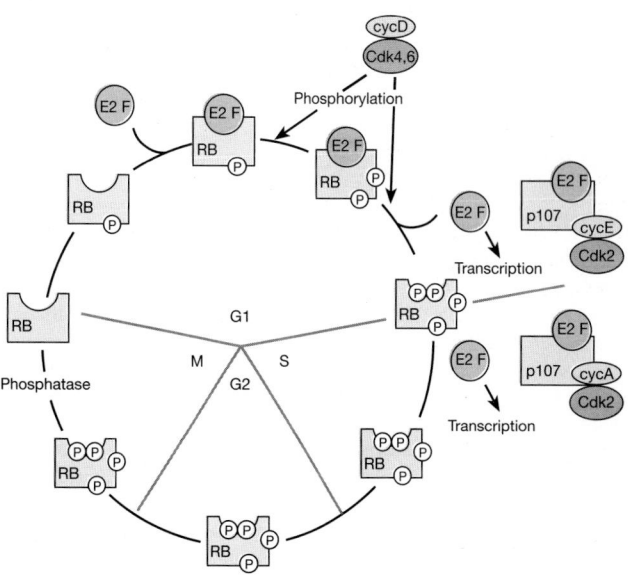

Fig. 12 Rb regulation of cell cycling. Cell cycle regulation by Rb and its association with E2F is depicted, as well as the regulation of the Rb/E2F association by cyclin D/Cdk4,6 phosphorylation of Rb on serine and threonine residues. Other potentially important kinase and transcription factor complexes involving E2F and Rb-like p107 are shown.

Cell cycle regulation: cyclin-dependent kinase inhibitors

Another layer of cell cycle regulation complexity has been revealed with the discovery of inhibitors of Cdk and cyclin/Cdk complexes. The first inhibitor identified and cloned was p21 (Waf1, Cip1, Sdi1) which binds several different cyclin/Cdk complexes and has been classified as a 'universal' inhibitor. While this and other properties of p21 (such as its ability to inhibit the process of DNA replication) account for its ability to induce cell cycle arrest, the regulation of p21 expression sheds the most light on its cellular function. Its expression is transcriptionally induced by p53 which is a transcription factor activated following DNA damage. This suggests that p21 is responsible for halting cell proliferation after DNA damage and allowing the cell time for damage assessment and repair. Other Cdk inhibitors similar to p21 exist. These include p27 (Kip1) which, like p21, bind and inhibit multiple cyclin/Cdk complexes. Upregulation of p27 is thought to mediate the growth arrest of cells under crowded conditions (contact-inhibition of cell growth) or after treatment with TGF-β, a growth arrest cytokine. Other Cdk inhibitors are more specific and inhibit specific Cdks. For example, p16 (INK4a, MTS1, Cdk4I) and p15 (INK4b, MTS2) are Cdk inhibitors that bind Cdk4 and Cdk6 exclusively, and binding inhibits their association with cyclin D and kinase activity. Since Rb is an important target of cyclin D/Cdk4,6 kinase activity, p15 and p16 may inhibit cell proliferation by preventing Rb phosphorylation by cyclin D/Cdk4,6. The observation that p16 overexpression inhibits proliferation of cells expressing Rb but not of cells devoid of Rb supports this idea.

Pathophysiological relevance

Evidence from a variety of spontaneously arising and experimental cancers indicate that Rb/E2F and their regulation by cyclin/Cdk play a central role in cell cycle regulation. In many types of human cancer cells, both copies of the *Rb* gene are disrupted, normal Rb protein is not made, and Rb regulation of E2F activity does not occur. The prototypic tumour in which Rb is pathogenically involved in this manner is retinoblastoma, but Rb abnormalities occur in other, more common cancers as well. Inactivation of Rb regulatory activity can also be achieved by means that do not alter the gene. In tumours induced by certain DNA tumour viruses, oncogenic proteins produced by the virus bind to and functionally inactivate Rb. Large T antigen (the transforming protein of SV40 virus), E1A (one of two transforming proteins of adenovirus), and E7 (one of two transforming proteins of human papilloma virus) proteins all bind Rb in its hypophosphorylated form and prevent it from inhibiting E2F activity. These examples of disruption of Rb cell cycle regulation by different viral oncoproteins provide compelling evidence that transforming viruses 'recognize' the importance of this pathway for maintaining normal cell behaviour and the need to disrupt it if they are to induce neoplasia.

Cell differentiation

Proliferation may provide organisms with the cells needed for growth, replacement, and repair, but differentiation endows these cells with the specialized characteristics and functions that make them useful. Cell differentiation to ultimate form and functionality does not occur in a single step but, rather, is an incremental process. In many tissues, cells, such as haematopoietic or intestinal epithelial cells, go through discernible stages of progressive lineage commitment leading up to full differentiation. In some differentiation lineages, the earliest cells are so-called 'stem cells' which display few if any signs of lineage commitment but have the potential for proliferation and self-renewal. Following cell division, progeny of stem cells undergo one of two fates—they either remain as stem cells or begin to commit to differentiate. The former path maintains the size of this critical pool of cells, while the latter supplies the organism's need for differentiated cells. Once stem cell progeny commit to differentiate, a process that may be progressive, incremental, and span several cell generations, they begin to express proteins that make them recognizable as 'blast cells' of their particular lineage. These remain largely undifferentiated but are fully committed and restricted to particular paths of differentiation. Though blast cells proliferate, they and their progeny inevitably acquire more differentiated characteristics and become fully differentiated cells of their type, that is they lack self-renewal potential and have limited or singular differentiation potential.

This model of progressive cell commitment and differentiation is well illustrated by haematopoietic differentiation. The elusive pluripotent haematopoietic stem cell is believed to divide infrequently, but when it does, it self-renews and gives rise to lymphoid progenitor cells and/or myeloid progenitor cells. These progenitors have the potential to develop into one of several lineages but, as their names imply, do not retain the full potential of the haematopoietic stem cell. Further along and perhaps some cell generations later, lymphoid and myeloid progenitor cells give rise to more committed progeny which are unipotential, that is they can differentiate only along one specific lineage, and show discernible features of differentiation. For example lymphoid progenitors may become T or B lymphocyte precursor cells (which are identifiable by evidence of T-cell receptor or imunoglobulin gene rearrangement), while myeloid progenitors give rise to erythroid, megakaryocytic, granulocytic, or monocytic precursors (which are identifiable as erythroblasts, megakaryoblasts, myeloblasts, monoblasts, etc. by special stains of bone marrow or *in vitro* colony forming assays). Even after reaching this stage, several days and a few cell divisions elapse before their progeny appear in the bloodstream as terminally differentiated blood cells. This multistep process of haematopoiesis clearly involves many fateful decisions about self-renewal, lineage commitment, restriction of potential, and differentiation. Through it, however, the stem cell pool is preserved as a resource for the life of the organism, and mitotic amplification of committed and differentiating cells supplies the body's huge requirement for the end products—an estimated 10^{10} to 10^{11} erythrocytes and granulocytes are normally produced every day.

The molecular switches that determine commitment, lineage-specification, and differentiation are incompletely understood. What is not in doubt is the involvement of transcriptional reprogramming of cells during this process, evidenced by the fact that cells committed to differentiate express a different complement of genes from their uncommitted counterparts. A stochastic model proposes that the stem cell decision to self-renew versus commit is based on probability. What determines this probability is unknown but, based on the likelihood that it involves transcriptional reprogramming, processes involved may include 'opening up' of critical regions of the genome so that they are permissive for gene transcription and binding of a requisite combination of transcription factors to their cognate sites in regulatory genes. When all these conditions are met, the cell may move to the next phase of differentiation (e.g. commit) but, otherwise, will remain as it was (e.g. self-renew). An alternative model is an inductive model of differentiation which suggests that environmental signals, perhaps originating from neighbouring cells and/or the cell stroma, induce stem cells to commit. However the decision is made, embarking on commitment and differentiation involves expression of lineage-specific genes. Among these genes are those encoding receptors for growth and survival factors pertinent to the development of that lineage. These may be crucial for the further progress of differentiation, because they provide the ability to receive instructions that promote the further proliferation, survival, and differentiation of cells of that lineage. For example erythropoietin signalling through its receptor promotes the survival, proliferation, and differentiation of cells of erythrocytic lineage, so that production of the erythropoietin receptor is an essential component of erythrocyte lineage-specific gene expression. The signals generated by these lineage-specific factors often provide an autocrine feedback loop by inducing specific transcription factors which activate *cis*-regulatory sequences and expression of additional genes that contribute to the survival and differentiation of cells committed to these, but not other, lineages.

Many of our current insights into the molecular basis and transcriptional regulation of cell differentiation have been gained from the study of cell culture systems and gene knockout mice to examine myogenic differentiation. *In vitro* studies of myogenesis indicated that certain mesenchymal cells without detectable features of myocyte differentiation could become myoblasts and differentiate into myocytes following treatment with agents (e.g. 5-azacytidine) that can derepress expression of certain silent cellular genes. Transfer of genomic DNA from these 5-azacytidine-induced myoblasts conferred myogenic differentiation on the parental cells, indicating that the myogenic phenotype was heritable. Identification of mRNAs expressed in myoblasts but not in the parental cells led to the cloning of the *MyoD* gene which was subsequently shown to be sufficient for myogenic conversion of the parental cells. MyoD is a basic–helix–loop–helix transcription factor that activates expression of muscle-specific genes by binding to consensus DNA sites present in enhancer elements of muscle-specific genes. It is a member of a family of myogenic transcriptional regulators, including Myogenin and Myf-5, that can induce development of the myogenic phenotype in certain undifferentiated mesenchymal cells. MyoD binds its DNA sites preferentially as a heterodimer with another basic–helix–loop–helix transcription factor, E2A. The ubiquitous presence of E2A suggested that myogenic differentiation and transcriptional regulation of muscle specific genes are regulated by the abundance of MyoD, but this was contradicted by the presence of MyoD in undifferentiated myoblasts. This led to the discovery of the *Id* (inhibitor of differentiation) gene whose protein resembles MyoD in having a helix–loop–helix domain that allows it to dimerize with MyoD or E2A, but differs from MyoD in that it lacks a basic region for binding DNA. Heterodimers containing Id are unable to bind DNA, and Id antagonizes myogenic differentiation by inhibiting the ability of MyoD to activate expression of muscle-specific genes. Expression of Id decreases in cells undergoing myogenic differentiation and cell cycle withdrawal, allowing MyoD to function unhindered in these cells. Neat though this model may be, myogenic differentiation is more complex, because other transcriptional regulators, such as Myogenin and Myf5, can also induce muscle differentiation programs *in vitro*. Furthermore, the finding that mice lacking either MyoD or Myf5 (generated by knocking out both germline copies of these genes) had normal skeletal muscle development, whereas those lacking both MyoD and Myf5 had no signs of skeletal muscle development indicated that MyoD and Myf5 either function redundantly or act in separate myogenic cell populations that can compensate for the other's absence. In mice lacking Myogenin, skeletal muscle differentiation is blocked, even though MyoD and Myf5 are expressed and myoblasts are present. Thus, Myogenin is needed to activate myocyte differentiation following myogenic commitment that seems to depend on MyoD and Myf5 activity.

Apoptosis (see also Chapter 4.6)

Apoptosis is the process of cell death, also called 'programmed cell death', in which the mechanism of cell killing is instituted from within the cell itself. Apoptotic cells undergo fairly stereotypic changes characterized morphologically by early compaction of nuclear chromatin and condensation into clumps at the nuclear periphery. Nuclear and cellular outlines become mildly convoluted, the nucleus fragments, and the dying cell sheds or breaks up into membrane-enveloped 'apoptotic bodies'. These bodies are taken up by adjacent cells or nearby phagocytic cells, and apoptosis typically engenders little or no inflammatory response *in vivo*. Biochemically, the genomic DNA of apoptotic cells undergo strand breaks due to cleavage between nucleosome loops. Since each nucleosome loop is about 180 base pairs in length, this fragmentation leads to a characteristic 'laddering' of DNA fragments in size increments of 180 base pairs on gel electrophoresis. The presence of so many free genomic DNA ends in apoptotic cells allows them to be detected sensitively by DNA end-labelling techniques.

Cell death by necrosis is different and generally occurs when cells are exposed to severe physical, thermal, or other injury imposed from without. In necrosis, nuclear clumping may also be evident, but the most obvious changes involve marked swelling of the cell and organelles, such as mitochondria, and eventual internal disintegration of the nucleus and other structures. Genomic DNA of cells undergoing necrosis is degraded without regard to nucleosomal organization and, upon electrophoresis, appears smeared (indicating random cleavage) rather than laddered. Necrosis tends

to be accompanied by inflammatory responses *in vivo*. It is important to point out that when pathologists use the term 'necrosis' to describe areas of cell death in tissues and organs, these terms are histopathology descriptors and are not generally meant to convey death mechanism, which may be apoptosis, necrosis, or a combination of the two. Indeed, apoptosis, rather than necrosis, is the most common mechanism by which cells die in the body, for example during tissue remodelling, after immunological attack, following cytotoxic chemotherapy or radiation therapy, and in pathological states such as congestive heart failure.

Cells can be induced to undergo apoptosis by a variety of factors and stimuli. Death programmes may be initiated following exposure of cells to toxic insults. The insults may be metabolic, such as severe hypoxia, acidosis, or a combination of the two stemming from ischaemia. They may be genotoxic, such as exposure to radiation that damages DNA beyond the point of repair. Chemotherapy-induced cell death is also attributed to apoptosis. Apoptosis can also be induced by factors unrelated to toxins and insults. Many cells thrive only in the presence of specific survival signals, and absence of these signals leads to apoptosis. These signals may come in the form of soluble factors, such as cytokines and interleukins, and 'permission' for cell survival may work hand in hand with cell differentiation mechanisms to establish specific populations of differentiated cells. For example erythropoietin induces development of late erythroid precursor cells but also promotes the survival of these precursors. Survival signals may also come from interaction of cell surface receptors, such as integrins, with specific components of the extracellular matrix in the cell's environment. Presumably, this insures that cells survive when they are in their 'correct' location or environment and not otherwise. In the last few years, specific receptor–ligand systems have been identified that function specifically to receive or stimulate cell death signals, and these provide another way that apoptosis can be induced. Among the best studied of these is the Fas/Fas ligand system. Fas is a member of the tumour necrosis factor (TNF) receptor 1 family of cell surface receptors which exist as trimers. Present only on certain cells, its interaction with crosslinking anti-Fas antibodies or Fas ligand (FasL; also a cell surface protein) induces apoptosis. Fas is conditionally expressed on lymphocytes and Fas/FasL interaction is known to be important for deletion of autoreactive lymphocytes (to prevent autoimmunity), following activation by antigen (to control immune responses and limit the number of antigen-reactive lymphocytes following antigen clearance), and in immunological sanctuary sites. The physiological importance of this system for maintaining lymphocyte and immune homeostasis is shown by the development of lymphoproliferative disease and autoimmunity in mice deficient in either Fas (*lpr* mice) or FasL (*gld* mice). Other members of this family of ligands and receptors, such as the prototypic TNF and TNF receptor 1, also generate apoptosis signals.

Cell killing during apoptosis is accomplished by members of the caspase family of cysteine proteases with specificity for aspartic acid residues in their substrates (Fig. 13). Upon activation of apoptosis, caspases cleave critical cellular proteins causing irreversible cell damage and death. Caspases exist in cells in inactive single-chain proenzyme form, and activation involves limited proteolytic cleavage of the proenzyme into a large and a small subunit, both of which are needed for catalytic activity. In some caspases, this proteolysis also removes an N-terminal regulatory domain, called the prodomain. Two large and two small caspase subunits assemble into a tetramer which form an active complex that possesses full proteolytic activity and executes cell death programmes. Caspases are activated in a hierarchical order, with caspases 8 and 9 activated first and cleaving procaspases 3, 6, and 7 to activate them so that they, in turn, can cleave and inactivate target cellular proteins (e.g. poly(ADP-ribose) polymerase or PARP, DNA-dependent protein kinase, actin, etc.). Thus the mechanism of caspase 8 and 9 activation provides the link between apoptosis stimulation and apoptosis execution. In the case of apoptosis signalling initiated by Fas ligation, a cytoplasmic domain of the receptor, termed the 'death domain', binds a similar domain in an adapter protein known as FADD. FADD also contains a 'death effector domain' which binds the prodomain of caspase 8.

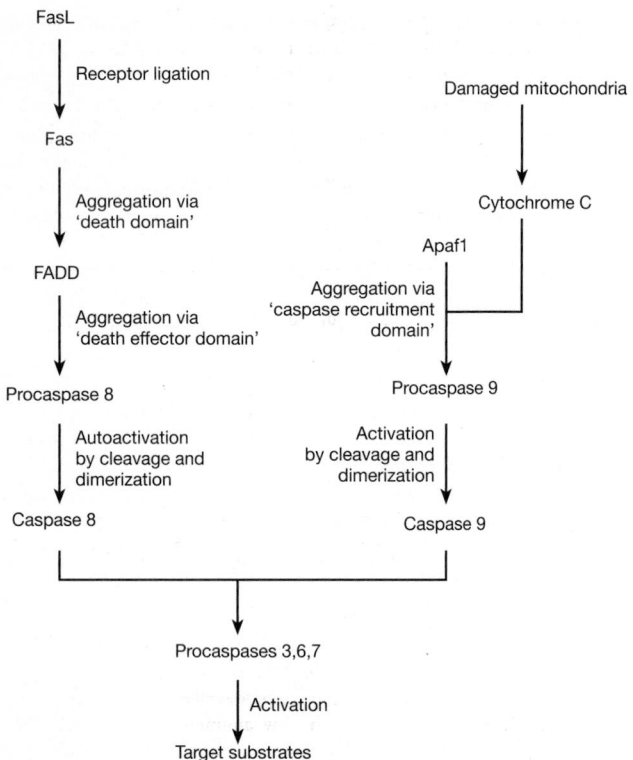

Fig. 13 Apoptosis mechanisms involving caspases. Apoptosis pathways leading from Fas death receptor activation and from cytochrome C release from damaged mitochondria to the hierarchical activation of different caspases are shown.

Assembly of this multiprotein complex brings several procaspase 8 molecules into close proximity, which may allow its very low level of proteolytic activity to cleave and activate nearby procaspase 8 molecules (i.e. 'autoactivation'). This would generate fully active, soluble caspase 8 and the subsequent cascade of downstream events. Procaspase 9, on the other hand, interacts via a 'caspase recruitment domain' in its prodomain with a similar domain in a protein called Apaf1 (apoptotic protease-activating factor 1). Apaf1 also self-associates, but this and procaspase 9-Apaf1 binding occur only in the presence of cytochrome c, which is made available by release from damaged mitochondria. Thus, mitochondrial release of cytochrome c triggers clustering and autoactivation of procaspase 9.

A system for activating efficient and irreversible self-destruction mechanisms cannot exist safely in cells without safeguards and regulators. A family of regulators exists in the Bcl-2 family of proteins. *Bcl-2* was identified as the gene juxtaposed to the immunoglobulin heavy chain gene in the t(14;18) translocation present in human follicular lymphomas. This type of lymphoma is characterized by a low growth fraction and indolent clinical behaviour early in its course. The accumulation of lymphoma cells in patients is attributable to their decreased rate of cell death due to decreased rates of apoptosis resulting from deregulated *bcl-2* expression. Bcl-2 is the prototypic member of a complex family of proteins, some of which are antiapoptotic (e.g. Bcl-2 and Bcl-X$_L$) and some of which are proapoptotic (e.g. Bax). Bcl-2 family proteins influence cellular responses to apoptosis signals by as yet poorly defined mechanisms but which may involve formation of solute channels in mitochondrial membrane and/or modulation of release of mitochondrial contents, including cytochrome c. Alternatively, certain antiapoptotic Bcl-2 proteins appear to bind Apaf 1, while certain proapoptotic Bcl-2 proteins dissociate this complex and allow Apaf 1 to activate caspase 9. Other proteins are also important in regulating apoptosis, including the tumour suppressor protein, p53. It is a regulator of gene transcription that becomes activated by DNA strand breaks and induces G$_1$ cell cycle arrest. Overexpression of p53 in cells has been associated with

enhanced apoptosis, while inactivation of p53 seems to confer resistance to apoptosis. However, p53 only appears to affect apoptosis induced by certain stimuli and not others, for example p53 null thymocytes undergo less apoptosis following ionizing radiation but have unchanged apoptosis following exposure to glucocorticoid. These observations suggest that some pathways to apoptosis are p53-dependent, while others are p53-independent. This has great clinical relevance to cancer therapy, because many chemotherapy agents kill tumour cells by inducing apoptosis. p53 is believed to be the most frequently inactivated gene in human cancers (an estimated 50 per cent), and the p53 status of tumours may be an important determinant of chemotherapeutic response. Other regulators of apoptosis may also exist, but the Bcl-2 family of proteins and p53 are clearly clinically important regulators of apoptosis.

Molecular basis of cancer (see also Chapter 6.3)

Molecular studies have been applied to the study of cancer pathogenesis with notable success. The knowledge gained has led to a much better understanding of the mechanistic basis of cell transformation and promises to improve our ability to categorize, diagnose, and treat cancer. The problem of cancer pathogenesis may be viewed from the perspective of cell fate determination. As described above, all cells in the body undergo one of three general fates: proliferate to produce more cells, differentiate to carry out specialized functions, or die by the process of apoptosis and be eliminated. Organisms require an appropriate balance of cells undergoing each of these fates for normal function and homeostasis, and neoplasia arises when proliferation consistently and aberrantly exceeds apoptosis in a clonal population of cells, leading to their inappropriate and pathological accumulation. To the extent that cell differentiation and proliferation are opposing cell fates, the deregulation of cell proliferation associated with neoplasia is generally accompanied by a loss of differentiation. While this reductionist view greatly oversimplifies the pathogenesis of cancer which proceeds through multiple stages (e.g. dysplasia, adenoma, carcinoma *in situ*, invasive carcinoma, etc.) and involves complex interactions with the host environment (e.g. induction of angiogenesis, invasion, metastasis, evasion of immune response, etc.), it has directed research towards mechanisms that deregulate cell proliferation and apoptosis. This effort has led to the discovery of a rich cache of cellular genes that normally regulate cell behaviour and have the potential to contribute to neoplastic transformation when they go awry (Table 1). The underlying lesson of these discoveries is that cancer has a genetic basis. It results when cells lose or deregulate the function of genes responsible for their normal behaviour and it is heritable. While the transformed phenotype is transmitted from cell to progeny cell, it is not done without modification. Genetic mutability is a characteristic of many, perhaps all, cancer cells, and evidence suggests that selective forces operate on these cells *in vivo* to allow those with selective growth advantage to thrive and predominate, much as 'natural selection' acts at the

Table 1 Cellular genes involved in human cancer pathogenesis

Transforming genes (oncogenes)

Genes involved in promoting cell proliferation
    receptor tyrosine kinases (*HER2/neu*, EGF receptor, etc.)
    ras (H-, K-, and N-*ras*)
    transcription factors (c-*myc*, N-*myc*, mutant *p53*)
    cell cycle regulators (cyclin D)
Genes involved in inhibiting cell apoptosis
    Bcl-2

Tumour suppressor genes

Genes involved in restraining cell proliferation
    Rb, APC, wild-type *p53, p16*^{INK4a}, *WT1* (Wilms' tumour suppressor)
Genes involved in repairing defective DNA
    hMSH2, hMLH1

organism and species levels. Cancer involves a cell evolutionary process in which the end product is the result of multiple genetic anomalies accumulated as once-normal cells progress to malignancy.

Oncogenes

Cellular genes potentially involved in neoplastic cell transformation have been identified by a number of approaches. Some were identified by their close relationship to transforming genes or oncogenes present in rapidly oncogenic retroviruses (e.g. *src* from Rous sarcoma virus, *myc* from avian myelocytomatosis virus, *ras* from Harvey and Kirsten sarcoma viruses, etc.). These retroviral oncogenes were originally derived from normal host genes present in infected cells by a process of gene capture ('retroviral transduction') that can occur during the retrovirus life cycle because they integrate into the host genome. This aetiology explains the close homology between retroviral oncogenes and their cellular precursors or 'proto-oncogenes' and makes the case that the latter have latent transforming potential. Cellular proto-oncogenes were also identified through study of genome integration sites of slowly transforming retroviruses. These retroviruses typically cause specific types of tumours in certain species (e.g. mouse mammary tumour virus or MMTV causes mammary tumours in mice, avian leukosis virus or ALV causes bursal or B cell lymphomas in chickens, etc.) but do not possess oncogenes. Instead, they transform by integrating into the host genome near specific cellular proto-oncogenes, deregulating their expression and activating their transforming potential (e.g. *int* in the case of MMTV mammary tumours, *myc* in the case of ALV bursal lymphomas, etc.). A different approach that identified cellular oncogenes employed experimental transfer of genomic DNA from cancer cells into phenotypically normal cells. Rare recipient cells acquired the transformed properties of the donor cells, and cloning of the donor genes in these recipients led to identification of the cellular oncogenes responsible. Finally, cancer cells commonly have chromosomal anomalies that are pathogenically significant because they are frequently or consistently associated with certain cancers (e.g. chromosomal translocations) or with aggressive clinical behaviour and advanced stage of disease (e.g. chromosomes with homogeneously staining regions, double minute, etc.). Cloning of the genes involved in these anomalies led to identification of additional oncogenes and proto-oncogenes.

The genes identified by the approaches outlined are transforming or have the potential to transform cells. One only has to consider that many proto-oncogenes produce proteins that participate in mitogenic signalling and cell cycling or are highly related to proteins that do to get a sense of their nature, that is proto-oncogenes are cellular genes whose products promote cell proliferation. More specifically, the types of genes that have been found to have oncogenic potential include genes that encode growth factors (e.g. platelet derived growth factor), growth factor receptors with tyrosine kinase activity (e.g. epidermal growth factor receptor or its homologue, Her2/neu), non-receptor tyrosine kinases (e.g. Src), Ras proteins (e.g. H-, K- and N-Ras), serine/threonine kinases (e.g. raf-1), transcription factors (e.g. Myc, Fos, Rel, etc.) and cyclins (e.g. cyclin D). While scores of candidate transforming genes have been revealed through the study of avian and rodent tumours and cells, only a few of these have actually been shown to

contribute to human cancer pathogenesis (*ras, myc, Her2/neu* are examples of these). As indicated previously, genes regulating cell death may also play a role in oncogenesis, and an inhibitor of cell apoptosis (*bcl-2*) is involved in the pathogenesis of certain human lymphomas.

The importance of proto-oncogenes for maintaining normal control of cell proliferation and apoptosis indicates that cell transformation is not an expected result of their normal function. Indeed, their oncogenic potential is only unveiled through 'gain-of-function' or activating gene mutations that release the proto-oncogene or its protein from normal regulation of their activity (Table 2). These genetic alterations tend to upregulate or deregulate gene expression or to enhance or alter the function of their protein products. For example deregulation can result from chromosome translocations which involve breakage and aberrant rejoining of chromosomes to link genetic segments that are not normally juxtaposed. If translocation breakpoints occur in the coding region of genes, it may result in the synthesis of truncated or chimeric proteins with altered regulatory or functional properties. Examples include the chimeric proteins produced by the *bcr–abl* [t(9;22) or 'Philadelphia' chromosome] translocation characteristic of chronic myelogenous leukaemia and the PML–RARα [t(15;17)] translocation characteristic of acute promyelocytic leukaemia. If the translocation breakpoint is outside the coding region of genes, it may bring genes under the regulation of alien transcriptional control elements and alter gene expression. Examples are common in B-cell and T-cell lymphomas where immunoglobulin gene or T-cell receptor gene enhancers and promoters, respectively, become juxtaposed to proto-oncogenes, such as *myc* and *bcl-2*. Other genetic alterations, such as gene amplification, produce multiple copies of genes which may augment or deregulate their expression and activate oncogenic potential. Clinically relevant examples include amplification and overexpression of N-*myc* in neuroblastoma and of *Her2/neu* in breast and ovarian cancer, both of which are associated with a worse prognosis. Point mutations in coding regions of genes can result in amino acid substitutions that alter protein functional properties. The oncogenic potential of *ras* proto-oncogenes typically become activated by this mechanism. Finally, viruses whose genomes integrate into the cell's genome as part of their life cycle (e.g. retroviruses) can activate nearby genes by insertion of their foreign transcription regulatory elements. While retroviral insertional activation of proto-oncogenes is important in the pathogenesis of several types of animal tumours, it has yet to be shown to be a significant mechanism of human oncogene activation.

Tumour suppressor genes

The transforming genes or oncogenes just described generally promote cancer by favouring cell proliferation. Tumour suppressors are entirely different kinds of genes involved in cancer causation. They are cellular genes that normally function to restrain cell proliferation and contribute to cell transformation only following 'loss-of-function' or inactivating mutations. Since the activity of only one copy of a tumour suppressor gene is generally sufficient for function in a diploid cell, the function of both copies must be lost before they promote transformation. Thus, tumour suppressor genes act recessively at the cellular level and stand in marked contrast to oncogenes, which act dominantly (only one activated copy of an oncogene has

Table 2 Mechanisms activating the transforming potential of human proto-oncogene

Mechanism	Effect	Examples
Chromosome translocation	Altered gene expression	*bcl-2* (follicular lymphoma t(14;18)), cyclin D
	Altered protein function Creation of fusion protein	*bcr–abl* (CML t(9;22)) *PML–RARα* (APL t(15;17))
	Altered gene expression Mutant protein with altered function	c-*myc* (Burkitt's lymphoma t(8;14))
Gene amplification	Altered gene expression	N-*myc* (neuroblastoma), *HER2/neu* (breast carcinoma)
Point mutations	Altered protein function	H-, K-, N-*ras*

to be present in a cell to promote transformation). Discovery and identification of tumour suppressor genes came much later than discovery of oncogenes because of the difficulties inherent in tracking down genes that produce effects only when they are absent or functionless. Almost all known tumour suppressor genes have been identified through laborious genetic mapping studies of cancer-prone kindreds. The telltale sign of tumour suppressor genes is loss of heterozygosity (LOH; loss of one of the two alleles normally present in diploid cells) at specific genetic loci in cancer cells that are not present in the normal cells of an individual with cancer. When the two copies or alleles of a gene in an individual's cells can be distinguished molecularly (e.g. by restriction fragment length polymorphisms (RFLP) or microsatellite repeat length polymorphisms), LOH can be detected by molecular analysis. A given LOH found in tumour cells can be an incidental occurrence of little or no pathogenic significance, because these cells tend to be genetically unstable and may have lost alleles of many cellular genes as a consequence. If, on the other hand, LOH at a particular genetic locus is found in tumour cells from many different patients, the probability is high that the loss is pathogenically significant. With LOH, the remaining alleles are physically present but, when these have been studied, they have been found to contain inactivating mutations (e.g. small deletions or premature termination and frameshift mutations). Thus, non-random LOH at specific loci in the cancer cell genome suggests the functional loss of tumour suppressor genes at these sites and provides the starting point for more precise localization studies and eventual cloning.

Inherited cancers and cancer-prone kindreds have been instrumental in providing insights into the presence and identity of tumour suppressor loci and genes. *Rb* (retinoblastoma susceptibility gene), *APC* (adenomatous polyposis coli gene), *WT1* (Wilms' tumour gene), *p16^{INK4a}*(melanoma susceptibility gene), and *BRCA1* and *BRCA2* (breast cancer susceptibility genes 1 and 2) are examples of tumour suppressor genes that were identified through study of families whose members had strong predispositions to developing the respective tumours. In each case, the inherited predisposition to cancer results from functional loss of one allele of the corresponding tumour suppressor gene in the germline (either through complete or partial deletion of the gene or the presence of inactivating mutations). Examination of the actual tumours in affected family members reveal that these have lost or inactivated the remaining, functional tumour suppressor allele and, thus, have undergone the obligate functional loss of both alleles for cancer pathogenesis. Thus, the high incidence of specific cancers in affected individuals in these kindreds is attributable to the pre-existing loss of one tumour suppressor allele, so that, as these individuals go through life, their cells have only to lose the remaining allele to embark on cancerous changes. Cells of normal individual, in contrast, need to lose both alleles before they embark on similar changes. While this obviously happens, attested by the fact that sporadic (non-familial) retinoblastomas consistently lose both copies of *Rb* and sporadic colon and breast cancers frequently lose both copies of *APC* and *BRCA2*, respectively, the likelihood must be substantially less given the much lower incidence of these tumours in the general population than in affected families. Finally, the vastly greater chance of cells losing one versus both tumour suppressor alleles accounts for the dominant inheritance pattern of cancer predisposition in families, despite the fact that the defect inherited resides in a gene that acts recessively at the cellular level. Thus, in familial retinoblastoma, children who inherit a defective *Rb* gene are virtually assured of developing these tumours, indicating that at least one retinoblast in their eyes will almost certainly lose its remaining good copy of *Rb*.

The number of known tumour suppressors is quite small compared to the number of putative oncogenes, but most if not all of the former have a role in human tumour pathogenesis. They are functionally diverse, act in seemingly distinct cellular pathways, and defy ready categorization. The function of Rb and p16^{INK4a} as a negative regulator of the cell cycle was described previously. WT1 is a transcriptional repressor that inhibits expression of genes that encode certain growth factors and growth factor receptors. The APC protein binds β-catenin (among other proteins) and targets it for degradation. β-Catenin is a protein with many functions, one of which is to interact with transcription factors of the Tcf (T cell factor)/Lef (lymphoid enhancer factor) family and activate transcription of genes that probably stimulate proliferation or inhibit apoptosis. In colon carcinoma cells deficient in APC, β-catenin levels are high and activity of β-catenin-transcription factor complexes is constitutive, which leads to activation of target genes and the beginnings of cell transformation and polyposis. Interestingly, the tumour suppressors responsible for hereditary non-polyposis colon cancer (HNPCC; a familial syndrome characterized by right-sided colon carcinomas without antecedent polyposis) are entirely different. Defects in several related genes and proteins are responsible for HNPCC, with defects in *hMSH2* and *hMLH1* being the most common. These proteins repair DNA that contain mismatches arising from errors during DNA synthesis, and defects in these proteins impede repair of these replication errors and allow them to accumulate. This 'mutator' phenotype presumably begins the process of cell transformation and colon carcinogenesis when errors affect genes that influence cell proliferation or apoptosis. These mismatch repair tumour suppressors differ from oncogenes and tumour suppressors, such as *Rb* and *APC*, in that the function of their products does not directly affect cell proliferation, apoptosis, or differentiation. Rather, they are responsible for maintaining the fidelity of genomic information transmitted from cell to progeny cell, and their absence contributes to tumourigenesis by favouring mutagenesis of genes that affect cell fate directly.

The relevance to cancer causation of genes that allow cells to repair defective DNA is reinforced by the role of the *p53* tumour suppressor in human cancers. Originally described as the gene producing a 53 kDa protein that is overexpressed in many transformed cells, *p53* was believed to be an oncogene, because overexpression of *p53* cloned from cell lines had transforming properties. Subsequently, comparison with normal *p53* cloned from fetal tissues revealed mutations in the *p53* genes previously used, and normal *p53* was found to suppress rather than promote cell transformation. These studies and findings of frequent *p53* LOH in tumours have led to the current view that *p53* is a tumour suppressor gene with a negative effect on cell proliferation. It is probably the most frequently deleted or mutated cancer-associated gene (involved in about 50 per cent of human tumours), and Li–Fraumeni syndrome kindreds, who are prone to developing a variety of cancers, are heterozygous for mutant *p53* in their germline. The observation that mutant *p53* transforms is explained by its 'dominant negative' effect: p53 modulates transcription of genes to which it binds as a tetramer, and mutant p53 not only loses this ability but prevents normal p53 from functioning when they are together in a mixed tetramer. Thus, a mutant *p53* allele may be transforming despite the presence of a normal *p53* allele in cells, especially since mutant p53 proteins are frequently longer lived and more abundant than normal p53 protein. Given the importance of p53 in preventing oncogenesis, it was somewhat surprising to find that mice with both their *p53* alleles deleted developed normally and were abnormal only in being prone to developing tumours. How p53 prevents tumourigenesis but is not essential for normal growth and development is explained by the conditional requirement for its activity. When DNA is damaged, for example by exposure to radiation or chemotherapy agents, p53 becomes functionally activated and modulates transcription of genes that induce cell cycle arrest, apoptosis, and repair of damaged DNA. Cell cycle arrest presumably allows the cell time to repair damaged DNA before it is replicated, passed on to progeny cells and becomes a ongoing source of genetic misinformation. Alternatively, induction of apoptosis presumably eliminates cells that are genetically damaged beyond repair. Cells without functional p53 fail to cell cycle arrest following DNA damage, are predisposed to genomic instability, and are less likely to be eliminated by apoptosis. These p53 functions obviously are not needed for normal growth and development but are needed for protection against DNA damage leading to cell transformation.

Fig. 14 Regulatory pathways targeted for deregulation in cancer. Three pathways important for the regulation of cell proliferation and apoptosis which are frequently deregulated during neoplastic cell transformation are shown. Components of these pathways that are frequently activated or inactivated by mutations in cancer cells are surrounded by ovals and rectangles. Rectangles designate tumour suppressor genes that are subject to loss-of-function mutations, and ovals designate proto-oncogenes that are subject to gain-of-function mutations.

Regulatory pathways disrupted during cell transformation

As more and more oncogenes and tumour suppressor genes are identified, the proteins of many have been found to interact with each other and function in the same cell regulatory pathways. This suggests that these regulatory pathways are important for maintaining normal cell behaviour and must be disrupted for neoplasia to occur and that cells undergoing transformation may achieve this by altering one pathway participant or another (Fig. 14). For example p53, activated by DNA damage, transactivates expression of a gene, *mdm2*, whose protein binds p53, promotes its degradation, and inhibits its transcription regulatory function—that is Mdm2 is a negative regulator of p53 activity. Interestingly, Mdm2 is an oncogene that induces cell transformation when overexpressed in cells, and in tumours that overexpress Mdm2, p53 is normal. Thus, inactivating p53 is important for cell transformation, but this can be achieved either by inactivating p53 directly or activating Mdm2 expression. More recently another protein, p19^{ARF}, has been found to interact with Mdm2 and inhibit its ability to counter p53. The genetic locus of p19^{ARF} (which coincides with the gene for the Cdk4,6 inhibitor, p16^{INK4a}, but is in an alternative reading frame) is disrupted in familial melanomas and other types of cancers, suggesting that it is a tumour suppressor gene affecting the p53 functional pathway.

The APC-β–catenin interaction provides another example of the importance of disrupting certain regulatory pathways during cell transformation, no matter the means. Many sporadic colon carcinomas resemble carcinomas arising in those with familial adenomatosis polyposis in that the tumour cells have no functional APC. In these carcinomas, both alleles have been inactivated by somatic mutations. Other cases of sporadic colon carcinoma, however, have normal APC. A substantial proportion of these cases have mutant β-catenin genes that produce proteins that do not interact with APC but retain the ability to interact and function with Tcf/Lef transcription factors, that is β-catenin is a mutationally activated oncogene in these cells. One can infer that deregulated expression of genes regulated by β-catenin–Tcf/Lef is important for colon carcinogenesis, and less important is whether this is achieved by eliminating APC, an inhibitor of β-catenin activity, or mutating β-catenin so that it is no longer susceptible to APC regulation.

The pathway of cell cycle regulation involving Rb perhaps best illustrates the importance of certain regulatory pathways for controlling cell behaviour and how these pathways may be subverted in a number of different ways during cell transformation. In many types of human cancer cells, both copies of the *Rb* gene are inactivated, and there is no functional Rb. While this may be the most effective way to eliminate Rb regulation, other events pushing cells towards neoplasia may achieve a similar effect without altering Rb itself. Enhanced cyclin D expression due to chromosome translocation is seen in certain neoplasms. As cyclin D/Cdk4,6 phosphorylates Rb and prevents it from regulating E2F, deregulating cyclin D expression pro-

duces an oncogenic effect resembling Rb inactivation. p16^{INK4a} inhibits Cdk4,6 function, and loss of this Cdk inhibitor has been shown to result from gene deletion or epigenetic mechanisms in different tumour types. Its loss eliminates a regulator of cyclin D/Cdk4,6 activity, allowing the latter to phosphorylate Rb when it should not and producing an effect similar to Rb inactivation (note that disruption of p16^{INK4a} is likely to disrupt the p19^{ARF} gene as well, in which case two important pathways, Rb and p53, are disrupted by one genetic event). The complexity of the Rb regulatory pathway—p16^{INK4a} inhibiting cyclin D/Cdk4,6 activity which inhibits Rb control of E2F function—allows inactivation of p16^{INK4a}, deregulation of cyclin D/Cdk4,6, or inactivation of Rb to effectively deregulate E2F function and cell cycling. Recall that DNA tumour viruses (SV40, certain adenoviruses, and certain human papilloma viruses) also know the importance of this pathway and produce viral proteins that neutralize Rb function. Together, these argue compellingly for the central importance of the Rb pathway for maintaining normal cell regulation and preventing neoplastic behaviour, and cells on the path to transformation need to find a way to subvert it.

Limitations and uses of the information available

No one questions that investigations into the molecular basis of cell transformation over the past two decades have radically altered and refined our view of cancer pathogenesis. Major concepts and important subtleties now known were not even suspected two to three decades ago. However satisfying this may be, clearly much more needs to be learned. Cancer as a clinical entity is the product of many changes undergone by the cancer cell, not only intrinsically but also in terms of how it relates to the host. Our understanding of the molecular mechanisms involved in cell transformation, the initial steps in pathogenesis, have outpaced our understanding of how the neoplastic cell masters its environment, the steps responsible for most of the symptoms, signs, and clinical character of cancer: how transformed cells evade the host immune system and invade the surrounding extracellular matrix, induce host blood vessel growth necessary to supply the demands of enlarging tumours, enter and exit lymphatic and blood vessels to initiate metastasis, and thrive in distant, ectopic sites to form metastases.

Despite these gaps in our understanding, the knowledge gained so far has proved clinically useful. Knowing the oncoproteins involved in cell transformation, specific inhibitors of their function are being developed. Fortunately, even though neoplastic transformation involves multiple steps and has many participants, interrupting only one of these steps may be sufficient to inhibit transformed behaviour. Perhaps the closest to clinical application are putative inhibitors of Ras function, the farnesyltransferase inhibitors. Ras and related G-proteins must attach to cell membranes to function and do so by adding lipid groups (e.g. farnesyl and geranyl moieties) post-translationally. Compounds that inhibit this modification prevent proper localization and function of Ras and relatives of Ras. Tumour suppressor proteins, in contrast, are generally missing in tumour cells, and consideration is being given to functional reinstatement of these proteins in tumour cells to reverse their neoplastic behaviour. Currently, most attempts have focused on gene transfer technologies ('gene therapy') to accomplish this goal. Tumour-associated proteins that are mutant or overexpressed in transformed cells are potential neoantigens and have been suggested as targets for tumour-specific immunological attack. Mutant Ras proteins, novel Bcr–Abl fusion proteins, overexpressed HER2/neu receptors, and abundant mutant p53 proteins have each been suggested as the basis for tumour vaccine formulations. Whether these ideas and approaches turn out to be practical and therapeutically useful will probably be determined with another decade of research, but, in that interval, many additional new ideas and approaches will undoubtedly surface.

The genetic changes and molecular participants in neoplastic transformation also may be used for diagnostic and classification purposes. With the extreme detection sensitivity of polymerase chain reaction (PCR) technology, genetic alterations characteristic of certain cancers may be detected even when they are present at extremely low frequency. For example this has been applied to the *bcr–abl* translocation that characterizes chronic myelogenous leukaemia and used to detect minimum residual disease in patients following therapy. The association between this translocation and this leukaemia is so strong that the presence of the *bcr–abl* translocation is considered diagnostic of chronic myelogenous leukaemia, whether or not a t(9;22) Philadelphia chromosome is detected on cytogenetic examination. For many cancers, the molecular 'genotype' may affect and even define clinical behaviour and, perhaps, therapeutic response. For example the t(15;17) *PML–RARα* translocation is responsible for the distinctive phenotype of acute promyelocytic leukaemia and its initial dramatic response to all-*trans* retinoic acid therapy. The influence of genotype on therapeutic response may be especially important with regard to the p53 status of tumours. Mutations in p53 are so common in human cancers and its influence on apoptosis seems so likely to affect the killing of cancer cells by certain chemotherapy agents that tumour p53 status may become an important factor in deciding between different types of cancer therapy. These examples just begin to illustrate the potential applications and utility of molecular genotyping of tumours in the future.

Molecular basis of dilated cardiomyopathy

Defining the molecular mechanisms by which cells respond to environmental stimuli and communicate with each other has led to greater understanding of the role played by intracellular signalling pathways in the pathogenesis of many common diseases. While it is intuitive that deregulated signalling might lead to uncontrolled cell growth, and hence malignancy, it is increasingly recognized that signalling cascades also play a significant role in the pathogenesis of many non-malignant conditions. For example the molecular events that culminate in dilated cardiomyopathy and congestive heart failure are mediated by signalling cascades initiated by increases in biomechanical stress.

Cardiomyocytes respond to increased biomechanical stress by increasing myocardial mass commensurate with the increase in work load. This increase in mass, or hypertrophy, is characterized by an increase in the number of contractile protein units contained in individual cardiomyocytes, but not an increase in the number of cells. Depending on the inciting event, the level of work required, and the physiological state of the functioning myocardium, this adaptive response can result in physiological hypertrophy (a proportional increase in the length and width of cardiomyocytes), concentric hypertrophy (increases in width of cardiomyocytes out of proportion to increased length), or eccentric hypertrophy (increased length relative to width). For example, in normal individuals, exercise can lead to physiological hypertrophy in response to increased cardiac workload. Loss of myocardium, as occurs following myocardial infarction, similarly increases the workload on residual cardiomyocytes and initiates compensatory hypertrophy. The magnitude of myocardial loss, and hence the level of biomechanical stress on residual cells, is a major determinant of whether the heart responds with physiological or eccentric hypertrophy. Increased biomechanical stress can also result from defects intrinsic to cardiac myocytes (e.g. genetic abnormalities of cytoskeletal proteins as seen in some forms of muscular dystrophy) or from extrinsic defects (e.g. haemodynamic overload resulting from chronic hypertension).

The molecular events that induce cardiac hypertrophy are only beginning to be defined. Biomechanical stress is known to induce release of a number of growth factors and cytokines, including proteins that activate G-protein-coupled receptors (e.g. endothelin-1 and angiotensin II), receptor tyrosine kinases (e.g. insulin-like growth factor I or IGF-1), and tyrosine kinase-associated receptors (e.g. the interleukin-6-related cytokine, cardiotrophin 1). Furthermore, each of these receptors transduce signals that induce cardiac hypertrophy. Receptors for endothelin-1 and angiotensin II induce hypertrophy by activating the heteromeric G_q protein, which, in turn, activates protein kinase A and specific isoforms of phospholipase (PLC-β and phospholipase D) and protein kinase C. Activation of these

Fig. 15 Signalling pathways activated by biomechanical stress that mediate cardiac hypertrophy and heart failure. Biomechanical stress activates multiple signalling pathways that converge to induce compensatory cardiac hypertrophy, including signals mediated by receptor tyrosine kinases, tyrosine kinase-associated receptors, and G-protein-coupled receptors. However, many of these same pathways can also stimulate apoptosis pathways. Loss of cardiomyocytes through apoptosis results in increased biomechanical stress on residual cell and leads ultimately to a dilated cardiomyopathy and congestive heart failure. The end physiological response to biomechanical stress depends on the balance of these two opposing signal transduction pathways.

pathways leads to transcriptional reprogramming of cardiomyocytes and produces compensatory hypertrophy through, as yet, poorly characterized mechanisms (Fig. 15). Factors activating receptor tyrosine kinases induce cardiac hypertrophy through multiple, different MAP kinases, including the ERKs and the stress-activated MAP kinases, JNK/SAPK and p38, each of which has been shown to be capable of activating hypertrophy programmes. The tyrosine kinase-associated receptor for cardiotrophin, gp130/LIF, activates specific JAK and STAT isoforms (JAK1, JAK2, and Tyk2; and STAT1 and STAT3) that regulate cardiac hypertrophy. These same growth factors and cytokines have pleiotropic effects in various other tissues, but they all activate signalling cascades that lead to hypertrophy in cardiomyocytes. Whether these different pathways represent functional redundancy and how they interact is unclear.

Prolonged, uninterrupted biomechanical overload ultimately leads to a dilated cardiomyopathy which is characterized by eccentric hypertrophy, loss of cardiac contractile function, and loss of cardiomyocytes due to apoptosis. The molecular events that tip the balance from adaptive hypertrophy to eccentric hypertrophy and heart failure are poorly understood, but increasing evidence implicates activation of apoptosis pathways in the development of dilated cardiomyopathy. Like most other cells, cardiomyocytes survival depends on activation of cell survival signals, and withdrawal of survival signals can induce apoptosis. This important property is highlighted by the unanticipated clinical observation that patients with metastatic breast cancer who received therapy with herceptin (a monoclonal antibody that blocks signalling via the receptor tyrosine kinase, ErbB2) had an approximately 15 per cent incidence of dilated cardiomyopathy, with patients previously exposed to anthracyclines being at greatest risk. The molecular basis of the heart failure seen in these trials is unclear, but was thought to result from apoptosis of cardiomyocytes. If true, this observation suggests that cardiomyocyte survival is dependent on ErbB2 signalling cascades and that apoptosis results when cardiomyocytes are deprived of these signals.

Interestingly, many of the signalling pathways that induce cardiac hypertrophy also regulate cell survival and cell death signals. The receptor for cardiotrophin-1, gp130/LIF, and the beta isoform of p38 transduce cell survival (antiapoptotic) signals, while the alpha isoform of p38, JNK/SAPK, and G_q all transduce proapoptotic signals. The balance of these pro- and antiapoptotic signals is likely to play a critical role in the adaptive response of the heart. When cell survival signals predominate, the heart responds with an adaptive hypertrophy, but a predominance of apoptotic signals induces cardiac decompensation with eccentric hypertrophy and heart failure. The magnitude and duration of biomechanical stress may play an important role in determining whether pro- or antiapoptotic signals predominate. For example moderate overexpression of G_q induces cardiac hypertrophy, but high expression results in cardiomyocyte apoptosis.

As heart failure progresses, signalling pathways are activated that appear to further exacerbate biomechanical overload and accelerate cardiac decompensation. To compensate for depressed cardiac function, β-adrenergic signalling pathways are activated in an attempt to augment cardiac contractility. While β-adrenergic signalling transiently improves contractility, prolonged stimulation depresses calcium fluxes resulting in impeded cardiac contractility. In this setting, β-adrenergic blockade improves calcium transport from the cytosol to the sarcoplasmic reticulum, and, in so doing, improves both cardiac relaxation and contractility. This observation provides the rationale for using β-adrenergic blockade in the treatment of patients with congestive heart failure.

Defining the signalling pathways that lead to cardiac hypertrophy has begun to provide a clearer understanding of the molecular basis for heart failure and the molecular events that link mechanical factors (e.g. workload) to biological effect. This understanding of what has traditionally been considered in mechanical and physical terms promises not only to provide important new mechanistic insights into these processes but also to suggest novel approaches for prophylactic and therapeutic intervention.

Further reading

Alberts B, *et al.*(2002). *Molecular biology of the cell*. New York, Garland Publishing, Inc.

Chien KR (1999). Stress pathways and heart failure. *Cell* **98**, 555–8. [Review.]

Lewin B, Lewin B (2000). *Genes VII*. New York, Oxford University Press, Inc.

Lodish H, *et al.* (1999). *Molecular cell biology*. New York, Scientific American Books, Inc.

4.4 Cytokines: interleukin-1 and tumour necrosis factor in inflammation

Charles A. Dinarello

The biology of cytokines

Cytokines are small, non-structural proteins with molecular weights ranging from 8000 to 40 000 Daltons. Originally called lymphokines and monokines to indicate their cellular sources, it became clear that the term 'cytokine' is the best description since nearly all nucleated cells are capable of synthesizing these proteins and, in turn, responding to them. There is no amino acid sequence motif or three dimensional structure that links cytokines; rather, their biological activities allow us to group them into different classes. For the most part, cytokines are primarily involved in host responses to disease such as infection and inflammation; involvement with homeostatic mechanisms is primarily at the level of host defence mechanisms in order to combat the constant challenge of micro-organisms from the environment. For example mice deficient in specific cytokines will spontaneously develop inflammatory bowel disease but when maintained in a germ-free environment, the disease does not occur.

It is not accurate to think of cytokines as hormones. First, hormones tend to be constitutively expressed by highly specialized tissues whereas cytokines are synthesized by nearly every cell. Hormones are the primary synthetic product of a cell (e.g. insulin, thyroid, ACTH), but cytokines account for a rather small proportion of the synthetic output of a cell. In addition, hormones are expressed in response to homeostatic control signals, many of which are part of a daily cycle. In contrast, most cytokine genes are not expressed unless specifically stimulated by noxious events. For example ultraviolet light, heat shock, hyperosmolarity, or adherence to a foreign surface activate cytokine gene expression. One concludes, then, that cytokines themselves are produced in response to 'stress' whereas most hormones are produced according to a daily, intrinsic clock.

Cytokine responses to infection and inflammation

There are at present 23 cytokines termed 'interleukin' (IL). Other cytokines have retained their original biological description such as 'tumour necrosis factor' (TNF). Most cytokines possess more than one biological activity and hence are often called 'pleiotropic'. Some cytokines clearly promote inflammation and are called proinflammatory cytokines whereas others suppress the activity of proinflammatory cytokines and are called anti-inflammatory cytokines. For example IL-4, IL-10, and IL-13 are potent anti-inflammatory agents. They are anti-inflammatory cytokines by virtue of their ability to suppress the expression of genes for proinflammatory cytokines such as IL-1 and TNF. Interferon-γ (IFNγ) is an example of the pleiotropic nature of cytokines. IFNγ is an activator of the pathway which leads to cytotoxic T cells. However, IFNγ is considered a proinflammatory cytokine because it augments TNF activity, upregulates vascular endothelial adhesion molecules, and induces nitric oxide (NO). Therefore, listing cytokines in various categories should be done with an open mind in that, depending upon the biological process, any cytokine may function differentially.

The concept that some cytokines function primarily to induce inflammation whereas others suppress inflammation is fundamental to cytokine biology and also to clinical medicine. The concept is based on the observation that during inflammation, the expression of genes coding for enzymes that synthesize small mediator molecules is upregulated. Examples of these proinflammatory enzymes are phospholipase A2 type-II, cyclo-oxygenase-2 (COX-2), and inducible nitric oxide synthase (iNOS), which synthesize platelet activating factor and leukotrienes, prostanoids, and nitric oxide. Another class of genes code for chemokines, small, proinflammatory peptides (8000 Daltons) that facilitate the passage of leucocytes from the circulation into the tissues. The prototypic chemokine is the neutrophil chemoattractant IL-8. IL-8 also activates neutrophils to degranulate and cause tissue damage. IL-1 and TNF are inducers of endothelial adhesion molecules, which are essential for the adhesion of leucocytes to the endothelial surface prior to emigration into the tissues.

Cytokine-mediated inflammation involves a cascade of proinflammatory gene products that are usually not produced in health. What triggers the expression of these genes? Although inflammatory products such as endotoxins can act directly, the cytokines IL-1 and TNF (and in some cases IFNγ) are particularly effective in stimulating the expression of these genes. Moreover, IL-1 and TNF act synergistically in this process. Whether induced by a infection, trauma, ischaemia, immune-activated T cells, or toxins, IL-1 and TNF initiate the cascade of inflammatory mediators by targeting the endothelium. Figure 1 illustrates the inflammatory cascade triggered by IL-1 and TNF.

IL-1 and TNF

The two cytokines discussed in detail here, IL-1 and TNF, have been selected because of their association with the pathogenesis and progression of disease, particularly autoimmune/inflammatory diseases such as rheumatoid arthritis and inflammatory bowel disease. IL-1 and TNF are the primary members of two 'families' of cytokines. Thus, seven cytokines have been identified as members of the IL-1 family; each has a different but related primary amino acid sequences and different but related receptors.

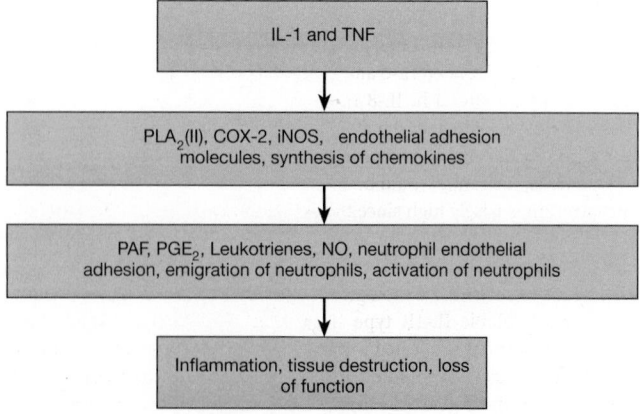

Fig. 1 The scheme of inflammatory cascade triggered by IL-1 and TNF.

The TNF 'family' and TNF receptor family is considerably larger (over 16 members). For the purposes of this chapter, IL-1 is used to denote IL-1β and IL-1α, the two major IL-1 agonists and TNF is used to denote TNFα, the major member of the TNF family. The case for a causative role of any cytokine in a particular disease can not be deduced from an association with production levels but can be proven only by specific inhibition of that cytokine in controlled, human trials. Fortunately, such trials are increasingly taking place since neutralizing antibodies to TNF and soluble receptors for TNF, which bind TNF in the extracellular space, have been approved for clinical use. The IL-1 receptor antagonist IL-1Ra is likely to be approved for use in patients with rheumatoid arthritis.

The biology of IL-1 relevant to disease

Although animal experiments revealed that IL-1 was a highly proinflammatory cytokine, a great deal of information has been learned from studies in which humans were injected with either recombinant IL-1α or IL-1β. Results from trials for treating cancer or bone marrow suppression in which humans received IL-1, suggested a role for IL-1 in those conditions. Although there was no reduction in tumour growth, IL-1 treatment resulted in a more rapid recovery of platelets in subjects given high-dose chemotherapy. However, patients receiving 30 to 50 ng/kg of IL-1 developed fever, hypotension, and profound systemic, flu-like symptoms. Acute toxicities of either IL-1α or IL-1β were greater following intravenous compared to subcutaneous injection; subcutaneous injection was associated with significant local pain, erythema, and swelling. Chills and fever were observed in nearly all patients, even in the 1 ng/kg dose group. The febrile response increases in magnitude with increasing doses and chills and fever were abated with indomethacin treatment. In patients receiving IL-1α or IL-1β nearly all subjects experienced significant hypotension at doses of 100 ng/kg or greater. Systolic blood pressure fell steadily and reached a nadir of 90 mmHg, or less, 3 to 5 h after the infusion of IL-1. At doses of 300 ng/kg, most patients required intravenous pressors. By comparison, in a trial of 16 patients given IL-1β from 4 to 32 ng/kg subcutaneously, there was only one episode of hypotension at the highest dose level. These results suggest that the hypotension is probably due to induction of NO and elevated levels of serum nitrate have been measured in patients with IL-1-induced hypotension.

At 30 to 100 ng/kg of IL-1 patients exhibited a sharp increase in cortisol levels 2 to 3 h after the injection. In addition, there were increases in ACTH and thyroid stimulating hormone but a decrease in testosterone. No changes were observed in coagulation parameters such as prothrombin time, partial thromboplastin, or fibrinogen degradation products. This latter finding is in contrasted to TNFα infusion into healthy humans which resulted in a distinct coagulopathy syndrome. Not unexpectedly, IL-1 infusion into humans significantly increased circulating IL-6 levels in a dose-dependent fashion. These elevations in IL-6 are associated with a rise in C-reactive protein and a decrease in albumin.

Patients receiving only 3 ng/kg IL-1, given by intravenous infusion over 30 min, exhibited elevated IL-6 and IL-8 levels after 1 to 2 h; IL-6 reached a peak of 25 pg/ml after 1 h, IL-8 reached a peak of 311 pg/ml at 2 h, and nitrite/nitrate peaked after 10 h at 89 μmol/l (all statistically significant). If one calculates the maximum possible plasma concentration of IL-1β in these patients, the range would be 50 to 65 pg/ml. However, this calculated concentration is falsely high since the cytokine was given as a 30-min infusion rather than a bolus injection. Nevertheless, at 3 ng/kg, maximal plasma levels of IL-1β is 3 to 4 pM which is the same concentration of IL-1β needed *in vitro* for a biological response. Of interest is that the concentration of soluble IL-1R type II in healthy subjects is about 175 to 200 pM. When IL-1β is injected intravenously, it immediately encounters a 50-fold molar excess of soluble receptor to ligand. Why is there any biological effect to IL-1β given the high affinity of IL-1β for the soluble receptor? And the biological effect is dramatic with fever, hypotension, increased IL-6, IL-1Ra, IL-8, etc. There are two possibilities: the soluble receptor is already bound or the biological response is seen even at low concentrations.

Effects of TNFα injected into humans

Similar to IL-1, TNF is a highly proinflammatory cytokine when injected into humans. Unlike IL-1, TNF induces cell death, particularly in tumour cells. TNF has been injected as part of anticancer protocols, either systemically or regionally, in order to bring about death of tumour cells. Similar to the effects of IL-1 in humans, TNFα induces fever, headaches, myalgias, nausea, vomiting, and profound hypotension. Similar to IL-1 administration, elevated levels of IL-6, other cytokines, soluble cytokine receptors, and acute phase proteins are observed. In fact, the systemic responses to TNFα and IL-1 are mostly indistinguishable. However, activation of the coagulation pathways is observed with TNFα but not IL-1. The injection of TNF, 50 μg/m² body surface area, induced an early and short-lived rise in circulating levels of the activation peptide factor X and an increase in prothrombin fragment F1+2. These findings demonstrate that a single injection of TNF elicits a rapid and sustained activation of the coagulation pathway, probably induced through the extrinsic route. In these subjects, TNF induced a short-term increase in circulating plasminogen activator activity with rises in the antigenic levels of urokinase-type plasminogen activator and tissue-type plasminogen activator. This was followed by an eight-fold increase in plasminogen activator inhibitor type I and a sustained coagulation activation for 6 to 12 h. These findings may explain the microvascular thrombosis seen in septicaemia. Sequential measurement of the plasma concentrations of von Willebrand factor antigen was determined after a bolus intravenous injection of TNF (50 μg/m²) in six healthy men. TNF induced a marked increase in von Willebrand factor antigen plasma levels, becoming significant after 45 min and peaking after 4 h (351 per cent increase). This increased von Willebrand factor secretion may explain the release observed in acute and chronic inflammatory disease and in systemic infection.

TNF also induced a transient stress hormone response, associated with an early and sustained rise in plasma glucose, free fatty acid, and glycerol concentrations. Resting energy expenditure showed a transient rise after TNF injection. In six healthy males, an intravenous bolus injections of TNF (50 μg/m²) produced the characteristic changes in circulating thyroid hormones and TSH observed in the sick euthyroid syndrome. In these subjects, TNF elicited a neutropenia after 15 min, followed by a neutrophilia. Decreased numbers of lymphocytes and monocytes were observed for several hours. There were increases in the concentrations of elastase–α1-antitrypsin complexes, lactoferrin levels, and neopterin, suggesting neutrophil and monocyte activation.

Diagnostic and prognostic value of measuring cytokines

Studies in human subjects have consistently revealed that circulating levels of pro- and anti-inflammatory cytokines as well as soluble cytokine receptors are elevated; moreover, levels may correlate with disease severity and outcome. In addition, spontaneous gene expression for certain cytokines in peripheral blood leucocytes or bone marrow cells are present in patients with various inflammatory and malignant disease whereas cells from healthy subjects rarely exhibited spontaneous cytokine production. A variety of animal models of infection, inflammation, or autoimmunity reveal that nearly all pro and anti-inflammatory cytokines are produced during disease and, as in humans, correlate with disease intensity. The best correlations of cytokine levels with disease activity are reported for IL-6 and IL-1Raα rather than with IL-1 or TNF; this includes patients with local infection, sepsis, and autoimmune diseases such as rheumatoid arthritis. Both IL-6 and IL-1Ra are considered 'acute phase reactants' and other correlate with C-reactive protein measurements. In addition, soluble receptors for IL-1 or TNF are better markers of disease intensity than the IL-1 or TNF itself. In patients with sepsis or septic shock, IL-6 and IL-1Ra levels correlated with mortality. In a study of patients with acute coronary artery syndromes, the admission and 48 h levels of IL-6 and IL-1Ra indicated which will undergo a corrective procedure such as angioplasty or by-pass graft and which patients will respond to conservative therapy and be discharged. In patients with rheumatoid arthritis who receive anti-TNF or anti-IL-1 therapy, the levels of IL-6 fall and are associated with a decrease in disease activity. Since IL-1 and TNF are the primary inducers of IL-6 and IL-1Ra, it is not surprising that therapeutic interventions to reduce IL-1 or TNF activity are associated with a decrease in IL-6 and IL-1Ra.

Reducing IL-1 and TNF activities in human disease

The reduction of the biological activity of any cytokine is based on a class of heterogeneous agents termed 'anticytokine-based therapies'. Treating patients with agents designed to reduce the production of cytokines or their biological effects has entered clinical medicine. Therapeutic strategies for reducing the effects of proinflammatory cytokines such as IL-1 or TNF are either specific or non-specific. This is an important distinction. For example corticosteroids inhibit the synthesis of proinflammatory cytokines but also suppress T-cell function as well as several metabolic pathways. Thalidomide also suppresses the synthesis of TNF, IL-1, and other cytokines and has been used to treat refractory multiple myeloma and the oral aphthous lesions of HIV-1 disease. IL-10, an anti-inflammatory cytokine, suppresses the synthesis of IL-1 and TNF but also of IL-6, IL-12, IFNγ, and the entire family of chemokines. In contrast, a specific anticytokine therapy targets only one cytokine or closely related members of a single cytokine family. Neutralizing antibodies, soluble cytokine receptors, or receptor antagonists have the advantage of specificity, preventing the activity of a single cytokine in a particular disease. The first anticytokine-based therapy for rheumatoid arthritis employed a monoclonal anti-TNFα antibody which neutralizes only TNFα. IL-1 receptor antagonist blocks the IL-1 receptor; in doing so, it prevents the binding of either IL-1α or IL-1β. Soluble IL-1R type I binds IL-1Ra as well as IL-1α. Nevertheless, soluble receptors for TNF, the IL-1 receptor antagonist, and soluble IL-1 receptors (either type I or type II) are examples of specific anticytokine therapies.

Specific anticytokine-based therapies usually require parenteral administration. Non-specific agents, even when their primary mode of action is anticytokine based, are usually administered orally. The precursors for IL-1β, TNFα, and IL-18 each require cleavage by specific proteases before they are active molecules. Therefore, inhibiting these proteases is a logical anticytokine-based, anti-inflammatory strategy. Cleavage of the IL-1β or IL-18 precursor molecules is carried out by the cysteine protease IL-1β converting enzyme (ICE, also known as caspase-1); inhibition of this enzyme is effective in reducing the secretion of biologically active IL-1β and IL-18. For cleavage of the TNFα precursor, a specific metalloprotease is needed. Small, orally-active molecules, which inhibit these proteases specifically, reduce disease activity in animals and are at present undergoing clinical trials.

In animals, blocking either IL-1 or TNF reduced disease severity despite the fact that several cytokines were overexpressed in the disease model. This finding led to the concept that IL-1 and TNF are 'upstream' from many of the other cytokines produced in disease. Thus, IL-1 or TNF, or the combination of IL-1 plus TNF acting synergistically, induce chemokines, IL-6, and several other 'downstream' cytokines. These observations explains why blocking just one cytokine (either IL-1 or TNF) reduces disease. Moreover, of these two cytokines, TNF induces IL-1 production. Thus, in patients with rheumatoid arthritis who receive neutralizing monoclonal antibodies to TNFα, there is a rapid fall in circulating IL-1β as well as IL-6 within 24 h of the initiation of the antibody treatment.

Treating rheumatoid arthritis with IL-1Ra

IL-1Ra was initially tested in a trial in 25 patients with rheumatoid arthritis. In patients receiving 4 mg/kg per day for 7 days, there was a reduction in the number of tender joints from 24 to 10, the erythrocyte sedimentation rate fell from 48 to 31 mm/h and C-reactive protein decreased from 2.9 to 1.9 μg/ml. In an expanded double-blind trial, IL-1Ra was given to 175 patients. After 3 weeks, a significant reduction in disease parameters such as number of swollen joints, the investigator and patient assessments of disease activity, pain score, and C-reactive protein levels. Optimal improvement was in patients receiving 70 mg/day.

A double-blind, placebo-controlled, multicentre trial of IL-1Ra in 472 patients has been reported. There were three doses of IL-1Ra, administered subcutaneously: 30, 75 and 150 mg/day for 24 weeks. After 24 weeks, 43 per cent of the patients receiving 150 mg/day of IL-1Ra met the criteria for response (the primary efficacy measure), 44 per cent met the Paulus criteria, and statistically significant (p=0.048) improvements were seen in the number of swollen joints, number of tender joints, investigator's assessment of disease activity, patient's assessment of disease activity, pain score on a visual analogue scale, and duration of morning stiffness. In addition, there was a dose-dependent reduction in C-reactive protein level, and erythrocyte sedimentation rate.

Importantly, the rate of radiological progression in the patients receiving IL-1Ra was significantly less than in the placebo group at 24 weeks, as evidenced by the Larsen score and the erosive joint count. The reduction in new bone erosions was assessed by two radiologists who were blinded to the patient treatment as well as blinded to the chronology of the radiographs. This finding suggests that IL-1Ra is blocking the osteoclast activating factor property of IL-1, as has been reported in myeloma cell cultures. This study confirmed both the efficacy and the safety of IL-1Ra in a large cohort of patients with active and severe rheumatoid arthritis.

A trial of IL-1Ra in combination with methotrexate in patients with rheumatoid arthritis has also been reported; 419 patients were randomized to receive either placebo or increasing doses of IL-1Ra. Patients were also being treated with methotrexate (mean 17 mg/week). After 24 weeks, patients taking IL-1Ra (1.0 mg/kg) had significantly decreased parameters of disease compared to the placebo. For examples the proportion of patients with a 50 per cent reduction in disease activity was significantly greater in the IL-1Ra treated group (24 per cent) compared to the placebo (4 per cent). These studies suggest that the addition of IL-1Ra to optimal methotrexate treatment results in a further decrease in disease.

Treating rheumatoid arthritis with soluble IL-1R type I

Soluble IL-1R type was administered subcutaneously to 23 patients with active rheumatoid arthritis in a randomized, double-blind study. Patients received subcutaneous doses of the receptor at 25, 250, 500, or 1000 μg/m^2 per day or placebo for 28 consecutive days. In patients receiving 1000 μg/m^2 per day, only one showed improvement in measures of disease activity. One possible explanation for the lack of clinical response despite efficacy in suppressing immune responses could be the inhibition of endogenous IL-1Ra. This was observed in volunteers receiving soluble IL-1R type I before challenge by endotoxin.

Neutralizing TNF in rheumatoid arthritis

Strategies for reducing the biological activity of TNF have focused on neutralization by either monoclonal antibodies or soluble TNF receptors. The initial studies on the efficacy of blocking TNF in rheumatoid arthritis were carried out with the monoclonal antibody cA2 which is specific for neutralization of TNFα. Using a double-blind, placebo-controlled trial, increasing amounts of the antibody clearly showed that specific neutralization of TNFα in rheumatoid arthritis reduced the severity of both clinical and laboratory parameters of the disease. There were dramatic reductions in the circulating levels of IL-1β, IL-6, soluble vascular adhesion molecules, and other markers of systemic inflammation such as C-reactive protein and erythrocyte sedimentation. When combined with methotrexate, the efficacy of monoclonal anti-TNFα in this disease is improved over either agent alone. The biological basis for the effectiveness of blocking TNFα in rheumatoid arthritis is experiments showing a unidirectional cascade of cytokines in explants of synovial tissues in which the presence of anti-TNFα antibody inhibited the spontaneous production of IL-1, IL-6, and IL-8. IL-1Ra reduced IL-6 and IL-8 production but not TNFα production.

Treating rheumatoid arthritis with soluble TNFR p75-Fc

There are two distinct receptors for TNF termed p55 and p75, based on their molecular size. The extracellular forms of these receptors (also termed 'soluble' receptor), which circulate in healthy humans, can be administered in pharmacological concentrations in order to neutralize TNF. To increase the affinity of TNFα and to prolong its plasma concentration, the p75 receptor was synthesized as a fusion protein linked to human Fc domain of the IgG1 (TNFR p75-Fc). A randomized, double-blind, placebo-controlled trial involving 234 patients with active rheumatoid arthritis was carried out using soluble TNFR p75-Fc administered twice-weekly by subcutaneous injection. After 3 months of treatment, there was a improvement in 62 per cent of the patients compared to 23 per cent of the placebo using a 20 per cent ACR response. After 6 months of treatment, 59 per cent of the treated group but only 11 per cent of the placebo group achieved a 20 per cent ACR response. Clearly, blocking TNF using this construct resulted in a significant and sustained benefit in patients with active rheumatoid arthritis. However, similar to monoclonal anti-TNFα, the inflammatory component of the disease returned upon cessation of therapy.

When combined with methotrexate, the use of TNFR p75-Fc resulted in a significant reduction in disease activity using a lower-dose of methotrexate. Eighty-nine rheumatoid arthritis patients were treated for 24 weeks with a stable dose of methotrexate and randomized to receive placebo or TNFR p75-Fc; 71 per cent of the patients receiving TNFR p75-Fc plus methotrexate but only 27 per cent of the placebo group plus methotrexate showed a reduction in the ACR 20 criteria. TNFR p75-Fc has also been used to treat patients with juvenile rheumatoid arthritis and Still's disease.

Treating patients with Crohn's disease with anti-TNFα

Animal and clinical studies suggest a role for TNF in the pathogenesis of inflammatory bowel disease, particularly Crohn's disease. During a 12-week multicentre, double-blind, placebo-controlled trial of a single infusion of anti-TNFα monoclonal antibody treatment in patients with moderate-to-severe Crohn's disease, 64 per cent of those given the antibody had a clinical response, as compared to 17 per cent of patients in the placebo group. Thirty-three per cent of the patients given the antibody went into remission. After 12 weeks, 41 per cent of the antibody-treated patients exhibited a clinical response as compared with 12 per cent of the patients in the placebo group. On the basis of this and other trials, the use of anti-TNFα monoclonal antibody to treat Crohn's disease was approved. In another study, 94 patients with enterocutaneous fistulas of draining abdominal or perianal fistulas of at least 3 months' duration were randomly assigned to receive placebo or anti-TNFα antibody; 38 per cent of the patients who received the antibody had closure of their fistulas compared to 13 per cent of the patients in the placebo group.

Neutralizing TNF in the treatment of congestive heart failure

Initial studies measuring biologically active TNF in the circulation of patients with severe (New York Heart Association class III and IV) congestive heart failure showed that the levels of TNF correlated with the severity

of cachexia and exercise tolerance. Therefore, treating patients with severe heart failure with strategies to block TNF activity were tested. To date, 18 (class III) heart failure patients have been treated with p75-Fc, given as a single intravenous infusion, in a randomized, double-blind trial. A significant overall increase in quality-of-life scores, 6-min walk distance, and ejection fraction was observed in the cohort that receiving p75-Fc. There was no significant change in these parameters in the placebo group. It should be noted that in these studies, the patients were already receiving optimal treatment for heart failure with ACE inhibitors and β-blockers.

The biological basis for TNF and IL-1 in heart failure is well-established. Using strips of human atrial heart tissue ex vivo, the presence of concentrations of TNFα or IL-1β as low a few pg/ml results in depression of contractility. Moreover, the effect of these two cytokines to depress myocardial function is highly synergistic.

Blocking IL-1 and TNF in patients in septic shock

The great promise of anticytokine therapy in human disease was to reduce the mortality of sepsis and particularly septic shock. Despite the impact of intensive care units and optimal physiological support, the mortality in septic shock remain high at 35 to 40 per cent. A great number of animal models of septic shock provided overwhelming data that blocking IL-1 or TNF activity would reduce mortality in these patients. Over 10 000 patients have been studied in carefully designed trials to examine IL-1Ra, neutralizing monoclonal antibodies to TNFα, soluble TNF receptor p55, and soluble p75 TNF receptor, the same agents described above as showing efficacy in the treatment of rheumatoid arthritis, Crohn's disease, and congestive heart failure. There has been no statistically significant improvement in all cause mortality 28 days after the onset of anticytokine treatment. However, in a meta-analysis of these trials, it was concluded that anticytokine intervention resulted in a small but consistent reduction (2–6 per cent) in all-cause 28-day mortality. In only one trial, mortality increased as a result of the anticytokine therapy. Some conclusions can be made from these trials since they offer insights into the effect of the same anticytokine agents as in patients with rheumatoid arthritis. First, despite being infected, the vast number of patients did not worsen or become vulnerable to more infection. There was one exception, the p75-Fc which is effective in treating rheumatoid arthritis was associated with a dose-dependent increase in 28 day all cause mortality. In each study, there was a subgroup with clear benefit but the overall group did not benefit significantly. The heterogeneity of the patients probably prevented the detection of a statistically significant improvement. Fortunately, these anticytokines are now receiving considerable attention for use in local inflammatory diseases.

Further reading

Bresnihan B, Alvaro-Gracia JM, Cobby M, et al. (1998). Treatment of rheumatoid arthritis with recombinant human interleukin-1 receptor antagonist. *Arthritis and Rheumatism* **41**, 2196–204.

Campion GV, Lebsack ME, Lookabaugh J, et al. (1996). Dose-range and dose-frequency study of recombinant human interleukin-1 receptor antagonist in patients with rheumatoid arthritis. *Arthritis and Rheumatism* **39**, 1092–101.

Elliott MJ, Maini RN, Feldmann M, et al. (1994). Randomised double-blind comparison of chimeric monoclonal antibody to tumour necrosis factor alpha (cA2) versus placebo in rheumatoid arthritis. *Lancet* **344**, 1105–10.

Moreland LW, Baumgartner SW, Schiff MH, et al. (1997). Treatment of rheumatoid arthritis with a recombinant human tumor necrosis factor receptor (p75)-Fc fusion protein. *New England Journal of Medicine* **337**, 141–7.

Torcia M, Lucibello M, Vannier E, et al. (1996). Modulation of osteoclast-activating factor activity of multiple myeloma bone marrow cells by different interleukin-1 inhibitors. *Experimental Hematology* **24**, 868–74.

4.5 Ion channels and disease

Frances M. Ashcroft

Ion channels are membrane proteins that act as gated pathways for the movement of ions across cell membranes. They are found in both surface and intracellular membranes, and play essential roles in the physiology of all cell types. An ever-increasing number of human diseases are found to be caused by defects in ion channel function. Ion channel diseases may arise in a number of different ways:

- From mutations in the coding region of the gene, or its control elements, leading to the gain, or loss, of channel function (Table 1). Diseases that result from ion-channel mutations are often known as 'channelopathies'. As with all single-gene disorders, their frequency in the general population is usually very low. Many channelopathies are genetically heterogeneous and the same clinical phenotype may be caused by mutations in different genes, as is the case for Long-QT syndrome. Conversely, mutations in the same gene may produce different phenotypes. For example, gain-of-function mutations in the epithelial Na$^+$ channel produce Liddle's syndrome, whereas loss-of-function mutations cause psuedohypoaldosteronism type-1. Disease severity may also vary with different mutations in the same gene.

- From defective regulation of channel activity by intracellular or extracellular ligands, or by channel modulators, due to mutations in the genes encoding the regulatory molecules themselves, or defects in the pathways leading to their production. For instance, glucokinase mutations cause one type of maturity-onset diabetes of the young (**MODY2**), by impairing the metabolic regulation of ATP-sensitive K$^+$-channels in pancreatic β-cells.

- From autoantibodies to ion channel proteins, which may either downregulate or enhance channel function (see Table 2). These diseases are discussed elsewhere.

- From ion channels that act as lethal agents. These are secreted by cells and insert into the membrane of the target cell to form large nonselective pores that cause cell lysis and death. Examples include bacterial toxins such as staphylococcal α-toxin and the amoebopore of *Entamoeba histolytica*. The membrane-attack complex of complement, perforin, and the defensins also act in this way.

To understand how ion channel defects give rise to disease, it is helpful to understand how these proteins work. The next section therefore considers what is known of ion channel structure, explains the properties of the single ion channel and shows how single-channel currents give rise to action potentials and synaptic potentials.

Properties of ion channels

Ion channel structure

Some ion channels consist of a single subunit, as in the case of the Ca^{2+}-release channel of the sarcoplasmic reticulum. In other cases, the channel pore is formed from a single (α) subunit but associated regulatory subunits may modify the ion channel properties, as in the case of voltage-gated Na$^+$ and Ca^{2+} channels. Yet other ion channels are multimeric and

several subunits are involved in pore formation—the nicotinic acetylcholine receptor comprises five subunits (2α, β, γ, δ), while the voltage-gated K$^+$ channels are composed of four subunits (which are sometimes, but not invariably, identical). Mutations in both pore-forming and regulatory subunits can cause disease.

The multimeric nature of an ion channel may influence whether or not a channelopathy is inherited in a dominant or recessive fashion. Individuals who are heterozygous for voltage-gated K$^+$ channel mutations will express both mutant and wild-type subunits in the same cell. If the mutant subunits co-assemble with wild-type subunits to form heteroligomeric channels that are non-functional, the resulting K$^+$ current will be much smaller than if heteromultimerization does not occur. This is known as the 'dominant negative' effect, and may give rise to a disease that is dominantly inherited.

Single-channel properties

An ion channel can either be open or closed. When it is open, permeant ions are able to move through the channel pore. The current flowing through the open pore is known as the single-channel current. Its magnitude is determined by the ion concentrations on either side of the membrane (the chemical gradient), by the membrane potential (the electrical gradient), and by the ease with which the ion can move thorough the channel pore (its permeability). At the equilibrium potential of an ion, the electrical and chemical gradients are equal in magnitude but opposite in direction, and thus there is no net ion flux. The single-channel conductance γ is a measure of the permeability of the ion and is given by the single-channel current (i) divided by the membrane potential ($\gamma = i/V$).

Ion channels are often highly selective in the ions they conduct. K$^+$ channels, for example, are about 100 times more permeable to K$^+$ than Na$^+$ ions, while Na$^+$ channels conduct Na$^+$ ions but discriminate against K$^+$ ions. Ion selectivity takes place within a narrow region of the pore known as the selectivity filter. The basis of ion selectivity is only just beginning to be understood, but it is clear that while some ions are excluded on the basis of their size or their charge, hydrophobic interactions and the energy required to remove the waters of hydration are also important.

The fraction of time the channel spends in the open state is known as the open probability. Some channels open and close at random, but gating is regulated in other channels. In voltage-gated channels, the open probability is determined by the membrane potential, whereas in ligand-gated channels it is regulated by the binding of extracellular or intracellular ligands. Gating may also be subject to modulation, a process in which channel opening or closing is modified, usually by one of a number cytosolic substances (for example, by Ca^{2+} binding, phosphorylation, etc.). Gating is believed to involve conformational changes in the channel structure that result in the opening or closing of the pore.

At the resting potential of the cell, most voltage-gated channels are closed. In response to a membrane depolarization, the open probability of the channel is increased. This voltage-dependent activation may be followed by a further conformational transition (inactivation) to an inactivated state in which the channel no longer conducts ions. Recovery from

Table 1 Ion-channel genes associated with disease

Gene	Chromosome location	Protein	Disease
Neuronal diseases			
SCN1A	2q24-33	Voltage-gated Na$^+$-channel α-subunit	Epilepsy (GEFS type-2)
SCN1B	19q13.1	Voltage-gated Na$^+$-channel β-subunit	Epilepsy (GEFS type-1)
KCNA1	12p13	Voltage-gated K$^+$ channel($K_{V1.1}$)	Episodic ataxia type-1
KCNQ2	20q13.3	Voltage-gated K$^+$ channel(I_{Km})	Epilepsy (BNFC)
KCNQ3	8q24	Voltage-gated K$^+$ channel(I_{Km})	Epilepsy (BNFC)
CACNL1A4	19p13.1	Voltage-gated Ca^{2+} channel(I_{ca}) (α-subunit or P/Q type)	Episodic ataxia type-2, familial hemiplegic migraine and spinocerebellar ataxia type-6
CACNB4	2q22-q23	Voltage-gated Ca^{2+} channel(I_{ca}) (β$_4$-subunit)	Juvenile myoclonic epilepsy
			Generalized epilepsy and praxis seizures
CHRNA4	20q13.2–13.3	nACh-receptor α$_4$-subunit	Epilepsy (nocturnal frontal lobe epilepsy type-1)
CHRNB2		nACh-receptor β-subunit	Epilepsy (nocturnal frontal lobe epilepsy type-3)
GLRA1	5p32	Glycine-receptor α$_1$-subunit	Hyperkplexia (startle disease)
GJB1	Xq13.1	Connexin 32	Charcot-Marie-Tooth disease
Cardiac muscle diseases			
SCN5A	3p21–24	Voltage-gated Na$^+$-channel α-subunit	Long-QT syndrome (LQT3)
			Congenital conduction defect
KCNQ1	11p15.5	Voltage-gated K$^+$ channel(I_{Ks})	Long-QT syndrome (LQT1)
			(Romano–Ward syndrome, Jervall–Lange–Nielsen syndrome)
HERG	7q35–36	Voltage-gated K$^+$ channel(I_{Kr})	Long-QT syndrome (LQT2)
KCNE1	21Q22.1-Q22.1	Voltage-gated K$^+$-channel(I_{Ks}) β-subunit (MinK)	Long-QT syndrome
			Jervall–Lange–Nielsen syndrome (LQT5)
KCNE2	21q22.1	Voltage-gated K$^+$-channel(I_{Kr}) β-subunit (MiRP1)	Long-QT syndrome (LQT6)
YR2	1q42.1-q43	Ca^{2+} release channel of cardiac SR	Ventricular tachycardia
Skeletal muscle diseases			
SCN4A	17q23–q25	Voltage-gated Na$^+$-channel α-subunit	HyperPP, PAM, paramyotonia congenita
CACNL1A3	1q32	Voltage-gated Ca^{2+} channel(I_{ca}) (α$_{1S}$-subunit or skeletal type)	Hypokalaemic periodic paralysis
			Malignant hyperthermia
KCNE3	11p13-14	Voltage-gated K$^+$-channel(I_{Kr}) β-subunit (MiRP2)	Hypokalaemic periodic paralysis
KCNJ2	17q23	Inward rectifier K$^+$ channel(Kir2.1)	Andersen syndrome
CLCN1	7q35	Voltage-gated Cl$^-$ channel	Myotonia congenita, generalized myotonia
RYR1	19q13.1	Ca^{2+}-release channel of SR	Malignant hyperthermia, central core disease
CHRNA1	2q24-q32	nACh-receptor α$_1$-subunit	Slow-channel syndrome
CHRNB1	17p12-p11	nACh-receptor β-subunit	Slow-channel syndrome
CHRND	2q33-q34	nACh-receptor δ-subunit	Slow-channel syndrome
CHRNE	17p13.1	nACh-receptor ε-subunit	Slow-channel syndrome, fast- channel syndrome
Kidney diseases			
KCNJ1	11q24	Inward rectifier K$^+$ channel(Kir1.1)	Bartter's syndrome (type II)
CLCNKB	1p36	Voltage-gated Cl$^-$ channel	Bartter's syndrome (type III)
CLCN5	Xp11.22	Voltage-gated Cl$^-$ channel	Nephrolithiasis (Dent's disease*)
SCNN1A	12p13	Epithelial Na$^+$-channel α- subunit	Pseudohypoaldosteronism (PHA-1)
SCNN1B	16p13-p12	Epithelial Na$^+$-channel β- subunit	Liddle's syndrome, PHA-1
SCNN1G	16p13-p12	Epithelial Na$^+$-channel γ- subunit	Liddle's syndrome, PHA-1
AQP2	12q13	Aquaporin 2 (water channel)	Nephrogenic diabetes insipidus
Other diseases			
KCNJ11	11p15.1	ATP-sensitive K$^+$ channel: Kir6.2 subunit	Congenital hyperinsulinaemia of infancy
SUR1	11p15.1	ATP-sensitive K$^+$ channel: SUR1 subunit	Congenital hyperinsulinaemia of infancy
CFTR	7q31	CFTR Cl$^-$ channel	Cystic fibrosis
CLCN7	16p13	Voltage gated Cl$^-$ channel	Osteopetrosis
CNGA1	4p12–cen	Cyclic nucleotide-gated channel α-subunit	Retinitis pigmentosa
GJB2	13q11-q12	Connexin 26	Deafness (DFNA3 and DFNB1)
			Vohwinkel's syndrome
GJB3	1p35.1	Connexin 31	Non-syndromal sensineural deafness (DFNA2)
			Erythrokeratodermia variabilis
GJB6	13q12	Connexin 30	Deafness (DFNA3)
			Ectodermal dysplasia type-2
GJA3	13q11	Connexin 46	Cataract (zonular pulverulent type-3)
			Ectodermal dysplasia type-2
GJA8	1q21.1	Connexin 50	Cataract (zonular pulverulent type-1)

BNFC, benign familial neonatal epilepsy; GEFS, generalized epilepsy with febrile seizures; HyperPP, hyperkalaemic periodic paralysis; PAM, potassium-aggravated myotonia; PHA-1, pseudohypoaldosteronism type 1.

*Dent's disease is now recognized to include X-linked recessive nephrolithiasis, X-linked hypophosphataemic rickets, and a renal tubular defect in Japanese children.

Table 2 Diseases resulting from autoantibodies to ion channels

Protein	Disease
Neuronal diseases	
Voltage-gated K$^+$ channel (K$_V$)	Acquired neuromyotonia
Voltage-gated Ca^{2+} channel (I$_{Ca}$, P/Q type))	Lambert–Eaton myasthenic syndrome
Glutamate receptor (GluR3)	Rasmussen's encephalitis
Skeletal muscle diseases	
nACh receptor	Myasthenia gravis, arthrogryposis multiplex congenita

inactivation occurs after a variable period following repolarization to the resting potential. Although most voltage-gated ion channels are opened by depolarization, a few types of voltage-gated channel are activated by hyperpolarization. Ligand-gated channels are opened (or more rarely closed) by binding of an appropriate ligand to a specific site on the channel protein, which induces a conformational change that allosterically opens the ion pore. The channel may open and close several times while the ligand remains bound to its receptor, but this intrinsic gating ceases on ligand dissociation.

There are numerous different types of channel. For example, even among the inwardly rectifying K$^+$ channels, there are seven subfamilies, most of which have several members. In general, ion channels are named after their gating and/or selectivity properties.

Single-channel currents summate to produce macroscopic currents

The cell membrane contains many hundreds of ion channels. The macroscopic current (I) flowing through all ion channels of the same type is determined by the product of the number of channels in the membrane (N), the channel open probability (P), and the single-channel current (i); in other words $I = NPi$. Disease-causing mutations may affect any or all of these parameters and thereby influence the macroscopic current.

Cell membranes also contain several different types of channel. The total current that flows across the cell membrane (the membrane current) represents the sum of the ion fluxes through all the different kinds of ion channel open in the membrane. If it is sufficiently large, the membrane current may cause a change in membrane potential. The size of this voltage change is given by Ohm's law ($V = IR$) and is therefore influenced by both the current amplitude (I) and by the membrane resistance (R) (which in turn reflects the number of open channels). A change in the membrane potential to a more positive value is known as 'depolarization'; 'hyperpolarization' is a change to more negative potentials. The resting potential of most cells lies between –60 to –100 mV.

Action potentials

In excitable cells, a depolarizing stimulus may elicit an action potential. In nerve axons and skeletal muscle fibres, the action potential results from the initial activation of voltage-gated Na$^+$ channels followed shortly afterwards by activation of voltage-gated K$^+$ channels. Because Na$^+$ channels open rapidly on depolarization, there is an initial inward Na$^+$ current. If this is greater than the outward current flowing through (voltage-independent) K$^+$ channels which are open at the resting potential, it will produce a further depolarization. This activates more Na$^+$ channels and depolarizes the membrane even more. In this way, a regenerative increase in membrane potential (an action potential) is produced. The membrane is returned to its resting level by inactivation of the Na$^+$ channels (which reduces the inward current) and the opening of K$^+$ channels (which produces an outward, hyperpolarizing current).

The potential at which the inward Na$^+$ current exactly balances the outward resting K$^+$ current through resting K$^+$ channels is known as the threshold potential. It is a critical potential: any increase in the Na$^+$ current

will elicit an action potential, while any reduction in the inward current (or increase in the outward current) will prevent action-potential generation. Ion channel mutations may increase nerve or muscle excitability either by enhancing the inward current (as in hyperkalaemic periodic paralysis), or by reducing the outward current (as in benign familial neonatal convulsions). This will produce a larger depolarization, so that the threshold potential is reached more easily and a subsequent action potential is initiated. Other mutations produce a depolarizing block of action-potential activity. This results from a maintained membrane depolarization of sufficient amplitude to inactivate the voltage-dependent Na$^+$ channels.

In some cells, additional types of ion channel contribute to the action potential—the ventricular action potential is mediated by voltage-dependent Na$^+$, Ca^{2+}, and at least four kinds of K$^+$ channel; several different kinds of K$^+$ channel contribute to the repolarization of action potentials in mammalian neurones; and chloride channels play an important role in the electrical activity of skeletal muscle. The functional importance of these different ion channels is exemplified by the fact that mutations in the genes which encode them produce a range of nerve and muscle diseases.

Synaptic potentials

When a nerve impulse arrives in the presynaptic terminal it opens voltage-gated Ca^{2+} channels, producing a rise in the intracellular Ca^{2+} concentration ([Ca^{2+}]$_i$) that triggers the exocytosis of synaptic vesicles. The amount of transmitter released varies with [Ca^{2+}]$_i$ and thus with the magnitude of the presynaptic Ca^{2+} current. In turn, this is influenced by the duration of the membrane depolarization and thus by the amplitude of the voltage-gated K$^+$ current that underlies membrane repolarization. A reduction in the presynaptic K$^+$ current therefore leads to excess transmitter release and postsynaptic hyperexcitability, as in episodic ataxia type 1 and acquired neuromyotonia. Conversely, a reduction in the presynaptic Ca^{2+} current is associated with reduced transmitter release, as occurs in the Lambert–Eaton myasthenic syndrome when the density of presynaptic Ca^{2+} channels is decreased by receptor internalization induced by the binding of autoantibodies.

Once released, the transmitter diffuses across the synaptic cleft and binds to receptors in the postsynaptic membrane. At the neuromuscular junction, for example, acetylcholine (**ACh**) binds to the nicotinic acetylcholine receptor (**AChR**), and opens an intrinsic ion channel. The resulting synaptic current produces a depolarization of the postsynaptic membrane (the endplate potential) which, if it is sufficiently large, triggers an action potential in the muscle fibre. A reduction in AChR density, as in myasthenia gravis, decreases effective transmission and leads to muscle weakness. Gain-of-function mutations in AChR may also induce myasthenia, by causing prolonged depolarization of the postsynaptic membrane and thereby Na$^+$ channel inactivation. This depolarizing block is the basis of the slow-channel syndromes. Mutations in the voltage-gated Na$^+$ channel of skeletal muscle may cause paralysis, or myotonia.

In skeletal muscle, the action potential is conducted into the interior of the fibre via invaginations of the surface membrane known as the transverse tubules (**T-tubules**). Depolarization of the T-tubule membrane stimulates the opening of Ca^{2+}-release channels (**RyR**) in the membrane of the sarcoplasmic reticulum (**SR**), the intracellular Ca^{2+} store. The T-tubule and SR membranes are not directly connected and the precise mechanism by which they interact is not fully understood. However, there is evidence that the α_1-subunit of the voltage-gated Ca^{2+} channel in the T-tubule membrane acts as the voltage sensor for the Ca^{2+}-release channels in the SR membrane. Mutations in the Ca^{2+}-release channel of skeletal muscles cause malignant hyperthermia and central core disease.

The channelopathies

This section provides brief descriptions of a range of channelopathies. Additional details may be found elsewhere in the *Oxford textbook of medicine* or in the books and Websites referenced.

Neuronal channelopathies

Generalized epilepsy with febrile seizures

Generalized epilepsy with febrile seizures (**GEFS**) has been linked to a mutation in the gene (*SCN1B*) that encodes the β_1-subunit of the voltage-gated Na^+ channel. Affected individuals exhibit febrile seizures in childhood and afebrile generalized epilepsy in later life. The presence of the β-subunit accelerates both the rate of inactivation, and the rate of recovery from inactivation, of the voltage-gated Na^+ channel. This modulatory effect is abolished if the β_1-subunit carries the GEFS mutation. It is predicted to cause a persistent inward Na^+ current that leads to neuronal hyperexcitability and seizures.

Benign familial neonatal convulsions

Benign familial neonatal convulsions (**BFNC**) is characterized by neonatal convulsions within the first 3 days after birth that show spontaneous remission by the third month of life. There is an increased risk of epilepsy in later life in 10 to 15 per cent of individuals. Mutations in the voltage-gated K^+ channel genes *KCNQ2* and *KCNQ3* are associated with BFNC.

KCNQ2 and KCNQ3 associate in a heteromeric complex to form the M-channel. This channel plays a critical role in determining the electrical excitability of many neurones. It is slowly activated when the membrane is depolarized to around the threshold level for action potential firing, thereby hyperpolarizing the membrane back towards its resting level. This reduces neuronal excitability by limiting the spiking frequency and decreasing the responsiveness of the neurone to synaptic inputs. All BNFC mutations studied to date result in reduced expression of the mutant protein. This may be expected to lead to neuronal hyperexcitability, accounting for the epileptic seizures. Because the M-channel is a heteromer of KCNQ2 or KCNQ3, mutations in either gene will disrupt channel function and cause BNFC.

Episodic ataxia type-1

Episodic ataxia type 1 (familial periodic cerebellar ataxia with myokymia) is an autosomal dominant disorder that causes ataxia accompanied by myokymia, nausea, vertigo, and headache. It results from mutations in the voltage-gated K^+ channel $K_V 1.1$, which is expressed in the synaptic terminals and dendrites of many brain neurones. These mutations either prevent the formation of functional channels or result in a reduced K^+ current. This is expected to prolong the neuronal action potential, inducing repetitive firing and excessive and unregulated transmitter release, and thereby produce the clinical symptoms of ataxia and myokymia.

Familial hemiplegic migraine, episodic ataxia type-2, and spinocerebellar ataxia type-6

There are three human diseases with different phenotypes that are associated with mutations in the same Ca^{2+}-channel gene, *CACNL1A4*. These are familial hemiplegic migraine (**FHM**), episodic ataxia type-2 (**EA-2**), and spinocerebellar ataxia type-6 (**SCA-6**). FHM is associated with missense mutations, EA-2 is caused by truncation of the protein within the third repeat, and SCA-6 is produced by expansion of a polyglutamine repeat in the C-terminal coding region of the protein. All three diseases result in progressive cerebellar atrophy, but they differ in the extent and rate of progression of neuronal degeneration, with SCA-6 showing the greatest, and FHM the least, atrophy. Migraine-like symptoms also occur in all three diseases, and are most severe in patients with FHM. EA-2 and SCA-6 are also characterized by ataxia and nystagmus. It remains unclear how the different mutations in *CACNL1A4* give rise to the different phenotypes.

Startle disease (hyperekplexia)

Glycine is the major inhibitory transmitter in the brainstem and spinal cord. It binds to a ligand-gated Cl^- channel, producing an increase in Cl^- permeability that reduces the membrane depolarization and neuronal firing induced by excitatory neurotransmitters. The glycine receptor is a pentamer of three α-subunits, which contain the glycine-binding site, and two β-subunits. In humans, two types of the α-subunit have been identified. Mutations in the gene encoding the α_1-subunit of the glycine receptor give rise to startle disease (hyperekplexia). This is an autosomal dominant, neurological disorder characterized by muscle spasm in response to an unexpected stimulus. It manifests as facial grimacing, hunching of the shoulders, clenching of the fists, and exaggerated jerks of the limbs. Startle disease mutations produce a dramatic decrease in glycine-activated currents. Because glycinergic interneurones are important for normal spinal cord reflexes, muscle tone, and the pattern of motor neurone firing during movement, this leads to excessive and uncontrolled movements.

Charcot-Marie-Tooth disease

Charcot-Marie-Tooth disease type 1 (CMT1) causes progressive degeneration and demyelination of the peripheral nerves. It is genetically heterogeneous, but the X-linked form of the disease results from mutations in the gap junction channel connexin 32 (Cx32). It shows incomplete dominant inheritance, with heterozygous females being affected less severely than hemizygous males. The phenotype may vary from mild, in which the patient has a normal gait, to a severe form which may necessitate the use of a walking stick or wheelchair.

Over a hundred mutations in *CX32* have been identified. These fall into two main groups–those in which the protein never reaches the plasma membrane, and those where the protein reaches the membrane but forms channels with altered functional properties. The former give rise to a severe phenotype, whereas the latter may be associated with either mild or severe phenotypes, according to whether they partially or completely disrupt channel function.

The Cx32 protein is primarily expressed in the Schwann cells of peripheral myelinated nerves, at the nodes of Ranvier and at Schmidt–Lanterman incisures. In these regions, the myelin is not complete and there is a thin layer of cytoplasm between each of the enveloping turns of the Schwann cell. This suggests that Cx32 may serve as short-cut pathway for nutrients and other substances moving to the innermost layers of the Schwann cell, and perhaps also to the axon itself. This might explain why loss of Cx32 function causes axonal degeneration and demyelination.

Cardiac muscle channelopathies

Long-QT syndrome is a congenital cardiac disorder associated with an abrupt loss of consciousness and sudden death from ventricular arrhythmia in children and young adults. It is characterized by an abnormally long QT interval in the electrocardiogram, which reflects the delayed repolarization of the ventricular action potential. The duration of the cardiac action potential is determined by the balance between the inward and outward currents flowing during the plateau phase. Prolongation of the action potential can therefore be caused by a persistent inward current or by a reduction in outward K^+ currents.

Some six different genetic loci for Long-QT syndrome have been mapped, five of which have been identified and shown to encode cardiac ion channels. The I_{Ks} channel is a complex of two different proteins, KCNQ1 and minK, and mutations in these genes cause LQT1. Likewise, I_{Kr} is a complex of HERG and Mirp1, and is associated with LQT2. Mutations in these four genes either abolish, or markedly decrease, the repolarizing K^+ currents I_{Ks} and I_{Kr}, and are therefore expected to prolong the cardiac action potential and increase the QT interval. Mutations in the cardiac muscle sodium-channel gene (*SCN5A*) cause LQT3. These mutations affect Na^+-channel inactivation, producing a sustained inward current that results in an increased action potential duration. The larger the component of non-inactivating current, the more severe the phenotype.

In many cases, LQT syndrome is not inherited but acquired. For example, drugs that block I_{Kr} or I_{Ks} currents prolong the cardiac action potential and induce the Long-QT syndrome. Among these are class III antiarrhythmic agents such as sotalol, dofetilide, and quinidine, which selectively block I_{Kr}, and the antihistamine H_1-receptor antagonists terfenidine and astemizole, which block HERG. In most people, terfenidine does not produce cardiac problems as it is rapidly broken down in the liver and its metabolite, terfenidine carboxylate, does not block I_{Kr}. However, if the activity of the P-450 enzymes that break down terfenidine is impaired (due to liver disease or drugs such as ketoconazole and the macrolide antibiotics), there is a risk of *torsade de pointes*.

Skeletal muscle channelopathies

Myasthenia and slow-channel syndromes

Myasthenia gravis is produced by autoantibodies directed against the nicotinic acetylcholine receptor (**nAChR**), as discussed elsewhere. These antibodies lead to receptor internalization and thus to a smaller endplate potential that fails to reach the threshold for action-potential initiation.

Slow-channel syndrome (**SCS**) is a congenital myasthenia that results from mutations in the muscle nAChR channel. These mutations have been found in all four types of adult nAChR subunits (α, β, δ, ε) and result in protracted channel activation by acetylcholine. The increase in channel open probability produces a prolonged synaptic current and endplate potential. Consequently, temporal summation of endplate potentials can occur at physiological rates of stimulation, leading to prolonged depolarization of the muscle membrane, inactivation of voltage-gated sodium channels, and failure of muscle excitability. This explains why patients with SCS experience muscle weakness and rapid fatigue. A similar 'depolarization block' is observed with acetylcholinesterase inhibitors or with AChR agonists like suxamethonium.

The prolonged endplate potential also causes enhanced Ca^{2+} entry, which may account for the progressive destruction of the postsynaptic neuromuscular junction observed in SCS—loss of junctional nAChRs and destruction of the junctional folds has been reported. Abnormal channel openings in the absence of acetylcholine may also contribute to the 'endplate myopathy'. This may explain why the SCS mutations that cause spontaneous openings are often associated with a more severe phenotype.

In contrast to myasthenic gravis, the symptoms of SCS are exacerbated by acetylcholinesterase inhibitors and patients do not respond to immunotherapies.

The periodic paralyses

Hyperkalaemic periodic paralysis, paramyotonia congenita, and the potassium-aggravated myotonias result from mutations in the α-subunit of the human skeletal muscle Na^+ channel. All are inherited as dominant traits and usually present within the first or second decade of life.

Hyperkalaemic periodic paralysis (**HyperPP**) may occur spontaneously, but attacks are commonly precipitated by exercise, stress, fasting, or eating K^+-rich foods. Paralysis is often preceded by signs of muscle hyperexcitability such as myotonia or fasciculations. The duration is variable (minutes to hours) and may be so severe that the patient is unable to remain standing. It is associated with a raised blood K^+ concentration (5–7 mM). Paramyotonia congenita is precipitated by cold and (in contrast to most classical myotonias) aggravated by exercise. In some patients, the myotonia may be followed by prolonged paralysis. Potassium-aggravated myotonia is characterized by myotonia without muscle weakness or paralysis. It can be distinguished from classical myotonias by the fact that the myotonia is exacerbated by a mild elevation of the plasma K^+ concentration.

All three types of disorder result from mutations in the α-subunit of the skeletal muscle Na^+ channel (*SCN4A*), which disrupt Na^+-channel inactivation. As a consequence, they produce a persistent inward current that causes a tonic depolarization of the muscle membrane (the larger the current, the greater the depolarization). The magnitude of the depolarization determines whether myotonia or paralysis occurs. A small depolarization causes membrane hyperexcitability by lowering the action-potential threshold, whereas a large depolarization can lead to Na^+-channel inactivation and thereby paralysis. It is still not understood how cold or an elevated plasma potassium level precipitate attacks.

Myotonia

Loss-of-function mutations in the gene (*CLCN1*) encoding the skeletal muscle Cl^- channel produce two forms of myotonia—the autosomal dominant myotonia congenita (Thomsen's disease) and the autosomal recessive generalized myotonia (Becker's disease). Clinical descriptions of the disease can be found elsewhere.

In normal skeletal muscle, the Cl^- conductance accounts for between 70 and 80 per cent of the resting membrane conductance. Mutations in *CLCN1* that result in a loss of functional Cl^- channels will therefore produce a marked increase in the input resistance of the muscle fibre. Consequently, muscle excitability will be enhanced (because a smaller Na^+ current will be sufficient to trigger an action potential). The elevated input resistance also produces a reduced rate of action potential repolarization, which enhances muscle excitability. An important role of the muscle Cl^- conductance is to counteract the depolarizing effect of K^+ accumulation in the transverse tubular (T-) system that accompanies muscle activity. During an action potential, K^+ ions leave the muscle fibre. In normal muscle, the amount of K^+ entering the T-system during a single action potential is not sufficient to alter the membrane potential, because the tubular Cl^- conductance is very high. But in myotonic muscle, the Cl^- conductance is very low and a small rise in tubular K^+ produces a significant depolarization following an action potential. If several action potentials occur in rapid succession, summation of the after-depolarizations may be sufficient to trigger spontaneous action potentials and thereby myotonia.

Mutations in *CLCN1* give rise to both recessive and dominant forms of myotonia. This may be because the muscle Cl^- channel comprises more than one subunit. In heterozygotes, mutant subunits might combine with wild-type subunits to form heteromeric channels. The extent to which the mutant subunit reduced the function of the heteromeric channel would thus dictate the severity of myotonia. Total inactivation of the channel by a single mutant subunit (the dominant-negative effect) would produce dominant myotonia, whereas recessive myotonia might occur if the heteromeric channel was unaffected by the mutant subunit.

Malignant hypothermia and central core disease

Mutations in the ligand-gated Ca^{2+} channel of skeletal muscle cause malignant hyperthermia and central core disease. This channel mediates Ca^{2+} release from the sarcoplasmic reticulum (SR), allowing Ca^{2+} to enter the cytoplasm and activate the contractile proteins. It is also known as the ryanodine receptor (or RYR1) because it binds the alkaloid ryanodine with high affinity.

Malignant hyperthermia (**MH**) is one of the main causes of death due to anaesthesia. In susceptible individuals, common inhalation anaesthetics or depolarizing muscle relaxants trigger accelerated skeletal muscle metabolism, muscle contractures, hyperkalaemia, arrhythmias, respiratory and metabolic acidosis, and a rapid rise in body temperature (as much as 1°C every 5 min). It is thought that this is due to stimulation of Ca^{2+} release from the SR, which produces a sustained increase in intracellular Ca^{2+}. This activates both metabolic and contractile activity; the former results in respiratory and metabolic acidosis and the latter produces the elevation in body temperature. The syndrome can be treated with dantrolene sodium, which blocks Ca^{2+} release from the SR. Malignant hyperthermia is genetically heterogeneous and is not linked to *RYR1* in all families.

Central core disease (**CCD**) is an autosomal dominant, non-progressive myopathy that presents in infancy as proximal muscle weakness and hypertonia. Diagnosis is by muscle biopsy, which reveals that regions of type 1 skeletal muscle fibres (known as 'central cores') are depleted of mitochondria and oxidative enzymes. The disease is often associated with a predisposition to malignant hyperthermia and results from mutations in *RYR1*. Thus CCD and MH are allelic disorders of the same gene. It is not clear how the different phenotypes arise, especially because the same mutation can give rise to MH in some individuals and CCD in others. Because all CCD patients are MH-susceptible, it is possible that additional factors are necessary for the development of central core disease.

Kidney channelopathies

Liddle's syndrome

Liddle's syndrome is a congenital form of salt-sensitive hypertension characterized by a very high rate of renal Na^+ uptake despite low levels of aldosterone, secondary hypokalaemia, and metabolic acidosis. It is caused by gain-of-function mutations in the epithelial sodium channel (**ENaC**). This channel consists of three subunits (α, β, γ), and disease-causing mutations have been identified in both the β- and γ-subunits. All are located in the C-terminus of the protein and result in constitutive channel hyperactivity.

The increase in ENaC current causes enhanced Na^+ uptake. This is accompanied by increased water uptake, thereby producing a chronic increase in blood volume and ultimately hypertension. An increased Na^+ uptake also has secondary consequences: in particular, K^+ secretion into the tubule lumen is stimulated because the apical membrane depolarizes and so increases the driving force for K^+ efflux. In addition, more K^+ enters the cell due to the enhanced activity of the Na+/K+-ATPase. This explains why excess ENaC activity in Liddle's syndrome is associated with hypokalaemia and, conversely, why reduced ENaC activity (as in pseudohypoaldosteronism type 1 (**PHA-1**) disease) is accompanied by hyperkalaemia.

Pseudohypoaldosteronism type 1

While gain-of-function mutations in ENaC cause enhanced Na^+ uptake and hypertension, loss-of-function mutations produce salt-wasting, hypotension, and dehydration in newborns and infants. Pseudohypoaldosteronism type 1 (PHA-1) results from loss-of-function mutations in the α, β, or γ ENaC subunits. The marked reduction in ENaC activity leads to decreased Na^+ absorption by the kidney. This stimulates renin and aldosterone secretion, but salt reabsorption cannot be augmented as ENaC is not functional. The high Na^+ concentration in the tubular fluid causes water to be osmotically retained in the tubule lumen, leading to diuresis and dehydration.

Bartter's syndrome

Bartter's syndrome is characterized by severe salt-wasting, with elevated plasma renin and aldosterone levels. The syndrome is both phenotypically and genetically heterogeneous, and several subtypes have been distinguished. Antenatal Bartter's syndrome or hyperprostaglandin-E syndrome presents *in utero* with a marked fetal polyuria. Newborns fail to thrive and show severe salt-wasting, moderate hypokalaemia, and metabolic acidosis, and elevated urinary excretion of prostaglandins. There is also marked calcinuria, osteopenia, and nephrocalcinosis.

Antenatal Bartter's syndrome results from loss-of-function mutations in the genes encoding proteins involved in salt transport in the cells of the distal kidney tubules. These include the inwardly rectifying K^+ channel Kir1.1 (*KCNJ1*; Bartter's syndrome type II), the NaK2Cl cotransporter (*SCL12A1*, Bartter's syndrome type I), and the voltage-gated Cl^- channel CLC-Kb (*CLCNKB*, Bartter's syndrome type III). These variants may be distinguished clinically, because hypokalaemia is less pronounced (3.0–3.5 mM) in patients with mutations in *KCNJ1*, and the course of the disease is less severe. And in contrast to patients with Bartter's syndrome types I and II, patients with mutations in *CLCNKB* do not suffer from nephrocalcinosis, despite elevation of the urinary calcium concentration.

Disease-causing mutations in Kir1.1 or CLC-Kb impair NaCl uptake in the distal tubules by impairing channel function or decreasing protein expression. This leads to a high salt concentration in the urine and thus to an osmotic diuresis, which accounts for the salt-wasting, polyuria, and low plasma volume characteristic of Bartter's syndrome. A similar phenotype is observed with loop diuretics, such as frusemide (furosemide), which inhibit the NaK2Cl cotransporter.

Nephrolithiasis

Mutations in the voltage-gated, renal chloride channel gene, *CLCN5*, cause Dent's disease, a congenital form of congenital nephrolithiasis. It is usually associated with proteinuria. Different mutations may produce phenotypically distinct syndromes (Table 1), but there is as yet no clear explanation for how this occurs. The mechanism by which mutations in a Cl^- channel impair calcium handling by the kidney is also not fully resolved.

Nephrogenic diabetes insipidus

Familial nephrogenic diabetes insipidus (**NDI**) results from impaired water uptake by the kidney tubules. The diseases manifests within the first few weeks of life and is characterized by the excretion of large amounts of hypotonic urine and excessive thirst. In early infancy these may not be noticed and the disease is often recognized by signs of dehydration, such as poor feeding, poor weight gain, irritability, and fever. In most cases, familial NDI is caused by a mutation in the vasopressin receptor, but in some families it results from loss-of-function mutations in the aquaporin 2 (*AQP2*) gene. AQP2 is expressed exclusively in the collecting duct of the kidney and plays a fundamental role in the production of a concentrated urine because it acts as a water channel. Vasopressin stimulates water uptake by causing the insertion of AQP2 channels into the apical membranes of the principal cells of the collecting duct, thereby enhancing water uptake. Loss-of-function mutations in *AQP2* result in a dramatic reduction in water channels, thereby accounting for the polyuria.

Other channelopathies

Cystic fibrosis

Of all the channelopathies, the best known is probably cystic fibrosis (**CF**). Its clinical features are described in Chapter 17.10. Cystic fibrosis results from mutations in an epithelial chloride channel known as the cystic fibrosis transmembrane conductance regulator (**CFTR**). Although its primary sequence is highly homologous to that of the ATP-binding cassette transporters, it is now well established that CFTR functions as a chloride channel. It also regulates the activity of the outwardly rectifying Cl^- channel and the epithelial Na^+ channel.

All disease-causing CF mutations result in the complete absence or a marked reduction in CFTR function. Those which result in the total loss of channel activity, either because the protein does not reach the plasma membrane or because it is present but completely inactive, give rise to a severe form of the disease. Mutations that result in a reduced Cl^- current are associated with a milder form of the disease. Compound heterozygotes carrying one allele with a severe mutation and another with a mild mutation will have significant residual channel activity and therefore a mild form of the disease.

While a large number of mutations (more than 450) have been identified in CFTR, it is still far from certain how the loss of Cl^--channel function gives rise to the clinical features of the disease, especially, in the lungs.

Congenital hyperinsulinaemia

Familial congenital hyperinsulinaemia (**CHI**) is characterized by an unregulated insulin secretion and profound hypoglycaemia that presents at birth or within the first year of life. Some patients respond to treatment with diazoxide, but in others the most effective treatment is resection of the pancreas (more than 90 per cent is usual). Many patients develop diabetes in later life.

CHI results from mutations in the genes encoding the pancreatic β-cell ATP-sensitive K^+ (K_{ATP}) channel. This channel plays a key role in glucose-stimulated insulin secretion. When the plasma glucose level is low (less than 3 mM), the channel is open and keeps the β-cell membrane potential at a hyperpolarized level. When plasma glucose levels rise, increasing glucose uptake and metabolism by the β-cell, the K_{ATP} channels close. This produces a membrane depolarization that activates voltage-gated Ca^{2+} channels, increases Ca^{2+} influx, and so stimulates insulin release. Two classes of therapeutic drugs modulate insulin secretion by interacting with K_{ATP} channels. Sulphonylureas inhibit channel activity and are used to enhance insulin secretion in patients with type 2 diabetes mellitus, whereas K-channel openers (for example, diazoxide) activate K_{ATP} channels, hyperpolarizing the β-cell and preventing insulin release.

The K_{ATP} channel consists of two types of subunit: a pore-forming subunit Kir6.2, and a regulatory subunit SUR1. Mutations in either subunit can cause CHI, but those in SUR1 are more common. CHI mutations result in the loss of K_{ATP} channel activity, even at low blood glucose levels. This results in a continuous depolarization of the β-cell, that leads to persistent Ca^{2+} influx and thus constitutive insulin secretion.

Non-syndromic deafness

About 70 per cent of all cases of prelingual deafness are non-syndromic. The disorder shows marked genetic heterogeneity, but in some families it results from loss-of-function mutations in the gene (*GJB2*) encoding the gap junction channel connexin 26. Both recessive and dominant mutations have been described. Connexin 26 (Cx26) is expressed in the cochlea, but the mechanism by which the lack of functional Cx26 leads to hearing loss remains obscure. In some individuals, mutations in Cx26 are associated with Vohwinkel's syndrome, a disorder characterized by keratoderma. Many patients also suffer from deafness.

Further reading

Ashcroft FM (2000). *Ion channels and disease* p.481. Academic Press, San Diego.

Lehmann-Horn F, Jurkatt-Rott K (1999). Voltage-gated ion channel and hereditary disease. *Physiological Reviews* **79**, 1317

Websites

http://www.ncbi.nlm.nih.gov/omim/ [Online Mendelian inheritance in man (**OMIM**), a database of human genes and genetic disorders.]

http://www.neuro.wustl.edu/neuromuscular/mother/chan.html [A website concerned with neurological and CNS disorders, including those associated with ion channel defects, maintained by the Neuromuscular Disease Center at Washington University School of Medicine, St Louis, USA.]

http://www.ncbi.nlm.nih.gov/ [The National Center for Biotechnology Information, providing access to genetic sequence databases (e.g. GenBank)]

4.6 Apoptosis in health and disease

Andrew H. Wyllie and Mark J. Arends

Introduction

Apoptosis is the process by which single cells die in the midst of living tissues. It is responsible for most—perhaps all—of the cell-death events that occur during the formation of the early embryo and the sculpting and moulding of organs. It continues to play a critical role in the maintenance of cell numbers in those tissues in which cell turnover persists into adult life, such as the epithelium of the gastrointestinal tract, the bone marrow, and lymphoid system including both B- and T-cell lineages. It is the usual mode of death in the targets of natural killer (**NK**)- and cytotoxic T-cell killing, and in involution and atrophy induced by hormonal and other stimuli. It also appears in the reaction of many tissues to injury, including mild degrees of ischaemia, exposure to ionizing and ultraviolet radiation or treatment with cancer chemotherapeutic drugs. Excessive or too little apoptosis plays a significant part in the pathogenesis of autoimmunity, infectious disease, acquired immunodeficiency syndrome (**AIDS**), stroke, myocardial disease, and cancer. When cancers regress, apoptosis is usually part or all of the mechanism involved.

Structural changes in apoptosis

Apoptosis can be recognized because of its characteristic, stereotyped sequence of structural changes (Fig. 1). The dying cells lose contact with their neighbours. They undergo a rapid loss of volume, often of the order of 50 per cent. There is explosive blebbing from the cell surface, in which

(a)   (b)   (c)

(d)   (e)

Fig. 1 The structure of apoptosis. (a) Scanning electron micrograph of a normal macrophage shows its surface sprouting many pseudopodia. In (b), the cell has been injured (in this case by oxidized lipid of the type often present in high concentration in atheromatous plaques) and is throwing out and retracting multiple surface blebs. In (c) the whole cell has fragmented into roughly spherical apoptotic bodies. Some of these are cratered by the orifices of the dilated endoplasmic reticulum. (d) Transmission electron micrograph of a thin section. The condensed chromatin (arrowheads), nucleolar remnant (arrow), and highly convoluted surface are clearly visible. The scale bar in μm. (Micrographs by courtesy of Dr Jeremy Skepper and Dr Jing Xia, Cambridge School of Biology Multi-imaging Centre.)

multiple cytoplasmic protrusions extend and are immediately withdrawn, and this is followed by fragmentation into a cluster of subcellular bodies (apoptotic bodies) each membrane-bounded and containing a variety of compacted cytoplasmic organelles. The nucleus undergoes similar distortion and fragmentation. Chromatin condenses under the nuclear membrane in granular aggregates with a knob-like, hemilunar or toroidal distribution. Nuclear membranes overlying residual uncondensed chromatin are rich in pores but these are absent adjacent to condensed chromatin, suggesting that redistribution takes place. The nucleolus segregates so that its argyophilic fibrillar centre lies close to the peripheral aggregates of chromatin, whilst the osmophilic particles that are associated with transcription complexes disperse in the central nucleoplasm. Eventually the nuclear membrane disappears and the entire nuclear remnant becomes a mass of condensed granular chromatin.

Within the cytoplasm, bundles of microfilaments often appear in a side-to-side configuration. Sometimes free ribosomes pack into semicrystalline arrays. There is dilatation of the endoplasmic reticulum. The cell surface loses any pre-existing microvilli or other indices of polarity. The shrunken cell and the apoptotic bodies into which it fragments tend to become spherical.

Isolated apoptotic cells lose the ability to maintain ionic homeostasis within an hour or so, lose density, swell in volume, and permit the entry of various dyes classically used to mark dead cells (such as Trypan blue and propidium iodide) to which they had been previously impermeable. Within tissues, however, this phase is seldom seen, because the apoptotic cell and its fragments undergo phagocytosis. Often this is undertaken by 'professional' phagocytes—the resident tissue macrophages—but where unusually large numbers of apoptotic cells are generated, other cell types share in ingesting them, including their viable neighbours. Once within the phagosome of the ingesting cell, the apoptotic cell and its fragments rapidly become indistinguishable from the contents of any other large secondary lysosome.

For reasons to be expanded later, the process of apoptotic-cell phagocytosis inhibits the neutrophil-dominated inflammatory reaction that is often seen when macrophages are activated in other circumstances. Cell loss by apoptosis can therefore be effected with little disruption of the tissue concerned. Moreover, apoptosis, once initiated, is completed swiftly. Although the interval from the initial application of a lethal stimulus to the first manifestations of shrinkage and blebbing can vary greatly, phagocytosis may be complete within an hour thereafter. Hence, the evidence for cell loss by apoptosis is transient and often surprisingly scanty relative to the reduction in cell number it effects.

Apoptosis is not the only mode of cell death. Dying cells sometimes show a very different pattern of change, dominated by volume overload and, eventually, plasma membrane breakdown and leakage of intracellular contents into the extracellular space. At first, the nucleus retains its general structure, although the chromatin patterns coarsen. Usually there is an associated acute inflammatory reaction. This pattern of death is frequently found when tissues are overwhelmed by high concentrations of toxic substances or in severe ischaemic damage, where vascular perfusion has been arrested. Classically, it is called necrosis.

Later, following equilibration of the cytosol with extracellular calcium, and the resultant widespread activation of degradative enzymes such as cathepsins, vestiges of nuclear structure fade away (karyolysis) and only ghost-like cellular outlines remain.

Caspases: effectors of apoptosis

Many of the morphological features of apoptosis are attributable to activation of a family of proteases called 'caspases', because of the presence of the amino acid **c**ysteine in their catalytic site, and their preferential cleavage of peptides immediately C-terminal to **asp**artate residues. There are at least 12 mammalian caspases. All are initially synthesized as relatively inactive proenzymes and undergo proteolysis to generate two fragments of around

Fig. 2 Schematic diagram of caspase activation. The proenzyme is on the left. Following processing, as shown on the right, the N-terminal sequence and the linker are lost. The active sites of the enzyme each contain elements from both p10 and p20 subunits.

10- and 20-kDa molecular weight, together with a fragment of variable length from the original N-terminus (Fig. 2). These 10- and 20-kDa fragments oligomerize in pairs to form a tetramer, which is the active enzyme. Long N-terminal sequences provide the opportunity for regulation through interaction with various binding proteins.

Caspases recognize 4-amino acid motifs that are present in many proteins. Significantly, such caspase target sites are often highly conserved between species, and frequently occur in strategic intramolecular locations, such that caspase cleavage would radically alter the function of the substrate protein. In particular, the cleavage of caspase substrates accounts for many of the structural changes of apoptosis already described. Particularly interesting substrates include proteases, structural proteins of the cytoskeleton, members of various signalling pathways, proteins involved in DNA damage and repair, and molecules of importance in the regulation of the cell cycle. Some caspase substrates appear to be intermediates in self-amplifying positive feedback systems required to complete the death process.

Caspases and proteases

For most caspases, the cleavage sites are themselves typical caspase target sequences, indicating that caspase activation might proceed by cascade-like autocatalysis. There is very good evidence for this, the initiator caspases with long N-terminal sequences (caspases 8–12 and probably 2, 4, and 5) being activated prior to the short effector caspases (3, 6, and 7). Caspases can also activate other proteases. There is, for example, a caspase site in the calpain-inhibitor protein, calpastatin. The inhibitor is rendered inactive by cleavage, so turning on calpain digestion within the dying cell.

Caspases and cytoskeletal proteins

Actin (the major protein of the cytoskeleton), fodrin (which provides the deformable shell underlying the plasma membrane), vimentin (an intermediate filament protein of the cytoskeleton), and the lamins (which form a major component of the nuclear envelope) are all caspase substrates. Caspase cleavage of these large polymeric proteins provides a means whereby they can be rapidly disassembled to the monomers of which they are composed. Gelsolin, a further caspase substrate, is an actin-binding protein that cleaves actin filaments in a calcium-dependent manner. Caspase cleavage of gelsolin separates the calcium-sensitive negative regulatory domain from the protease domain, and hence actin-filament cleavage is effected under normal intracellular calcium concentrations. These cytoskeletal proteolytic events probably contribute to the rounded shape of apoptotic bodies and to the eventual dissolution of the nuclear membrane.

Caspases and signalling proteins

The small G-protein, rho, regulates the mobility of the cell surface. Two rho-dependent kinases, PAK2 and ROCK-1, are rendered constitutively active by caspase cleavage, through excision of their negative regulatory domains. PAK2 activity is a factor in the early retraction of the apoptotic cell from its neighbours or from substrate attachment, whilst ROCK-1 activity is responsible for the enhanced action of a myosin light-chain kinase that drives the phase of cell-membrane blebbing that immediately precedes fragmentation of the apoptotic cell.

FAK^{P125} is the kinase associated with focal adhesion plaques. It is a critical element in the signalling pathway that links cellular awareness of substrate attachment (through integrins) to other cellular functions, including movement, attachment, and new transcription. FAK^{P125} is cleaved and inactivated by caspases, hence isolating the cell from such signals, many of which would normally promote survival. Somewhat similarly, the adenomatous polyposis coli protein (**APC**) and β-catenin are both elements in the wnt-1 signalling pathway, connecting cell-to-cell signals with regulation of cell function. Both are cleaved by caspases, although the precise significance of this is still speculative.

Certain members of the MAP kinase pathway are also targets of caspase cleavage. In particular, MEKK1 (MAPK/ERK kinase kinase; MAPK is mitogen activated protein kinase; ERK is extracellular signal-related kinase; all these enzymes form part of an autocatalytic cascade) a kinase upstream of the p38 stress-associated protein kinase, is activated through the removal, by caspase proteolysis, of an N-terminal inhibitory domain. As p38 itself initiates apoptosis, which would lead in turn to further activation of MEKK1, this could generate a positive feedback loop ensuring that the process of death is executed swiftly and effectively.

DNA damage and repair

ICAD (inhibitor of caspase-activated DNase) is a cytoplasmic chaperone that binds a double-stranded nuclease, **CAD** (caspase-activated DNase). The ICAD–CAD complex is normally cytoplasmic. ICAD, however, is a caspase substrate and once cleaved can no longer retain CAD in the cytoplasm. On translocation to the nucleus, CAD initiates the digestion of DNA, first to large fragments of around 50 kilobase pairs (**kbp**), and eventually—through cleavage of chromatin at internucleosomal sites—to a series of fragments that are multiples of the 180- to 200-bp unit wrapped around each nucleosome. These DNA fragments can be extracted from apoptotic cells and, on electrophoresis, produce the characteristic ladder pattern that historically was one of the distinctive signatures of apoptosis. Intranuclear DNA cleavage is still the basis of a variety of diagnostic methods that depend on the presence of large numbers of free double-stranded DNA ends. A further protein, acinus, also apparently activated by caspases, contributes to the extreme condensation of chromatin seen in the nuclei of apoptotic cells.

DNA-PK, ATM, PARP, and Rad51 are all DNA repair proteins concerned with the recognition and response to double-strand breaks. Significantly, all are cleaved in apoptosis at sites that separate their DNA-binding and catalytic domains, thus ablating their ability to effect non-homologous end-joining. This may be important in preventing re-ligation of the heavily digested DNA of the apoptotic nucleus, so avoiding the generation of large numbers of undesirable recombinant DNA molecules. Cleavage of PARP (poly-ADP-ribose polymerase) may have an additional function. PARP normally responds to DNA breaks by adding poly-ADP ribosyl tails. It is an abundant nuclear protein and has the capacity to exhaust cellular adenine nucleotide stores if presented with the large number of free DNA ends in the apoptotic nucleus. Apoptosis is an energy-requiring process, and it may therefore be advantageous to conserve adenine nucleotides, even during the process of death.

Caspases and cell-cycle proteins

Unexpectedly, several proteins that normally inhibit movement around the cell cycle are targets for caspase cleavage. These include p21^{WAF1} and p27^{KIP1}, inhibitors of cyclin-dependent kinases that catalyse movement through the G_1 and S phases of the cell cycle. Wee-1 is a further caspase substrate: normally it blocks movement from G_2 to mitosis. CDC27, a component of the anaphase-promoting complex which destroys cyclin B and hence inhibits entry into mitosis, is also subject to caspase cleavage. The purpose of this reactivation of elements of the cell cycle during the process

of death is still quite obscure. It occurs during the apoptosis of cells such as neurones which have long since ceased movement around the cycle.

Pathways that activate caspases

Two well-documented pathways converge on and activate the effector caspases, one leading from cytokine-activated, death-signalling receptors on the cell surface, the other from mitochondria.

Death-signalling receptors coupled to caspase activation

The death-signalling receptors are all members of the tumour necrosis factor-α (**TNF-α**) receptor family. They are type 1 membrane receptors (that is, with the N-terminus on the external surface), containing a series of cysteine-rich incomplete repeats in the ligand-binding domain, a single transmembrane domain, and a cytoplasmic moiety with one or more signalling domains (Fig. 3). Their ligands are homologues of the cytokine TNF-α. The prototype death-signalling receptor is fas (also called CD95 or Apo-1). On binding its ligand, FasL, this receptor trimerizes and immediately recruits to its cytoplasmic moiety a cluster of proteins collectively called the death-initiating signalling complex (**DISC**). The aggregation of DISC proteins is the result of protein–protein interaction at an α-helical region called the death domain (**DD**), because without it fas signalling is ineffective. Through the DD, fas interacts with an adapter protein called **FADD** (fas-associated protein with death domain) that contains a further interactive region called **DED** (for death-effector domain). Through DED, FADD recruits procaspase 8 to the DISC, an initiator caspase with two DEDs in its N-terminal sequence. Because they are at high local concentration in the DISC, the procaspase 8 molecules can catalyse their own activation, and so initiate the proteolytic cascade that ultimately turns on the effector caspases. Whilst fas is widely expressed in many tissues, fasL expression is largely restricted to cytotoxic lymphocytes and to cells in

Fig. 3 Death-signalling receptors, shown diagrammatically. The fas receptor, with its ligand and DISC, signalling exclusively to death, is shown on the left. The more complex TNF-α receptor 1 is shown in the centre. Both prosurvival and proapoptosis signals can emanate from this receptor. On the right is shown one of the decoy receptors for **TRAIL** (TNF-related apoptosis-inducing ligand), DcR1. This receptor has no membrane anchor and so competes for TRAIL with the death-signalling membrane receptors, DR4 and DR5.

immunologically privileged sites. In this way, the fasL/fas system plays a major role in cell killing by cytotoxic T-cells (**CTLs**) but can repulse CTLs at immunologically privileged sites. As will be described, upregulation of fas may play a much wider role in the sensitization of damaged cells to other types of apoptotic stimuli. Caspase 8 is not the only output from fas activation. A DISC component called daxx acts as an adaptor, connecting fas activation to the apoptosis signal-regulating kinase-1, **Ask-1**. This links fas signalling to the stress-activated kinases JNK and p38 (Figs 3 and 4).

TNFR1, the high-affinity TNF-α receptor, also trimerizes and signals to caspase 8 through FADD, in a DISC, but its action is substantially more complex. TNFR1 first recruits an additional DD-containing adaptor protein called TRADD. TRADD then recruits FADD, but can also bind other proteins into the DISC, including TRAF2 and a serine–threonine kinase called RIP. TRAF2 activates MEKK1 and Ask-1, elements of the MAP kinase pathway that transmit activation signals to JNK and hence the jun-containing transcription factor AP-1. RIP activates the transcription factor NFκB. NFκB provides a consistent survival signal, whilst JNK activation can be either prosurvival or proapoptosis. TNFR1 can also signal through yet another DD-containing adaptor protein, RAIDD, that in turn activates procaspase 2. Hence TNFR1-mediated signals can be interpreted as proapoptotic (through activation of caspase 8, caspase 2, or the p38 kinase), prosurvival (through NFκB), or ambivalent (through JNK and AP-1). This design means that incoming cytokine signals can be interpreted in opposite ways—for life or death—depending on precise conditions in the cell at the time.

DR3 is a receptor closely similar in structure to TNFR1 but with a narrower tissue distribution. Whereas TNFR1 is ubiquitous, DR3 is expressed predominantly in the lymphocytes of spleen, thymus, and peripheral blood. Interestingly, the expression of the ligands appears to adopt the opposite pattern, with TNF-α being a product predominantly of activated macrophages and lymphocytes, whereas the DR3 ligand (variously also called Apo3L and TWEAK) is expressed in many tissue types.

DR4 and -5 are similar receptors that bind a ligand called TRAIL (TNF-related apoptosis-inducing ligand). The downstream signalling appears to involve both FADD and caspase 8, although the possibility that certain cell types may couple DR4 and -5 to other signalling molecules is not excluded. Both TRAIL and its receptors are expressed in many tissue types. TRAIL has excited particular attention because it is frequently cytotoxic to tumour cells under conditions in which normal cells are unharmed. Variant receptors that lack the cytoplasmic signalling moieties are expressed in many normal tissues and appear to act as inhibitory decoys for TRAIL.

The death-signalling receptor pathway has the capacity to integrate several different types of environmental information in formulating its ultimate message to the caspases. Although its primary function is response, through the TNF-α family of receptors, to death-inducing ligands, its connection to the stress-activated kinases through Ask-1 also allows it to be sensitive to the redox status of the cell. Ask-1 binds to thioredoxin in a reversible, redox-sensitive manner. Hence the conditions under which Ask-1 is available for signalling are also redox-sensitive. Further, Ask-1 is inactivated, through binding to the chaperone 14–3–3, when serine phosphorylated. In this way the Ask-1 signalling pathway may be taken out of circuit by serine phosphorylation, as would pertain under conditions of growth-factor stimulation through raf kinase, PI3 kinase, and protein kinase B (Akt).

Mitochondrial signals coupled to apoptosis activation

The mitochondrial pathway depends upon the release of cytochrome *c*, together with dATP, from the intermembranous space of mitochondria. Cytochrome *c* and deoxyATP (**dATP**) bind to and effect a conformational change in a protein of the outer mitochondrial membrane, Apaf-1, so that it exposes a protein-binding domain (generically called a **CARD**, for caspase-activating recruitment domain) capable of recruiting and activating procaspase 9. This molecular assembly has been called the apoptosome, although other procaspase-containing complexes exist, including the DISC and probably others, referred to below. This then activates the effector caspases (Fig. 4). Triggers for the release of cytochrome *c* include reactive oxygen species, cellular redox stress, pH changes, and proteins of the BCL-2 family.

BCL-2 is a protein with a C-terminal hydrophobic domain that allows it to anchor to intracellular membranes, of which the outer mitochondrial membrane is one. It was first identified because of its consistent activation (through a chromosome translocation) in follicular B-cell lymphoma. In this sense, BCL-2 can function as an oncogene, but it differs from most other oncogenes in failing to stimulate cell proliferation—indeed, when expressed in isolation it inhibits cell-cycle progression. Its major role, however, is that of a survival factor, and thus it can cooperate with other oncogenes to sustain the life of clones of cells that otherwise might be deleted by apoptosis. This survival factor function appears to be a basic property of metazoan cells. The normal development of the nematode *Caenorhabditis elegans*, for example, depends on a BCL-2 homologue (ced 9), without which the embryo undergoes widespread apoptosis at an early stage. Transgenic mammalian BCL-2 can rescue the development of ced 9-deficient nematode larvae.

The mammalian BCL-2 family contains at least 15 members in three major branches, distinguished on the basis of their function, which can be either prosurvival or prodeath, and the presence or absence of certain conserved domains (called BH1–4). Amongst the prosurvival molecules are BCL-2 itself, BCL-xL, and BCL-w, all of which share all four BH domains, MCL-1 which lacks the BH4 domain, Boo which lacks BH3, and A1 which lacks both BH4 and BH3. In contrast, bax, bak, and bok form a branch of the BCL-2 family that possesses BH3, BH2, and BH1 domains but exerts prodeath functions. The third family branch consists of proteins whose sole

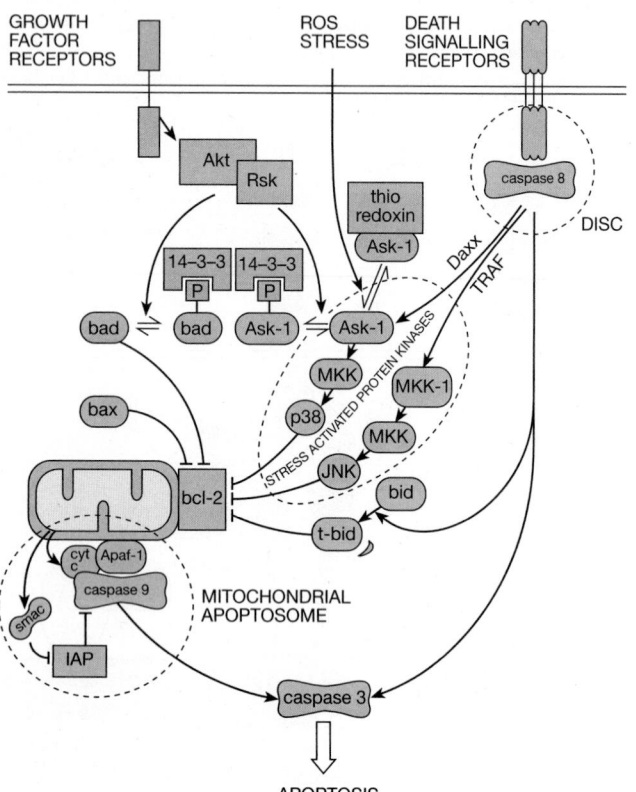

Fig. 4 Interaction between membrane receptors and mitochondrial signals coupled to apoptosis. In this summary diagram, proapoptotic elements are shown with rounded profiles, whilst prosurvival elements have rectangular borders. Cyt c, cytochrome *c*; t-bid, truncated bid.

region of homology with the others is a BH3 domain (sometimes amounting to no more than an 8-amino acid motif): bid, bad, bim, blk, hrk, and BNIP3. The BH1, BH2, and BH3 domains form part of a hydrophobic pocket in the molecule, into which another BH3 domain can fit in much the same way as a ligand binds to its receptor. Through this interdomain binding, BCL-2 family members can homo- and heterodimerize with each other. Whilst the prodeath action of the BH3-only proteins is known to depend upon such heterodimerization, the mechanism of action of the prolife and bax-related proteins is still uncertain.

Proteins in the prosurvival and bax-like prodeath branches of the BCL-2 family have a tertiary structure similar to bacterial haemolysins such as diphtheria toxin, suggesting that they could form transmembrane pore-like structures. Moreover, the majority of the members of the extended BCL-2 family possess C-terminal membrane anchors, and some (notably BCL-2 itself, BCL-xL, and bax under conditions of apoptosis activation) clearly localize to the mitochondrial outer membrane. Superficially at least, this could provide an explanation for the regulated escape of cytochrome *c* from mitochondria, through opening or closing of transmembrane channels formed from the BCL-2 proteins. This proposition is supported by the observation that BCL-2 family proteins can insert into artificial lipid membranes, thereby changing their electrical conductance. Further, the voltage gradient across the mitochondrial membrane ($\Delta\varphi$m) collapses around the time of apoptosis activation. There remains some doubt, however, both over the capacity of such channels to permit the exit of molecules as large as cytochrome *c* and whether the relationship between the collapse of $\Delta\varphi$m and the initiation of apoptosis is cause or effect. Another model proposes that BCL-2 family members modify the function of the mitochondrial permeability transition pore (a multimolecular transmembrane structure containing a voltage-dependent anion channel and an adenine nucleotide translocator) leading eventually to rupture of the outer membrane.

BCL-2 possesses an important regulatory serine site that, on phosphorylation, neutralizes the prosurvival function. This critical phosphorylation can be effected by the stress-activated kinase pathways mentioned above, that lead from Ask-1 to activation of the JNK and p38 kinases. In this way, cellular stresses of many kinds, including exposure to reactive oxygen species and ultraviolet light, can negate the survival functions of BCL-2 family members and so swiftly lower the cellular threshold for apoptosis.

The BH3-only, prodeath members of the family appear to play important roles in coupling the powerful mitochondrial pathway to lethal stimuli in the cellular environment (Table 1). Notably, bid is activated through cleavage by caspase 8 of a small peptide from its N terminus. The truncated, activated bid translocates from the cytosol to mitochondria and effects the mitochondrial release of cytochrome *c*. In this way, stimuli too small to activate the effector caspases directly can be amplified by recruitment of the mitochondrial pathway through bid. Put another way, bid can lower the threshold at which cytokines trigger apoptosis. Somewhat similarly, bad is involved in a mechanism to raise the threshold at which apoptosis is engaged, depending on the availability of cytokine growth factors. The bad protein is phosphorylated by the kinases Akt (protein kinase B) and Rsk, both in turn dependent on PI3 kinase and the growth factors responsible for its activation. Normally, phosphorylated bad is sequestered in the cytoplasm by the chaperone 14–3–3. In conditions of growth-factor deprivation, however, unphosphorylated bad becomes available, translocates to the mitochondria, and activates cytochrome *c* release. BNIP3 is a mitochondrial protein that accumulates under conditions of hypoxia. It may thus provide a trigger linking hypoxia to apoptosis. Normally, bim binds to the light chain of dynein, a cytoskeletal protein. It may act as a sensor, triggering apoptosis under conditions of cytoskeletal disruption.

Perhaps surprisingly, BCL-2 itself is a caspase substrate: caspase 9 can cleave it to produce a C-terminal peptide with proapoptotic function. This is a further example, along with activation of the mitochondrial pathway through caspase truncation of bid and activation of MEKK1 as a proapoptotic stress-responsive pathway, that emphasizes the subtle strategy embodied in the caspase cascade. Mechanisms of this type would have no meaning if activation of initiator caspases inevitably led to commitment to death through the effector caspases. Rather, the initiator caspases can adjust a threshold, influenced by and integrated with many other incoming stimuli, that determines whether the death sentence will be enacted or repealed. Cells under stress of various types may start nearer that threshold, but the system is designed to process and interpret the continuous arrival of potentially lethal stimuli from around and within the cell.

Additional pathways for caspase activation

Despite the importance of the mitochondrial and death-receptor pathways in activating the effector caspases, it is clear that other means of caspase activation exist. Procaspase 12 localizes to the endoplasmic reticulum, whilst procaspase 2 can be found in the Golgi apparatus and the nucleus. The nucleus also contains CARD-proteins, that are recruited to foci of DNA damage, and BCL-2 is anchored to nuclear and ER membranes as well as mitochondria. Thus the death and survival of the cell, as modulated by caspase activation, may depend upon the synthesis of signals arising at many intracellular sites: some resulting from cell injury, others reflecting physiological stimuli. Damage to nuclear DNA is a particularly important source of injury-related stimuli for caspase activation.

A remarkable set of DNA-binding nucleoproteins is responsible for the recognition of DNA damage of different types, and for the initiation of repair. Thus, separate molecular mechanisms exist for responding to the presence of inappropriately inserted bases (base excision–repair, **BER**), nucleotides that have become modified through crosslinking or the formation of covalently bonded adducts (nucleotide excision–repair, **NER**), nucleotide mismatch or abnormal methylation (mismatch repair, **MR**), and double-strand breaks (homologous recombination or non-homologous end-joining, **HR** or **NHEJ**). In MR, MSH-2 and MLH-1 are recruited sequentially into a molecular complex at the injury site, which activates

Table 1 The mammalian BCL-2 family*

	BH4	BH3	BH1	BH2	Membrane anchor
Prosurvival					
BCL-2	+	+	+	+	+
BCL-xL	+	+	+	+	+
BCL-w	+	+	+	+	+
MCL-1		+	+	+	+
A1			+	+	
Boo	+		+	+	+
BHRF1			+	+	+
KS-BCL2			+	+	+
Prodeath bax-like					
bax		+	+	+	+
bak		+	+	+	+
bok		+	+	+	+
Prodeath BH3 only					
bik		+			+
blk		+			+
hrk		+			+
BNIP3		+			+
bimL		+			+
bad		+			
bid		+			

* The order of the domains shown (BH4, 3, 1, 2, and the membrane anchor) reflect their orientation from N- to C-terminus in the molecules. All are endogenous cellular proteins except BHRF1 and KS-BCL2 which are encoded by herpesviruses (Epstein–Barr virus (EBV) and human herpesvirus-8 (HHV-8), respectively). Not all members with membrane anchors stay tethered to cell membranes. In particular, bax is usually cytoplasmic and migrates to the mitochondrial membrane as part of the cell's response to the apoptotic stimulus. This migration depends on conformational modification of the bax N-terminus, although the reason for this is not yet clear. The BH3 domain of BNIP3 is imperfect. Perhaps for this reason, the expression of this hypoxia-sensitive protein may not engender the classical phenotype of apoptosis, but structural changes more similar to necrosis.

p53, effects cycle arrest, and, in the meantime, initiates repair at the site of damage. Similarly, amongst the first molecules to bind to DNA double-strand breaks in NHEJ are the DNA kinases ATM, ATR, and DNA-PK. In turn, these recruit and activate p53 and other molecules (for example, chk1 and chk2). In surviving cells, these effect arrest at a variety of points around the cell cycle, so ensuring that there is an opportunity to load the repair machinery on to the damaged DNA template before this is further altered by passing through DNA replication or chromatid separation.

A profoundly different means of limiting the effect of genome damage, however, is to commit the damaged cell to apoptosis; activation of the repair complex in both MR and NHEJ can also do this. The molecular basis for the decision between apoptosis or survival with repair is still unknown: indeed, there are circumstances in which repair is activated despite clear evidence that the decision to engage the machinery of apoptosis has already been taken. Activation of p53 is common to both outcomes, and it is therefore reasonable to search in this molecule for clues to the nature of the life or death decision. Activated p53 alters the transcription of a large number of genes. Some are well-known inhibitors of cell-cycle progression, such as p21waf1/cip1, but others (for example bax, fas, and a membrane protein called PERP) are associated exclusively with apoptosis. The situation is further complicated by the fact that p53 also signals to the apoptosis effector process by non-transcriptional means, via an N-terminal sequence that does not appear to be instrumental in effecting cell-cycle arrest. Phosphorylation provides one of the critical signals for p53 activation, and there are several different phosphorylation sites that respond preferentially to the various kinases. Thus the precise phosphorylation status of p53 could provide a molecular signature indicative of the nature, and perhaps the outcome, of the DNA damage.

Another potential factor in controlling DNA injury is a kinase (called **DAP** kinase because it was originally discovered as a death-associated protein) that influences the selection of p14^{ARF} rather than p16^{INK4A}—alternative splice forms from the same gene. Whereas p16^{INK4A} is a cell-cycle regulator, inhibiting the cyclin-dependent kinases, p14^{ARF} displaces p53 from its inhibitor, MDM2, so generating a sustained p53 signal that may favour apoptosis. Curiously, DAP kinase normally docks on to the actin cytoskeleton. It is possible therefore that it affects the threshold at which apoptosis is triggered by DNA injury, depending on cytoskeletal-related factors such as cell-to-cell and cell-to-substrate contacts.

Further clues to the way in which a variety of factors may be integrated in the response to DNA injury have emerged from detailed study of the injured nucleus. Within an hour of DNA damage, very large molecular complexes form around the damaged site. The first arrival is the phosphorylated histone γH2AX, which may recruit later members. These complexes contain molecular species that appear to generate platforms on which many injury-response proteins can associate, including p53, ATM, MSH-2, and Rad50 and -51. One type of platform is constructed from a protein called **PML** (so-called because of its abnormal synthesis in association with promyelocytic leukaemia). PML polymerizes to form intranuclear bodies (called PML bodies) into which p53 and many other proteins in the DNA-injury response are recruited. Indeed, nuclei without PML cannot mount the expected p53-dependent responses to DNA damage, even though p53 itself is available. Another such injury-related subnuclear body (the BASC body) incorporates the large DNA helicases BRCA1 and -2, proteins often defective in inherited susceptibility to breast cancer. These molecular platforms may provide the means whereby complex decisions, including the appropriate response to injury, are informed and initiated.

The replicative status of the cell is a further important determinant of its sensitivity to apoptosis following DNA injury. The proto-oncogene c-*myc* is normally amongst the earliest gene products to be synthesized when cells are stimulated by growth factors to leave quiescence and enter their replicative cycle. Thereafter, continuous expression of c-*myc* is required to sustain repetitive re-entry to the cycle following each cell division, rather than return to quiescence. Paradoxically, however, c-*myc* expression is also a powerful factor lowering the threshold for apoptosis. In particular, c-*myc* expression without concurrent molecular evidence of external growth-fac-

tor stimulation (such as PI3 (phosphatidylinositol-3) kinase and Akt activation) is interpreted as a death signal. Similarly, other early regulators of cell-cycle entry, including inhibition of function of the retinoblastoma protein and the release of the transcription factor E2F-1 from its binding pocket, also trigger apoptosis in the absence of concurrent evidence of external mitogenic stimulation. Perhaps this represents a means whereby tissues are protected from autonomous cell replication: survival of replicating cells is made conditional on the presence of appropriate stimuli in the cellular environment. The benefits of removing cells that show a tendency for such replicative autonomy are obvious, but the precise mechanism that couples replication to death except in acceptable circumstances is far less clear. It seems probable that the cell cycle itself includes checkpoints at which the decision to engage the apoptosis machinery can be taken should any of the appropriate conditions for replication be absent. Indeed, it is possible that injured cells may force the activation of such checkpoints as one way to access their apoptosis programme. This might explain the paradoxical activation of cyclin-dependent kinases by caspases in cells such as neurones that normally do not engage in replicative cycles at all, as mentioned earlier.

Inhibitors of caspase activation

The role of the BCL-2 family proteins in the activation and inhibition of apoptosis has been described, but there are other powerful endogenous inhibitors of caspase-associated cell death. One is FLIP, a DED-containing version of procaspase 8 that lacks caspase activity. High local concentrations of FLIP compete with procaspase 8 for recruitment into the DISC and so inhibit further propagation of death signals originating from the TNF family of receptors.

The heat-shock proteins hsp70 and hsp90 inhibit caspase processing and block mitochondrial cytochrome *c* release. The hsp90 forms a complex with Apaf-1, which is required for the inhibition of procaspase 9 processing, and is reversed by exposure to lethal doses of DNA-damaging agents.

IAPs (inhibitors of apoptosis proteins) inhibit caspase activity after autocatalytic processing of the procaspase has begun. All contain an element called a BIR domain, that binds to the N-termini of the short fragment of partially processed caspases, in such a way that adjacent elements of the IAP molecule drape across the caspase active site and sterically hinder substrate attachment. There are several such proteins—IAP1 and -2, ILP, the neuronal NAIP, and an X-linked family member X-IAP, all of which possess several BIR domains, and livin and survivin which contain a single BIR domain. One manifestation of the importance of IAPs is the presence of an IAP inhibitor, variously called smac or DIABLO, which is released from mitochondria along with cytochrome *c* during caspase activation by the mitochondrial pathway. The inhibitor smac has an N-terminal sequence that competes with partially processed caspase for the binding site in the BIR domain, and so allows the caspase to escape from the inhibitory embrace of the IAP (Fig. 5).

The IAPs provide a further example of the extraordinary interconnections between the cell cycle and cell death. Survivin, apparently associated with caspase 9, forms a complex with and is phosphorylated by active **cdk1** (cyclin-dependent kinase-1) during mitosis. Loss of phosphorylation leads to dissociation of the survivin–caspase-9 heterodimer, activation of caspase 9, and apoptosis. As normal mitosis proceeds, survivin associates with kinetochore proteins, the spindle microtubules, and finally, at cytokinesis, with the mid-body. Complexes of survivin with cyclin-dependent kinases active earlier in the cycle (for example, cdk4) have also been identified and promote transit through G$_1$. Thus, survivin may form part of the cell-cycle checkpoint system postulated earlier, providing a means whereby apoptosis can be activated by abnormalities in progression through the cell cycle. Finally, IAPs are themselves potential substrates of caspase attack, transactivators of the survival factor NFκB, and downstream products of NFκB-directed transcription. They thus form part of positive-feedback systems for both survival and death.

Recognition of apoptotic cells

Macrophages recognize and bind to the surface of apoptotic cells by virtue of multiple molecular 'eat me' signals (Fig. 6). The disposition of phosphatidyl serine (**PS**) residues on the apoptotic cell surface is one of the most characteristic of these. Normally PS appears only on the inner leaflet of the cell membrane, but this strict polarity is lost very early in apoptosis: around the time of rounding up, substantially earlier than chromatin condensation and DNA cleavage, and probably prior to evidence of caspase activation. Macrophages possess a PS receptor that binds to the exposed PS residues. The exposed PS residues may also bind to molecules in the extracellular environment that then form linkers to receptors on macrophage surfaces. Thus thrombospondin helps bind PS on the apoptotic cell surface to β_1, β_3, and β_5 integrins on the macrophage surface. Similarly, the complement fragment iC3b links to macrophage β_2 integrins, whilst the near-ubiquitous extracellular molecule β_2 glycoprotein-1 links to a macrophage receptor specific for it. In the same way, extracellular complement component C1q links specific binding sites on the apoptotic cell surface to receptors on the macrophages. A group of scavenger receptors (SRA, CD36, CD68, LOX-1) may tether directly to poorly defined oxidized lipid groups (similar to those

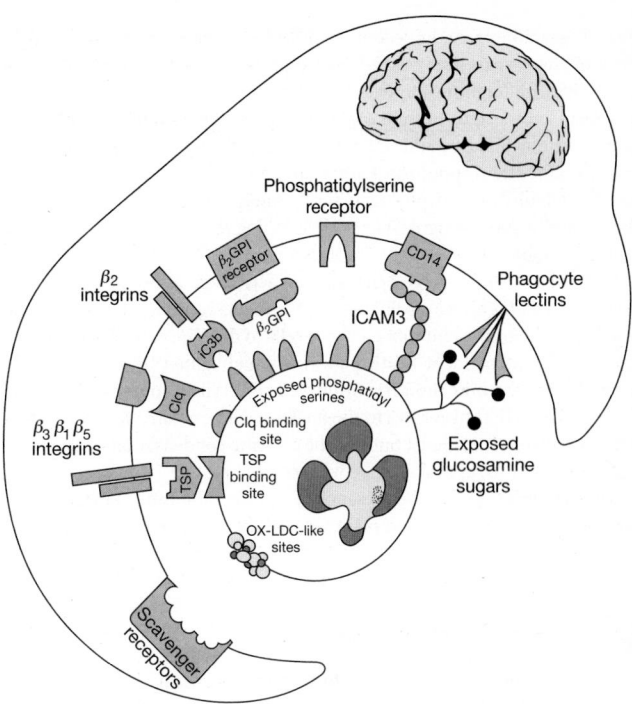

Fig. 6 Receptor–ligand interaction in the recognition of apoptotic cells by macrophages.

(a)

(b)

(c)

Fig. 5 Representation of the mode of action of IAPs. Following partial processing of the caspase, shown in (a), the IAP binds through its BIR domain, which identifies the newly exposed N-terminus of the linker region between the p20 and p10 caspase fragments. Thus bound, adjacent parts of the IAP molecule drape across the caspase active site (b). The inhibitor smac displaces the BIR domain, by presenting as a bait its own N-terminus, which is closely homologous to that of the partially processed caspase (c). With its active site now empty, the caspase can complete its processing and becomes fully active.

in oxidized low-density lipoproteins) exposed on the surfaces of apoptotic cells. CD14 on the macrophage binds to ICAM3, exposed on apoptotic cells. Endogenous macrophage surface lectins also bind to sugars (such as *N*-acetyl glucosamine) selectively exposed on apoptotic cell membranes.

A distinctive feature of macrophage binding to apoptotic cells is the concurrent effect on macrophage function. Macrophages that engage in the phagocytosis of particles opsonized by immunoglobulin or complement component C3b engage in a sharp increase in oxygen usage (the respiratory burst), generation of reactive oxygen species and nitric oxide, and the release of inflammatory cytokines such as TNF-α. These recruit other acute inflammatory cells to the site. In contrast, macrophages that ingest apoptotic bodies show suppression of proinflammatory responses, mediated through the release of different cytokines, such as TGF-β. The basis of these contrasting effector responses appears to be the different signalling pathways that are activated by the macrophage receptors engaged by apoptotic bodies as opposed to opsonized particles.

Are caspases necessary and sufficient for cell death?

Although caspase activation appears to play a dominant role in the effector phase of apoptosis, it is clear that it is not responsible for all the phenomena of apoptosis. One striking example is the surface exposure of 'eat me' signals described above: this is not affected by pharmacological blockade of caspases using inhibitors that are unquestionably effective in blocking other aspects of apoptosis. These inhibitors are usually molecules that jam the caspase catalytic site through presentation to it, in uncleavable form, of a motif similar to the caspase target tetrapeptide. Inhibitors of this type, applied to lethally injured cells *in vitro*, often prolong cellular lifespan, but seldom totally reverse the cellular commitment to death. Moreover, developmentally programmed cell death can sometimes occur on schedule in embryonic tissues in which caspases have been inhibited, or key members of the caspase activation system (such as Apaf-1) are rendered deficient through germline gene knockout. In all these circumstances, the morphology of the caspase-free death is not that of apoptosis. The nuclei swell rather than undergoing the widespread condensation of chromatin. The cytoplasm shows signs of fluid overload, sometimes with the formation of dramatic fluid-filled vacuoles. Some of these changes are reminiscent of necrosis rather than apoptosis. Rather similar changes take place during the developmental death of phylogenetically ancient multicellular organisms that do not possess recognizable close homologues to the caspases, such as the slime mould *Dictyostelium discoides*.

These observations suggest that caspase activation, although intrinsic to the subtle and highly co-ordinated death process recognized as apoptosis, may not be the only event that commits cells to die. The existence of at least one caspase-independent death pathway is highlighted by a flavoprotein released from the mitochondria of injured cells called 'apoptosis-inducing factor' (**AIF**). AIF translocates to the nucleus, where it can effect chromatin cleavage to large fragments, but not the extreme condensation observed in apoptosis. It also appears to reproduce the cellular volume overload described above, even in the presence of caspase inhibition. Phylogenetically it is found in bacteria and plants as well as invertebrate and vertebrate animals.

Apoptosis and disease

There are few disease processes in which apoptosis does not feature, but the examples below are chosen because they exemplify how various steps in the apoptosis pathways may be critical for, or are subverted in, the course of disease pathogenesis.

Immunity and its disorders

Apoptosis is used extensively in the normal function of the immune system to facilitate the process of clonal selection. Antigen stimulation of T-cell proliferation is usually followed by expression of both fas and fasL, a recipe for apoptosis on a grand scale (called activation-induced cell death, **AICD**) unless there is rescue by a survival stimulus. This can be provided by co-stimulation from the immediate environment—adhesion molecules or cytokine receptors. A particularly important route for co-stimulation is through CD28, a receptor on T cells for signals transmitted from antigen-presenting cells, which increases the expression of several cytokines and their receptors. Similarly, clonally expanded populations of stimulated B cells in the bone marrow or those undergoing affinity maturation in lymph-node follicle centres are deleted by fas signalling, but can be selectively rescued by co-stimulation through CD40.

Cytotoxic T cells (CTLs) kill their targets by delivering to them the contents of their granules. Amongst these are perforin, which creates regions in the target-cell membrane of enhanced permeability at the points of contact with the CTL, and granzyme B, a protease that directly activates the caspases of the target cell. In this way, CTLs induce target-cell apoptosis.

The importance of apoptosis for the normal function of the immune system is underscored by the effects of genetic defects. Strains of mice with deficiency in the fas or fas ligand (called *lpr* and *gld*, respectively) show similar immunological phenotypes, characterized by massive lymphoproliferation and autoimmune disorders. The human homologue is the rare condition of the Canale–Smith syndrome (childhood autoimmune lymphoproliferative syndrome or **ALPS**) in which there is a mutation in the DD of fas. Inherited deficiency in C1q also leads to an autoimmunity syndrome: affected individuals almost always develop systemic lupus erythematosus. The pathogenesis here appears to be ineffective recognition and phagocytosis of endogenous apoptotic cells, so that their intracellular antigens are inappropriately processed.

Infective disorders

Shigella dysentery is due to pathogenic strains of *Shigella flexneri*. Pathogenicity is conferred by plasmid-borne genes that neutralize the primary host defence: phagocytosis and destruction of the bacteria by macrophages in the intestinal lamina propria. The plasmid-encoded protein Ipa B activates macrophage caspase 1, so annihilating the defence by inducing macrophage apoptosis. This strategy appears to be successful, because the bacterium that would normally be destroyed if it persisted within the phagosome of the ingesting macrophage, can escape from the cytoplasm of macrophages that undergo apoptosis.

The initial response to *Trypanosoma cruzi*, the parasite responsible for Chagas' disease, is dominated by T-lymphocyte activation. The resultant AICD generates a population of apoptotic lymphocytes. These impinge upon the macrophages that, suitably armed by proinflammatory cytokine stimulation, would be one of the most effective elements in the host defence against the parasite. As described earlier, sustained macrophage phagocytosis of these large numbers of apoptotic cells leads to suppression of proinflammatory cytokine release. The parasite subverts this aspect of the physiology of apoptosis into a source of protection from the host-defence reaction.

Viruses engage with the machinery of apoptosis in many ways. Even lytic viruses have strategies designed to conserve the life of their host cells for some time. DNA viruses, in particular, require means to abort apoptosis, as they must activate the cellular DNA synthesis machinery in order to replicate their own genomes, yet must then avoid the apoptosis that would otherwise follow DNA synthesis unaccompanied by commensurate external stimuli. The *E6* gene of human papillomavirus 16 (**HPV16**) encodes a protein that targets p53 for ubiquitination and subsequent degradation, and so permits cellular survival as the viral *E7* gene inactivates Rb and initiates entry into S-phase. The transforming genes of adenoviruses pair up to effect rather similar outcomes: whilst E1A binds Rb and initiates DNA synthesis, the 55-kDa subunit of E1B binds and inhibits p53, and the 19-kDa subunit neutralizes proapoptotic members of the BCL-2 family. Human herpesviruses such as HHV8 encode their own version of FLIP (v-FLIP). They also have their own prosurvival BCL-2 family members, such as BHRF1 in the Epstein–Barr virus (**EBV**) and KS-BCL2 in HHV8. The HHV8 strategy is particularly subtle, because the virus also destroys the endogenous BCL-2. Unlike endogenous BCL-2, this viral surrogate lacks an internal caspase site, and cannot be converted into a killer peptide by caspase cleavage. Baculovirus encodes a 35-kDa protein with BIR domains that is a prototypical IAP.

Apoptosis plays a key role in the pathogenesis of AIDS. The progressive loss of circulating CD4+ T cells, by which the course of HIV-1 infection to clinical AIDS can be charted, involves numbers of cells that are several orders of magnitude greater than the numbers that ever carry the virus. It is therefore clear that the overwhelming majority of the dying cells must be bystanders, sensitized to apoptosis by the presence of infection but not infected themselves. Viral proteins, released from infected cells, effect this sensitization by several parallel routes. The HIV proteins Tat and Nef induce fas, fasL, and TRAIL. Tat alters the cellular redox equilibrium in a manner that may activate Ask-1. Vpr binds to the mitochondrial permeability transition pore. A type of AICD may be induced by stimulation of CD4 and the cytokine receptor CXCR4 (both of which bind HIV epitopes). In infected cells, however, Nef inhibits ASK-1, and so may selectively protect these from apoptosis. Rather similar mechanisms underlie the deletion of neurones in HIV-associated dementia.

Cardiovascular disease

Pathogenetic mechanisms that interface with apoptosis are relatively poorly understood in cardiovascular disease, but there are several observations of potential relevance. Laminar flow inhibits Ask-1 in endothelium, whilst the generation of reactive oxygen species (**ROS**) induces the p38 and JNK stress kinase pathways. Thus, turbulence and the presence of ROS generators such as oxidized low-density lipoproteins—both known risk factors in the genesis of atheroma—are liable to promote apoptosis in endothelium. Other elements of the vascular wall are also abnormal in atheroma. Vascular smooth muscle cells from atheromatous vessels express p53, induce fas, and undergo apoptosis in increased numbers, particularly in the shoulders of the plaque, thus weakening attachment of the fibrous cap and rendering plaque rupture more probable. Macrophages also undergo apoptosis in response to the oxidized lipids that are present in atheromatous plaques. Death of the lipid-filled macrophages (foam cells) produces extracellular depots of oxidized lipid in the plaque core, a key step in plaque progression.

Whilst necrosis is the pattern of the cell death that immediately follows episodes of infarction, there is now substantial evidence that apoptosis occurs in the surrounding tissue over several hours thereafter, probably in response to relative ischaemia and the local generation of ROS. In animal models of stroke, this apoptosis can be downregulated by a variety of manoeuvres, including caspase inhibition, with objective evidence of improved cerebral function. These observations have generated enthusiasm for the development of antiapoptotic drugs for use following stroke and myocardial infarction. Another approach, potentially applicable to ischaemic myocardium, is to promote angiogenesis, perhaps by the use of angiogenic stem cells. Experimental models suggest that this improves the remodelling of the peri-infarct tissue, including decreased apoptosis of myocytes and improved cardiac function.

CNS degeneration

Despite the importance of the subject, there is still much doubt over the role of apoptosis in the chronic degenerative disorders such as Alzheimer's and Parkinson's diseases. Much of the problem stems from the relative inaccessibility of the brain for sequential studies following injury. In both conditions there is clear evidence of a loss of neurones, and those that remain accumulate abnormal cytoplasmic material, such as presenilins 1 and 2, and amyloid protein Aβ in Alzheimer's disease. Cell culture and animal models suggest that the presence of these proteins may induce oxidative stress, which can lower the threshold for apoptosis. The protective effect of BCL-2 and caspase inhibition has also been recorded. The difficulties are compounded by the fact that neurones that undergo severe overstimulation (for example, by local high concentrations of the neurotransmitter glutamate) can also be induced to die (a phenomenon called excitotoxicity), but it is not clear whether the pathways involved overlap with or are identical to those of apoptosis.

Genetic studies of the inherited disorder, spinal muscular atrophy, provided what might have been the most definitive evidence linking the apoptotic pathways to CNS degeneration. A nearly consistent germline mutation has been identified that involves the IAP neuronal apoptosis inhibitory protein, **NAIP**. Unfortunately, another gene of quite different properties is also mutated in a high proportion of cases and it is still not clear which is responsible for the progressive loss of spinal motor neurones in this condition.

Tumour biology

Malignant tumours almost invariably show evidence of genomic instability. This commonly manifests itself as a tendency to undergo repeated episodes of chromosome breakage and recombination, or of mutation at microsatellite sites. The latter is due to defective function in the mismatch repair genes such as *MSH2* or *MLH1*, but there is less certainty over the basic causes of the former. Both can be associated with the loss of a p53-controlled checkpoint, chromosome instability more consistently so than microsatellite instability. Since MSH-2, MLH-1, and p53 are all connected to the activation of apoptosis, it follows that cancer cells inappropriately survive checkpoints normally controlled by these molecules. This gives cancer cells the opportunity to explore the consequences of genomic rearrangements that are denied normal cells. Some of these prove incompatible with continuing life but others lead to selective growth advantage (Fig. 7).

An apoptotic view of carcinogenesis has implications for tumour management. The earlier sections of this chapter have indicated how proapoptotic pathways can cooperate. The activation of p53, for example, increases

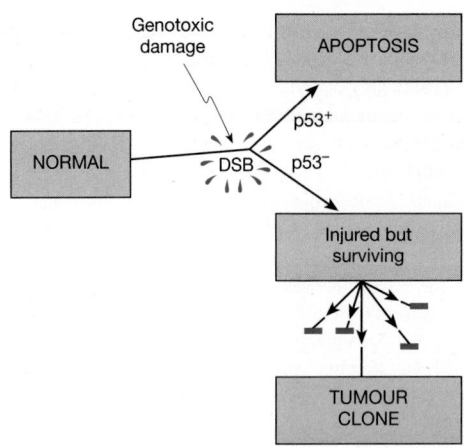

Fig. 7 Failure to activate apoptosis following damage by a genotoxic carcinogen, because of the absence of functional p53, leads to the inappropriate survival of clones of cells bearing double-strand breaks (DSB) and illegitimate recombination events. Whilst some of these clones may fail to proliferate further, others survive to become the founder clones of tumours. Constitutionally, these survivors have unstable genomes, as on further exposure to similar genotoxic stimuli they will again fail to enact apoptosis. Whilst the example given is for cells lacking p53, and hence unable to respond appropriately to DNA DSBs, exactly the same argument applies to cells that fail to identify nucleotide mismatch through defective MSH-2 or MLH-1. Such cells sustain extremely high mutations rates, as mismatches occur (and are normally recognized and repaired) in the course of normal DNA replication, even in the absence of genotoxic carcinogens.

fas expression and this in turn, perhaps through daxx, Ask-1, and p38 kinase, sensitizes cells to the action of many xenobiotics. By contrast, however, cells lacking a critical signal that couples DNA damage to apoptosis (in this case p53) may often survive further damage by these agents. Whatever other changes occur in the course of tumour progression, the entry to malignant behaviour is likely to involve the loss of one critical link to the apoptosis effector pathway rather than loss of the pathway itself. Thus there are few cancer cell lines, and no reported primary tumours, in which, for example, caspase activity is absent, and levels of caspases appear to bear no relationship to tumour chemoresistance. Restoration of the links that couple DNA damage and other cellular stresses to the effector pathways of apoptosis is thus a real objective for cancer drug discovery.

Further reading

Adams JM, Cory S (1998). The Bcl-2 protein family: arbiters of cell survival. *Science* **281**, 1322–5. [These three articles are part of a special issue in *Science* devoted to the biology of apoptosis, and include reference to many of the historic breakthroughs in this rapidly expanding subject.]

Bennett MR, Boyle JJ (1998). Apoptosis of vascular smooth muscle cells in atherosclerosis. *Atherosclerosis* **138**, 3–9. [A review, with new findings and speculation on therapeutic implications, on the role of apoptosis in atherogenesis.]

Cohen O, Kimchi A (2001). DAP-kinase: from functional gene cloning to establishment of its role in apoptosis and cancer. *Cell Death and Differentiation* **8**, 6–15. [A review of the discovery of a new family of death-regulating proteins, by the group leader concerned.]

Evan G, Littlewood T (1998). A matter of life and death. *Science* **281**, 1317–21.

Freire-de-Lima CG, *et al.* (2000). Uptake of apoptotic cells drives the growth of a pathogenic trypanosome in macrophages. *Nature* **404**, 904–6. [This paper shows how *T. cruzi* exploits macrophage handling of apoptotic cells to its own advantage, and how this might be approached therapeutically.]

Green DR, Reed JC (1998). Mitochondria and apoptosis. *Science* **281**, 1309–11.

Hengartner MO (2000). The biochemistry of apoptosis. *Nature* **407**, 770–6. [A racy introduction to some detailed cell biology. This article, together with those marked with an asterisk, form part of a special issue devoted to somewhat visionary reviews of apoptosis.]

Hilbi H, *et al.* (1998). Shigella-induced apoptosis is dependent on caspase-1 which binds to IpaB. *Journal of Biological Chemistry* **273**, 32895–900. [A good source paper on bacterial pathogenicity factors that interact with apoptosis effectors.]

Kang PM, Izumo S (2000). Apoptosis and heart failure. *Circulation Research* **86**, 1107–13. [Helpful literature-rich review of developing area.]

Kocher AA, *et al.* (2001). Neovascularization of ischemic myocardium by human bone-marrow-derived angioblasts prevents cardiomyocyte apoptosis, reduces remodelling and improves cardiac function. *Nature Medicine* **7**, 430–6. [A glimpse of the future in the use of circulating endothelial stem cells to repopulate tissues damaged by ischaemia.]

*Krammer PH (2000). CD95's deadly mission in the immune system. *Nature* **407**, 789–95.

Lin Y, *et al.* (2001). Laminar flow inhibits TNF-induced ASK1 activation by preventing dissociation of ASK1 from its inhibitor 14–3–3. *Journal of Clinical Investigation* **107**, 917–23. [A good introduction to ASK-1, with relevance to endothelial apoptosis.]

Mills JC, Stone NL, Pittman RN (1999). Extranuclear apoptosis: the role of the cytoplasm in the execution phase. *Journal of Cell Biology* **146**, 703–8. [A detailed account of the mechanisms underlying the classical structural changes of apoptosis.]

*Nicholson DW (2000). From bench to clinic with apoptosis-based therapeutic agents. *Nature* **407**, 810–16.

Ojala PM, *et al.* (2000). The apoptotic v-cyclin—CDK6 complex phosphorylates and inactivates Bcl-2. *Nature Cell Biology* **2**, 819–25. [Critical new information on phosphorylation of Bcl-2, in the context of the subtle strategy employed by HHV8 to ensure its own survival.]

*Savill J, Fadok V (2000). Corpse clearance defines the meaning of cell death. *Nature* **407**, 784–8.

Wellington CL, Hayden MR (2000). Caspases and neurodegeneration: on the cutting edge of new therapeutic approaches. *Clinical Genetics* **57**, 1–10. [Good review of potential role of apoptosis in CNS degenerative disease.]

Wyllie AH, Golstein P (2001). More than one way to go. *Proceedings of the National Academy of Sciences, USA* **98**, 11–13. [A brief review of non-caspase death.]

*Yuan J, Yanker BA (2000). Apoptosis in the nervous system. *Nature* **407**, 802–9.

Zhou B-B, *et al.* (1998). Caspase-dependent activation of cyclin-dependent kinases during fas-induced apoptosis in Jurkat cells. *Proceedings of the National Academy of Sciences, USA* **95**, 6785–90. [A classic paper on the controversial but intriguing subject of cell-cycle activation in apoptosis.]

5

Immunological mechanisms

5.1 Principles of immunology

A. J. McMichael

Introduction

There are two features which distinguished immune responses from the non-specific defence mechanisms such as inflammation. The first is the specificity of the reaction, which is easiest to appreciate in terms of antibody responses but it is also true of the cellular immune responses; an essential part of this specificity is the remarkable ability to distinguish between self and non-self. The second is memory by which a second challenge with a stimulus provokes a more rapid and more vigorous immune response. These concepts began to be formulated by Jenner and were developed by Pasteur, Erlich, Landsteiner, Medawar, Burnet, and many others. In the last 30 years, the cellular and molecular basis of these two characteristics has become much clearer.

Immune reactions play important roles in most disease processes. Much of what is observed at the bedside involves immune responses, although the visible, palpable, or audible end-result can be quite distant from the primary event. End-immune reactions can be divided into two: those dependent on antibody (humoral responses) and those on T lymphocytes (cell-mediated immune responses, CMI). Antibody reactions themselves are normally quite silent *in vivo* (e.g. neutralizing virus infectivity), but sometimes antibodies may trigger various secondary events that become literally visible (e.g. anaphylaxis) or revealed on investigation (e.g. haemolysis). Cell-mediated immune responses may also be silent (e.g. clearing of some virus infections by T cells lysing infected cells or releasing interferon) or visible (e.g. delayed hypersensitivity reactions in the skin) or revealed by investigation (e.g. kidney graft rejection).

These two different types of immune response are indicative of the basic division of lymphocytes into two types, B and T cells. They interact with each other and with a third important cell, the antigen presenting cell. The following sections explain how these cells work, as far as possible at a molecular level.

Antigens

Both B and T lymphocytes make the fundamental distinction between self and non-self. This is quite remarkable; for example each species will make antibody to cytochrome c of other species but not self, even though they are closely related proteins differing in very few amino acids. Similarly, T cells respond to all HLA (transplantation) antigens of other members of the species but not self. The mechanisms that underlie this self tolerance are complex and will be explained later. First, the nature of antigens recognized by B and T cells need to be examined, because there are important differences.

Antigens recognized by B cells

B lymphocytes recognize antigen through their surface antibody receptors. In chemical terms, the recognition is identical to that by secreted antibody. The antibody reacts with the native proteins. The availability of large amounts of purified antibodies, particularly monoclonal antibodies

secreted by hybridomas, has facilitated detailed analysis of how protein or carbohydrate macromolecules are recognized. By inhibiting antibody reactivity with polysaccharides with small sugars, Kabat was able to show that an antibody binds to a small part (epitope) of a macromolecule, about the size of seven sugars. For protein antigens, knowledge of their sequence has helped to define their epitopes. A good example is the haemagglutinin (HA) of influenza A virus. The amino acid sequence and three-dimensional structure of this molecule are known. In addition, the amino acid sequence of variant HA molecules that react with different antibodies are known. It is possible, thereby, to locate the parts of the molecule that bind to antibody. Four have been identified in this way, situated on the outside of the globular head of the molecule, each involving less than ten amino acids; because the antibodies bind to a folded molecule these amino acids are not in continuous sequence. Thus for both protein and polysaccharide the epitopes that react with antibodies and B cells are discrete and small.

A protein antigen must be greater than about eight amino acids in size to stimulate an immune response. It is possible, however, to make antibodies to smaller molecules if these are coupled to larger carrier proteins. In this way antibodies can be made to virtually all drugs and other small chemical (hapten) groups. This implies a further, very special feature of the humoral immune response; it can recognize molecules that do not occur in nature or that have not been previously synthesized. This is because of the spatial configuration of many small molecules may be similar in the sense that they fit antigen binding sites of antibodies. Such molecular mimicry has been invoked to explain some autoimmune reactions, for instance the cross-reaction between streptococcal and cardiac antigens in rheumatic carditis.

B cells can react with antigen in its natural form, and special processing is not required. However, the signal delivered to B cells by antigen is on its own insufficient to activate them to proliferate and secrete antibody. Growth and differentiation factors must be provided by helper T lymphocytes. As discussed below, T lymphocytes respond to processed antigen. Certain carbohydrate antigens, however, which have multiple repeating units that can function as epitopes, can stimulate B cells directly to divide and secrete IgM antibody. Some polysaccharide carbohydrate antigens facilitate this by non-specifically activating cells to which they bind (lipopolysaccharide from Gram-negative bacteria for example).

Antigens recognized by T cells

In principle, T cells can recognize as antigen the same range of molecules that are seen by antibodies. However, they are more fastidious about the nature of antigen and its presentation; they do not respond to soluble or free antigen, but to antigen at cell surfaces. On the presenting cells the antigen has to be associated with histocompatibility antigens, HLA (inappropriately standing for human leucocyte antigens) in humans. As foreign antigens are invariably presented *in vivo* with self HLA antigen, the T cells show specificity for self HLA plus foreign antigen. T cells so activated will not recognize the same foreign antigens if presented with foreign HLA *in vitro*. However, foreign HLA antigens provoke very strong immune reactions and these alloreactive T cells do not have to see foreign HLA in association with self HLA. There is therefore something very special about T cell recognition of HLA antigens.

Foreign protein antigens are presented to Th cells (helper T cells that will stimulate B cells to make antibody) by specialized antigen presenting cells. When the parts of the protein molecule that T cells respond to are analysed it is clear that these are often different from those seen by antibody. Using the same example as above, the T cells can recognize parts of the influenza A virus HA that are buried in the molecule. They respond well to short (15–20 amino acid residues) synthetic peptides that represent fragments of the known amino acid sequence. Experiments have indicated that if antigen presenting cells (macrophages) are lightly fixed with paraformaldehyde they will successfully present peptide fragments but not whole protein antigens to helper T cells. All this implies that helper T cells see digested fragments of protein antigens, rather than native proteins, in association with self major histocompatibility complex (MHC) antigens. The role of the antigen presenting macrophage or monocytes is to capture protein, or other antigen, ingest it, and present it in processed form on its surface in association with HLA antigen (Fig. 1). B lymphocytes, by binding antigen to their antibody receptors, can also process antigen and present to Th cells.

The other chief subset of T cells, the cytotoxic T lymphocytes, see foreign antigen at the surface of non-specialized presenting cells, particularly virus antigen at the surface of infected cells. Cytotoxic T cells recognize peptide fragments of virus antigens at the surface of target cells bound to HLA class I molecules. In this form, antigen would not be recognized by antibody specific for the intact protein. This suggests a reason for this apparently complicated process of T-cell recognition. If T cells could react with native antigen free from cell surfaces they would be inactivated because the receptor would be engaged but the secondary signals needed for T cell activation, provided by the antigen presenting cell, would be lacking.

Fig. 2 Gene map of the HLA complex on the short arm of chromosome 6, showing the immunologically important genes. Shown are the HLA class I loci, the related MIC A and B loci, genes relevant to inflammation including the complement components C2, C4, and Bf, the HLA class II loci, and genes relevant to antigen processing. The map is based on that published by Aguado *et al.* 1999.

Histocompatibility antigens

These antigens, HLA in humans, play a central role in T lymphocyte function because, as described above, they associate with foreign antigen to stimulate T cells. HLA antigens are controlled by the major histocompatibility complex (MHC) which is a cluster of genes on the short arm of chromosome 6 (Fig. 2). There are two types of MHC antigen: class I and class II.

Class I antigens are dimers with a 45 000 molecular weight heavy chain, encoded in the major histocompatibility complex (MHC) of genes on the short arm of chromosome six, and an invariant light chain, β_2-microglobulin (β_2m), that is coded on chromosome 15. In 1987, the three-dimensional structure of HLA A2 was determined by Bjorkman, Strominger, Wiley, and colleagues, a finding that has had a profound impact on our understanding of T cell recognition. The heavy chain is divisible into three extracellular domains of about 90 amino acids, of which the membrane-proximal α3 domain resembles an immunoglobulin domain. Together with β_2-microglobulin, which is also immunoglobulin like, these form a stalk on which sits a structure made up by the α-1 and -2 domains. The molecule is folded to form a groove, bounded on its sides by two alpha helices and on its floor by an eight-stranded beta sheet; nearly all of the amino acids that differ between different class I molecules contribute to the fine structure of this groove. The ends of the groove are closed and contain tyrosines and threonines that are conserved in nearly all class I molecules. The crystal structure showed that the groove contains bound peptides, now known to be derived from degraded cytoplasmic proteins. Because different class I molecules (HLA types) have different shaped grooves they bind different peptides. The peptides are usually nine amino acids in length and are bound as extended chains with the amino- and carboxy-termini bound in pockets at either end of the groove. Between two and four of the amino acids that make up the peptides are involved in binding to the HLA molecule with their side chains fitting into other pockets in the groove. These anchoring residues are different in different class I molecules; for instance all peptides that bind to HLA B27 have arginine at position two, those binding to HLA A2 usually have leucine at this position, compared to proline for peptides binding to HLA B35. The class I molecules on a given cell probably bind several hundred peptides, sharing the common anchor residues; these give the cell a 'signature' that is monitored by T cells which are tolerant to normal self peptides. If a foreign peptide, derived from an intracellular parasite or mutated self protein enters the system, T cells can react and destroy the cell. The class I molecules thus serve the function of displaying abnormalities within the cell at its surface.

Most nucleated cells express the classical class I HLA antigens (HLA-A, B, and C) although trophoblast is negative and very low amounts seem to

Fig. 1 Antigen processing: the two pathways are shown, through HLA class I on the left and through HLA class II on the right. For the class I route, cytoplasmic (e.g. virus) proteins are degraded to peptides in the cytosol. The peptides are transported to the lumen of the endoplasmic reticulum. Here, nonamer peptides bind to the newly synthesized class I molecules, stabilizing folding with β_2-microglobulin. The stable complex is translocated to the cell surface where foreign peptides, as well as self peptide, are displayed. For the class II route, foreign protein antigen is ingested by the cell and degraded to peptides in the endosome. The newly synthesized class II molecules fold in the endoplasmic reticulum and the groove is protected by binding to a polypeptide, 'invariant chain'. As the complex formed is transported towards the cell surface the invariant chain is digested away by proteases exposing the groove. HLA class II-containing endosomes fuse with peptide-containing vesicles and peptide binds to the class II HLA groove, stabilizing the structure. The HLA class II molecules reach the cell surface and display foreign peptides. (For further details see Townsend A and Trowsdale J (1993). The transporters associated with antigen presentation. *Seminars in Cell Biology* **4**, 53–61.)

be expressed on hepatocytes, muscle cells, and nerve cells. Some tumours are negative, which may be one way in which they evade T-cell immunity. However, expression on many cell types is increased by the action of γ-interferon released by activated T cells.

HLA class I heavy chains are encoded in the MHC. Products of two loci, HLA A and B, are expressed on cell surfaces in large amounts (10–100 000 molecules per cell); a third series, HLA C, is expressed at much lower levels. There are, in addition, three loci that express non-classical HLA class I molecules. HLA G is expressed almost exclusively on extra villous trophoblast and probably serves to inhibit natural killer cells and macrophages that might attack the foreign trophoblast. HLA E also inhibits natural killer cells; its surface expression is controlled by the availability of a particular peptide derived from the leader sequence of the classical HLA A, B, and C class I proteins, as well as HLA G. HLA E binds to a receptor CD94-NKG2 on natural killer (NK) cells that delivers inhibitory signals. Other receptors on NK cells (killer inhibitory receptors, KIR) detect the presence on classical HLA class I molecules, particularly HLA C, on the potential target cell but deliver an inhibitory signal that protects the target from lysis. Cells that fail to express HLA, such as certain tumour cells selected to evade T cell attack, are lysed by NK cells. Thus the HLA class I molecules are intimately involved in the maintenance of cell survival.

The HLA A, B, and C antigens are highly polymorphic with multiple alleles at each locus (Table 1). As their structure implies, class I antigens present peptide fragments of foreign antigens, usually virus, on the surface of normal cells to cytotoxic T lymphocytes (CTL). The polymorphism of HLA A, B, and C means that, when tested in vitro, cytotoxic T cells (primed to virus in vivo) will only recognize virus antigen on self cells or HLA matched cells (HLA restriction). It is likely that the extreme degree of HLA polymorphism results from evolutionary selection of multiple HLA alleles by pathogens. Individual HLA molecules show varying efficiency in presenting particular antigens to CTL, thus affecting the quality of the immune response to various intracellular pathogens.

HLA class II proteins have two chains, α and β. Each is around 30 000 daltons molecular weight and is composed of two extracellular domains (Fig. 2). At least four different members of the family are expressed on cells and most are polymorphic. The best studied series are the DR antigens, which have a highly polymorphic β-chain (encoded by the DRB1 locus) giving rise to over 20 DR types (Table 1). There is a second, less polymorphic DR-β chain that gives the specificities DR 51, 52, and 53, encoded by the DRB3, DRB4, and DRB5 loci respectively. The DQ molecules are polymorphic in both α and β chains, which means that hybrid molecules can occur in heterozygotes. The DP molecules are polymorphic in the β-chain and are expressed in smaller amounts. The HLA class II molecules are expressed on a limited set of cells that includes B lymphocytes, monocytes, dendritic cells, activated T cells, and some endothelial and epithelial cells. They can be induced on many more cell types by interferon-γ.

The crystal structure of HLA DR1 is remarkably similar to HLA class I. The main difference is that the groove is open-ended allowing the bound peptides to hang out; thus the peptides are longer, 12 to 16 amino acids. Like the peptides that bind class I, there are anchor residues, determined by the fine structure of the groove. There is a particularly prominent pocket in the floor at the left hand end of the groove which binds large aromatic side chains in some instances.

The function of the class II antigens is to present foreign processed antigen to helper T cells. As discussed above, this process is mediated by specialized antigen presenting cells, although the wider expression of class II antigens induced by interferon suggests that other cells may be able to process and present under certain circumstances. A particularly important antigen-presenting cell type is the dendritic cell; this expresses large amounts of HLA class II as well as important costimulatory molecules. Dendritic cells appear to be particularly good at processing antigen for both the class I and class II pathways.

Human individuals differ in the epitopes of an antigen that they recognize, according to their HLA class II type. The effects of this could be mani-

fest, for instance, in the degree of cross-reactivity between related viruses that stimulate antibody responses. Similarly, HLA class II type could determine whether antigens that differ from self in only a few epitopes are recognized. Self antigens that are slightly altered could fall into this category and it is striking that several organ-specific, autoimmune diseases are associated with HLA DR3. However, the exact reasons for this and other HLA and disease associations (Table 2) remain unresolved. It should be noted that the disease associations imply either a direct role for the HLA molecule or that there is a nearby disease-susceptibility gene in linkage disequilibrium with the HLA marker. In the case of HLA-DR3, there is strong linkage disequilibrium with HLA B8 and everything in between, including a complement C4 null allele and at least 50 other genes, most of which are non-polymorphic and many of unknown function.

The action of HLA class II antigens in presenting antigens to helper T cells gives them a key role in initiating immune responses. In contrast, class I antigens are involved at a later and more specialized stage. This is important in transplantation, where matching class II antigens is more important than matching class I, although the final damaging activity of cytotoxic T cells and antibody is directed at class I antigens.

Antigen processing

There are two pathways of antigen processing, generating the peptides that bind to HLA class I and II molecules, recognized by cytotoxic T lymphocytes (CTL) (which carry the CD8 surface marker) and Th (CD4 positive) respectively.

As indicated above, class I HLA molecules present short peptides derived from cytoplasmic proteins. The most likely pathway by which this happens is given in Fig. 1. Proteins in the cell are naturally turning over, broken down by cytoplasmic proteases. The multicatalytic proteasome complex is a major contributor to this process. It degrades cytoplasmic proteins that have been coupled to ubiquitin and digests them to small fragments. It is made up of 28 components; two of these are encoded in the MHC in the class II region, are interferon-γ inducible and they may affect the protease specificity. The peptides generated are transported by an ATP-dependent transporter (TAP, transporters associated with antigen processing), made up of two chains encoded in the class II region of the MHC, into the endoplasmic reticulum. Here the peptides are degraded further unless they bind to newly synthesized class I HLA molecules. The latter take the peptide to the cell surface bound in the groove. Expression of most class I molecules at the cell surface is dependent on the integrity of this pathway. Patients described recently who have a deficiency in the TAP, display very low levels of HLA class I molecules on their cell surfaces; interestingly, they suffer from recurrent bacterial infections and a severe granulomatous vasculitis with highly activated NK cells.

Processing of antigens to be presented by class II HLA takes place in specialized antigen-presenting cells, particularly monocytes, dendritic cells, and B lymphocytes. Protein antigens are taken into the cell from outside. Monocytes may take up antigen passively by endocytosis or by receptor-mediated uptake, acquiring proteins bound through complement or Fc receptors. The latter bind to the constant regions of antibodies and so mediate uptake of proteins bound to cells as immune complexes—antigen may bind to small amounts of 'natural antibody' or the early specific antibody (giving an early positive feedback). Also B lymphocytes with specific antibody receptors can bind foreign proteins directly, endocytose, and process antigen to present peptides bound to class II molecules. Digestion of proteins takes place in an endosome compartment; these fuse with class II HLA-carrying vesicles bringing class II molecules from the endoplasmic reticulum. The newly synthesized class II molecules do not bind peptides in the ER; instead they bind to a third chain the 'invariant chain'. This protects the groove from peptide binding and the complex is exported through the Golgi complex where glycosylation is completed and addition of sialic acid residues to both the class II molecules and the invariant chain takes place. In a late endosomal compartment, at low pH, the invariant chain is degraded and removed from the class II molecules. This process involves another HLA class II molecule, HLA DM that somehow facilitates the exchange of invariant peptide for foreign peptide. Binding of peptide stabilizes the class II structure and the class II molecule containing the peptide

Table 1 HLA antigens

A	B	C	DR (B1)	DR (Bx)	DQ	DP
A1	B5	Cw1	DR1	DR51	DQ1	DPw1
A2	B7	Cw2	DR103	DR52	DQ2	DPw2
A203	B703	Cw3	DR2	DR53	DQ3	DPw3
A210	B8	Cw4	DR3		DQ4	DPw4
A3	B12	Cw5	DR4		DQ5(1)	DPw5
A9	B13	Cw6	DR5		DQ6(1)	DPw6
A10	B14	Cw7	DR6		DQ7(3)	
A11	B15	Cw8	DR7		DQ8(3)	
A23(9)	B16	Cw9(w3)	DR8		DQ9(3)	
A24(9)	B17	Cw10(w3)	DR9			
A2403	B18		DR10			
A25(10)	B21		DR11(5)			
A26(10)	B22		DR12(5)			
A28	B27		DR13(6)			
A29(19)	B35		DR14(6)			
A30(19)	B37		DR1403			
A31(19)	B38(16)		DR1404			
A32(19)	B39(16)		DR15(2)			
A33(19)	B3901		DR16(2)			
A34(10)	B3902		DR17(3)			
A36	B40		DR18(3)			
A43	B4005					
A66(10)	B41					
A68(28)	B42					
A69(28)	B44(12)					
A74(19)	B45(12)					
	B46					
	B47					
	B48					
	B49(21)					
	B50(21)					
	B51(5)					
	B5102					
	B5203					
	B52(5)					
	B53					
	B54(22)					
	B55(22)					
	B56(22)					
	B57(17)					
	B58(17)					
	B59					
	B60(40)					
	B61(40)					
	B62(15)					
	B63(15)					
	B64(14)					
	B65(14)					
	B67					
	B70					
	B71(70)					
	B72(70)					
	B73					
	B75(15)					
	B76(15)					
	B77(15)					

This table shows the full listing of HLA serological specificities, grouped according to the locus for each allelic series. Some of the original types have been split into related types, shown with the original specificity in parentheses. (This is necessary because some of the older names persist in the literature (e.g. DR2, which is now DR15 or DR16)). The DR antigens are shown for specificities at the *BRB1* locus and the second locus *DRBx* (*x* = 3, 4, or 5 according to the haplotype).
(Data from Sasazuki T *et al.*, eds (1993). *HLA typing*. Oxford University Press.)

Table 2 HLA and disease associations: relative risks

Locus	Antigen	Disease	Percentage antigen frequency		Relative risk[a]
			Normal	Patients	
A	A3	Haemochromatosis	28	76	8
B	B5	Behçet's syndrome	10	41	6
	B27	Ankylosing spondylitis	9	90	87
		Reiter's syndrome	9	79	37
	B35	Subacute thyroiditis	15	70	14
C	Cw6	Psoriasis	33	87	13
D	DR2	Narcolepsy	26	100	>50
		Goodpasture's syndrome	26	88	16
		Multiple sclerosis	26	59	4
	DR3	Dermatitis herpetiformis	26	85	15
		Coeliac disease	26	79	11
		Sjögren's (sicca) syndrome	26	78	10
		Addison's disease	26	69	6
		Graves' disease	26	56	4
		Myasthenia gravis	26	50	2
		SLE	26	70	6
		Membranous nephropathy	26	75	12
		IDDM	26	56	3
	DR3 and/or 4	IDDM	57	99	8
	DR4	IDDM	20	75	6
		Rheumatoid arthritis	20	50	4
	DR5	Pernicious anaemia	6	25	5

Abbreviations: IDDM, insulin-dependent diabetes mellitus; SLE, systemic lupus erythematosus; RR, relative risk.

[a] Relative risk is the factor of increased risk of developing the disease by individuals with the HLA antigen. Data compiled from Svejgaard A, Platz P, Ryder LP (1983). *Immunology Review* **70**, 192.

reaches the surface. As for class I HLA, several peptides derived from normal proteins are displayed and elicit no T cell response because of tolerance. Foreign peptides that stimulate T cells with appropriate receptors initiate Th responses.

Priming the immune response

It is becoming clear that antigen presentation by class I or class II HLA on its own is insufficient to initiate a T-cell immune response. Specialized cells play a role, particularly B lymphocytes, dendritic cells, and others of the monocyte series. In addition to presenting peptides on their MHC molecules, they display other accessory molecules on their surface important for cell–cell interactions. In addition to the adhesion molecules, such as LFA-1 and CD2 that are also necessary for T cell recognition of target cells, the B7 molecule (CD80 and not to be confused with HLA B7) seems especially important. This binds to the T-cell marker CD28 and delivers a signal to naive T cells initiating the T-cell response. Once activated in this way these T cells can interact with antigen-presenting cells, such as virus-infected epithelial cells, and react; from here on, CD28 may be less crucial though it can inhibit activation-induced cell death and so ensure the responding T cell remains alive. The importance of the CD28–CD80 pathway is that there can be cells in the body that display antigenic peptides but because they lack CD80 do not initiate an immune response and suffer immune attack. However, a virus infection could sometime initiate a cross-reacting T-cell response and trigger an autoimmune response.

Antibodies

Structure

The basic structure of an antibody molecule is illustrated in Fig. 3. An IgG molecule consists of four chains, two identical heavy chains (50 000 daltons) and two identical light chains (25 000 daltons). The immunoglobulin molecule can be broken into segments by enzymes, giving the peptides

illustrated in Fig. 3. Sequence analysis of light and heavy chains and crystallographic studies have revealed that they are composed of domains of about 100 amino acids, held by a disulphide loop between two cysteines (a domain structure that has been found to be present in many other cell surface molecules). There are two for each light chain (L) and four for an IgGγ heavy chain (H). The N terminal domains of both L and H chains are highly variable when different antibody molecules are compared; they contain the antigen binding site. The constant domains of the heavy chain define the isotype of the antibody, IgG, A, D, M, or E, each of which has particular functions. The main differences between the various heavy chain

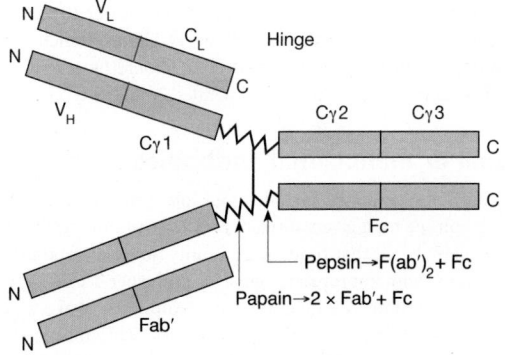

Fig. 3 Basic structure of an immunoglobulin, IgG, molecule. Two identical light (L) and two identical heavy (H) chains are shown. At the amino terminal (N) there is a variable (V) domain of 110 amino acids. In the light chain (L) this is connected to one constant domain of 100 amino acids which is one of the two types: λ or _. The heavy-chain variable domain links to three constant-region domains, Cl1, Cl2, and Cl3. Between Cl1 and Cl2 is the hinge region, which gives the binding site (VL+VH) flexibility and contains interchain disulphide (—S—S—) bridges (see Table 3.)

Table 3 Human immunoglobulins

Isotype	Chain structure[a]	Number of H domains	M_r (kDa)	Serum concentration (mg/ml)	t[b]	Clq[c]	Placenta[d]	Mast cells[e]
IgG1		4	146	9	21	+	+	±
IgG2		4	146	3	20	+	+	−
IgG3		4	165	1	7	+	+	±
IgG4		4	146	0.5	21	−	+	±
IgM		5	970	1.2	5	+	−	−
IgA1		4	160	2	6	−	−	−
IgA2		4	160	0.5	−	−	−	−
sIgA		4	405	0.5	−	−	−	−
IgD		4	170	0.06	3	−	−	−
IgE		5	190	0.0002	3	−	−	+

[a] To show light and heavy chains with disulphide bridges. (Derived from Nisonoff A. *Introduction to Molecular Immunology.* Sinauer, Massachusetts, USA.)

[b] Half-life in days.

[c] Binding of complement component Clq.

[d] Ability to cross the placenta.

[e] Ability to bind to and activate mast cells.

constant regions are described in Table 3. The isotypes determine essential properties of the antibodies, particularly binding of Clq of the complement system, binding of Fc receptors that enable antibody to cross the placenta, and binding of Fc receptors on macrophages, mast cells, and basophils. IgA binds to a specific Fc receptor, known as a secretory component, which is on epithelial membranes. The antibody can then be endocytosed and transported across these cells and released on the outside, that is the gut lumen, biliary tract, respiratory tract, or milk duct. Light chain constant regions are one of two classes, κ or λ, but there are no known differences in function between the two.

The N-terminal domains of L and H chains are variable regions. They vary between different antibodies to a remarkable degree. Sequence comparison of several variable regions has shown that there are three short, hypervariable patches between amino acids 28–34, 45–56, and 91–97 in both light and heavy chains. The crystalline structure of antibody indicates that these hypervariable regions form a surface to which antigen binds. In agreement with the studies on antigen epitopes, this is about the right area to bind to six amino acids on the surface of the antigen. Sequence analysis has also revealed that there are hundreds of genes for variable regions, explaining some of the enormous variability. Estimates, by various methods, agree that an individual must be capable of generating over several million different antibody molecules, probably nearer 10^8. As the variability is controlled by both the L and the H chains, which appear to associate independently, this means that there should be several hundred VL and VH sequences. How these are generated is discussed below.

Polyclonal or monoclonal antibodies

A normal antibody response includes multiple antibody molecules that bind to each epitope on a given antigen. B-cell activation requires binding of antigen, so any B cell that binds with affinity above a certain threshold stimulates B cells (with appropriate signals from helper T cells) and ultimately antibody secretion. A single antigen epitope can evoke a response comprising several hundred antibody molecules. This means that each antibody must be capable of binding more than one antigen, which is not surprising considering that antibodies recognize surfaces rather than sequences. An antiserum made up of hundreds or thousands of antibodies maintains its specificity because the immunogen is the common denominator. As each antibody molecule is the product of a single clone of B lymphocytes, and many are involved, this type of response is known as polyclonal (Fig. 4).

Under certain circumstances a monoclonal antibody response is generated. This may happen when the stimulating antigen is limited in its pre-

senting epitopes or when it is present in extremely low amounts, thus selecting out only cells with the receptor with the highest binding avidity. Oligoclonal responses are also found in the cerebrospinal fluid in multiple sclerosis, possibly as a consequence of limiting the immune response to the few clones of cells that manage to cross the blood–brain barrier. More commonly, a monoclonal antibody *in vivo* is the product of abnormal proliferation of a single clone of B cells or plasma cells.

Kohler and Milstein, in 1975, devised a way of fusing normal (mouse) B lymphocytes to cultured plasmacytoma cells to generate immortal hybrid cell lines (hybridomas) that secrete the antibody of the B-cell parent. Because the donor of the spleen cells can be immunized at will, these monoclonal antibodies can be generated to any antigen. They have been used to explore the structure of human cells, particularly their surfaces, because unlike polyclonal antibodies made in another species, each monoclonal antibody reacts with a single component of the immunogen. They also have a multitude of practical applications in the study of growth factors, cell surface receptors, micro-organisms, and many other antigens.

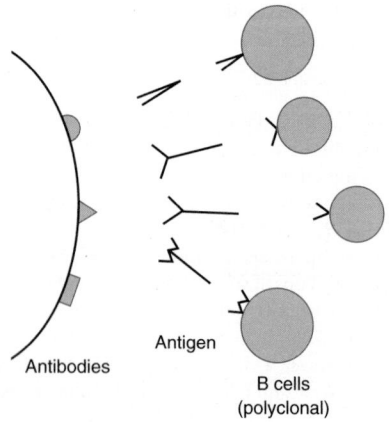

Fig. 4 Polyclonal antibodies. An antigen such as a protein has many antigenic sites (epitopes) on the surface of the molecule. To each can bind a set of antibodies with a range of affinity depending on the amino acid sequence of their variable regions. These are indicated diagrammatically by the shape of the binding site that binds to epitope. Each species of antibody is the product of one clone of B lymphocytes that can only make antibody with that shape, that is V-region sequence.

They have become routine tools for many diagnostic assays and are increasingly therapeutic applications are being developed, for instance the use of antitumour necrosis factor-α (anti-TNF-α) in the treatment of rheumatoid arthritis or the use of antibodies to respiratory syncitial virus to treat severe bronchiolitis in infants. For these clinical applications, it is possible to transplant the antigen binding sites of mouse antibodies into human immunoglobulins, retaining the antigen specificity. Antibodies that are 'humanized' in this way are less likely to provoke an immune response in recipients of the treatment.

Genetics of antibody production

The development of methods of DNA cloning, the use of the polymerase chain reaction, and sequencing have had a big impact on our understanding of immunoglobulin genes. The genes are arranged as shown in Fig. 5 on three chromosomes: 14 for heavy chain, 22 for _, and two for λ. The antibody genes are arranged in exons, each coding for a single immunoglobulin domain, variable and constant region, with further exons for the hinge and transmembrane regions. The constant region exons are grouped according to antibody class. There are additional exons for the leader sequences which take the newly synthesized antibody chains across the membrane (and is then cleaved off). The transmembrane exon is only expressed on antibody that is attached to cell surfaces.

The variable (V) genes are on the 5' side of the constant genes. (i.e. upstream, as DNA is read from 5' to 3'). There are many of these and it appears that any variable gene can combine with a constant gene on the same region of the chromosome. The antibody genes are therefore unusual and complex in their arrangement. Besides the multitude of variable genes there are also D (diversity) (for heavy chains but not light chains) and J (joining) genes which are short coding sequences (exons) found between V and C. The arrangement of the genes in B lymphocytes and plasma cells is different from that in all other cells. Early in B-cell development, a single heavy chain variable gene joins to a D and J gene to make a VDJ rearrangement. Similarly, in one light chain gene region a VJ rearrangement is made. Coupling of VDJ or VJ to the C gene occurs after transcription to nuclear RNA which is then processed to make messenger RNA, where, for both heavy and light chain transcripts, J is connected to C, and this is translated.

The D segment, which is one to three amino acids long, is in the third hypervariable and the very many combinations of VD and J that are possible contribute substantially to antibody diversity. In addition to this, breaks in this region may occur in early B cells and be repaired in a random fashion by an enzyme called terminal deoxynuceotide transferase, which again adds further diversity.

Further variation in both heavy and light chain variable regions occurs by somatic mutation as B lymphocytes proliferate in large numbers in the germinal centres of lymphoid organs. This involves selection by antigen and a mechanism that locates the mutations in particular sites in the antigen binding site. As the concentration of antigen declines, only high avidity B cell clones will be stimulated to divide and this exerts selective pressure on mutations in the hypervariable regions. It is now known that developing B lymphocytes divide rapidly in the germinal centres and that a large proportion die by apoptosis (programmed cell death), a process not unlike that occurring in the thymus as T cells develop.

The process of gene rearrangement described above occurs on only one of the chromosomes encoding the heavy chain, and a similar process occurs on one of the four chromosomes encoding a light chain (allelic exclusion). A B cell is therefore committed to making one antibody, one heavy chain VDJC and one VJC by the time it is immunocompetent. It is not clear why this only happens on one chromosome for each chain. It is possible that it is such a complex process that the chances of a single cell making two rearrangements successfully is extremely remote. Alternatively, there may be some suppressive signal generated once a successful VDJ arrangement has occurred. This property provides a useful way of determining whether proliferating or infiltrating lymphocytes (for example in a tissue section) are polyclonal or monoclonal. The latter will all express either a κ or λ chain; the former will include both light-chain types in roughly equal numbers.

The heavy chain VDJ sequence is attached to the C genes in an orderly progression during B cell development. The gene order is Cμ, Cδ, Cγ3, Cα1, Cγ1, Cγ2, Cγ4, Cε, and Cα2. All the B cells appear to go through a Cμ, stage, most go through Cδ and Cγ, but may end up at one of the γ subtypes, or α or ε, probably jumping segments in the process. This progression involves deletion of DNA coding the no-longer-used C genes as the B cell develops. It is therefore a one-way process. Switching of B cells from production of IgM to IgG is a striking and normal feature of a simple antibody response. The process is, in part, regulated by external factors, particularly the cytokines IL4 and IL5. IL4 drive switching to IgE and IL4-secreting T cells (Th2 cells) probably play a key role in the development of allergic responses. It is also of practical importance that fetal and cord B lymphocytes do not switch from IgM to IgG production.

The T-cell receptor

Although the T-cell receptor was elusive for many years it is now well understood and some crystal structures have been determined. Early studies with monoclonal antibodies revealed a two-chain glycoprotein of 85 000 molecular weight, reducing to two components of 40 000 and 45 000 daltons. When its DNA was cloned it was found to rearrange in ways very similar to that described above for B-cell immunoglobulin receptors. Unexpectedly, two families of T cell receptors were found, the α–β receptor present of all conventional T cells and the γ–δ receptor present on a subset of T cells whose function is still less clear.

Both chains of αβ T-cell receptors have been sequenced from multiple T-cell clones of known antigen specificity. Both chains are similar to immunoglobulin light chains with two external domains, each of about 100 amino acids. The N terminal domains of both α and β chains are variable. They include V and J segments, with a D segment for the β chain. Several families of Vβ, Jβ, Vα, and Jα have been identified. The genes for these rearrange as T cells develop, whilst the cells are in the thymus. There are two constant region classes for the β chain, Cβ1 and Cβ2, which are very similar in structure. The number of possible T-cell receptors has been estimated to be a staggering 10^{14}, generated by the multiple combinations of

Fig. 5 Arrangement of the immunoglobulin genes. These are arranged on three chromosomes, chromosome 2 for *L*κ, 22 for *L* λ, and 14 for the heavy chain. The basic arrangement of the human genes are shown. *L*κ is arranged with a large number (*n*) of V genes, each preceded for a gene for the leader sequence *L*. Downstream are five *J* genes and further on the one *C* gene. *L*λ is arranged in an unknown number (*n*) of sets, with a group of X (*?x > 20*) *L–V* pairs followed by one *J* and *C*. There may be six to nine such sets. *H* is arranged with a large number (>100) of *L–V* pairs followed by a set of *D* minigenes and a set of *J* genes. Downstream are the constant-region *C* genes, each split into separate exons for each domain, and an optional membrane segment, which are placed in the order shown.

the gene segments on the two chains. A substantial part of this diversity comes from the activity of the terminal deoxynucleotide transferase creating much variability at the V–(D)–J junction.

The crystal structure of the T-cell receptor shows that the three hypervariable regions (complementarity determining regions, CDR) form the MHC–peptide antigen binding site. This structure places the CDR-3 region, made up by the most hypervariable part of the T-cell receptor where the V–(D)–J join occurs, in a critical site to interact with the peptide part of the complex. The rules for this engagement are now being worked out. The T-cell receptor lies diagonally across the peptide binding groove of a class I MHC molecule and more at a right angle to the peptide in a class II MHC molecule. These orientations put the most variable parts of the receptor over the peptide and more conserved, but still variable, parts of the receptor over the MHC molecule.

Why do the T cells not simply use the antibodies as their receptor? The advantage of using MHC molecules as the antigen presenter is that it means that T cells do not see native antigen and thus cannot be inactivated by, for instance, free virus. In addition, by responding only to cell surface antigens the response can be controlled by signals derived from the presenting cell. Thus T cells that react with self-antigens in the thymus may be eliminated while those that react with foreign antigens in the periphery are stimulated.

The function of the T cells that carry the γ∂ T-cell receptor remains enigmatic. In mice they are abundant in the intestinal mucosa. In humans they have been found at sites of chronic inflammation, particularly mycobacterial infections. Some bind to non-classical MHC molecules including CD1 and MIC-1, but why is less clear. Some are probably important in antibacterial immunity. One particular subset of T cells that carry some natural killer cell markers express a particular receptor and interact with CD1d; these T cells are thought to play a role in regulating Th1 and Th2 responses (see below).

Lymphocytes

Lymphocytes mediate immune reactions and can be divided into two groups: B and T cells.

B lymphocytes

B lymphocytes are the precursors of antibody-secreting plasma cells. They express immunoglobulin on their surface, which acts as antigen receptor. The B cell expresses only one pair of immunoglobulin VH and VL gene products and thus antigen receptors of only one molecular type and sequence. The progeny, or clone, of this cell retains the same commitment

and the antibody secreted uses the same variable genes. Thus, antigen on first immune challenge selects B cells that already express appropriate receptors. These divide and some mature to antibody-producing cells while others develop into memory cells. The latter greatly exceed the original population in number and as they can in turn be activated by antigen to generate antibody-producing cells this provides a basis for the memory phenomenon. Immature B cells express IgM or IgM plus IgD antibody as their receptor. As the B cells differentiate they switch their heavy chain VDJ gene product to associate with a γ, α, or ε chain and thus switch secretion from IgM to IgA or IgE. Memory cells have γ, α, or ε receptors and secrete this class without an intermediate phase.

A number of B-cell differentiation antigens have been found using murine monoclonal antibodies raised against human lymphocytes. The best characterized of them are shown in Table 4. As has been the case with the T cell antigens described below, it is gradually emerging that these have important functions. Thus, antibodies to CD20 trigger B cells to divide, CD22 is involved in B-cell signalling, CD19 is part of the B cell antibody receptor complex, CD21 is the complement C3b receptor and is also the receptor for Epstein–Barr virus (EBV) which readily transforms B lymphocytes in vitro and probably in vivo. Another molecule that is crucial in B cell signalling is CD40; its ligand, CD40L, is expressed on T lymphocytes. In the hyper-IgM syndrome, where there is a failure of B cells to switch from IgM to IgG production, DC4L is mutated, implying a role for CD40 in immunoglobulin isotype switching. CD40 is also expressed on dendritic cells and is important for receiving signals from CD40-ligand bearing T-helper cells to make them efficient at stimulating primary CD8+ T-cell responses by releasing the Th1-inducing cytokine IL-12.

Activation of B lymphocytes requires antigen and a signal from helper T (Th) lymphocytes which are themselves responding to the same antigen. The T cells, of the Th2 subset (see below) release cytokines including IL-4 and IL-5 as well as initiating signals through CD40; these activate B lymphocytes in the presence of antigen to divide and differentiate. Note that two kinds of signal are needed, an antigen specific trigger through the antigen receptor and a second type mediated in a non-antigen specific fashion. Inappropriate signalling, such as an antigen signal in the absence of the second type, can lead to inactivation of the B cells.

Besides secreting antibody, B cells have a role in antigen presentation that is increasingly recognized as important. B cells can bind foreign antigen directly through their immunoglobulin receptor or as an immune complex through the Fc or complement (immune complexes bind complement—see Chapter 5.4) receptors. Such antigen can be internalized and digested in endosomes to generate peptides that bind to class II MHC. In this way, small amounts of circulating antibody can enhance primary

Table 4 Differentiation antigens on B cells

Antigen	Synonym	M_r (kDa)	Distribution	Function
Surface Ig		150	All B cells	Antigen receptor
CD9	BA2	24	Pre-B → Virgin B	
CD10	CALLA	100	Pre-B	
CD19	B4	95	Pre-B → P-blasts	Signalling
CD20	B1	35	Pre-B → P-blasts	Signalling
CD21		140	B subset	C3d and EBV receptor
CD22		135	All B cells	Adhesion, ligand CD45RO,CD75
CD23	B2	45	B subset	IgE receptor, signalling
CD24		45–55–65	All B cells	Signalling
CD37		40–52	Mature B cells	
CD40		50	Mature B cells	Ig-class switching
CD72		40	B cells	Activation, ligand CD5
CD80	B7,BB1	60	B subset, act-B	Priming T cells Ligand CD28

Abbreviations: act-B, activated B cells; EBV, Epstein–Barr virus; P-blasts, plasmablasts. Further concise details of leucocyte differentiation antigens can be found in Barclay et al. (1993).

T-cell responses by facilitating processing of antigen and, in the early immune response, can act as a positive feedback.

B cells have a complex life-cycle that includes a selection process in the germinal centres of lymphoid organs. Here, many cells die by apoptosis and there is selection by antigen in an environment that favours somatic mutation. The ontogeny of B lymphocytes is of some clinical relevance because various leukaemia and lymphomas express surface antigens characteristic of B cells at various stages of development. Figure 6 gives the scheme for B-cell differentiation indicating the corresponding leukaemias and lymphomas. Studies on the immunoglobulin light chains expressed indicate that these malignancies are monoclonal diseases.

Burkitt's lymphoma is a B-cell malignancy which is caused by Epstein–Barr virus (EBV). In addition to the presence of EBV DNA and protein in the malignant cells, there are some chromosomal rearrangements. The c-*myc* oncogene on chromosome 8 is translocated to chromosome 2, 14, or 22. There, it comes into close proximity with one of the three sets of immunoglobulin genes. It is likely that the tissue-specific enhancer that is present between the J and C exons activates the oncogene.

T lymphocytes

T lymphocytes require the thymus for their development and show a set of characteristic surface glycoproteins and their own form of receptor, as described above. They can be divided into types: cytotoxic T lymphocytes (CTL) that carry the CD8 marker and helper T cells that carry CD4. The latter can be divided according to the cytokines they release on antigen contact into Th1 (IL-2, IL-15, and interferon-γ) and Th2 (IL-4, IL-5, IL-10, and IL-13). There are also intermediate T cells, Th0 cells, and some claim for more immunosuppressive T cells in the gut which secrete transforming growth factor (TGF-β). T cells may also be divided into those in an inactive state (virgin T cells) and preactive state (memory T cells) by the CD45 isotype on the cell surface. The short version of the molecule CD45RO marks cells that have recently seen antigen; however, fully differentiated CD8+ T cells can revert to CD45RA expression. Another marker that characterizes a subset of memory T cells is the chemokine receptor CCR7. This is involved in the trafficking of T cells to lymph nodes and is present on the surface of long-term memory T cells but is lost as these are stimulated to become effector T cells, functional outside the lymphoid organs.

T-cell differentiation antigens

Hybridoma-generated monoclonal antibodies have been used to explore the surface of T lymphocytes and these have revealed a series of molecules that play essential, accessory roles in antigen recognition by T cells (Table 5). Monoclonal antibodies to these structures are now often used to define T-cell subpopulations or leukaemias and are being used therapeutically. Their expression on T cells as they develop is described in Fig. 7.

The T-cell receptor and CD3

The CD3 antigen is present on T-cell surfaces in association with the T-cell receptor. Antibodies to one will precipitate the other from detergent-solubilized cell membranes. The antigen is made up of three chains, which are closely associated with the T-cell receptor and form a complex on the inside of the T cell. When T-cell receptor binds antigen the receptors cluster on the cell surface in lipid rafts, bringing the coreceptors CD4 or CD8 (see below) with them. This activates a cascade of kinases within the cell, involving kinases such as Lck and Zap 70. Through a complex series of interactions between enzymes and a parallel flux of calcium into the cytosol, several genes are activated including IL-2 and interferon-γ. This causes a cytokine response within 6 h in memory T cells. Virgin T cells undergoing a primary T-cell response require additional activation through the cell surface glycoprotein CD28. This is activated by binding to its ligand CD80, which is expressed on dendritic cells, specialist antigen presenters. CD28 also sets up a kinase cascade important for T-cell activation and survival.

CD4

Recognition of processed antigen on antigen-presenting cells by helper T cells involves a specific binding interaction between CD4 and HLA class II molecules. Helper T cells carry the CD4 antigen. CD4 is also expressed at low levels on macrophages and some dendritic cells. The surface glycoprotein gp120 of human immunodeficiency virus (HIV) binds to CD4, giving the virus specificity for the cells that carry CD4, helper T cells, dendritic cells, and macrophages. The virus needs a second receptor to enter cells, either the chemokine receptor CCR5 or the chemokine receptor CXCR4. After high affinity binding to CD4, the gp120 undergoes a conformational change to expose the chemokine receptor binding site and then virus entry occurs. The cells targeted, with devastating consequences, by HIV are defined by the presence of these receptors, particularly CD4 which is restricted in its distribution to vital cells of the immune response.

CD8

This antigen is a glycoprotein of molecular weight 33 000. It is heavily glycosylated on a long stalk that holds an immunoglobulin domain away from the T-cell membrane. CD8 binds to the α-3 domain of HLA class I molecules and through its cytoplasmic domain recruits the tyrosine kinase Lck. It is the counterpart of CD4. In T-cell development in the thymus, immature T cells express both CD4 and CD8; if their receptor interacts strongly with self HLA antigens those T cells are deleted, if they react less strongly, but receive enhancing signals though CD4 or CD8, they are positively selected. In this process they lose expression of the inappropriate accessory molecule, CD4 or CD8, and become either CD4+ or CD8+ mature T cells.

Other important molecules on the surface of T lymphocytes are the chemokine receptors CCR5, CXCR4, and CCR7 which help to determine the trafficking of the T cells. The adhesion molecule LFA-1 (CD11a–CD18) is a two chain glycoprotein important for T and B cells to stick to endothelium and target cells. CD2 and CD44 have similar functions for different ligands. CD45 is an abundant glycoprotein that has several different isoforms and is expressed differently on lymphocytes at particular stages of differentiation; its cytoplasmic tail is a phosphatase that appears to control the state of activation of kinases such as Lck involved in T-cell activation.

Fig. 6 Expression of B-lymphocyte differentiation antigens on the surface of differentiating B cells. The circles represent developing B cells. The CD antigens are listed in Table 4

Table 5 T-lymphocyte differentiation antigens

Antigen	Synonym	M_r (kDa)	Distribution	Function
CD1	T6	47+12	Cortical thymocytes Langerhans cells	?Antigen presentation
CD2	T11, E-rec	50	T cells	Activation, adhesion Ligand LFA-3(CD58)
CD3/Ti	T3/TCR	26,21 19,30	T cells	Antigen receptor plus signalling (CD3)
CD4	T4	55	Th cells	Binds HLA class II HIV receptor
CD5	T1, Leu-1	60	T cells, B subset	Activation, ligand CD72
CD6	T12	120	T cells	Signalling
CD7		40	Pre-T and T cells	
CD8	T8, Lyt-2	33	CTL	Binds HLA class I
CD11a/18	LFA-1	180–95	All leucocytes	Adhesion, essential for T cell and leucocyte functions Ligands: ICAM-1, -2, -3.
CD25	IL-2R	35	Activated T cells	α-chain of IL-2 receptor
CD26		110	Activated T cells	Dipeptidyl peptidase IV
CD27		50	T cells	?activation, (nerve-growth factor receptor family)
CD28		44	T cells	Priming T cells; ligand B7
CD29		110	T_{mem}, activated leucocytes	Adhesion
CD45	LCA	180–240	All leucocytes	Activation, phosphatase
CD45RA			Virgin T cells	
CD45RO			Memory T cells	Binds CD22
CD40L			T cells	Binds CD40 on B cells

Abbreviations: CTL, cytotoxic T lymphocytes; ICAM, intercellular adhesion molecules; IL, interleukin; LFA, lymphocyte function-associated antigen; TCR, T-cell receptor; T_{mem}, memory T cells. Further concise details of leucocyte differentiation antigens can be found in Barclay et al. (1993).

T-cell subpopulations

Functionally, T lymphocytes can be divided into two major subtypes helper T cells (Th) which carry the CD4 glycoprotein and recognize antigens presented by class II HLA, and CTL which carry CD8 and respond to peptides presented by HLA class I. Th cells are divisible into two further major subtypes with different functions, Th1 and Th2. They differ in the cytokines they release on antigen activation. Th1 T cells release interferon-γ, IL-2, and IL-15. These have direct and indirect antiviral effects and some inflammatory activity. They are potent in successful T-cell responses to infectious agents including mycobacteria, most viruses, and a range of parasitic infections. In contrast, Th2 cells release IL-4, IL-10- and IL-13. IL-10 has some immunosuppressive properties, IL-4 and IL-13 favour B-cell responses, facilitating the IgG immunnoglobulin switching. The extreme of a Th2 response is the IL-4 mediated switching to IgE production, resulting in allergic reactions. Th2 cells also produce IL-5 which stimulates eosinophils. Th2 immune responses are in combating parasitic worm infestations.

The balance between Th1 and Th2 is of considerable pathological interest. The two extreme forms of leprosy exemplify this beautifully. In tuberculoid leprosy, there is a Th1 response, with a strong inflammatory response of the delayed hypersensitivity type. In lepromatous leprosy, there is a Th2 response, the infection is poorly controlled with abundant organisms despite a good antibody response. Similar polarization can be found in tuberculosis (minimal disease (Th1) versus miliary (Th2)) and leishmania infection (minimal disease where there is a Th1 response and kala azar with a Th2 response). Whilst Th2 responses appear bad in these contexts, there are other situations where Th1 responses can be harmful, particularly in autoimmune diseases such as juvenile onset diabetes and rheumatoid arthritis. The polarization is not always complete and a variety of intermediate CD4+ T cells (Th0) have been described. Also, a Th3 type associated with the intestinal tract has been claimed, predominantly secreting TGF-β and protecting against immunization against food proteins.

For many years there were claims that there were a distinct population of specialist suppresser T cells that carried the CD8 marker. These do not exist as such but there are clearly suppressive phenomena mediated by subsets of CD4 or CD8 T cells through their cytokines or cytolytic effects. The term 'suppressor T cell' should be rested for the time being.

Cytotoxic T lymphocytes (CTL)

The effector T cells that mediate cellular immune responses are the CTL and Th1 cells that secreted cytokines such as interferon-γ and tumour necrosis factor (TNF). Cytotoxic T cells recognize antigen plus class I HLA antigen on presenting cells. The antigen is peptide-derived, from intracellular proteins such as virus proteins. In fact, any cellular protein can enter the pathway that puts peptides into HLA molecules. The proteins are degraded by intracellular proteases, most important of which is the proteasome complex. The short peptides generated are transported by the transporter associated with antigen processing (TAP) into the endoplasmic reticulum

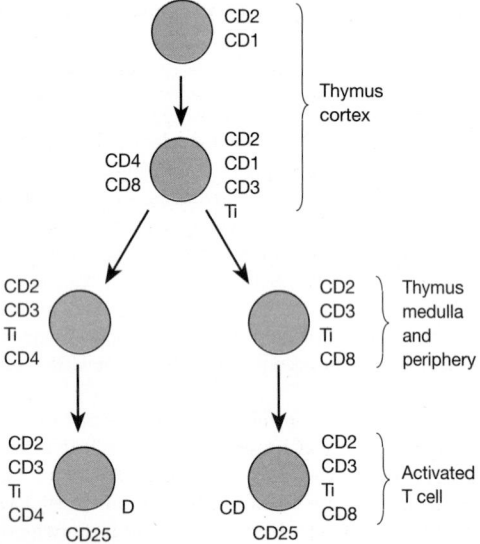

Fig. 7 Expression of T-lymphocyte differentiation antigens on differentiating T cells. The arrows indicate the probable pathway of T-cell development in the thymus and periphery. The CD antigens are described in Table 4

where most are further degraded, but some that have the right sequence characteristics to bind to HLA class I molecules, and are then presented on the cell surface. CTL monitor the surface of cells for abnormalities and react when their receptors bind. In the case of an acute virus infection, the magnitude of the CTL response is extraordinary. Before infection, T cells with specificity for any single epitope (antigenic region) on a virus are extremely rare, less than 1 in a million lymphocytes. In several acute virus infections they have now been recorded at between 2 and 20 per cent of all lymphocytes, a massive expansion. These T cells are functional, able to kill virus-infected cells, and release cytokines such as interferon-γ and TNF-α. The massive expansion is controlled by programmed cell death of the T cells and, as the virus antigen is removed, the number of antigen-specific T cells declines rapidly, leaving a memory T-cell response for rapid re-expansion should the virus attempt to reinfect.

There is considerable evidence that these T cells are crucial in clearing acute virus infections (such as measles, influenza) and controlling persistent infections, such as Epstein–Barr virus (EBV) or cytomegalovirus (CMV). Where CTL responses are impaired (e.g. by deliberate immunosuppression for transplantation) these viruses may escape control and cause disease, for example EBV-associated lymphomas. The CTL response is normally accompanied by a Th1 response that is important for initiating the CTL response and maintaining its functional activity and memory.

The CTL and Th1 responses, together often known as the 'cellular immune response' is central to the control of infections with intracellular pathogens that include not only viruses but some bacteria (e.g. *Listeria*, *Mycobacteria*) and protozoal infections (e.g. malaria liver stage). For some microbes, cytotoxicity is the important mediator of protection, for others interferon-γ release or chemokine release is crucial. The CTL response could well be important in the control of some cancers. For those caused by viruses (EBV lymphomas, HBV-associated liver cancers, HPV-associated cervical cancer) this is already clear. There is increasing evidence that CTL responses are generated to some solid tumours, melanomas being the best example. For tumours and also many viruses, particularly HIV, CMV, EBV and HCV, selection of escape pathways arises. Many tumours and several viruses can decrease expression of HLA class I molecules on cell surfaces, making them invisible to CTL. Some viruses and many tumours mutate the epitopes recognized by CTL. Viruses and tumours can also increase expression of Fas-ligand on the cell surface, triggering apoptosis in the attacking T cells that express the ligand Fas. The presence of such mechanisms implies that the T cells are worth escaping from.

Graft rejection is a classical cellular immune response that has a long history in immunology. Both CTL and Th1 cells are involved and infiltrate the graft. HLA class II is essential to induce T helper cells and thus to activate T cells, the CTL recognize the foreign HLA class I molecules.

The role of thymus in T-cell function

T lymphocytes by definition are thymus derived. Thymectomized or congenitally athymic animals lack mature T cells and T-cell-mediated functions. Athymic (nude) mice and human infants with thymic hypoplasia (Di George syndrome) show no cellular immune responses and impaired antibody responses. B cells, however, can respond by secreting IgM to some polysaccharide antigens in the absence of T cells. Normal thymocytes carry the T-cell differentiation antigens described above and also CD1, which has some similarities to an HLA class I molecule but is not MHC encoded and has an unknown function in the thymus; the molecules are, however, also expressed on dendritic cells where they are involved in presentation of glycolipid antigens to T cells.

Immature lymphocytes enter the thymus from the bone marrow and first rearrange their T-cell receptor β genes, expressing first a primitive receptor associated with a temporary second chain. Then the α chain genes rearrange and a functional receptor is expressed. At this point these thymocytes express both CD4 and CD8. Then two selection processes occur. The first is first deletion of any T cell that is self reactive (negative selection); dendritic cells enter the thymus from the periphery bringing in peptides from self tissues bound to self HLA class I and class II molecules. Self-

reacting T cells that carry both CD4 and CD8 die by apoptosis. The second selection step is positive selection; a repertoire of T cells that express either CD4 or CD8 and have receptors that can recognize non-self peptide bound to self HLA molecules is generated. It is thought that the receptors on these T cells react weakly with the self peptides on the self HLA molecules, enough to trigger a survival signal rather than the stronger apoptotic signal of negative selection. During this process either CD4 or CD8 is lost. The T cells that then populate the periphery have an affinity for self that is too low to trigger a signal but can respond to foreign peptides bound to the self HLA molecules. In addition to the active selection processes in the thymus, many T cells whose receptors confer neither negative nor positive selection, also die. Thus more than 90 per cent of thymocytes die.

Some self-reactive T cells may escape to the periphery. Many of these are probably deleted but some may instead be put into an inactive (anergic) state. Under some circumstances these cells may be activated, for instance by a cross-reactive microbial peptide antigen, and autoimmunity can result.

A third way of preventing autoimmunity is for the self cell to be immunologically inaccessible. This may occur at certain sites such as the eye. It can also occur on cells that fail to express the costimulatory molecule B7 (CD80) which is necessary to initiate immune responses.

Cytokines

A number of cytokines have already been referred to, particularly in the context of understanding the function of Th cells and immunoglobulin class switching. They are small polypeptides, released by immunocytes and other cells, with normally short-range functions on target cells that carry the appropriate receptor. Specificity is therefore conferred by the nature and state of activation of the cell that makes the cytokine and by the cell that bears the receptor. The actual effects of cytokines tend to be pleiomorphic—activating cells, triggering general differentiation, and activation of specific genes (e.g. co-ordinated expression of HLA class I and II genes plus antigen processing genes, TAP and components of the proteasome by interferon-γ). Of particular interest is the control of immunoglobulin isotype switching by cytokines (see Table 6) as well as by the CD40–CD40L interaction. Some cytokines, such as IL-12, seem more effective at orchestrating the others (the Th1 set for IL-12). Cytokine activity in terms of T-cell function can be described by the Th1–Th2 division. Also, Th3 cells that secrete the inhibitory cytokine TGF-β have been described. Although this is clear in mice it is more complex in human T cells, possibly because the original activation of the T cells *in vivo* is not under experimental control and also because the source of T cells, peripheral blood lymphocytes in man and spleen cells in mice, is different. In humans there are intermediate phenotypes known as Th0 cells. Nevertheless, it is a useful paradigm, implying that the response of Th cells may be set at the time of original activation and with implications for understanding disease processes. The cytokines relevant to the immune response are listed in Table 6. Some of these are being tried for therapy, for example interferon and IL-2. Also antibodies to some are useful, particularly anti-TNF for treatment of rheumatoid arthritis.

Accessory cells in the immune response

Antigen-presenting cells

Besides T and B lymphocytes, certain accessory cells play crucial roles in immune responses. Antigen-presenting cells are clearly important. B cells and CTL can react with antigen directly in native form or on altered cells, respectively, but both require signals from Th cells which are dependent on specialized presenting cells. The latter are either B lymphocytes or monocyte/ dendritic cells which can internalize antigen, degrade it, and display derived peptides in HLA class II molecules. They also carry specialized accessory molecules such as CD80 (also known as B7, not to be confused

Table 6 Cytokines important for T-cell function

Cytokine	M_r (kDa)	Made by:	Receptor on:	Function
IL-1($\alpha\beta$)	15.5	Monocytes	Type I: T,thy,fib,cho,syn, hep,end,ker	T activation, acute-phase reaction, inflammation
			Type II: B,mac,mono	
IL-2	15–20	Th1	Act-T, (B,mono)	T activation/ proliferation
IL-3	14–30	T	BM stem—all lineages	Growth, differentiation
IL-4	15–19	Th2	B,T,BM,fib,epi,end	Switch to IgG1, IgE macro activation
IL-5	2 × 21.5	Th2	eo,baso	Growth and differentiation
IL-6	21–28	Th2	act-B,PC (epi,fib,hep,neur)	Growth factor, acute-phase IgA selection
IL-7	25	T	Pre-B,thy,T,mono	Activation,proliferation
IL-8			N,baso,T subset, mono,ker	Chemotaxis, activation, adhesion
IL-9	32–39		T	Proliferation
IL-10	19	Th2	T,B,mono	Ig switch, T and B activation
IL-11	23		BM	Haemopoiesis
IL-12	35,40		T,B	IgE selection, T proliferation
IFN-γ	20–24	Th1,CTL	mac,mono,B,fib,epi,endo	Activation, proliferation → HLA I and II Ig2a (mice)
TNF	3 × 17	T	Most cells	Activation, apoptosis

The genes for all of the cytokines listed have been cloned, as have those for their receptors in most cases. The functions are summarized and in most cases are still under intense investigation. Abbreviations: act, activated; B, B cells; BM, bone marrow cells; baso, basophils; cho, chondrocytes; end, endothelial cells; epi, epithelial cells; eo, eosinophils; fib, fibroblast; hep, hepatocyte; ker, keratinocytes; mac, macrophages; mono, monocytes; neur, neuronal cells; PC, plasma cells; T, T cells; thy, thymocytes; TNF, tumour necrosis factor. For further details see Burke et al. (1993).

with HLA-B7) which binds to CD28 on T cells, delivering a cosignal. Dendritic cells are found not only in the T-cell areas of lymph nodes (see below) but also widely distributed in many organs. Here they may be important in activating local immune responses, for example to localized virus infection. Dendritic cells have to be activated to initiate CTL responses; this is achieved through the CD40 molecule recognized by CD40L on Th cells, although some viruses such as influenza may be able to activate directly. Dendritic cells seem to be able to internalize particulate antigens and can put these into the class I antigen presenting pathway. They are also able to take up apoptozing cells which may be an important pathway for initiating immune responses to viruses; macrophages are important for taking up necrotic cells and are not very effective in stimulating CTL responses. The requirements for initiating a primary CTL response are much more stringent than a secondary response, where the T cells may be able to respond and divide on contact with non-specialist cells that present antigen.

In the B-cell area of lymph nodes, the secondary follicles, there is a network of follicular dendritic cells. Unlike the dendritic cells referred to above, they are HLA class II negative but display receptors for C3b (of complement) and immunoglobulin Fc. They can therefore capture immune complexes which are particularly good at initiating primary immune responses. They are probably able to capture small amounts of antigen percolating through the sinuses of lymphoid organs. They can hold antigen at their surface for long periods, possibly months or years.

Adjuvants are chemicals given with antigen that are able to localize antigens at the site of injection, giving a local inflammatory response, activating macrophages, and antigen-processing cells and thus initiating immune responses more effectively. An example that was used clinically for several decades was potassium alum added to diphtheria and tetanus toxoids. By triggering a non-specific inflammatory reaction at the site of injection, an adjuvant may direct the type of immune response, Th1 or Th2, as well as enhancing the level. Recently, a hypothesis has been proposed by Matzinger, that non-specific danger signals are crucial in initiating immune responses to invading pathogens because self antigens do not provoke non-specific inflammatory responses and do not therefore provoke autoimmune reactions. Whilst the concept of the danger signal is probably correct, it is unlikely that the whole of self–non-self discrimination can be explained this way.

B cells are particularly important in priming Th cells. Because they carry antibody receptors, they can bind the foreign protein and internalize it for degradation. This can also be achieved if the antigen is bound to serum antibody; internalization occurs through the Fc receptor. In addition, complement receptors can facilitate presentation of antigen that is in immune complex form.

Natural killer cells

Interferon is a potent activator of natural killer cells. These are large, granular lymphocytes, neither classical T nor B cells, which lyse cultured tumour cells and virus-infected cells *in vitro* very efficiently. Their role *in vivo* is uncertain but they have been implicated in rejection of histocompatible bone marrow grafts, tumour immunity, antivirus immunity, and autoimmunity. They may thus form a general surveillance system, eliminating tumour cells and virus-infected cells as they arise. Although these effects are non-specific, antigen-specific T cells, by releasing γ-interferon, could activate them to give a vital enhancement of T-cell killing.

Recently, much has been discovered about the specificity of their function. It is clear that they are particularly effective at recognizing and killing cells that lack expression of classical HLA class I molecules. Two series of receptors have been identified that specifically bind HLA class I molecules and deliver inhibitory signals to NK cells. One series KIR (killer inhibitory receptors) interacts with particular HLA-C or B molecules—there are at least three series of these receptors and different isoforms with differing specificities in each series. Expression of these receptors is complex and seems to vary on different NK cells within one individual. In addition, there are receptors in a related series that deliver stimulatory signals to NK cells. The second type of receptor is the CD94/NKG2 series which recognize a non-classical HLA molecule, HLA-E, which is expressed on a cell surface only if it has bound a peptide derived from the signal peptide of classical HLA class I molecules. This means that HLA-E can signal to NK cells that the classical class I molecules are present and thereby inhibit NK cell attack. Although one of the CD94/NKG2 family is activating, the predominant effect is inhibition of NK cell activity. Thus NK cells express a variety of receptors with differing specificities for HLA class I molecules, most with inhibitory function but some activators. It would appear that these cells are controlled by a set of modulating receptors that signal the type of cell that is in contact with the NK cell.

Mast cells

In addition to antigen-presenting cells, there are other accessory cells at the other end of the immune response which might be termed enhancers. The best characterized of these is the mast cell which has a receptor for the Fc portion of the ε chain of IgE. When this antibody, bound by its Fc region to mast cells, binds antigen the cross linking of neighbouring Fc receptors triggers the cell to degranulate. This results in the release of histamine, kinins, and leucotrienes, which give the anaphylactic of type 1 allergic reaction. Mast cells also have receptors for some of the peptides released during complement activation.

Macrophages

Macrophages are derived from monocytes and are long-lived, potent phagocytic cells. Differentiation to macrophages and their activation is a response to local events such as contact with foreign material, lectins, and complement fragment C5a, but is also under the control of immune cells, with immune complexes and interferon-γ, which is released by antigen-specific T cells, being potent activators. Macrophages are larger than monocytes and differ in their surface glycoproteins with less HLA class II antigen and increased amounts of receptors for immunoglobulin Fc fragments and complement. Within the cells, lysosomes are increased in number.

The main function of macrophages, and also granulocytes, is phagocytosis. This is greatly enhanced (several thousand-fold) if the foreign material is coated with antibody and/or the complement fragment C3b. Ingested particles are taken into the cell in a phagosome which fuses to a lysosome. Similar processes in granulocytes and macrophages are associated with a respiratory burst; there is a sudden uptake of oxygen and generation of hydrogen peroxide and hydroxyl radicals which are toxic to micro-organisms. Nitric oxide production through activation of NO synthase is also of considerable importance. Activated macrophages also produce a variety of enzymes that are important in inflammatory processes, including proteases, elastase, collagenase, plasminogen activator, and procoagulants. The last may account for the deposition of fibrin, which is responsible for the characteristic induration of delayed-type hypersensitivity reactions.

Macrophages also release monokines and synthesize complement components. The former include interleukin-1 and tumour necrosis factor (Table 6). The latter may help to amplify the local inflammatory responses. Bioactive lipids, including prostaglandins and leucotrienes, are also made.

Macrophages are thus highly active cells which are crucially important in converting immune responses into inflammatory reactions. They feature prominently in granuloma formation where antigen persists or forms immune complexes. Mycobacteria are thought to inhibit fusion between phagosomes and lysosomes and thus evade the toxic mechanisms. Under these circumstances, the macrophages form epithelioid and giant cells in forming the granuloma.

Like natural killer cells, macrophages may be dangerous to the body and a number of inhibitory receptors have been identified. These include the 'immunoglubulin-like transcripts', ILT-2 and ILT-4, which bind HLA class I molecules, both classical and non-classical. Again normal cells deliver a 'hands off' signal whereas HLA-negative cells would be targets. A similar situation applies to the ligand for CD46, the latter is expressed on red cells and protects them from destruction by splenic macrophages in the white pulp.

Complement

The complement pathway is described in Chapter 5.4. This is an important, intrinsic pathway of immunity, activated directly by micro-organisms or by immune complexes. Complement can activate cells such as monocytes, macrophages, and neutraphils, contributing to inflammatory responses.

Organization of the immune system

The immunocytes are divided into those which are circulating in blood and lymph, and those localized in lymphoid organs: the thymus, bone marrow,

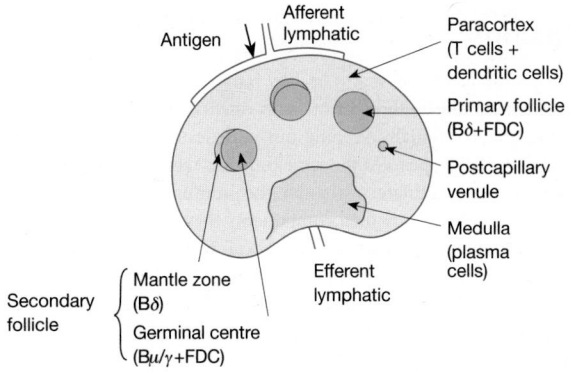

Fig. 8 Schematic representation of the structure of a lymph node. The drawing is not to scale but shows the main components. The cell types found in each region are indicated: Bδ, B cells expressing surface IgD; Bμ/γ, B cells expressing surface IgM or surface IgG; FDC, follicular dendritic cells; T, T cells (a few T cells are also found in the germinal centres where B cells may present antigen).

fetal liver, spleen, lymph nodes, and the gut-associated immune system of tonsils, Peyers patches, and intraepithelial lymphocytes.

The circulating lymphocytes follow precise routes. From the efferent lymph nodes they travel to the thoracic duct and thence to the venous blood. From the blood they return to lymph nodes or spleen through high-walled capillary venules. Gut-associated lymphocytes also circulate and tend to home back to gut lymphoid tissue, or bronchial or mammary tissue, thus distributing antigen-sensitive cells widely to all possible sites of entry of organisms.

The structure of a lymph node is shown in diagrammatic form in Fig. 8 (see also Chapter 23.1). The B cells are congregated in follicles. Primary follicles contain mostly early B cells with IgD on their surface. Activation of B cells by an immune response in a germinal centre results in division and accumulation of B cells to generate secondary follicles which contain mostly IgG-bearing B cells. Scattered through the follicle are helper T cells and follicular dendritic cells. From the follicles, stimulated B cells mature to plasma cells in cords in the medulla where they secrete immunoglobulin.

The majority of T cells in the lymph nodes are in the paracortex surrounding the follicles. The T helper cells and Tc/Ts are found there. They are clearly associated with the HLA class II-positive dendritic cells. Antigen enters by the afferent lymphatics and percolates through the lymph nodes, activating immune cells via the antigen presenting cells.

The spleen is similarly organized in the white pulp, which surrounds the end arterioles, whence the cells and antigen enter. Circulating lymphocytes leave by venous sinuses (Fig. 9).

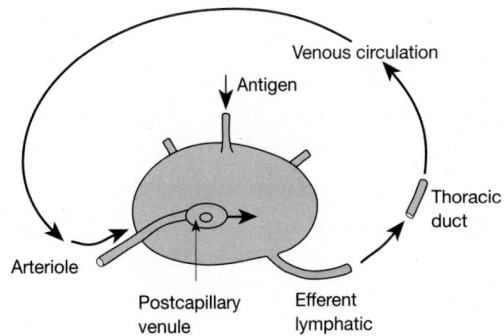

Fig. 9 Lymphocyte recirculation. Antigen enters the lymph node by the afferent lymphatics. Lymphocytes enter the lymph node through the walls of the postcapillary (high endothelial) venules. They leave by the efferent lymphatics, whence they go to the thoracic duct and the superior vena cava.

Conclusions

Immune responses are occurring in healthy individuals continuously. The immune system should be thought of as an essential part of the homeostatic mechanism, continually keeping out and destroying invaders and abnormal cells as they appear. At the same time it is regulating its own cells as they develop and circulate. Although the immune system has been described in terms of its individual components they do not react in isolation. Thus, an infecting virus, for instance, will evoke an antibody response, activate complement through the classical and alternative pathways, stimulate T-cell immunity involving both regulatory and effector T cells, stimulate lymphokine release, and activate natural killer cells. In a later chapter the consequences of abnormal immune responses are described, both where there is a deficiency in immune reactivity and where, for various reasons, the immune reaction itself is harmful.

Further reading

Aguado B *et al.* (1999). Complete sequence and gene map of a human major histocompatibility complex. *Nature* **401**, 921–23.

Alberts B *et al.* (1994). *Molecular biology of the cell*, 3rd edn. Garland, New York.

Barclay AN *et al.* (1993). *The leucocyte antigen facts book*. Academic Press, London.

Bjorkman PJ *et al.* (1987). Structure of the human major histocompatibility antigen, HLA-A2. *Nature* **329**, 506–12.

Burke F *et al.* (1993). The cytokine wall chart. *Immunology Today* **14**, 147.

Davis MM, Bjorkman PJ (1988). The T-cell receptor genes and T cell recognition. *Nature* **344**, 395–402.

Elliott T, Smith M, Driscoll P, McMichael AJ (1993). Peptide selection by class I molecules of the major histocompatibility complexs. *Current Biology* **3**, 854–66.

5.2 Allergy

L. M. Lichtenstein

Introduction

Approximately 20 per cent of the population suffers from allergy. In allergy, exposure to common environmental substances induces the production of specific antibodies of the IgE class that arm mast cells and basophils to initiate a complex response which leads to the tissue inflammation. It is believed that the IgE response originally developed to combat parasitic diseases but this has never been proved.

Allergens are antigens which induce IgE antibody responses. They may be large molecules, usually proteins, or they may be small molecules, 'haptens', such as penicillin, which link to protein molecules to induce the immune response. Not all individuals who develop an IgE antibody response develop allergic symptoms, but after exposure to the allergen most will suffer rhinitis, asthma, or anaphylaxis. The synthesis of allergen-specific IgE by B lymphocytes is thought to be mediated by activated CD4+ T lymphocytes. The IgE occupies high-affinity receptors on mast cells and basophils and the response is triggered when these cells bind allergen. Murine CD4 T-cell populations have been defined as T_{H1} cells, which produce interleukin 2 (**IL-2**) and γ-interferon, and T_{H2} cells, which produce IL-4 and IL-5. Both populations of cells secrete other cytokines. In humans, the distinctions between T_{H1} and T_{H2} cells are not so clear, but none the less help us to characterize allergic disease. Allergic individuals have much higher IgE levels than non-allergic individuals, which contribute to diagnosis. Allergen skin testing allows specific diagnosis.

Cytokines influence all phases of the allergic inflammatory response. IL-4 is required to initiate IgE synthesis, while ongoing synthesis is enhanced by IL-5. Other cytokines such as γ-interferon downregulate IgE synthesis. Granulocyte–macrophage colony-stimulating factor (**GM-CSF**) and IL-3, -4, and -9 promote the differentiation and expansion of mast cells, whereas γ-interferon interferes with their growth. Another group of recently discovered cytokines are the histamine-releasing factors, first identified in monocytes. Mast cells and, particularly, basophils, also synthesize cytokines which include IL-4 and IL-13. The stages of an allergic reaction are seen in Figs 1 to 3.

Allergens

Modern techniques have facilitated characterization of important allergens, many of which have enzymatic activities that may favour penetration of mucosal surfaces. In the past, the allergen preparations used for diagnosis and therapy have not been standardized, resulting in unacceptable inconsistencies in diagnosis and treatment. The current trend is to insist upon standardization of such preparations, based on their major defined allergens. The mapping of T-cell epitopes has allowed development of peptide vaccines for immunotherapy; some of these have clinical efficacy and merit further therapeutic exploration.

Genetic basis of atopic disease

There is a genetic basis to the allergic diathesis. Allergic susceptibility is clearly polygenic. For example, certain ragweed allergens such as Amb a V and Amb a V1 are recognized in association with HLA DR2, the W2 and HLA DR11 haplotypes, respectively. Lineage studies of large families have suggested autosomal dominant or recessive patterns of inheritance. Rather than focusing on atopic individuals, early studies sought associations with one or more criterion: high serum IgE, positive skin tests, or clinical allergic disease. Linkage data suggested the presence of a gene for atopy on the long arm of chromosome 11. This finding implied that non-MHC linked genes may determine the overall predisposition to allergic disease, while MHC gene products control the specificity of the allergic response.

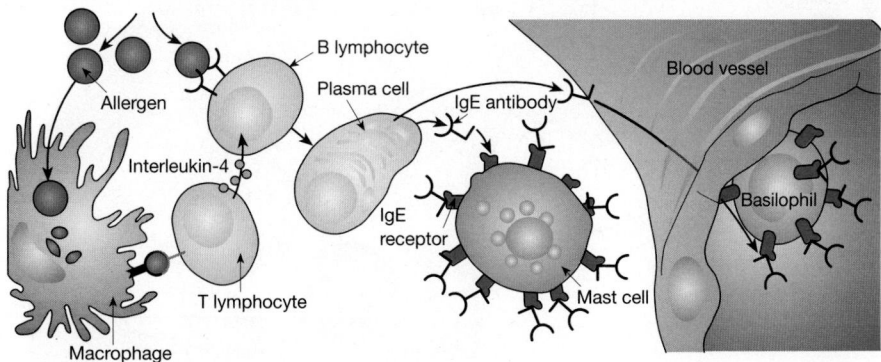

Fig. 1 Stages of an allergic reaction: sensitization. The initial meeting of an allergen and the immune system yields no symptoms; rather it may prepare the body to react promptly to future encounters with the substance. The sensitization process begins when macrophages degrade the allergen and display the resulting fragments to T lymphocytes (bottom left). The steps that follow are somewhat obscure, but in a process involving secretion of interleukin 4 by T cells, B lymphocytes mature into plasma cells able to secrete allergen-specific molecules known as immunoglobulin E (IgE) antibodies. These antibodies attach to receptors on mast cells in tissue and on basophils circulating in blood.

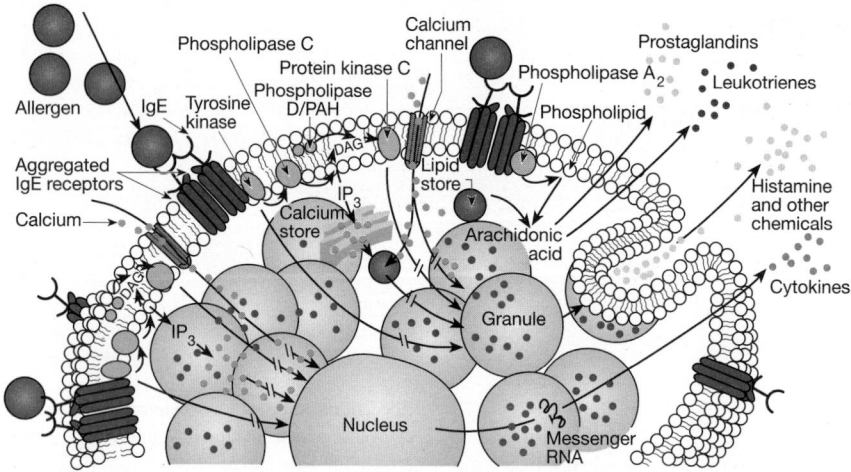

Fig. 2 Stages of an allergic reaction: activation of mast cells. In later encounters between the allergen and the body, allergen molecules promptly bind to IgE antibodies on mast cells (top left). When one such molecule connects with two IgE molecules on the cell surface, it draws together the attached IgE receptors, thereby directly or indirectly activating various enzymes (green spheres) in the cell membrane. Cascades involving tyrosine kinase enzymes, phospholipase C, protein kinase C, and an influx of calcium ions (black arrows) induce chemical-laden granules to release their contents. These cascades also appear to promote the synthesis and extrusion of chemicals known as cytokines (brown arrows). Other sequences of molecular interactions (green arrows) end in the secretion of such lipids as prostaglandins and leukotrienes. The various chemicals released by mast cells are responsible for many allergic symptoms. The reaction pathways shown are simplified and are only a few of those thought to occur; many are also only partly understood (broken arrows).

The cells involved in allergic disease

Mast cells and basophils

Tissue mast cells account for most acute allergic phenomena while the basophil, which infiltrates into the regions of an acute response, is responsible for chronic allergic manifestations. Both cell types originate in the bone marrow and have cytoplasmic granules. Tissue mast cells are found mostly in the lungs, skin, and gastrointestinal track, the location of most immediate hypersensitivity reactions. IL-3 and stem cell factor (**SCF**) are required for the growth, differentiation, and survival of basophils, while the added effects of SCF are critical for mast cell maturation and survival. The signal transduction events which are induced by cross-linking of cell-bound IgE by allergen have been studied with great interest, since interference with these signals would seem to be the best target for blocking the entire allergic response. Intracellular signals mediated by increased levels of

intracellular calcium and activation of protein kinase C lead to phosphorylation of granule membrane proteins. These signals lead to the release of preformed mediators such as histamine and to the production of arachidonic acid metabolites including prostaglandin D and leukotriene C. This mode of activation is associated with cytokine generation.

Eosinophils

Circulating and tissue eosinophilia are cardinal manifestations of allergic diseases. Eosinophils are derived from the bone marrow aided principally by IL-5 but also by IL-3 and GM-CSF, and normally constitute less that 3 per cent of the circulating granulocytes. Tissue retention of eosinophils is determined by chemotactic factors which include chemokines (e.g. eotaxin), leukotrienes (e.g. LTC_4), and platelet-activating factor. Eosinophils have very few if any IgE receptors on their surface. Eosinophils contain highly cationic proteins including the so-called major basic protein.

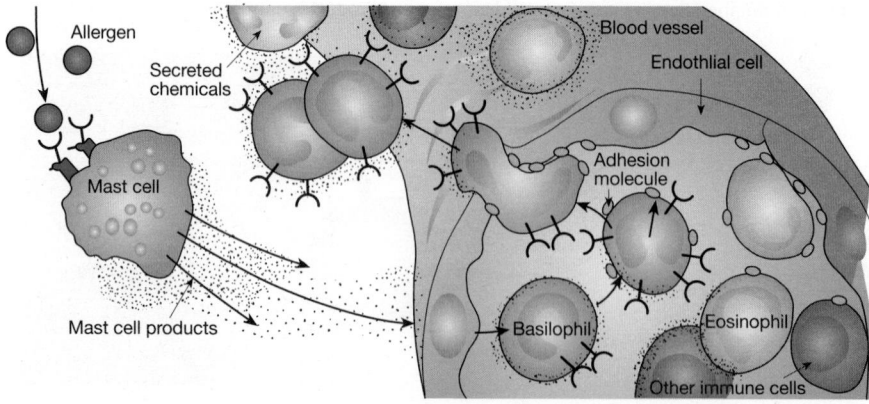

Fig. 3 Stages of an allergic reaction: prolonged immune activity. Chemicals emitted by activated mast cells (left) and their neighbours in tissue may induce basophils, eosinophils, and other cells flowing through blood vessels (right) to migrate into that tissue. The chemicals facilitate migration by promoting the expression and activity of adhesion molecules on the circulating cells and on vascular endothelial cells. The circulating cells then attach to the endothelial cells, roll along them, and eventually, cross between them into the surrounding matrix. These recruited cells secrete chemicals of their own (orange speckles), which can sustain immune activity and damage tissue.

These are highly toxic products which have been implicated in the denudation of bronchial epithelium in asthma and in other types of cellular injury.

Monocytes, macrophages, and lymphocytes

Monocytes and macrophages may be activated by allergen binding to a low-affinity IgE receptor and contribute thereby to the non-specific inflammation of allergic diseases. Stimulated monocytes and macrophages produce many proinflammatory mediators and cytokines, including lysosomal enzymes, superoxide anions, lipid mediators, and diverse cytokines. Lymphocytes contribute critically to allergic disease.

The mediators of allergic disease

Histamine

This is the principal mediator of immediate hypersensitivity reactions; it is produced by basophils and mast cells and reacts with three specific histamine receptors. The first recognized, H_1, mediates hypersecretion of mucus, pruritus, contraction of non-vascular smooth muscle, and relaxation of vascular smooth muscle. There are now several non-sedating H_1 antihistamine drugs which are useful in controlling the manifestations of allergic disease. The H_2 receptor mediates enhanced gastric acid, mucus secretion, and bronchodilatation. There are also specific H_2 antihistamines. An H_3 receptor mediates the synthesis and release of histamine and neurotransmitters; anti-H_3 drugs are not available.

Eicosanoids

Eicosanoids are synthesized by mast cells, basophils, and eosinophils by the oxygenation of arachidonic acid metabolites via two pathways: the cyclooxygenase pathway forms prostaglandins and thromboxanes and the 5-lipoxygenase pathway generates leukotrienes. Prostaglandin D_2 and thomboxane A_2 are bronchoconstrictors. Leukotriene A is an unstable intermediate in the formation of leukotrienes B, C, D, and E. Leukotriene B is a chemotactic for leucocytes and leukotrienes C, D, and E increase systemic vascular permeability, smooth muscle contraction, and mucus secretions. The recent introduction of leukotriene antagonists has been a useful adjunct to the control of allergic diseases.

Platelet-activating factor

Platelet-activating factor is a proinflammatory molecule whose true function in allergic phenomena is not clearly understood. It is derived from the membrane phospholipids of mast cells and other cell types. Inhalational challenge with platelet-activating factor promotes bronchoconstriction and airways hyperreactivity in both asthmatic and non-asthmatic individuals and increases vascular permeability and mucus release. Platelet-activating factor is also a chemoattractant for eosinophils and neutrophils.

Kinins

Kinins are generated by kallikrein action on serum kininogens. Their biological activities are quite similar to histamine.

Allergic diseases

Anaphylaxis

Anaphylaxis results from the rapid degranulation of mast cells and basophils, usually, but not always, caused by the parental administration of drugs such as penicillin, or insect stings. Anaphylaxis is a medical emergency that can result in death either by cardiovascular collapse, laryngeal oedema, and/or bronchial smooth muscle constriction and anoxia. Anaphylaxis can also be induced by several food allergens such as cow's milk,

shellfish, or peanuts. Anaphylactoid reactions, which do not act through IgE-related mechanisms, may follow ingestion of aspirin or other non-steroidal anti-inflammatory drugs or by the injection of radiocontrast media, metabisulphites, or opiates.

The clinical manifestations of anaphylaxis or anaphylactoid reactions are similar and may involve the skin (erythema, urticaria, angio-oedema), laryngeal oedema, bronchoconstriction, vascular shock, and gastrointestinal symptoms (abdominal pain, nausea, vomiting, or diarrhoea). These reactions cause tachycardia, arrhythmias, hypotension, and anoxia, leading to myocardial or cerebral damage. Treatment involves the removal of the inciting agent when possible with the immediate therapeutic use of adrenaline intravenously, if necessary. Antihistamines may be given but probably have little effect, and corticosteroids, while often recommended, are not useful in the acute phase. Attention to airway and cardiovascular support is crucial. After anaphylaxis, patients should be maintained under observation for a minimum of 24 h as the anaphylactic reaction may recur. Disseminated intravascular coagulation with widespread haemorrhage due to thrombocytopenia is a a severe late complication of anaphylaxis. Individuals allergic to insect venoms whose treatment is not complete, and patients who have food allergy should be advised to carry prepackaged adrenaline syringes.

Asthma (see also Section 17.4)

Extrinsic asthma is sometimes differentiated from intrinsic asthma. There is real doubt, however, as to whether intrinsic asthma exists or whether the causal allergen is simply not identified. Asthma affects 10 per cent of children and 3 to 5 per cent of adults and may range from a modest shortness of breath to a severe, life-threatening, obstructive ventilatory disease. By definition, asthma is characterized by widespread narrowing of the airways, which is reversible either spontaneously or as a result of treatment. However, chronic asthma may ultimately cause fixed airway obstruction. Asthma is usually associated with a personal family history of allergic disease and offending allergens may be known to precipitate attacks. However, a definitive clinical history and appropriate skin testing may be needed for diagnosis. Asthma may often be perennial, as a result of exposure to house dust mites or pet allergens.

Asthma is increasing all over the world, and this is especially true in inner-city African-American people. When wealth and environmental status are taken into account, the increase in African-American patients is still greater than that in Caucasian populations. The reasons for this are not known. Environmental pollution and cockroach allergy have been suggested to account for this, but evidence is lacking. The increase in asthma, for example, was shown to be greater in western Germany than in heavily polluted eastern Germany. The pathogenesis of asthma is exceedingly complex. When an atopic or asthmatic individual is challenged by bronchial allergens there is an early bronchocontraction, which is due to the release of mediators such as histamine and leukotrienes, followed by a recovery and a so-called late-phase response, which has been shown to be due to the infiltration of basophils, eosinophils, and other proinflammatory cells as well as the mediators of the acute phase. Asthmatic individuals have a heightened non-specific response to bronchoconstrictors such as histamine, methacholine, and especially, bradykinin.

The diagnosis and management of asthma are discussed in Section 17.4. However, a comment on a new therapy is appropriate here. A humanized anti-IgE antibody has been developed at Genentech and has been used in a variety of clinical trials. The use of this antibody in appropriate dosage intravenously decreases the serum IgE by more than 90 per cent. Moreover, as we predicted 20 years ago, based on the close correlation between serum IgE and mast cell and basophil IgE receptor number, it also decreases the IgE receptors on these cells. When this reduction is sufficient, there is a partial or complete inability to elicit basophil histamine release and the results of skin tests can be depressed or negative. The appropriate individuals for treatment with this regimen are just those who most need it:

asthmatic patients with sensitivities to multiple allergens. In these individuals, the number of allergen-specific IgE antibodies can be reduced below the necessary level for initiating mediator release. In most individuals with asthma caused by a single or a few allergens, anti-IgE therapy will not be helpful. Clinical trials in a mixed population, including those who should and should not be receiving anti-IgE, showed a modest amelioration of asthma. It seems likely that if therapy were limited to appropriate individuals, the relief may be greater.

Allergic rhinitis

Allergic rhinitis affects about 10 per cent of the population and may be seasonal, in response to the pollens of weeds, trees, and grasses, or perennial, usually linked to house dust mite sensitivity or animal dander. The symptoms are sneezing, nasal congestion, rhinorrhoea, and often pharyngeal and conjunctival pruritus. Inspection of the nasal passages usually reveals a pale mucosa with swollen turbinates. The disease may be diagnosed by the timing of symptoms since grass, tree, or weed pollination occurs at predictable times, or symptoms may appear in association with pet exposure. In order to induce allergy, the particles of pollens or dust mite must be in the range of 10 to 100 μm in diameter. Nasal polyps may accompany the mucosal oedema, particularly in perennial rhinitis. Vasomotor or non-allergic rhinitis has many of the same symptoms but it is not due to IgE-mediated events. The diagnosis of allergic rhinitis is made by clinical history and evidence of specific IgE antibodies by skin testing or by the presence of serum specific IgE detected in the laboratory. The former diagnostic test is preferable.

Insect venom allergy (see also Chapter 8.2)

Insect venom hypersensitivity can be demonstrated in approximately 20 per cent of individuals in the United States, although only 3 to 5 per cent have a history of an anaphylactic reaction. While the number of deaths caused by this sensitivity is few (perhaps 50 per year in the United States), the social morbidity induced by insect sensitivity is very significant and this condition is one of the few where allergen immunotherapy is clearly indicated and effective. The history of the treatment of insect sensitivity shows how misleading uncontrolled studies can be. The disorder was formerly treated with 'extracts' derived by grinding-up the entire insect and injecting it. When controlled studies were initiated, it was found that treatment with placebo and whole-body extract were identical, while, as noted, venom immunotherapy was almost completely effective.

Insect reactions are characteristic of the order Hymenoptera including honey bees and vespids, such as wasps, white and yellow hornets, and yellow jackets, as well as polistes and fire ants. Another form of response to an insect sting is a large local reaction which occurs immediately contiguous to the sting and does not involve any life-threatening response of blood vessels or airways. These individuals rarely develop systemic reactions and usually do not require specific treatment, but in some these reactions are very large, crossing a joint space and causing marked discomfort. Immunotherapy should be considered in these individuals because it is effective. Diagnosis, as with other allergies, can be established by history, skin testing, or by the measurement of specific IgE antibodies. Rarely, an individual will have an anaphylactic episode despite being unaware of the sting, so this possibility must be considered in all cases of idiopathic anaphylaxis. While patients are unprotected, as in early stages of immunotherapy, they should carry emergency kits containing adrenaline.

Since immunotherapy is extremely effective, it should be used in all adult patients. Immunotherapy is usually continued for 4 or 5 years and may then be stopped, although there is some risk even after the several years of therapy. There is a difference between adults and children with respect to the manifestations of insect hypersensitivity. In adults, most reactions involve the airways or vascular system and are life-threatening. This occurs only rarely in children, with most manifestations being cutaneous. Children who have had such a cutaneous reaction usually do not have a further reaction on re-sting and need not be treated.

Urticaria (see also Section 23)

Urticaria is characterized by well-defined areas of transient pruritic dermal oedema, demarcated by a red border, which usually resolve spontaneously within a few hours, although episodes may continue for days. If the oedema spreads through the underlying epidermis, then it is called angio-oedema. The latter occurs mostly in the periorbital regions, the lips, the tongue, and the oropharynx and does not itch. In these instances, the possibility of pharyngeal obstruction may develop rapidly. Urticaria is probably due to mast cell degranulation, whether this is immunologically or non-immunologically mediated. Basophils may play a role in the longer episodes. Biopsies of acute urticarial lesions simply show oedema, but infiltration with neutrophils and eosinophils with perivascular monocytes may occur. Most commonly, urticaria is 'idiopathic' as no offending allergen can be identified. However, certain foods such as eggs, shellfish, and peanuts, or drugs are implicated occasionally. There is also a syndrome caused by aspirin and other non-steroid anti-inflammatory agents. Underlying atopy is not usually associated with urticaria.

Acute urticaria usually resolves within hours or days. In urticaria which is protracted or recurrent, the causal agents are usually undiscovered. However, increasingly, antihypertensive drugs, antirheumatoid arthritis drugs, and hormone-based medications such oral contraceptives are identified as triggering agents. There are forms of urticaria that have physical triggers: dermatographism is the condition where individuals suffer from urticaria on scratching or pressure. Cholinergic urticaria is associated with a tendency to show symptoms due to perspiration. Urticaria may also be evoked by cold, heat, pressure, or sunlight. There is a rare condition called hereditary angio-oedema, which is an autosomal dominant disorder characterized by severe episodic attacks of intractable bowel, laryngeal, and cutaneous angio-oedema. A quantitative or qualitative defect of the C1 esterase inhibitor is associated with an uncontrolled activation of complement components, C4 and C2.

If attacks of urticaria are recurrent and without obvious precipitating factors, patients should keep a diary to document food, beverage, and drug intake. In this way, triggers may be identified. It should also be remembered that urticaria sometimes is associated with systemic diseases such as lymphoma or systemic lupus erythematosis.

Treatment at first is with antihistamines, and since they may have to be used quite vigorously, the non-sedating antihistamines are probably preferable. These may be ineffective and, if so, some of the other sedating H₁-antihistamines such as cyproheptadine or cetirizine should be used. Systemic corticosteroids may be required in very severe cases that do not respond to other treatments.

Food allergy

True IgE-mediated food allergy is far more rare in adults than is generally believed. As noted, this usually occurs with the ingestion of specific allergens such as eggs, nuts, or shellfish. Food allergy is far more common in children. Skin tests are rather ineffective and double-blind, controlled, oral challenge is usually necessary for diagnosis.

The diagnosis of allergic disease

Skin testing

Skin testing was first described in the 1860s by Charles Blackley. It may be performed at any site, but is usually on the lower aspect of the forearm. Allergen testing must be accompanied by saline as a negative control and histamine as a positive control. Methods differ with intradermal skin testing being most common in the United States while prick testing, a lancet through a drop of allergen extract, is in frequent use in the United Kingdom. Results are read at 15 to 20 min and are interpreted by several techniques which measure the magnitude of the weal and flare response. Large numbers of skin tests are not usually indicated; skin testing with 5 to 10 different allergens, based on history, is the proper clinical procedure. The identification of food allergies is less useful, since there are many false positives requiring appropriate double-blind ingestion of suspected foods.

In vitro tests for specific IgE antibodies

Such testing is necessary in certain conditions such as in dermatographism and in young children. Allergen extracts are immobilized on an insoluble particle and then are allowed to react with a patient's serum. After appropriate washing, antihuman IgE is added, either radiolabelled or conjugated to an enzyme.

The treatment of allergic disease

The most effective measure is allergen avoidance, and this should be rigorously attempted by scrupulous house-cleaning, impenetrable mattress and pillow covers, and the use of air conditioning and filters. The first line of medical treatment is with long-acting antihistamines. The standard antihistamines should be tried first as they are much cheaper than the nonsedating antihistamines and only a small percentage of the population are sedated by them. The next line in therapy is a topical corticosteroid spray. Used properly, these have no systemic side-effects and are very effective. Topical vasoconstrictors are not recommended as they cause a rebound chemical rhinitis.

For rhinitis unresponsive to these measures, immunotherapy involving weekly injections of gradually increasing doses of the allergens to which the patients are sensitive is effective, as shown by double-blind trials in the United Kingdom and the United States. The new standardized allergen extracts should be administered by an experienced physician. Immuno-therapy is not effective for asthma in children and has marginal utility in adults.

The underlying immunological mechanisms of successful immunotherapy have not been fully determined. There is an increase in specific IgG antibody to the allergen that is associated with successful immunotherapy, but this association is not felt to be causal. Other types of immunotherapy are being evaluated: in one, the relevant allergen peptides are determined by reaction with T lymphocytes. This has been shown to lead to significant clinical improvement unassociated with any changes in allergen-specific IgG or IgE. The method has been largely abandoned because it was shown to be less clinically effective than standard immunotherapy; however, only a single regimen was examined. The therapy has considerable potential as the peptides are completely unreactive with mast cells or basophils and is thus extremely safe. Another new therapy uses allergens linked to bacterial DNA, which leads to a complete switch of the established T_{H2} response to a T_{H1} response in mice. Recent experiments in primates shows a similar type of immune response to these materials and the results of clinical trials are eagerly awaited.

Further reading

Lichtenstein LM, Fauci AS, eds (1996). *Current therapy in allergy, immunology, and rheumatology*, 5th edn. Mosby-Year Book, Inc., St. Louis.

Marone G *et al.*, eds (1998). *Asthma and allergic diseases*. Academic Press, London.

Middleton E Jr *et al.*, eds (1998). *Allergy principles and practice*, 5th edn. Mosby-Year Book, Inc., St. Louis.

Naclerio RM, Durham SR, Mygind N, eds (1999). *Rhinitis mechanisms and management*, Marcel Dekker, Inc., New York. Vol 123 in the series, *Lung biology in health and disease*, Claude Lenfant, ed.

5.3 Autoimmunity

Antony Rosen

Introduction

The effector mechanisms that the immune system utilizes to destroy extracellular pathogens, or host cells that harbour intracellular foreign bodies (such as mycobacteria or viruses) must be appropriately targeted if indiscriminate damage to normal host tissue is to be avoided. Under most inflammatory circumstances, some bystander tissue damage is unavoidable. In most circumstances, this damage is self-limited, due to efficient clearance of the exogenous antigen source and appropriate down-modulation of the immune response. Tissue damage in autoimmune diseases differs fundamentally from bystander damage in that the host immune system is specifically activated and driven by self-components, focusing damaging immune effector pathways on host tissues expressing those components, in an autoamplifying and self-sustaining way. The danger inherent in initiating a self-sustaining, specific immune response directed against components of self-tissues is intuitively apparent, since antigen clearance under these circumstances is necessarily associated with complete tissue destruction.

It is now clear that an autoimmune component is a feature of many human diseases. Indeed, there are some estimates that autoimmune diseases afflict more than 3 per cent of inhabitants of Western countries, and impose a significant personal and economic burden on individuals and nations. This chapter will illustrate many of the principles unifying various autoimmune states, and will present a conceptual framework within which to understand their aetiology, pathogenesis, and pathology. The rapid advances in knowledge being made in this group of disorders predict that disease mechanisms will soon be more clearly understood, and will greatly impact therapeutics.

Definitions

Autoimmune disease occurs when a sustained, specific, adaptive immune response is generated against self-components, and results in tissue damage or dysfunction. Although a single immune effector pathway may predominate in generating tissue dysfunction and damage in some autoimmune diseases, it is much more frequent for multiple effector pathways to participate in generating the final phenotype. Those pathways which generate tissue damage or dysfunction include autoantibody binding to target cells, immune complex-mediated activation of complement and Fc receptor pathways, cytokine pathways, and lymphocyte-mediated cytotoxicity of target cells. The nature and sites of the tissue damage are what determine the pathological and clinical features of the specific diseases.

Tissue-specific autoimmune diseases (Table 1)

These occur where immune-mediated damage is restricted to a particular tissue or organ that specifically expresses the targeted antigen. Pertinent examples include: (i) Graves' disease (where autoantibodies bind to and stimulate the thyroid-stimulating hormone receptor, resulting in thyrotoxicosis); (ii) myasthenia gravis (where autoantibodies target the acetylcholine receptor at the neuromuscular junction, resulting in muscular weakness and fatigue due to the inefficient transmission of the acetylcholine signal); and (iii) insulin-dependent diabetes mellitus (where a cytotoxic T-cell response to the β-cells of the pancreatic islets results in destruction of the insulin-producing cells).

Systemic autoimmune diseases (Table 2)

These are frequently characterized by simultaneous damage in multiple tissues (such as kidney, lung, skeletal muscle, nervous system, and skin). Unlike tissue-specific autoimmune diseases which target tissue-specific antigens, autoantibodies in systemic autoimmune diseases are frequently directed against molecules expressed ubiquitously in multiple tissues. Examples include the tRNA synthetases targeted in autoimmune myositis, the small nuclear ribonucleoproteins (snRNPs) targeted in systemic lupus erythematosus, and topoisomerase-1 targeted in scleroderma. Each of these molecules is expressed in all cells, where they play critical roles in essential cellular processes (such as protein translation, mRNA splicing, and DNA replication and remodelling, respectively). Recent studies have suggested that novel forms of these ubiquitously expressed antigens are generated when cells undergo some forms of apoptotic death, and that apoptotic cells may represent an important source of immunogens in this group of disorders. While tissue damage is frequently mediated by numerous mechanisms in systemic autoimmune diseases, deposition of immune complexes at sensitive sites (such as skin, joints, and kidney) represents a prominent mode of tissue damage (see below).

Non-sustained autoimmune diseases

These are characterized by organ or tissue damage and dysfunction, which tends to be self-limited and resolve after the first attack, and are very unlikely to recur (e.g. epidemic Guillain–Barré syndrome). These processes typically occur in the setting of infection, and are associated with cross-reactive antibody responses that recognize both components of the infecting organism as well as the target tissue.

Epidemiology

Autoimmune diseases may affect individuals at all stages of life. In general, diseases have a predilection for beginning after the second decade, with peak incidence in the third to sixth decades. In many instances, females predominate, with the magnitude of this sex difference varying among the different diseases. Thus, for the systemic autoimmune diseases (such as systemic lupus erythematosus, rheumatoid arthritis, Sjögren's syndrome, scleroderma, and autoimmune myositis) and autoimmune thyroid disease, the female:male (F:M) ratio is approximately 4:1 to 9:1, whilst for insulin-dependent diabetes mellitus, multiple sclerosis, and myasthenia gravis, the female predominance is much less prominent (F:M ratio less than 2:1). The exact mechanisms underlying this female predominance remain unknown, but this striking biological difference provides a major clue to pathways underlying susceptibility to autoimmunity.

Aetiology

A general theme in the autoimmune diseases is that the diagnostic phenotype appears subacutely over weeks to months, even though non-specific symptoms and signs frequently predate this. Examples include the fatigue and constitutional symptoms that predate diagnosis of systemic lupus erythematosus and rheumatoid arthritis. The well-developed phenotype represents a highly driven immune response directed against self-antigens, which is amplified between the moment of initial immunization and development of diagnostic disease features. It is therefore operationally useful to divide autoimmune diseases into separate kinetic phases: (i) susceptibility (pre-disease, in which inherited or acquired defects in pathways required to maintain tolerance to self-antigens render the individual susceptible to disease initiation); (ii) initiation (the interface of susceptibility genes and unique environmental events, which initiate an immune response directed at and driven by self-antigens); and (iii) propagation (a self-amplifying phase in which the specific immune response to self-antigens causes damage of tissues, with the release of more antigens, which further drive the immune response). Although these phases are conceptually distinct, they probably overlap considerably *in vivo*. Diagnostic symptoms and signs

Table 1 Autoantigens targeted in several tissue-specific autoimmune diseases

Disease	Tissue target	Prominent autoantigen(s)	Disease mechanisms	Clinical features
Autoimmune haemolytic anaemia	Erythrocyte surface	Components of the Rh antigen, Band 3.1, glycophorin, and several unidentified molecules	Antibody-mediated destruction and clearance of erythrocytes	Anaemia
Autoimmune hepatitis	Hepatocytes	Smooth muscle cell cytoskeletal components Cytochrome P-450–2D6 ASGP-receptor	Multiple	Mild to severe chronic hepatic dysfunction in young women
Epidemic Guillain–Barré syndrome (Northern China)	Motor axons	Axonal gangliosides	Infection with *Campylobacter jejuni* induces cross-reactive antibody, which mediates axonal damage	Acute autoimmune axonopathy Flaccid paralysis with areflexia Elevated cerebrospinal fluid protein
Graves' disease	Thyroid gland	Thyroid-stimulating hormone (TSH) receptor	Antibody-mediated stimulation of TSH receptor, leading to excessive thyroid hormone secretion	Hyperthyroidism Goitre Graves' ophthalmopathy Localized dermopathy
Insulin-dependent diabetes mellitus	β-Cells of the islets of Langerhans	Glutamic acid decarboxylase (65 kDa form) Insulin Carboxypeptidase	Cytotoxic lymphocyte-mediated destruction of islet cells	Insulin deficiency and diabetes
Idiopathic thrombocytopenia	Platelet surface	Platelet integrins	Antibody-mediated platelet destruction and phagocytosis	Thrombocytopenia, bleeding
Inflammatory bowel disease	Gastrointestinal tract	pANCA	Cytokine- and lymphocyte-mediated epithelial damage	Chronic intestinal inflammation marked by remission and relapse
Multiple sclerosis	Myelinated nerve fibres	Myelin basic protein Transaldolase	Activated cytokine pathways Activated effector lymphocytes	Demyelinating disorder primarily affecting young adults: protean clinical manifestations depending on location and size of classic plaques
Myasthenia gravis	Neuromuscular junction	Nicotinic acetylcholine receptor	Antibody-induced blockade and down-regulation of acetylcholine receptor	Striated muscle fatigue and weakness
Myocarditis	Myocardium	Cardiac myosin Adenine nucleotide transporter Branched-chain ketodehydrogenase	Infection with Coxsackie virus induces myocardial damage and immunization with cardiac autoantigens	Subacute congestive heart failure
Pemphigus vulgaris	Hemidesmosome junctions	Desmoglein-3	Antibody-mediated disruption of epithelial cell junctions, with epidermal cell detachment	Blistering skin lesions
Rasmussen's encephalitis	Inhibitory neurones	Type 3 glutamate receptor	Antibody-mediated blockade of inhibitory neurotransmitter signalling	Severe epileptic seizures, progressive degeneration of a single cerebral hemisphere
Stiff man syndrome	GABA-ergic neurones modulating spinal cord reflexes	GAD67 Amphiplysin	Blockade of inhibitory neurotransmitter signalling, possibly autoantibody mediated	Rare disease characterized by severe, progressive stiffness with superimposed episodic muscle spasms, may be associated with autoimmune disease or malignancy
Vitiligo	Melanocytes	Tyrosinase	Cytotoxic lymphocyte-mediated damage of melanocytes	Skin depigmentation

pANCA, perinuclear-staining antineutrophil cytoplasmic antibodies; ASGP, asialoglycoprotein.

represent the highly amplified form of the phenotype generated by the immune system, and generally are kinetically widely separated from the initiating event. This has greatly complicated the study of events underlying disease initiation, since this phase is frequently non-specific and difficult to classify clinically.

Both genetic and environmental factors play important roles in initiation and propagation of autoimmune diseases. They probably play their central roles by regulating the activation, function, and targets of the host immune system. There is also evidence that stochastic processes play an important role in disease initiation, greatly complicating studies to define the causes and mechanisms of autoimmune disease (see below).

Genetic factors

There is accumulating evidence that numerous genes interact to determine the susceptibility threshold for initiating and propagating a self-sustaining autoimmune process in a given individual. Relevant genes include genes that: (i) regulate the immune response; (ii) facilitate efficient, non-inflammatory clearance of apoptotic cells (such as C1q and C-reactive protein); or (iii) influence the target tissue. Recent genetic studies in mice by Wakeland and colleagues in systemic lupus erythematosus (see below), and by Todd and colleagues in human and mouse insulin-dependent diabetes mellitus, have underscored several important observations.

1. Multiple genes interact to generate the final phenotype. Some of these genes render an individual susceptible to initiating an autoimmune response; others affect the target tissue and contribute to the fine disease phenotype.

2. Background genes can have a profound effect on the ability to generate a self-sustaining phenotype. The presence or absence of suppressor genes appears to be particularly important.

3. Genes in the MHC region as well as non-MHC genes appear to play critical roles. While there is a particularly striking contribution from MHC alleles (particularly MHC class II) to disease susceptibility and protection, the mechanisms underlying this phenomenon are still incompletely defined.

MHC class II genes

The associations of MHC class II alleles with disease susceptibility and phenotype can be grouped into the two broad categories that follow.

Association with an increased frequency of the disease itself

Some MHC class II alleles are found at increased frequency in patients with different autoimmune diseases. For example, patients with rheumatoid arthritis have an increased frequency of HLA DR4. HLA DR4 (initially defined serologically) encompasses numerous different alleles that have been defined by sequencing. Interestingly, not all subtypes of HLA DR4 are associated with an increased frequency of rheumatoid arthritis, but those alleles that are associated with this disease share a short amino acid sequence (QKRAA) at positions 70 to 74 of the β-chain of the HLA DR molecule. This sequence, termed the 'shared epitope' is located along the peptide-binding groove of HLA DR4, which presents peptides to the antigen receptor of T cells. Interestingly, this same 'shared epitope' is present in many individuals with rheumatoid arthritis who are positive for HLA DR1.

Table 2 Systemic autoimmune diseases

Disease	Prominent tissue target	Prominent autoantigen(s)	Disease mechanisms	Clinical features
Polymyositis (PM)/ dermatomyositis (DM)	Skeletal muscle	Mi-2 helicase tRNA synthetases DNA repair machinery	Complement activation (DM) Activated effector lymphocytes (PM)	Proximal muscle weakness (PM/DM) Heliotrope/skin rash (DM) Interstitial lung disease
Rheumatoid arthritis	Synovial joints	IgG Fc Citrullinated peptides Calpastatin	Activated cytokine pathways Activated effector lymphocytes Immune complex deposition	Symmetric, erosive polyarthritis
Scleroderma	Skin, lung, gastrointestinal, kidney, heart	Topoisomerase-1 (diffuse form) RNA polymerases (diffuse) Centromere proteins (CREST form)	Activated effector lymphocytes Anti-endothelial cell antibodies	Progressive fibrosis of skin, and multiple internal organs (including gastointestinal, lung, kidney and heart) Raynaud's phenomenon Vasculopathy
Sjögren's syndrome	Exocrine glandular epithelial tissue	Ro/SS-A; La/SS-B	Epithelial cell death induced by cytotoxic lymphocytes and other immune effector pathways	Keratoconjunctivitis sicca
Systemic lupus erythematosus	Numerous, including skin, kidney, joints, haematological elements, nervous system	dsDNA/nucleosomes Splicing ribonucleoproteins (e.g. Sm, U1-RNP) Ro/SS-A; La/SS-B Ribosomal P proteins Phospholipid–protein complexes	Autoantibody-mediated pathology Immune complex deposition	Multisystem inflammatory disease Skin lesions Arthritis Renal disease Anaemia, thrombocytopenia
Wegener's granulomatosis	Numerous, including upper airways, lungs, kidneys, and skin	Neutrophil proteinase-3 (cANCA)	cANCA binding to neutrophil surface induces degranulation in the vessel wall with consequent damage	Multisystem inflammatory vascular disease with predominance of sinus, middle ear, lung, and renal involvement

cANCA, cytoplasmic-staining antineutrophil cytoplasmic antibodies.

A similar principle appears to hold for patients with insulin-dependent diabetes mellitus, where there is a strong association of disease with a specific DQβ genotype. Whereas the DQβ sequence from most normal individuals has an aspartic acid at position 57, most patients with diabetes from the same population group had valine, serine, or alanine at that position.

Since MHC class II molecules function as a scaffold for presentation of specific peptides to T cells (see below), it is possible that this MHC-encoded susceptibility to disease reflects the ability of these alleles to present unique self-peptides to autoreactive T cells. Presentation of these specific peptides may play a critical role in disease initiation and propagation. It is important to note that an added level of complexity appears to be present that has not yet been accounted for. The presence of significant linkage disequilibrium within the MHC region (i.e. large stretches of DNA do not undergo recombination, generating functional cassettes of associated genes) also creates the potential for the disease association of particular MHC alleles to be influenced by additional genes on the extended haplotype in affected individuals.

Determination of which autoantibodies are produced in patients with a particular disease

In some autoimmune diseases, certain MHC class II alleles are strongly associated with the ability to mount a particular autoantibody response in that disease. For example, glutamate at position 34 and leucine at position 26 of the DQα1 and DQβ1 chains, respectively, have the strongest association with the ability to make antibodies to Ro and La (ribonucleoprotein antigens in systemic lupus erythematosus/Sjögren's syndrome). Similar observations have been made for numerous other autoantibody specificities, for example anti-DNA, antiphospholipid, and antiribonucleoprotein antibodies. This specificity may again reflect the ability of a particular MHC class II molecule to capture and present self-peptides to T cells. Where specific autoantibodies are associated with unique elements of disease phenotype (such as anti-DNA with renal disease, anti-Ro with photosensitive skin disease), MHC alleles may also be associated with specific disease phenotypes.

Non-MHC genes

Genes outside the MHC affect both susceptibility to, and the phenotypic expression of, autoimmune disease. For example, in studies performed by Wakeland and colleagues in lupus-prone mice, susceptibility and severity of lupus nephritis have been mapped to several different genetic intervals, including regions on chromosomes 1 (*sle1*), 4 (*sle2*), 7 (*sle3*), and 17 (*sle4*). While *sle1* mice exhibit loss of tolerance to chromatin and make autoantibodies to nucleosomes, they do not develop lupus nephritis. Similarly, mice having *sle3* exhibit low-grade polyclonal B- and T-cell activation, and only mild glomerulonephritis. Mice having both *sle1* and *sle3* and female gender show robust autoantibody response (targeting numerous antigens including nucleosomes), splenomegaly, and severe, fatal glomerulonephritis. The definition of the complex genetics underlying autoimmune diseases may

delineate those critical pathways required for development of self-sustaining disease, which might be amenable to therapy (see Fig. 1).

Similar types of observations have been made in insulin-dependent diabetes mellitus, where multiple non-MHC genes are associated with development of disease. There has also been the recent description of a single non-MHC gene (AIRE—for autoimmune response—that appears to be a transcription factor) which is strongly associated with the development of autoimmune polyendocrinopathy with candidiasis and ectodermal dysplasia (APECED) syndrome. The mechanisms whereby single or combinations of genes render individuals susceptible to development of autoimmune diseases are not yet clear, but major strides in this area are likely to be forthcoming within the next 5 to 10 years.

Environmental factors

That environmental insults and stochastic events influence the development of autoimmunity is clear from twin studies and in animal models, as individuals with an identical genotype may be variably affected by disease. For example, the concordance of systemic lupus erythematosus in identical twins is approximately 30 to 50 per cent, and for rheumatoid arthritis it is only about 15 per cent. Many potential environmental insults have been suggested to play a role in autoimmune diseases. These include infections, irradiation, and exposure to drugs and toxins. For example, exacerbations of systemic lupus erythematosus can follow sunlight exposure, and there are numerous reports that disease initiation may have a similar association with ultraviolet irradiation in rare patients. Numerous infections have been postulated to play a role in disease initiation across the spectrum of human autoimmune diseases (see below). In rare cases, the association between antecedent infection and subsequent development of disease is evident (for instance autoimmune myocarditis induced by Coxsackie virus infection, acute rheumatic fever following streptococcal infection, and Epstein–Barr virus infection with childhood systemic lupus erythematosus).

In the majority of autoimmune diseases an environmental connection has not been possible to confirm with any certainty. This does not imply that a causal connection does not exist in these instances, but rather reflects several features of the diseases that greatly complicate firm establishment of such a connection. These are (i) the kinetic complexity of the autoimmune diseases—since establishment of a recognizable disease phenotype often takes months, evidence of the initiating insult may have disappeared by the time the environmental component is sought for the first time; (ii) several different environmental insults may induce a similar response; and (iii) the environmental force may be extremely frequent in the population, and may only induce autoimmune disease in a unique subset of individuals with appropriate susceptibility genes.

How environmental forces influence initiation of autoimmune diseases is not yet known for most autoimmune diseases, but several plausible mechanisms have been advanced. These include: (i) the disruption of cell and tissue barriers, allowing previously sequestered antigens access to a

Fig. 1 Genetic susceptibility to autoimmune disease involves multiple interacting loci. Wakeland and colleagues have shown that numerous genes (*sle1*, *sle2*, *sle3*) interact to generate lupus-like autoimmunity in mice. By taking a non-autoimmune mouse (B6), and making a series of mouse strains carrying discrete disease susceptibility intervals, these investigators reproduce fully the phenotype in a lupus-susceptible host (NZM2410). In addition to genes that have a positive effect on generating the autoimmune phenotype, other 'suppressor' genes may counteract the effects of susceptibility genes. (Redrawn from Wakeland EK *et al.*, 1999, *Immunity* **11**, 131–9).

previously ignorant immune system (see below); (ii) inducing novel pathways of antigen presentation; (iii) alteration of the structure of self-antigens; and (iv) molecular mimicry. Some of these mechanisms are dealt with in more detail below.

Pathogenesis

Although extraordinarily complex in detail, the adaptive immune response operates by a set of relatively simple principles: (1) the immune system has the capacity to discern molecular structure in extremely fine detail; (2) it has a uniquely adapted set of signalling systems that computes the amount of antigen; and (3) it responds in a binary way to contextual information, that is, seeing an antigen in the setting of a dangerous context (such as infection) initiates an immune response, while seeing the antigen in the absence of such costimulatory signals leads to tolerance. Numerous studies over the past two decades have underscored that the sustained autoimmune response is extremely similar to adaptive immune responses directed against foreign pathogens, except that the driving antigens in autoimmune disease are self-molecules. For example, autoantibodies in most autoimmune diseases display evidence of isotype switching (for example from IgM to IgG or IgA), and show features of having undergone affinity maturation through somatic hypermutation. These properties of autoantibodies require the activity of antigen-specific CD4+ T cells, and have therefore focused much attention on defining the mechanisms whereby self-reactive T cells are activated in autoimmunity. Since this is such a central issue in the understanding of autoimmunity, and since there are numerous mechanisms employed by the normal individual to prevent activation of autoreactive T cells, it is important to review briefly the mechanisms that the normal immune system uses to maintain tolerance against self-proteins.

Thymic and peripheral T-cell tolerance purges the T-cell repertoire of receptor specificities that recognize self-peptide/MHC complexes

In order to prevent the survival of lymphocytes that will probably encounter their cognate antigens in healthy self-tissues, with potential autoimmune destruction of tissues, the immune system spends significant energy on testing the specificity of all receptors generated during antigen-independent development of lymphocytes, initially in the thymus and subsequently in the periphery. When the T-cell receptor generated through somatic recombination recognizes a peptide/MHC complex in the thymus with high affinity/avidity, cells expressing this receptor are negatively selected (since they are probably self-reactive, and will recognize their cognate antigens at additional peripheral sites). These self-reactive cells undergo apoptosis in the thymus, and never make it into the periphery. In contrast, those T-cell receptors that have some affinity for the selecting MHC molecule, but not for the peptide contained in the groove, are likely to recognize foreign peptides, and are positively selected. This process of establishing tolerance to self-proteins in the thymus is called 'central tolerance'.

T cells exiting the thymus therefore encompass cells which can recognize peptides within the scaffold of the MHC molecule used to select that T cell, but which have not encountered their specific peptide in the thymus. Since not all self-antigens are expressed in the thymus, there is still a chance that these T cells will encounter a self-peptide/MHC complex in the periphery for which they have high affinity. Since cells that have left the thymus no longer have the developmental context that is likely to denote a self-peptide (that is, recognition with high affinity of a peptide/MHC complex during development in the thymus), peripheral T cells utilize another binary system to define whether a high affinity interaction should lead to activation or inactivation. This binary system uses additional cell surface molecules (called costimulatory molecules) to denote context. Thus, when peripheral T cells recognize a peptide/MHC complex with high affinity in the absence of costimulation (through ligation of CD28 by surface B7.1 or B7.2 on the antigen-presenting cell), T cells are inactivated or tolerized. This is known as peripheral tolerance. In contrast, when peripheral T cells recognize a peptide/MHC complex with high affinity in the presence of costimulation, these T cells are activated.

In addition to T-cell tolerance, B-cell tolerance to self-components is also actively maintained. Thus, if B cells encounter either soluble or membrane-bound antigen during development in the bone marrow, these cells are either deleted (tolerance) or inactivated such that they become refractory to specific stimulation by their antigen (anergy).

Mechanisms which allow an immune response to be directed against self-antigens

Although tolerance to self-molecules is stringently maintained at the T- and B-cell levels, reactivity against self-molecules may still be possible for several reasons. These include the following.

Abnormal immunoregulation

There are numerous mechanisms used to establish and maintain T- and B-cell tolerance. There is accumulating evidence that defects in regulation of these pathways may result in the failure to eliminate autoreactive lymphocytes, or an altered activation threshold for lymphocytes. Examples include defects in the Fas/Fas–ligand system, a receptor–ligand pair which is required for removal of activated, self-reactive lymphocytes. Mice or humans with defects in this pathway manifest profound lymphadenopathy and a spectrum of autoimmunity. Similarly, defects in regulatory molecules which normally function to dampen the immune response (such as CTLA-4, the inhibitory T-cell receptor for the costimulatory molecules B7.1 and B7.2) may result in profound autoimmune responses. Mice lacking CTLA-4 develop fatal autoimmunity, with widespread T-cell infiltrates. Whether similar defects occur in human autoimmune diseases remains to be determined. It should be remembered that the immune system is a highly complex system, with interdependent regulation present at numerous levels. It is likely that many of the susceptibility genes in human autoimmunity impinge on these immunoregulatory pathways.

Existence of sites of immune privilege

Strict sequestration of tissue-specific antigens behind anatomical and immunological barriers prevents the development of tolerance to molecules expressed preferentially at these sites. Events (such as penetrating trauma) which breach this tight boundary may allow initiation of an immune response to these previously hidden self-molecules. Relevant examples include antigens within the eye, testis, and central nervous system. In the eye for instance, penetrating injury to one eye may be followed by development of inflammation in the contralateral eye (sympathetic ophthalmia) approximately 1 to 2 weeks after injury. Several mechanisms have been proposed to be responsible for maintaining the immune-privileged status of these tissues. One powerful mechanism appears to involve the constitutive expression of Fas–ligand in the relevant tissue (such as the eye). When this molecule binds to and activates its receptor on lymphocytes, these cells undergo apoptotic death, and are prevented from entering the tissue.

Cryptic determinants within self-molecules that are not normally revealed during antigen processing by default pathways, and allow the persistence of potentially autoreactive lymphocytes

Not all regions of a molecule are equally immunogenic. Regions of the molecule that are captured well by class II MHC molecules during natural processing of self-antigens are able to tolerize T cells (these determinants have been termed 'immunodominant' by Sercarz and colleagues). In contrast, regions of self-molecules that are not generated in significant amount during natural antigen processing (so-called 'cryptic determinants') cannot effectively tolerize T cells, since they are never seen by these cells either in the thymus or peripherally. This immunodominance appears to be influenced by the intrinsic affinity of the peptide for MHC class II, as well as by

Fig. 2 Dominant and cryptic T-cell epitopes in autoimmune disease. (a) The default processing pathway for intact antigen results in the preferential and reproducible loading of the 'dominant' peptide determinant into the antigen-binding groove of MHC class II. During establishment of thymic and peripheral tolerance, T cells recognizing this dominant epitope are purged from the repertoire, but T cells recognizing cryptic epitopes do not encounter their antigens, and are not deleted or anergized. (b) and (c) When the processing of self-antigens is altered (for example by novel proteolysis or through high-affinity binding to another molecule), a different hierarchy of epitopes is loaded on to class II MHC. If cryptic epitopes are loaded in sufficient amounts, these peptides can stimulate autoreactive T-cell responses directed against the cryptic self, and drive the autoimmune process.

neighbouring structural determinants on the antigen that may influence its binding to the peptide-binding groove. On self-molecules, two sets of determinants can therefore be defined (Fig. 2):

(1) those that are easily processed and presented (comprising the dominant self), which readily tolerize developing T cells.

(2) those that are not presented in appreciable amounts after natural processing (comprising the cryptic self), which do not tolerize.

There are unusual circumstances in which natural processing of self-antigens is altered from the default pathway. Examples include novel proteolysis of autoantigen (which destroys the dominant epitope or generates a new dominant epitope) prior to entry into the processing pathway, as well as high-affinity binding to specific receptors or antibodies, which can hinder access of the dominant epitope to the antigen-binding groove of MHC class II molecules, or optimize the loading of a previously cryptic epitope. Since T cells recognizing these cryptic peptides have not previously been tolerized, such 'autoreactive' T cells can now be activated (Fig. 3).

There are several clear demonstrations that autoreactive T cells recognizing cryptic epitopes can be activated *in vivo* through altered processing of self-molecules to reveal these previously immunocryptic epitopes. For instance, high-affinity binding of the HIV surface protein gp120 to CD4 alters the processing of CD4, and activates T cells which recognize epitopes of CD4 not generated during normal antigen processing. This mechanism may account for the autoimmune response to CD4 seen during HIV infection. Similarly, although intact mouse cytochrome c is not immunogenic in mice, cleavage of the molecule into smaller peptides induces a robust T-cell response to cryptic areas of cytochrome c, which were never previously presented by the natural processing pathway, and therefore did not induce tolerance.

The revelation of cryptic epitopes in self-antigens is likely to be a highly relevant mechanism in many human autoimmune diseases, but the studies to demonstrate the importance of this mechanism have only recently begun in earnest. Since the structure of autoantigens influences the hierarchy of dominant and cryptic and determinants generated when the molecule is processed, unique processes which alter the structure of molecules may play critical roles in initiation of autoimmune diseases. These unique events

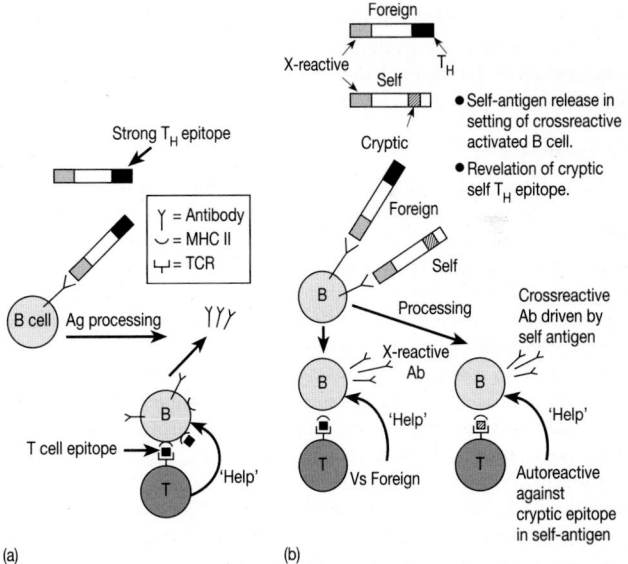

Fig. 3 Molecular mimicry. (a) Foreign antigens, which clearly differ from their homologous self-antigens in some areas, may nevertheless bear significant structural similarity to self-antigens in other regions. Initiation of an immune response to the foreign antigen may generate a cross-reactive antibody response that also recognizes the self-protein. When the self-antigen is a cell surface molecule, antibody-mediated effector pathways can lead to host tissue damage. Although the antibody response is cross-reactive with self-molecules, the T cells that drive this response are directed exclusively at the foreign antigen. (b) Under highly novel conditions, the simultaneous liberation of significant amounts of self-antigen in the setting of a cross-reactive antibody response may allow effective presentation of cryptic epitopes in the self-antigen to autoreactive T cells by activated cross-reactive B cells. These autoreactive T cells can now continue to drive an autoantibody response to the self-antigen. If continued release of self-antigen occurs as part of this process, a specific, adaptive immune response to self will be sustained.

are not likely to occur during normal homeostasis, but may occur preferentially during infectious or other pro-immune events at the host–environment interface. Relevant examples include the following.

1. Unique proteolytic pathways are activated that specifically alter the structure of autoantigens during immune effector pathways. It has recently been observed that the majority of autoantigens targeted across the spectrum of human autoimmune diseases are specifically cleaved by granzyme B during killing of infected target cells by cytotoxic lymphocytes. This cleavage generates unique molecular fragments never generated in the organism during development or homeostasis. Interestingly, this cleavage is a unique feature of autoantigens, and does not affect non-autoantigens. Although it has been proposed that these cleavage events allow the efficient presentation of previously cryptic epitopes, this remains to be formally demonstrated.

2. Additional post-translational modifications alter conformation of antigens and modify their subsequent processing. It is noteworthy that numerous post-translational modifications of autoantigens occur, and that in some cases the autoimmune response is strictly dependent on the occurrence of these modifications. Examples include phosphorylation, acetylation, deimination, and isoaspartyl formation, amongst others.

3. High-affinity complexes are formed between autoantigens and other viral or self-proteins.

In all these examples it should be remembered that the initiating event in autoimmunity requires that, on the background of appropriate susceptibility genes, several stringent criteria needed to initiate a primary immune response must be simultaneously satisfied. These include the generation of suprathreshold concentrations of self-molecules that have a structure not previously tolerized by the immune system, and the presentation of these unique molecular forms to T lymphocytes in the presence of costimulation (that is, in a pro-immune context).

Molecular mimicry

Foreign antigens, which clearly differ from their homologous self-antigens in some areas, may nevertheless bear significant structural similarity to self-antigens in other regions. Initiation of an immune response to the foreign antigen may generate a cross-reactive antibody response that also recognizes the self-protein (molecular mimicry). When the antigen is a cell surface molecule, antibody-mediated effector pathways can lead to host tissue damage. Although the antibody response is cross-reactive with self-molecules, the T cells that drive this response are directed at the foreign antigen (see below). Diseases involving this sort of 'antigen mimicry' therefore tend to be self-limited. It is important to realize that molecular mimicry alone cannot explain self-sustaining autoimmune diseases, which are driven by self-antigens and autoreactive T cells. In these cases, there is a requirement for overcoming T-cell tolerance to the self-protein. The simultaneous liberation of self-antigen in the presence of the cross-reactive antibody response is likely to play a critical role in this regard (see below).

Mechanistic insights into molecular mimicry: source of cross-reactive antibodies and potential role in overcoming T-cell tolerance to self-proteins
Although a number of microbial and viral antigens have regions of high homology with various human autoantigens, a causal link between exposure to these foreign antigens and the onset or exacerbation of autoimmune disease has been extremely difficult to establish. However, there are clear examples which suggest the existence of 'one-shot' autoimmune processes, in which cross-reactive antibodies directed against surface self-antigens are generated following infection, and result in tissue damage. This persists until infection is cleared, and the immune response wanes. Although the mechanistic details of this scheme are difficult to prove *in vivo*, several pertinent examples exist. One of these is a seasonal epidemic form of Guillan–Barré syndrome seen in northern China, which follows *Campylobacter jejuni* infection. Affected patients make antibodies recognizing ganglio-

sides, and the disease has a self-limited course, which rarely recurs. The anti-ganglioside antibodies generated are probably responsible for the pathological findings of acute motor axonal neuropathy. Another plausible example of this mechanism (although with meager *in vivo* evidence) is immune thrombocytopenia in children. This process characteristically: (i) follows an infectious process; (ii) demonstrates antiplatelet antibodies, and (iii) frequently shows durable remissions. The mechanistic details of this process have been difficult to prove *in vivo*, and cross-reactive epitopes on potentially initiating pathogens have not yet been defined.

The single episodes of tissue damage in the setting of a cross-reactive immune response must be contrasted to the sustained, autoamplifying disease frequently seen in other autoimmune syndromes. The central issues in this regard are: (i) how T-cell tolerance to self-antigens might initially be broken, and (ii) once this has occurred, why these antigens continue to drive the immune response to self. Examination of tolerance to cytochrome c, a ubiquitous protein that has regions of homology and divergence across different species, has been very useful in understanding molecular mimicry of cross-reactive epitopes. Mouse cytochrome c shares significant homology with human cytochrome c, although they are entirely different in other areas. When Mamula and colleagues used mouse cytochrome c to immunize mice, no T-cell or antibody response to the murine protein was observed. When human cytochrome c was similarly used to immunize mice, strong T-cell epitopes on the foreign cytochrome c were able to induce a strong antibody response to the foreign protein. The antibodies induced recognized both the murine and the human forms of cytochrome c, that is, cross-reactive antibodies that recognize the self-protein were produced. However, the T-cell response to cytochrome c was directed entirely against the foreign (human) form of the protein, and no T cells against the murine protein could be found. These cross-reactive antibodies disappear as the immune response to the foreign protein wanes.

Interestingly, when mouse cytochrome c was included with human cytochrome c during the immunization, a T-cell response to human cytochrome c, and a humoral response to the human protein that cross-reacts with the murine protein were induced. Within a few days, a strong helper T-cell response specific for murine cytochrome c was detected. This breaking of T-cell tolerance to murine cytochrome c was dependent on activated B cells specific for cytochrome c, which probably exert their effect through altering the processing of mouse cytochrome c, potentially uncovering previously cryptic epitopes in the self-protein (see Fig. 3). In the presence of continued release of self-antigen, this response may become self-sustaining—self-antigen driving autoreactive T cells, providing help to autoantibody-producing B cells (Fig. 3).

Molecular mimicry may therefore induce the production of cross-reactive antibodies, which in the absence of liberation of significant amounts of self-antigen, should disappear when the foreign pathogen is cleared. The form of epidemic motor axonopathy described above is probably representative of this scenario. Under highly novel conditions, the simultaneous liberation of significant amounts of self-antigen in the setting of a cross-reactive antibody response may allow effective presentation of cryptic epitopes in the self-antigen to autoreactive T cells by activated cross-reactive B cells. If continued release of self-antigen occurs, a specific, adaptive immune response to self will be sustained. Antigen release from tissues probably plays a critical role in driving this autoimmune process. Understanding the mechanisms of ongoing antigen release at sites of tissue damage in autoimmune disease (such as unique pathways of cell injury and death) is a high priority for future work, as it provides a novel target for therapy (see below).

It is clear from the above discussion that extraordinary complexity is operative in initiation of the human autoimmune diseases. The patient population is genetically heterogeneous, the human immune system is complex and extremely plastic, and it interacts with a plethora of environmental stimuli and stochastic events. The simultaneous confluence of susceptibility factors and initiation forces to set off the self-sustained and autoamplifying process is therefore an extremely rare occurrence. In contrast, once activation of autoreactive T cells has occurred, the ability of the immune system to respond vigorously to vanishingly low concentrations of antigen, to amplify the specific effector response to those antigens, and to spread the response to additional antigens in that tissue, greatly reduces the stringency that must be met to keep the process going (Fig. 4).

Effector mechanisms in autoimmune diseases

The initiation phase of autoimmunity requires co-operation between many different cell types, including antigen-presenting cells, T cells, and B cells, as well as numerous soluble mediators including antibodies, chemokines, and cytokines. The effector phase of autoimmunity uses the same immune and inflammatory effector mechanisms that the immune system has evolved for removing and destroying pathogens. These include activation of the complement cascade, which generates signals that effect inflammatory cell recruitment and activation. Similarly, ligation of activating Fc receptors on inflammatory cells by immune complexes activates macrophage and neutrophil effector function. Autoantibodies directed against cell surface antigens initiate antigen-dependent cellular cytotoxicity, probably mediated by macrophages and natural killer cells. Cytokines and chemokines play a central role in inflammatory cell recruitment and activation in the target tissue. Tissue damage can also be effected by cytolytic lymphocytes. The pathology characteristic of each autoimmune disease reflects the particular antigens targeted as well as the predominant effector mechanisms activated.

One principle of central importance in the effector phase of autoimmunity is autoamplification (Fig. 4), which appears to play a central role in the self-sustaining nature of the autoimmune process. Thus, immune effector pathways cause damage to cells in the target tissue, liberating antigen which further stimulates the immune response and effector pathways, thus liberating more antigen. Although this is probably an oversimplification, the view that the immune system plays a role in generating an ongoing supply of autoantigen is useful therapeutically, since it focuses

Fig. 4 Model of initiation and propagation of autoimmune disease. Autoimmune diseases are highly complex disorders which require the simultaneous co-operation of multiple factors for their development. Numerous susceptibility genes (some of which regulate the immune response) appear to determine the threshold for disease initiation. In many diseases, a discrete, pro-immune environmental trigger probably plays a role in disease initiation, but is infrequently recognized. A critical requirement for disease initiation is the generation of suprathreshold concentrations of self-antigen with novel structure. Development of a recognizable disease phenotype generally requires marked antigen-driven amplification of the autoimmune response, in which immune effector pathways play a role in generating the ongoing supply of antigen to sustain the process.

attention on controlling both the supply of antigen as well as immune effector pathways (see below).

Clinical features

The clinical features of the different autoimmune diseases are extremely diverse, and reflect the specific tissue dysfunction which results from activity of immune effector pathways. Almost all tissues may be affected, including prominent involvement of endocrine organs, nervous system, eye, bone marrow elements, kidney, muscle, skin, liver and gastrointestinal tract, blood vessels, lung, and joints. For tissue-specific autoimmune processes (such as insulin-dependent diabetes mellitus, immune thrombocytopenia, autoimmune haemolytic anaemia (AIHA)), symptoms may relate to tissue hypofunction resulting from: (i) target cell destruction (for insulin-dependent diabetes mellitus, destruction of the β-cells of the pancreatic islets; for immune thrombocytopenia and AIHA, destruction and phagocytosis of platelets and erythrocytes); or (ii) antibody-mediated interference with function or down-regulation of autoantigen expression (for example in myasthenia gravis, bullous pemphigus). In other cases, symptoms may arise from tissue hyperfunction (for example in Graves' disease) due to activating effects of antibody binding (where antibodies to the thyroid-stimulating hormone receptor induce non-physiological thyroid hormone secretion).

In the case of systemic autoimmune processes, symptoms frequently result from localized target tissue destruction (for example skeletal muscle in polymyositis, skin disease in systemic lupus erythematosus) as well as from the more general activities of inflammatory effector pathways. The latter result from: (i) immune complex deposition at multiple sensitive sites (such as joints, kidney, skin, and blood vessel walls) with activation of the complement cascade and recruitment and activation of myelomonocytic cells; and (ii) ongoing secretion of pro-inflammatory cytokines. In this regard, the profoundly positive effects of tumour necrosis factor inhibition recently observed on the inflammatory symptoms and joint destruction in rheumatoid arthritis underscore the central role of these general inflammatory mediators in generation and maintenance of the disease phenotype in systemic autoimmune diseases.

Prognosis

While the barriers that need to be overcome in terms of initiating an autoimmune disease are highly stringent, and are very difficult to satisfy even in the setting of appropriate susceptibility genes, the immune system is equipped with a powerful memory. The mechanisms of memory are still incompletely defined, but include the generation of a population of memory cells specific for the antigen that initiated the response, which respond vigorously (in terms of clonal expansion as well as effector function) to very low concentrations of antigen if they encounter it again. Since the autoimmune diseases are disorders driven by the ongoing release of self-antigen, this immunological memory constitutes a major barrier to complete cure. Autoimmune diseases therefore tend to be self-sustaining over long periods, and are often punctuated by clinical exacerbations (flares), which are probably due to re-exposure of the primed immune system to antigen (for example in systemic lupus erythematosus, autoimmune myositis, and rheumatoid arthritis). The possibility of disease recurring, even after long clinical remission, remains present in most of the autoimmune diseases. Tissue-specific autoimmune diseases may result in the complete destruction of the target tissue over time, with loss of function of that tissue accompanied by a waning immune response (for example in insulin-dependent diabetes mellitus). Interestingly, in cases where immune-mediated tissue pathology results from effector pathways being driven by a cross-reactive T-cell response to a foreign antigen (for example in epidemic Guillain–Barré syndrome), disease has a finite duration, and generally does not recur.

Therapy

It is not possible to discuss the therapy of this broad group of disorders in any detail in this chapter, but a few principles that underlie current approaches to therapy are discussed. Autoimmune diseases cause significant tissue dysfunction through: (i) inflammation, (ii) tissue destruction with loss of functional units, (iii) the consequences of healing, and (iv) functional disturbances (such as interference with acetylcholine signalling by autoantibody to the acetylcholine receptor and inducing receptor down-modulation in myasthenia gravis). Therapeutic interventions in auto-immune diseases are generally focused on controlling immune and inflammatory pathways, and at replacing or accommodating lost function.

Controlling the immune and inflammatory pathways responsible for ongoing damage

Since in the majority of instances, the critical autoantigens and effector pathways responsible for unique diseases have not been defined, this goal is frequently extremely challenging to accomplish. Thus, frequent use is made of anti-inflammatory and immunosuppressive therapies which broadly target many aspects of the immune response (such as steroids, azathioprine, cyclophosphamide, methotrexate, and mycophenolate). Since a robust immune response is required to protect the host from a myriad of infectious threats, this non-targeted suppression of the immune system can have deleterious consequences in terms of increased susceptibility to infection, with its attendant high morbidity and mortality. In this regard, therapeutic targeting of specific inflammatory pathways is extremely attractive, and there are recent examples in which this approach has been highly successful. In rheumatoid arthritis, the maintenance of chronic inflammatory joint pathology appears to be dependent on the activity of tumour necrosis factor. Specific inhibition of tumour necrosis factor through the use of either soluble tumor necrosis factor receptors or humanized monoclonal antibodies has led to an astonishing effect on disease activity in rheumatoid arthritis, with abolition of systemic symptoms, and a striking decrease in the rate of joint destruction. These positive effects were associated with only a minimal increase in susceptibility to infection, although this risk is certainly present. Inhibition or stimulation of specific inflammatory pathways as therapy for autoimmune diseases may well be more broadly applicable, and will certainly be tested in other autoimmune processes once critical roles of additional specific inflammatory pathways are defined.

Another example of specific targeting of pro-inflammatory pathways is that of intravenous immunoglobulin. This is prepared from pooled serum and its major component is immunoglobulin G. Intravenous immunoglobulin therapy has been used as a treatment for several autoimmune diseases, including immune thrombocytopenia, autoimmune myositis, and acute demyelinating polyneuropathy, but is only available at prohibitive cost. Recent data from mice have demonstrated that intravenous immunoglobulin induces surface expression of the inhibitory Fcγ receptor (FcγRII$_B$) on macrophages, and shifts the balance of signalling through Fc receptors towards inhibition, down-regulating the pro-inflammatory response to immune complexes. It is likely that continued identification of additional agents that precisely modulate specific inflammatory pathways will have a major therapeutic impact on this group of diseases.

Interventions aimed at replacing or accommodating lost function

The majority of autoimmune diseases are associated with loss of function of organs and tissues, many of which perform essential physiological functions. Indeed, recognition of the autoimmune phenotype in many instances requires that tissue damage is sufficiently severe to have led to characteristic loss of function. For example, loss of insulin-secreting β-cells of the pancreatic islets results in insulin-dependent diabetes mellitus, and blockade and down-regulation of the nicotinic acetylcholine receptor

causes striated muscle weakness and fatigue in myasthenia gravis. Similarly, chronic immune complex deposition in glomeruli causes renal inflammation and scarring in systemic lupus erythematosus. Where significant functional reserve is still present in a particular disease, a strong argument can be made for preventing further damage through specific or general immunosuppressive strategies described above. This is particularly relevant where the 'supply' of tissue that could be damaged is essentially inexhaustible (for example most instances of systemic autoimmune disease). Where functional impairment is already established, interventions aimed at replacing or accommodating lost function are indicated. For example, insulin replacement is required for insulin-dependent diabetes mellitus, and treatment for hyperthyroidism is indicated in Graves' disease.

Summary

Autoimmune disease results when the immune system becomes activated to recognize self-antigens. The response is antigen-driven and T cell-dependent, and is directed against highly specific autoantigens that are in many instances disease specific. The genetic contribution to autoimmunity is important, with MHC and non-MHC genes playing significant roles. MHC genes may confer susceptibility to disease in some cases, and determine the autoantibodies produced in others. The essence of sustained autoimmune disease is the breaking of T-cell tolerance to self-molecules, resulting in a sustained immune response to self, and consequent tissue damage. Although the mechanisms by which tolerance is broken remain unclear, it is likely that, in the genetically susceptible host, environmental influences play an important role in the initiation of an autoimmune response. Possible mechanisms include alteration of antigen structure, location, concentration, processing, presentation, and context. The pathology characteristic of each autoimmune disease reflects the particular antigens targeted as well as the immune effector mechanisms activated. Ongoing immune-mediated damage probably plays a central role in providing autoantigen to drive the continuing autoimmune response.

Further reading

Diamond B *et al.* (1992). The role of somatic mutation in the pathogenic anti-DNA response. *Annual Review of Immunology* 10, 731–57. [Comprehensive review of the evidence that autoantibodies are antigen driven and T-cell dependent.]

Feldmann M, Brennan FM, Maini RN (1996). Rheumatoid arthritis. *Cell* 85, 307–10. [Short review of the complex pathogenesis of rheumatoid arthritis.]

Gammon G, Sercarz EE, Benichou G (1991). The dominant self and the cryptic self: shaping the autoreactive T-cell repertoire. *Immunology Today* 12, 193–5. [Concise introduction to the concepts and consequences of immunodominance.]

Gianani R, Sarvetnick N (1996). Viruses, cytokines, antigens, and autoimmunity. *Proceedings of the National Academy of Science USA* 93, 2257–9. [Review of the pathogen–host interface and autoimmunity.]

Kotzin BL (1996). Systemic lupus erythematosus. *Cell* 85, 303–6.

Lanzavecchia A (1995). How can cryptic epitopes trigger autoimmunity? *Journal of Experimental Medicine* 181, 1945–8. [Important review of potential mechanisms of autoimmunity.]

Lin R-H *et al.* (1991). Induction of autoreactive B cells allows priming of autoreactive T cells. *Journal of Experimental Medicine* 173, 1433–9. [Important demonstration that autoreactive B cells may alter the processing of self-antigens to allow activation of autoreactive T cells.]

Morel L *et al.* (1999). Epistatic modifiers of autoimmunity in a murine model of lupus nephritis. *Immunity* 11, 131–9. [Clear definition of the complex genetics of systemic lupus erythematosus.]

Naparstek Y, Plotz PH (1993). The role of autoantibodies in autoimmune disease. *Annual Review of Immunology* 11, 79–104.

Radic MZ, Weigert M (1994). Genetic and structural evidence for antigen selection of anti-DNA antibodies. *Annual Review of Immunology* 12, 487–

520. [Comprehensive review of evidence that autoimmunity is driven by self-antigen.]

Rosen A, Casciola-Rosen L (1999). Autoantigens as substrates for apoptotic proteases: implications for the pathogenesis of systemic autoimmune disease. *Cell Death and Differentiation* **6**, 6–12. [Revew of role of altered autoantigen structure in autoimmune diseases.]

von Muhlen CA, Tan EM (1995). Autoantibodies in the diagnosis of systemic rheumatic diseases. *Seminars in Arthitis and Rheumatism* **24**, 328–58. [General review of autoantibodies and their specificities.]

Wicker LS, Todd JA, Peterson LB (1995). Genetic control of autoimmune diabetes in the NOD mouse. *Annuual Review of Immunology* **13**, 179–200. [Review of the complex genetics of mouse autoimmune diabetes.]

5.4 Complement

Mark J. Walport

Introduction

Jules Bordet first discovered complement as an activity in serum that complemented the activity of antibody in the killing of bacteria—hence its name. Complement comprises a group of more than 20 plasma and cell-bound proteins and is part of the innate immune system. The direct binding of particular complement proteins to potential pathogens activates a cascade of sequentially acting complement proteins.

Complement is a triggered enzyme cascade, initiated by the binding of any of three complement proteins, C1q, mannose-binding lectin, or C3, to acceptor molecules, especially on the surface of potential pathogens. The binding of these molecules may be direct or, in the case of C1q, to antibody bound to antigens (immune complexes). The binding of C1q to immune complexes represents an important bridge between the adaptive immune system and the innate immune system.

After initiation, the activation of complement is amplified by the sequential activation of a series of enzymes, which lead ultimately to the cleavage of C3 and C5. Thus a small initiating signal, for example from binding of a few mannose-binding lectin molecules to the surface of a bacterium, leads to cleavage of a large number of C3 and C5 molecules. These amplification steps in complement activation increase the effectiveness of complement as a host defence mechanism but also carry the risk to the host that inappropriate complement activation may cause bystander inflammatory injury to host tissues. To prevent this, there is a large array of regulatory mechanisms that prevent inappropriate complement activation and reduce the chance of complement injury to self tissues.

A detailed description of the biochemistry of complement is beyond the scope of this chapter; recent reviews that describe this are provided at the end of the chapter. This chapter will focus on the diseases associated with abnormalities of the complement system. We will first consider the different physiological activities of complement, which is necessary in order to understand the role of complement in disease. We will then review the diseases associated with hereditary disorders of complement, followed by diseases in which there are acquired complement abnormalities. The chapter will end with a consideration of when and how assays of the complement system should be performed in the assessment and management of disease.

Physiology of complement

The physiological activities of complement are summarized in Table 1. There are three overarching activities. The first is the role of complement in host defence against infectious disease. Complement provides mechanisms for the killing and clearance of micro-organisms; it does this by the covalent binding to their surface of C3 and C4 fragments that are ligands for receptors on phagocytic cells that ingest and kill the organism. The activation of complement also causes the generation of the anaphylatoxins, C5a and C3a, which have chemotactic activity and recruit leucocytes to sites of infection and inflammation. A further role of complement in host defence against infection is generation of the membrane attack complex. This may disrupt the cell membrane and kill the micro-organism.

The second activity of complement is as a bridge between the humoral adaptive immune system (antibody) and innate immunity. Activation of complement by immune complexes facilitates the clearance of antigen and thereby helps to prevent immune complexes from causing inflammatory damage to tissues, although, as we shall see, complement may contribute to inflammatory injury to tissues in circumstances when immune complexes persist. Activation of complement also augments antibody responses and thereby enhances host defence against pathogens. The binding of complement to antigens reduces the threshold of B lymphocytes for activation. It enhances antigen presentation and B cell memory by helping to localize antigen on antigen-presenting cells and on the follicular dendritic cells that are key to the maintenance of B cell memory for foreign antigens.

The third activity of complement is in the resolution of inflammatory responses. It is in this role that complement may prevent the development of systemic lupus erythematosus (SLE) by promoting the clearance of tissue debris.

Complement in disease

Hereditary disorders

Studies of the inherited abnormalities of the complement system have illuminated our understanding of the major roles of the complement system *in vivo*. There are three types of disease associated with hereditary complement deficiency. The first is immunodeficiency, which illustrates the role of complement in host defence against infection. The second is the association

Table 1 Physiological activities of the complement system

Activity	Complement proteins responsible for activity
Opsonin	Covalently bound fragments of C3 and C4
Chemotaxis and activation of leucocytes	Anaphylatoxins: C5a, C3a, and C4a
Lysis of bacteria and cells	Membrane attack complex: C5b-C9
Disposal of cellular debris	C1q, covalently-bound fragments of C3 and C4
Augmentation of antibody responses	C3b and C4b bound to immune complexes and to antigen

of systemic lupus erythematosus with deficiency of certain classical pathway proteins. This association has led to a greater understanding of the role of complement in the resolution of inflammation and in the waste disposal mechanisms of the body. The third category of disease is caused by deficiencies of proteins of the regulatory mechanisms of the complement system. This small group of diseases illustrate the effects of unrestrained activation of the complement system. We will consider each of these associations.

Complement deficiency and infection

Patients lacking C3 and the pathways leading to C3 activation show increased susceptibility to pyogenic infections with bacteria such as *Streptococci* and *Staphylococci*. There is a similar susceptibility to infections in patients lacking antibodies or normal phagocytic function (see Chapters 5.5 and 5.6). This shows that the normal pathway for host defence against such bacteria is binding of antibody, followed by complement, providing opsonins for uptake and bacterial killing by phagocytes. Disruption of any of the links in this chain causes increased susceptibility to infection by these pyogenic bacteria.

Neisserial infection and complement deficiency

Humans who lack one of the proteins of the membrane attack complex (C5, C6, C7, C8, or C9) display a unique susceptibility to neisserial infection, especially by *Neisseria meningitidis*, which is frequently recurrent (Fig. 1 and Plate 1). This pattern of infection shows that host defence against these bacteria, which are capable of intracellular survival, is mediated by their lysis by the membrane attack complex. Individuals lacking the earlier components of the complement system, which are the necessary precursors for the formation of the membrane attack complex, are also at increased risk of neisserial infection. Deficiency of properdin is also especially associated with neisserial infections. This protein stabilizes the alternative pathway C3 convertase enzyme and augments the cleavage of C3. It is encoded on the X chromosome and therefore properdin deficiency is found almost exclusively in males. Increased susceptibility to neisserial infections is also a feature of acquired complement deficiency, such as may be seen in patients with SLE or with C3 nephritic factor.

When should complement deficiency be suspected in a patient with infectious disease? Immunodeficiency should be suspected in any individual who has recurrent or unexplained major infections. The type of infection provides a clue to the relevant investigations of the immune system. Recurrent pyogenic infections imply a need to assay the activity of antibodies, the complement system, and phagocytic function.

In the specific case of meningococcal sepsis, factors that point to complement deficiency are recurrent attacks, a family history of meningococcal infection (especially if disseminated in time), or infection by unusual strains of *N. meningitidis*. Individuals with complement deficiency remain susceptible to neisserial infection throughout life and may present at any age.

Mannose-binding lectin deficiency

Mannose-binding lectin is a protein homologous in structure to C1q that initiates complement activation by a pathway similar to the classical pathway. Mannose-binding lectin binds to terminal mannose groups in a spatial orientation that is present on many micro-organisms, including certain Gram-positive and Gram-negative bacteria, mycobacteria, yeasts, and parasites, but absent on mammalian cells. It is one of the 'pattern-recognition' molecules of the innate immune system that binds molecules present on potential pathogens but not on the cells of the host. The importance of its role in host defence was identified when it was discovered that a group of children with recurrent bacterial infections in early childhood were deficient in the ability of their serum to opsonize yeast with C3 *in vitro*. It turned out that this *in vitro* opsonic deficiency was caused by a subtotal deficiency in the expression of mannose-binding lectin. The most important causes of this common deficiency are mutations of residues in the collagen domain of mannose-binding lectin, which cause misassembly of the

multimer and thereby have a dominant effect suppressing mannose-binding lectin levels.

The clinical effects of mannose-binding lectin deficiency are most apparent in young children from the ages of 2 to 5, when maternal passive immunity has waned and the antibody response has not yet matured. At this stage of life the innate immune system is of particular importance in host defence against infection.

Complement deficiency and autoimmune disease

A dramatically increased prevalence of SLE is found amongst patients with deficiencies of proteins of the classical pathway of complement. There is a hierarchy of susceptibility and severity of SLE according to the position of the missing protein in the pathway of classical pathway activation (Table 2).

These cases of SLE, associated with inherited complement deficiency are, *in toto*, extremely rare and only account for a tiny minority of the population of patients with SLE. However, they provide an important clue to the aetiology of the disease. They show that there is an important activity of the early classical pathway of complement that protects against the development of SLE. The source of the autoantigens that drive the autoimmune response in SLE is thought to be apoptotic cells. Complement has been

(a)

(b)

Fig. 1 Patient with hereditary deficiency of C6 who presented with meningococcal septicaemia. (a) a subconjunctival haemorrhage. (b) The deficiency of C6. Serum from the patient was placed in the central well of an agarose-coated plate. In each of the outer wells was placed antiserum to, respectively, C5, C6, C7, and C8. The antibody and antigen were allowed to diffuse in the gel and where the antibody encountered its antigen a precipitate formed, which was stained blue. No precipitate formed between the anti-C6 antibody and the patient's serum, indicating C6 deficiency. (See also Plate 1.)

Table 2 Association of complement deficiency with SLE

Complement protein deficiency	No of cases described	Prevalence of SLE
C1q	42	39/42 (93%)
C1r and C1s	14	8/14 (57%)
C4	24	18/24 (75%)
C2	>100	approx. 10%[a]
C3	23	3/23 (13%)

[a] C2 deficiency is the commonest hereditary homozygous classical pathway complement deficiency and is present in about 1:20 000 Western European Caucasoid individuals.

found to play a role in the disposal of apoptotic cells and in the processing of immune complexes. Loss of these activities might lead to abnormal processing of effete cells, that, in the context of an inflammatory response, could initiate and drive an autoimmune response leading to the development of SLE.

Hypotheses such as this may be tested in animal models of disease. A series of mice have been developed lacking molecules that have been implicated in the 'waste-disposal' mechanisms of the body. These include mice lacking C1q, serum amyloid P component (which coats and may mask extracellular chromatin from the immune system), DNase 1 (which digests extracellular chromatin), and IgM (which may augment the clearance of effete cells and cellular debris). Each of these spontaneously develops SLE and supports the hypothesis that effective mechanisms of cellular waste disposal are essential to prevent the development of SLE.

Abnormalities of complement regulation

C1 inhibitor deficiency

The disease hereditary angioedema is caused by deficiency of C1 inhibitor. This is inherited as an autosomal dominant disorder with partial penetrance. The disease is dominantly inherited because the production of C1 inhibitor from a single, normal allele is insufficient to maintain normal homeostasis of the complement and kinin pathways. The mutations may have two effects on protein production. In type 1 hereditary angioedema, which accounts for approximately 85 per cent of cases of the disease, the mutant prevents any expression of protein from the mutant allele. This variety of disease is therefore associated with reduced levels of C1 inhibitor.

Type 2 hereditary angioedema is caused by a series of point mutations in the C1 inhibitor gene that alter one of the amino acids at the active centre of the protein and abolish its activity as a serine proteinase inhibitor. These mutations allow expression of normal amounts of protein, which is nonfunctional, or even abnormally high C1 inhibitor levels, because the mutant protein is not consumed by normal interaction with activated serine proteinases. It is easy to miss the diagnosis of this variant of hereditary angioedema, if it is not appreciated that levels of C1 inhibitor can be normal or high in patients with the disease.

The clinical manifestations of hereditary angioedema are caused by vascular leakage of fluid that cause angioedematous swellings. The swellings are caused by the action of small peptides, called kinins, in particular bradykinin, that cause increased vascular permeability by their actions on vascular endothelium and smooth muscle. These kinins are produced by the action of serine proteinases that are ineffectively regulated in the presence of reduced activity of C1 inhibitor.

Allergy is much commoner than hereditary angioedema as a cause of angioedema. In hereditary angioedema, the swelling is not itchy and is not accompanied by other features of allergy such as asthma and urticaria. The disease is potentially life-threatening if there is major pharyngeal or laryngeal swelling, causing airways obstruction. Swelling of the submucosa of the intestines may cause severe abdominal pain and temporary obstruction of the bowel.

Diagnosis of hereditary angioedema is made on the basis of the clinical findings described above, the presence of family history, and blood tests. A

family history of angioedema makes diagnosis much easier but is not always present. This is because some cases of the disease are due to new mutations in the C1 inhibitor gene. In other families, other members with C1 inhibitor deficiency may have no clinical symptoms.

The abnormal blood tests associated with hereditary angioedema are reduced C1 inhibitor protein levels (usually below 30 per cent of normal levels) in patients with type 1 hereditary angioedema. However, in the 15 per cent of patients with type 2 disease, protein levels may be normal or high. In these patients functional assays of C1 inhibitor are necessary. These are based on the ability of C1 inhibitor to block cleavage of a chromogenic substrate by activated C1s. In addition to these abnormalities, levels of C2 and C4 are typically low. This is because the reduced C1 inhibitor activity allows C1s to cleave C4 and C2 in an unregulated fashion.

Treatment of the disease involves, firstly, the treatment of acute attacks and, secondly, prophylaxis to attempt to prevent their recurrence. Acute attacks of hereditary angioedema do not respond to epinephrine, though if there is any cause to suspect allergic rather than hereditary angioedema, then administration of epinephrine is unlikely to cause any harm. If attacks involve the airways, then respiratory support is the first priority. Acute attacks of angioedema may be arrested by infusion of purified C1 inhibitor concentrate. If this is not available, fresh frozen plasma may be infused. This is less satisfactory, as plasma not only contains C1 inhibitor but also kallikrein, C1r, and C1s, which may generate further kinin production. In patients with repeated attacks of angioedema or infrequent but life-threatening attacks of disease, prophylactic treatment should be given. C1 inhibitor levels originating from the single normal allele increase in response to treatment with impeded androgens, such as danazol and stanozolol. This is a moderately effective treatment, although these compounds still retain some virilizing activity. An alternative, though probably less effective therapy (there are no randomized trials), is the proteinase inhibitor tranexamic acid, which may reduce the consumption of C1 inhibitor by blocking the activity of the serine proteinases that interact with C1 inhibitor.

Diseases associated with unregulated C3 activation

Factor I and Factor H deficiency A key step in the regulation of complement activation is control of the fate of the C3 fragment, C3b. This acts as the nucleus for formation of further C3 convertase enzyme, unless it is catabolized by the serine esterase enzyme, Factor I, in conjunction with the cofactor protein, Factor H. Deficiency of either of these proteins allows the unregulated formation of C3 convertase enzyme and continuing cleavage of C3 (Fig. 2). Patients with deficiency of Factor I or H have a severe secondary deficiency of C3 and are susceptible to the pyogenic infections associated with this C3 deficiency. In addition, the enormous turnover of C3 associated with these deficiencies allows some C3 to deposit in glomerular basement membrane, which leads to the development of glomerulonephritis, which may proceed to renal failure. A number of families have been identified with inherited mesangiocapillary glomerulonephritis and some of these have mutations in just one Factor H allele, suggesting a dominant form of glomerulonephritis caused by partial Factor H deficiency. The mechanism of this form of nephritis is not understood.

Acquired disorders of complement

Complement is activated *in vivo* by many stimuli, which include invading organisms, the formation of immune complexes, and tissue necrosis. When complement activation occurs on a substantial scale, this causes depletion of complement proteins, which may be measured as a reduction in their antigenic levels or as a reduction in the activity of the classical and/or alternative pathway. The measurement of complement activation may be useful in both the diagnosis and monitoring of some diseases.

In the case of sepsis associated with endotoxic shock, the large-scale systemic activation of the complement system may play an important part in the pathogenesis of this lethal condition. Activation of the classical and alternative pathways by bacterial endotoxin causes the generation of large amounts of the anaphylatoxins, C3a and C5a, and of membrane attack complex which activate neutrophils and endothelial cells causing vascular and pulmonary injury, leading to death. Diagnosis of this condition is sadly all too easy and the measurement of complement in such patients does not play an important role in assessment or management.

Tissue necrosis is also an important cause of complement activation. Therapeutic studies of experimental models of myocardial infarction, and of ischaemia–reperfusion injury in other organs, including the brain, have shown that inhibition of complement causes a significant reduction in tissue injury and final infarct size.

The diseases associated with acquired complement activation may be divided into two categories. The first category is the diseases associated with abnormal regulation of complement, which is most commonly caused by certain autoantibodies to complement. Paroxysmal nocturnal haemoglobinuria is a further example of an acquired disorder of regulation of the complement system. The second category is the diseases in which infection or autoimmunity cause clinically important activation of the complement system.

(a)

(b)

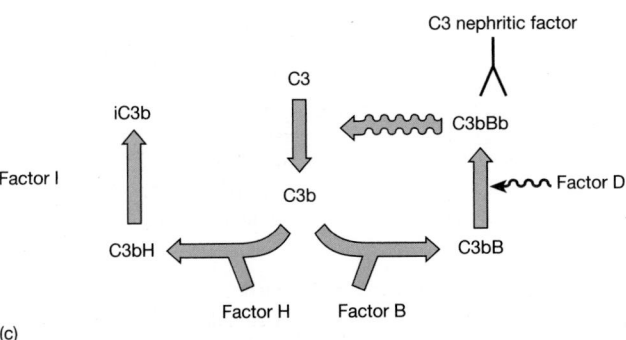

(c)

Fig. 2 Unregulated activation of C3 caused by Factor H or I deficiency, or by C3 nephritic factor. Panel A illustrates the normal control of C3 cleavage. In plasma and tissues any C3b that is formed by the normal low-grade turnover of C3 is bound by Factor H and catabolized by Factor I to inactive products. Panel B shows the effects of Factor H or Factor I deficiency. C3b can not be catabolized to inactive products. Instead there is increased formation of the alternative pathway C3bBb C3 convertase gene causing accelerated cleavage and depletion of C3. Panel C shows the effects of C3 nephritic factor. This antibody stabilizes the C3bBb C3 convertase enzyme. This results in accelerated cleavage and depletion of C3.

Diseases associated with abnormal complement regulation

We shall consider four diseases caused by acquired abnormalities of the regulation of complement. The first three of these are associated with the development of high-affinity autoantibodies to complement proteins, known as C3 nephritic factor, anti-C1q antibodies, and anti-C1 inhibitor antibodies. The fourth disease is paroxysmal nocturnal haemoglobinuria, in which a clone of haematopoietic cells loses expression of a family of cell surface molecules including regulatory proteins of the complement system.

Autoantibodies to complement proteins

C3 nephritic factor C3 nephritic factor is an autoantibody that binds to and stabilizes the C3bBb C3 convertase enzyme. This increased stability of the C3 convertase enzyme disrupts the normal regulation of C3 activation and leads to chronic consumption of C3 (Fig. 2). Patients with C3 nephritic factor have very low C3 levels in serum, accompanied by normal C4 levels. When serum from a patient with C3 nephritic factor is mixed with normal serum, the C3 in the normal serum is activated and converted to C3b, which forms the basis of an assay for C3 nephritic factor.

The presence of C3 nephritic factor is associated with three clinical manifestations. The first of these is partial lipodystrophy, in which there is disfiguring loss of fat from the face and upper part of the body. Adipocytes, or fat cells, produce several complement proteins including C3 and factor D, which was independently discovered in fat cells and named adipsin. It is thought that C3 nephritic factor stabilizes the assembly of a C3 convertase enzyme on adipocytes causing the activation of complement on these cells leading to their destruction. The second clinical feature is of mesangiocapillary glomerulonephritis type II, in which electron-dense deposits of unknown composition, associated with C3 deposited at the margins of the electron-dense deposits, are found in the glomerular basement membrane. This form of nephritis may be severe, leading to renal failure. The third clinical feature is of recurrent infections, caused by the severe acquired deficiency of C3 associated with this condition.

The conventional approach to treatment of patients with type II mesangiocapillary glomerulonephritis is the use of corticosteroids, often in combination with immunosuppressive agents such as azathioprine or cyclophosphamide.

Anti-C1q antibodies These autoantibodies react with a neoepitope, exposed in the collagenous region of C1q, which has dissociated from the other proteins of the C1 complex, C1r and C1s. Up to a third of patients with SLE develop anti-C1q autoantibodies. These are associated with activation of the classical pathway, causing very low C4 levels and, to a lesser extent, reduced C3 levels. The presence of anti-C1q autoantibodies is a marker for severe SLE, especially for the presence of lupus nephritis.

Anti-C1q antibodies are also found as the sole autoantibody in the uncommon disease hypocomplementaemic urticarial vasculitis (HUVS). In this condition, very high titres of anti-C1q antibodies are typically found, which may sometimes cause precipitation of C1q *in vitro*, hence they are known as C1q precipitins. The main clinical feature of HUVS is chronic urticaria, which is found on biopsy to be associated with a cutaneous vasculitis. Other clinical features of HUVS include glomerulonephritis, neuropathy, and chronic obstructive bronchitis. There is a considerable degree of overlap between the clinical manifestations of HUVS and SLE. This is analogous to the relationship between SLE and the primary antiphospholipid syndrome, discussed in Chapter 18.11.2.

Anti-C1 inhibitor antibodies The third disease associated with an autoantibody to a complement protein is angioedema associated with autoantibodies to C1 inhibitor. The symptoms and signs of this are very similar to the disease of hereditary angioedema, though typically occur with a late onset. Measurements of complement proteins in the serum from patients with this disease show a similar abnormal profile to that seen in the blood of patients with hereditary angioedema, with low C1 inhibitor and low C4 levels. Additional abnormalities are low C1q levels and the presence of autoantibodies to C1 inhibitor. This serious condition is frequently associated with the presence of a B cell lymphoma.

Paroxysmal nocturnal haemoglobinuria

Paroxysmal nocturnal haemoglobinuria (PNH) illustrates the role of membrane-bound complement regulatory proteins in protection against the activation of complement on normal cells. Haemolysis in this disease is caused by the loss of expression of a membrane protein named CD59. This prevents the formation and assembly of the membrane attack complex of complement in cell membranes and thereby inhibits the lysis by complement of autologous cells (see Chapter 22.3.12).

Complement in autoimmune disease

The measurement of complement is a useful diagnostic tool as part of the assessment of patients with vasculitis and glomerulonephritis (Table 3). Some of the causes of these conditions are associated with systemic activation of the complement system on a sufficient scale that plasma levels of classical pathway proteins and C3 are significantly reduced below normal. In these diseases, it is the formation of immune complexes, either in the circulation or *in situ* in tissues, that is responsible for the activation of the complement system.

SLE

The relationships between the complement system and SLE are complex. As we have discussed, inherited deficiency of classical pathway complement proteins causes SLE. However, the vast majority of patients with SLE do not have homozygous deficiencies of complement proteins. Indeed, in these patients, SLE is associated with large-scale activation of the classical pathway of complement. The deposition of complement proteins in tissues, associated with the presence of immune complexes, has been thought to play a role in causing inflammatory lesions in tissues in SLE. Deficiency of C1q protein is most strongly associated with the development of SLE, yet as we learnt above, approximately one-third of patients with SLE develop autoantibodies to C1q.

The explanation for these complex relationships between complement and SLE is partially understood. Studies in animal models of SLE show that the predominant manner in which immune complexes cause inflammation is by ligation of Fc receptors. Mice lacking Fc receptors were protected from glomerulonephritis caused by immune complexes, whereas mice lacking complement developed full-blown lupus glomerulonephritis. A key role of complement may be to protect against the development of tissue injury by immune complexes by promoting their clearance from tissues, rather than playing a major role in the causation of injury.

We have already discussed how C1q deficiency might cause the development of SLE. How might SLE cause the development of anti-C1q antibodies? The essential feature of SLE is the formation of autoantibodies to complexes of autoantigens, such as the spliceosome complex and chromatin. C1q binds to the cellular debris that is thought to be the source of the autoantigens that drive the autoimmune response in SLE. As part of the debris, C1q may become antigenic and evoke an autoimmune response. This is a situation analogous to the association in SLE, and the primary antiphospholipid syndrome, of the presence of anticardiolipin autoantibodies with anti-β2 glycoprotein I antibodies. β2-glycoprotein I is a plasma protein that binds to negatively charged phospholipids that are exposed on the cell membranes of apoptotic cells and may thereby become part of the cellular debris that drives the autoimmune response in SLE.

The measurement of complement and of anti-C1q antibodies in SLE is of clinical value in both the diagnosis and management of patients. Serum from patients with active disease typically shows evidence of classical pathway activation with reduced C4 and, to a lesser extent, reduced C3 levels. In patients with persistently very low C4 levels, there is a high likelihood that anti-C1q antibodies will be present and such patients are more likely to have, or to develop, glomerulonephritis. Patients with persistent, severe hypocomplementaemia are at increased risk of pyogenic infections and there are strong arguments for the use of prophylactic penicillin in such patients.

Haemolytic anaemia

There is sometimes sufficient systemic complement activation associated with the haemolytic anaemias caused by autoantibodies to erythrocyte surface antigens to cause reduction in the levels of complement proteins measured in serum. This is most prominent in cold agglutinin disease (see Section 22) in which IgM cold agglutinins, which bind to I antigen, cause the deposition of many thousands of C4 and C3 molecules per erythrocyte.

The accelerated clearance of erythrocytes in autoimmune haemolytic anaemias is mainly caused by ligation of cells bearing Fc receptors in the spleen, in the case of IgG autoantibodies. In the case of cold agglutinin disease, mediated by an IgM autoantibody which cannot bind to Fc receptors, there is typically low-grade intravascular haemolysis by complement.

Human red cells are well protected from complement-mediated lysis by complement regulatory proteins expressed on their cell membranes. As we have learnt, the activity of these proteins is illustrated dramatically by the disease PNH. Rarely, if there is extensive complement fixation, as in the case of a transfusion reaction caused by an ABO mismatch, then intravascular complement-mediated lysis of red cells may cause severe injury.

Infectious disease

We have already discussed the role of complement in the innate immune system and as an effector arm of humoral adaptive immunity by illustration of the infections that accompany hereditary or acquired complement deficiency. Complement is also involved in the pathogenesis of infections in other ways. For example several viral pathogens use the complement system in a subversive manner as part of their pathogenesis (Table 4). Several infections cause hypocomplementaemia through systemic activation of

Table 3 Levels of complement in patients with vasculitis and glomerulonephritis

Systemic vasculitis		Glomerulonephritis	
Normal complement	**Reduced complement**	**Normal complement**	**Reduced complement**
Polyarteritis nodosa	SLE	Minimal change glomerulonephritis	Poststreptococcal glomerulonephritis
Microscopic polyangiitis	Essential mixed cryoglobulinaemia	IgA nephropathy	Mesangiocapillary glomerulonephritis associated with factor H deficiency or C3 nephritic factor
Wegener's granulomatosis	HCV-associated vasculitis		
Henoch–Schönlein purpura	SBE-associated vasculitis		
	Hypocomplementaemic urticarial vasculitis		
	Waldenström's hypergammaglobulinaemic purpura		

Table 4 Viral subversion of the complement system

Activity	Virus	Host molecule	Viral molecule
Virus uses cell surface complement protein as receptor	Epstein–Barr virus	Complement receptor type 2 (CD21)	
	Measles	Membrane cofactor protein (CD46)	
Virus binds host complement protein to enter cell	HIV West Nile virus	C3b	
Virus expresses complement regulatory protein to avoid complement attack	Herpes simplex		Viral C3b receptor

complement in a similar fashion to autoimmune disease and we shall consider some examples.

Complement activation is a feature of chronic bacterial sepsis, for example in subacute bacterial endocarditis or ventriculoatrial shunt infection. In both of these conditions there is chronic release of bacterial antigens in the presence of an antibacterial antibody response that cannot eliminate the infection because of its relative inaccessibility to the immune system. This causes the chronic production of immune complexes with complement activation by the classical pathway, associated with low C4 and C2 levels and glomerulonephritis and small vessel vasculitis.

Chronic viral infection by hepatitis C is a further important cause of acquired hypocomplementaemia. This infection stimulates the production of large amounts of rheumatoid factor, which in some patients may lead to cryoglobulin production, causing complement consumption and vasculitis. In one survey in Japan of hypocomplementaemia in blood donations, infection with hepatitis C was the major cause.

Another example of hypocomplementaemia associated with infection is the complement activation associated with poststreptococcal glomerulonephritis. In this disease, which is thought to be due to an immune response to a pathogen cross-reacting with host tissues, there is marked complement activation, which includes activation of the alternative pathway, associated with low C3 levels.

Measurement of complement in clinical practice

Throughout this chapter examples have been given of diseases which are associated with abnormal levels of complement proteins in the blood. Complement levels and activity can be assayed in clinical practice. It is useful to consider the value of measuring complement proteins in two categories, firstly in diagnosis of disease and, secondly, measurement repeatedly to monitor the activity of particular diseases.

When to measure complement

Complement in the diagnosis of disease

There are four groups of diseases in which it is important to be able to measure complement activity in serum. The first is the immunodeficiencies—it is essential to measure complement in patients with recurrent pyogenic infections, particularly in the context of recurrent or familial meningococcal disease. In this group of diseases, simple antigenic measurement of C4 and C3 levels is insufficient—it is necessary to use tests that assay the activity of the whole complement system, preferably haemolytic assays of the classical and alternative pathways. If absent or severely reduced activity is detected, then the sample should be referred to a specialist laboratory to try to identify the precise nature of the deficient component. Treatment should comprise counselling, prophylactic penicillin, and vaccination against meningococci.

The second group of diseases is vasculitis and glomerulonephritis. We saw in Table 3 how a very useful diagnostic subdivision of these diseases can be made on the basis of whether or not there is evidence of systemic complement activation. It is in these diseases that it can also be helpful to use assays of complement to monitor disease activity.

The third group are the chronic infections, which may masquerade as primary systemic vasculitis and, in this context, there should be a high index of suspicion for the presence of bacterial endocarditis or hepatitis C.

The fourth group of diseases are those specifically associated with abnormalities of the complement system, including hereditary and acquired angioedema, the familial glomerulonephritis associated with factor H deficiency, and the syndrome of partial lipodystrophy with or without mesangiocapillary glomerulonephritis.

Complement in the monitoring of disease

There are very few diseases in which the repeated monitoring of complement levels is useful. In SLE, no single test acts as a reliable surrogate for the measurement of disease activity. However, there are some patients in whom fluctuation in complement levels correlates with the waxing and waning of disease activity and, in these individuals, it is useful to monitor regularly C4 and C3 levels. It can also be useful to measure complement levels regularly in patients with autoantibodies to complement proteins; in these individuals the complement levels are a useful surrogate marker for the continuing presence of the autoantibody.

How to measure complement

Complement can be measured in a several ways. The simplest is antigenic measurement of the concentration of individual proteins, and measurement of the levels of C3 and C4 are the most widespread assays in clinical use. The results of such assays need to be interpreted cautiously. The ranges of normality are wide, because there is substantial genetic variation in the levels of these proteins. Furthermore, protein levels are a product of both synthetic and catabolic rates and both of these may vary in health and disease. Both C3 and C4 are acute phase reactants and concentrations of these proteins may rise, in the case of C3 by as much as 0.5 g/l in response to acute phase stimuli.

Measurement of C4 and C3 levels act as very crude surrogate markers of classical and alternative pathway activation respectively. However, further measurements are needed if there is any suspicion of the possibility of inherited complement deficiency or of an abnormality elsewhere in the complement system. Functional assays of complement are fairly straightforward and have the advantage that they measure the activity of all of the proteins in the complement system between activation and the end point, which is the lysis of target erythrocytes. The classical pathway is usually measured by assessment of the lysis by serum of sheep erythrocytes coated with a rabbit polyclonal antisheep erythrocyte antibody. The alternative pathway is measured by assay of the lysis of guinea pig erythrocytes, which directly activate the alternative pathway of complement in the absence of antibody, in the presence of a buffer that prevents classical pathway complement activity. Results of these assays are normally expressed as CH50 or AP50 units, which are measurements of the haemolysis of 50 per cent of respective erythrocyte preparations.

Other approaches have been devised to assess the presence of complement activation *in vivo*. Many assays have been developed which identify the products of activation of the complement system. Although these assays are attractive in principle, the products of complement activation are only present in plasma very transiently and, in practice, assays of total C4 and C3 levels, together with measurement of CH50, have not been supplanted as the best 'rough and ready' estimates of complement activation in routine clinical practice.

Further reading

Janeway C Jr, Travers P, Walport MJ, Shlomchik MJ (2001). *Immunobiology: the immune system in health and disease*, 5th edn. Garland Publishing, New York.

Liszewski MK, Farries TC, Lublin DM, Rooney IA, Atkinson JP (1996). Control of the complement system. *Advances in Immunology* **61**, 201–83.

Moffitt MC, Frank MM (1994). Complement resistance in microbes. *Springer Seminars in Immunopathology* **15**, 327–44.

Morgan BP, Walport MJ (1991). Complement deficiency and disease. *Immunology Today* **12**, 301–6.

Pickering M, Botto M, Taylor P, Lachmann PJ, Walport MJ (2000). Systemic lupus erythematosus, complement deficiency and apoptosis. *Advances in Immunology* **76**, 227–324.

Ross GD, ed (1986). *Immunobiology of the Complement System*. Academic Press, Orlando.

Turner MW (1996). The lectin pathway of complement activation. *Research in Immunology* **147**, 110–15.

Volanakis JE, Frank MM, eds (1998). *The human complement system in health and disease*. Marcel Dekker, New York.

Walport MJ (2001). Complement. *New England Journal of Medicine*, **344**,1058–66, 1140–4.

Williams DG (1997). C3 nephritic factor and mesangiocapillary glomerulonephritis. *Pediatric Nephrology* **11**, 96–8.

5.5 Innate immune system

D. T. Fearon and M. Allison

Innate immunity is an ancient system of host defence found in invertebrates as well as vertebrates. There are similar mechanisms and parallels between aspects of the innate immune systems of the fruit fly, *Drosophila*, and man. The innate immune system can therefore be considered to have two general functions; first, as a mechanism of primary host defence and, secondly, as a means of priming the adaptive immune system. Innate immunity performs the first of these functions in both invertebrates and vertebrates, having evolved many systems that facilitate the recognition and elimination of pathogens. The second role of the innate immune system in vertebrates is the instruction of the adaptive immune system. The enhanced specificity of the adaptive response is guided by the uptake recognition mechanisms of the innate immune system with the consequent generation of immunological memory for components of infectious organisms.

A key concept in understanding why the innate immune system has evolved the way it has is that an essential requirement is fulfilled—recognition of the presence of foreign organisms and, in effect, the differentiation of infectious from non-infectious. During the evolution of the innate immune system certain properties of micro-organisms that differentiate them from the host have been identified and diverse ways of detecting pathogens have gradually developed. These recognition systems have evolved in association with a range of effector mechanisms, some innate themselves and others induced through the instigation of an antigen-specific, adaptive immune response. The innate recognition systems are described in this context.

Recognition systems, soluble and membrane-bound

The innate immune system has evolved several mechanisms for detecting the presence of 'infectious' substances as such, through the development of molecular species that recognize the lowest common structural denominators of invading micro-organisms. These receptors are both soluble proteins in blood and extracellular fluid and also membrane-bound species.

Complement

The complement system is an ancient system of host defence, found in invertebrates (e.g. sea-urchin) as well as mammals. The initial methods of activation and the specific members of the early component pathways differ between the classical pathway, the lectin pathway, and the alternative pathway. All, however, use as one of their effector arms the formation of the membrane attack complex, which forms a pore in the cell membrane, as the method of killing cells. The recognition reaction central to the tagging of surfaces of micro-organisms as infectious is the covalent attachment of activated C3 component to the microbial substance. This facilitates the elimination of the pathogen through recognition of the C3-coated surface by receptors which then phagocytose and kill the organism directly or indirectly, by formation *in situ* of the membrane attack complex and subsequent cytolysis (Fig. 1).

The complement system is essential for protective immunity against certain bacterial infections with polysaccharide antigens to which natural IgM reacts. In models of acute peritonitis, activation of the classical pathway of complement is required for the generation of an inflammatory response and resolution of the infection. The ability of complement-coated antigen to augment the antigen-specific response has also been proven through co-ordinated ligation of complement receptor 2 on B cells with the surface immunoglobulin within the B-cell receptor complex.

The complement system is thus essential for protective immunity to polysaccharide antigens against which natural IgM is reactive, in the generation of an effective inflammatory response in models of acute septic peritonitis, and in facilitating the production of an antigen-specific antibody response.

Soluble recognition molecules

In addition to the complement proteins, there are other secreted proteins that have a significant role in the systemic or local immune response (Table 1). In respect of local defence systems, there is increasing recognition that antimicrobial peptides may have a important role, particularly at mucosal surfaces. These include the defensins, which are polypeptides of 29

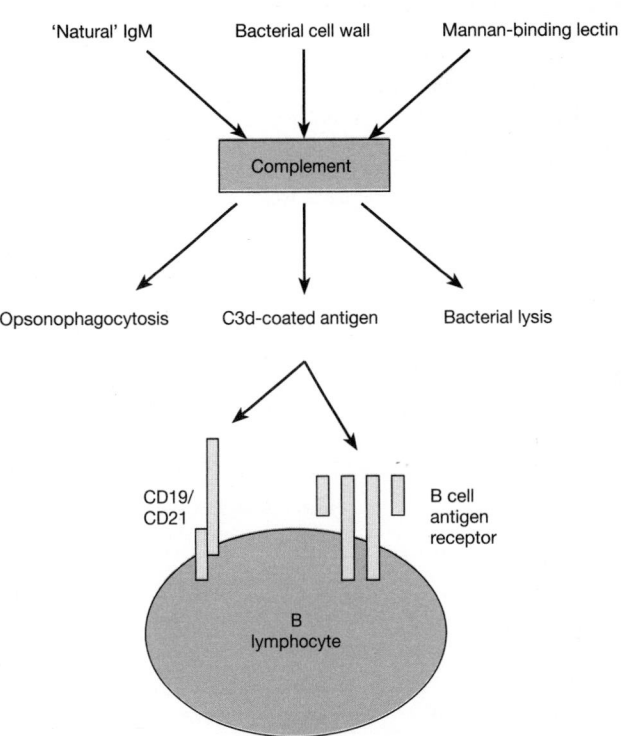

Fig. 1 The role of complement in the immune response.

Table 1 Recognition molecules—soluble receptors

Molecule	Site	Ligands	Functions
C3	Synthesis mainly in liver, induced in acute phase response	Hydroxyl groups on carbohydrates and proteins	Activated components bound by complement receptors for activation and clearance
Mannan-binding lectin (MBL)	Synthesis mainly in liver	Microbial cell wall saccharides	Bound by C1q receptor, complement activation phagocytosis
C-reactive protein (CRP)	Synthesis mainly in liver, induced in acute phase response	Microbial polysaccharides, DNA and ribonuclear proteins, phosphate esters	Complement activation, phagocytosis
Serum amyloid protein (SAP)	Synthesis mainly in liver, induced in acute phase response	Extracellular matrix proteins, microbial polysaccharides, DNA and ribonuclear proteins	Complement activation, phagocytosis, extracellular matrix protein stabilization
Lipopolysaccharide-binding protein (LBP)	Synthesis mainly in liver, induced in acute phase response	Binding and transfer of lipopolysaccharide to CD14, and from CD14 to serum lipoproteins	Increases sensitivity to lipopolysaccharide, clearance and inactivation of lipopolysaccharide

to 40 amino acids that exert microbicidal activity, most commonly by disruption of bacterial membranes. These proteins are able to augment the immune response by the activity of the human β-defensins 1 and 2, which are chemotactic for immature dendritic cells and memory T cells.

Mannose-binding protein recognizes carbohydrate moieties and has selectivity for foreign, as opposed to self, cell surfaces or glycoproteins as a result of the spacing of its terminal carbohydrate-recognition domains. Mannose-binding protein exists as an oligomer in the circulation and therefore achieves high-affinity interaction with multivalent carbohydrate molecular species, such as those found on microbial surfaces. Several different mutant alleles of mannose-binding protein have been described and individuals who are homozygous or heterozygous for the mutant alleles seem to be more susceptible to a certain infections, and exhibit a defect in opsonophagocytosis. There is evidence that other proteins, such as C1q, may act similarly since mannose-binding protein is recognized by a C1q receptor recently cloned from monocytes.

Mannose-binding protein is a member of the collection family of soluble proteins that also includes the surfactant proteins. These proteins possess collagenase domains and carbohydrate recognition domains. The latter mediate recognition of structures on the outer surface of micro-organisms. *In vitro*, surfactant protein-A and D bind carbohydrates on the surface of viruses, bacteria, and fungi and thereby may lead to the aggregation of the micro-organisms, thus encouraging phagocytosis by neutrophils and by alveolar macrophages. There is evidence that the surfactant proteins have a role in pulmonary defence; they bind to components of *Pneumocystis carinii* as well as *Cryptococcus neoformans*, which are important pathogens in

immunocompromised individuals. Furthermore, patients with cystic fibrosis, who are susceptible to repeated pulmonary infections, have diminished levels of surfactant protein-A and D; the deficiency correlates with reduced effective killing of pathogen.

A further family of soluble proteins that have an emerging role in the innate immune response are the pentraxins. The members of this family, which includes C-reactive protein and serum amyloid protein, exist as a radial pentameric structure in solution and recognize a variety of ligands such as phosphate esters and polysaccharides. Their production is induced by inflammatory cytokines, such as IL-1 and IL-6, and, as a consequence of being multimeric, they are able to activate the classical pathway of complement by directly binding C1q. In animal models, C-reactive protein has been found to have a role in protection against endotoxin-induced mortality. Recently, mice deficient in C-reactive protein have been found to develop autoantibodies, suggesting that C-reactive protein may also participate in the maintenance of immunological tolerance to self proteins, possibly by mediating the clearance of apoptotic cells.

Membrane-bound recognition receptors

In addition to soluble recognition systems, there are several cell-associated receptors whose cellular distribution reflects the effector arms of the immune system to which they are linked (Table 2). There are two broad types of receptor; those that have primarily an endocytic capacity and those that have signalling capacity.

The mannose receptor is an example of an endocytic recognition system and is expressed on tissue macrophages, immature dendritic cells, and

Table 2 Recognition molecules—surface receptors

Molecule	Expression	Ligands	Function
CR1 (CD35)	Macrophages, monocytes, polymorphonuclear cells, and lymphocytes	C3b, C4b	Augments cleavage of C3b and C4b
CR2 (CD21)	B lymphocytes, follicular dendritic cells	C3b degradation products	Enhanced B-cell activation
Mannose receptor	Tissue macrophages, dendritic cells, sinusoidal endothelial cells (liver), thymic epithelium	Microbial cell wall carbohydrates	Capture of antigen for presentation on class II and CD1b
DEC-205	Dendritic cell subset, thymic epithelium	Multiple carbohydrates	May capture antigen for class II presentation
CD14	Monocyte–macrophages, immature dendritic cells, polymorphonuclear cells	Lipopolysaccharide, various microbial cell wall constituents	Mediates response to lipopolysaccharide, microbial clearance
Toll-like receptors (Tlr)	Monocyte–macrophages	Lipopolysaccharide–LBP–CD14 complex?	Mediate response to lipopolysaccharide (Tlr 2 and/or T1r4)
Scavenger receptors			
Class AI/II	Macrophages, sinusoidal endothelial cells (liver), high endothelial venules	Lipopolysaccharide, lipotechoic acid and fungal cell walls	Microbial clearance, possible role in cell adhesion
Macrophage receptor with collagenous structure (MARCO)	Splenic marginal zone and medullary lymph node macrophages	Microbial cell walls	Bacterial clearance

some endothelial cells. This receptor recognizes saccharide residues commonly expressed on microbial surfaces but not those frequently found exposed on self glycoproteins. Hence this receptor is able to differentiate infectious from non-infectious and binds a large number of different organisms including *Mycobacteria*, *Trypanosoma*, yeast, and both Gram-positive and Gram-negative bacteria. Significantly, this receptor, which constitutively recycles to the cell surface through endosomal compartments, is able to target bound antigen for presentation on MHC class II molecules, and, in the case of a component of mycobacteria, lipoarabinomannan, on the non-classical MHC class I molecule, CD1b.

Within the same lectin family, but containing carbohydrate-recognition domains with a different structure, is DEC-205. Initially used as marker of dendritic cells but now known to be expressed on a subset of dendritic cells, DEC-205 may also be able to enhance presentation of antigen in the context of MHC class II molecules.

A further family of cell-surface receptors that is increasingly being recognized as having an important role in recognition and clearance of invading pathogens are the scavenger receptors. This group of recognition molecules is characterized by their broad ligand specificity; it was first identified by Brown and Goldstein in 1979 as responsible for binding modified, but not native, low-density lipoprotein. As well as binding acetylated and oxidized low-density lipoprotein, members of the scavenger receptor family also can recognize Gram-positive and Gram-negative bacteria, lipotechoic acid and lipopolysaccharide, and aldehyde-modified proteins. There are considered to be five classes of scavenger receptors, differentiated by structure and binding characteristics as well as the cells on which they are expressed. The class A scavenger receptors, expressed on macrophages, have a role in clearance of micro-organisms from the circulation. Mice deficient in two allelic forms of the class A scavenger receptors have increased susceptibility to herpes simplex virus and *Listeria*, as well as to the lethal effects of endotoxin.

A further exciting aspect of the biology of scavenger receptors is that they recognize apoptotic cells. This is achieved, at least in part, through their ability to bind phosphatidylserine, which becomes exposed on the surface of apoptotic cells during the process of cell death—a mechanism which may represent a means of clearing apoptotic cells in a way that avoids an inflammatory response.

Recognition of cell-surface components of pathogens is an important warning mechanism, indicating to the host the presence of foreign micro-organisms. It has long been recognized that a major constituent of the walls of Gram-negative bacteria, polysaccharide, is a potent inducer of an inflammatory response; lipopolysaccharide can be lethal through the induction of shock. The recognition of lipopolysaccharide, and hence the generation of an inflammatory cytokines in response to this stimulus, occurs through the CD14 surface receptor which binds lipopolysaccharide once lipopolysaccharide is itself bound by lipopolysaccharide-binding protein, a constituent of serum. The means of signalling upon ligation of lipopolysaccharide–lipopolysaccharide-binding protein by CD14 was, until recently, unclear, because CD14 is a glycophosphatidylinositol-linked membrane protein, and therefore would have no intrinsic signalling capacity. However, in 1997, Medzhitov and Janeway demonstrated the presence in humans of a protein homologous to the *Drosophila* protein Toll; they further showed that this facilitated the production of inflammatory cytokines by monocytes. Subsequently, four further members of the same family have been discovered and mutations in the gene encoding one of these toll-like receptors (Tlr4) have been found in two different strains of mouse that are lipopolysaccharide-non-responsive. Different members of the Tlr family can differentiate between various classes of micro-organisms—Tlr4 responds to Gram-negative organisms while Tlr2 is activated by Gram-positive pathogens and yeasts. Downstream consequences of ligation of CD14 and Tlr4 by lipopolysaccharide–lipopolysaccharide-binding protein, which include generation of inflammatory cytokines, are mediated through activation of the transcription factor, NFκB.

Cellular components of the innate immune system

Just as B and T lymphocytes are clearly constituents of the acquired response, macrophages, dendritic cells, and polymorphonuclear cells must be considered as key members of the innate response. Recently, greater attention has been given to the roles of these cells and the way they orchestrate an immune response, not just in their own right but also in co-ordinating the involvement of different arms of the adaptive immune system.

Macrophages

The monocyte/macrophage is beautifully adapted for its role of ingestion and intracellular killing of pathogens. It has several receptors that are able to recognize organisms or components of organisms and it is extremely active phagocytically—thus it can internalize bound micro-organisms and kill them after formation of phagosomes. In addition to the well-established production and activity of reactive oxygen species macrophages also produce reactive nitrogen intermediates (RNIs), including nitric oxide, by inducible nitric oxide synthase (iNOS or NOS2). Studies in mice deficient in NOS2 have demonstrated that the production of reactive nitrogen intermediates plays a non-redundant role in protection against viruses and intracellular pathogens. There is also synergy between nitric oxide formation and reactive oxygen intermediates, through the generation of peroxynitrite (ONOO⁻) which possesses additional microbicidal activity.

Dendritic cells

These cells are also bone-marrow derived (with the exception of a small subtype of dendritic cells). During maturation they pass through two functionally very different stages (Fig. 2). As immature dendritic cells, they populate various non-lymphoid tissues (e.g. Langerhans cells in the skin are immature dendritic cells) and actively sample their microenvironment through receptors, including the mannose receptor, DEC-205, and Fc receptors. Immature dendritic cells are thus well equipped to take up a large variety of antigens, and once activated by bacterial constituents, such as lipopolysaccharide and the CpG motifs within bacterial DNA, their surface phenotype changes and they are induced to migrate out of the tissues to

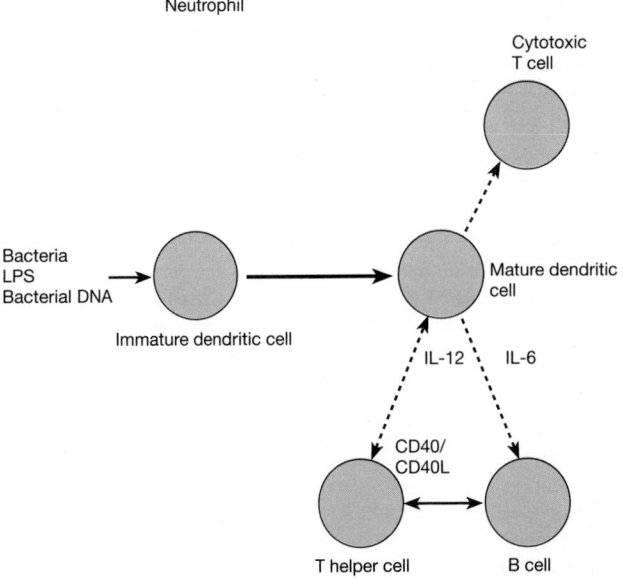

Fig. 2 The central role of the dendritic cell in the innate and acquired immune responses.

draining lymphoid tissue. By the time they reach the draining lymph nodes they acquire a fully mature phenotype; such antigen-capturing receptors as the mannose receptor and Fc receptor are down-regulated, and surface expression of MHC class II, as well as costimulatory molecules, CD80 and CD86, and, vitally, CD40, are up-regulated. At the same time, there is increased activity of the antigen-processing machinery within these cells, rendering them powerful 'professional' antigen-presenting cells.

The efficiency of dendritic cells is utilized by the immune system in several settings, and it is increasingly clear that they participate critically in the development of immune responses to certain tumours and viruses, both of which are mediated through CD8+ T cells. For some viral infections, the production of virus-specific CD8+ T cells requires the presence of antigen-specific CD4+ T cells. In this setting, activated dendritic cells provide the link, as these cells are able to stimulate CD4+ T cells, that then reciprocate by upregulating CD40 ligand on their surface. CD40 ligand then binds to CD40 expressed on the dendritic cells, giving a signal to these cells that enable them to activate antigen-specific CD+ T cells. Dendritic cells are absolutely required for initiation of antigen-specific CD8+ T cell responses to certain viral infections and tumours through a process called 'cross priming'. Antigens derived from one cell are captured by a second cell and this cell processes and presents antigenic determinants from the first cell in the context of surface MHC class I to CD8+ T cells. These CD8+ T cells are activated and expand clonally; they are then able to exhibit cytolyic activity for the first cell type, be it a tumour cell expressing the antigen or a virally-infected cell.

Neutrophils

Polymorphonuclear phagocytes constitute one of the principal arms of the innate immune system. As one of the first immune cells to arrive at the site of an infectious challenge, their response is important not only in the initial control of infection, but also in guiding the migration of other components to the local environment. Neutrophils, like macrophages, are phagocytically active and express receptors for bacterial peptides, complement components, and the constant regions of specific immunoglobulin isotypes. Hence, specific phagocytosis of either immunoglobulin- or complement-opsonized bacteria can occur. Signalling though some of these receptors induces activation of the neutrophil, with immediate release of reactive oxygen species and phospholipid-derived inflammatory mediators which exhibit microbicidal activity. The importance of this function in neutrophils and macrophages is reflected in the phenotype of individuals with chronic granulomatous disease who have a defect in the generation of the reactive oxygen species and who suffer from recurrent, non-resolving infections that are usually caused by organisms that express catalase.

Natural killer cells

Natural killer cells, although clearly related to T and B lymphocytes, are distinct in not expressing rearranged receptors for antigen or peptides fragments of antigen. First discovered as responsible for tumour cytolytic activity in mice devoid of lymphocytes, these cells can develop both from the bone marrow and from fetal thymocytes.

Natural killer cells act as a means of non-adaptive cellular cytotoxicity against tumour cells and some virally infected cells. Although these cells do not have antigen-specific receptors, a surface molecule, MICA, up-regulated on tumour cells and stressed cells (e.g. when virally infected) is recognized by a natural killer cell receptor, with consequent activation of the cell-killing machinery. Protection against lysis of healthy host cells is provided through the recognition by receptors on natural killer cells of self MHC class I molecules. Ligation of these receptors negatively regulates the natural-killer-cell-mediated lysis. Natural killer cell activation can be induced through ligation of CD16, the low affinity Fc receptor for IgG, on the surface of the cell leading to antibody-dependent cellular cytotoxicity. Inflammatory cytokines, including IL-15, TNF-α, IL-12, and IL-18, also trigger natural killer cell activation, with the concomitant production of interferon-gamma (IFN-γ).

Natural killer cells play an important and individual role in antiviral responses. For example adenovirus- and human cytomegalovirus-infected cells secrete proteins that inhibit surface MHC class I expression, which protect against antiviral cytotoxic T lymphocyte (CTL) activity, but these proteins also render the cells more susceptible to natural-killer-cell-mediated killing. A further protein, also produced by cytomegalovirus, however, is homologous to class I heavy chain and is able to bind to β$_2$-microglobulin. This protein facilitates transport of the complex to the cell surface and confers on the cell resistance to natural-killer-cell-mediated lysis.

Mast cells

Mast cells are most widely recognized for their role in allergic responses. They are bone marrow-derived cells whose proliferation and maturation are stimulated by a number of cytokines including, in particular, IL-3 and stem cell factor. The expression of FcεRI, the high affinity Fc receptor for IgE, is characteristic of mast cells. Once multiple molecules of IgE have bound to an allergen, ligation and cross-linking of this receptor can occur, which causes mast cell degranulation. The degranulating mast cell releases histamine, neutral proteases (for example tryptase), proteoglycans, and lipid mediators with diverse effects, including vasodilatation and increased vascular permeability, bronchoconstriction, and intestinal smooth muscle constriction.

Mast cells also aid the immune response to micro-organisms. They can phagocytose and, *in vitro* at least, present antigen in the context of MHC class I and class II molecules—although the functional importance of this in the host has not been demonstrated. These cells do, however, have a prominent role in the development of a protective response in animal models of acute septic peritonitis, in which they promote the clearance of organisms, in part by the production of TNF-α and the subsequent recruitment of neutrophils. In this setting, it is thought that mast cells are activated by complement products, and the generation of C5a anaphylatoxin induces mast cell degranulation as a result.

γδ T cells

These cells show features of both the innate and the adaptive immune systems. They have a limited ability to rearrange their T cell receptor genes, and *in vivo* are composed of prominent clones of γδ receptor combinations that respond to alkylamine components of micro-organisms.

The cytokines of the innate immune system

Interferons

The interferons (IFNs) were originally considered to have mainly antiviral activity. There are two groups—the type I interferons, IFN-α and IFN-β, and the type II, IFN-γ. While the type I IFNs are produced by virally-infected cells, IFN-γ is secreted by T lymphocytes and natural killer cells. The IFNs exert their antiviral activity through several mechanisms, that may be specific to the infected cell or involve the induction of broader host responses. The two groups of IFN inhibit cellular protein synthesis and induce activation of cellular RNAses, thereby destroying viral double-stranded RNA.

The broader actions of the IFNs affect innate as well as adaptive responses in host immunity. IFN-γ is produced by natural killer cells, once these are activated by IL-12. The IFN-γ itself activates the natural killer cell cytolytic machinery and also simulates macrophage microbicidal activity by inducing transcription of the *NOS2* gene and activating NADPH oxidase. Both classes of IFN, but particularly IFN-γ, can encourage the generation of the adaptive immune response, by inducing transcription of several genes that encode proteins involved in antigen processing and presentation. In these ways, interferons enhance humoral immune responses as well as antiviral T cell responses.

The inflammatory cytokines—TNF, IL-1, and IL-6

Tumour necrosis factor-alpha (TNF-α) plays a central role in the host response to bacterial infection, and while its production is essential for protection, excess TNF-α can also be lethal to the host. TNF-α is produced by macrophages when stimulated by bacterial products (including lipopolysaccharide) from Gram-negative bacteria, but can also derive from many other cell types from diverse tissues in response to inflammatory stimuli. TNF-α propagates the inflammatory response; it induces the microbicidal activity of macrophages, stimulates production of macrophage IL-1, IL-6, IL-8, as well as TNF-α, and augments the cytotoxic activity of natural killer cells. An additional feature of TNF-α is that it can induce the maturation of immature dendritic cells, that then leave the local environment where they have encountered micro-organisms and migrate to local lymphoid tissue to initiate an adaptive immune response. TNF-α can be considered as a double-edged sword because it also plays a role in the syndrome of septic shock, characterized by hypotension, capillary leak, and multiorgan failure.

IL-1 has many proinflammatory activities, most of which overlap with TNF-α. As well as influencing almost all cells of the immune system, it exerts activity in neuronal tissue, the liver, adipose tissue, and the endothelium. IL-1 results in the increased expression of adhesion molecules, accumulation of neutrophils at a site of inflammation, the hepatic acute phase response—and is involved, with IL-6 and PGE_2, in the generation of fever. Clearly, regulation of the activity of IL-1 is important; of the two types of IL-1 receptor, one (the type II IL-1 receptor) acts merely as an inactive ligand or decoy for IL-1, thereby preventing it binding to the type I IL-1 receptor. Furthermore, there is also an inactive analogue of IL-1 called IL-1 receptor antagonist (IL-1Ra) that binds to the type I IL-1 receptor but does not induce an activating signal.

IL-6 is produced by a large number of cell types, and its expression is increased in almost all tissues in response to infection. Inflammatory stimuli such as lipopolysaccharide, TNF-α, and IL-1 are responsible for the induction of IL-6 in infections. IL-6 is partly responsible for the hepatic acute phase response exemplified by enhanced transcription of the pentraxin C-reactive protein discussed earlier. IL-6 also induces B-lymphocyte differentiation and can induce activation of T cells.

IL-12 and IL-18

Both macrophages and dendritic cells possess further means by which they can stimulate their antimicrobial activity and that of other cells. IL-12 is a cytokine which is produced by macrophages and dendritic cells, either upon direct stimulation by certain microbial products, for example lipopolysaccharide or CpG motif-bearing DNA, or more commonly by stimulation of these antigen-presenting cells by CD4+ T cells, themselves activated by the antigen-presenting cells. The cognate interaction-medi-ating IL-12 generation by these cells is mediated by CD40 on the antigen-presenting cells, the stimulation of IL-12 production having a number of effects. IL-12 stimulates IFN-γ secretion by natural killer cells, which can then both stimulate CD8+ T cells and Th1-type CD4+ T cells. IL-12 also directly activates the microbicidal activity of macrophages by inducing the transcription of NOS2, with the consequent generation of reactive nitrogen intermediates as discussed earlier.

Another cytokine whose full role in the immune response to micro-organisms is still being elucidated, is IL-18. Initially described as a product of activated Kupffer cells and called IFN-γ-inducing factor (IGIF), IL-18 is now known to be produced by macrophages. IL-18 is synergistic with IL-12 in the induction of IFN-γ and, independently of IL-12, it also enhances natural killer cell activity.

Conclusions

The innate immune system, through various receptor species, is able to detect motifs common to pathogen subtypes, thus keeping the requirement for such receptors to a minimum. The receptors are linked to diverse effector mechanisms that facilitate inactivation or death of the micro-organism. An emerging pattern is that while the adaptive immune system recognizes protein structures, it is carbohydrate moieties that are the determinants for innate immune ligands.

Within the innate immune system, new components continue to be uncovered, and, at the same time, additional functions are being ascribed to previously characterized molecules. Thus, the field of innate immunity and especially its role in directing the subsequent adaptive response is one of the most active and exciting areas in contemporary immunology.

Further reading

Aderem A, Ulevitch RJ (2000). Toll-like receptors in the induction of the innate immune response. *Nature* **406**, 782–7.

Bogdan C, Rollinghoff M, Diefenbach A (2000). Reactive oxygen and nitrogen intermediates in innate and specific immunity. *Current Opinion in Immunology* **12**, 64–76.

Carroll MC (1998). The role of complement receptors in induction and regulation of immunity. *Annual Reviews of Immunology* **16**, 545–68.

Feizi T (2000). Carbohydrate-recognition systems in innate immunity. *Immunological Reviews* **173**, 79–88.

Jack DL, Klein NJ, Turner MW (2001). Mannose-binding lectin: targeting the microbial world for complement attack and opsonophagocytosis. *Immunological Reviews* **180**, 86–99.

Travis SM, Singh PK, Welsh MJ (2001). *Current Opinion in Immunology* **13**, 89–95.

5.6 Immunodeficiency

A. D. B. Webster

Introduction

The primary immunodeficiencies have provided a valuable insight into the critical components of the immune system for protection against infection. Although 10 years ago only two of these conditions were understood at a molecular level, over 80 defective genes causing a variety of clinical phenotypes have now been identified. This section focuses on lymphocyte disorders causing susceptibility to infection; defects in phagocytes and the complement pathways, which are important components of the innate immune system, are described in Chapter 5.4.

In the United Kingdom, there is still an unacceptable delay of 5 years on average for the diagnosis of some types of immunodeficiency, emphasizing a need for clinicians to be more aware of these disorders.

Classification

The primary immunodeficiencies (**PIDs**) are mostly inherited single-gene disorders presenting in infancy and early childhood. However, the one important exception is common variable immunodeficiency (**CVID**) that is still not precisely defined, most patients having a complex polygenic disorder of immune regulation which frequently presents in adults. PID includes a wide variety of cellular disorders of both the adaptive and innate immune systems, some causing autoimmunity rather than susceptibility to infection. The International Union of Immunological Societies (**IUIS**) supports a committee to meet every 5 years to review these classifications.

Secondary immunodeficiency occurs in a wide range of diseases, the immunodeficiency often being caused or exacerbated by therapy with immunosuppressive drugs.

History and examination

The family history is important, particularly since it may suggest X-linked or autosomal inheritance. There are few characteristic physical features, but the total absence of tonsils in infants and children is a feature of X-linked agammaglobulinaemia and severe combined immunodeficiency, the latter also being associated with failure to thrive and an absent thymic shadow on a chest radiograph. Signs of chronic otitis media, sinusitis, conjunctivitis, bronchitis, and bronchiectasis are typical, and splenomegaly is common in some types. Growth retardation, dysmorphic features, and severe skin disease (e.g. eczema, erythroderma) occur individually or in combinations in some of the PID syndromes. Chronic infection with atypical mycobacteria in young children suggests a defect in the γ-interferon and interleukin-12 signalling circuit. Massive lymphadenopathy and splenomegaly with autoimmune disease is a feature of lymphocyte apoptotic defects.

Primary immunodeficiency

Antibody-deficiency syndromes

Prevalence

The lifetime prevalence of the severe antibody-deficiency syndromes is about 16 per million of the Caucasian population in Western countries, but there is no reliable information on prevalence in developing countries; there are currently about 1000 diagnosed patients in the United Kingdom. However, selective IgA deficiency is common, occurring in about 1 in 700 of Caucasians, most of whom are healthy.

Aetiology

Most of the disorders are caused by single-gene defects leading to blocks at various stages of the maturation and differentiation of B lymphocytes (Fig. 1). However, common variable immunodeficiency, the most common of all the PIDs, appears to be a complex polygenic disorder of immune dysregulation.

Nomenclature (Table 1)

These follow IUIS guidelines, the individual types usually being referred to as a clinical description (e.g. X-linked agammaglobulinaemia), or alternatively by the molecular defect (e.g. CD40-ligand deficiency). The common use of acronyms by immunologists can be confusing for those outside the field.

Major types of antibody deficiency

Common variable immunodeficiency (CVID)

This is the most common of all the primary immunodeficiencies, affecting about 1 in 30 000 Caucasians. It is likely that the majority of patients labelled as CVID have a consistent combination of molecular abnormalities, the remaining few having as yet unidentified single-gene defects. Patients become symptomatic at any age, but usually in early childhood or late adolescence. Serum immunoglobulin levels are variable, but typically the serum IgA is below 0.1 g/l, the IgG below 2 g/l, and the IgM below 0.2 g/l. However, some patients have near-normal IgM levels and can occasionally make IgM antibodies. At least 20 per cent of patients with CVID can be shown to have a polygenic inherited disorder which is genetically linked to selective IgA deficiency. The pedigrees of affected families show a variable phenotype, even in affected siblings, ranging from IgG subclass defects, IgA deficiency, to CVID. Mothers with IgA deficiency and circulating antibodies to IgA are more likely to have affected offspring. The major predisposing genetic locus is located in the MHC region on chromosome 6, covering part of the class III and adjacent class II region. None of the genes has yet been identified, and there are at least three minor susceptibility genetic loci on other chromosomes.

A third of patients are lymphopenic, with circulating CD4+ T-cell counts between 0.15 and 0.4×10^9/l, often with a relative increase in CD8 T cells. Splenomegaly occurs in about 30 per cent of patients, and splenectomy may be necessary for those who develop hypersplenism. The spleen usually contains numerous non-caseating granulomas, with excessive numbers of activated macrophages in the surrounding tissue. A smaller number of patients develop granulomatous disease, requiring steroid therapy, in the lungs and liver; other organs such as the skin, brain, and kidneys are less commonly involved. Scandinavian patients are much less prone to granulomatous complications, suggesting an environmental factor is involved.

Chronic or recurrent diarrhoea, not related to known pathogens, occurs in at least 20 per cent of patients. This is often associated with a mild colitis and an excess of intraepithelial T lymphocytes. A minority have a Crohn's-like condition with a florid ileitis, and occasionally strictures. A few patients have upper intestinal villous atrophy with a florid inflammatory infiltrate; a minority of these will respond to a gluten-free diet, while the others need steroids to induce remission. About 10 per cent of patients have a pan-gastritis, sometimes with anaemia due to a lack of intrinsic factor and poor vitamin B12 absorption. Submucosal lymphoid nodules are common in the small bowel, but can occur elsewhere in the gut; this nodular lymphoid hyperplasia probably represents an aborted attempt at a local immune reaction to antigens in the gut.

The mechanism of CVID is complex and not well understood, but the evidence suggests that the fundamental abnormality is a failure to generate the appropriate microenvironment in the lymphoid apparatus for B-cell differentiation and antibody production. There is evidence of an excessive production of γ-interferon and interleukin-12 by lymphocytes and mono-cytes, respectively; this cytokine dysregulation is likely to cause a marked skewing towards a TH1-type response and increased susceptibility to chronic inflammatory disease. The antibody deficiency has recovered after HIV (human immunodeficiency virus) infection in five reported cases, probably by altering these abnormal cytokine patterns.

The differential diagnosis of CVID depends on excluding the other rarer single-gene PIDs and secondary immunodeficiency (see below).

Thymoma and hypogammaglobulinaemia

This has some distinctive features but many clinical and laboratory similarities with CVID. The thymoma, usually benign and well encapsulated, occurs in patients over 40 years of age, the hypogammaglobulinaemia being of varying severity. There may be autoimmune phenomena such as neu-tropenia, haemolytic anaemia, and red-cell aplasia. The disease has a poor prognosis, with most patients dying within 15 years from opportunistic viral or fungal infections due to deteriorating cellular immunity. Surgical removal of the thymoma has no effect on the immunodeficiency or the prognosis, but is usually necessary to exclude malignancy and/or involvement of neighbouring structures. The mechanism of the association with hypogammaglobulinaemia is not understood.

X-linked (Bruton's) agammaglobulinaemia (XLA)

Affected males usually develop recurrent infections in the first 2 years of life, often at about 6 months when maternal IgG is exhausted. Most patients have some residual IgG production (less than 50 mg/100 ml), but make no IgA and IgM. T-lymphocyte function is normal, but there are very few circulating B cells due to a block in the differentiation at the pre-B-cell stage in the bone marrow. The relevant gene on the X-chromosome codes for **Btk** (Bruton's tyrosine kinase), an intracellular signalling molecule involved in pre-B-cell development. A similar phenotype occurs in males and females with rare, autosomal recessive defects in critical molecules for B-cell differentiation upstream of Btk (see Table 1). Provided serious infection can be prevented, the patients have an excellent prognosis, and suffer from none of the chronic inflammatory/granulomatous complications seen in CVID. This may be partly explained by Btk having a role in the signalling cascade for macrophage activation, causing XLA patients to have a down-regulated inflammatory response.

Hyper-IgM syndrome (HIM)

There are three known rare molecular defects causing a failure of immuno-globulin class switching from IgM to IgG, and then to IgA and IgE. Two involve either the CD40 ligand (CD154), an activation-induced surface protein on CD4+ T lymphocytes, or its ligand CD40 on B cells. The CD154

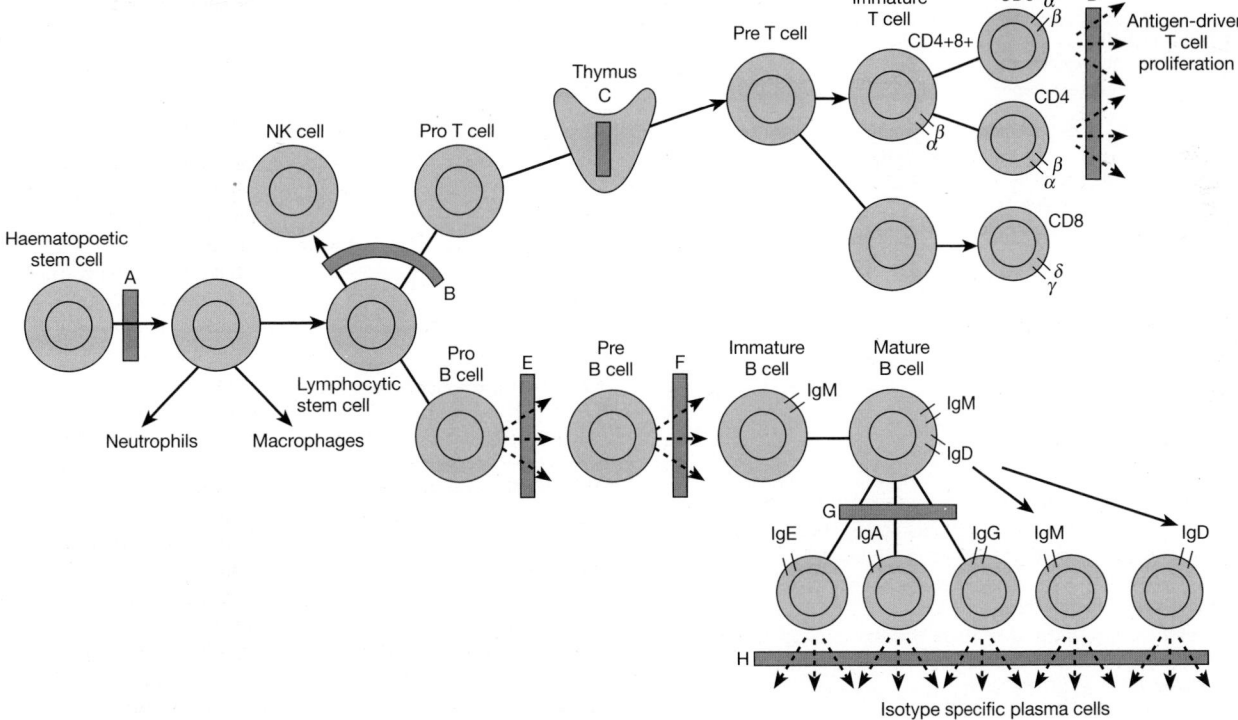

Fig. 1 Various blocks (hatched bars) in the maturation and differentiation of lymphocytes in the primary immunodeficiencies. (a) Reticular dysgenesis; B: X-linked severe combined immunodeficiency (**SCID**) (γc defect), JAK3 deficiency, adenosine deaminase (ADA) defects; C: purine nucleoside phosphorylase, *RAG1* and -2, *Artemis*, ZAP-70, CD45, IL-7Rα, and lymphocyte HLA class II defects; D: common variable immunodeficiency (CVID), p56[lck] defects. (b) E: defects in surface μ heavy-chain expression, Blnk, Igα, and λ5 surrogate light chain, RAG1 and -2, Artemis, ADA; F: XLA (Btk deficiency); G: X-HIM (CD40-ligand deficiency, CD40) and activation-induced cytidine deaminase deficiencies; H: CVID. Note that all defects causing SCID, other than those affecting B-cell development, will compromise antibody production through the lack of T-cell interactions in the lymphoid apparatus at stage G.

gene is on the X chromosome, affecting males who have a poor prognosis due to an unexplained susceptibility to sclerosing cholangitis, cirrhosis, and liver cancer. X-HIM patients are also prone to opportunistic infections with, for example, *Pneumocystis carinii* and *Cryptosporidium parvum*, suggesting that the failure to express CD40 ligand has wider implications for T-cell immunity. Sometimes female carriers of the genetic mutation can present with mild antibody deficiency due to incomplete Lyonization.

A rarer cause of HIM is caused by deficiency of a lymphocyte-specific cytidine deaminase, an enzyme involved in RNA editing in activated B cells. This autosomal recessive condition has a milder phenotype than X-HIM, resembling CVID and not being associated with opportunistic infections and liver disease.

X-linked lymphoproliferative syndrome (XLPS)

Affected males have a defect in the control of T-lymphocyte immunity to the Epstein–Barr virus (**EBV**), either dying during acute infectious mononucleosis or developing Burkitt's-like B-cell lymphomas and/or hypogammaglobulinaemia. XLPS is caused by mutations in the gene coding for **SAP** (surface lymphocyte activation molecule (SLAM) associated protein), a cytoplasmic protein that regulates the activation of cytotoxic CD8+ lymphocytes; those dying in the acute phase have a massive multi-organ infiltration by these cells. There appears to be a defect in the control of EBV reactivation leading to lymphoma in some survivors of acute infection. The mechanism of the immunodeficiency is not known, with some patients being misdiagnosed as having CVID.

Transient hypogammaglobulinaemia in infancy and childhood

Maternal IgG crosses the placenta in the last trimester of pregnancy and helps to protect the infant against infection for the first few months of life. Between 4 and 6 months of age the normal infant will develop an increasing repertoire of IgG antibodies, mainly of the IgG1 subclass. The capacity to make IgG2 and IgA is not fully developed until adolescence. This sequence may be retarded in some infants, who present in early childhood with infections and hypogammaglobulinaemia. There is no consensus on the

Table 1 Classification of primary immunodeficiency

	Molecular defect in:
Antibody deficiency	
X-linked agammaglobulinaemia (XLA)	Btk
Common variable immunodeficiency (CVID)	Unknown
X-linked hyper-IgM syndrome (XHIM)	CD40-ligand
Autosomal-recessive hyper-IgM	Activation-induced cytidine deaminase, CD40
Autosomal-recessive agammaglobulinaemia	Surface μ chain, Igα, BLNK, λ5
Selective IgA deficiency (IgAD)	Unknown
Selective IgG subclass deficiency	Mostly unknown (heavy-chain deletions rare)
Thymoma with hypogammaglobulinaemia	Unknown
Transient hypogammaglobulinaemia of infancy	Unknown
Functional antibody deficiency	Unknown
Severe T-cell deficiency	
(often with partial antibody deficiency)	
Thymic aplasia (Di George syndrome)	Gene(s) in chromosome 22q11
Purine-nucleoside phosphorylase deficiency	PNP
CD3-complex defects	γ or ε chain
Mixed T- and B-cell defects	
Severe combined immunodeficiency (SCID)	
Myeloid dysgenesis	Unknown
X-linked	Common γ chain (γc)
Autosomal recessive	Adenosine deaminase (ADA)
	Recombinase-activating gene 1 and 2
	Artemis gene
	Janus kinase-3 (JAK-3)
	HLA class II transcription factors
	(C11TA, RFX complex)
	Zeta-chain associated protein (ZAP-70)
	P56[lck] kinase
	Interleukin-7-receptor α chain
	CD45
Moderate mixed immunodeficiency	
Ataxia telangiectasia (A-T)	
Nijmegen breakage syndrome (NBS)	DNA repair genes
Ligase-1 defect	
Wiskott–Aldrich syndrome	WASP
Transporter for antigen presentation	TAP-2
X-linked lymphoproliferative syndrome (XLPS)	SLAM-associated protein (SAP)
Interferon-γ/interleukin-12 circuit defects	
Autosomal recessive	IL-12 p40 subunit
	IL-12-receptor β1 subunit
Heterozygous dominant-negative	Interferon-γ receptor (chain 1)
	STAT-1

See IUIS classification for additional rare defects causing severe or moderate combined immunodeficiency which are associated with major cytogenetic and generalized metabolic disorders.

precise definition of this disorder except that recovery should have occurred by 5 years of age. There is evidence that the mechanism has similarities with CVID.

Infections associated with hypogammaglobulinaemia

Patients are prone to bacterial septicaemia and respiratory infections, with a minority being also susceptible to mycoplasma and enteroviral infection (Fig. 2). There is usually uneventful recovery from most common childhood viral infections (e.g. measles, varicella, and mumps).

Bacteria

Patients may present with pneumococcal, *Haemophilus influenzae* (capsulated), or meningococcal septicaemia, but more often there is a history of recurrent respiratory infection, the main organism involved being non-encapsulated *Haemophilus influenzae*. This semi-commensal organism colonizes the upper respiratory tract of many normal individuals, spreading to involve the bronchi following common viral infections. Patients with antibody deficiency suffer from chronic infection in the ears, sinuses, and bronchi, often leading to bronchiectasis and deafness. *Pneumococcus* spp. and *Moraxella catarrhalis* are other common respiratory pathogens in these patients. Staphylococcal skin infection is common in children.

Mycoplasmas

Antibodies inhibit the growth of mycoplasmas on mucosal surfaces. About 10 per cent of XLA or CVID patients develop chronic mycoplasma arthritis with destruction of joints. Overgrowth of these organisms on mucosal surfaces (usually in the respiratory or genitourinary tracts) apparently leads to the uptake of viable organisms by phagocytes, which then transport them to joints where the microenvironment supports growth. A variety of myco-

plasma species have been implicated (e.g. *M. hominis* and *Ureaplasma urealyticum* from the urogenital tract, *M. pneumoniae* from the lungs). Rarely, infection can be acquired from animals as a zoonotic infection. Local infection can lead to chronic cystitis or urethritis, and there is the possibility that some species cause chronic bronchitis. Although methods based on the polymerase chain reaction (**PCR**) are being developed for rapid molecular diagnosis, very few laboratories can culture these organisms and provide antibiotic sensitivities. A working diagnosis of mycoplasma infection should be made in hypogammaglobulinaemic patients with arthritis, cystitis, or urethritis when samples taken for routine microbiological testing are negative; doxycycline should be given in the first instance, and specialist advice sought to confirm the diagnosis and provide antibiotic sensitivities in case the organism is resistant.

Viruses

Enteroviruses

These include polio-, coxsackie-, and echoviruses. Coxsackie- and echoviruses, of which there are many different strains, are a common cause of self-limiting mild enteritis and/or meningitis in normal individuals, but cause chronic meningoencephalitis and myositis in patients with severe hypogammaglobulinaemia. Echoviruses are usually involved, the classical features being convulsions, VIIIth nerve deafness, headache, and myositis, the last leading to fibrosis of the limb muscles with contractures. The diagnosis is usually made by culturing enteroviruses from the cerebrospinal fluid, or by a positive PCR for viral RNA. There is usually a gradual deterioration in the central nervous system features and death within 5 years; however, in a few people the disease can be modified or even cured by giving pooled immunoglobulin containing specific antibodies to the virus intravenously and into the cerebrospinal fluid on a regular basis. Standard prophylactic immunoglobulin therapy (see below) probably reduces the risk of enteroviral infection, but is not fully protective and often obscures the diagnosis by preventing culture of the virus from cerebrospinal fluid; patients in this situation may present with insidious mild symptoms of cerebral involvement such as altered personality and decreased mental ability. It is important to make the diagnosis because there is a new antienteroviral drug, pleconaril, which has cured most of treated patients.

There is a risk of paralytic poliomyelitis after live oral polio vaccination which is contraindicated in these patients. Fortunately, regular immunoglobulin therapy appears to prevent poliovirus infection from recently immunized family members, probably because enough neutralizing IgG leaks into the saliva and prevents faecal/oral transmission. However, rarely, a patient may become a chronic excreter of a virulent polio (vaccine related) strain. The World Health Organization, who are planning to discontinue routine polio immunization, are concerned about such patients who could start a new polio epidemic if immunity waned in the general population.

Other viruses

Patients with CVID are prone to recurrent *Varicella zoster* skin infection (shingles) but this rarely recurs after treatment with immunoglobulin. Reactivation of *Herpes simplex* (cold sores) or vaginal herpes is uncommon. The role of persistent picornavirus (e.g. rhinovirus, enterovirus) infection in the respiratory tract is unclear, but these viruses may have a role in the susceptibility to recurrent sinusitis and bronchitis.

Gastrointestinal infections/complications

Infections

Giardia lamblia

This is the only protozoal parasite to often cause symptoms in these patients. Mild to severe malabsorption may follow, with some patients complaining of abdominal distension, colicky pain, and flatulence. A secondary lactose intolerance may occur. The parasite may be difficult to eradicate with a standard course of metronidazole (2 g daily for 3 days),

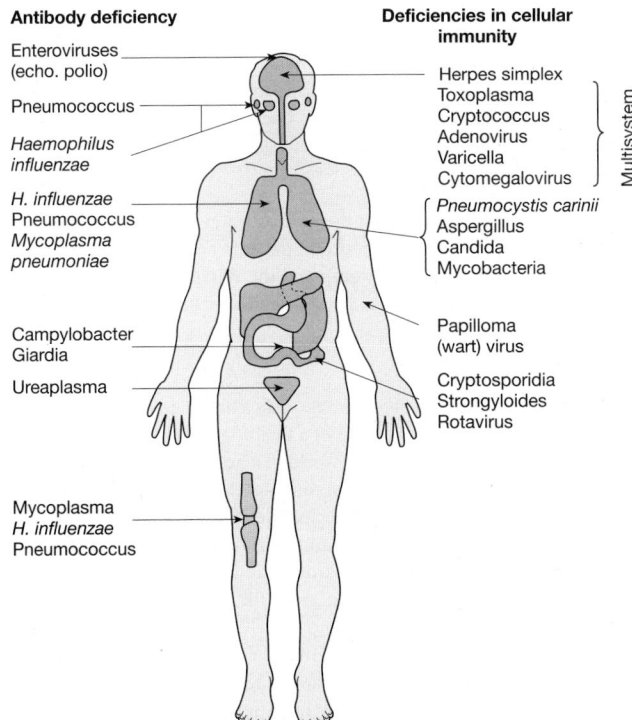

Antibody deficiency

Enteroviruses (echo. polio)

Pneumococcus

Haemophilus influenzae

H. influenzae Pneumococcus *Mycoplasma pneumoniae*

Campylobacter Giardia

Ureaplasma

Mycoplasma *H. influenzae* Pneumococcus

Deficiencies in cellular immunity

Herpes simplex Toxoplasma Cryptococcus Adenovirus Varicella Cytomegalovirus } Multisystem

Pneumocystis carinii Aspergillus Candida Mycobacteria

Papilloma (wart) virus

Cryptosporidia Strongyloides Rotavirus

Fig. 2 Pattern of infections associated with severe defects in antibody production or cellular immunity. Patients with severe combined immunodeficiency (**SCID**) disease suffer from all the infections listed, while those with the acquired immunodeficiency syndrome (**AIDS**) are prone mainly to infections shown in the right-hand column.

and tinidazole may be needed. It may be useful to give high-dose intravenous immunoglobulin therapy (2 g/kg body weight every 2 weeks) in resistant cases. Giardiasis is an uncommon complication nowadays in the Western world, probably because of higher dose immunoglobulin prophylaxis and improved cleanliness in the preparation of food.

Campylobacter

Campylobacter jejuni is the most frequent cause of bacteria-associated diarrhoea, usually responding to a course of a erythromycin (in adults, 500 mg four times a day for 10 days). Infection is currently uncommon in the United Kingdom, presumably because of improved hygiene. Stool culture will differentiate between shigella and salmonella infection, which occur no more frequently in these patients than in the general population.

Liver disease

The dependence on blood products led to a number of outbreaks of hepatitis C virus (**HCV**) infection before the early 1990s, with most infected patients dying from cirrhosis within 15 years. Hepatitis B virus (**HBV**) contamination of immunoglobulin products has not been a problem since the routine screening of blood donors started in the 1970s. No specific infection has yet been linked to the granulomatous hepatitis that occurs in at least 10 per cent of patients with CVID, the presinusoidal inflammatory reaction causing portal hypertension and oesophageal varices. The fact that about 30 per cent of patients with CVID in the United Kingdom have raised liver alkaline phosphatase serum levels is of concern as this is a good marker of liver involvement. This will lead to cirrhosis in some patients who should be considered for liver transplantation as their post-transplant survival is no worse than that for immunocompetent patients.

Sclerosing cholangitis is an important complication of X-HIM, and patients should be screened for abnormalities in liver function tests every 4 months, followed by cholangiography in those with persistently elevated liver enzymes. The cause is unknown, although cryptosporidial infection in the bile ducts may be the trigger in some cases. Affected patients should be considered for bone marrow transplantation, as well as liver transplantation for those with cirrhosis.

Malignancy

Apart from liver cancer and EBV-associated lymphoma in X-HIM and XLPS, respectively, malignancy is not a major complication of patients with hypogammaglobulinaemia. There is a small increase in lymphoma in XLA patients, with this being more impressive in patients with CVID (threefold increase over general population). However, a very high incidence of gastric carcinoma in patients with CVID was reported in the 1980s (50-fold increase over general population); this is now rare in the United Kingdom, possibly due to the wider use of prophylactic antibiotics for respiratory infection, which may have incidentally reduced the incidence of gastric infection with the cancer-promoting bacterium, *Helicobacter pylori*.

Prognosis

Recent surveys show that about 80 per cent of patients with CVID survive for 30 years, but morbidity and mortality depend on early diagnosis and management in an expert centre. The prognosis for X-linked agammaglobulinaemia is even better and is improving as patients are diagnosed earlier. Pneumonia and bronchiectasis remain the most common causes of death, liver and lung fibrosis being an additional complication in CVID. The overall prognosis for X-HIM and XLPS is poor, with most patients dying within 20 years of diagnosis.

Diagnosis

Diagnosing severe antibody deficiency is simple when the levels of serum IgG, IgA, and IgM are all very low or unrecordable. Death in childhood resulting from infection in a family member suggests one of the rare single-gene causes of immunodeficiency. For males presenting in childhood, blood should be sent to an expert laboratory to screen for Btk (XLA) and

SAP protein (XLPS) in lymphocytes by Western blotting, and for expression of CD40 ligand on activated lymphocytes (X-HIM); XLA is likely if there is an absence of circulating B lymphocytes. Other rare syndromes should be considered in those presenting in childhood (see Fig. 3(a)). The interpretation of low immunoglobulin levels in children under 1 year of age is difficult, and further follow up is always needed to confirm the presence of a significant antibody deficiency. In affected families with single-gene immunodeficiencies, a molecular diagnosis can be made at birth and the infant started on treatment. Similarly, fetal diagnosis can be offered at about 14 weeks' gestation by screening DNA from fetal blood, or amniotic or chorionic villous cells.

Diagnosis of mild/partial antibody deficiencies

Selective IgA deficiency (IgAD)

The class switch to IgA requires a co-ordinated sequence of events within the germinal centre, involving continuing B-lymphocyte proliferation and T/B-cell interactions. It is therefore not surprising that IgA deficiency is associated with a variety of defects in lymphocyte function. IgA deficiency, defined as a serum IgA level below 0.1 g/l, is the most common of the primary immunodeficiencies, and is often genetically linked to CVID with which it shares a major susceptibility genetic locus in the MHC region. It occurs mainly in Caucasians, with about 1 in 700 of the population affected in northern Europe; it is rare in Africans (~1:6000) and very rare in Japanese (1:18 000). IgA deficiency is also associated with inherited single-gene defects in DNA repair (for example, ataxia telangiectasia) and major cytogenetic defects in chromosome 18. Various antirheumatic and anticonvulsant drugs can induce IgA deficiency. Most patients with IgA deficiency are healthy, and the defect is discovered either by chance or during surveys of families with CVID. A small percentage are discovered during investigation for recurrent infections, but these patients usually have additional defects in IgG antibody production, and therefore have a mixed partial deficiency.

Some IgA-deficient individuals have high levels of serum anti-IgA antibodies, which may cause anaphylactic reactions during blood or blood product infusion. There is a slightly raised incidence of IgA deficiency in patients with coeliac disease, probably because of shared susceptibility genes in the MHC region.

Other selective class deficiencies

Complete selective IgM deficiency, the mechanism not being understood, is rare and usually discovered by chance in patients not susceptible to infection. Low IgM levels occur in Bloom's and the Wiskott–Aldrich syndrome (see below). Selective IgE deficiency has been described but is not clinically important.

IgG subclass deficiencies

The clinical significance of IgG subclass deficiency is controversial. As in IgA deficiency, the complete absence of a major IgG subclass is compatible with normal health in the Western world. There are four IgG subclasses: IgG1 having the highest serum level; and IgG2, IgG3, and IgG4 having sequentially lower levels. Many healthy individuals have IgG4 levels close to the limit of detection, and most immunologists in the United Kingdom no longer measure this subclass. Apart from rare individuals with inherited genetic defects in the constant-region genes for IgG1, 2, and 4, the mechanism of subclass deficiency is unknown, although some susceptibility genes are probably shared with CVID and IgA deficiency because all three types of defect can occur in the same family. IgG2 deficiency and IgA deficiency can occur together, particularly in patients with ataxia telangiectasia.

The four subclasses have different functional capacities in relation to activating the first component of complement (IgG2 being weak) and Fc-γ receptors on phagocytes. Specific IgG antibodies to bacterial components are also skewed towards certain subclasses, with those to polysaccharides being predominantly IgG2 in adults, and those to viral proteins being

Fig. 3 A scheme for the diagnosis of primary and secondary immunoglobulin (antibody) deficiency.

mainly IgG3. However, attempts to link subclass deficiencies with a predisposition to particular infections has been unsuccessful, probably because of the flexibility and redundancy in the immune system.

IgG subclasses can be measured in most routine immunopathology laboratories, but it is difficult to show that the results influence clinical management. Moreover, there is no official International Standard serum for the subclasses, making it difficult to compare results from different laboratories. Experience has shown that it is not worth measuring subclass levels in patients with total IgG levels above 8 g/l; furthermore, measuring them in children under 5 years is of little use because of the wide range of levels in healthy children in this age group. The current consensus is moving towards measuring the levels of functional IgG antibodies as a better indicator of immune status in those with recurrent infections.

Functional immunoglobulin deficiencies

Functional deficiency is defined as a complete or partial failure to produce antibodies to specific proteins or polysaccharides, in the presence of normal total serum immunoglobulin levels. The mechanism is not understood and its prevalence in the general population is not known. In practice, only functional IgG antibody deficiency is considered clinically important for protection against infection. The standard practice is to measure baseline levels of antibodies to proteins such as tetanus toxoid, and polysaccharides such as those purified from the capsules of pneumococci; if these are low then the response after immunization is measured. Antibodies to other antigens such as diphtheria toxin, measles and polio viruses can also be measured to provide a broader range of responses. There are workable normal values for baseline levels of antibodies to tetanus and diphtheria toxins, and for pneumococcal and *Haemophilus influenzae* B polysaccharides, but the interpretation of responses after vaccination is difficult because of the paucity of data from healthy age-matched individuals. Nevertheless, complete failure to respond following a second vaccination is evidence of an abnormality that may influence the clinical management.

Treatment

Immunoglobulin replacement therapy

Immunoglobulins for therapeutic use are manufactured from large pools of donor blood (about 20 000 donations). Those used for intramuscular (**IMIG**) or subcutaneous (**SCIG**) injection are approximately 16 per cent solutions, while those for intravenous use (**IVIG**) are less concentrated (6–12 per cent solutions). The manufacturing process involves alcohol precipitation of plasma to produce an IgG concentrate with very little IgA or IgM remaining. All preparations should be subjected to rigorous safety measures, which include screening donors for HIV, HBV, and HCV infection, and manufacturing procedures which inactivate a wide range of viruses. Fortunately, HIV is inactivated by alcohol, but there were outbreaks of HCV hepatitis caused by contaminated batches prior to the introduction of improved safety measures in the early 1990s.

Immunoglobulin prophylaxis protects against pneumococcal and *H. influenzae* septicaemia, parvovirus, and probably reduces the susceptibility to infection from *Giardia* and *Campylobacter* spp. However, it is much less effective in preventing infection with mycoplasmas and enteroviruses. It reduces the frequency of acute bronchitis in antibody-deficient patients, probably by preventing common respiratory viral infections. However, there is poor penetration into the respiratory mucosa with little effect on the growth of *H. influenzae* in the respiratory tract.

Indications and dose

Most patients with severe hypogammaglobulinaemia and a history of recurrent infections should be offered immunoglobulin replacement therapy. IVIG at a dose of 400 mg/kg every 4 weeks is usually given in the United Kingdom and the United States, but an alternative regime is to give SCIG at an equivalent total dose every week; this route is popular in Scandinavia. Intramuscular therapy is now rarely used because it is painful. With adequate training, many patients infuse at home, with a nurse or partner inserting the intravenous lines for IVIG, or using infusion pumps for SCIG. The aim is to maintain the preinfusion (trough) IgG level towards the lower limit of the normal range (~8 g/l). Failure to maintain this level on standard doses suggests an increased loss or hypercatabolism of IgG, the latter being a useful marker of chronic infection and/or inflammation. The majority of patients tolerate IVIG and SCIG well. About 10 per cent of patients experience mild 'reactions' during IVIG infusions (for example, headaches, mild fever, backache), but these can usually be controlled by reducing the infusion rate and/or giving an antihistamine; reactions needing adrenaline (epinephrine) and steroid therapy are rare. Changing the immunoglobulin product may be helpful in those with recurrent reactions. Some reactions are caused by high plasma levels of anti-IgA antibodies, although there is poor correlation between the level of these antibodies and susceptibility to reactions. Nevertheless, anti-IgA antibodies are usually measured routinely in patients with a serum IgA level below 0.1 g/l, and an immunoglobulin preparation chosen with minimal contaminating IgA for those with very high levels of anti-IgA. In practice, patients benefit from being referred to specialist centres for immunoglobulin therapy where the response to infusions can be assessed by experienced staff.

Reaching a decision on the treatment of patients with mild or moderate antibody deficiency is more difficult. It may be best to use prophylactic or intermittent courses of antibiotics, particularly in children. Objectively assessing the efficacy of immunoglobulin prophylaxis is not straightforward, particularly since there is likely to be a significant placebo effect.

General management

Patients should be encouraged to take antibiotics early to treat bronchitis, and those with structural lung damage may require long-term prophylaxis. The quinolones (for example, ciprofloxacin) are particularly effective because they are concentrated in the mucous layer lining of the respiratory tract and have a very low minimal inhibitory concentration for non-typable *H. influenzae*. Amoxicillin, alone or in combination with clavulanic acid, or cotrimoxazole, is a useful alternative. Postural drainage and regular exercise are useful in promoting the removal of secretions from the lungs. Patients should be encouraged to join support groups which provide educational literature in lay language and assistance for social problems.

Major defects in cellular (T cell) immunity

Thymic aplasia (Di George syndrome)

This rare condition (about 1 in 3500 live births) is caused by fetal malformation of the third and fourth branchial arches at about 7 weeks of gestation, apparently due to abnormal cephalic migration of neural crest cells into these regions. These cells contribute to the development of the skull, palate, thymus, and parathyroid glands, explaining why the syndrome is associated with dysmorphic facies, palatal abnormalities, and hypoparathyroidism—affected infants sometimes presenting with tetany and convulsions due to hypocalcaemia. Although originally thought to be caused by teratogens or maternal disease, the majority of cases are now known to be associated with a chromosomal deletion at 22q11. The condition overlaps with other genetic disorders such as the velocardiofacial syndrome and conotruncal anomaly face syndrome, the phenotype broadening into endocrine, cognitive, and neurological defects. The cardiac defects may require major cardiac surgery in infancy.

Most affected infants retain nests of thymic tissue in the neck and have only a moderate T-cell lymphopenia, mainly affecting CD8 T cells, which improves over the first few years of life. Antibody production is usually adequate, and there is an increased incidence of autoimmune disease such as thyroiditis and haemolytic anaemia. A minority of infants have a more severe T-cell defect and are prone to severe infections.

Treatment

Apart from treating the associated abnormalities (for example, hypocalcaemia), infants with circulating T-lymphocyte counts above 500/μl usually need no specific immunological intervention, but should be followed up regularly to confirm recovery of T-cell immunity. Those with a more profound T-cell lymphopenia may need either a bone marrow or thymic graft. Transplantation of partially HLA-matched postnatal thymic tissue has been successful, with the appearance of mature functional 'educated' host T cells in the blood a few months later. As for other patients with severe T-cell defects, live vaccines should be avoided and blood for transfusion irradiated to avoid graft-versus-host disease (**GvHD**). Infants with major cardiac defects should be screened for the condition before cardiac surgery.

Severe combined immunodeficiency disease (SCID)

These rare immunodeficiencies (about 1:30 000 live births) are caused by inherited mutations of genes that influence the maturation of lymphocytes, particularly T cells (Fig. 1). Those affected, who are usually infants or children, are susceptible to life-threatening infection with a wide range of pathogens and opportunistic microbes. The emphasis is on early diagnosis and transfer to a specialist centre for bone marrow transplantation. Most of the rare adult patients who present with severe infection associated with 'idiopathic CD4+ lymphopenia' have a 'leaky phenotype' of one of the known types of SCID.

Clinical features

Symptoms usually start before 7 months of age with failure to thrive, diarrhoea due to parasitic or viral infection (rotavirus, enteroviruses), *Pneumocystis carinii* pneumonia, and oral candidiasis. Other common viruses causing serious disease are adenoviruses, cytomegalovirus, human herpesvirus-6, and respiratory syncytial virus; systemic aspergillus or candida infections are less common but usually fatal. Routine immunization with live vaccines, particularly **BCG** (bacille Calmette–Guérin), may cause severe infection in patients with SCID. Most patients die within 2 years without a successful bone marrow graft. There are no specific features for any of the different types of SCID. The tonsils are usually absent and the thymic 'shadow' absent on a chest radiograph. Skin rashes due to a GvHD reaction, and more rarely lymphadenopathy and hepatosplenomegaly (Omenn syndrome), may confuse the diagnosis (see below).

Immunology

Most affected infants and children are lymphopenic, a characteristic finding which is often overlooked on the routine blood count. Table 2 outlines the differential diagnosis of lymphopenia in this age group. SCID can be classified into subgroups depending on the presence of T, B, and natural killer (**NK**) cells (Fig.4), those with no NK cells being more likely to engraft following bone marrow transplantation. The levels of serum immunoglobulins are of little diagnostic use during the first year of life. The proliferation of T lymphocytes in culture in response to mitogenic and antigenic stimulation is nearly always very depressed. The diagnosis may be obscured when there are normal numbers of circulating T lymphocytes, for example in the Omenn syndrome, or following engraftment by maternal cells *in utero* or cells from an unirradiated blood transfusion.

Molecular causes of SCID

There follows a brief description of the most frequent types of SCID, highlighting the contribution the discovery of the molecular defect has made to our understanding of the human immune system.

Table 2 Differential diagnosis, in order of probability worldwide, in patients with severe lymphopenia (adults <1.0 × 10^9/l, infants <3.0 × 10^9/l), normal immunoglobulin levels and opportunistic viral, fungal, and protozoal infections

Transient viral infection (e.g. varicella, measles)
AIDS
Severe nutritional deficiency
Cytotoxic/immunosuppressive drugs
Severe combined immunodeficiency (SCID)a
Inherited selective T-cell deficienciesb

aNearly always infants. bInfants/children only.

Defects of lymphocyte signalling It was surprising when mutations in the γ chain of the interleukin (**IL-2**) receptor were associated with X-linked SCID because the IL-2 'knock out' mouse had only a mild immunodeficiency. This led to a search for a wider role for the γ chain, now known to be the signalling chain for the IL-2, IL-15, IL-4, IL-9, and IL-7 receptors, the latter being critical in the early development of T lymphocytes. This common γ chain (γc) contains the appropriate tyrosine motifs on its cytoplasmic tail to facilitate the phosphorylation of Janus kinase-3 (JAK-3) which activates the signal cascade. Inherited defects in the IL-2-receptor α chain cause a multi-organ autoimmune disease, whereas defects in the IL-7-receptor α chain cause severe SCID. Failure to express HLA class II molecules on lymphocytes leads to severe SCID; research into the various molecular defects involved has improved our understanding of the factors that regulate class II gene transcription. Defects in the γ and ε chains of the CD3 complex are not always associated with severe immunodeficiency, suggesting some redundancy in the complex; inherited defects in ZAP (zeta chain-associated protein)-70 kinase, which interacts with the ζ chain, cause a predominantly CD8 lymphopenia. A defect in the p56^{lck} cytoplasmic kinase, which is important for signalling through the T-cell receptor, and complete absence of the surface protein tyrosine phosphatase receptor, CD45, are very rare causes of SCID.

Defects in VDJ (variable, diversity, joining) recombination Molecular defects in the recombinase activating genes (*RAG1* or *RAG2*) lead to a variable phenotype depending on the amount of residual RAG protein produced. In cases of complete RAG1 or -2 deficiency there is failure to express a functional T- and B-cell receptor, the result being severe SCID. Partial RAG expression is one cause of Omenn syndrome, characterized by severe skin rash, lymphadenopathy, hepatosplenomegaly, eosinophilia, and autoimmune disease. Recently, mutations in another gene (Artemis), which

appears to be involved in VDJ recombination and DNA repair, has been found in SCID infants who have a generalized sensitivity to ionizing radiation.

Defects in purine metabolism Lymphocytes need efficient salvage and interconversion pathways for purines and pyrimidines during rapid bursts of proliferation, particularly in the lymphoid germinal centres and fetal thymus. Adenosine deaminase (**ADA**) deficiency was the first established cause of SCID: the condition also being the first example of enzyme replacement therapy (initially using red cell transfusions which contain ADA) in clinical medicine, and later being the first disease to be treated by gene therapy, although with only partial success. ADA has an important role in the intermediate pathways of purine metabolism. Purine-nucleoside phosphorylase (**PNP**) is also active in this pathway, but is a much rarer cause of SCID. It is interesting that deficiencies in both these enzymes predominantly affect lymphocytes, despite their presence in most other cells of the body.

Diagnosis and early management

In most cases the clinical diagnosis is obvious, the infant failing to thrive with a severe infection and profound lymphopenia. Congenital HIV has to be considered in the differential diagnosis, but is easily excluded by PCR tests for the virus. A detailed family history is important, asking whether the parents are related and whether there have been early deaths from infection in family members. Lymphoreticular malignancy may need to be considered in patients with lymphadenopathy and hepatosplenomegaly; biopsies from bone marrow, skin, liver, and lymph nodes should be reviewed by a histopathologist with experience of SCID and GvHD; it may be necessary to confirm T-cell engraftment (maternal or otherwise) using chromosome markers.

Affected infants often present in respiratory distress due to a viral or fungal pneumonia; co-trimoxazole should be given immediately for possible *Pneumocystis carinii* infection and the patient transferred urgently to an expert paediatric centre where the diagnosis can be confirmed and specific treatment arranged; time should not be lost trying to diagnose and treat infection before transfer.

Subsequent management

Having identified and treated any current infection, the next priority is to confirm the diagnosis of SCID and then counsel the parents on the practicalities and risks of bone marrow transplantation (**BMT**), regardless of whether the molecular defect is identified. Screening tests for some SCIDs can be completed within a few days (ADA, PNP, HLA class-II defects) but others may take some weeks/months unless the molecular defect is already known in the affected family. BMT from an HLA-identical sibling is the ideal treatment and has close to 100 per cent success, but haploidentical sibling or HLA-matched unrelated marrow has about an 80 per cent success. Transplantation of stem cells from HLA-matched cord blood is an alternative. Unlike BMT in non-immunodeficient patients (e.g. for leukaemia), no preconditioning of the recipient is required to provide space within the marrow, but T-cell depletion of the donor marrow is necessary to minimize GvHD. The long-term outlook is good; there are now about 15 patients in the United Kingdom who have survived for between 12 and 20 years following BMT; the majority are healthy, although 20 per cent require regular immunoglobulin infusions because of failure to engraft donor B cells. For those rare adult patients who are diagnosed with SCID, bone marrow transplantation has previously been considered too risky; however, this view is changing since they rarely survive beyond a few years after presenting with severe infection. Some patients with ADA deficiency can be maintained on regular injections of bovine ADA, but this is very expensive and often does not completely correct the immune defect.

SCID is an ideal condition for gene therapy, but there have been problems in transfecting enough copies of the relevant gene into host bone marrow stem cells. However, this has been successfully achieved in at least four

This guide indicates the likely molecular defects depending on the results of lymphocyte subset analysis. The majority of these tests are best done in an expert paediatric centre

Fig. 4 Guide to the diagnosis of severe combined immunodeficiency (SCID) in infants and young children.

infants with X-linked (γc-deficient) SCID, possibly due to a selective advantage for the transfected stem cells; these patients now have normal immunity at up to 1 year of follow up.

Defects in the interferon-γ/IL-12 pathway and susceptibility to mycobacteria

The study of rare children with a familial susceptibility to fatal mycobacterial infection has confirmed animal studies showing the critical importance of interferon-γ (IFN-γ) in stimulating macrophages to kill mycobacteria. Affected children have mutations in components of the circuit involved in delivering the signal to macrophages: which are the IL-12 p40 subunit, the IL-12 receptor β1 subunit, both chains of the IFN-γ receptor (**IFN-γR**), and STAT1 (STAT, signal transducer and activator of transcription; a signalling component downstream of the IFN-γR). These are all autosomal inherited conditions in which the heterozygote carriers might be expected to be healthy; however, some families with heterozygotes for IFN-γR defects show a dominant inheritance pattern due to disruption of the receptor complex by non-functional chains. A similar dominant-negative effect has been described in a patient with a STAT1 defect because two functional molecules must be recruited to the cytoplasmic domain of the IFN-γR to provide a signal. Regular IFN-γ therapy is useful for those with normal IFN-γR function and downstream signalling, while the others require bone marrow transplantation. It is extraordinary that affected patients are so selectively susceptible to mycobacterial disease, particularly BCG and atypical strains such as *M. avium* and *M. fortuitum*. This suggests that this lymphocyte/macrophage interactive circuit has been selected by humans to specifically cope with mycobacterial infection (Fig. 5).

Inherited syndromes associated with immunodeficiency

Defects in DNA repair

Efficient repair of DNA damage is fundamental to cell survival. Our knowledge of the cascade involved in the excision of damaged nucleotides, insertion of new nucleotides, and rejoining (ligation) of the DNA strands is rapidly expanding, helped by the study of rare syndromes caused by genetic defects in this pathway. Ataxia telangiectasia (**A-T**) is an autosomal recessive disease characterized by progressive cerebellar ataxia, chromosomal instability, telangiectasia on exposed areas of skin, early death from cancer, and immunodeficiency of variable severity. About 80 per cent of patients

have IgA deficiency, with a third having complete absence of IgA; a minority have additional defects in IgG production, often IgG2 deficiency, while a few have severe panhypoimmunoglobulinaemia. T-lymphocyte function is often depressed. The relevant gene codes for a protein involved in the regulation of the cell cycle, probably having a role in the suspension of DNA replication after damage from ionizing radiation to allow time for repair. The defective gene in A-T leads to chromosomal instability and susceptibility to cancer, particularly lymphoma associated with translocations between chromosomes 4 and 7 involving the genes that code for immunoglobulin heavy chains and T-cell receptor α, β, γ chains. Most patients with A-T die before their third decade from either tumours or respiratory infection, the latter usually caused by a combination of immunodeficiency and progressive neurological deterioration. About 1 in 200 of the general population is heterozygous for the genetic defect, and there is some evidence that they are at an increased risk of malignancy. Furthermore, the gene is mutated in some types of leukaemia cells (e.g. T-prolymphocytic leukaemia), suggesting its product acts as a tumour suppressor.

The Nijmegen breakage syndrome (**NBS**) has a similar phenotype with additional craniofacial abnormalities, including progressive microcephaly. The normal physiological function of the *NBS* gene is not known, but like *ATM* leads to chromosomal instability following exposure to DNA-damaging agents. Other recessive chromosomal instability syndromes predisposing to cancer are caused by mutations in the DNA ligase-1 gene (with severe immunodeficiency and dwarfism), and the helicase mutated in Bloom's syndrome which is associated with moderately low immunoglobulin levels.

Wiskott–Aldrich syndrome

This X-linked disease is characterized by thrombocytopenia, moderate immunodeficiency, eczema, autoimmune disease (including vasculitis), and susceptibility to EBV-induced B-cell lymphomas. Patients have a dysregulated humoral response with depression of IgM antibody production to polysaccharides, and often a raised serum IgE. There is a milder variant resulting in only thrombocytopenia. The defective gene codes for a cytoplasmic protein (**WASP**, Wiskott–Aldrich syndrome protein) which is involved in cytoskeletal reorganization following the activation of platelets and T lymphocytes. The diagnosis is based on the presence of small platelets and on demonstrating the absence of WASP in white cells by Western blotting. Splenectomy may be needed to reduce the thrombocytopenia, and bone marrow transplantation is recommended for most patients because of the poor prognosis.

TAP deficiency

The transporter associated with antigen processing (**TAP**) is composed of two subunits (TAP-1 and -2) and facilitates the transport of HLA class I molecules from the endoplasmic reticulum to the *cis*-Golgi compartment. Inherited defects in TAP (so far only confirmed for TAP-2) lead to the failure to express class I molecules on the lymphocyte surface, preventing cytotoxic T and NK cells from recognizing antigen in the context of 'self' class I molecules. However, adequate cytotoxic function against virus-infected cells is retained using mechanisms that are not completely understood. Affected patients are prone to progressive bronchiectasis that is not entirely explained by infection. Some patients have developed nose and mid-face destruction, similar to midline granuloma, probably caused by a failure to inhibit NK-cell self-destruction via class I mediated inhibitory signals.

Other rare syndromes associated with severe infection

Chronic mucocutaneous candidiasis is a very rare sporadic disease of unknown cause, which in some patients is associated with multiple endocrine abnormalities. Patients have subtle defects in humoral and cellular immunity that do not explain the severity of the candida infection. Most patients can be managed satisfactorily with long-term antifungal therapy (fluconazole or itraconazole). The hyper-IgE (Job's) syndrome is another

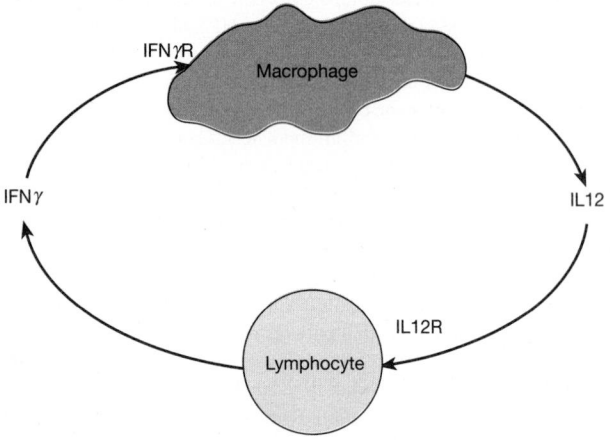

Fig. 5 This circuit is crucial for the effective killing of mycobacteria. Macrophages secrete IL-12 following uptake of bacteria, which amplifies the production of interferon-γ by sensitized T lymphocytes, which in turn stimulates the macrophage to kill the organism.

poorly defined disorder characterized by eczema, deep staphylococcal abscesses, and serum IgE levels usually in excess of 10 000 kU/l. Many patients have consistent facial features, delayed shedding of primary teeth, and hyperextensible joints suggesting they share the same underlying genetic defect. The Chediak–Higashi and Griscelli syndromes are autosomal-recessive diseases characterized by the presence of giant lysosomes in all granulated cells that compromises the function of neutrophils and NK cells. The relevant genes have been identified but their precise function is still unknown. Patients often die from infection or bleeding due to thrombocytopenia during an 'accelerated phase', which is similar to the virus-associated haemophagocytic syndrome. Bone marrow transplantation will correct the haematological abnormalities but not the other features, which include albinism and various neurological abnormalities.

Immunodeficiency associated with other congenital or inherited disorders

There are many rare disorders causing major multisystem disease in infants and young children that are associated with variable immunodeficiency states. Examples are inherited metabolic defects such as transcobalamin-2 deficiency (causing immunoglobulin deficiency secondary to severe vitamin B12 deficiency) and biotin-dependent carboxylase deficiency (causing a severe T-cell defect). A variety of skeletal (e.g. cartilage–hair hypoplasia), growth disorders (e.g. Schimke immuno-osseous dysplasia), and major dermatological abnormalities (e.g. ectrodactly ectodermal dysplasia) are associated with T-cell defects and early death from infection. (For a comprehensive list of these disorders see reference to the IUIS Report, 1999.)

Secondary immunodeficiencies (Table 3)

Lymphoid malignancies, immunosuppressive agents, and AIDS are common causes of severe immunodeficiency, while nutritional deficiencies, metabolic disturbances (for example, uraemia), and trauma have a less severe effect on the immune system. In many of these situations the primary disease usually overshadows the immunodeficiency, although attention to the latter can improve the patient's quality of life.

Recurrent pneumonia and bronchitis suggest antibody deficiency, whereas varicella-zoster and herpes-simplex reactivation, oral candida, and rapid growth of skin warts are often early indications of a defect in cellular immunity. The presence of lymphopenia, often overlooked, indicates that the immune system is compromised but is a poor guide to the clinical significance of the defect. In practice, measuring the numbers of circulating CD4+ T cells and serum immunoglobulins are useful simple tests for monitoring the severity of the immunodeficiency.

Lymphoid malignancy

Various types of lymphoreticular malignancy are associated with both humoral and cellular immunodeficiency, exacerbated by the use of cytotoxic drugs. There is no consistent pattern of immunodeficiency for any particular lymphoid malignancy, presumably the severity depending on the genetic background of the patient and immunomodulating factors released from the malignant cells. However, an important exception is chronic lymphatic leukaemia (**CLL**) in which the majority of patients develop hypogammaglobulinaemia during the course of their disease. Although the immunoglobulin deficiency in most patients is mild, a few have severe hypogammaglobulinaemia and suffer from recurrent infections, particularly of the upper and lower respiratory tract; these patients will benefit from regular immunoglobulin replacement therapy, while others can be managed with prophylactic or intermittent courses of antibiotics. The cause of the antibody deficiency is complex and seems to be due to a combination of inhibitory factors released by the malignant clone and inter-

ference with the normal traffic of T and B lymphocytes through the lymphoid apparatus by proliferating CLL cells.

Patients with myeloma often have antibody deficiency, which explains their predisposition to pneumococcal pneumonia and septicaemia. In the past, few haematologists paid attention to the immunodeficiency because of the very poor prognosis of the underlying condition. However, modern cytotoxic therapy can now induce prolonged remissions, during which the immunodeficiency recovers, so it may be worth treating the more severely immunocompromised patients with immunoglobulin during the induction period. There is evidence that the malignant plasma cells produce factors that inhibit normal antibody production.

The increasing use of bone marrow transplantation to treat leukaemia carries a legacy of persistent antibody deficiency in a minority of patients due to inadequate B-cell engraftment and/or the drugs used to prevent rejection. Follow-up protocols should include appropriate screening to identify those patients who may require immunoglobulin replacement.

Table 3 Classification of secondary immunodeficiency

Lymphoreticular malignancy
Chronic lymphatic leukaemia[a]
Myeloma[a]

Therapeutic agents
Anti-B-cell antibodies[a]
Anti-T-cell antibodies[b]
Azathioprine[b]
Bleomycin[b]
Captopril[a, +]
Carbamazepine[a]
Chloroquine[a, +]
Cyclosporin[b]
cis-Platinum[b]
Corticosteroids[b]
Cyclophosphamide[ab]
Fenclofenac[a, +]
Gold[a, +]
Methotrexate[b]
Penicillamine[a, +]
Phenytoin[a]
Sulfasalazine[a]
Valproate[a, +]
Vincristine[a, b]

Viruses
HIV[b]
Rubella[a]

Metabolic and vitamin deficiencies
Biotin-dependent carboxylase deficiency[a, b]
Burns[a]
Orotic aciduria[a, b]
Renal and liver failure[a, b]
Selenium[b]
Transcobalamin-II deficiency[a]
Trauma[a, b]
Vitamin A[a]
Zinc (acrodermatitis enteropathica)[b]

Hypercatabolism or increased loss of immunoglobulin
Nephrotic syndrome
Protein-losing enteropathy: primary and secondary lymphangiectasia
Inflammatory bowel disease
Dystrophia myotonica

Predominant effect on [a]antibody production or [b]cellular immunity.

+Only IgAD reported

Drugs

The extensive literature on the immunological effects of cytotoxic agents and steroids will not be reviewed here. Many of these drugs have a profound effect on cellular immunity, as shown by the severity of varicella infection in patients treated with corticosteroids, and the risk of cytomegalovirus and EBV reactivation in those on immunosuppression therapy to prevent graft rejection. Some of these drugs, particularly cyclophosphamide and azathioprine, may compromise antibody production after prolonged use. A variety of antirheumatic and anticonvulsant drugs induce a partial (often IgA) deficiency, and occasionally a severe antibody deficiency in a small minority of treated patients, probably due to their genetic susceptibility to the metabolic effects of the drug on B-cell differentiation and/or antigen presentation. The effects are reversible, but it may take up to 2 years for antibody production to recover after stopping the drug.

Viruses

HIV is the most common and important immunosuppressive virus, and is described in Chapter 7.10.21. Many other viruses cause moderate immunosuppression during active infection, particularly measles which depresses cellular immunity. Fetal infection with the rubella virus may, rarely, lead to prolonged depression of IgG and IgA antibody production after birth, sometimes with a high serum IgM level. Fetal cytomegalovirus infection can have a similar effect. There is evidence of prolonged alteration in the type of immune response after common childhood virus infections, some researchers suggesting that these events 'programme' the system towards a TH1 response and reduce the risk of allergy; the marked reduction in measles and other severe childhood infections due to vaccination has been suggested as one reason for the increase in childhood allergy, including asthma.

Immunodeficiency secondary to metabolic and nutritional defects

This is probably the most common cause of immunodeficiency worldwide and contributes to the high infant death rate in the Third World. Protein-calorie malnutrition and deficiency of vitamins and trace elements, particularly vitamin A, zinc, and probably selenium, can lead to significant depression of T-lymphocyte function and reduced antibody production. Poor nutrition in the very elderly in Western countries probably contributes to their poor antibody responses and an increased risk of pneumococcal pneumonia. Vitamin A supplementation has been shown to reduce childhood mortality from infection in New Guinea.

Prolonged metabolic disturbances associated with liver and renal failure will compromise immunity; this persists in about 10 per cent of patients on ambulatory peritoneal dialysis who have low IgG levels and are susceptible to infection, and may be due to a combination of persistent uraemia and hypercatabolism of IgG by activated peritoneal macrophages.

Severe trauma and major surgery often compromises both T- and B-lymphocyte function, but is usually clinically masked by the routine use of broad-spectrum prophylactic antibiotics and immunoglobulin provided in blood transfusions. Even full-thickness burns involving less than 10 per cent of surface area in young children appear to suppress IgG2 and IgG3 subclass production for at least a week. This observation provided an explanation for the high incidence of deaths from the toxic-shock syndrome in one centre and prompted the routine use of prophylactic antibiotics on admission. In major surgery, particularly when hypothermic cardiopulmonary bypass is used in elderly patients, attempts are being made to reduce the risk of postoperative infection by 'boosting' the nutritional requirements of the immune system with supplements such as L-arginine and nucleotides.

Increased catabolism/loss of immunoglobulin

Loss of immunoglobulin from the kidney or bowel is an important cause of mild/moderate hypogammaglobulinaemia, but is rarely of clinical significance. Serum IgM, being a larger molecule, is usually normal, with low IgA and IgG levels. The nephrotic syndrome and protein-losing enteropathy are the most common causes, the latter being difficult to diagnose when the serum albumin level is normal. Leakage of protein and lymphocytes occurs in primary or secondary intestinal lymphangiectasia—the combination of hypogammaglobulinaemia, low serum albumin level, and lymphopenia being a useful clue to this diagnosis. An increase in the catabolism of many proteins occurs in chronic infection/inflammation, but this is never severe enough to cause severe hypogammaglobulinaemia unless there is an associated primary defect in immunoglobulin synthesis. A selective increase in the catabolism of IgG occurs in dystrophia myotonica, but the mechanism is unknown.

Further reading

IUIS Scientific Committee (1999). Primary immunodeficiency diseases. Report of an IUIS Scientific Committee. *Clinical and Experimental Immunology* **118**(Suppl 1), 1–34.

Ochs HD, Smith CIE, Puck JM, eds (1999). *Primary immunodeficiency diseases. A molecular and genetic approach.* Oxford University Press, Oxford.

Webster ADB (2001). Common variable immunodeficiency. In: Roifman C, ed. *Immunology and Allergy Clinics of North America*, Vol 21, pp 1–22. WB Saunders, Philadelphia.

5.7 Principles of transplantation immunology

Kathryn J. Wood

Table 1 Terminology of transplantation

Autograft	Tissue from one part of the body transplanted to another Examples: skin grafts in patients with burns, vascular grafts
Isograft	Tissue transplanted between genetically identical members of the same species Examples: grafts between identical twins, grafts between members of the same inbred strain of mice or rat
Allograft	Tissue transplanted between non-identical members of the same species Examples: grafts between genetically disparate humans, grafts between different inbred strains
Xenograft	Tissue transplanted between individuals of different species Examples: pig to human, rat to mouse

Introduction

Transplantation of an organ, tissue, or cells between genetically disparate individuals within the same species, allografts, or between species, xenografts (Table 1), almost inevitably results in rejection of the graft if active steps are not taken to control the destructive immune response that is triggered immediately after transplantation.

Studies on the behaviour of tumour grafts in the early part of the twentieth century led Peter Gorer to formulate the concept of graft rejection in 1938. Gorer's description of what triggers rejection still holds today, even if the language he used does not fit with current immunological jargon: 'isoantigenic factors present in the graft tissue and absent in the host are capable of eliciting a response which results in the destruction of the graft'. The recognition that the immune system was involved came nearly 10 years later when Gibson and Medawar clearly identified specificity and memory as hallmark features of the rejection response.

The rejection process is complex. Many factors, including the nature of the tissue transplanted and the genetic disparity between the donor and recipient, the site of transplantation, as well as the immune status of the recipient, all contribute to determining the character of the rejection response (Table 2).

The events that lead to allograft rejection are summarized in Fig. 1. In brief, inflammation as a result of the removal of the graft from the donor and implantation into the recipient is always triggered as a result of the transplantation procedure itself, irrespective of whether the tissue is allogeneic or xenogeneic in origin. These 'danger' signals are responsible for activating both the innate and adaptive immune systems that act in concert to destroy the graft. For acute allograft rejection, activation of the adaptive immune system requires recognition of molecules that are mismatched or polymorphic between the donor and the recipient. Antigen recognition in combination with additional signals, termed costimulation, leads to the activation of donor reactive lymphocytes, both T cells and B cells. Clonal expansion, meaning proliferation of donor reactive lymphocytes, is triggered such that many more daughter cells with donor antigen specificity are produced rapidly. The environment created by such lymphocyte activation results in the differentiation of the activated donor reactive lymphocytes into effector cells, including cytotoxic T cells and mature B cells or plasma cells that secrete anti-donor antibodies. These antigen-specific effector cells in combination with activated components of the innate response, such as activated macrophages and natural killer cells, orchestrate the destruction of the graft (Fig. 1).

If immunosuppressive drugs such as cyclosporin, tacrolimus, mycophenolate mofetil, or azathioprine are administered at the time of transplantation, many of the events that lead to acute allograft rejection can be inhibited. As a result of the effective use of these drugs in clinical transplantation the short-term, 1-year, graft survival rates for all solid organ grafts have increased dramatically in the last 20 years (up-to-date summaries of graft survival data can be obtained from the websites listed at the end of this chapter). Unfortunately, this short-term success has not translated into significantly improved long-term, more than 10-year, graft survival outcome. Following the first year after transplantation there is still a steady attrition of grafts; this delayed or late graft loss occurs due to a variety of different processes and factors, only some of which are immunological. Late graft loss is often referred to as chronic allograft rejection (Table 2). Unfortunately, the drugs in use in clinical transplantation at present are

Table 2 Factors affecting the rejection response

	Allografts		Xenografts
Recipient status	**Naïve**	**Sensitized**	**Naïve**
Pre-formed antibodies	None	Yes Anti-donor HLA	Yes Natural Anti-carbohydrate
Hyperacute	No	Yes	Yes
Acute	Yes		
With immunosuppression			
Acute vascular		Yes	Yes
Chronic	Yes	Yes	?

relatively ineffective at preventing chronic stimulation of the immune system by the graft in the longer term after transplantation.

When tissues are transplanted between species (xenotransplantation) where the recipient species has preformed natural antibodies against the donor (so-called discordant species that include pig to human), additional immunological events contribute to the destruction of the graft, resulting in the very rapid elimination of the graft through a process known as hyperacute rejection (Table 2). In the pig to human species combination, preformed natural antipig antibodies bind to carbohydrate determinants present on pig cells. As a result the endothelial cell surface develops procoagulant activity causing leucocytes to accumulate in the vessels, complement is activated, and the tissue is rejected very rapidly. If hyperacute rejection can be inhibited, for example by removal of the preformed antibody before transplantation or by controlling complement-mediated damage to the graft, the downstream events involving the adaptive immune system will be triggered resulting in acute vascular or delayed xenograft rejection.

Hyperacute rejection can also occur when an allograft is transplanted into a recipient who has already been sensitized to the histocompatibility antigens of the organ donor (Table 2). In allotransplantation, anti-donor antibody formation can occur as a result of the rejection of a first graft, pregnancy, or blood transfusion. Rigorous screening processes, whereby sera from the recipient are cross-matched against tissue from the donor, ensure that the recipient does not have preformed antidonor antibodies and that hyperacute rejection of allografts hardly ever occurs in current clinical practice.

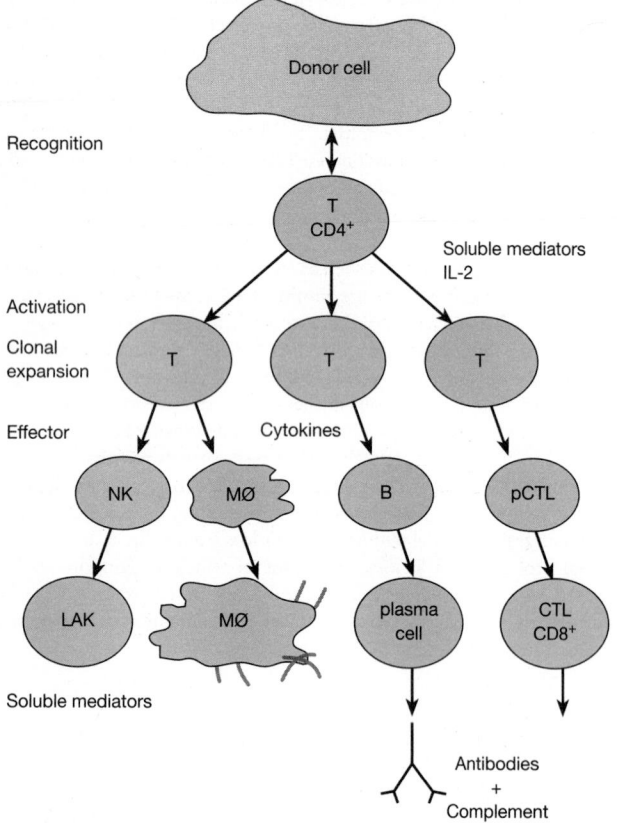

Fig. 1 Overview of allograft rejection. There are three phases to the responses—recognition (direct pathway allorecognition is illustrated), activation, and the generation of effector mechanisms. Each step involves the orchestrated interaction of cells and molecules to ensure that the response is driven towards an aggressive phenotype that will result in the destruction of the transplant. Immunosuppressive drug therapy is designed to interfere at different stages in the response to ensure effective inhibition of rejection.

This chapter will outline the key cellular and molecular events that lead to the destruction of a graft by the immune system of a naïve recipient. The events that lead to allograft rejection will be dealt with in most detail alongside a summary of the sequelae that also need to be considered when xenogeneic tissue is transplanted.

Transplantation sends danger signals to the host

The removal of tissue for transplantation from the donor and its implantation into the recipient will result in a series of changes in gene expression within the donor tissue that will markedly influence the way the recipient's immune system responds. When the organ or tissue to be transplanted is harvested from a cadaver donor some of these changes are a direct consequence of brain death. In addition, the trauma associated with the surgical procedures required to remove and transplant the tissue contributes to the very early events that initiate rejection. These factors are often referred to collectively as the events associated with ischaemia and reperfusion injury. Indeed, it has been suggested that there is a link between the ischaemia time and increasing immunogenicity of the graft.

The consequences of these events include the release of preformed P-selectin (CD62P) from the Weibel–Palade bodies contained within endothelial cells. This is an adhesion molecule responsible for the earliest step in leucocyte migration into the tissue. There is also *de novo* expression of a variety of genes, including those encoding chemokines (chemoattractant cytokines) and other adhesion molecules by the transplanted tissue. Expression of these molecules by the graft creates a proinflammatory environment and results in changes in endothelial cell function and the recruitment of inflammatory leucocytes into the graft, as well as the exodus of donor-derived passenger leucocytes from the graft and their migration to recipient lymphoid tissue. Thus the graft itself initiates a vicious circle of events that contribute to its own destruction.

It is important to note that some of these initial changes will occur even when there are no antigenic differences between the donor and recipient, as is the case when a graft is transplanted between genetically identical individuals—a syngeneic graft. These events are associated exclusively with organ retrieval and the transplantation procedure itself. Of themselves, they are not sufficient to lead to the destruction of the graft, as evidenced by the lack of rejection of autografts and isografts (Table 1). However, they can have a marked influence on early graft function and they will have a significant effect on the way in which the innate and adaptive immune responses to the graft are both triggered and evolve when an antigenic disparity does exist. Moreover, it has been suggested that these early events can predispose the graft to late dysfunction or chronic rejection, the distinctive feature of which is transplant vasculopathy (Fig. 2).

One way of thinking about the changes that arise as a direct result of the removal and transplantation of tissue is in terms of the trauma of these events initiating a series of 'danger signals'. Receipt and integration of these signals by the host immune system, along with information about the genetic disparity of the tissue transplanted with the recipient, will determine whether and how the recipient immune system is triggered.

Role of the innate immune system

The innate immune system is used by the host as the first line of defence against any adverse event, including transplantation. It comprises a series of cells and molecules that are poised for action as soon as the normal resting situation in the body is perturbed. Elements of the innate immune system will be triggered by the danger signals arising from the trauma associated with the transplantation procedure. The nature of the components of the innate immune system involved in this phase of the rejection response are relatively poorly characterized but are likely to include the components of

Fig. 2 Histological features of vascular rejection—the hallmark of chronic graft rejection. A normal and rejected vessel are shown in the cartoon. The rejected vessel (right) exhibits severe intimal proliferation compared with the normal vessel (left) as a result of the proliferation of smooth muscle cells.

the complement system, particularly C3, and phagocytic cells such as macrophages.

The complement system is a cascade of proteolytic enzymes whose activation leads to opsonization of targeted cells as well as the generation of a membrane attack complex that can initiate cell lysis. Complement can be activated in a variety of ways, including by some of the proteolytic enzymes produced by the clotting cascade, as well as by contact with damaged or altered endothelial cells. Once activated the enzymes of the complement cascade release soluble mediators, such as C3a and C5a, that will attract leucocytes to the site of the graft, and also produce molecules that can bind covalently to the cells within the graft forming a focus for the damaging events that follow.

Macrophages express a series of pattern recognition receptors, including those that recognize carbohydrate structures, reactive oxygen species, and activated complement components. When these receptors engage their ligands the macrophage is triggered to release a battery of inflammatory cytokines—including tumour necrosis factor (**TNF**), interleukin-1 (**IL-1**), and IL-6 amongst others—that further augment the proinflammatory environment and promote the activation of the adaptive response.

Role of the adaptive immune system

Antigens that stimulate allograft rejection

The degree of histocompatibility (tissue compatibility) between the donor and recipient determines whether a graft is rejected or accepted when transplanted between two members of the same species. In molecular terms this arises from a series of molecules, both cell surface and intracellular, that are polymorphic or variant between different members of the species—so-called histocompatibility antigens. These were originally classified as either major or minor depending on the location of the gene encoding the polymorphic molecule in the genome.

A series of cell surface molecules encoded by genes present within one region of the genome, the major histocompatibility complex (**MHC**), are known as the major histocompatibility antigens or MHC antigens. Many of these molecules are well characterized. Any other polymorphic molecules that trigger rejection are called minor histocompatiblity (**miH**) antigens. The genes for miH antigens are scattered throughout the genome.

Incompatibility or mismatching for either MHC or miH antigens can trigger graft rejection. In general, in naïve recipients the greater the number of incompatibilities for MHC and miH antigens, the more vigorous the rejection response. However, the type of tissue transplanted as well as the site of transplantation will have a marked influence on graft outcome, even when the matching for MHC and miH antigens between the donor and the recipient is identical. For solid organ grafts such as the kidney, matching for MHC antigens between the donor and the recipient improves graft outcome in immunosuppressed recipients. However, in bone marrow transplantation even grafts transplanted between individuals who are identical for MHC antigens can still trigger an immune response, either rejection or graft-versus-host disease, as a result of mismatching for miH antigens.

MHC class I and class II molecules

The MHC encodes a series of polymorphic genes in every species of vertebrate (Fig. 3). Within any one species a large number of variant forms of each of these genes exists within the population as a whole. Of the genes present in the MHC there are two families that code for cell surface molecules known as the MHC class I and MHC class II molecules (Fig. 3). Some of the loci that form part of the class I and class II families have been well characterized and in humans these are called HLA A, HLA B, and HLA C, and HLA DR, HLA DQ, and HLA DP, respectively. Additional class I and class II genes are present in the MHC, but they are less well characterized than those mentioned above and polymorphisms in these molecules are not considered routinely before either organ or bone marrow transplantation at present and they will not be discussed further here.

MHC class I molecules are cell surface glycoproteins comprising two polypeptide chains; the polymorphic α chain (molecular mass, **MM**, 45 kDa), which is anchored in the plasma membrane and encoded by a gene in the MHC, and β_2-microglobulin (MM: 12 kDa), which is not anchored in the membrane and is encoded by a gene on another chromosome (Fig. 3). MHC class I molecules are expressed on virtually all somatic nucleated cells, albeit at different levels in the resting state. Their expression is rapidly upregulated in response to cytokines such as interferon-γ (IFN-γ) and tumour necrosis factor-α (TNF-α) that are produced during an immune response. After transplantation, mismatched intact donor MHC class I molecules expressed by donor cells can be recognized and trigger the activation of recipient CD8+ T cells.

Class II molecules are also cell surface glycoproteins built up of two polypeptide chains. However, in contrast to class I, both chains—α and β (MM: 35 and 28 kDa, respectively)—are anchored in the plasma membrane. The two chains are encoded by genes found in the MHC; class II A and B genes for the α and β chains, respectively. Both genes can be polymorphic. MHC

Fig. 3 Outline map of the major histocompatiblity complex (MHC) in man. The HLA gene complex maps to the short arm of chromosome 6. It is divided into regions and subregions that in simple terms each contain a family of genes. Only the well characterized loci are shown in this representation: HLA A, HLA B, and HLA C class I α-chain genes, and HLA DR, HLA DQ, and HLA DP class II A and B genes. Additional class I and class II genes have been described. A full map for the HLA region is available at the website attached to *Nature* (1999) **401**, 921–3.

class II molecules are not expressed by all cells in the body, their tissue distribution is therefore much more restricted than for class I molecules and expression is only found constitutively on some cells, including dendritic cells, B lymphocytes, macrophages, and some endothelial cells. Importantly, expression of MHC class II molecules can not only be increased on the cells that already express class II molecules but can be induced on other cell types during an immune response. After transplantation, mismatched MHC class II molecules expressed by donor cells can be recognized and trigger the activation of recipient CD4+ T cells.

During the biosynthesis and transport of MHC molecules to the cell surface they become associated with short peptides derived from both intracellular and extracellular proteins. This process is known as antigen processing and presentation. As a result of these antigen processing pathways, MHC class I and class II molecules expressed at the cell surface report the status of the internal and external environment of a cell to the immune system. When the cell is functioning normally the peptides associated with MHC molecules are derived from self proteins, that is, the proteins belonging to the tissue itself, and including peptides derived from the MHC molecules themselves. However, when there is an adverse event such as a pathogen invading either the cell itself or its local environment, the MHC molecules will become loaded with peptides derived from the invader. It is this peptide–MHC complex that is recognized by T cells.

In the context of transplantation the situation is slightly more complex. Before transplantation, donor MHC molecules expressed by the transplanted tissue will contain peptides of donor origin. After transplantation, these donor-derived MHC–peptide complexes can be recognized by recipient T cells via the so-called direct pathway of allorecognition (Fig. 4). How-

ever, recipient antigen-presenting cells also come into contact with donor cells and molecules (see below) and through the normal pathways of antigen processing and presentation peptides of donor origin become associated with recipient MHC molecules in just the same way as any other foreign antigen. Recipient MHC–donor peptide complexes can then be recognized by recipient T cells via the so-called indirect pathway of allorecognition (Fig. 4), and this pathway is also used for recognition of mismatched miH antigens. Thus, after transplantation there are two routes of presentation of donor MHC molecules to the recipient immune system, the direct and the indirect pathways of allorecognition.

Two pathways for presentation of donor antigens to recipient T cells

Bone marrow-derived passenger leucocytes are present in non-lymphoid tissues throughout the body and have the characteristics of immature dendritic cells. After transplantation, in response to inflammatory cytokines and other danger signals, the donor-derived passenger leucocytes migrate out of the graft very rapidly and end up in the recipient lymphoid tissue. The migration process results in the passenger cells acquiring the phenotype and function of mature dendritic cells. Mature dendritic cells are often referred to as professional or immunostimulatory antigen-presenting cells as they express high levels of MHC class I and class II molecules as well as other cell surface and soluble molecules that enable them to stimulate naïve CD4+ and CD8+ T cells to respond (Fig. 5). The additional molecules required for an antigen-presenting cell to stimulate the activation of naïve T cells include costimulatory molecules such as members of the B7 family, in particular CD86, CD40, and adhesion molecules. Thus the donor passenger leucocytes that end up in the recipient lymphoid tissue have all of the attributes required for them to present any donor MHC molecules that were mismatched between the donor and the recipient to recipient T cells via the direct pathway of allorecognition.

Evidence that the donor-derived passenger leucocytes play an important role in initiating rejection comes from studies showing that in certain situations removal of the passenger cells from grafts before transplantation can

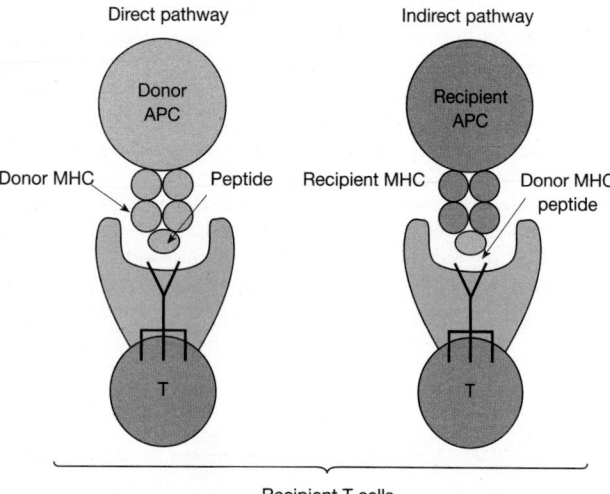

Fig. 4 Direct and indirect pathways of allorecognition. (1) Direct pathway: Donor MHC–peptide complexes are presented to recipient T cells by donor-derived antigen-presenting cells. Two hypotheses have been proposed to explain the high frequency of T cells, between 1 and 10 per cent of the repertoire, that can respond to alloantigens presented in this way. (i) High determinant density: the similarity in structure between MHC molecules results in T-cell receptors exhibiting cross-reactivity for donor MHC molecules irrespective of the peptide that is bound to each molecule. When donor molecules are expressed at high levels, as is the case on donor-derived passenger leucocytes, a sufficient number of T-cell receptors will engage the molecule to trigger a response. (ii) Multiple binary complexes: each donor MHC–peptide complex can be recognized by a different clone of T cell in the recipient giving rise to a high overall frequency of responding cells. (2) Indirect pathway: Donor MHC and miH antigens are processed by recipient antigen-presenting cells and presented as peptides by recipient MHC molecules. Each recipient MHC–donor peptide complex can be recognized by T cells in the recipient. The frequency of responding cells is of the same order of magnitude to T cells responding to other nominal antigens, such as viral antigens.

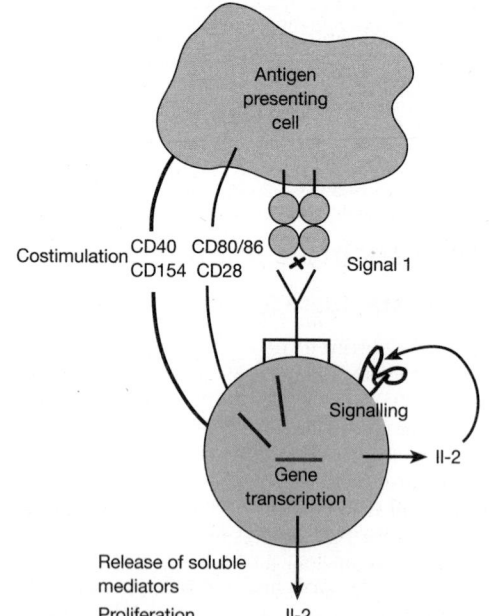

Fig. 5 Antigen presentation to naïve T cells. In conjunction with antigen recognition, additional signals or costimulation are required to trigger T-cell activation. Some of the molecules involved are illustrated, including on the T-cell side CD28 and CD154 (CD40L) and on the antigen-presenting cell side CD86 and CD40.

result in prolonged graft survival. However, this is not the case in every situation and the second route of antigen presentation—the indirect pathway—has also been shown to contribute to acute rejection as well as playing a significant role in the evolution of chronic rejection.

At the same time that donor antigen-presenting cells are migrating from the graft, recipient leucocytes are being attracted to the graft in response to chemokines (along with other mediators) released by the transplanted tissue. Amongst the cells recruited into the graft are circulating antigen-presenting cells. These take up debris arising from the tissue damage caused by the transplantation procedure itself, and then migrate to the draining lymphoid tissue. In addition, soluble antigens released as a result of damage to the tissue at the time of transplantation are also transported to the draining lymphoid tissue where they can be picked up by resident antigen-presenting cells. The captured antigens are then processed and presented as peptides with recipient MHC molecules to T cells in the T-cell areas of the recipient lymphoid tissue. In the context of transplantation this route of presentation is known as the indirect pathway of allorecognition (Fig. 4). It is clearly the more physiological of the two pathways that are used to trigger the activation of the response after allotransplantation. Moreover, indirect presentation of donor antigens is likely to continue in the long term after transplantation. Once all of the donor-derived passenger leucocytes have migrated from the graft they are obviously not replaced and therefore only so-called 'non-' or less-professional antigen-presenting cells, such as endothelial cells of donor origin, are available for the continued stimulation of direct pathway T cells.

It has been shown recently that migrating antigen-presenting cells are drawn to the correct area within the lymphoid tissue by chemokines, thereby ensuring that they come into contact with naïve T cells maximizing the chances of antigen presentation. Similarly, once a T cell has been triggered it migrates to other areas of the lymphoid organ, notably the B-cell area, in order to propogate the response and initiate the development of effector cells (Fig. 1).

Activation of recipient T cells

Recipients deprived of T cells either through manipulation of the immune system or through genetic mutations are unable to reject allografts. T cells are therefore a key element of the rejection response. The relative roles of CD4+ and CD8+ T cells in the initiation of the response will depend on the donor–recipient combination and the context in which the activation takes place.

As has become clear in the preceding sections, for T cells to become activated they need to recognize antigen. Every T cells bears a recognition structure, the T-cell receptor (**TCR**). The majority of T cells in the peripheral lymphoid organs and peripheral blood express a TCR comprising an α and β chain—the recognition structure—that is associated with a complex of polypeptides which form the signalling moiety known as CD3 (Fig. 5). αβTCRs can recognize MHC–peptide complexes with exquisite specificity, each being specific for one MHC–peptide complex. Once recognition has taken place, signals are delivered to the intracellular machinery by CD3.

At this stage in the process the cell membrane in the vicinity of the TCR–CD3 complex becomes very active and reorganization of the molecules in the membrane occurs to form an immunological synapse. This results in all of the elements required for productive T-cell activation being brought into close proximity with the TCR, including the accessory molecules, CD4 or CD8, and molecules required for the delivery of costimulation or second signals to the T cell, CD28 and CD154. Other structures that are important for adhesion of the antigen-presenting cell and the T cell localize to the edges of the synapse, thus ensuring that the two remain in close contact with one another for long enough for information to be transmitted in both directions.

The localization of CD4 or CD8 in the immunological synapse brings them into close proximity with the TCR–MHC–peptide complex. CD4 is expressed by T cells that recognize MHC class II–peptide complexes (class

II-restricted T cells) and CD8 by T cells that recognize MHC class I–peptide complexes (class I-restricted T cells). Each of these molecules can interact with conserved elements of the class II or class I structure, respectively, and they fulfil both an adhesion and signalling function when antigen recognition occurs.

In addition to signals coming through the TCR–CD3 complex and accessory molecules—also known as signal 1—additional signals arising from other cell surface receptors are required to ensure that the responding T cell is activated. These additional signals are often referred to as signal 2 or costimulation. In the presence of signal 1 but the absence of signal 2, T cells become unresponsive or anergic and fail to proliferate in response to further signals from antigen-presenting cells. Thus, during the initial phase of activation it is important that the antigen is presented by a professional antigen-presenting cell that can provide costimulation in addition to presenting donor antigen, either as the intact molecule or as recipient MHC–donor peptide complexes.

Costimulation is a complex process involving many cell surface structures. In strict terms costimulatory molecules can be defined as those that are essential for the initiation of a response from naïve T cells. The best characterized of these on the T-cell side is a molecule known as CD28 (Fig. 5). This is expressed by naïve T cells at rest, interacts with two cell surface ligands on antigen-presenting cells (CD80 and CD86), and is reported to have a preferential interaction with CD86 at the initiation of the response. CD86 is expressed at low levels by immature antigen-presenting cells, but upregulated rapidly during maturation of the antigen-presenting cell and following contact with T cells. By contrast, CD80 is expressed at lower levels than CD86 at the beginning of the response, but once expressed can also interact with CD28. The current interpretation of these data suggests that CD86 is more important for interaction with CD28 during the initiation of the response and that CD80 participates more actively in the downregulation of the response by preferentially interacting with another T-cell molecule, CD152 or CTLA4 (see below).

Signals delivered through CD28 result in increased cytokine synthesis by the responding T cell resulting from the stabilization of cytokine mRNA species. Signals through CD28 are independent of those delivered through the TCDR–CD3 complex and can be blocked independently by different immunosuppressive drugs. However, when the two signalling pathways occur in the same context the signals are integrated by the responding T cell, resulting in an augmented response. The complex series of phosphorylation and dephosphorylation events that take place results in the production of transcription factors, including nuclear factor of activated T cells (NF-AT), that translocate the nucleus of the T cells and switch on transcription of genes such as that for IL-2.

Regulation of immune responses is always critically important: dysregulated immune responses can have very dramatic and harmful consequences for the host. A pathway that counterbalances the positive signals coming through CD28 therefore exists to ensure that the process of T-cell activation does not continue indefinitely in an uncontrolled manner. Later during the course of T-cell activation a new molecule, CD152, is expressed by the activated T cells and acts as a negative regulator of the response. Evidence for this has been obtained by analysing mice that have a targeted disruption in the CD152 gene, so-called CD152 knockout mice. These mice have uncontrolled T-cell expansion when they are housed under normal environmental conditions where they are exposed continuously to a wide variety of antigenic stimuli. CD152 has been shown to have a higher binding affinity for CD86 and CD80 than CD28. Once it is expressed by the activated T cell it can therefore compete for binding with these molecules on the antigen-presenting cell. In addition, the interaction of CD152 with CD80 has been shown to deliver a negative signal to the T cell, shutting down further clonal expansion.

The construction of a fusion protein from the extracellular domains of CD152, CTLA4Ig or CTLA4Fc, and its use as a therapeutic agent has provided evidence that blocking costimulation through CD28 is sufficient to inhibit graft rejection, and confirming that T-cell costimulation through this pathway is a critical step in the activation steps of the rejection response.

Following the initial stages of T-cell activation, CD4+ T cells also express another cell surface molecule, CD154 or CD40L, that can provide additional costimulatory signals for the responding cell. CD154 interacts with its ligand CD40, which is expressed by antigen-presenting cells, including dendritic cells, B cells, and monocytes (Fig. 5). Non-haematopoietic cells can also express CD40, including endothelial cells, fibroblasts, and epithelial cells. Interestingly, signalling through this pathway is a two-way event, not only leading to modification of the functional capabilities of the T cell but also those of the antigen-presenting cell. Thus, signalling through CD40 results in the augmented expression of CD86 and CD80 by antigen-presenting cells, potentially setting up an amplification loop for augmenting the response. For example, in the kidney, tubular epithelial cells have been shown to express CD40 and engagement by CD154 results in the increased production of chemokines, including IL-8 and Rantes.

CD40 and CD154 are members of the TNF and TNF receptor families, respectively. They utilize different signalling molecules to both the TCR–CD3 and CD28 pathways. Blockade of CD154 by a monoclonal antibody has been shown, either in combination with CTLA4Ig or at high doses alone, to prevent acute allograft rejection and lead to long-term rejection-free survival of vascularized as well as non-vascularized grafts. This pathway is therefore also critical for the early events in T-cell activation. Although CD4+ T cells are highly dependent on it for activation, evidence is emerging that activation of CD8+ T cells is much less dependent upon or independent of the CD154–CD40 pathway. Thus in some donor–recipient combinations rejection can still be initiated by CD8+ T cells even in the presence of high doses of anti-CD154.

Determining the character of the rejection response

The character of the downstream response is critically dependent on the context in which the initial activation and restimulation of donor antigen-specific T cells takes place. Once activated, T cells recruit other cells into the response and play a role in determining how these differentiate into effector cells. The antigen-presenting cells involved, the cytokine environment, and the immune status of the host will all have a marked influence on the downstream response. Following chronic antigen stimulation, such as will occur with time after transplantation, a marked divergence in cytokine production by the responding cells can take place. This was first noted following chronic stimulation of antigen-specific mouse T cells *in vitro*, but has subsequently been demonstrated to occur in humans as well.

T-cell activation in the presence of IL-12 has been shown to result in the differentiation of T cells that secrete IFN-γ and IL-2. By contrast, if the initial contact between the T cell and antigen takes place in the presence of IL-4, then the cell will differentiate along a different pathway and secrete IL-4, IL-5, and IL-10, so-called signature cytokines (Fig. 6). The two types of T cell have been referred to as T_{H1} and T_{H2} or T_{C1} and T_{C2} depending on whether they express CD4 or CD8. T cells secreting IFN-γ and IL-2 orchestrate cell-mediated immunity, resulting in the activation of cytotoxic T cells (T_C) and macrophages predominantly, whereas T cells secreting IL-4 and IL-10 trigger the differentiation of B cells into plasma cells producing certain isotypes of immunoglobulin (humoral immunity) and the activation of eosinophils. Both types of T-cell response have been shown to lead to rejection. Therefore the hypothesis that a T_{H1} response is aggressive and results in rejection whereas a T_{H2} response promotes tolerance—the T_{H1}–T_{H2} paradigm for transplantation—is not clear cut and the context in which the response evolves will have a marked influence on whether rejection occurs.

Migration of activated leucocytes into the graft

Once activated, the donor-specific leucocytes must migrate from the recipient lymphoid tissue back to the graft if they are going to be effective in destroying the transplanted tissue. To enter the graft the leucocytes have to cross the donor vascular endothelium. Leucocyte extravasation is a multistep process, controlled by the production of chemokines by the transplanted tissue and multiple interactions between cell surface molecules expressed by the endothelium and the migrating leucocytes. Chemokine receptors involved in the recruitment of leucocytes into tissues are only expressed at low levels on resting leucocytes, therefore activation of the different leucocyte populations that participate in either the innate or adaptive immune response to the graft is a key step in the recruitment process.

Characterization of the chemokines and chemokine receptors involved in recruiting leucocytes to the graft is currently in progress. Chemokines produced within the tissue can be tethered to endothelial cells by interaction with carbohydrate structures on the endothelial cell surface as well as secreted from the tissue. Thus leucocytes flowing in the blood through the vessel can become attracted to the endothelial cells as a result of chemotactic gradients being established from the vessel wall into the tissue. Cell–cell interactions between the leucocytes and the endothelial cells are initiated such that the leucocytes flowing past the tissue in the blood are taken out of the flow and begin to roll along the vessel endothelium. As the leucocytes roll they sample the environment of the endothelial cells. If there is nothing wrong with the endothelial cell surface, then the leucocytes detach and return to the blood flow. However, in the presence of 'danger' signals the leucocytes express new cell surface structures, including P-selectin. The rolling leucocytes then becomes tethered to the endothelial cell. As a result

Fig. 6 T-cell differentiation. The microenvironment present when a T cell is activated will have a marked influence on the way in which it differentiates upon restimulation with antigen. T cells that are activated in the presence of IL-12 will differentiate into cells that secrete the signature cytokines IFN-γ and IL-2, whereas T cells that encounter antigen in the presence of IL-4 will differentiate into cells producing IL-4, IL-5, and IL-10.

of interaction between additional families of cell surface molecules, both on the endothelial cell and the leucocytes, including integrins and immunoglobulin superfamily members, firm adhesion of the leucocytes to the endothelial cell surface occurs, allowing the cells to transmigrate between endothelial cell junctions into the tissue along the chemokine gradient.

Graft destruction

Unlike some immune responses, for example to certain viruses, where a single effector mechanism dominates the final stages of the process, for allograft rejection the immune system uses many strategies to destroy the graft (Fig. 1). Once the vascular endothelium of the graft has been damaged by one or more of the mechanisms outlined below, the blood supply to the graft will be lost and rapid necrosis of the transplanted tissue will occur. Later in the rejection process the parenchymal cells of the graft will also become targets for these destructive mechanisms.

Antibody

Alloantibodies have been shown to play a role in hyperacute, acute, and chronic rejection. As mentioned above, hyperacute rejection of allografts is very rarely seen in clinical transplantation as rigorous screening of recipients for antidonor reactive antibodies is carried out before transplantation to eliminate any patients who have preformed antibodies against the donor. Hyperacute rejection of xenografts is the first immunological barrier that needs to be overcome if xenotransplantation is to be successful in the future. Different approaches are being investigated with varying degrees of success. Understanding how antibodies can trigger the destruction of a graft is clearly one of the important pieces of information required to facilitate the design of effective strategies to prevent antibody-mediated damage.

Antibodies that react with the graft can trigger its destruction in two ways: by activating complement or through antibody-dependent cellular cytotoxicity via killer cells.

Complement is a cascade of proteases that are triggered sequentially following the initial activating event. The system can be activated when antidonor antibodies formed as a result of T-dependent B-cell activation (Fig. 1) bind to donor antigens. As a result, inflammatory mediators will be released, increasing the vascular permeability of vessels in the graft and thereby facilitating the migration of leucocytes into the graft. The graft will become coated with antibody and activated complement components, targeting donor cells for opsonization by phagocytic cells which express receptors both for complement components and antibody. The membrane attack complex of the complement system is then formed, resulting in the lysis of donor cells. Many of the pathological changes that are associated with acute rejection, such as arteriosclerosis, interstitial haemorrhage, and fibrinoid necrosis of arteriolar cell walls, may result from the binding of antibodies and complement activation.

Antibody-dependent cellular cytotoxicity is cell dependent and occurs when the antibodies act as a bridge between the graft and killer cells, activating their lytic machinery. Killer cells are heterogeneous and many different types of leucocyte can participate in antibody-dependent cellular cytotoxicity when they are present in the correct microenvironment.

Although the appearance of antidonor antibodies can trigger rejection, their appearance does not necessarily mark the rejection of the graft. Indeed, the presence of antidonor antibodies may be perfectly compatible with continued graft survival. The specificity and the effector properties of the antibodies produced hold the key to whether particular antidonor antibodies are destructive.

Donor-specific cytotoxic T cells

Donor-specific cytotoxic T cells (TC) mature from precursor T_C (pTC) following activation of donor-specific T-helper cells (TH) (Fig. 1). T_C are activated either as a result of the formation of a three-cell cluster with the helper cell and the antigen-presenting cell, or as a result of the activated T_H cell 'licensing' the antigen-presenting cell to activate the pT_C. Once mature, effector T_C exhibit potent, antigen-specific cytotoxic activity. Their cytotoxic activity arises through a variety of mechanisms: these include the release of proteases called granzymes; the deposition of perforins, proteins that punch holes in the membrane of the target cell; the triggering of Fas-dependent cytotoxicity; and the release of soluble molecules such as tumour necrosis factor (TNF). The exact mechanism that is used *in vivo* may vary depending on the conditions that prevail within the graft.

There is considerable evidence to suggest that T_C can be involved in graft rejection. Most convincingly, when CD8+ cells are eliminated from the recipient before transplantation (most T_C recognize donor class I molecules and express CD8), graft rejection is often delayed or prevented. However, the presence of T_C is not mandatory for rejection as in some circumstances this has been shown to occur in the absence of demonstrable T_C activity. Moreover, the demonstration that donor-specific T_C activity can be detected *ex vivo* is not a guarantee that rejection is taking place. Again, the precise microenvironment in the graft markedly influences the ability of the effector cells to elicit graft destruction.

Natural killer cells

Natural killer (**NK**) cells form part of the innate immune response and are a potent source of cellular cytotoxicity. They are only triggered to kill when certain non-polymorphic MHC class I molecules, HLA E molecules, are missing from the target cells. In other words, NK cells are not used to destroy normal cells of the host unless they have been modified such that they no longer express HLA E molecules.

The receptors involved in NK-cell activation have been characterized and under normal circumstances these receive both positive and negative signals from both activating and inhibitory receptors when they engage their ligands on the target cell. Only when the inhibitory signals are missing do the cells exhibit cytotoxic activity. The role of NK cells in the rejection of solid organ allografts is still uncertain. NK cells with the ability to kill target cells *ex vivo* can be found in rejecting allografts, but to date there has been no direct demonstration that they play a role in rejection. By contrast, NK cells have been shown to be capable of rejecting bone marrow cells that express very low levels of MHC class I molecules and are thought to be very important in the rejection of xenografts where the graft will express no human class I.

Macrophages, eosinophils, and cytokine release

When T cells are activated they can elicit a non-specific effector mechanism referred to as a delayed-type hypersensitivity reaction (**DTH**). DTH reactions are characterized by the infiltration of leucocytes, including lymphocytes, macrophages, and eosinophils into the target site, in this case the graft. Damage to the graft occurs as a result of the production of non-specific mediators, such as nitric oxide, reactive oxygen species, IL-1, and TNF-α by the infiltrating cells. This activity is triggered in an antigen-specific manner by the T_H cell, but the effector mechanisms that lead to the destruction of the graft are non-specific. DTH reactions have been shown to be capable of playing a role in acute and chronic allograft rejection.

Conclusion

The immune response to a transplant is complex. The precise nature of the response will depend on many factors: the donor–recipient incompatibility, the type of graft, the site of transplantation, and not least the cocktail of immunosuppressive drugs that are used to try and prevent or control the response.

Further reading

Bach F *et al.* (1995). Barriers to xenotransplantation. *Nature Medicine* **1**, 869–73.

Banchereau J, Steinman R (1998). Dendritic cells and the control of immunity. *Nature* **392**, 245–52.

Brent L (1997). *A history of transplantation.* Academic Press, San Diego.

Cyster J (1999). Chemokines and cell migration in secondary lymphoid organs. *Science* **286**, 2098–102.

Ginns L, Cosimi A, Morris P, eds. (1999). *Transplantation.* Blackwell Science, Oxford.

Gould D, Auchincloss H (1999). Direct and indirect recognition: the role of MHC antigens in graft rejection. *Immunology Today* **20**, 77–82.

Matzinger P (1994). Tolerance, danger and the extended family. *Annual Reviews of Immunology* **12**, 991–1045.

Medzhitov R, Janeway C (2000). Innate immune recognition: mechanisms and pathways. *Immunological Reviews* **173**, 89–97.

Transplantation Websites

The Eurotransplant Foundation. _ HYPERLINK http://www.eurotransplant.org __http://www.eurotransplant.org_

Anthony Nolan Bone Marrow Trust. _ HYPERLINK http://www.anthonynolan.com __http://www.anthonynolan.com_

United Network of Organ Sharing. _ HYPERLINK http://www.unos.org __http://www.unos.org_

6

Principles of clinical oncology

6.1 Epidemiology of cancer

R. Doll and R. Peto

Introduction

All cancers have certain pathological and clinical characteristics in common, but those arising in different organs often have very different causes. The epidemiology of cancer, by which is meant the study of the incidence of the disease in people under different conditions of life, is, therefore the epidemiology of specific types of cancer, usually, but not always, defined as cancers of specific organs. In this sense, the subject has a history dating back nearly 300 years to Ramazzini's observation that cancer of the breast occurred more often in nuns than in other women of similar age and to Pott's observation, 200 years ago, that scrotal cancer in young men occurred characteristically in chimney sweeps. The high risk in nuns (which largely reflected the protective effect of multiple pregnancies in the general population) helped the realization that hormonal factors can substantially affect the incidence of several types of cancer, while the latter led to the recognition that the combustion products of coal to which sweeps had been exposed could cause cancer on any part of the skin with which they came into repeated contact and to the isolation of the first specific chemical carcinogen. Many other similar observations were made over the next 150 years, mostly as a result of the acumen of individual doctors who were struck by the observation that clusters of cases of a particular type of cancer occurred in patients with a similar occupational or cultural background. Lip and tongue cancers were found in pipe smokers, bladder cancer in certain aniline dye workers, buccal cancer in those who habitually chewed mixtures of tobacco and betel in India, lung cancer in miners of particular ores (who, it was subsequently realized, were heavily exposed to radon and its daughter products), and skin cancer in the early radiologists and radiographers who were heavily exposed to X-rays and in farmers and seamen heavily exposed to sunlight. Gradually, however, clinical anecdotes were replaced by statistics as the epidemiological methods that are described below began to be applied to the study of cancer and other noninfectious disease. As a result, many other causes were identified with sufficient certainty to justify preventive action and data were obtained to suggest hypotheses that could be tested in the laboratory.

Preventability of cancer

Perhaps the most important result of such observations has been the realization that any type of cancer that is common in one population is rare in some other, and that the differences between populations are mostly not genetic. Hence, where they are common these cancers occur, in large part, as a result of the way people behave and the circumstances in which they live and they are, therefore, at least in principle, preventable. This does not mean that we can at present envisage a society in which any of the common cancers are completely eliminated (although this may prove to be possible when we understand more clearly the mechanisms by which they are produced). What it does mean is that we can envisage a society in which the age-specific risk of developing any type of cancer is low.

Differences in incidence between communities

Reliable evidence of variation in the incidence of particular types of cancer between different communities was slow to emerge because of differences in the standards of medical care, and hence in the extent to which any cancers are diagnosed, the absence of population-wide systems for the registration of any cases that were diagnosed, and differences in the reliability with which cases were reported when registration systems were established. Nowadays, however, the large differences that are reported between good cancer registries throughout the world are, for the most part, real, particularly if comparisons are restricted to the limited range of ages between 35 and 64 years. This excludes the youngest ages, at which cancer is rare, and the oldest ages, at which the records of the incidence of the disease are least reliable.

Table 1 shows, for selected types of cancer, the range of variation recorded by cancer registries that have produced data sufficiently reliable for the purpose of international comparison (International Agency for Research on Cancer, 1992) or, in a few instances, the range determined by special surveys. Types of cancer have been included if they are common enough somewhere to have a cumulative incidence among men or women of at least 1 per cent by 75 years of age. The ranges of variation shown are for incidence rates between 35 and 64 years (see above). The range of variation is never less than seven-fold and is sometimes more than a hundred-fold. Despite the selection of reasonably reliable registries, some of this tabulated variation may still be an artefact, due to different standards of medical service, case registration, and population enumeration; but in many cases the true ranges will be greater. First, there are still gaps in the cancer map of the world, so that some extreme figures may have been omitted because no accurate surveys have been practicable in the least developed areas and it is just these areas that are likely to provide the biggest contrasts (both high and low) with Western society, as Chen *et al.* (1990) have shown in rural China. Secondly, the figures cited refer, with one exception, to cancers of whole organs and do not distinguish between different histological types or different locations within an organ and the more one learns about each type of cancer the more disadvantageous this is found to be. It is obvious in the case of skin cancer, which includes melanomas that have increased in incidence dramatically in the last 50 years, basal-cell carcinomas of the face, which affect more than half the fair-skinned population of Queensland by 75 years of age, scar epitheliomas of the leg, which develop on the site of old ulcers in some African populations and account for 10 to 20 per cent of all cancers seen in some hospitals in Malawi and Rwanda Burundi, 'dhoti' cancers of the groin in India, and occupational cancers on the forearm due to exposure to tar and oil in industrialized countries. But it also applies, to a greater or lesser extent, to most of the cancers listed in Table 1.

The variation in incidence is not limited to the common cancers, but is also shown by many others. Burkitt's lymphoma, for example, never affects more than 1 in 1000 of the population, but it is at least 100 times as common among children in parts of Uganda as it is in Europe and North America; while Kaposi's sarcoma, which was extremely rare in most of the world until the advent of the acquired immunodeficiency syndrome (AIDS), was

Table 1 Range of incidence rates of common cancers (men, unless specified otherwise)

Site of origin of cancer	High-incidence area	Cumulative incidence (%) in high incidence area[1]	Low-incidence area	Ratio of rates in high- and low-incidence areas[2]
Skin	Australia[3] (Queensland)	>20	India (Bombay)	>200
Oesophagus	Iran, N.E.[3]	20	Nigeria	300
Lung	US (blacks)	12	Nigeria	35
Stomach	Japan (Hiroshima)	10	Uganda	25
Cervix uteri[4]	Columbia (Cali)	10	Israel (non-Jews)	15
Prostate	US (blacks)	10	China (Shanghai)	70
Breast[4]	US (whites)	10	China (Qidong)	7
Liver	China (Qidong)	9	England	90
Colon	US (whites)	4	India (Madras)	13
Corpus uteri[4]	US (whites)	3	Thailand (Kha Koe)	14
Bladder	US (Connecticut)	3	Philippines (Manila)	7
Larynx	Spain (Basque region)	3	Japan (Yamagata)	11
Nasopharynx	Hong Kong	3	England	100
Buccal cavity	France (Bas Rhin)	2	Israel (Jews)	20
Rectum	Denmark	2	Thailand (Kha Koe)	20
Ovary[4]	Denmark	2	China (Qidong)	10
Pharynx	India (Ahmedabad)	2	Denmark	8
Pancreas	Czech Republic	1	India (Ahmedabad)	10
Penis[3]	Parts of Uganda[3]	1	Israel (Jews)	30

[1] By age 75 years, in the absence of other causes of death.

[2] At ages 35–64 years, standardized for age.

[3] Special survey.

[4] Women.

so common in children and young adults in parts of Central Africa, even before 1970, that it accounted for 10 per cent of all tumours seen in one of the African hospitals surveyed by Cook and Burkitt. Some few cancers occur with approximately the same frequency in all communities; but all of these are uncommon. Acute myeloid leukaemia at 15 to 25 years of age is an example; nephroblastoma is another, except that it appears to be only half as common in Japan as elsewhere.

The figures that have been cited so far all refer to the incidence of cancer in different communities defined by the area in which they live. Communities, can, however, be defined in other ways and no matter what method is used, including categorization by ethnic origin, religion, or socioeconomic status, substantial differences may be found. Jewesses, for example, have a low incidence of cervical cancer irrespective of the country in which they live, and the Mormons of Utah and the Seventh Day Adventists of California suffer fewer cancers of the respiratory, gastrointestinal, and genital systems than members of other religious groups living in the same American states.

Few of the large differences observed between communities can be explained by genetic factors, apart from some of the differences observed in the incidence of cancer of the skin, the risk of which is much greater for whites than blacks, and possibly also for some of those in the incidence of testis cancer, which rarely affects black populations, and in the incidence of chronic lymphocytic leukaemia, which rarely affects people of Chinese or Japanese descent. Genetic factors cannot explain the differences observed on migration or with the passage of time, which are discussed below, nor can they explain the correlations observed between the national rates for particular types of cancer and some measures of the lifestyle of the different countries.

Changes in incidence in migrant groups

That changes in the incidence of cancer occur on migration is certain. Many groups have been studied, including Indians who went to Fiji and South Africa, Britons who went to Fiji and Australia, and Central Europeans who went to North America. Among the most reliable data are those for the black Africans whose ancestors were taken to America and the Japanese who went to Hawaii. The former now experience incidence rates for

internal cancers that are generally much more like those of white Americans than those of the black populations in West Africa from which most of their ancestors came, while the latter have experienced rates that are much more like those of the Caucasian residents in Hawaii than those of the Japanese still living in Japan (Table 2). The ancestors of black Americans and Hawaiian Japanese will have come from many different parts of West Africa and Japan, some of which are likely to have cancer rates somewhat different from those that have been cited in Table 2. Nevertheless, the contrasts are so great that there can be no serious doubt that new factors were introduced with migration.

Changes in incidence over time

Within one population there may be substantial changes in the incidence of a particular type of cancer over a period of a few decades that provide conclusive evidence of the existence of preventable factors. Changes in incidence over time may, however, be difficult to assess reliably, chiefly because it is difficult to compare the thoroughness of the selection and registration of particular types of cancer at different periods and partly because few incidence data have been collected for long enough, so we often have to fall back on changes in mortality rates even though these may be influenced by changes in treatment as well as by changes in incidence.

There are no simple rules for deciding which of the many changes in recorded cancer incidence and mortality rates are reliable indicators of real changes in incidence. Each set of data has to be assessed individually. It is relatively easy to be sure about changes in the incidence of cancer of the oesophagus, as the disease can be diagnosed without complex investigations and its occurrence is nearly always recorded, at least in middle age, because it is nearly always fatal. It is much more difficult to be sure about changes in the incidence of many other types. The common basal-cell carcinomas of the skin, for example, are also easy to diagnose, but they seldom cause death and can be treated effectively outside hospital, so they often escape registration. What appears to be a change in incidence may, therefore, be a change only in the completeness of registration. Cancers of the pancreas, liver, and brain, and myelomatosis, in contrast, usually cause death, but even when they do they may be misdiagnosed as another disease (for example brain tumours in old people could frequently in the past be

Table 2 Comparisons of cancer incidence rates in migrants and residents in homelands and adopted countries (men, unless otherwise specified)

Primary site of cancer	Annual incidence per million persons[1]					
	Japan[2]	Hawaii		Nigeria	US	
		Japanese	Caucasians	(Ibadan)	Blacks[2]	Whites[2]
Oesophagus	131	46	75			
Stomach	1311	397	217			
Colon	83	371	368	34	351	315
Rectum	93	297	204	34	204	225
Liver				272	77	36
Pancreas				55	225	124
Larynx				37	193	141
Lung	268	379	962	27	1532	981
Prostate	14	154	343	134	651	275
Breast[3]	315	1221	1869	337	1187	1650
Cervix uteri[3]	364	149	243	559	569	276
Corpus uteri[3]	26	407	714	42	222	568
Ovary[3]	53	160	274			
Non-Hodgkin's lymphoma				133	8	4

[1] Rates are standardized for age among men aged 35–64 years unless otherwise specified. Data are provided only for those types of cancer where there are marked differences in incidence between residents of countries of origin and of adoption.

[2] Average of rates in two regions.

[3] Women.

misdiagnosed as other neurological conditions), so that an increased incidence or mortality rate may be wholly or partly due to improvements in diagnosis, in the availability of the medical services, or in the readiness of physicians to inform cancer registries of the cancers they find. Such changes are particularly likely to affect the rates recorded for people over 65 years of age, as many old people who were terminally ill used not to be intensively investigated.

Despite these difficulties, some of the decreases and increases in the recorded rates of particular types of cancer have been so gross that there must have been real changes in their incidence. Examples include the increase in oesophageal cancer in the black population of South Africa, the increase in lung cancer throughout most of the world (and its recent large decrease in men in the United Kingdom), the increase in mesothelioma of the pleura in men in industrialized countries, the decrease in cancer of the tongue in the United Kingdom, and the decrease in cancers of the cervix uteri and stomach throughout western Europe, North America, and Australasia. For a fuller account see *Trends in the incidence of cancer*, Doll et al., 1994.

Identification of causes

Finally, it has been possible to obtain evidence of the preventability of cancer by defining agents or circumstances that are a cause of the disease and are capable of control. In general, reliable evidence of causality (and particularly of the magnitude of any risks) has to come from epidemiology and not from laboratory experiments, although the latter can often provide reinforcement of epidemiological findings and essential guidance or completely novel hypotheses for epidemiological study. Reliable epidemiological evidence does not require randomized trials within particular populations, but it does require the study of different individuals within populations and not just the comparison of incidence rates in different populations. Non-randomized epidemiological studies of individuals have often yielded proof of causation beyond reasonable doubt (like that required to convict in a court of law). Action based on such evidence has, moreover, often been followed by the desired result—for example a reduction in the incidence of bladder cancer in the chemical industry on stopping the manufacture and use of 2-naphthylamine and, on a national scale, the reduction in the incidence of lung cancer in men in the United Kingdom following the decrease in smoking over the previous half century.

Cancer research workers have, therefore, accepted that the type of human evidence that has been obtained (often, but not invariably, combined with laboratory evidence that the suspected agents are carcinogenic in animals) is strong enough to conclude that a cause of human cancer has been identified and that, as a corollary, the disease can be prevented if this cause is controlled.

Biological factors

Speculations about the causes of cancer and the mechanisms that lead to its occurrence have been constrained by some of its biological characteristics. These include the relationships between incidence and genetic susceptibility, age, sex, and the delay (which is sometimes misleadingly called the 'latent period') that occurs between exposure to a causative agent and the appearance of clinical disease.

Genetic susceptibility

Genetic differences in susceptibility are discussed in Chapter 6.3. We note here only the role of epidemiology in (i) detecting familial clusters that are so marked that no statistical analysis is needed to show the reality of their existence, or (ii) demonstrating by large studies that if one member of a family develops a specific type of cancer, other members are somewhat more likely to develop that same type than would be expected in the population as a whole.

The first has shown that several rare genes have such a great effect on susceptibility that bearers of one such gene (if it is dominant) or two (if they are recessive) almost invariably develop a particular type of cancer. Examples include the dominant genes for polyposis coli and Gardner's syndrome that lead to cancer of the large bowel, and the recessive genes for retinoblastoma and xeroderma pigmentosum that lead (in the latter case) to squamous carcinoma and (less commonly) melanoma of the skin. Similar evidence has shown that other genetic syndromes frequently, but not invariably, lead to cancer, such as von Recklinghausen's neurofibromatosis leading to fibrosarcoma, the Peutz–Jeghers syndrome leading to carcinoma of the small bowel, the Wiskott–Aldrich syndrome leading to non-Hodgkin's lymphoma, and ataxia telangiectasia, Bloom's syndrome, and Fanconi's anaemia leading to leukaemia. The recognition of these syndromes is important to the individual, as it may provide an opportunity for prophylactic surgery, or enable the diagnosis of malignancy to be made at an early stage when treatment is more likely to be effective, or (rarely) enable precautions to be taken to prevent exposure to the relevant carcinogens, as in the case of sufferers from xeroderma pigmentosum or albinism, who can be protected against sunlight. The proportion of all cancers that occur in people who are highly susceptible to cancer in this way is, however, very small.

The second sort of epidemiological evidence has shown that there is no material tendency for cancer as a whole to cluster in families and that there are no common genetic polymorphisms that substantially increase the risk of developing cancer in all organs (although mutations in the p53 gene may increase the risk in many). It has also shown, however, that several of the common types of cancer do tend to cluster in families to some extent. Differences of this sort do not necessarily imply that the familial clusters are genetic in origin; they could be due to familial similarities of behaviour. Nor, however, do they necessarily imply that any genetic difference in susceptibility is particularly small. Calculations show that they are compatible with 50- to a 100-fold differences in genetic susceptibility if the genes for high susceptibility have an appropriate prevalence in the population. That socially important genetic variants exist is demonstrated by the greatly increased risk of developing basal-cell and squamous carcinomas of the sun-exposed skin in fair-skinned populations compared with dark-skinned, and there may be other genes associated with localized populations, which, for example, diminish the risk of chronic lymphatic leukaemia and myelomatosis in Chinese, Japanese, and Indians. Other genes may have only a minor effect, such as the gene for blood group A, the possession of which increases the risk of gastric cancer by about 20 per cent over that of people belonging to blood groups O or B.

Discovery of genetic factors that affect particular types of cancer is unlikely to explain much of the social and geographical differences in the distribution of cancer other than skin cancer, but it should help to elucidate mechanisms and in extreme cases may help to focus health education and costly methods of early diagnosis on the sections of the populations that are most at risk.

Age

Some risk of cancer occurs at every age, but the risk of developing any particular type varies with age. The most common relationship with age is a progressive increase in incidence from near zero in childhood and adolescence to a high rate in old age. This type of relationship is shown by carcinomas of the skin, lung, and gastrointestinal and urinary tracts, and by myelomatosis and chronic lymphatic leukaemia. The rate of increase is rapid, being typically proportional to the fourth, fifth, or sixth power of age in years, so that the annual incidence may be 100 or 1000 times greater above age 75 than before age 25. With most of these cancers, the recorded incidence may stabilize, or even decrease, in the oldest age groups; but this is partly or wholly an artefact due to incomplete investigation of the terminal illnesses of old people. This pattern is observed for skin carcinoma due to exposure to ultraviolet light and for bronchial carcinoma, both in non-smokers and in men who regularly smoke a constant number of cigarettes a day, and can, under certain circumstances, be observed in the laboratory in skin-painting experiments on mice. It is probable that it reflects the cumulative effect of processes that operate steadily throughout life, starting at around the time of birth (or, for lung cancer among habitual smokers, in adolescence).

A less common pattern is a peak incidence early in life, which may be followed either by a decline virtually to zero or by a slow rise in middle and old age. Retinoblastomas and nephroblastomas occur only in childhood, with peak incidences (respectively) in the first and second years of life. Teratomas and seminomas of the testis have peak incidence rates at about 20 and 30 years of age, respectively, and later almost cease to occur, while osteogenic sarcomas have a peak incidence in adolescence and then show a slow increase with age from a lower rate in young adult life.

The remaining cancers show a variety of patterns. Carcinomas of the breast and cervix uteri of women, for example, begin to appear in adolescence and become rapidly more common up to the menopause. After the menopause the incidence of carcinoma of the breast may remain approximately constant, or may even become slightly reduced for a few years, before increasing again with age, though at a slower rate. Carcinoma of the cervix continues to increase fairly steeply for a few years after the menopause, before showing a stable or declining rate. Hodgkin's disease, on the other hand, appears in childhood and then continues to occur more or less evenly throughout life with only minor peaks in young adult life and in old age, while connective tissue sarcomas become progressively more common from childhood on, but with a much slower rate of increase than is shown by the common carcinomas.

Some of these relationships with age, like that for retinoblastoma in early childhood, seem to be invariant everywhere and, as far as is known, at all times. Others vary from community to community, or from time to time. In postmenopausal women, for example, cancer of the breast becomes progressively less common with increasing age in parts of Asia, but more common in Europe, while carcinoma of the lung used to show a peak incidence at about 60 years of age in the United Kingdom, which gradually moved to older ages, as a generation that had not smoked substantial numbers of cigarettes throughout adult life was replaced by one that had, and the same process is now being repeated in many developing countries.

These various patterns provide information, either about the period of activity of the stem cells from which the cancers derive, or about the period when the main exposure to causative agents occurs and the duration of that exposure. Some of this variation has already helped to explain some of the causes of cancer, as was the case with the shift in the peak incidence of bronchial carcinoma; but much of it still awaits elucidation.

Sex

Cancer used to be more common in women than in men in many countries due to the great frequency of carcinoma of the breast and of the cervix uteri and to the rarity of bronchial carcinoma, and this is still the case in populations for which similar conditions persist, as in parts of Latin America. Elsewhere, cancer is now more common in men, among whom lung cancer often predominates. This overall male preponderance hides, however, a wide range of sex ratios for cancer of different organs. If the sites of cancer that are peculiar (or almost peculiar) to one sex are ignored, the sex ratio varies (in Britain) from a male excess of about 6 to 1 for pleural mesothelioma and carcinoma of the larynx, through many types of cancer with only a small male preponderance, to carcinomas of the right side of the colon, thyroid, and gallbladder, which may be up to twice as common in women.

For many types of cancer the sex ratio is much the same in different countries and at different times. For some, however, and particularly for cancers of the mouth, oesophagus, larynx, and bronchus, the sex ratio is extremely variable—not only between countries and at different times, but sometimes also between different ages at the same time and in the same country. The most marked variation is shown by cancer of the oesophagus, which may affect both sexes equally or be 20 times more common in men than in women. As with the various patterns of incidence with age, these different sex ratios and their variation can provide useful clues to the causation of the particular type of cancer, not all of which have yet been successfully followed up.

Delay between cause and effect

One reason why it has been difficult to recognize causes of cancer in humans is the long delay that characteristically occurs between the start of exposure to a carcinogen and the appearance of the clinical disease. This 'latent period', as it is commonly, but rather misleadingly, called is often several decades, although it may be as short as 1 year or as long as 60. The exact relation between the date of exposure and the date of the appearance of different cancers is still uncertain, partly because the interval is subject to random factors, partly because few cancers are induced by a single, brief exposure, and partly because there are still very few sets of quantitative data with detailed information about the dates when exposure began and ended.

When cancer is induced by short but intensive exposure to ionizing radiation, as following the explosions of the atomic bombs in Hiroshima and Nagasaki or in patients treated by radiotherapy, the excess incidence of solid tumours rises for 15 to 20 years and then may continue to rise, level off, or decline. In the case of acute leukaemia, however, a peak incidence occurs much earlier (about 5 years after irradiation) and relatively few cases appear after more than 30 years.

Short, intensive exposure to a carcinogen is, however, exceptional. The more usual situation is for sporadic or continuous exposure to a carcinogen to be prolonged for years—a decade or two in the case of occupational exposure, several decades in the case of tobacco smoking, and a lifetime in the case of ultraviolet sunlight. In this situation the incidence of cancer increases progressively with the length of exposure. In the last two cases cited, the incidence appears to increase approximately in proportion to the fourth power of the duration of exposure so that the effect after (say) 40 years is more than 10 times as great as that after 20 years, and more than 100 times as great as that after 10 years. Whether the same holds for occupational exposure is not known; but it has been shown to hold in some experiments in which chemicals were repeatedly applied to the skin of genetically similar mice and it may prove to be a general biological rule for many types of carcinoma and many carcinogens.

There is still less quantitative information about what usually happens when exposure ceases; but in the case of cigarette smoking the rapidly rising annual risk among those who continue to smoke stabilizes for one or two decades after smoking ceases before increasing again slowly. The exsmoker consequently avoids the enormous progressive increase in risk suffered by the continuing smoker.

These delayed effects accord with the idea that the appearance of clinical cancer is the end-result of a multistage process in which several mutations have to be produced in a single stem cell to turn it into the seed of a growing cancer. From the practical point of view, the important conclusions are that cancer may be very much more likely to occur after prolonged exposure to a carcinogen than after short exposure, that it is seldom likely to appear within a decade after first exposure (except in the case of leukaemia and the specific cancers of childhood), that it commonly occurs several decades after first exposure, and that some excess risk may continue to occur for decades after exposure has ceased. The exact relationship may, however, differ for different carcinogens and different types of tumour. Bladder tumours, for example, began to appear within 5 years of intensive exposure to 2-naphthylamine in the dye industry, while mesotheliomas of the pleura have seldom, if ever, appeared within 10 years of exposure to asbestos, but they continue to increase in incidence for up to 50 years after first exposure, even if the exposure was relatively brief.

Luck

There remains the influence of luck, which is commonly ignored; yet it is important for the individual as it is the reason why two animals of identical genetic constitution that have been treated in the same way do not, in general, develop cancer in the same place at precisely the same age. It reflects the element of chance that determines whether a particular series of events all occur in one particular stem cell out of the many thousands of stem cells that exist that don't give rise to a malignant clone. For any one individual the role of good or bad luck in determining the occurrence of cancer may be large (just as luck plays a substantial part in whether or not an individual driver has a traffic incident); but in a large population luck has little net effect on the incidence of cancer and only nature and nurture are important.

Avoidable factors

Tobacco

Tobacco is by far the most important single cause of cancer in developed countries. Chewed it can cause cancers of the mouth and oesophagus; smoked it is a major cause of cancers of the mouth, pharynx (other than nasopharynx), oesophagus, larynx, lung, pancreas, renal pelvis, and bladder. For these eight cancers, epidemiological evidence indicates that pro-

Table 3 Per cent of deaths from cancer attributable to smoking, 1975 and 1995, by sex: various countries

Country	Male		Female	
	1975	1995	1975	1995
Australia	39	32	4	14
Finland	46	37	1	4
France	33	38	0	2
Hungary	36	53	5	15
UK	52	40	12	20
US	42	43	10	25

longed smoking of average numbers of cigarettes per day increases the risk 3 to 20 times. It is, however, now clear that cigarette smoking also causes a proportion of several other types of cancer, increasing the incidence up to twice that in non-smokers: namely, cancers of the lip, nose, nasopharynx, stomach, liver, and renal body and also myeloid leukaemia. Although the proportional increases are not large, the consistency of the findings in different countries, the evidence of dose–response relationships, the lower mortality in exsmokers than in continuing smokers, the lack of evidence for important confounding, and the presence in the smoke of many different carcinogens provide strong grounds for believing that most or all of these observed associations are causal.

In sum, smoking is estimated to have caused 30 per cent of all fatal cancers in the United Kingdom in 1995, down from 34 per cent 20 years earlier. The reduction was substantial in men (down from 52 per cent to 40 per cent) but it was largely counteracted by the increase in women (from 12 per cent to 20 per cent). Comparable figures from the United States and from some other developed countries are shown in Table 3. In men, there have been decreases in some developed countries, but increases in others, particularly in Central and Eastern Europe. In women, the proportion of cancer deaths attributed to smoking was generally low in 1975, but has subsequently increased in all developed countries and must be expected to increase further. It was, however, still small in countries such as France, where few middle-aged or elderly women had been smoking for long enough for any material effect to be produced.

In developing countries, the effects of smoking have only recently begun to be studied systematically and much remains unclear. In general, women in developing countries do not smoke (or if they do they smoke very little). In men, however, there has been a very large increase in cigarette consumption, the full effects of which have yet to materialize. China, with 20 per cent of the world's population, smokes 30 per cent of the world's cigarettes and by 1990 smoking was already responsible for about 20 per cent of male cancer deaths. In India, where many men have smoked 'bidis' (small home-manufactured cigarettes) for decades, the proportion may be even greater (chiefly because smoking can act as a cofactor for the production of cancers of the mouth, oesophagus, or stomach in those who habitually chew quids containing betel and tobacco). In some parts of South America, the male lung cancer rates from smoking are already as high as in developed countries. Overall, tobacco may be causing about as many cancer deaths in developing as in developed countries, in which case it would be responsible for about 20 per cent of cancer deaths throughout the world.

Alcohol

At least six types of cancer are caused in part by the consumption of alcohol. One, liver cancer, is produced only secondarily to the production of liver cirrhosis and is, consequently, caused only by heavy and prolonged consumption. Four are causally related to smoking as well as to alcohol: namely, cancers of the mouth, pharynx (other than nasopharynx), oesophagus, and larynx. The two agents act synergistically, increasing each other's effect, so that the risk from alcohol in non-smokers or long-term exsmokers is very small, while that in heavy smokers is disproportionately large. The remaining type, cancer of the breast, has been shown to be related to alcohol only within the last decade or so. Cohort studies show that the risk increases progressively with the amount drunk (at least up to moderately high levels) and laboratory studies that show that alcohol increases the level of oestrogen in the blood suggest a plausible mechanism.

Cancers of the large bowel have also been associated with alcohol in many studies, but the relationship is weak and its nature uncertain: it could be due to confounding with smoking and diet.

Ionizing radiations

Ionizing radiations, of whatever sort, share the characteristic of being able to penetrate animal tissues and damage DNA. It is not surprising, therefore, that they have been found to increase the incidence of cancer in practically every organ. It has not been possible to detect by direct observation the effect of the small amounts that adults receive as a result of exposure to (for example) radiological examination, atmospheric pollution, and normal levels of natural background; but it has been possible to make an estimate of their effect by extrapolating from the observed effects of the much larger doses received by the survivors of the atomic explosions at Hiroshima and Nagasaki, patients given radiotherapy or repeatedly screened radiologically, and people exposed occupationally to radium or to high concentrations of radon in mines or exceptionally in houses. Theoretical considerations and the dose–response relationship observed with these relatively large doses both indicate that there is unlikely to be any threshold below which no effect is produced. This conclusion is reinforced by the discovery that children who received doses of 10 to 20 mGy *in utero* (because their mothers were irradiated for diagnostic purposes whilst they were pregnant) were subject to an added risk of developing cancer in childhood of approximately 1 in 2000. At low doses (less than about 20 mGy) it seems probable that the carcinogenic effect is linearly proportional to the dose; at higher doses the same is true for most cancers other than leukaemia, for which the risk is approximately proportional to the square of the dose. It is unlikely, however, that we should be far out in our estimate if we accepted the conclusions of the International Committee on Radiological Protection (1991) and assumed that the lifetime risk of developing a fatal cancer is approximately 10 per cent per Gray (or per Sievert) to the whole body if the radiation dose is moderate and given acutely and about half that if the dose is low and spread out over time (that is 5 per 100 000 per mGy (or mSv)) with corresponding reductions if only part of the body is exposed.

People are exposed to different amounts of radiation in different countries, depending principally on the build up of radon in the air in domestic houses and the medical use of radiation for diagnosis and therapy. In the United Kingdom, the average annual dose is about 2.6 mSv, which, in a population of about 55 million, is estimated to cause about 7000 deaths a year from cancer, about 5 per cent of the total. In the United States, the average annual dose is about 50 per cent greater. The estimated hazard depends critically on the effects of chronic exposure to radon in houses, which, in the United Kingdom, contributes about half the total dose from all forms of radiation. In some parts of the country, however, most notably Devon and Cornwall, the average domestic radon dose is three or four times greater and in a few houses may be 10 or even 100 times greater. Its effect is discussed later under lung cancer. Nearly all the rest comes from other sources of natural radiation (35 per cent) and medical uses (14 per cent). The last, however, causes less cancer than would be deduced from the dose, as a large proportion is received by old or ill people who will not survive for long enough for a radiation-induced cancer to appear or because the doses given radiotherapeutically are so large that most of the cells that might have been made cancerous are destroyed. Less than 0.5 per cent of the average annual dose from all sources can be attributed to occupational exposure, fall-out from past bomb tests, and man-made products or radioactive waste.

Ultraviolet light

Photon energies in the ultraviolet (UV) range are sufficient to excite electrons in atoms to chemically active higher energy states permitting the formation of pyrimidine dimers between adjacent pyrimidine bases in DNA

and these may, as a result of misrepair, be the origin of mutations. UV does not penetrate much below the skin, so that it is chiefly within the skin that it is directly carcinogenic. Within the skin, however, it is the principal cause of all types of cancer, other than Kaposi's carcinoma. Whether it has any indirect carcinogenic effect on other tissues (notably the lymphopoietic tissue) by (for example) destroying Langerhans cells and so modifying immune reactions, has yet to be proved.

Infection

Infection, principally viral, but also in some cases bacterial and parasitic, is a major cause of avoidable cancer.

Viral Viruses that are known to cause human cancers, or suspected of doing so, are listed in Table 4, along with the types of cancer with which they are associated. Not all infected people develop the disease. In some cases the proportion doing so is quite small, unless other factors are also present. These include heavy malarial infection for Burkitt's lymphoma, the consumption of a type of salted fish for nasopharyngeal cancer, and the consumption of aflatoxin, a metabolic product of fungal infection with *Aspergillus flavus*, for liver cancer. What they are for the cancers produced by the human papilloma virus is not known.

Quantitatively, chronic infection with hepatitis B virus is one of the most important causes of cancer in many parts of the world. In China, for example, liver cancer accounts for about 20 per cent of all cancer deaths, the large majority of which are due to chronic lifelong infection with the virus. Infant vaccination against the virus is now being introduced and will protect the new generation, but will not provide retrospective protection for those born previously.

Bacterial Only one bacterial infection has been closely linked with the development of cancer: namely, *Helicobacter pylori*. Persistent infection acquired early in life leads to chronic gastritis in the antrum of the stomach and increases the risk of gastric cancer two to three-fold. Non-specific chronic infection in the bladder may also increase the risk of bladder cancer by the local formation of carcinogenic nitrosamines.

Parasitic In parts of Africa and Asia, parasitic infection is a major cause of cancer. Infestation with *Schistosoma haematobium*, which excretes its eggs through the bladder wall, causes a high incidence of bladder cancer in Egypt and East Africa while infestation with *Schistosoma japonicum*, which excretes its eggs through the wall of the large bowel, is responsible for a high incidence of intestinal cancer in parts of China. Liver flukes (*Clonorchis*

Table 4 Viral causes of cancer

Virus	Cancer
Hepatitis B	cancer of liver
Hepatitis C	cancer of liver
Human papilloma types 16, 18, and others	cancers of cervix, vulva, vagina, penis, anus; some skin cancers
Human herpes type 4 (EBV)	Burkitt's lymphoma
	immunoblastic lymphoma
	nasal T-cell lymphoma
	Hodgkin's disease
	nasopharyngeal cancer
Human herpes type 8 (Kaposi associated herpes virus)	Kaposi's sarcoma
	body-cavity lymphoma
Human T-cell leukaemia type 1	adult T-cell leukaemia/lymphoma
Human immunodeficiency virus[1]	Kaposi's sarcoma
	non-Hodgkin's lymphoma
	conjunctival carcinoma
Simian virus 40-like[2]	ependymoma
	choroid plexus tumours
	mesothelioma
	bone tumours

[1] In most cases, if not all, by facilitating the effect of other viruses.
[2] Causal nature of observed association unproved.

sinensis and *Opisthorcis viverrini*) are similarly responsible for the high incidence of cholangiosarcoma of the bile ducts in parts of South East Asia. The parasites may not cause cancer directly but chronic infection may start a chain of events that leads to cancer in other ways, such as chronic bacterial infection and the local formation of nitrites and nitrosamines.

Medical drugs

Apart from ionizing radiations, some 20 agents have been used therapeutically that are known to cause cancer in humans. These are listed in Table 5. That so many carcinogenic agents should have been prescribed medically is not surprising when it is borne in mind that treatment often requires modification of cellular metabolism and is sometimes intended to interfere with DNA. The hazard of cancer, however, need not necessarily be a bar to the use of a drug if the risk to life due to iatrogenic cancer is materially less than the chance of saving life that is achieved by its use—as is commonly the case with antineoplastic agents, immunosuppressive drugs, and radiotherapy.

Some of the chemotherapeutic agents listed in Table 5 were soon abandoned, while others have continued to be used for the treatment of uncommon conditions, and the sum of the cancers that these now produce cannot amount to more than a 100 or so a year in the United Kingdom.

Three of the listed drugs are, however, used extensively: hormonal replacement therapy (HRT) for postmenopausal women, selected steroids for contraception, and tamoxifen for the treatment of hormone-sensitive breast cancer. The first two increase the risk of breast cancer and all three can increase the risk of endometrial cancer, but HRT does so substantially only when given in the form of oestrogen alone and steroid contraceptives do so only in the form (now abandoned) in which oestrogen and progestogen are given sequentially. The combined steroid contraceptives currently in use can also rarely cause liver cancer and they may possibly increase the risk of cervix cancer. In contrast to these effects, tamoxifen reduces the incidence of breast cancer, and combined steroid contraceptives reduce the incidence of endometrial cancer and halve the risk of ovarian cancer for many years after they have been used. HRT and the combined steroid contraceptive are, moreover, associated with a reduction of some 20 per cent in

the risk of colorectal cancer, but whether this is causally related to their use remains to be proved.

Other drugs that may inhibit cancer rather than cause it are the non-steroidal analgesics, most notably aspirin, the prolonged use of which may somewhat reduce the risk of colorectal cancer.

Taken altogether it seems unlikely that medically prescribed drugs can be responsible for more than 1 per cent of all today's fatal cancers and may, in total, reduce the risk by somewhat more.

Occupation

In the years that followed Pott's observation that chimney sweeps tended to develop cancer of the scrotum, many other groups of workers were found to suffer from specific hazards of cancer and more substances that are known to be carcinogenic to humans have been unearthed by the search for occupational hazards than by any other means. These hazards, many of which are described in relation to individual types of cancer, are listed in Table 6. Many of the hazards that have been recognized caused large, or at least relatively large, risks, albeit for limited populations, and it may well be that other occupational hazards exist that have not yet been detected, either because the added risk is small in comparison with that due to other causes, or because only a few workers have been persistently exposed, or simply because the hazards have not been suspected and so not looked for. It must also be borne in mind that cancer in humans seldom develops until one or more decades after exposure to the carcinogen first occurs and it is, therefore, too soon to be sure whether agents that have been introduced into industry only during the last 20 years are carcinogenic or not.

Many groups of workers not listed in Table 6 have been suspected of having a special risk, but it has not been possible to decide whether the risk is real and attributable to their work. Many types of cancer have been examined in these groups and, in these circumstances, some differences that are conventionally 'statistically significant' are bound to have arisen by chance alone. Such differences can provide substantial evidence of a hazard only if highly significant ($p<0.001$), or if excess rates are confirmed in other studies, or if a risk of the specific type of cancer could be predicted from the nature of the agent to which they were exposed.

Other excess rates may be due to confounding; that is, they may be produced by social factors that are associated with the occupation in question rather than by the occupation itself. The potential importance of such confounding was illustrated by Fox and Adelstein's analysis of the occupational mortality statistics for England and Wales over the period 1970 to 72. They aggregated the occupations of men aged 15 to 64 years into 25 major categories and found that the lung cancer rates in these categories differed up to two-fold, a spread that was far too wide to be attributed to chance alone. However, data obtained from random samples of the general population showed that the proportions of men who smoked in each of these 25 large occupational categories varied from about 65 per cent of the national average to about 130 per cent, and that the differences in these proportions could account for most of the variation in the mortality from lung cancer.

Given sufficient details and the ability to repeat the observations, it is usually possible to obtain a fairly clear idea of whether or not an excess incidence in an occupational group does or does not reflect an occupational hazard by (for example) seeing whether the effect is related to the length of employment, the time after first exposure, and a specific type of work within the industry. Unfortunately these details are not always available and the reasons for many of the moderate excesses of cancer that have been reported in certain industries are still uncertain.

At present it seems unlikely that occupational hazards account for more than 2 or 3 per cent of all fatal cancers in developed countries such as the United Kingdom; but the quantitative evidence is uncertain and this estimate could be out by a factor of two. The three principal causes are probably asbestos dust (lung and pleural cancer), the combustion products of fossil fuels (skin and lung cancer), and ionizing radiations (any cancer).

Table 5 Carcinogenic agents used in medical practice (other than ionizing radiations)

Agent	Type of cancer
Antineoplastic agents:	
Busulphan	Leukaemia[1]
Chlorambucil	Leukaemia[1]
Chlornaphazine	Bladder
Cyclophosphamide	Bladder, leukaemia[1]
Melphalan	Leukaemia[1]
MOPP[2]	Leukaemia[1]
Thiotepa	
Treosulfan	Leukaemia[1]
Arsenic	Skin, liver (angiosarcoma), lung
Immunosuppressive drugs:	
Azathioprine	Non-Hodgkin's lymphoma
Cyclosporin	
Methoxypsoralen (plus UV light)	Skin
Phenacetin	Renal pelvis
Polycyclic hydrocarbons (coal-tar ointment)	Skin
Oestrogens:	
Unopposed	Endometrium, breast
Transplacental	Vagina (adenocarcinoma)
Steroids:	
Oxymetholone	Liver (hepatoma)
Oral contraceptives (combined)[3]	Breast, liver (hepatoma)
Tamoxifen[3]	Endometrium

[1] Acute non-lymphocytic.

[2] Combination of nitrogen mustard, vincristine, procarbazine, and prednisone.

[3] See text for value in preventing cancer.

Pollution

The idea that pollution might be an important cause of cancer has been in the forefront of the minds of cancer research workers since it was realized that the incidence of lung cancer tended to be higher in towns than in the countryside and that the combustion products of coal, which used to produce a pall of smoke over all large cities in Britain, contained carcinogenic hydrocarbons. Subsequently, with the rapid expansion of the chemical industry and the discovery that some of its products are mutagenic *in vitro* and carcinogenic in laboratory animals, anxiety increased about the possible effects of distributing such products ubiquitously in the air we breathe, the water we drink, and the food we eat.

The effects of pollution of this sort are, however, peculiarly difficult to assess directly by epidemiological methods, as pollutants are likely to be present in most areas, the absolute risk from each is likely to be small, and there may be little difference in the extent to which individuals are exposed over a wide area. Reliance is, therefore, often placed on two indirect methods: extrapolation from the effects of chronic exposure to much larger amounts in an occupational setting, and prediction of the effects on humans from laboratory tests. Both, however, (but particularly the latter) involve substantial uncertainties.

So far as atmospheric pollution is concerned, the epidemiological picture is complicated by the personal pollution produced by tobacco smoke and the social distribution of smoking habits; but, despite this complication, the various methods that have been discussed under lung cancer all lead to the conclusion that the pollution of the past may have contributed to the production of a few per cent of all lung cancers; but that the levels over the last three decades (principally from the combustion of fossil fuels, but also from asbestos, dioxins, and various other materials) are unlikely to be responsible for more than a fraction of 1 per cent of future cancers—although there may be exceptions awaiting discovery in the neighbourhood of particular factories. The greater effect of the modern type of pollution with ultra fine particles and of the intense indoor pollution with smoke that occurs in parts of China is examined later under lung cancer.

The effect of polluted drinking water and food is more obscure. Until recently no serious consideration had been given to the possibility that either might be important, except for the possible effect of the contamination of food with smoke from urban air. Now, however, analytical techniques permit the detection of chemicals at concentrations of less than 1 p.p.b. in both food and water and, in consequence, many have been detected that might arguably be carcinogenic, including pesticide residues and a variety of halogenated organic materials produced by the chlorination of water supplies. Relationships have been reported between the concentrations of some of these compounds in water and the mortality from cancers of the bladder and, possibly, the large intestine, in different localities; but it is extremely difficult to know what these relationships mean as there are many potentially confounding factors.

Mortality rates from cancers of the gastrointestinal and urinary tracts are, for the most part, stable or decreasing in early middle age, when the effects of new agents might be expected to show themselves first, and, in the absence of more specific evidence, it seems unlikely that chemical pollution of water and food could have a greater effect than the small effect already estimated for pollution of the air. It is important, however, to monitor the situation and, in particular, to seek an explanation for any increase in incidence (as has occurred with testis cancer and with non-Hodgkin's lymphoma not attributable to AIDS) and for any irregularities in the geographical distribution of any type of the disease.

Diet

For many years there has been suggestive evidence that most of the cancers that are currently common could be made less so by modification of the diet; but, with few exceptions, there is still little reliable evidence as to the modifications that would be of major importance. If we define diet to include all materials that occur in natural foods, are produced during the processes of storage, cooking, and digestion, or are added as preservatives or to give food colour, flavour, and consistency, the ways in which diet could influence the development of cancer are legion.

Ingestion of preformed carcinogens The most obvious is the ingestion of small amounts of powerful carcinogens or precarcinogens. Several have been identified in foodstuffs but only two have been related at all clearly to the production of cancer in humans: that is aflatoxin, a metabolic product of *Aspergillus flavus*, which contaminates stored or oily foods in many countries, and is a major cause of liver cancer in the tropics among those individuals who are also chronic carriers of the hepatitis B (or less commonly hepatitis C) virus. Likewise, the salted fish eaten extensively in South China, probably acts synergistically with EBV to cause nasopharyngeal cancer. A third possible source is bracken fern, an extract of which is carcinogenic in animals. It is eaten extensively in Japan and has been tentatively

Table 6 Occupational causes of cancer

Agent	Site of cancer	Occupation[1]
Aromatic amines:	Bladder	Dye manufacturers
4-Amino-diphenyl		Rubber workers
Benzidine		Coal-gas manufacturers
2-Naphthy-lamine		Some chemical workers
Arsenic	Skin, lung	Copper and cobalt smelters
		Pesticide manufacturers
		Some gold miners
Asbestos	Lung, pleura, peritoneum	Asbestos miners
		Asbestos textile manufacturers
		Insulation workers
		Shipyard workers
Benzene	Marrow	Workers with glues and varnishes
Beryllium[2]	Lung	Beryllium refiners and machiners
Bis-chloromethyl ether	Lung	Makers of ion-exchange resins
Cadmium[2]	Lung	Cadmium refiners
Chromium[2]	Lung	Manufacturers of chromates from chrome ore; pigment manufacturers
Ionizing radiations	Lung	Uranium and some other miners
	Bone	Luminizers
	Marrow, all sites	Radiologists, radiographers
Mustard gas	Larynx, lung	Poison-gas manufacturers
Nickel[2]	Nasal sinuses, lung	Nickel refiners
Polycyclic hydrocarbons in soot, tar, oil	Skin, scrotum, lung, and sometimes bladder	Coal-gas manufacturers, roofers, asphalters, aluminium refiners, and many groups exposed to tars and selected oils
Silica, when crystalline as quartz or cristobalite	Lung	Miners, stone workers, refractory brick workers
Sulphuric acid mists (strong acid)	Nasal sinuses, larynx	Many industries, isopropanol manufacture, 'steel pickling'
Ultraviolet light	Skin	Farmers, seamen
Vinyl chloride	Liver (angio-sarcoma)	PVC manufacturers
?	Nasal sinuses	Hardwood furniture manufacturers
?	Nasal sinuses	Leather workers

[1] Typical occupations with proven hazards.

[2] Certain compounds or oxidation states.

linked with the development of oesophageal cancer. The polycyclic hydro-carbons and other mutagens that are produced in food by grilling or smoking have often been suspected of playing a role, but intensive investigation has failed to detect one.

It seems, therefore, that if diet does affect the incidence of cancer in the Western world in any material way, it is likely to do so by more indirect means, such as those described in Table 7.

Overnutrition That overnutrition could affect the incidence of cancer was first suggested by Tannenbaum's experiments on mice during the Second World War. These showed that the incidence of spontaneous tumours of the lung and breast and of a variety of tumours produced experimentally could be halved by moderately restricting the intake of food without modifying the proportions of the individual constituents. This protective effect has subsequently been demonstrated repeatedly, but has attracted little attention (perhaps because reports of such results emphasized the benefits of restriction rather than the harm of overeating). It is now clear, however, that what is considered normal nutrition in developed countries increases the risk of breast cancer (by bringing forward menarche and increasing body size) and possibly also that of testis cancer. With greater consumption obesity (that is a BMI greater than 25 kg/m²) has been estimated to be responsible for 5 per cent of all incident cases in Europe and 10 per cent of all cancer deaths in non-smokers in the United States (Peto, 2001): most notably cancer of the breast in women after the menopause and cancers of the endometrium, large bowel, pancreas, gallbladder, prostate, and kidney and myelomatosis. For some of these increases, the explanation is obvious: namely, those of the two female cancers, which in postmenopausal women are attributable to the formation of oestrogen from androstenedione in adipose tissue while the increased risk of gallbladder cancer may be due to a greater secretion of bile salts. For others, the explanation is obscure.

Meat and fat Figures for food consumption and cancer incidence and mortality rates in different countries show fairly close correlations between the consumption of fat and, to a less extent, the consumption of meat and the incidence of several types of cancer. The correlations are closest for breast cancer and cancer of the large bowel and are less strong for cancers of the endometrium, pancreas, and prostate. When, however, attempts are made to associate the consumption of either type of food with the disease in individuals within a country the evidence is commonly conflicting. This could be because the international correlations are misleading, indicating only that the risks are correlated with something that is correlated with fat and meat consumption (for example some other aspect of a high gross national product), but it could be partly because of the inaccuracy of dietary histories and partly because people in developed countries, and particularly in North America, eat such similar diets. Overviews of the published data, however, do suggest that a high consumption of fat is associated with a high risk of colorectal cancer, but the claim that a high consumption of fat (or of particular types of fat) is associated with high risks of breast and endometrial cancer after the menopause, other than by providing a high calorie diet leading to obesity, is controversial.

Whether meat increases the risk of any type of cancer, apart from the contribution it makes through its calorie content, is also uncertain. The low incidence of several types of cancer that is commonly observed in vegetarian communities is not necessarily due to the absence of meat from the diet, as it can generally be explained by the increased consumption of protective foods (vegetables and fruits) and commonly by associated behavioural characteristics (below average use of tobacco and alcohol). Some studies that make allowance for these confounding factors have claimed that meat specifically increases the risk of large-bowel cancer, but the evidence is weak and the increase in risk, if any, is small.

Fibre That fibre may play a part was suggested by Burkitt's observation that several intestinal diseases, including cancer of the colon, were common in countries in which cereals were processed to remove the fibre and rare in rural Africa and Asia where they were not. The idea was attractive, as 'fibre' passes through the small bowel unchanged and serves as pabulum for the colonic bacteria, thus increasing faecal bulk and possibly protecting against the development of cancer mechanically by diluting any carcinogens present and hastening their transit through the bowel. The idea was, however, too simple and has not been confirmed (using the original definition of fibre) by either epidemiological studies on individuals in developed countries or by experiments aimed at reducing the recurrence of colorectal adenomas. In fact, fibre is difficult to define and the term is better replaced by 'non-starch polysaccharides' as there are many that share the characteristics of passing through the small bowel unchanged and being, for the most part, partially or wholly degraded by bacteria in the large bowel. Some starch, moreover, known as 'resistant starch' and found in green bananas and cold potatoes, has similar physiological characteristics. Further studies that take these complexities into account are, therefore, needed before 'fibre' in any of its manifestations can be considered as having any place in protecting against the development of cancer.

Retinoids and carotenoids Experiments on animals and on cell cultures *in vitro* have suggested that vitamin A (retinol) and its esters and analogues (retinoids) may, in appropriate circumstances, reduce the risk of cancer by reducing the probability that partially transformed cells become fully transformed and proliferate into clinically detectable tumours, although in other circumstances they appear to have opposite effects. Human studies, however, fail to support the idea that serum levels of retinol are related to the risk of any type of cancer, at least in countries in which clinical symptoms of vitamin A deficiency seldom or never occur. Such studies suggested that the risks were inversely related to the serum level of β-carotene, which acts as an antioxidant and is broken down to produce retinol. When, however, β-carotene was put to the test of clinical trials it provided no benefit and the

Table 7 Some indirect ways in which diet may influence the incidence of cancer indirectly

Possible ways	Example
Affecting the formation of carcinogens in the body	Providing substrates for the formation of carcinogens (e.g. nitrites, secondary amines)
	Inhibiting formation of carcinogens (e.g. vitamin C in the stomach)
	Altering intake or excretion of cholesterol and bile acids and hence the production of carcinogenic metabolites in the bowel
	Altering the bacterial flora and hence the capacity to produce carcinogenic metabolites
Affecting contact of carcinogens with stem cells	Altering transport of carcinogens (e.g. alcohol, fibre)
	Altering concentration of carcinogens (e.g. effect of fibre on faecal mass)
Affecting activation or deactivation of carcinogens	Induction or inhibition of enzymes that affect metabolism of carcinogens (e.g. indoles in Brassica)
	Deactivation or prevention of formation of short-lived intracellular species (e.g. by selenium and vitamin E, by otherwise trapping free radicals, or by antioxidants used as preservatives)
Affecting secretion of hormones	Increasing amount of adipose tissue

inverse relationship commonly observed in epidemiological studies is presumably due to confounding with some other protective factors in vegetables.

Other components Many other components of the diet, including lycopene in tomatoes, indoles in cabbages and sprouts, vitamins C, D, and E, and calcium and selenium have also been proposed as protective agents; while nitrates, nitrites, secondary amines, and the preservation of food by salting, have been thought to increase the risk of cancer. For some the evidence is strongly suggestive: notably for vitamin C as protective against gastric cancer and for salt-preserved foods predisposing to it. In general, however, the evidence of benefit or harm is too weak to justify any firm conclusion.

Conclusion Some of the uncertainties about the effect of diet could be resolved only by means of controlled trials in which volunteers are allocated at random micronutrient supplements (such as vitamin C, lycopene, calcium, and selenium) or a dietary schedule that requires a substantial reduction in the consumption of fat. Several such studies are under way and if any such factors affect the later stages of cancer induction, clear answers may be obtained to some of the outstanding questions within a few years. Practicable modifications of the diet may well provide the means for reducing cancer deaths in developed countries by a third; but the range of uncertainty about this figure is large. Meanwhile the only dietary changes that can be recommended with confidence in developed countries are a general increase in the use of fresh fruit and vegetables and a sufficient limitation of calories to avoid obesity.

Reproduction and other factors affecting secretion of reproductive hormones

Epidemiological observations have shown clear relationships between a woman's reproductive history and the risk of cancers of the sex organs, which are generally thought to reflect changes in hormonal secretions; but which hormones are concerned and the mechanisms by which they act are, for the most part, still uncertain. An exception is endometrial cancer, the risk of which is directly related to the degree of exposure to oestrogen not followed after an appropriate interval by progestogen. Proof that oestrogenic stimulation of the mammary tissues is a cause of most cases of breast cancer in developed countries has been provided by randomized trials of tamoxifen, an antioestrogenic drug that blocks the oestrogen receptors in the cells of the normal breast. The effect is large and rapid: 5 years of tamoxifen approximately halves the incidence of breast cancer not only while the drug is being taken but also for some years afterwards. Exogenous oestrogen also increases the risk of breast cancer when given as hormonal replacement therapy and endogenous oestrogen accounts for the increased risk associated with adiposity after the menopause, as androstenedione, which continues to be produced by the adrenals, is converted to oestrogen in adipose tissue. It is presumably oestrogens, too, that cause a small increase in risk of breast cancer during and immediately after pregnancy and the oestrogen component of the steroid contraceptives that causes a similar small increase in risk during their use and for a few years after their use is stopped. It is, however, unclear which hormone-related processes are involved in reducing the long-term risk for the rest of a woman's life that occurs some years after the occurrence of each pregnancy and it is equally unclear why the use of oral contraception and the consequent suppression of ovulation reduces the long-term risk of ovarian cancer.

Hormones, it is thought, must also be involved in producing cancers of the testis and prostate in men, but the epidemiological evidence is, as yet, unhelpful. Randomized trials of the effects of physical or medical castration in men who already have prostate cancer have, however, shown that progression of the disease can be slowed substantially, presumably by the reduction of androgenic stimulation.

Physical inactivity

Physical inactivity contributes to the risk of cancer indirectly by increasing the risk of obesity but it may also contribute directly to the risks of cancers of the colon and breast. An association with colon cancer has been consistently reported, which may be due to a reduction in colonic mobility with corresponding prolonged exposure of the colonic mucosa to faecal carcinogens. An association with breast cancer may simply be due to confounding, but it may also reflect an effect on hormone secretion.

Interaction of agents

Attribution of the risk of cancer to different causes is complicated by the fact that some agents interact with others to produce effects that are much greater than the sum of the separate effects of each on its own. An example is provided by smoking and asbestos, which multiply each other's effects so that, compared with non-smokers in general, the incidence of cancer of the lung was increased six-fold among a group of asbestos insulation workers in the United States who did not smoke, but were heavily exposed to asbestos dust in the 1940s, 10- to 20-fold among cigarette smokers in general who did not work with asbestos, and nearly 90-fold among such asbestos insulation workers who also smoked cigarettes regularly. Other examples are provided by smoking and radon (which interact similarly, though somewhat less than multiplicatively, to produce cancer of the lung), by smoking and alcohol (which interact to produce cancers of the mouth, pharynx, larynx, and oesophagus), and by infection with the hepatitis B virus and aflatoxin (which interact to produce cancer of the liver).

Such interactions may come about through some analogue of the dual mechanism of initiation and promotion that was suggested 60 years ago by the experiments of Rous and Kidd and Berenblum and Shubik. They could, however, also be produced in many other ways, some of which have been discussed in the section on diet (see above). From a statistical point of view, they complicate the attribution of risk, as we may find ourselves appearing to claim that more cancer can be prevented than actually occurs by attributing, say, 80 per cent of lung cancers in men heavily exposed to asbestos to their occupational exposure and 90 per cent of the same cancers to cigarette smoking.

Conclusion

Estimates of the proportions of fatal cancers that can be attributed to environmental and behavioural factors are given in Table 8, along with the proportions that are now known to be avoidable in practicable ways. For this purpose, individual causes (such as the various carcinogenic drugs and occupational hazards) have been grouped into 12 main categories. The evidence on which these estimates are based is summarized in this chapter and for earlier periods in greater detail by Doll and Peto (1981) and the International Agency for Research on Cancer (1990).

The sum of the best estimates in Table 8 amounts to less than 100 per cent, despite the fact that some of the listed agents interact with one another to augment each other's effect and that some fatal cancers are consequently counted twice. The total would be somewhat more than 100 per cent, however, if the true proportions attributable to some of the categories turn out to be nearer the upper end of the acceptable estimates and it would be a great deal more than 100 per cent if it had been possible to characterize the factors that have been classified as 'other and unknown'.

The estimates in columns two and three of Table 8 do not distinguish between factors (such as tobacco) that are sufficiently understood to enable specific action to be taken with a guarantee of success and those (such as diet) that are not. They should not, therefore, be taken as guides to the proportion of cancer deaths that can now be prevented by practicable means, without reference to the paragraphs in which they are individually discussed. This is illustrated by the fourth column in Table 8, which shows the proportions of United Kingdom cancer deaths in 1995 that are reliably known to be avoidable by practicable means. The only percentage that is both large and reliably known is that attributed to tobacco and that is more than twice the sum of the percentages reliably attributable to other specific factors for which practicable preventive measures are available: and tobacco causes about twice as many deaths from other diseases as it does from cancer. The position is different in countries such as China, where hepatitis B virus causes about as many cancer deaths as tobacco and the hazard for

Table 8 Proportion of cancer deaths attributable to different environmental and behavioural factors in the United Kingdom and the proportion known to be avoidable in practicable ways

Factor or class of factors	Percentage of deaths		
	Best estimate of attributable proportion	Range of acceptable estimates	Known to be avoidable in practicable ways
Tobacco	30	27–33	30
Alcohol	6	4–8	6[1]
Ionizing radiation	5	4–6	<1
Ultraviolet light	1	1	<1
Infection (virus 3%, bacteria 2%)	5	4–15	1[2]
Medical drugs	<1	0–1	<1
Occupation	2	1–5	<1
Pollution	2	1–5	<1
Diet	25	15–35	2[3]
Reproduction[4]	15	10–20	<1
Physical inactivity	<1	0–1	<1
Other and unknown	?	?	?

[1] The total avoidance of alcohol would increase the age standardized mortality in the UK, as the increase in mortality from vascular disease would be greater than the reduction in mortality from cancer.

[2] By sexual hygiene and regular cervical screening.

[3] By reduction of obesity.

[4] and other factors affecting the secretion of reproductive hormones.

future generations can be avoided in a cost-effective way by infant vaccination.

Epidemiology of cancer by site of origin

In the following account of the epidemiology of cancers arising in specific organs, the description of each type is preceded by notes showing its importance in England and Wales. One figure gives the proportion of all cancers that arise in the site, as indicated by the national cancer register for England and Wales for 1994 (Office of National Statistics, 2000) and another gives the proportion of all cancer deaths allocated to the site in the national mortality statistics for 1998 (Office of National Statistics, 1999). A third gives the ratio of the age-standardized incidence rates for each sex. The way in which the incidence of the disease varies with age is shown for males and females in a series of graphs, using the data for England and Wales over a 5-year period (International Agency for Research on Cancer, 1992). Under 25 years the numbers of most types of cancer that occur in a 5-year age group, even in a 5-year calendar period, are small and the rates are consequently unreliable due to chance variation of small numbers. Trends in incidence and mortality for each type, along with the trends in possible causative factors, are given by Swerdlow *et al.* (2001). Major differences between Britain and other countries are commented on in the text and are described more fully in the report on *Cancer causes, occurrence and control* by the International Agency for Research on Cancer (1990).

Lip

- 0.1 per cent of all cancers and 0.02 per cent of cancer deaths.
- Sex ratio of rates 5.0 to 1. Age distribution like skin (non-melanoma).

Carcinoma of the lip was one of the first types of cancer to be related to an extrinsic cause when, more than 200 years ago, it was noted to occur characteristically in pipe smokers. Many years later it was realized that the disease could also be produced by smoking cigarettes, although much less readily, so that it must be produced by the chemicals in smoke rather than by the non-specific effect of local heat. It is also much more common in outdoor than in indoor workers and is induced by ultraviolet light in the same way as other cancers of the exposed skin. Ultraviolet light and tobacco account, between them, for the great majority of all cases in Britain, probably multiplying each other's effects. The disease is much less common than

it used to be, because of the decrease in both pipe smoking and outdoor work.

Oral cavity and pharynx (excluding salivary glands and nasopharynx)

- 1.0 per cent of all cancers and 1.2 per cent of cancer deaths.
- Sex ratio of rates 2.3 to 1. Age distribution, see Fig. 1.

Cancers of the tongue, mouth, and pharynx (other than nasopharynx) are all related to smoking (of pipes, cigars, and cigarettes) and to the consumption of alcohol. The two factors act synergistically and cancers in these sites are extremely rare in non-smokers who do not drink alcohol.

Cancer of the tongue is much less common in Britain than it was early this century, but the reason for the sharp decline in incidence is unknown. One explanation could be the decrease in syphilis, which was commonly believed to be a predisposing factor because of the clinical association with

Fig. 1 Annual incidence of cancers of the oral cavity and pharynx by age and sex (excluding cancers of the salivary glands and nasopharynx).

syphilitic leucoplakia. Recent increases in oral and pharangeal cancer in men are partly due to increased consumption of alcohol and possibly, in the case of pharyngeal cancer, to human papilloma virus infection.

Cancers that occur low in the hypopharynx are distinguished by a tendency to affect women who have suffered from iron-deficiency anaemia and dysphagia.

Cancers of the mouth and pharynx (excluding nasopharynx) are particularly common in South-East and Central Asia where tobacco smoking is largely replaced by chewing tobacco, betel nut or leaf, and lime (calcium hydroxide). A close association with such chewing habits has been established by studies that have shown that the cancers tend to originate in the part of the mouth in which the quid is usually held—a characteristic that varies both between individuals and between areas. The materials chewed differ in different places and, although the disease is commonly described as 'betel chewer's cancer', betel is not invariably a component of the quid and the most characteristic constituent seems to be a small amount of lime and, in most cases, some form of tobacco. In parts of Asia, the disease is so common that it accounts for 20 per cent of all cancers and in those populations the abandonment of chewing would be the single most effective means of reducing the total incidence of cancer—so long as the habit was not replaced by an increase in tobacco smoking. Among habitual quid chewers, the risks are particularly elevated in those who both chew and smoke—indeed, in parts of India the majority of deaths from 'betel chewer's cancer' could have been avoided if those affected had not also smoked. The incidence might also be reduced by improved nutrition, as the disease in Southern Asia tends to be associated with vitamin A deficiency.

In parts of India where women tend to smoke local cigars and cigarettes with the burning end inside the mouth to prevent them going out, the habit is associated with cancer of the palate.

Salivary glands

- 0.2 per cent of all cancers and 0.1 per cent of cancer deaths.
- Sex ratio of rates 1.3 to 1. Age distribution like non-Hodgkin's lymphoma.

The salivary glands are not common sites for cancer anywhere. They are, however, relatively more common in the Asiatic populations of Hawaii and in Canadian Indians than elsewhere. A small proportion of cases occurs specifically in families that also have a high incidence of breast cancer. No causative factors are known and no notable changes in incidence over time have been reported.

Nasopharynx

- 0.1 per cent of all cancers and of cancer deaths.
- Sex ratio of rates 2.0 to 1. Age distribution, see Fig. 2.

Cancers of the nasopharynx, unlike those in other parts of the pharynx, are not related to alcohol and are only weakly related to tobacco. They are rare in most populations but are common in those that originated from parts of Guangdong, in southern China, where the disease is the most common type of cancer. Moderately high rates have been observed in Alaskan Eskimos and American Indians, with intermediate rates in Malaysia, Kenya, and North Africa. A weakly significant relationship with HLA type has been reported from Singapore, but the existence of a specific genetic predisposition remains to be proved. Incidence rates appear to have been decreasing among Chinese Americans.

DNA characteristic of the Epstein–Barr virus (EBV) has been detected in the nuclei of nasopharyngeal cancer cells and patients with the disease tend to have unusually high antibodies against EBV-related antigens. Among adults, sudden increases in certain EBV antigens in the blood often precede by a few years the appearance of a pathological cancer. Infection with the EBV is, however, almost universal and can be only one of several agents that act in combination to produce the disease. One such agent in Southern China occurs in the 'salted fish' on which children are commonly weaned.

Nasopharynx, 1983–1987

Fig. 2 Annual incidence of cancer of the nasopharynx by age and sex.

This strongly flavoured delicacy bears little relation to the salted fish eaten elsewhere, and might better be described as decomposing fish: it contains various mutagens, and exposure to it in childhood when infection with EBV first occurs may alter the usual lifelong balance between host and virus in some hazardous way.

Oesophagus

- 2.3 per cent of all cancers and 4.4 per cent of cancer deaths.
- Sex ratio of rates 2.0 to 1. Age distribution like gastric cancer.

Cancer of the oesophagus, like other cancers of the upper respiratory and digestive tracts, is closely related to prolonged smoking and the consumption of alcohol. All types of smoking have comparable effects and, so it appears, do all alcoholic drinks, although spirits may be slightly more effective per gram of ethyl alcohol than other alcoholic drinks. Alcohol and tobacco act synergistically and, in the absence of either, the incidence of the disease in Britain would be greatly reduced. In France, where the consumption of alcohol is greater than in Britain, it would be reduced even more. A few cases originate from the scars produced by poisoning with corrosive substances and a very few in conjunction with a particular hereditary form of tylosis (presenting with keratoses of the palms and soles). The relatively small excess in men probably reflects the existence of other unknown causes in women, possibly nutritional in origin and similar to those responsible for cancers of the hypopharynx. Mortality (which, because of the high fatality rate, approaches incidence) fell progressively in the first half of the twentieth century in line with the fall in the consumption of alcohol, and rose again after 1950 when the trend in the consumption of alcohol reversed. Since pipe smoking affects oesophageal cancer risks at least as strongly as cigarette smoking, no large effects on male oesophageal cancer trends could be predicted from the male switch from pipes to cigarettes, although the switch by females from non-smoking to cigarettes should, other things being equal, produce a large upward trend. It appears, however, that other things were not equal and some other, possibly nutritional, cause of oesophageal cancer seems to have decreased, for any upward trends in oesophageal cancer are moderate. In men, in contrast, the rates have increased when they might have been expected to decrease. To some extent this can be accounted for by the increased consumption of alcohol and possibly by an increase in the nitrosamine content of tobacco smoke, which has resulted from changes in the method of curing tobacco and which could have a specific effect on the oesophagus. A small part of the increase is due to an increased risk of adenocarcinoma at the lower end of the oesophagus, which may be associated with a decreased prevalence of *Helicobacter pylori* and gastritis, and an increase in oesophageal reflux.

In Africa and Asia, the epidemiological features are quite different and present some of the most striking unsolved problems in the field of cancer epidemiology. In parts of China (particularly in North Henan but also elsewhere) and on the east coast of the Caspian Sea in Turkmenistan and Iran, oesophageal cancer is the most common type of cancer, with incidence rates in both sexes that are equal to the highest rates observed for lung cancer in men in European cities. Within China, the disease varies more than 10-fold from one county to another; alcohol and tobacco cannot account for these geographic differences, but when people within one particular Chinese county or city are compared with each other the disease is more common among those who smoke. In parts of Africa, particularly in the Transkei region of South Africa and on the east coast of Lake Victoria in Kenya, extremely high rates are also observed, sometimes equally in both sexes and sometimes only in men. In these and several other areas, as in Asia, the high incidence zones are strictly localized and the incidence falls off rapidly over distances of 200 or 300 miles.

When tobacco and alcohol are used, they increase the hazard, but they are not the principal agents in these high-incidence areas. Many causes have been proposed, including molybdenum deficiency in the soil (resulting in a deficiency of the plant enzyme nitrate reductase and a build-up of nitrosamines), contamination of food and pickled vegetables by fungi (particularly by species of *Fusaria*) with the production of carcinogenic metabolites, an agent associated with the production of beer from maize, and the residues left behind in pipes from smoking opium (which are commonly swallowed). None, however, is supported by any impressive epidemiological data. The high incidence area in Iran, which has been intensively investigated, is characterized by extreme poverty and a restricted diet consisting chiefly of home-made bread and tea, with some sheep's milk and milk products, and very little meat, vegetables, or fruit. In this area the disease has been common for centuries. In Southern Africa, however, it seems to have become common only since the First World War. In China, where cancer of the oesophagus was the second most important neoplastic cause of death in the 1970s, the high incidence has persisted.

Stomach

- 3.7 per cent of all cancers and 4.7 per cent of cancer deaths.
- Sex ratio of rates 2.5 to 1. Age distribution, see Fig. 3.

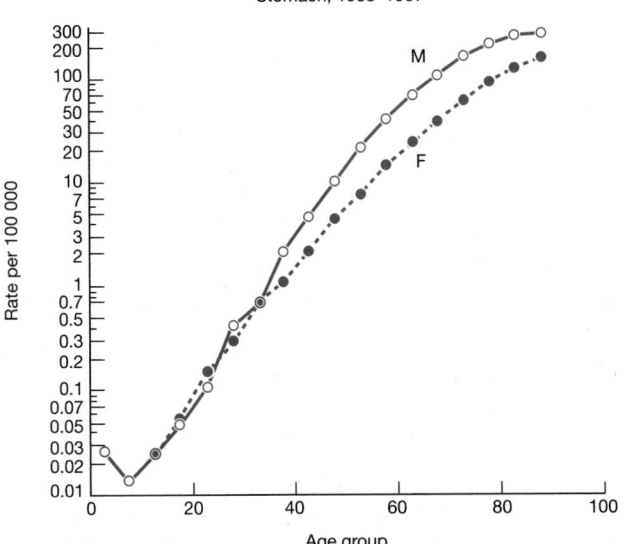

Fig. 3 Annual incidence of cancer of the stomach by age and sex.

Until about 1980, gastric cancer was responsible for more deaths from malignant disease world-wide than any other. Over the last 50 years, however, the incidence has declined in Western Europe, North America, and Australasia and recently it has begun to do so in South America and Japan. High rates are now confined to China, Japan, Russia and other countries of the old Soviet Union, and Central and South America, while the lowest rates are found equally in North America, Australasia, and some of the least developed parts of Africa. Irrespective of whether the incidence is high or low, the sex ratio is between 1.5 and 3 to 1.

Within Britain, cancer of the stomach is most common in North Wales and becomes progressively less common from north to south and from west to east. Over the last 70 years it has consistently been some five times more common in unskilled labourers than in members of the major professions, a gradient with socioeconomic status that has been one of the most marked for any disease. Relatively high rates have been observed in coal miners and in some chemical workers; but no specific occupational hazards have been identified and the excess in coal miners was paralleled by a similar excess in their wives. A hazard has been suspected from exposure to asbestos, but the apparent excess may be due to misdiagnosis of lung cancer and mesothelioma.

Four factors are known to predispose to the disease: blood group A constitution, gastritis associated with infection by *Helicobacter pylori* (sometimes leading to atrophic gastritis), a diet deficient in fruit and green and yellow vegetables, and a poor diet with large amounts of salt and salt-preserved food. Chronic infection with *H. pylori* is a major cause of peptic ulcer, a finding that is of considerable practical value in patients with ulcers, because the infection can generally be eliminated from the stomach by a short course of appropriate antibiotic therapy and this provides long-term protection against recurrence. Whether such treatments will have any material effect on the incidence of stomach cancer remains, however, to be shown. How these various factors influence the production of the disease is unclear. One possibility is that they encourage or discourage the formation of carcinogens *in vivo*, particularly perhaps the production of nitrosamines; but if they do, the intake of nitrates (which can be converted into nitrites by bacterial enzymes) is not a rate-limiting factor. Changes in the prevalence of the three environmental factors could have contributed to the decline in the incidence of the disease, but they could not have brought about such a large and widespread reduction in risk, and it seems probable that the better preservation of food, resulting from the extensive use of refrigeration, has played the major part.

No risk has been detected from the consumption of mutagens produced by the different methods of cooking meat and fish, nor from food additives or pesticide residues. Some food additives may, on the contrary, have served to reduce risk (by avoiding food spoilage and hence improving nutrition, by avoiding contamination by carcinogen-producing micro-organisms, or by some antioxidant or other protective effect on the gastric epithelium).

Large bowel

- 11.1 per cent of all cancers and 11.0 per cent of cancer deaths.
- Sex ratio of rates 1.4 to 1. Age distribution, see Fig. 4.

Cancers of the colon and rectum ought to be considered separately, as their causes are not identical. Cancer of the colon, for example, tends to occur more often in women than in men, particularly when it occurs on the right side, while cancer of the rectum is nearly twice as common in men. The geographical distribution also differs slightly, colonic cancer varying in incidence more than rectal cancer. Separate consideration may, however, sometimes be misleading as cancers commonly occur at the rectosigmoid junction and the site of origin of these cases is not recorded consistently. Moreover, there is a growing tendency to describe both diseases merely as 'cancers of the large bowel', which, according to the internationally agreed rules, are classed as cancers of the colon. The two diseases will, therefore, be considered together.

Fig. 4 Annual incidence of cancer of the large bowel by age and sex.

Fig. 5 Annual incidence of cancer of the liver by age and sex.

Over the past few decades the male incidence rates in both the United Kingdom and the United States have been approximately constant, while the female rates have decreased slightly. More recently, decreases in early middle age have begun to be seen in both sexes. In contrast, the incidence in Japan, which used to be very low, has begun to increase and the disease in Japanese migrants in Hawaii has become as common as in Caucasians. In most other parts of Asia, and in Africa and Eastern Europe, large-bowel cancer continues to be relatively uncommon (except in areas where chronic schistosomal infestation of the large intestine is prevalent; for example, high rectal cancer rates are found in Chinese counties in which *S. japonicum* was, until recently, a major cause of death). Incidence rates in different countries correlate closely with the per capita consumption of fat and meat and crudely with the consumption of processed foods from which the natural fibre has been removed. Ways in which these and other dietary constituents might influence the development of the disease have been discussed under diet. Other factors increasing risk are obesity and physical inactivity. A weak association with smoking has been observed in several cohort studies, which may be the result of confounding with the consumption of alcohol and a high fat diet. It is possible, however, that smoking may cause a few cases indirectly by causing the diet to be modified in the direction of a higher fat content.

Within Britain, there is no clear relation to socioeconomic status and no occupational hazard has been established. The association that has been reported with exposure to asbestos may be due to misdiagnosis as in the case of cancer of the stomach. Cases in childhood or early adult life occur as a complication of polyposis coli or (more rarely) Gardner's syndrome. These conditions are determined by dominant genes, which increase the susceptibility to the disease so much that it almost invariably develops before middle age. Many other cases develop from adenomatous polyps and a few occur as a complication of long-standing ulcerative colitis.

Anal intercourse causing infection with types 16, 18 or some other specific types of the human papilloma virus is a probable cause of some anal carcinomas, but patients who have sexually transmitted anal warts that are due to other types of human papilloma virus are not for this reason at special risk of anal cancer.

Liver

- 0.6 per cent of all cancers and 1.4 per cent of cancer deaths.
- Sex ratio of rates 2.1 to 1. Age distribution, see Fig. 5.

Incidence rates have tended to be overestimated in developed countries because the primary condition is often confused with metastases to the liver from cancer in various other organs, particularly over 65 years of age when carcinomas of the gastrointestinal and respiratory tracts are common. Recently, however, there has been a small increase in the United Kingdom and the United States from the very low level that had come to be recorded, which is probably due to an increased prevalence of infection with hepatitis C.

The disease is much more common in South-East Asia and tropical Africa; in China it accounts for about 20 per cent of all cancer deaths and in parts of Africa it is the most common cancer in men. Most cases derive from the main cells of the organ (hepatocellular carcinomas) and are attributable primarily to chronic active infection, established early in life, with the hepatitis B virus, exacerbated by consumption of some specific metabolite (e.g. aflatoxin) of particular types of fungi that contaminate stored foods. Neonatal vaccination against the virus produces a marked decrease in the proportion of children who, at 5 years of age, are chronically infected. This has begun in Japan, Taiwan, and parts of China and tropical Africa and has already produced a decreased risk of hepatocarcinoma at young ages. Some cases, however, are caused by the hepatitis C virus, which is an RNA virus spread by blood transfusion, and these cannot be avoided by immunization.

In developed countries, some cases are also due to infection with hepatitis B and C viruses, but more arise as complications of cirrhosis of the liver attributable to heavy and prolonged consumption of alcohol or, rarely, to haemochromatosis. Occasionally, liver cancer is produced by drugs. A few cases have occurred in young men who have taken androgenic-anabolic steroids to increase their muscular strength and a few from the use of steroid contraceptives, either arising *de novo* or from benign adenomas, which are themselves rare complications of the use of steroid contraceptives. Some can be attributed to smoking for an association has been observed in parts of China where little alcohol is drunk and case–control studies in Europe have shown an association after alcohol consumption has been taken into account.

A second histological type (cholangiosarcoma) arises from the intrahepatic bile ducts, tends to occur at a somewhat later age than hepatocellular carcinoma, and, although generally less common than hepatocellular carcinoma, nevertheless accounts for an appreciable proportion of cases. In China, Thailand, and other parts of Asia it can be produced by chronic infection with liver flukes (*Clonorchis sinensis* or *Opisthorchis viverrini*).

A third histological type that is extremely uncommon everywhere has been variously described as reticuloendothelioma or angiosarcoma. It was first recognized as a complication of the use of 'Thorotrast' as a contrast agent in neuroradiology, a long-abandoned practice that led to chronic retention of insoluble thorium radionuclides in the marrow, spleen, and liver. In 1973, the disease was found to be an occupational hazard for men exposed to vinyl chloride monomer. A few hundred cases have occurred throughout the world in men who were heavily exposed in the manufacture of vinyl chloride polymer, and it seems improbable that the minute amounts that have leached out of the plastic consumer products can have caused more than a dozen or so cases altogether in the general public, if indeed they have produced any. A third, and even rarer, cause is prolonged exposure to inorganic arsenic, such as used to result from the medical pre-scription of Fowler's solution. Despite these multiple causes only one case of hepatic angiosarcoma normally occurs annually in some 10 million people, which is why the recognition of new causes has been easy.

The relative rarity of cancer of the liver in most developed countries is intriguing, since most of the carcinogens thus far discovered in experimen-tal animals induce, perhaps with other cancers, tumours of the liver. The lack of any high or increasing liver cancer rate in Britain and America con-sequently suggests that, on average, people have not been substantially exposed to the sort of chemical carcinogens that are currently recognized by such studies.

Gallbladder and extrahepatic bile ducts

- 0.5 per cent of all cancers and 0.4 per cent of cancer deaths.

- Sex ratio of rates 1.0 to 1. Age distribution like colorectal cancer.

Cancers of the gallbladder and extrahepatic bile ducts are nearly always classed together, which is unfortunate as the causes differ. The former is more than twice as common in women as in men, is strongly associated with obesity, and is usually preceded by (and probably caused by) chol-elithiasis. The latter is slightly more common in men and is increased in incidence by clonorchiasis and (to a less extent) by long-standing ulcerative colitis. Both types are uncommon, and their aggregate varies only slightly from one population to another. Relatively high rates are recorded among Jewesses in Israel, especially among those born in Europe and America.

The incidence of cancer of the gallbladder has fallen sharply in the United States in the last 25 years, which may be partly due to the decreased consumption of animal fat and, perhaps more importantly, to an increase in the rate of cholecystectomy in people who, having gallstones, are at greatest risk of cancer of the gallbladder.

Pancreas

- 2.3 per cent of all cancers and 4.3 per cent of cancer deaths.

- Sex ratio of rates 1.5 to 1. Age distribution like stomach cancer.

Cancer of the pancreas is two to three times more common in regular cigarette smokers than in lifelong non-smokers. The chemicals in cigarette smoke that specifically cause pancreatic cancer have not been identified, but the volatile nitrosamines in smoke that are absorbed from the alveoli and carried to the pancreas in the bloodstream are likely candidates. The disease is twice as common in diabetics as in the population as a whole. It is, therefore, not surprising that the highest rate is recorded among New Zealand Maoris, who smoke heavily and are prone to obesity, hypertension, myocardial infarction, and diabetes.

Cancer of the pancreas is generally regarded as a disease of the developed world, but the diagnosis is difficult in the absence of a well-developed med-ical service and some of the relatively small geographical and temporal vari-ations may be due to variation in diagnostic standards. Mortality rates in Britain and the United States have begun to decrease under 65 years of age, and this is more likely to reflect a reduction in incidence from reduction in smoking than to any improvement in treatment, as the 5-year survival rate remains well under 10 per cent.

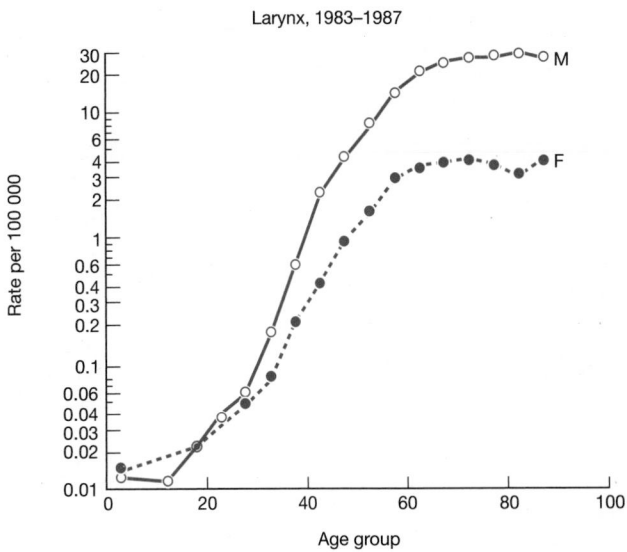

Fig. 6 Annual incidence of cancer of the larynx by age and sex.

Nose and nasal sinuses

- 0.1 per cent of all cancers and of cancer deaths.

- Sex ratio of rates 2.0 to 1. Age distribution like non-Hodgkin's lymphoma.

Surprisingly, in view of the widespread exposure of the human nose to tobacco smoke and other airborne toxins, cancers of the nasal cavity itself are extremely rare. Most arise from the paranasal sinuses. Several occu-pational hazards have been recognized, including the refining of nickel, processes giving rise to exposure to strong sulphuric acid mists, and the manufacture of hardwood furniture and leather goods. It would be wrong, however, to conclude that all contact with nickel, hardwood dust, and lea-ther creates a hazard. The hazards have been observed in special occupa-tional situations in which exposure has been intensive and prolonged. The nickel-refining hazard was first observed in South Wales where the nickel carbonyl process was used, but similar hazards were subsequently observed with other refining processes in Canada, Norway, and the Soviet Union. In the Welsh refinery the workplace exposures were much heavier before the Second World War, and (despite the continued use of the nickel carbonyl process in Wales) no hazard of nasal sinus cancer has been observed among men first employed there since 1950. The hazard in furniture workers was first observed in High Wycombe and appears to have followed the intro-duction of high-speed wood-working machinery early in the twentieth cen-tury. A hazard certainly affects some other groups of wood-workers, but should not be assumed to affect furniture workers in general.

Most nasal and nasal sinus cancers are squamous carcinomas, but the hazard from hardwood dust characteristically produced adenocarcinomas. In some of the groups exposed to this hazard, as many as 5 per cent of the men developed the disease. This meant that the risk of adenocarcinoma was increased 1500 times (as this histological type of the disease is normally very rare) and the hazard was, in consequence, easy to confirm once sus-picion had been aroused.

Chromate workers are sometimes said to experience a hazard of nasal cancer, but this may be an error due to confusion with the characteristic 'chrome ulcer' of the nasal septum. Such ulcers have not generally been found to become malignant.

Larynx

- 0.8 per cent of all cancers and 0.5 per cent of cancer deaths.

- Sex ratio of rates 5.7 to 1. Age distribution, see Fig. 6.

Cancers of the larynx, like cancers of the oesophagus and buccal cavity, are closely associated with tobacco smoking and with the consumption of alcohol. The two agents act synergistically and in the absence of either the disease is rare. The different parts of this small organ are, however, related to the two agents differently. Cancers of the glottis are strongly related to smoking, particularly to cigarette smoking, and only weakly to alcohol; while cancers of the epilarynx resemble cancers of the neighbouring hypopharynx and are strongly related to both agents and to pipe and cigar smoking equally with cigarette smoking.

In Scandinavia, the incidence has increased in line with the increase in cancer of the lung. A similar increase has not, however, been seen in Britain and it seems probable that some other aetiological factor, perhaps nutritional in character, has become less prevalent. That there are other causal factors is evident from the relatively high incidence rates in parts of India, Turkey, North Africa and Brazil, which cannot be accounted for by tobacco and alcohol.

The disease has also occurred as an occupational risk in the manufacture of mustard gas and in processes that cause exposure to strong sulphuric acid mists.

Lung

- 13.6 per cent of all cancers and 22.2 per cent of cancer deaths.
- Sex ratio of rates 3.2 to 1. Age distribution, see Fig. 7.

Nearly all lung cancers are bronchial carcinomas and should properly be so described. The term 'lung cancer' is, however, in such common use that it is used here as synonymous with bronchial carcinoma, although it actually includes a very small proportion of alveolar-cell carcinomas and other rare types of cancer with different characteristics.

Until the 1920s, lung cancer was uniformly rare (except in the Hartz mountains, see below). In the next two decades, German and then British pathologists began to comment on an apparent increase, but this tended to be dismissed as an artefact of the greatly improving methods of diagnosis and the establishment of special centres for thoracic disease. Gradually, however, the increase became so pronounced and the change in the sex ratio so marked that the increase could no longer be dismissed as wholly artefactual and, by the late 1940s when the age-standardized mortality rate in men in the United Kingdom had increased 20 times, it was clear that the developed world had begun to see an epidemic of lung cancer comparable in severity to, though with a longer time scale than, the epidemics of infectious disease of the past. Until the 1940s, the increase among British women

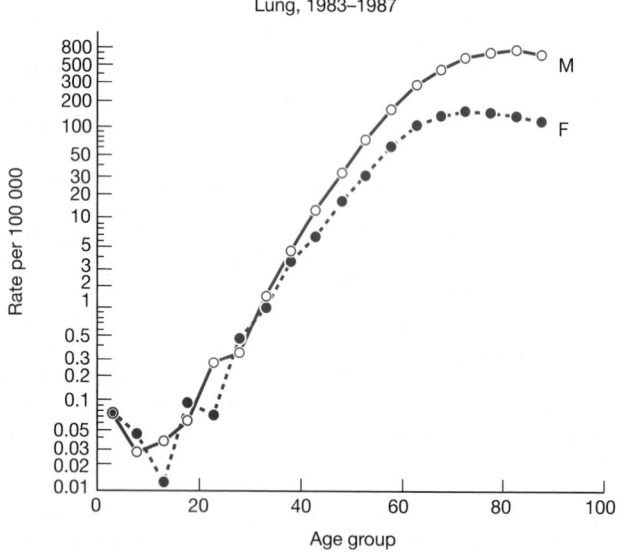

Fig. 7 Annual incidence of cancer of the lung by age and sex.

was largely a diagnostic artefact, and so provides a useful indication of the quantitative extent to which such artefacts may have affected the male rates. Since 1950, however, diagnostic standards in middle age have changed very little, the increase in British men has been replaced by a decrease, while the increase among middle-aged women has continued for longer, before also reversing. As a result, the sex ratio (male rate divided by female rate) at, for example, 50 to 54 years of age, which rose from 1.8 after the First World War to 8.9 after the Second World War, was reduced to 1.6 in 1998. In the first quarter of the twentieth century, the male excess may have been largely due to the effects of pipe smoking which was an almost exclusively male habit in the nineteenth century.

Smoking

Changes in treatment have had little effect on the fatality rate, which remains extremely high, and real changes in mortality closely reflect real changes in incidence. These can be explained almost entirely by the effect of smoking tobacco, particularly in the form of cigarettes, which caused more than 90 per cent of all lung cancers in Britain in the early 1990s. Evidence of this effect was first obtained in the middle of the last century by comparing the smoking histories of patients with different diseases. It was found that the proportion of patients who had never smoked was much smaller if they had lung cancer than if they had some other disease, and the proportion who had smoked heavily was correspondingly greater.

Further evidence was obtained by asking large numbers of apparently healthy men and women what they smoked and then following them up to determine the causes of death of those that had died. Cohort studies of this type—in over a million American men and women studied by the American Cancer Society, in 34 000 male British doctors, in a regional population of nearly 300 000 Japanese, and in a random sample of the Swedish population—have all shown similar results, the risk increasing with the amount smoked, but varying quantitatively depending on the length of time cigarettes had been smoked. If attention is restricted to populations in which most cigarette smokers had been smoking cigarettes regularly since early adult life, lung cancer is about 20 times more common in regular cigarette smokers than in lifelong non-smokers and up to 40 times more common in very heavy smokers. At first the relationship was less marked in women than in men, but this was because female smokers who were old enough to have a high risk of cancer either had not begun smoking cigarettes so early in adult life or had smoked them less intensively when they began, and the sex differences in behaviour and risk have both been progressively eliminated with the passage of time.

No other exposure has been identified that can account for the extreme difference in lung cancer risk between regular cigarette smokers and lifelong non-smokers and most or all of the excess must have been caused by smoking. Further quantitative studies have found that the relative risk of lung cancer has increased with decreasing age of starting to smoke and decreased with the number of years that smoking has been stopped; that the national increases in incidence have appeared at appropriate times after the increase in cigarette sales (after due allowance is made for a spurious increase due to improved diagnosis and appropriate differences in consumption by men and women), and that there is a general parallelism between the incidence of the disease in different countries and social and religious groups and the prolonged consumption of cigarettes. Furthermore, it has been found that when extracts of cigarette smoke are applied repeatedly to the skins of laboratory mice many tumours develop. Finally, and most encouragingly, the trend in mortality has reversed following reduction in smoking. By 1998, the mortality from lung cancer among men in their 30s in Britain was only about a quarter of that of men of the same ages some 40 years earlier, corresponding to the earlier changes in the prevalence of smoking. The reduction in tar delivery between 1939 and 1965 contributed to the reduction in lung cancer in young men after the war, but the later reduction had little effect because of changes in the way cigarettes were manufactured and in the way they were smoked to ensure an adequate intake of nicotine. At older ages the decreases are less striking, but they are now seen at all ages in British men, and up to 60 in British women.

Occupation

Several other causes of lung cancer have been discovered as a result of observations in industry. Many thousands of men and women have experienced significant hazards from exposure to asbestos or to polycyclic hydrocarbons (from the combustion of fossil fuel). The former has given rise to hazards in asbestos mines, asbestos textile works, and insulation work in the shipbuilding and construction industries and the latter to specific hazards in the manufacture of coal gas in coking ovens, in steel works, in aluminium foundries, and wherever substantial amounts of incompletely combusted fumes were released into the working environment. Much smaller numbers of men have experienced substantial hazards from radon in the air of mines (not only when mining radioactive materials, but also when mining haematite and fluorspar under conditions in which radon seeped into the mine air from streams and the surrounding rock), from the manufacture of chromates and chrome pigments, from the refining of nickel, from arsenic (in the manufacture of arsenical pesticides and in the refining of copper, which is always contaminated with arsenic), from the manufacture of mustard gas, and, to a small extent, from exposure to silica if sufficient to cause silicosis. In one extreme situation, the absolute risk of contracting lung cancer due to the occupational hazard of radon was so large that more than half the workers contracted the disease (in the cobalt mines of the Hartz mountains in Central Europe, that were subsequently mined for radium and uranium). In several other situations with heavy exposure to asbestos or the early stages of nickel refining, the occupational hazard has affected as many as 20 to 30 per cent of the exposed men.

Atmospheric pollution

Some of the materials responsible for these occupational hazards—particularly the combustion products of fossil fuels—are or have been widely distributed in the air of towns and it is still uncertain how far they have, in this way, contributed to the production of the disease in the general population. That lung cancer was more common in big towns than in small towns and rural areas is certain, but this held as strongly for Oslo and Helsinki, two relatively unpolluted cities, as it did for London, Birmingham, Manchester, Chicago, Los Angeles, and Pittsburgh. Differences between the largest towns and the least populated areas have seldom been more than three-fold and much of the difference can be accounted for by past differences in cigarette smoking, a habit which has tended to spread outwards from the major cities. Attempts to 'allow for' cigarette smoking have usually been inadequate, as it is impossible to take full account of such factors as the age of starting to smoke cigarettes, the amount smoked daily at different periods, and the method of smoking (number of puffs, depth of inhaling, etc.). It is clear, however, that in the absence of cigarette smoking any effect of urban pollution in developed countries is relatively small. Estimates, based on extrapolation from the heavy pollution with coal-smoke that used to occur in large towns, suggest that in such towns it may have contributed, in synergism with smoking, to as much as 10 per cent of the risk of lung cancer, but would have caused very little risk in non-smokers. On this basis, the present levels of pollution with benzo(a)pyrene and the other known lung carcinogens in town air can be only very small. Modern pollution with ultra-fine particles (<10 μm diameter) may, however, be more hazardous. Study of residents in six contrasting cities in the United States in which information about personal smoking habits had been obtained suggests that the risk in the most polluted city compared to that in the least polluted could be increased by about a quarter in both smokers and non-smokers. The position in some developing countries is different: notably in parts of China, where intense indoor pollution with smoke and fumes from heating and cooking more than doubles the risk of lung cancer in non-smokers.

The effect of another form of pollution—that of house air with radon leaked from underground rocks and building materials—can be estimated by extrapolation from the effects of the much larger doses to which some groups of underground miners have been exposed and by direct observation in case–control studies of people with and without lung cancer. Both methods suggest that indoor radon may contribute to about 6 per cent of lung cancers in the United Kingdom and 12 per cent in the United States. Most cases are caused in synergism with smoking, so that in the absence of smoking only few cases would be produced.

Geographic differences

The development of the male lung cancer epidemic and the early signs of its departure have been most prominent in Britain and Finland, since the switch of young men to cigarettes was largely complete in these countries by the 1920s. In the United States, where cigarette consumption doubled during the Second World War, the benefits of recent reductions in tobacco exposure are superimposed on the increasing lung cancer rates due to the delayed effects of past increases in smoking in early adult life by those who are now reaching middle and old age. Hence, it is thus far only among younger men in the United States that the benefits of reduced smoking and a switch to low-tar cigarettes are causing net decreases in lung cancer mortality. In some other developed countries, the development of the epidemic is still further behind and it is only just beginning to appear in many developing countries. Chinese males, for example, who now consume about 30 per cent of the world's cigarettes, experienced a three-fold increase in cigarette consumption during the 1980s that may well eventually cause almost a million cancer deaths a year when the young men of today reach middle age.

In women, the development of the epidemic has been later than in men. Only in the Maori population of New Zealand did it occur at the same time. In the United Kingdom, United States, and a few other developed countries, the female lung cancer rates are already substantial, but in others, such as France and Spain, the epidemic in women has scarcely begun. A relatively high risk has long been noted in Chinese women who are non-smokers, irrespective of their country of residence, which is probably due to their exposure to mutagens in the fumes from oils used in cooking with a wok and from the coal smoke with which many Chinese homes are heavily polluted.

Pleura and peritoneum

- 0.5 per cent of all cancers and 0.4 per cent of cancer deaths.

- Sex ratio of rates 6.0 to 1. Age distribution like laryngeal cancer.

The existence of a specific type of tumour arising from the pleura, or less commonly the peritoneum, was debated by pathologists until 1960 when Wagner and his colleagues reported that six African patients with a similar type of 'peripheral lung cancer' had all lived in villages that were heavily polluted with dust produced by the mining of blue asbestos (i.e. crocidolite). Since then, many cases have been reported throughout the world, the great majority of which have been specifically associated with exposure to asbestos at work. They are much less likely to be produced by white asbestos (chrysotile) than by brown asbestos (amosite) or blue, as the two last persist for longer in the lungs. A few cases arise from neighbourhood pollution with asbestos or secondary contamination (e.g. from household contact with asbestos workers) and some in Turkish villages are due to the weathering into the general atmosphere of mineral fibres in local rock that are physically similar to, but chemically different from, asbestos. A few cases have been caused by radiotherapy and natural ionizing radiations may be responsible for most of those that are not associated with asbestos. An SV-40 like virus has been found in some tumours; but it is uncertain whether it plays a part in causing the disease.

Mesotheliomas seldom occur less than 15 years after first exposure to asbestos, commonly occur 25 to 30 years afterwards, and may be delayed for 50 years or more. Almost all cases are fatal, so that the mortality would reflect incidence, if all cases were correctly diagnosed. Due to confusion with lung or other types of cancer, it is still uncertain how many cases have

Fig. 8 Annual incidence of cancer of bones by age and sex.

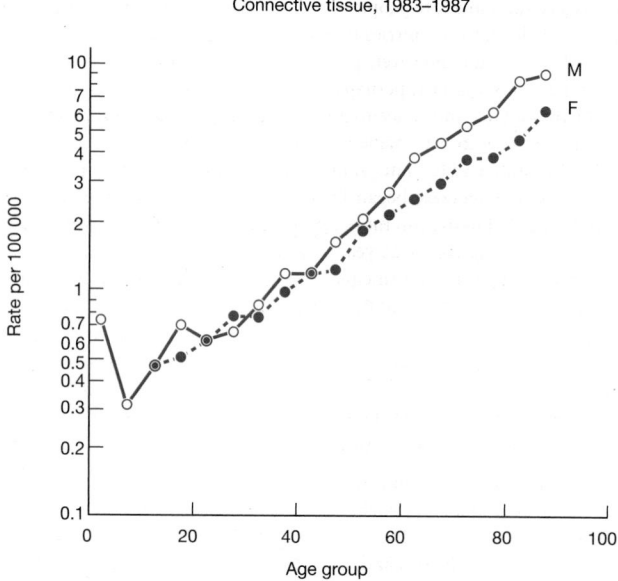

Fig. 9 Annual incidence of connective tissue sarcoma by age and sex.

occurred each year and some of the large increase since 1960 may be arte-factual. In the last few years, the recorded mortality under 70 years of age has begun to decrease.

Pleural mesothelioma is not related to cigarette smoking and the occu-pational hazard affects smokers and non-smokers alike.

Bone

- 0.1 per cent of all cancers and of cancer deaths.

- Sex ratio of rates 1.3 to 1. Age distribution, see Fig. 8.

Sarcomas can affect any bone, but characteristically affect the long bones in adolescence. After 45 years of age they occur most commonly in bones affected by Paget's disease (osteitis deformans), which predisposes to sarcoma so strongly that as many as 1 per cent of all people affected by the disease eventually develop a bone tumour.

Many different histological varieties occur, some of which appear to have different causes. Osteogenic sarcomas and chondrosarcomas are the most common, the former accounting for nearly all the adolescent peak. One rare type (Ewing's tumour) occurs only in childhood and adolescence and is almost unknown in black people, irrespective of the society in which they live.

Ionizing radiations are the only known extrinsic cause. Cases have been produced after intensive radiotherapy or the medicinal use of thorium (a bone-seeking radionuclide). In industry they have occurred in 'luminizers' who, in previous decades, used delicate paint brushes to apply radium compounds, and ingested radium, possibly as a result of 'pointing' the paint brushes in their mouths.

National statistics record a reduction in mortality over the last 50 years, but are unreliable indicators of incidence as many deaths attributed to tumours of bone are due to cancers that have metastasized from other sites. The recorded decrease in mortality is, therefore, largely an artefact due to improved diagnosis (though it has been contributed to in recent years by higher survival rates in childhood) and the true incidence may have remained roughly constant.

Connective tissues

- 0.4 per cent of all cancers and 0.5 per cent of cancer deaths.

- Sex ratio of rates 1.3 to 1. Age distribution, see Fig. 9.

Sarcomas of the soft tissues include a variety of different diseases, all of which are rare everywhere. Some are genetic in origin and others are caused by ionizing radiations. A few may be caused by intensive immunosuppres-sion or exposure to chlorophenols, but the evidence is inconclusive.

Skin (melanoma)

- 1.8 per cent of all cancers and 1.0 per cent of cancer deaths.

- Sex ratio of rates 0.6 to 1. Age distribution, see Fig. 10.

The incidence of the disease varies inversely with the amount of skin pigmentation. In white people the tumour occurs most commonly on the legs (in women) and the trunk, head, and neck (in men). It is extremely rare in blacks in the United States, but is more common in Africa, where it occurs at the junction of the pigmented and unpigmented skin on the sole of the foot. Like basal-cell and squamous carcinoma of the skin, it is par-ticularly common in sufferers from xeroderma pigmentosum.

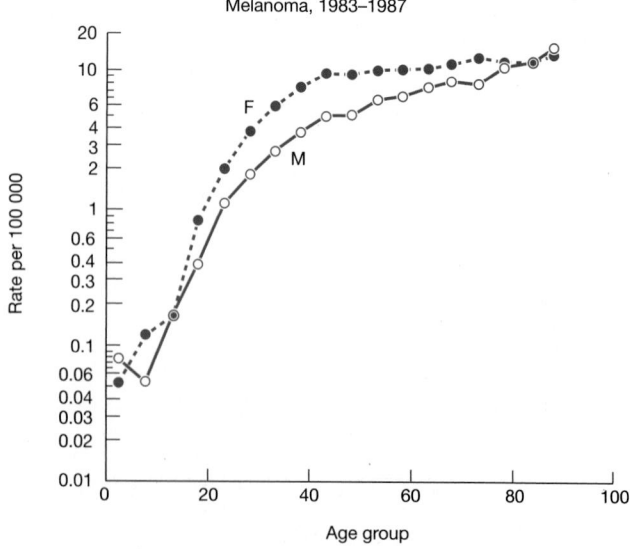

Fig. 10 Annual incidence of melanoma of the skin by age and sex.

Incidence rates in white people vary roughly in proportion to the flux of ultraviolet light in the countries in which they live. For all sites combined, the incidence is not, however, greater in outdoor than indoor workers (rather the reverse, in fact, perhaps due to the protective effects of a semi-permanent suntan) and it seems to be associated with periodic bouts of sunbathing and sunburn. Incidence and mortality rates have increased in Britain, the United States, and in many other countries with mainly white populations. The increase began in cohorts born early this century, who exposed their skin to the sun more than their predecessors had done, and it still continues at ages over 60 years. The totality of the evidence suggests that ultraviolet light is the principal cause, but the relationship is not simple and other factors may also be important.

Skin (non-melanoma)

- 14.1 per cent of all cancers and 0.3 per cent of cancer deaths.

- Sex ratio of rates 1.5 to 1. Age distribution, see Fig. 11.

Non-melanomatous skin cancers are of two main types, basal-cell and squamous carcinomas. The former, also known as rodent ulcers, are produced by ultraviolet light. They occur mainly on parts of the body that are regularly exposed to the sun and, in particular, on the face, head, and neck. They are more common in outdoor workers, such as seamen and farmers, than in indoor workers, more common in fair-skinned than in dark-skinned people, and are almost unknown in blacks (except those who suffer from albinism). Some few cases have been produced by exposure to X-rays, but the risk is very small unless the dose is very large and they seldom occur after normal courses of radiotherapy. People who suffer from xeroderma pigmentosum, a hereditary condition in which there is a defect in the enzyme responsible for the repair of the damage done to DNA by ultraviolet radiation, develop large numbers of skin tumours at an early age in response to even quite mild exposure to diffuse sunlight (see Chapter 23.1).

Squamous carcinoma is also produced by ultraviolet light, but less easily, so that it accounts for only about 20 per cent of cancers on the exposed skin. It is, however, the principal type of skin cancer produced by various carcinogenic chemicals, and particularly by polycyclic hydrocarbons in the combustion products of coal. These chemicals have been responsible for the scrotal cancers of chimney sweeps, who accumulated soot in the folds of the scrotum, of mule spinners, whose clothes were saturated with carcinogenic oils, and of various other groups of workers whose clothes were con-

taminated with tar. They have caused (and still do cause) cancers of the forearm in industrial workers whose arms are regularly splashed with tar or carcinogenic oils, cancers of the groin in India, localized by the continued friction of the *dhoti* cloth, and cancers of the abdomen in Kashmir associated with the habit of carrying a *kangri*, or small stove, inside the clothes in winter to keep warm.

Squamous carcinoma has also been due to prolonged exposure to arsenic, which is excreted by the skin and in the hair, when it may be accompanied by arsenical pigmentation and keratoses. All these conditions have been produced by prolonged medical treatment with inorganic arsenic, which used to be prescribed for a variety of chronic conditions, by the consumption of well water from arsenic-rich soils, and by occupational exposure, sometimes to as much as 1000 μg of arsenic/m³ of air, in the smelting of copper and cobalt (the ores of which often contain arsenic), and in the manufacture of arsenical pesticides.

How large a part human papilloma viruses play in the development of squamous carcinoma of the skin is unclear. The type 5 virus is responsible for the warty lesions of epidermodysplasia verruciformis, some of which progress to cancer, and other types of the virus may contribute to the increased risk that follows the intensive immunosuppression given to permit the survival of organ transplants.

A third type is Kaposi's sarcoma, which is now classed as a skin cancer. It is associated with AIDS when AIDS results from homosexual intercourse, but probably only when this is accompanied by orofaecal contact. Frequent at first, particularly in the United States, the association has become progressively less common. Before the advent of AIDS, Kaposi's sarcoma was common in some parts of Central Africa, where it occasionally affected children, progressed rapidly, and could account for as many as 10 per cent of all hospital patients with cancer. Elsewhere it was rare, but indolent cases occurred occasionally in developed countries, principally on the legs of middle-aged and elderly men. The disease is initiated by infection with the human herpes virus type 8, but cofactors are required for tumour development.

Breast

- 12.2 per cent of all cancers and 8.6 per cent of cancer deaths.

- Sex ratio of rates 0.01 to 1. Age distribution, see Fig. 12.

Cancer of the breast was the most common fatal cancer in women throughout most of the developed world, but is now being displaced by

Fig. 11 Annual incidence of non-melanomatous skin cancer by age and sex.

Fig. 12 Annual incidence of breast cancer in women by age.

lung cancer in the United Kingdom and the United States. It is less common in Eastern Europe and much less common in Asia and in black African populations south of the Sahara. Incidence rates have tended to rise slowly in many countries, but the changes have been relatively small and decreases have recently been recorded in young age groups. The geographical differences are unlikely to be chiefly due to genetic factors, as black women in the United States and Japanese women in Hawaii have rates that are similar to those in their white American compatriots and much greater than those in their countries of origin.

Hormonal factors are important in the production of the disease, particularly oestrogens, but others may also be important. The duration of ovarian activity is relevant, as the disease is particularly common in women who have an early menarche and a late menopause (the former being more important than the latter). Pregnancy produces a short-term increase in risk, followed after a few years by a lifelong decrease, particularly after teenage or early adult pregnancies. The incidence in later life increases progressively with a woman's age at the time of her first full-term pregnancy, being about three times greater when the first birth occurs after 35 years of age than when it occurs before 18 years. Full-term pregnancies after the first have an additional protective effect. Pregnancies that end in abortion have little or no effect, however, suggesting that the effects of pregnancy depend on the induction of lactation. The duration of lactation has an additional protective effect but is not marked unless it continues for a year or more.

Parity and menstrual differences are insufficient to account for the large variations in the incidence of the disease in different countries, which seem to be correlated with a 'high' standard of living: that is, with life in a developed country. Diet may play an important part, but the evidence is complex and inconclusive. Obesity is associated with a reduced risk before the menopause, as it tends to be associated with ovarian dysfunction. After the menopause, obesity increases both the incidence and probably the fatality of the disease. Oestrogens prescribed medically, as hormone replacement therapy (HRT) after the menopause, increase the risk by about 2 per cent for each year of use; combined with progestogens in the contraceptive pill they increase it by about 25 per cent during use, but the increased risk gradually disappears over 10 years, when use is stopped, as it does after HRT is stopped. Tamoxifen, an antioestrogen prescribed for the treatment of breast cancer, reduces the subsequent incidence of the disease in the unaffected breast.

Much of the recent increase in incidence is the result of intensive case finding in association with mammography and there is no reason to attribute it to any form of environmental pollution.

Cervix uteri

- 1.2 per cent of all cancers and 1.1 per cent of cancer deaths.
- Confined to women. Age distribution, see Fig. 13.

Carcinoma of the cervix is the most common type of cancer throughout much of Africa, Asia, and Latin America, and used also to be common in Europe and North America. It has always been rare in Jewesses and has tended to be less common in Muslim women than in women of other faiths living in the same country (as, for example, Hindus in India).

Changes in incidence have been difficult to assess, partly because mortality data have not always distinguished between deaths due to cancer of the cervix and those due to cancer of the corpus (or endometrium), partly because the introduction of screening programmes has made it possible to diagnose and treat premalignant lesions (see below), and partly because hysterectomy for benign conditions has become progressively more common, with a corresponding reduction in the number of uteri in which the disease could occur. Despite these complications there can be no doubt that the disease has become substantially less common in Europe and North America than it was before the Second World War.

The rarity of the disease in Jewesses and its relative rarity in Muslims suggest that male circumcision may reduce the risk of its development, but this is unlikely as the state of circumcision of her husband has no substan-

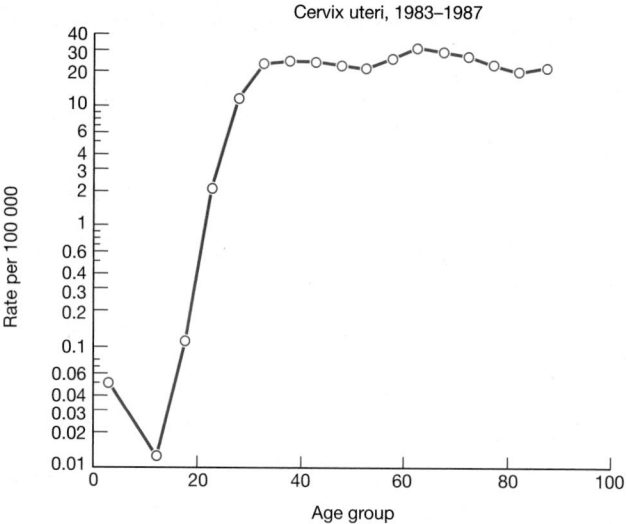

Fig. 13 Annual incidence of cancer of the cervix uteri by age.

tial effect on a woman's risk of developing the disease in communities in which only some men are circumcised. Cleanliness is likely to be protective, as the disease is relatively uncommon in communities that practise ritual ablution before and after intercourse and, within each community, it becomes less common with rising socioeconomic status.

Squamous carcinoma, which constitutes the vast majority of all cases, is intimately connected with sexual activity. It almost never occurs in virgins and increases in frequency with the number of sexual partners that a woman or her partner has had. The great majority of cases are attributable in part to infection with some types of the human papilloma virus, most notably types 16 and 18.

The development of squamous carcinoma is preceded by pathological changes limited to the epithelium, known as cervical intraepithelial neoplasia (CIN) types I, II, and III. CIN III is associated with the same types of virus as squamous carcinoma, but CIN I and CIN II generally are not. The changes may progress from one to another, finally leading to carcinoma, but the early lesions (CIN I and II) commonly regress and even CIN III (previously known as carcinoma *in situ*) may do so occasionally. The lesions can be recognized in cervical smears and destroyed by lasers or extensive biopsy and the occurrence of clinical disease can be greatly reduced by the examination of all sexually active women every 2 or 3 years and the treatment of advanced CIN lesions.

Other factors associated with the production of the disease are the use of oral contraceptives and cigarette smoking. Both tend to be associated with behaviour conducive to venereal infection, but it is uncertain whether this tendency can wholly account for their association with the disease. That smoking may be responsible for some cases is suggested by the presence of mutagens in the cervical mucus of smokers that are not present in the secretions of non-smokers.

Adenocarcinoma of the cervix uteri is generally rare, but may have become somewhat more common recently. Its causes are unknown.

Endometrium (corpus uteri)

- 1.5 per cent of all cancers and 0.7 per cent of cancer deaths.
- Confined to women. Age distribution like cancer of ovary.

The epidemiological features of endometrial cancer are in many respects the opposite of those of cervical cancer. Histologically, it is nearly always an adenocarcinoma. It is common in developed countries, rare in poor populations, and is, if anything, becoming more common with the passage of time. It is inversely related to parity, but not otherwise related to coitus, and is unaffected by the number of sexual partners. Like cancer of the breast, it is positively associated with early menarche and late menopause.

The one factor known to produce the disease is regular exposure to oestrogens, unopposed by progestogens. This leads to endometrial hyperplasia and eventually, in some cases, to cancer. Known causes include oestrogen-secreting tumours of the ovary, the use of oral contraceptives in which oestrogens and progestogens are prescribed sequentially (types that have now been abandoned), the use of 'natural' conjugated oestrogens to relieve menopausal and postmenopausal symptoms, and adiposity. The last causes the disease because oestrogens are produced in the body after the menopause in adipose tissue from the adrenal hormone, androstenedione. Tamoxifen, an analogue of the natural oestrogens, which blocks oestrogen receptors in the breast and hence acts as an antioestrogen, can, due to differences between the hormone receptors in different tissues, have a pro-oestrogenic effect in some other organs, and slightly increases the incidence of endometrial cancer.

It is improbable that oestrogens are initiating agents. They are not mutagens *in vitro* and the changes that took place in the incidence of the disease in the United States following the increase and the subsequent reduction in the use of premarin (a conjugated oestrogen) for the treatment of menopausal symptoms occurred so quickly that they make sense only if oestrogens act on some late stage(s) of the carcinogenic process.

Ovary

- 2.0 per cent of all cancers and 2.9 per cent of cancer deaths.

- Confined to women. Age distribution, see Fig. 14.

Cancer of the ovary is not a uniform disease, but has many types defined by their histological appearance. Most are too rare to have been considered separately in epidemiological studies and the few characteristics that have been recognized may refer only to the common adenocarcinoma. These mostly resemble the characteristics of endometrial cancer, in that the risk of developing the disease is greatest in countries with a high standard of living, increases with duration of time from menarche to menopause, and decreases progressively with increasing number of children. The incidence of the disease is, however, reduced by the use of oral contraceptives and seems to depend on the number of ovulations.

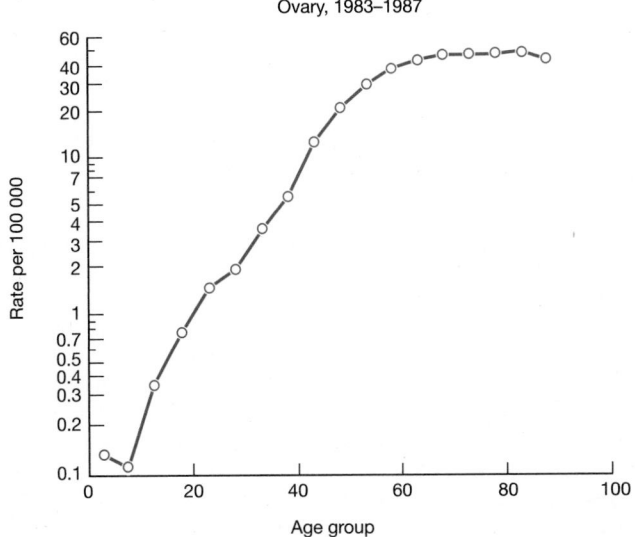

Fig. 14 Annual incidence of cancer of the ovary by age.

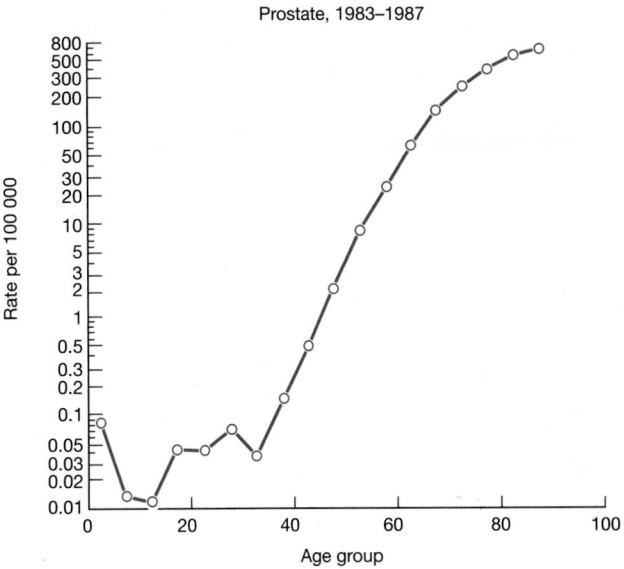

Fig. 15 Annual incidence of cancer of the prostate by age.

Prostate

- 7.4 per cent of all cancers and 6.3 per cent of cancer deaths.

- Confined to men. Age distribution, see Fig. 15.

Cancer of the prostate is more characteristically a disease of old age than any other cancer, so that it comes to play a much larger part in clinical experience as the proportion of old people in the population increases. It is unusual in that foci of cells resembling cancer can be found in a high proportion of clinically normal prostates, so that the recorded incidence is drastically increased by increasing the number of prostatic biopsies. Some increase in mortality has been recorded in Britain and North America, but the weight of evidence suggests that the disease is principally due to factors that have affected society for many years. What these factors are remains obscure. Associations have been reported with both increased and decreased sexual activity. On general grounds it seems likely that the disease is dependent on hormonal imbalance (particularly as castration slows the progression of clinical disease) but the nature of the imbalance is unknown. Vasectomy was thought to increase the incidence of the disease, but probably does not.

Two epidemiological observations stand out: the high incidence in black populations throughout the world, and the low incidence in Japanese. Both may be partly due to genetic factors, but they are not wholly so, as both Japanese and blacks have higher rates in the United States than they have in Japan and Africa.

Testis

- 0.5 per cent of all cancers and 0.1 per cent of cancer deaths.

- Confined to men. Age distribution, see Fig. 16.

Testicular cancers are of two main types. Seminomas, which are the more common, have a peak incidence at about 30 years of age and teratomas, commonly called embryomal carcinomas in the United States, which have a peak incidence about 10 years earlier. Tumours after 50 years of age are mostly lymphomas and are now classed as such. Both genetic and environmental factors are important. On the one hand, the disease is uniformly rare in black populations, whether in Africa or in the United States. On the other, it has increased in incidence in many countries, notably in Denmark and Britain. In Britain, the increase began in the 1920s and affected first the higher socioeconomic groups. The increase trebled the mortality at 15 to 34 years of age and produced a sharp peak in young adult

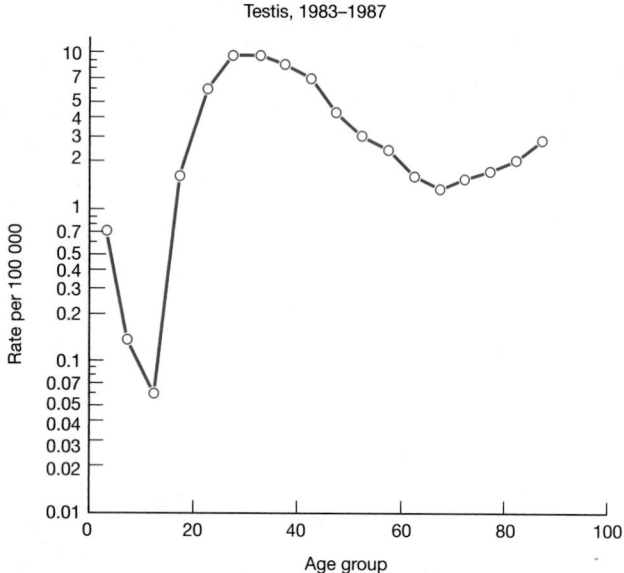

Fig. 16 Annual incidence of cancer of the testis by age.

life that had not previously been present. In the United States, the increase started later and has been less marked. The disease is much more likely to occur in an undescended than in a normal testis, but otherwise its causes are unknown.

Penis

- 0.1 per cent of all cancers and of cancer deaths.
- Confined to men. Age distribution like skin (non-melanoma).

Carcinoma of the penis is at all common only in some parts of tropical Africa and Brazil, where it has accounted for 10 per cent of all cancers in men. It is avoided almost entirely by circumcision at birth and is very rare if circumcision is carried out in boyhood. In developed countries it is rare even in the absence of circumcision if the glans, coronary sulcus, and foreskin are kept clean.

The oncogenic types of the human papilloma virus (principally types 16 and 18) can usually be identified in the malignant cells and are important causes of the disease.

Bladder

- 4.5 per cent of all cancers and 3.3 per cent of cancer deaths.
- Sex ratio of rates 3.6 to 1. Age distribution like gastric cancer.

Cancer of the bladder can be produced by cigarette smoking, occupational exposure to a group of chemicals classed together as aromatic amines, infestation of the bladder with *Schistosoma haematobium*, and the medical prescription of chlornaphthazine (*N,N′*-bis(2-chloroethyl)-2-naphthylamine) and cyclophosphamide. Most bladder cancers are transitional cell carcinomas, but those associated with schistosomiasis are characteristically squamous carcinomas. It is not surprising that the bladder should be affected by many chemicals, as any noxious small molecules in the blood will tend to be found at greatly increased concentration in the urinary tract. Cigarette smoke contains several mutagenic chemicals that enter the bloodstream and thence the bladder, so that when tested *in vitro* on bacterial DNA the urine of cigarette smokers is found to be mutagenic, while that of non-smokers is barely active.

Occupation

An occupational cause was first suspected in 1898 in Germany, when Rehn commented on a cluster of cases in men using aniline for the manufacture

of dyes. Aniline, however, is not carcinogenic in experimental animals, more recent studies have failed to incriminate it epidemiologically, and it seems likely that other carcinogenic chemicals were present as impurities. Four aromatic amines that are carcinogenic in experimental animals have been shown to cause bladder cancer in humans: 2-naphthylamine, benzidine, 3,3′-dichlorobenzidine, and 4-aminobiphenyl. The first is one of the most powerful human carcinogens yet known and was responsible for the development of bladder cancer in all the 19 men who were employed in distilling it in a British factory. Its manufacture in Britain was stopped in 1949; but small amounts continued to be imported until the 1960s. Other aromatic amines that may cause bladder cancer include auramine, magenta, and, perhaps, 1-naphthylamine. The last is dubiously carcinogenic in experimental animals and it seems probable that the cases associated with its use have been due to a few per cent of 2-naphthylamine present as an impurity in the commercial material. These chemicals were used in the manufacture of dyes, in the rubber industry as antioxidants (1-naphthylamine and 4-aminobiphenyl) and hardeners (benzidine), and in laboratories as a reagent (benzidine). 2-Naphthylamine is also found in the combustion products of coal and may have been responsible for the hazard of bladder cancer in men who made coal gas. As many as 10 per cent of cases were, at one time, attributable to occupational causes in Britain and North America; but the proportion should now be much less.

Smoking

The most important cause numerically is cigarette smoking, which probably accounts for about half the total number of cases in Britain and North America. 2-Naphthylamine and 4-aminobiphenyl are present in cigarette smoke, but whether the amounts are sufficient to account for the carcinogenic effect is uncertain.

Medicines

The two medicinal causes have, by contrast, been responsible for only a handful of cases. Chlornaphthazine was used briefly for the treatment of myelomatosis, until it was found to be metabolized into 2-naphthylamine. Cyclophosphamide is used primarily for the treatment of malignant disease, but it is also used as an immunosuppressant. In large doses it may cause sloughing of the bladder mucosa and, occasionally, cancer.

Parasitic infection

Heavy infection of the bladder with *Schistosoma haematobium* has been found to be a cause of the disease, most notably in Egypt and Tanzania.

Diet

The evidence linking bladder cancer to diet is weak. Several case–control studies suggested a positive relation with the consumption of coffee, but the results were inconsistent and it is difficult to exclude the effect of confounding by the stronger relation with cigarette smoking. Artificial sweeteners came under suspicion because of the results of animal experiments in which, first, mixtures of cyclamates and saccharin and then saccharin alone were shown to cause bladder cancer in rats. The human use of cyclamates was banned before saccharin came under suspicion and it now appears that the 'positive' results of animal experiments with cyclamates alone were due to impurities. Saccharin has been shown to cause bladder cancer in rats in feeding experiments, especially when given over two generations and when given after a single instillation into the bladder of a powerful carcinogen. In both instances the quantities that had to be given were large, constituting a few per cent of the feed. The human evidence is extensive and could hardly be more negative, except that it does not cover lifelong use.

Kidney

- 1.8 per cent of all cancers and 2.0 per cent of cancer deaths.
- Sex ratio of rates 2.1 to 1. Age distribution, see Fig. 17.

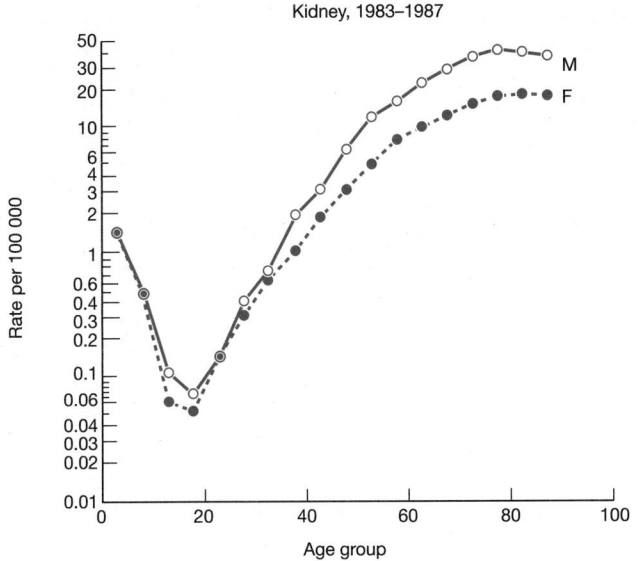

Fig. 17 Annual incidence of cancer of the kidney by age and sex.

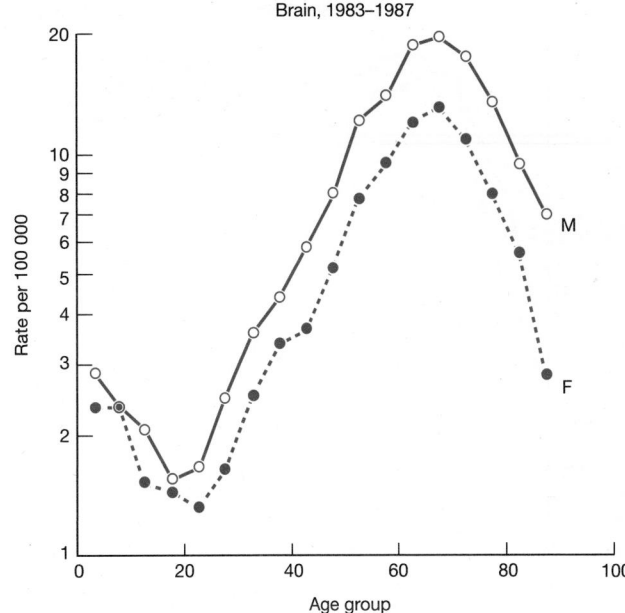

Fig. 18 Annual incidence of cancer of the brain by age and sex.

Cancers of the kidney are of three main types: nephroblastomas (or Wilms' tumours), adenocarcinomas (or hypernephromas), and transitional- and squamous-cell carcinomas of the renal pelvis. The first are limited to childhood, occur with almost equal frequency everywhere, and apart from a few of genetic origin, are of unknown aetiology. The second constitute by far the majority of all cases, are more common in Western Europe and North America than in Africa and Asia, and have been slowly increasing in incidence. Cigarette smoking is one cause, but the association is weak and it does not account for more than about a quarter of the cases.

The third type of renal cancer (carcinoma of the pelvis) constitutes some 10 per cent of all cases. Three established causes are occupational exposure to the chemicals that cause cancer of the bladder, smoking, and the consumption of phenacetin in large enough amounts to produce analgesic nephropathy. In all three cases the hazards are relatively small (two to three-fold). A fourth cause, Balkan nephropathy (see Section 20.7) increases the risk several hundred-fold.

Brain

- 1.3 per cent of all cancers and 2.1 per cent of cancer deaths.
- Sex ratio of rates 1.4 to 1. Age distribution, see Fig. 18.

Tumours of the brain and nervous system are of several different histological types, some of which may not be clearly either benign or malignant. One type occurs characteristically in childhood (medulloblastoma), another in adult life (glioblastoma), and a third (astrocytoma) at all ages. Despite the overall male excess, one type (meningioma) is more common in women.

A moderately large increase in incidence in old age has been recorded in many countries, which can be attributed to improved diagnosis with computerized tomographic scans and nuclear magnetic imaging. Little or no increase in mortality has been reported in or before middle age and the recorded increases in incidence are certainly largely, and possibly wholly, artefactual. No new environmental cause has been established, but many have been suspected, including electromagnetic fields associated with the use of electricity (50–60 Hz) and mobile phones.

Thyroid

- 0.4 per cent of all cancers and 0.2 per cent of cancer deaths.
- Sex ratio of rates 0.5 to 1. Age distribution, see Fig. 19.

The thyroid is particularly sensitive to ionizing radiation in childhood. Substantial numbers of cases have occurred among the survivors of the atomic explosions in Hiroshima and Nagasaki, children who were exposed to large amounts of radioactive iodine following the Chernobyl accident, and young people whose necks were irradiated in infancy for the treatment of an enlarged thymus (a condition now considered to be perfectly normal, but at one time thought to be a cause of sudden death). Fortunately, the thyroid tumours produced by ionizing radiations are nearly all of the papillary and follicular types, which respond well to treatment. No causes are known of the medullary and anaplastic types, which have a high fatality and occur only in adult life.

The disease is several times more common in Iceland, northern Norway, Hawaii, Fiji, and Israel than elsewhere.

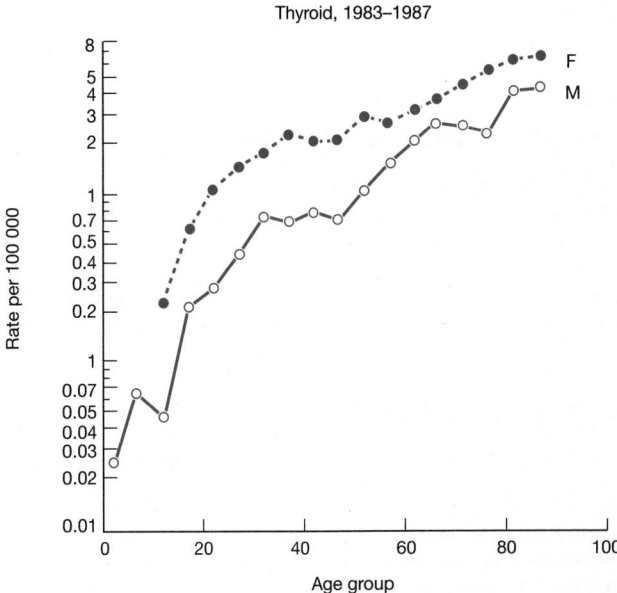

Fig. 19 Annual incidence of cancer of the thyroid by age and sex.

Fig. 20 Annual incidence of Hodgkin's lymphoma by age and sex.

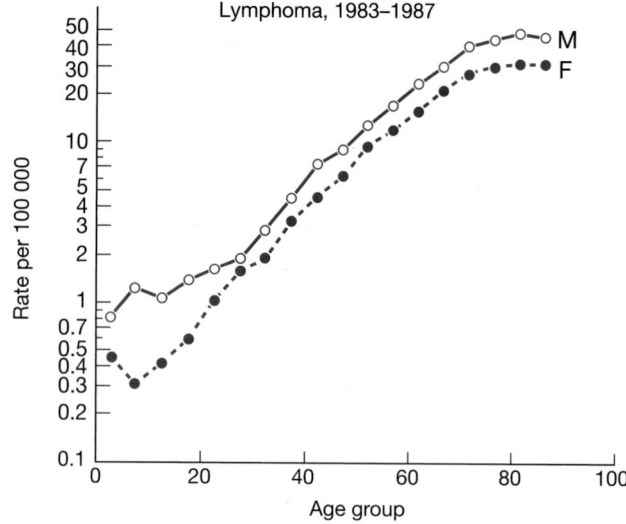

Fig. 21 Annual incidence of non-Hodgkin's lymphoma by age and sex.

Hodgkin's disease (Hodgkin's lymphoma)

- 0.5 per cent of all cancers and 0.2 per cent of cancer deaths.
- Sex ratio of rates 1.6 to 1. Age distribution, see Fig. 20.

Hodgkin's disease is best thought of as at least two diseases, one affecting primarily youths and young adults, the other primarily the middle aged and elderly. This division is suggested partly by the existence of two peaks in the age-specific incidence rates, partly by the histological appearances (younger patients tending to have the nodular sclerotic form of the disease and older patients the mixed cellular form), and partly by the clinical distinction that young patients show mediastinal involvement in more than 50 per cent of cases and infradiaphragmatic involvement in less than 5 per cent, while the reverse tends to be true in the elderly.

There are several reasons for thinking that the type characteristic of young people is infective in origin. In developing countries, Hodgkin's disease occurs in childhood, but as the standard of living rises, the childhood cases disappear and are replaced by a larger number in young adults. This is reminiscent of what happened to poliomyelitis in the first half of the century and suggests that the disease may be due to a ubiquitous infective agent that becomes less widespread as hygiene improves. That the agent was likely to be the Epstein–Barr virus (EBV or human herpes virus type 4) was suggested by the finding that the incidence was increased 5 to 20 years after a clinical attack of infectious mononucleosis and the virus has now been found in the DNA of the malignant cells characteristic of the tumour (the Reed–Sternberg and tumour reticulum cells). As with other virus-induced cancers, there are likely to be cofactors (at present unknown) that determine whether cellular infection leads to the production of a malignant clone.

Non-Hodgkin's lymphoma

- 2.8 per cent of all cancers and 2.9 per cent of cancer deaths.
- Sex ratio of rates 1.5 to 1. Age distribution, see Fig. 21.

Non-Hodgkin's lymphoma is a non-specific term that embraces several diseases with different histological appearances. The histological classification has, however, varied from place to place and from time to time, and it has been difficult to collect epidemiological information about the individual types.

One type that has been clearly distinguished is Burkitt's lymphoma, derived from B lymphocytes. This affects children everywhere, but is common only in a few areas in which malarial infection is both heavy and widespread. In parts of Uganda, Tanzania, and Nigeria the disease is 100 times more common than in Europe and North America. In high incidence areas, EBV can nearly always be recovered from the lymphomatous cells and part of its genome is identifiable in the cells' DNA. Infection with the virus is, however, not necessary for the development of the disease, as some cases occur in its absence; nor is it sufficient, as infection is almost universal and occurs at a very young age in high incidence areas. It seems, therefore, that EBV is a potential cause and that its carcinogenic effect is precipitated by the intense stimulation of the reticuloendothelial system that is characteristic of heavy and chronic malarial infection.

Another type occurs as part of the adult T-cell leukaemia–lymphoma syndrome that follows infection with the human T-cell leukaemia–lymphoma virus (HTLV-1). The disease is common in South Japan and the Caribbean, but may occur occasionally anywhere.

A third type, primary upper small-intestinal lymphoma (PUSIL), affects young people in many populations with a low standard of living, not only in North Africa and the Middle East (where its frequency gave it the earlier name of Mediterranean lymphoma) but also in South Africa and Central and South America. Malnutrition is not, however, a sufficient cause as it is uncommon in Bangladesh and several other malnourished populations.

A fourth type, the mucosa-associated lymphoid tissue tumour known as a maltoma, occurs in the stomach as a result of *H. pylori* infection and can be cured by aggressive treatment of the infection.

The remaining lymphomas, which constitute the majority in developed countries, should probably be divided further. Some in childhood might be better classed with acute lymphatic leukaemia from which they are distinguished arbitrarily only by the number of lymphocytes in the blood. At present, however, they have to be considered as a group. As such they constitute one of the few types of cancer that have been increasing in incidence at all ages.

Two factors that have contributed to the increase, but which cannot account for it all, are the use of immunosuppressive drugs and the spread of AIDS. Intense immunosuppression is followed within 1 or 2 years by an increase in the incidence of the disease of the order of 50- to 100-fold, and smaller increases follow the less intensive use of immunosuppressive drugs for the medical treatment of patients with arthritis, Crohn's disease, and other similar conditions. Many, but not all, of the lymphomas that occur in these circumstances are associated with EBV and some of these may, unusually, arise in the brain. Greatly increased incidence rates are also seen in a variety of rare hereditary disorders characterized by major immunological impairment, such as the Wiskott–Aldrich syndrome.

The rare hairy-cell leukaemia, of unknown aetiology, is now regarded as another type of lymphoma rather than as a leukaemia.

Myelomatosis

- 1.1 per cent of all cancers and 1.6 per cent of cancer deaths.
- Sex ratio of rates 1.5 to 1. Age distribution like large bowel cancer.

Myelomatosis has been much easier to diagnose since marrow puncture and then serum electrophoresis became standard diagnostic tools and since the improvement in the management of renal failure, which is often the presenting symptom. As a result it is difficult to be sure whether the increase that was recorded until recently, in both incidence and mortality rates, was due solely to improved diagnosis, or whether it also reflects the introduction of major new causes into Europe and North America between the two World Wars. In southern Sweden, where there has been a long-standing interest in, and search for, cases of myelomatosis, no large increase was seen over the same period; the rates were higher than in other developed populations, but in recent decades those in other populations have caught up.

The disease is uncommon in undeveloped areas, where it is almost certainly underdiagnosed. Genetic factors could be important, as it is twice as common in blacks in the United States as in whites and is rare in Japanese irrespective of where they live.

Leukaemia

- 2.1 per cent of all cancers and 2.6 per cent of cancer deaths.
- Sex ratio of rates 1.5 to 1. Age distribution, see Fig. 22.

Leukaemia may be divided primarily into chronic lymphatic leukaemia (CLL), chronic myeloid leukaemia (CML), acute myeloid leukaemia (AML), and acute lymphatic leukaemia (ALL). CML, AML, and ALL are, in turn, amalgams of two or more different types, with different causes, different age distributions, and different prognoses, but the distinctions between them are still undergoing evolution and, with the exception referred to later, the epidemiological descriptions of each subtype are unclear.

CLL increases progressively with age in the same way as myelomatosis and most of the common epithelial cancers. It is extremely rare in Chinese, Japanese, and Indians, which is presumably due to genetic differences in susceptibility as it continues to be rare in these racial groups even when they migrate to other countries.

Fig. 22 Annual incidence of leukaemia by age and sex.

AML occurs at all ages. It becomes slowly, but progressively, more common from childhood on and is the most common type in young adult life. In this age group, its incidence is probably less variable throughout the world than that of any other reasonably common type of cancer. CML, by contrast, is very rare in youth, but becomes more common than AML in later middle age. The few cases that occur in childhood should perhaps be regarded as constituting a separate disease, as they lack the Philadelphia chromosome that normally characterizes CML in adult life.

ALL is the most common type of childhood cancer. Three main types can be distinguished. Common (c) ALL arises from B-lymphocyte precursors and is responsible for a peak incidence of the disease at 2 to 3 years of age. Null ALL also arises from B-cell precursors, but lacks the common antigen and accounts for most cases in the first year of life. T-cell ALL occurs more or less equally at all ages in childhood. ALL in adult life can be either B cell or T cell.

Many causes of leukaemia are known. The most important is ionizing radiation, which causes all types except CLL. The sparing of CLL may be because the relevant stem cells are so radiosensitive that they are killed by small doses that would otherwise be carcinogenic. The other main types are induced by ionizing radiation more easily than most other types of cancer and constitute about 10 per cent of all fatal cancers from exposure of the whole body to moderate doses.

Whether extremely low frequency non-ionizing radiation can cause leukaemia, particularly ALL in childhood, is uncertain. There is evidence to suggest that the risk of ALL is approximately doubled by exposure to power frequency magnetic fields of an intensity greater than 0.4 μT that occurs rarely in the United States but only very rarely in the United Kingdom. The evidence for a causal relationship is, however, inconclusive.

One type of the disease (adult T-cell lymphoma/leukaemia) is caused by a virus (HTLV/1) and has been described under non-Hodgkin's lymphoma.

Other causes include smoking, which causes a small increase in myeloid leukaemia, several chemicals, and genetically determined diseases. The most important chemical is benzene, which is used widely in industry. Prolonged occupational exposure to large amounts has caused a substantial risk of AML (particularly one of its subtypes, erythroleukaemia) and, less commonly, acute lymphatic leukaemia. Many cases are preceded by periods of aplastic anaemia and there is still some doubt whether leukaemia can be caused by small doses.

Two other chemicals, melphalan and busulphan, are used in the treatment of cancer and the small risk of AML that follows their use is unimportant in comparison to the benefit obtained if they are used appropriately. Melphalan is an alkylating agent and so presumably mutagenic. Busulfan, however, has been observed to produce a substantial risk of leukaemia only after being given in such high doses that it produces aplastic anaemia.

Of the hereditary causes, Down's syndrome is the most common and is probably responsible for the greatest number of cases, although the relative risk in some of the other rarer syndromes may be greater than the 20-fold increase in childhood leukaemia that occurs with Down's disease. Ataxia telangiectasia and Bloom's syndrome predispose to ALL, while Fanconi's anaemia predisposes to AML.

Further reading

Chen J, Campbell TC, Li J, Peto R (1990). *Diet, life-style, and mortality in China: a study of the characteristics of 65 Chinese counties*. Oxford University Press.

Dockery DW, Pope III CA, Du X, Spengler JD, Ware JH, Martha EF, Ferris BG, Speizer FE (1993). An association between air pollution and mortality in six US cities. *New England Journal of Medicine* **329**, 1753–9.

Doll R, Peto R (1981). The causes of cancer: quantitative estimates of avoidable risks of cancer in the United States today. *Journal of the National Cancer Institute* **66**, 1191–308. (Reprinted Oxford University Press, 1981.)

Doll R, Fraumeni J, Muir C, eds (1994). *Trends in cancer incidence and mortality. Cancer surveys*, Vol. 19 and 20. Cold Spring Harbor Laboratory Press, New York.

Hammond EC, Selikoff IJ, Seidman H (1979). Asbestos exposure, cigarette smoking, and death rates. *Annals of the New York Academy of Sciences* **330**, 473–90.

International Commission on Radiological Protection (1991). Recommendations of the International Commission on Radiological Protection. Publication 60. *Annals of the ICRP* **21**, Nos. 1–3.

Office of National Statistics (1999). *Review of the Registrar General on deaths by cause, sex and age, in England and Wales, 1998*. Stationery Office, London.

Office of National Statistics (2000). *Registrations of cancer diagnosed in 1994, England and Wales*. Stationery Office, London.

Parkin DM, Muir CS, Whelan SL, Gao Y-T, Ferlay J, Powell J, eds (1992). *Cancer incidence in five continents*, Vol. 6. International Agency for Research on Cancer, Lyon.

Peto R (2001). Cancer epidemiology in the last century and the next decade. *Nature* **411**, 390–5.

Peto R, Darby S, Deo H, Silcocks P, Whitley E, Doll R (2000). Smoking, smoking cessation, and lung cancer in the UK since 1950, combination of national statistics and two case-control studies. *British Medical Journal* **321**, 323–9.

Swerdlow A, Dos Santos Silva I, Doll R (2001). *Cancer incidence and mortality in England and Wales: trends and risk factors*. Oxford University Press, Oxford

Tomatis L, ed. (1990). *Cancer causes, occurrence and control*. IARC Scientific Publications No. 100. International Agency for Research on Cancer, Lyon.

6.2 The nature and development of cancer

Andrew Coop and Matthew J. Ellis

Introduction

The disruption of proteins with pivotal roles in cell growth, death, and the regulation of gene expression is the underlying cause of cancer. The most common causes of these disturbances are somatic mutations that accumulate in cellular DNA over time, induced by chemicals in the environment (carcinogens), radiation, or simply the background rate of error in DNA replication. On occasion, carcinogenic mutations are inherited ('germline' mutations). The study of individuals with a genetic predisposition to cancer ('inherited cancer') has contributed greatly to our understanding of malignancy by pinpointing individual genes involved in this process (see Chapter 6.3). In a several instances, including Burkitt's lymphoma, Kaposi's sarcoma, cervical cancer, and hepatocellular carcinoma, cancer is initiated by viral infection, not somatic mutation ('endemic cancer'). 'Tumour viruses' encode proteins that either mimic or disrupt the functions of essentially the same set of cellular proteins whose genes are targeted by mutation in sporadic and inherited cancers.

Extensive functional and epidemiological studies of the genes responsible for cancer show that they can be broadly divided into two operational classes: oncogenes and tumour suppressor genes. Oncogenes are associated with mutant proteins demonstrating a gain in function, which overstimulate cell division or support the survival of genetically aberrant cells. In contrast, tumour suppressor genes are characterized by mutations that cause a loss of function. Typically, tumour suppressor genes encode proteins that suppress cellular proliferation, activate cell death pathways, or protect the integrity of the genome in the presence of DNA damage. In general, inactivation of both alleles of a tumour suppressor gene is required before aberrant cellular behaviour is evident. In contrast, gain-of-function mutations in oncogenes act in a dominant manner, so that typically only one allele is mutated. To qualify as an oncogene or tumour suppressor gene, there must be evidence for cancer-specific mutations in the gene concerned. Furthermore, introduction of the gene in question into appropriate recipient cells should either generate cellular responses typical of cancer cells (in the case of an oncogene) or suppress malignancy in cells that harbour defects in both alleles of the gene (in the case of a tumour suppressor gene).

In addition to cell growth and death, mutation in a oncogene or tumour suppressor gene causes disturbances in cellular physiology that ultimately lead to all the characteristics of a lethal tumour. These include an ability to acquire a blood supply (angiogenesis), tumour extension across anatomical boundaries (invasion), and growth in tissues beyond the organ of origin (metastasis). For several decades now, cancer researchers have focused on identifying the key genes responsible for these cellular processes. Their key assumption has been that the identification of so-called 'cancer genes' will lead to rational and more effective therapies. Today this is reality, with gene-targeted treatments a routine aspect of cancer management and clinical cancer research.

Cancer as a defect in cellular society

Unlike unicellular species, cells within a multicellular organism must co-operate in a way that favours the survival of the whole organism rather than that of the individual cell. If cellular co-ordination is disrupted, the unrestrained growth of even a single cell, by competing with its neighbours for space and nutrients, will eventually cause the death of the organism. Cancer is the term used to describe this breakdown in cellular society. Multicellular organisms must depend on complex gene networks that ensure full cellular co-operation. Unfortunately somatic mutation causes these networks to degrade over time, ultimately leading to cancer. Current research on the pathogenesis of cancer therefore focuses on the identification of genes that serve to maintain cellular order. Research has been greatly assisted by the recognition that cancer genes are organized into gene families that are conserved in evolution, from the simplest worm through to *Homo sapiens*. This observation has profoundly influenced the investigation of human cancer because the results of gene manipulation in experimentally tractable lower organisms, such as the nematode worm *Caenorhabditis elegans*, the fruit fly *Drosophila melanogaster*, mice, yeast, and even bacteria, have direct implications for their human homologues.

Cellular transformation

In many instances cancer cells can be grown in tissue culture, which has greatly facilitated the study of this disease. Unlike their healthy counterparts, cancer cells have been found to have some or all of the following *in vitro* characteristics:

1. Reduced requirement for growth stimulatory molecules, termed 'growth factors'.

2. Loss of contact inhibition, so that the cells tend to pile up and form foci.

3. Anchorage-independent growth, usually manifest as an ability to grow in soft agar.

4. The ability to divide indefinitely, a characteristic termed 'immortalization'.

When a cell has acquired these *in vitro* characteristics, it is referred to as 'transformed'. Empirically, cellular transformation can be achieved in human cells in tissue culture by disabling or disrupting the activities of four cellular components (Fig. 1). However, the process of becoming a cancer cell begins, not ends, with transformation. Not all experimentally transformed cells are capable of establishing a tumour when transplanted into a suitable host, and fewer still are capable of metastasis. The process of becoming a lethal, angiogenic, invasive, and motile cancer involves the activities of additional families of genes that serve these cellular programmes. For research purposes, the pathways involved in cancer tend to be categorized along functional lines, i.e. transformation, genetic instability, aberrant growth and survival, angiogenesis, tissue invasion, and cellular motility. While this provides an excellent framework for discussion, these distinctions are somewhat artificial because many of the genes implicated in cancer serve not one but several of these processes.

Somatic mutation and clonal evolution

The theory that cancer is a multistep or multigene process is supported by epidemiological evidence. The incidence of common cancers increases as individuals age, with kinetics dependent on the fourth or fifth power of elapsed time. This observation implies that a minimum of four to five events must take place before a tumour is evident clinically. If each event

Fig. 1 *In vitro* experiments demonstrate that at least four events are required to convert a normal human cell into a tumour cell. Addition of the catalytic hTERT subunit of telomerase (event 1) prevents telomere shortening (normal telomerase expression results in progessive telomere shortening, until further replication cannot be sustained and the cells become senescent). Introduction of SV40 large T antigen (LT), an oncoprotein from simian virus 40, disrupts the Rb and p53 protein pathways, which are essential for normal cell proliferation control (events 2 and 3). Finally, introduction of the oncogene *ras* is sufficient to cause malignant transformation (event 4). That the cells are indeed malignant can be demonstrated by their ability to form tumours in nude mice and colonies in soft agar.

represents a somatic mutation, how does tumour evolution occur at the cellular level? Estimates of the rate of somatic mutation in normal tissues indicate that for any gene there is a one in a million chance of a somatic mutation each time a cell divides. The baseline somatic mutation rate is therefore very low and a somatic mutation that significantly affects the function of a 'cancer gene' must be a very rare event. In fact, the background rate of somatic mutation appears to be too low to be the driving force behind cancer. However, carcinogenic mutations favour the growth or survival of a cell at the expense of neighbouring cells. As a result, cancer-promoting mutations are subject to a powerful positive selection process that magnifies the impact of these low-frequency events. In the model depicted in Fig. 2, a mutation has occurred that stimulates growth. As a result, a clone of cells has arisen that has replicated the initial mutation thousands of times. As the size of the clone approaches 10^6 cells, the chance of a second growth-stimulating mutation in one of the cells in the clone increases significantly. When a second mutation does occur, the cell with two growth-promoting mutations begins to outgrow the original clone. In this way a tumour evolves continuously, with each successive mutation adding a new facet to the repertoire of cellular properties required for a cell to be malignant. This process continues after diagnosis, with treatment resistance also driven by somatic mutation. Evidence for the 'clonal selection' theory of cancer abounds in the literature. For example, in Barrett's oesophagitis, where normal tissue, premalignant lesions, and cancers often coexist in the distal segment of the oesophagus, genetic analysis of oesophageal biopsies over time reveals multiple competing cell clones evolving simultaneously, each with a different complement of somatic mutations.

Gatekeepers and caretakers

As already pointed out, cancer-inducing mutations are rare events and despite the amplifying effect of clonal selection, the rate of somatic mutation in normal cells may still be insufficient to generate cancer at a high frequency. However, the evolution of cancer is also accelerated by 'genetic instability'. This term implies an increase in the rate of mutation in cancer cells when compared with normal cells, not simply that cancer cells possess a large number of mutations. A detailed mutational analysis of human tumours indicates that there are at least two general categories of genetic instability. In a minority of cancers there is instability at the nucleotide level, with a higher rate of nucleotide substitution, deletion, or insertion

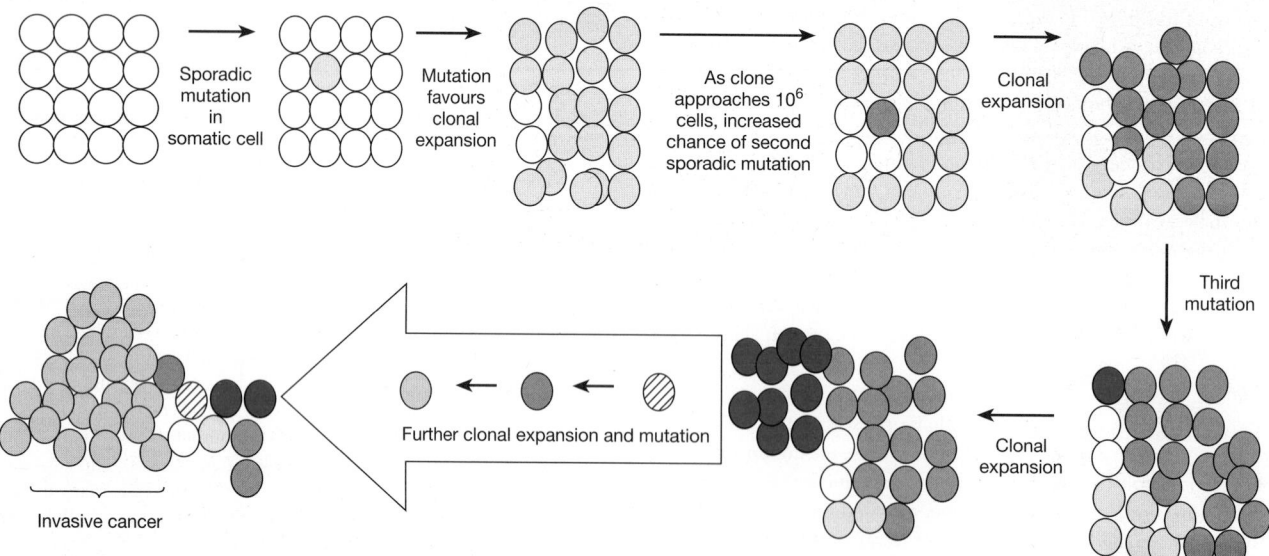

Fig. 2 Sporadic mutations which give a somatic cell a selective growth advantage encourage the outgrowth of mutated clones. Successive clones continue to accumulate growth-favouring mutations and outgrow preceding clones. The process of clonal expansion and mutation eventually results in a clone of cells with a malignant phenotype (invasive cancer). Even after the emergence of a malignant clone, the process of clonal expansion and mutation continues.

than in normal cells. More commonly, instability is observed at the level of the chromosome, with large-scale deletions, duplications, translocations, and amplification of entire chromosomal regions (Fig. 3 and Plate 1).

How does genetic instability arise? The integrity of DNA is protected by two classes of genes referred to as 'caretaker' and 'gatekeeper' genes. Caretaker genes are involved in recognizing and/or participating in the repair of damaged nucleotides or DNA strand breaks. Gatekeeper genes have a cell cycle arrest function that is triggered by DNA damage. Cell cycle arrest is coupled to DNA damage so that caretaker proteins can repair DNA before replication is reinitiated. If gatekeeper functions fail, replication continues through tracts of damaged DNA, generating mutations that are passed on to daughter cells, courting disaster in the form of cancer-promoting mutations.

Gatekeepers function through 'checkpoint' signal transduction pathways that operate at transition states in the cell cycle, when the cell normally pauses for an analysis of DNA integrity and an integration of internal and external signals that either promote or inhibit progression of the cell cycle. Activation of gatekeeper pathways can prevent the onset of DNA synthesis (G_1 checkpoint) or entry into mitosis (G_2 checkpoint) or prevent completion of chromosomal segregation after chromosomes are aligned on the mitotic spindle (spindle checkpoint). Importantly, gatekeepers can also trigger cell death, so that if genetic damage is so extensive that it cannot be repaired, or the repair process fails in some way, genetically altered cells with the potential to become malignant are deleted. Cancer cells that possess both gatekeeper and caretaker defects can have astonishing rates of genetic instability and often display rapid progression towards a lethal tumour phenotype.

Genetic instability at the nucleotide level

Subtle nucleotide changes are frequently observed in cancer cell genomes and cause 'gain-of-function' or 'loss-of-function' mutations in oncogenes and tumour suppressor genes. The majority of these mutations are probably not due to defects in gatekeeper and caretaker functions, but reflect the impact of environmental carcinogens or the background rate of somatic mutation. Under two circumstances, however, defective DNA repair leads to errors in nucleotide replication at an abnormally high rate. Nucleotide excision repair is responsible for restoring the correct DNA sequence after damage by exogenous mutagens, particularly ultraviolet light. Individuals with inherited nucleotide excision repair defects (xeroderma pigmentosum, see Chapter 6.3) have a marked increase in the incidence of skin cancer. Interestingly, the incidence of internal cancer is not increased to the same degree as in the skin. Furthermore, xeroderma pigmentosum heterozygotes are not at increased risk for cancer. Thus, nucleotide excision repair appears to be relevant to genetic instability only in the rare circumstance of an inherited cancer predisposition syndrome.

In contrast to nucleotide excision repair, mismatch repair defects accelerate the mutation rate in both hereditary and sporadic cancers of the colon, stomach, and endometrium. Conclusions concerning mismatch repair defects originated from the observation that a group of colorectal tumours have frequent alterations in short polynucleotide tracts in their genomes ('microsatellites') and the term 'microsatellite instability' arose to refer to this type of error. The similarity of these changes to mismatch repair defects in bacteria and yeast led to the identifications of six human homologues of bacterial mismatch repair genes (*mutS* and *mutL*) which, when inactivated by mutation, cause human tumours with microsatellite instability. A mismatch repair defect can be detected in about 13 per cent of all colorectal, stomach, and endometrial cancers, and in virtually all tumours arising in individuals with inherited *mutS* and *mutL* defects (hereditary non-polyposis colon cancer). Microsatellite sequences can be found throughout the genome, frequently in non-coding regions. It is noteworthy that some genes with roles in growth suppression have been found to be

(a)   (b)

Fig. 3 In a spectral karyotype (SKY), each normal chromosome stains homogeneously with a single distinct colour, making translocations evident by the presence of more than one colour in a single chromosome. (a) Forty five chromosomes are visible in this karyotype (left) from a patient with Turner's syndrome. Despite the loss of the X chromosome, the spectral karyotype (right) clearly shows the homogeneous chromosomal staining pattern typical of normal chromosomes. (b) In contrast, SKY analysis of a metaphase spread prepared from a breast cancer cell line displays both numerical and structural chromosomal aberrations. (By courtesy of Dr Bassem Haddad, Department of Oncology, Georgetown University Medical Center.) (See also Plate 1.)

Table 1 Examples of genes containing microsatellite sequences, and neoplasms in which the gene has been demonstrated to contain mutations within its microsatellite sequence

Gene	Microsatellite sequence	Neoplasms
TGF-β1 type II receptor	AAAAAAAA	Gastrointestinal (HNPCC, colorectal, gastric and ampullary adenocarcinoma and Barrett's oesophagus). Glioma. Endometrial
IGFIIR	GGGGGGGG	Gastrointestinal (HNPCC and Barrett's oesophagus)
BAX	GGGGGGGG	Gastrointestinal (HNPCC and colorectal)

HPNCC: hereditary non-polyposis colon cancer.

mutated at microsatellite sequences within their coding sequences (Table 1).

Instability in chromosome number

In contrast to the relative rarity of nucleotide excision repair and mismatch repair defects, another form of genetic instability, characterized by gains and losses of large segments of chromosomes, occurs in most human tumours. True chromosomal instability appears to underlie this observation, since the rate of losses and gains of chromosomal material in cancer cells with aneuploid genomes (more or less DNA than the normal diploid DNA complement) are at least tenfold higher than in cells with a normal chromosomal complement. The 'average' aneuploid cancer cell of the colon, breast, or prostate loses up to 25 per cent of its alleles, with the figure exceeding 50 per cent in some cases. Interestingly, in colon cancer and endometrial cancer, there is an inverse relationship between chromosomal instability and mismatch repair defects, suggesting that the two routes to genetic instability are somewhat mutually exclusive. In both cases, the hallmarks of genetic instability can be detected early in tumorigenesis and increase markedly over time, as each wave of cell clones arises bearing a new set of mutations, with a relentless progression in tumour size, aggression, and the degree of genomic disorganization. The molecular basis of chromosomal instability is heterogeneous, and unlike mismatch repair defects, no unifying mechanism has been proposed. However, defects in several cell cycle checkpoints have been implicated. In one example, an aberrant mitotic spindle checkpoint is proposed in which an abnormal mitosis is tolerated despite the presence of a lagging chromosome, causing an imbalance in chromosomal segregation. Several 'spindle checkpoint' genes have been isolated, and in the case of hBUB1 or hBUBR1, somatic mutations in tumours have been detected. Defects in a second checkpoint, referred to as the 'DNA damage checkpoint', is probably a more frequent cause of chromosomal instability. As discussed earlier, DNA damage checkpoints exist because gross structural alterations in chromosomes will occur if DNA replication occurs in the presence of single or double DNA strand breaks. As with mismatch repair defects and nucleotide excision repair, many of the genes within the 'DNA strand break pathway' have been identified through an association with an inherited predisposition to cancer and are further discussed below. A third, and by no means final, potential mechanism concerns disruption of centrosome function. Centrosomes nucleate the ends of the mitotic microtubule spindle along which the sister chromosomes segregate into two daughter cells. An abnormal number of centrosomes (i.e. more than two) have been observed in a variety of common cancers. When more than two poles form during mitosis, the potential for abnormal chromosomal segregation is high. Recently, overexpression of two centrosome-associated kinase genes, STK15 and PLK1, both homologues of Drosophila genes known to regulate centrosome function, have been associated with an increase in centrosome number and defective chromosome segregation in human cancer cells. Despite considerable insights into these complexities, it is fair to state that for the majority of

cancers the cause of aneuploidy is unclear. There are a number of pathways that lead to chromosomal instability, and perhaps this is the reason why chromosomal instability is so common in human tumours.

Chromosome translocation

There are two types of chromosomal translocations in human cancers. The first type is common and is without any clear pattern of repetition within tumours of the same histopathological type. The driving force behind this so-called 'complex' type of translocation is probably the same set of gatekeeper and caretaker defects that are a frequent cause of chromosomal instability. A favoured postulate is that these complex translocations reflect cells that enter mitosis before double-strand breaks are repaired, leading to random joining of free DNA ends through non-homologous recombination. The second pattern of translocation is referred to as the 'simple' type. These are common in leukaemia, lymphomas, and in a subset of sarcomas. The breakpoints in these translocations have been analysed and several distinct types of molecular effect have been identified. For example, when an oncogene is repositioned next to transcription regulatory sequences, overexpression occurs. In other cases, translocation generates a fusion gene that combines a coding sequence from the two genes at each end of the break point (Table 2).

Genetic instability is not thought to be the cause of simple translocations. In lymphoid cells, DNA strand breaks are generated as part of the normal recombination process that generates diversity in immunoglobulin genes and the T-cell receptor. The translocations characteristic of lymphoid malignancies are therefore thought to reflect low-frequency aberrations in physiological recombination events. The genesis of simple translocations in sarcoma is more enigmatic, however, as physiological gene rearrangement does not occur in the soft tissues from which sarcomas arise.

Gene amplification

Gene amplification occurs in late stage cancers and almost certainly reflects an aspect of genetic instability, because these aberrations occur at a higher rate in cancer cells than normal cells. Gene amplification is also thought to represent a relatively late step in the evolution of cancer and can lead to massive overexpression of oncogenes. It has been argued that the key defect underlying amplification concerns an inability to trigger a cell suicide or 'apoptosis' signal that usually deletes cells with amplified chromosomal segments. Table 3 lists a series of genes that are commonly amplified in human cancers.

Cell cycle deregulation

The cell cycle is governed by the activities of cyclin/cyclin-dependent protein kinases that oscillate through the cell cycle, orchestrating the complex process of cell division (Fig. 4). The activities of cyclin and cyclin-dependent protein kinase are closely regulated through checkpoint pathways that exist to monitor the integrity and replication status of DNA. Genes encoding proteins that promote cell cycle progression often operate as oncogenes, and are subject to activation in human cancers through gain-of-function mutations or gene amplification. In contrast, genes encoding the components of checkpoint pathways are tumour suppressors that may be inactivated during tumorigenesis. The importance of the restraining influence of cell cycle checkpoints is underscored by the finding that the tumour suppressor genes involved are amongst the most frequently mutated in human cancer.

The G₁/S checkpoint

Transition through the G_1/S checkpoint is promoted by the cyclin D family and their partner kinases, cyclin-dependent protein kinase 4 and 6 (Fig. 5). The cyclin D/cyclin-dependent protein kinase complex ('Rb kinase'), after activation by a cyclin-dependent protein kinase-activating kinase (**CAK**), phosphorylates the retinoblastoma tumour suppressor gene product, Rb. An increase in Rb phosphorylation releases a set of transcription factors

Table 2 Translocations observed in specific malignancies. In the case of gene fusion, a chimeric protein under the influence of a cell-specific promoter allows abnormal expression of a transcriptionally active product. A transcription factor (**TF**) gene is frequently affected

Neoplasm	Description	Associated translocations	Genes disrupted in translocation
Lymphoma	Burkitt's lymphoma	t(8;14), t(2;8), t(8;22)	*myc* (TF) overexpression under control of immunoglobulin promoter sequences
	Follicular lymphoma	t(14;18)	*BCL2* overexpression under control of immunoglobulin promoter sequences
AML*	Acute promyelocytic subtype	t(15;17)	Fusion of *PML* and *RARα* (TF)
CML†	90 per cent of all CML	Philadelphia chromosome t(9;22)	Fusion of *BCR* and *ABL*
ALL‡	Pre-B ALL	t(1;19)	Fusion of *PBX1* and *E2A* (TF)
Sarcoma	Ewing's sarcoma	t(11;22)	Fusion of *EWS* and *FLI1* (TF)
	Clear cell sarcoma	t(12;22)	Fusion of *EWS* and *ATF1* (TF)
	Alveolar rhabdomyosarcoma	t(2;13)	Fusion of *PAX3* (TF) and *FKHD* (TF)
	Synovial sarcoma	t(X;18)	Fusion of *SYT* (TF) and *SSX1* or *SSX2* (TFs)
	Myxoid liposarcoma	t(12;16)	Fusion *FUS* and *CHOP* (TF)

*Acute myeloid leukaemia.
†Chronic myeloid leukaemia.
‡Acute lymphoid leukaemia.

termed E2F. E2F proteins stimulate the expression of genes required for the S phase, for example the nucleotide biosynthetic genes dihydrofolate reductase and thymidine kinase. E2F also activates the functions of cyclins A and B to promote further cell cycle progression. Finally, E2F activates a negative feedback loop through a gene called *CDKN2A*. The p16*CDKN2A* protein inhibits Rb kinase by interfering with CAK activity and disrupting the cyclin-dependent protein kinase 4/Rb complex. Mutations in these regulatory genes are frequently present in cancer cells, underscoring the importance of this pathway in the regulation of normal cell growth. Gain-of-function mutations may occur in cyclin-dependent protein kinase

4, or cyclin D may be subject to gene amplification, deregulating Rb kinase activity and increasing E2F-dependent transcription. Loss-of-function mutation in *Rb* or *CDKN2A*, both common events in tumorigenesis, also result in deregulated E2F.

The G₁/S checkpoint is also under strict control from a gatekeeper pathway activated by DNA strand breaks. The components of this pathway have recently been put together as a result of research on a series of inherited cancer predisposition syndromes (Fig. 6). Perhaps the most critical component of the DNA strand break pathway is the tumour suppressor gene *p53*. Mutations in *p53* are possibly the most frequent genetic lesion in cancer cells. This, and the critical role of p53 in the DNA damage pathway, has inspired the name 'the guardian of the genome'. In fact, *p53* is a member of a regiment of 'genome guards' that act in concert to protect the integrity of DNA. At the apex of the DNA strand break pathway is the ataxia telangiectasia gene product ATM. ATM is a phosphatidylinositol-3 kinase that is activated by double-strand DNA breaks and orchestrates the function of proteins that repair DNA and arrest the cell cycle. To achieve this, ATM directs the phosphorylation of a series of targets, including p53, CHK2, NBS1, and BRCA1. When p53 is activated through the ATM-dependent kinase CHK2, the expression of p53-regulated genes is greatly increased. It is the spectrum of p53-regulated genes that actually conduct the caretaker and gatekeeper functions associated with p53. For example, p53 activates the expression of ribonuclease reductase, the enzyme responsible for a rate-limiting step in the production of deoxyribonucleotide triphosphates, 'sending' nucleotides to repair DNA. The G₁/S checkpoint function of p53 is mediated by *CDKN1* gene activation. The p21*CDKN1* protein acts in a

Table 3 Examples of malignancies where gene amplification has been observed

Gene product	Description	Cancer type
Epidermal growth factor receptor	Receptor tyrosine kinase	Breast
		Head and neck
		Urogenital
		Glioblastoma multiforme
ErbB2/Her2	Related to epidermal growth factor receptor	Breast
		Ovarian
		Bladder
		Cervical
		Head and neck
Fibroblast growth factor 4 or Hst-1	Growth factor	Oesophageal carcinoma
		Breast
Fibroblast growth factor 3 or Int-2	Growth factor	Breast
		Lung
		Gastric
		Oesophageal carcinoma
		Head and neck
Cyclin D1	Cell cycle regulation	Breast
		Oesophageal carcinoma
		Urogenital
		Head and neck
N-myc	Transcription factor	Neuroblastoma
		Small cell lung cancer
		Ovarian adenocarcinoma
Retinoic acid receptor	Transcription factor	Breast
		Prostate
Androgen receptor	Transcription factor	Breast
Topoisomerase IIa	Enzyme involved in DNA replication	

Fig. 4 Following growth stimulation, resting cells (G₀) move into and through the cell cycle. Cycle progression is tightly regulated by the temporal expression of cyclins and cyclin-dependent kinases, which are not expressed in the resting state.

Fig. 5 Growth factor stimulation of cells promotes accumulation of cyclin D and the assembly of cyclin D and cyclin-dependent protein kinase 4 or 6 into complexes. Phosphorylation of the cyclin-dependent protein kinase component by CAK activates the complex, which phosphorylates the Rb protein. Phosphorylated Rb releases a transcription factor of the E2F family. E2F drives transcription of genes required for cell cycle progression as well as the gene *CDK2NA*, from which the inhibitory protein p16*CDKN2A* is translated. In a negative feedback mechanism, p16 disrupts activity of CAK and cyclin D/cyclin-dependent protein kinase complexes, marking the completion of the initial phase of the cell cycle.

similar fashion to p16*CDKN2A*, inhibiting Rb kinase and preventing E2F activation. p53 is also instrumental in activating cell death after DNA damage. This is achieved in part by activating the expression of the cell death protein BAX (see below). *p53* mutations are therefore a major contributor to DNA instability since the cell continues to replicates in the presence of DNA strand breaks and fails to undergo cell death after DNA damage.

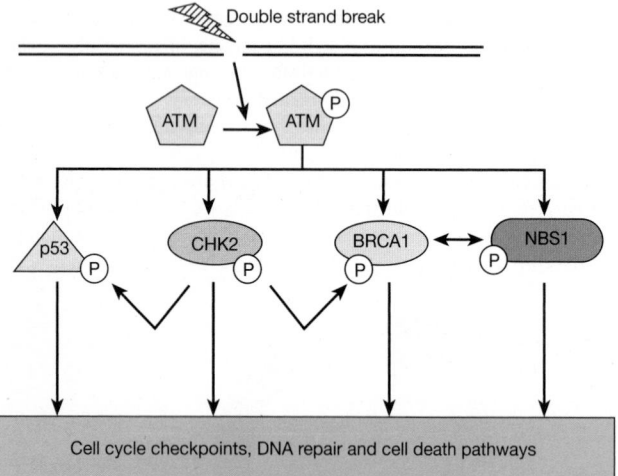

Fig. 6 Double-strand DNA breaks result in the activation of ATM. ATM activates, by phosphorylation, a variety of proteins (including p53, CHK2, BRCA1, and NBS1) whose checkpoint and repair functions prevent propagation of DNA damage. Each of the depicted proteins was identified as a product of a gene mutated in familial cancer syndromes. p53 (Li–Fraumeni syndrome), also activated by the ATM-dependent kinase CHK2 (Li–Fraumeni), increases the expression of genes including p21*CDKN1* and *BAX*. Interaction between BRCA1 (familial breast and ovarian cancer) and NBS1 (Nijmegen breakage syndrome) may co-ordinate DNA repair.

The G$_2$/M checkpoint

Normal cells arrest in G$_2$ in the presence of DNA damage. Cells mutant for p53 do not maintain arrest at G$_2$ and enter mitosis in the presence of DNA strand breaks or other types of chromosomal damage. A major component in sustaining p53-dependent G$_2$ arrest is the p53-regulated signalling protein 14-3-3σ, an inhibitor of the cyclin B/cyclin-dependent protein kinase 2 complex required for the initiation of mitosis. The integrity of these biochemical events is thought to have a major impact on the action of cytotoxic drugs, because agents that disrupt the G$_2$ checkpoint selectively potentiate the cytotoxic effects of DNA-damaging agents on p53 mutant cancer cells.

The discovery of oncogenes

A major feature of cancer cells is a loss of dependence on growth factor stimulation as a result of mutations in growth factor signal transduction pathways. Signal transduction genes were the first oncogenes identified, initiating the genetic revolution in cancer research in the late 1970s and early 1980s. In experiments initiated by Peyton Rous, retroviruses were isolated from chicken and rodent tumours that were capable of rapidly inducing cancer in infected animals. DNA sequence analysis of these 'acutely transforming' retroviruses showed that the transforming activity was due to a growth-stimulating 'oncogene' of non-viral origin that had been picked up in a rare recombination event from a host cell. The study of acutely transforming retroviruses led to the identification of a family of oncogenes that when subjected to gain-of-function mutations or overexpression induce aberrant signal transduction, cellular transformation, and tumour formation (Table 4).

Plasma membrane receptors as oncogenes

Ligand-activated, tyrosine kinase-linked plasma membrane receptors (receptor tyrosine kinases, **RTKs**) that operate as oncogenes include erbB2 and epidermal growth factor receptor. Amplification of the genes for these receptors occurs in a wide spectrum of common malignancies, including breast, lung, pancreatic, and head and neck cancer. Receptor overexpression reduces or bypasses the requirement for the presence of a ligand, removing dependence on external growth signals. For example, erbB2 normally signals as a heterodimer in partnership with a second member of the erbB2 family, because erbB2 cannot bind to a ligand directly. When overexpressed, erbB2 is forced into homodimers that are active in the absence of ligand. The RTK oncogenes c-*met* and c-*ret* are involved in a more limited spectrum of tumours, including papillary renal cancer (c-*met*) and medullary thyroid cancer (c-*ret*). In these cases, missense mutations introduce cysteine residues in the extracellular binding domain, resulting in inappropriate disulphide bond formation, dimerization, tyrosine kinase activation, and ligand-independent growth.

Plasma membrane receptors as tumour suppressor genes

The transforming growth factor β (**TGF-β**) pathway provides an example of a plasma membrane receptor that suppresses cell growth (Fig. 7). Transforming growth factor β is a peptide growth factor with complex effects on both tumour cells and on host stromal cells. Responses to TGF-β include inhibition of tumour growth, induction of cell death, extracellular matrix synthesis, and angiogenesis. Transforming growth factor β signals through a heterodimer of two receptors, TGF-β RI and TGF-β RII, both plasma membrane serine–threonine kinases. TGF-β RII binds TGF-β and then dimerizes with and phosphorylates TGF-β RI. TGF-β RI in turn phosphorylates the signal transduction proteins Smad2 and Smad3. Cytoplasmic Smad proteins then migrate to the nucleus to activate gene expression in concert with a third Smad protein, Smad4. One of the genes activated is p27*kip1*, a cyclin-dependent kinase inhibitor in the same family as p21*CDKN1* and p16*CDKN2A* with roles in both cell cycle arrest and the

Table 4 Examples of acute retroviruses and the oncogenes they harbour

Retrovirus	Oncogene(s)	Oncogene product
Avian erythroblastosis virus	*erbB2, erbB3, erbB4*	Members of EGF receptor family
	erbA	Related to thyroid hormone receptor
Simian sarcoma	*sis*	Growth factor
Rous avian sarcoma	*src*	Protein kinase
Abelson murine leukaemia	*abl*	Protein kinase
3611 murine sarcoma	*raf*	Protein kinase
Harvey murine sarcoma	H-*ras*	G-protein
Avian sarcoma virus 17	*jun*	Transcription factor
FBJ murine osteosarcoma	*fos*	Transcription factor
Avian MC29 myelocytomatosis	*myc*	Transcription factor
Avian sarcoma	*ski*	Component of TGF-β signalling pathway
Avian reticuloendotheliosis	*rel*	Component of NFκB transcription complex

EGF, epidermal growth factor; TGF, transforming growth factor.

induction of programmed cell death. Loss-of-function mutations, characteristic of tumour suppressor genes, occur in the TGF-β/Smad pathway. TGF-β RII is inactivated in 20 per cent of colorectal cancers with mismatch repair defects because of a vulnerable poly(A) microsatellite in the TGF-β RII coding sequence (Table 1). In addition, Smad4 is inactivated in up to 50 per cent of pancreatic cancers.

Cytoplasmic signal transduction components as oncogenes (*ras*)

When an RTK is activated by dimerization, the cytoplasmic portion of the receptor becomes autophosporylated and a variety of intracellular docking proteins are recruited to the cell membrane. These docking proteins create a scaffold in the inner surface of the plasma membrane around which signalling components congregate further downstream. Critical amongst these components is the 'Ras' family of proteins (K-, N-, and H-Ras). *ras* genes are frequently mutated in human cancer and at least partially bypass the need for RTK signalling in cell growth. Ras proteins operate a GTP-dependent switching mechanism that alternates between a GTP-bound active form and a GDP-bound inactive form. When an RTK is activated, docking proteins, together with a protein called SOS, stimulate the release of GDP from Ras, replacing it with GTP. Activated, GTP-bound Ras then signals to a host of downstream targets to stimulate multiple cellular changes, including activation of DNA synthesis, and changes in lipid metabolism, cellular morphology, cell adhesion, and gene expression (Fig. 8). The system is switched off by GTPase-activating proteins that stimulate the hydrolysis of Ras-bound GTP to GDP. Mutations in *ras* genes cause the protein to be held in the GTP-activated form, generating a continuous unregulated signal. K-*ras* and N-*ras* mutations are found in common solid tumours including lung, brain, colon cancer, and nearly 95 per cent of pancreatic cancers and 30 per cent of acute leukaemias. H-*ras* mutations are found only in a small subset of bladder and head and neck tumours.

Cytoplasmic signal transduction components as tumour suppressor genes

Neurofibromatosis is caused by germline mutation of the tumour suppressor neurofibromin (**NF1**), a GTPase-activating protein. Loss of NF1 increases Ras activity; however, NF1 is not commonly targeted for mutation in common solid malignancies. The oncogenic consequences of NF1 inactivation are tissue specific since patients with type 1 neurofibromatosis do not have a marked increase in the incidence of common solid malignancies. The adenomatous polyposis coli (**APC**) gene product is a stronger example of a cytoplasmic tumour suppressor gene that operates to downregulate a growth regulatory pathway (Fig. 9). The *APC* gene is mutated in most human colon cancers and germline mutations are associated with

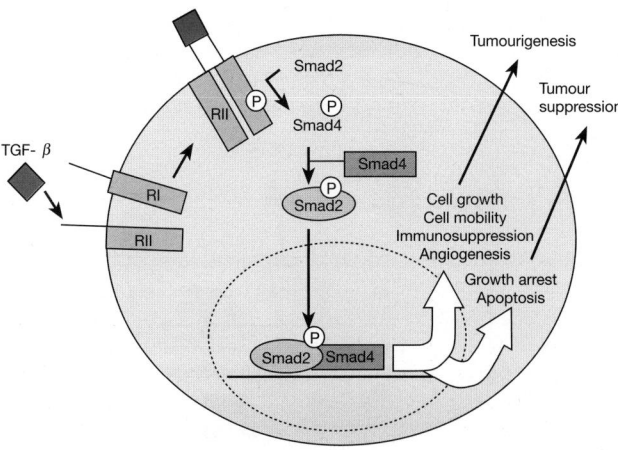

Fig. 7 On TGF-β binding to TGF-β RII, this receptor dimerizes with and phosphorylates TGF-β RI. Activated TGF-β RI phosphorylates the cytoplasmic proteins Smad2 and Smad 3 (not shown), which in turn interact with Smad4. The Smad complex migrates to the cell nucleus where, in concert with various transcription factors, it drives transcription of genes involved in both tumorigenesis and tumour suppression.

Fig. 8 Dimerization and activation of most cell surface receptor tyrosine kinases (RTKs) is dependent on ligand binding. The ligand-activated receptor autophosphorylates specific tyrosine residues in the cytosolic domain. These phosphotyrosine residues act as binding sites for a variety of proteins. GRB2 binds to both activated RTK and a protein called SOS. SOS facilitates the exchange of GDP for GTP, converting inactive Ras/GDP to active Ras/GTP. Active Ras binds to Raf (a serine/threonine kinase), and this complex binds to and phosphorylates the kinase MEK. MEK phosphorylates MAP kinase; MAP kinase subsequently activates proteins important for cell growth.

Fig. 9 (a) In the presence of a growth signal, cytoskeleton-associated β-catenin migrates from the inner plasma membrane to the nucleus, where it increases the activity of TCF/LEF transcription factors. APC binds β-catenin and targets it for degradation by the ubiquitin pathway. (b) Certain APC mutations disrupt interaction between APC and β-catenin. This prevents ubiquitin targeting, so that β-catenin accumulates and migrates to the nucleus, where the increased levels drive excessive transcription of TCF/LEF-regulated genes. (c) In a similar manner, certain β-catenin mutations disrupt interaction with functional APC, with the same consequences.

familial colon polyps and cancer. APC normally regulates the signal transduction protein β-catenin by targeted degradation, so that in an APC mutant cell, β-catenin accumulates abnormally. β-catenin is an essential component of a signal transduction pathway that connects cell adhesion and the extracellular matrix to the cell nucleus. β-catenin operates by activating the TCF/LEF family of transcription factors, leading to gene transcription and cell cycle progression. For example, in APC mutant cells, overexpression of cyclin D1 occurs because of deregulated β-catenin /LEF activity. β-catenin is also subject to somatic mutation, particularly in colon cancers without germline APC mutations, as well as melanoma, prostate cancers, gastric cancer, hepatocellular carcinoma, and medulloblastoma. Mutations in the β-catenin gene tend to stabilize the β-catenin protein, increasing TCF/LEF activity and cyclin D expression.

Transcription factors as oncogenes and tumour suppressor genes

Transcription factors regulate the rate of transcription by binding to specific DNA motifs in non-coding sequences, thereby recruiting a multicomponent protein complex that promotes (or represses) the activity of RNA polymerase. A broad spectrum of mutations activates the oncogenic potential, or disrupts the tumour suppressor functions, of transcription factor genes. In examples discussed already, point mutations inactivate or alter the functions of the transcription factors p53, β-catenin, and Smad4. In other instances, transcription factor genes are subject to activation through gene amplification, including c-*myc*, a gene required for cell cycle progression and cyclin expression, and amplified in breast cancer-1 (*AIB1*), a gene encoding a protein that boosts the transcriptional activity of steroid receptors.

Perhaps the most remarkable examples of aberrant transcription factors in cancer result from translocations that create transcription factor gene fusions (Table 2). For example, in promyelocytic leukaemia, the retinoic acid receptor α gene (*RARα*) on chromosome 15 is involved in a translocation with a gene on chromosome 17 termed *PML*. The resulting fusion

transcription factor, RARα/PML, demonstrates aberrant localization within the cell nucleus where it acts as a 'decoy', binding normal retinoic acid receptor family members and inhibiting their role in myeloid differentiation. High doses of retinoic acid induce remission of PML by inducing the degradation of the RARα/PML fusion protein, thereby releasing normal retinoic acid receptors to activate the terminal differentiation of leukaemic cells. Ewing's sarcoma family of tumours provides further examples of transcription factor gene fusion, in this instance between the *EWS* gene and the ETS family of transcription factors, either FLI1 or ERG (95 per cent and 5 per cent of Ewing's tumours respectively). In these cases, the fusion ETS transcription factor becomes hyperactive because of the anomalous presence of *EWS* gene sequences. In a further example of transcription factor overactivity, the c-*myc* gene becomes overexpressed in Burkitt's lymphoma as a result of an 8→14 translocation that places the c-*myc* gene under the influence of immunoglobulin gene sequences.

Mutations in cell death pathways (Fig. 10)

Programmed cell death or apoptosis is an essential aspect of the ability of a multicellular organism to develop and survive (see Chapter 4.6). For example, during embryogenesis the targeted removal of cells in tissue remodelling is achieved through cell death programmes, generating digits and body cavities. In the immune system, apoptosis deletes lymphocytes that recognize 'self-antigens', thereby preventing the growth of B- and T-cell clones capable of autoimmune damage. Apoptosis is also essential for the deletion of cells with DNA damage, chromosomal aberrations, and abnormalities of mitotic spindle formation. These events stimulate the release of cytochrome C from mitochondria. Cytoplasmic cytochrome C activates a cascade of 'caspase' proteases that effect DNA fragmentation, plasma membrane destruction, and the characteristic morphological features of apoptosis (see *section 4.6*). Receptor tyrosine kinases play a critical role in cell survival by activating the signal transduction enzyme phosphatidylinositol-3-kinase. Phosphatidylinositol-3-kinase in turn activates a serine threonine kinase, AKT (an oncogene, discovered through the study of acutely transforming retroviruses). AKT promotes survival by phosphorylating and inactivating BAD, a protein that promotes mitochondrial release of cytochrome C. Excess phosphatidylinositol-3-kinase activity and aberrant survival are also consequences of loss-of-function mutations in a tumour suppressor termed PTEN (phosphatase tensin homologue deleted in chromosome 10). The *PTEN* gene encodes a protein phosphatase mutated in a wide spectrum of cancers, including breast, thyroid, lung, and a small proportion of lymphomas. When PTEN is lost through somatic mutation,

Fig. 10 Apoptosis is triggered by cytochrome C release from the mitchondrion which activates caspase proteases that destroy the cell. Cytochrome C release is therefore a tightly regulated process that is under the control of several signal transduction pathways that operate through the BCL2 family of cell death regulators.

AKT becomes constitutively active, holding the cell death-promoting protein BAD in an inactive conformation. The activity of BAD is also tightly controlled through the BCL2 family of BAD dimerization partners. BAD and BCL2 are members of a family of at least 15 proteins that promote or suppress cell death. BCL2 itself is an oncogene activated by a translocation that increases expression in indolent lymphoma. BCL2 is a very potent cell survival factor that binds to BAD (and other proapoptotic partners, BAX, BID, and BCLX$_L$) to prevent cytochrome C release, and when overexpressed BCL2 potently inhibits cell death. The tumour suppressor gene *p53* is also a key regulator of apoptosis. When *p53* is activated, the transcription of the proapoptotic gene *BAX* is increased, also promoting mitochondrial cytochrome C release after DNA damage.

Genetic programmes serving tissue invasion

Tissue invasion is a complex process that, like all other aspects of the malignant phenotype, is driven by a complex array of genetic lesions. Like many of the pathways described thus far, the molecular details of the cancer invasion pathway are incompletely resolved. Since non-invasive tumours are essentially benign, how tumour cells acquire an invasive phenotype is at the core of understanding what makes a tumour benign or malignant. Invasion requires tissue degradation and several classes of enzyme have been identified that are expressed by invasive tumours, including metalloproteinases and collagenases. Inhibitors of these enzymes are currently in clinical trial as antimetastasis or anti-invasion agents.

Another important aspect of invasion is increased cell motility, required for a malignant cell to migrate away from its site of origin. Excess growth factor signalling, typical of cancer cells, promotes motility, and specific motility genes, for example the *C-MET* 'scatter factor' receptor, are subject to activation through somatic mutation. Building on the concept of cell cycle checkpoints, a checkpoint for invasion has recently been proposed based on a receptor–ligand pair termed amphoterin/RAGE (receptor for advanced glycation end products). Amphoterin assists in the generation of the protein-degrading protein plasmin, which then activates metalloproteinases. RAGE is the receptor for amphoterin, which promotes, through MAP kinase, motility, 'adhesion' receptors, and growth pathways. While genetic lesions in this pathway have yet to be described, the outline of a motility and invasion pathway is emerging. As part of this developing concept, 'invasion suppressor genes' are being identified. Mutations in the E-cadherin gene have been described in breast, colon, and gastric cancers and are associated with changes in cell morphology, increased motility, and activation of the β-catenin/LEF transcriptional pathway discussed in the context of the *APC* tumour suppressor gene.

Genetic programmes serving angiogenesis

Angiogenesis is also a critical aspect of the cancer phenotype. Due to the limitations of tissue diffusion, a tumour cannot increase beyond 1 mm in size without a blood supply. Exactly how a tumour manipulates the process of angiogenesis is beginning to be understood, and once again mutations in regulatory genes are at the root of the issue. Normal cells respond to hypoxia by increasing the expression of a set of hypoxia-inducible genes, of which that for vascular endothelial growth factor (**VEGF**) is a prime example. VEGF profoundly stimulates the growth of the endothelial cells that line blood vessel walls. The transcription factors concerned, hypoxia-inducible factors 1α and 2α (**HIF1α** and **HIF2α**), are tightly regulated by oxygen tension. Unlike normal cells, tumour cells may show HIF activity even when oxygen tension is adequate, i.e. the connection between hypoxia and HIF activity is severed. In tumours that arise in the cancer predisposition syndrome von Hippel–Lindau syndrome, as well as in sporadic renal cell carcinoma, uncoupling of hypoxia-inducible gene expression from hypoxia is due to loss-of-function mutations in the von Hippel–Lindau gene, *VHL*. The VHL protein normally targets HIF1α and HIF2α for degradation. When VHL activity is lost, excess HIF1α and HIF2α activity drives increased VEGF expression and excessive blood vessel formation. Of course, aberrant angiogenesis also occurs in tumours in which VHL is not mutated. VEGF is only one of many angiogenic factors. For example, fibroblast growth factors are also angiogenic, and the fibroblast growth factor-3 gene is subject to gene amplification in breast cancer, squamous cell carcinoma of the head and neck, and nasopharyngeal cancer.

Human cancers caused by infection

Up to 20 per cent of cancers worldwide may be due to viral infection. The discovery of infectious agents that induce cancer has proved invaluable for the identification of genes implicated in tumorigenesis. The insights gained from the study of acutely transforming retroviruses (RNA tumour viruses) were discussed earlier. As the name implies, these viruses are capable of causing tumours in the affected species within a few weeks to months of infection. As far as we know, such viruses are not a cause of human cancer. However, endemic retroviruses are strongly implicated in several malignant diseases of humans. Unlike the acutely transforming retroviruses, endemic retroviruses do not contain host (human) gene sequences and are associated with cancer only after a long latency period of years to decades. The most prominent example is the HTLV-I virus, associated with endemic T-cell leukaemia in Caribbean and Japanese populations. An HTLV-I viral protein essential for T-cell transformation, Tax, activates the transcription factor NFκB.

The immune system normally provides a considerable measure of protection from a class of viruses termed 'DNA tumour viruses'. By weakening this immune surveillance, the human immunodeficiency virus (**HIV**) is responsible for a significant cancer burden. Three DNA tumour viruses are prominently responsible for HIV-associated malignancies: Epstein–Barr virus (**EBV**), human herpesvirus 8 (**HHV-8**), and human papilloma virus (**HPV**). These viruses can also cause disease in individuals with apparently normal immune systems.

It has long been appreciated that EBV is capable of immortalizing B cells, thereby stimulating polyclonal populations of B cells in which secondary transforming events occur. In HIV-infected patients, lack of a T-cell-dependent antiviral response allows proliferation of EBV-infected polyclonal B-cell populations, from which highly aggressive lymphomas evolve. Through a similar mechanism, EBV is a cofactor in endemic childhood Burkitt's lymphoma in Africa. In this case, poor nutrition and malarial infection deplete the immune system, allowing an EBV-expanded population of lymphocytes to proliferate. Eventually a c-*myc*/immunoglobulin gene translocation generates an aggressive, poorly differentiated Burkitt's-type lymphoma. Finally, EBV is implicated in the pathogenesis of nasopharyngeal cancer, an endemic malignancy of the nasal sinus epithelium in southern China. The genome of EBV encodes up to 100 potential genes and several have oncogene-like properties, including BHRF1, a BCL2-like protein. While the exact role of all EBV-encoded proteins in transformation has yet to be elucidated, viral gene products are likely to initiate the malignant process, even if EBV genes may not be required for the continued growth of the malignancies that ultimately arise.

Like EBV, HHV-8 is a herpesvirus that is associated with malignancy, including Kaposi's sarcoma, primary effusion lymphomas, multiple myeloma, angioimmunoblastic lymphadenopathy, and Castleman's disease. Kaposi's sarcoma is an indolent sarcoma affecting the skin (and more rarely internal organs). At least 95 per cent of Kaposi's sarcoma lesions can be shown to contain the HHV-8 virus. While first recognized in eastern European males at the beginning of the twentieth century, Kaposi's sarcoma became a common problem only after the onset of the HIV epidemic. Sequencing of the HHV-8 genome reveals several genes that may be associated with malignant transformation, including a cyclin-like gene that inhibits the function of Rb, and a BCL2-like protein that inhibits apoptosis. Therefore, like EBV, HHV-8 may initiate Kaposi's sarcoma and other malignancies by encoding proteins that mimic several steps in the multistep carcinogenesis process.

HIV-infected individuals are also prone to develop squamous carcinoma of the anus and, in women, cervical cancer. Both diseases are caused by infection with HPV. Cervical cancer is an endemic disease that does not require an immunodeficient state for the virus to be pathogenic. The viral genome of HPV has been extensively examined, and two viral genes in particular have been implicated in HPV-induced cellular transformation, *E6* and *E7*. The E6 protein interferes with the function of p53 by targeting the protein for degradation. The E7 protein binds to and interferes with Rb. Thus, HPV mimics two of the most common loss-of-function mutations in human malignancy.

Another example of a strong link between malignancy and viral infection is the hepatitis B virus. In several parts of the world, including parts of China, hepatocellular carcinoma is the most common malignancy and reflects the very high incidence of hepatitis B infection in these areas. Portions of the hepatitis B virus can be found integrated into the genome of hepatocellular carcinomas. These hepatitis B virus 'X gene' fragments may be critical to carcinogenesis by providing viral promoter sequences that activate neighbouring oncogenes.

Epigenetic gene silencing in cancer

Epigenetic gene silencing is another non-mutational pathway for inactivation of tumour suppressor genes that has recently come into focus. In a number of instances, expression of tumour suppressor genes is lost in cancer cells, even though genetic analysis had shown that the sequence of the gene is intact. Tumour suppressor genes subject to gene silencing in cancer cells include *VHL*, *hMLH1* (a mismatch repair gene) *CDKN2A*, and *E-cadherin*. The mechanism for gene silencing involves methylation of cytosine residues in CpG dinucleotide sequences found within gene regulatory sequences. Methylation is believed to hold the gene in a closed conformation that cannot be accessed by RNA polymerase. How epigenetic gene inactivation is faithfully passed on to daughter cells during cellular replication is not clear. The mechanism may represent an aberration of the process that suppresses the expression of genes on the inactive X chromosome in females.

In addition to epigenetic gene silencing, there is also evidence for epigenetic oncogene activation due to loss of methylation. A good example is the gene for insulin-like growth factor 2 (**IGF2**). IGF2 is a potent growth factor that signals both cell growth and survival. Normally in adult tissues only the paternal IGF2 allele is expressed. The maternal allele is silenced through methylation, in an embryonic process termed 'imprinting'. In paediatric tumours (Wilm's tumour, rhabdomyosarcoma, and hepatoblastoma) the imprinting pattern is lost, with the occurrence of biallelic IGF2 expression and excess IGF2 activity in these malignancies. In these instances, loss of imprinting has been found to be due to mutation in the *H19* locus that is usually targeted for imprinting on chromosome 11p15, the vicinity of the *IGF2* gene.

Cancer therapy in the twenty-first century

The completion of the human genome project represents an enormous opportunity in medicine. Cancer therapy is likely to be an early beneficiary from this triumph because detailed information on the genetic nature of cancer will be translated into new, less toxic, and more effective cancer treatments. The recent development of a gene-targeted treatment for chronic myeloid leukaemia illustrates this potential well. Chronic myeloid

Table 5 Cancer therapies that target somatic mutations

Genetic lesion	Therapeutic compound/therapy
BCR/ABL fusion gene due to 9→22 translocation	Oral Abl tyrosine kinase inhibitor
erbB2 gene amplification	Humanized anti-erbB2 antibody and oral tyrosine kinase inhibitor
Loss of *VHL* gene, leading to VEGF overexpression	Humanized anti-VEGF antibody
EGFR gene amplification	Humanized anti-EGFR antibody and oral EGFR tyrosine kinase inhibitor
p53 gene mutation	Adenovirus that selectively replicates in p53 mutant cells
BCL2 overexpression due to 14→18 translocation	BCL2 antisense oligonucleotide
RARα/PML fusion gene due to 15→17 translocation	All-*trans* retinoic acid
ras gene mutation	Farnesyl transferase inhibitor (prevents Ras plasma membrane attachment)

VEGF, vascular endothelial growth factor; EGFR, epidermal growth factor receptor..

leukaemia is characterized by excess proliferation of cells from the myeloid lineage. The hallmark of this disease is a reciprocal translocation between chromosomes 9 and 22 creating the so-called 'Philadelphia chromosome'. The molecular consequence of this translocation is to fuse the c-*abl* gene, a nuclear tyrosine kinase, with the *BCR* gene. The fusion BCR–ABL gene product has enhanced tyrosine kinase activity. Having identified the enzyme target that drives chronic myeloid leukaemia, selective ABL tyrosine kinase inhibitors were developed that were able to cure up to 90 per cent of mice with human chronic myeloid leukaemia cells in their bone marrow and circulation. In early clinical trials with chronic myeloid leukaemia patients, the ABL tyrosine kinase inhibitor was highly effective, and certainly less toxic than the alternatives that include chronic treatment with interferon or allogeneic bone marrow transplant.

Like gene translocation, gene amplification also provides an opportunity for gene-targeted therapy. For example, a humanized antibody against the *erbB2* oncogene produces a 40 per cent response rate in breast tumours with *erbB2* gene amplification. Exposure to the erbB2 antibody downregulates erbB2 tyrosine kinase activity by internalization of the receptor/antibody complex. These early successes have spurred the development of new inhibitors of essentially the entire spectrum of signal transduction enzymes discussed in this chapter. Promising gene-specific therapeutic approaches are summarized in Table 5.

Further reading

Kaelin WG (1999). Choosing anticancer drug targets in the postgenomic era. *Journal of Clinical Investigation* **104**, 1503–6.

Lengauer C, Kinzler KW, Vogelstein B (1998). Genetic instabilities in human cancers. *Nature* **396**, 643–9.

Tycko B (2000). Epigenetic gene silencing in cancer. *Journal of Clinical Investigation* **105**, 401–7.

6.3 The genetics of inherited cancers

Andrew Coop and Matthew J. Ellis

Introduction

The description of families with multiple members afflicted by cancer provided an early and persuasive argument that the aetiology of cancer has a genetic component. This conclusion is now beyond doubt, since germline mutations responsible for inherited cancer syndromes have been identified, and a role for the encoded proteins in malignant transformation established. While the development of essentially every cancer is influenced by the genetic complement of the patient, only in these inherited cancer syndromes is the effect of a single gene mutation powerful enough to generate a mendelian pattern of cancer predisposition. The study of these diseases, despite their rarity, has provided critical insights into the genesis of more common forms of cancer because the same genes are frequently affected. In the case of sporadic cancer, however, mutations are not present in the germline but arise entirely through the process of somatic mutation and selection, whereby mutations that enhance cellular survival or proliferation accumulate in tissues over prolonged periods. DNA-based diagnostic tests are now available for gene abnormalities underlying inherited cancer predisposition syndromes. A positive test may mandate intensive cancer screening and, in carefully selected cases, surgery to remove organs at risk. Researchers are also examining the use of medications designed to prevent cancer (chemoprevention), allowing cancer-prone individuals to 'escape' their genotype. This chapter is intended to provide insights that will facilitate the recognition of cancer predisposition syndromes, help in understanding the clinical implications of the diagnosis, and render further study comprehensible. For a completely exhaustive list of familial cancer syndromes the reader is referred to the section on further reading at the end of the chapter.

The identification of cancer predisposition genes

Hereditary retinoblastoma: a classical example of a cancer predisposition syndrome

The first cancer predisposition genes were identified through the careful analysis of rare but remarkable syndromes. Hereditary retinoblastoma provides a classical example. A cancer of retinal cells, retinoblastoma usually occurs before the age of 3 years. One in 13 500 to one in 25 000 children are affected, with an equal sex distribution. About 40 per cent of patients have a family history of the disease, with an autosomal dominant pattern of inheritance. Eighty-five per cent of retinoblastomas presenting at less than 6 months of age affect both eyes and are likely to be the inherited form. The proportion of bilateral cases declines to 6 per cent by 24 months, when most cases are of the sporadic type, with no risk of genetic transmission. Overall only 10 per cent of patients with single tumours transmit susceptibility to the next generation. Individuals with hereditary retinoblastoma are at an increased risk of developing a variety of cancers (especially osteosarcoma). Retinoblastoma illustrates the cardinal clinical features of inherited cancer predisposition syndromes: early onset, bilateral or multifocal cancer, and an association with similarly affected close relatives (see Table 1).

In a series of now classical studies, Knudson carefully examined family histories and tumour characteristics from patients with retinoblastoma and generated a 'two-hit' model to explain his statistical observations (Fig. 1). He hypothesized that the gene for retinoblastoma, *Rb*, is a tumour suppressor gene, whose function must be lost for a retinoblastoma to develop. In familial cases, he postulated that affected individuals had inherited an inactive mutant *Rb* allele. In these individuals every cell in the retina, indeed every cell in the body, carries an inactive copy of the *Rb* gene. As a result, a single second somatic mutation, or 'hit', in the remaining *Rb* allele is sufficient to inactivate *Rb* function and initiate a tumour. The barrier to the development of retinoblastoma in the absence of an inherited *Rb* mutant allele is much higher, as the coincidence of two somatic mutations (two hits) in a single cell to inactivate both *Rb* alleles is considerably less likely. This explains the low incidence, later onset, and absence of multiple tumours in non-familial retinoblastoma. The experimental verification of Knudson's model arose from studies that identified a region of chromosome 13 that was consistently lost in both inherited and non-inherited retinoblastoma. By examining multiple cases, investigators were able to identify the common region of loss on chromosome 13q14, and ultimately the gene concerned. True to Knudson's model, germline loss-of-function *Rb* mutations were present in familial cases, and the loss of chromosome 13 in familial tumours always eliminated the remaining wild type allele. Furthermore, sporadic adult onset cancers, for example of the lung, breast, and bladder, also have *Rb* mutant alleles, acquired as somatic mutations. This testifies to the importance of *Rb* in the formation of not just a rare childhood tumour, but common tumours as well. The final proof that *Rb* is a tumour suppressor gene came from studies that showed that malignant tumour formation can be suppressed when *Rb* function is returned to *Rb*-null cancer cells in gene transfer (transfection) experiments. These seminal studies on inherited retinoblastoma defined key experimental approaches and concepts that were subsequently used to identify other cancer predisposition genes.

Familial clustering of common cancers

Retinoblastoma is striking because cancer is a rare event in childhood, but up to 5 to 10 per cent of adults with cancers at commonly affected sites, such as breast and colon, have a family history of similar cancers. How

Table 1 Features of inherited cancer predisposition syndromes

Earlier onset than sporadic cancer
Bilateral or multifocal cancer
Rare cancers in unusual anatomical locations
Phenotypic abnormalities indicating a disorder of tissue formation/regulation
Multiple benign tumours
Usually an autosomal dominant pattern of inheritance
New germline mutations may account for new cases where there is no family history

Fig. 1 Knudson's hypothesis. (a) In individuals with an inherited predisposition to retinoblastoma every somatic cell contains one intact *Rb* allele and one mutant *Rb* allele. A single somatic mutation is therefore sufficient for loss of *Rb* activity, with subsequent clonal expansion of the double mutant cell and tumour formation. (b) In normal individuals both copies of *Rb* must be targeted by somatic mutation for *Rb* function to be disrupted. Since the somatic mutation rate is low the risk of two *Rb* mutations occurring in the same cell is low. This explains the later onset and unifocal nature of retinoblastoma cases that occur in the absence of a family history.

many of these instances of 'familial clustering' are due to germline mutations in tumour suppressor genes? Careful analysis of many of these family trees suggests that cancer predisposition is inherited in an autosomal dominant fashion. However, locating the genes associated with familial clustering is a daunting prospect. The presence of a family history of cancer alone is not particularly reliable evidence for an inherited cancer predisposition gene because many cases of familial clustering may be due to common exposure to environmental risk factors (smoking or poor diet for example). Other issues that frustrate the geneticist include small family size, incomplete knowledge of a relative's medical problems, or, in the case of breast and ovarian cancer, lack of female relatives in which the phenotype can be expressed. Geneticists also define the twin problems of 'incomplete penetrance' and 'phenocopy' as particularly awkward because they mask a mendelian inheritance pattern (Fig. 2). Incomplete penetrance refers to the situation where an individual has inherited a mutated tumour suppressor gene but does not develop cancer. By masking the presence of a mutant allele, incomplete penetrance generates confusing phenomena such as 'generation skipping'. The phenocopy problem arises because 'common cancers occur commonly'. A sporadic tumour can occur in an individual in a family with cancer predisposition who did not inherit the predisposing mutation. These false negative and false positive situations led to the development of statistical tools to predict the likelihood of mutations in tumour suppressor genes in any particular family. These models are now frequently used to help decide who should undergo expensive genetic testing. An example of one approach for breast cancer is provided in Table 2. A history of early onset or bilateral disease is used to weight these analyses, as these features substantially increase the likelihood that a cancer predisposition gene is present. Ethnic background is also taken into account. For example, certain mutations in the breast cancer genes *BRCA1* and *BRCA2* are more common in individuals with Jewish ancestry. These statistical approaches are critical because, unlike retinoblastoma, there were initially no cytogenetic clues from tumour analysis to help identify the chromosomes that contained the

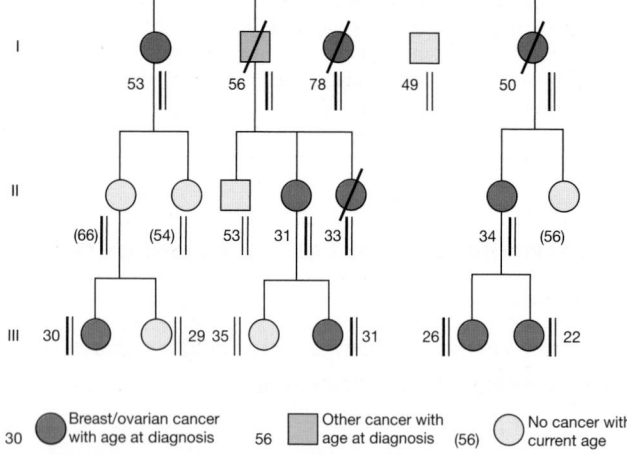

Fig. 2 Incomplete penetrance and phenocopies obscure mendelian inheritance patterns for cancer predisposition genes. In this hypothetical family, cancer predisposition is due to a mutant *BRCA1* allele on chromosome 17 (represented by the thick black line). Molecular analysis identified a 66-year-old woman in generation II who carries a mutant *BRCA1* allele but has not yet developed cancer. None the less she did transmit a mutant allele to one of her daughters who developed breast cancer at the age of 30. This is an example of incomplete penetrance that caused hereditary breast cancer to 'skip' a generation. In generation I, a 78-year-old woman developed breast cancer, but did not carry the mutant *BRCA1* allele. In this instance breast cancer was of the sporadic type, typically occurring in an older patient population. This case is referred to as a 'phenocopy' that mimicked the consequences of inheriting a disease allele.

Table 2 Estimated prior probabilities of a particular constellation of cases being due to a mutant ***BRCA1*** allele

Criterion	Cancer	Age at diagnosis	Prior probability case has *BRCA1* mutation
Single affected	Breast	< 30	0.12
	Breast	< 40	0.06
	Breast	40–49	0.03
	Ovarian	< 50	0.07
Sister pairs	Breast/breast	Both < 40	0.37
	Breast/breast	Both 40–49	0.20
	Breast/ovarian	Both < 50	0.61
Families	Breast, ≥ 3 cases diagnosed	All < 50	0.40
	≥ 2 breast with ≥ 1 ovarian		0.82
	≥ 2 breast with ≥ 2 ovarian		0.91

genes responsible for familial clusters of common tumours. Tumour chromosomes from common solid malignancies often show multiple gains and losses of chromosomal material, and no obvious single change associated with cases that arose in families with multiple affected members can be identified.

Inherited cancer predisposition syndromes

These classical syndromes can be distinguished from the problem of familial clustering of common cancers because the frequent occurrence of cancer is not the only feature of these unusual but instructive diseases. A diagnosis of one of these syndromes should be considered when cancer arises in organs not commonly affected by sporadic cancer or when tumours have unusual 'premalignant' manifestations or other disease characteristics that suggest the presence of a disorder of tissue regulation or formation. An example that illustrates these concepts is neurofibromatosis type 1. In excess of 90 per cent of the individuals who inherit a mutated neurofibromatosis type 1 gene (*NF1*) develop *café au lait* spots and skin neurofibromas. Other clinical manifestations may also be present, but with much lower frequency, for example learning difficulties, skeletal abnormalities, and more deforming 'plexiform' neurofibromas. Cancer is actually fairly uncommon and occurs in less than 5 per cent of cases. Tumours arise at unusual sites, including the adrenal medulla (phaeochromocytoma), the central nervous system (optic nerve gliomas, ependymomas, and meningiomas), and also within neurofibromas (neurofibrosarcomas). The reason for the extreme variability in the clinical features of neurofibromatosis is unclear. The effects of other genes (modifier genes) segregating within an affected family probably enhance or suppress the consequences of an *NF1* mutation. In addition, *NF1* mutations are diverse and lead to highly variable losses of coding sequence. Future studies may therefore define a relationship between the site of the mutation in the *NF1* gene and the clinical severity of the syndrome.

Linkage analysis

An effective, although labour intensive, approach to identifying genes that cause cancer predisposition is called DNA linkage analysis. Scattered throughout the human genome are sequence polymorphisms that are frequently heterozygous. Examples of these markers are single-nucleotide polymorphisms ('snips') or repetitive sequences (microsatellites) that can be identified through DNA sequencing or restriction fragment length polymorphisms. To identify the chromosomal location of a cancer predisposition gene these polymorphic markers are used in a genome-wide search to find a marker that cosegregates, or is 'linked' to the diagnosis of cancer

because it is on the same chromosome. Once the chromosome carrying the cancer predisposition gene is identified, the segregation of further markers along the chromosome in question is determined. Because DNA is exchanged between chromosomes (recombination), the statistical association between a marker and the presence of cancer increases the closer the marker in question is to the disease locus. Eventually a marker is identified that is considered (statistically) close enough for the investigator to clone the segment of DNA that encompasses the marker and look for 'candidate genes'. Ultimately the gene is identified by sequencing each gene candidate to identify mutations that are present in individuals that have developed cancer but are not present in unaffected family members. Tumour DNA is examined for evidence for loss-of-function somatic mutations in the remaining wild type allele to confirm Knudson's postulate. The number of families necessary for linkage analysis depends of the nature of the disorder. For the breast and ovarian cancer genes *BRCA1* and *BRCA2*, a large number of families were required to generate sufficient linkage information because of the family history problems discussed above. For inherited cancer syndromes with characteristic clinical features and high penetrance, fewer families are required because affected and unaffected individuals within a family can be more reliably identified (which is just as well considering how rare these diseases are).

A classification of inherited cancer syndromes based on gene function

Textbook descriptions have classified cancer predisposition syndromes by mode of inheritance (dominant or recessive), by site of organ involvement (for example breast and ovarian cancer syndromes or colon cancer syndromes), or by the presence of associated clinical features (for example gastrointestinal polyps or neurofibromas). However, there is now sufficient insight into the function of genes associated with cancer predisposition to use a mechanistically based, rather than clinical, classification. This functional approach has the advantage of illustrating the relationship between gene function and the clinical manifestations of these disorders. The conversion of a normal cell to a cancer cell requires multiple mutations in genes that control the fundamental cellular processes of proliferation, cell death, and differentiation. An inherited mutation can therefore contribute to the process of malignant transformation by disrupting signal transduction, regulation of the cell cycle, chromosome stability, or DNA repair. All known cancer predisposing mutations, in which the function of the encoded protein has been established, involve one, or more than one, of these four cellular processes.

Cancer predisposition syndromes associated with mutations in signal transduction proteins (Table 3)

Signal transduction is the key to normal tissue homeostasis, and mutations in genes that encode components of these pathways are extremely common in cancer cells. Many cancer predisposition syndromes could really be considered inherited 'signal transduction disorders' because germline mutations in signal transduction proteins generate not only malignant tumours but also benign growths and unusual syndrome stigmata that represent the effects of abnormal signal transduction on the formation of normal tissue. Furthermore, tumours induced by mutant signal transduction proteins tend to arise in an organ-restricted manner, presumably reflecting the tissue-specific roles of the signalling pathways concerned. Examples of signalling proteins disrupted in these diseases include plasma membrane tyrosine kinases, cytoplasmic protein kinases, protein phosphatases, GTPase activating proteins, and transcription factors. All the conditions discussed in this section are autosomal dominant, but with variable penetrance, except ataxia telangiectasia, which is autosomal recessive.

Table 3 Inherited cancer syndromes caused by mutations in genes encoding signal transduction proteins (all exhibit dominant inheritance patterns except ataxia telangiectasia which is autosomal recessive)

Syndrome	Gene locus	Gene symbol	Gene function
Multiple endocrine neoplasia type 2	10q11.2	RET	A tyrosine kinase plasma membrane receptor
Renal papillary cancer, familial	7q31.1–q34	MET	A tyrosine kinase plasma membrane receptor
Basal cell naevus syndrome (Gorlin's syndrome)	9q22.3	PTCH	A transmembrane receptor involved in body patterning and growth
Familial adenomatous polyposis	5q21–q22	APC	APC gene product is a negative regulator of β-catenin signalling
Cowden's disease	10q23	PTEN	PTEN (a protein phosphatase) opposes the phosphoinositol-3-kinase pathway thereby inhibiting cell survival and growth
Neurofibromatosis type 1	17q11.2	NF1	GAP protein (neurofibromin), regulates RAS-related signal transduction
Neurofibromatosis type 2	22q12.2	NF2	Schwannomin, may be involved in maintenance of cytoskeleton
Tuberous sclerosis	9q34	TSC1	Hamartin, function unknown. Tuberin, a putative GTPase activating protein
	16p13.3	TSC2	
Von Hippel–Lindau disease	3p25–p26	VHL	Transduction of growth signals generated by tissue hypoxia
Peutz–Jeghers syndrome	19p13.3	STK11	Serine threonine kinase with a negative role in signal transduction
Wilm's tumour	11p13	WT1	Transcription factor that regulates growth factor and growth factor gene expression
	11p15.5	WT2	Unknown
	Unmapped	WT3	Unknown
Ataxia telangiectasia	11q22.3	ATM	Member of phosphoinositol-3-kinase family, involved in DNA damage recognition and cell cycle control

Mutations in peptide growth factor receptors

Cell growth is regulated by peptide growth factors that bind and activate plasma membrane receptors. These receptors are enzymes that activate downstream cytoplasmic signal transduction proteins to alter gene expression and regulate the cell cycle. Four syndromes have been identified that are associated with activating mutations in either the RET or MET growth factor receptors, i.e. the mutation activates the receptor in the absence of the cognate peptide ligand (constitutive activation). These syndromes represent a major exception to Knudson's model, because the mutations concerned are 'gain-of-function'. As a result, there are no second mutational events in the remaining wild type allele. A fifth syndrome involves the PTCH gene that encodes a transmembrane receptor involved in body patterning. In this case the gene does conform to Knudson's postulate with respect to a 'second hit' and the germline and somatic mutations are all 'loss-of-function' in nature.

Multiple endocrine neoplasia types 2A and 2B and familial medullary thyroid cancer

Three disorders are due to activating mutations in the RET tyrosine kinase-linked cell surface receptor encoded by the *RET* gene at 10q11.2. RET is a neurotrophic pepide receptor and is predominantly expressed in cells of neural crest origin. Medullary thyroid cancer is common to all three conditions and about 20 per cent of all cases of this rare cancer are associated with a germline *RET* mutation. When no other stigmata are present, a diagnosis of familial medullary thyroid cancer is made. In the case of multiple endocrine neoplasia types 2A and 2B, additional unusual tumours arise including phaeochromocytoma and parathyroid adenomas (particularly in multiple endocrine neoplasia type 2A). Multiple endocrine neoplasia type 2B is associated with ganglioneuromas of the gastrointestinal tract and mucosal neuromas. In 95 per cent of cases of multiple endocrine neoplasia type 2A, mutations affect cysteine residues in the extracellular binding domain of RET, resulting in inappropriate disulphide bond formation, dimerization, and constitutive (ligand independent) activation of the RET tyrosine kinase. Familial medullary thyroid cancer results from mutations which similarly involve cysteine residues in the majority of cases but at different sites. The mutation found in multiple endocrine neoplasia type 2B is distinct and involves a methionine to threonine substitution in the ATP binding site of the receptor tyrosine kinase, leading to excessive receptor activity.

Familial papillary renal cell carcinoma

Some cases of this recently recognized syndrome, characterized by multiple bilateral papillary renal cell carcinomas, are due to germline mutations in the gene for MET tyrosine kinase at 7q31.1–q34. MET is a transmembrane tyrosine kinase receptor for hepatocyte growth factor or scatter factor, a peptide with essential roles in embryogenesis, cell motility, and tumour invasion. Germline *MET* missense mutations in cysteine residues, homologous to those involved in aberrant dimerization and activation of the RET receptor, are associated with familial papillary renal cell carcinoma. Monoallelic activating mutations in *MET* are also found the sporadic form of the disease. The spectrum of mutations found in sporadic papillary renal cell carcinoma is wider and includes activating mutations in the MET tyrosine kinase domain. However, recent studies have indicated that *MET* mutations occur in only about 15 per cent of sporadic papillary renal cell carcinomas.

Basal cell naevus syndrome (Gorlin's syndrome)

This condition should be considered in any patient presenting with a basal cell carcinoma before the age of 30, or with a personal or family history of multiple basal cell naevi/carcinomas. Associated abnormalities include abnormalities of skin, bone, and tooth formation (including polyostotic bone cysts, odontogenic keratocysts (jaw cysts), ectopic calcification, and palmar or plantar pits). An increased incidence of other cancers, including medulloblastoma, ovarian carcinoma, and sarcomas, may also occur. The incidence has been estimated at one in 55 600 in the United Kingdom. The gene believed to be responsible in the majority of cases, *PTCH* on 9q22.3, is a homologue of the *Drosophila* patched gene that encodes a transmembrane receptor for an extracellular ligand (hedgehog). This pathway is unrelated to classical peptide growth factor signalling and controls the fate of cells, body patterning, and growth by forming gradients in embryonic tissues. Initial analysis indicates that the *PTCH* gene behaves as a classical tumour suppressor gene.

Mutations in cytoplasmic signal transduction proteins

Plasma membrane receptors are linked to a highly complex array of cytoplasmic signal transduction proteins that transmit signals generated by an activated receptor to the nucleus to activate the cell cycle and alter gene expression. A number of highly characteristic syndromes are the result of loss-of-function mutations in proteins that have a negative role in signal transduction. The molecular genetics of these disorders generally conform to Knudson's model. However, disorders of tissue formation in these syndromes may occur in the absence of a second mutation, presumably because two normal functioning copies of the gene are required to maintain tissue homeostasis. In some cases, syndrome stigmata may arise because the mutated signal transduction protein interferes with the function of the wild type protein (a dominant negative effect).

Peutz–Jeghers syndrome

This autosomal dominant disorder has an incidence of one in 120 000. The syndrome stigmata are obvious with multiple pigmented spots on the lips and buccal mucosa, and multiple benign hamartomatous polyps throughout the gastrointestinal tract, most frequently affecting the jejunum. Malignant transformation of the gastrointestinal polyps is not common but may account for the increased incidence of colon cancer in these patients. In addition there is an increased risk of other cancers, including ovarian, cervical, testicular, and pancreatic cancer. The gene for Peutz–Jeghers syndrome, *STK11*, a serine threonine kinase, is located on 19p13.3. *STK11* is a tumour suppressor gene because germline mutations are predicted to disrupt the kinase domain of the protein. Molecular studies of hamartomas and gastrointestinal cancers associated with Peutz–Jeghers syndrome suggest that additional somatic mutation events are required for the transition of a hamartoma to an adenocarcinoma.

Neurofibromatosis type 1

The clinical features of neurofibromatosis were described in the introduction. The *NF1* gene (located on chromosome 17q11.2) encodes a guanosine triphosphatase activating protein known as the NF1-GAP-related protein, or neurofibromin. GAP proteins downregulate the activity of RAS, a critical mediator of the mitogenic response. An association between neurofibromin and the tropomyosin fibres of the cytoskeleton indicates a role in RAS-related signal transduction from the cell membrane to the cytoskeleton. A variety of mutations have been identified, and most result in a truncated protein. The rate of new germline mutations in *NF1* is high, with one-third to one-half of cases arising without affected parents. The *NF1* gene is prone to new mutational events because of its extremely large size (59 exons).

Neurofibromatosis type 2

This disease has an autosomal dominant pattern of inheritance. The neurological effects of neurofibromas predominate in neurofibromatosis type 2. There is a predisposition to development of tumours of the central nervous system, including schwannoma of the eighth cranial nerve ('acoustic neuroma'), meningioma, spinal cord schwannoma, and malignant gliomas. Deafness and tinnitus due to acoustic neuromas as well as muscle weakness and wasting due to spinal cord compression are not unusual. The *NF2* gene, located at 22q12.2, encodes a protein named schwannomin (or merlin). The majority of mutations within *NF2* result in the synthesis of a truncated protein. Schwannomin shows a close relationship to the family of ezrin–radixin–moesin proteins that link membrane proteins to the cytoskeleton and thus may function to maintain cytoskeletal organization. The incidence of neurofibromatosis type 2 is one in 35 000, of which half represent new germline mutations.

Tuberous sclerosis

Tuberous sclerosis is a disease of variable severity characterized by the development of multiple hamartomas involving many organs. Characteristic skin lesions often suggest the diagnosis. Often there is no family history since as many as 60 per cent of cases are due to a new germline mutation. There is a 5 to 15 per cent incidence of childhood brain tumours in affected individuals, mostly subependymal giant cell astrocytomas. In addition a weak association with renal cell cancer has been reported. A wide variety of benign tumours, including hamartomas, angiofibromas, and renal lesions, occur. Linkage studies have identified two genes, *TSC1* at 9q34 and *TSC2* at 16p13.3. *TSC1* encodes a protein called hamartin. Most mutations described within this gene result in a truncated protein. *TSC2*

encodes tuberin, a protein showing some homology to GTPase activating proteins.

Von Hippel–Lindau disease

The diagnosis of von Hippel–Lindau disease depends on the presence of either coexisting central nervous system and retinal haemangioblastoma or one or other of these features, plus multiple renal, pancreatic or hepatic cysts, phaeochromocytoma, or clear cell renal cancer. Only one of these clinical features need be present if there is a family history of von Hippel–Lindau disease. The incidence of the disease in the United Kingdom has been estimated as one in 36 000, with near complete penetrance by the seventh decade of life. Life expectancy is markedly reduced with death usually due to haemangioblastoma (benign vascular tumours) or renal cell cancer. The *VHL* gene at 3p25–p26 contains three exons that encode a 213 amino acid protein. The von Hippel–Lindau protein plays a role in the transduction of growth signals generated by changes in oxygen tension, promoting the translation of target genes that include vascular endothelial growth factor. *VHL* is a classical tumour suppressor gene, with a second, somatic mutation required for the development of cancer. Mutations in *VHL* are common in sporadic renal clear cell carcinoma.

Familial adenomatous polyposis or adenomatosis polyposis coli including Turcot's syndrome and Gardener's syndrome

Familial adenomatous polyposis (alternatively referred to as adenomatosis polyposis coli) has an incidence of one in 6000 to one in 13 000. Adenomatous polyps of the colon appear at an early age, with multiple polyps present in more than 90 per cent of cases by the age of 20 years. The polyps are premalignant, with the risk of adenocarcinoma of the colon approaching 100 per cent by the fifth decade of life. There is an increased risk of gastrointestinal carcinomas at other sites, thyroid cancer, childhood hepatoblastoma, and central nervous system tumours. Sometimes the combination of these tumours generates a recognizable syndrome. For example, multiple adenomatous colonic polyps in combination with a medulloblastoma is referred to as Turcot's syndrome. There is also an increased frequency of benign neoplasms including duodenal polyps, gastric polyps, and lipomas. In addition, there is an elevated risk for desmoid tumours. The gene for these disorders, *APC*, is located on chromosome 5q21–q22. Up to a third of cases are due to new germline mutations that usually cause protein truncation. Mutations mostly occur in the middle of *APC*, causing multiple colonic polyps appearing at puberty. *APC* mutations outside of this region are associated with fewer polyps and later onset. Some mutations correlate with the presence of unusual extracolonic syndrome stigmata, including congenital hypertrophy of the retinal pigment epithelium and benign bone tumours (osteomas). When these features are present the condition is referred to as Gardener's syndrome. These abnormalities occur in the absence of second mutations and may be due to the ability of mutant APC protein to interfere with the function of the remaining wild type protein (dominant negative effect). The APC protein is a negative regulator of β-catenin, a critical component of a signal transduction pathway that regulates cell–cell adhesion, cellular polarity, and tissue architecture.

Cowden's disease (gingival multiple hamartoma syndrome)

This autosomal dominant condition is most often recognized on the basis of characteristic skin lesions and intestinal hamartomas. Craniomegaly and mental subnormality occur in about 50 per cent of affected individuals. The pathognomic mucocutaneous lesions include trichilemmomas, acral keratoses, papillomatous papules, hyperkeratoses, and oral fibromas. Breast cancer occurs in 30 per cent of female gene carriers. Thyroid cancer is also prevalent (3 to 10 per cent), as well as glial masses that may present as cerebellar ataxia and seizures (Lhermitte–Duclos disease). The gene concerned, 'phosphatase tensin homologue deleted in chromosome 10' or *PTEN*, is located on 10q23 and is frequently deleted in sporadic breast cancer and glioblastoma. The PTEN phosphatase, by operating in opposition to the phosphoinositol-3-kinase pathway, inhibits cell survival and growth.

Table 4 Hereditary cancer syndromes caused by mutations in genes encoding cell cycle regulators (all autosomal dominant)

Syndrome	Gene locus	Gene symbol	Gene function
Li–Fraumeni syndrome	17p13.1	p53	Mediates cell cycle arrest and apoptosis in response to cell stress and DNA damage
Breast/ovarian cancer syndrome 1	17q21	BRCA1	Tumor suppressor with a 'p53 like' role in cell cycle arrest in response to DNA damage
Breast/ovarian cancer syndrome 2	13q12–q13	BRCA2	Homologous to BRCA1 and presumably serves a similar function
Familial melanoma, with or without dysplastic naevi	1p36	CMM1	Unknown
	9p21	CMM2	Cyclin-dependent kinase inhibitor p16
	12q14	CMM3	Cyclin-dependent kinase 4
Hereditary retinoblastoma	13q14	Rb	Negatively regulates transcription factors required for G_1/S transition in proliferating cells

Ataxia telangiectasia

This rare recessive condition (one in 30 000 to one in 100 000) is not easily classified. Traditionally ataxia telangiectasia has been grouped with Fanconi's anaemia, Bloom syndrome, and other disorders associated with an increased rate of somatic mutation. Ataxia telangiectasia patients, however, have a distinct signal transduction defect, hence the inclusion of ataxia telangiectasia in this section. The AT gene, at 11q22.3, encodes a 350 kDa protein which contains a domain sharing homology to members of the phosphatidylinositol-3-kinase family. The AT gene product is believed to be a signal transduction protein that regulates cell cycle checkpoints. In the presence of DNA damage, cells with an AT mutation fail to activate p53-dependent cell cycle arrest (see next section). Although the precise connection to p53 and other cell cycle regulators is unclear, it is understood that AT-deficient cells exhibit extreme sensitivity to agents which damage DNA, genetic instability, and spontaneous chromosome aberrations. There is a 30 to 40 per cent lifetime risk of malignancy including epithelial tumours, solid tumours, chronic T-cell leukaemia, and lymphoma. Ataxia telangiectasia patients exhibit multiorgan defects including progressive cerebellar degeneration, general neuromotor dysfunction, and humoral and cellular immune defects. In fact, neurological problems and infection dominate the clinical picture. AT heterozygotes do not exhibit any of these defects, but may suffer a two- to threefold increase in the risk of cancer.

Mutations in transcription factors that control tissue-specific gene expression

The signal transduction pathways discussed above ultimately have an impact on the activity of DNA binding transcription factors that either activate or suppress transcription from target genes. At the time of writing there is only one example of a transcription factor involved in tissue-specific gene expression that functions as a tumour suppressor, the Wilm's tumour gene WT1. It is unclear why mutations in transcription factors that regulate tissue formation are rarely the cause of familial cancer, while mutant transcription factors occur frequently in sporadic cancer. One can extrapolate from transgenic experiments in mice that this disparity is explained by fact that the regulatory functions encoded by transcriptional suppressors are essential for normal embryogenesis.

Wilm's tumour (nephroblastoma)

Wilm's tumour is a poorly differentiated tumour of the kidney associated with developmental abnormalities of the genitourinary tract. Males and females are equally affected and usually present early in childhood, most often with an abdominal mass. Two sites of loss of heterozygosity have been identified in Wilm's tumours, WT1 at 11p13 and WT2 at 11p15.5. There are also rare familial cases in which linkage to neither 11p locus has been established (referred to as the 'WT3' group). In 10 to 30 per cent of patients, the disease is bilateral or multifocal, but less than 1 per cent of all cases are truly familial. Most cases of bilateral nephroblastoma are due to new germline mutations in WT1. The protein encoded by the WT1 gene is a 'zinc finger' DNA-binding transcription factor. WT1 interacts with another tumour

suppressor, p53, to bind and suppress transcription from the epidermal growth factor receptor and insulin-like growth factor 2 gene promoters. When WT1 function is compromised, transcription from these growth- and survival-promoting proteins is increased, initiating tumour development. WT1 is not, however, a strictly Knudson-type tumour suppressor. Statistical analysis of age at diagnosis and proportion of bilateral and unilateral tumours does not follow the pattern described for retinoblastoma. Furthermore, the children of patients who survive Wilm's tumour are at lower risk of the disease than would be expected from a dominant-acting tumour suppressor gene. There is evidence that 'genomic imprinting' may explain some of these anomalies. Imprinting is a process of gene inactivation through DNA methylation that preferentially favours expression from genes inherited from one or other parental lineage. The reader is referred to the list of further reading for a comprehensive discussion of this complex issue.

Cell cycle checkpoint defects (Table 4)

Cell cycle checkpoint defects and cancer

The entry of a cell into the cell cycle is regulated by a 'G_1/S' checkpoint that controls the transition of cells from a resting (G_0/G_1) state into a DNA synthetic or S phase. When S phase is complete, cells enter premitosis (G_2). A second major checkpoint, G_2/M, regulates entry into mitosis (M phase). A major component of these two checkpoints is a family of regulatory proteins called cyclins that regulate the activity of enzymes called cyclin-dependent kinases. As the cell cycle progresses, cyclin and cyclin-dependent kinase activities oscillate, with peak activities corresponding to transition through each cycle checkpoint. Cyclin-dependent kinase activity is subject to negative regulation by Rb, p53, and a family of cyclin-dependent kinase inhibitors. These proteins operate to arrest the cell cycle in response to a wide variety of signals, including inhibitory factors, radiation, and other 'genotoxic' stresses. By blocking the cell cycle in cells that have undergone DNA damage, cell cycle inhibitory genes provide important protection against the development of cancer. Without this protection, cells exhibit genetic instability, with the accumulation of chromosomal deletions, translocations, and duplications. Cancer predisposition syndromes that are due to mutant cell cycle regulators are not generally associated with obvious clinical stigmata because cell cycle proteins do not regulate tissue-specific gene expression. Premalignant tumours may occur, however. Despite the fundamental role these genes have in cell cycle regulation, the pattern of tumour development is surprisingly restricted. This may be due to a major role for environmental stresses as a cofactor in tumour development (ultraviolet irradiation of the skin for example) or poorly understood tissue-specific roles for the genes concerned.

The retinoblastoma gene product Rb

The clinical features of retinoblastoma were described in the introduction. The Rb-1 gene encodes a 928 amino acid protein. Rb functions by binding to the 'E2F' family of transcription factors. When Rb becomes phosphorylated by a cyclin-dependent kinase, E2F transcription factors are released to drive transcription from genes required for DNA synthesis. In addition, transcription of cyclins that stimulate entry into S phase is activated. Mutations in Rb therefore disrupt the ability of Rb to interact with and inhibit E2F. As a result, the G_1/S checkpoint is lost and cells initiate unscheduled DNA replication.

Li–Fraumeni syndrome

This uncommon autosomal dominant disease exhibits a high incidence of a wide variety of early onset tumours, including rhabdomyosarcoma, osteogenic sarcoma, breast cancer, brain cancer, leukaemia, and adrenal corticoid carcinoma. Penetrance is high, with almost half of genetically affected individuals developing cancer by the age of 30 (compared with 1 per cent in the general population), rising to almost 90 per cent by the age of 70. Cancer at multiple sites is common. The clinical diagnosis is made by a patient with sarcoma under the age of 45, a first-degree relative under the age of 45 with cancer (not specified), and a third affected family member (first- or second-degree relative) with either sarcoma or any cancer under the age of 45. Approximately half of Li–Fraumeni syndrome families have mutations within the *p53* gene located at 17p13.1 resulting in a truncated p53 protein. *p53* is a classical tumour suppressor that stimulates transcription of cyclin-dependent kinase inhibitors in response to cellular stress. *p53* has been referred to as the 'guardian of the genome' because of a critical role in arresting the cell cycle in the presence of DNA damage.

Familial melanoma with or without dysplastic naevi

An autosomal dominant susceptibility to melanoma occurs in some families. Affected individuals in these families tend to have a large number of moles and are at risk for development of multiple melanomas and dysplastic naevi at a young age. Linkage to three loci, *CMM1*, *CMM2*, and *CMM3*, has been established. *CMM2* (9p21) encodes the cyclin-dependent kinase inhibitor 2A (known as p16). *p16* mutations are associated with a markedly elevated risk of both melanoma and pancreatic cancer and mutations occur frequently in a wide variety of sporadic tumours. Two transcripts are encoded by the same gene. One transcript, p16 (INK4a), induces a G_1 cell cycle arrest by inhibiting the phosphorylation of the Rb protein by cyclin-dependent kinases 4 and 6. The second (β) transcript encodes p14 (ARF), and is believed to function as a tumour suppressor by stabilizing p53 and leading to p53 accumulation. Mutation in the gene for cyclin-dependent kinase, identified as the gene at the *CMM3* locus 12q14, generates a dominant acting oncogene that promotes cell cycle progression. The gene responsible for the locus at chromosome 1p36, termed *CMM1*, has not been identified.

Hereditary breast/ovarian cancer (*BRCA1*)

In this condition there is an autosomal dominant predisposition to breast and/or ovarian cancer. Cancer occurs at a young age and is more frequently bilateral. Several hundred deletions, insertions, and point mutations have been identified within the *BRCA1* gene, with most predicted to result in truncated protein. The risk of breast cancer for individuals inheriting mutant forms of *BRCA1* is 3 per cent by the age of 30 years, 19 per cent by 40 years, and 85 per cent by 70 years. The risk for ovarian cancer is not as dramatic, but is increased greatly over that of the general population. An increased risk for colon and prostatic cancer is also present. The *BRCA1* gene on 17q21 has a role in the maintenance of genetic stability and the cell cycle response to DNA damage. This genetic surveillance role is similar to that of p53; BRCA1 and p53 are known to directly interact with each other.

Hereditary breast/ovarian cancer (*BRCA2*)

As in *BRCA1*, *BRCA2* mutations cause an autosomal dominant pattern of early onset breast and/or ovarian cancer predisposition. The onset of breast cancer in *BRCA2* families tends to occur earlier than in *BRCA1* families. Unlike *BRCA1*, there is an increased frequency of male breast cancer and pancreatic cancer in *BRCA2* patients. *BRCA2* has been localized to 13q12–q13. BRCA1 and BRCA2 share some homology and presumably serve simi-

Table 5 Hereditary cancer syndromes due to DNA helicase defects (autosomal recessive)

Syndrome	Linkage	Gene symbol	Gene function
Bloom syndrome	15q26.1	*BLM*	RecQ DNA helicase
Werner's syndrome	8p12–p11.2	*WRN*	RecQ DNA helicase
Rothmund–Thompson syndrome	8q24.3	*RECQ4*	RecQ4 DNA helicase

lar functions in cell cycle checkpoint control and response to DNA damage.

Increased somatic mutation due to DNA helicase defects (Table 5)

The following recessive chromosome instability syndromes are rare and distinct from the classical cancer predisposition syndromes. There is no evidence for somatic mutation in these genes in tumours and so Knudson's model is not pertinent. The clinical features of these disorders overlap, with all three showing features of premature ageing. On a molecular level these syndromes are due to recessive mutations in a family of helicases that operate to maintain DNA topography during replication, recombination, and DNA repair.

Bloom syndrome

This an autosomal recessive disease of unknown incidence, more common in Ashkenazi Jews. Manifestations include growth retardation, sensitivity to the sun, skeletal abnormalities, and susceptibility to infection. An increased frequency of malignant neoplasms occurs throughout life, with dramatically reduced life expectancy. Lymphoma and leukaemia predominate before the age of 25; those that survive into their fourth and fifth decades are prone to a variety of common solid tumours. The age at diagnosis for these carcinomas is usually 20 or more years earlier than usually expected in the general population. Multiple mutations have been documented in the gene responsible, *BLM*, located on chromosome15q26.1. Loss of BLM, a RecQ DNA helicase, generates genetic instability with spontaneous chromosomal abnormalities and increased sensitivity to radio- and/or chemotherapeutic agents. Males are infertile due to a defect in meiosis. Heterozygotes do not seem to have an increased cancer risk, reflecting apparently normal genetic stability.

Werner syndrome

Werner syndrome is characterized by a multisystem premature aging phenotype also due to a RecQ helicase defect. The incidence is one in 50 000 to one in 100 000. Affected individuals have an excess of neplasms (especially osteosarcoma, meningioma, and thyroid cancer). A variety of loss-of-function mutations in the *WRN* gene located at chromosome 8p12–p11.2 have been identified. Loss of WRN helicase function leads to inappropriate expression of inhibitors of DNA synthesis, early cellular senescence, and genetic instability.

Rothmund–Thompson syndrome

This is the third recessive cancer predisposition syndrome due a defect in a RecQ-type DNA helicase (in this case, *RECQ4* at 8q24.3). The clinical features are similar to Werner and Bloom syndromes, comprising poikiloderma (marbleized pigmentation), telangiectasia, growth deficiency, cataracts, some aspects of premature ageing, and a predisposition to malignancy, especially osteogenic sarcomas and skin tumours.

Table 6 Hereditary cancer syndromes caused by mutations in DNA repair genes (may be autosomal recessive or dominant, depending on the rate of somatic mutation in heterozygotes)

Syndrome	Linkage	Gene symbol	Gene function
Xeroderma pigmentosum (autosomal recessive)	9q34.1	XP-A	Involved in excision repair of ultraviolet radiation-induced DNA pyrimidine dimers
	2q21	ERCC3	
	3p25.1	XPC	
	19q13.2	ERCC2	
	11p12–p11	XPE	
	16p13.2–p13.1	ERCC4	
	13q32–q33	ERCC5	
Fanconi's anaemia (autosomal recessive)	16q24.3	FA-A	Functions are unknown but all are believed to be 'caretakers' protecting against chromosomal instability in the presence of DNA damage
	Unmapped	FA-B	
	9q22.3	FA-C	
	3p26–p22	FA-D	
	Unmapped	FA-E	
Hereditary non-polyposis colon cancer (autosomal dominant)	3p21.3	hMLH1	All participate in repair of errors that occur during DNA replication though recognizing nucleotide 'mismatch'
	2p22–p21	hMSH2	
	2q31–q33	hPMS1	
	7p22	hPMS2	
	2p16	hMSH6	

Increased somatic mutation due to DNA repair defects (Table 6)

The fourth major class of cancer predisposition syndromes involves defects in DNA repair. Some of these defects cause severe problems in childhood and others are associated with a delayed onset, with cancer in adult tissues the major phenotype. These conditions can be recessive or dominant, depending on the consequences of the heterozygous state on the rate of somatic mutation. All promote the development of cancer by increasing the rate of somatic mutation. The genetics of these conditions is very complex—since DNA repair involves multiple protein components, a defect in any one will generate essentially the same phenotype.

Xeroderma pigmentosum

This is a spectrum of autosomal recessive disorders, with an incidence of one in 1 000 000 in the United States. Childhood onset of photosensitivity and freckling leads to progressive degenerative skin changes and early development of skin and eye cancers. Approximately one-quarter of affected patients have concurrent neurological abnormalities. Basal cell and squamous cell carcinomas of the skin are increased 2000-fold and so the differential diagnosis includes Gorlin's syndrome. An increased risk of melanoma has also been observed. An increased risk of other tumours has been reported, including brain, lung, stomach, and haematological tumours. Benign neoplasms include conjunctival papillomas, actinic keratoses, lid epitheliomas, keratoacanthomas, angiomas, and fibromas. Defects of several enzymes involved in excision repair of ultraviolet light-induced pyrimidine dimers are responsible for this syndrome including XPA on chromosome 9q34.1, ERCC3 on 2q21, XPC on 3p25.1, ERCC2 on 19q13.2, XPE on 11p12–p11, ERCC4 on 16p13.2–p13.1, and ERCC5 on 13q32–q33.

Fanconi's anaemia

Fanconi's anaemia is another spectrum of recessive diseases characterized by a complex variety of developmental abnormalities, progressive marrow failure, and a predisposition to acute myeloid leukaemia (15 000 times that of the general population). Fanconi's anaemia commonly presents in early to middle childhood with anaemia and bruising. Progressive pancytopenia and chromosome breakage, worsened by exposure to alkylating agents, is characteristic. Fanconi's anaemia homozygotes may develop a wide range of common cancers occurring at an early age, and are vulnerable to the hepatocarcinogenic effects of androgens used to treat Fanconi's anaemia.

Squamous cell carcinomas, especially of the head and neck, oesophagus, cervix, vulva, and anus, occur with increased frequency, as do liver adenomas. Life expectancy is poor, around 12 years, with most deaths resulting from marrow failure and cancer. Approximately one-fifth of childhood aplastic anaemia is associated with Fanconi's anaemia. The heterozygote frequency is estimated to be one in 300 to one in 600, and is even commoner in Ashkenazi Jews. At the cellular level, Fanconi's anaemia homozygotes display chromosomal instability in response to DNA damage and reactive oxygen species and increased sensitivity to DNA crosslinking agents such as mitomycin C. Spontaneous chromosome aberrations are seen in a variety of cell types and an increase in chromosome deletion is seen. Five genes have been defined by complementation studies: FA-A at 16q24.3, FA-C at 9q22.3, and FA-D at 3p26–p22; FA-B and FA-E are currently unmapped. Several mutations have been found for FA-C and FA-A. The FA-C gene has been cloned but the function of the gene product is still not understood as it is a novel protein with no recognized functional motifs. However, the cellular phenotypes strongly suggest a role in DNA regulation or repair. Most studies have shown that Fanconi's anaemia heterozygotes do not display spontaneous genetic instability and do not have an increased risk of malignancy.

Hereditary non-polyposis colon cancer

This autosomal dominant condition may account for 6 to 10 per cent of all colorectal cancers. Clinically a diagnosis of hereditary non-polyposis colon cancer requires the following: three cases of colon cancer in a family in which two of the affected individuals are first degree relatives of the third; colorectal cancers occurring in two generations; and one colon cancer diagnosed before the age of 50 years. Five genes have so far been identified (located at 3p21.3, 2p22–p21, 2q31–q33, 7p22, and 2p16), each encoding proteins that participate in multimeric DNA mismatch repair complexes. Two of the genes, hMLH1 and hMSH2, account for more than 90 per cent of cases of hereditary non-polyposis colon cancer. Most characterized mutations yield truncated gene products. The dominant inheritance pattern of these repair defects clearly distinguishes hereditary non-polyposis colon cancer from xeroderma pigmentosum and Fanconi's syndrome. Heterozygotes have 50 per cent expression of the mismatch repair protein in question, which presumably raises the somatic mutation rate sufficiently to increase the risk of cancer. Tumours that arise in patients with hereditary non-polyposis colon cancer exhibit very dramatic genetic instability in

Table 7 Other important Inherited cancer predisposition syndromes

Syndrome
Gastric cancer, familial
Prostate cancer, familial
Carcinoid, familial
Hodgkin's disease, familial
Pancreatic cancer, familial
Testicular cancer
Oesophageal cancer with tylosis
Carney syndrome
Familial chordoma
Renal cancer, familial (non-papillary, clear cell)
Multiple endocrine neoplasia type 1
Familial paraganglioma
Osteochondromatosis, multiple

nucleotide repeat sequences (microsatellites). In fact, microsatellite instability can be used as a clinical test to distinguish adenomatosis polyposis coli from hereditary non-polyposis colon cancer. The lifetime risk of colon cancer for patients with hereditary non-polyposis colon cancer is 80 per cent, the average age at diagnosis is 45 years, and most cancers occur in the right side of the colon. Hereditary non-polyposis colon cancer is associated with an increased risk of other cancers, in particular endometrial adenocarcinoma, but also ovarian, gastric, small intestine, hepatobiliary tract and pancreatic cancer, skin cancer (sebaceous carcinomas), and transition cell cancer of the renal collection system. Glioblastoma multiforme is associated with hereditary non-polyposis colon cancer. 'Turcot's syndrome' of hereditary brain and colon cancer can therefore occur with both adenomatosis polyposis coli and hereditary non-polyposis colon cancer.

Syndromes in which the underlying gene defect has not been identified or the function of the gene has not been fully established (Table 7)

This review has focused on syndromes with established genetic aetiologies. Of course there are many other instances of familial clustering of common cancers that are under investigation, including those for prostate cancer, gastric cancer, carcinoid tumour, Hodgkin's disease, pancreatic cancer, and testicular cancer. In addition there are cancer predisposition syndromes with unusual phenotypes that should yield to genetic investigation soon, including oesophageal carcinoma with tylosis, Carney syndrome (hereditary myxoma), familial chordoma, osteochondromatosis, and familial paraganglioma. Again, the reader is referred to the further reading list.

Interventions for patients with inherited cancer predisposition

The role of clinical genetic testing in the management of cancer predisposition syndromes is in a constant state of flux. When the genetic basis for an inherited cancer syndrome is established there is an immediate opportunity to develop a reliable genetic test. However, genetic testing is fraught with methodological, psychological, and clinical difficulties and should not be applied without careful genetic counselling of the entire family concerned. In general, genetic testing is most rationally applied when the patient can be offered an intervention to prevent the cancer. This may simply be increased surveillance, a strategy most successfully applied when the target organ is easily accessible. For example, melanoma screening with regular skin examinations and sun avoidance for patients with hereditary melanoma syndromes is almost certainly successful in reducing the incidence of lethal melanoma. In contrast, for patients with Li–Fraumini syndrome, a condition in which cancers arise in a variety of internal organs with a high frequency, surveillance strategies are cumbersome and patients are generally reluctant to comply. A genetic test can be used to establish an indication for prophylactic surgery. For example colectomy should be offered to patients with adenomatosis polyposis coli or hereditary non-polyposis colon cancer and mastectomy and ovariectomy for patients with BRCA1 or BRCA2. These are not easy decisions, however, since prophylactic surgery is disfiguring and/or is associated with significant functional and/or psychological impairment. The most hopeful approaches to these conditions involve the application of chemoprevention. Here a positive genetic test is an indication for a medication that attenuates the effect of a cancer predisposing mutation. The use of tamoxifen, an anti-oestrogen, to prevent breast cancer for patients with BRCA mutations is under investigation and inhibitors of prostaglandin synthesis have been shown to inhibit the development of polyps for patients with adenomatosis polyposis coli.

In the future it may be possible to develop preventative drugs specifically designed to interfere with the deregulated enzymatic activity generated by a mutant protein. For example, it is conceivable that RET or MET specific tyrosine kinase inhibitors could be employed to prevent the onset of cancer in multiple endocrine neoplasia type 2 and familial papillary renal cancer. Finally, using gene therapy strategies it may be possible to restore tumour suppressor function. Recent reports on p53 gene therapy certainly offer hope in this regard.

Further reading

Foulkes WD, Hodgson SV, eds (1998). *Inherited susceptibility to cancer: clinical, predictive and ethical perspectives.* Cambridge University Press, Cambridge.

Lindor NM, Greene MH (1998). The concise handbook of family cancer syndromes. *Journal of the National Cancer Institute* **90**, 1039–71.

Ponder BAJ (1997) Inherited cancers. In: Cox TM, Sinclair J, eds. *Molecular biology in medicine*, pp 172–90. Blackwell Science, Oxford.

6.4 Tumour metastasis

V. Urquidi and D. Tarin

Introduction

Tumour dissemination with colonization of distant sites in the body and the formation of secondary tumours, termed metastasis by Recamier in 1829, is an enigmatic phenomenon. It is also by far the most common cause of death in cancer patients, because of the failure of vital organs replaced by deposits of disorganized, malfunctioning tumour tissue.

In the human embryo, progenitor cells undergo complex migrations and interactions during the formation of body structure, but after arriving at their final positions, they remain fixed throughout adult life. The only normal cell lineages exempt from this fate are leucocytes which continue to patrol the blood vessels, tissues, and lymphatics. Neoplastic non-haematological cells can acquire the capability to do likewise, and the characteristic patterns of colonization displayed by specific types of tumours and cell lines derived from them demonstrate that tumour metastasis is not a random process. Such programmed disorderly behaviour by a subpopulation of host cells, compromising the regimented anatomy of the other cell lineages, is a unique phenomenon in animals. Its mysterious quality and its grave clinical implications both hinge upon the failure thus far to identify any properties unique to metastatic cells that can illuminate the mechanisms involved or help treatment to control or eliminate disseminated malignant disease.

The metastatic process

Formation of a secondary tumour colony in a new site is the culmination of a complicated series of sequential and highly selective events. It begins with the emergence within the expanding tumour cell population of one or more clones whose descendants can cross tissue boundaries and infiltrate adjacent cellular populations, progressively disrupting the structure and function of the organ. As the tumour grows it induces blood vessels to penetrate and arborize within it to supply its metabolic needs. This in turn provides opportunities for tumour cells with appropriate properties to break into the circulation and be carried away to seed distant sites. Survivors that attach to the vascular endothelium at a distant site gain access to the resources of the tissue or organ where they have alighted by diapedesing through the endothelium and focally destroying the surrounding sleeve of basement membrane. To complete the process and produce a secondary tumour or metastasis in this site they then proliferate and attract a new fibrovascular scaffolding from the host organ, to sustain growth and prepare for the next metastatic event.

Clinicopathological correlations of metastasis

Not only are molecular events within the spreading tumour cells responsible for the phenomenon of metastasis, but microenvironmental conditions within the mixed tumour cell populations, composing the organ in which the secondary deposits are established, also play an important role.

This interaction between tumour and host cells causes characteristic patterns of organ distribution of secondary tumours, linked to the site of origin of the primary tumour, that are clinically well recognized. Thus, for instance, the distribution of metastatic deposits in patients with breast cancer most commonly involves the regional lymph nodes, the long bones, the lungs, and the liver. Similar, largely predictable, patterns of spread are seen in patients with colon cancer, prostate cancer, and many other common malignancies. These patterns are exceptionally useful clinically, in guiding physicians where to search in order to stage the degree of spread of the disease and seek early evidence of recurrence.

Many studies in animals and humans have demonstrated that these distribution patterns result primarily from preferential colonization of some sites rather than from simple vascular drainage patterns, although such mechanical factors can be superimposed on the biological processes involved. This 'seed and soil' synergy between the properties of the spreading tumour cells and the cells comprising the colonized organ dictating the distribution of secondary deposits, first recognized by Paget in 1889, has been corroborated by many converging lines of evidence in recent years and finally proven by studies in ambulatory humans. The cumulative evidence shows that the disseminating tumour cells are not omnipotent, and are still dependent upon co-operative interactions between them and the cells of the stroma and vasculature of the host organ in order to establish a secondary colony.

The routes of dissemination are also clinically and experimentally important in that the tumour cells sometimes preferentially go by lymphatic or transcoelomic pathways rather than by the blood vascular system. Additionally it has been shown that certain types of mouse tumours suppress the growth of dispersed micrometastases by the release of blood-borne antiangiogenic molecules that inhibit the growth of the secondary tumours. Removal of the primary tumour can result in the simultaneous and sudden growth of many secondaries in these model systems. However, although some anecdotal literature suggests that similar phenomena have been observed in humans, it is certainly not accorded sufficient clinical credence to alter the current best standard of clinical practice, which is to excise as much tumour tissue as one can without compromising vital functions of the patient.

Clinical consequences of metastasis

The clinical effects of metastasis relate to the exponentially increasing tumour burden in scattered locations, which ultimately leads to the failure of organs vital for survival of the host. These effects are compounded by the proven capability of the progeny of cells in metastatic colonies to metastasize again. This makes it impossible to effectively focus treatment on the expanding and leap-frogging tumour population and therefore increases the risk of collateral damage to surrounding normal tissue. The idiosyncratic metabolic and physical effects of this increasing tumour load, such as paraneoplastic effects, pain, anxiety, haemorrhage, pathological fractures, and compressed or eroded vital structures, also need to be alleviated. Furthermore, the significant possibility of recurrence of disease in a distant site long after successful eradication of a locoregional tumour necessitates careful and prolonged monitoring, sometimes assisted by appropriate tumour markers.

Therapeutic considerations relating to metastasis

The current practice of tailoring combined therapeutic approaches, incorporating various radiotherapeutic and/or chemotherapeutic regimens, after surgical excision to staging of disease in the patient is increasingly effective for some cancers. Spectacular successes can result if multimodality therapy is used fairly early in the course of the disease. However, the main difficulty of treating widely disseminated metastatic cancer remains intractable and its solution is the 'Holy Grail' of oncology. New research on genetic mechanisms offers the best currently available hope of finding target molecules for rational drug design, gene therapy, and novel approaches to biological therapy, all aiming specifically at the eradication of late stage disease. Meanwhile, however, some significant and useful advances in treatment of such patients have been made by:

(1) combining therapeutic regimens (for example surgery and hormone therapy and/or chemotherapy for patients with breast cancer)

(2) delivering chemotherapy by appropriate routes (for example intrathecally for cerebral deposits, intraperitoneally for ovarian carcinomatosis peritonei), and

(3) increasing dose intensity within a short period.

Although very high-intensity chemotherapy with subsequent (autologous or heterologous) bone marrow transplantation has been effective for some haematological malignancies, recent trials have failed to show clear evidence of benefit in patients with breast cancer or other solid cancers. Radiotherapy, like surgery, remains more suitable for the management of locoregional disease or isolated secondaries.

The problem of deciding how much treatment is needed to eradicate dormant micrometastases (small collections of clinically undetectable tumour cells sprinkled in many sites), otherwise known as minimal residual disease, without exposing non-neoplastic stem cells in many of the patient's tissues to irreversible toxicity, is a continually present dilemma. The detection and treatment of metastatic tumour deposits in the brain, leptomeninges, bone marrow, and bones pose particularly difficult challenges. In the neural axis, treatment is fraught with the problems of delivery of chemotherapeutic agents across the blood–brain barrier and the difficulty of adjusting the dose of radiation therapy to be effective without damaging sensitive, normal nervous tissue. Sampling difficulties complicate evaluation of whether the marrow is involved in a patient and recent advances in purging it of malignant cells using monoclonal antibodies vary in their efficacy, depending on the type of tumour. Bony involvement is effectively controlled by radiotherapy if it is localized, but widely scattered deposits are refractory to reduction or elimination by most therapeutic regimens.

Current metastasis research and its importance for clinical oncology

There is, therefore, a real need for novel research to identify special characteristics of metastatic cells that could render them susceptible to therapies controlling further spread. The prevention of escalating dissemination whilst the existing tumour deposits are attacked would be a valuable contribution to the therapeutic armoury. Current research on the mechanisms of tumour cell metastasis is opening promising avenues for such advances. These are still in their infancy, but new observations on cellular, genomic and postgenomic (gene expression) aspects of the metastatic phenotype permitted by recent technological advances (i.e. cDNA microarray and proteomic methods) are providing clues to the mechanisms involved. At the cellular and biochemical level, the data demonstrate that tumour-induced angiogenesis, proteolytic activity by tumour-derived matrix metalloproteases, and epithelial–mesenchymal interactions, dependent on specific growth factor receptor–ligand binding events, facilitate the metastatic process in many experimental tumour systems. Other studies have indicated the presence of putative metastasis suppressor genes on a variety of chromosomes, depending on the tumour system under investigation. Interestingly, to date, comparable information on metastasis promoting genes is less abundant, although some studies have provided data supporting this concept. Additionally, a substantial body of data has been published indicating that expression of individual effector molecules, such as integrins, selectins, CD44, and cadherins, may accomplish various parts of the metastatic process under the direction of co-ordinating genes, as yet unknown. Despite decades of research, no single consistent marker or effector of metastatic behaviour has yet been identified and modern emphasis has shifted to using high-throughput gene expression analysis, such as gene chips and spotted microarrays, to identify whether co-ordinated patterns of expression of clusters of genes are involved in this complex process.

As the basic events in the metastatic process are comparable in many different species and in individuals with tumours of differing histogenetic origin, it seems likely that the underlying causal mechanisms will be initiated and driven by the same group of regulatory genes. If this interpretation is correct, the recognition of patterns of gene expression meaningfully correlated with metastatic phenotypes should guide investigators to the identity of the co-ordinating genes governing the phenotype and more effective targets for therapy. Results from our own laboratory using gene chips and other methods of genome-wide expression analysis support this view and are revealing previously invisible reliable differences in mRNA species between metastatic and non-metastatic tumour cells cloned from a patient with breast cancer. Computational analysis of several such datasets, utilizing clustering algorithms, to screen for commonalities in gene expression within the metastatic versus the non-metastatic phenotype should facilitate identification of the functional implications of such associations. Using such methods, genes at ascending levels in the hierarchy of regulation of the phenotype will be catalogued. The ultimate objective of modern clinical cancer research is to identify better markers for reliable evaluation of prognosis and detection of disease recurrence and to develop improved targets and strategies for novel therapies.

Summary

Although considerable progress has been made in the clinical management of patients with cancer, the best immediate hope of surviving the grim sequelae of metastatic spread of cancer still lies in early detection of the primary tumour, before it has started to shed cells into the circulation. The hunt for molecules or combinations of molecules which indicate the imminent onset of malignancy and which are released into easily accessible body fluids (blood, saliva, sputum) and waste products (urine and faeces) therefore has practical and scientific appeal, although success may not necessarily provide much information on the underlying mechanisms of the metastatic process. For new methods to contain or eradicate cancer that has already begun to disseminate, we still need to understand the mechanisms involved. Suffice it to say for the present, however, that understanding the fundamental basis of the metastatic process will also profoundly illuminate how cellular societies, which compose all metazoan and especially vertebrate organisms, are assembled and kept in strict topographical and developmental order. Such an intellectual 'spin-off' adds a further level of interest to the challenge of finding a practical solution to the vexing and challenging biological problem of human malignant disease.

Further reading

Fidler IJ (1999). Critical determinants of cancer metastasis: rationale for therapy. *Cancer Chemotherapy and Pharmacology* **43** (Suppl.), S3–S10.

Fidler IJ, Kripke ML (1977). Metastasis results from preexisting variant cells within a malignant tumour. *Science* **197**, 893–5.

Tarin D (1992). Tumour metastasis. In: McGee, JO'D, Isaacson PG, Wright NA, eds. *Oxford textbook of pathology*, Vol. 1, pp 607–33. Oxford University Press, Oxford.

Tarin D (1997). Prognostic markers and mechanisms of metastasis. In: Anthony PP, MacSween RNM, eds. *Recent advances in histopathology*, Vol. 17, pp 15–45. Churchill Livingstone, Edinburgh.

Tarin D, Matsumura Y (1994). Recent advances in the study of tumour invasion and metastasis. *Journal of Clinical Pathology* **47**, 385–90.

Tarin D *et al.* (1984). Mechanisms of human tumour metastasis studied in patients with peritoneovenous shunts. *Cancer Research* **44**, 3584–92.

Welch DR, Wei LL (1998). Genetic and epigenetic regulation of human breast cancer progression and metastasis. *Endocrine-related Cancer* **5**, 155–97.

6.5 Tumour immunology

P. C. L. Beverley

Historical perspective

The strategies that have been tried in tumour immunology are based on the idea that tumour cells harbour differences that can be detected by the immune system. The first is to use antibodies to distinguish between tumour and normal cells; this difference can then be exploited for diagnostic, prognostic, or therapeutic purposes. The second is to stimulate the host by specific or non-specific immunization to react more vigorously to autologous tumour. All these avenues have been pursued for close to a hundred years so that it is pertinent to ask why it is that immunology has had such a minor impact in oncology, and particularly in cancer therapy.

The early attempts involved experiments in tumour transplantation and the description of tumour rejection. Unfortunately, the tumour rejection experiments were carried out in outbred animals and it was later realized that allograft, rather than tumour rejection, was being demonstrated. Nevertheless, the experiments did show the power of the immune response to destroy a large, growing tumour mass. Non-specific stimulation with bacterial products (Coley's toxin) was also tried as therapy but later more rigorous examination of the effect of immunostimulation showed that the success rate was extremely low. After the second world war, the development of inbred animals allowed properly controlled experiments on tumour-specific immune responses to be performed and the theory of immune surveillance provided a stimulus and a basis for a new wave of experiments in tumour immunology. Nevertheless, although tumour-specific immune responses were soon detected, it remained difficult to define their target antigens until the development of monoclonal antibodies and methods for gene cloning. One other advance was also essential for understanding of antitumour immune responses, the realization that thymus-derived (T) lymphocytes can only recognize antigens processed inside cells and displayed at the cell surface in association with major histocompatibility complex (MHC) antigens (Fig. 1).

Here are discussed immune surveillance, the evidence for immune responses to tumours, and aspects of immune function relevant to immunotherapy. Current understanding of the nature of tumour antigens recognized by the host immune system and how differences between tumour and normal cells may be exploited for diagnostic and therapeutic purposes are also reviewed.

Immune surveillance

The theory of immune surveillance postulated that tumours arise frequently but that most are eliminated by the immune system before becoming clinically apparent. Diverse evidence was adduced in support of the theory (Table 1) and many experiments performed to test it. Most of these were studies of the effects of immunosuppression, since the strongest prediction of the theory was that tumours should arise with overwhelming frequency in the absence of an immune response. Examination of congenitally immunodeficient or deliberately immunosuppressed mice supported the theory, since a higher frequency of tumours was observed than in controls. However, many tumours were characteristic of those caused by mur-

Fig. 1 Antigens recognized by T lymphocytes may be extracellular, in which case they are captured and internalized by antigen presenting cells to enter the exogenous antigen processing pathway. The antigens are broken down to peptides for loading on to newly synthesized MHC II molecules and translocated to the cell surface. Antigens synthesized within cells, which may originate from viral or self proteins, enter the endogenous pathway. They are broken down to peptides by proteasomal enzymes and the peptides are transported into the endoplasmic reticulum for loading and translocation to the cell surface.

Table 1 Evidence for immune surveillance

- Tumours arise frequently in the young and old, periods of relative immunoincompetence.
- Tumours arise frequently in genetically immunodeficient individuals.
- Tumours arise frequently in immunosuppressed individuals.
- Tumours usually show infiltrating lymphocytes.
- Immune responses to tumours can be demonstrated *in vivo* and *in vitro*. Spontaneous regression occurs associated with lymphoid infiltration.

Table 2 Tumours and immunosuppression

Tumour type	Approximate relative risk
Kaposi's sarcoma	50–100
Non-Hodgkin lymphoma	25–45
Carcinoma of the liver	20–35
Carcinoma of the skin	20–50
Carcinoma of the cervix	2.5–10
Melanoma	2.5–10

ine oncogenic viruses. Similarly, in man, deliberately immunosuppressed individuals or AIDS sufferers do have a greatly increased risk of tumours (Table 2) but not the most common types. Strikingly, viruses are implicated in the aetiology of most of the tumours types arising in immunocompromised individuals (Table 3). These data are clearly not in accord with a straightforward immune surveillance mechanism, since this would postulate an increased frequency of all tumours but in practice the strongest effects attributed to surveillance against tumour cells are most probably due to immune responses against potentially oncogenic viruses.

In spite of strong immune responses against oncogenic viruses, these agents do cause tumours in normal individuals as well as the immunocompromised. This may be because the virus-transformed cells adopt several strategies for escaping from immune attack (see below). In turn, this leads to the suggestion that the most effective means of preventing these tumours is by prophylactic immunization against the oncogenic virus, preventing infection and therefore transformation. Immunization against hepatitis B virus has already been demonstrated to decrease the incidence of liver cancer in endemic areas and vaccines against Epstein–Barr virus (EBV) and papillomaviruses are areas of active research.

In the case of many of the most common tumours, there is no evidence for a viral aetiology so that for these tumours the existence and importance of immune responses to tumour-associated antigen remains questionable. This is discussed below.

Tumour-specific immunity

The first convincing evidence that there were tumour-specific antigens came from experiments with inbred mice using chemically-induced tumours. Animals immunized with irradiated tumour cells or by grafting and then excising tumour, were protected against rechallenge with the same, but not a different, tumour line. Immunity could be transferred to naïve animals with cells but not serum. Notably, spontaneous tumours were usually much less immunogenic, raising the possibility that non-viral as well as virus-induced tumours may exhibit escape mechanisms.

In man, the evidence was rather slower to accrue but the development of the colony inhibition test, in which tumour cells were cocultured with patients' lymphocytes and the number of growing colonies counted, allowed an analysis of antitumour responses. Early studies showed that many patients were resistant to tumour and it was also suggested that 'blocking factors' present in serum might be responsible for the progressive growth of tumours in the face of a cellular colony-inhibiting response.

Table 3 Viruses and human tumours

Tumour	Virus
Burkitt lymphoma	EBV
Nasopharyngeal carcinoma	EBV
Lymphomas in the immunocompromised	EBV
Carcinoma of the liver	Hepatitis B and C viruses
Carcinoma of the cervix	Human papillomaviruses
Carcinoma of the skin	Human papillomaviruses
Adult T cell leukaemia	HTLV-1
Kaposi's sarcoma	HHV 8

Later results threw doubt on the specificity of the early research and it became clear that both normal and cancer patients' lymphocytes could often inhibit the growth of tumour targets. This led to the definition of natural killer cells. These cells play a role in the early innate (non-specific) response to infectious agents but there is little to suggest that they play an important role in protection against non-viral tumours.

More persuasive evidence of specific T-cell responses to tumours became available following the realization that T cells can only recognize antigen in the context of self MHC (Fig. 1) and that specific immune responses can often only be revealed following an in vitro boost. Since that time, a number of authors have shown that both MHC class II restricted tumour-specific T-helper and class I restricted T-cytotoxic responses can be generated by coculture of lymphocytes and autologous tumour cells. Although it is clear that these responses occur in many tumour-bearing patients, the fact that they have been difficult to detect reproducibly indicates that they are often weak, in other words that there is a low frequency of responding T cells. That these responses may nevertheless play a role in host protection is suggested by the observation that loss of MHC molecules is very common in tumours. At least 50 per cent of human tumours show either down regulation of all class I or allele-specific loss. Clearly loss of MHC molecules which could present a tumour antigen is a very effective mechanism of tumour escape.

What are the tumour antigens recognized by T cells?

The nature of the tumour-specific antigens of non-viral experimental tumours and of most human tumours remained inaccessible until the development of gene expression cloning methods. In the 1980s Boon and his colleagues set out to identify tumour antigens of a mouse tumour, P815. The tumour was initially non-immunogenic in syngeneic DBA/2 mice, so that it grew readily even in preimmunized mice. A set of tumour variants were produced by treating the tumour with a mutagen. Some of these were highly immunogenic and unable to grow in preimmunized mice (tum– variants). From mice immunized with tum– cells, it was possible to isolate cytotoxic T-cell clones, which could kill only the immunizing tumour variant and not parental P815 or other tum– variants. The cytotoxic T-cell clones were used to screen parental P815 cells, which had been transfected with a cosmid library constructed from tum– variant cells. Eventually tum– antigen-positive transfectants were identified, the cosmid recovered, and, after subcloning, transfecting the subclones, and rescreening, the gene coding for the cytotoxic T-cell target antigen could be identified. Several different tum– antigens have now been cloned in this way and it has become clear that they fall into two categories (Table 4). The first is due to a genetic alteration in the coding sequence of a gene and the second to altered expression of a normal gene product.

Table 4 The properties of tumour antigens recognized by T cells

Altered antigen	'Normal antigen'
Tumour sequence has a point mutation (or other genetic alteration)	Sequence identical to normal gene
Not necessarily expressed at a high level	Expressed at higher than normal level or in an aberrant site
Non-mutated version of the gene expressed in one or many cell types in normal tissues	Normally expressed at very low level or in inaccessible sites
The antigens are short peptides recognized in association with MHC molecules	The antigens are short peptides recognized in association with MHC molecules

Table 5 Properties of a human melanoma antigen.

- MAGE 1 tumour sequence is identical to genomic MAGE 1
- MAGE 1 has no homology to known genes
- MAGE 1 is an internal cellular antigen
- MAGE 1 is part of a large gene family
- One or another family member are expressed in most melanomas and some other tumours
- MAGE 1 is only expressed in testis among normal tissues surveyed
- The epitope detected by MAGE 1-specific CTL is HLA-A1 restricted.

Boon and his colleagues also investigated human tumour antigens in a similar fashion. Melanoma has long been recognized as capable of stimulating a relatively strong host T-cell response. Melanoma-specific cytotoxic T-cell clones were therefore produced and used to screen a melanoma cDNA library. They first identified MAGE-1 (melanoma antigen 1), belonging to the category of over-expressed, unaltered tumour antigens (Table 5). More remarkably, the antigen belongs to a large, previously undiscovered gene family which is widely expressed in tumours and seldom in normal tissues. Subsequently, Boon's group and others have cloned several other melanoma antigens as well as antigens of other tumours (Table 6). The majority of antigens identified by this methodology are unaltered. However, mutations and genetic rearrangements creating new sequences are common in tumours (Table 7) and computer analysis has shown that many of the neoepitopes formed could bind to common HLA alleles such as HLA A2. It has been shown also that some tumour patients and mice can respond to peptides of mutant *ras* oncogene and some cancer patient can generate cytotoxic T cells to the HER2/*neu* oncogene product. This work also established that most tumour antigens recognized by T cells are similar to other antigens recognized by T cells (Fig. 1, Table 4), that is they are short peptides presented by MHC molecules.

One other form of T-cell antitumour response is noteworthy. Mucins are heavily glycosylated molecules which are expressed at the surface of many epithelial cells and corresponding tumours. However, the glycosylation of the molecule is frequently altered in tumour cells leading to the detection of new epitopes by monoclonal antibodies on the tandem repeat structure

Table 6 Some human tumour associated molecules recognized by T lymphocytes

Antigen name(s)	Tumour types	Normal tissue Distribution
Cancer/testis antigens		
MAGE 1	Some	Testis
MAGE 3	melanomas	
BAGE	and other	
GAGE	tumour	
NY-ESO-1	types	
Other antigens		
MelanA/	Melanoma	Normal melanocytes
MART-1		
Tyrosinase		
gp100/Pmel 17		
gp75/TRP-1		
Her-2/neu	Breast and ovary	Some normal epithelial cells
Prostate specific antigen (PSA)	Prostate	Prostate
Carcino-embryonic antigen (CEA)	Colon and other carcinomas	Colon
Mutated ras	Many carcinomas	Mutated ras not present

Table 7 Some genetic alterations in human tumours

Alteration	Function of protein	Tumour type
Point mutations		
ERB B2 (HER 2/neu)	Growth factor receptor	Breast carcinoma
FMS	CSF-1 receptor	AML, myelodysplasia
ras	GTP-binding protein	Carcinomas and others
p53	Tumour suppressor cell cycle control	Many including lung, colon, bladder
RB1	DNA binding protein	
Chromosomal translocations		
BCR-ABL	Tyrosine kinase	CML, ALL
EZA-PRL	Transcription factor	Pre-B cell ALL
H4- RET	Growth factor receptor tyrosine kinase	Thyroid Carcinoma
MYL-RAR	Retinoic acid receptor	APL
TPR-MET	Growth factor receptor tyrosine kinase	Gastric carcinoma
L MYC-RLF	Transcription factor	SCLC
NPM/ALK	Tyrosine kinase	Lymphoma
Deletion mutations		
ERB-B	Growth factor receptor	Gliomas

of the protein core of the molecule. Cytotoxic T cells generated from breast cancer patients lyse tumour cells expressing the mucin but in a MHC-unrestricted fashion. The cytotoxic T cells may be CD4 or CD8 and have an αβ T-cell receptor but unusually killing can be blocked a mAbs to the mucin tandem repeat. Exactly how these unusual cytotoxic T cells recognize their antigen remains to be determined.

The demonstration that many tumour patients make a cellular immune response to their tumour raises the question as to why tumours continue to grow and suggests that the response to tumours may be weak. This is discussed below.

Why are the responses to tumour antigens weak?

Just as for other T-cell-recognized antigens, several factors will determine whether a tumour antigen stimulates an immune response in the host. The first is that processed peptides from the molecule must reach the cell surface in association with MHC molecules. Whether a particular peptide does so depends on the amount produced by processing enzymes, the ability of the peptide to reach intracellular compartments where it may bind to MHC molecules, and its affinity for the MHC alleles expressed by the cell.

The second factor determining whether there is a response is that there must be T cells capable of responding. During normal development of T lymphocytes in the thymus, those cells that react with high affinity to self antigens are deleted to prevent the development of autoimmunity. It is, therefore, somewhat surprising that so many human tumour antigens detected by T cells appear to be unaltered self molecules. The most likely explanation is that thymic deletion and T-cell responsiveness in the periphery are governed by the affinity of the interaction of the T-cell receptor with peptide–MHC complexes. The thymic deletion mechanism selects against the highest affinity cells, while cells with lower affinity for self escape to the periphery. If the antigen is up-regulated, there may now be enough peptide–MHC complexes to stimulate lower affinity cells that have escaped deletion in the thymus. For antigens containing new sequences introduced through genetic alteration, there is in principle no reason why there should not be responsive T cells in the periphery. However, the frequency of T cells able to respond to a single epitope will be low (contrast this situation with that of a pathogen which has many proteins and even more peptide epitopes).

There is a second reason why responses to tumours may be poor. This is the need for 'danger signals' in initiation of immune responses. Recently, it

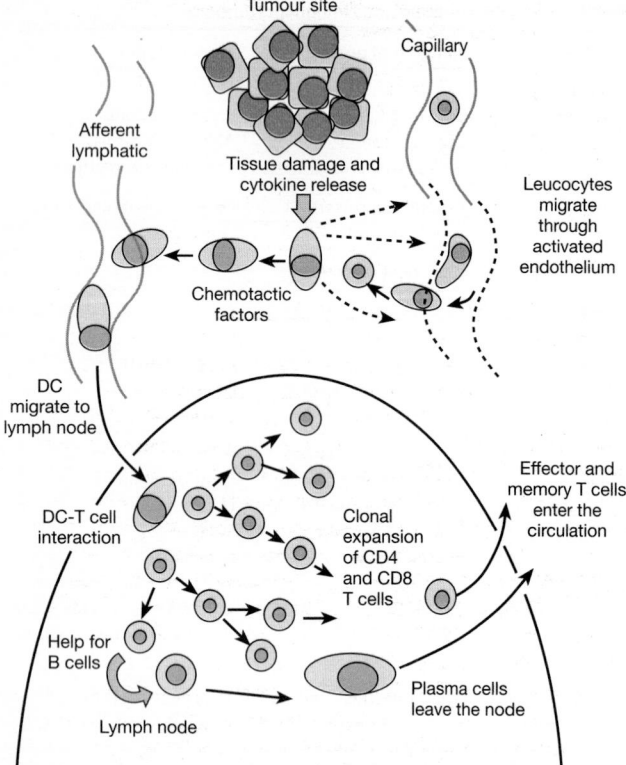

Fig. 2 Initiation of immune responses to pathogens is dependent on 'danger' signals carried by micro-organism, which stimulate production of cytokines by tissue cells and tissue-resident dendritic cells and macrophages, leading to influx of more leucocytes and migration of antigen-loaded dendritic cells to the draining node. Tumour sites are unlikely to stimulate these events until tissue damage and cell death occur as a relatively late event, so that the immune response to tumours may be delayed.

has been recognized that activation of the innate immune system is essential for development of a subsequent, specific immune response. Pathogens carry 'danger signals' which perform this function. These are conserved structures such as bacterial carbohydrates, lipopolysaccharides, and signature DNA and RNA sequences that are recognized by conserved host receptors including complement components, receptors for carbohydrates (mannose and scavenger receptors) and lipopolysaccharides (CD14), and as yet ill defined recognition systems for nucleic acid sequence motifs. Interaction of danger signals with these conserved receptors leads to the production of cytokines by dendritic cells, macrophages, natural killer, and tissue cells that are essential for initiation of immune responses (Fig. 2).

In the case of a tumour it is not clear what would provide such danger signals during the early stages of growth; later, tissue damage and repair processes would be expected to lead to cytokine production. Tumours may therefore be immunologically silent until a relatively late stage, by which time the tumour burden may be too great for the immune system to deal with, especially in the face of tumour escape mechanisms.

An important second stage in initiation of immune responses, induced by T-cell receptor–peptide–MHC contact, is the up-regulation of costimulatory molecules on both T and antigen presenting cells (usually dendritic cells) (Fig. 3). The interaction between CD28 and B7 is particularly important in promoting T-cell proliferation and that between CD40 and CD40 ligand has recently been shown to play a key role in differentiation of cytotoxic T cells. It has also been shown that T-cell receptor–peptide–MHC interaction in the absence of costimuli may lead to inactivation rather than activation of T cells. Since most tumour cells lack costimulatory molecules, they are usually poor antigen-presenting cells. Even when activated effector

cells return to the tumour site, the lack of costimuli may provide a mechanism for tumour escape, as may the production by tumour cells of down-regulatory cytokines, such as transforming growth factor-β (TGF-β). T lymphocytes isolated from tumour-bearing patients have been reported to show defects in signalling through the T-cell receptor, supporting the idea that tumours are indeed immunosuppressive.

Tumour antigens defined by antibodies

The exquisite specificity of antibodies has long persuaded investigators that it should be possible to use them to distinguish between tumour and normal cells. However, until the development of monoclonal antibodies (mAbs) there had been few successful examples. Many mAbs have now been raised against tumours and the vast majority recognize not tumour antigens but normal differentiation antigens. There are a few exceptions—antibodies to the idiotype of T and B cell tumours are tumour specific and antibodies to mutant forms of the p53 tumour suppressor gene product identify this as a tumour-associated molecule. In spite of this apparent failure, mAbs have proved extremely useful in studying the biology of tumours and lack of absolute specificity for tumour cells does not preclude their use as diagnostic or therapeutic agents.

More recently, serological analysis of tumour antigens by recombinant cDNA expression cloning (SEREX) has been developed. Sera from patients are used to screen cDNA expression libraries from fresh tumour material. Isolation of antigens detected by high titre IgG or IgA antibodies implies that there is a T helper cell response to the same antigen, as immunoglobulin class switching does not occur without this. That there is often a concurrent T-cell response when antibody to autologous tumour is present, is confirmed by the finding that some SEREX-defined antigens are identical to those recognized by T cells (see Tables 6 and 8). The SEREX method has

Fig. 3 Most T cells responses are initiated by contact between T cells and dendritic cells, which are specialized for antigen presentation and express key costimulatory molecules such as B7 and CD40. Many tumour cells lack these and are therefore likely to be poor antigen-presenting cells.

Table 8 Examples of antigens defined by SEREX

Name	Source	Type of Antigen
HOM-Mel-40	Melanoma	Cancer testis antigen
NY-ESO-1	Melanoma	Cancer testis antigen
MAGE 1	Melanoma	Cancer testis antigen
Tyrosinase	Melanoma	Differentiation antigen
Galectin-9	Hodgkin's disease	Over-expressed normal gene product
Carbonic anhydrase	Renal carcinoma	Over-expressed normal gene product
Proliferating cell nuclear antigen (PCNA)	Melanoma	Cell cycle gene
HERV-K10	Renal carcinoma	Endogenous retroviral env
p53 (mutated)	Colon carcinoma	Tumour suppressor gene

the disadvantage that it may not detect all conformational epitopes of a protein and does not identify carbohydrate antigens. Nevertheless, over 900 sequences of genes cloned using the SEREX method have already been deposited in a data base set up for this purpose. These include previously identified antigens such as MAGE-1 and tyrosinase, sequences identical (or nearly identical) to known genes not previously identified as eliciting an autoantibody response (e.g. kinectin, a transporter of golgi vesicles), and a large group of previously unknown genes (Table 8). A full description of the expression patterns of these genes in normal and tumour tissue, let alone a analysis of their functions, will be a major undertaking, but will eventually identify many new targets for immunotherapy.

The potential for immunodiagnosis and immunotherapy

Monoclonal antibodies have already found a place in the diagnosis of malignant disease (summarized in Table 9) although they seldom play a role in deciding whether a cell is malignant (although antibodies to some of the gene products identified by SEREX may eventually change this). So far, they have been most useful in cell identification. MAbs readily allow identification of single gene products in sections or smears and this is often a simple way of assigning a cytologically undifferentiated cell to a cell lineage. A relatively small panel of mAbs (Table 9) allows the identification of most tumours, which might otherwise cause diagnostic confusion. An extension of this is the detection of rare malignant cells. Thus, mAbs have been used to identify micrometastases in lymph nodes, blood, bone marrow, or cerebrospinal fluid, which are below the limit of detection by conventional histology or cytology. This data indicates that the presence of micrometastases at the time of diagnosis is much more common for many carcinomas than had been appreciated before. The clinical importance of this observation remains to be determined.

MAbs may also be used to provide prognostic information. Estimation of the proportion of cells expressing molecules associated with progression through cell cycle, such as the transferrin receptor or nuclear cyclins, cor-

relates to some degree with the malignancy of tumours. However, it is not to be expected that expression of any single marker will correlate absolutely with tumour behaviour since one result of studies with mAbs is to reinforce the view that tumours are very heterogeneous. Nevertheless, as understanding of the function of gene products expressed in tumour cells improves, studies of tumours with carefully designed panels of mAbs will provide increasingly useful prognostic information.

Serological tests for a number of cancer-associated molecules have been developed; examples are carcinoembryonic antigen, α-fetoprotein, and prostate specific antigen. These are useful confirmatory diagnostic tests and can be used for follow up after treatment. A rise in serum antigen may indicate a recurrence of tumour.

Antibodies *in vivo*

As discussed above, there are few antibodies against molecules which are truly tumour specific. For *in vivo* use it is also necessary that the target antigen should be at the cell surface. In spite of these limitations, many mAbs have been used *in vivo* for diagnostic or therapeutic purposes. For both uses, the problems are similar. The first is to obtain sufficient penetration of antibody into tumour to give a useful signal-to-noise ratio. Penetration depends on the size of the molecule, its half-life in the serum, the vascularity of the tumour, and the abundance and availability of the antigen. The second problem is that heterologous antibody is immunogenic as are most of the larger molecules which are commonly attached to it, such as plant toxins. Both of these problems have been addressed by immunochemical or molecular engineering methods. It is possible to produce a variety of sizes of antibody fragments and to replace most of a rodent immunoglobulin by human sequences. This reduces greatly the immunogenicity of the antibody (although the idiotypic epitopes associated with the antibody binding site may remain immunogenic) but will not affect the ability of attached toxins to generate an antibody response. Strategies designed to circumvent this problem include further engineering of toxin moieties to render them less immunogenic, induction of tolerance to immunogenic molecules, and the use of a succession of different antibody–toxin or drug conjugates. Some of these strategies have now been explored in human clinical trials (see below). It should also be noted that the anti-idiotype response to an antitumour mAb can generate a further anti-idiotypic response (Ab3) which may react with the original tumour antigen. The presence of Ab3 has been associated with a favourable outcome in some studies.

Experience in man with antibodies for diagnosis suggests that their sensitivity is of the same order as that of computer assisted tomography. However, optimization of the antibody and radioisotope selection and coupling procedures will undoubtedly yield improvements.

For therapy, the problem of penetration into large tumour masses may dictate that antibodies are most useful in an adjuvant setting. In a randomized trial of a murine mAb to an epithelial differentiation antigen given at the time of surgery to colon cancer patients, treated patients showed significantly increased survival. Here the target is micrometastases, which would be expected to be relatively easily reached by serum antibody, and

Table 9 Antibodies for tumour typing

Antibody specificity	Tumour example	Tissue recognized
Vimentin	Connective tissue	Sarcoma
Cytokeratins	Epithelia	Carcinoma
Epithelial membrane antigen	Epithelia	Carcinoma
Neurofilaments	Nervous tissue	Neuroblastoma
Desmin	Glia	Glioma
Leucocyte common antigen (CD45)	Leucocytes	Lymphoma
S100	Nervous tissue	Melanoma
Placental alkaline	Germ cells	Teratoma, choriocarcinoma

indeed it could readily be demonstrated that antibody had bound *in vivo* to tumour cells in the bone marrow. A number of other trials of antibodies have been carried out. In perhaps the most promising, a humanized antibody to the *neu* antigen (a member of the epidermal growth factor (EGF) receptor family) has been used alone or combined with chemotherapy to treat metastatic breast cancer; increased objective response rates have been reported. The antibody has received a licence from the Federal Drug Administration. Trials of anti-CD20 (a B lymphocyte differentiation antigen) mAb in lymphoma have also shown encouraging results.

CD20 antibody has also been used as a carrier for a radioisotope, as has an antibody to the mucin, MUC1, to deliver high doses of yttrium to the peritoneal cavity in ovarian cancer patients with minimal residual disease after chemotherapy. In the latter trial, a significant benefit was seen compared to historical controls. A phase three trial is underway.

One possible avenue of progress in achieving antibody penetration is to target not the tumour itself but tumour vasculature. Endothelial cells respond to their microenvironment by changes in surface phenotype and the vessels of tumours may therefore express molecules which could be targeted. Initial animal experiments are encouraging. So also is the successful treatment of melanoma by limb perfusion with very-high-dose tumour necrosis factor (TNF-α), in which the tumour vasculature appears to be susceptible while normal endothelium remains unscathed.

T-cell immunotherapy

For those tumours in which a virus is implicated (Table 3), prophylactic vaccination would be the most obvious long-term solution. For other common cancers where there is no obvious viral target, T-cell-based therapy, if it does have a role, will have to be directed at established tumours. Viral antigens may also be targeted for active immunotherapy as has been tried in the case of carcinoma of the cervix, where the human papillomavirus transforming proteins E6 and E7 have been used (Table 10).

As discussed above, there is now good evidence for a specific T-cell response to at least some human tumours. In principle, it seems that any altered and expressed gene product, or even a normal but over-expressed product, may be recognized as a tumour antigen. It seems likely that most tumours will accumulate several possible tumour antigens during their evolution, though not all will be immunogenic in a particular individual because of the necessity for peptides of the tumour antigen to bind to self HLA molecules (genetic restriction). Although cataloguing the target epit-

opes present in tumours is a major task, it is certainly now possible and methodology will continue to improve. Given this increasing list of target epitopes, how can it be exploited?

Active immunization

One possibility will be to attempt active immunization against the antigens identified. This can be done using whole cells expressing the antigen, with recombinant viruses (most commonly recombinant vaccinia virus; see Table 10), with proteins or peptides, and most recently with DNA. Animal experiments have indicated that transduction of tumour cells with costimulatory molecules such as CD80 (B7) or cytokines (particularly GM-CSF and IL-2) reduces their tumorigenicity and renders them better able to immunize against subsequent tumour challenge. Recombinant viruses and DNA offer the possibility of introducing similar costimuli along with antigen and also ensure that the antigen can enter the class I pathway of antigen processing so that cytotoxic T cells should be induced. A related strategy is to isolate dendritic cells from patients and load them *in vitro* with tumour antigen before reintroducing them into the patient. Tumour antigen can range from tumour cell lysate, through recombinant antigens, to peptides, DNA, or RNA. Table 10 summarizes some of the approaches and antigens that have been tried in at least phase 1 trials. Inevitably, most of these trials have been performed in patients with advanced disease who have often received chemo- and radiotherapy. These patients are unlikely to make optimal immune responses, often have a large disease burden, and their tumours often show loss of HLA antigens. Nevertheless, objective clinical responses have been demonstrated in several trials.

Non-specific immunotherapy

Once cytokines became more readily available through the introduction of recombinant technology, several clinical studies were carried out. So far, the overall results have not been dramatic although high-dose IL-2, with or without lymphokine activated killer cells, does appear to cause some remissions in renal carcinoma and melanoma, but not without considerable toxicity. In retrospect, it is perhaps not surprising that the effects of high-dose cytokine therapy have been less than dramatic. Few cytokines are directly cytotoxic to tumour cells, although they may be cytostatic, and their effects are often transient because of receptor down-regulation. In addition, the indirect *in vivo* effects of high doses of cytokines are little understood.

Table 10 Clinical trials of immunotherapy

Mode of therapy	Target tumour and antigen	Method
Active non-specific	Bladder	BCG
	Melanoma and RCC	IL-2
Passive antibodies	Colon	Anti-epithelial antigen mAb
	Breast, HER-2/neu	Anti-HER-2/neu mAb
	Ovary, MUC 1	Anti-MUC 1 mAb.
	Leukaemia and	Campath-1, CD20 or anti-idiotype mAbs
	Lymphoma	
	Surface Ig or other antigens	
	Lymphoma, Surface Ig	Idiotypic Ig + adjuvant or Ig gene DNA
Active immunization	Colon, CEA	Recombinant VAC-CEA +/– GM-CSF.
	Breast, MUC 1	Sialyl Tn antigen-KLH conjugate or VAC-MUC 1-IL-2
	Prostate,	
	PSA	Liposome encapsulated PSA
	PMSA	Antigen pulsed dendritic cells
	Globo H Hexasaccharide	Synthetic antigen-KLH conjugate with QS21 adjuvant
	Melanoma, various melanoma antigens	Whole cells transduced with cytokines or peptides
	Cervix	Recombinant VAC-HPV 16/18 E6E7

Much more work on the biology of cytokines is needed if they are to be used for tumour therapy in a rational fashion.

Cytokines have found application in cancer therapy, since colony stimulating factors can significantly shorten the period of aplasia following bone marrow transplantation. Another possibility is to use cytokines as vehicles for targeting. A recombinant IL-2–diphtheria toxin molecule has been engineered and shows some promise as an immunosuppressive agent. In principle, such a recombinant molecule can be used to target IL-2-receptor-bearing tumours such as those caused by HTLV-1.

Non-specific immunotherapy has a long history, dating back to the experiments of Coley. More recently Matthé used BCG to treat leukaemia, though with uncertain effect. However, there is now good evidence that intravesical BCG is an effective treatment for bladder cancer. Large-scale clinical trials have show that BCG can give very high response rates in recurrent superficial transitional cell carcinoma and the duration of remission is significantly prolonged. The mechanism of action of BCG remains incompletely understood but is presumed to be a consequence of altered local cytokine production in the tumour environment.

Passive immunotherapy

An alternative may be to develop passive immunotherapy. T-cell lines can be grown to very large numbers *in vitro* and in animal models tumour-specific cells can be effective especially when given with recombinant interleukin-2. Definition of tumour antigens will make it easier to isolate human tumour-specific clones and grow the large numbers of cells required for this strategy. Initial experiments using marker genes have shown some localization of *in vitro* expanded tumour infiltrating lymphocytes. More encouragingly, cytotoxic T cells against EBV antigens have been demonstrated to be effective in eliminating post-transplant lymphoma. To circumvent the difficulty of growing tumour specific T cell clones, methods are being developed for introducing genes for tumour-antigen-specific receptors into normal lymphocytes using retroviral vectors. A potential advantage of *in vitro* grown cells is that they might also be used to carry damaging molecules to the tumour. A disadvantage is that this method will always be labour intensive and will have to be carried out individually for each patient.

Conclusions

In non-malignant disease, immunological manoeuvres have been most effective when applied prophylactically. It is not expected that immunotherapy of established tumours will be easy. Antibody-based therapy shows promise and some antibodies may become standard adjuvant therapy in the near future. The future of T-cell-based therapy is less clear. Although active immunization against tumour antigens is now possible, its effectiveness will depend on the frequency of responding T cells and how quickly tumour escape mutants develop. Much work remains to be done to optimize immunization schedules and methods for monitoring the success of immunological approaches in cancer patients. New methods, such as the use of MHC tetramers and sensitive elispot assays, will help in enumerating tumour-antigen-specific cells.

Further reading

Boon T (1995). Tumor antigens and perspectives for cancer immunotherapy. *Immunologist* 3, 262–3.

Lee MS *et al.* (1998). Hepatitis B vaccination and reduced risk of primary liver cancer among male adults: a cohort study in Korea. *International Journal of Epidemiology* 27, 316–19.

Matzinger P (1998). An innate sense of danger. *Seminars in Immunology* 10, 399–415.

Riethmuller G *et al.* (1998). Monoclonal antibody therapy for resected Dukes' C colorectal cancer: seven-year outcome of a multicenter randomized trial. *Journal of Clinical Oncology* 16, 1788–94.

Schoenberger SP *et al.* (1998) T-cell help for cytotoxic T lymphocytes is mediated by CD40–CD40L interactions. *Nature* 393, 480–3.

Sheil AG (1998). Cancer in immune-suppressed organ transplant recipients: aetiology and evolution. *Transplantation Proceedings* 30, 2055–7.

6.6 Cancer: clinical features and management

R. L. Souhami

Introduction: cancer in general medical practice

Cancer is a common disease—approximately 20 per cent of the population of the United Kingdom will die of cancer. It is a source of concern and perplexity to oncologists that so many of their patients are referred to them late in the disease. Symptoms may have been present for a long time, during which their significance has been overlooked, or multiple (and sometimes futile) investigations have been performed with a failure to appreciate the need for speed. To this delay can be added a frequent lack of understanding of the possibilities of treatment and a failure to inform patients either of the nature of the diagnosis or of its implications and possibilities for therapy.

Almost every specialist sees patients with cancer affecting their particular field; unfortunately, these specialists may not have been taught the principles of cancer medicine. Oncologists therefore frequently see patients with advanced disease, who have not had a proper explanation of their illness, and who have little idea of what treatment might involve. Many patients dying with lung cancer in the United Kingdom have never seen a specialist in cancer medicine at any stage in their illness. While some will have had disease so far advanced that nothing but palliative treatment was needed, others may have been denied the opportunity for treatment and prolongation of life. The principles of cancer management are important for every physician.

Management of suspected cancer would be improved greatly if the following simple rules were adhered to:

1. Cancer should be suspected with any unexplained illness, especially in the elderly.

2. Imaging with isotopic and computed tomography (**CT**) and magnetic resonance imaging (**MRI**) (see Chapter 6.5), will often accelerate diagnosis. However, a tissue diagnosis cannot be made by these means and every attempt should be made to make a histological or cytological diagnosis expeditiously.

3. Patients with many tumours should start a planned programme of treatment within days and not weeks of diagnosis. The need for speed in diagnosis and treatment is tacitly recognized in specialist centres for breast cancer where patients can, in well-regulated clinics, reasonably expect to have a diagnosis made within a few days of first consultation and to begin definitive treatment within 2 weeks. This admirable efficiency should be attainable for nearly all cancers.

Common symptoms and signs of cancer

Many of the symptoms and signs of cancer are due to the local effects of the tumour infiltrating surrounding tissues and causing pressure and distortion of neighbouring structures. Tumours also produce symptoms that are, to some extent, common to all cancers. These are general symptoms due to the metabolic disturbances caused by the tumours and specific symptoms related to hormonal effects and immunological effects of the particular tumour—so-called paraneoplastic syndromes.

Pain

Most patients with cancer experience pain at some stage in their illness, either as a direct result of the tumour or of its treatment. Pain is a feature at presentation in about 30 per cent of patients with cancer, but the incidence varies greatly with the site of the tumour. For example, over 90 per cent of patients with primary bone tumours or with metastases to bone have pain, and this has the characteristic feature of being worse at night-time. In contrast, only 5 per cent of patients with leukaemia develop pain. Pain also varies according to the rate of progression of the disease and is more likely to occur with rapidly growing tumours. No symptom of cancer causes greater demoralization than unremitting pain. Any patient with unexplained, persistent pain should be suspected of having malignant disease and appropriate investigations performed. In pain clinics, 80 per cent of patients seen with cancer have pain due to direct tumour infiltration. If the pain is due to neurological infiltration it may be felt at the distribution of the nerve root. Certain pain syndromes are sufficiently common and misleading to warrant separate consideration.

Direct tumour infiltration of bone

The origin of the pain that occurs with tumour infiltration of bone is not fully understood. The periosteum is a pain-sensitive structure and may be the source in many patients. It is probable that osteolytic processes involving prostaglandins are also involved. Pain is a common feature of metastasis at the base of the skull. If the tumour is situated around the jugular foramen, pain is often referred to the vertex of the head and the ipsilateral shoulder and arm. Movement of the head may exacerbate the pain and, later, cranial nerve involvement may cause hoarseness, dysarthria, and dysphasia. Involvement of the 9th to the 12th cranial nerves, and the development of ptosis and Horner's syndrome indicates involvement of the sympathetic nervous system extracranially adjacent to the jugular foramen. When metastases occur in the sphenoid sinus, severe headache, usually felt in both temples or retro-orbitally, is a common feature. There may be a full sensation in the head, nasal stuffiness, and a 6th nerve palsy.

When metastases occur in vertebral bodies the pain frequently precedes neurological signs and symptoms. Persistent thoracic vertebral pain and a positive bone scan is an indication for urgent investigation and treatment. In small-cell lung cancer, for example, a patient with thoracic vertebral pain and a positive bone scan has a 30 per cent chance of developing a paraplegia. Ninety per cent of patients who have epidural spinal cord compression have vertebral body metastasis as the source of the epidural tumour (the management of spinal compression is described later). With metastasis to the odontoid process, patients complain of severe neck pain and stiffness radiating over the skull, up to the vertex. This is then followed by progressive neurological signs, often associated with autonomic dysfunction. In the lower cervical vertebras pain is felt as an aching sensation, often radiating over both shoulders. If nerve root compression occurs at this site, there will be pain in the root distribution felt in the back of the arm, the elbow, and the ulnar aspect of the hand. The association with Horner's syndrome suggests involvement of the paravertebral sympathetic system. Lumbar metastases are associated with local pain, worse on lying or sitting and relieved by standing. In lesions in L1 the pain is often felt over the superior iliac crests. In the sacrum, pain may be accompanied by neurological signs with symptoms of bowel and bladder dysfunction and perianal sensory loss and impotence.

When tumours infiltrate peripheral nerves they are often accompanied by an alteration in sensation, with hyperaesthesia, dysaesthesia, and sensory loss. This is a particularly common presentation when tumours invade the paravertebral or retroperitoneal region. Here the pain is often in a root distribution and is unilateral. Another common site is when a metastasis in a rib entraps the intercostal nerves. When tumour infiltrates the brachial plexus the pain is felt in the C7 or T1 distribution. Pain in this site is frequent with the Pancoast syndrome, where an apical lung cancer infiltrates the lower brachial plexus roots. Pain in the C5 distribution occurs with upper root infiltration.

Visceral pain is a frequent symptom of cancer; it can cause diagnostic confusion and be difficult to control when a tumour has already been diagnosed. Poorly localized abdominal pain is a frequent feature of ovarian and pancreatic cancer and of peritoneal carcinomatosis. Retroperitoneal pain may be particularly difficult to diagnose. It may vary greatly in position (being relieved on leaning forwards) and be felt variably in the back. Left upper quadrant pain may be a presenting feature of carcinoma of the tail of the pancreas involving the mesentery of the splenic flexure of the colon.

Weight loss

Weight loss is an invariable accompaniment of advanced cancer and also a frequent presenting symptom. Often it results from the physical presence of the tumour interfering with gastrointestinal function, such as in carcinoma of the stomach, pancreas, or colon, or with peritoneal carcinomatosis. Mechanical obstruction of the bowel and loss of appetite commonly accompany these tumours. Loss of appetite is a frequent symptom of any cancer that has metastasized to the liver and usually appears at a point when metastasis is replacing much of the normal liver tissue. The mechanism is not known. Pancreatic cancers, and cancers metastatic to the porta hepatis, cause weight loss from a malabsorption syndrome due to obstructive jaundice or blockage of the pancreatic ducts.

Nevertheless, many tumours cause weight loss without direct involvement of digestive organs. It is well recognized that a weight loss of more than 5 per cent is a very adverse prognostic feature in almost all cancers. Usually it indicates that the disease is more widespread than is apparent on clinical investigation, but the mechanisms of this symptom, which is often accompanied by alteration of taste, anorexia, and a general feeling of ill health, are obscure. Sometimes quite profound weight loss can accompany non-metastatic tumours, which are relatively small. As with advanced cancer, the cachexia syndrome is then accompanied by anorexia and altered taste. These tumours may produce circulating factors responsible for the weight loss and loss of appetite. Tumour necrosis factor-α and interleukin 1β have both been shown to produce cachexic syndromes experimentally. Tumours may themselves contribute to weight loss by alteration in protein and energy metabolism. Negative nitrogen balance has been frequently documented in patients with cancer, particularly when advanced. An increase in whole-body glucose recycling via pyruvate and lactate has also been described in patients with cancer.

The loss of body weight is therefore due to an accumulation of events involving direct interference with digestive function, production of factors leading to weight loss and anorexia by the tumour, and possible alteration in protein and energy metabolism. Later in the course of the illness, antineoplastic treatment with chemotherapy, radiation, and surgery may exacerbate weight loss.

Tumour mass

It is astonishing that patients sometimes report the appearance of a swelling only to have the significance of the finding overlooked by their doctors. The appearance of any mass should lead to prompt investigation. Although imaging techniques can sometimes distinguish benign from malignant swellings, a biopsy will usually be necessary and should be taken without delay. Nowadays it is often unnecessary to undertake surgical excision biopsy. Indeed, doing so may sometimes make subsequent management almost impossible. Where there is doubt about the nature of a swelling the correct procedure will usually be needle biopsy. Biopsy is in general preferable to aspiration cytological diagnosis because the precise diagnosis of many cancers depends on architecture as well as on cytology. The great advantage of early biopsy diagnosis is that a planned approach to treatment can then be undertaken by oncologists, radiotherapists, and surgeons together. Injudicious, and often marginal, surgical excision may lead to a greatly increased risk of local recurrence of the tumour. This is a particularly frequent occurrence in sarcomas where an avoidable amputation may then be necessary or the local recurrence provoked by inadequate excision prove uncontrollable and fatal. Furthermore, for some tumours chemotherapy may be the first line of treatment and will allow assessment of response to drug treatment before surgery is undertaken; a good response may modify the need for surgery.

Fever

In cancer, fever is usually caused by infection. However, about 30 per cent of patients with cancer develop fever at some stage in their illness and it may be the presenting feature of some tumours, particularly lymphomas, renal carcinoma, and any cancer metastatic to the liver. The fever may be accompanied by sweating, particularly at night. The characteristic feature of the sweats that accompany malignant lymphomas and other cancers is that the patient falls asleep and wakes in the middle of the night to find themselves drenched with sweat. Rigors are very uncommon with febrile episodes in cancer, and should always lead to a suspicion that an infective complication is present. Characteristic patterns of fever are seldom observed; usually it is of a low-grade remittent type. The Pel–Ebstein fever of Hodgkin's disease, in which febrile periods are interspersed with several days of normal temperature, is well known but very uncommon.

The cause of the fever of malignant disease is unknown. Endogenous pyrogens may be liberated from mononuclear phagocytes in the liver or bone marrow. Tumour cells have also been shown to produce 'pyrogens'. The nature of the cytokines responsible is not clear. Exogenously administered tumour necrosis factor and interleukin 2 both produce fever and may be secreted in patients with cancer.

The fever of malignant disease may respond to simple antipyretics such as aspirin or paracetamol. In malignant lymphoma it will disappear with successful treatment of the tumour. In advanced cancer non-steroidal anti-inflammatory agents may also help, but corticosteroids are more effective, at least for a short period.

Anaemia

The anaemia of malignant disease is multifactorial (see Section 22). Chronic blood loss may occur in cancer of the gastrointestinal tract, as a result of vaginal bleeding, or because of malabsorption of iron. Usually the anaemia is normochromic, or slightly hypochromic in nature, and the plasma transferrin and serum iron are low. The iron stores are not reduced as judged by stainable iron in the bone marrow. The mechanism is discussed in Section 22.

Hypercalcaemia

Malignant disease is responsible for most of the very severe cases of hypercalcaemia seen in clinical practice. The patient will usually have widespread skeletal metastases, but occasionally the syndrome is paraneoplastic (see below). Parathyroid hormone-related protein (PTH-rP) may contribute to the pathogenesis of both paraneoplastic hypercalcaemia and that produced by bone metastases. For some cancers it appears that metastases in bone release PTH-rP locally and stimulate osteoclastic resorption of bone. Resorption releases cytokines such as transforming growth factor-β and insulin-like growth factor 1 which, in turn, provokes more release of PTH-rP from the metastatic tumour. These cytokines may also cause proliferation of the tumour. Bisphosphonates may arrest the process by decreasing the activity of the osteoclasts. In the same way, bisphosphonates interrupt the activity of PTH-rP when this is liberated from a non-metastatic tumour as a paraneoplastic phenomenon. Bisphosphonates are important both for the treatment of hypercalcaemia and containing growth of bone metastases.

Hypercalcaemic symptoms include anorexia, weight loss, and mental confusion, all of which may simulate metastatic disease. The symptoms and signs of hypercalcaemia and its management are discussed in Sections 12 and 22.

Paraneoplastic syndromes

Many patients with cancer have complications that are not due to direct invasion of adjacent tissues by the cancer or its metastases. The tumour produces hormones or cytokines, which are responsible for symptoms at a remote site. Alternatively, the tumour provokes an immune response to altered cellular constituents and the paraneoplastic syndrome arises from the resulting immunological reaction. Paraneoplastic syndromes are not rare but each syndrome only occurs in a minority of patients with cancer. Furthermore, although some syndromes, such as the production of parathyroid hormone-related peptide, are found in many cancers, others, such as Cushing's syndrome, are found in a few neuroendocrine tumours.

It is important to be aware of paraneoplastic syndromes because their appearance may be the first sign of malignant disease. Furthermore, they may lead the physician into believing that the patient has metastases and thus alter management inappropriately. The syndromes themselves may cause considerable disability, which is amenable to treatment. The diversity of paraneoplastic syndromes is such that only a brief description can be given in this chapter. A summary is shown in Table 1.

Cancer can cause almost any clinical syndrome, however bizarre, and should, therefore, enter the list of differential diagnosis in any unusual clinical disorder. There are, however, dangers in making a diagnosis of a paraneoplastic syndrome as a cause of symptoms. For example, most neurological problems in cancer are not due to paraneoplastic manifestations but to the local presence of the tumour. This means that spinal cord signs in a patient with cancer are much more likely to be due to direct compression of the cord than due to transverse myelitis as a paraneoplastic syndrome. Prompt treatment of the space-occupying lesion is essential and a mistaken diagnosis of paraneoplasia is potentially disastrous. Similarly, endocrine syndromes from cancer are often caused by resectable endocrine cancers themselves. Anaemia or thrombosis may be paraneoplastic in origin but more frequently a deep venous thrombosis is due to a direct compressive effect of cancer in the pelvis and iron-deficiency anaemia should always raise the possibility of occult bleeding. Unless obviously paraneoplastic in nature, symptoms from cancer should, in the first instance, be regarded as likely to be produced by a direct effect of the tumour since this distinction has important therapeutic consequences. Some of these syndromes are described in detail in later sections: endocrine in Section 12, renal in Section 20, and neurological in Section 24.

Investigation and staging

Histopathological diagnosis

The foremost investigation of a cancer is to verify that the diagnosis is correct. Oncologists are completely dependent on the quality of the histopathological examination. Errors are not common but may be very serious, as they may lead to inappropriate investigation or the denial of curative treatment. The latter merits fuller consideration.

Misdiagnosis of a lymphoma

Lymphomas may present with histological appearances that resemble anaplastic or undifferentiated carcinoma. The diagnosis should therefore always be considered when this is the pathology report. Nowadays diagnosis of lymphoma has been made much easier as a result of immunohistochemical techniques. An example is shown in Fig. 1. The use of antibodies to leucocyte common antigen, or a combination of B-cell and T-cell markers are invaluable in diagnosis. If tumour cells do not stain, it makes lymphoma unlikely, but does not rule out the possibility. If positive, the diagnosis of lymphoma is virtually certain. Nevertheless, histologists may have difficulty either because the immunohistochemical technique is not sufficiently standardized in the laboratory, or because they mistake infiltrating lymphocytes for the tumour cells. Some undifferentiated pleomorphic lymphomas may be negative for leucocyte common antigen. These present formidable diagnostic difficulties, which may be resolved by examination of the tissue by molecular genetic techniques looking for rearrangement of the T-cell receptor genes or for immunoglobulin gene rearrangement. Other situations in which lymphoma may be overlooked, or a mistaken diagnosis made, are in the pulmonary lesions (or metastases) from small-cell carcinoma, which may be mistaken for lymphoma, or in biopsies from gastric ulcers where malignant lymphoma cells may wrongly be regarded as a chronic inflammatory cellular infiltrate. As non-Hodgkin's lymphomas can present in many different sites, where the diagnosis is not clear a prudent physician will always ask the pathologist whether the diagnosis of lymphoma has been firmly excluded when a diagnosis of chronic inflammation is made in an atypical clinical setting.

Mediastinal or metastatic germ cell tumours

These tumours may be mistaken for anaplastic carcinoma, but the recognition of a germ cell tumour is exceedingly important because many of them are curable. Mediastinal germ cell tumours typically present in young adults and with cervical node metastases. Special stains or serum tests for α-fetoprotein or β-human chorionic gonadotrophin may be very helpful, but if negative, do not exclude the diagnosis. Several reports have indicated that the use of intensive combination chemotherapy, as for germ cell tumours at other sites, may result in lasting remissions of mediastinal poorly differentiated tumours in young adults, even when there were no other features of the germ cell nature of the neoplasm. In contrast, poorly differentiated adenocarcinoma in the mediastinum of young adults can seldom be ascribed to germ cell tumour, although occasional cases may respond dramatically to chemotherapy.

Investigating the local extent of the tumour

Following diagnosis, clinical staging is the most important first procedure. Clinical examination will often establish the likely extent of the tumour. This may require specialized techniques such as ear, nose, and throat examination and bronchoscopy. The extent of infiltration and fixation to surrounding structures is assessed. CT scanning and MRI have greatly improved the preoperative determination of tumour extent. They have largely replaced more invasive techniques such as angiography and lymphangiography. MRI is particularly valuable in the staging of sarcomas and central nervous system tumours. Both techniques show the extent of the tumour and infiltration of surrounding structures (Figs 2(a and b)). CT scanning is a particularly valuable aid to needle biopsy diagnosis of deep-seated tumours.

Staging of lymph node spread

Spread to adjacent lymph nodes may be noted clinically or on straightforward investigations, such as chest radiography. Lymphangiography was used formerly to examine pelvic and lower para-aortic nodes but has largely been supplanted by CT. In fact the two techniques give slightly different information, as a CT scan will show enlarged lymph nodes (the assumption being that these are replaced by tumour when the lymph nodes become more than 2 cm in size), while lymphangiography may show abnormal appearances even when the nodes are not enlarged but contain foci of tumour cells within them.

Table 1 Paraneoplastic syndromes

Syndrome	Clinical features	Tumour	Comments
*Endocrine syndromes**			
Cushing's syndrome	Metabolic features (BP ↑ K$^+$↓ glucose ↑) are severe. Obesity, etc. occur in slower growing SCLC tumours	SCLC, carcinoid, other neuroendocrine tumours	Pro-opiocortin produced by tumour. Occurs in 0.5% of cases. Immunoreactive ACTH ↑ in many more. In SCLC, chemotherapy may help the syndrome. In other tumours resection is curative
Antidiuretic hormone excess	Low plasma sodium (less than 130 mmol/l with continued urine sodium excretion; below 120 mmol/l altered mental state, confusion, fits, coma, death)	SCLC	Tumour produces ADH. Slightly low plasma Na is common feature of all advanced cancer (due to pituitary ADH release). Treatment is by water restriction and demeclocycline. Hypertonic saline in emergency
Hypercalcaemia	Symptoms of hypercalcaemia often very severe	Squamous cancers	Immunoreactive PTH-related peptide. Possibly release of cytokines (IL-1β, osteoclast activating factors) in some cases. Treatment described in Chapter 12.6
		T-cell leukaemia Some lymphomas	
Gonadotrophin excess	Gynaecomastia in men, oligomenorrhoea, thyroid overactivity	Gestational trophoblastic tumours	β-hCG produced in excess. Clinical syndromes are uncommon. Mechanism of clinical syndrome is incompletely understood
		Germ cell tumours Adenocarcinoma of the lung Hepatoblastoma Other adenocarcinomas	
Hypoglycaemia	Clinical features are of hypoglycaemia	Sarcoma	Major mechanism is non-suppressible insulin-like activity (NSILA, somatomedins) and insulin-like growth factors. Mesothelioma is usually abdominal
	Tumours are usually large	Mesothelioma Hepatoma Adrenal carcinoma	
Osteomalacia	Vitamin-D-resistant rickets with bone pain, phosphaturia	Benign mesenchyme tumours, fibromas, haemangiomas in soft tissue and bone	Low 1,25-OH vitamin D, low PTH. Treatment requires large doses of vitamin D and removal of tumour
Neurological syndromes			
Dementia	Variable-onset dementia	Lung cancer (SCLC)	May be due to vascular endothelial disorder induced by the tumour
Cerebellar degeneration	Subacute and progressive associated with dementia	Hodgkin's disease, uterine and ovarian cancer	CSF[1] protein raised and lymphocytosis
Limbic 'encephalitis'	Dementia	SCLC	Pathologically there is hippocampal degeneration
		Hodgkin's disease	
Optic neuritis	Visual failure, papilloedema often bilateral	SCLC	Produced by antibodies (? to altered tumour-related proteins) which bind to retinal ganglion cell
Myelopathy	Rapid-onset cord degeneration often mid-thoracic. Usually quickly fatal	SCLC	CSF[1] protein elevated
Amyotrophic lateral sclerosis	Lower motor neurone weakness combined with spasticity fasciculation. Mostly in men. Slow course	Various	Cancer found in 5–10% of cases of ALS
Peripheral neuropathy	Either pure sensory neuropathy or a severe sensorimotor neuropathy	SCLC. Other intrathoracic tumours (thymoma, oesophageal cancer, lymphoma)	CSF[1] protein may be elevated. May antedate tumour. Often does not improve if tumour removed. Sensory neuropathy is due to dorsal root ganglion degeneration and specific antibodies have been found
Guillain–Barré syndrome	Typical clinical features	Lymphomas	Association frequently noted but ? genuine
Dermatological syndromes			
Acanthosis nigricans	Hyperkeratosis and pigmentation in axillas, neck, and flexures	Gastric, other intra-abdominal	There is a congenital form which must be distinguished
Seborrhoeic keratoses	Sudden onset of keratoses (Leser–Tralat syndrome)	Gut, non-Hodgkin's lymphoma	Keratoses appear quickly in large numbers

Table 1 *Continued*

Syndrome	Clinical features	Tumour	Comments
Exfoliative dermatitis	Severe erythema and scaling	Lymphomas, especially T-cell type	Common cause of exfoliative dermatitis Responds to steroids and treatment of lymphoma
Migratory erythema	Blistering, necrotic erythema	Glucagonoma	
Panniculitis	Crops of tender, subcutaneous lesions which look like erythema nodosum	Pancreas	Probably due to fat inflammation caused by liberation of pancreatic lipases
Porphyria cutanea tarda	Nodular or erythematous skin lesions. Photosensitive	Hepatocellular carcinoma	Very uncommon
Ichthyosis	Dry scaly skin with hyperkeratosis of palms and soles	Lymphomas	Different from congenital form, which may be accompanied by carcinoma of oesophagus
Musculoskeletal syndromes			
Finger clubbing and hypertrophic pulmonary osteoarthropathy	Clubbing of finger nails. Tenderness over distal ends of radius and ulna, and tibia and fibula. Periosteal reaction on radiography	Bronchial carcinoma (not SCLC), benign mesothelioma, diaphragmatic neurilemmoma	One of the great unsolved mysteries of medicine. Cause unknown
Dermatomyositis	Erythema of face—cheeks, eyelids— and over backs of hands	Wide variety of cancers, especially adenocarcinoma	May precede cancer by 6–24 months. In middle age approx. 30% of cases have underlying malignancy
Lambert–Eaton syndrome	A myasthenic syndrome with muscle weakness, especially in thighs and pelvis. Ptosis, dysarthria, double vision occur. EMG shows increase in action potential with repeated stimulation	SCLC	Syndrome often antedates cancer. Muscle strength does not deteriorate with exercise. An IgG autoantibody to voltage-gated calcium channels reduces acetylcholine release. Responds to treatment of tumour and to guanidine
Haematological syndromes			
Autoimmune haemolytic anaemia	Anaemia may be the presenting symptom. Splenomegaly may occur. Response to steroids is poor. May be associated with ITP	Non-Hodgkin's lymphoma (B-cell type), wide variety of epithelial cancers	Antibodies to red cell antigens.

? cross-react with altered tumour surface antigens. Remits with successful treatment |
Microangiopathic haemolytic anaemia	Mild forms are common, clinically apparent cases rare	Mucin-producing adenocarcinomas	May respond to anticancer treatment. Procoagulant appears to be produced by the tumour
Thrombocytosis	Usually asymptomatic. Mild elevation of platelet count is common. Thrombosis of haemorrhage is rare	Carcinoma, Hodgkin's disease	The tumour-associated cytokine has not yet been identified
Granulocytosis	Usually asymptomatic. Modest elevations frequently found with liver metastases	Adenocarcinomas, melanoma	Blood film does not show immature forms. CSFs[2] are assumed responsible, but IL-1 and IL-3 have been implicated in some tumours
Erythrocytosis	Elevated Hb with normal	$P_{a}o_2$ and Hb electrophoresis	Renal carcinoma, Wilms' tumour, adrenal tumours, hepatomas

Erythrocytosis resolves with removal of primary. Erythropoietin is made by the tumour or its release is stimulated |

These are some of the most common paraneoplastic syndromes.

*The endocrine syndromes are those where the hormonal syndrome is produced by a non-endocrine cancer.

ACTH, adrenocorticotrophic hormone; ADH, antidiuretic hormone; ALS, amyotrophic lateral sclerosis; BP, blood pressure; CSF[1], cerebrospinal fluid; CSF[2], colony-stimulating factor; EMG, electromyography; Hb, haemoglobin; hCG, human chorionic gonadotrophin; IL, interleukin; ITP, idiopathic thrombocytopenia

Staging for distant metastases

Bone metastases are usually demonstrated by $^{99}Tc^m$-polyphosphate isotopic scanning. The sensitivity of the examination is high and abnormalities frequently precede detectable changes on plain radiography. However, the specificity is rather lower because any traumatic or inflammatory disorder in bone can give areas of increased uptake. When areas of increased uptake are seen on technetium scanning it is important to follow up with plain skeletal radiography, particularly in the long bones of the limbs. This is because isotope scanning gives no indication of the structural integrity of the bone and the risk of pathological fracture in a limb cannot be assessed on an isotope scan.

Liver metastases are detected by an increase in circulating enzyme levels, particularly alkaline phosphatase and serum glutamic oxaloacetic transaminase. Lactic dehydrogenase is also elevated in a somewhat greater frequency. Nevertheless, liver metastases can be present without alteration in serum enzyme levels and ultrasound scanning is an invaluable non-invasive method of detecting liver metastases. CT and modern ultrasound scanning are approximately equal in sensitivity. Metastases down to 1 cm in size can be detected reliably.

Pulmonary metastases may be detected on chest radiograph but may be present even when the chest radiograph is normal if they are below 1.5 cm in size. Metastases larger than this may also be overlooked if they are situated behind the heart or behind the diaphragm. CT scanning is the best

(a)

(b)

Fig. 1 (a) Section stained with haematoxylin and eosin of excision specimen of a retroperitoneal mass. The tumour is poorly differentiated, with fibrosis and infiltration of retroperitoneal fat. (b) Immunostaining with an antibody of CD20 (a B-lymphocyte marker) shows intense staining of tumour cells confirming that this is a B-cell non-Hodgkin's lymphoma.

method for demonstrating pulmonary metastases and lesions as small as 0.4 cm in diameter may be seen. CT scanning is therefore an essential investigation in patients who are to undergo extensive or mutilating surgery, such as for sarcomas where metastases to the lungs are particularly frequent and the presence of metastases may influence the surgical decision.

Brain metastases are detected by CT scanning or, more reliably, by MRI. In a patient who is neurologically normal there is only a low chance of detecting asymptomatic cerebral metastasis by these methods (about 5 per cent). For this reason the technique is not worthwhile as a routine investigation of most cancers.

Surgical staging of cancer

Surgery specifically for staging rather than treatment is reserved for a few specific tumour sites. In lung cancer, investigation of the mediastinum is extremely important in deciding whether a tumour is operable. CT scanning may demonstrate inoperability either because the tumour is infiltrating the mediastinum or because there is lymph node spread to both ipsilateral and contralateral hilar nodes. However, in other patients, the mediastinum may appear normal and a mediastinoscopy may reveal tumour in mediastinal nodes implying the inoperability of the condition. Staging laparotomy used to be performed in localized Hodgkin's disease, but is now reserved for specific indications. In ovarian cancer thorough surgical staging is performed at the time of the initial resection, but surgical

staging is in this case (as in many other tumour resections) part of the treatment.

An important recent development has been the introduction of so-called 'sentinel node' biopsy. In this technique a radioactive tracer, or a blue dye, is injected in the vicinity of the tumour, or into the tumour itself, and the lymph node at the first adjacent site of uptake is sampled, either by biopsy or surgical removal. In the case of breast cancer, the disease in which the technique is exciting most interest, the sampling may be at the time of operation. The presence or absence of tumour cells in the lymph node is taken as an indication of whether lymphatic spread has occurred and surgery, and subsequent treatment, can be modified accordingly. There are unresolved issues about accuracy of the technique, and the confidence with

(a)

(b)

Fig. 2 (a) Longitudinal MRI of lower thigh. A large, soft tissue mass is seen displacing the muscle groups posteriorly. It lies behind the femur and the femoral artery is in close proximity to the mass, which at one point surrounds it. (b) CT scan of abdomen. A carcinoma of the body of the pancreas is shown (arrowed). The liver contains numerous small metastases.

which the results can be used to plan therapy, but it is likely that the procedure will become part of the lymph node staging of some cancers.

The use of a staging notation

This has been valuable in the reporting of results of cancer treatment and is also helpful, in an individual patient, in focusing attention on the extent of the disease and the subsequent planning of treatment. A widely used system is the **T** (tumour) **N** (nodes) **M** (metastasis) system. This is particularly valuable for tumours that follow an orderly progression of spread from the primary site to adjacent lymph nodes and then to metastatic sites. Thus, tumours of the head and neck, breast, non-small-cell lung cancer, renal carcinoma, bladder carcinoma, and rectal carcinoma are all well-defined by this means. In addition to the TNM system, many classifications contain a stage grouping, by which tumours with varying TNM assignments are grouped together because of equivalence of prognosis or similar approaches to management. An example of the TNM staging system and stage grouping for lung cancer is given in Table 2.

Not all tumours can be summarized by the TNM system. For example, small-cell lung cancer is usually widely metastatic at the time of presentation and a simpler classification into limited (confined to one side of the thorax with ipsilateral supraclavicular node) or extensive (disease that is bilateral within the chest or metastatic) is used. This simple classification serves to separate patients in whom radiation treatment may be worthwhile and those in whom it is unlikely to have any benefit. In leukaemia and myeloma, other staging criteria, which are based on prognostic factors and are not related to anatomical stage, have been developed. In Hodgkin's disease and non-Hodgkin's lymphoma, the presence (B) or absence (A) of constitutional symptoms is added to the anatomical staging system, which is used to define the degree of lymph node spread. These additions were made because the presence of constitutional symptoms confers an adverse prognostic significance in addition to the prognosis related to the anatomical stage (see also Section 22).

Principles of cancer management

The principles and details of cancer chemotherapy are discussed elsewhere. This section summarizes an integrated approach towards cancer management.

Nowadays the management of cancer will nearly always involve more than one specialist and more than one type of treatment. Increasingly,

Table 2 Staging of non-small cell lung cancer

T_1	< 3 cm diameter		
T_2	> 3 cm diameter but		
	> 2 cm distal to carina, may be visceral pleural invasion		
T_3	Involves chest wall or mediastinum		
T_4	Invades heart, great vessels, trachea or oesophagus, malignant pleural effusion		
N_0	No involved nodes		
N_1	Ipsilateral peribronchial or hilar nodes		
N_2	Ipsilateral mediastinal or subcarinal		
N_3	Contralateral nodes or supraclavicular nodes		
M_0	No distant metastases		
M_1	Distant metastases		
Stage grouping			
Stage 1	$T_{1, 2}$	N_0	M_0
Stage 2	$T_{1, 2}$	N_1	M_0
Stage 3a	$T_{1, 2}$	N_2	M_0
	T_3	N_{0-2}	M_0
Stage 3b	Any T	N_3	M_0
	T_4	Any N	M_0
Stage 4	Any T	Any N	M_1

Table 3 The management of tumours

Chemotherapy (including endocrine therapy)	Radiotherapy
May be curative in:	*May be curative in:*
Hodgkin's disease	Localized Hodgkin's disease
Non-Hodgkin's lymphoma	Non-Hodgkin's lymphoma
Germ cell tumours	Stage II seminoma
Wilm's tumour	Head and neck cancer
Ewing's sarcoma	
Osteosarcoma	
Rhabdomyosarcoma	
Leukaemia	
Adds to cure rate in:	*Adds to cure rate in:*
Stage II breast cancer	Ewing's sarcoma
? Colorectal cancer	Localized breast cancer
Ovarian cancer	Small-cell lung cancer
Small-cell lung cancer	Anal cancer
	Cervical cancer
	Skin cancer
	Rectal cancer
Produces remission and/or prolongs survival in:	*Produces remission and/or prolongs survival in:*
Small-cell lung cancer	Non-small cell lung cancer
Advanced breast cancer	Glioma
Prostate cancer	Prostate cancer
Ovarian cancer	Biliary tract cancer
Myeloma	
Palliates:	*Palliates:*
Non-Hodgkin's lymphoma (when incurable)	Small-cell lung cancer (extensive)
Bone metastases	Non-small-cell lung cancer
Brain metastases	Rectal cancer
	Oesophageal cancer

patients with cancer are being seen in joint clinics where surgeons, medical oncologists, and radiotherapists plan treatment. Often there will be several possible approaches towards treatment, and these require discussion and assessment by the appropriate experts. It is of inestimable value if a patient is referred for expert opinion before any definitive procedure is undertaken. For example, more information about gynaecological malignancy can often be obtained if a patient with abdominal swelling and ascites and an ultrasound-demonstrable mass in the pelvis is assessed preoperatively by a gynaecological oncologist. The subsequent laparotomy is likely to reveal much more information than if it is carried out as an emergency by an inexperienced surgeon. Similarly, a mass on a limb should be investigated thoroughly, including a biopsy diagnosis, before surgery is undertaken, because the nature of the histological diagnosis may profoundly alter management in the case of a sarcoma. Table 3 lists tumours in which radiotherapy and chemotherapy have an important part to play in management and where these modalities of treatment may sometimes be curative.

Surgery

Surgeons see over 80 per cent of patients presenting with cancer for the first time. Following diagnosis and staging to exclude metastases, curative surgery may be undertaken, for example in breast or colorectal cancer. The aim of the operation is complete excision of the tumour with a margin of normal, uninvolved tissue around the main tumour mass. The risk of local recurrence is very high with a marginal excision in which a tumour has been 'shelled out' because the pseudocapsule around the tumour is likely to be infiltrated with tumour cells. Removal or sampling of the draining lymph nodes will often be undertaken, for example in breast cancer and other tumours where involvement of regional lymph nodes is likely (see the discussion of sentinel node biopsy above). In some cancers, such as breast cancer, it has become clear that very extensive primary tumours are usually accompanied by distant metastasis. In this situation the role of surgery is to prevent local recurrence rather than to be curative. With other tumours, for example of the head and neck, extensive surgery may be the only means of gaining effective control and in these cases a considerable degree of surgical expertise is necessary. In some situations the tumour may be approached either by surgery or by radical radiotherapy and there may be little to choose between the results. An example is in early prostate cancer where the results of radical radiation and surgery are probably equivalent, and in operable oesophageal cancer, particularly of squamous histology, where long-term results of radiation may be the same as those of surgery. In these situations the benefits of local control, survival, and long-term side-effects have to be judged together in making a decision.

Nowadays local treatment frequently involves surgery and radiation to maximize the chances of local control. Wide local excision is increasingly practised in carcinoma of the breast and radiation to the breast and to axillary nodes is used as an adjunct. Radiation reduces the risk of local relapse, both in the breast and in the axilla. 'Lumpectomy' and radical radiotherapy have now replaced mastectomy for many patients with small primary breast cancers. Preoperative radiation of soft tissue sarcoma may increase the chance of successful compartmental excision of the tumour, and postoperative radiation decreases the risk of local recurrence in patients in whom the excision has been marginal. These are two examples of the way in which the definitive local management of the primary tumour is a matter of discussion between surgical and radiation oncologists.

Optimum local management has become further complicated by the successful use of chemotherapy in many tumours. An example is the treatment of Ewing's tumour. In this highly malignant round-cell tumour of childhood, initial chemotherapy usually produces a prompt regression of the main tumour mass, both in the bone and in the surrounding soft tissues. However, the tumour permeates widely through the bone, and local irradiation, given after initial chemotherapy, is a standard means of maintaining local control. There is an increasing tendency to continue both chemotherapy and radiation synchronously. However, in large tumours, even with full-dose radiation, the risk of local relapse is still present. For this reason surgery is being used increasingly, provided that the cosmetic and functional results are reasonable. Surgical excision alone may be successful after chemotherapy, but frequently, because of the permeating nature of the tumour, viable tumour is present right up to the resection margins of the bone. In this situation radiation will be needed in addition to the chemotherapy and surgery. In these tumours, very detailed planning of the approach to treatment by experienced specialists is essential for optimum results.

Specific management problems

Spinal cord and cauda equina compression

Cord and cauda equina compression are common and devastating complications of metastatic cancer. For successful management it is essential to remember one rule—every hour counts. Even if early treatment is not always successful, delay ensures that the patient will end his or her days bed- or chair-bound, paralysed, and incontinent.

The metastasis often develops in a vertebra, from which it spreads directly or via the intervertebral foramina to compress the cord (or cauda equina below L1) from the extradural space (Fig. 3). Alternatively, the malignant mass may originate in a mass of retroperitoneal nodes, or the primary tumour (for example a bronchial carcinoma) may be in the posterior mediastinum or retroperitoneum (Fig. 3). Damage to the cord is by direct compression and by interruption of the arterial supply leading to infarction. It is uncommon for the tumour to be metastatic to the cord itself, although meningeal spread occurs and may cause compression (see carcinomatous meningitis, below). Cord compression may be the first manifestation of cancer but more commonly arises with metastases from a known primary.

Fig. 3 MRI of thoracic vertebras showing destruction of the body of T10 by a mass of Hodgkin's disease. The tumour extends posteriorly and compresses the spinal cord. The tumour mass has passed to the side of the vertebra (not shown), and is also compressing the cord posteriorly after infiltrating into the intervertebral foramen.

Pain often precedes the onset of neurological symptoms. In the case of cord compression it is felt in the thoracic and cervical vertebras. It is worse on coughing. An exceedingly sinister symptom is vertebral pain with a root distribution. A patient with this symptom needs urgent investigation, as cord compression may be imminent. The next symptom is usually weakness of the legs combined with sensory loss, of which loss of proprioception is especially characteristic. Loss of bladder and bowel sensation is late and once weakness and bladder disturbance begins, progression to irreversible paraplegia occurs in hours or a few days.

The patient often has a sensory level, motor weakness, brisk leg reflexes, and extensor plantar responses. The bladder may be palpable. Radiography of the spine often shows vertebral destruction—loss of a pedicle or compression of the body being typical. Myelography will demonstrate the block, but MRI (and, less reliably, CT scanning) is very valuable and has now largely replaced myelography. Treatment usually consists of surgical decompression, although for radiation-sensitive tumours such as lymphoma or Ewing's sarcoma, high-dose corticosteroids and radiation will produce quick relief of compression. If there are multiple sites of block, radiation and steroids may be the only feasible option. The surgical approach to decompression varies according to the nature of the lesion—whether anterior or posterior, cervical or thoracic. Anterior decompression may involve removal of part of the vertebral body, but the risk of destabilization of the spine means that immediate stabilization may be necessary. It is not clear whether radiation is inferior to surgical decompression in patients with tumours that show sensitivity to radiation. Radiation is, in any event, usually given after laminectomy.

Outcome is crucially dependent on the functional state of the patient before treatment. Less than 10 per cent of those who are paraplegic before treatment will be able to walk later, 25 per cent will do so if they have some motor function preserved, while almost all patients who can still walk will continue to be able to do so.

Cerebral metastasis

Cerebral metastasis is clearly a serious complication of cancer occurring in about 30 per cent of all patients. Metastases are over 10 times as common as primary brain tumours. About 15 per cent of patients with cancer will develop symptomatic brain metastases during life. Thus, there will be approximately 15 000 deaths each year in the United Kingdom of patients with symptomatic cerebral metastasis. Metastasis at this site is life-threatening and disabling, causing severe deterioration in quality of life and great difficulty for the patient and his or her carers.

Most cerebral metastases are intradural, usually in the substance of the brain extending to the meningeal surface. About 80 per cent of these are situated in the cerebrum and the rest in the cerebellum and other regions. Lung cancer and breast cancer are the most common primary sites, and certain tumours are particularly associated with single metastases (cancer of the breast, ovary, and kidney). Usually cerebral metastases occur following diagnosis and treatment of a primary tumour.

In the brain substance, the metastases are vascularized from the cerebral circulation, but there is no evidence that a vascularized metastasis maintains a 'blood–brain' barrier—the vascularization is, after all, of non-nervous tissue without the tight endothelial junctions which characterize cerebral capillaries. Indeed, capillary leakiness appears to be a feature of cerebral metastasis and is responsible for the substantial amount of oedema of the brain, which typically accompanies cerebral metastasis. The blood–brain barrier may, however, be an important impediment to cytotoxic treatment when the metastasis is being established before it is vascularized and at the periphery of an established metastasis. It will be a very significant factor in failure of treatment of leptomeningeal cancer.

Symptoms and signs

The typical signs are headache, disturbance of cognitive function and effect, focal fits or grand mal convulsions, and limb paresis. Headache usually reflects a rise in intracranial pressure. It is typically present in the morning and increases in duration and frequency until other signs of raised intracranial pressure become apparent. Focal weakness is present in about half of all patients, and disturbance in higher cerebral function in about 60 per cent.

Investigation

CT scanning or MRI is the essential diagnostic investigation. On a CT scan most metastases appear hypodense but enhance with contrast material. Typically there will be oedema around the metastases. Occasionally CT scans may be normal even in patients whose symptoms strongly suggest cerebral metastasis and where cerebral metastasis is sometimes proved by further scanning some weeks later or at autopsy. In these patients there may be multiple small metastases without oedema or leptomeningeal spread. MRI has a greater degree of sensitivity and is particularly valuable in detecting leptomeningeal spread of tumour. In the presence of a known primary it is not usually necessary to subject patients to histological confirmation of the tumour. However, after a very long disease-free interval, or where the primary is unknown, histological diagnosis will be essential.

Treatment

Dexamethasone is started as soon as the diagnosis is made. The usual dose is approximately 16 mg/day, although higher doses can be used if the patient does not respond. The clinical effects are rapid and usually noticeable within 24 h. The maximum effect is achieved in about 4 days. Approximately 80 per cent of patients will respond. Phenytoin or carbamazepine are used to control focal fits.

The most useful non-surgical treatment is radiation therapy. The therapeutic doses depend on the likely primary site, but usually consist of 30 Gy in 10 fractions in 2 weeks, or 40 Gy in 15 fractions in 3 weeks. The former is the most widely used schedule in the United Kingdom and no schedule has been proved to be superior over another. Solitary cerebral metastases may be removed if they are in an accessible site. The criteria for operation are usually that a solitary metastasis is present, that the diagnosis is uncertain, or that the response to radiation is unpredictable because of doubt about the nature of the primary tumour. The patient must be clinically fit in other respects to undergo surgery, and without life-threatening metastatic disease elsewhere.

There has been recent interest in the use of chemotherapy in the treatment of cerebral metastasis, as it is now clear, for example in small-cell lung cancer, that the response to chemotherapy in cerebral metastases is equal to that in metastases at other sites. Responses to chemotherapy in tumours such as small-cell lung cancer may be rapid and dramatic but cranial radiation will usually be necessary as an adjunct to chemotherapy.

Prognosis

The prognosis depends on the clinical setting. If there is a solitary metastasis with no disease elsewhere then a long disease-free interval may result, particularly if the metastasis has occurred after a considerable interval following the primary treatment. In other tumours, where multiple metastases occur either synchronously with the primary tumour or after a short disease-free interval, and where the tumour is a particularly difficult type to treat (such as melanoma and non-small-cell lung cancer), the prognosis is very poor indeed. Overall, only 30 per cent of patients will be alive at 1 year and the median survival is about 7 months. A small randomized trial has suggested that surgical resection of a solitary metastasis adds to survival when compared with radiation and steroids alone.

Carcinomatous 'meningitis'

Leptomeningeal spread of cancer seems to be increasing in frequency. In autopsy series about 4 per cent of patients dying of advanced cancer have leptomeningeal spread. The frequency is higher in breast cancer (5 to 10 per cent). This complication is increasing in lymphoma, small-cell lung cancer, ovarian cancer, and some sarcomas. Curiously, adenocarcinomas seem to have a greater propensity for this form of metastasis than other epithelial tumours. There may or may not be intracerebral metastasis at the same time. Malignant cells may enter the cerebrospinal fluid from intracerebral tumour via the arachnoid, or from vertebral deposits growing along nerve roots into the subarachnoid space. However, the most likely source of seeding appears to be directly from the bloodstream. Tumour is present as a thin covering of malignant cells, but in some cases the tumour cells penetrate deeper into the substance of the brain along blood vessels. The tumour may also penetrate cranial and spinal cord nerves as they pass through the subarachnoid space.

Clinical features

The onset is usually over a few weeks and may be subtle at first. Headache is often severe and is due to raised intracranial pressure. Cranial nerve dysfunction is frequent, with diplopia, hearing loss, and facial numbness. There is often back pain and sometimes bladder and bowel dysfunction. A change in mental state may occur. Focal fits are uncommon. On examination there may be an abnormal mental state, signs of raised intracranial pressure, and extensor plantar responses. Focal neurological signs in the limbs are uncommon. Cranial nerve weaknesses are frequent, the most common being ocular muscle palsy, facial weakness, and hearing loss.

Diagnosis and treatment

The diagnosis is made by examining the cerebrospinal fluid. Typically, the opening pressure is high, the white count is raised, the cerebrospinal fluid sugar low, and the protein increased. Cytological confirmation on the first lumbar puncture is obtained in about 60 per cent of patients, but a negative examination does not exclude the diagnosis. Myelography may show typical appearance of multiple small tumour seeds in the subarachnoid space, but MRI is proving invaluable and is now the preferred initial investigation if cerebrospinal fluid cytology is negative and the diagnosis strongly suspected.

Treatment is difficult and often unsuccessful. Temporary improvement can be obtained by the insertion of an intraventricular reservoir to deliver chemotherapy. Chemotherapy administered by lumbar puncture is uncomfortable and may not be effective if there is meningeal invasion supratentorially, since the drugs do not penetrate in high concentration beyond the foramen magnum. In breast cancer and lymphoma, intrathecal methotrexate is effective and may be administered in combination with thiotepa or, in the case of lymphoma, cytosine arabinoside. In addition, whole-brain irradiation is often given if the patient is improving and the clinical situation indicates that this treatment would produce further benefit. In general, however, the prognosis is poor when the meningeal infiltration is from an epithelial tumour, with a median survival of only 4 months.

Pleural effusion

Malignant pleural effusions occur either as a sign of metastasis or due to direct invasion of the pleural space from an underlying primary bronchial carcinoma, or pulmonary metastasis. The effusions are typically exudates with a protein content of more than 3 g/dl. There is increased capillary permeability through inflammation and abnormal capillary endothelium in the tumour lining the pleural space. Typical primary sites are: breast and ovarian cancer, as common epithelial tumours metastasize into the pleural space; lung cancer, as a cause of pleural effusion with underlying lung disease; and sarcomas, as a cause of pleural effusion due to invasion of the pleura by pulmonary metastasis.

Clinical features

The typical features are dyspnoea, which is directly related to the size of the effusion, dry cough, and chest wall discomfort. Even a small effusion may cause dyspnoea in a patient who has underlying lung disease such as chronic bronchitis and emphysema. Many patients have asymptomatic pleural effusions detectable on chest radiograph. The sequence of radiological appearances includes blunting of the costaphrenic angle (with volumes of 2 to 3 ml), increasing effusion, and, finally, mediastinal shift, which usually occurs when amounts in excess of 2 litres have accumulated. Ultrasound examination may assist in localizing the effusion and any loculi, which may influence the procedure for aspiration.

Diagnosis

The diagnosis, if the primary tumour is not known, is made by demonstrating malignant cells in the pleural fluid. The rate of positivity, in patients known to have an underlying cancer, is about 60 per cent with a low false-positive rate. If pleural cytology is negative on the first aspiration it should be repeated using fresh aspirates. Occasionally, pleural biopsy will be necessary to make a diagnosis, and the combination of the two increase the diagnostic yield to about 90 per cent. If both techniques fail, thoracoscopy is more successful, but is, of course, more invasive.

Treatment and prognosis

The primary tumour should be treated if possible. When a pleural effusion persists after treatment of the primary tumour, or if such treatment has been unsuccessful, treatment may need to be directed to the effusion itself. Frequently the effusion will need to be aspirated in order to make the patient comfortable, and pleural sclerotherapy considered. For best results of sclerotherapy it is important to drain the pleural cavity as completely as possible. A small flexible chest drain is ideal and is left in place for some time (12 to 24 h if possible) to allow the fluid to drain as far as possible. If there has been loculated effusion, the insertion of the drain is best done under ultrasound control. Sclerosis of the two pleural surfaces can be achieved by a variety of means; all give approximately equivalent results. The most favoured techniques are the instillation of talc, tetracycline, bleomycin, or *Corynebacterium parvum*. They all cause an inflammatory reaction in the pleural space and have an approximately 60 per cent success rate in preventing immediate recurrence of the effusion. When pleural effusion complicates an underlying bronchial carcinoma it is more difficult to control than when it is a metastatic manifestation of a distant neoplasm, such as ovarian cancer. If the effusion is recurrent and is the major cause of morbidity, pleuroperitoneal shunting can be carried out, whereby the pleural fluid drains into the peritoneal cavity.

Pericardial effusion

The most common malignancies to cause pericardial effusion are breast, lung, ovary, and gastrointestinal cancers and non-Hodgkin's lymphomas. Pathologically, the pericardium may be infiltrated with tumour or diffusely nodular. The accumulation of fluid is due to obstruction of lymphatic and venous drainage of the pericardium.

Symptoms and signs

The symptoms are usually vague in onset, including orthopnoea, dyspnoea, and cough. Fatigue and dizziness also develop. If cardiac tamponade occurs it is associated with severe dyspnoea, vague central chest pain, and anxiety. The physical signs are usually minimal, although when tamponade occurs there will be jugular venous distension, pulses paradoxus, hypotension, and tachycardia.

Investigation

Investigations include a chest radiograph, which shows enlargement of the cardiac silhouette, and echocardiography, which is a rapid non-invasive technique for demonstrating pericardial effusion.

Diagnosis and management

The diagnosis is made by finding malignant cells in the pericardial fluid. False negative results occur and the test may need to be repeated. Once the diagnosis has been established, the pericardial fluid may need drainage using a small rubber catheter. Installation of sclerosants can be carried out as for pleural effusions, but troublesome pericardial effusions can be controlled by the formation of a pericardial window through a small left anterior thoracotomy. Some patients, particularly those who have lymphoma, will respond to external-beam radiation with a dose of approximately 30 Gy given in 15 fractions over a 2- to 3-week period. Radiation is also considered for control of chronic pericardial effusion in breast cancer. The management of cardiac tamponade is discussed in Section 15.

Metastatic cancer from an unknown primary site

Approximately 3 per cent of patients present with a metastasis from a cancer where the primary site is not known after full history, physical examination, blood count, and chest radiograph. This clinical situation requires considerable clinical expertise, as the diagnosis creates especial anxiety for the patient. The clinician has to decide on the most effective therapy and to sustain the patient without indulging in futile, invasive, and expensive investigations which will not alter management. The problem with extensive investigations is that they seldom alter management and the overall prognosis in this position is poor (4 to 6 months median survival). As one investigation after another fails to reveal the primary site, the patient and the doctor may come to consider this a failure and confidence can be badly shaken. Nevertheless, some tumours are potentially curable and, for these, investigation is justified. The common primary sites, when one is discovered, are cancers of the lung, pancreas, liver, gut, and stomach. The tumours for which therapy is possible, and which therefore must not be overlooked, are listed in Table 4.

Presentation

If the presentation is exclusively in cervical nodes, a full ear, nose, and throat examination is mandatory as local treatment with surgery and/or radiation may produce prolonged survival or even cure. The higher the cervical node, the more likely it is that and ear, nose, and throat tumour is the primary source. Supraclavicular lymph nodes carry a worse prognosis because the likely primary site on the right-hand side is the lung or breast, and on the left-hand side intra-abdominal malignancy via the thoracic duct. Patients presenting with lymph node enlargement in the axilla are likely to have breast cancer as the primary site and this may not be excluded even with normal mammograms. Malignant melanoma is another possibility at this site and a careful examination for skin lesions should be made. Inguinal lymph nodes usually point to a primary site in the pelvis, vulva or

Table 4 Metastasis from an unknown primary site. Possibilities for treatment

Potentially curable tumours
Germ cell tumours
Lymphomas
Trophoblastic tumours
Effective palliative chemotherapy
Breast cancer
Small-cell lung cancer
Ovarian cancer
Palliative hormonal therapy
Prostate cancer
Breast cancer
Endometrial cancer
Effective (potentially curative) local therapy
Head and neck cancer

rectum, or prostate. Malignant melanoma may present with an inguinal mass. Cutaneous metastasis typically occurs from carcinomas of the lung, breast, and melanomas. A pulmonary metastasis may arise from a variety of different sites, including breast, kidney, gut, melanoma, and sarcoma. In the liver, the likely source for the primary will be the gastrointestinal tract, although breast and lung primaries are other possibilities. A metastasis presenting in bone is particularly likely to occur from a cancer of the lung, breast, or prostate, the last being particularly likely if there is a mixed lytic and osteoblastic radiological appearance.

Investigation

The most important single investigation is a review of the histology. The clinician should discuss the diagnosis with the pathologist so that appropriate tests can be carried out. It is absolutely essential to distinguish between an epithelial tumour, a sarcoma, and a lymphoma. Immunohistochemistry may be invaluable in this respect. If there is any question of a germ cell tumour, the section should be stained for α-fetoprotein, β-human chorionic gonadotrophin, and placental alkaline phosphatase. If the histology is that of adenocarcinoma, the diagnosis will be more difficult and special stains may not serve to elucidate the diagnosis further. Where possible, the tissue should be examined for the presence of oestrogen or progesterone receptor, as this would make carcinoma of the breast or ovary more likely. The protein S100 is typically present in melanoma and may be invaluable in distinguishing this diagnosis from anaplastic carcinoma.

Further investigation and management

Investigation must be selective. Since there is specific treatment available for breast and prostate cancer, these diagnoses must always be considered when the histology is adenocarcinoma. Mammography is therefore justifiable, and measurement of serum acid phosphatase and prostatic specific antigen are simple and non-invasive. A pelvic ultrasound may show an ovarian mass, which may influence management as platinum-based combination chemotherapy might then be used, whereas it would not be contemplated in many patients with metastasis from an unknown primary site in view of its toxicity. The possibility of a germ cell tumour must always be considered in a young person, and in these circumstances full investigation is necessary if this diagnosis is possible.

Treatment follows pragmatic lines. Locally troublesome or painful metastases are treated with irradiation. If breast cancer seems a possible diagnosis a trial of hormone therapy is fully justified and, similarly, hormone treatment of prostatic cancer should be introduced if this seems a likely diagnosis. As mentioned above, radiation is frequently given to patients with enlarged cervical nodes when the diagnosis is poorly differentiated carcinoma, even if a head and neck primary has not been found.

The use of combination chemotherapy when the primary site is not known is much more controversial. In general, responses are infrequent and are not long lasting. This drug treatment should be reserved for patients with more than one lesion and particularly when symptoms occur. It is important not to be dogmatic about this issue because many patients find it quite unacceptable to be told that no treatment of any kind is available to them, and are willing to accept the possible toxicities of chemotherapy in exchange for the chance of response. Most chemotherapy programmes will include an alkylating agent and some include doxorubicin or a taxane.

Supportive care of the patient with cancer (see also Section 31)

Psychological support

Nearly everyone will have had friends or relatives who have had cancer and who may have died of it, and they will have read articles and seen television programmes about cancer and its management. Many patients will have been worried about the possibility of cancer before they ever consult their general practitioner, or are subjected to a series of diagnostic tests, the effect of which may be to increase their anxiety. At each stage in the diagnostic process physicians should be aware of patients' feelings and be prepared to talk openly to them about why investigations are being performed. When the diagnosis is established it is essential for the physician to sit quietly with the patient, explaining the nature of the diagnosis and the broad principles that treatment will follow. Sometimes patients will like to have a member of the family with them during this conversation, in case they forget aspects of what is said. The conversation should take place quietly, not on a ward round, with both the patient and the physician seated and the physician calm and unhurried in approach. Avoidance of the word 'cancer', body language that indicates discomfiture or embarrassment, and evasion and vagueness are very likely to be interpreted by the patient as signs of a serious or hopeless outlook.

Many patients will be unable to take in all that is said in the first conversation, and the physician needs to make it quite plain that he or she will be very pleased to talk again the next day, to go over points that need further clarification. There is much useful literature for the patient to take home, there are professional and expert support groups that the patient can contact and, in many hospitals, skilled counsellors who can provide follow-up support after the physician has outlined the basis of treatment. It is essential that all members of the medical team understand what was said and what words were used. The members of the family also need to understand exactly what information has been imparted. It may be necessary to hold back on a precise prognosis; first, because one may not be known until treatment starts, and second, because patients naturally tend to become fixated on the numerical prognosis, which is likely to be extremely inaccurate. If referral to an oncologist is to be made it is critical to indicate exactly what has been said to the patient. Oncologists are put in an extremely difficult position when patients arrive with a diagnosis of cancer, without any indication at all of whether they know the diagnosis, or what words have been used.

A new difficulty in communication is now displacing that which formerly arose from concealment of the diagnosis. Modern cancer management is often complex, with equivalent results sometimes being obtained from approaches that have different early and late effects. A well-intentioned wish to 'share' the treatment decisions with the patient, and an increasing resort to litigation when events don't turn out well, has led doctors sometimes to present treatment options as a series of uncertainties in which the outcome will be strongly influenced by chance and fate. It is bad enough to be told you have cancer. Worse still if your treatment seems mired in uncertainty. For some patients, treatment options will have been made even less clear by access to unfiltered advice on the internet, from reputable sources, charlatans, and cranks. There is nothing paternalistic in sensible advice from a well-informed, kind, sensitive, and experienced specialist. Questions which arise from complexity of choice and outcome in management increase the need for competent advice; they are not answered by passing the problem to the patient. Much distress, and a feeling of being abandoned, can come from lack of clear guidance.

When treatment is to be palliative, after relapse or with widespread metastatic disease, it should none the less be made clear to the patient that it is 'treatment'. Patients dislike feeling that they are being abandoned. Indeed, many wise oncologists see their patients more frequently when they are having palliative treatment than they do during routine treatments or follow-up. They do this because palliative treatment requires great attention to detail, especially with respect to control of pain and other symptoms, and also to provide psychological support for the patient and the family. One of the most common reasons for patients seeking second opinions is that they have been given no feeling that there are possibilities for treatment in their case. Continuity in management is one of the most rewarding aspects of cancer medicine for the physician and for the patient. There is no place for impersonal clinics where patients see different doctors each time they attend, and where the emotional component of their illness cannot be properly explored.

Management of cancer pain

Pain is a common and distressing feature of cancer. A careful history is essential to determine the exact site and nature of the pain and to establish a close and trusting relationship with a patient who feels that the symptom is being taken seriously. Exacerbating factors should be noted and an anatomical diagnosis made as far as possible. If the pain is arising in a bone it may be quickly and effectively helped by radiation treatment. The primary tumour or metastasis may be responsive to treatment with irradiation or chemotherapy. If specific antitumour treatments of this kind are not appropriate, then the only approach is to control the pain with analgesics.

Non-narcotic analgesics are used for mild or moderate pain. Useful agents include aspirin, paracetamol, and non-steroidal anti-inflammatory drugs such as ketoprofen or naproxen. A combination may be useful. Combination drugs such as co-proxamol or co-dydramol are also helpful. Although prescribing each drug separately allows greater control over the constituents, in practice this may not be helpful, particularly for elderly patients who often find it difficult to take multiple medication. The aim of treatment should be to prevent pain as far as possible by taking regular analgesics, and to have additional analgesics on hand for an acute exacerbation. Side-effects of non-opiate analgesics include gastric irritation (and they should therefore be used cautiously if steroids are being used at the same time), nausea, and constipation, particularly with codeine, oxycodone, or propoxyphene.

If these analgesics do not control the pain, opiate analgesics are essential. Two preparations have made an enormous contribution to pain relief. The first is long-acting morphine sulphate, which can be given twice daily, and the second is short-acting morphine sulphate (Sevredol). The former has a duration of action of 8 to 12 h and the latter of about 4 h. One curious feature of the use of morphine-like drugs is that the dose required to control pain varies greatly from person to person. It must therefore be found by trial and error and the patient must be prepared to increase the dose under medical supervision. The aim is to produce background pain relief for most of the day and night. Sevredol is particularly useful for dealing with acute exacerbations of pain.

If oral opiates are unable to control pain fully, continuous subcutaneous infusion is a useful alternative. This approach is particularly valuable in patients who cannot tolerate oral analgesics because of gastrointestinal symptoms, or where the tumour causes nausea or intestinal obstruction. Many pumps are now available, which are designed for continuous infusion through a small-gauge butterfly needle implanted subcutaneously. Patients can manage at home with these infusion pumps, with a nurse calling daily to change the infusion mixture.

Specialized forms of analgesia

A detailed discussion is beyond the scope of this chapter. Amongst the specialized techniques available are continuous epidural and intrathecal opiate infusion, nerve block procedures (including coeliac plexus block, peripheral nerve block, and epidural blocks), neurosurgical procedures, such as ablation of the peripheral nerve by neurectomy or, more radically, interruption of pain pathways by cordotomy. Each of these procedures has its value and limitations and the advice of specialists in the field of pain relief will be necessary.

Further reading

deVita VT, Hellman S, Rosenberg SA (1998). *Cancer: Principles and practice of oncology*, 5th edn. Lippincott, Philadelphia.

Souhami RL *et al.* (2001). *Oxford textbook of oncology*, 2nd edn. Oxford University Press.

6.7 Cancer chemotherapy and radiation therapy

Michael L. Grossbard and Bruce A. Chabner

The last two decades have brought significant improvements in cancer therapy. Patients with previously fatal diseases, including acute leukaemia, non-Hodgkin's lymphoma, Hodgkin's disease, and germ cell tumours, can have a reasonable expectation of cure. For patients with commonly occurring solid tumours, including lung cancer and breast cancer, several new chemotherapeutic agents have been developed which offer improved treatment options and enhanced survival. An increased understanding of tumour biology and the explosion in knowledge in molecular biology have paved the way for new developments in cancer treatment.

Nevertheless, cancer remains the second leading cause of death in the United States. Although exciting advances continue to be made in cancer therapeutics, nearly 40 per cent of patients diagnosed with cancer will die of their disease. An estimated 1.2 million new cancer cases will occur in the United States in 2000 and 552 000 patients will die cancer-related deaths. Virtually all patients diagnosed with advanced stage solid tumours will succumb to their tumour or complications of its therapy. Because a medical oncologist and radiation oncologist will manage many patients diagnosed with cancer only after initial referral from an internist or surgeon, it is critical for the primary care physician to understand the general principles of cancer therapy. The dramatic increase in the number of effective chemotherapy agents since nitrogen mustard was introduced more than 50 years ago has made this challenge greater.

Chemotherapy and radiation therapy, together with surgery, are the major modalities of cancer therapy. Chemotherapy has the advantage of targeting tumour cell throughout the patient, while external beam radiation therapy acts to provide local control. Often, the two modalities are combined to take advantage of synergistic cytotoxicity. This chapter will describe major principles of chemotherapy and radiation therapy.

Chemotherapy

A knowledge of cancer chemotherapy requires an appreciation of some general principles of tumour biology. Cancer results from the uninhibited growth of a single clone of cells. As cancer cells grow, they move through the cell cycle, characterized by several phases: resting (G0), pre-DNA synthesis (G1), DNA synthesis (S), post-DNA synthesis (G2), mitosis (M). Most chemotherapy drugs are active in the S phase of the cell cycle, although some directly block cells entering mitosis and most directly promote apoptosis (programmed cell death).

Chemotherapy can be used in several different settings (Table 1). Foremost, chemotherapy is applied as primary therapy for the treatment of advanced-stage cancer. A few diseases, including leukaemias, lymphomas, and advanced-stage germ cell tumours are sensitive to multiple chemotherapy agents and can be cured with combination chemotherapy. More often, combinations of therapeutic agents are used to diminish tumour-related symptoms, improve the quality of life, and extend survival in patients with advanced-stage tumours. For example randomized clinical trials of chemotherapy versus best supportive care have demonstrated a survival advantage and quality of life improvement when patients with advanced-stage lung cancer receive chemotherapy.

Second, chemotherapy can be used as neoadjuvant therapy, given prior to radiation or surgery for locally advanced disease. In this setting, the drugs are used to decrease the tumour mass, reduce the extent of the subsequent surgery or radiation, and to determine disease sensitivity to drugs. Clinical trials have identified a potential role for neoadjuvant therapy in the treatment of lung cancer, oesophageal cancer, and locally advanced breast cancer, among other diseases. In the case of osteosarcomas, neoadjuvant therapy can provide important information about tumour sensitivity, thereby permitting a more tailored approach to further management. Finally, the drugs can be used as adjuvant therapy, administered after the completion of local definitive surgery and/or radiation therapy in order to decrease the risk of recurrence. For instance adjuvant chemotherapy reduces the risk of tumour recurrence and improves survival in node-positive colon cancer and in breast cancer following surgical resection. In all of these settings, chemotherapy can be administered in conjunction with radiation therapy to optimize local effects of treatment.

Only in rare circumstances, such as the use of methotrexate as therapy for choriocarcinoma, can therapy with single agents cure advanced-stage cancer. Single agents tend to select for drug resistant cells. Most often, therapy with multiple drugs has been required to effect cure. In combining drugs, it is imperative to employ agents that have independent activity, have toxicities that do not overlap significantly, and that can be used at an optimal dose and schedule. Chemotherapy schedules are designed to permit marrow recovery prior to the next dose administration. Typically, peripheral blood counts will reach a nadir at 5 to 10 days post-therapy, with recovery seen by day 21.

Combinations of drugs may circumvent tumour cell resistance, so treatments have been designed in which non-cross-resistant drugs are administered either together or in sequence. One of the earliest combination

Table 1 The role of chemotherapy in cancer management

Primary therapy (curative)
Acute lymphoblastic leukaemia, acute myeloblastic leukaemia
Hodgkin's disease
Non-Hodgkin's lymphoma
Germ cell tumours
Ewing's sarcoma
Small cell lung cancer (with radiation therapy)

Adjuvant therapy
Breast cancer
Colon cancer

Neoadjuvant therapy
Oesophageal cancer (with radiation)
Stage III non-small cell lung cancer
Head and neck cancer

Palliative therapy
Lung cancer
Breast cancer
Pancreatic cancer
Colorectal cancer

therapy programmes to cure a cancer was the use of MOPP (mechlorethamine, vincristine, prednisone, and procarbazine) for the treatment of Hodgkin disease. Similarly, acute lymphoblastic leukaemia can now be cured in 80 per cent of children using multidrug chemotherapy administered at frequent dosing intervals to avoid the development of resistant cells. Alternatively, extremely high doses of therapy can be used to overcome tumour resistance, but this may obligate the use of stem cell support to overcome the resulting profound bone marrow toxicity.

Because of the potentially severe toxicities of chemotherapy, physicians should administer regimens that have been reported in the peer-reviewed medical literature. Alternatively, the development of new regimens in the context of well-designed institutional review board approved clinical trials can permit the development of novel investigational treatment programmes. Clinicians should not routinely administer drug combinations based on anecdotal evidence.

Classes of chemotherapy agents

There are several distinct classes of chemotherapy agents (Table 2). Because these drugs can have major side-effects, only physicians knowledgeable in their dosing and side-effects should administer them. In order to reduce variability in exposure to drugs, doses of most chemotherapy agents are administered based on the patient's body surface area, a calculation determined by the patient's height and weight. In addition, doses of chemotherapy need to be adjusted for renal (methotrexate, bleomycin, fludarabine) and hepatic function (anthracyclines, vinca alkaloids, taxanes).

Adequate intravenous access must be secured since many of the drugs are vesicants and extravasation can lead to tissue necrosis. Similarly, patients must be adequately hydrated prior to the administration of cisplatin and cyclophosphamide, to prevent renal toxicity and bladder toxicity, respectively. Careful attention must be given to fluid and electrolyte balance with the administration of many agents. Cisplatin renal toxicity can cause profound hypomagnesaemia.

Antimetabolites exert their cytotoxicity by serving as substrates in pathways vital to cellular function and replication. Many of these agents are incorporated into DNA or RNA or act on enzymes involved in the synthesis of nucleic acids. Methotrexate acts by inhibiting the enzyme dihydrofolate reductase, which maintains intracellular pools of reduced tetrahydrofolates required for the synthesis of purine nucleotides and thymidylate. 5-Fluorouricil is another commonly used antimetabolite. A metabolite of this drug, fluorodeoxyuridine monophospate inhibits thymidylate synthase, an enzyme required for the synthesis of deoxythymidine triphosphate and DNA. In addition, fluorodeoxyuridine triphosphate is incorporated into RNA, interfering with its function, and fluorodeoxyuridine triphosphate is incorporated into DNA, leading to strand breakage.

Table 2 Cancer therapy agents

Chemotherapy
Alkylating agents and platinating drugs
Anthracyclines
Antimetabolites
Topoisomerase inhibitors
Mitotic inhibitors
Hormone therapy
Biological therapy
Monoclonal antibodies
    unconjugated antibodies
    radioimmunoconjugates
    immunotoxins
Cytokines
    interferons
    interleukin-2
Antisense oligonucleotides
Gene therapy

A third important antimetabolite is cytarabine (ara-C) which is converted to cytarabine triphosphate (ara-CTP) in the cell. Cytarabine triphosphate is incorporated into DNA and serves as a chain terminator. A related deoxycytidine analogue, gemcitabine, has the additional actions of inhibiting the conversion of ribonucleotides to deoxyribonucleotides, which are DNA precursors. Prolonged exposure of tumour cells to some of the antimetabolites, such as 5-fluorouracil and cytosine arabinoside, through continuous intravenous infusion may be more effective than bolus injections alone.

Purine analogues also have important roles as antimetabolites; 6-mercaptopurinre (6-MP) and 6-thioguanine (6-TG) are converted in the cell to monophosphates which inhibit the first step of purine synthesis. Moreover, the triphosphate nucleotides of 6-mercaptopurinre and 6-thioguanine are incorporated into DNA resulting in an increase in strand breaks. Another purine analogue is fludarabine phosphate, which serves as an adenosine analogue. Fludarabine is converted to 2-fluoro-ara-A in plasma and subsequently is phosphorylated intracellularly. The resulting triphosphate inhibits DNA polymerase and ribonucleotide reductase, interfering with DNA and RNA synthesis.

Alkylating agents exert their cytotoxicity by binding to DNA and forming DNA adducts which alter DNA structure and function enough to disrupt DNA replication and transcription. They act throughout the cell cycle, but have their greatest activity on rapidly proliferating cells. These agents, including cyclophosphamide, nitrogen mustard, melphalan, busulfan, and chlorambucil were among the first chemotherapy drugs and remain important agents in cancer therapy, with particular activity in haematological malignancies and breast cancer. In a similar manner, the platinum derivatives bind to and cross-link DNA, leading to DNA breaks and apoptosis.

The anthracyclines intercalate into DNA and disrupt DNA synthesis. The antitumour activity of doxorubicin and daunorubicin, the two most commonly used agents in this drug class, results in part from triggering of topoisomerase II dependent DNA breaks. Etoposide also inhibits topoisomerase II. In a similar way, other topoisomerase inhibitors interfere with topoisomerase I, which is critical in the repair of normal DNA; these agents include irinotecan and topotecan. Vinca alkaloids interfere with microtubule formation and disrupt cell division. In contrast, the taxanes stabilize microtubule assembly, also inhibiting mitosis.

Along with the traditional cytotoxic agents, hormone-directed therapy can be critical in the regulation of tumours. The growth of many normal tissues and tumours is influenced by hormone exposure. Many breast cancers express receptors for oestrogen and progesterone and most prostate cancers have androgen receptors. Depriving these tumours of the hormonal stimulus can exert both cytocidal and cytostatic effects on the cell. Thus, more than 50 per cent of breast cancers expressing the oestrogen receptor will respond to treatment with tamoxifen, an antioestrogen. Similarly, the use of luteinizing hormone releasing hormone (LHRH) agonists (which reduce testosterone synthesis) or antiandrogens can have dramatic effects on prostate cancer growth.

Chemotherapy resistance

Unfortunately, there are several mechanisms by which tumours may become resistant to the effects of cytotoxic chemotherapy (Table 3). Decreased accumulation of drug in the cell through alteration in transport mechanisms permits resistance to methotrexate. Alternatively, the intracellular target for methotrexate may be altered, as in the case of amplification of dihydrofolate reductase. Similarly, with 5-flurouracil, the target enzyme thymidylate synthase may be amplified. Altered drug metabolism, as occurs with ring reduction of 5-fluorouracil, can contribute to drug resistance. In tumours resistant to alkylating agent, the alkylating agents may be inactivated through reactions with thiol-containing compounds or through enhanced DNA repair.

A particularly important mechanism of resistance, conferred by a P-glycoprotein, leads to resistance to multiple drugs. Multidrug resistance

Table 3 Mechanisms of chemotherapy resistance

Drug	Mechanism of resistance	Biological effect
Methotrexate	Decreased drug uptake	Increased expression of folate transporter
	Decreased drug activation	Decreased folylpolyglutamyl synthetase
	Altered drug target	Altered dihydrofolate reductase
Doxorubicin	Altered drug target	Altered topoisomerase II
	Increased drug efflux	Increased MDR expression or gene amplification
Alkylating agents	Increased detoxification	Increased glutathione or glutathione transferase
	Enhanced DNA repair	Increased nucleotide excision repair
Cisplatin	Defective recognition of DNA adducts	Mismatch repair defect
	Enhanced DNA repair	Increased nucleotide excision repair
Etoposide	Increased drug efflux	Increased MDR expression or gene amplification
	Altered drug target	Altered topoisomerase II
Most anticancer drugs	Defective checkpoint function and apoptosis	P53 mutations
5-Fluorouracil	Increased drug target	Amplified thymidylate synthase

MDR, multidrug resistance.

results from enhanced drug efflux from the cell secondary to P-glycoprotein over-expression. In this setting, the cancer cells becomes resistant to anthracyclines, vinca alkaloids, taxanes, etoposide, and other drugs simultaneously. Several agents currently in clinical trials are designed to inhibit the multidrug resistance pump. A different type of multidrug resistance can occur with the topoisomerase inhibitors where quantitative and qualitative changes in topoisomerase II activity have been associated with decreased tumour sensitivity.

Side-effects of chemotherapy

The commonly used chemotherapy agents have several side-effects in common (Table 4). Myelosuppression occurs with virtually all agents, although the timing of its onset and its duration differs with different groups of drugs. Cyclophosphamide causes an acute, short-onset depression in counts, affecting the white blood cell count more than platelets. By contrast, the nitrosoureas lead to delayed-onset reductions in both neutrophils and platelet with nadir counts typically reached 4 to 6 weeks after therapy.

Nausea and vomiting remain a troubling side-effect of chemotherapy, though the present use of serotonin uptake inhibitors has diminished the incidence of vomiting with the most emetogenic agents, including cisplatin. Alopecia is a major cause of concern to patients and occurs uniformly with some agents such as doxorubicin, but rarely with agents such as methotrexate and fludarabine. Profound neuropathy frequently accompanies the use of vinca alkaloids, and occurs less frequently with cisplatin and paclitaxel.

Moreover, many of the agents have unique side-effects that are of concern to the practising internist. Doxorubicin can cause cardiac toxicity, including an acute syndrome characterized by arrhythmias and congestive heart failure. In addition, doxorubicin can cause a cumulative, dose-dependent decline in left ventricular ejection fraction, with a higher incidence of myocardial dysfunction seen in patients receiving a cumulative dose of greater than 500 mg/m^2. Bleomycin causes lung toxicity, including pneumonitis, which can progress to interstitial fibrosis. The carbon mon-

oxide diffusing capacity of the lung diminishes with increasing cumulative bleomycin doses. Methotrexate in high doses can cause acute renal failure due to drug precipitation in the renal tubules. The administration of paclitaxel can cause anaphylaxis in response to cremaphor, the vehicle in which it is delivered. Hence, premedication with dexamethasone and antihistamines is required to reduce the risk of adverse reactions. Cytarabine administered in high single doses (3 gm/m^2 or greater) can cause irreversible cerebellar dysfunction, so a neurological exam should be performed daily on patients receiving therapy so that it can be discontinued at the earliest sign of such toxicity.

A major, delayed side-effect of cancer chemotherapy is the development of secondary leukaemias due to therapy. These are most commonly seen in patients receiving therapy with multiple alkylating agents, as was the case for the treatment of Hodgkin disease with MOPP chemotherapy. Five to six per cent of patients receiving this therapy developed leukaemia as a consequence of therapy. Newer regimens for Hodgkin disease treatment avoid this devastating complication of therapy. More recently, topoisomerase II therapy (etoposide, anthracyclines) in high total doses has been associated with a risk of secondary leukaemias. High-dose therapy followed by autologous stem cell infusion has a risk of secondary leukaemias that exceeds 10 per cent. As survival rates are improved with combination chemotherapy regimens used in the treatment of diseases such as leukaemia and lymphoma, the long-term complications of cancer chemotherapy become more evident.

Finally, infertility occurs with many chemotherapy regimens, especially when patients are treated with alkylating agents or high-dose therapy. While reduced sperm counts may occur only transiently in males, most alkylating-induced azoospermia is irreversible, and a discussion should be initiated regarding the possibility of banking sperm for any patient at risk. For premenopausal woman, the risk of infertility and early menopause increases with age. These fertility issues must be addressed with patients prior to the administration of chemotherapy.

Biological therapy

Cancer chemotherapy not only refers to the traditional, cytotoxic agents but also encompasses novel biological therapies including monoclonal antibody-based treatments and cytokine therapies. Currently, two unconjugated monoclonal antibodies are available for commercial use in the United States. Rituximab binds to the CD20 antigen that is expressed on the surface of both normal and malignant B lymphocytes. Nearly 50 per cent of patients with low-grade B-cell lymphoma respond to this targeted therapy, which lacks the typical myelosuppressive side-effects of chemotherapy as well as the typical alopecia and emesis. The most common side-effects with antibodies are infusion-related fevers, chills, and hypotension. Another biologically active antibody is herceptin, which binds to the Her-2 receptor that is over-expressed in 15 to 20 per cent of breast cancer cases.

Table 4 Side-effects of chemotherapy

Adverse effect	Representative agents
Nausea/ vomiting	Cisplatin, doxorubicin
Alopecia	Cisplatin, adriamycin, taxol
Neuropathy	Taxol, cisplatin
Renal toxicity	Cisplatin, methotrexate
Pulmonary toxicity	Bleomycin, BCNU, methotrexate
Cardiotoxicity	Doxorubicin, daunorubicin
Bladder toxicity	Cyclophosphamide, ifosfamide
SIADH	Cyclophosphamide, vincristine
Mucositis	5-FU, Methotrexate, doxorubicin
Nail changes	Bleomycin, cyclophosphamide, 5-FU

When given in conjunction with paclitaxel, the combination appears to prolong survival for patients with metastatic breast cancer.

The two most extensively studied cytokine therapies are interferon and interleukin-2 (IL-2). The interferons are a class of proteins produced by the body in response to viral infections. These agents have relatively disappointing antitumour activity, although they can induce major responses in patients with low-grade lymphoma and hairy cell leukaemia. Toxicities include fevers, chills, liver function test abnormalities, and cytopenias. IL-2 is a cytokine produced by activated T cells that plays a role in triggering the immune system. IL-2 has activity in renal cell carcinoma and melanoma, with occasional patients achieving long-duration remissions. However, its toxicities include fevers, renal dysfunction, and capillary leak syndrome.

Recent advances in molecular biology have led to the development of additional therapies which are currently in clinical trials. Antisense oligonucleotides of 15 to 20 bases in length can be used to target specific messenger RNAs. A bcl-2 antisense compound has shown biological activity against low grade non-Hodgkin's lymphoma (which over-express the bcl-2 protein). Another exciting class of compounds target new blood vessel formation, which may be critical for the implantation and growth of tumour cells. These antiangiogenic compounds also are in clinical trials.

Radiation therapy

Understanding the cytotoxicity of radiation therapy requires knowledge of radiation physics and tumour biology. Over the last two decades, the ability of CT scans and MRI scans to carefully localize the tumour within the patient, along with technical improvements in treatment machines, have radically improved the accuracy of radiation therapy.

Electromagnetic radiation, used most commonly in patient care, consists of roentgen (X-rays, photons) and gamma radiation. In general, gamma rays are produced by the degradation of nuclear isotopes while electrical machines produce photons. Alternatively, electron beams can be used for the treatment of superficial tumours (such as cutaneous lymphoma) because of the sharp reduction in dose that occurs beyond a certain tissue depth. Proton beam therapy can be used to delivery high treatment doses to a highly localized lesion because of its very sharp margins of dose deposition, and has particular relevance in the treatment of spinal tumours and some central nervous system tumours.

The dose of irradiation is defined as the unit of energy absorbed by each kilogram of tissue. This is conventionally expressed in 'Grays' (Gy). As the dose of radiation is increased the percentage of cells that is killed increases.

Radiation used for the treatment of patients generally consists of either external beam irradiation delivered from outside the body or brachytherapy, in which the radiation device is placed within or near the target tumour. Brachytherapy has been used effectively in the treatment of head and neck cancer, cervical cancer, and endometrial cancer. At some centres, intraoperative radiation therapy can be used to deliver a single, large fraction of radiation directly to the tumour bed. In some circumstances, radioisotopes themselves can be used for systemic treatment. For example iodine-131 is taken up by thyroid tissue both locally and at sites of metastatic disease.

The target for radiation-induced cytotoxicity is DNA. Radiation therapy generates free radicals that damage DNA. Because the presence of oxygen is important in the generation of free radicals, hypoxic tissues are less sensitive to the toxic effects of radiation. Thus, well vascularized tissues are most sensitive to radiation therapy. A theoretical advantage of preoperative radiation is the chance to treat a tumour while its vasculature remains intact. However, resection of a larger, poorly vascularized tumour may improve the chances of curing a locally advanced head and neck cancer with irradiation.

The delivery of radiation therapy requires careful planning. CT scans or MRI scans are used to identify the target tissue and surrounding normal tissues accurately. Next, treatment technique and volume are tested on a radiation simulator. The simulator duplicates the treatment plan, but uses only superficial radiation for imaging and accurately assessing the location of the treatment beam. To make certain that treatments are delivered to the same tumour volume each day, tattoos are placed on the patient. Blocks are made to exclude treatment from normal tissue such as the heart and lungs. Often the maximum tolerated dose of radiation is administered to the total treatment volume with a boost administered to the treatment bed.

Radiation doses are usually delivered in a number of daily fractions with the total fractionated dose dependent on tumour sensitivity and normal tissue tolerance. Seminoma is an exquisitely radiation sensitive tumour and requires a lower therapy dose (30 Gy) than solid tumours such as lung cancer (60 Gy). Some tumours, such as melanoma, are relatively radioresistant.

Within 6 h after radiation, cells begin to recover from the effects of therapy. Thus, fractions placed too close together can offer increased toxicity to normal tissues, but those too far apart can permit repair of sublethal damage. While conventional therapy usually provides a daily radiation fraction of 1.8 to 3 Gy over 15 to 35 treatments, to total doses of 40 to 65 Gy, alternative schemes have been investigated. In hyperfractionated therapy, a smaller fraction size is used, and more fractions are administered. This permits a higher total radiation dose to be administered. For palliation of painful bone metastases, radiation therapy can be given in either a single large dose or four to five moderate doses to minimize the patient's travel to the treatment centre. More recently, radioisotopes such as iodine-131 have been conjugated to antibodies, with radiation delivered directly to the surface of the targeted cell. In this scenario, low-dose continuous radiation therapy is effectively delivered at the tumour site.

Complications of radiation therapy

Adverse effects of radiation therapy can be considered with respect to both acute and delayed toxicities. Tissues that normally proliferate rapidly, such as skin, mucosal linings, and bone marrow, are most susceptible to radiation cytotoxicity. Thus, erythema and desquamation are important acute, local effects of therapy. For patients receiving radiation therapy for gastrointestinal tumours, diarrhoea, nausea, and vomiting are common. If a significant radiation dose is delivered to the bone marrow, patients may develop cytopenias. In the case of whole body irradiation, the lymphocyte count falls and significant immune suppression occurs. On occasion, these acute side-effects are severe enough to require delays in treatment to allow the normal tissues to repair themselves. When patients receive irradiation to the lung, a resultant radiation pneumonitis may occur characterized by fevers, cough, dyspnoea, and pulmonary infiltrates. Occasionally, this may require treatment with corticosteroids.

Long-term sequelae are tissue specific and occur most commonly if normal tissue tolerance is exceeded. Thus, careful dosimetry and radiation planning must be done to verify that tissues do not receive treatment beyond their maximum tolerated dose. For example radiation doses to the spinal cord in excess of 45 Gy can cause myelitis, doses to the small bowel in excess of 45 Gy can cause strictures, and doses to the kidney above 20 Gy can cause renal dysfunction. The liver tolerates radiation therapy poorly. Accelerated coronary artery disease has been seen in patients with Hodgkin disease who received radiation to the heart in an effort to encompass a mediastinal mass.

Perhaps the most severe side-effect of radiation therapy is the development of secondary tumours. Ordinarily, this is not an issue for patients with metastatic cancer receiving radiation therapy for palliation of disease related symptoms since their survival will be short. However, in patients with Hodgkin disease, who can be cured with radiation therapy, the development of second solid tumours in the radiation field, including sarcomas, lung cancers, and oesophageal cancer, can limit survival.

Role of radiation therapy in cancer treatment

In the clinical management of patients, radiation therapy is used as primary therapy for tumour treatment, as an adjuvant or neoadjuvant therapy

Table 5 Role of radiation therapy in cancer treatment

Curative therapy alone
Hodgkin's disease
Non-Hodgkin's lymphoma (early stage, indolent histology)
Laryngeal carcinoma
Prostate cancer
Central nervous system tumours (e.g. medulloblastoma)
Cervical cancer
Breast cancer (postsurgery)
Curative in conjunction with chemotherapy
Small cell lung cancer (limited stage)
Non-Hodgkin's lymphoma (early stage aggressive histology)
Anal carcinoma
Adjuvant therapy
Rectal cancer (with 5-FU)
Gastric cancer (with 5-FU)
Neoadjuvant therapy
Oesophageal carcinoma
Lung cancer (stage III)

either alone or in conjunction with chemotherapy (which often acts as a radiation sensitizer), and as palliative therapy for advanced stage treatment (Table 5).

Radiation therapy has a role in the management of several acute complications of cancer. Radiation can be valuable in the treatment of bone metastases, both to decrease painful lesions and to diminish the risk of pathological fractures. Radiation therapy can be delivered as an emergency procedure in patients with spinal cord compression to reduce the risk of permanent neurological toxicity. Likewise, radiation has an important role in the management of brain metastases, either as primary therapy for patients with multiple lesions or as a prophylactic therapy for patients undergoing excision of a solitary brain metastasis. In lung cancer, radiation can be used to palliate obstructive symptoms. In bleeding tumours, radiation therapy can often assist in local control of haemorrhage.

In the management of several tumours, radiation therapy can serve as the definitive treatment. In early-stage Hodgkin's disease, patients can be cured with either mantle radiation therapy alone or with mantle and para-aortic radiation. Similarly, 35 to 50-Gy doses of radiation therapy can induce long-term remissions in 50 to 60 per cent of patients with stage I/II low-grade non-Hodgkin's lymphoma. Seminoma is an exquisitely radiation sensitive tumour and early stage disease can be cured in a high percentage of patients with radiation therapy alone. Radiation therapy can provide equivalent long-term survival to surgery in patients with prostate cancer and laryngeal cancer, with potentially reduced morbidity as compared with surgery. Finally, in early-stage breast cancer, lumpectomy and radiation therapy provides an equivalent survival outcome to a modified radical mastectomy.

In other diseases, such a squamous cell carcinoma of the anus, combined modality therapy using radiation therapy in conjunction with 5-FU and mitomycin C chemotherapy yields a high cure rate without surgery. Similarly, in patients with limited stage small cell lung cancer, combined modality therapy using cisplatin-based chemotherapy and radiation therapy reduces local tumour recurrence and improves survival. Likewise, in cervical cancer, a combination of cisplatin and radiation post-resection reduces tumour recurrence.

Radiation therapy also has an important role in adjuvant therapy. In the adjuvant treatment of rectal cancer, randomized clinical trials have demonstrated that radiation therapy administered in conjunction with 5-FU chemotherapy can reduce local recurrence and systemic recurrence and can improve both disease free and overall survival. In node-positive gastric cancer, a combination of 5-FU based chemotherapy administered as adjuvant therapy can reduce the risk of recurrence and improve survival. Recent studies have demonstrated that the administration of prophylactic cranial irradiation to patients with small cell lung cancer who achieve a complete

remission can reduce the risk of central nervous system spread of disease and improve survival. In the neoadjuvant setting, radiation in combination with cisplatin-based chemotherapy has been shown to improve survival in patients with stage IIIA lung cancer and oesophageal cancer.

As noted earlier, the gamma radiation from radioactive isotopes also can be used to treat tumours. Well-differentiated thyroid cancer metastases take up iodine-131 which then can offer tumour-specific toxicity. Antibodies have been conjugated to iodine-131 and yttrium-90 to deliver targeted radiation therapy to the surface of lymphoma cells.

Conclusions

Advances in radiation therapy and chemotherapy have revolutionized the care of cancer patients. Significant improvements in supportive care and the development of new, active anticancer agents have improved the prospects for long-term survival even for patients with metastatic disease. The internist has a pivotal role in co-ordinating care for such patients and should be aware of these advances and new option for patients.

Further reading

DeVita VT Jr (1997). Principles of cancer management: chemotherapy. In: DeVita VT Jr, Hellman S, Rosenberg SA, eds. *Cancer: principles and practice of oncology*, pp. 333–73. Lipincott-Raven, Philadelphia. [Describes general aspects of chemotherapy and concepts of drug resistance, cell cycle biology, and dose intensity.]

Goldie JH (1987). Scientific basis for adjuvant and primary (neoadjuvant) chemotherapy. *Seminars in Oncology* 14, 1–7. [Discusses principles of adjuvant and neoadjuvant therapy as well as theoretical benefits and concerns.]

Greenlee RT, *et al.* (2000). Cancer statistics, 2000. *CA: a Cancer Journal for Clinicians* 50, 7–33. [Summarizes data on incidence and survival for all types of cancer in the United States.]

Hellman S (1997). Principles of cancer management: radiation therapy. In: DeVita VT Jr, Hellman S, Rosenberg SA, eds. *Cancer: principles and practice of oncology*, pp. 307–32. Lipincott-Raven, Philadelphia. [Overview of biological and physical properties of radiation therapy.]

Leibel SA, Phillips TL, eds (1998). *Textbook of radiation oncology.* WB Saunders, Philadelphia. [Comprehensive textbook describing current techniques in radiation oncology and their clinical application.]

Marino P, *et al.* (1994). Chemotherapy vs supportive care in non-small-cell lung cancer. *Chest* 106, 861–5. [A meta-analysis demonstrating improved survival and quality of life for patients with metastatic lung cancer receiving chemotherapy.]

Mauch PM, *et al.* (1996). Second malignancies after treatment for laparotomy staged IA-IIIB Hodgkin's disease: long-term analysis of risk factors and outcome. *Blood* 87, 3625–32. [Describes risk of secondary haematological malignancies and solid tumours in 794 patients receiving either radiation therapy or combined modality therapy.]

Multani PS, Grossbard ML (1998). Monoclonal antibody-based therapies of hematologic malignancies. *Journal of Clinical Oncology* 16, 3691–710. [Provides an overview of this developing field.]

Perez CA and Brady LW, eds (1997). *Principles and practice of radiation oncology*, 3rd edn. Lippincott-Raven, [New York. Comprehensive textbook of radiation oncology.]

Pinedo HM, Longo DL, Chabner BA, eds (1999). *Cancer chemotherapy and biological response modifiers: annual 18.* Elsevier, New York. [Up-to-date text on mechanisms of action and resistance of chemotherapy agents and their major indications for use.]

Walsh TN *et al.* (1996). A comparison of multimodal therapy and surgery for esophageal adenocarcinoma. *New England Journal of Medicine* 335, 462–7. [Improved survival for patients receiving preoperative chemotherapy and radiation versus surgery alone in a phase III trial.]

7

Infection

7.1 The clinical approach to the patient with suspected infection

David Rubenstein

Presentation of illnesses and the history

Most systemic infections produce fever but not all fevers are, at cause, infectious. Patients with systemic infections range symptomatically from apparent full fitness to near moribund and initial appearance will indicate the speed of clinical response required. Appearances can be deceptive and many serious, potentially fatal infections do not present acutely. This gives time for more careful assessment although not for too much delay.

The standard undergraduate history produces a reliable range of questions covering all systems, which usually indicates the system or systems at fault (except perhaps for over- and underactivity of the thyroid) and should always be completed thoroughly. Where infection is common or possible, the addition of a detailed travel history can be invaluable, particularly as some infections occur in local geographical pockets, for example schistosomal infection from swimming in Lake Malawi, histoplasmosis along the Ohio river valley, and coccidioidomycosis in the San Joaquin Valley, California. Also air passengers may contract illness either during travel, from air droplet transmission, and even after a very brief stop-over. A detailed drug history is also most important. Not only do drugs produce fever but prophylactic agents may themselves be the cause of illness. As general physicians, in parallel with the rest of humanity, we have blind areas and ours are ear, nose, and throat, gynaecology, and sexually transmitted diseases, all of special importance when considering infection sites, if not obvious on initial history taking. The past and social history rarely give a pointer to the cause of infection, but previous surgery has commonly created a site of infection even weeks or months after operation, and social and sexual contacts and their illness may offer an important clue—HIV infection now occurs worldwide.

Examination

A complete and well learned and rehearsed examination system is an essential component of a clinician's skill. With time this becomes almost second nature and will prevent serious omission. ('The more I practise the better I get'—Arnold Palmer, but also variously attributed.)

The initial history almost invariably focuses the examiner on the likely site of infection, but occasionally a clinical finding will add to the clinical picture. If so, this will guide further management, but if not, it is essential to assess lymph nodes carefully at all common sites, and listen to the heart for murmurs. Careful examination of the skin may give important clues. The ear, nose, and throat region and the pelvis may hide infection as can the abdomen and re-examination should be performed daily to include these and the 'physician's blind areas' of the midline—the epigastrium, umbilical, and suprapubic regions. I have on first examination missed enlarged lymph nodes, heart murmurs, suprapubic masses, splenic enlargement, scrotal ulcers, and circinate balanitis—and probably many other signs, but the chance of missing a key sign is greatly reduced by repeated examination and by different observers.

Key investigations

'Ned, why do you keep robbing the banks?'
'Well, Judge, that's where all the money is'
(Ned Kelly, Australian bush ranger, nineteenth century and
variously attributed.)

The history and examination findings usually point to the system involved and often the diagnosis and investigation is aimed at confirming clinical suspicion. This is rarely a problem as most patients present with both a fever and some other marker, such as rash, vomiting, diarrhoea, cough, and sputum. It becomes more difficult when there are no key features other than fever. In all cases it is worth rechecking the drug and travel history, particularly if malaria is suspected, and all patients require a full blood count, blood cultures, a routine urine check, and a chest radiograph. At the same time and for future reference, studies may reveal early evidence of dehydration, a common feature of acute infectious diseases.

The white blood count is of particular value in septicaemia/bacteraemia and also in returning travellers, as the neutrophil count is not raised in malaria. The presence of a neutrophilia does not exclude malaria but suggests bacterial or amoebic infection. Some returning travellers have both. Blood cultures will allow confirmation of bacterial blood infection and guide antibiotic therapy, particularly alteration in antibiotic cover if the initial choice is ineffective. Routine urine testing and culture is often revealing even in the absence of urinary tract symptoms. As it is now simple, it is often omitted—even on renal units. In fairness, blood may not be sent for culture prior to treatment even on specialist infectious disease wards. A chest radiograph in the absence of respiratory symptoms may reveal tuberculosis, an abscess, or hilar lymph node enlargement, this being the first indication of tuberculosis, lymphoma, or sarcoid. If the diagnosis remains uncertain, more detailed studies including serology and ultrasound CT or MR scanning should be guided by clinical suspicion and probability, followed if indicated, by guided biopsy. Persistent fever has many causes, some of which are non-infectious and investigation of these should continue in parallel if clinical suspicion is sufficient (see Chapter 7.2).

Management

This is guided by the clinical picture and investigation findings. It becomes more difficult if the patient is too ill to wait for results or if these initially fail to reveal the diagnosis. This is commonly encountered in 'ill' patients with suspected septicaemia. This is a medical emergency and treatment should not be delayed until results are through. Antibiotics chosen to cover the likely infective organisms should be given intravenously as soon as key investigations, including blood and urine for culture, have been taken. Results and the patient's progress may change the plan, but delay may have serious consequences.

It is essential not to forget the important general supportive measures of rehydration and short-term anticoagulation for bed-bound and dehydrated patients. Good communication and reassurance are also very important, but nothing like as important as getting the right answer and starting the right treatment.

The future

New infectious diseases

These continue to appear and Lassa fever, legionnaire's disease, Lyme disease, and HIV infection were little recognized or unknown 30 years ago. Remaining alert to new diseases is critical but almost impossible for any single clinician, who must remain up to date with the literature and particularly the regular and superb publications from the Centers for Disease Control, Atlanta, the Public Health Laboratory Service in London, the World Health Organization, and the Pro Med web site.

Prevention

This is the key to future success and currently at a very exciting phase. Smallpox is we hope eradicated, although some of us remain slightly nervous in the era of biological warfare. Current research, if fruitful, may produce successful vaccines against a wide range of infections—malaria, leishmaniasis, and even HIV are all good candidates.

Advanced diagnostic technique

It is impossible for our generation to appreciate the 'miracle' of chest radiography. Likewise, those of us who practised prior to scanning, particularly CT and now MR scanning, still remain amazed at the detail and accuracy of current radiology and the great improvement in diagnostic accuracy which can be quickly, safely, and almost atraumatically achieved. No doubt future advances, and greater availability with lowered cost, will make these techniques much more widely available. The polymerase chain reaction is now well established, but not universally available. Of perhaps even greater diagnostic help may be results of research into the use of 'antigen strips'. If the example of urine dipsticks is a guide, these may become a universally available, accurate, inexpensive, and possible bedside aid.

Final thoughts

Given sufficient knowledge and experience, your initial diagnosis is probably right and investigation will be aimed at confirmation. If the answer remains obscure after careful reassessment of history, examination, and clinical notes, seek a second opinion. In the hour of need, microbiologists and dermatologists make excellent friends.

Always consult with ease but selectively, remembering that colleagues who refer everyone or no one might have something to hide. Working alone makes clinical medicine a scary occupation and the best clinicians hunt in packs. It makes for more certain diagnosis, finer tuned investigation, better overall therapy, and peace of mind.

Further reading

Web sites

Pro Med

Mobile texts

Chin J, ed. (2000). *Control of communicable diseases manual*, 17th edn. American Public Health Association, Washington DC.

Wilkes D, Farrington M (1975). *The infectious diseases manual*. Blackwell Scientific Publications, Oxford. [2nd edn—2002.]

Essential reviews

Morbidity and Mortality Weekly Reports. United States Department of Health and Human Diseases, Washington DC.

Communicable Disease Report Weekly. PHLS (Communicable Disease Centre), London NW9 5EQ.

Ethics

Cronin AJ (1996). *The citadel*. Victor Gollancz, London.

7.2 Fever of unknown origin

David T. Durack

Febrile episodes are common, often transient, and often due to an obvious cause. In many cases the cause is obvious, such as an upper respiratory infection in a child. In a few cases, fever is persistent and the cause is not easily diagnosed. Such episodes are termed 'fever of unknown origin' (**FUO**) or 'pyrexia of unknown origin'.

Definitions and terminology

Normal body temperature is 37.0 °C or 98.6 °F. The normal range is quite wide, being affected by site of measurement, diurnal variation, heavy exercise, hormonal and menstrual status, individual variation, and environmental factors. A patient's body temperature is often estimated by measurements taken in the mouth for reasons of convenience, but oral temperatures can be affected by mouth-breathing, by the respiratory rate, and by recent drinking of hot or cold liquids. Many modern thermometry instruments take readings from the ear canal, so that the temperature is not affected by these factors. The core body temperature is more closely reflected by rectal measurements, which are usually 0.3 to 0.6 °C higher than oral measurements. Heavy exercise can temporarily raise the core temperature of healthy people by 2 °C or more. Another factor is normal circadian variation, which cycles through a range of approximately 0.5 °C (0.9 °F) daily, with the lowest temperatures occurring between 0400 and 0600 h and the highest between 1600 and 2000 h. The normal circadian rhythm varies between individuals and is likely to be affected by jet travel between time zones, by work and sleep patterns, and by illnesses. The menstrual cycle alters the baseline temperature of normal women by 0.3 to 0.5 °C, with a small spike at ovulation and higher temperatures from about the 15th to the 25th days of a 28-day cycle. In addition to these factors, there is considerable variation in normal temperature patterns between individuals. Some normal young people, especially women, persistently exhibit slightly 'high' temperatures that are of no pathological significance. This common normal variant, which does not require investigation, may be termed 'habitual hyperthermia'.

Fever and hypothermia may be defined, respectively, as core body temperatures above or below the normal range, allowing for all the factors listed above. For practical clinical purposes, oral or rectal temperatures falling outside the range of 35.5 to 38.0 °C (95.9–100.4 °F) can be regarded as abnormal. Specific circumstances should be considered; for example, an oral temperature of as low as 37.5 °C taken at 0600 h in an elderly patient could represent a clinically significant fever.

FUO has many possible causes. To help classify these, four distinct types of prolonged fever have been defined: classical FUO, nosocomial FUO, neutropenic FUO, and human immunodeficiency virus (**HIV**)-associated FUO.

Symptoms and signs of FUO

The symptoms and signs of FUO are highly variable. Some patients have mild feverish symptoms, while others may be incapacitated by debilitating chills, rigors, and sweats. The clinical findings may be limited to manifest-

ations of the fever itself, or may also reflect the underlying disease. The physician should evaluate every symptom or sign, especially new ones, as potential clues to the primary diagnosis.

Certain diseases can produce characteristic patterns of fever, notably malaria, brucellosis, typhoid fever, and some lymphomas, but in practice the shape of the fever curve is seldom of major value in the diagnosis of FUO. Individual host reactions to disease and the common use of antipyretic analgesic drugs confuse the picture. There is a common misconception that drug-induced fevers are usually low-grade ones, with relatively little variation from peak to trough and a relatively low pulse rate, but in fact the clinical characteristics of drug-induced fevers are highly variable.

Classical FUO

Most of the many causes of classical FUO can be classified into five categories: infections, malignancies, connective tissue diseases, miscellaneous conditions including factitious fever and habitual hyperthermia, and undiagnosed cases. Within the first three categories, certain diagnoses predominate (Tables 1 and 2). The leading infectious aetiologies for classical FUO are intra-abdominal infections, complicated urinary tract infections, tuberculosis, and infective endocarditis. The leading malignancies are lymphomas, leukaemias, and some solid tumours, including adenocarcinomas and hypernephromas. Vasculitides, including the temporal arteritis–polymyalgia syndromes, Still's disease, systemic lupus erythematosus, and rheumatic fever, are important among the connective tissue diseases. Among the miscellaneous conditions that can cause FUO, alcoholic hepatitis and granulomatous conditions such as sarcoidosis or granulomatous hepatitis are important. Self-induced or factitious fever is surprisingly common. Some of the many other miscellaneous, uncommon, or rare diseases that can cause FUO are listed in Table 2. In all published series, a sizeable subgroup of patients with FUO remains undiagnosed.

FUO in children

The proportion of cases of FUO due to infections is higher in children, and the proportion due to malignancy is correspondingly lower. Viral syndromes and urinary tract infections are particularly common infections in children. Still's disease and rheumatic fever are more likely to cause FUO in children than in adults, and children are less likely to have factitious fever. The overall mortality of FUO in children is lower than in adults.

FUO in the elderly

In patients over 65 years of age, intra-abdominal abscesses including hepatic abscesses, malignancies, and vasculitides cause a higher proportion of cases of FUO. The proportion of FUOs that remain undiagnosed in the elderly is lower, being only about half that in children and younger adults. The higher rate of underlying malignancies in any series of elderly patients with FUO means that the long-term prognosis is less favourable than in a younger group. The temporal arteritis–polymyalgia rheumatica syndromes are particularly important because they are common in the elderly, and their many non-specific symptoms may be missed or misdiagnosed. This diagnosis is easily suspected if the erythrocyte sedimentation rate (**ESR**) is over 100 mm/h, but is easily overlooked if an ESR is not obtained. Another hint is a high platelet count. Other connective tissue diseases are less common than in younger patients. Bacterial prostatitis and related urinary tract infections are more common in elderly men due to prostatic hypertrophy. In developed countries, infective endocarditis has become more common in older patients. Occult pulmonary emboli always should be considered in the differential diagnosis. Factitious fever is rare in the elderly.

Nosocomial FUO

Fever that develops after a patient has been admitted to hospital, and which remains undiagnosed, is termed 'nosocomial FUO'. These patients are usually being treated for one or more major pre-existing conditions, and have multiple possible reasons for developing fever. Several of these factors may be contributing simultaneously to the development of fever. After common bacterial infections such as pneumonia, urinary tract infection, and bacteraemia have been excluded, many other conditions remain in the differential diagnosis: for example, local or disseminated candidiasis, *Clostridium difficile* diarrhoea or colitis, cytomegalovirus infection, hepatitis, sinusitis (especially if the patient is intubated), intravascular catheter-related local or bloodstream infections, and infective endocarditis. The possibility that a non-infectious inflammatory condition such as acalculous cholecystitis,

gout, or pseudogout has flared during hospital admission for another condition should be considered. Occult pulmonary emboli are an important cause of nosocomial FUO. Drug fever is especially common in this patient group.

Neutropenic FUO

The number of patients with neutropenia caused by cytotoxic chemotherapy for various diseases is increasing, although the duration of neutropenia is now often curtailed by the timely administration of colony-stimulating factors. Fevers in neutropenic patients are very different from the classical FUO defined above. The leading causes of neutropenic FUO are bacteraemias, pneumonias, and skin/soft tissue infections. Urinary tract infections are less common than in nosocomial FUOs (above). Focal bacterial infections of intravascular lines and puncture wounds, skin folds, and the perianal area all are common, and often associated with bacteraemia. In the early stages of neutropenia, fevers are usually caused by bacteria, but if neutropenia persists, fungal, viral, and other conditions become relatively more common. However, this well-known sequence loses diagnostic value when the patient has received multiple cycles of chemotherapy and antimicrobial drugs.

Table 1 Summary of definitions and major features of four types of FUO

	Classical FUO	Nosocomial FUO	Neutropenic FUO	HIV-related FUO
Definition	>38.0 °C, >3 weeks, >2 physician visits or 3 days in hospital	>38.0 °C, >72 h, not present or incubating on admission	>38.0 °C, >72 h, <1000 PMNs/mm³, negative cultures after 48 h	>38.0 °C, >3 weeks for outpatients, >3 days for inpatients, HIV infection confirmed
Patient location	Community, clinic, or hospital	Acute-care hospital	Hospital or clinic	Community, clinic, or hospital
Leading aetiologies	Malignancies, infections, inflammatory conditions, undiagnosed cases, habitual hyperthermia	Nosocomial infections, postoperative complications, drug fevers	Majority due to infections, but aetiology documented in only 40–60%	HIV, typical and atypical *Mycobacteria* spp., CMV, lymphomas, toxoplasmosis
History emphasis	Travel, contacts, animal and insect exposure, immunizations, family history	Operations and procedures, devices, anatomical considerations, drug treatment	Stage of chemotherapy, drugs administered	Drugs, exposures, risk factors, travel, contacts, staging of HIV infection
Examination emphasis	Abdomen, lymph nodes, spleen, joints, muscles, arteries	Wounds, drains, devices, sinuses, urine	Skin folds, IV sites, lungs, perianal area	Mouth, skin, lymph nodes, eyes, lungs, perianal area
Investigation emphasis	Imaging, biopsies, ESR, tuberculin skin test	Imaging, bacterial cultures	Chest radiograph, bacterial cultures	Blood and lymphocyte count; serologies; chest radiograph; stool examination; biopsies of lung, bone marrow, liver; cultures and cytologies; brain imaging
Management	Observation, outpatient temperature chart, investigations, avoid empirical drug treatments	Depends on situation	Antimicrobial treatment protocols	HAART, antimicrobial treatment protocols, revision of treatment regimens, nutrition
Time course of disease	Months	Weeks	Days	Weeks to months
Tempo of investigation	Weeks	Days	Hours	Days to weeks
Mortality (attributable to the cause of FUO)	Moderate	Moderate	Low	High

Adapted with permission from Durack and Street (1991).

FUO, fever of unknown origin; PMNs, polymorphonuclear neutrophils; HIV, human immunodeficiency virus; CMV, cytomegalovirus; IV, intravenous; ESR, erythrocyte sedimentation rate; HAART, highly active retroviral therapy.

The duration of neutropenic FUOs tends to be much shorter than that of classical FUOs. The onset of fever often occurs within days of the onset of neutropenia; immediate empirical antimicrobial treatment is usually given, and improvement is frequently rapid. The aetiology of these FUOs often remains unconfirmed. In the majority of neutropenic FUOs the fever is probably due to infection, but the aetiological organism(s) will be identified in only 40 to 60 per cent of cases. Recurrent episodes are likely to occur for as long as the patient remains neutropenic.

HIV-associated FUO

A self-limited episode of fever often occurs during primary HIV infection. After a long asymptomatic interval, fevers and FUOs become extremely common during the later stages of HIV infection. This justifies the introduction of the term 'HIV-associated FUO' in the definitions listed above. The single most common cause of FUO in this setting is mycobacterial infection (tuberculosis in developing countries, *Mycobacterium avium* complex (**MAC**) in the developed world). MAC infection eventually affects up to 40 per cent of patients with acquired immunodeficiency syndrome (**AIDS**) in developed countries. Many other diagnoses must be considered, especially *Pneumocystis carinii* infection, cytomegalovirus infection, disseminated cryptococcosis, toxoplasmosis of the central nervous system, lymphomas, and nocardiosis. In the appropriate geographical regions, disseminated leishmaniasis, histoplasmosis, coccidiodomycosis, and *Penicil-*

lium marneffei infection must be considered. Recently, *Bartonella* species, which cause bacillary angiomatosis and peliosis hepatitis, have also been found to cause febrile bacteraemic syndromes and endocarditis in patients with AIDS.

Investigation of FUO

At the first encounter with the patient, a meticulous history should be taken and a complete physical examination performed. The theme should be attention to detail: for example, careful ophthalmoscopy after dilating of the pupils could reveal Roth spots or retinal tubercles in patients with classical FUO, retinal candidiasis in those with nosocomial FUO, or cytomegalovirus retinitis in cases of HIV-associated FUO. Routine test results (chest radiograph, routine blood count, differential cell count, erythrocyte sedimentation rate, and serum biochemistry) should be scanned for clues. A raised serum uric acid level could signal rapid cell turnover in lymphoma, and a raised alkaline phosphatase level can indicate liver involvement. The peripheral blood smear should be carefully examined for abnormalities such as thrombocytosis, leukaemoid reactions, the presence of nucleated red blood cells, and other clues that the marrow is reacting to a pathological stimulus. The initial findings should be reviewed in relation to the tempo of disease progression before deciding upon the next round of investigations. What major tests have already been performed elsewhere? Repetition of costly radiographs and scans may be unnecessary. Can further

Table 2 Various causes of FUO

Leading causes of FUO (by category and approximate frequency)	Uncommon or rare causes of FUO (in alphabetical order)
Infection (30–50%)	Alcoholic hepatitis
Bacterial abscesses (especially intra-abdominal)	Aortic dissection
Mycobacterial infections (human and atypical)	Atrial myxoma
Urinary tract infections	Behçet's syndrome
Infective endocarditis	Castleman disease
Viral infections (HIV, CMV, EBV)	Chronic meningitis
Amoebic abscess	Carcinomatous meningitis
Leishmaniasis	Cyclic neutropenia
Brucellosis	Drug fever and other hypersensitivities
Schistosomiasis	Erythema multiforme
	Fabry's disease
Malignancy (15–20%)	Familial Mediterranean fever
Lymphoma	Granulomatous hepatitis
Leukaemia	Granulomatous peritonitis
Other haematological malignancies	Haemoglobinopathies
Solid tumours	Haemolytic anaemias
	Histiocytosis X
Connective tissue diseases (10–20%)	Inflammatory bowel disease
Temporal arteritis/polymyalgia rheumatica	Lymphomatoid granulomatosis
Still's disease	Pancreatitis
Systemic lupus erythematosus	Paroxysmal haemoglobinurias
Polyarteritis nodosa	Pericarditis
Rheumatic fever (including recurrences)	Periodic fever
	Phaeochromocytoma
Miscellaneous (see right-hand column) (10–15%)	Pulmonary emboli
	Postpericardiotomy syndrome
Undiagnosed (10–25%)	Retroperitoneal fibrosis
	Sarcoidosis
	Serum sickness
	Sjögren's syndrome
	Thrombophlebitis
	Thrombotic thrombocytopenic purpura
	Thyroiditis and thyrotoxicosis
	Vogt–Koyanagi–Harada syndrome
	Wegener's granulomatosis
	Whipple's disease

FUO, fever of unknown origin; HIV, human immunodeficiency virus; CMV, cytomegalovirus; EBV, Epstein–Barr virus.

testing be safely postponed? Sometimes more will be learned by waiting, or the FUO may resolve spontaneously.

The next level of investigation will usually involve blood cultures, skin testing for delayed hypersensitivity to tuberculosis, and selected serological tests for infections and connective tissue diseases. In older patients, tests for prostate-specific antigen and carcinoembryonic antigen should be obtained. Echocardiography should be performed if any clues are found that increase the pretest probability of infective endocarditis (for example, unexplained heart murmurs or emboli).

Selection of further investigations requires careful consideration of the likely yield, risks, and costs of each. Because many FUOs are associated with intra-abdominal conditions, computed tomography (**CT**) of the abdomen often is valuable. Sinus radiographs and pulmonary CT can reveal the lesions of Wegener's granulomatosis. Radiographs of the bowel with contrast can reveal abnormalities needing further investigation. Gastrointestinal endoscopy with biopsy is often appropriate if symptoms or imaging studies suggest enteric conditions such as inflammatory bowel disease or cancer. Adjunctive imaging with magnetic resonance imaging scan and/or ^{67}gallium- or ^{111}indium-labelled leucocytes can be helpful, but these tests should be used selectively because they are costly and of limited sensitivity; the chance that one of these will reveal a diagnosis is quite low if radiographs and CT scans are negative. Positron-emission tomography using isotopic fluorodeoxyglucose (**FDG-PET** scan) is a new imaging technique which may prove better than older scanning methods. Transoesophageal echocardiography should be performed if the transthoracic echocardiogram is normal or indeterminate but endocarditis still seems likely.

Biopsies of bone marrow, lymph nodes, lung tissue, liver, skin, and temporal arteries or other vessels are essential for the diagnosis of many FUOs. Exploratory laparotomy, previously often performed for the diagnosis of FUO, is now rarely necessary because of improved imaging techniques and directed biopsies. Abnormalities of cytokine levels in blood occur in over two-thirds of patients with FUO, but this finding has not yet proven useful in diagnosis.

For HIV-associated FUO, if the chest radiograph is abnormal or the patient is hypoxic, bronchial washings or biopsy may reveal *Pneumocystis* spp. *Mycobacteria* spp. *Cryptococcus* spp. or cytomegalovirus infection. Direct staining of stool may reveal the presence of *Mycobacteria* spp. If the patient is stable, the results of blood cultures for *Mycobacteria* spp. and unusual bacteria such as *Rhodococcus* or *Bartonella* spp. should be awaited before further invasive tests are done. If the fever remains undiagnosed at this stage, bone marrow and liver biopsies are most likely to be informative.

Approach to treatment

Treatment of the fever itself is indicated if fever distresses the patient, exacerbates heart failure, or is severe enough to cause catabolism and wasting. Otherwise, the temperature curve can be observed in the absence of treatment, often yielding useful new information while investigations continue. If the fever must be treated, aspirin, paracetamol, or a non-steroidal anti-inflammatory drug in standard doses will usually suffice. A regular dosage schedule rather than occasional or 'as required' dosing is recommended.

Treatment of classical FUO

If an aetiological diagnosis cannot be made at first, it is usually best to withhold treatment while observing the patient's progress at frequent intervals. Ideally, a diagnosis will eventually be made, so allowing specific therapy. If an undiagnosed patient is too ill to permit prolonged observation, empirical treatment for FUO may be considered. The most common choice for an empirical therapeutic trial is a corticosteroid. The recommended dose for an adult is prednisone 30 mg orally twice daily initially, or the equivalent dose of another corticosteroid. The possibility that the fever may be eliminated by empirical corticosteroid therapy while the primary disease

is unaffected (or even exacerbated) should be kept in mind. The next most common choice for empirical therapy is a broad-spectrum antibiotic such as oral amoxicillin or a fluoroquinolone, or a parenteral regimen such as ampicillin plus gentamicin. In patients who are desperately ill, a combination of parenteral corticosteroid plus antibiotics may be administered. Less commonly, empirical therapy for possible tuberculosis may be tried.

Treatment of neutropenic FUO

After performing a focused physical examination, obtaining a chest roentgenogram, and sending two blood samples and a urine sample for cultures, empirical broad-spectrum antibacterial therapy should be started immediately, before the results of laboratory tests are available. If initial cultures are positive, an antibiotic regimen specific for the aetiological micro-organism can be chosen. If necessary, antifungal or antiviral therapy may be added or substituted, according to the patient's progress and the results of investigations.

Treatment of HIV-associated FUO

HIV-infected patients with an acute onset of fever and hypoxia will usually be treated immediately for possible *Pneumocystis carinii* infection, even if the chest radiograph is normal. Ideally, a diagnosis should be made as soon as possible through standard investigations. Once the cause of HIV-associated FUO has been diagnosed, specific treatment regimens as described in Chapter 7.10.21 can be prescribed. For patients who remain undiagnosed, various empirical treatments may be tried. Antimycobacterial drugs are commonly included because of the high prevalence of both tuberculous and non-tuberculous mycobacterial infections in HIV-infected subjects.

Prognosis

Classical FUO is a serious condition. Although most of the causes of this type of FUO can be treated, the 1-year mortality is still between 20 and 30 per cent. Obviously, the prognosis varies depending upon the underlying disease and the age of the patient. If FUO persists undiagnosed for more than 6 to 12 months, the likelihood that a specific diagnosis will ever be made decreases, and the prognosis improves greatly, to less than 5 per cent mortality.

The prognosis for nosocomial FUO depends largely on the underlying diagnoses. The short-term prognosis for neutropenic FUO is excellent, with over a 90 per cent response to initial empirical antimicrobial therapy (with appropriate modification as laboratory results return). Again, the long-term prognosis is determined largely by the underlying disease.

Most of the causes of HIV-associated FUO can be treated, but these patients have a relatively poor prognosis, with death likely within 2 years because HIV disease is usually advanced by the time the patient has FUO. The prognosis has improved somewhat with the introduction of highly active antiretroviral therapy. Atypical *Mycobacteria* spp. (which are the commonest cause of HIV-associated FUO) can be suppressed but seldom eliminated, and are likely to develop resistance during therapy.

Further reading

Armstrong WS, Katz JT, Kazanjian PH (1999). Human immunodeficiency virus-associated fever of unknown origin: a study of 70 patients in the United States and review. *Clinical Infectious Diseases* **28**, 341–5.

Blockmans D, *et al* (2001). Clinical value of (18F) fluoro-deoxyglucose positron emission tomography for patients with fever of unknown origin. *Clinical Infectious Diseases* **32**, 191–6.

Durack DT, Street AC (1991). Fever of unknown origin—reexamined and redefined. In: Remington JS and Swartz MN, eds. *Current clinical topics in infectious diseases*, Vol 11, pp 35–51. Blackwell Scientific, Boston.

Cunha BA (1998). Fever of unknown origin. In: Gorbach SL, Bartlett JG, and Blacklow NR, eds. *Infectious diseases*, 2nd edn, pp 1678–89. WB Saunders, Philadelphia.

Hughes WT, *et al* (1997). 1997 guidelines for the use of antimicrobial agents in neutropenic patients with unexplained fever. *Clinical Infectious Diseases* **25**, 551–73.

Kazanjian PH (1992). Fever of unknown origin: review of 86 patients treated in community hospitals. *Clinical Infectious Diseases* **15**, 968–73.

Kjaer A, Lebech AM (2002). Diagnostic value of (111)In-granulocyte scintigraphy in patients with fever of unknown origin. *Journal of Nuclear Medicine* **43**, 140–4.

Knockaert DC, Bobbaers HJ (1996). Long-term follow-up of patients with undiagnosed fever of unknown origin. *Archives of Internal Medicine* **156**, 618–20.

Knockaert DC, Vanneste LJ, Bobbaers HJ (1993). Recurrent or episodic fever of unknown origin. Review of 45 cases and survey of the literature. *Medicine* **72**, 184–96.

Mackowiak P, ed. (1997). *Fever: basic mechanisms, and management*, 2nd edn. Raven Press, New York.

Maschmeyer G (1999). Interventional antimicrobial therapy in febrile neutropenic patients. *Diagnostic Microbiology, and Infectious Diseases* **34**, 205–12.

Norman DC (2000). Fever in the elderly. *Clinical Infectious Diseases* **31**, 148–51.

Petersdorf RG, Beeson PB (1961). Fever of unexplained origin: report on 100 cases. *Medicine* **40**, 1–30.

Sepkowitz KA (1999). FUO and AIDS. *Current Clinical Topics in Infectious Diseases* **19**, 1–15.

7.3 Biology of pathogenic micro-organisms

T. H. Pennington

Why clinicians need to know about the biology of pathogens

Joseph Lister in Glasgow in the late 1860s was the first successfully to apply a hypothesis about the biology of pathogenic micro-organisms to the management of individual patients. It was that 'putrefaction.... as it occurs in surgical practice'. is caused by the 'germs of various low forms of life' that could be 'deprived of energy' by various chemicals without seriously injuring patients. The subsequent development of microbiology paved the way for the replacement of his antiseptic method by aseptic procedures—one of the most successful innovations in direct patient care that has ever happened—as well as the rational development of vaccines. Antibiotics followed. All of these have been enormously successful. But, even in the richest countries, the current importance of nosocomial infections, the long list of organisms for which vaccines are still desired, and increasing antibiotic resistance show that, despite a successful track record, much unfinished business remains. In poor countries, infections such as tuberculosis are still common causes of premature death. Capping all these things is the regular— but unpredictable—appearance and intercontinental spread of totally new pathogens such as HIV.

Progress towards resolving these problems will very often depend on achieving a better understanding of the relevant pathogens. Genomics promises much. Equally important for practitioners and for medicine, however, is the more effective application of the science that is already known. Both of these considerations explain why a general understanding of the biology of pathogens is important in clinical practice.

The ecology of pathogens

For a parasite to be successful, it must be capable of invading and maintaining itself in a host population. For it to spread, its basic reproductive rate— the average number of progeny that it produces— must be greater than one. Our aim for pathogens is to reduce this below unity, both in patients and in human communities. World-wide, polio may be eradicated soon, but smallpox is our sole success so far. Only infecting humans, it had a low efficiency of transmission which could effectively be interrupted by isolating patients and surrounding them with a ring of individuals made resistant to infection by immunization— which had already reduced the number of susceptibles to a very low figure. These factors— host range, patterns of transmission, and those affecting susceptibility—are key biological parameters for understanding why infections occur and for devising countermeasures. Knowledge about them enables us to explain why, for example, the pattern of *Salmonella* infections has undergone such a dramatic change in Britain since the end of the nineteenth century. It is a reasonable estimate that the overall incidence of human infections with species of this genus was much the same in 1880 as 1990. But infections with *S. typhi*—which accounted for nearly all those contracted in 1880—have almost completely disappeared to be replaced by those caused by *S. enteritica* serovars. This is because the human-to-human faecal–oral spread of *S. typhi* has been interrupted by the provision of clean water and safe sewers, while the recent cultivation of poultry on a massive scale in crowded hen houses with ample opportunities for faecal–oral spread, and subsequent processing that contaminates carcasses with gut contents, has provided bacterially contaminated food on a grand scale.

The lists of important transmission routes and sources of pathogens are short. Person-to-person skin contact, sex, mother to fetus transmission, inoculation of pathogens by arthropod or animal bites and other wounds and by needles, ingestion in food and water, inhalation in droplet nuclei, and transmission by fomites are the important routes. Exogenous sources of infection are other individuals, animals, the environment, and arthropods (as an intermediate but replicative step in transmission from other humans or animals). Many bacteria and viruses are facultative pathogens. Organisms such as *Staphylococcus aureus* and *Streptococcus pneumoniae* spend most of their time living harmlessly on the skin or in the throat, and a significant proportion of the clinically important infections they cause are endogenous, in that they occur in the individuals who carry them. Consideration of these factors provides explanations as to why some public health measures have been much more successful than others, and why current problems, such as nosocomial infections, still occur. Thus, it is easier to filter and chlorinate water than to change human sexual behaviour. The difficulty of changing human behaviour has also provided a major obstacle to the implementation of the critically important safety measure in preventing person-to-person spread and in food safety—hand washing.

The classification of pathogens

Many different bacteria and viruses cause disease in humans. Biodiversity is their hallmark. The modern classification of bacteria is based on DNA sequence data. So far, only a few genomes have been completely sequenced and relationships have been worked out using data from limited regions of the genome, particularly those coding for 16S ribosomal RNA—a relatively stable molecule from an evolutionary standpoint (Fig. 1). Viruses are classified according to schemes which take account of the nature of the nucleic acid in the virus particle—DNA or RNA—and its size and dispositions, particle structure—particularly crystallographic symmetry, size, and the presence or absence of a lipid envelope—and the pathways of virus messenger RNA synthesis (Fig. 2). Only a few general rules emerge from these groupings. Thus, the ability to form spores (which drives the need for autoclaves) only occurs in two medically important Gram-positive genera, *Clostridium* and *Bacillus*. Gram-negative and Gram-positive bacteria have different cell wall structures which play an important role in determining the different antibiotic sensitivities of organisms in these categories. Endotoxin, a major virulence factor, is the lipopolysaccharide component of the Gram-negative cell wall.

Only viruses with DNA genomes (such as herpesviruses) or with RNA genomes that are copied into DNA as part of the infection cycle (such as

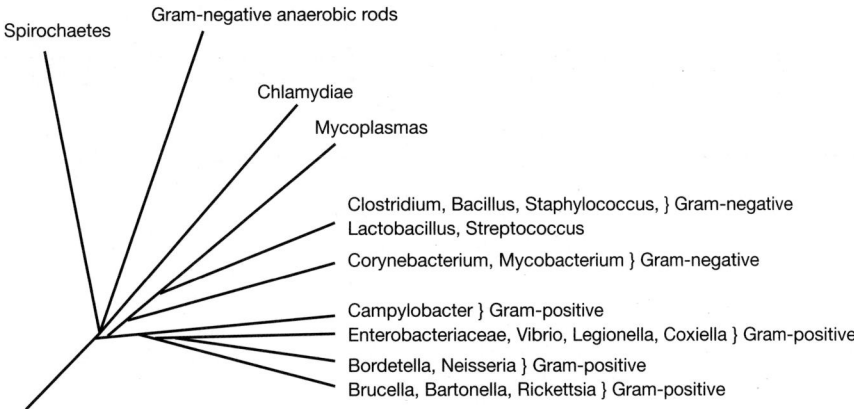

Fig. 1 Phylogenetic tree of medically important bacteria based on 16S rRNA sequence comparisons.

retroviruses) set up long-term or permanent residence in the host; sometimes this is associated with the formation of malignant tumours. Genome size is inversely proportional to the rate of evolution of natural populations. A small genome, coupled with high mutation and replication rates and high yields, explains why the evolution of some viruses proceeds millions of times faster than that of the human host. In one or two cases, notably HIV, the evolution rate is so great that the virus population in a patient comprises a 'quasispecies' made up of a 'cloud' of variants a few mutational steps away from a master sequence—the sequence of highest fitness—and the master sequence itself. For the influenza viruses a high evolution rate is facilitated by a high recombination rate (strictly speaking a reassortment of segments of its naturally fragmented genome). Other RNA viruses, such as measles virus and poliovirus, show much less genetic variation during natural infections—one reason why their empirically developed vaccines continue to be successful many years after their development.

The fact that they have not been designed, but have evolved, explains why pathogens are so diverse and why so few general principles can be drawn from the groupings that emerge from their classification. Neverthe-

less, important guides to practice do emerge from evolutionary considerations. Thus the use of antibiotics, antiviral drugs, and vaccines exert strong selection pressures on pathogens and so should only be used in the context of evolutionary thinking. Evolutionary theory also generates explanations as to why virulence has evolved to certain levels; these may in turn generate hypotheses about how to reduce it.

Virulence determinants

Just as pathogens show enormous biodiversity, so many different mechanisms—virulence determinants—are involved in the causation of disease by them. The coincidental operation of multiple factors is nearly always needed to cause disease. A classical and notable exception is botulism, where the ingestion of preformed exotoxin in food is sufficient.

For most pathogens our knowledge of which virulence factors they possess and how they work together is significantly incomplete. The practical impact of this on clinical work is that it often limits the help that laboratory tests can provide in assessing the virulence of organisms isolated from

Fig. 2 Grouping of viruses by genome composition and pathway of mRNA synthesis.

patients. Indeed, tests for the production, or capability of producing, exotoxins, as in the cases of *Corynebacterium diphtheriae* and enterohaemorrhagic *E. coli* (such as *E. coli* 0157 H7), provide about the only examples where routine laboratory testing for virulence factors is used to distinguish between virulent and avirulent strains of the same species. Lack of knowledge about virulence factors and how they work in concert is a particularly important deficiency in the area of emerging and rapidly evolving pathogens such as influenza virus, and antibiotic resistant bacteria such as MRSA (methicillin-resistant *Staphylococcus aureus*). Thus it is still not possible, confidently, to predict from the details of its genetic structure whether an influenza virus will be more or less virulent—despite the very great depth of knowledge accumulated over many years about the sequence, function, and variation of the genes of the virus, and its structure, replication, and natural history in general. Likewise, laboratory tests have not helped to resolve the debate about whether—drug resistance apart—MRSA have added clinical importance because they are more virulent than other *Staphylococcus aureus* strains.

Adhesion and cell entry

To cause disease after being transmitted to its host, a pathogen must adhere to cells or other structures such as connective tissue or foreign bodies. Some bacteria produce clinically apparent effects when growing extracellularly; for others, entry into cells is an essential part of the disease process. Obligate intracellular parasites such as viruses and some bacteria must go through this step in order to replicate. The rates and extent of subsequent local or distant growth are usually important determinants of disease outcomes. Specialized structures, molecules, and processes are used to carry out these steps. For bacteria, surface structures and molecules important for adhesion include fimbriae (pili)—hair-like structures synthesized by Gram-negative bacteria—, flagella (in *Vibrio cholerae* and *Campylobacter jejuni*), outer membrane proteins (particularly in *Neisseria gonorrhoeae*), exopolysaccharides (in cariogenic streptococci and some staphylococci), and collagen, fibronectin, and fibrinogen binding proteins (as in *Staphylococcus aureus*). Many important pathogens employ molecular mimicry. In some, their adhesion molecules may mimic natural ligands, such as the *Bordetella pertussis* haemagglutin which mimics integrins. In others, the organism binds to host ligands which then bind to their natural receptors, as with *Legionella pneumophila* which becomes coated with complement components which then bind to complement receptors.

One of the main functions of a virus particle is to optimize the likelihood of infection by providing structures that interact with molecules on the surface of host cells and prepare the way for virus entry into them. All animal viruses carry multiple attachment proteins or sites on their surface. In some, these are discrete structures, such as the glycoprotein spikes on the surface of influenza virus. In others, such as picornaviruses, receptor binding sites are created at the interfaces between different viral polypeptides. In some large viruses, such as *Herpes simplex*, an initial low-affinity interaction with one receptor is followed by a slower, tighter, binding to another. Viruses enter cells either by fusing their envelopes with the cell membrane and internalizing the nucleocapsid, or by receptor-mediated endocytosis into endosomes, subsequent fusion of the virus with the endosome membrane, and entry of its genome into the cytoplasm.

The bacterial species that enter cells when infecting humans are all important pathogens. They include *Mycobacterium* species, *Salmonella*, *Shigella*, pathogenic *E. coli*, *Yersinia*, *Legionella*, and *Listeria*. For *Yersinia* and *Listeria* internalization correlates with a strong adhesion of bacteria to the cell surface (mediated in *Yersinia* by interactions between bacterial invasion and multiple integrins, and in *Listeria* by its internalin interacting with cellular E-cadherin). Cellular pseudopods extend around the bacterium and engulf it in a tight phagosome. *Shigella* and some pathogenic *E. coli* inject proteins into cells which cause rearrangements which promote and lead to entry. The *Shigella* Ipa protein enters the cell and associates with vinculin. A major rearrangement of the host cytoskeleton follows in which actin linked to the cell membrane causes the formation of projections which engulf the bacterium, cell entry occurring by micropinocytosis. Other pathogens, as taxonomically diverse as *Listeria* and vaccinia virus, also associate with the cytoskeleton. They use actin cables to move about the cell during the intracytoplasmic part of their life cycles.

Spread of pathogens within the body

Local, restricted spread is sufficient for some pathogens to cause common and self-limiting or, with a few bacterial species, lethal conditions. The commonest clinically apparent staphylococcal infections—boils—fall into the first category, as do rhinovirus infections of the upper respiratory tract. Localized infections may be life threatening because of the productions of exotoxins that act at a distance, as with *Clostridium tetani*, or exotoxins that act locally as well, as with *Corynebacterium diphtheriae*, *Clostridium perfringens* when causing gas gangrene, and *Streptococcus pyogenes* when causing necrotizing fasciitis. A few bacterial pathogens, such as *Salmonella typhi* or *Treponema pallidum*, invade and grow in organs such as the brain, bones, and skin as a matter of course. For the majority of common bacterial pathogens such outcomes occur in only a small minority of infected individuals. Thus the number of individuals that develop meningitis or septic arthritis is much smaller than the number who carry *Neisseria meningitidis* in their throats or suffer from gonorrhoea. Nevertheless, all these pathogens must possess mechanisms—many of which are poorly understood at present— that allow them to reach blood vessels, traverse the endothelial lining, and use the circulation to travel to distant organs. Similar considerations apply to viruses. While some remain localized, others spread widely. The circulation is the most important route. Viruses enter either via lymphatics or are shed from infected endothelial cells or circulating mononuclear leucocytes. Then they circulate free in the plasma or associated with formed elements. During this process some replicate in monocytes, T or B lymphocytes, or, occasionally, erythrocytes. A particularly important example is HIV, which infects CD4+ T lymphocytes and monocytes in the blood, particularly the former. Some viruses are disseminated in the body by spreading along peripheral nerves, an essential route for rabies and certain herpesviruses, and a supplementary one (to viraemia) for polio- and reoviruses.

Factors that neutralize host defences

Many pathogens employ mechanisms which optimize their chances of establishing themselves and growing in a host. Some bacteria that live in the respiratory tract, such as *Streptococcus pneumoniae*, *Haemophilus influenzae*, and *Neisseria meningitidis*, produce a protease that selectively destroys host secretory IgA. Bacterial polysaccharide capsules protect against phagocytosis— unless opsonized by the attachment of specific antibody— and against the activity of the alternative complement pathway. Some bacteria evade the host immune response by taking up an intracellular location; it is considered that *Mycobacterium tuberculosis* can survive inside macrophages for long periods, setting up a latent infection which can reactivate and cause disease many years after the initial infection. Large DNA viruses code for proteins that interfere with host mechanisms that respond to infection. A major herpes simplex glycoprotein binds the C3b and iC3b components of the complement cascade protecting against complement-mediated virus neutralization and lysis of infected cells; likewise the vaccinia virus complement control protein binds to C4b—mutations in this gene result in reduced virulence. Poxviruses also induce the synthesis of many other proteins that interfere with host cytokine functions, including soluble receptors for interleukin-1β (IL-1β), interferon γ, and tumour necrosis factor (TNF), serpins that inhibit cytokine activation, and proteins that inhibit the expression of MHC-1 antigens at the cell surface.

Factors that damage the host

Bacterial infections damage hosts in three different ways. Bacterial cell components are directly toxic; some bacterial species produce exotoxins which damage cells, cell function, or physiological processes; and the host response to infection may itself contribute to pathology.

The lipopolysaccharide component of the cell walls of Gram-negative bacteria, particularly its core region lipid A, is an important virulence factor. Lipid A stimulates the production of cytokines such as IL-1 and TNF by macrophages. Gram-positive cell wall and other surface structures components may also be toxic. A diversity of bacterial species produce exotoxins. They are important because their toxicity can be very great and because medical measures can be targeted against them by developing toxoids for prevention, and antitoxins for treatment. The former have been much more successful in practice than the latter. Exotoxins are nearly all medium sized to large proteins. Multicomponent ones, such as cholera toxin with one A subunit and five B subunits, are the exception. Some are inactive when produced and need to be cleaved by proteolysis, such as cholera toxin, the *Clostridium botulinum* toxins, and diphtheria toxin. The B region of the latter molecule, for example, binds to cells and is proteolytically nicked to release another part, the A region, which enters the cell and exerts its toxic effect. Some exotoxins cause very different diseases but have similar actions at the molecular level. Thus both the cholera toxin and a pertussis toxin activate adenylate cyclase by enzymatically ribosylating its GTP-binding regulator, and diphtheria toxin causes the ADP ribosylation of elongation factor 2. The end result of these actions on individuals is, of course, quite different. Activation of adenylate cyclase by pertussis toxin damage inhibits the functions of immune effector cells, while in cholera it stimulates chloride secretion and the inhibition of sodium uptake in villus and crypt gut cells causing profuse, watery diarrhoea. In diphtheria, cell protein synthesis is turned off. Some toxins are highly organ specific, such as the neurotoxins of *Clostridium botulinum* which cause flaccid paralysis by acting presynaptically at neuromuscular junctions where they inhibit the exocytosis of vesicles containing acetylcholine. Others have a more widespread effect, such as the staphylococcal toxins that act directly on cell membranes, the α toxin causing cytotoxic damage by creating transmembrane channels, and the β toxin, a phospholipase active on sphingomyelin, being cytolytic for red cells, platelets, and macrophages.

Viruses do not produce exotoxins, neither do their virions contain toxic components such as endotoxins. They produce disease by killing cells (directly or indirectly), by altering patterns of cell growth, and by immunopathological mechanisms. The irreversible inhibition of host cell protein synthesis is a common consequence of infection. A variety of mechanisms selectively turn off cell protein synthesis. They include host mRNA degradation and the inactivation and subversion of components involved in the translation of capped mRNAs. The induction of apoptotic cell death by virus infection has been clearly shown in experimental models. Its role in the causation of human disease is not clear. The induction of benign or malignant tumours by viruses is not uncommon. Representatives of all the major subdivisions of viruses with double-stranded DNA have been implicated in neoplasia, and it has been estimated that up to 20 per cent of human tumours have a viral risk factor. Oncogenes occur in retroviruses and some DNA viruses; the association of other virus infections with tumour formation is indirect and usually associated with cofactors such as malaria in the case of Epstein–Barr virus and Burkitt's lymphoma. The mechanisms responsible for virus-induce immunopathology are exemplified by hepatitis B, where the destruction of virus-infected hepatocytes can follow attack by CD8 T cells, and rashes, glomerulonephritis, and polyarteritis nodosa can be caused by immune complexes.

Why do pathogens cause disease in particular patients?

The possession of virulence factors by a pathogen are necessary, but not usually sufficient, for it to cause disease. In other words, infections with most pathogens are asymptomatic in at least a minority of patients. Factors which may increase the probability of host damage include pathogen dose and route of transmission, particularly if the latter by-passes host defences. In individual patients, it is hardly ever possible to measure pathogen dose and prognostic attention usually focuses on host factors. Many are important, including the efficiency of non-specific and immunological host defences in neutralizing virulence factors and inhibiting pathogen growth. Previous infections can play roles through immunosuppressive effects, as in HIV and AIDS, or by causing tissue damage, as in the bacterial pneumonia that sometimes follows influenza. Genetically determined host susceptibilities to infection include various immunodeficiencies, and conditions which enhance the ability of pathogens to cause tissue damage. Human B19 parvovirus infections provide a good example. The much shortened red cell survival times in sickle-cell disease and hereditary spherocytosis combine with the preferential replication of this virus in erythroid precursor cells to lead to complete red cell aplasia in individuals with these conditions, in contrast to the transient reduction in reticulocyte count seen in normal individuals.

Age is also an important factor in determining the outcome of infection. Although as a general rule disease severity is more severe in the very young and the very old, pathogen-specific features such as the severe organ damage produced by rubella in the first trimester of pregnancy are also important. The biological basis of age-determined susceptibility is not known for most pathogens, even when the effect is consistent and marked. In untreated typhus, for example, mortality rates increase steadily with age, being negligible in children, about 5 per cent in young people under 20, 50 per cent in 50-year olds, and 100 per cent in those over 60.

All the factors discussed in this chapter are the result of evolution. Evolutionary studies on pathogenicity have only just started but they are beginning to provide explanations about how organisms evolve towards virulence. Bacteria reproduce asexually and so have clonal population structures. Horizontal gene exchange is not infrequent, however, and genomes have mosaic structures built up of a basic clonal framework peppered with DNA regions derived from other organisms. These include 'pathogenicity islands'—stretches of DNA containing many virulence genes. Toxin genes also move around on bacteriophages and plasmids. Viruses have incorporated virulence genes, such as oncogenes, from their hosts. Why organisms become pathogens is much less certain.

Further reading

General

Anderson RM, May RM (1991). *Infectious diseases of humans. Dynamics and control.* Oxford University Press.

Collier L, Balows A, Sussman M, eds (1998). *Topley and Wilson's microbiology and microbial infections.* Vol. 1 Chapters 1–13, Vol. 2 Chapters 1–12, Vol. 3 Chapters 1–11. Arnold, London.

Stearns SC, ed (1999). *Evolution in health and disease.* Oxford University Press.

Specific reviews illustrating general principles

Abu Kwaik Y (1998). Fatal attraction of mammalian cells to *Legionella pneumophila. Molecular Microbiology* **30**, 689–95.

Frankel G *et al.* (1998). Enteropathogenic and enterohaemorrhagic *Escherichia coli*: more subversive elements. *Molecular Microbiology* **30**, 911–21.

Hinton JCD (1997). The *Escherichia coli* genome sequence: the end of an era or the start of FUN? *Molecular Microbiology* **26**, 417–22.

O'Brien V (1998). Viruses and apoptosis. *Journal of General Virology* **79**, 1833–45.

Petit L, Gilbert M, Popoff MR (1999). *Clostridium perfringens*: toxinotype and genotype. *Trends in Microbiology* **7**, 104–10.

Smith DB *et al.* (1997). Virus 'quasispecies': making a mountain out of a molehill? *Journal of General Virology* **78**, 1511–19.

Sokurenko EV, Hasty DL, Dykhuisen DE (1999). Pathoadaptive mutations: gene loss and variation in bacterial pathogens. *Trends in Microbiology* **7**, 191–5.

Wallinga J, Edmunds WJ, Kretzschmar M (1999). Perspective: human contact patterns and the spread of airborne infectious diseases. *Trends in Microbiology* **7**, 372–7.

7.4 The host response to infection

Leszek K. Borysiewicz

Introduction

The expansion in our knowledge of the pathogenesis of infectious diseases over the last two decades is principally a consequence of the development of analytical techniques for investigating biological molecules. Our greater understanding of the biology of infectious agents, including complete genomic sequences of pathogens, as well as the nature of the host response, provides new opportunities for therapeutic research. The interdependence of host and parasite shows the importance of selective pressure from microbes on the evolution of human immune responses. None the less, the central and perplexing question confronting clinicians remains unanswered—what are the principal determinants of disease in an individual patient? This chapter cannot answer this question, but it does describe developments in the field and how they may impact on our understanding of infectious diseases.

The nature of the host–pathogen interaction

Although the parasite–host interaction is often portrayed as a balance of host and parasite factors (Fig. 1), the full range of interactions is large and complex. Symbiosis occurs in the gastrointestinal tract even though factors involved in pathogenesis, such as bacterial adherence and colonization, also operate—but usually with benefit to the host. True pathogenic effects are seen when the host–parasite interaction is modified, such as antibiotic-associated colitis. The survival advantage to a pathogen of host damage is variable and often the best-adapted parasites find an ecological niche and disseminate with minimal disturbance to the host.

Pathogen factors

The molecular basis of microbial pathogenicity has advanced significantly through a genomic approach. Since the sequence of *Haemophilus influenzae* was reported in 1995, more than 50 complete bacterial genomes have now been sequenced. They range from 0.58 Mbp for *Mycoplasma genita-*

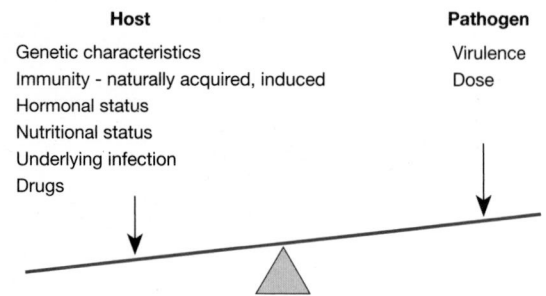

Host	Pathogen
Genetic characteristics	Virulence
Immunity - naturally acquired, induced	Dose
Hormonal status	
Nutritional status	
Underlying infection	
Drugs	

Fig. 1 Factors affecting the host/parasite balance.

lium to 4.4 and 4.6 Mbp for *M. tuberculosis* and *Escherichia coli*, respectively. Analysis of these genome sequences supports earlier work suggesting that bacterial populations are derived from clonal lineages. This concept implies that genetic exchange (through recombination or horizontal exchange using mobile genetic elements) occurs at low frequency, otherwise a greater heterogeneity of bacterial populations would be observed. However, horizontal transfer is an important source of diversity in bacterial genomes (~18 per cent in *E. coli*). Some pathogenic bacteria are remarkably homogeneous; there are few clonal populations of *Shigella sonnei* and *Bordetella pertussis* in which a single clonal type represents the whole species. Other species such as *Neisseria gonorrhoeae* and *N. meningitidis* show random chromosomal rearrangement, although, during outbreaks of meningitis, a few clonal types dominate the bacterial isolates. Multiple clones of *E. coli* are present during colonization but pathogenic clones persist, suggesting a process of selection within the host environment.

Virulence factors

Observations based on genome analysis combined with information on pathogenic factors, suggest that three mechanisms, each operating on a different time-scale, permit the acquisition of pathogenicity within a clonal subpopulation of bacteria:

- Transfer of virulence genes on mobile genetic elements, such as bacteriophages and plasmids, is rapid, and in the clinical context that allows the acquisition of antibiotic resistance in a population of bacteria during a single episode of infection. Other virulence factors are similarly transferred: for example, cholera toxin is encoded by a vibriophage, which integrates into the *Vibrio cholerae* chromosome.

- Random chromosomal transfer and bacterial transformation allows the acquisition of factors by *N. gonorrhoeae* to replicate in a host.

- The above mechanisms may be coupled with chromosomal relocation of genes in pathogenic bacteria to create 'pathogenicity islands'. These are segments of the bacterial genome (up to 200 kbp) that are flanked by repeat or insertion elements. The segments encode clusters of virulence genes including adhesion molecules, toxins, and secretory and regulatory proteins.

Bacterial virulence factors are regulated such that they are expressed in particular environmental circumstances. Common factors triggering expression include: changes in ionic concentration, pH, iron concentration, and temperature: for example, induction of K-88 and K-99 and pyelonephritis-associated fimbriae in uropathogenic *E. coli*. The factors regulating transcription of these genes are often aggregated into 'regulons' as exemplified by *Bordetella pertussis*. The bacterium expresses a number of virulence factors, such as pertussis toxin, haemagglutinin, fimbrial protein, and pertactin, regulated in a co-ordinated manner by the *bvgAS* chromosomal locus. The locus encodes a BvgS protein that spans the periplasmic membrane. At 37 °C, BvgS autophosphorylates with later transfer of the phosphorylation signal to BvgA, a bacterial regulator that can bind to specific regions of *Bordetella* DNA, thereby promoting the specific transcription of virulence factors as well as amplifying its own signal and repressing other genes. Thus a single signalling cascade can induce a variety of changes responding to several environmental stimuli in a co-ordinated manner.

Although many virulence factors are secreted, others are surface molecules that promote adhesion and bacterial entry by intracellular pathogens as well as interfering with specific host immunity. Intermittent expression of such factors on bacterial pili in *N. gonorrhoeae* reduces the ability of the host to mount a neutralizing antibody response. The mechanisms regulating antigenic variation at this locus and the correct orientation of such factors in pili are the consequence of gene rearrangements in chromosomal DNA and are essential for immune evasion by *N. gonorrhoeae*. Similar mechanisms operate in larger parasites such as *Trypanosoma brucei*.

Route of entry

Invasion of the host to access its environmental niche requires a pathogen to overcome physical barriers, as well as specific defence mechanisms, to establish itself. Many organisms have more than one phase in their lifecycle, either in another host (for example, malaria) or persisting outside a host by an alteration of its lifecycle (for example, encystment in *Amoeba* spp. or spore formation in *Clostridia* spp.). The skin is a relatively impermeable barrier which the pathogen must bypass. This can be achieved for some pathogens by insect vectors or direct trauma with penetrating wounds: for example, a needlestick injury for transmission of the human immunodeficiency virus (**HIV**) and hepatitis C. Even those organisms that produce local skin infections have to either penetrate the skin at sites of injury to gain access to susceptible cells in the basal layers of the epithelium (for example, human papillomaviruses) or infect adnexal structures (for example, staphylococcal folliculitis).

Alternatively, pathogens enter at mucosal surfaces; but here again physical barriers limit the ability of the pathogen to be retained, let alone replicate at such sites. Many pathogenic factors encoded by bacteria are adhesion molecules that interact with specific host receptors, for example to enable the pathogen to avoid the mucociliary carpet of the respiratory tract or the urothelial/gastrointestinal tract. However, such interactions are not inert because receptor–ligand binding may trigger cellular activation, which itself can be utilized to promote pathogenicity.

For intracellular parasites such as viruses, host interactions also provide the mechanism of entry to the intracellular environment. One of the best-studied mechanisms for the initiation of infection is the interaction of the haemagglutinin of orthomyxoviruses, such as influenza A, with sialic acid. The influenza haemagglutinin (**HA**) is present in the viral envelope as homotrimers of 550 amino-acid chains attached to a membrane-spanning and a short cytoplasmic domain. The molecule has a globular head that includes a conserved receptor pocket in the HA_1 globular region and a long stalk that incorporates an HA_2 domain. Depending on minor variations in HA_1, there are preferences between influenza strains for the optimum configuration of the presented sialyl residues that are bound. After the virus has bound to the cell surface, it is endocytosed and transferred to the endosomal compartment where the pH is reduced to between 5 and 6. Acidification results in an irreversible conformational change, which exposes a hydrophobic domain of amino acids in HA_2, normally concealed in the stalk of the intact molecule. The hydrophobic domain interacts with the lipid bilayers to result in membrane fusion and release of the viral genome into the intracellular environment to initiate virus replication. This mechanism of entry is blocked by amantadine, which can inhibit virus replication by raising the pH within cellular endosomes thus preventing haemagglutinin cleavage and exposure of the hydrophobic domain. Influenza mutants resistant to amantadine have been identified, these are characterized by changes in the hydrophobic region to initiate membrane fusion at higher pH, thereby bypassing the action of this drug.

The molecular structure of the binding domain for the host cell receptor is central to the process of infectivity and the establishment of virus infection. It is a common structural feature of viruses that this domain is often shielded by numerous loops—giving rise to the concept of a receptor 'canyon', first promulgated in the context of rhinovirus infection and its inter-

action with the intercellular adhesion molecule, **ICAM-1**. Such loops can enhance the specificity of a receptor–ligand interaction, but they also deflect the generation of antibodies from the receptor-binding site itself. This is an important virus evasion mechanism, since greater variation in these loops can be accommodated than in the sterically sensitive receptor site.

Adhesion is essential for bacterial pathogenesis. This is usually achieved through fimbriae or pili, present as 100 to 1000 2- to 7-nm rod-like structures often identified as virulence factors. Uropathogenic *E. coli*, express so-called P-fimbriae in up to 90 per cent of patients with pyelonephritis. These *E. coli* bind to uroepithelial cells through glycolipids expressing a galactose–galactose (**Gal–Gal**) carbohydrate moiety. P-fimbriae genes are expressed from the *pap* gene operon in *E. coli*—*papA* gene products form the core of the fimbrial rod, attached to the membrane through *papH*, and this assembly is protected by two-pap operon-encoded chaperones. The ends of the P-fimbriae consist of fibril-associated proteins, with the *papG* product at the tip acting as the Gal–Gal binding unit. There are at least three 'alleles' of *papG* with slightly different affinities for Gal–Gal, which in turn affect disease association in the urinary tract. However, there is added complexity, in that the whole P-fimbriae complex is regulated, possibly by the *papI* and *papB* units of the operon, enabling the detachment and migration of bacteria to new sites. Therefore local pathogenicity and transmission in a single host may be regulated in response to environmental change.

The ability to interfere with bacterial–host cell binding is attractive for prophylaxis or therapy. The presence of excess soluble Gal–Gal subunits blocks bacterial adhesion, and immunization with *E. coli* bearing class-II PapG protects primates against pyelonephritis by the development of P-fimbrial antibodies. However, protection is limited to a specific allele on the P-fimbriae and little cross-protection against other strains of *E. coli* is observed.

The adhesion of *E. coli*, in particular enteropathogenic types, alters epithelial-cell morphology to facilitate bacterial colonization. Binding of the bacterial adhesin intimin to a membrane receptor (**Tir**, translocated intimal receptor), results in the host membrane developing pseudopodia or 'pedestals', via a cytoskeletal modification process, to aid bacterial attachment but not cell invasion. This is regulated through a bacterial pathogenicity island—'locus for enterocyte effacement'. However, this effacement is unusual in that the 'cell' receptor is also of bacterial origin. Tir is secreted from the bacterial cell through a specialized secretory pathway along with other molecules that cause the epithelial cell to phosphorylate Tir, as well as producing other changes in the activation state of the epithelial cell. Other gastrointestinal pathogens induce similar epithelial-cell adaptations such as the epithelial ruffling associated with *Salmonella* spp., in this instance facilitating bacterial uptake into the optional intracellular environment.

Bacteria also colonize surfaces as 'biofilms'—arrangements of populations of bacteria, which coexist on an inert surface surrounded by a matrix that contains microchannels which facilitate the circulation of micronutrients required for colony survival. Microfilms have evolved to promote bacterial survival in adverse environmental conditions; they occur naturally in dental plaque. Microfilms have assumed great importance because of the bacterial biofilm contamination of indwelling devices including intravenous catheters, peritoneal dialysis tubing, urinary catheters, mechanical valves, and orthopaedic prostheses. The formation of biofilms is associated with a 500-fold enhanced antibiotic resistance related to the presence of the matrix encapsulating the micro-organisms. *Staphylococcus epidermidis*, a common skin commensal, is often associated with the development of such films on indwelling devices. The initial adherence to plastic is through fimbrial adhesion proteins SSP-1 and SSP-2, which is followed by bacterial replication. Secretion of a polymer of β1–6-linked, 2-deoxy-2-aminoglucopyranosyl residues, in a structure that resembles cellulose, is regulated by a bacterial operon, and this allows the formation of bacterial colonies in the biofilm.

Pathogen dose

One important pathogenicity factor, frequently forgotten, is the dose of pathogen that is delivered at the portal of entry. The numbers of organisms required for the development of clinical syndromes are dependent on the site of entry as well as on the nature of the pathogen. Conclusions are often drawn from experimental infections that use inappropriate routes of infection, and excessive pathogen doses. It is difficult to establish the infectious dose needed to produce disease through natural routes in humans. Studies rely entirely on volunteers, which in some instances have been held as unethical. The infectious doses for respiratory virus based on direct inoculation studies suggest that 1 $TCID_{50}$ is sufficient to produce infection via the nasal cavity but that a higher dose is required at the posterior pharyngeal wall.

Large doses ($>10^8$ bacteria) of water-borne pathogens such as *Vibrio cholerae* are needed to produce a gastrointestinal infection, this is because many bacteria are inactivated by gastric acidity—the infectious dose administered with bicarbonate is reduced to 10^4 bacteria. About 10^5 salmonellae are required for infection, while only 10 to 100 shigellae are needed because of their resistance to gastric acid.

Encysted forms of organisms are particularly resistant to gastric acid—mathematical modelling of a water-borne outbreak of cryptosporidiosis in Milwaukee suggested that ingesting a single oocyst may have been sufficient to produce disease.

Host factors

The susceptibility of the host to infection is dependent on the ability of a pathogen to break down or bypass host barriers, physical and non-specific defence mechanisms which developed early in phylogeny.

Mechanical and local barriers to infection

Skin and epithelial surfaces

Provided the morphological integrity of local epithelial surfaces is maintained, epithelia represent a harsh environment for micro-organisms. Skin is dry and slightly acidic (pH 5–6) due to fatty acids, which are often produced by the local bacterial microflora from the hydrolysis of triglycerides. In addition, secretions such as sebum may be protective, while physical desquamation itself prevents effective colonization by adherent pathogenic species.

Mucosal barriers are more inviting to micro-organisms because of humidity, but this is offset by an established microflora and secretions with antimicrobial properties: for example, lysozyme and N-acetyl muramyl-L-alanine amides which cleave the amino-acid backbone of the peptidoglycans found in Gram-positive organisms. Each anatomical site has specific antimicrobial barriers, as discussed below.

Respiratory epithelium

- Air filtration provided by the upper respiratory tract and large bronchi ensures that larger particles are deposited on bronchial mucus and that penetration to the bronchioles and alveoli only occurs with particles smaller than 5 μm in diameter. The large numbers of suspended bacteria in air (approximately 400–900 organisms/m^3 in buildings, resulting in 10^4–10^5 organisms inhaled and cleared each day) emphasizes the efficiency of this barrier.

- A mucociliary blanket clears 90 per cent of surface-deposited material in less than 1 h

- Secretion of defensins and collectins in alveoli help in the opsonization of organisms for clearance by alveolar macrophages.

Intestinal epithelium

- Gastric acidity provides a direct barrier—bacteria penetrate more readily to intestinal sites in the presence of achlorhydria.

- Pancreatic, biliary, and intestinal secretions contain antimicrobial agents, including enzymes and defensins.

- Peristalsis—use of atropine-like agents can prolong the duration of infection with *Shigella* spp.

- Normal bowel flora

Genitourinary epithelium

- Urinary pH and osmolarity is inhibitory to bacterial growth.

- Tamm–Horsfall protein may compete for bacterial binding to the epithelium.

- Urinary voiding—bacterial urinary tract infection is more common where there is a genitourinary obstruction.

- Lactobacilli, present at 10^8/ml in the vaginal microflora, degrade glycogen to lactic acid thereby producing an acidic environment.

The role of commensal microflora at epithelial surfaces

This important barrier to pathogenic micro-organisms is acquired from the environment after birth and is modified throughout life. Although the bacterial interactions in this environment are poorly understood, perturbations caused by the therapeutic use of antibiotics that bring about the establishment of an inappropriate flora readily exemplify its importance. The precise mechanisms of protection are unknown, but commensal bacteria may:

- compete for adhesion sites with pathogenic organisms;

- produce antibacterial compounds to limit bacterial expansion from outside the ecosystem;

- compete with pathogens for nutrients;

- produce metabolic products that limit the growth of other species: for example, lactobacilli in vaginal secretions;

- induce generation of 'natural' antibodies.

Non-specific protective immunity

This involves several defensive mechanisms mediated through cellular and humoral mechanisms.

Complement

Complement is an evolutionary conserved cascade of proteins that not only provides direct protection against invading micro-organisms but also augments the effector functions of specific immune responses (Chapter 5.4). These include:

- *Complement-mediated lysis* is largely dependent on the presence of antibody; polysaccharide-coated bacteria can directly activate this alternative pathway, as can certain virus-infected cells (for example, measles), but this is seldom enough to mediate direct damage. There is little direct evidence that complement lysis in isolation is protective, although deficiency of the terminal pore-forming C8/9 components predisposes to neisserial infection.

- *Opsonization and neutralization.*

- *Induction of inflammation.*

Febrile response

Although body temperature is tightly regulated, no single 'temperature centre' has been identified in the central nervous system. A series of structures in the reticular formation, limbic system, and lower brainstem, including the hypothalamic preoptic region with thermosensitive neurones, can initiate behavioural thermoregulatory responses. These regions become responsive by increasing the rate of neuronal firing to a variety of interactive cytokines, either by direct receptor interactions or through intermediary mediators, such as prostaglandins. Micro-organisms induce the release of pyrogenic cytokines from macrophages, including interleukin (**IL**)-1α and -1β, IL-6, tumour necrosis factor-α (**TNF-α**), and interferon-γ

(**IFN-γ**). Unfortunately, because of their complex interaction and involvement of intermediaries, it is difficult to dissect individual roles. Although cytokines may not cross the blood–brain barrier, they can alter the thermoregulatory setpoint either by inducing phospholipase A_2 to release prostaglandin E_2 or using a common pathway involving IL-6.

Acute-phase response

Similar stimuli generating a febrile response also induce acute-phase proteins, which may modulate inflammation and tissue repair: for example, the C-reactive protein (**CRP**) binding of phospholipids on damaged cells or micro-organisms. It may also activate the complement cascade and promote anti-inflammatory products. Serum amyloid A may potentiate the inflammatory response by improving adhesion between effector cells and lipid uptake. Complement components and proteins, such as haptoglobin, with antioxidant activity are increased alongside a number of protease inhibitors (for example, α_1-antichymotrypsin).

Acute inflammatory responses and the role of the polymorphonuclear leucocyte

Polymorphonuclear neutrophils are produced at the rate of 10^{11} cells daily, with a marrow reserve allowing a 10-fold increase in the presence of infection. Neutrophils circulate in rapid flow as a marginated population of cells through transient endothelial interactions. Following establishment of an infection, polymorphs are recruited to the site by their interaction with specific endothelial and chemokine receptors. There are four distinct phases of migration recognized—rolling adhesion, integrin activation, firm adhesion, and transmigration—mediated, respectively, by selectins, integrins, immunoglobulin-like proteins, and mucin-like selectin ligands. The process is active both in the endothelial cell and neutrophil, necessitating the differential expression of receptors as well as an altered affinity of receptors. This is regulated by multiple interacting signals requiring accessory molecules and signalling through chemokines such as IL-8.

Phagocytosis of microbes is enhanced by receptor-mediated entry, especially if the microbe is opsonized by antibody or complement components. Once the microbe is ingested, the changes in the cytoskeletal architecture adjacent to the vacuole allow the orderly fusion of cellular proteins to ensure a sequential transfer to the phagosome and, ultimately, fusion with neutrophil granules. The pH in the granules falls to 3.5, and enzymes aiding the breakdown of bacteria are released. A distinct microbicidal mechanism is the generation of a respiratory burst enabling the production of reactive oxygen species that are toxic to bacteria. In addition, non-oxygen-dependent killing also occurs through a variety of mediators, including pH, enzymes, defensins, bactericidal/permeability-increasing protein (BPI), lactoferrin, and a range of cationic proteins. This complex interaction has resulted in the identification of numerous clinical syndromes associated with a failure of neutrophil function, all of which enhance susceptibility to infection.

A neutropenia of less than 1000 cells/mm^3, regardless of its clinical cause, carries a significant risk of Gram-positive and Gram-negative bacterial sepsis. More specifically, defects in intracellular killing as found in chronic granulomatous disease caused by different mutations in the NADPH-dependent oxidase complex, can have multiple effects, often depending on the severity of the impairment of the oxidative burst. In its most severe form, there is increased susceptibility to staphylococcal with Gram-negative bacterial infections which normally would be low-grade pathogens for example, *E. coli*, *Klebsiella*; failure to clear the pathogen often results in granuloma formation with viable pathogens in the presence of accumulated polymorphs and macrophages. The selective nature of the defect is illustrated by the observation that most neutropenic patients have minor problems with streptococcal infection. A mild counterpart in the family of neutrophil deficits is myeloperoxidase deficiency. Previously thought to be rare, this disorder is now identified as one of the most common gene defects (1 in 2–4000 of the population), but as yet has not been associated with susceptibility to infections, except perhaps an increased frequency of candidiasis.

While identification of these defects underlines the importance of the polymorph in host protection, their cellular nature does not render them easily accessible to passive replacement therapy—thus antibiotic prophylaxis is the mainstay of treatment. However, in the future, gene therapy-based approaches may offer the best option for cure.

Natural killer (NK) cells

These cells have long been recognized by their ability to kill both virus-infected and tumour cells *in vitro* without the requirement of MHC restriction. This activity is markedly enhanced by the presence of cytokines such as IFN-γ during infection *in vivo*. The capacity of NK cells to recognize transformed or infected target cells does not depend on conventional antigen presentation. NK cells carry receptors which are C- type lectins that bind diverse carbohydrates or inhibitory receptors interacting with MHC molecules, that is to say killing occurs when MHC is downregulated. The specificity of the three immunoglobulin-like receptors is being defined, but their role in protective immunity may be broader. Human NK-cell defects are rare, but in one that was identified, the deficit was only identified as a result of an enhanced susceptibility to herpesvirus infections. Therefore, although the direct protective role may be limited, recent studies suggest that the initial NK response at sites of infection may be important for initiating local-early specific responses to the pathogen. Such initiation may represent a fundamental link between innate and specific immunity.

Specific immune responses

Vertebrates, and especially mammals, have evolved specific immunity, probably in response to the selective pressure of exposure to intra- and extracellular pathogens. Although originally protective, enhanced immunity may render some responses detrimental (for example, atopy and asthma) or occasionally augment the effect of an infection by immune-mediated injury. Each effector mechanism is tightly regulated to minimize this possibility and immune responses show unique properties of: specificity for antigens; the ability to turn off the response once an exposure is cleared; and memory with augmentation, such that repeated exposure results in a more rapid and augmented response. These detailed aspects and associated pathology are discussed elsewhere (Section 5), and only mechanisms associated with protective antimicrobial immunity are considered here.

Antibody-mediated protection

Antibodies consist of glycoprotein immunoglobulin molecules secreted in response to infection by T-cell regulated B cells. Antigenic specificity is provided by the primary protein structure at one end of the heavy and light chains that make up the molecule. These specificities are produced by a recombination to bring one of a large number of variable gene segments alongside constant-region genes before transcription and translation of the resultant complex. The biological properties of antibodies are a property of the heavy chains, and immunoglobulins are divided into classes based on the genes that encode the heavy-chain polypeptides. The molecules are invested with unique protective properties against microbial pathogens:

- *Neutralization of toxins and viruses.* One of the earliest observations of the clinical role of antibodies was the recognition that a soluble factor could block both bacterial toxins as well as pathogen entry, especially with viruses. This has led to the use of passive immunotherapy where antibodies can be administered postexposure in toxin-mediated disease (for example, tetanus) or in susceptible patients to block infection (for example, varicella-zoster virus infection in immunocompromised children). However, a wider utility of this approach with the development of monoclonal-antibody technology has not proved successful, for example the use of anti-J5 antibody in *E. coli* bacteraemia. Neutralization is often viewed as steric hindrance consequent on an antibody binding close to a receptor/ligand domain. But, particularly in the context of virus neutralization, this view is simplistic. Titration analysis of picornaviruses has shown that one or two antibody molecules may neutralize poliovirus infectivity despite the presence of 60 potential receptor-binding sites. The exact mechanism of inactivation is unknown, but it could be due to antibody-induced changes in the virion capsid or an inability of the virus to uncoat on entry into the cell.

- *Agglutination.* This may be considered another form of neutralization but is a result of polyvalent antibodies of IgM, IgA, and IgG classes crosslinking particles, thereby blocking adherence and infectivity—as well as enhancing susceptibility to phagocytosis.

- *Complement activation.* IgM and IgG are able to bind complement through the classical pathway via C1q, particularly when there is aggregation of IgG on the surface of the microbe. Binding of complement augments local inflammation and enhances phagocytosis consequent on opsonization.

- *Opsonization and phagocytosis.* Antibodies together with any bound complement components enhance phagocytosis by promoting receptor-mediated entry into phagocytes. Such interactions may also trigger cytokine release, as well as promoting enhanced bactericidal activity in the phagocyte by direct activation of the oxidative burst in these cells.

- *Antibody-dependent cellular cytotoxicity.* Binding through the Fc receptor on leucocytes can kill the target cell, which has been well described with NK cells and the low-affinity FcγRIII. However, the relative importance of this mechanism in host protection is unknown.

Perhaps the best measure of the importance of antibody-mediated protection against microbes is from naturally occurring deficiency diseases. These include X-linked agammaglobulinaemia, common variable immunodeficiency, and the X-linked hyper-IgM syndrome (Chapter 5.6). These diseases present with common clinical features of early-onset recurrent pulmonary infections with *S. pneumoniae* and *H. influenzae* often complicated by chronic sinusitis and middle-ear infections, with gastrointestinal infections caused by common pathogens, such as *Salmonella* spp., *Shigella* spp., and *Campylobacter* spp., as well as more chronic infection with *Giardia* spp. Increased susceptibility to viral infection is limited to rotavirus and enteroviral infection. The latter are unusual in that they can induce a chronic viral meningitis in the face of immunoglobulin-replacement therapy. Enteroviruses are also associated with an unusual polymyositis syndrome.

Cell-mediated immunity

Specific cell-mediated immunity to infection is mediated by T cells of thymic origin, which recirculate to specific sites because of specific cell-surface receptors. Naïve T cells first encounter antigen that has been processed by professional antigen-presenting cells such as dendritic cells. As has been shown by cannulation of lymphatic vessels draining to and from local lymph nodes following local visna virus infection, these cells pick up antigen locally, are activated, and then migrate to the lymph nodes. Here the cells mature and express the processed antigen in the context of MHC class I and II molecules, as well as numerous accessory molecules (for example, CD40 and B7) required for efficient maturation of specific T cells. Specific T cells leave the lymph node after 4 to 5 days and aggregate at sites of infection and/or inflammation. Here the T cells encounter processed antigen either in infected cells or in local antigen-presenting cells. CD8 T cells may act by directly killing infected cells through perforin or the FAS–FASL (FAS ligand) interaction, with the consequential activation of apoptotic pathways. CD4 and, to a lesser extent, CD8 T cells release a range of cytokines such as the interleukins, IFN-γ, TNF-α and -β, granulocyte–macrophage colony-stimulating factor (**GM-CSF**), etc., which may have a direct anti-infective action but that also allow the development of delayed-type hypersensitivity, particularly important for the control of intracellular

bacteria. Cytokines and their specific functions are discussed in Chapter 4.4.

One feature of the specific cell-mediated response is the development of memory T cells. These cells are characterized by the expression of specific cell-surface proteins and their ability to recognize antigen without the need for priming through professional antigen presentation. It has been shown for a number of specific cell-mediated immune responses, notably CD8 T-cell responses to the lymphocytic choriomeningitis virus (**LCMV**), that a circulating pool of memory T cells is established following the first *in vivo* encounter with antigen. Subsequent encounter with the virus results in the more rapid activation from this pool of memory T cells, which are often retained for the lifetime of the host. Numerous studies are currently focusing on the nature of the memory T-cell pool: whether it can be augmented; whether antigen is required to sustain this T-cell population; and whether continuous exposure can result in specific depletion. These issues are of particular importance to the development of effective subunit vaccines, as well as to the development of optimum methods of vaccination for maximum protection especially against weaker antigens.

Mucosal immunity

Since the primary encounter with antigen occurs at mucosal surfaces, the nature of the local response can often determine whether infection is initially established. Various elements of the innate immune response are active at surfaces, including cytokines, complement, lysozyme, lactoferrin, NK cells, and phagocytes, as well as specific immune responses such as secretory IgA (**sIgA**). IgA is secreted at most surfaces (including in colostrum) by the addition of a 'secretory piece' to dimeric IgA. Its secretion follows initial encounter of antigen by a mucosal B cell, which circulates to localize at distant mucosal sites, such as salivary glands. Their mucosal localization is determined by specific receptors to endothelial cells at these locations. This has given rise to the concept of a mucosal, as distinct from a systemic, immune system. This system permits the use of active vaccines to block the entry of pathogens at mucosal sites.

Evasion of the host immune response

To establish effective parasitism, it is essential to bypass the immune response in the host. Several strategies are used, such as the speed of replication—the organism replicates rapidly and spreads to infect the next host before an effective specific immune response can be generated (for example, picornaviruses). If a specific locally active antibody response is generated, then some organisms can bypass it by destroying the antibody through IgA proteases. Alternatively, the antibody may be deflected to components of a pathogen that are irrelevant: for example, failure to develop neutralizing antibodies or even antibodies that may facilitate the entry of the micro-organism to optimum sites of replication as in dengue infection. Some viruses may coat themselves with antibody by expressing Fc receptors to block the development of neutralizing activity.

Similarly, the infected cell can be 'masked' by pathogens so that it becomes invisible to the immune response; for example, DNA viruses, especially herpesviruses, downregulate the expression of MHC class I molecules and block antigen processing/presentation so that specific CD8 cytotoxic T cells cannot recognize the infected cell. Inhibition of cytokine action is similarly employed by viruses, notably vaccines that interfere with cytokine action by virally encoded inhibitors and decoy cytokine receptors (for example, for IL-1, IL-8, TNF).

Alternatively, many pathogens such as *Trypanosoma brucei* vary their antigenicity. The parasite is surrounded by a surface coat of carbohydrate and a 67-kDa glycoprotein. The trypanosome genome consists of a large number of chromosomes, including around 150 mini-chromosomes. The coat glycoprotein is encoded by basic copy genes lying near telomeric sites and also internally within chromosomes, so that more than 200 copies of these genes exist. In humans, trypanosomes express one copy of the protein which is transcribed from a telomeric site. Variation occurs by gene conversion, replacing the gene at the active transcription site by a silent copy from elsewhere in the genome, although additional novel sequences may be created. During infection, changes in the basic copy gene expressed occur spontaneously once in 10 000 organisms, resulting in an antigenic change that can always bypass the host immune response generated. Although the organism commits approximately 10 per cent of its genome to this evasion mechanism, it ensures its long-term survival in the host in the presence of an otherwise effective immune response.

Antigenic variation also occurs outside the host to ensure pathogen survival within the population. This is exemplified by influenza whose mode of entry via haemagglutinin and sialic acid interaction has been described. During virus replication in the host, point mutations are introduced into haemagglutinin which result in the virus bypassing the prevalent immune response to the original infecting virus type. Hence, a small number of hosts will always be susceptible to such changes. As the immune response in the population naturally wanes, the population again becomes susceptible to the parental strain every 4 years, resulting in local outbreaks of influenza. This phenomenon is termed 'antigenic drift'. However, influenza A also demonstrates 'antigenic shift', which is the consequence of the genetic recombination of large segments of the genome in an intermediary host such as birds. If such recombination involves the haemagglutinin gene, against which most neutralizing antibodies are directed, then the host population is severely exposed and global pandemics of influenza A as occurred during 1918, 1957 (Asian 'flu), and 1968 (Hong Kong 'flu) can result.

The ability to maintain a reservoir of pathogen in the face of an active immune response, either in the host or the population, is a prerequisite for the effective survival of many pathogens. Each of the mechanisms briefly considered requires elaborate genomic mechanisms or the utilization of a considerable part of the genome to be committed to this end—for example, a trypanosome utilizes approximately 10 per cent of its genome by encoding multiple copies of the surface glycoprotein, while human cytomegalovirus, in the more restricted genome of viruses, utilizes at least six open-reading frames for genes that interfere with MHC class I antigen presentation in the infected cell. Such genomic commitment, of itself, recognizes the importance of evading immunity for parasite survival.

Pathogen persistence and latency

Pathogens, especially DNA herpesviruses, have evolved a virus cycle that enables them to remain dormant at anatomical sites with little virus gene expression, thereby minimizing the potential for immune activation. Following primary infection with herpes simplex, multiple cutaneous lesions develop and virus is shed. An effective immune response develops that clears most of the infectious virus, and the skin lesions heal. However, virus passes to nerve ganglia where it enters a latent state. Periodically it can be triggered to reactivate; infectious particles track down axons with epithelial reinfection and temporary shedding until the immune response again clears the cutaneous site. Therefore a virus–host equilibrium is established, although the relationship is never symbiotic. Not only can activation of the virus by non-specific triggers alter the equilibrium, but immunosuppression can result in the more widespread peripheral dissemination of reactivation. The virus gains two major advantages from this virus cycle: evasion of the immune response and a host reservoir that enables it to bypass a host generation for horizontal transmission, thereby sustaining itself in small isolated populations in the face of an active immune response.

Immune-mediated injury

In most instances the development of an active immune response is beneficial to the host and results in pathogen clearance or the establishment of persistent or latent infection, in which a host–parasite equilibrium is established that minimizes damage to the host. Occasionally, the infectious agent may not itself be as damaging to the host as the immune response that is generated against it.

Immunopathology

At the simplest level, many clinical features of infection are the result of the host's response to the infectious agent; fever is caused by the release of cytokines to the infectious agent. However, in some circumstances the phenotype of clinical disease is altered depending on the nature of the immune response. *Mycobacterium leprae* infection results in a spectrum of disease phenotype with lepromatous and tuberculoid leprosy at either extreme. In the former, the host is relatively 'anergic' to the infectious agent or products of *M. leprae*, with the result that the clinical lesions are less physically destructive but contain high levels of viable organisms, allowing easier spread of infection. In the tuberculoid form, the cell-mediated response to *M. leprae* is strong, with local mononuclear infiltrates at sites of infection and few organisms but more intense tissue destruction and local injury.

Similarly, respiratory syncytial virus infection can result in bronchiolitis in young infants. An immunopathological explanation for this condition was suggested following a failed vaccination campaign using an alum-precipitated killed virus, which resulted in vaccinated children suffering worse disease. The mechanism was thought to be a failure to induce neutralizing antibody, but a T_H2 response capable of releasing IL-3, IL-4, and IL-5 was generated. On infection, release of these cytokines resulted in bronchospasm and local inflammation with eosinophil infiltration. Similar changes can be observed in experimental murine infection.

Autoimmunity

If immunopathology can be induced by an infecting agent through the generation of an aberrant or misdirected immune response, the question arises of whether such a response could be sustained and result in end-organ damage as in autoimmune disease. While attractive as a hypothesis, the 'hit and run' nature of infectious triggers for common autoimmune disorders is difficult to establish. However, in the experimental setting autoimmunity is induced using bacterially derived adjuvants in genetically susceptible hosts. In such circumstances the infectious agent may break tolerance, although direct evidence for this mechanism in humans is lacking.

Alternative mechanisms have been proposed that include molecular mimicry, in which an immune response is generated against an antigen from an infectious agent to trigger a crossreactive response to a host-cell protein, due to its structural similarity. Experimentally transgenic mice expressing the LCMV nuclear protein under an insulin promoter (such that it is expressed only in β cells in the Islets of Langerhans) do not generate a response against the protein and do not develop diabetes. However, if the mouse is infected with the virus then the CD8 T cells generated will destroy the islets and render the mouse diabetic. Evidence for this phenomenon in humans is lacking; infection with *Streptococcus* spp. elicits crossreactive antibodies resulting in rheumatic fever, but even in this case there is little evidence that the response can be sustained. Similarly, the demonstration of prior chlamydial infection in the identification of a specific MHC type and late Reiter's syndrome with reactive arthritis is suggestive but not conclusive.

Host susceptibility to infection

In addition to specific and non-specific immune mechanisms, there are several other host factors that mediate susceptibility to infection.

Genetic factors

The overall impact of genetic factors in host susceptibility to infection is difficult to estimate. Perhaps the best evidence comes from twin studies—susceptibility to infections ranging from malaria to *Helicobacter pylori* are inconclusive, with associations being established for disease severity rather than a global susceptibility to an infectious agent. However, a Swedish study of adoptees reported a sixfold increased risk of an infectious cause of death where a biological, as opposed to an adoptive, parent had also died from an infectious illness. Alternatively, the role of candidate genes in specific infections has been suggested.

MHC and infection

The central position of the MHC in regulating specific immunity make this locus an obvious candidate. However, studies have required large numbers of subjects because this locus is highly variable. Perhaps the best known association is the linkage of HLA-B*5301 with resistance to severe malaria in children in The Gambia. This study was given additional impetus with the identification of a malaria-derived peptide that shows variability and can be presented by HLA-B*5301. An MHC class II locus *HLA-DRB1*1302* was also associated with disease resistance. Taken together with the observation that the HLA-B53 association did not pertain in East African populations, this suggests that the association is complex and that there could be geographical variation in the pathogen which could influence susceptibility to infection by affecting the presentation of microbial peptides by different MHC molecules.

Other associations have been described including: HLA-DQ with cervical cancer associated with human papillomavirus infection (**HPV**); and HLA-DRB1 with the clearance of hepatitis B infection. Numerous studies have been performed to try to establish an association of resistance or disease progression with HIV infection but none are conclusive to date. The subtleties of such associations are exemplified by the association of HPV infection and cervical cancer. While an MHC class II association has been recognized, differences in the survival of patients with invasive cervical cancer have been linked to HLA-B7. This is not evident when all patients with HLA-B7 who have the disease are studied. However, in cervical cancer, there is selective loss of expression of individual MHC class I alleles on the surface of tumour cells. In this instance, patients who lost only HLA-B7 expression on tumour cells had a reduced survival rate. This could be the result of tumour-specific MHC class I-restricted immune responses, but whether the restriction affects the initial infection with HPV or the maintenance of the oncogenic process, is unknown.

The recognition that infections are associated with specific antigens in the host's MHC is important. With improved knowledge of the regulation of cellular immunity and an ability to generate specific immunity with peptides that bind to appropriate MHC molecules, it is possible to develop a new range of vaccines for the treatment and prevention of a range of infectious diseases. However, the vaccine-based approach must take into account possible protective and adverse associations to ensure that the real risk of immunopathology is minimized.

Other genetic factors

A range of other candidate genes have been identified that predispose to specific susceptibility. Blood groups are well described; peptic ulceration is associated with blood-group secretor status, which may confer susceptibility to *H. pylori* infection. Mutations in haemoglobin, particularly in heterozygotes, results in resistance to malaria, which may allow the persistence in the population of what would otherwise be a detrimental defect. Several authors have reported alterations in receptor and chemokine and cytokine genes and susceptibility to infection: elevated TNF concentrations consequent on a mutation in the promoter of TNF-α have been associated with cerebral malaria in Africa, mucocutaneous leishmaniasis in South America, and lepromatous leprosy in India. Mutations in chemokine CCR5 receptors are associated with a reduced susceptibility to HIV infection. Other molecules that may be linked to immune or inflammatory responses are also associated with susceptibility to infection, for example mannose-binding lectin may be associated with invasive disease by encapsulated bacteria, although enhanced susceptibility to individual pathogens has not been demonstrated. The natural resistance-associated macrophage protein type 1 (**NRAMP1**) protein is found on macrophages. The gene encoding NRAMP1 is homologous to a murine gene that has been associated with a

susceptibility to leishmania and salmonella infection in defined strains, but mutations in the human gene product are associated with severe pulmonary tuberculosis. Mutations in the human vitamin D receptor also appear to be associated with severe *Mycobacterium tuberculosis* infections.

Conclusions

Despite a number of interesting associations with widely disparate molecules, it is difficult to draw conclusions with respect to pathogenesis at this stage. As the most intriguing associations are with the MHC complex, it is tempting to infer that microbial infections are a powerful evolutionary driver to polymorphism at these loci. Although the specific examples described here are intriguing, it is likely that the factors that determine susceptibility and resistance to individual pathogens in the general population are highly polygenic.

Environmental and intercurrent susceptibility to infection

Several additional factors that operate in a patient have to be considered as influencing susceptibility, severity, and the likelihood of recovery from infection.

Age

Common infectious diseases occur more frequently in older patients: for example, pneumonia (twofold), bacteraemia (threefold), urinary tract infections (fivefold), reactivation of varicella-zoster virus (**VZV**), and tuberculosis (**TB**). The explanation is frequently given that cell-mediated immunity declines with age and that this is reflected in the increased incidence. While this may be the case with VZV and TB, it is difficult to reconcile this alongside other common physical problems of ageing, such as urinary obstruction due to prostatic hypertrophy, and confounding variables such as relative malnutrition, social isolation, and socioeconomic deprivation.

Hormonal influences

Hormones can affect immunity and impact on infections. 'Stress' is often cited as an important factor in the severity of infection. Chronic stress and 'life events' are strongly associated with the increased duration of virus shedding and the intensity of symptoms in upper respiratory tract infections. Pregnancy is associated with an increased severity of poliomyelitis and influenza (among other viral infections) during the third trimester.

Malnutrition

Worldwide, calorie malnutrition is the most common cause of increased susceptibility to infections such as bacterial septicaemia, middle-ear infection, dental caries, and perioral infection. Enhanced severity of measles has been widely reported, although the effect of overcrowding, which frequently accompanies malnutrition in developing countries, may also contribute. However, improvement in diet has historically been associated with reduced mortality from several infectious diseases. Specific nutrients are difficult to identify, although the best evidence supports a role for vitamin A; deficiency of this vitamin in pregnancy has been associated with enhanced vaginal HIV shedding and increased perinatal transmission.

Intercurrent illness and infections

Many severe illnesses, including other infections, can impair host immunity. Although the obvious example is HIV infection, impairment can also be associated with many conditions such as alcoholism, liver failure, renal failure, and late-stage cancer. Some specific examples are also well documented: measles infection is associated with the loss of delayed-type hypersensitivity in the Mantoux response, with the possibility that tuberculosis may be exacerbated.

Therapy

There are obvious examples of immunosuppressive drugs that render the host susceptible to numerous opportunistic infections.

Altering the host response to prevent and treat infection

Vaccination

The decline in common infectious diseases throughout the last 150 years can be attributed to improved public health measures (sanitation and hygiene) and the development of cheap and effective vaccines. The success of mass vaccination was highlighted by the eradication of smallpox in 1980, and may soon be followed by the eradication of poliomyelitis. However, the vaccination programme has also controlled important childhood infections such as measles, mumps, rubella, diphtheria, haemophilus meningitis, etc. The development of these vaccines has relied primarily on empiricism based on the principle of producing a mild form of the illness, either by using a low infecting dose or an attenuated live agent. Killed vaccines are effective where the appropriate immunity can be generated to a pathogenic toxin, for example antitetanus toxoid.

With a greater understanding of the nature of immunity induced by vaccination, a rational basis exists to pursue the more difficult pathogens that remain major targets for vaccine development, including: malaria, schistosomiasis, hookworm, tuberculosis, infantile diarrhoea, pneumonia, and HIV infection.

A successful vaccine not only has to induce effective immunity, but it must also be acceptable to the public. Such acceptability is difficult to gauge and varies from one community to another. Public acceptance may be partly based on a relative-risk perception between the hazards of vaccination and the burden of morbidity and mortality. There are several examples of difficulties in implementing vaccination programmes such as the *Bordetella pertussis* vaccine and the recent difficulties of sustaining high levels of immunity against measles due to a suggested link between autism and the triple vaccine. Failure to sustain high levels of herd immunity result in resurgent epidemics of diseases previously held under control, for example the diphtheria outbreaks in the former Soviet Union. In addition, for worldwide use a vaccine has to be stable, cheap, and easy to administer. Thus the development of a theoretically effective immunogen may not necessarily translate directly to a successful vaccine for clinical use.

None the less, improvements in technology utilizing the nature of T- and B-cell interaction have seen the development of cellular conjugate vaccines such those undergoing trial against *S. pneumoniae*. Adjuvant technology is also improving to enhance immune responsiveness, and cytokines have been shown to enable vaccine non-responders to generate effective immunity to hepatitis B. Furthermore, DNA vaccines are being produced and undergoing efficacy testing alongside appropriate delivery systems; such as prime–boost immunization—where two different vaccines are administered in sequence: for instance DNA vaccination followed by a booster of the same agent in another recombinant form or the pure cognate protein. Similarly, specific antigens are being delivered to different anatomical sites to enhance mucosal immunity utilizing isolated properties of pathogens, for example the fimbrial proteins of *S. typhimurium*.

This expansion in the utilization of new methods for vaccine development has raised our expectations of tackling difficult pathogens—especially those where a persistent or latent state can be established in the host. There is also the possibility that vaccines may be able to alter the immune response against established infections to control clinical disease. In infections such as leprosy, leishmaniasis, and schistosomiasis, cytokine therapy may modify the effects of the infection, especially where the disease itself is mediated by immune events. Some viruses that persist or even transform cells may continue to express a range of proteins in the transformed state; these products too may serve as appropriate targets for eliminating the infected or transformed cell.

Passive immunotherapy

Perhaps one area that has still not seen the full exploitation of its potential is passive immunotherapy. Passive antibody is used to prevent disseminated varicella in immunocompromised subjects and in the treatment of tetanus; it is also used as an adjunct to the postexposure prophylaxis of rabies. The ability to modify heterologous antibodies to render them less immunogenic, alongside the ability to select the antibody repertoire *in vitro*, makes passive immunotherapy an attractive option for the control of established infection or for modifying immunopathology. In addition, the adoptive transfer of specific cell-mediated immunity in specific circumstances, such as following bone marrow transplantation to prevent human cytomegalovirus pneumonia, may be coupled with the modification of cellular responses including the repertoire of T-cell receptors. Currently, these approaches are still experimental but they may soon be explored in clinical trials.

Conclusions

Although there have striking advances have been made in the control of infectious disease by modifying host responses, many challenges remain. Common childhood infections pose major difficulties for healthcare in many parts of the world, and here the availability of effective prophylaxis must engender greater international effort for its effective implementation. Finally, a greater understanding of the nature of the host–parasite relationship will, coupled with increased knowledge of immune mechanisms, be required to develop new methods to prevent and treat the more intractable common infections.

Further reading

Costerton JW, *et al.* (1995). Microbial biofilms. *Annual Review of Microbiology* **49**, 711–45. [Review of formation and factors involved in biofilm formation.]

Cotter PA, Miller JF (1998). *In vivo* and *ex vivo* regulation of bacterial virulence gene expression. *Current Opinion in Microbiology* **1**, 17–26. [Description of regulation of the control of virulence island genes.]

Gander S (1996). Bacterial biofilms: resistance to antimicrobial agents. *Journal of Antimicrobial Chemotherapy* **37**, 1047–50. [Antibiotic resistance in biofilms.]

Hill AVS (1998). The immunogenetics of human infectious diseases. *Annual Review of Immunology* **16**, 593–617.

Mackowiak PA (1998). Concepts of fever. *Archives of Internal Medicine* **158**, 1870–81. [Discussion of major factors in the regulation of temperature.]

Mims C, Nash A, Stephen J (2001). *Mims' pathogenesis of infectious disease*, 5th edn. Academic Press, San Diego. [A full and readable account of major factors involved in microbial pathogenesis.]

Nicholson KG, Webster RG, Hay AJ (1998). *Textbook of influenza*. Blackwell Science, Oxford. [A detailed account of the virology and pathogenesis of influenza infection in man and associated species, including a good section on the development and problems of influenza vaccines.]

Plotkin SA, Orenstein WA (1999). *Vaccines*, 3rd edn. WB Saunders, Philadelphia. [The standard reference work to currently used vaccines, future developments, as well as regulatory and delivery issues.]

Rosen FS, Cooper MD, Chapel HM (1995). The primary immunodeficiencies. *New England Journal of Medicine* **333**, 431–40.

Rossman MG (1989). Neutralisation of small RNA viruses by antibodies and antiviral agents. *FASEB Journal* **3**, 2335–43. [A good discussion of the mechanisms of virus neutralization and drugs that block entry of picornaviruses.]

Sorenson TI, *et al.* (1988). Genetic and environmental influences on premature death in adult adoptees. *New England Journal of Medicine* **318**, 727–32. [Suggestion of global genetic susceptibility to infection.]

'Vaccines and immunology' (2001). *Science* **293**, 233–56. [A series of articles defining the current issues in immunology impacting on future vaccine development.]

Van der Woude M, Braaten B, Low D (1996). Epigenetic phase variation of the *pap* operon in *Escherichia coli*. *Trends in Microbiology* **4**, 5–9. [Discussion of the regulation of expression of pathogenicity-associated fimbriae in *E. coli*.]

Ziegler E, *et al.* (1991). Treatment of Gram-negative bacteraemia and septic shock with HA-1A human monoclonal antibody against endotoxin: a randomised, double blind, placebo-controlled trial. *New England Journal of Medicine* **324**, 429–36. [Failure of monoclonal antibody immunotherapy to protect against bacteraemia.]

7.5 Physiological changes in infected patients

P. A. Murphy

All of us are exposed to potentially lethal infectious agents from shortly after birth until we die. And while there are viral, bacterial, fungal, and parasitic infections, there is no doubt that the most dangerous organisms are bacteria. Bacteria in logarithmic phase divide every 15 to 20 min: no eukaryotic cell can match that rate, nor can any virus, fungus, or parasite. The immune system evolved primarily to deal efficiently with bacterial infections. It is true that the immune system has minor effects on some tumours, but if mice with severe inherited immune defects are maintained in a sterile environment they have a normal lifespan and do not have an unusual incidence of cancer. Out of the plastic bag, they last a week or two before dying of overwhelming infection.

The immune system is divided into the natural immune system and the acquired immune system. The natural immune system is a series of defences against bacteria and other infections which is present from birth. None of its mechanisms depend on previous experience with the organism, and they do not improve with experience. It is so efficient that the overwhelming majority of bacteria are destroyed shortly after entry into tissue without eliciting any noticeable host response. There are responses, but they function at a microscopic, sometimes a molecular, level. The only infectious diseases of which we become aware are those in which the natural immune system has failed, the population of invading organisms has become large, and inflammatory reactions become sufficiently pronounced to cause symptoms that we can feel and signs that we can see. A healthy adult may go months or years between clinically apparent infections.

Acquired immunity is called on when the initial battle has gone badly and bacterial populations have become large. Initiating an immune response of any kind usually requires antigen concentrations in the microgram range. Since a bacterium weighs about a picogram, specific acquired immune responses are only likely to occur when bacterial populations are measured in millions or billions. Organisms which can multiply to these levels in healthy people generally have some feature, such as a capsule, which enables them partially to evade the natural immune response. Small numbers of B and T lymphocytes which can respond to essentially any immunodeterminant exist in everyone. Uncontrolled infection leads to rapid clonal expansion of specific B and T cells which mediate immunity to the pathogen, most usually by antibody formation. Antigen is maintained in tissue depots so that antibody secretion is prolonged long after the initiating infection has resolved. Both B and T cells generate long-lived memory cells which can initiate secondary immune responses if the organism is encountered again. Secondary immune responses require ten to a hundred times less antigen to elicit them, and occur faster than do primary immune responses. The increased efficiency means that many clinical infections occur only once. Lifelong immunity is often, but not always, maintained by periodic asymptomatic rechallenge with virulent organisms.

Bacteria and fungi are recognized as foreign by the natural immune system. Both classes of organism have thick cell walls which have no counterpart in mammalian cells. The recognition molecule is C3; one important foreign structure is a hydroxyl group on each of two adjacent carbon atoms, which is found in most sugar residues. C3 has a very low but finite rate of spontaneous activation to C3a and nascent C3b. Nascent C3b has an unstable thioether bond which has about 60 μs to find a carbohydrate before it reacts with water and is inactivated. Binding to carbohydrate results in covalent attachment of a molecule of C3b to the bacterial or fungal surface. This is the primary activator of the alternative pathway of complement fixation, which causes fixation of C3b to the foreign surface in amounts which are opsonic for phagocytic cells. Mammalian glycoproteins have carbohydrate groups but many of the hydroxyl residues on terminal sugars are oxidized to carbonyl groups which do not react with C3b.

There are whole families of proteins, both soluble and cell bound, which recognize specific sugar residues such as mannose. Since many fungi have cell walls which are largely polymannose, some of these are likely to be important for antifungal defence.

Bacteria are prokaryotic and present many more foreign labels than do fungi. Probably most important are the major cell wall constituents, endotoxin in Gram-negative organisms and peptidoglycan in Gram-positive organisms. These are recognized as foreign by many systems, both soluble proteins such as lysozyme and cell bound proteins. The key cell in initial defence against organisms is clearly the macrophage. Every tissue contains macrophages which are often organized anatomically in ways which facilitate defence against infection. Alveolar macrophages patrol the alveoli, Kupffer cells have processes which stretch across hepatic sinusoids, and splenic macrophages inspect the blood which filters past them in the red pulp. Most normal tissues contain few or no polymorphonuclear leucocytes. CD14 protein is exposed on macrophage membranes. It contains two high-affinity binding sites, one for endotoxin and one for peptidoglycan. These sites are not identical, but they are so close together that monoclonal antibodies exist which can block binding of both ligands. This single protein is a bacteria detector, and binding of its ligand activates the macrophage to secrete interleukins IL-8 and IL-1 and tumour necrosis factor. IL-1 and tumour necrosis factor act on capillary endothelium to initiate the cascades which result in increased permeability and display of receptors for polymorphonuclear leucocytes. IL-8 is powerfully chemotactic for polymorphonuclear leucocytes. Thus recognition of bacteria by the CD14 protein initiates the natural immune response.

Additional properties of bacteria which initiate inflammation are their ability to fix complement and the fact that bacterial proteins start with an N-formyl methionine residue rather than the methionine employed by eukaryotic cells. Almost all bacteria fix complement in the cell wall, though pathogenic species may fix complement in deep layers which are not accessible to polymorphonuclear leucocytes. The soluble complement component C5a is strongly chemotactic for polymorphonuclear leucocytes and even though the bacteria are not opsonized, if polymorphonuclear leucocytes are attracted to their vicinity the bacteria may be destroyed by surface phagocytosis. Similarly, there is a high-affinity receptor for N-formyl methionyl peptides in the membranes of polymorphonuclear leucocytes; binding to this receptor initiates a chemotactic response which may be useful in the same way.

Some bacteria, such as mycobacteria, and some fungi, such as *Histoplasma capsulatum*, can evade the natural immune response and the antibody mediated arm of the acquired immune response. These infections tend to be chronic, asymptomatic at first, but progress to extensive destructive reactions such as caseous necrotic cavitation and scarring. The destructive reactions are mediated by macrophages highly activated by parasite-specific T cells.

In general, viruses do not contain components which are directly inflammatory, but typically produce inflammation by killing cells. Some viral infections are not cytolytic; symptoms occur only when the acquired immune response is activated and large populations of virus-specific T cells have been generated. When these T cells kill cells infected by virus, inflammation is induced. In measles, cells can be replaced and the rash signals the end of the disease. If the cells are not replaceable (for example neurones) the immune response may be lethal.

Parasites which live in tissue are almost never directly inflammatory, and they invariably have some mechanism for suppressing or evading the acquired immune response.

A few organisms have specific properties which determine most of the features of the illness. Sore throat due to diphtheria bacilli would be inconsequential if it were not for the toxin which binds to cardiac muscle cells, stops protein synthesis, and leads to heart failure. Many diarrhoeal syndromes are mediated by bacterial toxins, and the absence of toxin means absence of disease. However, even where there are distinctive features some symptoms are shared with other infections—there is almost always fever and inflamed areas hurt.

The general characteristics of infections are explained by the features discussed above. The vast majority of infections are dealt with at a microscopic level by the natural immune system and never give rise to any clinical symptoms. The relative importance of natural and acquired immunity is given by observations on untreated individuals born with congenital defects of one or other system. A child born with no B cells will generally die of infection at about the age of 6, a child born with no T cells will generally die at 2 or 3. A child born with no neutrophils will last a few weeks, and no child with congenital absence of macrophages has ever been described. Admittedly, that may have more to do with the role of macrophages in remodelling tissues during fetal development than with resistance to infection.

Bacterial infections are characterized by acute onset, intense local general inflammation, rapid progression to severe local and general symptoms, and resolution towards death or recovery in a week or two. Infections by slowly dividing organisms like mycobacteria are characterized by less initial inflammation but deterioration over months or years. Fungal infections are far less inflammatory than bacterial ones, though there may be intense inflammation in the later course due to acquired immunity. Viral infections are not usually serious unless, as in poliomyelitis, the virus grows in a population of cells which cannot be replaced. Patients with fungal and viral infections may be highly febrile, but are-notably less generally ill than those with bacterial infections, because the infecting organisms are less inflammatory.

Whether or not an infection becomes established depends on the balance between the host's ability to mobilize an adequate inflammatory response and the parasite's ability to evade that response. Numbers are crucial: it is highly improbable that one organism by itself can initiate a serious or lethal infection. There is good evidence that many infections begin with the survival of a single organism from the initial inoculum, and that all the myriad of organisms which eventually overwhelm the patient are descendants of that one bacterium. However, the probability of that happening is so low that it is almost never observed. As a practical matter, most experimental infections in small groups of animals are initiated by inocula of many millions of organisms so that the individual tiny probabilities are multiplied to a level which can be observed. Spontaneous infections in people are ordinarily initiated by small inocula, but there are hundreds of millions of people. Even though serious infection is improbable, the number of people at risk is so huge that some serious infections are observed.

If there is a defect in host defences, the probability of a serious infection initiating from a small inoculum is greatly increased. Worldwide, the most common cause of poor immune performance is malnutrition, especially lack of adequate protein. Every component of the natural and acquired immune system depends on proteins, and if the building blocks are not available these components cannot be made. Premature infants and elderly patients have serious defects of T-cell function; in one case the system has not completely developed and in the other it has atrophied. There are also numerous acquired immune defects in people who have had transplants, been given chemotherapy for malignancy or immunosuppressive treatment for diseases such as lupus erythematosus and rheumatoid arthritis, and infected with HIV. All these people frequently develop infections with organisms which rarely or never trouble normal people because they cannot control bacterial populations at a low level.

Large numbers of bacteria are inherently inflammatory. If bacterial populations reach hundreds of millions, inflammation will occur whether the bacteria are alive or dead. It makes no difference whether or not the species is 'pathogenic'; the response is to the cell wall components which are found in all bacteria. Pathogenic species possess some attribute such as a capsule or a leucocidin which enables them to evade the initial natural immune response and to multiply in tissue. Multiplication to large numbers does several things. Local inflammation is induced wherever the organisms are, and one sees a clinical sore throat, a boil, pneumonia, or a urinary tract infection. Initially mediators of inflammation leak out of the inflamed area into the circulation and induce a systemic inflammatory response. The systemic inflammatory response includes new aspects of protection by the natural immune response. Generally speaking, bacteria in numbers which induce a systemic inflammatory response also initiate acquired immune responses. Bacteria may invade the bloodstream from the local lesion; they may be able to grow in the bloodstream (sepsis), or they may set up distant foci of infection such as endocarditis, a septic joint, or a splenic abscess. Finally, certain aspects of the systemic inflammatory response are deleterious and may progress to circulatory failure (septic shock) or multiple organ failure.

The concept that large numbers of essentially any bacterium in tissue will cause serious or fatal inflammatory reactions explains a number of clinical situations: aspiration of saliva containing 10^8 bacteria/ml causes pneumonia; a burst appendix causes peritonitis. Infusion of infected fluids intravenously has caused fatal shock in otherwise healthy people. Most of the fatal cases have been due to Gram-negative species; if the organism is Gram positive high fever is common but death is rare. This corresponds to the fact that endotoxin is more inflammatory than peptidoglycan by a factor of 10 to 1000, depending on the test used. In all these cases, most of the bacteria are of species which are ordinarily not pathogenic, This is particularly clear with infected blood transfusions, where the selective factor is the ability to grow in a refrigerator at 4 °C, not the ability to evade the immune response.

It is possible to explain, at least in general terms, almost all the changes which we see in infected patients. The most common reaction to infection in normal people is to develop no clinical symptoms. However, a great deal is going on unobserved. The natural immune system controls and eliminates most invading pathogens. However, the natural immune system has as its key cell the macrophage, which is also a key cell for the acquired immune response. Macrophages display pieces of dismembered bacteria on their cell membranes, in the context of major histocompatibility determinant and IL-1. This is recognized by T cells, which help B cells to make antibodies. Only about 1 per cent of healthy people can remember an attack of pneumococcal pneumonia, but every healthy adult has serum antibodies to 30 or 40 pneumococci, as well as antibodies to common bacteria of most other species. Most infections result in symptomless seroconversion.

If the infection is not controlled at a low population, local inflammation will develop. The classical signs of local inflammation are redness, warmth, swelling, pain, and loss of function. As mentioned above, inflammation is initiated by macrophages which secrete tumour necrosis factor-α, IL-1, IL-6, and IL-8 in response to sensing bacteria through the CD14 protein.

Macrophages secrete a powerful thromboplastin which initiates thrombosis and fibrinolysis. Local vasodilatation (redness) is caused by many molecules: in no particular order some of them are histamine from local mast cells, several arachidonic acid derivatives from the membrane phospholipids of activated cells of many types, kinins from serum kininogens activated by Hageman factor exposed to endotoxin, and nitric oxide generated by capillary endothelial cells. There are two distinct waves of nitric oxide synthesis, both induced by IL-1 and tumour necrosis factor acting synergistically. In the first few hours preformed enzyme is activated. After about 12 h newly synthesized enzyme becomes most important.

Local warmth (heat) occurs because of increased blood flow, which raises the temperature of the skin closer to aortic blood temperature. In the fingers this is very obvious because the temperature of the skin of the hand is normally about 30 °C. However, even shoulder skin normally has a temperature of about 35 °C and covered skin such as that on the stomach is still a degree or so below central temperature. The increased rate of local metabolism must contribute something to local warmth, but the effect is thought to be trivial.

Swelling occurs because of local accumulation of extravascular fluid. Normally the amount of albumin in blood is just sufficient to pull back into the low-pressure venous end of the capillaries almost all the fluid which passes into the extracellular space under the higher pressure of the arterial end of the capillary. The rate of lymph flow from a resting non-inflamed tissue is almost zero, and the albumin content is less than 0.5 per cent. Inflamed capillary endothelium is leaky; initially IL-1 and tumour necrosis factor synergize to cause retraction of the cell edges so that gaps develop between adjacent cells. Later, polymorphonuclear leucocytes bound to integrins and palisaded along the endothelial cells may degranulate directly onto the endothelial cell surface and may cause further endothelial cell damage due to lipid peroxidation by generation of reactive oxygen derivatives such as superoxide and hydroxyl radicals. Eventually, there is widespread death of endothelial cells, some of which seems to be due to apoptosis. The increased capillary permeability is of extraordinarily rapid onset—1 h after injecting Gram-negative bacteria into the veins of a dog, pulmonary lymph flow had quadrupled, and the albumin content of pulmonary lymph was over 2 per cent.

Pain appears to be relatively simple. In experiments in which various inflammatory mediators were dropped onto denuded blisters in people, bradykinin was by far the most effective at eliciting pain.

Pus forms when so many polymorphonuclear leucocytes accumulate locally that their secreted proteases are able to overwhelm the local concentrations of antiprotease control proteins such as α_1-antitrypsin. Pus has a thick consistency because it contains large amounts of DNA from the nuclei of broken down polymorphonuclear leucocytes, and it is sometimes greenish because of the presence of large quantities of myeloperoxidase. Pus formation causes local tissue destruction, and, although bacteria do not grow well in it, spontaneous or surgical evacuation of pus often brings an infection to an end.

In serious infections, cytokines such as IL-1, IL-6, and tumour necrosis factor leak out of the local lesion and cause a generalized inflammatory response. This is characterized by fever, polymorphonuclear leucocyte lecocytosis, a striking lowering of serum iron and zinc, and major changes in hepatic protein synthesis. All these changes are adaptive, systemic aspects of the natural immune response which often enable survival in serious infections for long enough to allow production of specific antibody so that the host can recover. A most striking example of this was sometimes found in untreated pneumococcal pneumonia, in which the patient was desperately ill for 6 or 7 days and then, if lucky, had an almost miraculous recovery in a 24-h period. This crisis corresponded to the appearance of free antipneumococcal antibody in the serum, indicating that enough antibody had been made to opsonize all the pneumococci and leave some unbound antibody in the serum.

Fever is due to resetting of the anterior hypothalamic thermostat by IL-1, IL-6, and tumour necrosis factor. The body temperature is controlled just as precisely as it is in health, but the set point is higher. These three cyto-

kines probably work by inducing hypothalamic synthesis of prostaglandin E_2 or a similar compound; aspirin and other non-steroidal anti-inflammatory drugs are antipyretic because they inhibit prostaglandin synthesis. The adaptive value of fever in infectious illness appears to be that it potentiates the immune response.

Polymorphonuclear leucocyte leucocytosis is largely induced by IL-1; initially they are mobilized from the reserve pool of mature polymorphonuclear leucocytes in bone marrow. In a healthy person, this reserve contains about 100 times more polymorphonuclear leucocytes than there are in the blood. Blood smears show more polymorphonuclear leucocytes than average with an increased proportion of band forms. In serious infections, the mature pool of polymorphonuclear leucocytes in the bone marrow is exhausted, and production of polymorphonuclear leucocytes is stimulated from earlier levels. Development is hurried and polymorphonuclear leucocytes are allowed into blood with markers of rushed development. 'Toxic granules' are large, blue perfectly normal polymorphonuclear leucocyte tysosomal granules; the cell did not have time to make the specific granules which would ordinarily have covered them up. 'Dohle bodies' are bluish patches in the cytoplasm of a polymorphonuclear leucocyte; they are pieces of endoplasmic reticulum which the cell did not have time to discard. Vacuoles are not markers of immaturity: polymorphonuclear leucocytes with vacuoles are cells which have had a 'near miss' with bacteria and have partially degranulated into their own cytoplasm. Vacuoles are highly correlated with the presence of bacteraemia. The adaptive value of mobilization of polymorphonuclear leucocytes is obvious.

The specific granules of polymorphonuclear leucocytes contain lactoferrin an iron binding protein which has a dissociation constant two orders of magnitude less than that of transferrin, the normal serum iron transport protein. Polymorphonuclear leucocytes exposed to bacteria are 'messy feeders' and much of their lactoferrin is released into the surrounding fluid. Lactoferrin finds its way into the circulation, strips iron off transferrin, and the lactoferrin–iron complex is taken up and stored in the reticuloendothelial system. Iron is not available for haemoglobin synthesis, and so the 'anaemia of chronic disease' develops in prolonged infections. More important, iron is not available for bacterial growth. There are many organisms which become highly virulent in iron-overloaded individuals. An example is Vibrio vulnificus septicaemia, which is very rare. More than half of the published cases have occurred in people with haemochromatosis.

Normally, the liver makes mostly albumin. It also makes smaller amounts of plasma proteins such as complement components and coagulation cascade proteins, both participating proteins such as fibrinogen and control proteins such as protein C. During serious infections, there is a switch. Little or no albumin is made, and the production of complement and coagulation proteins is increased. Serious infections in individuals with extensive atherosclerosis are often punctuated or terminated by thrombotic events such as strokes and myocardial infarctions. The increased erythrocyte sedimentation rate found in acute infections is mostly due to increased plasma fibrinogen. The adaptive significance of increased levels of complement is obvious; the adaptive significance of faster blood clotting is not so obvious. In addition, the liver makes huge quantities of two proteins, C reactive protein and serum amyloid associated protein, which are not found at all in normal serum. C reactive protein is a phosphoryl choline binding protein which binds to the cell walls of many bacteria. Once bound, it fixes complement, and the bacterium becomes opsonized. Serum amyloid associated protein behaves in a similar way. These proteins act in a non-specific and low-affinity manner, and the protection they provide against any one organism is far inferior to that provided by specific antibody. But their non-specificity is their virtue: they provide low-grade protection against a wide variety of bacteria, and they are available in quantity early in infection. In 24 h, the liver can synthesize 15 g of C reactive protein. The main inducer of changes in liver protein synthesis is IL-6, with assistance from IL-1.

If infection becomes overwhelming, especially if bacteraemia is present, a generalized inflammation of capillaries occurs which is clearly maladaptive. The inducers of the sepsis syndrome are the same as those which induce local inflammatory changes; sepsis is simply inflammation writ large and affecting every tissue in the body. The shock of sepsis is due to peripheral circulatory failure—there is generalized vasodilation in all the vascular beds of the body. Patients with normal hearts attempt to compensate by tachycardia and increased left ventricular stroke volume, The cardiac output in a young man may be 15 to 20 litre/min, with a blood pressure of 80/50 and a systemic vascular resistance of about 4×10^7 N s/m^{-5}. This pattern is completely different from either shock due to left ventricular failure or shock due to major blood or fluid loss. In both of these, the blood pressure may be identical, but the cardiac output is very low, and the peripheral resistance is high. The circulatory pattern is so reliable that the diagnosis of sepsis can be made with virtual certainty if it is present. The only real differential diagnosis is anaphylaxis, which can generally be ruled out on the history.

The capillaries become leaky, and there is a steady loss of fluid and albumin from the blood into the extravascular space ('third spacing'). Unless fluid is replaced, the contracting intravascular volume exaggerates the shock state because the heart cannot maintain a high cardiac output and cardiac output eventually falls below normal. By this time the patient is well into multiple organ failure—the lungs are heavy and waterlogged and Po_2 plunges to levels which require supplemental oxygen. Eventually, the lungs become so stiff that the patient cannot sustain the work of breathing and needs intubation. Even then very high inflation pressures, high positive end expiratory pressure, and high concentrations of inspired oxygen may be necessary. This is full-blown adult respiratory distress syndrome and carries a 50 per cent mortality because the measures required to keep the patient alive themselves induce progressive pulmonary damage.

Other organs react to the anoxia in their own ways. Delirium is an early sign of sepsis: neurones are adapted to a lower pH and slightly different electrolyte concentrations from those found in serum. When the blood–brain barrier becomes leaky, the concentrations of constituents of the cerebrospinal fluid approach those in serum and there is clouding of consciousness. Initially, septic patients are lethargic and inattentive, but can be roused. Late in sepsis patients are usually stuporous. The kidney stops making urine, the liver may stop conjugating bilirubin, and the intestine may become permeable to the endotoxins and bacteria in its lumen. There is lactic acidosis, probably because of glycolysis in ischaemic tissues. Eventually the heart stops beating.

Sepsis has for 40 years carried a mortality of about 30 per cent. If there is adult respiratory distress syndrome the mortality is 50 per cent, and if three or more organs fail the mortality is 85 per cent. For most of this time the treatment has been with antibiotics to eliminate bacteria, fluid replacement to restore intravascular volume, vasoconstrictors if necessary to get the mean arterial pressure above 70, provision for oxygenation by whatever means necessary, correction of obvious electrolyte disorders, hypoglycaemia, and perhaps extreme acidosis, and support for organ failure. In 28 clinical trials, attempts have been made to lower the mortality of sepsis using antagonists of known septic mediators such as tumour necrosis factor, IL-1, platelet activating factor, etc. And it has not worked: the mortality of sepsis has not changed over that 40-year period.

Recently some progress may have occurred. First, experiments in animals have made it clear that the high flow rates in early sepsis are deceptive: much of the bloodflow is bypassing the tissues, and from the outset there is tissue ischaemia. The most convincing demonstration of this was in septic rats: their livers showed strong fluorescence when illuminated with ultraviolet light, indicating that most of the cellular NAD was in the reduced state, and therefore that the hepatocytes were anoxic. Livers of normal rats had low fluorescence. Second it was realized that at least some of the progressive capillary obliteration, which underlies multiple organ failure, is due to exhaustion of clotting control proteins and widespread thrombosis.

Septic patients were shown to have very low or zero levels of activated protein C, and the lower the level the worse the outlook. Replacement with human recombinant activated protein C was shown to reverse some of the circulatory disorder. A placebo controlled double blind multicentre trial of the efficacy of human recombinant activated protein C in 1000 septic patients with at least one organ failing has just been published. For the first time in 40 years, a significant change in mortality was demonstrated. Mortality fell from 30 per cent to 25 per cent—not much, but significant in this number of patients. Where this will lead is difficult to say, but a way has been found to start attacking the capillary dysfunction which is the main problem in septic people.

Further reading

Bernard OR *et al.* (2001). Efficacy and safety of recombinant human activated protein C for severe sepsis *New England Journal of Medicine* **344**, 699–709.

Djiarski R, Tapping RI, Tobias PS (1998). Binding of bacterial peptidoglycan to CD14. *Journal of Biological Chemistry* **273**, 8680–90.

Moxon ER, Murphy PA (1978). *Haemophilus influenzae* bacteremia and meningitis resulting from survival of a single organism *Proceedings of the National Academy of Sciences of the USA* **75**, 1534–6.

7.6 Antimicrobial chemotherapy

R. G. Finch

Introduction

The discovery and clinical application of antibiotics and antimicrobial chemotherapeutic agents is one of the major achievements in medicine. Life-threatening infections such as meningitis, endocarditis and typhoid fever are now treatable, whereas before they were generally fatal. Likewise, the morbidity associated with many infectious diseases of a less life-threatening nature, such as urinary tract infections, skin and soft tissue infections, and bone and joint sepsis, has been substantially reduced. Perioperative prophylactic use of antibiotics has reduced the risk of infections complicating surgical procedures, such as large bowel and gall bladder surgery, vaginal hysterectomy, and implant surgery, such as the insertion of prosthetic heart valves, joints, and neurosurgical shunting devices.

Antimicrobial chemotherapy is the use of antibiotics and chemotherapeutic substances to control infectious disease. The term 'antibiotic' was coined by Waksman to describe a substance derived from naturally occurring micro-organisms and possessing antimicrobial activity in high dilution. The latter characteristic is essential in defining its selective toxicity to other micro-organisms. True antibiotics include penicillin, derived from the mould *Penicillium notatum*; streptomycin from *Streptomyces griseus*, and the cephalosporins from *Cephalosporium* spp. Many chemotherapeutic substances with antimicrobial activity have been artificially synthesized, such as the sulfonamides, quinolones, and isoniazid. However, the term 'antibiotic' is loosely applied to both the true antibiotics and other antimicrobial agents.

Antibiotics are among the most widely prescribed drugs, accounting for an international expenditure of $25b. In the United Kingdom, some 80 per cent of all prescribing is in the community where the emphasis is largely on oral agents; the remainder are used in hospitals where there is a greater emphasis on injectable drugs. More than 125 different antibiotics are available, but a relatively small number is necessary to deal with most prescribing needs. It is important that clinicians who prescribe are familiar with the principles of antimicrobial chemotherapy and that they adopt a continuous learning approach throughout their professional lives to ensure safe and effective prescribing. Table 1 summarizes the agents available for the treatment of bacterial, mycobacterial, fungal, viral, protozoal, and helminthic infections. More agents have been developed for the treatment of bacterial infections, but globally viral, fungal, and parasitic infections predominate. In recent years, there have been major advances in the availability of antiviral drugs particularly for the treatment of the herpesviruses and HIV. Likewise, safe and effective systemic antifungal agents have resulted from the discovery of azoles and triazoles.

The very success of antimicrobial chemotherapy has led to widespread and often excessive use, particularly in community practice where prescribing is largely empirical and clinical distinction between viral and bacterial infections is difficult. Antibiotics are used extensively in animal husbandry both for the treatment and prevention of infectious disease and, more controversially, as growth-enhancing agents among commercially raised poultry and swine. This has raised concerns about the emergence and spread of antibiotic resistance which affects many classes of antibiotic, may be intrinsic to a particular pathogen, or may result from genetic mutation. Resistance may be caused by enzymatic inactivation (β-lactamase), failure of drug penetration into the bacterial cell (porin mutation), alteration of the target binding site (e.g. penicillin-binding protein alteration in penicillin-resistant *Streptococcus pneumoniae*), or from efflux resistance whereby the drug is extruded from the bacterial cell (e.g. chloroquine-

Table 1 Antimicrobial agents available by class or indication effective against bacterial, fungal, viral, protozoal, and helminthic infection (indicative number of agents available[a])

Antibacterial (78)	Antifungal (9)	Antiviral (18)	Antiprotozoal (16)	Anthelminthics (8)
penicillins	polyenes	nucleoside analogues	antimalarials	antithreadworm/hookworm
cephalosporins	flucytosine	non-nucleoside agents	amoebicides	ascaricides
carbapenems	azoles	protease inhibitors	trichomonacides	taenicides
tetracyclines	triazoles	tribavirin	antigiardials	schistosomicides
aminoglycosides	terbinafine	amantadine/rimantadine	leishmaniacides	filaricides
macrolides		neuraminidase inhibitors	trypanocides	antihydatid agents
clindamycin			antipneumocystis agents	antistrongyloidiasis
chloramphenicol				anticutaneous larva migrans
sodium fusidate				
glycopeptides				
sulfonamides				
trimethoprim				
antituberculous				
antiherpetic				
nitroimidazoles				
quinolones				
urinary antiseptics				

[a]Based on agents listed in the British National Formulary.

resistant *Plasmodium falciparum*). Organisms can also develop alternative metabolic pathways which by-pass drug inactivation. Resistance may be transferable between the same species or genera but may also spread between genera. Coding for multiple antibiotic resistance has been increasingly observed and results from a number of mechanisms, in particular plasmid transfer.

Despite the advances in antimicrobial chemotherapy, fresh challenges remain. These include the treatment and prevention of viral causes of enteric infection, meningitis, and hepatitis which are still without effective chemotherapy. Tuberculosis and malaria are among the world's major infectious disease killers and here problems of antibiotic resistance and, in the case of tuberculosis, the continuing need for long and complex regimens continue to frustrate disease management.

Among the more worrying trends in antibiotic resistance is the emergence within hospitals of methicillin-resistant *Staphylococcus aureus* (MRSA) and vancomycin-resistant enterococci (VRE). Among community pathogens, *Strep. pneumoniae* has rapidly become less sensitive to penicillin causing clinical failures in the treatment of meningitis and otitis media. Internationally, multidrug resistant tuberculosis and multidrug resistant salmonellae, including *Salmonella typhi*, are of major concern.

Resistance is not confined to bacteria. Fungal resistance is increasing (e.g. of *Candida albicans* and *C. krusei.* to fluconazole). Resistance by the human immunodeficiency virus (HIV) to the nucleoside, non-nucleoside, and protease inhibitors is rapidly emerging. Within a decade of the introduction of antiviral agents, failure of chemotherapy may become a major factor responsible for progression of HIV disease.

Pharmacology

Mode of action

Knowledge of the pharmacological mode of action of an antimicrobial agents permits an understanding of the diverse mechanisms of microbial inhibition and the opportunities for drug resistance. This is best established for antibacterial and antiviral agents. In the case of antifungal, and especially antiparasitic agents, the modes of action are less well defined. This reflects the process of drug discovery whereby an understanding of the biochemical and molecular action of agents derived from natural or chemical sources has not always been a priority in establishing efficacy and safety.

Antibacterial drugs

Antibacterial agents may affect cell wall or protein synthesis, nucleic acid formation, or may act on critical metabolic pathways (Table 2).

The β-lactams (penicillins, cephalosporins, and monobactams (aztreonam)) and the glycopeptides (vancomycin and teicoplanin), inhibit cell wall synthesis. The β-lactams, which share the common β-lactam ring, act on cell wall transpeptidases to inhibit cross-linking of peptidoglycan. The glycopeptide antibiotics act at an earlier stage of cell wall synthesis by binding to acyl-D-alanyl-D-alanine. Despite their similar mode of action, they are less efficient bactericides than the β-lactams.

Inhibitors of protein synthesis

Antibacterial agents that inhibit protein synthesis act on the 30S ribosomal subunit responsible for binding mRNA, or the 50S subunit which binds aminoacyl tRNA. The aminoglycosides, tetracyclines, and macrolide antibiotics are the most widely used inhibitors of protein synthesis. Chloramphenicol, clindamycin, and the recently introduced agent quinupristin/dalfopristin (Synercid) also act at this site.

Inhibitors of nucleic acid

Nucleic acid synthesis is targeted by quinolones, metronidazole, and rifampicin. The bacterial DNA gyrase is essential for the supercoiling of bacterial DNA. This, together with the enzyme topoisomerase IV, are the major targets for the quinolones. These enzymes are absent in humans, explaining the selective activity of these drugs. Rifampicin and other rifamycins interfere with DNA-dependent RNA polymerase, preventing chain initiation.

Metabolic inhibitors

The best known metabolic inhibitors are the sulfonamides and trimethoprim which interfere with folic acid synthesis by sequentially inhibiting the enzymes pteroic acid synthetase and dihydrofolate reductase. By acting sequentially, a combined bactericidal effect results. The selective activity of these compounds is dependent upon the fact that humans are unable to synthesise folic acid and require preformed folic acid in their diet.

Antiviral agents

Viruses live and replicate within the host cell. Antiviral chemotherapy therefore presents a particular challenge if it is to be selectively toxic. The cycle of viral replication provides a number of opportunities for therapeutic intervention. Most available antiviral agents are nucleoside analogues, largely used in the treatment of HIV or herpesvirus infections (Table 3). The recent growth in numbers of antiviral agents has benefited greatly from HIV related research through the identification of new drug targets (Fig. 1). Interference with cell surface attachment through ligand blockade of surface receptors provides a theoretical, as yet unfulfilled, target. Penetration into the host cell may be through a process of translocation or direct fusion between the outer lipid membrane of the virus and the cell membrane, before uncoating and release of viral nucleic acid. Replication differs among viruses, thereby providing a number of therapeutic options.

Table 2 Microbial site of action and targets for selected antibacterial drugs

Site of action	Drugs	Target
cell wall peptidoglycan	penicillins	transpeptidase
	cephalosporins	transpeptidase
	vancomycin	acyl-D-alanyl-D-alanine
	teicoplanin	acyl-D-alanyl-D-alanine
ribosome	chloramphenicol	peptidyl transferase of 50S subunit
	clindamycin	50S ribosomal subunit transpeptidation
	macrolides	50S ribosomal subunit
	tetracyclines	ribosomal A-site
	aminoglycosides	initiation complex and translation
	fusidic acid	elongation factor G
nucleic acid	quinolones	DNA gyrase
	metronidazole	DNA strands
	rifampicin	RNA polymerase
folic acid synthesis	sulfonamides	pteroic acid synthetase
	trimethoprim	dihydrofolate reductase

Viral mRNA becomes translated into multiple copies of viral proteins encoded by the viral genome either as a result of virus-specific enzymes or by co-opting host-derived protein. HIV, for example, employs its own reverse transcriptase to convert RNA to DNA before integration into the host cell chromosome. Transcription and translation follow. Before the virus can be released, new viral particles must be assembled for which host cell proteins and mechanisms of phosphorylation and glycosylation may be recruited. The protease inhibitors act at this stage and have been particu-

Table 3 Mode of action of selected antiviral drugs

Drug	Target virus	Antiviral activity
aciclovir	HSV	nucleoside analogue
famciclovir	VZ	nucleoside analogue
foscarnet	CMV	inhibits DNA polymerase
ganciclovir	CMV	nucleoside analogue
amantadine	influenza A	uncoating and assembly
rimantidine	influenza A	uncoating and assembly
zidovudine	HIV	nucleoside reverse transcriptase inibitors
zalcitabine	HIV	nucleoside reverse transcriptase inibitors
didanosine	HIV	nucleoside reverse transcriptase inibitors
stavudine	HIV	nucleoside reverse transcriptase inibitors
lamivudine	HIV	nucleoside reverse transcriptase inibitors
abacavir	HIV	nucleoside reverse transcriptase inibitors
delavirdine	HIV	non-nucleoside reverse trancriptase inhibitors
nevirapine	HIV	non-nucleoside reverse transcriptase inhibitors
efavirenz	HIV	non-nucleoside reverse trancriptase inhibitors
saquinavir	HIV	protease inhibitors
ritonavir	HIV	protease inhibitors
indinavir	HIV	protease inhibitors
nelfinavir	HIV	protease inhibitors

larly successful. Virus release is either the result of transportation and budding, or host cell lysis.

Antifungal agents

The polyene antifungals (amphotericin B and nystatin) act on ergosterol within the fungal cell membrane. Ergosterol is largely absent from bacteria and humans, explaining the selective toxicity of these agents. The azole antifungals include the imidazoles (e.g. clotrimazole, miconazole, ketoconazole) and the triazoles (fluconazole and itraconazole) which bind preferentially to fungal cytochrome P450 to inhibit 14-α-methylsterol demethylation to ergosterol.

Antiparasitic agents

The mechanism of action of many antiparasitic drugs is only partially known. Among the antimalarials, chloroquine interferes with the digestion of haemoglobin taken up by *Plasmodia*. Quinine is thought to act in a similar manner. Metronidazole is active against a number of protozoa such as *Entamoeba histolytica* as well as anaerobic bacteria. It acts as an electron sink, by reducing of its 5-nitro group and activated by nitroreductase within the target pathogen, thus interrupting DNA synthesis.

Among the antihelminthic drugs, piperazine and paraziquantel act by selectively inducing muscle paralysis in the target helminth. Others, such as thiabendazole, inhibit parasitic ATP synthesis and energy production.

Antimicrobial spectrum of activity

The antimicrobial spectrum of an agent is dependent upon target site susceptibility among pathogenic organisms at clinically achievable drug concentrations. Some micro-organisms are intrinsically resistant to certain antibiotics. For example the aminoglycosides are inactive against anaerobic bacteria because cell entry is an energy dependent process relying on respiratory quinones, which are absent in anaerobic bacteria. Certain strains of *Pseudomonas aeruginosa* are resistant to the aminoglycosides as a result of altered protein porin channels which inhibit antibiotic penetration.

The antimicrobial spectrum of a drug in part dictates its clinical indications. While information on this spectrum is more easily determined *in*

Fig. 1 Sites of inhibition of HIV replication by current antiretroviral drugs.

vitro, in vivo efficacy can only be confirmed through clinical use, which can be supported by animal model data during drug development. For example *in vitro Salmonella typhi* is susceptible to gentamicin, but the drug is not effective clinically.

Narrow spectrum and broad spectrum agents

There are few truly narrow spectrum agents. Fusidic acid, mupirocin, and the glycopeptides (vancomycin and teicoplanin) target specific pathogens and are mainly used to treat microbiologically confirmed infections.

Broad spectrum agents, such as the quinolone antibiotics and the parenteral cephalosporins, such as cefotaxime and ceftriaxone, are active against many Gram-positive and Gram-negative pathogens. Metronidazole has activity against a large number of anaerobic bacteria and, because of this restricted activity, is considered to have a narrow spectrum. The aminoglycosides, although active against staphylococci and aerobic Gram-negative bacilli are inactive against streptococci and anaerobes and are therefore frequently prescribed in combination. The carbapenems (imipenem and meropenem) possess the broadest spectrum of activity which includes most aerobic and anaerobic bacterial pathogens. Broad spectrum agents are often used empirically in the initial management of severe infection. However, they frequently affect the normal flora so that super-infection with *Clostridium difficile* and yeasts are more likely to arise.

Susceptibility testing

Antibiotic susceptibility testing of clinical isolates is important for appropriate prescribing and for gathering epidemiological data. It is determined *in vitro* by using either broth- or agar-based methods. Pathogens are exposed to known concentrations of an antibiotic and their degree of inhibition compared to a standard control. Disk susceptibility testing is the most widely used method. Zones of inhibition around the antibiotic-containing disk are measured, compared to a standard, and the pathogen designated sensitive, resistant, or of intermediate susceptibility to the drug. Currently, such methods require the isolate to be tested in pure culture. It is therefore difficult to obtain information on the susceptibility of a pathogen in less than 36 to 48 h from sample collection.

The minimal inhibitory concentration (MIC) in mg/l provides more precise *in vitro* information on the activity of a drug against bacterial pathogen. It is more time consuming and costly to determine although automated systems and commercial strip tests are available (Fig. 2). Defining susceptibility by MIC determination permits greater predictive benefit in the treatment of certain infections such as gonorrhoea, bacterial endocarditis, and pneumococcal meningitis. Knowledge of the *in vitro* susceptibility of common pathogens to antimicrobial agents (Fig. 3) is helpful in selecting drug therapy but is only relevant to the achievable drug concentrations, which is important in predicting performance as discussed below.

Combined drug therapy

In hospital practice, it is common to combine agents when dealing with mixed infections or where initial broad spectrum empirical therapy is required. Another important reason for combining drugs is to prevent the emergence of antibiotic resistance, such as in the treatment of tuberculosis and HIV infections. Antituberculosis regimens have been developed to ensure that naturally occurring minority populations of *Mycobacterium tuberculosis* resistant to isoniazid or rifampicin do not emerge during therapy. By combining isoniazid and rifampicin with pyrazinamide and ethambutol for the initial phase of therapy (2 months), resistance is usually avoided. Therapy can be restricted to isoniazid and rifampicin for the continuation phase (4 months). The regimen is extended in those patients unable to tolerate pyrazinamide and in the treatment of tuberculous meningitis (Table 4).

HIV infection is treated with multidrug regimens. The success of highly active antiretroviral therapy, in which nucleoside analogues and protease inhibitors are combined in a three-drug regimen, is not only based on greater potency of the combined regimen but also on its ability to slow the emergence of drug-resistant mutants. The more recently introduced nonnucleoside reverse transcriptase inhibitors, such as efavirenz, appear to be equally potent in combination with nucleoside analogues and can delay the need for using protease inhibitors. This may increase the period of time in which antiretroviral therapy remains effective in an individual. The options for treating HIV infection are summarized in Table 5 (see also Chapter 7.10.21).

Occasionally, drugs are combined for the purpose of achieving a synergistic effect based on evidence that the *in vitro* activity of the combination is shown to be greater than the sum of the activity of the individual agents. Most drugs in combination will simply be additive in effect. One of the more frequently prescribed synergistic combinations is that of penicillin (or ampicillin) and streptomycin (or gentamicin) in the treatment of endocarditis caused by *Enterococcus* spp. The aminoglycoside alone is generally inactive against enterococci but in combination with ampicillin achieves synergistic killing (Fig. 4). A similar effect is employed in the treatment of viridans streptococcal endocarditis with this combination.

Another widely used example of synergistic inhibition is the combined effects of an antipseudomonal β-lactam, such as ceftazidime or piperacillin, and an aminoglycoside, such as gentamicin, tobramycin, or amikacin. This combination is used to treat documented or suspected *Pseudomonas aeruginosa* infections occurring in neutropenic states complicating bone marrow transplantation, cytotoxic chemotherapy, and burn wound infections.

Antibiotic resistance

General considerations

Antibiotic resistance has been recognized since the introduction of effective antibiotics. For example penicillin-resistant strains of *Staphylococcus aureus* became widespread shortly after the introduction of this agent; penicillin sensitive strains are now uncommon. Resistant strains of Gram-negative bacteria, such as *Klebsiella*, *Enterobacter*, *Acinetobacter*, and *Pseudomonas* spp. are commonly found in high dependency units where they may cause epidemics. The international emergence of epidemic MRSA infections, primarily within hospitals and nursing homes, is very worrying. Conventional approaches to controlling these infections have been largely unsuccessful. The emergence of MRSA together with multiple-antibiotic-resistant coagulase-negative staphylococci has rapidly increased the use of vancomycin. Vancomycin-resistant enterococci has emerged in specialist hospital facilities such as dialysis and haematology units; therapeutic options are

Fig. 2 *Staphylococcul aureus* resistant to penicillin (minimum inhibitory concentration 8 mg/l) on the left and sensitive to vancomycin (minimum inhibitory concentration 1.0 mg/l) on the right as demonstrated by a commercial strip test.

limited. Other problems include the emergence of penicillin-resistant pneumococci and β-lactamase producing *Haemophilus influenzae*.

At present, there is great international concern among professionals, politicians, and, increasingly, the public about antibiotic resistance. In the United Kingdom, the House of Lords published an influential document in 1998 reviewing the issues surrounding this problem. This has led to a number of initiatives: reducing the use of antibiotics, particularly in the treatment of minor upper respiratory tract infections in the community; education strategies for prescribers and the public; and better enforcement of infection control policies. Within the European Union, similar measures have been proposed together with a ban on the use of antibiotics as growth promoters in livestock animals. However, antibiotic resistance is a global problem. An increasing number of multidrug resistant infections caused by *Salmonella* spp. and *Mycobacterium tuberculosis* are being imported from developing countries where the availability or prescribing of antibiotics is less controlled.

Antibiotic resistance drives changes in patterns of prescribing and is a major impetus to the pharmaceutical industry in its search for new therapies. Micro-organisms differ in their ability to develop resistance, which may affect a particular drug, a class, or multiple classes of antibiotics. Genetic mutations select for antibiotic resistance which frequently occur under the influence of antibiotic pressure. The major mechanisms of resistance are summarized in Table 6. Resistance to single or multiple antibiotics may be either chromosomally, or plasmid mediated, or both. In turn, genes may code for resistance to a single or multiple antibiotics. In addition to plasmid-mediated resistance, other transposable genetic elements (transposons), and insertion sequences incapable of self-replication, may exist within a chromosome, plasmid, or bacteriophage.

Resistance genes are most frequently transferred between organisms by conjugation. This occurs between the same or different species of bacteria and also between different genera. Other mechanisms of transferring resistance include transduction via a bacteriophage, and less commonly transformation in which naked DNA released during cell lysis is taken up by other bacteria.

Transposon-mediated resistance reflects transfer of discreet sequences of DNA between chromosomes or plasmids whereby individual or groups of genes can be inserted to the host bacterial cell. More recently, molecular structures known as integrons have been identified which facilitate new combinations of resistance genes within the bacterial chromosome, plasmid, or transposons. The antibiotic resistance genes are bound on each side by conserved segments of DNA. These individual resistance genes can be inserted or removed between the conserved structures and act as an expression vector for antibiotic resistance genes.

While the molecular mechanisms of antibiotic resistance are legion, the ability of drug-resistant micro-organisms to survive, disseminate, and cause disease varies widely. In many instances, antibiotic resistance may give a survival advantage only in the presence of continued antibiotic exposure to such agents. This is reflected in the occurrence of epidemic disease in high-dependency units such as intensive care facilities where antibiotic usage is often high. However, it is also clear that once the genetic mechanism for evading antimicrobial activity has been acquired, it is rarely lost and adds to the continuously expanding genetic memory that has steadily eroded the efficacy of many antimicrobial drugs.

Enzymatic inactivation

Aminoglycoside-modifying enzymes include adenylating, acetylating, and phosphorylating enzymes. Gentamicin is the most susceptible and amikacin the least susceptible to such inactivation. However, the largest group of inactivating enzymes are the β-lactamases which hydrolyse the β-lactam ring common to all penicillins and cephalosporins. Penicillinase was the

Fig. 3 Sensitivity of selected pathogenic bacteria to some common antibacterial agents.

Table 4 Tuberculosis treatment regimens for pulmonary and non-pulmonary[a] tuberculous infection caused by *Mycobacterium tuberculosis*

Initial phase (2 months)	Continuation phase (4 months)
isoniazid	isoniazid
rifampicin	rifampicin
pyrazinamide[b]	
ethambutol	

[a]CNS and tuberculous meningitis should be treated for 10 months after the initial phase of four drugs.

[b]If pyrazinamide contraindicated or not given the continuation phase is extended to 7 months.

first β-lactamase to be identified and is the reason why most strains of *Staphylococcus aureus* are resistant to this drug. Another important β-lactamase is that known as TEM-1 which is responsible for resistance to ampicillin by *Haemophilus influenzae*. The major impetus to the development of the penicillins and cephalosporins was to extend their spectrum of activity by resisting inactivation by β-lactamases present in many aerobic Gram-negative bacilli. However, new inactivating enzymes continue to emerge, including the extended spectrum β-lactamases, which are now

Table 5 HIV infection—treatment regimens for drug-naïve patients[a]

2 nucleoside reverse transcriptase inhibitors + non-nucleoside reverse transcriptase inhibitor

2 nucleoside reverse transcriptase inhibitors + protease inhibitor

2 nucleoside reverse transcriptase inhibitors + 2 protease inhibitors[b]

3 nucleoside reverse transcriptase inhibitors

[a]See Table 3 for agents available.

[b]Ritonavir + another agent.

Fig. 4 Effects of ampicillin (0.5 mg/l) and gentamicin (2 mg/l) alone and in combination on a strain of *Enterococus faecalis* from a patient with infective endocarditis. A synergestic effect is observed with the combined agents.

limiting the clinical utility of third-generation cephalosporins, and the carbapenemases which hydrolyse imipenem.

Impermeability resistance

Drug uptake of antibiotics such as the penicillins, tetracyclines, and quinolone antibiotics by bacteria is through protein channels (porins) which cross the outer membrane. Alterations in the permeability of the outer membrane of Gram-negative bacteria is an increasingly important mechanism of drug resistance. Mutations in porin structure are responsible for resistance among pathogens such as *P. aeruginosa* and *Serratia marcescens*.

Alterations in target site

Another important mechanism of resistance is mutational modification of drug binding sites. This affects susceptibility to β-lactams, erythromycin, chloramphenicol, and rifampicin. Erythromycin and chloramphenicol bind to the bacterial 50S ribosomal subunit which is subject to genetic mutation. In contrast, the quinolones target DNA gyrase which is subject to subunit structure alteration resulting in one variety of resistance to drugs such as ciprofloxacin. The increasing resistance to penicillin among *Streptococcus pneumoniae* is the result of reduced binding of penicillin to several binding proteins (PBP-2a and PBP-2x). *Staph. aureus* resistance to methicillin is due to the presence of penicillin binding protein (PBP-2a) which has reduced affinity for methicillin and other β-lactams and is encoded by the *mecA* gene.

The recently recognized problem of vancomycin resistant enterococci, which largely affects *Enterococcus faecium*, is the result of the production of enzymes (ligases) which permit continued cell wall synthesis despite the presence of vancomycin. To date, five different genes have been found responsible for this phenomenon (Van A-E) which result in different phenotypic patterns of resistance to the glycopeptides vancomycin and teicoplanin.

Metabolic bypass resistance

Bacteria must synthesize folic acid from the precursor *p*-aminobenzoic acid. The sulfonamide antibiotics competitively inhibit the enzyme dihydropteroate synthetase. Trimethoprim acts on the same metabolic pathway by inhibiting dihydrofolate reductase. The sequential inhibitory effects of trimethoprim and sulfamethoxazole (co-trimoxazole) result in synergistic bactericidal activity against many pathogens. Resistant organisms are able to synthesize their own enzymes thereby evading such competitive inhibition.

Surveillance of antibiotic resistance

Information on the susceptibility of pathogenic micro-organisms is important. Such data can provide information on the relative frequency of pathogens and the pattern of susceptibility to prescribed agents. Surveillance, therefore, has a role in guiding prescribing, in developing prescribing policies and in identifying and monitoring organisms which are subject to infection control measures. On a broader front, surveillance is also of value in alerting industry and health-care planners to the need for new drug and vaccine strategies for disease control.

To be of maximum benefit, surveillance needs to be sensitive to a defined geographical base which may simply reflect the catchment area of specimens submitted to a particular laboratory, providing information on the

Table 6 Examples of resistance mechanisms for selected antibiotics

Enzymatic/inactivation	Altered target site	Altered permeability	Efflux	Metabolic bypass
aminoglycosides	erythromycin	β-lactams	tetracycline	sulfonamides
β-lactams	chlor-amphenicol	quinolones	quinolones	trimethoprim
chloramphenicol	fusidic acid		β-lactams	
	streptomycin			

trends in community and hospital isolates. Within hospitals, more specific information can be provided about susceptibility patterns in high dependency units, where antibiotic consumption is often greater, and more resistant pathogens, such as *Klebsiella, Serratia, Enterobacter, Acinetobacter spp.*, and *Pseudomonas aeruginosa* are found. Among Gram-positive pathogens, *Staphylococcus aureus* and enterococci present an increasing challenge to prescribing and infection control practice.

National networks of surveillance often vary in their focus and include data on enteric pathogens, *Staphylococcus aureus*, penicillin resistance among pneumococci, and, more recently, vancomycin resistant enterococci. There are important international networks which collect information on such pathogens as *Legionella pneumophila* and *Mycobacterium tuberculosis*. Drug resistant tuberculosis is increasingly prevalent in the United Kingdom and overseas.

Surveillance of resistance to antiviral agents is rudimentary. Patient-specific data is increasingly sought in those with HIV infection, to assess drug failure, guide change in management, and direct primary therapy in selected cases of person-to-person and mother-to-infant transmission. Determination of phenotypic resistance is still costly and time consuming and most data relate to genotypic patterns of resistance to antiretroviral drugs among HIV isolates.

Pharmacokinetics

To be effective, antimicrobial agents must achieve therapeutic concentrations at the site of the target infection. This may be localized to a single anatomical site, such as the bladder or the cerebrospinal fluid, or involve a major organs such as the lung. Infections may also be generalized and affect many body sites. Drug selection must take into consideration the fact that pathogens such as *M. tuberculosis, Legionella pneumophila*, and *S. typhi* replicate intracellularly. Antimicrobial drugs may be administered parenterally, orally, or topically to the skin, external auditory meatus, conjunctiva, and by intraocular application. In the case of systemically active agents, the effective drug concentrations are determined by the standard pharmacokinetic parameters of absorption, distribution, metabolism, and elimination. Since selective toxicity is crucial to safe prescribing, the dose regimen for each agent aims to avoid concentrations toxic to the host but inhibitory to the micro-organism. This 'therapeutic window' varies by drug.

Bioavailability

The rate and degree of absorption from the gastrointestinal tract is not only important for plasma concentrations reflected in the pharmacokinetic parameters of C_{max} and T_{max} of a drug, but also for potential adverse effects on the bowel (Table 7). For example ampicillin, the first of the aminopenicillins, commonly caused gastrointestinal side-effects, most notably diarrhoea. These effects have been reduced by increasing the bioavailability of the active drug through the introduction of hydroxy-ampicillin (amoxicillin) and various esters and prodrugs of ampicillin.

Some agents such as cefalexin, doxycycline, and a number of the quinolone antibiotics are extremely well absorbed, achieving 80 to 100 per cent bioavailability. In the case of some recent quinolones, the excellent bioavailability has raised the possibility of treating with oral antibiotics some severely ill patients who might normally require parenteral therapy. In contrast, drugs which are poorly bioavailable, such as cefixime and cefuroxime axetil, not only have a higher incidence of gastrointestinal side-effects but are also more likely to select for *Clostridium difficile* associated large bowel disease.

Distribution

Most drugs are distributed in the blood via the plasma before gaining access to the extracellular fluid. Tissue concentrations of a particular agent are affected by pH, drug ionizability, lipid solubility, and the presence of an inflammatory reaction whereby the capillary fenestrations are increased in size. In the case of agents administered intravenously by infusion or by bolus injection, the distribution phase is rapid in comparison with orally, rectally, or intramuscularly administered drugs. Drugs which are poorly lipophilic, such as the β-lactams and aminoglycosides, achieve low concentrations in tissues such as the brain. However, the β-lactams achieve therapeutic concentrations in the cerebrospinal fluid as a result of the inflammatory reaction which accompanies meningitis.

Drugs may also be taken up intracellularly, as in the case of macrolides and quinolones, resulting in a large volume of distribution compared to drugs confined to the extracellular space, such as the β-lactams and aminoglycosides. This is important in relation to the treatment of intracellular pathogens such as *Mycoplasma pneumoniae, Legionella pneumophila,* and *Mycobacterium tuberculosis* which can only be effectively treated by drugs which are concentrated and remain biologically active intracellularly.

Table 7 Bioavailability and intestinal elimination of some commonly prescribed antibacterial drugs after oral administration

Drug	Bioavailability (%)	Intestinal elimination
Penicillins		
Amoxicillin	80–90	Concentrated up to 10-fold in bile
Ampicillin	50	Concentrated up to 10-fold in bile
Flucloxacillin	80–90	Negligible
Cephalosporins		
Cefalexin	80–100	Concentrated up to 3-fold in bile
Cefuroxime axetil	30–40	Bile concentrations of up to 80 per cent of serum
Cefixime	40–50	Concentrated up to 50-fold in bile
Quinolones		
Nalidixic acid	90–100	Biliary concentrations similar to serum
Ciprofloxacin	70–85	Concentrated up to 10-fold in bile; additional enteral secretion
Other antibacterials		
Erythromycin	18–45	Concentrated up to 300-fold in bile
Metronidazole	80–95	Concentrations in bile similar to serum
Rifampicin	90–100	Concentrated up to 1000-fold in bile
Sulfamethoxazole	70–90	Concentrations in bile 40–70 per cent of serum
Tetracycline	75	Concentrated up to 10-fold in bile
Trimethoprim	80–90	Concentrated up to 2-fold in bile

Note that drugs which are well absorbed may still achieve high concentrations in the faeces because of secretion into bile or other enteral secretions.

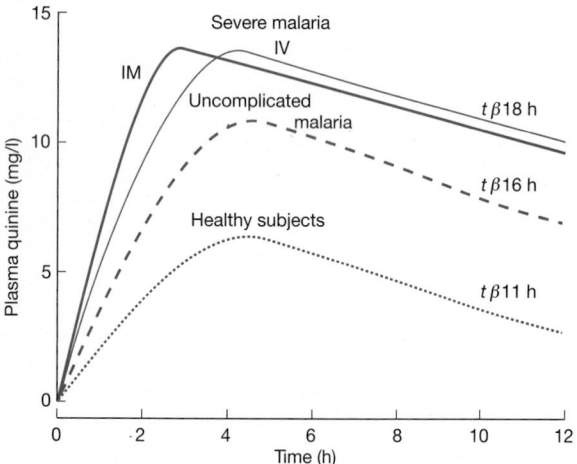

Fig. 5 Average plasma quinine concentrations following administration of a loading dose of 20 mg (salt)/kg to patients with severe and uncomplicated malaria, compared with those predicted to occur in normal subjects. (Reproduced from White (1992), with permission.)

The plasma half-life ($T^{1/2}$), which is the time required for the concentration of a drug in the plasma to fall by half, is affected by drug distribution and, in particular, its rate of elimination as a result of metabolism and excretion. This in turn affects the time taken to reach steady state. In the treatment of life-threatening infections, it is important that steady state kinetics are achieved rapidly. This may require the administration of a loading dose. This applies to the use of agents such as gentamicin for the treatment of serious Gram-negative infections and intravenous quinine in the case of life-threatening malaria where the pharmacokinetic behaviour can be altered by the severity of the disease in comparison with healthy subjects (Fig. 5).

Drugs are commonly distributed in the blood and tissues bound to plasma proteins, largely albumin. Drugs vary in their degree of protein binding. With agents such as flucloxacillin and ceftazidime it exceeds 95 per cent. The importance of protein binding lies in the fact that the active moiety is the unbound drug. Dissociation from the bound to the unbound state is usually rapid but this equilibrium may affect drug performance at certain sites such as the joints. The relationship between protein binding and drug performance has been emphasized in recent studies of the pharmacodynamics of drug activity (see below).

Metabolism

Antibiotics, like other drugs, are degraded at various sites in the body but, predominantly within the liver. Degradation involves conjugation, hydrolysis, oxidation, glucuronidation, or dealkylation, according to the particular drug. Members of the hepatic cytochrome P450 group of enzymes play a dominant role in this process. Drug metabolites are usually but not always biologically inactive. For example cefotaxime is degraded to desacetyl-cefotaxime and clarithromycin to hydroxy-clarithromycin, both of which are biologically active and contribute to the overall antibacterial activity of these agents.

Excretion

Most drugs are excreted in the urine by glomerular filtration, tubular secretion, or a combination of these mechanisms. Thus high concentrations of drug will often be present in the urine; this has therapeutic importance in the treatment of urinary tract infections. Urinary pH affects the biological activity of many drugs; for example the activity of ciprofloxacin is markedly reduced at pH 5.5. Tubular excretion can be blocked by probenecid. This was formerly used to ensure higher plasma concentrations of penicillin and is still recommended in the treatment of gonorrhoea with single doses of

amoxicillin, ampicillin, or intramuscular procaine penicillin. It is also important to note that any reduction in glomerular filtration rate will not only affect urinary concentrations of drug but also the plasma half-life and, in turn, serum concentrations of drugs which are primarily excreted by this route. In the case of antibiotics such as the aminoglycosides and vancomycin, the dose must be reduced in renal failure.

Biliary excretion is another important route for drug elimination either as the active compound or as a microbiologically active or inactive metabolite. Reabsorption from the gastrointestinal tract can result in enterohepatic recirculation, which in turn may affect plasma half-life. Drugs which achieve high concentrations in the bile are effective in the treatment of infections at this site such as cholecystitis. However, biliary obstruction or hepatic impairment may reduce therapeutic efficacy and require dose reduction to avoid toxic effects. Examples include clindamycin, efavirenz, mefloquine, and tetracyclines.

Therapeutic drug monitoring of some antibiotics is essential in order to ensure therapeutic yet non-toxic concentrations. This applies particularly to aminoglycosides which have a relatively narrow therapeutic index. Trough concentrations of gentamicin in excess of 2 mg/l, if sustained, can result in nephrotoxicity and ototoxicity. The target cells for such toxicities are the renal tubular lining cells and the cochlear hair cells of the inner ear respectively. Vancomycin is also frequently monitored, particularly in patients with impaired renal function.

Pharmacodynamics

The inter-relationship between drug, micro-organism, and the infected host creates an important pharmacological dynamic. Antibiotics are unique in therapeutics in that they are targeted at an invading micro-organism which may be present at a particular site or be more widely distributed in the body. The host's response to infection may modify the pharmacokinetic handling of a drug. Many antibiotics have a measurable effect on a variety of bacterial and host cell functions, even at subinhibitory concentrations. It is difficult to establish the exact role that these factors play clinically, but they are likely to contribute to the overall effect of an antibiotic. Macrolides, such as erythromycin, illustrate this point since they affect a variety of virulence characteristics (Table 8) as well as affecting the host's response to infection.

Exposure of micro-organisms to sublethal concentrations of an antibiotic may temporarily inhibit growth which recommences following removal of the drug. The time to recovery is known as the postantibiotic effect. This varies with the drug and the micro-organism; for example the quinolones have a longer postantibiotic effect than β-lactams (Table 9). The relevance of this observation to the *in vivo* situation, where plasma drug concentrations are often well above the inhibitory concentration and are sustained through repeat dosaging, remains uncertain. It may have greater relevance to tissue concentrations which tend to be lower than plasma concentrations. Postantibiotic effect certainly contributes to the effects of agents that are administered once daily, such as gentamicin.

The relationship between the pharmacokinetic characteristics of a drug and bacterial inhibition is critical to therapeutic outcome (Table 10). In the

Table 8 Effect of macrolides on bacterial virulence at subinhibitory concentrations

Factor	Effect	Factor	Effect
adhesins (pili, fimbriae)	↓	exoenzyme production	
fibronectin binding	↓	elastase	↓
alginate production	↓	protease	↓
extoxin A production	↓	DNase	↓
β-haemolysin activity	↓	coagulase	↓
serum susceptibility	↑	leucocidin	↓
		flagellar function	↓

Shyrock *et al.* (1998). *Journal of Antimicrobial Chemotherapy.*

Table 9 Postantibiotic effects (hours) of selected drugs agains *Staph. aureus, Escherichia coli,* and *Pseudomonas aeruginosa*

Drug	S. aureus	E.coli	Ps. aeruginosa
Ampicillin	1.7	0.1	NT
Cefotaxime	1.4	0.2	−0.3
Ciprofloxacin	2.0	2.1	2.4
Imipenem	2.6	0.5	1.5
Gentamicin	2.0	1.8	2.2
Vancomycin	2.2	NT	NT
Erythromycin	3.1	NT	NT
Rifampicin	2.8	4.2	NT

NT = not tested

case of agents such as penicillins and cephalosporins, the time that drug concentrations are maintained above the minimum inhibitory concentration (MIC) predicts the response. This contrasts with agents such as the quinolones and aminoglycosides, where it is more important to achieve high C_{max} to MIC ratios. Modelling the MIC of a particular organism against the dose response curve for a drug (Fig. 6) has established a number of important pharmacodynamic parameters which have been supported by studies in animal models and man. For example dosage regimens of quinolones, such as ciprofloxacin and levofloxacin, have been based on pharmacodynamic data. The ratio of C_{max}:MIC has been refined in the parameter, area under the inhibitory concentration, which is the ratio of the area under the time curve (AUC):MIC. This is more predictive of outcome. The importance of protein binding for drug performance has also emerged as an important modifying factor in this modelling. The AUC:MIC of the free drug is the most sensitive predictor of response. The manner in which these ratios differ for selected quinolones is shown in Table 11.

Principles of use

In comparison with many other classes of drugs, antimicrobial agents are usually prescribed in short courses ranging from a single dose to a few days. Prolonged therapy is required for certain infections such as tuberculosis and bone and joint sepsis, and for HIV infection, treatment is usually lifelong.

Most antibiotic prescribing, especially within community practice, is empirical. Even among patients in hospital, where there are greater opportunities for diagnostic precision based on laboratory investigations, the exact nature of the infection is established in only a minority of cases. Most therapeutic prescribing requires a presumptive clinical diagnosis which, in turn, is linked to a presumptive microbiological diagnosis based on know-

ledge of the usual microbial causes of such infections. Among the most widely treated infections are those affecting the upper and lower respiratory tracts, the urinary tract and skin and soft tissues for which the likely microbial aetiology is restricted. For example urinary tract infections arising in the community are usually caused by *Escherichia coli* and other Gram-negative enteric pathogens and, less commonly, by enterococci or *Staphylococcus saprophyticus*. Local knowledge of the susceptibility of these pathogens to commonly used agents such as trimethoprim, ampicillin, and a quinolone such as norfloxacin is helpful in recommending initial empirical antibiotic management.

In more severe infections, such as community-acquired pneumonia, prompt empirical therapy is essential. Although the range of possible pathogens is more extensive (Table 12) *Streptococcus pneumoniae* predominates and must always be targeted. Assessment of severity, based on validated criteria, assists in defining the initial empirical antibiotic regimen. This is illustrated by the British Thoracic Society's recommendations for the initial empirical antibiotic management of community acquired pneumonia (Table 13).

The use of empirical therapy depends on the ease with which a clinical diagnosis can be made, disease severity, and toxicity. In the case of herpes-virus infections, the empirical use of aciclovir for the treatment of mucocutaneous herpes simplex infections or of shingles in the elderly is now common. However, it would be inappropriate to start treatment for HIV or CMV infections without laboratory support for these diagnoses in view of the toxicity and cost of the antiviral agents used to treat these infections.

Antibiotic prophylaxis

Antibiotics are used widely in the prevention of infection, in association with surgery and in a range of medical conditions (see above). Antibiotic prophylaxis is used for selected surgical procedures where the risk of infection, although relatively low, is of serious import should it occur. Examples include prosthetic joint implantation and cardiac surgery in which prosthetic valves and intracardiac patches are inserted.

The principles of antibiotic prophylaxis are based on the selection of an agent active against the known potential target pathogen(s). The drug should be present in high concentrations at the site and time of surgery and be relatively free from adverse reactions. One or two doses are generally effective depending on the length of the procedure. No regimen can be effective against all potential pathogens hence the importance of postoperative follow-up.

An important medical indication for the use of prophylactic antibiotics is the prevention of bacterial endocarditis in those with established valvular heart disease undergoing selected dental, urinary tract, or gastrointestinal

Table 10 Summary of major pharmacodynamic differences between aminoglycosides and β-lactams

Pharmacodynamic measurement	Aminoglycosides	β-lactam
Rate of bacterial killing	Rapid and dose related	Slower with little or no increase in higher doses
Number of bacteria killed per dose administered	Concentration-dependent over a wide concentration range	Little increase in degree or rate of killing at concentrations above minimum bactericidal concentration (MBC)
Postantibiotic effect	Concentration-dependent over a wide concentration range for Gram-positive and Gram-negative pathogens	Unpredictable in Gram-negative bacteria, always short (' 3 h) with little or no increase related to concentration
Experimental models	Large, infrequent doses more effective than smaller, more frequent doses which supports once-daily dosing for Gram-negative infections	Frequent (hourly) injection or constant infusion most effective
Clinical trials	High peak serum concentration to *in vitro* minimum inhibitory concentration (MIC) ratio is strongly related to treatment outcome for Gram-negative bacteraemia or pneumonia. Clinical trials with amikacin, gentamicin, and netilmicin have shown single daily dosing to be effective	Limited supportive data in patients with neutropenia or nosocomial pneumonia with dosing regimens that keep serum concentrations above the MIC throughout therapy

Fig. 6 Relationship between the MIC of a drug and its pharmacokinetic profile.

procedures during which transient bacteraemia carries the risk of endo-cardial infection. Here again, the principles governing the selection of the regimen are based on the recognition of the likely target pathogens, their pattern of susceptibility, and the necessity to ensure high bactericidal concentrations of drug at the time of the procedure. In community dental practice, single-dose oral therapy with high-dose amoxicillin/clavulanate (co-amoxiclav) or in those allergic to this agent, clindamycin, are currently recommended. Another example of effective prophylaxis is the use of low-dose suppressive therapy to prevent *Pneumocystic carinii* pneumonia in those with advanced HIV infection. Co-trimoxazole is the preferred agent. Dapsone and inhaled pentamidine are also used.

Anatomical or functional asplenia is associated with a 12.6-fold increased incidence of severe sepsis compared with the general population. This risk is related to the patient's age and, in those splenectomized, the reason for surgery and the period of time that has elapsed. Young children are particularly at risk but this declines substantially after the age of 16 years. Hence the recommendation for prophylactic oral penicillin (ery-thromycin for the intolerant) to prevent fulminant pneumococcal sepsis which predominates. It will not offer protection against other pathogens such as *Escherichia coli* and *Pseudomonas aeruginosa*. Apart from good evidence for the benefit of prophylaxis in children with sickle cell disease, there is poor support for efficacy in splenectomized patients.

There remain, therefore, differences of opinion about the recommendation for the continued use of chemoprophylaxis in adults. Issues of cost, compliance, and drug resistant pathogens add further fuel to the debate. What is clear is that the patient or legal guardian(s) should be educated concerning this risk.

Dose selection

Few antibacterial drugs are specific to a single pathogen, hence the dosage regimen must capture a range of susceptibilities of the various target micro-organisms to ensure a successful response. The dosage regimen is determined initially by pharmacokinetic studies in healthy volunteers. This

is supplemented by information from standardized animal models which simulate infections such as peritonitis, endocarditis, meningitis, thigh abscess, otitis media, pneumonia, and sepsis complicating neutropenia. In man, information on drug penetration into CSF, bile, joint fluid, and cuta-neous blisters can be supplemented by data from biopsy specimens from sites such as tonsils, bronchus, and prostate. The role of pharmacodynamic assessment is of increasing importance in defining dose and predicting out-come as discussed earlier. Despite all this information, the definitive dosage regimen still requires support from large clinical trials in which the endpoints of response are precisely determined.

Bactericidal versus bacteristatic agents

In the treatment of many common community infections which are usually of mild or moderate severity, the choice of either a bacteristatic or bacteri-cidal antibiotic is of limited importance. However, in patients with severe infection, particularly when complicating an immunocompromised state, a bactericidal agent must be used. This applies particularly to those with severe granulocytopenia which is a common accompaniment of cytotoxic chemotherapy, especially in the treatment of haematological malignancies and following bone marrow transplantation. Another important indication for selecting a bactericidal regimen is in the treatment of infective endo-carditis; although the infected vegetations are in the bloodstream, they are relatively protected from host phagocytic control. Effective penetration into the fibrin–platelet mass requires high concentrations of a bactericidal drug to sterilize the infected vegetations.

Duration of treatment

The duration of therapy for many common infections has not been rigor-ously determined. The treatment of many common conditions is based on custom and practice and often varies internationally. The duration of treat-ment has been more thoroughly determined in the following cases:

- Gonococcal urethritis responds promptly to single dose treatment with agents such as ceftriaxone, spectinomycin, or a quinolone antibiotic such as ciprofloxacin or ofloxacin.

- Uncomplicated urinary tract infection, particularly when affecting women of child bearing years, responds promptly to single dose and 3-day treatment regimens with selected agents such as trimethoprim and norfloxacin, although bacteriuria can be eliminated with a single dose, the symptoms of dysuria and frequency take longer to subside, hence a 3-day course is preferred.

- Pharyngitis caused by *Streptococcus pyogenes* improves symptomatic-ally within a few days of antibiotics such as penicillin but eradication of the infecting organism from the throat often takes up to 10 days. It is acknowledged that this presents major difficulties with regard to drug compliance.

- Pulmonary tuberculosis—the current recommendation of 6-months treatment with rifampicin, isoniazid, pyrazinamide, and ethambutol, reducing to isoniazid and rifampicin for a further 4 months provided the isolate is confirmed to be susceptible, is based on extensive clinical trials (Table 4).

Table 11 Pharmacokinetic and pharmacodynamic parameters of some recent quinolone antibacterial drugs

Drug (dose mg)	Protein binding (%)	MIC90 S.pneu-moniae	AUC total (mg/h per l)	AUC free (mg/h per l)	AUIC (total drug)	AUIC (free drug)
Trovafloxacin (200)	78	0.25	34.4	7.6	137.6	30.2
Levofloxacin (500)	25	2.0	72.5	54.4	36.2	27.2
Moxifloxacin (400)	48	0.25	26.9	14.0	107.6	56.0
Gatifloxacin (400)	20	0.5	51.3	41.0	102.6	82

AUC = area under the concentration curve.

MIC = minimum inhibitory concentration active against 90 per cent of isolates tested.

AUIC = AUC/MIC ratio or area under the inhibitory concentration of total and free (unbound) drugs.

Table 12 Microbiological aetiology (%) of adult community-acquired pneumonia in the United Kingdom[a]

Pathogens	Community (n = 236)	Hospital (n = 870)	ICU (n = 185)
S. pneumoniae	36.0	36.1	21.6
H. influenzae	10.2	4.5	3.8
Legionella spp.	0.4	3.7	17.8
Staph. aureus	0.8	2.1	8.7
Enterobacteriaceae	1.3	1.0	1.6
M. pneumoniae	1.3	13.1	2.7
C. psittaci	1.3	2.6	2.2
C. burnetii	0	1.4	0
Viruses	13.1	9.1	9.7
Influenza A and B	8.1	8.1	5.4
Mixed	11.0	10.3	6.0
Other	1.7	2.2	4.9
None	45.3	32.4	32.5

[a]Based on published studies (*Thorax* 2001, in press).

ICU = intensive care unit.

- Bacterial endocarditis—knowledge of the *in vitro* susceptibility of the infecting organism is crucial in determining dose, duration, and outcome of therapy. Highly penicillin-sensitive strains (MIC < 0.1 mg/l) of viridans streptococci are treated effectively with a 2-week regimen of parenteral penicillin which may be supplemented with sequential high-dose oral amoxicillin for a further 2 weeks. Less sensitive strains should be treated with parenteral penicillin and gentamicin for a total of 4 weeks, which is essential if the infecting organism is an enterococcus.

Infections caused by *Staph. aureus* are a particular challenge since the severity is highly variable and yet the potential for metastatic infection and chronicity as in the case of osteomyelitis must be kept in mind. The isoxazolyl penicillins, such as flucloxacillin are preferred with, or without, the addition of fusidic acid. Clindamycin is a useful alternative agent. Many *S. aureus* of the skin and soft tissues respond promptly to 7 to 14 days oral therapy. Where there is a severe systemic response to infection, parenteral therapy is appropriate initially. Where there is evidence of dissemination, treatment should be extended for periods up to 4 weeks.

In the case of septic arthritis, antibiotics should be given promptly and joint aspiration carried out, sometimes repeatedly, to avoid damage to the articular cartilage. The duration of therapy has not been rigorously determined. Most infections will resolve in 2 to 3 weeks. One of the most challenging infections is staphylococcal osteomyelitis. To avoid chronicity, it is customary to treat for 4 to 6 weeks. Treatment is generally administered parenterally. In centres where skill, experience, and administrative support exist, patients are increasingly being managed in the community by parenteral administration through peripherally inserted venous catheters. Under these circumstances, a glycopeptide such as teicoplanin is convenient since it is administered once daily.

For most infections, the duration of therapy remains uncertain. However, many mild to moderate uncomplicated infections will defervesce within a 3 to 5-day period suggesting that 5 to 7-days treatment is usually adequate. There is little evidence to suggest that treatment periods of 7 to 14 days, or longer, are any more effective and are likely to be associated with an increased risk of side-effects, superinfection, and the selection of antibiotic resistant organisms, apart from being more costly.

The parenteral administration of antibiotics is appropriate in the management of severe life-threatening infections and when oral therapy is contraindicated, such as in the postoperative period, if the patient is vomiting, or where gastrointestinal absorption cannot be relied upon. However, the need for continued parenteral therapy should be reviewed regularly. In the treatment of many common infections, the acute features of infection such as temperature, tachycardia, and an elevated circulating neutrophil count usually improve within a period of 48 to 72 h. Provided there is no contra-indication to oral therapy, this should be considered early in the course of patient management. The advantages are not just in the reduced cost of

Table 13 Preferred and alternative initial empirical treatment regimens for community-acquired pneumonia as recommended by the British Thoracic Society

Home-treated, not severe[†]		
Preferred		amoxicillin 500 mg–1.0 g three times daily PO
Alternative[*]		erythromycin[a] 500 mg four times daily PO
Hospital-treated, not severe and ward treated		
Preferred	either oral	amoxicillin 500 mg–1.0 g three times daily PO *plus* erythromycin 500 mg four times daily PO *or* clarithromycin 500 mg twice daily PO
	or if IV needed	ampicillin 500 mg four times daily IV *or* benzylpenicillin (penicillin G) 1.2 g 6-hourly IV
		plus erythromycin 500 mg four times daily IV *or* clarithromycin 500 mg twice daily IV
Alternative[*]	or	levofloxacin 500 mg once daily PO[b]
Hospital-treated, severe and ICU treated		
Preferred		amoxicillin/clavulanate 1.2 g three times daily IV *or* cefuroxime 1.5 g three times daily IV *or* cefotaxime 1 three times daily IV *or* ceftriaxone 2 g once daily IV
		plus erythromycin 500 mg four times daily IV *or* clarithromycin 500 mg twice daily IV ± rifampicin 600 mg once or twice daily IV
Alternative[*]		levofloxacin 500 mg[b] once daily IV or PO *plus* benzylpenicillin 1.2 g 6-hourly IV

[†]Also includes persons admitted for non-clinical reasons and previously untreated in the community.

[*]Alternative regimen is provided for those intolerant of preferred regimen.

[a]Clarithromycin may be substituted for those intolerant of oral erythromycin. IV clarithromycin is preferred to IV erythromycin due to reduced side-effects.

[b]Fluoroquinolones with Gram-positive activity currently include levofloxacin 500 mg once daily, PO or IV and in future may include gatifloxacin, gemifloxacin, and moxifloxacin.

[c]Alternative regimen is provided for those intolerant of preferred regimen.

ICU = intensive care unit; IV = intravenous; PO = oral.

medication. The risk of intravenous line associated complications, such as infection, is also eliminated and discharge from hospital may be hastened.

Adverse drug reactions

Overall, antimicrobial agents have an outstanding record of safety. Nonetheless, no drug is without the potential for side-effects. The risk varies by agent, sometimes dose, while host genetic factors and pathophysiological status can also be important.

Oral antibiotics are largely used in the community where they are generally well tolerated and used in the treatment of minor infections in large populations. Injectable agents selected for short course perioperative prophylaxis have a well established safety record. However, agents such as the antiretroviral drugs and amphotericin B carry a higher risk of more serious adverse drug reactions which must be balanced against the life-threatening nature of their target infections.

While drug safety is assessed during drug development, the full repertoire of adverse reactions becomes apparent only during widespread clinical use, hence, the importance of adverse drug reaction reporting systems. In the United Kingdom, the 'yellow card' system has been very successful and relies on voluntary reporting of possible adverse drug events to the Medicines Control Agency by physicians and, more recently, pharmacists. It is important to distinguish between adverse event reporting and adverse drug reaction reporting. The latter is more difficult to establish with certainty and may require rechallenge which raises medical and ethical concerns.

It is essential to enquire about previous drug reactions as well as other forms of drug toxicities before prescribing. The relationship to a previously prescribed drug requires careful assessment. Hypersensitivity is among the more common of drug reactions and, in the case of β-lactam drugs, appears to be more a function of the five-membered thiazolidine ring (Fig. 7) of the penicillin molecule since hypersensitivity reactions are less common with the cephalosporins which have a six-membered dihydrothiazine ring. The monobactam, aztreonam, has neither ring structure and hypersensitivity reactions appear to be rare. However, it is important to note that accelerated systemic hypersensitivity reactions (anaphylaxis) can be life-threatening such that any previous association with a β-lactam drug is an absolute contraindication to the use of all β-lactams.

Some drug toxicities are genetically determined. For example people who are genetically slow acetylators of isoniazid are more at risk of side-effects such as peripheral neuropathy. Those genetically deficient in the enzyme glucose-6-phosphate dehydrogenase are at risk of drug-induced haemolysis. This risk is more common in those of African, Mediterranean, or Far Eastern descent. Hence, it is important to screen for this red cell enzyme deficiency before the administration of oxidant drugs such as primaquine.

Adverse drug reactions may not always be acute in their presentation but reveal themselves after prolonged drug exposure. Oral flucloxacillin and co-amoxiclav when administered for several weeks, particularly in the elderly, are more likely to induce drug-associated hepatotoxicity. Likewise, parenteral formulations of selected drugs may be more toxic than their oral formulation, as is the case with a fusidic acid where prolonged parenteral administration frequently gives rise to hepatotoxicity.

Concentration-dependent adverse reactions (Table 14) are more likely to occur in the presence of organ system failure. Aminoglycoside toxicity is more common in the elderly, in those with pre-existing renal failure, and after repeated aminoglycoside doses or other nephrotoxic drugs. Concentration-dependent bone marrow suppression characterizes the use of chloramphenicol whereby pancytopenia arises when plasma concentrations are in excess of 25 mg/l. This is to be distinguished from the idiopathic aplastic anaemia that is a rare accompaniment of chloramphenicol use, but unfortunately is rarely reversible.

Much has been learned about the structure activity determinants of drug toxicity. For example the quinolone antibiotics as a class have the potential

to induce phototoxicity, arthrotoxicity, CNS toxicity, cardiotoxicity, and interact with agents such as caffeine, theophylline, and non-steroidal anti-inflammatory drugs (Fig. 8). Knowledge of such predictors has lead to the selection of agents with safer structural profiles. Despite this, adverse drug reactions have led to the withdrawal or modification of the licensed indications for several quinolones, notably temafloxacin, trovafloxacin, sparfloxacin, and grepafloxacin, emphasizing the importance of clinical recognition and reporting of adverse events.

Few infectious conditions require life-long therapy. The management of HIV infection has challenged this tenet. To date, drugs directed at the causative viruses or complicating opportunistic infections are suppressive rather than achieving eradication. It is also important to note that the drugs used in the treatment of HIV and AIDS are often licensed with limited information concerning their long-term safety. The potential for adverse reactions and especially interactions is considerable and requires careful attention to their detection and management. This has become an increasingly important challenge as life expectancy for those with HIV infection improves. It is important to balance drug safety while encouraging compliance and the maintenance of a reasonable state of health.

Failure of antibiotic therapy

Antimicrobial therapy may fail for a number of reasons. The agent selected may be inappropriate for the particular infection and fail to inhibit the

Fig. 7 Chemical structure of the β-lactam antibiotics (penicillins, cephalosporins, and monobactams) identifying the common β-lactam ring component which is subject to hydrolysis by β-lactamases.

target organism, or fail to reach the site of infection in sufficient concentration. For example drugs such as nitrofurantoin and norfloxacin, while achieving high urinary concentrations, fail to deal adequately with parenchymatous infection of the kidney or bacteraemia which may complicate acute pyelonephritis.

The prostate also presents a chemotherapeutic challenge owing to the relatively low pH, of about 6.4, in chronic bacterial prostatis. Drugs which are weak bases, such as trimethoprim either alone or in combination with sulfamethoxazole (co-trimoxazole), are preferred, especially since they are also lipid soluble. Ciprofloxacin has similar characteristics and has also produced favourable results. However, treatment of acute bacterial prostatitis sometimes needs to be prolonged (4–6 weeks and occasionally for longer duration), especially if there is a history of chronic relapsing infection.

The drug may be appropriate, but the dose selected may be inadequate. This may apply to such conditions as unsuspected bacterial endocarditis where high-dose parenteral antibiotic is required. Likewise, the concentration of penicillin required to deal with pneumococcal meningitis greatly exceeds that effective in the treatment of pneumococcal pneumonia; occasionally the two diseases may coexist. Infections caused by *Legionella pneumophila* and *Chlamydia* spp. require drugs that achieve high intracellular concentrations such as the macrolides, tetracyclines, or quinolones.

Resistance emerging during treatment is an uncommon cause of clinical failure but should be considered. Drug resistant *Mycobacterium tuberculosis* can develop on therapy as a result of the emergence of minority populations of organisms resistant to such first-line drugs as rifampicin and isoniazid. The current multidrug regimens are, in part, designed to avoid this occurrence. Likewise, in those with HIV infection, drug resistant virus is an increasingly important cause of treatment failure and requires good compliance with multidrug regimens to slow its rate of emergence.

Mixed infections are commonly associated with intrabdominal sepsis and occasionally with infections of the lung. They may fail to respond to treatment unless the regimen covers the full range of bacterial pathogens. In the case of intrabdominal sepsis, the regimen should be active against anaerobic as well as aerobic bacterial pathogens.

Another important cause of antibiotic failure is the continued presence of a focus of infection. This may be an abscess which requires surgical drainage or the removal of an implanted medical device such as an intravascular catheter. Much more serious is infection of a prosthetic heart valve, hip joint, or CNS shunt where revision surgery carries significant risks. Many antibiotics fail to achieve therapeutic concentrations within abscess cavities, or are pH sensitive. Implant-associated infections present a similar challenge since bacteria often replicate slowly within a biofilm that is protective against normal host defences.

Finally, it should be remembered that a persistently elevated temperature in the presence of what appears to be adequate antibiotic treatment can reflect drug fever or indeed fever complicating a non-microbial diagnosis. This emphasizes the importance of monitoring the response to treatment and repeated patient assessment.

Table 14 Dose-related adverse effects of selected antimicrobials

Drug	Adverse effect	Comment
Antibacterial drugs		
	Superinfection by yeasts or *Clostridium difficile*; selection of drug-resistant bacteria from the normal flora	These are universal adverse effects of antibacterial drugs and are generally related to the duration of exposure
β-Lactams	Myelosuppression	Neutropenia may occur after 1–2 weeks high-dose IV therapy
	Drug fever	Occurs during prolonged (> 1 week), high-dose IV therapy (e.g. endocarditis)
	Central nervous stimulation/ convulsions	Can occur with overdose in renal failure
Aminoglycosides	Nephrotoxicity; ototoxicity	Monitoring of serum concentrations minimizes but does not avoid toxicity
		Risk of toxicity is related to the duration of the dose and concomitant therapy
Vancomycin	Nephrotoxicity; ototoxicity	May potentiate aminoglycoside nephrotoxicity
Macrolides (e.g. erythromycin)	Gastrointestinal stimulation	This is a prokinetic effect of erythromycin which does not occur with all macrolides
	Ototoxicity; cardiac arrhythmias	Only with high-dose IV therapy
	Drug interactions	Increased serum concentrations of theophylline and cyclosporin
Quinolones (e.g. ciprofloxacin)	Central nervous stimulation	Quinolones are weak GABA antagonists; this effect is potentiated by coadministration with NSAIDs, especially fenbufen
	Drug interactions	May inhibit metabolism of theophylline
Antifungal/ antiprotozoal/ antiviral drugs		
Amphotericin B	Nephrotoxicity	Decreased creatinine clearance and renal potassium wasting are universal at clinically effective doses
	Rigors/ hyperthermia/ hypotension	Related to the rate of infusion
Ketoconazole	Inhibition of steroid synthesis	Occurs with prolonged (> 1 week) high-dose therapy
Aciclovir	Central nervous adverse effects; crystalluria	Rare except with high-dose IV therapy
Quinine	Hypoglycaemia	

GABA = γ-aminobutyric acid; NSAID = non-steroidal anti-inflammatory drug.

Fig. 8 Structure:activity side-effect relationships of the fluoroquinolone antibacterial drugs (redrawn after Domagala 1994).

Practice guidelines and formularies

The plethora of therapeutic agents currently available presents a considerable challenge to the prescriber. Guidance on the choice of agent and the management of disease is becoming increasingly important. This is not only to ensure that the selection of treatment is appropriate for the target infection and consistent with current patterns of antimicrobial susceptibility but that it reflects an acceptable safety profile as well as being sensitive to the appropriate use of health-care resources. Such guidance is increasingly provided within formularies designed for local use, either within a hospital or community practice. These frequently offer information on preferred and alternative regimens for particular infections. Formularies should include drugs currently tested by the diagnostic laboratory since changing patterns of susceptibility may require modification of recommended drugs.

Within hospital practice, it is common for such formularies to identify drugs which may be prescribed freely according to specific indications, and those for which expert advice from a clinical microbiologist or infectious disease specialist should be sought. The latter applies particularly to drugs that require specific skill and experience in their use, need drug levels to be monitored, or are expensive. For example the treatment of deep-seated fungal infections with amphotericin B requires careful clinical assessment and guidance on dosage and monitoring. Likewise, the treatment of HIV infection is increasingly a specialist area. Antibiotics which are expensive to prescribe such as parenteral quinolones, third generation cephalosporins, and the carbapenems may be restricted. The policy may also have recommendations for the timing of transfer from parenteral to oral therapy in order to minimize the use of injectable agents.

Formularies are educational and allow the prescriber to become familiar with indications and safety of the most commonly used agents. Their use should be supported by educational activities both at undergraduate and postgraduate level.

Ideally, the selection of agents for inclusion in the formulary should be based on sound evidence of efficacy, safety, and economic benefit. However, such evidence-based medicine is often lacking or incomplete for commonly treated infections, since clinical trials of antibiotics, although increasingly robust in their design, are largely conducted to support licensing requirements rather than to address clinical use. They generally demonstrate the equivalence of a new agent in comparison with existing therapies. As a result, the recommendations of formularies and practice guidelines are based on a matrix of information derived from knowledge of the *in vitro*

profile of an agent, its pharmacokinetic parameters, its clinical and microbiological efficacy, and safety profile. This in turn is modified by custom and practice which explains why there is local and, sometimes, national and international variation in recommendations for some common indications such as community-acquired pneumonia and bacterial meningitis.

In developing countries where medical resources are much more limited, greater reliance is placed on low-cost agents. The World Health Organization regularly updates its list of recommended essential drugs which includes anti-infective agents (Table 15). Despite the emphasis on low cost agents, the drugs offered cover the majority of infections and prescribing needs of developing countries. The agents available in individual countries often vary according to local interpretation of the needs for these 'essential' drugs.

Recent developments in economically advanced countries have included an assessment of health-care technologies for current management, national need, and the resources available. In the United Kingdom, the National Institute of Clinical Excellence (NICE) was established in 1999 to assess a variety of health-care technologies including procedures as well as new therapies. At the time of its initial assessment by NICE, zanamavir, a recently licensed drug effective in the treatment of influenza virus infection, lacked sufficient evidence of efficacy in people known to be at higher risk of

Table 15 The WHO model list of essential drugs (anti-infectives)

Antihelminthics	Antibacterials (cont.)
albendazole	ethambutol
levamisole	isoniazid
mebendazole	isoniazid + ethambutol
niclosamide	pyrazinamide
praziquantel	rifampicin
pyrantel	rifampicin + isoniazid
diethylcarbamazine	rifampicin + isoniazid + pyrazinamide
ivermectin	streptomycin
suramin sodium	thioacetazone + isoniazid
praziquantel	**Antifungals**
triclabendazole	amphotericin
oxamniquine	griseofulvin
Antibacterials	ketoconazole
amoxicillin	**Antivirals**
ampicillin	flucytosine
benzathine	potassium iodide
benzylpenicillin	zidovudine
cloxacillin	**Antiprotozoals**
phenoxymethylpenicillin	diloxanide
procaine benzylpenicillin	metronidazole
amoxicillin + clavulanic acid	meglumine
ceftazidime	pentamidine
ceftriaxone	amphotericin
imipenem + cilastatin	chloroquine
chloramphenicol	primaquine
ciprofloxacin tablet	quinine
doxycycline	doxycycline
erythromycin	mefloquine
gentamicin	sulfadoxine + pyrimethamine
metronidazole	artemether
nalidixic acid	chloroquine
nitrofurantoin	mefloquine
spectinomycin	proguanil
sulfadiazine	pentamidine
sulfamethoxazole + trimethoprim	pyrimethamine
trimethoprim	sulfamethoxazole + trimethoprim
chloramphenicol	melarsoprol
clindamycin	pentamidine
vancomycin	suramin sodium
clofazimine	eflornithine
dapsone	benznidazole
rifampicin	nifurtim

complicated influenza virus infection. Such assessments place greater emphasis on ensuring that new technologies are evaluated in a manner that more closely resembles clinical practice as well as demonstrating economic benefit, in contrast to drug licensing which addresses the quality, safety, and efficacy of new therapies. This new emphasis is likely to require a greater partnership between health-care systems and pharmaceutical companies to ensure that the place of new technologies is not only rapidly assessed but that they are consistent with health-care strategies.

Further reading

Bennett WM, Aronoff GR, Golper TA, Morrison G, Brater DG, Singer I (1994). *Drug prescribing in renal failure: Dosing guidelines for adults*, 3rd edn. American College of Physicians, Philadelphia.

Combined Working Party (1998). Revised guidelines for the control of methicillin-resistant *Staphylococcus aureus* infection in hospitals. *Journal of Hospital Infection* **39**, 253–90.

Davey PG, Parker SE, Malek MM (1993). Pharmacoeconomics of antimicrobial prophylaxis. *Journal of Antimicrobial Chemotherapy* **31** (Suppl. B), 107–18.

Domagala JM (1994). Structure–activity and structure–side-effect relationships for the quinolone antibacterials. *Journal of Antimicrobial Chemotherapy* **33**, 685–706.

Finch RG and Williams RJ (1999). *Bailliére's clinical infectious diseases: antibiotic resistance*. Bailliére Tindall, London.

Joint Tuberculosis Committee of the British Thoracic Society (1998). Chemotherapy and management of tuberculosis: recommendations. *Thorax* **53**, 536–48.

Kerr KG (1999). The prophylaxis of bacterial infections in neutropenic patients. *Journal of Antimicrobial Chemotherapy* **44**, 587–91.

Kucers A, Crowe S, Grayson ML, Hoy J (1997). *The use of antibiotics*, 5th edn. Butterworth Heinemann, Oxford.

Macfarlane J, et al. (2001). The British Thoracic Society Guidelines for the Management of Community Acquired Pneumonia in Adults. *Thorax* (in press).

O'Grady FW, Lambert HP, Finch RG, Greenwood D (1997). *Antibiotic and chemotherapy*, 7th edn. Churchill Livingstone, Edinburgh.

Raviglione MR, Snider DE, Kochi A (1995). Global epidemiology of tuberculosis—morbidity and mortality of a world-wide epidemic. *Journal of the American Medical Association* **273**, 220–6.

Read RC and Finch RG (1994). Prophylaxis after splenectomy. *Journal of Antimicrobial Chemotherapy* **33**, 4–6.

Russell AD and Chopra I (1996). *Understanding antibacterial action and resistance*, 2nd edn. Ellis Horwood, London.

Shyrock TR, Mortensen JE, Baumholtz M (1998). The effects of macrolides on the expression of bacterial virulence mechanisms. *Journal of Antimicrobial Chemotherapy* **41** 505–12.

Simmons NA (1993). Recommendations for endocarditis prophylaxis. *Journal of Antimicrobial Chemotherapy* **31**, 437–8.

Standing Medical Advisory Committee Subgroup on Antimicrobial Resistance (1998). *The path of least resistance*. Department of Health, London.

Wenzel RP and Edmond MB (1998). Vancomycin-resistant *Staphylococcus aureus*: infection control considerations. *Clinical Infectious Diseases* **27**, 245–51.

White NJ (1992). Antimalarial pharmacokinetics and treatment regimens. *British Journal of Clinical Pharmacology* **34**,1–10.

Wise R and Honeybourne D (1999). Pharmacokinetics and pharmacodynamics of fluoroquinolones in the respiratory tract. *European Respiraatory Journal* **14**, 221–9.

7.7 Immunization

D. Goldblatt and M. Ramsay

Introduction

Infectious diseases remain a major cause of mortality and morbidity worldwide. The prevention of certain infectious diseases by effective immunization programmes represented one of the major triumphs of twentieth-century medicine. Most of this was achieved in the final third of that century during which rapid strides in the understanding of the biology and causality of infectious agents and improved techniques for the purification of infectious agents or their components led to the development of safe and effective vaccines. The greatest triumph in the field of immunization was the eradication of smallpox. In 1959 the World Health Organization (**WHO**) declared its intention to eradicate smallpox, and in 1966 began to allocate sufficient resources to accomplish this ambitious goal. Thirteen years later, in 1979, the global eradication of smallpox was officially declared. Effective vaccines can eliminate infectious diseases, but to do this they must be implemented and used appropriately. Over 12 million children under the age of 5 years die annually. Two million of these deaths are from diseases that could be prevented by vaccines already available through the WHO's Expanded Programme of Immunization (**EPI**). While rapid advances in vaccine science have introduced new techniques such as DNA vaccines, delivering vaccines to those most at risk must remain a priority.

Immunology of active immunization

Both non-specific (innate) and specific adaptive immune systems are responsible for protecting humans against infectious diseases. The ability of the adaptive immune system to refine its antigen recognition domains and establish immunological memory is the basis of successful active immunization. The specific immune system contains both cellular and humoral elements whose relative importance differs depending on the nature of the infecting organism. Cell-mediated immune responses depend on T lymphocytes and their secreted factors derived from the thymus, while humoral responses involve B lymphocytes derived from the bone marrow which produce antibodies (immunoglobulins IgG, IgM, IgA, IgD, or IgE).

Cellular responses are induced when antigen-presenting cells, such as dendritic cells, present antigens to T cells. T cells do not respond to soluble, unmodified antigens but only recognize peptide antigens in association with self major histocompatability complex (**MHC**) molecules. Two major forms of MHC molecules exist. The majority of nucleated cells express MHC class I molecules, which stimulate a subset of T cells expressing the CD8 differentiation antigen. These T cells recognize and lyse infected target cells, hence their designation as cytotoxic T lymphocytes. In contrast, MHC class II molecules are expressed on cells that participate in the immune response, and are recognized via a subset of T cells expressing the CD4 differentiation antigen. A major role of such T cells is to augment the immune response and so they are known as T helper cells. At least two subsets of T helper cells have been described: T helper 1 cells are involved in cytotoxic and delayed hypersensitivity type responses, while T helper 2 cells support antibody production.

Immunoglobulin receptors on the surface of B cells are able to recognize soluble antigens and so initiate the process of B-cell activation and differentiation. During differentiation, naïve B cells become antibody secreting plasma cells. In addition, there is endocytosis of antigen bound to surface immunoglobulin, and processed antigen in the form of small peptides is re-expressed on the surface of the B cell in the context of MHC class II molecules. Thus B cells act as antigen-presenting cells and recruit T-cell help. The signals and soluble factors that result from such T-cell help drive the B-cell process of affinity maturation and memory formation. This takes place in the germinal centres of lymph nodes where there is intimate contact between B cells, T cells, and dendritic cells. It is here that memory B cells are formed and then migrate to the bone marrow, spleen, and the submucosa of the respiratory tract and gut. On re-encounter with antigen, memory B cells undergo rapid activation and differentiation into plasma cells and secrete large amounts of switched, high-affinity antibody.

Thus, the ideal vaccine antigen will lead to the activation, replication, and differentiation of T and B lymphocytes. Ideally, the antigen will persist, conformationally intact, in lymphoid tissue to allow the continuing production of cells that secrete antibody of high affinity and the generation of memory cells.

Vaccine antigens

The ideal vaccine antigen is safe with minimal side-effects, promotes effective resistance to the disease (although it does not necessarily prevent infection), and promotes immunity that is lifelong. It needs to be stable and remain potent during storage and shipping and also has to be affordable to allow widespread use. Most currently licensed vaccines contain live or killed bacterial or viral constituents, bacterial polysaccharides, or bacterial toxoids (Table 1).

Live vaccines are ideal for certain diseases as replication in the body mimics natural infection thereby inducing appropriate and site-specific immunity. Live vaccines must be attenuated to produce the beneficial effects of inducing immunity without the danger of clinical disease. Some live vaccines may be spread from person to person and thus enhance herd immunity although such spread may endanger immunocompromised individuals in whom live vaccines should be avoided. Live vaccines are inherently less stable than killed vaccines and the possibility of reversion of vaccine virus to wild type exists (as in polio). Killed vaccines do not carry the risk associated with person-to-person spread and are inherently more stable, but often require two or three doses to induce optimal immunity, especially when used in the first year of life.

New developments in vaccine antigens

Developments in molecular biology have begun to revolutionize the field of vaccine science and provide a glimpse of the future when traditional reliance on live attenuated viral vaccines or purified bacterial or viral products as vaccine antigens may be reduced. The first licensed vaccine to contain

Table 1 Currently licensed vaccines for use in humans

Vaccine type	Live vaccines	Killed vaccines
Viral	Rubella	Poliomyelitis (Salk)
	Measles	Influenza
	Poliomyelitis (Sabin)	Rabies (Human diploid cell)
	Yellow fever	Hepatitis A
	Mumps	Hepatitis B
	Varicella zoster	Japanese encephalitis
	Rotavirus	
	Japanese encephalitis	
Bacterial	BCG	Cholera
	Typhoid	Typhoid
	Cholera	Pertussis
		Borrelia burgdorferi
		Anthrax
		Plague
Bacterial polysaccharides		*Haemophilus influenzae* type b
		Neisseria meningitidis group A and C
		Streptococcus pneumoniae
Rickettsial		Typhus
Bacterial toxoid		Diphtheria
		Tetanus

recombinant genetic material was the hepatitis B vaccine. Despite the licensing of highly effective plasma-derived hepatitis B vaccines in the early 1980s, fears about safety and their high cost led to the search for other hepatitis B vaccines. Several vaccine manufacturers used recombinant DNA technology to express hepatitis B surface antigen in other organisms, which has led to the development of new vaccines.

Recent developments have focused on the use of DNA as a vaccine antigen. The utility of naked DNA as a vaccine antigen was discovered by chance in 1989 during a gene therapy experiment when it was shown that a gene inserted directly into a mammalian cell could induce the cell to manufacture (express) the protein encoded by that gene. In early experiments, DNA was injected directly into muscle and the resulting immune response was measured (see Fig. 1).

DNA vaccines can induce protective immunity in animals to a variety of pathogens, but data in humans are limited. As DNA has the theoretical potential to be incorporated into the host genetic makeup and subvert the genetic working of cells, safety concerns have delayed studies in humans. Phase I studies, however, have assessed DNA vaccines designed to protect against hepatitis B, herpes simplex type 1 and 2, HIV, influenza, and malaria. So far clinical trials have proved disappointing, either because the level of the response was inadequate or because excessive doses of DNA were required to achieve an adequate response. To improve the response to DNA vaccines, a number of newer techniques have been developed. These include:

1. Incorporation of DNA into microprojectiles that are then shot into the target cell via the skin (the so-called 'gene gun' technique).

2. The coating of DNA with cationic lipids or other material that neutralizes its charge; the lipids facilitate cellular uptake and membrane transfer.

3. Delivery of DNA by incorporating it into a viral delivery system using disabled viruses.

4. Delivery of DNA by incorporation into a bacterial delivery system such as attenuated *Salmonella typhimurium*.

5. Delivery of DNA together with traditional adjuvants such as alum.

6. Improving immunogenicity by including a cytokine gene in the plasmid, adjacent to the gene encoding the protective antigen. Local expression of the appropriate cytokine (for example granulocyte–macrophage colony stimulating factor) may augment the immune response in a fashion similar to that seen with adjuvants.

7. Combination of 'priming' immunization with DNA vaccine with subsequent 'boost' with recombinant vaccine.

The huge potential of DNA vaccines, which offer the promise of cheap and stable vaccines that do not require a cold chain for distribution, will stimulate further development of these exciting products.

New developments in vaccine delivery

Research into different routes of vaccine delivery has been driven by the limitations of the parenteral route. These include the difficulty associated with the use of live viral vaccines in the first 6 to 9 months of life (due to the neutralizing effect of passively transferred maternal antibody) and the difficulty and expense of delivering mass immunization by injection. Mucosal delivery of vaccine via the intranasal route has been studied for a number of antigens including measles, influenza, rubella, varicella, and *Streptococcus pneumoniae*. The induction of local immunity for pathogens that either enter the body via the nasopharynx (measles, influenza) or are commonly carried in the nasopharynx (*S. pneumoniae*) is attractive.

Edible vaccines are attracting increasing attention, providing as they do both a means of antigen production and delivery. Studies in animals and

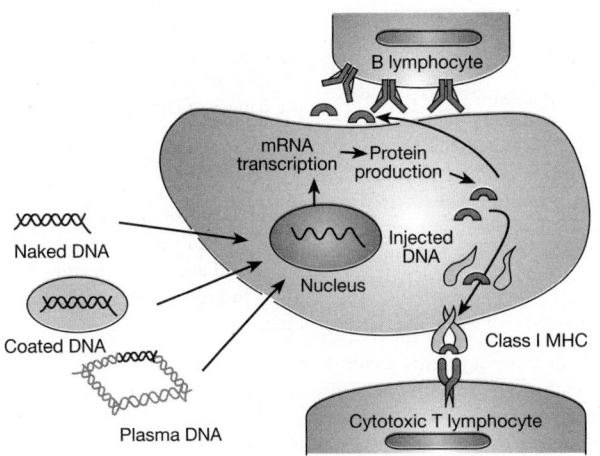

Fig. 1 Injection of DNA encoding a foreign protein can elicit antibodies and a cytotoxic T-lymphocyte response.

Phase I studies in humans have demonstrated their potential. Mice fed with potatoes expressing a non-toxic fragment of the cholera toxin developed mucosal antibodies to the toxin which reduced diarrhoea on challenge with whole cholera toxin. Humans fed raw potatoes expressing the B subunit of enterotoxigenic *Escherichia coli* also showed mucosal immune responses and an increase in neutralizing antibody levels. There are some problems with stability, but edible vaccines are a potentially simple and convenient method of vaccine delivery on a wide scale.

The aim of immunization programmes

Once a vaccine has been developed and shown to be effective it can be used in different ways. Many vaccines are used selectively in groups of the population who are at increased risk of infection (for example because of occupation or travel) or of the severe consequences of the disease that results from infection (because of an underlying medical condition for example). Other vaccines are employed for mass immunization targetting the whole population. Mass immunization can aim to eradicate, eliminate, or to control an infectious disease. Eradication, the state where a disease and its causal agent have been removed from the natural environment, has been achieved only for smallpox. Once eradication has been certified, mass immunization programmes can cease and resources can be transferred to other programmes.

The next target for the WHO is the global eradication of poliomyelitis. Characteristics that favour eradication are the absence of an animal host, the absence of a carrier state, and lifelong protection from vaccination. Poliovirus infection has now been eliminated from the Pan American and Western Pacific WHO Regions although there was a recent resurgence in Haiti. In recently endemic countries, wild poliovirus transmission has been interrupted by a series of National Immunization Days—where live attenuated polio vaccine is delivered to a high proportion of the childhood population on a single day. In 1997, almost 450 million children under 5 years of age were immunized during National Immunization Days. In addition to the resources within each country, this effort has required massive financial support from international donors. Between 1988 and 1998, the number of reported cases of polio worldwide had fallen from 35 251 to 3228 and only three major foci of transmission remain—South Asia and West and Central Africa.

For some infections, eradication by immunization is not possible. A good example is tetanus where the agent is distributed widely in the environment. For these programmes, the aim is to control infection to the point where it no longer constitutes a public health burden. To maintain control, immunization will need to be continued indefinitely.

For diseases that are transmitted from person to person, a good immunization programme provides protection by conferring both individual and herd immunity. For many vaccines, herd immunity can be achieved by vaccinating a high proportion of the childhood population—older individuals are generally immune from previous natural infection. If such a situation can be sustained, transmission of the infection may be interrupted and elimination or eradication becomes possible. If vaccine coverage or efficacy is suboptimal, however, then, in the absence of natural transmission, the number of susceptible people will gradually increase. Eventually the proportion of susceptible people (those who did not receive vaccine or who failed to respond to it) may reach a level sufficient to support an epidemic. Although the size of these epidemics may be small by prevaccine standards, the average age of those infected will be higher than in the prevaccine era. For infections that have more severe consequences in older individuals the morbidity associated with such outbreaks can be substantial. A tragic example of this has been recently observed in Greece where mass vaccination with rubella in childhood has been recommended since 1975. Implementation was poor, however, and during the 1980s coverage was below 50 per cent. The low level of coverage, however, was sufficient to interrupt transmission for several years. By the time rubella infection recurred in 1993, a high proportion of pregnant women were susceptible to rubella and an epidemic of congenital rubella syndrome occurred.

Table 2 Immunization schedule for infants recommended by the WHO EPI

Age	Vaccines	Hepatitis B‡	
		Scheme A	Scheme B
Birth	BCG, OPV	HB1	
6 weeks	DTP1, OPV1	HB2	HB1
10 weeks	DTP2, OPV2		HB2
14 weeks	DTP3, OPV3	HB3	HB3
9 months	Measles		
	Yellow fever†		

Abbreviations: OPV = oral polio vaccine; DTP = diphtheria, tetanus, pertussis; HB = hepatitis B.

†In countries where yellow fever poses a risk.

‡Scheme A is recommended where perinatal transmission is frequent (for example in Southeast Asia). Scheme B may be used where perinatal transmission is less frequent (for example in sub-Saharan Africa).

The Expanded Programme of Immunization

In 1974, the WHO, in recognition of the major contribution of vaccines to public health, launched the EPI. At the start of the programme fewer than 5 per cent of the world's infants were immunized against the six target diseases—diphtheria, tetanus, whooping cough, polio, measles, and tuberculosis. Between 1990 and 1997, around 80 per cent of the 130 million children born each year were immunized by their first birthday—preventing around 3 million deaths each year. Each year, over 500 million immunization contacts occur with children and these have provided an opportunity for the delivery of other primary health care interventions.

During the 1990s, EPI has added immunization against yellow fever and hepatitis B to its target (see Table 2) The introduction of these vaccines, however, has been less impressive, particularly in those poorest countries in greatest need. Of 33 African countries at risk of yellow fever, only 17 have included the vaccine in the childhood schedule. By 1998, hepatitis B vaccine had been incorporated into the national programmes of 90 countries, but it is estimated that 70 per cent of the world's hepatitis B carriers live in countries without programmes. The major barrier to using new vaccines in the developing world is likely to be sustainable funding.

Delivery of immunization programmes

For mass immunization to achieve its aims, high and uniform coverage of immunization must be reached and sustained. Coverage of immunization is associated with a variety of factors including sociodemographic characteristics of the population, organization of health services, knowledge among health professionals, and parental attitudes.

Sociodemographic factors that may influence vaccine coverage include deprivation, maternal education, and family size. Centrally co-ordinated health services with few barriers to access and standard record systems with facilities for call and recall are likely to achieve higher vaccine coverage. Health professionals with accurate knowledge of the indications and true contraindications to immunization are important. Excessive lists of contraindications for DTP immunization in the newly independent states of the former USSR contributed to a massive resurgence of diphtheria in the early 1990s. The number of cases rose from 2000 in 1990 to over 47 000 in 1994; 2500 deaths from diphtheria occurred between 1990 and 1995.

Whether or not parents decide to have their children vaccinated depends on their perceptions of the severity of the disease and of the safety and effectiveness of the vaccine. Knowledge of parental perceptions can be used successfully to target health promotion campaigns. When coverage is high, the incidence of vaccine preventable disease declines and parental perception of the severity of that disease may decrease. In this situation, concerns about the safety of vaccine become paramount and can lead to a decline in

Fig. 2 Whooping cough cases and vaccine coverage in England and Wales between 1940 and 1998.

vaccine coverage. Such a situation arose in the United Kingdom in the early 1970s when concern about the safety of pertussis vaccine led to a fall in vaccine coverage. This resulted in resurgence of disease with consequent mortality and morbidity (see Fig. 2). Over the next decade, vaccine coverage improved again and the incidence of disease fell to the lowest levels ever.

A more recent example of where largely unsubstantiated concerns about vaccine safety have damaged the success of a vaccination programme have occurred in France. Anecdotal reports of multiple sclerosis following hepatitis B vaccine produced a fall in vaccine coverage in France. Although the number of reports were in line with expected numbers, in October 1998, the French Ministry of Health decided to suspend the schools programme but to continue immunization in general practice. Three case–control studies failed to confirm the link and it is clear that the risk of hepatitis B infection always outweighs the potential risk of adverse events. The WHO and the national committees of several neighbouring countries have reviewed the data and concluded that there is no evidence of a causal association. Despite this, coverage of hepatitis B vaccine has continued to fall in France and in French-speaking Belgium.

In the United Kingdom, speculation that the combined measles–mumps–rubella (**MMR**) vaccine produced bowel problems which in turn could result in autism was published in *The Lancet* in February 1998. This anxiety was based upon a case-series of only 12 patients and the validity of the study was questioned in an accompanying editorial. Subsequent population-based studies of children with autism in the United Kingdom have failed to demonstrate a link with measles-containing vaccines - a finding which is supported by data from Finland. Despite the lack of scientific evidence, a majority of mothers in the United Kingdom now believe the MMR vaccine to be unsafe. This, together with a low proportion of mothers who believe that measles is a severe disease, has resulted in a small but sustained fall in MMR vaccine coverage in the United Kingdom.

Evaluation of immunization programmes

Evaluation of an immunization programme may include the measurement of vaccine coverage, surveillance of disease incidence, assessment of prevalence of immunity, and the monitoring of adverse events.

Vaccine coverage

Timely measurement is important for monitoring trends in vaccine coverage and to identify pockets of low coverage. Low coverage may be apparent before any increase in disease incidence is observed. Since the late 1970s, three outbreaks of poliomyelitis have been observed amongst groups with religious objection to immunization in The Netherlands. Despite national coverage of 96 per cent for MMR vaccine, the same group has recently been the focus of a large epidemic of measles. Between April and December 1999, 1750 cases of measles occurred in The Netherlands compared with only nine in the whole of 1998.

Disease surveillance

Once an immunization programme has been implemented, disease incidence data can be used to monitor the effectiveness of that strategy. For example, the dramatic decline in the incidence of invasive *Haemophilus influenzae* infection described in both The Netherlands and the United Kingdom can be used to demonstrate the impact of conjugate vaccination. The age distribution of infection may change as children above or below the target age will form an increasing proportion of those infected. Various epidemiological methods, including case–control studies, cohort studies, and the screening method, can be used to estimate the efficacy of the vaccine in the field.

Seroprevalence studies

Seroprevalence studies are used to assess population immunity to infection. Such immunity results either from immunization or from natural infection. This can detect groups including a high proportion of susceptible individuals who may be the focus of future outbreaks. In 1991, seroprevalence studies in the United Kingdom identified that a large proportion of school-age children was susceptible to measles and therefore that an epidemic of measles was likely. A large campaign was mounted to immunize children from 5 to 16 years of age in November 1994. The number of cases of measles fell rapidly and remained at low levels over the next 5 years.

Adverse events

Monitoring of adverse events is important in maintaining public confidence in an immunization programme and for detecting rare events that could not be identified before licensing the vaccine. The detection of such events may lead to the withdrawal of certain vaccines. In August 1998, rotavirus vaccine was licensed for use in the United States and recommended for mass immunization of infants. During prelicensing studies, five cases of intussusception had been reported in around 10 000 recipients, compared with only 1 in almost 5000 controls; this difference was not statistically significant. During postlicensing surveillance, however, 15 cases were reported to the Vaccine Adverse Event Reporting System. On 22 October 1999, a review of scientific data concluded that there was an increased frequency of intussusception in the 1 to 2 weeks after vaccination which led to withdrawal of the vaccine in the United States.

Further reading

Chen RT (1999). Vaccine risks: real, perceived and unknown. *Vaccine* **17**, S41–S46.

Czerkinsky C *et al.* (1999). Mucosal immunity and tolerance: relevance to vaccine development. *Immunological Reviews* **170**, 197–222.

Leitner WW, Ying H, Restifo NP (1999). DNA and RNA-based vaccines: principles, progress and prospects. *Vaccine* **18**, 765–77.

Orenstein WA, Bernier RH, Hinman AR (1988). Assessing vaccine efficacy in the field. Further observations. *Epidemiologic Reviews* **10**, 212–41.

Tacket CO *et al.* (1998). Immunogenicity in humans of a recombinant bacterial antigen delivered in a transgenic potato. *Nature Medicine* **4**, 607–9.

World Health Organization and the United Nations Children's Fund (1996). *State of the world's vaccines and immunization*. WHO, Geneva.

World Health Organization (1997). *Polio. The beginning of the end*. WHO, Geneva.

7.8 Travel and expedition medicine

C. P. Conlon and D. A. Warrell

United Kingdom citizens make 56 million visits abroad each year, 8 per cent of these to developing countries which carry a higher risk of illness (600-fold risk in Mexico, 1835-fold in the Indian subcontinent) than travel to continental Europe (for example, to France).

Pretravel advice

This can be obtained from medical practitioners interested in travel medicine, embassies of the countries to be visited, travel agencies, organizations, specialist travel clinics, and the internet (see below). Members of immigrant communities in Western countries, especially from the Indian subcontinent and West Africa, are vulnerable to endemic diseases, including malaria and typhoid, when they return on holiday to their country of origin, perhaps to visit their families. This group of travellers is less likely to receive good pretravel advice and perhaps less willing to seek or accept it. A certificate of vaccination against yellow fever may be needed for entry to some countries. Details of other immunizations, allergies, blood group, and regular medications should also be carried by the traveller. Adequate insurance is essential. The geographical area to be visited, the age and health of the traveller, and any special risks of the journey (for example, mountain climbing) are taken into account. In remote areas or those with inadequate health facilities the travel insurance policy must cover repatriation.

General advice about health

The basic first-aid kit should include: a topical antiseptic solution; bandages; plasters; proprietary drugs for pain relief, diarrhoea, dyspepsia, allergy, and itch; sunscreen preparations; water purification tablets; and insect repellents.

For motion sickness, antiemetic drugs such as cyclizine are effective, but they may cause sedation and a dry mouth. Long-acting transdermal skin patches containing scopolamine are preferable. Long-haul air flights lead to jet lag: sleep disturbance, fatigue, a feeling of light-headedness and unreality, and poor concentration. These symptoms may be attributable to a 'hangover' if excessive alcohol has been drunk on the flight! A short-acting benzodiazepine, such as temazepam, taken for the first couple of nights after flying, helps to re-establish a regular sleeping pattern. Some travellers have found that melatonin is helpful (Chapter 12.13), but a recent trial demonstrated no efficacy for this product. People with diabetes may need advice on adjusting their insulin regimen or diet for changes in time zones.

Climatic and environmental extremes

At high altitudes, snow blindness and severe sunburn can occur under clear skies even at very low ambient temperatures. Those going to high altitudes should acclimatize slowly and build up their level of physical activity gradually (see Chapter 8.5.4). They should be aware of the symptoms and signs of altitude sickness. Acetazolamide ('Diamox'), in an adult dose of 250 mg twice a day, starting 12 h before starting the ascent, is effective prophylaxis for mild mountain sickness, especially if the traveller has to ascend rapidly (e.g. flying from sea level to more than 3000 m). But gradual ascent, allowing acclimatization is preferable and, if severe symptoms develop, there is no substitute for rapid descent. In the tropics, heat, dehydration, and salt depletion may cause problems. Several days of relative inactivity are needed to acclimatize safely to hot climates.

Strict food and water hygiene are important in countries with relatively poor sanitation. 'Boil it, peel it, or forget it'; is a useful adage for the traveller. Water purification tablets and many types of portable water filters are available. Beverages made with boiled water are generally safe, whereas bottled water and, particularly, ice cubes are unreliable. Treated water should be used even for tooth cleaning.

In many developing countries, blood-borne pathogens, such as hepatitis B and C viruses, human immunodeficiency virus (**HIV**), human T-cell leukaemia/lymphoma virus type 1 (HTLV-1), and, in some areas, malaria, trypanosomiasis, and other infections are prevalent. Screening of donated blood may not be rigorous and needles are commonly reused, sometimes without adequate sterilization. As a result, travellers have been advised to take 'AIDS kits', usually containing needles, cannulas, intravenous giving sets, syringes, and artificial plasma expanders. These are too bulky and expensive for most travellers, but it is worth taking a few 21-gauge needles and 10-ml syringes in case blood must be taken for a laboratory test or an injectable drug is needed. A covering letter from a doctor may allay the suspicion of customs officials that they are to be used for drug abuse.

Travellers seem to become unusually disinhibited and foolish and are particularly likely to engage in promiscuous unprotected sexual activity, especially if they are taking alcohol or other recreational drugs. Since sexually transmitted diseases, including HIV, are highly prevalent in many holiday resorts (not only in prostitutes), good-quality condoms, often not available when travelling, should be carried and used.

Patients with chronic illnesses, such as diabetes or asthma, should take plenty of their current medications as these may not be available abroad. It is a good idea to carry separate supplies in case of luggage loss or theft.

Immunizations

The record of routine childhood immunizations should be reviewed. Many adults will require booster doses for tetanus, polio, and diphtheria.

Yellow fever is only endemic in tropical Africa and South America, not in Asia. Recently, a Belgian tourist acquired fatal yellow fever in The Gambia, emphasizing the continuing importance of this immunization. Cholera vaccine is no longer recommended by the World Health Organization as its adverse effects outweigh its usefulness, but a new oral vaccine is promising. Other immunizations may be recommended after considering the travel itinerary and risk of exposure (Table 1).

The risk of hepatitis A in developing countries ranges from 300 to 2000/100 000 unprotected travellers per month of stay. Active immunization is safe, effective, and durable (see Chapter 7.10.19).

In the 'meningitis belt' of sub-Sahelian Africa, from Senegal east to the Sudan, and in some other areas, dry season meningococcal meningitis outbreaks are so common that immunization is recommended.

Pre-exposure rabies vaccination is being used increasingly. Although the risk of transmission is fairly low, the lack of effective treatment for rabies encephalitis and the fear engendered by a dog bite justifies considering immunization.

Plague vaccine is effective but may give rise to serious side-effects. An alternative in endemic areas is prophylactic or postexposure doxycycline treatment (see Chapter 7.11.16). Anthrax is endemic in many tropical countries, but, despite anxieties raised by its use for bioterrorism in the United States, vaccination or chemoprophylaxis are unnecessary. Japanese (B) encephalitis vaccine is safe and there is a risk of infection in many parts of Asia (see Chapter 24.14.2). Hepatitis B is a risk for medical staff, whose work involves contact with human blood and to those receiving unscreened blood transfusions in some developing countries (see Chapter 7.10.19). It is also a risk of unprotected sexual activity.

Prevention of malaria

Both travellers and non-specialist physicians must be educated about the prevention and recognition of malaria (see Chapter 7.14.2).

Travellers' diarrhoea (Table 2)

This is the most common health problem of travellers. Symptoms are usually mild, lasting only about 3 to 5 days, but holiday and business plans may be disrupted. The most common cause is enterotoxigenic *Escherichia coli* (**ETEC**). *Salmonella* spp., *Campylobacter* spp., *Shigella* spp., and other pathogenic *E. coli* are also common. Protozoan pathogens, such as *Giardia lamblia*, *Entamoeba histolytica*, *Cryptosporidium parvum*, and viruses are less common causes. Fish and shellfish poisoning cause similar symptoms starting within minutes or hours of exposure.

Table 1 Immunizations

Vaccine	Type	Route[1]	Primary course	Booster
Routine				
Diphtheria	Adsorbed toxoid	IM/SC	3 doses at monthly intervals	Single low dose if under 10 years old
Polio (Sabin)	Live virus (attenuated)	PO	3 doses at monthly intervals	10 years
Polio (Salk)	Killed virus	IM/SC	As above	10 years
Tetanus	Adsorbed toxoid	IM/SC	3 doses at monthly intervals	10 years (maximum 5 doses)
Haemophilus influenzae b	Conjugated polysaccharide	IM	2–3 doses, every 2 months	Single dose
Influenza	Killed virus	IM	Single dose	Yearly
Pneumococcal	23-valent polysaccharide	IM/SC	Single dose	Repeat in those at high risk
Travel				
Hepatitis A[2] (Havrix Monodose)	Killed virus	IM	2 doses 2–4 weeks apart	6–12 months, then every 3 years
Hepatitis B	Adsorbed	IM[3]	0, 1, and 6 months	Single booster at 5 years
Japanese (B) encephalitis (JE Vax Aventis-Pasteur; Jap B encV Korea)	Killed virus	SC	3 doses on days 0, 7, and 28	1 year, then every 4 years
Meningococcal	Polysaccharide types A, C, (Y, W)	IM or SC	Single dose	Every 3 years
Rabies	Killed virus	IM or ID[4] (1/10 dose)	3 doses on days 0, 7, and 28	Every 2–3 years
Tick-borne encephalitis	'Encepur' (Chiron)	IM	0 and 4 weeks, then at 9–12 months	Every 3 years
Tuberculosis: BCG	Attenuated	ID	Single dose	None
Typhoid	Killed bacteria	IM	2 doses a month apart	Every 3 years
Typhoid	Live Ty21a strain (attenuated)	PO	3 doses on alternate days	Every 5 years
Typhoid[2]	Capsular Vi polysaccharide	IM	Single dose	Every 3 years
Yellow fever	Live virus (attenuated)	SC	Single dose	Every 10 years

[1]PO, oral; IM, intramuscular; SC, subcutaneous; ID, intradermal

[2]Combined HepA and typhoid vaccines are available.

[3]Should not be given into buttock; deltoid or anterior thigh preferred. Double the dose for immunocompromised patients or those on dialysis.

[4]Efficacy reduced if given with chloroquine antimalarial prophylaxis.

Table 2 Travellers's diarrhoea: some causes

Aeromonas, Plesiomonas
Enterotoxigenic *E. coli* (ETEC) ~50%
Campylobacter jejuni
Cryptosporidium parvum
Cyclospora cayetanensis
Entamoeba histolytica
Rotavirus/Norwalk virus
Salmonella spp.
Shigella spp.
Schistosoma mansoni
Strongyloides stercoralis
Vibrio parahaemolyticus

(*Plasmodium falciparum, S. typhi*, irritable and inflammatory bowel disease, tropical sprue, drug side-effects,
Clostridium difficile toxin, fish/shellfish toxins)

Strict food and water hygiene reduces the risk of gastroenteritis. Heating water to 100 °C will kill most pathogens, as will chemical treatment with chlorine or iodine (iodine is contraindicated in pregnant women and some patients with thyroid disease). Water filters are useful additions. Antimicrobials such as co-trimoxazole, doxycycline, and the 4-fluoroquinolones are protective to some extent but are not cheap, may cause side-effects, cannot be taken for prolonged periods, and may encourage antimicrobial resistance. Colloidal bismuth salts are cheaper, safer, and reasonably effective, but the large volumes are inconvenient. An effective vaccine against ETEC may soon be available.

Treatment is by maintaining an adequate fluid intake and using sachets of oral rehydration salts that can be made up with boiled water. Eating solid food may stimulate bowel action by the gastrocolic reflex. Antidiarrhoeal agents, such as codeine phosphate, imodium, or loperamide, often relieve symptoms sufficiently for normal activities to be continued. Short courses of empirical antimicrobials, for example ciprofloxacin (500 mg for 3 days, adults only), can be useful, particularly for patients with underlying diseases. Localized abdominal pain or bloody diarrhoea are indications for seeking medical help immediately.

Immunocompromised travellers

Except for asplenic patients, immunocompromised travellers—including those who have received radiotherapy for lymphomas—should not be given live vaccines such as yellow fever, oral polio, and oral typhoid. Killed or synthetic vaccines are safe. Those patients with mild to moderate immune suppression, including those with early HIV infection, will probably make a reasonable response to immunization; those with more severe immunosuppression may still make a useful, though less durable, response. Influenza, pneumococcal, and *Haemophilus influenzae* b (**Hib**) conjugate vaccines are recommended, as the risk of respiratory infection and bacteraemia is increased. Gammaglobulin is the preferred prophylaxis against hepatitis A in these patients, as the response to hepatitis A vaccine may be unreliable. Asplenic individuals should be on prophylactic antibiotics, such as amoxicillin, particularly if travelling, and should be dissuaded from travelling to areas with high rates of malaria transmission.

Immunocompromised patients should carry antimicrobials with them for treating respiratory or gastrointestinal infections, should seek medical help when abroad, and should carry a letter from their physician outlining their condition and medication.

Pregnant travellers

Commercial airlines will not normally convey a woman who is 36 weeks or more pregnant without a covering letter from her physician. Insurance to cover the costs of delivery abroad should be considered.

The risk–benefit assessment of immunizations and chemoprophylaxis is of particular importance for the pregnant woman and the fetus. Live vaccines should be avoided, but if there is a genuine risk of yellow fever the vaccine should be given as there is no recognized associated teratogenicity. Inactivated polio vaccine may be given parenterally and tetanus immunization is safe. Heat-killed typhoid vaccine is best avoided as it might cause a febrile reaction, stimulating premature labour. However, the modern polysaccharide capsular Vi vaccine should be safe. Pneumococcal, meningococcal, and hepatitis B vaccines are safe in pregnancy, as is gammaglobulin.

Malaria is specially dangerous in pregnant women (see Chapter 7.14.2). Chloroquine and proguanil are safe chemoprophylactic drugs, and quinine, in normal therapeutic doses, is safe for treatment. Mefloquine is best avoided in pregnancy. Pregnant women should take special care with food and drink when abroad, as dehydration may threaten the fetus. There are concerns about congenital goitre when pregnant women use iodine to purify water—the maximum recommended daily intake is 175 µg. Loperamide as an antidiarrhoeal agent is safe, but antimicrobials such as tetracyclines and quinolones should be avoided.

Extremes of age

Young children should have completed their routine immunizations before travelling. Malaria chemoprophylaxis is recommended for all ages. Yellow fever vaccine should only be given to children older than 9 months as a few cases of vaccine-associated encephalitis have occurred in younger children. Most other vaccines, including rabies, are safe. Hepatitis A is rarely symptomatic in children under 5-years old. Families planning to live in developing countries should be offered BCG vaccination for their children to reduce the risk of tuberculous meningitis.

The elderly should have the same immunizations as younger adults and should take antimalarial drugs. They are more prone to respiratory infection and should, therefore, be given influenza, pneumococcal, and *Haemophilus influenzae* vaccines. Jet lag and changes in time zones may be very disturbing. Older people are more likely to have an underlying medical condition requiring medication. It is important that sufficient supplies of medicines are taken abroad and that the patient has a detailed list of these medicines and their dosages, in case the tablets are lost or stolen, and the name and contact address of their physician at home in case of emergency.

Explorers and expeditions

Because of their adventurous aims, expeditions are likely to involve exposure to greater environmental extremes and hazards than ordinary travel. Expeditions usually take place in areas remote even from rural health centres, and so a greater responsibility for dealing with medical problems will devolve on the expedition members. The explorer's greatest fear may be to fall victim to a lethal tropical disease or an attack by a wild animal, but the reality is more mundane: road traffic accidents, mountaineering disasters, drowning, and attacks by humans. Prevention and treatment of medical problems must be planned well in advance. Detailed advice and information can be obtained from a number of organizations, such as the Expedition Advisory Centre of the Royal Geographical Society in London (Tel: 0207–581–2057; Fax: 0208–584–4447), from clubs specializing in mountaineering, cave exploring, diving, and other activities, and from books, journals, and websites. All expeditions should have a designated medical officer and all their members should receive first-aid training, aimed ideally at the particular needs of the expedition. The basics are clearing the airway, controlling bleeding, treating shock, relieving pain, and moving the injured person without causing further damage. Expedition medical kits should be more comprehensive than those carried by ordinary tourists and travellers. Lists of essential drugs are given in Anderson and Warrell (2002). Scissors, and a generous supply of large triangular and crêpe bandages, adhesive plasters, and an 'AIDS kit', to reduce the risk of infection from dirty needles and intravenous fluids are important. Lightweight emergency insulation must be taken if there is any risk of exposure in severe weather conditions, a lightweight collapsible stretcher for mountaineering, and an adequate water supply must be assured or taken if the expedition is into desert areas. A covering letter on official notepaper, signed by a doctor, may be helpful in getting drugs, even apparently innocuous ones such as codeine, through Customs (for example, the Russian Federation) and explaining the need for needles and syringes. The medical facilities nearest to the site of the expedition must be identified and contacted in advance. An emergency plan must be drawn up for the first-aid treatment and evacuation of severely ill or injured expedition members. In some areas, 'Flying doctor' and air evacuation services (such as AMREF in East Africa) are available. Medical insurance must be generous and comprehensive, to include repatriation of the injured. Before leaving their home country, expedition members should have a thorough dental check and treatment for outstanding medical or surgical problems. Control of chronic medical problems such as diabetes mellitus, hypertension, and asthma should be stabilized. In selecting members for an expedition, the most important attributes are experience, possession of the necessary skills (for example, diving and mountaineering), physical fitness, and proven psychological stability under stress. It is advisable always to appoint a reliable local agent in the country where the expedition will take place.

Illness in returning travellers

Details are needed about the countries visited, activities while travelling, immunizations, and antimalarials taken. Common problems are fever, rash, diarrhoea, and eosinophilia (Tables 3, 4, and 5).

In travellers with acute diarrhoea, a dietary history, assessment of hydration state, stool microscopy and culture, abdominal films, and sigmoidoscopy may be needed. There are many possible causes (see Table 2). Patients with chronic diarrhoea may be infected with *Giardia* spp., *Cryptosporidium* spp., *Entamoeba histolytica*, shigellae, or salmonellae. Investigations should

include a search for *Clostridium difficile* and its toxin, especially if the patient took antimicrobials while abroad. A minority of patients may develop a postinfective enteropathy, the most common problem being a secondary lactose intolerance. Rarely, bacterial overgrowth or tropical sprue develop.

The commonest causes of eosinophilia are allergy and helminths (see Table 5).

Further reading

Anderson S, Warrell DA (eds) (2002). *Expedition medicine*, 2nd edn. Profile Books, London.

Auerbach PS (1995). *Wilderness medicine. Management of wilderness and environmental emergencies*, 3rd edn. Mosby, St Louis.

Backer HD, et al. (eds) (1998). *Wilderness first aid. Emergency care for remote locations*. Jones and Barlett, Boston.

Bradley DJ, Bannister B (2001). Guidelines for malaria prevention in travellers from the United Kingdom for 2001. *Communicable Diseases and Public Health (PHLS)* 4 (2), 82–101.

Dawood R (2002). *Travellers' health*. Oxford University Press, Oxford. [New edition in press]

Department of Health (2001). *Health information for overseas travel*, 2nd edn. London, Stationary Office.

Forgey WW (2000). *Wilderness medicine. Beyond first aid*. Globe Pequot Press, Guilford, Connecticut.

Freedman DO, eds (1998). Travel medicine. *Infectious Disease Clinics of North America* 12, 249–554.

Journal of Wilderness Medicine (1990–). Published for the Wilderness Medical Society by Chapman and Hall Medical, London.

Milne AH, Siderfin CD, eds (1995). *Kurafid. British Antarctic Survey medical handbook*. British Antarctic Survey, Natural Environment Research Council, Cambridge, UK.

Monath TP, Modlin JF (2002). Prevention of yellow fever in persons traveling to the tropics. *Clinical Infectious Diseases* 34, 1369–78.

Table 4 Causes of rash in returning travellers

Infective	Non-infective
Cutaneous larva migrans, myiasis	Contact allergy
	Drug reaction
Cutaneous leishmaniasis	Erythema multiforme
Dengue	Insect bites
Dermatophytes	Sunburn
Lyme disease	
Meningococcus	
Mycobacterial	
Scabies/lice	
STDs[1]	
Tick/scrub typhus	
Tinea versicolor	
Typhoid/paratyphoid	

[1]STD, sexually transmitted disease.

Table 5 Infective causes of eosinophilia in travellers

Angiostrongylus	Pulmonary eosinophilia
Ascaris	Schistosomiasis
Echinococcus spp.	Strongyloides
Filaria (onchocerciasis)	Trichinosis
Gnathostoma	Trichuris
Hookworm and other gut nematodes	Visceral larva migrans

Table 3 Causes of fever in returned travellers

Tropical (short incubation; <3 weeks)	Tropical (long incubation; >3 weeks)
African trypanosomiasis	Amoebic abscess
Brucellosis	Brucellosis
Dengue	Coccidioidomycosis
Haemorrhagic fevers (Lassa)	Filariasis
Hepatitis A	Hepatitis A, B, or C
Malaria	HIV (?incubation)
Relapsing fevers	Leishmaniasis
Tick/scrub typhus	Malaria
Typhoid	Schistosomiasis (Katayama fever)
Leptospirosis	Tuberculosis
Malaria	Typhoid
Other infections	*Non-infective causes of fever*
Endocarditis	Connective tissue disease
Pneumonia	Drug reaction
Prostatitis	Factitious inflammatory bowel
Sexually transmitted disease	disease
Sinusitis	Malignancy
UTI[1]	

[1]UTI, urinary tract infection.

Potter SA, ed. (1992). *Anare Antarctic field manual*, 4th edn. Australian Antarctic Division, Kingston, Tasmania.

Salisbury DM, Begg NT, eds (1996). *Immunisation against infectious disease.* HMSO, London. [New edition in press]

Steedman DJ (1994). *Environmental medical emergencies.* Oxford University Press, Oxford.

Voluntary Aid Societies (1997). *First aid manual*, 7th edn. Dorling Kindersley, London.

Ward MP, Milledge JS, West JB (1989). *High altitude medicine and physiology.* Chapman and Hall Medical, London.

Internet sites

www.cdc.gov/travel/

www.who.int/ith/

www.the-stationery-office.co.uk/doh/hinfo/index.htm

www.isid.org/

www.premedmail.org

www.doh.gov.uk/traveladvice/index.htm

www.istm.org/

7.9 Nosocomial infections

I. C. J. W. Bowler

Definitions

Hospital-acquired or nosocomial (Greek νοσοκομειον, hospital) infections are distinct from community-acquired infections. They may affect patients and hospital staff. A useful epidemiological tool for the study of these infections is to define them as any infection manifesting more than 48 h after admission. However, some nosocomial infections may not be so easily identified as hospital acquired; for example hospital-acquired hepatitis B infection may not become clinically apparent until months after the patient has been discharged because of the prolonged incubation period. **Iatrogenic infections** are acquired as the direct consequence of a therapeutic intervention (e.g. insertion of a urinary catheter). **Opportunistic infections** are caused by organisms that do not ordinarily harm healthy people; they occur in people with impaired defences. **Endogenous (autogenous) infections** are produced by the patient's normal flora, while **exogenous infections** result from transmission of organisms to the patient from elsewhere. Although in practice it may not always be possible to distinguish endogenous from exogenous infections, this differentiation must be attempted because of important implications for control. Rapid changes in health-care provision in hospitals mean the frequency and nature of nosocomial infection are also changing. The increasing trend to early discharge, particularly for surgical patients, can lead to an under assessment of the burden of nosocomial infection. New interventions provide new opportunities for infection. For instance flexible endoscopes, which have revolutionized the investigation and management of a wide variety of diseases, can transmit Hepatitis B between patients if they are not decontaminated.

Nosocomial infections are preventable. Systematic surveillance to assess the size of the problem and an organized programme aimed at preventing or minimizing the impact of nosocomial infection should be an important part of the hospital's quality assurance system. Hospital managers must ensure appropriate staffing and resources. The programme involves surveillance, feedback of data on infections to staff, plans for outbreak management, and agreed policies for antibiotic prophylaxis, the management of patients with infections, and for carrying out procedures likely to increase the risk of infection. Staff should be educated, through an organized teaching programme, and results should be systematically audited.

Scale and costs of nosocomial infections

The World Health Organization (WHO) recognizes the serious global problem of nosocomial infections. Epidemic nosocomial infections frequently receive greater attention because of the alarm caused by the obvious spread of an infectious disease. A common point source or person-to-person spread are usually involved. Immediate application of control measures to prevent transmission often curtails such outbreaks. However, only about 3 per cent of nosocomial infections are accounted for by epidemic infection. Prevention of the other 97 per cent of (endemic) nosocomial infections requires a systematic approach based on careful surveillance. Host susceptibility, the infectious risk of medical procedures, and the type of hospital environment (e.g. intensive care units) are responsible.

The risk of endemic nosocomial infections is reduced, for example, by using prophylactic antibiotics for contaminated surgical procedures.

Rates of nosocomial infections between 5.7 and 8 infections per 100 admissions have been reported. The urinary tract, surgical wounds, and the lower respiratory tract are the most common sites, in that order (Table 1). In the United States, it is estimated that, of 200 000 deaths in patients with nosocomial infections, 20 000 were directly attributable to the infection. In a further 60 000, it contributed to death. Costs were estimated at $4.5 billion in the USA in 1992 and approximately £120 million in England and Wales in 1987, based on an average additional stay of 4 days for each hospital-acquired infection. These are likely to be underestimates. The WHO published comparative world-wide costs in 1984 based on an extra 5 days of admission per infection and a minimum cost of a hospital stay, per day, of $45.00 (Table 2). For developed countries, this hospital stay cost is too low.

Host factors

The principal risk factor is the severity of the underlying disease (e.g. neutropenia, organ system failure). In multivariate analysis, the number of medical diagnoses on admission, especially diabetes, renal failure, or alcohol abuse, are most strongly associated with risk. Treatment itself may lower host defences, for example surgical incisions, bladder catheterization, mechanical ventilation, and neutropenia following cancer chemotherapy. Pathogens are able to form biofilms on the increasingly used prosthetic devices (totally implantable, e.g. hip replacement, or transcutaneous, e.g. intravascular devices) subverting normal host clearance mechanisms.

Patients with similar clinical problems, who are likely to share similar risk factors for infection, tend to be nursed together for convenience but the introduction of a micro-organism into such a group can infect a number of patients. A good example is the rapid spread of small round structured virus gastroenteritis in geriatric wards. A poorly maintained hospital environment is a threat to vulnerable patients; an example is outbreaks of legionellosis in units caring for patients with solid organ transplants, resulting from defective ventilation and hot water systems.

Table 1 Rates and sites of nosocomial infection in three countries

	Canada (1976)	UK (1994)	USA (1986)
Rates	8.2[1]	9.0[1]	5.7[2]
Sites (% of all infections)			
UTI	39	23	42
SWI	24	11	24
LRI	26	23	11
Other	11	43	23

[1]Cases/100 admissions (prevalence)

[2]Cases/100 admissions/year (incidence)

UTI, urinary-tract infection; SWI, surgical wound infection; LRI, lower respiratory-tract infection.

Table 2 Estimated cost to countries of nosocomial infections

Continent[1]	Average no. of patients	5% of patients with nosocomial infections	Cost estimated for 5 days ($US)
Africa	4 900 000	245 000	55 125 000
America	46 500 000	2 325 000	523 125 000
Asia	17 500 000	875 000	196 875 000
Europe	56 000 000	2 800 000	630 000 000
Oceania	490 000	24 500	5 512 500
Total	125 390 000	6 269 500	1410 637 500

[1]Statistical data are not available from 16 countries in Africa—Egypt, Equatorial Guinea, Ethiopia, Kenya, Mali, Mauritania, Mozambique, Namibia, Niger, Nigeria, Réunion, Seychelles, Sierra Leone, Somalia, United Republic of Cameroon, and Zaire; 15 countries in the Americas—Anguilla, Argentina, Belize, Bolivia, Brazil, Dominica, Guadelupe, Haiti, Mexico, Antilles, Paraguay, Peru, Surinam, US Virgin Islands, and Venezuela; 14 countries in Asia—Afghanistan, Bangladesh, China, Democratic Kampuchea, East Timor, India, Korea, Lebanon, Nepal, Oman, Pakistan, the Philippines, Qatar, and Yemen; eight countries in Europe—Albania, Belgium, Bulgaria, German Democratic Republic, Isle of Man, Malta, Rumania, and the USSR; five countries in Oceania—Australia, New Hebrides, Tuvalu, Papua New Guinea, and Solomon Islands.
Reproduced from Kereselidze T and Mangay Maglacas A (1984). *Journal of Hospital Infection* **5** (Suppl. A), 7–11, with permission.

Micro-organisms

Bacteria (*Escherichia coli*, *Staphylococcus aureus*, *Enterococcus* spp., *Pseudomonas* spp., and coagulase-negative staphylococci, in decreasing order of frequency) are the most important. Viruses, fungi, and protozoa play a minor part.

Whether endogenous or exogenous, the organisms causing nosocomial infection are usually part of a patient's colonizing flora. It may be difficult to distinguish infecting from colonizing organisms using bacteriological tests alone. They are frequently multidrug resistant. Empirical antibiotic therapy must accommodate the shift towards more resistant colonizing flora occurring in hospitals, particularly in burns and intensive care units. For example *Pseudomonas aeruginosa*, methicillin-resistant *Staph. aureus* (MRSA), and enterococci exhibit multiresistance to antimicrobials, making them difficult and expensive to treat.

Principles of hospital infection control

The main goal of hospital infection control is to prevent nosocomial infection. First, hospital-acquired infections must be identified as endemic or epidemic by clinical and epidemiological investigations. The identification and typing of isolates causing nosocomial infection allows recognition of organisms that are epidemiologically linked. Invasive multiresistant organisms, such as MRSA, often require infection control measures to prevent their spread, and so minimize the use of expensive, sometimes toxic, antibiotics required for their prophylaxis and treatment.

Epidemic outbreaks are usually amenable to measures that interrupt the spread of infection, such as use of gowns and gloves and careful hand washing by those attending patients. Transfer of colonized or infected patients to a single room or an isolation ward is a physical means of preventing spread. Patients infected with the same organism can be grouped together and attended to by a cohort of nurses not involved with uninfected patients. Identification of additional carriers and elimination of colonization may be necessary for some epidemic outbreaks. Controlled trials demonstrating the efficacy of such measures have not been made, but many observational studies support their use.

Endemic nosocomial infections are less straightforward to control. The size of the problem may not be apparent because attack rates in individual units may be low or because some infection is seen as a normal consequence of certain interventions. It is important that information about endemic infections is collected systematically, analysed, disseminated, and discussed so that preventive strategies can be improved. Control measures are applied to selected patients according to risk; for example correctly timed antimicrobial prophylaxis and meticulous sterile technique in prosthetic joint replacement surgery.

Site of nosocomial infections

Urinary tract

A bacterial count of 10^5 organisms or more per ml in cultured urine indicates infection. However, counts as low as 10^2 organisms/ml are included by some. Urinary-tract infection accounts for 30 to 40 per cent of all nosocomial infections. Most patients remain asymptomatic, but 20 to 30 per cent develop the symptoms of urinary-tract infection, about 1 in 100 of whom develop bacteraemia. Causes of nosocomial urinary-tract infections are listed in Table 3.

Indwelling urinary catheters account for 80 per cent of nosocomial urinary-tract infections; 50 per cent of patients catheterized for longer than 7 to 10 days develop bacteriuria. Most of the others result from instrumentation of the urinary tract. The main source of organisms is the periurethral flora. Bacteria gain access to the bladder, usually by spreading up the outside of the lumen of the catheter. Occasionally, infection is acquired exogenously during an epidemic of nosocomial infection. Most symptomatic or bacteraemic infections occur within 24 h of the organisms gaining access to the bladder. Early recognition, by daily urine culture, of a urinary-tract infection before it becomes symptomatic is not helpful.

Treatment is with broad-spectrum antimicrobials administered empirically after obtaining appropriate cultures and later adjusted after receiving results of bacteriological studies. Asymptomatic patients need not be treated.

Since the important risk factor is the duration of catheterization, prevention is by avoiding catheterization or reducing the period of catheterization. Catheters should be inserted aseptically, and closed sterile drainage

Table 3 Micro-organisms causing nosocomial urinary tract infections (%)

	UK	USA
Escherichia coli	43	32
Proteus spp.	13	7
Klebsiella spp.	8	9
Enterococci	7	14
Pseudomonas aeruginosa	5	11
Coagulase-negative staphylococci	3	3
Enterobacter spp.	1	4
Other	14	22

systems, uninterrupted gravity drainage, or intermittent or suprapubic catheterization employed. Prophylactic antimicrobial treatment is not useful.

Surgical wound infection

One acceptable definition requires the presence of a purulent discharge in, or exuding from, a wound. *Staph. aureus* (15–33 per cent of all wound infections) and *E. coli* (12–19 per cent) are leading causes. Many other aerobic and anaerobic bacterial may be implicated.

The main risk factor is the degree of wound contamination at operation. Operations may be 'clean' (e.g. herniorrhaphy), 'clean contamination' (e.g. appendicectomy which requires incision of bowel), or 'contaminated' (e.g. gross spillage from the gastrointestinal tract during surgery). *Staph. aureus* causes most infections complicating clean surgery. 'Contaminated' surgery is associated with polymicrobial infections, especially with *E. coli* and mixed anaerobes. Other risk factors include the length of the operation, obesity, a remote infection, and underlying disease. Most wound infections follow direct inoculation of organisms into the wound at surgery or spread of bacteria to open wounds such as burns.

Wound infections present with local symptoms and signs (pain, erythema, pus, dehiscence) with general features of infection such as fever. Appropriate cultures, including blood cultures, are taken, pus is drained, and broad-spectrum antimicrobials are given empirically, directed at the likely flora but later adjusted according to bacteriological results. Prevention is by meticulous aseptic surgical technique. Prophylactic antimicrobials, given no more than 2 h before the surgical incision, are indicated for clean-contaminated and contaminated procedures, and in clean surgery when a prosthesis is inserted (e.g. vascular grafting).

Nosocomial pneumonia

Pneumonia is defined clinically by production of purulent sputum, chest signs, a fall in arterial Po_2 and the appearance of new infiltrates on the chest radiograph not ascribable to pulmonary emboli, collapse, or pulmonary oedema. Between 0.55 and 1.5 per cent of patients admitted to hospital develop lower respiratory-tract infections. Crude case fatalities of between 20 and 30 per cent are quoted but death may be due to underlying disease. Intubated and ventilated patients have the highest risk of acquiring pneumonia. Bacteria colonizing the gastrointestinal and upper respiratory tracts are probably aspirated. This flora is often acquired after admission to hospital. Organisms cultured from bronchoscopic samples are listed in Table 4.

Culture of expectorated sputum or tracheal aspirate is poorly predictive of the bacterial cause of nosocomial pneumonia, which is best determined by quantitative culture of specimens obtained by sampling the terminal airways (e.g. by bronchoalveolar lavage). Initially, broad-spectrum antimicrobials appropriate for likely infecting flora should be given empirically. Once the susceptibility of the causative pathogen has been determined, specific antimicrobial treatment can be instituted. Selective decontamination of the digestive tract has reduced occurrence of nosocomial pneumonia but

Table 4 Causative organisms identified in samples drained at bronchoscopy by protected specimen brush (percentage of all pneumonias)

	France	Spain
Pseudomonas aeruginosa	31	35
Acinetobacter spp.	15	30
Proteus spp.	15	
Moraxella catarrhalis	10	
Haemophilus spp.	10	
Staphylococcus aureus	33	25
Streptococci	15	20
Other species	37	60
Polymicrobial	21	50

there has been no reduction in the mortality of ventilated patients. Epidemic nosocomial pneumonia usually results from bacterial contamination of respiratory equipment such as nebulizers, ventilators, or bronchoscopes and can be prevented by cleaning and disinfection of the equipment and hand washing after patient contact.

Intravascular device-associated infections

The most important result of intravascular device-associated infection is bacteraemia, varying in incidence from about 0.04 per cent for subcutaneous central venous ports, to about 0.2 per cent for peripheral intravenous cannulae, and approximately 10 per cent for central venous haemodialysis catheters.

Duration of intravascular cannulation is the greatest risk factor. Bacteria usually gain access to the blood by direct spread from the skin surface along the subcutaneous catheter tunnel to its tip in the blood vessel. Bacteraemia from intraluminal bacteria results from contamination of connecting devices. This is particularly important in catheters with subcutaneous cuffs, such as Hickman catheters, where the periluminal route of infection is less likely. The leading organisms causing intravenous device-related sepsis are *Staph. aureus, Pseudomonas* spp., and *Candida* spp. In patients with haematological malignancies, coagulase-negative staphylococci and enterococci are also frequently implicated.

Line-related sepsis presents with local inflammation or signs of thrombophlebitis but usually with features of bacteraemia. Blood cultures are obtained, the affected catheter is removed and cultured, and empirical antimicrobials are given. Sometimes, long-term intravenous catheters, such as Hickmen lines, can be 'sterilized' by giving parenteral antibiotics down the line. Exit site infections involving these devices can usually be treated with antibiotics with the line *in situ*. Tunnel infections usually require line removal for resolution. Prevention is by using aseptic technique when inserting catheters, maintaining a high standard of line care, and removing catheters as soon as possible. The insertion site should be disinfected with a reliable disinfectant such as an iodine-containing agent, 70 per cent alcohol, or 2 to 4 per cent chlorhexidine. At the time of insertion the operators should wash their hands and for long-line insertion, wear sterile gloves, gown, face mask, and hat. Removal of peripheral intravascular devices should be considered after 3 days. Central venous catheters are usually only removed if blocked or suspected as a source of sepsis. The skin at the exit site should be checked daily and the device removed if sepsis is suspected. Subcutaneous tunnelling, insertion of a subcutaneous cuff (Hickman line), burying them subcutaneously (e.g. portacaths), and incorporating antimicrobials on to the surface of the device can all reduce the infection rate significantly. Replacing the entire intravenous delivery set every 72 h is sufficient to reduce sepsis secondary to intraluminal contamination of 'giving' sets.

Prosthetic device-related infection

Infections of prosthetic devices such as heart valves, vascular grafts, cerebrospinal fluid shunts, artificial lenses, and joints are usually caused by the normal skin flora, for example coagulase-negative staphylococci. The devices become coated with a layer of host-derived macromolecules such as fibronectin and fibrin which have specific adhesion receptors for bacteria, particularly staphylococci. Once attached, these organisms multiply on the surface of the coated prosthesis forming a biofilm in a state physiologically different from rapidly dividing, 'free' micro-organisms. They are inherently more resistant to antimicrobials, which explains the frequent failure of antimicrobial treatment. Bacteria gain access to prosthetic devices by direct inoculation, usually at surgery, or by settling on a prosthesis after bacteraemic spread. Direct inoculation at surgery is responsible for prosthetic-device infections occurring more than 1 year after insertion since the organisms involved are usually skin commensals of low virulence. Except for organisms that are exquisitely susceptible to antimicrobials, these infections are seldom cured with antimicrobial agents. Surgical removal of the device is frequently necessary. However, infection of artificial lenses in the eye are frequently cured by antimicrobial treatment.

Prevention is by avoiding contamination of the wound at surgery, by using strict aseptic surgical technique. Sometimes, as when inserting prosthetic joints, there is an advantage in providing operating theatres with ultra-clean air. Prophylactic antimicrobials reduce the risk of some prosthetic devices becoming infected during insertion.

Antibiotic-associated diarrhoea

Up to 30 per cent of patients treated with antibiotics will develop diarrhoea as a result of the disturbance of the complex gut flora. In a few, loss of 'colonization resistance' predisposes to acquisition of *Clostridium difficile*. Faecal/oral colonization by this organism is usually harmless, but in about a third, particularly the elderly, the organism may overgrow, produce a cytotoxin and causing colitis. The clinical picture varies from mild diarrhoea with fever to fulminating toxic megacolon requiring colectomy. *Clostridium difficile* related diarrhoea entails a delay in discharge of about 3 weeks. Since attack rates in the elderly are around 5 per cent, the disease can have a major impact on hospital resources. Diagnosis is by detection of the cytotoxin in stool, but the test has poor disease specificity since toxin may be found for many weeks after full recovery. Patient management includes adequate rehydration, avoiding drugs which inhibit gut motility, and stopping the provoking antibiotics. More severe cases will require metronidazole or vancomycin given by mouth and surgical review. Prevention is by restricting the use of antibiotics according to agreed and audited protocols. Hand washing after patient contact, isolation of patients with diarrhoea, and cleaning the ward environment are employed on microbiological grounds, despite a lack of prospective studies showing their efficacy.

Nosocomial bacteraemia

Bacteraemia may occur secondarily to the infections mentioned above. The incidence is approximately 3/1000 hospital discharges. The case fatality is about 40 per cent, but varies with the severity of the underlying disease, being as low as about 2 per cent in obstetric patients. The focus must be identified and, if possible, removed surgically. Appropriate antimicrobials are given after obtaining blood and other relevant cultures.

Other nosocomial infections

These include viral infections such as varicella-zoster, hepatitis C, hepatitis B, Norwalk, and rotaviruses, bacterial infections such as tuberculosis and legionellosis, and fungal infections such as aspergillosis.

Further reading

Ayliffe GAJ, Lowbury EJL, Geddes AM, Williams JD, eds (1992). *Control of hospital infection: a practical handbook*, 3rd edn. Chapman and Hall, London.

Bennett JV and Brachman PS, eds (1992). *Hospital infections*, 3rd edn. Little, Brown, New York.

Emmerson AM, Enstone JE, Griffin M, Kelsey MC, Smyth ETM (1996). The second national prevalence survey of infection in hospitals—overview of the results. *Journal of Hospital Infection* 32, 175–90.

Haley RN, Culver DH, White JW, *et al.* (1985). The efficacy of infection surveiellance and control programs in preventing nosocomial infections in US hospitals. *American Journal of Epidemiology* 121, 182–205.

Infection Control Standards Working Party (1993). *Standards in infection control*. HMSO, Southampton, UK.

Meers P, Jacobsen W, McPherson M (1992). *Hospital infection control for nurses*. Chapman and Hall, London.

Wenzel RP, ed. (1997). *Prevention and control of nosocomial infections*, 3rd edn. Williams and Wilkins, Baltimore.

7.10 Viruses

7.10.1 Respiratory tract viruses

Malik Peiris

Introduction

Infections of the respiratory tract are one of the most common afflictions of mankind. In economically developed countries, acute respiratory infections account for 20 per cent of all medical consultations, 30 per cent of work absences, and 75 per cent of antibiotic prescriptions. Viruses account for the majority of acute respiratory infections, although when they occur, bacterial infections tend to be more severe. Longitudinal family studies suggest that an individual has on average 2.4 respiratory viral infections per year, a quarter of them leading to a medical consultation. With the exception of influenza, these infections are not a major cause of mortality in the developed world, but it is estimated that they contribute to 20–30 per cent of the 4.5 million deaths annually associated with acute respiratory infection in the developing world.

The term 'respiratory virus' is imprecise, but for the purpose of this discussion it will include those that have the respiratory tract as their primary target. Taxonomically, they belong to diverse virus families (Table 1) and are global in distribution. Other viruses cause systemic disease with respiratory tract involvement as part of an overall disseminated disease process in immunocompetent (e.g. measles, Hantavirus pulmonary syndrome) or immunocompromised (e.g. cytomegalovirus) patients. These are dealt with elsewhere.

A respiratory virus may cause a range of clinical syndromes. Conversely, a respiratory syndrome may be caused by more than one virus. The major viral respiratory syndromes and their common aetiological agents are shown in Table 2. The pattern seen in tropical countries is similar, a notable difference being the role of measles as a major cause of lower respiratory tract infections and fatality.

Table 1 Respiratory tract viruses: summary of classification, incubation period, duration of infectivity, and diagnostic options

Virus	Classification	Subgroups, serotypes, and subtypes	Incubation period (days)	Duration of virus shedding in immunocompetent patients (days)	Options for laboratory diagnosis
Rhinovirus	Picornaviridae Non-enveloped RNA viruses	>115 serotypes	1–2 days	5–6 days	Viral culture
Coronavirus	Coronaviridae Enveloped RNA virus	2 types (OC43 and 229E)	4–5 days	5–8 days	Laboratory diagnosis not routinely available
Respiratory syncytial virus (RSV)	Paramyxoviridae Enveloped RNA virus	Subgroup A and B	5 days	6–7 days	Culture Rapid antigen detection* Serology: useful in adults but less so in infants
Parainfluenza	Paramyxoviridae Enveloped RNA virus	Type 1, 2, 3, 4a, 4b	3–6 days	7 days	Culture Rapid antigen detection* Serology: useful in adults but less so in infants
Influenza	Orthomyxoviridae Enveloped RNA virus	Types A, B, C Human influenza A subtypes currently in circulation are H1N1 and H3N2	Average 2–3 (range 1–7)	~ 5 days in adults ~ 7 days in children	Culture Rapid antigen detection* Serology
Adenovirus	Adenoviridae Non-enveloped DNA virus	Subgroups A–F Types 1–49	Average 10 (range 2–15)	Days–weeks (from respiratory tract), weeks–months (in faeces)	Culture Rapid antigen detection* Serology

* Best sensitivity from nasopharyngeal aspirates or nasopharyngeal swabs (in that order). Throat swabs give lower sensitivity.

Table 2 Viral aetiology of common respiratory syndromes

Virus	Coryza	Pharyngitis	Croup	Bronchiolitis	Pneumonia
Rhinovirus	+++*	++	+	+	Rare
Coronavirus	++	+			
Adenoviruses	(+)	++	++	++	++ (all ages)
RSV	++	+	++	+++	+++ (children); + (elderly)
Parainfluenza 1	+	++	+++	+	
Parainfluenza 2	+	++	++	+	
Parainfluenza 3	+	++	++	++	++ (children)
Influenza A/B	+	++	++	+	++ (all ages)

* Frequency of cases caused by the virus: +++ the major cause (>25%); ++ a common cause (5–25%); + an occasional
cause; blank, rare cause or not reported.
(Data adapted from Treanor 1997).

The anatomical demarcation between upper and lower respiratory tract infections is the larynx. Influenza and adenoviruses are well-recognized lower respiratory tract pathogens in adults as well as in children. Respiratory syncytial virus and parainfluenza viruses, hitherto diseases associated mainly with children, are now being increasingly recognized as important lower respiratory tract pathogens in adults and the elderly.

Transmission

The routes of respiratory virus transmission are through direct contact, contaminated fomites, and large airborne droplets (mean diameter >5 μm, range of transmission <1 m). Influenza may be spread over longer distances by small particle aerosol (mean diameter <5 μm), but even here, direct contact, fomites, and large droplets are more important. Adenoviruses are transmitted by the faeco-oral route as well as by direct contact and large droplets.

Factors increasing transmission of respiratory viruses include the time of exposure, close contact (e.g. spouse, mother), crowding, family size, and lack of pre-existing immunity (including lack of breast-feeding). School-age children often introduce an infection into the family and the commencement of school term may affect transmission patterns in the community. Infected children shed higher titres of viruses than adults. The duration of virus excretion is shown in Table 1. Infectivity usually precedes the onset of clinical symptoms. Immunocompromised patients shed virus for a longer time.

Seasonality

Some respiratory viruses have a predictable seasonality, which varies regionally. For example in temperate regions, influenza A is a typically winter disease while in tropical regions it is a spring/summer disease (e.g. Hong Kong) or occurs all year round (e.g. Singapore, India). Similarly, respiratory syncytial virus (RSV), a primarily winter disease in temperate countries, is a summer disease in Hong Kong. Rhinoviruses occur year round (with increases in the spring and fall) in temperate climes while adenoviruses have no predictable seasonality. The basis for seasonality is unclear but climatic factors such as high humidity may help virus survival and transmission. Factors affecting population congregation such as commencement of school-term and seasonal effects on social behaviour may also play a role.

Laboratory diagnosis

A well-collected specimen is the first (and often most important) determinant in successful laboratory diagnosis. Nasopharyngeal aspirates (secretions aspirated from the back of the nose into a mucus trap) or nasopharyngeal washes are superior to nasopharyngeal or throat swabs for the isolation of many respiratory viruses. They offer the advantage that rapid ('same day') diagnosis for a number of viruses is possible provided the appropriate methods are available. Swabs for viral culture are placed in viral transport medium immediately upon collection and kept cool (around 4°C) until processed. More invasive specimens such as endotracheal aspirates, brochoalveolar lavage or lung biopsy, when available, usually provide better information. However, the likely site of pathology must be kept in mind—the more invasive specimen is not always better.

The laboratory methods used for detecting a virus in the clinical specimen/s are viral culture, antigen detection, and, more recently, nucleic acid detection. Serology is an option for diagnosing some respiratory virus diseases, but is impractical for others such as rhinoviruses where the large number of antigenically distinct serotypes have no common immunodominant antigen/s. On the other hand, adenoviruses (or influenza viruses), though having many antigenic types or variants, have common antigen/s and a single antigen can detect serological responses to many of them. IgM assays are not routinely available for diagnosis of respiratory viral diseases and paired sera are required so that significant increases in antibody titres can be documented. Complement fixation tests are widely used for this purpose though their sensitivity is not ideal. Haemagglutination inhibition tests are more sensitive for diagnosis of influenza and ELISA tests (though still only available in research settings) provide better sensitivity for diagnosis of RSV and parainfluenza infections.

'Near patient testing' is becoming a reality for some viruses (e.g. influenza) with availability of tests that can be performed in a general practice setting. These become more relevant with the greater availability of antiviral drugs.

Rhinoviruses

Rhinoviruses are adapted to replicate at temperatures of 33–35°C, as found in the external airways. There are over 115 distinct serotypes, but only a few will circulate in a region at any given time. Most rhinoviruses use ICAM-1 on the cell surface as the receptor for attachment but a minority of rhinoviruses use other receptors.

Epidemiology

Rhinoviruses remain one of the most common infections of humans, with 0.5 infections per person per year being a conservative estimate. Secondary attack rates in a family setting may be around 50 per cent overall and 70 per cent in those who are antibody negative.

Immunity

In experimental challenges, immunity is serotype specific, and homologous type specific protection lasts for at least 1 year and correlates with serum IgA, IgG, and secretory IgA antibody levels.

Pathogenesis

Viral replication occurs predominantly in the ciliated epithelial cells of the nasopharynx. The structure of the epithelium is preserved. Mucosal secretions associated with coryza appear to be due to the release of inflammatory mediators and neurogenic reflexes.

It was thought that the preference of the virus for a lower temperature for replication restricted it to the upper respiratory tract, however, this is not strictly true. The temperature of the mucosa of the trachea and bronchi is also lower than core body temperature and does not preclude rhinovirus replication. The virus has been isolated from the lower respiratory tract (including bronchial brushings) and viral RNA has been demonstrated by in situ hybridization in bronchial epithelial cells. Rarely, the virus has been isolated from post mortem lungs of immunocompromised patients.

Clinical manifestations

Rhinorrhoea, nasal obstruction, pharyngitis, and a cough are common features of rhinovirus infections. Fever and systemic symptoms are rare, but more common in the elderly in whom disease can be more severe. Rhinoviruses are a major cause of exacerbations of asthma and chronic obstructive respiratory disease. Lower respiratory tract symptoms are uncommon in the healthy young adult, but may occur in children (bronchiolitis), the immunocompromised, and the elderly.

Treatment and prevention

There are no established antiviral drugs for treatment. Topical interferon-α prevents symptoms if given before onset of disease, but cannot be used for prophylaxis over prolonged periods because of side effects. A viral capsid-binding agent (pleconaril) blocks viral attachment and uncoating and is undergoing clinical trials at present. Antibiotics are ineffective in preventing bacterial complications of the common cold. Mucopurulent discharges are part of the natural course of the common cold and are not an indication for antimicrobial treatment, unless it persists (e.g.>10 days). Given the large number of rhinovirus serotypes, vaccination is not an option.

Coronaviruses

There are two distinct serotypes of respiratory coronavirus—0C43 and 229E. They cannot be cultured from primary specimens and laboratory investigations rely on serology or molecular methods which are only available for research.

Epidemiology

Infection occurs in early childhood and 85 to 100 per cent of adults have antibody to both virus types.

Immunity

Volunteer reinfection studies show that 1 year after initial infection protection from reinfection and illness following a challenge from the homologous virus is incomplete.

Pathogenesis

In common with rhinoviruses, coronaviruses induce little or no damage to the respiratory mucosa. The mucosal discharge is caused by the release of mediators from affected host cells.

Clinical findings

Coronaviruses typically cause upper respiratory tract infections and the common cold. Involvement of the lower respiratory tract is probably more frequent than with rhinoviruses. The virus contributes to exacerbation of asthma in children and adults, but is less important in this role than rhinoviruses. Coronaviruses are also significant pathogens of the elderly.

Treatment and prevention

There are presently no options for antiviral treatment or prevention.

Adenoviruses

Adenovirus subgroups A to D cause respiratory, ocular, hepatic, genitourinary, or gastrointestinal system disease in immunocompetent or immunocompromised individuals. Only respiratory diseases are considered here.

Productive replication and excretion of infectious virus can occur for a prolonged period (see below). In addition, adenoviruses can establish chronic persistence or 'latency', the virological basis and clinical significance of which is poorly understood.

Epidemiology

Adenovirus infections are common during childhood (usually serotypes 1, 2, 5 in early childhood, 3 and 7 during school years or later), but continue to occur throughout life. Reinfection with the same serotype occurs but is usually asymptomatic. Serotypes 1,2,5, and 6 are typically endemic, types 4 and 7 more typically associated with outbreaks, and type 3 can occur in either situation.

Clinical features

Adenovirus respiratory illness often leads to upper respiratory tract disease with coryza and sore throat. Fever may last up to 2 weeks. The sore throat may be exudative and clinically difficult to differentiate from streptococcal infection. Adenoviral infection may present as pharyngoconjunctival fever. Otitis media is a complication in children. Unlike other respiratory viral infections, adenoviruses may be associated with elevated white blood cell counts (>15 × 10^9/l), C-reactive protein, or ESR and thus more easily confused with bacterial diseases.

Though uncommon, pneumonia may occur sporadically or in epidemics (caused by serotypes 4 and 7 for example), particularly in closed communities such as the military where stress and physical exertion may predispose to lower respiratory tract involvement. Community outbreaks of adenoviral pneumonia have been reported. Radiological appearance varies from diffuse to patchy interstitial infiltrates and pleural effusion may be present. Adenovirus type 7 pneumonia can lead to permanent lung damage, including bronchiectasis, bronchiolitis obliterans, and unilateral hyperlucent lung syndrome.

Adenoviral infection may disseminate and present as 'septic shock' in the newborn baby. Manifestations in the immunocompromised patient includes hepatitis (especially in liver transplant recipients), colitis, and haemorrhagic cystitis (in renal and bone marrow transplant recipients) in addition to pneumonia. The serotypes associated with disease in these patients may differ from those typically found in the immunocompetent patient, and include the subgroup B2 serotypes 11, 34, and 35. With improving control of other common viral diseases of the immunocompromised (e.g. cytomegalovirus), the role of adenoviruses infections is being increasingly appreciated.

Isolation of an adenovirus from a clinical specimen presents a challenge in interpretation. Adenoviruses are excreted for a prolonged period after initial infection, especially, but not exclusively, from faeces. In children, one-third of patients shed viruses longer than 1 month and 14 per cent longer than 1 year. The clinical significance of a positive result depends on the specimen, the method, and the serotype. Isolation of viruses from the respiratory tract carries greater significance than that from faeces. Patients who have symptomatic adenoviral diseases have higher viral loads than those with asymptomatic carriage. Thus, a rapidly growing virus, a positive antigen detection test (both reflecting higher virus load), or a detectable serological response all point to greater clinical significance. Antigen detection applies only to nasopharyngeal aspirates or bronchial washings.

The above guidelines may not apply to immunocompromised patients who may be infected with unusual serotypes. The presence of the virus in multiple body sites or in peripheral blood possibly points to clinical significance, although further data are needed.

Treatment and prevention

Most adenoviral infections in immunocompetent patients are self-limited and require no specific therapy, however, some infections, especially but not exclusively in the immunocompromised, are severe and life threatening. Ribavirin, vidarabine, cidofovir, and ganciclovir are active against adenoviruses *in vitro*. There are anecdotal reports of their therapeutic use with variable success. However, there are no clinical trials on which to base firm recommendations.

Live attenuated oral vaccines containing serotypes 4 and 7 (associated with outbreaks in military conscripts) are safe and effective, but not licensed for general use.

Respiratory syncytial virus (RSV)

Respiratory syncytial virus (RSV) infects human and non-human primates and was first isolated from a chimpanzee with a 'cold'. Related viruses affect cattle and sheep but do not directly affect humans. The virus has two surface glycoproteins on its envelope (G and F) and the immune responses to them correlate with protection. Two subgroups (A and B) are recognized on the basis of antigenic differences of the G glycoprotein.

Epidemiology

Over two-thirds of infants acquire RSV infection during the first year of life. Of patients hospitalized with RSV disease, 75 per cent are younger than 5 months. The peak of morbidity occurs around 2 months of age, a time when passive maternal antibodies protect against most other viral infections. Primary infection does not lead to solid immunity and reinfection is common. The first reinfection can still be associated with lower respiratory tract involvement. Subsequent reinfection occurs throughout life leading to asymptomatic or upper respiratory tract infections. However, significant diseases may result in the immunocompromised or elderly.

Immunity

Both antibody and cell mediated immunity are important in protection. Antibody to the G proteins prevents attachment of viruses to the cellular receptor, but immunity to the F protein is required to prevent cell to cell spread via fusion of virally infected cells. Cell mediated immunity is important in eliminating established viral infection.

Pathogenesis

The virus leads to a ballooning degeneration of the ciliated epithelial cells, lymphocytic infiltration, and necrosis of the epithelium. There is oedema and increased secretion from the mucous cells and the formation of plugs of mucous and cellular debris in the bronchioles. This results in obstruction and air trapping leading to collapse or over-distension of the distal alveoli. Cells throughout the respiratory tract are affected but the alveoli are spared unless there is RSV pneumonia. Degranulation products of mucosal eosinophils and mast cells and cytokines released by infected macrophages contribute to disease pathogenesis. The cell-mediated immune response contributes to immunopathology in some circumstances. For example when patients with severe combined immunodeficiency and chronic RSV infection receive a bone marrow transplant (for correction of the immuno-deficiency), engraftment may be associated with exacerbation of the lung pathology, sometimes with fatal consequences.

Severe RSV bronchiolitis is strongly associated with subsequent childhood asthma. RSV appears to promote type-1 hypersensitivity responses following subsequent exposure to unrelated antigens.

Clinical features

RSV infections of infants may lead to bronchiolitis and pneumonia. Bronchiolitis in infants is associated with expiratory wheeze, subcostal recession, hyperinflation of the chest, nasal flaring, and hypoxia with or without cyanosis. Fever is not prominent in half of the patients. Complete obstruction of a small airway leads to subsegmental atelectasis. Apnoea may occur (particularly in premature infants or in those <3 months of age) and may precede the development of bronchiolitis. Interstitial pneumonitis is uncommon but carries a bad prognosis. Otitis media is a common complication of RSV infection in children. Infants at highest risk from severe RSV disease are those under 6 months, those with pre-existing congenital heart disease, chronic lung diseases (e.g. bronchopulmonary dysplasia), and those born premature.

Infection in adults is often asymptomatic or leads to upper respiratory tract infection. During the RSV season, it is an important cause of lower respiratory tract infection in adults and the elderly—estimated to cause 2 to 9 per cent of the hospitalizations and deaths associated with pneumonia in the elderly. Much of this morbidity is clinically indistinguishable from influenza.

RSV (as well as parainfluenza and influenza) infections in the immunocompromised patient can be life threatening. They usually occur during community outbreaks, but a significant proportion are nosocomially acquired. Once infected, immunocompromised patients have a prolonged period of viral shedding and pose a risk of transmission to other high-risk patients. The disease typically commences as an upper respiratory tract infection but may progress to involve the lower respiratory tract with more serious consequences. Factors that increase risk of disease progression appear to include bone marrow transplant recipients who acquire the infection in the period prior to engraftment and oncology patients with neutrophil counts less than 0.5×10^6/l. Those immunocompromised by HIV appear to tolerate community acquired respiratory viruses better than oncology patients and transplant recipients. This may, however, reflect inadequacy of data rather than reality.

Treatment and prevention

Ribavirin has activity against RSV *in vitro*. Aerosol administration is recommended because it results in much higher concentrations in the respiratory tract than can be achieved by intravenous administration. A number of controlled clinical trials in patients with severe RSV disease have reported clinical benefits associated with its administration by small particle aerosol via a mist tent, mask, oxygen hood, or ventilator, but these findings remain controversial.

In adult bone marrow transplant recipients, an uncontrolled study of ribavirin together with intravenous immune globulin (selected batches with high neutralizing antibody titre) appeared to be beneficial when compared to historical controls. More information is required for deciding the best management strategy.

Monthly intravenous administration of human hyperimmune RSV immunoglobulin during the RSV season, protects against disease of the lower respiratory tract and otitis media in patients with pre-existing risk factors, but is not yet widely available. It did not confer benefits to children with cyanotic heart disease and is not recommended for this group. Side-effects included reversible fluid overload, decrease in oxygen saturation, and transient fever. High titre RSV intravenous immunoglobulin by itself is ineffective in treatment of established RSV disease.

Candidate vaccines for RSV are undergoing clinical trials at present but none is yet available for routine use. Experience of early trials with inactivated RSV vaccines that led to enhanced RSV disease, rather than protection, continues to haunt the field.

Parainfluenza virus

Parainfluenza viruses, despite their name, are not related to influenza viruses, and are more akin to respiratory syncytial virus with which they are classified. They carry two envelope glycoproteins; HN containing both haemagglutinin and neuraminidase activity and F carrying fusion activity.

Epidemiology

The total impact on hospitalization of children by all four types of parainfluenza viruses taken together is comparable to that of RSV but, in contrast to RSV, their impact is in later infancy and childhood. In temperate countries, parainfluenza virus type 3 occurs annually and infects two-thirds of all infants in their first year of life. Parainfluenza type 1 and 2 tend to occur in alternate years and infection is acquired more slowly over childhood. Reinfection with parainfluenza viruses occurs, but rarely leads to lower respiratory tract infection.

Pathogenesis

The virus is confined to the respiratory epithelial cells, macrophages, and dendritic cells within the respiratory tract. Dissemination, even in immunocompromised patients, is rarely documented.

Immunity

Reinfection with parainfluenza viruses continues throughout life. Presence of virus specific IgE in nasopharyngeal secretions has been implicated in the development of parainfluenza croup or bronchiolitis.

Clinical features

Parainfluenza type 1 predominantly causes croup, while type 2 and 3 also cause bronchiolitis and pneumonia. Croup (or laryngotracheobronchitis) is associated with fever, hoarseness, and a barking cough and may progress to inspiratory stridor due to narrowing of the subglottic area of the trachea. The differential diagnosis is epiglottitis due to *Haemophilus influenzae* type b. Parainfluenza type 4 infection is rare, but causes bronchiolitis and pneumonia in children, often in those with underlying disease.

Reinfection in adults, when symptomatic, is a coryzal illness with hoarseness being prominent. Parainfluenza viruses (type 3 in particular) are significant causes of lower respiratory tract disease in adults when the virus is active in the community.

Parainfluenza viruses cause problems in immunocompromised patients (see section on RSV). Lower respiratory tract involvement is associated with wheezing, rales, dyspnoea, and diffuse interstitial infiltrates, and a fatal outcome in one-third of patients. When pneumonia occurs, the histological appearance of the lung is that of a giant cell or an interstitial pneumonia.

Treatment and prevention

The need for specific antiviral therapy arises, particularly in the immunocompromised. Ribavirin is effective *in vitro* but there are no controlled trials documenting its clinical efficacy. There are anecdotal reports of clinical efficacy as well the lack of it.

There are no options for prevention at present, either using vaccines or passive immunization. A live attenuated bovine-derived vaccine strain is currently undergoing clinical trials.

Influenza viruses

Influenza viruses contain a segmented RNA genome. Types A, B, and C are antigenically distinct; of these, types A and B are important in human disease. The viral envelope contains two glycoproteins, the haemagglutinin (H) and neuraminidase (N), which are critical in host immunity. Influenza viruses are designated by the virus type, place of isolation, strain designation, year of isolation, and the H and N antigen subtype, for example A/Sydney/5/95 (H3N2).

Epidemiology

The H and N genes of influenza types A, B, and C undergo mutational change resulting in the emergence of antigenic variants ('antigenic drift'). Every few years, a variant successful in evading the prior immunity of the human population emerges, to cause a global epidemic.

Fifteen H and 9 N subtypes of influenza A are found in aquatic birds, the natural reservoir of the virus. Human influenza A viruses in the first half of this century carried H1N1 surface antigens. In 1957, this virus acquired the genes for different H and N antigens (H2N2) by reassortment of its segmented genome with an avian virus ('antigenic shift'). The human population had no immunity to these new antigens and the virus caused the 'Asian flu' pandemic. A similar reassortment event gave rise to the H3N2 virus and the 'Hong Kong influenza' pandemic of 1968. While all three influenza pandemics this century resulted in significant morbidity and mortality, the toll exacted by the 'Spanish flu' of 1918 was horrendous—over 20 million deaths, greater than that of both World Wars combined. Since influenza B and C have no significant zoonotic reservoirs, antigenic shift and pandemics do not occur.

Avian viruses (e.g. subtype H5N1, H9N2) can occasionally infect humans without undergoing prior reassortment with existing human strains. The H5N1 virus that recently emerged in Hong Kong clearly had the potential to cause disease of unusual severity. However, such non-reassorted avian viruses do not appear to be efficiently transmitted between humans, a prerequisite for a pandemic virus. What might have happened had the H5N1 virus had the opportunity to undergo reassortment and adapt to transmission in humans is too horrifying to contemplate.

Pathogenesis

Viral replication occurs in the columnar epithelial cells leading to its desquamation down to the basal cell layer. The pathology involves the entire respiratory tract. Infection results in decreased ciliary clearance, impaired phagocyte function, and increased adherence of bacteria to viral infected cells, all of which promote the occurrence of secondary bacterial infection.

While there are differences in viral virulence (e.g. current H1N1 strains cause milder disease than H3N2), pre-existing cross-reactive immunity is a major determinant in reducing disease severity. Virus dissemination outside the respiratory tract is uncommon in humans, though it has been occasionally detected in the brain, heart, and fetus.

Immunity

Infection by an influenza virus results in long-lived immunity to homologous reinfection. However, the continued antigenic change in the virus allows it to keep ahead of the host immune response. Cross-immunity to 'drifted' strains within the same H or N subtype may provide partial protection, but there is little cross protection between different subtypes. Local and systemic antibody responses and cytotoxic T cells contribute to host protection.

Clinical features

Influenza ranges from asymptomatic infection, through the typical influenza syndrome, to the complications of influenza. While it cannot always be distinguished from other viral infections on clinical grounds, the typical influenza syndrome is relatively characteristic. It is associated with fever, chills, headache, sore throat, coryza, non-productive cough, myalgia, and sometimes prostration. The onset of illness is abrupt and the fever lasts 1 to 5 days. The pharynx is hyperaemic but does not have an exudate. Cervical lymphadenopathy is often present and crackles or wheezing are heard in around 10 per cent of patients. While the acute illness usually resolves in 4 to 5 days, the cough and fatigue may persist for weeks thereafter.

Common (>10 per cent of symptomatic patients) complications of influenza include otitis media (in children) and exacerbation of asthma, chronic obstructive airways disease, and cystic fibrosis. Less common complications are acute bronchitis, primary (viral) and secondary (bacterial) pneumonia, myocarditis, febrile convulsions, encephalopathy, encephalitis, and myositis (especially in patients with influenza B infection). Age, prior immunity, virus strain, the presence of underlying diseases, pregnancy, and smoking all influence morbidity and severity.

Treatment and prevention

Antiviral therapy

Antiviral drugs with proven clinical efficacy for treatment of influenza A are amantadine, rimatadine and a new class of antivirals, the neuraminidase inhibitors (e.g. zanamivir, oseltamivir). The neuraminidase inhibitors are also active against influenza B, while amantadine and rimatadine are not. All these drugs have maximal efficacy if administered early (within the first 48 h) in the illness.

Rimatadine has fewer neurological side-effects than amantadine. The former is mainly eliminated by the liver while amantadine is excreted by the kidney, a point relevant for patients with compromised renal or liver function. These drugs may be used for containing institutional outbreaks. However, the prophylactic efficacy may be lost if the index case is also treated, probably due to the emergence and transmission of resistant strains.

Preliminary data suggests that antiviral resistance may be less of a clinical problem with the neuraminidase inhibitors. Zanamivir is administered by inhalation, oseltamivir orally. There is limited clinical data suggesting efficacy of aerosolized ribavirin in therapy of influenza A and B.

Aspirin should be avoided in children with influenza because of the increased risk of Reye's syndrome.

Vaccines

Influenza vaccines contain antigens from the two subtypes of human influenza A (H3N2 and N1N1) and B viruses. To keep abreast of change in the surface antigens of the virus, its composition must be modified on an annual basis and annual reimmunization is required. To make global recommendations on vaccine composition and to maintain surveillance for emergence of influenza viruses with pandemic potential, the World Health Organization maintains a global network of collaborating laboratories.

Vaccines in use hitherto have been made from egg-grown viruses and contain: (a) inactivated whole virus, (b) detergent-treated virus (split virus vaccines), or (c) purified surface antigens (subunit of surface antigen vaccines). Split virus and subunit vaccines are associated with fewer side-effects in children (<12 years) and are therefore preferable. Previously unvaccinated children require two doses at least 1 month apart, whereas a single dose appears adequate for adults. These vaccines are generally safe, the most common side-effect being soreness at the injection site lasting a few days. Efficacy is best when there is a good antigenic match between the vaccine and outbreak virus. Immunogenicity and clinical protection are better in healthy young adults compared to patients with chronic renal failure, the immunocompromised, and the elderly (all groups most at need of the vaccine). However, the vaccine is still effective in reducing influenza and pneumonia-related hospitalization and mortality in the elderly and is cost-saving. In young adults, vaccination is associated with decreased absenteeism from work. The duration of protection is limited and therefore vaccine administration should be timed to precede the expected peak of influenza activity.

Influenza vaccine is recommended to those groups at highest risk of morbidity. Recommendations vary from country to country, but they usually include patients in chronic care facilities (especially the elderly), those with chronic cardiopulmonary, lung, or renal diseases, diabetes mellitus, haemoglobinopathies, and the immunocompromised. Some countries, such as the United States, extend the recommendation to all persons over 65 years, pregnant women who will be in the second or third trimester during the influenza season, children receiving long-term aspirin therapy (potentially at risk from Reye's syndrome if they acquire influenza), healthcare workers (particularly those in contact with the high-risk patient groups above), and household members of persons in high-risk groups. Currently, there is no consensus on the use of influenza vaccine in HIV infected patients.

An intranasally administered, cold-adapted, live attenuated vaccine has undergone clinical trials with promising results and may in future offer advantages of easier administration and greater patient acceptability.

Nosocomial infection

Respiratory viruses are efficient nosocomial pathogens. Although influenza and RSV are the most notorious, even rhinoviruses cause problems when transmitted to immunocompromised patients. Though paediatric units face the brunt of the problem, adult wards are not exempt. Transmission may occur from patient to patient, patient to staff, and staff to patient, with visitors making their own contribution.

While transmission occurs by large respiratory droplets gaining access to the mucosa of a susceptible individual, their dispersal range is short (<1 m). Much of the transmission occurs by direct hand contact. Adherence to strict hand-washing is the most critical preventive measure. Gloves are useful in reinforcing the 'hand-washing message', but will only be effective if they are changed between patients. Cohorting infected patients, either by symptoms (during the outbreak season) or by rapid viral diagnostic results, is useful. Influenza A vaccination of health-care workers, especially those caring for high-risk children, is to be recommended. Staff education is vital, including awareness of the fact that some of these viruses manifest themselves as a mild 'cold' in adults, and that infected staff members can transmit to patients under their care.

Further reading

Centers for Disease Control and Prevention (2001). *Prevention and control of influenza: recommendations of the Advisory Committee on Immunisation Practices* (ACIP). MMWR 50 (No.RR-4), pp. 1–65. Atlanta, GA. [Reviews the use of vaccines and antiviral therapy for influenza prophylaxis.]

Dolin R, Wright PF, eds (1999). *Viral infections of the respiratory tract.* Marcel Dekker, Basel, pp. 1–432. [Comprehensive monograph with chapters on each of the respiratory viruses, antiviral therapy, and on infections in immunocompromised patients.]

Dowell SF, ed (1998). Principles of judicious use of antimicrobial agents for pediatric upper respiratory tract infections. *Pediatrics* 101 (Suppl.), 163–84. [Journal supplement reviewing the use and abuse of antibiotics in upper respiratory tract infections.]

Gem JE, Busse WW (1999). Association of rhinovirus infections with asthma. *Clinical Microbiology reviews* 12, 9–18.

Han LL, Alexander JP, Anderson U (1999). Respiratory syncytial virus pneumonia among the elderly: An assessment of disease burden. *Journal of Infectious Diseases* 179, 25–30. [Key paper reviewing data on the role of RSV in respiratory disease of the elderly.]

Jacob John I, *et al.* (1991). Etiology of acute respiratory tract infections in children in tropical Southern India. *Reviews in Infectious Diseases* 13 (Suppl. 6), S463–9. [Describes the epidemiology of respiratory viruses in a tropical setting.]

Madeley CR, Peiris JSM, McQuillin J (1996). Adenoviruses. In: Myint S, Taylor-Robinson D, eds. *Viral and other infections of the human respiratory tract*, pp.169–90. Chapman and Hall, London. [Reviews the adenoviral respiratory disease and laboratory diagnosis.]

Nicholson KG, Webster RG, Hay AJ, eds. (1998). *Textbook of influenza*. Blackwell Scientific, Oxford. [Comprehensive review of the ecology, clinical features, and control of influenza.]

Shortridge KF (1995). The next pandemic influenza virus. *Lancet* **346**, 1210–12. [Reviews the genesis of pandemic influenza viruses in the context of its zoonotic origin.]

Siddell S, Myint S (1996). Coronaviruses. In: Myint S, Taylor-Robinson D, eds. *Viral and other infections of the human respiratory tract*. Chapman and Hall, London, pp. 141–67.

Treanor J (1997). Respiratory infections. In: Richman DD, Whitley RI, Hayden FG, eds. *Clinical virology*, pp. 5–33. Churchill Livingstone, New York. [Reviews viral respiratory infections.]

Yuen KY, *et al.* (1998). Clinical features and rapid viral diagnosis of human disease associated with avian influenza A H5N1. *Lancet* **351**, 467–71. [Describes the clinical features of an avian influenza outbreak with high morbidity and mortality.]

7.10.2 Herpesviruses (excluding Epstein–Barr virus)

J. G. P. Sissons

Human herpesviruses

General introduction

The family of Herpesviridae is widely distributed in the animal kingdom. More than 100 herpesviruses have been isolated from humans, primates, and other mammals, and from reptiles and fish. Comparative sequence analysis suggests they have been coevolving with their individual hosts for millions of years. To date, eight human herpesviruses have been identified, as summarized in Table 1. Herpesviruses have been assigned to three subfamilies, the alpha-, beta-, and gammaherpesvirinae, on the basis of shared genomic and biological properties. All the herpesviruses are characterized by a linear double-stranded DNA genome, contained inside an icosahedral capsid, which is surrounded by a protein tegument and an outer lipid envelope containing virus glycoprotein spikes. They are large viruses whose genomes consist of unique segments of DNA flanked by repeat sequences and encode most of the proteins needed for replication. Although differing in many of their biological properties, all herpesviruses share an important biological feature: their capacity to produce latent infection in their natural host, during which the viral genome persists in cells as a closed circular episome, only a limited subset of virus genes being expressed. Although individual viruses establish latency in different types of cell, this property is key to their ability to produce persistent lifetime infection of the host, and thus to persist in the population. The individual human herpesviruses, and their associated diseases are described in the succeeding chapters: these diseases may result from primary infection, or reactivation of the virus from latency, and tend to be more severe in immunosuppressed patients. The gammaherpesviruses can induce cell transformation and are associated with specific tumours.

Herpes simplex virus infections

Historical introduction

Herpes is a word derived from the Greek meaning to creep or crawl, apparently used since antiquity to describe the evolution of the skin lesions caused by herpes simplex virus (**HSV**) and varicella zoster virus (**VZV**). HSV was the first of the herpesviruses to be isolated, during the 1930s, after the infectious nature of the mucous membrane lesions it causes had been demonstrated by transmission to animals in 1919. The serological distinction of the two types of HSV, HSV-1 and HSV-2, and the association of HSV-2 with genital herpes was made in the 1960s. HSVs are now some of the most intensively studied human viruses.

Aetiology

HSV has a genome size of 150 kbp and codes for some 80 proteins. The genomes of HSV-1 and HSV-2 are largely colinear, but have different restriction endonuclease sites. Gene expression occurs in three temporally regulated phases of immediate-early, early, and late genes. Immediate-early proteins are largely regulatory proteins which prepare the cell to produce further virus, the early genes code particularly for enzymes involved in the replication of virus DNA, and the late genes for the structural proteins of the virion. Antigenic differences in the surface glycoprotein G are used to distinguish between HSV-1 and HSV-2. Release of progeny virus is normally accompanied by host-cell death—that is, the infection is lytic. The virus infects a relatively wide range of cells *in vitro*, and can also infect experimental animals thereby allowing studies of its pathogenesis.

Epidemiology

HSV is a ubiquitous virus, widely distributed in all populations of the world. Although the virus can produce experimental infections of animals, there are no natural animal hosts and humans are the only reservoir for the virus. Transmission occurs by direct contact of a susceptible individual with infected secretions from an HSV carrier. This is usually via transmission from oral, genital, or skin lesions to mucous membranes or abraded skin of the recipient. HSV carriers can excrete virus asymptomatically, and 1 to 15 per cent of adults excrete HSV at any one time. The prevalence of infection is conventionally assessed by the demonstration of antibody to HSV-1 or HSV-2. The prevalence of HSV-1 increases with age, although the time of acquisition of HSV-1 antibody varies depending on socioeconomic factors. There is a higher seroprevalence in lower socioeconomic groups in

Table 1 The human herpes viruses

Common name	Designation	Subfamily	Genome size (kb pairs)	Site of latency and persistence
Herpes simplex virus 1	Human herpesvirus 1	α	152	Neurones (sensory ganglia)
Herpes simplex virus 1	Human herpesvirus 2	α	152	–
Varicella zoster virus	Human herpesvirus 3	α	125	–
Epstein-Barr virus	Human herpesvirus 4	γ	172	B lymphocytes (oropharyngeal epithelium)
Human cytomegalovirus	Human herpesvirus 5	β	235	Blood monocytes (probably epithelial cells)
	Human herpesvirus 6	β	170	Monocytes, T lymphocytes
	Human herpesvirus 7	β	145	–
Kaposi sarcoma associated herpesvirus	Human herpesvirus 8	γ	230	Uncertain

early life: 70 to 90 per cent of individuals have antibodies by the age of 10 years, whereas only about 30 per cent of higher socioeconomic groups have antibody by this time. By mid-life 80 to 90 per cent of all individuals have antibody to HSV-1.

HSV-2 infection is usually acquired through sexual contact: consequently seroconversion correlates with the onset of sexual activity, and there is a progressive increase in seroprevalence to HSV-2 beginning in adolescence. The number of sexual contacts is a major risk factor for acquisition of HSV-2. Cumulative seroprevalence rates in adults vary from 10 to 80 per cent depending on the population and risk factors.

HSV can be transmitted to the neonate by infection (usually HSV-2) from maternal genital secretions at the time of delivery. Neonatal HSV infections usually occur in children born to mothers who are asymptomatic excretors of the virus and have no history of genital herpes.

Pathogenesis

HSV infects and replicates in epithelial cells at the site of inoculation on to mucous membranes or abraded skin, with an incubation period of between 4 and 6 days before clinical lesions appear. There is a marked local inflammatory response, but viraemia and dissemination may occur in the immunocompromised host. Following local epithelial replication, HSV enters the peripheral sensory nerves innervating the site of epithelial replication, and ascends the axons by retrograde transport to reach the dorsal root ganglia, or the trigeminal ganglion in the case of oral or conjunctival inoculation. The virus then becomes latent in sensory ganglia, but, despite extensive study, the mechanism of virus latency remains uncertain. Latent HSV-DNA is in an inactive state with minimal gene expression. RNA species called 'latency-associated transcripts' (**LATs**) are the only detectable transcripts. LATs have no detectable protein product and their deletion from the genome does not prevent the establishment of latency, although reactivation is impaired. Latent HSV is carried for the lifetime of the host, but may reactivate in response to certain stimuli including stress, menstruation, ultraviolet light, and immunosuppression. Upon reactivation, infectious virus is produced, travels down peripheral nerves by anterograde transport, and replicates in epithelial cells at the nerve ending. The neuronal latency of HSV and VZV is an extremely effective method of virus persistence. Latent virus in neuronal cells appears to be inaccessible to the immune response, and as it does not replicate, is not susceptible to the action of antiviral drugs. In addition to specific antibody, normal HSV carriers mount a cytotoxic T-lymphocyte response to the virus, which is presumed to control reactivation at local sites. HSV encodes genes which interfere with antigen processing by the class I MHC pathway, and are presumed to help the virus to evade the T-cell immune response. There is no good evidence that the immune response to HSV of people who have symptomatic reactivation episodes differs from that of asymptomatic carriers.

Clinical features

Primary infection with HSV is often asymptomatic: in a recent study of sexually active subjects, only 60 per cent of primary infections with HSV-1, and 40 per cent with HSV-2, were symptomatic. HSV-1 is the predominant cause of orofacial infections and HSV-2 the predominant cause of genital HSV infection, but the clinical manifestations overlap.

Gingivostomatitis

This is the commonest clinical form of primary infection with HSV-1. It is most often seen in children and has an incubation period of 2 to 12 days. Primary infection may be associated with a considerable systemic reaction, with fever, sore throat, pharyngeal oedema, and redness. Painful vesicles appear a few days later on the pharynx and the oral mucosa, lips, and the skin around the mouth: there may be cervical lymphadenopathy. Affected patients may have difficulty in eating, and the lesions last from 3 days to 2 weeks. The differential diagnosis includes other causes of pharyngitis including bacterial pharyngitis and herpangina (due to coxsackie A virus

infection): anterior vesicles and ulceration affecting the lips and skin around the mouth are more suggestive of HSV infection. Stevens–Johnson syndrome and severe aphthous ulceration may appear similar, and staphylococcal impetigo affecting the skin around the mouth can give a similar external appearance, but is not associated with oral ulceration.

Reactivation of HSV may give rise to recurrent orolabial lesions: appearing as intraoral mucosal ulcers, but more frequently as the classical 'cold sore' on the lips or skin around the mouth (Plate 1). Patients may first experience a tingling sensation in the area of impending ulceration 1 to 2 days prior to the appearance of vesicles. The lesions usually recur in the same site in individual patients. Around 25 per cent of HSV-1 seropositive people develop recurrent orolabial lesions: the majority have only one or two reactivation episodes per year, although a minority (less than 10 per cent) have more than one attack a month. These episodes are not associated with systemic symptoms and diagnosis is usually straightforward.

Infection at other cutaneous sites

Herpetic whitlow

HSV infection of the finger (herpetic whitlow) may complicate primary oral or genital herpes by autoinoculation of virus, or may occur through occupational exposure (for instance, in nursing, medical, and dental staff). There is oedema, erythema, and local tenderness of the infected finger. Lesions at the fingertip may be confused with pyogenic bacterial paronychias and incised (which is contraindicated for herpetic whitlow, and may even spread infection).

Herpes gladiatorum

This is a term which refers to mucocutaneous HSV infection occurring by transmission of infection through skin trauma, resulting from wrestling or other contact sports.

Eczema herpeticum

HSV infections of the skin are more severe in patients with pre-existing skin disease. In patients with eczema, burns, or other blistering skin diseases, HSV infection may become disseminated.

Cutaneous HSV infection can be confused with herpes zoster, although the latter is usually easy to diagnose by its unilateral dermatomal distribution.

Herpes simplex and erythema multiforme

About 15 per cent of all cases of erythema multiforme are preceded by a symptomatic attack of recurrent herpes simplex, and in susceptible individuals the characteristic rash can be induced by the intradermal inoculation of inactivated herpes simplex virus antigen. The rash of erythema multiforme starts several days after the onset of the herpetic vesicles, and in severe cases can involve the mucous membranes (Stevens–Johnson syndrome). The frequency of these attacks can be reduced by aciclovir prophylaxis.

Keratitis

HSV keratitis is characterized by the acute onset of pain, blurred vision, conjunctival injection, and dendritic ulceration of the cornea. HSV keratitis can cause corneal blindness and its treatment is urgent. Topical aciclovir is the drug of choice, for topical steroids may make the infection worse. HSV can also cause an acute necrotizing retinitis, usually seen in immunosuppressed subjects such as those with HIV infection, but rarely in immunocompetent people.

Genital herpes

Primary genital HSV infection is sexually transmitted and may be associated with systemic symptoms such as fever, headache, and myalgias. Symptoms tend to be more severe in women than in men. There is local pain and itching, dysuria, and vaginal discharge with inguinal lymphadenopathy, with vesicles and ulcers on the vulva, perineum, vagina, and cervix, and sometimes on the skin of the buttocks (Plate 2). In males, primary HSV lesions are seen as vesicles on the shaft or glans of the penis and there may be an associated urethritis. Most genital HSV infections are due to HSV-2, with a variable smaller proportion due to HSV-1. Only 40 per cent of primary HSV-2 genital infection is symptomatic: in patients who have had prior HSV-1 infection, the symptoms of primary genital herpes tend to be less severe. HSV has been isolated from the urethra in 5 per cent of women with the 'urethral syndrome', in the absence of obvious genital lesions. Other manifestations of genital tract disease due to primary HSV infection are, rarely, endometritis and salpingitis in women, and prostatitis in men.

HSV proctitis may follow rectal intercourse. There is anorectal pain and discharge with ulcerative lesions visible on sigmoidoscopy. Perianal lesions are seen in immunosuppressed patients, and spreading perianal HSV infection and HSV proctitis occur in patients with human immunodeficiency virus (**HIV**) infection.

Recurrent genital herpes is frequent in the first year following primary genital infection (90 per cent for HSV-2 and 55 per cent for HSV-1). Thereafter the recurrence rate tends to decrease with time and is around 3 or 4 attacks per year for HSV-2, but less for HSV-1. Severe recurrent genital herpes is particularly troublesome to women.

Complications of primary genital HSV infection include a sacral radiculomyelitis with urinary retention and hyperaesthesia of the perineal area, which usually resolves over several weeks. Aseptic meningitis requiring admission to hospital occurs in up to 7 per cent of women and 2 per cent of men, although suggestive symptoms are more common. Occasionally, and more seriously, transverse myelitis may occur.

HSV encephalitis (see also Viral infections of the CNS)

Encephalitis is the most serious type of disease produced by HSV in the normal immunocompetent host, and has an estimated annual incidence of 2 or 3 cases per million of population. It is the commonest identified cause of acute sporadic encephalitis in Western countries, with the great majority of cases due to HSV-1. There is a reported biphasic age incidence, with higher rates between the ages of 5 and 30 and in those over 50 years. The clinical presentation is that of a focal encephalitis, with an acute onset of fever, confusion and unusual behaviour, impaired consciousness, and possibly focal neurological abnormalities. However, as there are no clinical features specific to HSV encephalitis, the diagnosis should be considered in any patient who presents with clinical features that could indicate an encephalitis.

The cerebrospinal fluid (**CSF**) shows lymphocytic pleocytosis, although neutrophils and red cells may also be present, with a raised protein level. Computed tomographic (**CT**) scans of the brain may show changes in the temporal lobe: magnetic resonance imaging (**MRI**) is a more sensitive method of detection. The electroencephalogram (**EEG**) classically shows spike- and slow-wave activity localized in the temporal lobes. The most definitive way of establishing the diagnosis is by brain biopsy: in the original trial of aciclovir for the treatment of HSV encephalitis, brain biopsy was an entry criterion and confirmed the diagnosis in only 50 per cent of clinically suspected cases. Brain biopsy is very rarely used now, since the advent of non-toxic effective chemotherapy for HSV. There is good correlation between a positive polymerase chain reaction (**PCR**) test for HSV-DNA in the CSF and the diagnosis of HSV encephalitis by brain biopsy and virus isolation. Evidence for intrathecal production of specific HSV antibody is also diagnostic, but as it usually becomes positive a week after onset, PCR-based diagnosis is more useful. Serum or CSF titres of antibodies to HSV do not usually increase in the first week of the illness. In practice, the diagnosis is established by a compatible clinical picture, evidence of characteristic temporal lobe involvement on CT or MRI imaging and EEG, and by PCR-based detection of HSV-DNA in the CSF.

The pathogenesis of HSV encephalitis remains uncertain. Up to half of patients have primary infection and in the rest the disease is presumed to result from reactivation. However, where HSV has been isolated from the brain and the mouth simultaneously in the same patient, the two isolates differ by restriction endonuclease analysis in about 30 per cent of the patients, suggesting a new exogenous virus infection in an already seropositive patient. HSV-DNA can be detected in the brain at autopsy of normal virus carriers, but the factors precipitating HSV encephalitis are not known. Immunosuppression is not usually associated with HSV encephalitis, which predominantly affects normal immunocompetent adults, and very rarely patients with advanced HIV infection. The pathology is that of a focal haemorrhagic necrotizing encephalitis, affecting the temporal lobes.

Treatment

Treatment should be started immediately with intravenous aciclovir (in doses as given below) in any patient in whom HSV encephalitis is clinically suspected, without waiting for confirmation of the diagnosis. Prior to effective antiviral therapy, the mortality from HSV encephalitis was over 70 per cent with very few patients making a full neurological recovery. Intravenous aciclovir was established to be more effective than the previous best therapy of vidarabine in a randomized trial reported in 1986. Mortality in the aciclovir-treated group was 28 per cent, although a lower Glasgow Coma Score on entry carried a higher risk of mortality. However, only 38 per cent of those who received aciclovir had fully recovered at 6 months: there is thus still a high incidence of permanent neurological events, particularly seizures, defects of memory, and personality changes and the prognosis of HSV encephalitis remains serious.

Meningitis

HSV can cause an aseptic meningitis which is quite independent of, and not associated with progression to, HSV encephalitis. The commonest association is with primary genital HSV-2 infection: the incidence of proven HSV meningitis is 7 per cent in women, and 2 per cent in men, with primary genital HSV. There is a pleocytosis, usually lymphocytic, but neutrophils may predominate in early meningitis. HSV may be isolated from CSF by culture, but is now more reliably detected by PCR for HSV-DNA.

In a high proportion of patients with Mollaret's meningitis (a recurrent aseptic meningitis of unknown aetiology), HSV-DNA is reported to be detectable in cerebrospinal fluid by PCR.. The role of HSV in this syndrome remains uncertain.

An association of HSV with Bell's palsy has been reported, but a recent Cochrane review considered the evidence was inconclusive.

Neonatal HSV infection and pregnancy

The incidence of neonatal HSV infection is approximately 1 in 3500 deliveries per annum in the United States, but appears to be rarer in the United Kingdom at 1.65 in 100 000 live births. About 70 per cent of cases are caused by HSV-2 and result from fetal acquisition of HSV-2 from maternal genital secretions during delivery. Most infants with neonatal HSV are born to mothers without clinically evident HSV infection. The risk of transmission from a woman with symptomatic primary HSV infection is about 50 per cent, and 20 per cent from a woman with clinically evident recurrent HSV-2 infection. A small proportion (about 10 per cent) of infections are acquired postnatally by contact with other family members with active lesions.

Neonatal HSV infection appears as lesions on the skin, eye, and mouth or may present as encephalitis or disseminated visceral infection. Although initial superficial infection may progress to visceral infection, visceral infection can present with no evidence of cutaneous lesions, and the diagnosis should be considered in severely ill neonates. Untreated, visceral infection has a high mortality (around 60 per cent).

Primary infection in early pregnancy can lead to congenital HSV infection. This is rare, but can produce serious congenital abnormalities.

HSV in the immunosuppressed patient

HSV infections in immunosuppressed subjects are usually due to reactivation rather than primary infection. They tend to be more severe, are more likely to progress, and take longer to heal than in the normal immunocompetent host. Clinical manifestations in patients with HIV infection include severe perineal, orofacial, and oesophageal infection. HSV pneumonitis, hepatitis, and colitis are also described in immunosuppressed patients.

Pathology

The histological appearance of HSV infection is identical whether infection is primary or recurrent. There is ballooning of infected cells with condensed chromatin in the cell nuclei. Intranuclear inclusion bodies (Cowdrie type A bodies) may be seen and multinucleated giant cells form. VZV produces similar appearances.

Laboratory diagnosis

Definitive diagnosis is made by isolation of virus: swabs from vesicular fluid or other body fluids in virus transport medium can be inoculated into tissue culture and typical cytopathic effects seen. Virus from vesicle fluid can also be identified rapidly as a herpesvirus by electron microscopy after negative staining. The use of PCR-based techniques to detect viral DNA is becoming more widespread. It is particularly applicable to the detection of HSV-DNA in cerebrospinal fluid.

Serological tests for antibody to HSV are only useful in making a retrospective diagnosis. Seroconversion provides proof of primary infection and absence of antibody to HSV-1 or HSV-2 rules out a diagnosis of recurrent HSV infection. However, making a diagnosis of reactivation by demonstrating rising antibody titres is of limited value.

Treatment

The introduction of aciclovir heralded a new era of targeted antiviral drugs and superseded other drugs previously used for the treatment of HSV infections such as vidarabine and idoxuridine. Aciclovir is an acyclic nucleoside which is preferentially phosphorylated in HSV-infected cells by the virus-encoded thymidine kinase to aciclovir monophosphate. Cellular kinases then phosphorylate the aciclovir monophosphate to the triphosphate, which is incorporated into nascent HSV-DNA where it acts as a chain terminator; aciclovir also directly inactivates the HSV-DNA polymerase. Two newer related drugs with the same mechanism of action are famciclovir, a prodrug of penciclovir, and valaciclovir, the valyl ester of aciclovir, which has greater bioavailability and requires less frequent dosage. All these drugs are relatively free of side-effects, although intravenous aciclovir can crystallize in the renal parenchyma and produce renal impairment: it should be given by infusion over 1 hour, and patients should be adequately hydrated. The doses should be reduced in patients with renal impairment.

Primary mucocutaneous infection

In primary oral and genital infection aciclovir 200 mg, 5 times daily, given orally for 10 to 14 days from the onset, reduces the severity of infection, the duration of symptoms, and the duration of viral shedding. There is little evidence that treatment of primary infections reduces the incidence of subsequent symptomatic reactivation episodes. If swallowing is difficult, intravenous aciclovir (5 mg/kg, every 8 h) may need to be given. Famciclovir, 250 mg thrice daily, or valaciclovir, 500 mg twice daily, are alternatives.

Symptomatic reactivation of mucocutaneous infection

Treatment of recurrent infections in the immunocompetent host is often unnecessary as the symptoms are usually very mild. However, aciclovir can shorten the duration of symptoms if it is given very early in the course of the recurrence, preferably during the prodrome before vesicles appear. Oral aciclovir is effective and anecdotal reports suggest that topical aciclovir is effective symptomatically. The same dosage as above for treating a primary infection can be given for 5 days: famciclovir and valaciclovir can be used as alternatives.

Long-term suppressive therapy

This can be considered in immunocompetent patients with genital herpes who have frequent reactivation episodes. Trials of aciclovir in recurrent genital herpes have shown that a dose of 400 mg twice a day significantly reduces the frequency of attacks. However, patients may be able to find a lower effective dose, and in some 200 mg daily prevents attacks. Although it is advised that treatment is discontinued for a month every 6 to 12 months, there is little evidence that resistant virus is a problem in this population. Valaciclovir, 500 mg daily, or famciclovir, 250 mg twice daily, are alternatives.

CNS infection

For HSV encephalitis intravenous aciclovir (10 mg/kg, every 8 h for 10–14 days) should be given to any patient in whom the diagnosis is clinically suspected (see above).

For HSV meningitis intravenous aciclovir (5 mg/kg, every 8 h) can be used with conversion to oral valaciclovir (1 g, twice daily) when improvement occurs, for a total of 10 days.

Systemic infection in the immunosuppressed

Oral treatment as for primary HSV can be used for mild mucocutaneous infection, but for more severe infection and for visceral involvement intravenous aciclovir 5 mg/kg every 8 h should be used. After resolution, continued prophylaxis is usually necessary until immunocompetence is restored, particularly in patients with HIV.

Aciclovir resistance

Resistance of HSV to aciclovir develops readily *in vitro* but is clinically rare: it is due to mutations in the HSV thymidine kinase or DNA polymerase gene. It is seen almost exclusively in immunocompromised patients who have received prolonged aciclovir prophylaxis, especially those with HIV infection, and is manifest as unresponsive or worsening HSV disease despite treatment with aciclovir. There is usually cross-resistance to famciclovir and valaciclovir, and intravenous foscarnet (more usually used to treat human cytomegalovirus infection, see the HMCV section) is the most useful alternative drug for use in severe infection due to resistant HSV.

Prevention and control

There is no vaccine yet available for HSV, although several candidates are approaching phase III trials. There is particular interest in the use of vaccines for postinfective immunization to reduce the frequency of recurrent genital HSV attacks (which has been shown to be possible experimentally in guinea-pigs).

Special problems in pregnant women

Prevention of neonatal HSV infection is best achieved by preventing genital HSV infection late in pregnancy. There is no reason to give aciclovir prophylactically to women with a history of recurrent genital herpes who are asymptomatic, as the incidence of neonatal HSV infection is low in their children. However, women with clinically apparent genital herpes during the last trimester (and probably at any other time in pregnancy) can be treated with aciclovir (although the drug is not licensed for treatment in pregnancy). Women with no clinical lesions may have a vaginal delivery, but the presence of active lesions at the time of labour is regarded as an indication for Caesarean section. Babies born to mothers with clinically apparent genital HSV infection or with a history of recurrent genital HSV infection should be screened for HSV by cultures from the nasopharynx and eyes after birth.

Proven neonatal HSV infection should be treated with high-dose intravenous aciclovir (60 mg/kg per day in three divided doses for 21 days).

Varicella zoster virus infection

Historical introduction

There are clinical descriptions of varicella (chickenpox) and herpes zoster (shingles) in very early medical literature, although the skin lesions of herpes simplex and herpes zoster were grouped together under the term 'herpes'. The similarities between the exanthematous rashes associated with smallpox and with varicella meant they were not distinguished until the latter part of the nineteenth century. Because of its characteristic clinical appearance in a dermatomal distribution, shingles was recognized as a discrete entity in the early Greek literature: the term 'zoster' is said to derive from the Greek term for a girdle, and shingles from the Latin *cingere* meaning to encircle. Von Bocquet in 1892 observed that children developed varicella after contact with adults who had herpes zoster, and in 1925 it was shown that vesicular fluid from patients with zoster produced chickenpox in susceptible individuals when directly inoculated. The idea that zoster resulted from reactivation of latent virus remaining in the individual following childhood varicella was put forward by Garland in 1943, and was strengthened by the work of Hope-Simpson, a British general practitioner. Varicella zoster virus (VZV) was isolated in 1958, and Weller and colleagues showed the similarity of the viral isolates from varicella and zoster. Identity by restriction endonuclease analysis has been shown between the isolates from chickenpox and from later zoster in the same individual, although this was an immunocompromised patient: the long interval between the two illnesses in normal subjects means such studies have never been conducted in this population.

Aetiology

VZV is structurally similar to other members of the Herpesviridae family. The genome is a linear double-stranded DNA of 125 kilobase pairs. The virus is closely cell-associated and spreads from cell to cell in tissue culture. VZV is an alphaherpesvirus, and encodes sets of genes which are largely colinear to those of HSV, and are also expressed in immediate-early, early, and late phases.

Epidemiology

VZV only infects humans, who are thus the only reservoir. The virus is presumed to spread by the respiratory route. Varicella is predominantly a disease of childhood affecting both sexes: 90 per cent of cases occur in children under the age of 13. The incubation period of varicella from exposure to VZV to development of the initial rash is about 2 weeks (with a range of 10–20 days). Patients with varicella are infectious for about 48 h before the vesicles appear, and remain so for 4 or 5 days afterwards until all the vesicles have crusted over. Secondary attack rates in susceptible contacts where there is an index case in the household are between 70 and 90 per cent. The prevalence of VZV varies in different ethnic groups. After 15 years of age only about 10 per cent of subjects in Europe are seronegative for, and consequently susceptible to, infection, although in tropical countries only 50 per cent of young adults may be seropositive. Varicella in adulthood is uncommon in Europe, with less than 2 per cent of all cases occurring in patients older than 20 years.

After primary infection, VZV becomes latent in dorsal root ganglia. Reactivation appears clinically as herpes zoster (shingles), which is a common disease that can affect all age groups but particularly the elderly: about 20 per cent of the population will experience an attack. There is no evidence that exposure to people with active VZV infection predisposes to herpes zoster in their contacts, but a seronegative subject may catch varicella from contact with the vesicles of a patient with shingles. As nosocomial varicella infection is well recognized, isolation of patients with varicella and immunocompromised patients with herpes zoster should be ensured in hospitals. Local unidermatomal zoster is less likely to cause infection and consequently to need isolation. Subclinical infection is unusual and accounts for less than 5 per cent of all infections, but the disease may be mild and in some surveys only 10 per cent of people with a negative history were in fact seronegative for VZV. One attack of chickenpox usually confers life-long immunity.

Pathogenesis

Upon primary infection, initial virus replication probably occurs in the epithelial cells of the upper respiratory tract mucosa, followed by a phase of viraemia during which VZV can be isolated from leucocytes. This blood-borne spread is associated with the production of the disseminated rash. In the skin, the virus infects capillary endothelial cells and adjacent fibroblasts and epithelial cells. During the viraemic phase virus may spread to visceral organs, the lung including alveolar epithelial cells, and transient subclinical hepatitis is probably a normal feature of varicella. Infection of the brain can occur, and VZV encephalitis may be a feature of primary infection, particularly affecting the cerebellum. The encephalitis usually recovers completely (unlike that associated with HSV), and it has been suggested it may have an immune-mediated pathogenesis. Following recovery from primary infection, the virus persists for life in a latent state in dorsal root ganglia. VZV reaches the ganglia by retrograde axonal transport from the lesions in the skin during primary infection, and all dorsal root ganglia and the trigeminal ganglion can potentially carry latent VZV in neurones and possibly in satellite cells.

As for other herpesviruses, the host response is critical in containing the initial infection. The cellular immune response is of particular importance since varicella may be progressive in patients with severely impaired T-cell immunity. Both CD4 and CD8 cytotoxic T lymphocytes specific for VZV are present in normal people carrying latent VZV. The cellular immune response presumably plays a part in controlling reactivation, since impaired T-cell immunity is associated with an increased risk of developing zoster, with zoster in multiple dermatomes, and with cutaneous dissemination of reactivated virus. The increasing risk of herpes zoster with age may reflect waning cellular immunity to VZV.

Clinical features

Primary infection and varicella (chickenpox)

The most striking feature of varicella is the rash, which is centripetal (mainly on the trunk) in distribution (Plate 3). Initially, lesions are present on the face and scalp, before progressing to the trunk and later to the limbs. A macular erythematous rash, papules, and vesicles may all be present together. Individual lesions progress from being papular to vesicles to pustules and then crust over. The scabs normally separate after 10 days without scarring. The systemic symptoms associated with varicella vary considerably. In the majority of children there is a mild illness with fever. Adults characteristically have a more severe illness with myalgias, headache, arthralgias, malaise, and higher fever, with the complications listed below. Symptoms may precede the rash by 1 to 2 days.

The principal complications of varicella in the immunocompetent person are pneumonitis and encephalitis.

Pneumonitis

A prospective study showed that 6 per cent of young adults with chickenpox had respiratory symptoms, but 16 per cent had changes on chest radiography, although the rate of admission to hospital with pneumonia in adults with varicella is only about 0.3 per cent. Patients present with dyspnoea, cough, hypoxia, and bilateral infiltrates on the chest radiograph occurring 1 to 6 days after the appearance of the rash. Hypoxia may be more severe than expected from the physical signs or the chest radiograph. The interstitial pneumonitis can progress to respiratory failure requiring artificial ventilation and intensive care, but it is more commonly transient and resolves completely within 2 to 3 days. Varicella pneumonia is said to be commoner in smokers. Fatalities do occur but the great majority of patients survive, and VZV pneumonia is not associated with long-term respiratory problems. Benign nodular calcification throughout the lung occasionally follows.

Encephalitis

Central nervous system involvement during varicella infection most commonly presents as an acute cerebellar ataxia within a week of the onset of the rash, although it may present as late as 21 days after the rash: it resolves completely over 2 to 4 weeks. A frequency of 1 in 4000 cases of children under the age of 15 years has been quoted. The cerebrospinal fluid of these patients shows a lymphocytosis and elevated protein concentration.

A more serious encephalitis can occur in between 0.1 and 0.2 per cent of cases of varicella. This begins earlier in the course of infection than the cerebellar ataxia, with headache, vomiting, confusion, and impaired consciousness. There is evidence of diffuse cerebral oedema but no defined pattern of CT or MRI abnormality. The encephalitis may be progressive and the mortality is between 5 and 20 per cent with neurological sequelae in up to 15 per cent of survivors.

A meningitis can occur with varicella. Other rare neurological complications reported include optic neuritis, transverse myelitis, and Reye's syndrome.

Other complications

Other complications of primary VZV infection include acute thrombocytopenia with petechiae and purpura and haemorrhage into vesicles and other haemorrhagic manifestations. The platelet count can remain low for weeks after the illness has resolved. Secondary infection of the skin lesions with *Staphylococcus aureus* or *Streptococcus pyogenes* can occur. Purpura fulminans is a rare complication associated with arterial thrombosis and haemorrhagic gangrene. Nephritis and arthritis have been reported as rare complications and myocarditis, pericarditis, pancreatitis, and orchitis are even more rare.

Special problems in pregnant women

Varicella in pregnant women can be severe, with a quoted maternal mortality of 1 per cent. Varicella in the first trimester can cause 'varicella embryopathy': in affected infants there may be a scarred atrophic limb, microcephaly, and cortical atrophy, as well as eye defects, including chorioretinitis, micro-ophthalmia, and cataracts. The autonomic nervous system may be damaged. Varicella embryopathy is rare in recent reported series, giving a risk of about 1 to 2 per cent in mothers with varicella in the first 20 weeks of pregnancy. Varicella zoster immune globulin (**VZIG**) should be considered for pregnant women in contact with varicella (see below), and varicella during pregnancy should be treated with aciclovir on a named patient basis. Neonatal varicella occurs in babies whose mothers contract varicella just prior to or after delivery, and is more severe when the maternal onset is from 2 days before to a week after delivery.

Herpes zoster

The clinical syndrome associated with reactivation of VZV from sensory ganglia is herpes zoster (shingles). This typically presents with pain followed by erythema and vesicular lesions occurring in a dermatomal distribution. The thoracic dermatomes, especially T5 to T12, are involved in about 50 per cent, lumbosacral dermatomes in about 16 per cent, and cranial nerves, mainly the Vth, in 14 to 20 per cent of patients. The first symptoms are usually paraesthesias and shooting pains in the affected dermatome, which precede the eruption of vesicles by several days and occasionally a week or more. Erythematous maculopapular lesions then appear and quickly evolve into a vesicular rash, nearly always in a unilateral dermatome with no vesicles beyond the midline. The vesicles usually form scabs after 3 to 7 days and these separate after 2 weeks or so. There is a risk of secondary infection, particularly with *Staphylococcus aureus*. There may be malaise and low-grade fever, but there are usually no abnormalities of laboratory investigations, although up to 40 per cent of patients with uncomplicated zoster may have lymphocytes and elevated protein concentrations in the CSF. Involvement of the mandibular branch of the Vth cranial nerve can give intraoral lesions on the palate, floor of the mouth, and tongue. Involvement of the geniculate ganglion results in the Ramsay Hunt syndrome, with pain and vesicles in the external auditory meatus, a loss of taste in the anterior two-thirds of the tongue, and a lower motor neurone VIIth cranial nerve palsy.

Complications of zoster

Ophthalmic zoster VZV reactivation from the trigeminal ganglion can affect the ophthalmic division of the trigeminal nerve resulting in ophthalmic zoster (Plate 4). The features include conjunctivitis, anterior uveitis, a keratitis, and sometimes iridocyclitis with secondary glaucoma and panophthalmitis. However, these latter sight-threatening complications of ophthalmic zoster are unusual. A rare association of ophthalmic zoster is granulomatous cerebral angiitis, which can be associated with arterial thrombosis: cerebral angiography shows segmental narrowing in cerebral arteries on the side of the ophthalmic zoster. CT scanning may show cerebral infarcts, particularly in the distribution of the middle cerebral artery.

Motor zoster Weakness or paralysis can sometimes be associated with zoster, and is due to involvement of the anterior horn cells in the same segment of the spinal cord as the involved dorsal root ganglion. Depending on the segment involved, this can lead to a monoparesis affecting the upper or lower limb or to diaphragmatic palsy (with involvement of C5/6). Paralysis usually recovers completely, although the outlook for recovery of facial nerve palsy is more variable. It is suggested VZV may be responsible for some cases of 'idiopathic' VIIth nerve (Bell's) palsy.

Autonomic zoster Lumbosacral herpes zoster can be associated with a neurogenic bladder and acute retention of urine, which may be accompanied by haemorrhagic cystitis due to vesicles on the bladder wall. Intestinal ileus and obstruction may occur.

Zoster meningoencephalitis A meningoencephalitis may accompany zoster at any site and is characterized by impaired consciousness, headache, photophobia, and meningism. The interval from the onset of skin lesions to symptoms of encephalitis is around 9 days, but may be as long as 6 weeks. Symptomatic encephalitis usually lasts around 2 weeks and is nearly always followed by full recovery without neurological sequelae.

A transverse myelitis, although rare, can occur at any level of the spinal cord.

Postherpetic neuralgia The incidence of postherpetic neuralgia rises with increasing age of the patient. It is uncommon in young people, but can occur in 50 per cent of patients over the age of 50 years. It is characterized by pain in the affected dermatome persisting for 1 month or more after the acute attack of zoster has resolved. The pain may be steady and burning or paroxysmal and stabbing in nature: it may occur spontaneously or be triggered by stimuli such as temperature or touch.

Zoster sine herpete This term refers to a syndrome characterized by radicular pain, similar to that experienced in zoster, but without any antecedent skin lesions of zoster. It was originally applied to patients who did have obvious zoster, but had dermatomal pain in areas distinct from those areas where there was rash: however, subsequently it has usually been applied to patients with radicular pain and no rash at all. There are more recent reports describing the use of PCR testing for the detection of VZV-DNA in the CSF of patients with presumed zoster sine herpete. The literature is anecdotal, and it is difficult to regard zoster sine herpete as a diagnostic entity unless there is good evidence for VZV involvement, for instance as shown by the detection of VZV-DNA in CSF and/or blood mononuclear cells. It should be kept in mind, however, as a possible explanation for radicular pain of unknown cause: any possible mechanism is speculative.

Varicella zoster virus infection in the immunosuppressed patient

In patients with immunosuppression, particularly of cellular immunity, varicella can be much more severe (Plate 3). The skin lesions are more diffuse and can take up to three times as long to heal. There may be visceral dissemination to the lungs, liver, and central nervous system. Patients with lymphomas being treated with chemotherapy are particularly susceptible.

Herpes zoster in immunosuppressed patients is also more severe than in normal subjects. Prior to the availability of effective antiviral therapy, skin lesions were more extensive and could take several weeks longer to heal. Dissemination, presumably due to viraemic spread, with widespread skin lesions as in varicella, occurs in 10 to 40 per cent of patients. Cutaneous dissemination is more likely to be associated with visceral dissemination to the same sites as those associated with varicella.

Patients with HIV infection and the acquired immunodeficiency syndrome (**AIDS**) are prone to multidermatomal zoster, which can be one of the defining features of AIDS.

VZV retinitis

This presents with pain and blurred vision in one eye, with progressive necrotizing retinitis seen on ophthalmoscopy. Adjacent cutaneous zoster indicates the diagnosis, but occasionally VZV retinitis can present in immunocompetent patients as the sole manifestation of VZV reactivation. VZV retinitis may be difficult to distinguish from cytomegalovirus (**CMV**) retinitis. A severe form of the disease, seen particularly in patients with HIV infection, is known as progressive outer retinal necrosis: it is associated with a high incidence of retinal detachment and may require treatment with ganciclovir as aciclovir is often ineffective.

Differential diagnosis

Varicella is usually recognized relatively easily. Other causes of a vesicular rash are generalized herpes simplex in the immunosuppressed patient and enterovirus disease, particularly hand, foot, and mouth disease due to coxsackievirus infection, but the rash on the hands and feet is unlike that of varicella which has a centripetal distribution. Human cases of infection with animal pox viruses (monkey pox and camel pox) have rarely been described.

Pathology

Histological appearances of VZV infection are similar or indistinguishable from those of HSV infection.

Laboratory diagnosis

The diagnosis of varicella and herpes zoster are usually made on clinical criteria alone. Virus can be seen in vesicular fluid by electron microscopy or isolated in culture. Serological diagnosis of varicella can be made by demonstrating seroconversion or VZV-IgM antibody. Urgent serology is needed to confirm the seronegative status of contacts at risk of severe VZV infection, to determine the need for VZV immunoglobulin (see below). PCR-based tests for the detection of VZV-DNA are available, and are most useful in testing CSF in cases of suspected central nervous system disease.

Treatment

Pruritus may be alleviated in patients with chickenpox by calamine lotion and antihistamines. Fingernails should be closely cut to minimize scratching. Skin care is important to prevent secondary bacterial infection in patients with varicella and zoster. Aspirin should be avoided in children with chickenpox because of the risk of Reye's syndrome. Strong analgesia may be needed in patients with zoster.

VZV is sensitive to the nucleoside analogues, aciclovir (aciclovir), famciclovir, and valaciclovir: as for HSV, VZV encodes a thymidine kinase which preferentially phosphorylates these drugs in infected cells. The median 50 per cent inhibitory concentration of aciclovir against HSV is 0.1 μmol/l, but it is 2.6 μmol/l against VZV and consequently 800 mg orally is necessary to achieve inhibitory concentrations against VZV.

Treatment recommendations for varicella and herpes zoster are summarized in Table 2.

Varicella

Whether to treat normal children with varicella (who are the great majority of patients) has been much debated. The argument can be made that it is not possible to predict which child may have a severe case and the disease is not always mild. Therapy with aciclovir is safe and, although it has been suggested that widespread treatment with antivirals might result in viral resistance or failure to develop normal immune responses, there is no evidence of this in controlled trials. Treatment with aciclovir begun within 24 h of the onset of rash leads to a 25 per cent decrease in the duration and

Table 2 Use of aciclovir in varicella zoster infections

Indications for intravenous aciclovir (10 mg/kg, every 8 h)
Chickenpox:
Immunocompromised patients
Neonatal chickenpox
Chickenpox with systemic complications
Severe chickenpox in adults and during pregnancy **(5 mg/kg, 8-hourly)**

Shingles:
Severe shingles in immunocompromised patients
Multidermatomal shingles
Shingles complicated by ocular, motor, autonomic, or systemic involvement
v2v retinitis (severe forms in AIDS may require foscarnet or ganciclovir)

Indications for oral aciclovir (800 mg, 5 times daily)
Uncomplicated chickenpox
Uncomplicated shingles in patients over 45 years
Uncomplicated shingles in immunosuppressed patients
Shingles presenting with severe pain

Infections not requiring active antiviral treatment
Uncomplicated, mild chickenpox in children
Patients presenting more than 48 h after appearance of last lesion or when all lesions have crusted
Uncomplicated shingles in patients under 45 years
Postherpetic neuralgia

severity of chickenpox. The argument for treating all adolescents and adults is easier, as chickenpox is more severe for them than it is for young children. Chickenpox in neonates, children with leukaemia, and transplant recipients, should always be treated with aciclovir: intravenously administered aciclovir limits the visceral spread of the virus if given immediately on diagnosis. Treatment in these immunosuppressed patients can be changed from intravenous to oral aciclovir once the fever has settled, if there is no evidence of visceral varicella.

Herpes zoster

The major justification for the antiviral treatment of herpes zoster in immunocompetent patients has been to limit postherpetic neuralgia. Although there are difficulties in accurately and objectively quantifying the pain of postherpetic neuralgia, trial data indicates that acyclovir, valaciclovir, and famciclovir can limit the duration of zoster-associated pain and that valaciclovir is slightly more effective. Acyclovir, valaciclovir, and famciclovir accelerate the healing of cutaneous lesions by 2 days over placebo. Valaciclovir and famciclovir have the advantage of more convenient dosage, as well as being probably slightly more effective.

Patients with zoster over the age of 50 are at the highest risk of postherpetic neuralgia and should consequently be offered antiviral treatment. Patients younger than this may warrant treatment if they have marked pain. All patients with ophthalmic zoster should be treated with antiviral agents, even if they present relatively late, as acyclovir reduces the incidence of keratitis. Immunosuppressed patients with herpes zoster should receive intravenous acyclovir to prevent cutaneous and visceral dissemination of VZV. Valaciclovir and famciclovir may be used if zoster presents in a localized form in less severely immunosuppressed patients.

Corticosteroids have been advocated in patients with herpes zoster, in order to reduce the severity of postherpetic neuralgia. However, in recent trials the addition of oral prednisone to acyclovir resulted in a slightly increased rate of healing of skin lesions but did not affect the incidence of postherpetic neuralgia. The place of corticosteroids thus remains unproven.

Prevention and control

Varicella zoster immune globulin (VZIG), prepared from high-titre immune human serum, has been shown to prevent or ameliorate varicella in seronegative individuals at high risk, such as immunocompromised patients and pregnant women. Seronegative immunodeficient patients (including those on high-dose corticosteroid treatment) and pregnant women with definite contact with varicella are candidates for VZIG administration. It should be administered within 10 days (preferably 2–4) of exposure. Neonates whose mothers have had varicella less than a week before delivery or within 28 days after delivery are also recommended for VZIG administration.

A vaccine is available for VZV. This is the Oka strain of VZV, which is a live attenuated vaccine developed in Japan. It induces 90 per cent protection from natural varicella when administered to non-immune immunosuppressed individuals (such as patients with leukaemias and lymphomas treated with chemotherapy), but it can produce a vaccine-induced rash in up to 40 per cent of such recipients. In immunized healthy children the risk of subsequent varicella after community exposure is reduced to less than 5 per cent, and vaccine-induced rash is much less common (about 5 per cent of recipients). This vaccine is licensed in Japan, some European countries, and the United States, where it is recommended for routine immunization in children aged between 12 and 18 months, but not in the United Kingdom where it is available on a named patient basis only for use in non-immune immunosuppressed subjects. Trials are in progress to assess whether postinfective immunization with the vaccine can diminish the incidence of zoster in those over the age of 50 years: it has already been shown to boost pre-existing cell-mediated immunity to VZV in this age group.

Nosocomial transmission of VZV from those patients with varicella who require admission to hospital is a significant risk as 10 per cent of adults are seronegative. The nursing and management of inpatients with varicella should be restricted to those staff known to be seropositive for VZV. Patients with varicella in hospital should ideally be isolated in negative-pressure rooms to prevent airborne transmission.

Human cytomegalovirus infection

Historical introduction

The syndrome of congenital cytomegalovirus infection 'cytomegalic inclusion disease' was described in children with fatal infection in 1904, but the intranuclear inclusions were attributed to a protozoan parasite. In 1921, the pathologist Goodpasture suggested the inclusions in the parotid glands of infants were caused by a virus, because a filterable agent produced similar histology in guinea-pig salivary glands, and the lesions were attributed in 1926 to 'salivary gland virus'. Human cytomegalovirus (**HCMV**) was finally isolated in 1956, and so named by Weller for the characteristic 'owl's eye', or cytomegalic, inclusions it produces in the nucleus of infected cells.

HCMV produces little morbidity in the immunocompetent, but can produce severe disease in the fetus if infection is acquired *in utero*, and in the immunosuppressed patient.

Aetiology

HCMV is the largest human herpesvirus with a linear double-stranded DNA genome of 250 kb encoding over 200 proteins. It can be grown in tissue culture in human fibroblasts. Mammalian cytomegaloviruses are species-specific, and so HCMV cannot be studied in animal models. The most widely studied laboratory strain, AD169, shows significant genomic variation from recent clinical isolates which possess an additional 15 kb of DNA. They can infect and replicate in macrophages, which are probably an important site of latency for this wild-type virus. HCMV replicates slowly compared to other herpesviruses: gene expression occurs in sequential immediate-early, early, and late phases.

Epidemiology

Following primary infection, HCMV persists for life as a latent infection with periodic asymptomatic excretion of virus in saliva, breast milk, urine, semen, and cervical secretions. Infection is spread by close contact with

these body fluids. In less developed countries HCMV is usually acquired in childhood and seropositivity is nearly 100 per cent in young adults. In more developed countries seropositivity increases with age, but seroprevalence is higher in lower socioeconomic groups. Overall, about 50 per cent of adults are seropositive. During childhood, HCMV is acquired from breast milk or contact with other infected children excreting virus in their saliva or urine: studies in day nurseries have shown transmission between children as well as to susceptible adult carers. Later, sexual transmission becomes a major route of infection: seroprevalence approaches 100 per cent in homosexual men and sex workers.

Blood and blood products from seropositive donors can transmit HCMV. Transfusion recipients at risk of HCMV disease now usually receive screened seronegative blood, otherwise the risk of transfusion-related HCMV infection is 2.5 per cent per unit of blood. Transmission results from virus in leucocytes, but leucodepletion of blood (now being widely adopted as a preventive measure against transmissible spongiform encephalopathies) greatly reduces the risk of HCMV transmission. Finally, solid organ and bone marrow transplants from seropositive donors can transmit HCMV, and produce particularly severe disease in seronegative recipients.

Pathogenesis

Current evidence suggests myeloid lineage cells are a principal site of HCMV latency, and that virus may be reactivated when monocytes acquire a permissive phenotype as they differentiate into macrophages. Other cells, including endothelial cells and possibly epithelial cells, may also be sites of latency.

The immune response is critical in controlling infection in the normal host. Normal immunocompetent infected individuals mount a strong T-cell response, with very high frequencies of cytotoxic (CD8+) T lymphocytes in the peripheral blood particularly targeted at the HCMV major tegument protein (pp65) and the major immediate-early protein (IE1). Impairment of this response is associated with the risk of disseminated infection. HCMV possesses at least four genes whose products interfere with the class I MHC antigen-processing pathway, and a number of other potential 'immune evasion' genes, which may help the virus reactivate by delaying immune recognition of infected cells. Natural killer cells may be active early in the infection. Antibody probably limits the blood-borne dissemination of HCMV, as maternal IgG appears to be especially important in preventing viral transmission to the fetus. Subclinical reactivation occurs frequently in the normal host but is controlled by the immune response. Immune deficiency, particularly of the T-cell response, as occurs with iatrogenic or disease-induced immunosuppression, may allow uncontrolled replication and result in HCMV disease. Pathology is presumably produced by direct cytopathic effects of the virus, although indirect effects produced by soluble virus-encoded proteins or the host response are also possible. The presence of HCMV in a diseased organ does not necessarily implicate the virus as a cause of disease, because reactivation of virus may sometimes be non-pathogenic and a 'bystander' effect to some other pathogenic process.

This difficulty in unequivocally attributing disease to HCMV is illustrated by its postulated role in arterial disease. HCMV has been detected in atherosclerotic lesions by immunohistology. A more recent study associated HCMV with the smooth muscle cell proliferation responsible for coronary artery restenosis following angioplasty, although subsequent reports failed to confirm this. Other microbial agents have now been described in atherosclerotic lesions in humans, and Marek's disease virus (also a herpesvirus) is associated with atherosclerosis in chickens. The association thus remains plausible but speculative.

Clinical features of HCMV disease

Primary infection in immunocompetent subjects

Primary infection in children and adults is asymptomatic in most cases, but HCMV can produce an illness clinically indistinguishable from infectious mononucleosis caused by primary Epstein–Barr virus (**EBV**) infection, characterized by fever, myalgia, cervical lymphadenopathy, and mild hepatitis. Tonsillopharyngitis is much less common than in primary EBV infection, and lymphadenopathy and splenic enlargement are less prominent features. The fever lasts 2 to 3 weeks, but it can persist for up to 5 weeks. In more developed countries an increasing proportion of HCMV seroconversion illness is seen in older adults, and the diagnosis should still be considered in patients over 50 or 60 years of age. Myocarditis, pneumonitis, and aseptic meningitis are rare complications. A proportion (5–10 per cent) of patients with Guillain–Barré syndrome (**GBS**) show serological evidence of primary HCMV infection: they are more likely to have antibodies to the GM2 ganglioside than other patients with GBS, and a causal relationship is postulated.

Primary HCMV infection acquired from blood transfusion is characterized by a similar clinical picture occurring 3 to 6 weeks after transfusion, and is usually self-limiting in the normal host. The distinction of primary HCMV infection from other causes of mononucleosis syndromes (such as EBV and toxoplasmosis) depends on serological testing (the Paul-Bunnell and Monospot tests are negative in HCMV mononucleosis).

HCMV disease in the immunosuppressed patient

HCMV produces its most severe disease in immunosuppressed patients, particularly solid organ and bone marrow transplant (**BMT**) recipients, and those with AIDS, all characterized by impaired T-lymphocyte function: this strongly supports the importance of T cells in controlling infection.

Disease in solid-organ transplant recipients

The risk of HCMV disease is three- to fivefold greater in a seronegative recipient receiving a graft from a seropositive donor than in a seropositive recipient, and disease is much more severe. Many centres 'match' seronegative donors to seronegative recipients, although this is often thwarted by organ shortage. Disease presents with specific organ involvement not seen in the normal subject. Interstitial pneumonitis due to HCMV carries a poor prognosis; gastrointestinal disease includes oesophagitis, gastritis and peptic ulceration, and colitis; HCMV retinitis may occur in severely immunosuppressed patients. HCMV has been reported to be associated with increased graft rejection and renal artery stenosis in renal transplant recipients, with accelerated coronary artery stenosis in heart transplant recipients, and with 'vanishing bile duct' syndrome in liver transplant recipients. However, none of these associations is definitively established as causal.

Disease in bone marrow transplant (BMT) recipients

HCMV disease is a major problem in allogeneic BMT recipients, with a 30 to 50 per cent incidence of clinically significant infection. It is a lesser problem in autologous BMT. Seropositivity in donor or recipient, or both, carries a risk of HCMV disease, but the risk can be eliminated when both donor and recipient are seronegative if HCMV seronegative blood products are used to support the patient. Pneumonitis is the most serious manifestation of HCMV infection after BMT, occurring in 10 to 15 per cent of allogeneic BMT recipients, with a mortality of 80 per cent without antiviral therapy. There is interstitial pneumonitis in the absence of any other identifiable pathogen, with increasing arterial hypoxaemia, and progression to respiratory failure. It is suggested that graft-versus-host disease (**GvHD**) may contribute to the lung injury in HCMV pneumonitis in BMT recipients. The relationship of HCMV to GvHD is controversial, with propositions that HCMV may predispose to GvHD, and vice versa.

Disease in patients with AIDS

HCMV disease is one of the most frequent opportunistic infections in patients with advanced HIV infection, of whom 40 per cent develop sight- or life-threatening HCMV disease. A CD4 count below 50/µl carries a high risk of disease, although the widespread use of antiretroviral therapy in developed countries means that relatively few patients now have such low CD4 counts, and the incidence of HCMV disease in patients with AIDS has consequently declined significantly.

HCMV retinitis was seen in up to 25 per cent of patients with AIDS prior to effective antiretroviral therapy (Plate 5). Characteristically, haemorrhagic retinal necrosis spreads along retinal vessels and threatens sight when disease encroaches on the macula. Patients present with visual impairment and have an increased risk of retinal detachment and haemorrhage: hence those with low CD4 counts should undergo regular examination of the optic fundi to detect retinitis before it becomes symptomatic. Diagnosis is made by the ophthalmological detection of typical retinal changes, preferably with accompanying evidence of HCMV viraemia. Without treatment, HCMV retinitis almost invariably progresses to affect both eyes and destroy vision.

HCMV is reported to produce a diffuse encephalitis in AIDS patients but, although the virus is sometimes seen in neuronal cells at autopsy, encephalitis attributable to HCMV is relatively rare in clinical practice in comparison to the other causes of encephalitis in those with AIDS. HCMV can also produce a progressive radiculopathy causing low back pain, which radiates to the area supplied by the affected spinal nerve root, and the development of flaccid paraparesis.

In the gastrointestinal tract, HCMV is associated with oesophagitis, gastritis, and enterocolitis. Virus can be seen in biopsies from these sites, usually in shallow ulcers.

HCMV pneumonitis is rare in patients with AIDS, suggesting there must be additional factors to account for its frequency in BMT recipients.

Congenital and neonatal HCMV infection

HCMV infection of the neonate may be congenital from intrauterine infection, perinatal transmission during birth, or postnatal from breast milk. The frequency of congenital HCMV infection in developed countries is around 0.5 to 1 per cent of live births: it results from either primary maternal infection in pregnancy, or from reactivation of HCMV during pregnancy in a previously infected mother. The risk of primary maternal infection in pregnancy is about 1 per cent, and it carries a 40 per cent risk of congenital infection. Fetal infection is more likely to occur, and to be severe, when a seronegative mother acquires primary infection in early pregnancy. The risk of symptomatic congenital infection from reactivation of maternal HCMV in pregnancy is much lower, although not absent. Pre-existing maternal immunity limits spread to the fetus.

Approximately 5 to 20 per cent of congenitally infected babies are symptomatic at birth: the higher figure applies to babies of mothers with primary infection, who are also more likely to have serious disease. In its most severe form congenital HCMV infection is associated with microcephaly, chorioretinitis, nerve deafness, hepatitis with jaundice and hepatosplenomegaly, and thrombocytopenia with petechiae: such classical 'cytomegalic inclusion disease' has a high mortality, and 80 per cent of all infants symptomatic at birth who survive have serious sequelae such as mental, visual, and hearing impairment. However, the majority of congenitally infected babies are asymptomatic at birth: only 5 to 15 per cent subsequently develop sequelae on long-term follow-up, the commonest being sensorineural deafness, which occurs in isolation in otherwise normal babies.

Perinatal or postnatally acquired HCMV infection is rarely symptomatic or associated with long-term sequelae, if the mother is seropositive.

Malignancy

Although associations between HCMV and malignancy have been postulated in the past, there is currently no good evidence to associate the virus with any human malignancy.

Pathology

On light microscopy, typical HCMV-infected cells appear large with a relative reduction in cytoplasm, and nuclei that contain prominent intranuclear inclusions, surrounded by a clear halo (described as 'owl's eye' inclusions). These cells contain replicating virus and are associated with active infection and disease. They are diagnostic when seen in biopsies of affected organs. In patients dying of severe disease, histological evidence of

HCMV involvement can be found in most organs, whereas it infects a restricted range of cells *in vitro*.

Laboratory diagnosis

Primary infection is usually diagnosed by the detection of IgM antibody to HCMV in the absence of IgG antibody: there is a marked atypical lymphocytosis (mainly due to increased CD8+ T cells) but heterophile antibody (as detected in primary EBV infection by the Monospot or Paul-Bunnell tests) is absent. Serology is of limited use in confirming HCMV disease in the immunosuppressed patient: IgG antibody is a useful marker of HCMV carriage, but titres do not rise reliably in disease. IgM antibody is found during primary infection, and also sometimes with reactivation in patients who are immunosuppressed. Culture of virus from urine may only indicate asymptomatic reactivation; culture from the blood buffy coat is more definitively associated with HCMV disease as virus can never be cultured from the blood of normal HCMV carriers, and culture from an organ site (such as bronchoalveolar lavage fluid) may indicate locally active disease. Rapid culture methods, such as the **DEAFF** (detection of early antigen fluorescent foci, by a monoclonal antibody against an immediate-early viral protein) or shell vial tests facilitate virus isolation. The HCMV antigenaemia assay detects the presence of the HCMV pp65 protein in peripheral blood neutrophils (where it may be taken up passively, rather than expressed by natural infection): the number of positive cells correlates with the level of viraemia. PCR-based techniques are increasingly used to detect and quantitate the HCMV load in blood or plasma, and in many laboratories are now the standard assay for detecting HCMV. As virus can never be detected in plasma (as opposed to leucocytes) in normal carriers, the presence of HCMV-DNA in plasma indicates active viral replication. Detection of virus in biopsy specimens by histological and immunohistological techniques implies organ disease due to HCMV.

In practice, HCMV disease is usually diagnosed by the combination of an appropriate clinical syndrome, and HCMV detection in blood or plasma, or in biopsies from involved organs, in the absence of any other likely causal microbial pathogen.

Treatment

Several drugs are now available for the treatment of disease due to HCMV. Aciclovir has little *in vitro* activity against HCMV, which, unlike HSV, does not possess a thymidine kinase (see above), and has no place in its therapy (although it is used in prophylaxis—see below). Ganciclovir, another nucleoside analogue, is monophosphorylated in infected cells by the *UL97* gene product of HCMV, and is active against HCMV: its most limiting side-effect is myelotoxicity with leucopenia and thrombocytopenia, but it has many other potential side-effects including azoospermia in males. Intravenous administration is necessary since an oral form of ganciclovir has bioavailability of only about 10 per cent, restricting its use to prophylaxis (oral valganciclovir, a new valyl ester of ganciclovir, has much higher bioavailability: it also produces equivalent plasma concentrations to intravenously administered ganciclovir, which initial trials suggest it may replace). Resistance to ganciclovir results from mutations in the drug target, the HCMV-DNA polymerase, or in the *UL97* gene, and is seen mainly in AIDS patients in whom prolonged use is necessary. An alternative drug to ganciclovir is foscarnet (trisodium phosphonoformate), which is a competitive inhibitor of the viral DNA polymerase and shows no cross-resistance with ganciclovir. This also has to be given intravenously and its side-effects include renal impairment and hypocalcaemia. Cidofovir, a nucleotide analogue acting on the viral DNA polymerase is also licensed for use in the United Kingdom, but is highly nephrotoxic (probenecid has to be given concurrently to prevent irreversible renal damage) and therefore relatively little used.

Primary infection

In the immunocompetent host, this requires no specific antiviral treatment.

HCMV disease in the immunosuppressed (due to primary or secondary infection, or reactivation)

This is usually treated with ganciclovir or foscarnet for 2 to 3 weeks of full-dose induction intravenous therapy: for ganciclovir this is 5 mg/kg body weight every 12 h; and for foscarnet 60 mg/kg every 8 h. Secondary prophylaxis may well be needed if immunosuppression persists (see below).

HCMV pneumonitis in BMT recipients

HCMV pneumonitis responds poorly to ganciclovir or foscarnet alone, but the combination of full-dose ganciclovir with intravenous immunoglobulin has been shown to reduce mortality. Although specific anti-CMV immunoglobulin was initially used, recent trials suggest normal pooled intravenous immunoglobulin is equally effective. Many centres monitor BMT recipients, especially of allogeneic grafts, for CMV viraemia and if detected commence 'pre-emptive therapy' with ganciclovir prior to the development of symptomatic or obvious organ disease.

HCMV retinitis in patients with AIDS

This is treated with an induction course of ganciclovir or foscarnet (both drugs have also been used in combination). Continued prophylaxis is needed to prevent relapse unless significant recovery of the CD4 count can be induced with antiretroviral therapy: for this, intravenous ganciclovir—5 mg/kg per day for 5 days per week—is effective, but high-dose oral ganciclovir (1000 mg three times per day) may be adequate if retinal disease is peripheral to the macula. Given the difficulty of these regimes, implantable intraocular devices giving a sustained release of ganciclovir into the vitreous humor have also been used. The use of combination antiretroviral therapy in HIV-infected patients is associated with a much improved long-term control of HCMV infection.

However, the syndrome of 'immune recovery vitritis', characterized by posterior segment inflammation, can occur in patients with inactive treated CMV retinitis as their CD4 count reconstitutes on antiretroviral therapy.

Congenital HCMV infection

In a phase II evaluation of ganciclovir (8 or 12 mg/kg body weight daily for 6 weeks) for the treatment of symptomatic congenital HCMV infection, excretion of CMV in the urine decreased: however, after cessation of therapy viruria returned to near-pretreatment levels. Hearing improvement occurred in 5 out of 30 babies at 6 months or later, suggesting some efficacy, but the role of antiviral therapy in congenital HCMV infection remains to be established.

Prevention and control

The problem posed by HCMV in immunosuppressed patients has led to several approaches to prophylaxis.

Antiviral prophylaxis

Ganciclovir has been used for primary prophylaxis in solid-organ and BMT recipients, particularly those at high risk of disease (seronegative recipients of a seropositive graft, or seropositive recipients), and in AIDS patients with less than 100 CD4 cells/µl. Oral ganciclovir has been shown to be effective in many of these settings. Despite their limited *in vitro* activity against HCMV, and lack of efficacy as therapy, oral aciclovir and valaciclovir have also been shown to provide significant prophylaxis against HCMV disease in renal transplant recipients. Moreover, valaciclovir prophylaxis was also associated with a lower rate of graft rejection. This evidence, combined with their lack of toxicity compared to ganciclovir, has led to their widespread use.

Passive immunization

CMV hyperimmune globulin has been reported to reduce the risk of HCMV disease in renal transplant recipients but is expensive and little used in practice.

There are initial reports that HCMV-specific T-cell immunity can be reconstituted in BMT recipients by the adoptive transfer of virus-specific T lymphocytes from the immune donor, but this is still a research therapy.

Active immunization

A live laboratory (Towne) strain of HCMV has been tested as an experimental candidate vaccine in renal transplant recipients and found to have some evidence of protective immunity, perhaps equivalent to having previous natural HCMV infection. However, there is currently no available licensed vaccine, although some candidates are in early development.

Special problems in pregnant women

Pregnant women who are seronegative should avoid contact with possibly infected children in day nursery settings, although this may be impractical. This population would be the target for a vaccine were one available. Ganciclovir must not be used in pregnancy.

Human herpesvirus-6 and -7

Human herpesvirus-6

Introduction

Human herpesvirus-6 (**HHV-6**) was originally isolated in 1986 from cultured human lymphocyte lines and initially named 'human B lymphotropic virus'. However, it was subsequently shown to be tropic principally for T cells, although it can also replicate in macrophages, glial cells, and EBV-transformed B cells. HHV-6 is widely distributed in humans and primary infection is associated with roseola infantum (also known as exanthem subitum or sixth disease), an aetiological association first described in Japanese children by Yamanishi and colleagues in 1988.

Aetiology

HHV-6 has typical herpesvirus morphology and is genetically classified in the betaherpesvirus subfamily. Two groups of HHV-6 isolates, HHV-6A and HHV-6B, are now clearly distinguished by their genetic sequence and some variation in their biological properties. HHV-6B is associated with roseola, whilst HHV-6A has not been clearly associated with human disease.

Epidemiology

There is high seroprevalence of HHV-6 in all populations. More than 90 per cent of children are seropositive at 2 years of age. The virus (usually the HHV-6B variant) can be detected in peripheral blood mononuclear cells by PCR in nearly all healthy people. It is most probably transmitted via maternal saliva, although intrauterine and perinatal transmission could occur. The virus is not detectable in breast milk.

Pathogenesis

Upon primary infection with HHV-6, the virus probably replicates in regional lymphoid tissue in the oropharynx and can be found in circulating lymphocytes. HHV-6 replicates *in vitro* in CD4+ T-cell lines. However, during persistent infection in a normal adult, the virus can be detected by PCR in both CD4+ T cells and in monocytes/macrophages in peripheral blood. Monocytes/macrophages are probably the principal site of carriage during persistent infection. The mechanism of viral latency is uncertain. HHV-6 induces CD4 expression on CD4− lymphocytes, and *in vitro* may thus facilitate HIV entry into previously CD4− cells.

Although HHV-6 cannot normally be isolated in culture from the peripheral blood of normal individuals, it is easy to detect HHV-6 DNA in the peripheral blood of immunosuppressed subjects: this and other evidence indicates immunosuppression is associated with reactivation of HHV-6. Mechanisms by which HHV-6 may produce clinical manifestations remain unclear.

Clinical features

Primary infection with HHV-6 in young children is associated with roseola and also with a febrile illness without rash.

Roseola infantum (exanthem subitum, sixth disease)

Roseola is an acute illness of infants and young children, characterized by 3 to 5 days of high fever with upper respiratory tract symptoms and sometimes cervical lymphadenopathy. As the fever defervesces, a rash appears and lasts for 1 to 3 days. The rash is diffuse, macular or maculopapular, and appears similar to that of rubella. The illness is accompanied by mild atypical lymphocytosis and there may be neutropenia. Rarely, infections are complicated by febrile convulsions, meningitis, encephalitis, and hepatitis, which is usually mild but occasionally severe.

Roseola has been estimated to occur in only 10 to 20 per cent of children, as primary HHV-6 infection is commonly subclinical.

Febrile illness

Fever without rash is a more usual manifestation of primary HHV-6 infection than roseola. In one major study of 1600 children under the age of 3 years presenting to a North American hospital emergency department with acute febrile illness, 10 per cent of cases were ascribed to primary HHV-6 infection. In children between the ages of 6 and 12 months within this study, 20 per cent of acute febrile illness was due to HHV-6, but only 17 per cent of all these children with documented primary HHV-6 infection had clinical roseola.

Febrile convulsions

There is accumulating evidence that HHV-6 has a major association with febrile convulsions in young children. In the study quoted above, 13 per cent of all the children under 3 years of age had febrile convulsions associated with acute HHV-6 infection, and the infection was reported to account for one-third of all febrile seizures in children up to the age of 2 years. It is believed that this association is not solely because HHV-6 induces high fever, but because it also specifically infects the nervous system. HHV-6 DNA can be detected in the cerebrospinal fluid of children with primary infection.

HHV-6 infection in immunosuppressed patients

A number of studies have shown increases in antibody titres to HHV-6 and increased HHV-6 DNA levels in peripheral blood by PCR in immunosuppressed solid-organ and bone marrow transplant recipients. In bone marrow transplant recipients, HHV-6 has been associated with fever, skin rash, graft-versus-host disease, encephalitis, delayed engraftment, marrow suppression, and pneumonitis: however, it is not clear whether HHV-6 plays a specific aetiological role in these syndromes. In the case of pneumonitis, BMT recipients have higher levels of HHV-6 DNA in the lung, but other opportunist infections such as human cytomegalovirus were not always excluded as the cause.

There is good evidence that HHV-6 reactivates in patients with advanced HIV infection and AIDS. However, there is no firm evidence for any HHV-6 associated disease in patients with AIDS.

In summary, current evidence suggests HHV-6 is infrequently associated with disease in immunosuppressed patients, but that it could be responsible for occasional cases of pneumonitis in BMT recipients.

Other disease associations

Some studies have associated HHV-6 with the chronic fatigue syndrome and with multiple sclerosis. The present consensus is that there is no convincing evidence for any significant aetiological association between HHV-6 and these illnesses.

Malignancy

HHV-6 DNA has been detected in the blood of patients with a number of lymphoproliferative disorders, but this probably reflects reactivation rather than any causal association with the tumour. There are reports of HHV-6 DNA being detected in some tumours, such as the nodular sclerosis variant of Hodgkin's disease, but there is no convincing aetiological association between HHV-6 and any tumour.

Differential diagnosis

Primary HHV-6 infection may be confused with many febrile childhood illnesses associated with a rash. The rash associated with roseola may mistakenly be attributed to sensitivity to recent antibiotic treatment. Other virus infections (EBV, HCMV) may also be associated with atypical lymphocytes and a mononucleosis syndrome.

Pathology

HHV-6 replicates in cells of central nervous system origin, particularly glial cell lines, *in vitro*. HHV-6 DNA can be detected in the brain of apparently normal individuals, suggesting viral persistence in the central nervous system. No distinctive histopathology has yet been attributed to HHV-6.

Laboratory diagnosis

Commercial assays for HHV-6 antibody do not distinguish between antibody to HHV-6A and HHV-6B and may cross-react with antibodies to HHV-7. Seroconversion is evidence of primary infection. IgM assays for HHV-6 antibody are not reliable indicators of primary infection as some HHV-6 carriers may have IgM antibody periodically.

Although HHV-6 can be cultured from peripheral blood mononuclear cells during acute primary infection, few laboratories will undertake this. PCR-based techniques for the detection of HHV-6 DNA in plasma and cerebrospinal fluid are the method of choice for clinical diagnosis, and are becoming increasingly available.

Treatment

HHV-6 sensitivity to antiviral drugs corresponds to the sensitivity of cytomegalovirus. Thus, HHV-6 replication is inhibited *in vitro* by ganciclovir and foscarnet but not aciclovir, but there are no controlled clinical trials of these agents. Their use may be considered for an immunosuppressed patient in whom HHV-6 associated pneumonitis is suspected.

Prevention and control

There is currently no place for measures to prevent HHV-6 transmission. It seems unlikely there will be a case for the development of a vaccine because infants may be infected so early in life, while they still have maternal antibody.

Special problems in pregnant women

Nearly all pregnant women will be carriers of HHV-6. There is no evidence to associate HHV-6 with a specific risk to the fetus or neonate.

Human herpesvirus-7

Human herpesvirus-7 (HHV-7) was isolated in 1990. It is also a betaherpesvirus, similar to but distinct from HHV-6. HHV-7 predominantly infects CD4+ T cells and can be reactivated from latency upon T-cell activation.

Although there is serological cross-reactivity between HHV-6 and HHV-7, the evidence is that HHV-7 infects nearly all humans during childhood (but later than HHV-6), with greater than 90 per cent of children being infected by the age of 5 years. The virus is excreted in saliva.

HHV-7 has been associated with some cases of roseola, and in a Japanese study was reported to cause roseola in infants who had already had a previous episode of roseola proven to be due to HHV-6. The similarity between HHV-7 and HHV-6 suggests that they may be associated with a similar range of diseases, but the association with roseola is the only one so far identified.

The best method of diagnosis is by PCR on serum or CSF. Laboratory tests for HHV-6 often also test for HHV-7 in a multiplex PCR. In the

absence of any disease associations, apart from that with roseola, there is no reason to consider any treatment for HHV-7.

Human herpesvirus-8

Introduction

Human herpesvirus-8 (HHV-8) is the most recently isolated of the human herpesviruses. In 1994 Chang and colleagues, using the technique of representational difference analysis (which selectively amplifies DNA present in diseased tissue, but not the corresponding normal tissue), reported the detection of novel DNA sequences with homology to herpesviruses in Kaposi's sarcoma tissue. This herpesvirus is most closely related genetically to a well-characterized simian herpesvirus (herpesvirus saimiri) and less so to EBV, and it was consequently assigned to the γ2-herpesvirus subfamily. It was initially named Kaposi's sarcoma-associated herpesvirus (**KSHV**), but was subsequently designated HHV-8. Current culture techniques are unreliable, but the virus can be detected by PCR. Serological assays depend on the use of infected cell lines or synthetic antigens from predicted open-reading frames. The seroepidemiology, biology, and disease associations of the virus are still being analysed, but HHV-8 is clearly closely associated with Kaposi's sarcoma, a tumour which has long been suspected of having a viral aetiology, with primary effusion lymphoma, and with Castleman's disease. Reported associations with multiple myeloma and other cancers are unconfirmed.

Aetiology

HHV-8 has the characteristic morphology of a herpesvirus. The viral genome is composed of a 141-kbp long unique segment flanked by multiple 801-bp direct repeats. Sequence analysis suggests that HHV-8, like other herpesviruses, is an ancient human virus, with several major subtypes reflecting the migrationary divergence of human populations. HHV-8 contains eight genes homologous to mammalian genes encoding cell-cycle regulatory proteins (the cyclins), chemokines, and inhibitors of apoptosis. Comparative genetic analyses show a high rate of amino acid variation in *ORF-K1* and another gene, *K15*. Analysis of the variable genes indicates there are at least four virus subtypes, A–D. On the evidence to date the normal cellular site of latency of HHV-8 almost certainly includes the B cell.

Epidemiology

The emerging epidemiology of HHV-8 suggests it is less ubiquitous than other human herpesviruses. Initial serological assays using indirect immunofluorescence on infected cell lines to detect antibodies to a latent nuclear antigen (**LANA**), give a seroprevalence of approximately 80 per cent in patients with Kaposi's sarcoma, and 25 to 30 per cent in HIV-positive homosexual men without Kaposi's sarcoma. Seroprevalence in normal adults is reported as being more than 50 per cent in African adults in West Africa, 20 per cent in Black South African blood donors, and less than 5 per cent in blood donors in the United Kingdom and United States, with intermediate rates in Italy and other Mediterranean countries. Seroprevalence in HIV-positive and -negative adults in Uganda was equal at 53 per cent. HHV-8 can be detected by PCR in nearly all cases of Kaposi's sarcoma, so the failure of this assay to detect antibody in all cases of Kaposi's sarcoma implies it has limited sensitivity. An assay using lytic-cycle antigens gave higher rates of seroprevalence, but these may result from cross-reaction with EBV antibodies. Newer assays using multiple HHV-8 antigens are currently being applied.

The normal route of transmission of the virus is unknown, but sexual transmission occurs between homosexual men. A LANA-based assay detected seroconversion to HHV-8 in HIV-infected homosexual men at a median of 33 months before they subsequently developed Kaposi's sarcoma. HHV-8 infection in children correlates with seropositivity in their mothers, but whether this reflects vertical or horizontal transmission is unknown.

Pathogenesis

There has been much uncertainty over the cell of origin of Kaposi's sarcoma, but the spindle cells of which the tumour is largely composed are thought to be of lymphatic endothelial origin. In Kaposi's sarcoma tumour tissue, HHV-8 DNA and LANA are present in every spindle cell, suggesting an aetiological role for the virus.

In HIV-associated Castleman's disease, the HHV-8 LANA antigen is present in immunoblasts in the mantle zone of the tumour. HHV-8 is present in the tumour cells of all cases of primary effusion lymphoma so far studied, although so also is EBV. HHV-8 latently infected cell lines derived from these tumours can be induced *in vitro* to release infectious virus, and are used to detect antibodies to the virus.

These clear associations of virus DNA with tumour cells suggest a definite oncogenic role for HHV-8. The possession of the genes encoding cyclin and antiapoptotic protein homologues suggests they may be involved in cellular transformation and oncogenesis by HHV-8.

It has been suggested that HHV-8 may be involved in the pathogenesis of multiple myeloma. The virus has been reported in bone marrow dendritic stromal cells of myeloma patients, but not in myeloma cells; however, this putative association remains speculative. The individual HHV-8 subtypes are not associated with any distinct pathology.

Clinical features

Apart from these malignancies, the only reported clinical syndrome accompanying primary or reactivated HHV-8 infection is fever and bone marrow failure in immunosuppressed transplant recipients.

Kaposi's sarcoma

Kaposi's sarcoma manifests clinically as purplish brown macules, papules, or plaques. It is described in four characteristic clinical settings: the classic form in elderly Mediterranean or Jewish males, the endemic African form (accounting for 10 per cent of cancer in equatorial Africa), in patients with immunodeficiency states such as transplant recipients, and the AIDS-associated form. The classic and African forms are characterized by lesions on the extremities, systemic and mucosal involvement is rare, and the disease is indolent. In immunosuppressed patients (other than those with AIDS) lesions are more widespread and more rapidly progressive, although visceral involvement is still unusual, and lesions may regress if immunosuppressive drugs are stopped. AIDS-associated Kaposi's sarcoma is seen predominantly in homosexual men in Western countries, but is commonly associated with heterosexually acquired HIV infection in African countries: it is characterized by widespread cutaneous lesions with involvement of the oral mucosa (Plate 6), and visceral lesions may occur in the lungs or gastrointestinal tract. Progression can be much more rapid than the other forms. HHV-8 has been isolated from all these forms of Kaposi's sarcoma.

Primary effusion lymphomas

Previously known as body cavity-based lymphomas, these are a rare and aggressive type of B-cell lymphoma presenting in patients with AIDS as lymphomatous effusions of the peritoneal, pleural, or pericardial spaces, usually with no identifiable tumour mass. HHV-8 is present in the tumour cells of all cases so far studied, although so also is EBV.

Castleman's disease

Also known as angiofollicular lymph node hyperplasia, Castleman's disease can be localized and is amenable to curative excision. However, a multicentric form is seen particularly in HIV-infected patients and is more aggressive: HHV-8 is found in a high proportion of these multicentric cases, especially those associated with HIV.

Pathology

No distinctive histopathology, independent of the pathology of the tumours with which it is associated, has been identified as attributable to HHV-8 infection in cells.

Laboratory diagnosis

HHV-8 can best be detected by PCR-based tests. Antibody assays are described above, and may become commercially available in the near future.

Treatment

Assays based on the HHV-8 infected lymphoma cell lines suggest that HHV-8 replication is moderately sensitive to foscarnet, ganciclovir, and cidofovir. It has been suggested that patients with AIDS treated with foscarnet and ganciclovir may have been less likely to develop Kaposi's sarcoma. There is no established use of antiviral drugs in treating HHV-8 tumours.

The treatment of Kaposi's sarcoma is discussed in Chapter 7.10.24. Kaposi's sarcoma confined to the skin can be treated with radiotherapy or with intralesional interferon-alpha. More widespread cutaneous or visceral disease can be treated with single-agent or combination chemotherapy.

Kaposi's sarcoma lesions may regress with antiretroviral treatment, possibly due to the improved cellular immunity that occurs with a reduction of the HIV load.

Prevention and control

Given limited knowledge of the epidemiology and disease associations of HHV-8, no prevention or control measures are used. No special problems of infection have been identified in pregnant women.

Cercopithecine herpesvirus-1 (herpes B virus)

Introduction

Cercopithecine herpesvirus-1 is the formal name now given to herpes B virus (also previously known as herpesvirus simiae, a term no longer used), whose natural hosts are members of the *Macaca* genus of Old World monkeys. It produces minimal disease in its natural host, but its transmission to humans results in a high incidence of severe disease. Although more than 30 other herpesviruses have been isolated from non-human primates, none of these have been unequivocally associated with a disease in humans. The virus was first isolated in 1932 from the brain of Dr WB who died of encephalitis after a bite from a macaque monkey (hence the name herpes B virus). There have since been about 45 cases of human infection resulting from accidental transmission from captive monkeys.

Aetiology

Herpes B virus is an alphaherpesvirus closely related to HSV and appears to behave in an analogous manner to HSV in its natural primate host. Herpes B virus can also infect and produce disease in other non-human primates and small mammals.

Epidemiology

Herpes B virus is enzootic in Old World macaque monkeys, principally rhesus (*Macaca mulatta*) and cynomolgus (*Macaca fascicularis*) macaques. The epidemiology in its primate host is similar to that of HSV in humans, with 80 per cent or more of natural and captive adults monkeys being infected. Infected monkeys may develop vesicular oral lesions and can shed virus intermittently from oral, conjunctival, and genital secretions.

Rhesus and cynomolgus macaques have been quite widely used in medical research, particularly for polio vaccine development during the mid-

1950s and for studies of retroviruses from the late 1980s following the AIDS epidemic. Nearly all the reported human cases resulted from occupational exposure through bites and scratches in workers handling monkeys, but transmission from needlestick injuries and a splash in the eye have also been reported. One case of human-to-human transmission apparently occurred by inoculation on to inflamed skin.

Two clusters of infections have been described in the United States (in 1987 and 1989), the earlier one involving the case of human-to-human transmission. A seroprevalence study of over 300 monkey handlers revealed no seropositive subjects, and asymptomatic infection documented by seroconversion appears to be extremely uncommon.

Clinical features

The incubation period from occupational exposure to the development of symptoms has been 3 to 5 days in most cases, but it can range from 3 to 30 days. Cutaneous vesicles may occur at or near the site of inoculation accompanied by regional lymphadenitis. A prodrome of fever, malaise, headache, and abdominal pain occurring in the first 2 weeks is common, but the dominant and characteristic feature of reported cases is a progressive myelitis and encephalitis. Herpes B virus produces a multifocal haemorrhagic myelitis and encephalitis. Visceral spread is recorded in fatal cases. Before the advent of aciclovir and later antiviral drugs, the mortality rate was 70 per cent.

It is not clear whether herpes B virus can establish latency and then reactivate in humans. Viral shedding has recurred when antiviral treatment was stopped relatively early, so most patients have been maintained on antivirals for long periods.

Laboratory diagnosis

Herpes B virus is a category IV pathogen and only a few designated laboratories can undertake culture and isolation of the agent. In the United Kingdom the designated laboratory is at the Central Public Health Laboratory, Colindale, London, and in the United States at the South West Foundation for Biomedical Research, San Antonio, Texas. Suspected infected monkeys should be bled to determine seropositivity. Serodiagnosis in humans is made difficult because of antigenic cross-reactivity between herpes B virus and herpes simplex virus. The inoculation site should preferably be biopsied for possible culture and analysis. PCR-based methods are available in specialized centres and are the standard for definitive diagnosis.

Treatment

Suspected injuries from macaques carry the risk of herpes B virus infection, although most captive macaque colonies are now maintained free of the virus. A suspected contaminated wound should be debrided and cleaned with chlorhexidine or iodine soap. There may be a case for initiating immediate antiviral treatment if infection in the monkey is suspected or for a deep wound. Otherwise presumptive therapy may be initiated if the monkey is subsequently shown to be positive for herpes B virus, although the report of transmission by an eye splash favours early presumptive treatment.

Aciclovir and ganciclovir both inhibit herpes B virus replication *in vitro*. For presumptive therapy, oral aciclovir 800 mg, 5 times daily, or preferably valaciclovir in equivalent dose can be given for at least 2 weeks.

If symptomatic disease is suspected, intravenous aciclovir should be used (10 mg/kg body weight every 8 h for peripheral disease, and 15 mg/kg every 8 h for central nervous system involvement). If progression occurs, ganciclovir (5 mg/kg every 12 h) should be considered as an alternative. Treatment has been associated with limitation of disease and recovery in some patients.

Prevention and control

Those working with macaques should follow standard procedures to avoid infection. Screening of newly imported monkeys, and the creation of colonies of macaques free of herpes B virus, are now becoming standard practice.

Further reading

Herpes simplex virus infection

Balfour HH, Jr (1999). Review article: drug therapy: antiviral drugs. *New England Journal of Medicine* **340**, 1255–68. [A good review of antiviral therapy including coverage of drugs for HSV.]

Lakeman FD, Whitley RJ (1995). Diagnosis of herpes simplex encephalitis: application of polymerase chain reaction to cerebrospinal fluid from brain-biopsied patients and correlation with disease. NIAID collaborative antiviral study group. *Journal of Infectious Disease* **171**, 857–63. [Study showing detection of HSV-DNA by PCR in 98 per cent of 54 patients with brain-biopsy proven HSV encephalitis.]

Langenberg AGM, *et al.* (1999). A prospective study of new infections with herpes simplex virus type 1 and type 2. *New England Journal of Medicine* **341**, 1432–8. [A recent study of incident HSV-1/2 infections (undertaken for an unsuccessful vaccine trial), which reports the proportion of symptomatic infections.]

Roizman B, Pellett PE (2001). Herpesviridae. In: Knipe DM, Howley PM, eds. *Fields virology*, pp 2381–48. Lippincott, Williams and Wilkins, Philadelphia. [Authoritative chapter on the herpesviruses in major virology text, accompanied by another on the basic virology of HSV.]

Tookey P, Peckham CS (1996). Neonatal herpes simplex virus infection in the British Isles. *Paediatric and Perinatal Epidemiology* **10**, 432–42. [Comprehensive survey of neonatal HSV in the UK over a 5-year period.]

Whitley RJ (2001). Herpes simplex viruses. In: Knipe DM, Howley PM, eds. *Fields virology*, pp 2461–510. Lippincott, Williams and Wilkins, Philadelphia. [Chapter on clinical aspects of HSV in major authoritative virology text.]

Whitley RJ *et al.* (1986). Vidarabine versus acyclovir therapy in herpes simplex encephalitis. *New England Journal of Medicine* **314**, 144–9. [The classic original trial showing efficacy of aciclovir in, and probably the largest case series of, HSV encephalitis.]

Varicella zoster virus infection

Arvin AM (2001). Varicella-zoster virus. In: Knipe DM, Howley PM, eds. *Fields virology*, pp. 2731–68. Lippincott, Williams and Wilkins, Philadelphia. [Chapter in major authoritative virology text, accompanied by another by JI Cohen and SE Straus on the basic virology of VZV.]

Enders G, *et al.* (1994). Consequences of varicella and herpes zoster in pregnancy: prospective study of 1739 cases. *Lancet* **343**, 1547–50. [Large study from Germany and the UK assessing risk of varicella embryopathy.]

Gilden DH, *et al.* (2000). Medical progress: neurologic complications of the reactivation of varicella-zoster virus. *New England Journal of Medicine* **342**, 635–46. [A good recent review of the subject including postherpetic neuralgia.]

Pastuszak AL, *et al.* (1994). Outcome after varicella infection in the first 20 weeks of pregnancy. *New England Journal of Medicine* **330**, 901–5. [A North American study of 106 women with varicella in pregnancy.]

Wallace MR, *et al.* (1992). Treatment of adult varicella with oral acyclovir—a randomized placebo-controlled trial. *Annals of Internal Medicine* **117**, 358–83. [Describes the influence of aciclovir on the course of varicella in young adults.]

Wood MJ, *et al.* (1994). A randomised trial of acyclovir for 7 days or 21 days with and without prednisolone for treatment of acute herpes zoster. *New England Journal of Medicine* **330**, 901–5. [UK study showing that longer courses of aciclovir and prednisone do not reduce the frequency of postherpetic neuralgia.]

Human cytomegalovirus infection

Crumpacker CS (1996). Review article: drug therapy: ganciclovir. *New England Journal of Medicine* **335**, 721–9. [A comprehensive review of the use of ganciclovir in the treatment of HCMV.]

Fowler KB, *et al.* (1992). The outcome of congenital cytomegalovirus infection in relation to maternal antibody status. *New England Journal of Medicine* **326**, 663–7. [United States study of sequelae of congenital HCMV infection in relation to primary infection.]

Lowance D, *et al.* (1999). Valacyclovir for the prevention of cytomegalovirus disease after renal transplantation. *New England Journal of Medicine* **340**, 1462–70. [Trial showing efficacy of valaciclovir for HCMV prophylaxis in this group.]

Minton EJ, Sinclair JH, Sissons JGP (1995). Biological aspects of cytomegalovirus infection in marrow transplantation. In: Sullivan KM, Koppa SD, eds. *Marrow Transplantation Reviews 1991–1994*, pp 171–5. Kluge, Virginia. [Review of HCMV biology in relation to marrow transplantation.]

Ramsay ME, Miller E, Peckham CS (1991). Outcome of confirmed symptomatic congenital cytomegalovirus infection. *Archives of Diseases in Childhood* **66**, 1068–9. [United Kingdom study of congenital HCMV outcome.]

Pass RF (2001). Cytomegalovirus. In: Knipe DM, Howley PM, eds. *Fields virology*, pp. 2675–706. Lippincott, Williams and Wilkins, Philadelphia. [Chapter in major authoritative virology text, accompanied by another by ES Mocarski on the basic virology of HCMV.]

Ross R (1999). Atherosclerosis—an inflammatory disease. *New England Journal of Medicine* **340**, 115–26. [A review which includes discussion of the possible role of HCMV and other microbial pathogens in the aetiology of arterial disease.]

Whitley RJ, *et al.* (1998). Guidelines for the treatment of CMV diseases in patients with AIDS in the era of potent antiretroviral therapy. *Archives of Internal Medicine* **158**, 957–69. [Recommendations of an international panel on treatment of CMV disease in AIDS.]

Human herpesvirus-6 and -7

Hall CB, *et al.* (1994). Human herpesvirus-6 infection in children: a prospective study of complications and reactivation. *New England Journal of Medicine* **331**, 432–8. [A comprehensive study of primary HHV-6 infection in children presenting with febrile illness to a hospital emergency department.]

Knox KK, Carrigan DR (1994). Disseminated active HHV-6 infections in patients with AIDS. *Lancet* **343**, 577–8. [Provides evidence for HHV-6 reactivation in AIDS.]

Pellett PE, Dominguez G (2001). Human herpesvirus 6. In: Knipe DM, Howley PM, eds. *Fields virology*, pp. 2769–84. Lippincott, Williams and Wilkins, Philadelphia. [Chapter in major authoritative virology text, including the basic virology of HHV-6.]

Yamanishi K (2001). Human herpesvirus-6 and 7. In: Knipe DM, Howley PM, eds. *Fields virology*, pp. 2785–802. Lippincott, Williams and Wilkins, Philadelphia. [Description of the clinical disease associations of HHV-6 and 7.]

Human herpesvirus-8

Antman K, Chang Y (2000). Medical progress: Kaposis sarcoma. *New England Journal of Medicine* **342**, 1027–39. [Review of Kaposi's sarcoma and the association with HHV-8, including review of therapy of Kaposi's sarcoma.]

Cesarman E, *et al.* (1995). Kaposi's sarcoma-associated herpesvirus-like DNA sequences in AIDS-related body-cavity-based lymphomas. *New England Journal of Medicine* **332**, 1186–91. [Describes the association between HHV-8 and primary effusion lymphomas.]

Chatlynne LG, Ablashi DV (1999). Seroepidemiology of Kaposi's sarcoma-associated herpesvirus (Kaposi's sarcomaHV). *Seminars in Cancer Biology* **9**, 175. [Summarizes current knowledge of seroepidemiology of HHV-8.]

Hayward GS (1999). Kaposi's sarcomaHV strains: the origins and global spread of the virus. *Seminars in Cancer Biology* **9**, 187. [Summarizes current molecular evidence for the evolution of the virus.]

Martin JN, *et al.* (1998). Sexual transmission and the natural history of human herpesvirus 8 infection. *New England Journal of Medicine* **338**, 948–54.

[Provides evidence for sexual transmission of HHV-8 and association with Kaposi's sarcoma in homosexual men.]

Moore PS, Chang Y (1995). Detection of herpesvirus-like DNA sequences in Kaposi's sarcoma in patients with and those without HIV infection. *New England Journal of Medicine* **332**, 1181–5. [The original detection of HHV-8 in Kaposi's sarcoma.]

Cercopithecine herpesvirus-1 (herpes B virus)

Davenport DS, *et al.* (1994). Diagnosis and management of human B virus (*Herpesvirus simiae*) infections in Michigan. *Clinical Infectious Diseases* **19**, 3. [Review of clinical aspects of herpes B virus infection.]

Holmes GP, *et al.* and the B Virus Working Group (1995). Guidelines for the prevention and treatment of B virus infections in exposed persons. *Clinical Infectious Diseases* **20**, 421–39. [Current US recommendations for management of human herpes B virus infection.]

Sabin AB, Wright AM (1934). Acute ascending myelitis following a monkey bite, with the isolation of a virus capable of reproducing the disease. *Journal of Experimental Medicine* **59**, 115–36. [The original description of herpes B virus and the case of Dr WB.]

Straus SE (2000). Herpes B virus. In: Mandell GL, Bennett JE, Dolin R, eds. *Principles and Practice of Infectious Diseases*, pp. 1621–4. Churchill Livingstone, Edinburgh. [Recent chapter in major textbook of infectious disease.]

Whitley RJ, Hilliard JK (2001). Cercopithicine herpesvirus (B virus). In: Knipe DM, Howley PM, eds. *Fields virology*, pp. 2835–48. Lippincott, Williams and Wilkins, Philadelphia. [Review of herpes B virus and disease.]

7.10.3 The Epstein–Barr virus

M. A. Epstein and Dorothy H. Crawford

Background

The virus

Epstein–Barr virus (**EBV**), discovered in 1964, is one of the eight herpesviruses of man. It consists of an outer envelope, a protein capsid, and an inner double-stranded linear DNA genome.

Viral infectious cycle

Natural infection is limited to man and susceptible target cells are circulating B lymphocytes and, in certain circumstances, squamous epithelial cells of the oropharynx. Lytic infection of these cell types leads to production of viral progeny and cell death. The virus also causes a latent infection of B cells *in vivo* and can transform normal B lymphocytes *in vitro* into continuously growing, latently infected, immortalized lymphoblastoid lines. Specific sets of virus-coded proteins are expressed in each type of infection.

Virus-coded proteins

EBV-coded proteins are categorized according to the time of their appearance during the infectious cycle as latent, early, or late antigens. Most elicit cytotoxic T-cell responses and serum antibodies; both are important for controlling the infection and the latter are used in diagnosis.

General epidemiology

The virus is widespread in all human populations. Primary infection usually occurs in early childhood, at which age it is clinically silent, but leads to the generation of antibodies to the virus-determined antigens and of specific cytotoxic T lymphocytes. A lifelong carrier state ensues, in which both humoral and cellular immune responses are maintained continuously. The virus persists as a latent infection in a few circulating B lymphocytes and as a productive, lytic infection in intraepithelial B cells of the mouth and pharynx, and perhaps also the urogenital tract and salivary glands. EBV is shed into the buccal fluid in considerable amounts in about 20 per cent of those who have been infected and in small amounts in the remainder; the virus has also been detected in genital secretions. Virus in the buccal fluid provides the main source for transmission of the infection in the population; in children this occurs via droplets or when objects are casually contaminated with saliva and sucked, whereas amongst the sexually active, transmission is by salivary transfer during kissing. In developing countries, 99.9 per cent of children are infected by the second to the fourth year of life but in industrialized countries with high standards of hygiene many do not meet the virus as young children. The percentage of teenagers or young adults remaining free of infection in Western societies depends on socio-economic group—the higher the standard of living, the greater the percentage; 50 per cent of very affluent young adults may escape childhood infection (Fig. 1).

Infectious mononucleosis

Infectious mononucleosis occurs in about 50 per cent of those who miss EBV infection in childhood when, sooner or later, they undergo delayed primary infection; the other 50 per cent of delayed infections are symptom free. Because teenagers and young adults in the affluent classes of Western countries escape infection as children, infectious mononucleosis is a disease of upper socio-economic groups; conversely it is exceptionally rare in developing countries (Fig. 1). Although most cases occur in adolescents and young adults, children and the middle aged may sometimes develop the disease, and rarely also the elderly. Infectious mononucleosis is associated with kissing and is acquired when a healthy carrier, who is shedding virus in his/her saliva, passes this during close buccal contact directly into the oropharynx of a partner who has not been primarily infected in the usual way as a child. This explains why case-to-case infection and epidemics are not seen and why the incubation period, perhaps 30 to 50 days, is difficult to calculate. Primary EBV infection giving infectious mononucleosis-like symptoms may also be transmitted by blood transfusion or organ grafting from an infected donor to a previously uninfected recipient.

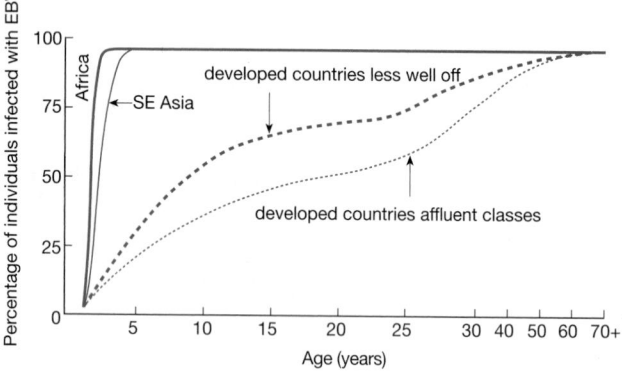

Fig. 1 Comparison of the ages at which individuals in different populations become infected with EBV. In developing countries, almost all children have acquired the virus by 2 to 4 years of age, depending on geographical region. In developed countries with high standards of living and hygiene, the time of infection is delayed for many, more markedly among the affluent than the less well off. Amongst the very rich, as many as 50 per cent may reach adolescence or young adulthood without having encountered the virus and will undergo delayed primary infection with a high risk that this will be accompanied by the symptoms of infectious mononucleosis. (Reprinted with permission from Epstein MA (2002). Infectious mononucleosis. In: *Encyclopedia of life sciences*, vol. 10, pp.211–16. http://www.els.net, London: Nature Publishing Group.)

Fig. 2 Percentage of patients with infectious mononucleosis showing various clinical features during the course of the disease, and the timing and average duration of each. (Reprinted with permission from Epstein MA (2002). Infectious mononucleosis. In: *Encyclopedia of life sciences*, vol. 10, pp.211–16. http://www.els.net, London: Nature Publishing Group.)

Symptoms

Classic infectious mononucleosis may follow some days of vague indisposition or may start abruptly. It presents with sore throat, fever with sweating, anorexia, headache, and fatigue, together with malaise quite out of proportion to the other complaints. Dysphagia may be noticed and also brief orbital oedema. Erythematous and maculopapular rashes occur in a small number of untreated patients, but in many more who have been taking ampicillin for sore throat before infectious mononucleosis has been diagnosed. Tonsillar and pharyngeal oedema can rarely cause pharyngeal obstruction (Fig. 2).

Signs

The fever may rise to 40°C but high levels and swings are not seen. There is redness and oedema of the pharynx, fauces, soft palate, and uvula, and about half the patients develop greyish exudates. Generalized lymphadenopathy is almost always present, most marked in the cervical region; the glands are symmetrical, discrete, and slightly tender, and are accompanied by splenomegaly in about 60 per cent of cases and an enlarged liver in 10 per cent. There is usually a moderate bradycardia. Besides the rash, characteristic palatal enanthematous crops of reddish petechiae are found in about one-third of patients, and jaundice occurs in about 8 per cent (Fig. 2).

Clinical course

Mild cases may resolve in days, but 1 to 2 weeks is more usual, followed by a period of lethargy. The duration of this convalescence is influenced by psychological factors, particularly the speed with which patients are encouraged to resume full activity. About 1 case in 2000 may continue in a truly chronic or recurrent form for several months or years, and here exhaustive investigations have shown immunological defects. Most other cases of so-called chronic infectious mononucleosis are in reality manifestations of 'chronic fatigue syndrome', but it is highly controversial as to whether this is a true entity rather than a form of depression or a belief disorder; credible connections with EBV have not been established. In contrast, there is an extremely rare, genetically determined, X-linked, lymphoproliferative condition (XLP disease, or Duncan syndrome after one of the first families to be recognized) in which the affected young males of certain kindred die from infectious mononucleosis owing to a specific inability to respond normally to EBV during primary infection; the disease progresses inexorably, with necrotic destruction of vital organs and multisystem failure. There is evidence that an aberrant immune response to EBV in XLP results in unregulated cytotoxic T-cell activity being directed against the normal cells of vital organs instead of targeting solely on EBV-infected cells displaying EBV antigens. The gene responsible for this defect has recently been cloned.

Complications

Minor non-specific complications may occur; rare more serious complications include secondary bacterial throat infections, traumatic rupture of the enlarged spleen, asphyxia from pharyngeal oedema, massive hepatic necrosis, Guillain–Barré syndrome, and autoimmune manifestations such as thrombocytopenia and haemolytic anaemia.

Differential diagnosis

Classic infectious mononucleosis is diagnosed on the basis of the clinical picture considered in conjunction with serological and haematological laboratory investigations (see below). An infectious mononucleosis-like disease can occur in primary cytomegalovirus infection and in toxoplasmosis, but in both conditions the sore throat is much less severe and with cytomegalovirus the lymphadenopathy may be minimal or absent.

Laboratory diagnosis

A rapid screening test (Monospot test) can be used to detect the presence of heterophil antibodies in the patient's serum. Although these heterophil antibodies are not directed against viral-coded proteins they are present in up to 85 per cent of acute infectious mononucleosis sera. Cases of Monospot-negative infectious mononucleosis tend to be those outside the classic 15- to 25-year age range, and false-positive tests may occur in pregnancy and autoimmune disease. However, the presence of serum IgM antibodies to EB virus capsid antigen (**VCA**) are diagnostic of infectious mononucleosis. An additional important feature of infectious mononucleosis is the presence of lymphocytosis of up to $15 \times 10^9/1$, with the majority of cells having an 'atypical' morphology.

Treatment

Bed rest and aspirin for headache and pharyngeal discomfort are the only treatments required. When the fever resolves the patient should be encouraged to get up and resume some activities as fast as is practicable, but violent exercise should be avoided for 3 weeks after an enlarged spleen ceases to be palpable. Only complications need active therapy: splenic rupture requires surgery, bacterial infections call for appropriate antibiotics, airway obstruction must be relieved by tracheostomy, and corticosteroids should be given for life-threatening pharyngeal oedema and for neurological and haematological complications.

Pathogenesis

Why children do not have symptoms during primary EBV infection whereas adolescents and young adults frequently react by developing infectious mononucleosis is not fully understood. The immunological reactions of young adults on first encountering EBV are more exuberant than those of children reflecting physiological differences in responsiveness. The mode of infection and consequent size of infecting dose also play an important part; children come into contact with small amounts of virus in saliva from a shedder in droplets or casually contaminating some sucked object, whereas a young person may take in large amounts of virus-containing saliva from a carrier during kissing so that virions reach susceptible cells in large numbers. Intraepithelial B cells become productively infected in infectious mononucleosis and at this stage EBV can easily be found in patients' saliva. The newly replicated virus infects masses of B lymphocytes which are released from the throat into the blood and lymphatics from where they accumulate in lymphoid tissue throughout the body. In response, there is a generation of even greater numbers of cytotoxic T cells specifically directed against EBV-determined antigens displayed by the infected B lymphocytes. An exaggerated immunological response thus

underlies the changes seen in infectious mononucleosis since all these lymphoid cells present in the circulation, in lymph nodes, in tonsils, in lymphoid centres in the mouth and pharynx, and in spleen and liver are responsible for causing the sore throat, fever, malaise, lymphadenopathy, and hepatosplenomegaly by immunopathological mechanisms.

Endemic (or 'African') Burkitt lymphoma

The classic form of this B-cell tumour, first described by Burkitt in 1958, is found in certain parts of Africa and Papua New Guinea where the temperature does not fall below 16°C or the annual rainfall below 55 cm. Endemic Burkitt lymphoma is distinct from the 'Burkitt-like' tumours that occur sporadically everywhere in the world (sometimes called 'American' Burkitt lymphoma) and that have a different age incidence, anatomical distribution, and response to therapy, and arise from B cells with different phenotypic characteristics.

The association between EBV and endemic Burkitt lymphoma is so close that it is generally accepted that the virus is an essential link along with cofactors in a complicated chain of events which leads to the malignancy. Hyperendemic malaria has been identified as the important cofactor, and its spread by anopheline mosquitoes requiring warmth and moisture explains the climate dependence of Burkitt lymphoma.

Burkitt lymphoma is a disease of childhood, is extremely rare over the age of 14 years, and in the endemic areas it is more common than all other childhood tumours added together.

Symptoms

The tumour is usually multifocal and the symptoms depend entirely on the anatomical location. Jaw tumours are present in 70 per cent of patients, are the usual presenting feature, may be multiple in up to all four quadrants, and are almost always accompanied by tumours elsewhere. They give a rapidly growing mass with loosening of teeth and exophthalmos from orbital spread. Abdominal tumours involve retroperitoneal nodes, liver, ovaries, intestines, and kidneys. Burkitt lymphoma sometimes presents in thyroid, the adolescent female breast, testicles, and salivary glands; extradural tumours in the spine cause rapid paraplegia, and skeletal tumours also occur. Characteristically Burkitt lymphoma does not involve the spleen or peripheral lymph nodes.

Signs

The tumours are firm, very rapidly growing, painless, and cause minimal constitutional disturbance. Their sites determine the clinical signs.

Clinical course

Tumour growth is relentless and death ensues within a few months in the absence of treatment.

Differential diagnosis

In endemic areas Burkitt lymphoma can be diagnosed from the clinical picture. Unlike Burkitt lymphoma, retinoblastoma is intraocular, rhabdomyosarcoma is extraorbital and does not involve teeth, nephroblastoma is not multifocal, and neuroblastoma and ovarian tumours can be distinguished histologically. Paraplegia of tuberculous origin causes vertebral collapse and acute transverse myelitis is preceded by pain and fever. Other lymphomas have a markedly dissimilar anatomical distribution.

Laboratory diagnosis

Histological examination of a biopsy sample gives ready confirmation. Antibodies to EBV antigens show a unique pattern and titres rise or fall with disease progression or response to therapy. IgG anti-VCA titres are around 10 times higher than in controls and antibodies to EBV-restricted early antigens (EA-R) and membrane antigens (MA) are also detectable.

Treatment

Surgery and radiotherapy are ineffective, but moderate courses of chemo-therapy give excellent results with cyclophosphamide being the drug of choice.

Pathogenesis

The molecular pathways whereby EBV-coded antigens transform normal B lymphocytes *in vitro* into continuously growing immortalized cell lines are partially understood. There are now credible explanations as to how EBV combines with cofactors such as hyperendemic malaria to cause the tumour. The virus is a necessary, but not on its own sufficient, element in the aetiology of the disease.

Lymphoproliferations in immunosuppressed states

In primary and secondary suppression of cellular immunity there is dimin-ished immune control of persisting EBV infection which leads to increased virus replication in the oral cavity, increased numbers of circulating, virus-carrying B lymphocytes, and increased levels of serum antibodies to EBV antigens. This is sometimes described as a 'reactivated infection' although the condition is clinically silent. However, on occasions the loss of control leads to the development of EBV-associated lymphoproliferations.

In transplant recipients

Transplant recipients who receive lifelong immunosuppressive drugs to prevent graft rejection have a 28 to 100 times increased risk of developing lymphoproliferative disease and lymphoma compared with normal con-trols; most of these conditions are of B-cell origin, contain the EBV gen-ome, and express viral antigens in their cells. Lymphoproliferative disease has two forms. About 50 per cent of cases are associated with primary EBV infection in patients who were seronegative at the time of grafting, occur within the first year after transplantation in a young age group, and have infectious mononucleosis-like symptoms. The remainder of the cases occur in older patients late after transplantation as a localized mass, commonly in the gut, central nervous system, or transplanted organ; biopsy shows large-cell lymphoma, which is usually monoclonal. Reduction of immunosup-pressive therapy, with or without acyclovir therapy, is the first line of treatment, with cytotoxic drugs and/or radiotherapy being used only where there is no response or after recurrence. Recently, experimental treatments with EBV-specific cytotoxic T-cell infusions have shown encouraging results.

In acquired immunodeficiency syndrome (AIDS)

Two types of lymphoma are seen in patients with AIDS; large-cell lymph-oma and Burkitt lymphoma, and both may be associated with EBV.

Large-cell lymphomas similar to those found in transplant recipients (see above) occur in severely immunocompromised patients with AIDS; their distribution is extranodal, involving many unusual sites, most com-monly the central nervous system. These lymphomas show a strong associ-ation with EBV which reaches 100 per cent in cerebral tumours; the progress is rapid, with a mean survival time from diagnosis of 3 to 4 months. Treatment (radiotherapy) is disappointing because patients with terminal AIDS are in such poor general health.

Burkitt lymphoma occurs earlier in the course of human immunodefi-ciency virus (HIV) disease while the immune system is still relatively intact and is therefore more amenable to treatment. About 50 per cent of these lymphomas contain EBV DNA.

Hodgkin's disease and T-cell lymphomas

There has long been a suspicion that EBV is involved in the induction of Hodgkin's disease because of the similar socio-economic epidemiology of Hodgkin's disease and infectious mononucleosis, and because within 5 years of infectious mononucleosis there is a four- to sixfold increase in the likelihood of developing Hodgkin's disease. There is now evidence that in Hodgkin's lymphomas EBV DNA is carried and expressed in both the Reed–Sternberg and the mononuclear Hodgkin's cells. These findings are as yet insufficient to implicate EBV in the aetiology of Hodgkin's disease, but point to the need for further investigation. A similar situation exists with oral T-cell lymphoma in patients with AIDS, and nasal T-cell lymphomas.

Nasopharyngeal carcinoma

This tumour is restricted to the postnasal space where it arises from squa-mous epithelial cells. The tumour is seen rarely throughout the world but has a remarkably high incidence in southern Chinese, and in the Inuit and related circum-Arctic races. In high incidence areas, nasopharyngeal car-cinoma is the most common cancer of men and the second most common of women. A rather high incidence of nasopharyngeal carcinoma is seen amongst Malays, Dyaks, Indonesians, Filipinos, and Vietnamese people, and a medium-high incidence belt stretches across North Africa, through the Sudan, to the Kenya highlands. The tumour usually occurs in middle or old age, but in North Africa it has bimodal age peaks, one involving young people up to 20 years of age and a second much later in life. Irrespective of geographical region, nasopharyngeal carcinoma cells always carry the EBV genome.

Symptoms

Nasopharyngeal carcinoma causes nasal obstruction, discharge, or bleed-ing; deafness, tinnitus, or earache; headache; and ocular paresis from tumour spread to involve cranial nerves. Patients may present with a single symptom caused locally by the tumour or with several symptoms, and about one-third complain only of cervical lymph-node enlargement due to metastatic spread from an occult primary tumour.

Signs

Direct spread from the primary tumour may involve the soft tissues, bone, parotid gland, buccal cavity, and oropharynx. The neoplasm may extend into the nasal fossas, the paranasal sinuses, or the orbit, and can invade the eustachian canal or the parapharyngeal space where cranial nerves IX, X, XI, and XII can be involved. Invasion of the skull or cranial foramina may damage cranial nerves II, IV, V, and VI. Lymphatic spread causes enlarged cervical lymph nodes and subsequently extends to the supraclavicular glands. If bloodborne metastases occur, they are most frequent in the bones, liver, and lungs, but may be in any organ.

Clinical course

Untreated nasopharyngeal carcinoma progresses inexorably to death.

Differential diagnosis

Nasopharyngeal carcinoma must be distinguished from other tumours of the nasal cavities, namely adenocarcinomas, sarcomas, malignant lymph-omas, and rare malignancies such as chordoma, teratoma, and mela-noma.

Laboratory diagnosis

The diagnosis of nasopharyngeal carcinoma is made histologically on a biopsy sample either from the primary tumour or from an enlarged cer-vical lymph node. In addition, serum antibody titres to EBV antigens show a characteristic reaction pattern—IgG and IgA antibodies to VCA and diffuse early antigen (EA-D) are raised, with the titre correlating with the tumour burden. Uniquely, IgA antibodies to VCA and EA are also found in the saliva from patients.

Treatment

Nasopharyngeal carcinoma responds well to radiotherapy, which is the treatment of choice. In the earliest stages of the disease, radiotherapy gives 5-year survival rates of 50 per cent or more, and of those surviving 5 years, 70 per cent remain permanently free of relapse. More advanced stages of nasopharyngeal carcinoma have correspondingly worse prognoses.

Pathogenesis

EBV is now widely accepted as necessary for the causation of nasopharyngeal carcinoma, but is not sufficient on its own. Besides the racial predisposition there is also a genetic predisposition since southern Chinese people with an A2BW36 haplotype are four to six times more likely to have nasopharyngeal carcinoma than those without. Epidemiological studies suggest that important environmental cofactors associated with the Chinese way of life play a role and two likely candidates are: traditional herbal medicines, taken as snuff, and containing tumour-promoting substances of phorbol ester type; and traditional salt fish which has been shown to contain carcinogenic nitrosamines.

Hairy leukoplakia in AIDS

This lesion occurs in people with HIV and in other immunosuppressed individuals; it usually presents as painless white patches on the tongue or on the lateral buccal mucosa. The lesions are slightly raised, poorly demarcated, and have a 'hairy' or corrugated surface; the patches are usually multiple and measure up to 3 cm in diameter.

The squamous epithelial cells of this condition contain large amounts of actively replicating EBV, providing an unusual example of the production of the virus by such cells. Treatment with acyclovir arrests the EBV replication and the lesions regress, but only for as long as the drug is continued.

Smooth muscle tumours and gastric carcinoma

Recently EBV has been implicated in various types of gastric carcinoma and in leiomyomas and leiomyosarcomas in children immunosuppressed by AIDS or after organ transplantation. Much further study of these relationships is required.

Further reading

Bar RS *et al.* (1974). Fatal infectious mononucleosis in a family. *New England Journal of Medicine* **290**, 363–7. [The first account of an XLP (Duncan) syndrome family.]

Burkitt D (1958). A sarcoma involving the jaws of African children. *British Journal of Surgery* **46**, 218–3. [The first description of Burkitt lymphoma.]

Burkitt D (1963). A lymphoma syndrome in tropical Africa. *International Review of Experimental Pathology* **2**, 67–138. [An early comprehensive review of Burkitt lymphoma.]

de Thé *et al.* (1978). Epidemiological evidence for a causal relationship between Epstein-Barr virus and Burkitt's lymphoma: results of the prospective Ugandan study. *Nature* **274**, 756–61. [A massive investigation linking EBV to the causation of Burkitt lymphoma.]

Epstein A (1999). On the discovery of Epstein-Barr virus: a memoir. *Epstein-Barr Virus Report* **6**, 58–63. [Details of how EBV was discovered.]

Epstein MA, Achong BG, eds (1979). *The Epstein–Barr virus.* Springer Verlag, Berlin. [A complete survey of the first 15 years of EBV research.]

Greenspan JS *et al.* (1985). Replication of Epstein-Barr virus within the epithelial cells of oral hairy leukoplakia, an AIDS-associated lesion. *New England Journal of Medicine* **313**, 1564–71. [The first description of the condition.]

Henle G, Henle W, Diehl V (1968). The relation of Burkitt's lymphoma tumor-associated herpesvirus to infectious mononucleosis. *Proceedings of the National Academy of Sciences (USA)* **59**, 94–101. [The account of the original findings identifying EBV as the cause of infectious mononucleosis.]

Herbst H, Niedobitek G (1994). Epstein–Barr virus in Hodgkin's Disease. *Epstein–Barr Virus Report* **1**, 31–5. [A very useful review.]

Hoagland RK (1955). Transmission of infectious mononucleosis. *American Journal of Medical Science* **229**, 262–72. [The first recognition of infectious mononucleosis as the 'kissing disease'.]

Rickinson AB, Kieff E (2001). Epstein–Barr virus. In: Fields BN *et al.* eds. *Fields virology*, 4th edn, Vol 2, pp 2575–627. Lippincott, Williams and Wilkins, Philadelphia. [A comprehensive review of recent work on EBV.]

Rickinson AB *et al.* (2001). T-cell recognition of Epstein–Barr virus associated lymphomas. *Cancer Surveys* **13**, 53–80. [An excellent survey.]

Schlossberg D, ed. (1989). *Infectious mononucleosis*, 2nd edn. Springer Verlag, Berlin. [A multiauthor work covering many aspects of the disease.]

Shanmugaratnam K (1971). Studies on the etiology of nasopharyngeal carcinoma. *International Review of Experimental Pathology* **10**, 361–413. [An excellent review.]

Sprunt TP, Evans FA (1920). Mononuclear leucocytosis in reaction to acute infections ('infectious mononucleosis'). *Bulletin of the Johns Hopkins Hospital* **31**, 410–17. [The first description of infectious mononucleosis.]

Thomas JA, Allday MJ, Crawford DH (1991). Epstein–Barr virus-associated lymphoproliferative disorders in immunocompromised individuals. *Advances in Cancer Research* **57**, 329–80. [A good review.]

7.10.4 Poxviruses

Geoffrey L. Smith

Poxviruses are large DNA viruses that replicate in the cell cytoplasm. The most infamous was variola virus, which caused smallpox, a disease responsible for devastating epidemics with up to 40 per cent mortality. Smallpox was eradicated (1977) by immunoprophylaxis with vaccinia virus, a related orthopoxvirus. Poxvirus infections in humans have since been restricted to molluscum contagiosum and rare zoonoses such as monkeypox, cowpox, orf, pseudocowpox, yaba tumour virus, and tanapox.

Classification

The chordopoxviruse subfamily is subdivided into eight genera, of which the orthopoxviruses have been the most important (Table 1). Viruses within different genera are antigenically distinct, while those within a genus are cross-reactive and cross-protective. Four of the nine poxviruses that infect humans are orthopoxviruses: cowpox, variola, monkeypox, and vaccinia virus. Different orthopoxviruses are distinguishable by their biological properties such as pock type, ceiling temperature on the chorioallantoic membrane, or by the restriction pattern of genomic DNA. Following the sequencing of several virus genomes, species-specific DNA probes are becoming available. Vaccinia virus has no known natural animal reservoir and its origin remains a mystery. It caused human disease only as a rare complication after vaccination against smallpox. Cowpox and monkeypox viruses were named after the species from which they were isolated

Table 1 Poxvirus classification

Subfamily	Genus	Species
Entomopox		
Chordopox	orthopox	*variola virus
		*vaccinia virus
		*monkeypox virus
		*cowpox virus
		ectromelia virus
		rabbitpox virus
	capripox	sheeppox virus
		goatpox virus
		lumpy skin disease virus
	parapox	*orf virus
		*pseudocowpox virus
	avipox	fowlpox virus
		canarypox virus
	suipox	swinepox virus
	leporipox	myxoma virus
		Shope fibroma virus
		malignant rabbit virus
	molluscipox	*molluscum contagiosum virus
	yatapox	*yaba tumour virus
		*tanapox virus

* Viruses that infect man.

Fig. 1 Electron micrograph of material from smallpox lesion, viewed by negative contrast, showing a clump of poxvirus particles. (By courtesy of the late Henry Bedson.)

but the natural reservoir of each virus may be rodents. Infections in cows or monkeys, like the occasional transmission to man, are rare. Cowpox, monkeypox, and vaccinia virus have a broad host range, while variola virus infected only humans and the lack of an animal reservoir aided the smallpox eradication campaign.

Poxvirus biology

Poxviruses replicate in the cytoplasm, encode enzymes for transcription and DNA replication, and have large, complex virions (Fig. 1) and double stranded DNA genomes of 150 to 300 kb. Vaccinia virus is the most intensively studied poxvirus. It encodes about 200 genes of three classes (early, intermediate, and late) that are expressed in a strictly regulated manner. Transcription of each class is dependent upon the prior expression of the previous class.

Virus morphogenesis is complex (Fig. 2(a)) and produces two forms of infectious virion: intracellular mature virus (IMV) and extracellular enveloped virus (EEV). IMV remains within the cell until it is lysed and forms most of the progeny, whereas EEV is released from the cell before death and represents less than 1 per cent of infectivity (Fig. 2(b)). EEV possesses an additional lipid envelope with which several virus and cellular proteins are associated, giving it distinct immunological and biological properties. EEV is necessary for virus dissemination *in vitro* and within the infected host. Immunity to EEV-specific antigens, which are highly conserved among orthopoxviruses, is required for protection against disease.

Pathogenesis

Poxvirus infections cause a local skin lesion or generalized pustular rash. Detailed experimental analysis of human smallpox was impossible, but generalized poxvirus infections have been studied in experimental models, namely monkeypox in monkeys, rabbitpox (a neurovirulent vaccinia virus) in rabbits, and ectromelia virus in mice. The spread of variola virus in man was probably similar to that of ectromelia virus in mice and is characterized by sequential phases of virus infection, replication, and release accompanied by cell necrosis.

Virus enters through skin abrasions (ectromelia and cowpox) or inhalation of airborne virus and establishes a respiratory infection (ectromelia, rabbitpox, and variola). In smallpox, the respiratory route was most important and sometimes the only possible route of transmission from index cases to contacts; also patients became infectious only after enanthem developed. A respiratory infection was established in the epithelial cells of the alveoli and small bronchioles. Here, alveolar macrophages became infected and transmitted the virus via lymphatics to the local lymph node, where further virus replication occurred. Virus released into the blood (primary viraemia) was mostly cell-associated and spread to other organs of the reticuloendothelial system, notably the liver, spleen, and lymph nodes.

Extensive replication here released larger amounts of virus into the blood (secondary viraemia) enabling the virus to infect other organs such as the kidneys, lungs, and intestines and to reach the skin and produce the skin lesions with the characteristic centrifugal distribution (Fig. 3) (Plate 1). Lesions started with a papule that became pustular and then crusted. After 2 to 3 weeks the scab was shed leaving a scar. The incubation period of smallpox was approximately 12 days. Symptoms included headache, fever, malaise, vomiting, and, in severe cases, prostration, toxaemia, and hypotension. Delayed onset of the skin eruptions usually correlated with a grave prognosis. Haemorrhagic or flat confluent-type smallpox had very high mortality rates.

The outcome of infection depended upon the age and physiological and immunological status of the patient and the strain of virus. Variola major was more virulent and produced fatality rates in unvaccinated patients of between 5 and 40 per cent, while the milder variola minor, called alastrim in the Americas, caused only 0.1 to 2 per cent mortality. Morphologically, the viruses were indistinguishable, and vaccination with vaccinia virus was equally effective against both. However, alastrim virus was consistently more thermolabile and had a lower ceiling temperature of 37.5°C compared to 38.5°C for variola major, 39°C for monkeypox, 40°C for cowpox, and 41°C for vaccinia virus.

Very young and elderly patients were most susceptible to smallpox and those aged 5 to 20 years most resistant. Pregnancy and immunological deficiency, particularly in cell-mediated immunity, increased the severity of infection. Pregnant women were more likely than any other group to develop haemorrhagic-type smallpox, which was usually fatal. The greater importance of cell-mediated immunity rather than antibody in recovery from poxvirus infections was illustrated in several ways. Firstly, in children with severe defects in cell-mediated immunity there was a progressive and uncontrolled virus replication from the vaccination site that was usually fatal. In contrast, defects in antibody production were usually tolerated if the cell-mediated immune response was normal. Secondly, passive administration of antivaccinia virus serum had little effect on mice infected with ectromelia virus, whereas prior infection with vaccinia virus was protective. Thirdly, in mice infected with ectromelia virus, the effective mechanisms that combated infection in the liver and spleen were operative by 4 to 6 days postinfection and coincided with the maximum levels of cytolytic T cells, but preceded the development of systemic antibody.

Fig. 3 Smallpox in a 9-month-old boy in Pakistan, photographed on the eighth day of the rash. (By courtesy of the World Health Organization.)

The eradication of smallpox

Early attempts to control smallpox relied upon variolation or inoculation, in which material isolated from a mild case of smallpox was administered by sniffing or scratching. This was replaced by vaccination in 1798 after Jenner noticed that milkmaids, who often acquired cowpox infections on their hands from the teats of cows, were protected from smallpox. Jenner infected a boy (James Phipps) with poxvirus material (probably cowpox), derived from a cow via a milkmaid (Sarah Nelmes), and subsequently challenged him with smallpox. Protection was achieved and due to the efficacy and greater safety of this procedure it rapidly replaced variolation. Sometime between 1798 and the twentieth century vaccinia virus replaced cowpox as the smallpox vaccine. In 1959, the World Health Organization (WHO) adopted a recommendation to achieve the global eradication of smallpox. With fresh funding and a plentiful supply of potent freeze-dried vaccine this goal was achieved in 1977. Two years later, the WHO certified that eradication was complete. This triumph of preventive medicine justifies the saying 'prevention is better than cure' but also demonstrates that prevention is best achieved by eradication.

Sequencing of poxvirus genomes

The genomes of vaccinia virus strains Copenhagen, Western Reserve and modified virus Ankara (MVA), variola virus strains India-1967 and Bangladesh-1975, and camelpox virus have been determined. In addition, regions of variola virus Harvey-1947, Garcia-1966, Congo-1970, and Somalia-1977, rabbitpox, and cowpox virus GRI-90 have been sequenced. These analyses showed that the central region of these orthopoxvirus genomes are very closely related with greater than 96 per cent nucleotide identity between vaccinia and variola viruses, but that there is significant divergence in the terminal regions. A notable difference between the vaccinia and variola genomes is the fragmentation of several genes in variola that are intact in vaccinia virus. It is possible that the disruption of genes of an ancestral

(a)

(b)

Fig. 2 Electron micrographs showing (a) a cytoplasmic vaccinia virus factory containing maturing virus particles with stages of morphogenesis numbered 1 to 4 and (b) fully enveloped virus particles, one of which is leaving the cell.

poxvirus may have contributed to the evolution of variola major as a highly pathogenic virus for man. The retention of these non-functional genes in the variola virus genome suggests that they became non-functional in the relatively recent evolutionary past, and perhaps that variola virus is a 'recent' human pathogen that never became fully adapted to man.

Other poxvirus genomes that have been sequenced are molluscum contagiosum virus, Shope fibroma virus and myxoma virus, yaba-like disease virus, and the *Melanoplus sanguinipes* entomopoxvirus.

Poxvirus expression vectors

Vaccinia virus recombinants expressing foreign genes were developed in 1982 and have become a widely used laboratory expression system and have potential as live vaccines for infectious disease and cancer. Infection with a recombinant vaccinia virus allows expression and simultaneous delivery of the foreign antigen to the immune system. Moreover, the large capacity of vaccinia virus allows expression of multiple foreign genes from a single virus so creating polyvalent vaccines. Safer vaccinia virus strains that do not cause vaccination complications (eczema vaccinatum, generalized vaccinia, progressive vaccinia, encephalopathy (<2 years), or encephalitis (>2 years)) are being developed by deletion of virulence genes from conventional vaccinia virus strains. An alternative strategy is to use poxviruses that establish only abortive infections in human cells, such as MVA or the avipoxviruses fowlpox virus and canarypox.

Human monkeypox

Monkeypox was discovered in captive primates in 1958, but in 1970 was isolated in tropical rain forests of West and Central Africa from humans who had suffered generalized poxvirus rashes visibly very similar to smallpox. The virus is distinct from variola in pock morphology, ceiling temperature, genomic restriction endonuclease pattern, lesion morphology on rabbit skin, and its ability to be passaged indefinitely in mouse brain. However, although monkeypox produced a very similar disease to smallpox in man, person-to-person transmission was too inefficient for establishing epidemics. Thus human monkeypox infections are single or multiple sporadic cases restricted to dense tropical rain forests in Central and West Africa. Clinically, human monkeypox closely resembles ordinary, discrete-type smallpox except that there is a pronounced lymph node enlargement (Fig. 4). Mortality rates in unvaccinated patients between 1970 and 1986 were 11.2 per cent but these were all in children less than 8 years old and the highest rate (18.7 per cent) was in infants less than 2 years. The virus is probably acquired from infected monkeys or rodents such as squirrels.

Cowpox and pseudocowpox

Cowpox virus has a broad host range including cattle, humans, large felines, and even elephants, but it is not enzootic in cattle and its natural hosts are rodents. It is distinguishable from vaccinia virus by the pock type, ceiling temperature, rate of replication in tissue culture, genome size and restriction pattern, and the production of cytoplasmic A-type inclusion bodies. Pseudocowpox is enzootic in cattle, unlike cowpox. Historically, it was important since it was sometimes used mistakenly for vaccination and, being a parapoxvirus, was ineffective in preventing smallpox. Its misuse compromised Jenner's correct assertion that true cowpox was an effective smallpox vaccine.

In man, cowpox produces an acutely inflamed, local lesion, similar to a primary smallpox vaccination. There is usually fever, enlargement of the local lymph nodes, and pain. Unlike vaccinia virus, which occasionally produced a generalized infection, cowpox lesions are always local. Human lesions caused by pseudocowpox virus (milker's nodules) are extremely rare and are less painful than those caused by cowpox.

Fig. 4 Moderately severe monkeypox in a girl of 7 years from Equateur Province, Zaire. (By courtesy of the World Health Organization.)

Tanapox and yaba tumour virus

Tanapox virus was first isolated from the Tana valley in Kenya from humans suffering from localized skin lesions typical of poxviruses (Plate 2). Subsequently, a similar virus was found in humans in Zaire during surveillance for monkeypox. It is a rare zoonosis of monkeys, that in Kenya may have been transmitted by mosquitoes. Serologically, it is related to yaba-like disease virus and yaba tumour virus. In man it usually produces a solitary lesion that is preceded for a few days by a mild fever. The lesion takes 5 to 6 weeks to clear and is distinguished from other poxvirus lesions by its failure to become pustular. This virus cannot be cultured on the chorioallantoic membrane.

Yaba tumour virus is a monkey virus that can cause histiocytomas if injected subcutaneously or intradermally into man. The lesions are not neoplastic and are cleared by the immune response.

Cutaneous poxviruses (orf and molluscum contagiosum)

See Chapters 7.10.25 and 7.10.26.

Further reading

Binns MM (1992). *Recombinant poxviruses.* CRC Press, Boca Raton, Florida.

Fenner F, Wittek R, Dumbell KR (1989). *The orthopoxviruses.* Academic Press, London.

Moss B (1996). Poxviridae: the viruses and their replication. In: Fields BN, Knipe DM, Howley PM, Chanock RM, Melnick J, Monath TP, Roizman B, Straus SE, eds. *Virology*, 3rd edn, pp. 2637–71. Lippincott-Raven, Philadelphia.

7.10.5 Mumps: epidemic parotitis

B. K. Rima

Aetiology

Mumps is an acute, generalized, communicable infection of children and young adults, caused by a paramyxovirus. Almost any organ can be infected—salivary glands, pancreas, testis, ovary, brain, mammary gland, liver, kidney, joints, and heart. Swelling of the face is only one of the symptoms of the disease, albeit the most common and important one for diagnosis.

Epidemiology

The incubation period lies between 14 and 18 days. In any outbreak, 30 to 40 per cent of those exposed infected have subclinical illness. Mumps is highly infectious. Transmission depends on close personal contact with a patient who is excreting virus in the saliva and spreading it in droplets. In the prevaccine era, the peak incidence was in the late winter or early spring, in 3- to 7-year cycles. Most morbidity is associated with meningitis and orchitis. Case fatality is about 2 per 1000.

Virology

Mumps virus (**MuV**) can be grown in tissue cultures of chick embryo, monkey kidney, human amnion, or HeLa cells. Cytopathic changes may be seen as early as 24 h postinfection. With immunofluorescence the virus can

be detected in a matter of hours. The virus can also be cultured in the yolk sac or embryonic cavity of chick embryos.

MuV is thermolabile. It can be stored for years at −70°C but infectivity is lost in a few days at room temperature. Treatment with ether or paraformaldehyde inactivates the virus rapidly, but neither of these processes destroys the antigens responsible for the complement fixation, haemagglutination, or reactivity in the skin test.

A patient excretes culturable MuV in the saliva for between 2 and 6 days before parotitis develops and for up to 4 days afterwards. Virus can be cultured from the urine for up to 14 days around the onset of disease. It is almost as easily cultured from ultracentrifugates of urine as from saliva. There is, however, no evidence of viral spread of the virus by urine. During the acute disease MuV can also be cultured from throat washings or a swab of the orifice of Stensen's duct and be detected by reverse-transcriptase polymerase chain reaction (**RT-PCR**), in saliva, throat swabs, and urine. In the blood it can be cultured only for a day or two around the start of disease. Virus can be isolated from cerebrospinal fluid for the first 3 or 4 days of the meningeal illness.

MuV is an enveloped RNA virus with a genome of 15 384 nucleotides. Its inner core is a ribonucleoprotein complex (the nucleocapsid) containing the non-segmented, negative-strand, RNA molecule encapsidated by the major nucleocapsid protein (N). The nucleocapsid has the herring bone structure characteristic of paramyxoviruses (Fig. 1(a)). Attached to this are two further proteins involved in transcription and replication of the RNA genome: the phosphoprotein (P) and the large replicase protein (L). The nucleocapsid is surrounded by a lipid bilayer membrane derived from the host cell (Fig. 1(a, b)). On the inner leaflet there is a membrane or matrix protein (M) that plays an essential role in virus budding. On the outer surface are two glycoproteins, one carrying the haemagglutinin-neuraminidase activity (HN), the other responsible for fusion activity (F). A non-structural, small, hydrophobic protein (SH) has been described in the

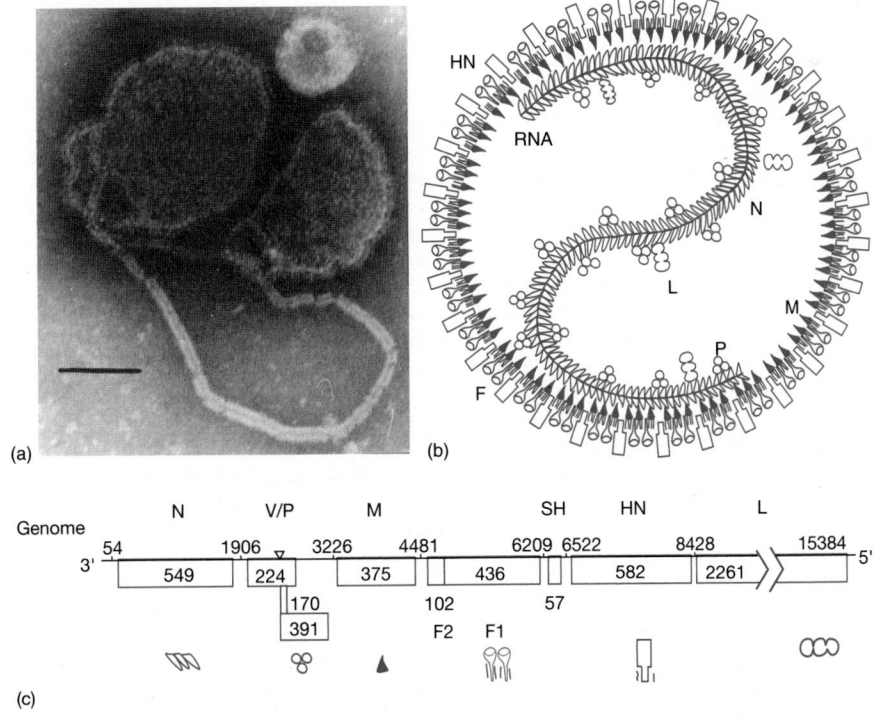

Fig. 1 Structure and genome organization of mumps virus. (a) A disrupted, negatively stained, mumps virion. The viral nucleocapsid protrudes from the particle and the fringe of viral spikes is visible (bar = 100 nm). (b) Diagram of the localization of the nucleocapsid (N), phospho- (P), large (L), matrix (M), haemagglutinin-neuraminidase (HN), and fusion (F) proteins in the mumps virion. (c) Structure of the genome of mumps virus indicating the localization of the genes, the nucleotide number of their starting and stopping position, and (in boxes) the number of amino acid residues in each of the viral proteins.

membrane of MuV-infected cells. The sequence of the SH protein is hyper-variable. This has been exploited in molecular studies of the epidemiology of MuV. The functions of V, and other non-structural protein, and SH are unknown. The gene order (Fig. 1(c)) leads to an expression gradient in which the abundance of mRNAs decreases with increasing distance to the promoter at the 3_ end of the genome so that the N mRNA is more abundant than the L mRNA.

Pathogenesis and pathology

MuV causes an infection of the upper respiratory tract that spreads to draining lymph nodes. The subsequent viraemia and infection of the lymphocytes and macrophages causes spread to many organs, but because mumps is so rarely lethal, details are scant. Lymphocytic infiltration and destruction of periductal cells lead to blockage of the ducts both in salivary glands and in the seminiferous tubules of the testes. The lymphatics in the tissues surrounding and overlying the parotid glands become obstructed, producing a gel-like oedema that may spread down over the chest wall, especially when the swelling of the salivary glands is severe.

MuV frequently invades the nervous system: changes can be detected by electroencephalography or by examination of the cerebrospinal fluid in at least half the patients. However, in most of these cases there are no neurological symptoms or signs. Mumps virus is one of the most common known causes of lymphocytic meningitis. Neuronal damage probably does occur, explaining the occurrence of quadriplegia or single-nerve paralysis in some patients. Apart from transient weakness of the facial nerve, which may be due to pressure of a swollen gland or damage by mumps virus, these complications are very rare.

Mumps encephalitis is a different entity; cerebrospinal fluid is normal and contains no virus. At autopsy there is perivascular demyelination as in other forms of postinfectious encephalitis (see Chapter xxxx).

Clinical features and diagnosis

Parotitis

A patient with mumps parotitis may have a fever without rigors (40 to 40.5°C) as well as pain near the angle of the jaw. The face and neck become distorted with swelling. The skin over the gland is hot and flushed but there is no rash, unlike in the swelling of erysipelas. If the swelling is severe, the mouth cannot be opened for pain and tightness, and is dry because the flow of saliva is blocked. This discomfort lasts for 3 or 4 days. Sometimes as one side clears, the parotid on the other side swells. When there is bilateral parotitis, clinical diagnosis is usually obvious. One condition that must be excluded is bull-neck diphtheria (see Chapter 7.11.1), which can look very like mumps.

Rarely, the submaxillary and sublingual salivary glands may also be affected. The symptoms are similar to those in parotitic mumps, but it is difficult or impossible to distinguish the swelling from other forms of sub-maxillary swellings, especially inflammation of various groups of lymph nodes and Ludwig's angina. In mumps, the neck swelling is ill defined and the angle of the jaw is impalpable. To determine if cervical lymph nodes are swollen from some other cause, the pharynx must be examined carefully. The fauces must be examined for signs of tonsillitis that might cause cervical adenitis. The lymph nodes in contact with the submaxillary and sublingual salivary glands drain the corner of the eye, the side of the nose, the cheeks, the lips, and the floor of the mouth, all of which must be explored, before a diagnosis of submaxillary or sublingual mumps can be made. Laboratory tests are needed to confirm the diagnosis.

In infectious mononucleosis, the glands stand out distinctly and the parotid is not affected. In septic parotitis there is more parotid tenderness; there may be fluctuation, and pus exudes from the orifice of Stensen's duct. Calculus causes spasmodic pain and swelling and may be detected radiographically. Recurrent parotitis and Mikulicz's syndrome are unlikely to be confused with mumps except in the earliest stages, nor are uveoparotid fever and tumours of the gland, as they are chronic conditions.

Orchitis

Orchitis may occur 4 or 5 days after the onset of parotitis. Quite often it occurs without preceding parotitis. It is an acute condition, with chills, sweats, headache, and backache, and a swinging temperature as well as severe local testicular pain and tenderness. The scrotum is swollen and oedematous, and the testicles are impalpable. Usually only one testicle is affected but sometimes both: the second testicle may become affected just as the swelling of the first is subsiding. The illness lasts 3 or 4 days before the swelling begins to subside. Orchitis is unusual before the age of puberty, though it has occurred in young boys and even in infants. In adolescent and young males it develops in 1:5 cases. Some degree of atrophy of the testicle occurs in at least one-third of patients with orchitis. Azoospermia after mumps is rare and only temporary. The fear of sterility after mumps orchitis has been exaggerated, so the doctor can reassure the patient. Orchitis when it occurs without parotitis is difficult to distinguish from gonococcal epididymo-orchitis unless there has been contact with mumps. The rare case of orchitis in infancy may resemble torsion of the testis and perhaps it is safer to operate than risk a serious misdiagnosis.

Meningitis and encephalitis

Lymphocytic or viral meningitis may develop a few days after the start of parotitis, but almost as often it occurs in the absence of parotitis. In the cerebrospinal fluid, protein and lymphocytes are increased. Occasionally the patient develops transient paralysis of limbs. Polyneuritis, neuritis of the trigeminal or facial nerve, and retrobulbar optic neuritis have been described in mumps but all are rare. The meningitis is usually mild and self-limiting. In encephalitis the outlook is different. The patient is confused and may lapse into coma and remain comatose for days, weeks, or months. Almost 2 per cent of the encephalitis cases are fatal.

Other complications

Deafness is sometimes reported after mumps, but it is rarely permanent. Women sometimes complain of ovarian pain during an attack of mumps, but it is rarely as severe as in men with orchitis. There is no evidence that it affects fertility. Mastitis occurs in 15 per cent of the cases, both in females and males, but it is usually mild and fleeting. Mild upper abdominal pain in about 50 per cent of the cases may be related to viral changes in the pancreas. The amount of amylase in duodenal fluid may be less than normal. This is probably caused by a blockage of the ducts in the pancreas. Although there are anecdotal reports of diabetes occurring after an attack of mumps, there is no virological or immunological evidence for a direct link.

Mumps in the fetus and infant

Abortion may occur in women with mumps in the first trimester of pregnancy. It is not common and probably not caused by viral damage to the fetus. The connection between primary endocardial fibroelastosis, which is declining in incidence, and mumps is rather vague, but recent evidence indicates that by RT-PCR viral RNA could be amplified from myocardial samples in more than 70 per cent of the cases. Mumps virus has not been isolated from heart tissue at autopsy and these infants have no mumps antibody in their blood. They may show a delayed hypersensitivity response to the skin test. This has not been explained, but may reflect some immune defect in the fetus which could cause myocarditis and fibroelastosis.

In the normal infant, maternal IgG passes to the fetus and seems to protect the infant against mumps during the first year of life. The typical disease of mumps in infants is a rare clinical finding even in populations with no previous experience of the disease. Orchitis has been reported in infants, and mumps virus may be isolated in vague respiratory infections in infants.

Laboratory diagnosis

In patients without parotitis, especially meningitis, and in the absence of contact history, serological tests, RT-PCR, and virus isolation are the only means of reaching a firm diagnosis. MuV isolation is now rarely used. MuV contains several different antigenic components, which provoke distinct antibodies that are useful for laboratory confirmation. The most important are the HN protein (V antigen) and the N protein (S antigen). S antibody rises in the first 2 weeks of infection but then declines rapidly. V antibody appears at the end of the first week, usually in high titre: it may persist for years and indicates past infection. Neutralizing antibodies also develop. Nowadays, sensitive enzyme immunoassay (EIA) allows early diagnosis by detection of mumps-specific IgM and IgA. IgA can be detected in saliva or mouth washings on about the fourth day after infection, and in the serum early in the disease. Measurement of antibodies in acute and convalescent sera is a reliable method for diagnosis, especially in patients who have no parotitis. Viral antigen produces a tuberculin-like reaction when injected into the skin of people who have been infected with mumps virus before, with or without clinical symptoms. The test is of value in assessing immunity or the need for vaccination.

Treatment

There is no specific treatment. Symptomatic treatment includes simple analgesics, but for the severe pain of orchitis, morphine (15 to 30 mg) may be required for a day or two. Corticosteroids are worth trying in severe cases of parotitis, more especially in orchitis. An adult dose of 60 mg prednisolone daily for 2 or 3 days sometimes gives dramatic relief from pain though it may not reduce the swelling.

Prevention and control

The mainstay of prevention is vaccination of susceptible individuals. Isolation is not effective as the patient has been infectious for days before parotitis occurs and inapparent cases are frequent. Attenuated live vaccine, licensed since 1967, gives 95 per cent seroconversion, and protection lasts for at least 15 years. In developed countries, mumps vaccine is currently given between 14 and 16 months of age as one component of a trivalent mumps/measles/rubella (**MMR**) vaccine, using live attenuated strains of all three viruses. This has succeeded in suppressing the incidence of mumps by more than 98 per cent in the United States and in the United Kingdom. Mumps vaccination is contraindicated in pregnant women and patients with immunodeficiency due to immunosuppressive therapy or disease. However, HIV seropositive children should be vaccinated with the MMR vaccine.

Further reading

Christie AB (1980). *Infectious diseases: epidemiology and clinical practice*, 3rd edn. Churchill Livingstone, Edinburgh.

Feldman HA (1989). Mumps. In: Evans AJ, ed. *Viral infections of humans*, 3rd edn, pp 471–91. Plenum Medical, New York.

Rima BK (1999). Mumps virus. In: Webster RG, Granoff A, eds. *Encyclopedia of virology*, 2nd edn, pp 988–94. Academic Press, London.

Wolinsky JS (1996). Mumps virus. In: Fields BN, Knipe DM, Howley PM, eds. *Virology*, 3rd edn, pp 1243–65. Lipincott–Raven Publishers, Philadelphia.

7.10.6 Measles

H. C. Whittle and P. Aaby

Measles is an acute, highly transmissible viral infection of man spread by aerosolized droplets, which causes much death and suffering, especially among children of the so-called Third World. Its severity varies according to host and socioeconomic factors, not to antigenic variation or alteration in virulence of the virus. There is no reservoir of infection other than in man and no evidence of a carrier state. The virus causes a generalized infection coupled with severe immunosuppression. The chief clinical features result from infection of the skin, mucous membranes, and respiratory tract. Attack rates in home contacts are very high (of the order of 90 per cent), subclinical infection is infrequent, and children are the main victims. Long-life immunity follows the disease. Although global coverage by measles immunization in 1998 was 72 per cent, at least 36 million children are infected annually and 1 million die mainly in sub-Saharan Africa where immunization coverage is low.

Epidemiology

The epidemiology of this global infection varies markedly between developed and developing countries.

In the West, most children are infected between 3 and 6 years of age, when they attend nursery and primary schools. Mortality is low (under 0.05 per cent) and morbidity, although considerable when compared to many other common viral infections, is limited. Most cases occur in the winter and spring, with a biannual epidemic pattern. Recently the epidemicity has been influenced by widespread immunization (Fig. 1), which has dramatically reduced both the number of cases and complications. However, even in the United States, which has the longest experience of systematic immunization, there is now evidence of a resurgence of measles with a higher case fatality in non-immunized subgroups of the population, such as religious minorities who do not believe in vaccines, refugees, illegal immigrants, and the poor in the inner cities.

In the Third World, measles is severe and different: it kills between 3 and 15 per cent of children in the community and some 10 to 20 per cent of those admitted to hospital. Mortality from measles is considerably higher in Africa (5–15 per cent) than in Asia or South America (1–3 per cent); within Africa, West Africa has the highest case-fatality rates. Contrary to the early European experience, when the highest mortality was among the overcrowded urban poor, studies from the developing world indicate a higher mortality in rural rather than urban populations. In communities where females tend to stay at home and are more constrained in their social contacts, mortality is higher in girls than boys. There is a high fatality rate in children with chronic disease, including kwashiorkor, tuberculosis, and human immunodeficiency virus (**HIV**) infection.

There are many reasons for this increase in severity: children are infected at a young age (median age, 12–24 months); severe malnutrition leads to prolonged, severe measles that kills up to 40 per cent of those infected. Overcrowding is another strong determinant of outcome, for secondary and tertiary cases in large families are at great risk of death. Exposure to a large dose of the virus when in close contact with the index case may be an important factor. Furthermore, the severity of measles and the chances of the secondary case dying are dependent on the severity of disease in the index case. Transmission of measles from one sex to the other has been found to increase mortality two- to threefold compared to transmission from the same sex. The high mortality found in West Africa is probably due to the very large, polygamous, and extended families, which increase the risk of intense exposure.

The epidemiology of measles used to vary according to the degree of urbanization, but now the coverage of immunization may be a more important determinant. In remote villages, outbreaks were less frequent

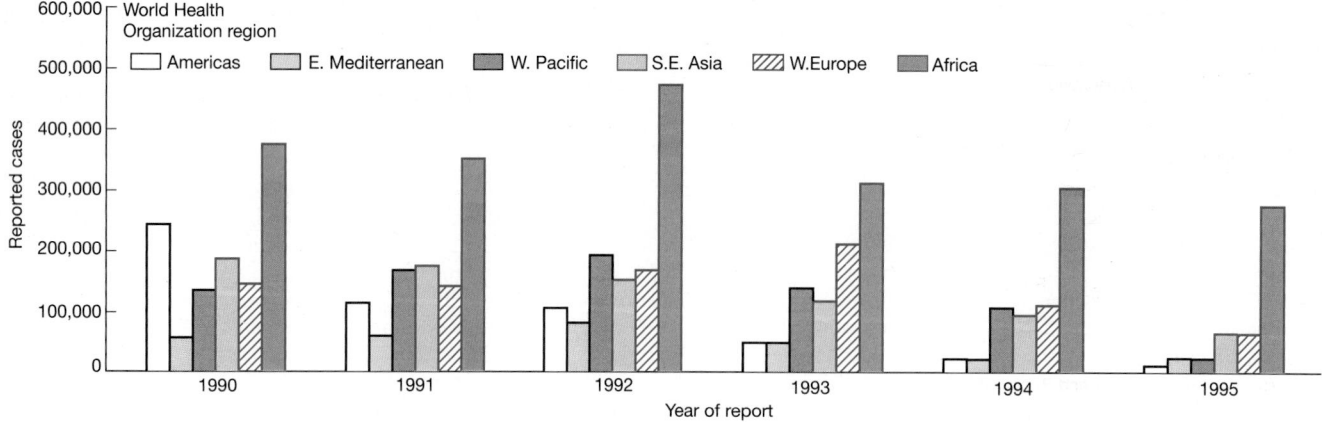

Fig. 1 Reported incidence of measles—World Health Organization regions, 1990–1995.

and with more susceptible children in each family the risk of intensive exposure and severe disease was increased. These outbreaks resembled the severe epidemics that in the past have devastated the remote island populations of the Faeroes, Fiji, Greenland, and Tristan da Cunha and killed more than 80 per cent of the Inca people in the wake of the Conquistadors in fifteenth-century Middle America. In urban areas, migration, and overcrowding have led to a hyperendemic pattern of infection with a low age of infection but fewer cases per family, the case fatality therefore being lower than in rural outbreaks. Hospital wards and clinics in the developing world are usually important centres of infection; in a hospital in the north of Nigeria, 35 per cent of children with measles had acquired the infection by attending the outpatient clinic 2 to 3 weeks before.

Acute measles is often less severe among children under 6 months of age, among previously immunized children, and among those who have received immunoglobulin when exposed. In these cases the course of infection is characterized by a prolonged incubation period, a short prodrome, mild symptoms, and a favourable outcome. Recent research has provided limited support for the previous belief in a general increase in long-term morbidity and mortality after the first 6 weeks of measles infection. These long-term consequences may have been due to the initial severity of infection as secondary cases have a higher long-term mortality than index cases. However, nowadays in areas with high vaccination coverage the disease is milder. This is particularly true for index cases who tend to be older than the secondary cases and have a lower mortality than uninfected children (suggesting that there is a beneficial effect of mild measles). Long-term morbidity is most likely to be experienced by young children who have severe measles following intensive exposure.

The severity and mortality of measles in developing countries has decreased dramatically as a consequence of measles immunization, which reduces the severity of infection, increases the number of subclinical cases, and lessens the likelihood of transmission. However, even if coverage is maintained, the epidemiology of measles alters as a result of changes in herd immunity from exposure to natural measles, and subclinical infection is important in maintaining protective antibody levels among vaccinated individuals. Thus, as antibody levels fall and the number of unvaccinated and unexposed subjects rise, there will be an increasing potential for epidemics among young adults. This is particularly true in developing countries where fertility rates are high; for measles is severe in young pregnant women and may attack both mother and child at the same time.

Popular beliefs

In most cultures, measles has a specific local name and is a much feared disease. Popular understanding is centred around the rash, which if it stays within the body will lead to severe disease. This belief has some basis in truth for the prodrome is prolonged in severe cases, and a proportion of deaths reportedly occur before the appearance of the rash during very severe epidemics. Therapeutic practices, such as rubbing the skin with palm oil or kerosene, are aimed at eliciting the rash quickly. In West Africa it is believed that cooling keeps the rash within the body, so the child may be bedded in warm sand or covered with blankets, and is not washed or given cold water to drink. Such customs may aggravate dehydration. In West Africa, as a result of popular awareness of measles, good correspondence exists between parental diagnosis and that based on clinical and immunological assessments. The mother's diagnosis, which can be used for epidemiological surveillance, is nearly always correct.

The virus and its antigens

Measles mainly infects humans, but like the other closely related morbilliviruses (such as rinderpest or canine distemper virus) it is able to cross species to infect other primates and, on occasions, dogs. It contains a single strand of RNA, is highly pleomorphic, and ranges from 100 to 300 nm in diameter. The virus propagates by budding from the cell membrane, from which it acquires an envelope. The membrane of infected cells and the virion envelope contain two surface glycoproteins, the haemagglutinin (**H**) and fusion (**F**) proteins, and a non-glycosylated matrix (**M**) protein, which forms the inner layer. The H protein, which allows attachment of the virus to cells, via the CD46 or CDw150 receptors, is the main target for neutralizing antibodies; the F protein is responsible for fusion and syncytium formation of infected cells. CD46 is a ubiquitous membrane cofactor protein, which together with five other proteins, protects cells from complement activation and lysis. Vaccine strains of measles virus bind to CD46 to downregulate the protein, resulting in complement-dependent cell lysis which limits viral replication. Some wild-type viruses, but not all, bind to the receptor but do not downregulate it, thus preventing lysis and allowing efficient viral replication. The CDw150 receptor (also known as signalling lymphocyte-activator molecule or **SLAM**) is expressed on immature lymphocytes and on effector memory T cells, and is rapidly induced on T and B cells after activation. The internal components or nucleocapsid consist of RNA, the nucleoprotein (**N**), which is the major protein, the phosphoprotein (**P**) and the large protein (**L**). The F protein is remarkably stable, the H protein shows minor antigenic variation, but the N protein, which contains a variable region in the C terminus, is highly divergent among different strains of virus. Genetic analysis of *H* and *N* genes allowed molecular surveillance of the measles virus in the United States, which suggested that the majority of cases were the result of international spread of the virus. There is also variation in the M protein, which some claim is related to persistent infection. The replication and assembly of measles virus is shown in Fig. 2.

- F-protein ▼ M-protein
- H-protein ⚬ RNA+NP–,L- and P- proteins

Fig. 2 Replication and assembly of measles virus. (Reproduced by courtesy of van Binnedijk RS (1992). T-cell function in measles. PhD thesis. University of Utrecht, Holland.)

Pathogenesis and the immune response

The course of infection and the immune response to this invasion are shown in Fig. 3. The measles virus, which is thermolabile and survives best at low humidities, is spread to susceptible contacts in droplets during sneezing and coughing. First it infects and multiplies in the epithelium of the upper respiratory tract or the conjunctivas. Some 4 to 6 days later the virus is found in the reticuloendothelial tissue of the liver and the spleen after passage through lymph nodes and spread via the blood. Here it multiplies, causing fusion of cells to form giant cells with many nuclei. Viral antigens, which can be found by immunofluorescent techniques in and on the surface of both these cells and lymphocytes, now induce the immune response. First, natural killer cells and cytotoxic T cells mount a cell-mediated reaction that contains the virus and limits its spread within cells. Later, B cells are primed to produce antibody. Defects in the cellular immune system, as in severe malnutrition, cancer or primary immunodeficiencies,

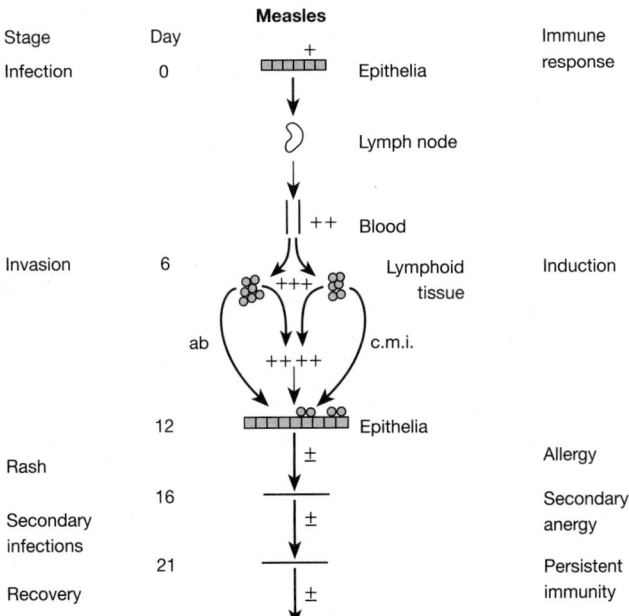

Fig. 3 Pathogenesis of measles. + Denotes amount of virus; ab, antibody. (Reproduced with permission from Parry EHOP (1984). *Principles of medicine in Africa*, 2nd edn. Oxford University Press, Oxford.)

allow widespread multiplication of the virus to cause fatal giant-cell pneumonia.

Around day 8, the measles virus is carried by the blood, either free or in mononuclear cells, to the target tissues, which are the epithelia of the eye, lung, and gut. Again, the agent multiplies to cause a bright redness of the mucosa and Koplik's spots (see below), which are foci of viral multiplication. At this stage, measles virus may be cultured from nasopharyngeal secretions, and antigen can be detected by immunofluorescent techniques in the characteristic giant cells of the buccal mucosa, in epithelial cells, and in both B and T lymphocytes in the blood.

The rash, appearing around days 14 to 16, is the sign of a strong and complicated allergic reaction to the virus in the epithelia. The extent and severity of the rash, which reflects the clinical severity of the disease, is determined by the number of target cells infected. Histological examination shows virus in the disrupted epidermis, in the corium, and in capillary endothelium. These tissues are infiltrated by mononuclear cells together with antibody, immune complexes, and complement. An intact cell-mediated immune response is essential to generate the rash and clear the virus, for if impaired, as in the case of children with leukaemia, or occasionally in severe kwashiorkor, the virus multiplies unchecked and no rash appears. Some 2 or 3 days after the start of the rash, around day 17 or 18, the virus can no longer be cultured in the epithelia, for infected cells have been disrupted and the free virus neutralized by antibody. The first antibody to appear is to the nucleoprotein antigens. The second, which is largely responsible for neutralization of the virus, is to the haemagglutinin. Finally, the antibody to the fusion glycoprotein appears in a low titre. This antibody stops cell-to-cell spread of the virus. At this stage the child is markedly immunosuppressed and thus susceptible to secondary infections of the eyes, mouth, gut, and lungs. Latent viruses, such as herpes simplex or cytomegalovirus, may be reactivated and in turn cause further immunosuppression. The delayed hypersensitivity reaction, as measured by skin tests to old tuberculin or candida antigen, is absent or severely impaired.

By the third week, day 21, as the patient recovers, antibody is in full production. Levels remain elevated for the rest of the patient's life, either because of repeated subclinical infections or because the virus persists in latent form in the spleen and other organs, so stimulating antibody. Occasionally the virus persists in the brain in a damaging form to cause subacute sclerosing panencephalitis (see below). In this rare condition, virus can be isolated from the brain up to 8 years after measles, and antibody levels to all but the M protein antigen are raised in the cerebrospinal fluid and blood. The immune system, for unknown reasons, has failed to clear the virus, which is probably aberrant, for such strains are unable to produce normal amounts of protein.

The mechanisms of immunosuppression are complex. The cytotoxic T-cell response, which is exuberant, may result in the destruction of infected T cells and dendritic cells thus leading to their depletion, deficient antigen processing, and generalized immunosuppression. Crossbinding of the CD46 cellular receptor downregulates IL-12, a crucial cytokine in the development of TH-1 and delayed hypersensitivity responses (Fig. 4). Infection of CDw150+ lymphocytes, which are predominantly of the T_{H0}/T_{H1} type, results in suppression of lymphoproliferation and cell death. Thus measles ultimately dampens the TH1 response, resulting in a skewing towards a TH2 cytokine response and susceptibility to intracellular and other pathogens. However, this immunosuppression may be in the interest of the host by limiting further autoallergic damage of infected tissues.

Pathogenesis in the underprivileged, in the malnourished, and in the HIV-infected

Measles in the children of the Third World, as was formerly the case in the underprivileged in Europe, is severe, prolonged, and carries a high case-fatality rate due to secondary infections. Two explanations are offered. Crowding leads to a high dose of measles virus and also increases the

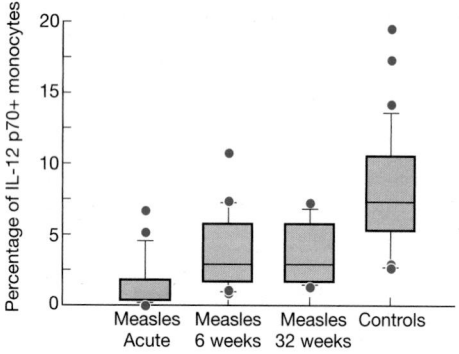

Fig. 4 Production of interleukin-12 by monocytes is depressed long after measles. (Reproduced with permission from Atabani SF et al. (2001). Journal of Infectious Diseases **184**, 1–9.)

chances of secondary infection. The period of incubation has been found to be short in severe and fatal cases, which is consistent with the emphasis on infecting dose as a mechanism of severe disease. Alternatively, or in tandem, malnutrition diminishes the immune response to the virus, allowing great proliferation of virus and subsequent damage to the host. There is experimental evidence, although only in severely malnourished children with marasmus or kwashiorkor, that the lymphocytes of these patients may be more readily infected during the induction phase. A normal immune response follows, which generates a severe and widespread rash followed by prolonged immunosuppression. Secondary bacterial infections with, for example, Streptococcus pneumoniae, or latent infections such as herpes simplex or Mycobacterium tuberculosis follow in the wake of this intense immunosuppression, often killing or maiming the child. Virus persists in lymphocytes and epithelial cells for up to 30 days after the start of the rash. Antibody production occasionally fails and secretory IgA is deficient, which may explain why the virus persists for so long in the gut. Anorexia, increased catabolism, protein loss from the gut, and further malnutrition exaggerate the problem, which is worst in the weanling child (Fig. 5).

Over 1 million children under the age of 5 years are living with HIV infection in sub-Saharan Africa. The impact of measles and measles vaccination on disease and death in this population will probably depend, as in malnutrition, on the degree of immune damage at the time of infection. The death rate after measles in hospitalized infants is higher in HIV-infected children, and prolonged viral shedding, as detected by the polymerase chain reaction (**PCR**), occurs in the majority of these children. Thus, in regions of high prevalence, HIV-infected children may be important unrecognized transmitters of the virus. Asymptomatic HIV-infected children respond normally to vaccination, but those with **AIDS** (acquired immunodeficiency syndrome) are less likely to respond and may be threatened by persistent infection. Further research is needed on the interaction of the two infections and their impact on the epidemiology and eradication of measles.

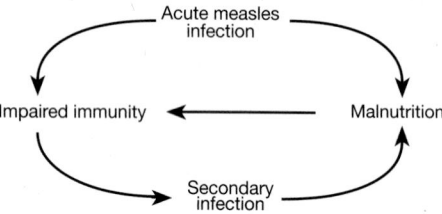

Fig. 5 The complex interaction between infection, nutrition, and impaired immunity seen in measles. (Reproduced with permission from Greenwood BM (1996). The host's response to infection. In: Weatherall DJ, Ledingham JGGL, Warrell DA (1996). Oxford Textbook Medicine, 3rd edn, p. 282. Oxford University Press.)

Clinical features

There is a spectrum of severity that ranges from mild in the privileged and well nourished to severe in the blatantly malnourished or immunosuppressed. However, the rule is not inviolate and other factors such as the age and dose of infection are probably as important in determining the severity of disease. Measles, often severe, occasionally infects unvaccinated young adults or individuals who have lived in isolated communities. The clinical features of measles and some complications are shown in Fig. 6 and discussed below.

Prodrome (days 10–14)

A diagnosis of measles is often missed at this stage, when fever coupled with a runny nose, and sometimes complicated by convulsions, is the main feature. Other signs are mild conjunctivitis, red mucosa, Koplik's spots, and diarrhoea. Koplik's spots are found in the buccal mucosa. They are 'small irregular spots of bright-red colour; in the centre of each spot is seen a minute bluish-white speck'. A useful diagnostic test is to scrape the buccal mucosa with a spatula, place the scraping on a microscope slide, stain with Leishman's stain, and examine for giant cells under a microscope. The prodrome is prolonged in severe cases, and reduced in individuals with modified measles due to maternal antibodies or the prophylactic use of immunoglobulin.

Rash (days 14–18)

The morbilliform rash first appears on the forehead and neck and then spreads, over a period of 3 to 4 days, to involve the trunk and finally the limbs (Plate 1).

In children in Africa and other parts of the developing world the rash is often red, confluent, raised, very extensive, and sometimes accompanied by bleeding into the skin and gut (Plate 2). Later the rash blackens, then the skin peels causing extensive desquamation. Other epithelial surfaces are inflamed, the severity matching that of the rash. Cough, a cardinal sign, may be hoarse and coupled with inspiration difficulty if the larynx and trachea are inflamed. Signs of pneumonitis are apparent, which in severe cases may cause cyanosis or be complicated by mediastinal and subcutaneous emphysema. Conjunctivitis, especially in those who are vitamin-A deficient, can be severe; enteritis may cause profuse diarrhoea with a resulting loss of protein, and malabsorption of food and water. The mouth is painful and red, which adds to the misery of the child, who becomes anorexic and may even refuse to suck the breast. In the uncomplicated case, as is usual in the West, the convalescent period is short, usually lasting less than a week. Complications should be suspected if fever persists while the rash is fading or desquamating.

Complications

Early complications (days 18–30)

As a result of the widespread, severe allergic reaction to the measles virus signified by the rash, the patient is left severely immunosuppressed and is susceptible to infection.

Pneumonia

This causes the most deaths (Table 1) and is heralded by a rise in fever, leucocytosis, and respiratory difficulties. Lobar pneumonia is usually caused by S. pneumoniae, but bronchopneumonia, which is more common, results from other bacteria, such as S. aureus, or secondary viral infections with, for example, herpes simplex or adenovirus. A variety of other organisms such as Gram-negative bacteria, cytomegalovirus, fungi, M. tuberculosis, and Pneumocystis carinii should be considered as potential lung pathogens in the malnourished or immunocompromised child.

Stomatitis and enteritis

Chronic diarrhoea and a sore mouth caused by candidal infection are common complications of measles in children in the Third World. The gut is often superinfected with *Bacteroides* spp., *Escherichia coli*, *Pseudomonas* spp., and *S. aureus*, which results in malabsorption and protein loss. Deep ulcers caused by herpes simplex virus erode the corners of the mouth, gums, and inner surface of the lips causing much misery, illness, and pain (Plate 3).

Eye infections

Corneal ulceration leading to impaired vision or blindness is common after measles, especially in malnourished and vitamin A-deficient children (Plate 4). Several studies from Africa have shown that more than half of childhood blindness is related to measles. The mechanisms are still under discussion. In northern Nigeria, herpes simplex was found in 47 per cent of active corneal ulcers after measles, and measles virus in 12 per cent: the children often had evidence of oral herpes. In a study in Tanzania, blindness precipitated by measles was associated with vitamin A deficiency (50 per cent), *herpes simplex* infection (21 per cent), and the use of traditional eye medicine (17 per cent).

Skin and other infections

Pyoderma is common after measles. In the malnourished patient, deep eroding ulcers may bore through the skin even into bone. When originating in the mouth they are know as cancrum oris or noma (Plate 5). Otitis media is also common.

Encephalitis

This is a rare, but much feared, complication found in approximately 1 to 2 per 1000 cases. The onset is usually between 4 and 7 days after the start of the rash, but, rarely, it may occur within 48 h or up to 2 weeks from the onset. In addition to seizures, there is often fever, irritability, headache, and a disturbance in consciousness that may progress to profound coma. The disorder is probably attributable to a neuroallergic process: lymphocytes from the cerebrospinal fluid have been shown to respond to myelin basic protein, as in experimental allergic encephalomyelitis. The virus cannot be isolated from cerebrospinal fluid, which contains lymphocytes and raised levels of IgG but normal levels of measles antibody. Mortality and morbidity is high: 10 to 15 per cent of victims die and 25 per cent of children are left with permanent brain damage. Treatment is supportive; dexamethasone has no convincing beneficial effect.

Late complications

Malnutrition

This is the most frequent complication, for children of the developing world often lose a lot of weight during measles and may take many weeks to regain it. Those originally underweight, who have had severe measles, are at greatest risk, for anorexia in these children is prolonged, much protein is lost from the gut, and secondary infections, which lead to marasmus or marasmic kwashiorkor, are frequent. Measles has been shown to persist in the epithelia and lymphocytes of the severely malnourished for 30 or more days after the rash.

Persistent infection

Pneumonitis

A giant-cell pneumonia is found in patients with defects in cell-mediated immunity; children with leukaemia or kwashiorkor are particularly vulnerable as are those with symptomatic HIV infection. The lung disease may develop weeks after measles, and in most cases the rash of measles has been

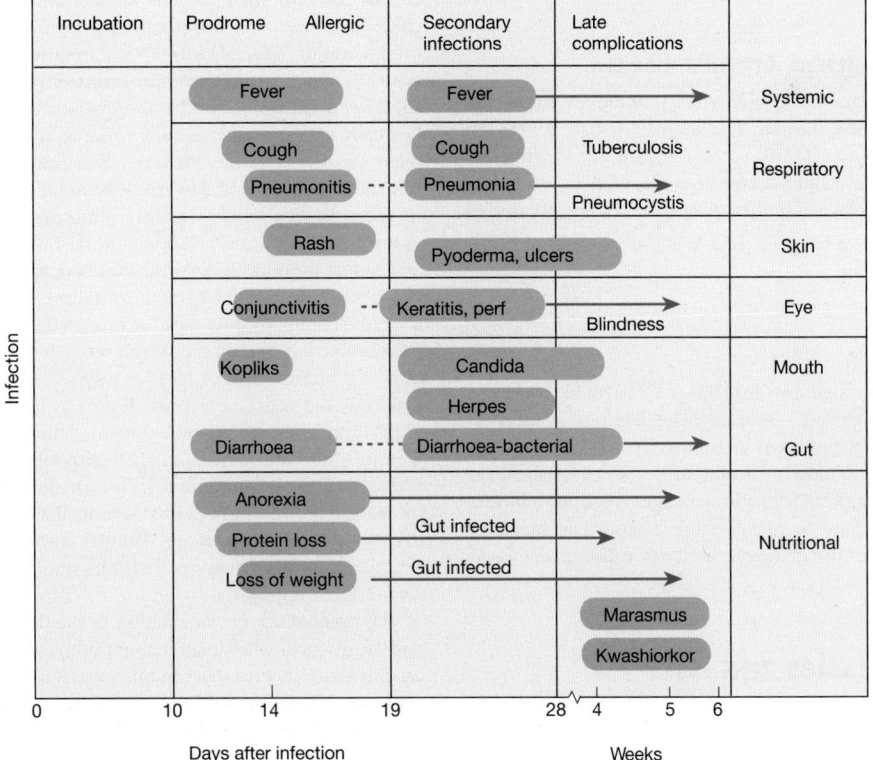

Fig. 6 Clinical features of measles and some of its complications. (Reproduced with permission from Parry EHOP (1984). *Principles of medicine in Africa*, 2nd edn, Oxford University Press, Oxford.)

Table 1 Complications and mortality in inpatients with measles, northern Nigeria, July–December 1978

	No.	Died	Percentage dead
Pneumonia	169	32	18.9
Gastroenteritis	65	9	13.8
Marasmic kwashiorkor	25	6	24.0
Laryngotracheobronchitis	21	4	19.0
Encephalitis	10	4	40.0

Reproduced with permission from Parry EHOP (1984). *Principles of medicine in Africa*, 2nd edn. Oxford University Press, Oxford.

absent and thus the diagnosis may not be suspected. The diagnosis is made by virological and/or histological examination of lung tissue. Most of these children die.

Subacute sclerosing panencephalitis (SSPE)

Persistent measles virus infection is responsible for this rare, progressive disease of the brain, which is found in 0.1 to 1.4 per million children after measles. The virus is detected in the brain by electron microscopy and by immunofluorescent methods, and has only been isolated using cocultivation techniques. The child with SSPE has usually experienced normal measles, albeit at a young age, 5 to 10 years earlier. The first indication is a disturbance in intellect and personality; behaviour disorders and deterioration in school work are frequently mentioned. There then follows, over a period of weeks and months, myoclonus-like seizures, signs of extrapyramidal and pyramidal disease, and finally a state of decerebrate rigidity followed by death. The electroencephalogram shows a characteristic regular series of high-amplitude, spike-like waves. Very high titres of measles complement-fixing and haemagglutinin-inhibiting antibody are present both in serum and cerebrospinal fluid; the haemagglutin-inhibiting antibody is probably produced within the nervous system. Treatments for SSPE have included the use of transfer factor, plasmapheresis, and antiviral drugs, but to no avail.

Multiple sclerosis, autism, Crohn's disease

There is no convincing evidence that measles virus or immune responses to it have a causative role in these diseases. The alleged association between the measles, mumps, and rubella (**MMR**) vaccine, autism, and Crohn's disease was based on weak science and has now been convincingly refuted by larger and stronger epidemiological studies. Subsequent molecular studies have failed to confirm the original finding of measles virus and genomic RNA in diseased bowel.

Diagnosis

This is primarily clinical, although signs may be less clear-cut in vaccinated subjects. Thus in areas of high vaccine coverage the detection of measles-specific IgM antibody by enzyme-linked immunoassay (**ELISA**) or, better still, the detection of measles antigen in saliva or urine may clinch the diagnosis if the rash is mild or atypical. Subclinical measles is common in vaccinated children after exposure to measles: the diagnosis is made by detecting a fourfold or greater rise in measles antibody within 2 to 6 weeks of exposure. It is not clear if such cases are infectious.

Treatment of measles and its complications

No effective antimeasles drug exists, yet some children do benefit from treatment in hospital. The following criteria indicate severe measles and a need for hospital admission: a widespread, confluent rash darkening to deep red or purple; signs of laryngeal obstruction; subcutaneous emphy-

sema; marked dehydration; blood in the stool or more than five stools a day; convulsion or loss of consciousness; severe secondary pneumonia; corneal ulceration; or severe ulceration of the mouth and skin. These signs should be taken particularly seriously when the child is underweight or frankly malnourished.

Hydrate the child orally or intravenously. Treat lobar pneumonia with benzylpenicillin, and bronchopneumonia with combined antibiotics such as gentamicin and cloxacillin, or with co-trimoxazole. Antibiotic eye ointments relieve discomfort and possibly prevent secondary infections of measles conjunctivitis. Antibiotics (topical and systemic) and vitamin A should be given routinely for the treatment of eye ulcers. If *herpes simplex* virus is the cause, use aciclovir topically or, when severe, systemically. Candidal infections of the mouth or gut often respond dramatically to nystatin. Feeding, by tube if necessary, needs careful planning and presentation, for the anorexic infected child will be in severe negative energy balance due to a greatly increased catabolic rate. Case fatality rates are 30 to 50 per cent lower in those children in hospital treated with vitamin A. This should be given orally at the time of diagnosis in a dose of 100 000 IU for children below 12 months of age and in a dose of 200 000 IU for older children. If eye signs of vitamin A deficiency are present, the initial dose should be repeated the next day and again 1 to 4 weeks later.

No specific effective treatment for encephalitis or SSPE exists.

Prevention

Passive immunization with human immunoglobulin is highly effective if given within 2 or 3 days of exposure, in a dose for children of 0.2 ml/kg. Immunoglobulin should be given to those in whom vaccination is contraindicated: children immunosuppressed by kwashiorkor, by malignancies such as leukaemia or lymphoma, or by steroids or cytotoxic drugs. Passive immunization may also be used to protect pregnant women, those with active tuberculosis, and those with AIDS.

The currently used vaccines are live strains, attenuated by culture in chick fibroblasts. The complications of vaccination are few and generally mild. Fever of moderate severity is infrequent, and a mild rash with some signs of upper respiratory tract infection occurs rarely. Encephalitis or SSPE is exceedingly rare after vaccination. Underweight children respond normally to the vaccine, as do ill children attending the outpatient department and those on the ward. As clinics and hospitals are major sites of transmission of the virus in the developing world, all susceptible children in these places—unless seriously immunocompromised because of, for example, leukaemia, kwashiorkor, or AIDS—should be vaccinated.

The first measles vaccines introduced in the United States and Europe in the 1960s were inactivated with formalin. Although they produced high levels of H antibody, they failed to raise antibody to the F protein. This gave poor protection, and on exposure a severe local reaction at the site of injection or a bizarre form of measles resulted. The rash was unusual, having urticarial and vesicular features, fever was high, oedema of the limbs frequent, and severe pneumonia present. This syndrome is still occasionally seen in adults who were vaccinated with killed vaccine during childhood. Rhesus macaques immunized with formalin-inactivated vaccine followed by challenge with measles virus developed an atypical rash and pneumonitis accompanied by immune-complex formation and eosinophilia. This experiment shows that atypical measles results from a non-protective type-2 CD4 T-cell response.

The optimal age for vaccination in the developed world is between 14 and 16 months, when maternal antibody, which neutralizes the virus to cause vaccine failure, has disappeared. This recommendation does not apply to children in the Third World, because there measles infects at an early age. The World Health Organization (**WHO**) recommends vaccination at 9 months of age but, by then, 5 to 15 per cent of children may have had measles. Edmonston–Zagreb, a different strain of vaccine, passaged in human diploid cells, and given in high dose (in excess of 10^5 infectious particles) subcutaneously, has proved to be immunogenic at the age of 4 to

6 months. Subsequently, the WHO recommended its use at 6 months of age in areas of the world with a high incidence of measles occurring below 9 months of age. However, long-term follow-up demonstrated lower survival rates among female recipients of high-titre vaccine than among female recipients of standard-dose measles vaccine. Although the biological explanation for this unexpected finding is unknown, the use of high-titre vaccines is now no longer recommended.

Some scientists have argued that measles vaccines will have a limited impact on childhood survival—for disadvantaged children, saved from measles by vaccination, will only die at a later date from other infections or malnutrition. However, a variety of epidemiological studies has documented remarkable reductions in mortality after standard measles vaccine. In Bangladesh, measles vaccination was associated with a 36 per cent reduction in all-cause mortality from the age of 9 months, despite the fact that acute measles accounted for only 4 per cent of deaths in the community. The reason for this unexpected benefit is unknown but it is not related to the prevention of measles. The benefit is particularly marked for girls and is most likely due to non-specific immune stimulation.

Primary vaccine failure may occur because maternal antibody neutralized the vaccine, or it may be due to heat-inactivation of improperly stored vaccine. Secondary vaccine failure may occur because the children are intensively exposed or because protective antibody levels wane. This has not been a problem in developed countries where most children have received their vaccine after 15 months of age, but in developing countries early vaccination at 6 to 9 months of age may increase the likelihood of antibody concentrations declining to non-protective levels.

Waning immunity may become an increasing problem as vaccine coverage increases: because more mothers will have been vaccinated and since they have not been exposed or had natural measles, they will transmit lower levels of maternal antibody. Thus their babies become susceptible to measles by 3 to 5 months of age. This increases the problem of measles control: the two groups of children, born to vaccinated or naturally infected mothers, will have low or high levels of maternal derived antibody, respectively, and thus will need to be vaccinated at different ages.

...or eradication?

Measles eradication has yet to be made an official global policy. However, several regions are pursuing a policy of measles elimination. The United States has been successful with a policy of obligatory vaccination before school entry. The Pan-American Health Organization (**PAHO**) has pursued a successful but expensive policy of national immunization days for all children aged between 1 and 14 years, high routine vaccination coverage, and periodic follow-up campaigns during which all children aged 1 to 4 years are vaccinated. However, the real test of global measles eradication will be in Europe and Africa. Europe, which at best has a coverage of 85 to 90 per cent, has no tradition of an obligatory use of vaccines and an increasing proportion of the population are averse to vaccination. Africa will be a stern test of the PAHO strategy, for due to political instability it is difficult to maintain a sufficiently high coverage for a long period. In addition, because of high fertility rates there will be a constant renewal of susceptible children, combined with an accumulation of susceptible young adults due to waning immunity.

New vaccines, which can be given in early infancy, or two-dose strategies using the standard vaccine at 6 and 9 months of age, will be necessary to contain measles in the developing world. Coverage of at least 95 per cent of all susceptible children, including those between 3 and 9 months of age, with a vaccine that is at least 95 per cent effective will be necessary if the virus is to be eradicated. Current vaccines do not meet these standards. New vaccines such as the Modified Vaccinia Ankara recombinant virus, a non-replicating mutant of horsepox made to express the F and H proteins, or a DNA vaccine expressing these proteins may possibly fulfil such exacting requirements, for they have been shown to protect macaques from measles. However, in those countries with a high child mortality rate where measles vaccine has been shown to have non-specific beneficial effects, vaccination programmes may need to be continued even if measles is eradicated.

Further reading

Aaby P, *et al.* (1983). Measles mortality, state of nutrition, and family structure. A community study from Guinea-Bissau. *Journal of Infectious Disease* **147**, 693–701.

Aaby P, *et al.* (1995). Non-specific beneficial effects of measles immunization: analysis of mortality studies from developing countries. *British Medical Journal* **311**, 481–5.

Cutts FJ, Steinglass R (1998). Should measles be eradicated? *British Medical Journal* **316**, 765–7.

Fenner F (1948). The pathogenesis of the acute exanthems. An interpretation based on experimental investigations with mouse-pox (infectious ectromelia of mice). *Lancet* **ii**, 915–20.

Karp CL (1999). Measles immunosuppression, interleukin 12, and complement receptors. *Immunological Reviews* **168**, 91–101.

Morley D (1969). Severe measles in the tropics. *British Medical Journal* **1**, 297–300; 363–5.

Polack FP, *et al.* (1999). Production of atypical measles in rhesus macaques: evidence for disease mediated by immune complex formation and eosinophils in the presence of fusion—inhibiting antibody. *Nature Medicine* **5**, 629–34.

Whittle HC, *et al.* (1979). Severe ulcerative herpes of mouth and eye following measles. *Transactions of the Royal Society for Tropical Medicine and Hygiene* **73**, 66–9.

Whittle HC, *et al.* (1999). Effect of sub-clinical infection on maintaining immunity against measles in vaccinated children in West Africa. *Lancet* **353**, 98–101.

7.10.6.1 Nipah and Hendra viruses

James G. Olson

Nipah virus

Introduction

An outbreak of severe, febrile encephalitis associated with human deaths occurred in Malaysia, beginning in September 1998. Initially recognized near Ipoh in the northern state of Perak, it was attributed to an endemic mosquito-borne viral encephalitis caused by Japanese encephalitis virus which is amplified by swine. Veterinary and public health measures for control of Japanese encephalitis failed to have an impact on the encephalitis in humans. In January 1999, the outbreak spread to the state of Negri Sembilan and cases increased dramatically.

Aetiology

A new virus of the family Paramyxoviridae, genus *Megamyxovirus*, shows characteristic syncytia and giant cell formation in Vero cell culture. Nipah virus, named for the location where the first isolate was obtained, is approximately 1.1 µm in length with an average diameter of 21 nm. Extracellular, pleomorphic virus particles average 500 nm but vary greatly in size. Surface projections along the envelope are seen only sporadically and measure 10 nm in length. Nipah virus differs genetically from its closest relative, Hendra virus, at the nucleotide level in the phosphoprotein (11 per cent), nucleoprotein (26 per cent), and matrix protein (31 per cent) genes, respectively.

Epidemiology

Nearly all patients had a history of direct contact with pigs. Exposures were primarily occupational and frequently included close contact with pigs with respiratory disease. Since late 1996, a new disease of swine has spread among pig farms in Malaysia. It was not identified as a new syndrome because morbidity and mortality were not considered excessive, and the clinical signs were not markedly different from those of a range of other swine diseases. Transmission of virus among pig farms was by trade and movement of asymptomatic pigs. Other species have become infected with Nipah virus, but only in circumstances where they were exposed to infected pig farms. Serological studies have implicated two species of pterapid fruit bats (flying foxes) as possible wildlife reservoirs of infection (Plate 1).

Clinical features (see also Chapter 24.14.2)

Nipah virus encephalitis is a severe, acute, febrile disease with prodrome of fever, headache, and drowsiness. On admission, patients have fever (70 per cent), drowsiness (50 per cent), disorientation (18 per cent), neck stiffness (12 per cent), myoclonus (10 per cent), unresponsiveness or coma (9 per cent), and seizures (6 per cent). Most (58 per cent) cerebrospinal fluid white blood cell counts were normal, while cerebrospinal fluid protein levels were increased (68 per cent). Platelet counts were mildly decreased (median, 137×10^9/l). Of patients who had CT scans; 16 per cent showed cerebral oedema and 14 per cent had focal hyper densities. MRI scans of brain revealed multiple small hyper intensity signals on T2-weighted images. New findings following admission include hypotension (40 per cent), signs of autonomic dysfunction (26 per cent), seizures (22 per cent), and myoclonus (20 per cent). Almost half (49 per cent) of patients became unresponsive or comatose and 50 per cent required intubation. The case fatality ratio was 43 per cent, with the median time from admission to death of 4 days. Intubation, seizures, myoclonus, hypotension, and autonomic dysfunction were grave prognostic indicators.

Pathology

Histological and immunohistochemical findings at autopsy included a systemic vasculitis with fibrin thrombi and fibrinoid necrosis. Endothelial cells of affected vessels showed occasional multinucleated syncytial giant cell formation. Endothelial cells also showed lytic necrosis and sloughing into the lumen of the blood vessels. In the central nervous system, the vasculitis was diffuse involving cerebral cortex and brain stem and was associated with extensive areas of rarefaction necrosis. In these areas, neuronal degeneration and death, neuronophagia, microglial nodules, and mild perivascular inflammatory infiltrates were present. Eosinophilic, mainly intracytoplasmic, viral inclusions were seen in affected neurons and parenchymal cells.

Laboratory diagnosis

Enzyme immunoassay and immunohistochemical tests for Nipah virus infections are sensitive and specific methods for laboratory confirmation of clinical illness. Viral isolation in Vero cells can be successful using throat washings, serum, and urine from acutely ill patients and from brain of patients who die. Isolation of Nipah virus is not recommended for laboratory confirmation because of the extreme hazard (biosafety level 4) of the virus.

Treatment

Clinical management of patients is primarily supportive. Most patients required intubation. Patients with hypotension were treated with intravenous fluids and pressor agents, while those with seizures and myoclonus received anticonvulsive drugs. Oral tribavirin (ribavirin) was administered to several patients but data are not available on its efficacy.

Prevention and control

Control areas with active disease were identified, all pig farms within the designated areas were culled, and the pigs buried. This broke the cycle of transmission to humans. Serological testing of swine showed that on infected farms most of the adult pig population had been exposed, an observation which formed the basis of a national testing and eradication programme. Serum samples from every pig farm in Malaysia outside the control were sampled twice at a minimum interval of 3 weeks. Nipah virus should be eradicated from the Malaysian pig herd.

Hendra virus

Since its first description in Australia in 1994, there have been two outbreaks of fatal disease in horses and humans in Queensland, caused by Hendra virus (formerly known as equine morbillivirus). This is closely related to Nipah virus (see above) and Menangle virus, which was responsible for disease in pigs and humans in New South Wales in 1997. Clinical features of Hendra virus infection in humans were pneumonitis and meningoencephalitis. The natural hosts of Hendra, Menangle, and Nipah viruses and Australian bat Lyssavirus (see Chapter 7.10.10) are species of flying foxes (genus *Pteropus*). In eastern Australia, 20 per cent of flying foxes (*P. poliocephalus* and *P. alecto*) were seropositive for Hendra virus. In these bats, the disease is usually subclinical. Virus is found in uterine fluid and is transmissible oronasally to horses, cats, and other mammals.

Further reading

Chua KB, Goh KJ, Wong KT, *et al.* (1999). Fatal encephalitis due to Nipah virus among pig-farmers in Malaysia. *Lancet* **354**, 1256–9.

Department of Health (UK) (2000). *Hendra virus and Nipah virus. Management and control.* www.doh.gov.uk/jointunit/jip.htm.

Goh KJ, Tan CT, Cheu NK, *et al.* (2000). Clinical features of Nipah virus encephalitis among pig farmers in Malaysia. *New England Journal of Medicine* **342**, 1229–35.

Halpin K, Young PL, Field HE, Mackenzie JS (1999). Newly-discovered viruses of flying foxes. *Vetinary Microbiology* **68**, 83–7.

Halpin K, Young PL, Field HE, Mackenzie JS (2000). Isolation of Hendra virus from Pteropid bats: a natural reservoir of Hendra virus. *Journal of General Virology* **91**, 1927–32.

Lee KE, Umapathi T, Tan CB, *et al.* (1999). The neurological manifestations of Nipah virus encephalitis, a novel paramyxovirus. *Annals of Neurology* **46**, 428–32.

Paaton NI, Leo YS, Zaki SR, *et al.* (1999). Outbreak of Nipah-virus infection among abattoir workers in Singapore. *Lancet* **354**,1253–6.

7.10.7 Enterovirus infections

Ulrich Desselberger and Philip Minor

Enteroviruses are a major group of viruses causing systemic infection in man. They form two genera of the Picornaviridae family (the Enterovirus and Parechovirus genera) and occur in at least 66 serotypes in humans. They infect via the gastrointestinal tract and are mostly clinically inapparent. However, viraemia can be followed by infection of organs distant from the site of entry with often devastating affects in the form of meningitis, encephalitis, myopericarditis, and also rashes and conjunctivitis.

The viruses

Viruses of the Picornaviridae are unenveloped icosahedral particles of 27 to 30 nm in diameter, containing single-stranded RNA of positive polarity and approximately 7.5 kb size as their genome. The nucleic acid is poladenylated at the 3′ end and carries a small protein, VPg, covalently linked at its 5′ end. The enteroviruses and parechoviruses form two of the six current genera of the Picornaviridae family, the other four being rhinoviruses, cardioviruses, aphthoviruses, and hepatoviruses. Three serotypes of poliomyelitis virus (polio virus), 23 types of Coxsackie A virus, six types of Coxsackie B virus, and various types of enterocytopathic human orphan (echo) viruses are recognized within the enterovirus genus. The parechoviruses comprise echoviruses 22 and 23 and were established as a separate genus on the basis of the highly distinctive nature of the sequence of their genomes. Other classical features of the enteroviruses, such as their stability at acid pH (in contrast to rhinoviruses or aphthoviruses), their buoyant density in caesium chloride gradients, and the nature of their broad clinical effects and persistence in the environment are also shared by the parechoviruses.

The three-dimensional structure of the poliovirus particle has been elucidated by crystallographic analysis. The viral capsid consists of 60 protein subunits, each containing the four unglycosylated viral proteins VP1 to VP4. The capsid proteins are arranged in such a way that VP1 molecules form the apices at the five-fold symmetry axis of the icosahedron whereas two other proteins, VP2 and VP3, are arranged in the centre of the triangular face near the three-fold axis of symmetry. VP4 is an internal protein. All proteins interact with each other. The N terminus of VP4 is myristilated.

Viruses initiate replication by attaching to their cellular receptors, and some of these have been characterized. The poliovirus receptor is a member of the immunoglobulin superfamily. Transgenic mice expressing the human poliovirus receptor become susceptible for poliovirus infection with a pathology similar to that of infected primates. They may eventually replace primates for vaccine testing (see below). Other enterovirus receptors are the decay accelerating factors (DAF; receptor for echovirus 7), implicated in the complement pathway, and the integrin VLA-2 (echovirus 1). Other cell surface molecules may be involved in the virus–cell receptor interactions of many enteroviruses, as the expression of an identified receptor is not always sufficient to make a previously resistant cell line susceptible to productive infection. It is also of interest that some strains of poliovirus, mainly of serotype 2, are able to paralyse mice if injected. The receptor involved in mice has not been identified.

The positive sense RNA genome acts as a messenger molecule. All enterovirus RNAs have a long 5′ end untranslated region (UTR) of approximately 750 nucleotides length, containing an internal ribosomal entry site (IRES) which is important for binding of ribosomes and translation of RNA into protein. Downstream of the 5′ UTR is a large single open reading frame containing three parts: P1, coding for structural proteins VP1 to VP4; P2, coding for proteins 2A, 2B, and 2C; and P3, coding for proteins 3A to 3D. Protein 3C is a viral protease and protein 3D the RNA-dependent RNA polymerase. P2 and P3 proteins (with the exception of VPg = 3B) are only found in infected cells. The P1 to P3 proteins are synthesized as one large precursor, from which the individual proteins are produced by a complex autocleavage and cleavage cascade. RNAs replicates via double-stranded replicative intermediates. The ratio of positive to negative stranded RNA molecules in infected cells is approximately 100:1. Naked enterovirus RNA is infectious upon transfection, and can be transcribed from full length cDNA clones permitting biochemical manipulation and studies of structure and function at the molecular level.

The extensive antigenic variation of enterovirus capsid proteins allows typing into polio-, Coxsackie-, and echoviruses using type-specific neutralizing antisera, but there is some cross-reactivity. The main antigenic sites are located on all three major virion proteins (VP1–VP3), and some involve sequences from more than one protein.

Comparison of complete RNA genome sequences of many enteroviruses show a very close relationship between some enterovirus and rhinovirus sequences. Within the echoviruses, however, there is great diversity, for example echovirus 22 shows a very low degree of homology with any other enteroviruses.

Four subdivisions of human enteroviruses have been proposed according to genomic relatedness:

- Group 1: polioviruses, Coxsackie viruses A1, A11, A13, A17, A18, A21, and A24;
- Group 2: enterovirus types 68–70;
- Group 3: Coxsackie viruses B1–B6, A9, all echoviruses except types 22 and 23, and enterovirus 69;
- Group 4: Coxsackie viruses A2, A3, A5, A7, A8, A14, and A16, and enterovirus 71.

Hepatitis A virus has previously been designated enteroviruses 72, but is now in its own genus Hepatovirus. Echoviruses type 22 and 23 form the Parechovirus genus.

Pathogenesis

The most widely accepted model of the pathogenesis of enterovirus infection is based on that developed by Bodian for poliovirus, in which the virus infects via the gastrointestinal tract and undergoes primary replication in lymphoid cells lining the alimentary tract (oropharyngeal, intestinal). A viraemic phase follows, allowing infection of distant target organs: spinal cord and brain, meninges, myocardium, skeletal muscles, skin, mucous membranes. Other tissues, for example lymph nodes and brown fat tissue, can also become infected. Intensive multiplication in the CNS leads to the destruction of motor neurones and results in paralysis.

A slightly different and more subtle model of poliovirus pathogenesis was proposed by Sabin, in which the virus infects the mucosal surface, so accounting for the fact that virus can be shed in faeces long after it has become undetectable in lymphoid tissues and when neutralizing antibody is detectable in the blood. The primary replication creates a viraemia which seeds distant, still unknown, sites and virus replication there results in a second viraemia which may be detected about 1 week postinfection and can lead to systemic infection including CNS involvement.

Shedding of virus occurs from the throat and faeces for many weeks and even months after infection and thus ensures transmission (see below). Virus replication in sites distant from the port of entry normally terminates with the appearance of neutralizing antibody, first IgM at 8 to 12 weeks after infection, and then IgG. Children with B cell immunodeficiencies may develop persistent infections.

Most enterovirus infections are silent or produce a 'minor illness' with the symptoms of a mild upper respiratory tract infection with or without fever. In a minority of infections (1 per cent or less) a systemic 'major disease' may develop:

- paralytic poliomyelitis and aseptic meningitis (polioviruses);
- aseptic meningitis, herpangina, conjunctivitis, hand, foot and mouth disease (Coxsackie A viruses);
- aseptic meningitis, myopericarditis, encephalitis, pleurodynia (Coxsackie B viruses; enterovirus 71);
- aseptic meningitis, rashes, conjunctivitis (echoviruses);
- polio-like illness, aseptic meningitis, hand, foot and mouth disease, epidemic conjunctivitis (enterovirus types 68–71).

Symptoms of clinical illness caused by enteroviruses are summarized in Table 1 and are discussed in more detail below.

Clinical symptoms

Central nervous system infections

Poliomyelitis

While there is evidence of poliomyelitis as an ancient human disease as shown on a funerary stele from Middle Kingdom Egypt, about 1300 BC, there is little documentation of its occurrence until near the end of the nineteenth century, when it appeared in epidemics in children (hence the alternative name 'infantile paralysis'). The appearance of poliomyelitis

Table 1 Clinical symptoms and their possible enteroviral causes

Clinical symptom (phenotype)	Poliovirus			Coxsackievirus															Echovirus									Entero-virus	
	Type			Group A type										Group B type					Type									Type	
	1	2	3	2	4	5	6	7	9	10	16	21	24	1	2	3	4	5	1	2	4	6	9	11	16	19	30	70	71
Aseptic meningitis (rarely encephalitis)	✓	✓	✓	✓	✓			✓	✓	✓				✓	✓	✓	✓	✓	✓	✓		✓	✓	✓	✓		✓	✓	✓
Paralysis	✓	✓	✓					✓	✓						✓	✓	✓	✓	✓	✓	✓	✓	✓	✓			✓		✓
Severe systemic infection (neonates)														✓	✓	✓	✓	✓				✓	✓	✓	✓				✓
Myo(peri)carditis					✓					✓				✓	✓	✓	✓	✓				✓	✓			✓			
Epidemic pleurodynia								✓						✓	✓	✓	✓	✓				✓	✓						
Exanthemata, enanthema				✓	✓	✓		✓	✓	✓				✓	✓	✓	✓	✓				✓	✓			✓			✓
Conjunctivitis												✓	✓	✓			✓											✓	
Respiratory symptoms (herpangina)								✓		✓	✓	✓	✓	✓			✓	✓		✓		✓	✓						
Diarrhoea																								✓					

coincided with improvement in standards of public hygiene and is explained by the consequent exposure of infants to infection at a later age. Maternal antibody is capable of confining infection to the gut, where the virus can persist until the immune response develops to eliminate it. In contrast, when maternal antibody has declined in older infants, the virus can spread to sites outside the intestine, causing paralysis.

Even under modern conditions of hygiene, infection with all three poliovirus types is normally inapparent, but illness with neurological symptoms results in about 1 per cent of infections. This can present as aseptic meningitis with neck stiffness, usually recovering after 10 days (abortive or non-paralytic poliomyelitis). Meningitis is also caused by several other enteroviruses (see below). The more serious presentation is paralytic poliomyelitis, appearing 5 to 10 days after a mild upper respiratory tract infection ('minor illness') and progressing to flaccid paralysis resulting from motor neurone destruction ('major illness'). This may be accompanied by spasms and inco-ordination of non-paralysed muscles. Various forms of the 'major illness' reflect infection of different parts of the CNS. Paralysis of limbs results from destruction of motor neurones in the lower part of the spinal cord ('spinal form'), while the more life threatening bulbar poliomyelitis ('bulbar form') involves infections of the medulla oblongata or bulb. Respiratory functions can be affected in both the spinal and bulbar forms of the disease. Encephalitis is rare. In children under 5 years old, paralysis of one leg is most common; in children 5 to 15 years of age, weakness of one limb or paraplegia are frequent; quadriplegia is most common in adults, often accompanied by urinary bladder and respiratory muscle dysfunction. Muscular function in limbs may return slowly but there is residual paralysis in 90 per cent of survivors. Ten to 25 per cent of paralytic cases have bulbar symptoms with hypertension, shock, and dysphonia. Complications are nosocomial pneumonias (by staphylococci or Gram-negative bacteria), urinary tract infections, and emotional problems. The mortality from paralytic polio is 2 to 5 per cent among children and 15 to 30 per cent among adults. Muscle weakness may develop many years after the initial polio disease (postpolio syndrome or postpolio neuromuscular atrophy). A persistent poliovirus infection as cause of this has been assumed, based on the presence of viral RNA in cerebrospinal fluid and neural tissue. However, such RNA has also been found in patients with other neurological and non-neurological diseases and is therefore less likely to be related to the postpolio syndrome. The alternative view is that the postpolio syndrome is anatomical in origin, such that the initial attack of polio destroys motor neurones and reduces the backup available as the patient ages.

Aseptic meningitis

Aseptic meningitis is the most frequent clinical presentation of enterovirus infection and can be caused by Coxsackie viruses of both groups A and B, and echoviruses, mainly types 4, 6, 11, 14, 16, 25, 30, and 31 (see Table 1). The disease starts with fever, headache, neck stiffness, and photophobia. Sensory or motoric deficits are unusual but confusion is common. The symptoms may persist for 4 to 7 days. The CSF usually shows pleocytosis consisting of 10 to 500 leucocytes per µl, mainly lymphocytes. Polymorphonuclear cells may predominate at the onset, but, should they persist, bacterial infection and possibly abscesses should be considered. The protein concentration in CSF may be normal or slightly increased; the glucose level is normal. Complete recovery is the usual outcome of aseptic meningitis.

Encephalitis

Enterovirus encephalitis is rare but may follow aseptic meningitis. Enterovirus infection in patients with hypo- or agammaglobulinaemia may persist for years with chronic meningitis or encephalitis as sequelae, and a high mortality.

Enterovirus 71 infection which is normally associated with hand, foot, and mouth disease has been found to cause severe meningoencephalitis (with brain stem involvement), polio-like acute flaccid paralysis, and a high case fatality rate in children during several recent outbreaks in Bulgaria, Taiwan, and Malaysia. In some of the fatal cases there may have been coinfections with a species B adenovirus. Enterovirus 71 occurs in three genotypes and is rapidly evolving; it is most closely related to Coxsackie virus A16.

Neonatal infections

Neonatal infection followed by severe, generalized disease may be caused by Coxsackie B viruses and echovirus, mainly of types 6, 7, and 11. These viruses seem to be transmitted late in pregnancy, perinatally, or postnatally by the mother or other virus-infected infants in neonatal wards or special care baby units. The infants develop heart failure due to a severe myocarditis, or a meningoencephalitis. Hepatitis and adrenalitis may also occur.

The mortality is high. Viruses may be recovered from brain, spinal cord, myocardium, and liver at autopsy.

Bornholm disease (epidemic pleurodynia)

This is usually caused by Coxsackie B viruses but also by echoviruses of types 1, 6, 9, 16, and 19, and by Coxsackie A viruses of types 4, 6, 9, and 10. The disease can strike families in small outbreaks. It typically starts abruptly with fever and chest pain due to the involvement of the intercostal muscles, or abdominal pain resulting from involvement of muscles of the abdomen. There may be severe frontal headache. The symptoms last 3 to 14 days, followed by complete recovery.

Myopericarditis

Enterovirus-induced myocarditis is mostly due to infection with Coxsackie B viruses in the young. The onset of disease is usually acute, very severe, and may be fatal in neonates, however in adolescents and adults it is normally mild. The virus may persist after the initial infection and cause dilated cardiomyopathy. In fatal cases (usually neonates 2–11 days after onset of disease) there is cardiac dilatation, myocyte necrosis, and an inflammatory reaction. The diagnosis is often difficult, particularly in older patients, as pericarditis, coronary artery occlusion, or heart failure may have been diagnosed initially. Typical clinical findings are often tachycardia, arrhythmias, murmurs, rubs, and cardiomegaly.

Besides causing acute myocarditis, chronic enterovirus infection can lead to chronic myocarditis and dilated cardiomyopathy, possibly due to immunopathologial mechanisms. In chronic disease, neither infectious virus nor viral antigens are normally detected in heart biopsies; however, viral RNA is regularly found in cardiac muscle, suggesting that the viral genome persists. The true significance of the presence of the viral genome in such cases is still under discussion.

The disease can be produced with Coxsackie B viruses in mice. In this animal model there is also initial viraemia and replication in myocytes, but this is followed by disappearance of infectious virus and destruction of myocytes, possibly by autoimmune mechanisms.

Herpangina

This is caused by Coxsackie viruses of types A1 to 6, 8, 10, and 22. Children and young adults between 2 and 20 years of age are mainly affected. The disease presents with acute onset of fever, sore throat and pain on swallowing, also vomiting and abdominal symptoms. Small vesicular lesions or white papules surrounded by a red halo can be seen on the fauces, pharynx, palate, uvula, and tonsils. The disease is mild and self-limiting.

Exanthemata

Rubella-like rashes can be produced by echoviruses of types 4, 9, and 16, but also Coxsackie viruses A9, A16, and B5. Those usually occur in the summer and may be accompanied by fever, malaise, cervical lymphadenopathy, and aseptic meningitis.

Hand, foot, and mouth disease

A typical distribution of vesicular lesions in hands, feet, and mouth (but also buttocks and genitalia) is produced by infection with Coxsackie virus type A16 and enterovirus 71, less frequently with Coxsackie viruses A4, A5, A9 and A10, B2, and B5. Enterovirus 71 may produce more severe clinical symptoms (see above).

Foot and mouth disease

The aphthovirus causing foot and mouth disease in cloven hoofed animals, is endemic in Africa, Asia, and South America. Virus is secreted before blisters of mouth and feet appear in animals. The zoonosis in humans is very rare, with about 37 recorded cases. Human infection occurs from virus entering through broken skin, drinking unpasteurised milk, or by inhal-ation of droplets. A 2 to 6-day incubation period is followed by blisters of hands, feet, and mouth, fever and sore throat. Complete recovery ensues. No person-to-person spread is recorded.

Conjunctivitis

Several enterovirus types cause conjunctivitis, often affecting large numbers of people epidemically. Most notable causes are echovirus types 7 and 11, Coxsackie virus A24 and B2, and enterovirus 70 that often produces a haemorrhagic conjunctivitis.

Diabetes and pancreatitis

Insulin-dependent diabetes mellitus (IDDM, or type 1 diabetes) is likely to be an autoimmune disorder in which the insulin-secreting pancreatic islet cells (beta cells) are destroyed. The human disease has long been thought to be caused by infectious agents, particularly since association between enterovirus infection and the development of IDDM has been shown in animal model studies (infection of mice with Coxsackie B3–B5 viruses). However, there is also a strong genetic component in the development of IDDM.

Chronic fatigue syndrome (CFS)

Chronic fatigue syndrome (CFS), also known under the names of myalgic encephalomyelitis (ME), Royal Free disease, Iceland disease, postviral fatigue syndrome, and neuromyasthenia, can occur both sporadically and epidemically. The main clinical feature is excess fatiguability of skeletal muscle, accompanied by pain. Other symptoms include headaches, inability to concentrate, paraesthesia, and impairment of short-term memory. A major problem in diagnosis is a clear definition of the clinical entity. Several virus infections have seemed to precede the development of CFS. Those are mainly enterovirus infections, chronic Epstein–Barr virus (EBV) infection and also infections with Toxoplasma and Leptospira species. The stringency of the association of chronic enterovirus infection with the appearance of CFS is controversial. A recent report of a joint working group of the Royal Colleges of Physicians, Psychiatrists and General Practitioners has concluded that persistence of enteroviruses is unlikely to play a role in the development of CFS. Similar conclusions have been drawn for the possibility of a causal link between chronic EBV infection and CFS (see Chapter 7.10.3).

Gastroenteritis

Although enteroviruses infect via the gastrointestinal tract and readily replicate there, they very rarely cause diarrhoea. Outbreaks of diarrhoea with echovirus type 11 have been reported. In Japan, an entervirus termed Aichivirus which is proposed as the type species of a new genus of the Picornaviridae family has been identified as the cause of multiple outbreaks of gastroenteritis in humans, mostly associated with the consumption of raw oysters. This virus seems to circulate widely in populations of Japan and other South-east Asian countries, with subclinical infections likely to be common (see Chapter 7.10.8).

Laboratory diagnosis of enterovirus infections

Virus isolation

Virus isolation is an excellent procedure to diagnose enterovirus infections. Virus is shed for weeks, and sometimes months, from the primary infection sites (cells lining the gut, see above). Starting from a few days after infection, virus can be found in concentrations of 10^5 to 10^6 tissue culture infectious doses 50 per cent per g faeces ($TCID_{50}$/g faeces). Throat swabs are also a good source for virus, particularly early in infection and when there are respiratory symptoms. In cases of meningitis, enteroviruses can be propagated in cell culture from the CSF, but the method is much less sensitive than genome detection (see below). Viruses are readily isolated in secondary cultures of monkey kidney cells, or in cultures of permanent cell lines derived from human embryonic kidney, human amnion, or human fetal lung. The cytopathic effect (CPE) produced by enteroviruses is non-specific. Typing of a cytopathic agent is carried out using antiserum pools or in multistep procedures. Most Coxsackie A viruses (with the exception of Coxsackie virus A9) do not grow well in cell culture but can be readily isolated by intracerebral, intraperitoneal, or subcutaneous infection of mice, causing flaccid paralysis and death. In contrast, Coxsackie B viruses cause spastic paralysis. Polio- or echoviruses do not usually grow in mice although polioviruses will replicate in transgenic animals that have appropriate receptors (see above).

Serology

Neutralization assays are the method of choice for typing enteroviruses. These tests are labour intensive and not apt for rapid diagnosis. They are mainly used for seroepidemiological studies. Recurrent enteroviruses infections during a lifetime often result in elevated serum antibody titres which obscure diagnostic changes. Significant antibody rises are therefore rarely observed in paired sera (taken at the onset of and during convalescence from disease).

A Coxsackie B virus-specific IgM test (using an IgM antibody capture technique) has been developed for rapid diagnosis. However, there is cross-reactivity between the IgM responses to different enteroviruses, including different genera of the picornaviruses, and so this test is not very specific. Prolonged presence of enterovirus-specific IgM has also been observed. Thus, in summary, the usefulness of serology for the diagnosis of enterovirus infection is limited.

Genome detection

Hybridization techniques and, more recently, reverse transcription polymerase chain reaction (RT-PCR) techniques have been applied to test for the presence of enterovirus genomes. This approach has been very productive, particularly in diagnosing CNS infections from CSF specimens, and has become the 'gold standard' of diagnosis, surpassing viral culture. Enterovirus RNAs have also been detected in myocardial biopsies from patients with myocarditis and dilated cardiomyopathy, in muscle of people with inflammatory muscle disease and chronic fatigue syndrome, and in brain biopsies. The significance of these findings is not clear as infectious virus can rarely be isolated, and viral antigen cannot be detected. Highly conserved sequences in the 5′ UTR of enterovirus genomes have allowed the design of PCR primers detecting most enterovirus RNAs. As the echovirus 22 genome is very different from that of the other enteroviruses, tailor-made primers have to be added in a multiplex RT-PCR to include these viruses, which occur particularly in neonates and infants. A modified RT-PCR procedure can differentiate between wild-type and vaccine-derived poliovirus infections.

Epidemiology of enterovirus infections

Enteroviruses are mainly transmitted by the faecal–oral route, due to the fact that viruses are shed in faeces for weeks or months after infection. Spread is particularly intense within families, usually starting from young children's primary infection. In temperate climates, there are seasonal peaks (July–September in the northern, and December–February in the southern hemisphere), whereas in subtropical/tropical climates enterovirus infections occur all the year round. The vast majority of primary human enterovirus infections occur during the first decade of life. Type-specific surveillance in several geographical regions has shown that Coxsackie viruses A9, A16, B4, and echovirus types 6, 9, 11, 19, 22, and 30 are most frequently found.

Prevention of enterovirus infections

As there are only three poliovirus types and no significant animal reservoir, it has been possible to develop very successful poliovirus vaccines. In 1954, a formalin-inactivated poliovirus vaccine (IPV) was introduced by Dr Jonas Salk in the United States, and in 1962 Dr Albert Sabin introduced a vaccine consisting of attenuated strains of the three poliovirus types which could be given orally (OPV). Protection by the live-attenuated vaccine is effected mainly at the site of entry by eliciting locally virus-specific IgAs and IgGs. Inactivated vaccine mainly elicits serum IgGs which prevent infection of the CNS and other sites distant of the port of entry by neutralization of viraemic virus. The main characteristics of IPV and OPV are summarized in Table 2.

Inactivated poliovirus vaccine

This vaccine was and is used with high acceptance rates in Scandinavia and Holland and has virtually eliminated poliomyelitis in these countries. There was a small outbreak of poliomyelitis due to poliovirus type 3 in Finland in the early 1980s, which seemed to be possible due to the fact that type 3 antibody levels in the community were comparatively low. However, the poliovirus strain isolated during the outbreak was antigenically unusual

Table 2 Characteristics of poliovirus vaccines

Characteristic	Live attenuated poliovirus vaccine (OPV)	Inactivated poliovirus vaccine (IPV)
Virus source	Attenuated virus (Sabin strains)	Virulent virus strains
Primary course	3 doses at monthly intervals starting at age of 2 months (temperate climates; more doses in tropics)	Three doses at 2-month intervals
Administration route	Oral	Parenteral (injection)
Immunity produced–systemic	IgA, IgM, IgG	IgM, IgG, (IgA)
–local	IgA	(IgA, minimal)
Booster doses required	1. at school entry 2. between 15 and 19 years 3. in adult life when exposed (last dose 10 years or more ago)	Yes (every 3–5 years or when exposed)
Efficacy	good in temperate climates, variable in tropics	good
Spread to contacts	Yes	No
Vaccine-associated paralysis (revertance)	0.5–3.4 cases/million first doses in susceptible children	No
Production cost per dose	$0.07	$0.7
Requirement on personnel	Not highly trained	Trained and skilled
Requirement of 'cold chain'	Yes	Less than OPV
Combination with other vaccines	No	Possible
Use in immunodeficiency	No	Possible

and less well neutralized by antisera to the reference strains of type 3 poliovirus. IPV is the vaccine of choice in cases of immunodeficiency.

Live attenuated poliovirus vaccine

This vaccine has a number of advantages compared to the inactivated vaccine as it:

- parallels the natural infection;
- stimulates both local secretory IgA in the pharynx and alimentary tract, and systemic circulating virus-specific IgG antibody;
- is easy to administer as an oral vaccine;
- is more cost effective.

The disadvantage is that in a few cases the attenuated vaccine strains have reverted to virulence. Since the early 1980s, all cases of polio in the United States and Europe were found to be caused by vaccine-related, that is reverted poliovirus, or were imported from endemic countries and were not indigenous, original wild-type strains. The risk of vaccine-associated poliomyelitis is between 0.5 and 3.4 cases per million of susceptible children immunized. Vaccine-related polio is mostly caused by type 2 or type 3 viruses, probably due to the fact that the number of point mutations in type 1 vaccine virus compared to wild type is much higher than in type 2 and type 3 vaccine viruses. However, this finding raises the question of whether oral vaccination should be continued. In the United States, guidelines have been developed recently which replace the oral vaccination programme by a mixed procedure, initially using inactivated vaccine, followed by booster doses of oral vaccine. For a variety of reasons many countries (United States, France, Germany) have either subscribed to the exclusive use of IPV or are likely to do so in the near future. The decision was influenced by the good progress made towards the eradication of polio due to wild-type virus.

OPV is the vaccine of choice for people travelling into poliovirus endemic areas if their immune status is unknown or in doubt. The vaccine should be given at least 2 weeks before departure.

Polio eradication and surveillance

For many years it was thought that the Sabin oral poliovaccines were ineffective in tropical countries. While many reasons were put forward, the lack of impact of polio vaccination programmes was probably due to loss of vaccine potency through failure to maintain storage at cool temperatures, and also the epidemiology of poliovirus infection. In temperate countries, poliomyelitis is seasonal with infections peaking in the summer months. A strategy of vaccination based on immunization of young children at a set age (usually a few months) is therefore able to build up a highly immune population in the winter so that transmission of the wild-type virus becomes more difficult. In tropical countries, where exposure is year round, it is a matter of chance whether a child is first naturally infected, or immunized. This was recognized by Sabin in 1960, but not acted upon until some 20 years later, when the strategy of National Immunization Days was developed in South America. This approach involves immunizing all children below a certain age in a country within a very short period, so that all susceptible children's intestinal tracts are occupied by vaccine virus and are therefore resistant to infection by the wild type. Transmission of wild-type virus is therefore broken, and the virus dies out.

WHO have pronounced the intention of eliminating poliomyelitis due to wild-type virus. The Americas have been free of polio since 1992, but vaccine-derived poliomyelitis occurred in Haiti and the Dominican Republic in 2000/1. The last case of polio in South East Asia occurred in March 1997. In 2000, the Western Pacific Region was declared polio-free by WHO, and polio is now endemic in only 30 countries (Fig. 1). The scale of the undertaking is colossal, and the progress towards eradication is extraordinary. For example in 1992 in China, all children aged 5 or less were immunized over a 1-week period. This amounts to one-quarter of the world's children. At the time of writing, virus was still known to be endemic in

India and surrounding countries, countries of West and Central Africa, and of the Eastern Mediterranean region, but eradication before long is a real possibility.

Part of the challenge is to demonstrate that the virus has in fact been eliminated, and this depends on rigorous, effective surveillance. One approach is to obtain data on cases of acute flaccid paralysis of whatever cause, including the Guillain–Barré syndrome. All cases should be investigated to see whether they are due to poliovirus infection or not, and it is considered that the background rate in the absence of poliomyelitis should be one case per 100 000 members of the population, providing a control for the adequacy of the surveillance scheme. Alternative approaches include the investigation of poliovirus isolates to establish whether they derived from vaccine or wild-type strains. There are possible concerns over the adequacy of either approach.

Once wild-type poliovirus has been eradicated, the only sources of the virus will be manufacturers of vaccines, laboratories holding stocks, and recipients of live attenuated vaccine. While manufacturers and laboratory workers can be required to work under high containment level conditions to avoid escape of virulent virus, vaccinees pose a particular problem. The vaccine works by establishing an infection in the recipient but the virus may adapt to the gut and eventually undergo major molecular changes to improve its fitness. In principle, such viruses could spread to others forming a focus for a return of poliovirus infections and poliomyelitis. In practice, the vaccine virus seems to be poorly transmissible compared to the wild type. In countries such as Cuba where it has been given only in the early part of the year as a matter of policy, virus is not detectable after 6 months. Thus, it might be possible to stop vaccinating with no further precautions, as the vaccine strain of poliovirus will die out more rapidly than susceptible individuals will accumulate to provide a population to maintain it. However, people with B cell immunodeficiency can remain infected but apparently healthy for up to 15 years. During this time the virus may adapt to an extent that neurotropism is regained, and an unvaccinated population will again be highly susceptible. The numbers or geographical distribution of such long-term excretors are unknown. One possible approach to the problem would be to use inactivated vaccine for some unspecified period. The fact that serious consideration has to be given to how to deal with the cessation of vaccination is a tribute to the extraordinary progress which has been made towards polio eradication.

Further reading

Centers for Disease Control (2000). Progress toward global poliomyelitis eradication, 1999. *Morbidity and Mortality Weekly Report* **49**, 349–54.

Joint Working Group of the Royal Colleges of Physicians, Psychiatrists and General Practitioners (1997). *Chronic fatigue syndrome*, pp. 58. Royal College of Physicians, Publication Unit, London.

King AMQ, Brown F, Christian P et al. (2000). Picornaviridae. In: van Regenmortel MHV, Fauquet CM, Bishop DHL, et al. eds. *Virus taxonomy. classification and nomenclature of viruses. Seventh report of the International Committee on Taxonomy of Viruses*, pp, 657–78. Virology Division, International Union of Microbiological Societies. Academic Press, San Diego.

Melnick JL (1996). Enteroviruses: polioviruses, coxsackieviruses, echoviruses, and newer enteroviruses. In: Fields BN, Knipe DM, Howley PM et al., eds. *Fields virology*, 3rd edn, pp. 655–712. Lippincott-Raven, Philadelphia.

Mendelsohn C, Wimmer R, Racaniello VR (1989). Cellular receptor for poliovirus: molecular cloning, nucleotide sequence and expression of a new member of the immunoglobulin superfamily. *Cell* **56**, 855–65.

Minor PD (1990). Antigenic structure of picornaviruses. *Current Topics in Microbiology and Immunology* **161**, 122–54.

Minor PD (1996). Poliovirus. In: Nathanson N, Ahmed R, Gonzalez-Scarano F, et al., eds. *Viral pathogenesis*, pp. 555–74. Lippincott-Raven, Philadelphia.

Minor P (1999). Picornaviruses. In: Mahy BW, Collier IL, eds. *Topley and Wilson's microbiology and microbial infections*, Vol. 1: Virology, 9th edn, pp. 485–509. Arnold, London.

Racaniello VR and Baltimore D (1981). Cloned poliovirus complementary DNA is infectious in mammalian cells. *Science* **214**, 916–19.

Yamashita T *et al.* (2000). Application of a reverse transcription-PCR for identification and differentiation of Aichi virus, a new member of the picornavirus family associated with gastroenteritis in humans. *Journal of Clinical Microbiology* **38**, 2955–61.

7.10.8 Virus infections causing diarrhoea and vomiting

Ulrich Desselberger

Introduction

Acute gastroenteritis and vomiting in humans is a well-characterized clinical entity caused by several different agents (viruses, bacteria, parasites, etc.). Viral gastroenteritis is a global problem, particularly in infants and young children.

Many viruses are found in the gut but not all of them produce acute gastroenteritis (Table 1). Viral infections normally associated with gastroenteritis are caused by: rotaviruses; enteric adenoviruses; small, round structured viruses (**SRSVs**) and classic human caliciviruses; and astroviruses. Other viruses found in the gastrointestinal tract (enteroviruses, reoviruses, non-group F adenoviruses, toroviruses, coronaviruses, parvoviruses) are not regularly associated with diarrhoeal disease in humans. Finally, there are viruses found in the gut of immunosuppressed patients (most often those with human immunodeficiency virus (**HIV**) infection), including herpes simplex virus (**HSV**), cytomegalovirus (**CMV**), and picobirnaviruses. HIV itself can also infect the gut directly.

Only the major virus groups regularly causing gastroenteritis in man are described here separately. Clinical symptoms, diagnosis, treatment, epidemiology, and vaccine development are reviewed under common headings.

Table 1 Virus infections of the human gut

Viruses found as:	Genus (Family)
Regular cause of diarrhoea and vomiting	Rotaviruses (*Reoviridae*)[a]
	Group F adenoviruses (*Adenoviridae*)
	Small, round structured viruses (SRSVs; *Caliciviridae*)[a]
	Classical caliciviruses (*Caliciviridae*)
	Astroviruses (*Astroviridae*)
Occasional cause of diarrhoea and vomiting	Enteroviruses (*Picornaviridae*)[b]
	Reoviruses (*Reoviridae*)
	Adenoviruses other than Group F (*Adenoviridae*)
	Toroviruses (*Coronaviridae*)
	Coronaviruses (*Coronaviridae*)
	Parvoviruses (*Parvoviridae*)
Cause of diarrhoea in immunodeficient patients	Human immunodeficiency virus (*Retroviridae*)
	Herpes simplex virus (*Herpesviridae*)
	Cytomegalovirus (*Herpesviridae*)
	Picobirnaviruses (*Birnaviridae*)

[a] Not all infections cause disease (see text).
[b] Outbreaks of diarrhoea caused by echovirus type 11 infections have been reported (see Chapter 7.11.8).

Rotaviruses

Structure

Rotaviruses are the major cause of infantile gastroenteritis worldwide and also of acute diarrhoea in the young of many mammalian species. They are members of the Reoviridae family, with a genome of 11 segments of double-stranded RNA encoding six structural viral proteins (VP1–4, VP6, and VP7) and six non-structural proteins (NSP1–NSP6). The structural proteins VP1–3 are located in the inner or core layer, VP6 forms an inner shell or intermediate layer, and VP7, and VP4 are components of the outer shell or outer layer (VP4 protrudes as spikes). Thus, a double-shelled/triple-layered particle, 75 nm in diameter, appears in a characteristic form on electron micrographs (Fig. 1), the name of the virus being derived from *rota* (Latin = wheel).

Classification

Rotaviruses are classified according to the immunological reactivities and genomic sequences of three of their structural components.

1. Specific epitopes on the inner-shell protein VP6 allow five groups (A–E) to be distinguished, and two more groups (F, G) probably exist. Within group A rotaviruses, there are at least four subgroups. Group A rotaviruses constitute the vast majority of human infections.

2. Both surface proteins, VP4 and VP7, elicit neutralizing antibodies and thus confer type-specificity. A dual-type classification system has been devised for group A rotaviruses, which differentiates G types (VP7-specific, G for glycoprotein) and P types (VP4-specific, P for protease-sensitive protein)—for example, G1P1A[8] is G serotype and genotype 1, P serotype 1A, P genotype 8. At least 11 G types and 9 P types have been found in humans (see reviews by Estes 1996 and Desselberger 2000). As group A rotaviruses reassort readily in doubly infected cells, various combinations of VP4 and VP7 types occur in natural isolates.

Replication

Rotaviruses replicate in the mature epithelial cells at the tips of the villi of the small intestine. Viruses enter cells either by receptor-mediated endocytosis or directly, and single-shelled subviral particles (devoid of VP4 and VP7) produce and protrude large numbers of mRNAs from all 11 segments

Fig. 1 Rotavirus particles in the faeces of a child admitted to hospital with acute gastroenteritis. Negative staining with aqueous 2 per cent potassium phosphotungstate, pH 7.0. The scale bar represents 100 nm. Four different morphologies of particles are shown: (a) double-shelled (ds) particles containing RNA; (b) ds particle without RNA (empty; core penetrated with stain); (c) single-shelled (ss) particle containing RNA; (d) single-shelled empty particle. (Figure by courtesy of M. Jenkins, Regional Virus Laboratory, East Birmingham Hospital). (Taken from U. Desselberger, Reoviruses. In: *Medical Microbiology*, 14th edition, (eds. D. Greenwood, R. Slack, J. Peutherer), page 620. Churchill Livingstone, Edinburgh, 1992, with permission of the publisher.)

into the cytoplasm. Viral proteins are synthesized from mRNAs, and morphogenesis proceeds in a complex fashion. Mature rotavirus particles are released from cells by lysis, resulting in very high concentrations of up to 10^{11} virus particles per ml of faeces at the peak of the acute diarrhoea.

Pathogenesis

The diarrhoea arises by cellular necrosis and atrophy of the epithelium, leading to a reduction in the breakdown and absorption of carbohydrates and to increased osmotic pressure in the gut lumen. The villous damage is repaired by cells emerging and differentiating from the crypts of the gut epithelium, which show a reactive hyperplasia. This is accompanied by increased secretion, which also contributes to the diarrhoea. Several viral proteins have been shown to be determinants of the pathogenicity of rotaviruses and VP4 is of major significance. Most recently, the non-structural protein NSP4 (= VP10) has been characterized as the first viral enterotoxin.

Immune response

A serotype-specific humoral immune response is elicited after neonatal or primary rotavirus infection. However, during the first 2 years of life children are repeatedly infected with rotaviruses, leading to multiple serotype-specific, but also partially heterotypic, protection. The presence of rotavirus-specific secretory IgA coproantibodies seems to correlate best with protection against disease, although the exact correlates remain to be determined. There are also rotavirus-specific cytotoxic T-cell responses whose exact role in immunity is unknown.

Enteric adenoviruses

Structure and classification

Adenoviruses are non-enveloped icosahedral viruses possessing a genome of linear double-stranded DNA approximately 35 000 bp in size. Their capsid is between 70 and 80 nm in diameter and consists of 240 hexons and 12 pentons that stand out as projecting fibres at the corners of the icosahedral virus particle. Human adenoviruses occur in 51 distinct serotypes, ordered in six different subgroups (A–F). Those adenoviruses regularly associated with gastroenteritis are classified as subgroup F, serotypes 40 and 41. Adenoviruses of different groups (causing respiratory tract infections) are also found in the gut, but are not regularly associated with diarrhoea.

Replication

Adenoviruses attach to susceptible cells via the fibre proteins, and enter via receptor-mediated endocytosis. Phased early and late gene transcription of the viral DNA in the cellular nucleus is followed by translation and mor-

phogenesis in the cytoplasm, and numerous particles are released after cell death. The early protein E1A is a potent blocker of apoptosis and of interferon-α and -β expression. Late adenovirus gene expression blocks cellular DNA expression. Some adenoviruses seem to decrease the expression of MHC class 1 antigens on the surface of infected cells, thus reducing susceptibility to adenovirus-specific cytotoxic T cells. There is a serotype-specific humoral immune response providing homotypic protection.

Small, round structured viruses (SRSV)

Structure and classification

These viruses were first recognized as the cause of gastroenteritis during outbreaks in Norwalk, Ohio, in the late 1960s. Norwalk virus (**NV**) particles are spherical and measure 27 to 35 nm in diameter. NV and Norwalk-like viruses (**NLVs**) are all members of the Caliciviridae family. Their 7.7-kb genome consists of single-stranded RNA of positive polarity. Cup-shaped depressions on the surface of virions have given the name to this viral family (Latin *calix* = goblet, cup). Phylogenetic trees of full-length sequences of caliciviral cDNA demonstrate at least three genogroups (Norwalk virus representing genogroup 1; Lorsdale virus, genogroup 2; and Manchester virus, genogroup 3). The SRSVs and typical caliciviruses that infect humans are shown in Table 2. Genogroup 3 viruses have been termed 'classical' caliciviruses as their structure is better preserved on electron microscopy, and the genomes of some show greater homology with several animal caliciviruses which are possible sources of human infection.

Replication

Details of the replication of human caliciviruses can only be deduced from those of animal caliciviruses as there is no reproducible *in vitro* cell-culture system for the human SRSVs. The viruses seem to interact with species-specific receptors and a single protein precursor is co- and post-translationally cleaved in a way similar to that observed in enteroviruses.

Immune response

Although SRSV infections elicit human immune responses, they do not seem to give full protection against subsequent infection. On the contrary, higher pre-existing antibody levels seem to predispose to more severe illness upon reinfection.

Astroviruses

Structure and classification

Astroviruses are members of the newly defined family Astroviridae. They possess a 6.8-kb genome of single-stranded RNA of positive polarity. So far,

Table 2 *Caliciviridae* causing human infection and diarrhoeal disease

Virus	Abbreviation	Name derived from morphology	Calicivirus genogroup
Norwalk virus	NV	SRSV[a]	I
Southampton virus	SV	SRSV	I
Desert shield virus	DSV	SRSV	I
Hawaii agent	HA	SRSV	II
Snow Mountain agent	SMA	SRSV	II
Mexico virus	MV	HuCV[b]	II
Lorsdale virus	LV	HuCV	II
Hu CV VK1-UK4		Hu CV UK1-UK4	II
Toronto virus	TV	Minireovirus	II and untyped
Sapporovirus	SaV	Hu CV Sapporo	III
Manchester virus	MaV	Hu CV Manchester	III
Plymouth virus	PlV	Hu CV Plymouth	III

[a] Small, round structured virus.

[b] Human calicivirus.

eight different serotypes have been distinguished, which correlate well with major differences in genome sequences (that is, genotypes).

Replication

Human astroviruses grow well in particular cell cultures. After viral absorption to unidentified cellular receptors and uncoating in the cytoplasm, full-length and subgenomic RNAs are made. These direct the production of protein precursors which are post-translationally cleaved. Replication takes place purely in the cytoplasm.

Illness

The onset of acute viral gastroenteritis follows a short incubation period of 1 to 2 days. It is sudden, with watery diarrhoea lasting between 4 and 7 days, vomiting, and varying degrees of dehydration. Over one-third of children with rotavirus infection have a fever of more than 39 °C. Fewer have a high fever after infection with SRSVs. The duration of diarrhoea after infection with SRSVs is as a rule shorter (1–2 days) than after infection with rotaviruses or enteric adenoviruses (4–7 days). Disease due to SRSV infection may be accompanied by abdominal cramps, headache, and myalgia. In rotavirus infection all degrees of severity are seen. Inapparent infections are not infrequent, particularly in neonates where the infection is caused by so-called 'nursery strains'. It is not clear whether the asymptomatic nature of rotavirus infection in neonates is due to infection with particular strains or depends on the presence of maternal antibodies that provide partial protection. Rotavirus infections are frequently accompanied by respiratory symptoms; but there is no strong evidence that rotavirus replicates in the respiratory tract. In immunodeficient children, chronic gut infections with rotaviruses, adenoviruses, and astroviruses have been observed, accompanied by virus shedding over weeks and even months.

Diagnosis

The diagnosis of rotavirus, astrovirus, and enteric adenovirus infections is relatively easy as large numbers of particles are shed during the acute phase of the illness. In contrast, SRSVs replicate for a shorter period and are shed at lower concentrations. Diagnosis is by electron microscopy of negatively stained specimen suspensions ('Catch-all method'), by passive particle agglutination tests, virus-specific enzyme-linked immunosorbent assays (**ELISAs**), and more recently by viral genome detection using the polymerase chain reaction (**PCR**) (for adenoviruses) and reverse transcription-PCR (**RT-PCR**) (for rotaviruses, caliciviruses, and astroviruses). The morphological appearances of the main viruses pathogenic for humans are shown in Fig. 2. PCRs are extremely sensitive diagnostic tools, allowing both viral detection and typing. Aliquots of PCR amplicons can also be sequenced and the information used to establish phylogenetic trees. Such trees are becoming increasingly important not only for virus classification but also for epidemiological studies and surveillance (see below).

Treatment

Treatment is mainly by oral rehydration or, in more severe cases, intravenous rehydration. In severe rotavirus infections, treatment with oral immunoglobulins has shown to affect the duration of diarrhoea and virus shedding. This is not, however, a routine treatment. Otherwise treatment is symptomatic, but the use of antimobility drugs (codeine phosphate, diphenoxylate, coperamide) in children is not advised. Specific antiviral agents have been tested in animal models of rotavirus infections but are not used for human treatment.

Fig. 2 Electron micrographs of (a) rotavirus, (b) enteric adenovirus, (c) SRSV, (d) calicivirus, (e) astrovirus, (f) enterovirus, and (g) parvovirus. Negative staining with 3 per cent phosphotungstate, pH 6.3; bar represents 100 nm (Figures by courtesy of Dr J. Kurtz, Oxford Public Health Laboratory (astroviruses) and Dr J. Gray, Clinical Microbiology and Public Health Laboratory Cambridge (all other viruses)). Reproduced from *Principles and practice of clinical virology*, 4th edn (eds. A. Zuckerman, J. Banatvala, J. Pattison), p. 236. J. Wiley and Sons, Chichester, 2000, with permission of the publisher.

Epidemiology

Rotaviruses

Rotavirus infections occur endemically worldwide and cause over 800 000 deaths annually in children below the age of 2 years, mainly in developing countries. Therefore development of vaccine candidates has been a major goal since the early 1980s (see below). The epidemiology of rotaviruses is complex. Besides children, elderly patients and patients with immunodeficiencies can be affected. There is a strict winter peak of rotavirus infections in temperate climates, but infections occur year round in tropical and subtropical regions. Transmission is by the faeco-oral route. Nosocomial infections on infant hospital wards occur and are difficult to eliminate. Group A rotaviruses of different G and P types are found to cocirculate in various populations within the same geographical location, and the relative incidence of different types changes over time. Various surveys have shown that usually more than 90 per cent of cocirculating strains in temperate climates are types G1 to G4 and occur in combination with different P types as types G1P1A[8], G2P1B[4], G3P1A[8], and G4P1A[8]. Other G types may also be represented, seen particularly in tropical and subtropical areas but increasingly in temperate climates. For instance, G9 strains have caused outbreaks with increasing frequency in the United States and Europe. Most mammalian, as well as avian species, harbour a large diversity of rotaviruses and may act as a reservoir for human infections. An animal source is suspected for many of the more unusual human group A rotavirus isolates, and possibly for group B rotavirus isolates. The latter caused outbreaks in children and adults in China during the 1980s and have recently been isolated from patients with diarrhoea in Calcutta. Group C rotaviruses are associated with small outbreaks in humans.

Small, round structured viruses

Age-related seroprevalence studies of SRSVs have recently shown that infection is much more frequent and occurs from younger ages onwards than previously thought. Approximately 50 per cent of infants have been infected by the age of 2 years. The rate of inapparent infection is high, particularly in the young. In contrast to rotavirus infections, SRSVs cause outbreaks of acute gastroenteritis, mostly due to contamination of food or water. Contaminated oysters and green salads are often implicated as sources of infection. Outbreaks occur in older children and adults in recreational camps, hospitals, nursing homes, schools, cafeterias, hotels, cruise ships, at banquets, etc. SRSV outbreaks occur worldwide throughout the year, in contrast to the regular winter peaks of rotavirus infections in temperate climates. The viruses are highly infectious and spread rapidly. Transmission is spread by the faeco-oral route and also by projectile vomiting, scattering viruses into the environment by aerosol. At least seven different genotypes cocirculate, which have been confirmed as serotypes. Type 1 and 2 viruses are most frequent.

Astroviruses

Infections with astroviruses occur in infants and the elderly as endemic infections, but they can also cause food-borne outbreaks of diarrhoea. There are at least eight genotypes, correlating well with known serotypes which cocirculate. Serotype 1 is most frequently found, followed by serotypes 2 to 4 at intermediate and serotypes 5 to 7 at low frequencies. Seroprevalence studies have indicated that infection by more than one serotype is not unusual.

Vaccine development

Vaccines have been found to be the best individual and also population-based tools to restrict infection with epidemic viruses. Of the gastroenteritis-inducing viruses, vaccine development has only been intensely directed towards rotaviruses. After many trials with variable success, a live-attenuated, rhesus rotavirus (**RRV**)-based, human reassortant vaccine eliciting immunity to human rotavirus strains G1 to G4 has recently been found to confer significant protection (70–80 per cent) from severe disease including dehydration, whereas protection from infection alone was only moderate (40–50 per cent). This vaccine was recommended by the Advisory Committee on Immunization Practices (**ACIP**) in the United States in 1998. However, after 1.5 million doses had been used, the rare complication of gut intussusception was found to be apparently significantly associated with vaccination. In 1999 the ACIP withdrew the recommendation, and the vaccine has been taken off the market by the manufacturer. Studies of the epidemiological findings and possible mechanisms of pathogenesis are underway.

As a result, other approaches to immunization against rotavirus infection have gained interest, such as the use of virus-like particles obtained from baculovirus-recombinant coexpressed rotavirus proteins, enhancement of rotavirus immunogenicity by microencapsidation, DNA-based candidate vaccines, and possibly 'edible vaccines'.

No vaccines against other viruses causing gastroenteritis in humans have been developed so far. For NV-like viruses this is unlikely to happen, as long-term immunity does not usually seem to follow natural infection.

Outbreak control

Nosocomial rotavirus outbreaks among paediatric populations (on hospital wards and in day-care centres) are common. There have been numerous reports of outbreaks of diarrhoea and vomiting occurring in adults and children due to infections with Norwalk-like viruses, acquired from banquets, travel on cruise ships, cafeterias, schools, hotels, fast-food restaurants, etc.

Outbreak control measures should focus on the interruption of person-to-person transmission and the removal of common sources of infection (food, water, etc.) in conjunction with measures to improve environmental hygiene (by food-handlers, etc.).

Further reading

Ball JM, *et al.* (1996). Age-dependent diarrhoea induced by a rotaviral nonstructural glycoprotein. *Science* **272**, 101–4.

Desselberger U (1992). Reoviruses. In: Greenwood D, Slack R, Peutherer J, eds. *Medical microbiology*, 14th edn, pp 619–33. Churchill-Livingstone, Edinburgh.

Desselberger U (2000). Viruses causing gastroenteritis. In: Zuckerman A, Banatvala J, Pattison J, eds. *Principles and practice of clinical virology*, 4th edn, pp 235–52. Wiley, Chichester.

Estes MK (1996). Rotaviruses and their replication. In: Fields BN, *et al.*, eds. *Fields virology*, 3rd edn, pp 1625–55. Lippincott-Raven, Philadelphia.

Kapikian AZ, Estes MK, Chanock RM (1996). Norwalk group of viruses. In: Fields BN, *et al.*, eds. *Fields virology*, 3rd edn, pp 783–810. Lippincott-Raven, Philadelphia.

Matsui, SM, Greenberg HB (1996). Astroviruses. In: Fields BN, *et al.*, eds. *Fields virology*, 3rd edn, pp 811–24. Lippincott-Raven, Philadelphia.

Offit PA (1994). Rotaviruses. Immunological determinants of protection against infection and disease. *Advances in Virus Research* **44**, 161–202.

Shenk T (1996). Adenoviridae: the viruses and their replication. In: Fields BN, *et al.*, eds. *Fields virology*, 3rd edn, pp 2111–2148. Lippincott-Raven, Philadelphia.

7.10.9 Rhabdoviruses: rabies and rabies-related viruses

M. J. Warrell and D. A. Warrell

Virology

The Rhabdoviridae are a family of more than 100 rod- or bullet-shaped RNA viruses found in vertebrates, insects, and plants (Fig. 1). Two genera infect animals: *Vesiculovirus* and *Lyssavirus*. Vesicular stomatitis virus is a *Vesiculovirus* of cattle and horses, which occasionally causes an influenza-like illness in farmers or laboratory workers. The genus *Lyssavirus* comprises seven genotypes: rabies and six genotypes of rabies-related viruses.

30nm

Fig. 1 Rhabdoviruses. Virion of rabies virus. (Electron micrograph by courtesy of Mr C. J. Smale and Dr Joan Crick.)

The rabies virion is approximately 180 × 75 nm. Its core is a single strand of negative non-segmented RNA, associated with a nucleoprotein, a phosphoprotein, and an RNA polymerase to form a helical ribonucleoprotein complex (RNP). This is enveloped in a matrix protein covered by a coat of glycoprotein (G) and host cell-derived lipid. The G protein forms numerous spikes or knobs, 10 nm long, and its composition determines viral virulence.

The virus is readily inactivated by ultraviolet light, drying, boiling, most organic lipid solvents including more than 45 per cent ethanol, soap solution, detergents, hypochlorite, and glutaraldehyde solutions.

Typing by means of monoclonal antibodies or genetic sequencing techniques allows the identification of strains of rabies and rabies-related viruses from different geographical areas and vector species, revealing the diversity of rabies virus strains.

Epidemiology

Rabies is a zoonosis that remains endemic in most parts of the world (Fig. 2). Currently, the following countries are rabies free: Iceland, Norway, Sweden, Finland, Switzerland, Portugal, Italy, Greece, Cyprus and other Mediterranean islands, Singapore, Sabah, Sarawak, Bali, New Guinea, New Zealand, Antarctica, Oceania, Hong Kong islands (but not the New Territories), Japan, South Korea, Taiwan, and Caribbean islands with the notable exceptions of Cuba, the Dominican Republic, Grenada, Haiti, Trinidad, and Tobago. Some other countries have no indigenous rabies but infected animals cross land borders.

Primarily an infection of wild mammals, rabies is spread by bites and rarely by inhalation of aerosols in bat caves and by ingestion of infected prey. The ecology of rabies virus can be divided into urban and sylvatic phases, which overlap to a varying extent in different countries.

In a particular area, transmission in the sylvatic phase tends to occur predominantly within a single species in separate ecological compartments. Each vector has a separate virus strain and a distinctive method of transmission. The wild-mammal reservoir species varies in different geographical areas: in the United States, striped skunks (*Mephitis mephitis*) and to a lesser extent spotted skunks (*Spilogale putorius*) in the central States and California; raccoons in the east; the grey fox (*Urocyon cineroargenteus*) in central areas and red fox (*Vulpes vulpes*) in the east; coyotes in the south; and in the arctic, the fox *Alopex lagopus*.

Bat rabies in the Americas is all due to genotype 1 virus, whereas in the rest of the world bats have rabies-related lyssaviruses. In North America insectivorous bats are the vectors, including the Mexican free-tailed bat (*Tadarida brasiliensis mexicana*), the red bat (*Lasiurus borealis*), the big brown bat (*Eptesicus fuscus*), and the silver-haired bat (*Lasionycteris noctivagans*), whose virus is the main cause of human rabies infections in the United States (see below). Bat infection has been found in every state except Alaska and Hawaii.

The three species of true vampire bats, *Desmodus rotundus*, *Diaemus youngi*, and *Diphylla ecaudata* (Desmodontinae), occur from sea level to over 3500 m but usually below 1500 m, only in Mexico, Central and South America, and some Caribbean Islands (Fig. 3). The common vampire bat, *D. rotundus* is the main vector of vampire bat rabies in Trinidad, Mexico, and Central and South America. Carnivorous bats of the family Megadermatidae, such as the Indian 'vampire' (*Megaderma lyra*), are usually responsible for the myth that vampires occur outside this area. In Latin America vampire bat-transmitted paralytic rabies (derriengue) has locally serious economic consequences. In Brazil 50 000 head of cattle are estimated to die annually.

In Grenada and Puerto Rico mongooses (*Herpestes auropunctatus*) are vectors of sylvatic rabies; in most of Africa and Asia, wolves, jackals, and small carnivores of the families Mustelidae and Viverridae (e.g. the yellow mongoose *Cynictis penicillata* in South Africa and the palm civet *Paradoxurus hermaphroditus* in Indonesia); and in Europe, foxes, wolves, raccoon dogs (*Nyctereutes procyonoides*), and insectivorous bats (see rabies-related viruses). There are reports of rabies virus being isolated from wild rodents in many countries including the Russian Federation, Germany, Egypt, Nigeria, Thailand, and the United States, but the significance of this finding is uncertain.

Humans are occasionally infected by wild mammals, but domestic dogs and cats, the principal vectors of urban rabies, are responsible for more than 90 per cent of human cases worldwide. Domestic dogs are the principal reservoir in many parts of Africa and Asia, and in urban areas elsewhere. Rabies control programmes can reduce the risk of rabies in domestic animals to such an extent that wild animals, for example, bats in the United States, become the principal vectors of infection to humans.

Cyclical epizootics of rabies, such as the fox epizootic in Europe, result from an uncontrolled increase in the population of the key reservoir species. This epizootic started in Poland at the end of the Second World War. Initially it advanced at a rate of about 40 km a year across France, but recently has retreated. Although the fox is one of the most susceptible species to rabies, about 3 per cent of animals survive the infection and become immune. In the Caribbean island of Grenada, almost half of the mongooses have serum neutralizing antibody against rabies. Seropositive raccoons, bats, and very occasionally dogs have also been found.

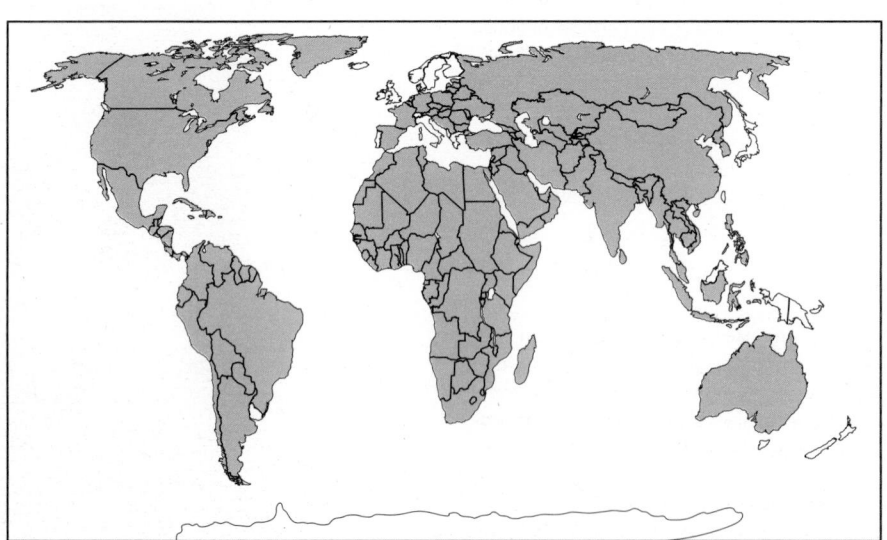

Fig. 2 Global distribution of rabies. Rabies-free areas shown in white.

Fig. 3 Distribution of the three species of true vampire bats (Desmodontinae).

Fig. 4 Child bitten on the face by a rabid dog. This wound carries a high risk of rabies with a short incubation period. (Copyright D.A. Warrell.)

Incidence of human rabies

The true incidence of human rabies throughout the world is not reflected in official figures, such as those reported by the World Health Organization. In 1998, in India alone, the estimated mortality was 30 000, in Bangladesh, it was 2000 ($1.6/10^5$ population) and in Sri Lanka, 110. The true mortalities were probably considerably higher. High mortalities also occur in Nepal, Pakistan, and Ethiopia, but there are very few data from Africa. In the United States in 10 years since 1990, 27 human cases occurred, seven of whom were infected by dogs (two from Asia). Twenty (74 per cent) patients were infected by bats, and 15 (75 per cent) of the bat infections were due to a rabies strain associated with silver-haired (*Lasionycteris noctivagans*) and pipistrelle bats (*Pipistrellus subflavus*). The Russian Federation reported 11 deaths from rabies in 1999. Rabies was eradicated from Britain by 1903 but in November 2002 a man died of European bat lyssavirus infection (see below) in Scotland.

Transmission

Virus can penetrate broken skin and intact mucosa. Humans are usually infected when virus-laden saliva is inoculated through the skin by the bite of a rabid dog or other mammal (Fig. 4). Saliva from a rabid animal can infect if the skin is already broken, by the animal's claws for example. In the United States infective contact with bats may be unnoticed: only one of 20 patients had a history of a bat bite. Animals can be infected through the gastrointestinal tract, but there is no evidence that this happens in humans.

Inhalation of aerosolized virus created by bats' infected nasal secretions may be an important method of transmission among cave-dwelling bats. In Texas, two men died of rabies after visiting caves inhabited by millions of Mexican free-tailed bats, many of which were rabid. Two laboratory workers in the United States developed rabies after inhaling fixed strains of rabies virus during the preparation of vaccines. The accidental use of vaccine in which the virus was not inactivated has led to fixed virus rabies (*rage de laboratoire*): for example, in Fortaleza, Brazil in 1960.

Transmission of rabies from one person to another has been proved in six patients who received infected corneal grafts (Fig. 5). The donors had died of undiagnosed neurological diseases. Twenty-two to 39 days after transplantation, the recipients developed retro-orbital headache on the side of the graft and died of rabies. In a seventh recipient, in Morocco, rabies was prevented by vigorous postexposure prophylaxis. Other infections spread by corneal grafts are Creutzfeldt–Jacob disease and cryptococcosis.

Considering that the saliva, respiratory secretions, and tears of patients with rabies contain virus it is surprising that the disease has not been spread to relatives and nurses.

Transplacental infection has been observed in animals but only once reported in humans. A number of women with rabies encephalitis have given birth to healthy babies. The transmission of rabies from mother to

Fig. 5 Corneal transplant graft (by courtesy of Professor A. Bron).

suckling infant via the breast milk has been suspected in at least one human case and is well known in animals.

Pathogenesis

The mechanism by which the highly neurotropic rabies virus enters the nervous system, travels into the brain, and out again to many organs is intriguing. The virus may replicate locally in muscle cells or attach directly to the nerve endings. Its preferential attachment to nicotinic acetylcholine receptors at motor end-plates is blocked by α-bungarotoxin, whose structure has a homologous sequence with rabies glycoprotein. Once inside peripheral nerves, virus travels in a retrograde direction within the axoplasm. This progression can be blocked experimentally by local anaesthetics, metabolic inhibitors, and nerve section. No virions are detectable in the axons. A current hypothesis is that the virus travels in an incomplete form, perhaps as naked ribonucleoprotein complexes, at this stage. Rabies virus is experimentally inaccessible to antibodies while inside the peripheral nerve.

On reaching the central nervous system, there is massive viral replication on membranes within neurones and direct transmission of virus from cell to cell occurs across synaptic junctions. There is neuronal dysfunction without significant pathological change. Centrifugal spread of virus from the central nervous system in the axoplasm of somatic and autonomic efferent nerves deposits virus in many tissues including skeletal and cardiac muscle, adrenal medulla, where infection may be clinically significant, and in kidney, retina, cornea, pancreas, and nerve twiglets in the hair follicles (see below). At this stage, productive viral replication occurs, with budding from outer cell membranes in the salivary and other glands. This is the means of the further transmission of rabies by bites to other mammals. In humans, virus is also delivered to the lacrimal glands, taste buds, and respiratory tract. Viraemia has very rarely been detected in animals and is not thought to be involved in pathogenesis or spread.

Immunology

Immunological response to rabies infection in humans

There is no detectable immune response until encephalitic symptoms develop, suggesting that rabies virus avoids or suppresses the immune system. Neutralizing and other antibodies become detectable in serum after about 7 days and in cerebrospinal fluid a little later. They may rise to high levels in patients whose lives are prolonged by intensive care. A small amount of rabies-specific IgM is sometimes detectable, but is not useful as a means of diagnosis.

There is little evidence of a lymphocyte-mediated immune response to rabies encephalitis. A pleocytosis appears in only 60 per cent of patients, with a mean leucocyte count of 75×10^3/mm. Peripheral-blood lymphocyte transformation has been shown in a few patients with furious rabies, but not in those with paralytic disease. Experimentally, in fatal rabies there is suppression of the cytotoxic T-lymphocyte response to unrelated viral antigens and a T-cell response is associated with survival in mice.

Interferon is induced by rabies infection, but appears to be at a very low level in human patients. In animals, latent infections can be reactivated by corticosteroids and stress. This provides a possible explanation for occasional reports of long incubation periods.

Rabies nucleoprotein is a weak superantigen, as it directly stimulates CD4 type 2 T lymphocytes bearing Vβ8 T-cell receptors without intermediary antigen-presenting cells. The development of paralytic rabies in mice is dependent on the presence of the specific T-cell receptors. In humans the effect might be an inefficent polyclonal antibody response, preventing a specific immune response and eventually resulting in anergy.

Immunological response to rabies vaccination

Neutralizing antibody may be detectable as early as 7 days after the start of primary immunization. The surface glycoprotein of the virus induces neutralizing antibody, which protects against subsequent challenge with rabies virus in animals. The titre of these antibodies shows a better correlation with protection than any other measure of immune response.

Rabies nucleoprotein antigens also stimulate protective immunity in animals, through non-neutralizing antibody, helper T lymphocytes, and interferon-α induction. This protection is effective against a variety of rabies and rabies-related strains, unlike the glycoprotein-mediated immunity.

In human vaccinees, peripheral-blood lymphocyte transformation occurs in response to a variety of rabies and rabies-related virus antigens. The role of helper and cytotoxic T lymphocytes in protection against disease is unclear.

Neutralizing antibody is undoubtedly protective in the early stages after inoculation of virus, but in experimental animals the 'early death phenomenon' is due to a very low level of rabies antibody which accelerates the terminal phase of the encephalitis.

A low level of interferon may be induced briefly after the first dose of rabies vaccine. In animals, interferon induced by viruses or synthetic inducers, or the administration of exogenous interferon, was effective postexposure prophylaxis against rabies.

Rabies in animals

Any warm-blooded animal (mammal or bird) can be infected with rabies. In dogs the incubation period ranges from 5 days to 14 months, but is usually between 3 and 12 weeks. The first symptom, as in many humans, is intense irritation at the site of the infection. Despite the popular idea of the 'mad' rabid dog, only 25 per cent develop furious rabies. Clinical features include an early and marked change in behaviour, dysphagia, ptosis, altered bark, paralysis of the jaw, neck, and hind limbs (Fig. 6), hypersalivation, congested conjunctivas, pruritus, shivering, trembling, snapping at imaginary objects, pica, and extreme restlessness, causing the animal to wander miles from home. Dogs with furious rabies attack inanimate objects, often seriously injuring their mouths in the process. Virus may be excreted in the saliva 3 days before symptoms appear, and the animal usually dies within the next 7 days. This is the basis for the traditional 10-day observation period for dogs that have bitten humans. There are rare reports, from India, Ethiopia, and elsewhere, of chronic excretion of virus in the saliva of apparently healthy dogs. *Oulou fato* is a clinical variant of canine rabies with

Fig. 6 Dog with paralytic rabies showing paralysis of the limbs and hypersalivation. (Copyright D.A. Warrell.)

apparently reduced virulence for humans, seen in West Africa 50 years ago.

Rabid foxes lose their fear of humans and the majority develop the paralytic form of the disease. An extreme degree of furious rabies is seen in 75 per cent of infected cats. Cattle usually develop paralytic symptoms, with dysphagia, hypersalivation, groaning, trembling, colic, diarrhoea, tenesmus, and rectal prolapse. Most other domestic ungulates develop paralytic symptoms. Horses often show furious features with sexual excitement. Most wild animals, like foxes, lose their fear of humans and may appear tame. Rabid skunks, raccoons, badgers, martens, and mongooses may become very aggressive. Dysphagia and inability to drink is common in rabid animals, but they do not exhibit hydrophobia.

Clinical features in humans

The incubation period ranges from 4 days to many years, but it is between 20 and 90 days in three-quarters of cases. It tends to be shorter after bites on the face (average 35 days) than after those on the limbs (average 52 days).

Prodromal symptoms

In many patients, the first symptom is itching, pain, or paraesthesia at the site of the healed bite wound (Fig. 7). Non-specific prodromal symptoms include fever, chills, malaise, weakness, tiredness, headache, photophobia, myalgia, anxiety, depression, irritability, and symptoms of upper respiratory tract and gastrointestinal infections. Subsequently, symptoms of either furious or paralytic rabies will develop, depending on whether the spinal cord or brain are predominantly infected.

Furious rabies

Furious rabies is the more commonly diagnosed form. Most patients have the diagnostic symptom of hydrophobia: a combination of inspiratory muscle spasm, with or without painful laryngopharyngeal spasm, associated with terror (Fig. 8). Initially provoked by attempts to drink water, this reflex can be excited by a variety of stimuli including a draught of air ('aerophobia'), water splashed on the skin, irritation of the respiratory tract, or ultimately, the sight, sound, or even mention of water. The inspiratory spasm is violent and jerky. The neck and back are extended, the arms thrown up, and the episode may end in generalized convulsions with cardiac or respiratory arrest.

Patients experience hyperaesthesia and generalized arousal, during which they become wild, hallucinated, fugitive, and aggressive, alternating with lucid intervals. Despite these symptoms, attributable to brainstem encephalitis, neurological examination may prove surprisingly normal. Abnormalities include meningism, cranial-nerve lesions (especially III, VI, VII, IX, X, XI, and XII), upper motor-neurone lesions, fasciculation, and involuntary movements. Disturbances of the hypothalamus or autonomic

Fig. 8 Hydrophobic spasm in a 14-year-old Nigerian boy with furious rabies. Note the violent contraction of inspiratory muscles: sternomastoids and diaphragm (depressing xiphisternum). (Copyright D.A. Warrell.)

nervous system cause hypersalivation (Fig. 9), lacrimation (Fig. 10), sweating, hypertension or hypotension, hyperthermia or hypothermia, inappropriate secretion of antidiuretic hormone, or diabetes insipidus and, rarely, priapism with spontaneous orgasms. Hypersexuality suggests similar aetiology to Klüver-Bucy syndrome.

Without supportive treatment, about one-third of the patients will die during a hydrophobic spasm in the first few days. The rest lapse into coma and generalized flaccid paralysis, and rarely survive for more than a week without intensive care.

Fig. 9 Hypersalivation in a Thai woman with furious rabies. (Copyright D.A. Warrell.)

Fig. 7 This man developed intense itching in the left leg, provoking scratching and excoriation, 6 weeks after being bitten in that limb by a mad dog. He died with furious rabies a few days later (by courtesy of Professor Sornchai Looaresuwan).

Fig. 10 Lacrimation in a Thai patient with furious rabies. (Copyright D.A. Warrell.)

Fig. 11 Vampire bat bite inflicted on the ear of a sleeping child in Tapirái, São Paulo, Brazil (by courtesy of Dr João Luiz Costa Cardoso, São Paulo).

Paralytic or dumb rabies

This is the clinical pattern in less than a fifth of human cases except in the case of vampire bat-transmitted rabies (Fig. 11), which is invariably paralytic. The largest reported outbreak was in Trinidad between 1925 and 1935, when there were 89 human cases; others have been described from Mexico, Guyana, Brazil, Peru, Bolivia, and Argentina. The paralytic form of rabies was also seen in patients with postvaccinal rabies, in the two patients who inhaled fixed virus, and is said to be more likely to develop in patients who have received antirabies vaccine. After the usual prodromal symptoms, especially fever, headache, and local paraesthesiae, flaccid paralysis develops, usually in the bitten limb, and ascends symmetrically or asymmetrically with pain and fasciculation in the affected muscles and mild sensory disturbances. Paraplegia and sphincter involvement then develop, and finally fatal paralysis of deglutitive and respiratory muscles. Hydrophobia is unusual, but may be represented by a few pharyngeal spasms in the terminal phase of the illness. Even without intensive care, patients with paralytic rabies have survived for up to 30 days.

Other manifestations and complications

Respiratory system

Asphyxiation and respiratory arrest may complicate the hydrophobic spasms or generalized convulsions of furious rabies and the bulbar and respiratory paralysis of dumb rabies. Bronchopneumonia is an expected complication and a primary rabies pneumonitis may occur. Various abnormal patterns of respiration have been described, including cluster and apneustic breathing. There are some similarities to respiratory myoclonus. Pneumothorax may complicate inspiratory spasms.

Cardiovascular system

A variety of dangerous cardiac arrhythmias has been reported, including supraventricular tachycardias, sinus bradycardia, atrioventricular block, and sinus arrest. Hypotension, pulmonary oedema, and congestive cardiac failure are attributable to myocarditis.

Nervous system

Raised intracranial pressure resulting from cerebral oedema or internal hydrocephalus has been reported in a few cases, but spinal-fluid opening pressure is usually normal and papilloedema rarely found. Evidence of diffuse axonal neuropathy is consistent with histological appearances of degeneration of peripheral nerve ganglia and axons.

Gastrointestinal system

'Stress' ulcers and Mallory–Weiss syndrome are possible explanations for the haematemesis often reported in rabies.

Differential diagnosis

Rabies should be suspected whenever a patient develops severe neurological symptoms after being bitten by a mammal in a rabies endemic area. Some patients fail to remember that they have been bitten. Hydrophobia is pathognomonic of rabies and is unlikely to be mimicked accurately by the hysteric. Inspiratory spasms with associated emotional response are produced by asking the patient to swallow accumulated saliva or by directing a draught of air on to their face. Patients are sometimes misreferred to otolaryngologists or psychiatrists.

Tetanus, which can also follow an animal bite, is similar to rabies in some respects, especially the pharyngeal form of cephalic tetanus ('hydrophobic tetanus'). It is distinguished by its shorter incubation period (usually less than 15 days), the presence of trismus, the persistence of muscle rigidity between spasms, the absence of meningoencephalitis (cerebrospinal fluid is universally normal), and a better prognosis. Hydrophobia does not occur in other encephalitides; the combination of intense brainstem encephalitis and furious behaviour in a conscious patient would be most unlikely except in rabies. Delirium tremens and some plant toxins (e.g. *Datura fastuosa*) and drugs (phenothiazines and amphetamines) may enter the differential diagnosis.

Paralytic rabies can be confused with other causes of ascending (Landry-type) paralysis. Postvaccinal encephalomyelitis (see below) usually develops within 2 weeks of the first dose of the older types of rabies vaccines. In poliomyelitis, objective sensory disturbances are absent and fever rarely persists after paralysis has developed. Examination of cerebrospinal fluid may help to distinguish acute inflammatory polyneuropathy (Guillain–Barré syndrome). *Herpesvirus simiae* (B virus) encephalomyelitis is transmitted by monkey bites, but the incubation period (3 to 4 days) is usually shorter than in rabies. Vesicles may be found in the monkey's mouth and at the site of the bite, and a diagnosis can be confirmed virologically.

Pathology

The brain, spinal cord, and peripheral nerves show ganglion-cell degeneration, perineural and perivascular mononuclear cell infiltration, neuronophagia, and glial nodules. Inflammatory changes are most marked in the midbrain and medulla (Fig. 12) in furious rabies and in the spinal cord in paralytic rabies. The diagnostic Negri bodies (Fig. 13 and Plate 1) are eosinophilic, intracytoplasmic inclusions predominantly consisting of masses of viral ribonucleoprotein, with a basophilic inner body, containing fragments of cellular organelles including ribosomes and occasional virions. They can be demonstrated by haematoxylin and eosin or Schleiften's stains in histological sections of grey matter in up to 75 per cent of human cases, especially in hippocampal pyramidal cells and cerebellar Purkinje cells.

In view of the appalling prognosis of rabies encephalitis, neuronolysis is often surprisingly mild and patchy, and death can occur without any inflammatory response. Vascular lesions such as thrombosis and haemorrhage have also been described. The brainstem, limbic system, amygdaloid nuclei and hypothalamus appear to be most severely affected. Outside the nervous system, there is focal degeneration of salivary and lacrimal glands, pancreas, adrenal medulla, and lymph nodes. An interstitial myocarditis, with round-cell infiltration, is found in about 25 per cent of cases.

Fig. 12 Inflammatory cells around neurones in the central medulla (para-ambigualis region) of a patient who died of rabies encephalitis (× 400). (Reproduced by courtesy of Dr P. Lewis, London.)

Fig. 14 Diagnosis of human rabies during life. Vertical section through a hair follicle and shaft (H) showing fluorescence of nerve cells around the follicle (R) indicating the presence of rabies antigen (× 250). (Copyright M.J. Warrell.)

Laboratory diagnosis

A suspect rabid animal that might have infected a patient should be killed and the brain examined without delay. Rabies antigen detection by a direct immunofluorescent antibody test on acetone-fixed brain impression smears is usually used or alternatively, if no fluorescent microscope is available, by rapid enzyme immunodiagnosis. Virus isolation takes up to 3 weeks by intracerebral inoculation of mice, or about 4 days in murine neuroblastoma cell culture.

In humans, rabies can be confirmed early in the illness by demonstration of viral antigen by a direct immunofluorescent antibody test in nerve twiglets in skin biopsies (Fig. 14). This rapid method is positive in 60 to 100 per cent of cases, and no false-positive results have been reported. Antigen can also be detected in brain biopsies but tests on corneal impression smears are usually falsely negative. The polymerase chain reaction is being used increasingly to identify rabies antigen in secretions.

During the first week of illness virus may be isolated from saliva, brain, cerebrospinal fluid, and very rarely urine. Rabies antibodies are not usually detectable in serum or cerebrospinal fluid before the eighth day of illness in unvaccinated patients. Antibody may leak into the cerebrospinal fluid in patients with postvaccinal encephalomyelitis, but a very high titre suggests a diagnosis of rabies. A specific IgM test has not proved useful diagnostically.

Treatment

Patients with rabies must be sedated heavily and given adequate analgesia to relieve their pain and terror. If intensive care is undertaken, the aim is to prevent complications such as cardiac arrhythmias, cardiac and respiratory failure, raised intracranial pressure, convulsions, fluid and electrolyte disturbances including diabetes insipidus and inappropriate secretion of antidiuretic hormone, and hyperpyrexia. Antiserum, antiviral agents, interferon-α, corticosteroid, and other immunosuppressants have proved useless.

Prognosis

Rabies was formerly regarded as a universally fatal disease, but there are reports of five cases of recovery or prolonged survival, following intensive care. Two patients who recovered had had nervous-tissue vaccine treatment, and the diagnoses were made serologically. Three patients were given pre- or postexposure tissue-culture vaccine and they never recovered from profound neurological deficits.

Despite intensive care, the prognosis of rabies encephalomyelitis is still virtually hopeless. At the time of the bite, however, before virus has invaded the nervous system, correct cleaning of the wound (see below) and the use of optimum postexposure immunization reduce the risk of rabies developing from about 35 to 65 per cent in untreated cases to near zero. The risk varies with the biting species and the site and severity of the bites. It is

Fig. 13 Street virus in human cerebellar Purkinje cells as seen with the light microscope. Several Negri bodies can be seen (one is arrowed) (× 615). (By courtesy of the Armed Forces Institute of Pathology 73–12330.) (See also Plate 1.)

highest following head bites by proved rabid wolves, when the mortality in unvaccinated people may exceed 80 per cent.

Prevention and control

In countries where rabies is endemic

Control strategy is based on gathering information about the prevalence and host range of rabies in wild and domestic animals. This requires laboratory facilities for confirming the diagnosis. Domestic animals can be protected by yearly vaccination. Dogs are muzzled and kept off the streets; strays are eliminated. People should be discouraged from keeping wild carnivores, such as skunks, raccoons, coatimundis, and mongooses, as pets. Unnecessary contact with mammals should be avoided (e.g. stroking stray dogs, exploring bat-infested caves). Reduction of wild-animal reservoir populations may be attempted, but this is difficult to achieve and likely to cause ecological chaos. An alternative approach is to attempt the vaccination of key reservoir species by using live oral vaccines distributed in bait. An oral vaccinia-recombinant rabies glycoprotein vaccine has successfully controlled fox rabies in Western Europe, and is also used in North American raccoons and coyotes. Rabies is most likely to be controlled or eradicated where the principal reservoir is the domestic dog, as in nineteenth-century Britain, Malaysia, and Japan.

Education and publicity about rabies is always needed. Clinics and dispensaries must be adequately supplied with vaccine and antiserum to provide postexposure prophylaxis, but difficulties over expense, supply, and preservation often preclude this. In dog-rabies endemic areas, pre-exposure vaccination is advisable but rarely used.

In countries where rabies is not endemic

Importation of potential vectors, especially domestic dogs and cats and wild bats and carnivores, should be strictly controlled and, where feasible, imported mammals should be vaccinated against rabies and kept in quarantine for an adequate period.

Postexposure prophylaxis may be required for people who were exposed to the risk of rabies while abroad. Travellers should be educated to seek local medical help if they are bitten, scratched, or licked by animals. Many travellers wait until they return to their homeland, sometimes weeks or months after the bite, before asking for medical advice.

Pre-exposure immunization regimens

Pre-exposure vaccination is the most effective form of rabies prevention. No rabies deaths have been reported in anyone who had pre-exposure vaccine followed by postexposure booster doses. In rabies-free areas it is needed by those who handle imported animals before and during quarantine in kennels, zoos, and laboratories; those who work with rabies virus in laboratories; and those who are resident in or intend to travel to dog rabies-endemic areas. In endemic areas others particularly at risk in certain areas include veterinarians, dog-catchers, cave explorers, naturalists, and animal collectors.

A course of three doses of tissue-culture rabies vaccine (see below) is given on days 0, 3, and 28 (or 21) intramuscularly or 0.1 ml intradermally into the deltoid or the anterolateral thigh in children, preferably into the same limb. If chloroquine is being taken for malaria prophylaxis, or in other cases of suspected immunosuppression, the intramuscular route must be used. If sharing an ampoule for intradermal injections, a sterile needle and syringe must be used for each patient. The neutralizing antibody response is enhanced and prolonged by a booster dose after 1 year. A prompt secondary response to booster injections then occurs after many years. Repeated booster doses are only needed if the risk of infection is high.

The antibody response is so predictable that it need not normally be checked, unless there is immunosuppression. An antibody level above 0.5 IU/ml indicates immunity, and serological monitoring can prevent

unnecessary booster doses for rabies laboratory staff and others at continuous risk.

Postexposure prophylaxis

The decision to give postexposure treatment depends on the precise geographical location of the exposure; when it occurred; its severity—whether it was a bite or lick on broken skin; the nature, appearance, behaviour, and fate of the biting animal and if possible, whether it had been vaccinated against rabies within the last year. This information may allow proper assessment of risk; but if there is any doubt the patient should be given full postexposure prophylaxis, even if the bite is several months old.

The aim is to neutralize inoculated virus before it can enter the nervous system. Wound cleaning and active and passive immunization must be implemented as soon as possible.

Wound cleaning

This is effective in killing virus in superficial wounds, but is often neglected. First aid consists of scrubbing the wound with soap and water for several minutes. Foreign material should be removed and a viricidal agent such as povidone iodine, or 40 to 70 per cent alcohol, should be applied liberally. Quarternary ammonium compounds, such as benzalkonium chloride, are inactivated by soap and so are no longer recommended. Hospital treatment of wounds involves thorough exploration, debridement, and irrigation of deep wounds, if necessary under local or general anaesthetic. Suturing should be avoided or delayed and the wound left without occlusive dressings. Attention should be given to tetanus prophylaxis and the range of bacterial and other pathogens, particularly associated with mammal bites. Most of the bacteria are sensitive to amoxicillin/clavulanic acid, cephoxitin, or tetracycline.

Specific prophylaxis

This consists of active and passive immunization. The indications are given in Table 1.

Active immunization

Tissue-culture vaccines

Human diploid cell vaccine (**HDCV**) (Imovax rabies™ Aventis Pasteur), purified chick embryo cell vaccine (Rabipur/Rab Avert™ Chiron Behring), and purified vero cell vaccine (**PVRV**) (Verorab™ Aventis Pasteur) are now the tissue-culture vaccines of choice.

The intramuscular postexposure regimen of these vaccines is 5×1 ml doses into the deltoid on days 0, 3, 7, 14, and 28, although for PVRV each dose is only 0.5 ml. An economical eight-site intradermal regimen can be used with vaccines which have an intramuscular dose of 1 ml. On day 0, eight intradermal injections of 0.1 ml are given (deltoids, suprascapular, lower-quadrant abdominal wall, and thighs) using a whole ampoule in a Mantoux-type syringe. On day 7, four intradermal injections of 0.1 ml are given (deltoids and thighs), and single intradermal doses of 0.1 ml are given on days 28 and 91. Advantages of the eight-site method are: fewer hospital attendances; a rapid induction of neutralizing antibody, making it the treatment of choice when no rabies immunoglobulin is available; a wide margin of safety; using a whole ampoule on day 0, which avoids sharing ampoules of vaccine between patients during the emergency treatment; and finally, giving a large antigenic stimulus on day 0 gives the best chance of survival to patients who are 'low responders' to the vaccine and to those who fail to return on time for subsequent doses.

The two-site intradermal regimen was designed for use with PVRV. A dose of 0.1 ml for PVRV and 0.2 ml for the other two vaccines is given intradermally at two sites (deltoids) on days 0, 3, and 7 and a one site on days 28 and 90. Both of these intradermal regimens use a similar total amount of vaccine per course, about 40 per cent of that of the intramuscular regimen, but the antibody response following the eight-site method is significantly earlier and higher than that after the two-site regimen.

Table 1 Specific postexposure prophylaxis for use in a rabies endemic area[1] following contact with a domestic or wild rabies vector species, whether or not the animal is available for observation or diagnostic tests

Minor exposure (including licks of broken skin, scratches, or abrasions without bleeding)	Start vaccine immediately
	Stop treatment if animal remains healthy for 10 days
	Stop treatment if animal's brain proves negative for rabies by appropriate laboratory tests
Major exposure (including licks of mucosa, minor bites on arms, trunk, or legs, or major bites—multiple or on face, head, fingers, or neck)	Immediate rabies immune globulin and vaccine
	Stop treatment if domestic cat or dog remains healthy for 10 days
	Stop treatment if animal's brain proves negative for rabies by appropriate laboratory tests

[1] This scheme is a simplification of the recommendations of the WHO Expert Committee on Rabies (1997).

Side-effects of tissue-culture vaccines are mild and transient: local itching, redness or pain at the site of injection, influenza-like symptoms, and occasionally a rash. More serious allergic reactions include rare, type I immediate hypersensitivity during primary courses. Type III immune-complex hypersensitivity was reported in 6 per cent of those receiving booster doses of HDCV in the United States and consisted of urticaria, rash, angio-oedema and arthralgia 3 to 13 days after injection, but none has been fatal. A few cases of polyneuritis, Guillain–Barré syndrome, or local limb weakness have been reported in patients receiving tissue-culture vaccines. These events are very rare and no more frequent than for other commonly used virus vaccines.

Nervous-tissue vaccines

Semple vaccine, a 5 per cent sheep or goat brain suspension, and suckling mouse brain (Fuenzalida) vaccine are still used in Asia and the latter also in Africa and South America. The abdomen is often used as a suitable target for the daily subcutaneous injections. These vaccines produce neurological reactions, including postvaccinal encephalomyelitis.

Postvaccinal encephalomyelitis

Neurological reactions to nervous-tissue vaccines occur in up to 1 in 220 courses of Semple vaccine, with a 3 per cent mortality, and are an allergic response to myelin and related neural proteins in the vaccine. In Latin America, neuroparalytic reactions complicated 1/7865 to 1/27 000 courses of suckling mouse brain vaccine with a 22 per cent mortality. Most reactions to Semple vaccine affect the central nervous system, whereas at least 70 per cent of those following suckling mouse brain vaccine involved the peripheral nervous system.

The incubation period ranges from 3 to 35 days after the first injection of vaccine, but it is usually between 7 and 14 days. Clinical forms include a rapidly reversible mononeuritis multiplex involving particularly the cranial, radial, brachial, and sciatic nerves; a dorsolumbar transverse myelitis with fever, paralysis, and sensory loss in the lower limbs, with sphincter involvement, loss of tendon reflexes, extensor plantar responses, and severe girdle and thoracic pain; an ascending paralysis (Landry type), which ends in fatal bulbar paralysis in a third of cases; and meningoencephalitic and meningoencephalomyelitic reactions. The overall mortality of these reactions is 15 to 20 per cent. Most survivors make a complete recovery in 2 to 3 weeks, but a few are left with permanent neurological sequelae.

A moderate lymphocyte pleocytosis and elevated cerebrospinal fluid protein is usual. Pathological changes consist of swelling and chromatolysis of neurones with extensive perivascular demyelination and lymphocytic infiltration in the spinal cord. These features resemble experimental allergic encephalitis, postvaccinal encephalomyelitis after vaccinia vaccine, postinfectious encephalomyelitis, and acute multiple sclerosis. Corticosteroids, for example, prednisolone at 40 to 60 mg/day, are thought to be helpful, and the use of cyclophosphamide has been suggested. Vaccination should be stopped as soon as symptoms appear and the course continued with a tissue-culture vaccine.

Passive immunization

Rabies immune globulin (**RIG**) has proved valuable in protection, presumably by neutralizing rabies virus during the first week after initial vaccination, before neutralizing antibody has appeared, and it enhances the T-lymphocyte response to vaccine experimentally. Its use is recommended at the start of all primary postexposure courses of rabies vaccine, but it is vital following severe bites (on the head, neck, hands, and multiple or deep bites).

The dose of human RIG is 20 IU/kg body weight, and 40 IU/kg for equine RIG. Serum sickness has not been reported after human RIG treatment, but hypersensitivity reactions to equine RIG occur in 1 to 6 per cent of those treated; however, these are not reliably predicted by a previous intradermal test. RIG must be given even if the test is positive, and the skin test is unnecessary. Adrenaline should always be available in case of reactions.

The RIG is infiltrated into the tissues around the bite wound, and any remaining is injected intramuscularly into the thigh, not the buttock. If RIG is given hours or days before the first dose of vaccine, the immune response will be impaired. RIG is prohibitively expensive and is not available or affordable to more than 95 per cent of patients receiving postexposure treatment in developing countries.

Postexposure prophylaxis in people who have received previous vaccination

If a complete pre- or postexposure course of a modern potent tissue-culture vaccine has been given, or if the neutralizing antibody level has been over 0.5 IU/ml, only two intramuscular doses of tissue-culture vaccine should be given on days 0 and 3. The first dose of the vaccine can be divided between four or eight intradermal sites on day 0. Passive immunization is not required. Otherwise, full postexposure treatment must be given.

Failures of postexposure prophylaxis

Deaths from rabies have occurred despite vaccine treatment. These may be attributable to the use of low-potency nervous-tissue vaccines, delay in starting vaccination, an incomplete vaccine course, omission of passive immunization, failure to infiltrate RIG around the wound, injection of vaccine into the buttock, or decreased immune responsiveness of the vaccinee. So far, in the few cases in which the virus strain could be typed, tissue-culture vaccine failures could not be attributed to failure of neutralization of the particular infecting strain of virus by antibody induced by the vaccine. However, vaccine protection against rabies-related viruses may be less efficient than against genotype 1 rabies viruses (see below).

A reduced or delayed immune response to vaccine can sometimes be predicted. If treatment is started late (e.g. more than 2 days after exposure), no RIG is available for severe bites, the patient is immunocompromised, or a rabies-related virus infection is suspected, the immune stimulus can be enhanced either by doubling the initial dose of vaccine, or by dividing the first dose of tissue-culture vaccine between eight sites intradermally, as for the economical eight-site regimen (see above).

Rabies-related viruses known to infect humans

Mokola virus, Duvenhage virus, European bat lyssavirus, and Australian bat lyssavirus are rabies-related viruses that have been proved to infect humans. Three genotypes are only found in Africa. Genotype 2, Lagos bat virus has not been detected in humans. Mokola virus (genotype 3) has been isolated from shrews (*Crocidura* spp.) in Nigeria and Cameroon, and mainly from cats in South Africa, Zimbabwe, and Ethiopia. It was isolated from a child with meningitis who recovered, and from another with fatal encephalitis. Duvenhage virus (genotype 4) caused a fatal illness, with clinical features identical to furious rabies, in a South African of that name who was bitten by a bat and had then received a full course of rabies vaccine. The rabies fluorescent antibody test was negative in the Duvenhage case and weakly positive in the Mokola cases.

Rabid bats had been found occasionally in Europe since 1954. In 1985, a woman was bitten by a rabid, insectivorous bat in Denmark, and an extensive search revealed many rabid bats there and across Europe. The European bat lyssavirus (**EBL**) group comprises genotype 5 (**EBL 1**) and genotype 6 (**EBL 2**), which are each subdivided into phylogenetically distinct groups a and b. The vector species of EBL 1 is *Eptesicus serotinus*. Type 1a is found in Russia, Poland, Germany, Denmark, and the Netherlands; type 1b in France, the Netherlands, and Spain. Two Russian girls died of rabies following bat bites. Myotis bats harbour EBL 2: EBL 2a in the Netherlands and the United Kingdom (three isolates including the human fatality in 2002), and EBL 2b in Switzerland. A fatal human case in Finland was due to EBL 2b.

The identification of a lyssavirus in fruit bats (genus *Pteropus*) in eastern Australia was an unexpected finding in 1996. This Australian bat lyssavirus (**ABL**) (genotype 7) has since caused a fatal rabies-like encephalitis in two women who had handled bats.

The G protein of rabies vaccine strains is very similar to that of all genotype 1 viruses, but shows a variable degree of antigenic homology to rabies-related viruses. Tissue-culture rabies vaccines have not protected animals against challenge with Mokola virus and their effect against Duvenhage virus is uncertain. Protection against EBL viruses may be slightly less efficient, but ABL is closely related to genotype 1 strains and so protection should be undiminished.

Further reading

Baer GM *et al.* (1988). Research towards rabies prevention. *Reviews of Infectious Diseases* **10** (Suppl. 4), S1–815.

Centers for Disease Control (1999). Human rabies prevention—United States, 1999. Recommendations of the Advisory Committee on Immunization Practices. *Morbidity and Mortality Weekly Report* **48** (Suppl) RR –1.

Dietzschold B, Morimoto K, Hooper DC (2001). Mechanisms of virus-induced neuronal damage and the clearance of viruses from the CNS. *Current Topics in Microbiology and Immunology* **253**, 145–55.

Helmick CG, Tauxe RV, Vernon AA (1987). Is there a risk to contacts of patients with rabies? *Reviews of Infectious Diseases* **9**, 511–18.

Jackson AC, Wunner WH, eds. (2002). *Rabies.* Academic Press, San Diego.

Smith JS (1996). New aspects of rabies with emphasis on epidemiology, diagnosis and prevention of the diease in the United States. *Clinical Microbiology Reviews* **9**, 166–76.

Warrell DA *et al.* (1976). Pathophysiologic studies in human rabies. *American Journal of Medicine* **60**, 180–90.

Warrell MJ, Warrell DA (1995). Rhabdovirus infections of humans. In: Porterfield JS, ed. *Exotic viral infections*, pp 343–83. Chapman & Hall, London.

Warrell MJ *et al.* (1985). Economical multiple-site intradermal immunisation with human diploid-cell-strain vaccine is effective for post-exposure rabies prophylaxis. *Lancet* **i**, 1059–62.

WHO (1997). WHO Recommendations on rabies post-exposure treatment and the correct technique of intradermal immunization against rabies. WHO/EMC/ZOO.96.6.

7.10.10 Colorado tick fever and other arthropod-borne reoviruses

M. J. Warrell and D. A. Warrell

Within the large family of Reoviridae human pathogens are found in four genera: *Reovirus*, *Rotavirus*, and two arthropod-borne genera *Coltivirus* and *Orbivirus*. Colorado tick fever is a group A coltivirus, together with Eyach virus, from Europe. Group B comprises coltiviruses from South-east Asia and Indonesia and Banna virus from China. This group may be reclassified as the *Seadornavirus* genus. Banna virus has been isolated from patients with encephalitis. The four pathogenic orbivirus serogroups are Kemerovo, Changuinola, Orungo, and Lebombo.

Colorado tick fever

The virus responsible for Colorado tick fever or 'mountain fever' is an 80-nm, double-shelled particle, covered with capsomeres. The icosahedral core contains 12 segments of double-stranded, negative-sense RNA. The virus has the ability to infect human erythrocytes and this may also occur with the other colti- and orbiviruses.

Colorado tick fever is a zoonosis involving hard (ixodid) ticks (principally *Dermacentor andersoni*, but also *D. occidentalis*, *D. variabilis*, *D. parumapertus*, *D. albipictus*, etc.) and wild mammals including porcupines, coyotes, squirrels, chipmunks, deer, mice, and other rodents. Ticks pass Colorado tick fever virus trans-stadially, but not transovarially.

Epidemiology

Colorado tick fever is acquired from tick bites in western and north-western parts of the United States (including California), British Columbia, and Alberta. Very rarely, it has been caused by an infected blood transfusion. Several hundred cases are reported each year in the United States, but the true incidence is thought to be at least 10 times higher than that. Hikers and campers are at special risk in rodent and tick-infested terrain. The prevalence of antibody to Colorado tick fever among shepherds was 32 per cent. The highest incidence is from May to July when ticks are most active. Infection usually confers lasting immunity.

Clinical features

In adults the infection is nearly always mild, but in children it is occasionally severe or even fatal. Three to six days after the tick bite (extreme range, 1 to 19 days) there is a sudden fever with rigors, generalized aches, myalgia, headache, and backache. In half the patients there is a biphasic fever. A maculopapular or petechial rash appears in about 10 per cent of cases and gastrointestinal symptoms in 20 per cent. Laboratory findings include leucopenia with relative lymphocytosis, occasional thrombocytopenia, and mild lymphocyte pleocytosis.

The illness usually resolves in about 10 to 14 days, but convalescence may be prolonged. Severe manifestations include meningism and drowsiness, sometimes associated with gastrointestinal symptoms, spontaneous bleeding, thrombocytopenia, and disseminated intravascular coagulation. Late, possibly immunological effects, include myocarditis, pericarditis, pleurisy, arthritis, and epididymitis. Colorado tick fever infection may precipitate abortion, but the transplacental infection and teratogenic effects reported in mice have not been observed in man.

Diagnosis

Viral antigen may be detected in erythrocytes by immunofluorescence 1 to 120 days after the start of symptoms. Erythrocyte precursors are infected in the marrow, but their survival is apparently not affected. Virus can be isolated from the blood, and if there is central nervous system involvement, the cerebrospinal fluid. Colorado tick fever virus produces a cytopathic effect on several cell lines, but intracerebral injection of ground blood clot, or preferably washed erythrocytes, into suckling mice is more sensitive for diagnostic isolation. An indirect fluorescent antibody test can provide early serodiagnosis, but acute infections can be diagnosed by polymerase chain reaction detection of antigen. Neutralizing antibody and specific IgM enzyme immunoassays become positive after 14 to 21 days and the IgM disappears after 45 days.

Differential diagnosis

Many other tick-borne acute febrile illnesses, some with rashes and nervous system involvement, can be acquired in the endemic area for Colorado tick fever. These include Rocky Mountain spotted fever, tularaemia, Lyme disease, and relapsing fever. Tick paralysis caused by *D. andersoni* and other ixodid ticks presents as a poliomyelitis-like, ascending, flaccid paralysis that is unlikely to be mistaken for the meningitic or encephalitic syndromes of Colorado tick fever.

Treatment

The symptomatic treatment of fever and pain should exclude salicylates in case of thrombocytopenia. Tribavirin (ribavirin) inhibits the replication of Colorado tick fever virus experimentally but its use in humans has not been reported.

Orbivirus serogroups

Kemerovo

The orbivirus serogroup Kemerovo contains three viruses isolated from *Ixodes* and *Hyalomma* ticks in Russia and Central Europe. They cause benign febrile illnesses and, occasionally, meningitis or encephalitis in spring and early summer, when ticks are active. Rodents and birds are involved in the zoonotic cycle. Oklahoma tick fever is another Kemerovo virus rarely causing febrile illness in the United States.

Changuinola

There is a single report of human febrile illness with the orbivirus Changuinola in Panama. The virus has been isolated from phlebotomine flies and mammals in that area.

Orungo

Orungo virus is found mainly in West Africa but also in Uganda and the Central African Republic. Up to 75 per cent of some populations are seropositive. The clinical effects are unknown but fever and diarrhoea occur in some people, perhaps with encephalitis, as in experimental mice. There is no rash or jaundice. It is transmitted by *Anopheles*, *Aedes*, and other mosquitoes. Monkeys, sheep, and cattle may be infected.

Lebombo

This reovirus was isolated from one febrile child in Nigeria. Lebombo is also found in mosquitoes and rodents.

Further reading

Brown SE, Knudson DL (1995). Coltivirus infections. In: Porterfield JS, ed. *Exotic viral infections*, pp 329–42. Chapman & Hall, London.

Burgdorfer W (1977). Tick-borne diseases in the United States: Rocky Mountain spotted fever and Colorado tick fever. A review. *Acta Tropica* **34**, 103–26.

Libikova H *et al.* (1978). Orbiviruses of the Kemerovo complex and neurological diseases. *Medical Microbiology and Immunology* **166**, 255–63.

Monath TP, Guirakhoo F (1996). Orbiviruses and coltiviruses. In: Fields BN *et al* eds. *Fields virology*, 3rd edn, Vol 2, pp 1735–66. Lippincott-Raven, Philadelphia.

7.10.11 **Alphaviruses**

L. R. Petersen and D. J. Gubler

Introduction

The genus Alphavirus of the family Togaviridae comprises 27 registered viruses, 16 of which cause human infection (Table 1). Alphaviruses are lipid-enveloped virions with a diameter of 50 to 70 nm whose genome is a molecule of single-stranded, positive-sense RNA approximately 12 000 nucleotides in length. Most alphaviruses are maintained in nature in complex transmission cycles between wild or domestic animals and one or more mosquito species. Humans become infected from infective mosquitoes that take a bloodmeal. Patients develop high viraemias with some alphaviruses and may contribute to the transmission cycle by infecting mosquitoes. The epidemiology and geographic distribution of the alphaviruses depend on several factors, including the requirements for and presence of suitable amplifying hosts, the presence and feeding behaviour of a suitable arthropod vector, and the frequency of exposure of non-immune reservoir hosts and humans to infected vectors. Alphavirus infections are not communicable.

Most infections in humans are asymptomatic, but alphaviruses can cause a spectrum of clinical illness ranging from non-specific febrile illness, often with rash, myalgia, or arthralgia, to frank encephalitis and death (Table 1). No specific therapy is available. Vaccines for some alphaviruses are used in animals, although none have been licensed for humans.

Laboratory diagnosis

Alphavirus infections are diagnosed serologically by detection of immunoglobulin M (IgM) and G (IgG) responses. All alphaviruses have common antigenic determinants that result in cross-reactions in immunodiagnostic tests. Neutralization tests may be necessary for serological confirmation in areas where multiple alphaviruses are endemic/enzootic. Isolation of virus from acute-phase serum is possible with some alphaviruses, but they are seldom recovered from the central nervous system, including cerebrospinal fluid, except from fatal cases. Virological diagnosis may also be made using polymerase chain reaction and immunohistochemistry on tissue samples.

Specific alphavirus infections

Chikungunya

Aetiology and epidemiology

Chikungunya virus is found in Africa and Asia and is transmitted primarily by *Aedes* mosquitoes. Non-human primates such as monkeys and baboons may be the primary maintenance hosts in sylvan settings in Africa. In urban settings in Africa and Asia, the virus is transmitted from human to human via *Aedes aegypti* mosquitoes. Explosive urban epidemics occur during the rainy season. One epidemic, in Madras in India, caused an estimated 300 000 cases. Serosurveys have shown antibody prevalences greater than 90 per cent in some areas of Africa.

Clinical characteristics

The sudden onset of fever and crippling arthralgia follows an incubation period of 2 to 3 days (range 1 to 12). The fever may remit for 1 to 2 days and then recur ('saddle back' fever). Arthralgias are polyarticular, migratory, and mostly involve the small joints. Papular or maculopapular skin rashes, typically on the trunk and limbs, occur, usually during the second to fifth day of illness. Most infections are probably asymptomatic. Arthralgia may last several months; a few patients may have symptoms 5 years after infection. Children are less likely to present with arthralgia and rash, and more likely to have headache, injected pharynx, and gastrointestinal symptoms.

Diagnosis

Leucopenia is the only likely laboratory finding. Viraemia usually is present in the first 48 h of illness. Haemagglutinin-inhibition and IgM antibodies will be present in nearly all patients by the seventh day of illness. IgM anti-bodies detectable in serum by IgM antibody capture enzyme-linked immunosorbent assay (MAC-ELISA) may persist 6 months after infection.

Prevention, control, and treatment

Prevention and control can only be achieved by reducing *Ae. aegypti* populations in the large urban centres of the tropics and by avoiding mosquito bites. No licensed vaccines currently exist. There is no specific treatment. Anti-inflammatory drugs may relieve arthralgia. Chloroquine phosphate may be helpful for refractory arthralgias.

Eastern equine encephalitis

Aetiology and epidemiology

The virus is widely distributed throughout North, Central, and South America and the Caribbean; however, little is known about the epidemiology of eastern equine encephalitis outside North America. In the United States, human infections are usually sporadic and small outbreaks occur each summer, mostly along the Atlantic and Gulf Coasts. In recent years, one to 14 cases have been reported annually. In North America, wild birds and *Culiseta melanura* mosquitoes maintain the virus.

Clinical characteristics

The incubation period exceeds 1 week and the onset is abrupt with high fever. About 2 per cent of infected adults and 6 per cent of children develop encephalitis. Eastern equine encephalitis is the most severe of the arboviral encephalitides, with a mortality of 50 to 75 per cent. Symptoms and signs include dizziness, decreasing level of consciousness, tremors, seizures, and focal neurological signs. Death can occur within 3 to 5 days of onset. Sequelae, common in non-fatal encephalitis, include convulsions, paralysis,

Table 1 Alphaviruses known to cause human disease

Virus	Geographical distribution	Disease in humans	Outbreaks	Other features
Babanki	West and Central Africa	SFI, arthropathy	No	
Barmah Forest	Australia	SFI, arthropathy	Yes	Clinically similar to Ross River virus infection
Bebaru	Malaysia		No	Lab infection only
Chikungunya	Tropical Africa, India, South and Southeast Asia, Philippines	SFI, arthropathy	Yes	Large outbreaks in urban settings
Eastern equine encephalitis	North and South America on Atlantic and Gulf Coasts, Caribbean	SFI, encephalitis	Yes	Isolated cases or small outbreaks occur mainly in North America
Everglades	Florida	SFI, encephalitis	No	Variant of Venezuelan equine encephalitis
Mayaro	Trinidad, Brazil, Bolivia, Surinam, French Guyana, Peru, Venezuela	SFI, arthropathy	Yes	
Me Tri	Vietnam	Encephalitis	Unknown	Virus not registered, possible variant of Semliki Forest virus
Middleburg	South, West, and Central Africa	Not described	No	
Mucambo	Trinidad, Brazil, Surinam, French Guiana, Colombia, Venezuela	SFI	No	Proposed species in the Venezuelan equine encephalitis antigenic complex
O'nyong-nyong	East and West Africa, Zimbabwe	SFI, arthropathy	Yes	Igbo-ora virus is a subtype of o'nyong-nyong
Pixuna	Brazil	SFI	No	Laboratory infection only
Ross River	Australia, South Pacific	SFI, arthropathy	Yes	Periodic epidemics in South Pacific
Semliki Forest	Subsaharan Africa	SFI, encephalitis	No	
Sindbis	Africa, East Mediterranean, South and Southeast Asia, Borneo, Philippines, Australia, Sicily, Scandinavia	SFI, arthropathy	Yes	
Tonate	French Guiana, Surinam	SFI	No	Proposed species in the Venezuelan equine encephalitis antigenic complex; fatal encephalitis in one infant
Venezuelan equine encephalitis	Northern South America, Central America, Mexico	SFI, encephalitis	Yes	
Western equine encephalitis	North and South America	SFI, encephalitis	Yes	Human disease rare outside of North America and Brazil

SFI = systemic febrile illness.

and mental retardation. Illness due to eastern equine encephalitis in South America appears to be less severe.

Diagnosis

Cerebrospinal fluid pressure may be raised, with slightly increased protein, normal sugar, and up to 2000 cells/mm³. IgM antibodies are readily detected in serum or cerebrospinal fluid by ELISA. Paired serum samples can be tested by haemagglutinin inhibition, ELISA, or neutralization tests. Horse or pheasant deaths and the proximity to swamps provide clues to the diagnosis.

Prevention control and treatment

Prevention depends on the avoidance of mosquito bites and mosquito control in suburban areas. Inactivated vaccines have been used successfully in horses, and an inactivated vaccine has been used experimentally in laboratory workers and others at high risk of exposure. No specific treatment is available.

Ross River virus

Aetiology and epidemiology

This virus causes 'epidemic polyarthritis' in Australia, south-western Pacific islands, and Fiji. *Ae. vigilax* is an important vector in Australia and *Ae. scutellaris* complex mosquitoes in some south Pacific islands, although the virus has been isolated from more than 30 mosquito species. An epidemic in various Pacific islands in 1979 to 1980 affected more than 50 000 people. An average of 4800 cases is reported annually from Australia. Explosive outbreaks and viraemias in humans suggest virus transmission from human to human by certain mosquitoes.

Clinical characteristics

The illness begins suddenly with arthralgia in the small joints of the hands and feet. A maculopapular rash occurs in about half of patients within 2 days of onset and is most prominent on the trunk and limbs, but can cover the entire body. The rash may progress to small vesicles. Myalgia, headache, anorexia, nausea, and tenosynovitis are common, but the temperature is only slightly elevated. The arthralgia may be prolonged. Symptomatic infection is rare in children.

Diagnosis

Isolation of virus from serum is possible for the first few days of illness. IgM antibodies will be detected by MAC-ELISA within 5 to 10 days of onset. Complement fixation, haemagglutinin inhibition, and neutralization tests may be useful, particularly when paired serum samples are available.

Prevention, control, and treatment

Avoidance of mosquito bites and peridomestic mosquito control can effectively reduce the risk of infection. No specific treatment is available. Non-steroidal anti-inflammatory drugs may relieve symptoms.

Venezuelan equine encephalitis complex

Aetiology and epidemiology

Six subtypes (I–VI) within the Venezuelan equine encephalitis virus complex have been identified. Five antigenic variants exist within subtype I (IAB, IC, ID, IE, IF). These subtypes and variants are classified as epizootic or enzootic, based on their apparent virulence and epidemiology. Epizootic variants of subtype I (IAB and IC) cause equine epizootics and are associated with more severe human disease. Enzootic strains (ID-F, II (Everglades), III (Mucambo, Tonate, Paramana), IV (Pixuna), V (Cabassou), VI (unnamed)) do not cause epizootics in horses, but may produce sporadic disease in man. Large epizootics (IAB and IC) have occurred in equines in northern countries of South America and Central America, sometimes reaching the United States. In 1969 to 1972, a massive epizootic extending from Ecuador to Texas killed more than 200 000 horses and caused several thousand human infections. In 1995, a large epizootic, which began in Venezuela and spread to Colombia, affected thousands of horses and caused approximately 90 000 human infections. Epizootic strains are carried by a wide variety of mosquitoes including *Aedes*, *Mansonia*, and *Psorophora* spp. Horses are the principal amplifying hosts during epizootics but are not amplifying hosts for enzootic transmission. Enzootic strains are maintained in a cycle involving *Culex* (*Melanoconion*) mosquitoes and rodents.

Clinical characteristics (epizootic virus infections)

After an incubation period of 1 to 6 days, there is a brief febrile illness of sudden onset, characterized by malaise, nausea or vomiting, headache, and myalgia. Acute symptoms last 2 to 5 days; generalized asthenia up to 3 weeks. Among those with clinical illness, less than 0.5 per cent of adults and less than 4 per cent of children develop encephalitis. Nausea and vomiting, nuchal rigidity, ataxia, convulsions, paralysis, and death may occur. Long-term sequelae following encephalitis are uncommon.

Diagnosis (epizootic virus infections)

A marked leucopenia is universal, often accompanied by neutropenia and thrombocytopenia, with moderate lymphocytosis in the cerebrospinal fluid. Virus isolation from serum or throat swab is possible within the first few days of illness. Paired sera can be tested by HI and neutralizing tests. Specific IgM can be detected by MAC-ELISA in the second week of illness.

Prevention, control, and treatment

Equine immunization is effective in controlling epizootic disease. Venezuelan equine encephalitis is highly infectious by the aerosol route; many laboratory infections have occurred. Live attenuated and inactivated vaccines have been used in laboratory workers. People in affected areas should avoid mosquito bites. No specific treatment is available.

Western equine encephalitis

Aetiology and epidemiology

This is a complex of closely related viruses found in North and South America, but human disease is rare outside North America and Brazil. Summer outbreaks may be precipitated by flooding, which increases breeding of *Culex* mosquitoes (particularly *Culex tarsalis* in the western United States). Large outbreaks of western equine encephalitis in humans and horses occurred in the western United States in the 1950s and 1960s; however, a declining horse population, equine vaccination, and improved vector control have reduced the reported number of human cases to zero, in most years during the last decade.

Clinical characteristics

The ratio of apparent to inapparent infection in adults is less than 1 in 1000; however, this ratio increases to 1:1 in infants under 1 year of age. Following an incubation period of about 7 days, headache, vomiting, stiff neck, and backache are typical; restlessness and irritability are seen in children. Weakness and hyporeflexia are common. Convulsions occur in 90 per cent of affected infants and 40 per cent of children between 1 and 4 years, but are rare in adults. Recovery in 5 to 10 days is common, but convalescence may be protracted. Although rare in adults and older children, sequelae are common in infants, with half of those with encephalitis left with convulsions, and/or severe motor or intellectual deficits. The case fatality rate is 3 to 7 per cent.

Diagnosis

Clinical laboratory findings in western equine encephalitis are often not remarkable. IgM antibodies are readily detected in serum by ELISA. Paired sera can be tested by HI, IgG ELISA, or neutralization tests. Virus can occasionally be isolated from serum or cerebrospinal fluid.

Prevention, control, and treatment

Prevention of western equine encephalitis relies on mosquito control and the avoidance of mosquito bites. Vaccine is available for horses. An inactivated vaccine has been used for laboratory staff and others at high risk of exposure. No specific treatment is available.

Other alphavirus infections

Barmah Forest virus

Since its first recognition as a cause of human disease in 1988, the geographical distribution of Barmah Forest virus has expanded recently in Australia. It causes sporadic disease and epidemics, with up to 300 serologically confirmed cases. The disease resembles that of Ross River virus infection, although the rash tends to be more florid and true arthritis is less common. The illness is prolonged in some patients. Little is known about the ecology of Barmah Forest virus, although outbreaks have coincided with Ross River virus outbreaks, and the virus has been identified in the same mosquito species.

Mayaro virus

Mayaro virus has been isolated from humans and various mosquito species (mostly *Haemagogus*) in Trinidad, Brazil, Bolivia, French Guiana, Surinam, Peru, and Venezuela. Several outbreaks have been identified, most recently in Venezuela in 2000. The disease is characterized by an abrupt onset with fever, chills, headache, myalgia, and arthralgia, mostly in the small joints of the extremities. A maculopapular rash may occur 2 to 5 days after defervescence. Arthralgia may persist for several months.

O'nyong-nyong virus

From 1959 to 1962, this virus caused epidemics in Uganda, Kenya, Tanzania, and Malawi, involving approximately 2 million people. The virus was isolated in 1978 from *Anopheles funestus* mosquitoes in Kenya after a long period of no apparent o'nyong-nyong virus activity. In 1996 to 1997, an outbreak occurred in Uganda. O'nyong-nyong is closely related to chikungunya and produces a similar illness, although fever is less pronounced and lymphadenopathy is more common. *Anopheles funestus* and *A. gambiae* transmit the virus.

Sindbis

Sindbis virus is widely distributed in Africa, India, tropical Asia, Australia, and northern Europe but is only rarely associated with human disease. The clinical features include fever, rash, arthralgia, myalgia, malaise, and headache. The fever, if present, is not high. The maculopapular rash progresses from trunk to extremities and vesicles can occur on the palms and soles. Virus has been isolated from vesicle fluid.

In northern Europe, symptomatic disease is recognized from Sweden, through Finland, to the former Karelian SSR, where it is known as Ockelbo disease, Pogosta disease, or Karelian fever, respectively. Prominent rheumatic complaints, sometimes persisting for several years, have been noted in Europe and South Africa. The virus has been isolated most often from ornithophilic *Culex* mosquito species. High antibody prevalences in Africa suggest that human exposure is common. Several outbreaks have been noted.

Further reading

Gubler DJ, Roehrig JT (1998). Arboviruses (Togaviridae and Flaviviridae). In: Collier L, *et al.*, eds. *Topley and Wilson's microbiology and microbial infections*, 9th edn, Vol. 1, Virology, Ch. 29, pp. 579–600. Arnold, London.

Johnston RE, Peters CJ (1996). Alphaviruses. In: Fields BN, Knipe DM, Howley PM, *et al.*, eds. *Fields virology*, 3rd edn, pp. 843–98. Lippincott-Raven, Philadelphia.

7.10.12 Rubella

P. A. Tookey and S. Logan

Introduction

Rubella infection usually causes a mild exanthematous disease of little clinical significance. However, in early pregnancy, infection may result in multiple congenital abnormalities. As a result of the widespread use of rubella vaccine, congenital rubella is now uncommon in most countries with developed health services.

The enveloped RNA virus of rubella is classified in its own genus, *Rubivirus*, within the family Togaviridae. Little variation has been detected among rubella isolates.

Epidemiology

Humans are the only known host for rubella virus. In temperate zones the infection is seen predominantly in spring and early summer. Before the introduction of rubella vaccine, rubella was endemic in virtually all countries. Epidemics were superimposed on the endemic infection every 4 to 9 years, and pandemics every 10 to 30 years. In most populations, in the absence of a mass immunization programme, around 10 to 20 per cent of women reach child-bearing age still susceptible to rubella infection. Infection is rare in infancy, incidence rises slowly in early childhood and then rapidly, peaking between 5 and 9 years of age.

Postnatally acquired infection

The rash usually begins on the face and spreads to the trunk and then the extremities; the pink maculopapular lesions are initially discrete but later tend to coalesce. The suboccipital and posterior cervical lymph nodes are characteristically enlarged. Mild fever, sore throat, coryza, cough, and conjunctivitis may be present; symptoms are usually mild and last 3 to 7 days. There may be a prodrome with malaise and fever, especially in adults. There is no specific treatment.

Arthralgia is a common complication in older patients, but frank arthritis is unusual; both are normally transient but recurrent or persistent symptoms have been reported, mainly in women. Less common complications include purpura, thrombocytopenia, postinfectious encephalitis, transverse myelitis, and the Guillain-Barré syndrome.

Rubella is clinically indistinguishable from a number of other infections and at least half of all infections are clinically inapparent or non-specific; a history of clinically diagnosed rubella infection is unreliable.

The incubation period is 14 to 21 days. The exact mode of transmission is uncertain but airborne spread by the respiratory route is likely and close contact is usually necessary for transmission. Individuals are infectious from about 5 to 7 days before to 3 to 5 days after the start of symptoms. Infectivity is highest immediately before, and on the first day of, symptoms. Congenitally infected infants shed large amounts of virus from the oropharynx and may be a source of infection for many months.

Infection usually produces lifelong immunity but reinfection has occasionally been reported.

Congenital infection

Congenital rubella is typically associated with cataracts, cardiac anomalies, and sensorineural hearing loss. The teratogenic effects may result in a wide range of defects (Table 1), but sensorineural hearing loss alone or combined with other abnormalities is most common. The earlier the stage of pregnancy at which infection occurred, the more likely it is that the child will have severe, multiple problems. The risk of damage following primary maternal infection in the first 10 weeks of pregnancy is around 90 per cent; this drops rapidly thereafter, and after 16 weeks' gestation even sensorineural hearing loss and growth retardation are rare; no abnormalities have been demonstrated following serologically confirmed maternal infection after 18 weeks' gestation.

Some defects, particularly sensorineural hearing loss, may not develop or reveal themselves until later infancy or childhood. Other reported late-onset problems include diabetes mellitus, thyroid dysfunction, and possibly autism and other behavioural and psychiatric disorders. A rare progressive rubella panencephalitis has been reported.

Maternal rubella infection is not always transmitted to the fetus. Transmission is most likely during the first trimester, the rate then declines until the last few weeks of pregnancy when it rises again. Most prospective studies of the risk to the fetus have been carried out on women with symptoms, but asymptomatic primary infection is thought to carry a similar risk. The risk of transmission following maternal reinfection in the first trimester is estimated to be about 8 per cent, but the likelihood of damage is low. Symptomatic maternal reinfection is rare, but in these circumstances viraemia is more likely and the risk to the fetus may be greater.

Table 1 Defects associated with congenital rubella

Classic triad
Sensorineural deafness
Abnormalities of the cardiovascular system:
    Patent ductus arteriosus
    Pulmonary stenosis
    Aortic and renal artery stenosis
    Tetralogy of Fallot
    Ventricular septal defect
    Myocarditis
Abnormalities of the eye:
    Retinopathy
    Cataracts
    Microphthalmos
    Glaucoma
Other defects
Growth retardation
Microcephaly
Mental retardation
Other signs in infancy and the neonatal period
Hepatosplenomegaly
Jaundice
Rash
Purpura
Thrombocytopenia
Osteopathy
Hypogammaglobulinaemia
Pneumonitis

The diagnosis of congenital rubella infection is relatively easy if suspected early, but more difficult to confirm later. Virus can be isolated or detected by polymerase chain reaction (PCR) from multiple sites including the oropharynx, urine, and conjunctival fluid during the first months of life; viral shedding occasionally persists for years, but only about 10 per cent of infants are still shedding virus at 12 months. The presence of rubella IgM antibody in early infancy is virtually diagnostic of congenital infection because acquired infection is rare at this age. The presence of IgG antibody alone is not diagnostic since it is likely to indicate passively transferred maternal antibody, but persistence of IgG beyond 6 months is strongly suggestive of congenital infection. When abnormalities present late, a presumptive diagnosis can be made based on a compatible clinical picture and the presence or persistence of rubella IgG antibodies in a young child who has not yet been vaccinated.

Management of rubella-like illness during pregnancy

Routine antenatal rubella testing is not designed to identify infection in pregnancy, and specific diagnostic investigations are needed. Pregnant women with a rubella-like rash should be investigated simultaneously for rubella and parvovirus B19, since they are clinically indistinguishable. Even women previously reported to be immune should be investigated in case of laboratory error or reinfection. Blood should be tested for IgG and IgM antibodies, with a repeat test after 2 weeks if the results are equivocal. Rising IgG or detectable IgM antibody indicates recent infection. Investigations must be done in consultation with a virologist, who should be aware of the date and type of contact, stage of pregnancy, and history of previous immunization and testing.

Vaccination

Three strains of live, attenuated rubella vaccine were licensed in 1969. The RA27/3 strain is commonly used. Protective antibody levels are produced in around 95 per cent of recipients; protection is probably lifelong in most individuals.

In children, rubella vaccine causes few side-effects. Low-grade fever and rash are occasionally reported, and transient arthralgia has been seen in about 3 per cent of vaccinees; there have also been rare reports of myositis and vasculitis. Joint symptoms are common in adult women, affecting up to 40 per cent of vaccinees. They are less frequent and less severe than following naturally acquired rubella infection. Symptoms are generally mild and transient but a handful of cases of apparently recurrent or persistent arthritis after rubella immunization have been described.

Different vaccine strategies have been pursued. In some countries, including the United States, there was mass immunization of all children early in their second year in an attempt to eliminate rubella from the community. This strategy not only protects those who are vaccinated but also reduces the risk of infection in susceptible pregnant women. However, if there is low vaccine uptake in childhood the spread of wild virus is slowed down but not eliminated: the effect is to push up the peak age of incidence of infection, which could, paradoxically, increase the number of congenital rubella cases.

In the United Kingdom, concern about low vaccine uptake and the duration of vaccine-induced immunity led initially to the adoption of a selective strategy of immunizing schoolgirls after the age of peak incidence. Routine testing and immunization of nursing and other staff who might be in contact with pregnant women was introduced, as well as antenatal screening for rubella susceptibility, with postpartum vaccination of susceptible women to protect subsequent pregnancies. The continued circulation of wild virus ensured that most women were protected by natural immunity acquired during childhood, with most of the remainder being covered by the schoolgirl and adult immunization programmes.

A third method was implemented in Sweden in 1982, when measles, mumps, and rubella (**MMR**) vaccine was introduced for all 1-year olds with a second dose at 12 years in order to reach those who did not receive vaccine previously or failed to respond, and to boost antibody status in the rest.

In 1988, in the United Kingdom, reassuring data on the persistence of immunity after vaccination and high vaccine uptake levels led to the introduction of mass immunization for all children in the second year of life with MMR; in 1996 this was supplemented by a preschool booster, and the schoolgirl vaccination programme was abandoned. Antenatal screening for rubella susceptibility continues, but the delivery of postpartum vaccination is not routinely monitored. Uptake of MMR by the age of 24 months averaged about 92 per cent between 1988 and 1992, but declined to about 88 per cent by 2000. Although the circulation of wild virus has dropped to very low levels since MMR was introduced, if the decline in vaccine uptake is not reversed it is possible that outbreaks of rubella could occur once again, putting susceptible pregnant women at risk.

Vaccination has led to dramatic declines in the numbers of susceptible pregnant women, rubella-associated terminations, and children born with congenital rubella. In the United Kingdom less than five congenitally infected infants were reported on average each year between 1990 and 2000, compared with 58.5 per year in the 1970s (when diagnostic methods and case ascertainment were less efficient). Terminations of pregnancy for rubella disease or contact averaged 612 a year in England and Wales during the 1970s, but during the 1990s the annual average was less than 10.

The strategy to be adopted in any country seeking to control congenital rubella by vaccination must depend on the projected uptake of vaccination and the long-term prospects for continuing the programme. An important element should be the screening and immunization of susceptible health personnel, particularly those in contact with pregnant women.

Vaccination in pregnancy

There have been persistent concerns that the vaccine virus might be teratogenic if given during pregnancy. Although vaccinees cannot infect other susceptible individuals, the virus can cross the placenta. Data pooled from studies of children born to several hundred women inadvertently vaccinated up to 3 months before conception or during pregnancy show less than 3 per cent with serological evidence of congenital infection, and no reported case of abnormalities attributable to congenital rubella. Over 80 of these infants were born to women vaccinated in the month of conception, probably the period of greatest vulnerability. These data suggest that the likely maximum theoretical risk is less than 5 per cent.

Further reading

Banatvala JE, Best JM (1998). Rubella. In: Mahy BWJ, Collier L, eds. *Topley and Wilson's microbiology and microbial infections: virology*, 9th edn, pp 551–77. Arnold, London.

Cooper LZ, Preblud SR, Alford CA (1995). Rubella. In: Remington JS, Klein JO, eds. *Infectious diseases of the fetus and newborn infant*, 4th edn, pp 268–311. W.B. Saunders, Philadelphia.

Miller E (1990). Rubella infection in pregnancy. In: Chamberlain G, ed. *Modern antenatal care of the fetus*, pp 247–70. Blackwell Scientific, Oxford.

Miller E *et al.* (1997). The epidemiology of rubella in England and Wales before and after the 1994 measles and rubella vaccination campaign. Fourth joint report from the PHLS and National Congenital Rubella Surveillance Programme. *Communicable Disease Report* **7**, R26–32.

7.10.13 Flaviviruses

L. R. Petersen and D. J. Gubler

Introduction

The genus Flavivirus of the family Flaviviridae comprises 68 registered viruses; 35 of which cause natural human infection (Table 1). Flaviviruses are small (37–50 nm), spherical particles whose genome is a molecule of single-stranded, positive-sense RNA approximately 11 000 nucleotides in length. Based on epidemiological and phylogenetic characteristics, the flaviviruses are classified into three groups: those that are mosquito-borne, tick-borne, and those in which no arthropod vector has been demonstrated. All flaviviruses of human importance belong to the first two groups; the last group contains a few viruses found in vertebrates.

Most flaviviruses are maintained in nature in complex transmission cycles between wild or domestic animals and one or more haematophagous arthropod vectors. Humans become infected from infected arthropod vectors that take a bloodmeal, but for most of the flaviviruses, humans do not usually develop high viraemias and are not thought to contribute to the transmission cycle. However, some flaviviruses of world-wide importance, including the dengue and yellow fever viruses, do produce high-level viraemias in humans and can be maintained in urban settings through a mosquito–human–mosquito transmission cycle.

The epidemiology and geographical distribution of the flaviviruses depend on several factors, including the presence of suitable amplifying hosts, the presence and feeding behaviour of a suitable arthropod vector, and the frequency of exposure of non-immune reservoir hosts and humans to infected vectors. Globalization of trade and travel, human population growth, and neglect of mosquito control programmes have produced conditions conducive for increasing incidence and geographic expansion of the flaviviruses. A recent dramatic example is the introduction and subsequent spread of the West Nile virus in the western hemisphere. Flavivirus infections are not communicable.

Flavivirus infection in humans can result in asymptomatic infection or a spectrum of clinical illness ranging from non-specific febrile illness, fever with rash or arthralgia or both, haemorrhagic fever, hepatitis, encephalitis, and death. The same virus can cause a variety of syndromes, and often the majority of those infected are asymptomatic. Although no specific therapy is available, prompt supportive treatment and proper management may substantially reduce mortality from some flavivirus infections. Ribavirin has been shown to have antiviral activity against several RNA viruses, but it has low *in vitro* and *in vivo* activity against flaviviruses.

Laboratory diagnosis

All flaviviruses have common group epitopes on the envelope protein that result in extensive cross-reactions in serological tests. The specificity of antibody detected should therefore be confirmed by cross-neutralization tests in areas where multiple flaviviruses are endemic/enzootic.

The IgM antibody capture enzyme-linked immunosorbent assay (MAC-ELISA) is widely used for diagnosis of flaviviruses. IgM antibody is usually detectable 5 to 8 days after infection. Because detectable IgM antibody persists for one or more months after infection with most flaviviruses, its presence is not confirmatory of current infection. Therefore, people with detectable IgM antibody are considered presumptive cases. Confirmatory laboratory diagnosis of most flaviviruses requires isolation of the virus, detection of specific viral RNA or specific antigen in a clinical sample, or virus-positive immunohistochemistry in autopsy tissues. A four-fold or greater rise in specific neutralizing antibody is confirmatory in some infections.

Important mosquito-borne flavivirus infections

Dengue and dengue haemorrhagic fever

Aetiology and epidemiology

There are four closely related, but serologically distinct dengue viruses, called DEN-1, DEN-2, DEN-3, and DEN-4. Since there is only transient, weak cross-protection among the four serotypes, persons living in an area of endemic dengue can be infected with three, and probably four, dengue serotypes during their lifetime.

Dengue fever is the most widespread and has the highest incidence of all the flaviviruses; with an estimated 50 to 100 million infections, and 200 000 to 500 000 cases of dengue haemorrhagic fever per year throughout most tropical regions of the world depending on epidemic activity (Fig. 1). The case fatality rate of dengue haemorrhagic fever cases averages 5 per cent. Over 2.5 billion people live in areas where dengue is endemic. The transmission cycle of most importance is the *Aedes aegypti*–human–*Ae. aegypti* cycle in large urban centres of the tropics. Multiple virus serotypes often cocirculate within the same city (hyperendemicity), causing periodic epidemics, especially in south-east Asia.

Humans are infected with dengue viruses by the bite of an infective mosquito. *Ae. aegypti*, the principal vector, is a highly domesticated tropical mosquito that lays its eggs in artificial water containers commonly found in and around homes. The adult mosquitoes rest indoors and prefer to feed on humans during daylight hours, with peak biting activity in the early

Table 1 Flaviviruses known to cause human disease

Virus	Geographical distribution	Disease in humans	Incidence[a]	Outbreaks	Other features
Mosquito-borne viruses					
Banzi	S and E Africa	SFI	<1	No	2 cases only
Bussuquara	Brazil, Colombia, Panama	SFI	<1	No	1 case only
Dengue types 1–4	World-wide in the tropics	SFI, HF	>50 000 000	Yes	>200 000 dengue haemorrhagic fever
Edge hill	Australia	SFI	<1	No	Polyarthalgia prominent
Ilheus	C and S America	SFI, ME	<10	No	
Japanese encephalitis	E, SE, and S Asia, W Pacific	SFI, ME	45 000	Yes	
Kedougou	Africa	Not described	<1	No	
Kokobera	Australia	SFI	<1	No	Polyarthralgia prominent
Kunjin	Australia, Sarawak	SFI, ME	<5	Yes	Polyarthralgia prominent
Murray Valley	Australia, New Guinea	SFI, ME	<5	Yes	
Rocio	Brazil	SFI, ME	<10	Yes	
Saint Louis	N America, Panama, Jamaica, Trinidad, Brazil, Argentina	SFI, ME	<100	Yes	
Sepik	New Guinea	SFI	<1	No	1 case only
Spondweni	E, W, and S Africa	SFI	<1	No	
Usutu	E, W, and C Africa	SFI	<1	No	1 case only
Wesselsbron	E, W, and S Africa, Thailand	SFI, ME	<5	No	
West Nile	E, W, and S Africa, India, Pakistan, Mediterranean area, Central Asia, E United States, Europe	SFI, ME	>100	Yes	Incidence and geographic distribution increasing, newly introduced to North America
Yellow fever	W, C, and S Africa, and S America	SFI, HF	>200 000	Yes	
Zika	E and W Africa, Uganda (1 case), Malaysia, Philippines, Indonesia	SFI	<1	No	
Tick-borne viruses					
Koutango	Africa	SFI	<1	No	Laboratory infection only
Kyasanur-Forest disease	Karnataka India, Saudi Arabia	SFI, HF, ME	>200	Yes	
Langat	Malaysia, Thailand, Russian Federation	SFI, ME	<1	No	Experimental infection only
Louping-ill	British Isles	SFI, ME, HF	<5	No	Most infections laboratory acquired
Negishi[b]	Asia	SFI, ME	<1	No	
Omsk	Central Russian Federation	SFI, HF	<10	No	
Powassan	Canada, United States	SFI, ME	<1	No	
Tick-borne encephalitis[c]	Europe, E Europe, W Russian Federation	SFI, ME	>1000	Yes	Small outbreaks from milk ingestion
No known arthropod vector					
Apoi	Japan	SFI, ME	<1	No	Laboratory infection only
Dakar bat	W, E, and C Africa, Madagascar	SFI	<1	No	2 cases only
Modoc	California	SFI, ME	<1	No	1 naturally acquired infection known
Rio Bravo	United States, Mexico	SFI	<1	No	

[a] Reported incidence of disease. As surveillance is not systematic for most flavivirus infections, the true incidence of disease may be much higher than that reported.

[b] Never isolated from ticks, but antigenically and phylogenetically related to the tick-borne group.

[c] Absettarov, Hanzaolva, Hypr, and Kumlinge are registered separately but have been shown to be identical to the western subtype of the tick-borne encephalitis virus.

SFI = systemic febrile illness; ME = meningoencephalitis; HF = haemorrhagic fever.

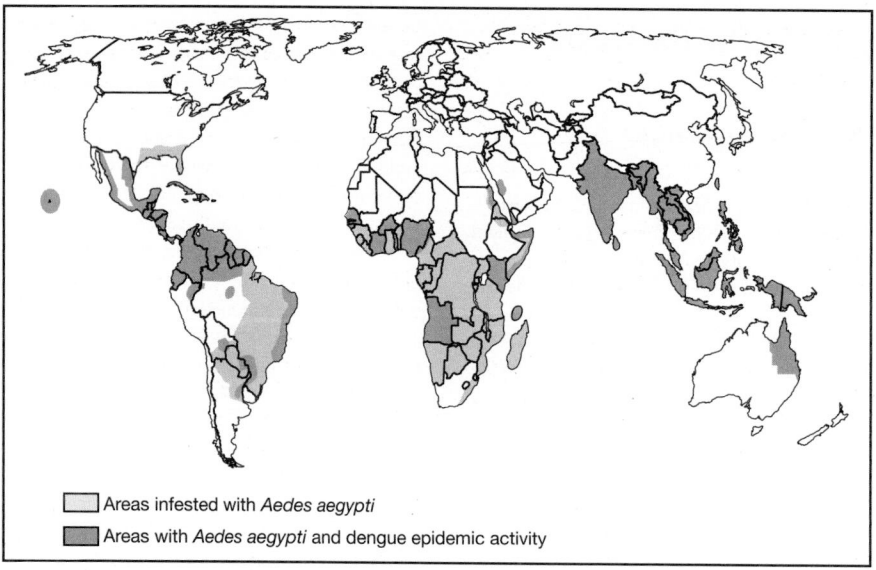

Fig. 1 The geographical distribution of dengue fever.

morning or late afternoon. The adult female mosquitoes are nervous feeders and, if their feeding is interrupted, will return to the same person or different persons to continue feeding. Thus, during a single blood meal, several persons may become infected, making *Ae. aegypti* a highly efficient epidemic vector.

Clinical characteristics

Dengue virus infection in humans causes a spectrum of illness ranging from inapparent or mild febrile illness to severe and fatal haemorrhagic disease. The incubation period averages 4 to 7 days, with a range of 3 to 14 days. There are two major clinical syndromes: classic dengue fever and dengue haemorrhagic fever.

Dengue fever

Classic dengue fever, primarily a disease of older children and adults, is characterized by sudden onset of fever, frontal headache, retro-orbital pain, lumbrosacral pain, severe malaise, myalgias, bone pain, nausea, and vomiting. Patients may be anorectic, have altered taste sensation, and have a mild sore throat. Initial temperature may rise to 41°C and fever may last 2 to 7 days; a relative bradycardia may be present. Up to half the patients may have a transient rash or skin mottling in early illness. Defervescence occurs between days 3 and 6. A second, non-pruritic skin rash, varying in form from scarlatiniform to maculopapular and usually lasting an average of 2 to 3 days, may appear on the trunk, spreading to the face and extremities, sparing palms and soles, and often resolving with desquamation. The fever may rise again (saddleback pattern) with the presence of the rash.

Other findings associated with dengue fever include generalized lymphadenopathy and haemorrhagic manifestations. Skin haemorrhages, including petechiae and purpura, are the most common, along with gum bleeding, epistaxis, menorrhagia, and gastrointestinal haemorrhage. Haematuria is uncommon and jaundice is rare. Clinical laboratory findings include a neutropenia followed by a lymphocytosis, often marked by atypical lymphocytes. Liver enzyme levels may be mildly elevated, but in some patients serum alanine aminotransferase and aspartate aminotransferase levels reach 500 to 1000 U/l. Thrombocytopenia is not uncommon.

Classic dengue fever is rarely fatal, but weakness and depression may last several weeks following the acute illness, particularly in adults. There are no permanent sequelae.

Dengue haemorrhagic fever

During the last 50 years, dengue haemorrhagic fever has been recorded in south-east Asia, where all four dengue serotypes have circulated, but the first epidemic of dengue haemorrhagic fever in the Americas appeared in 1981 in Cuba, associated with the arrival of a new Asian virus of different genotype.

Pathogenesis The characteristic development of dengue haemorrhagic fever during a heterotypic dengue infection, is presumed to result from pre-existing cross-reactive immunity. Subneutralizing levels of dengue antibodies enhance the infectivity of the virus by increasing the efficiency of binding and uptake of virus–antibody complexes through Fc receptors on blood monocyte or tissue macrophage cells, the chief site of replication in humans. This phenomenon of antibody-dependent enhancement is demonstrable *in vitro*. Cellular components of the primed immune response are probably also involved, and the resulting complement activation and release of cytokines and other mediators cause capillary leakage and coagulopathy, the hallmark of dengue haemorrhagic fever. The contribution of viral factors and variations in the host's immune response to the development of dengue haemorrhagic fever is unknown.

Clinical features Although dengue haemorrhagic fever can occur in adults, it is primarily a disease of children under the age of 15 years. It is associated with all four virus serotypes. Dengue haemorrhagic fever is characterized by sudden onset of fever, usually lasting 2 to 7 days, and non-specific signs and symptoms. During this acute phase, it is difficult to distinguish dengue haemorrhagic fever from dengue fever and other illnesses found in tropical areas. However, at the critical time of defervescence, signs of circulatory failure or haemorrhagic manifestations may occur, the most common being petechiae, purpuric lesions, and ecchymoses. Epistaxis, bleeding gums, gastrointestinal haemorrhage, and haematuria occur less commonly. In its most severe form, dengue shock syndrome, occurring in approximately one-third of dengue haemorrhagic fever cases, patients experience hypotension, narrowing of the pulse pressure (≤ 20 mmHg), and circulatory failure. Patients may complain of abdominal pain shortly before the onset of shock.

Physical findings associated with dengue shock syndrome include cool, blotchy, and congested skin, cyanosis, diaphoresis, tachypnia, and oliguria. Hepatomegaly, pulmonary effusion, and oedema are common, as is leucopenia. By definition, patients with dengue haemorrhagic fever/dengue shock syndrome must have objective evidence of plasma leakage such as a haemoconcentration (haematocrit elevated by 20 per cent), and thrombo-cytopenia with a platelet count of 100 000/mm³ or less. Liver enzymes in serum may be elevated. The duration of shock is usually short. The mortality rate in aggressively treated patients is 1 per cent or less.

Differential diagnosis and diagnosis The differential diagnosis during the acute phase of illness includes influenza, measles, rubella, typhoid, leptospirosis, rickettsia, malaria, and other arboviral infections with rash. Other viral haemorrhagic fevers and meningococcaemia should be considered in patients with haemorrhagic manifestations.

A definitive diagnosis depends on isolating the virus, detecting viral antigen or RNA in serum or tissues, or a rising titre of specific antibodies. The MAC-ELISA is the most widely used serological test for dengue diagnosis. Because antidengue IgM antibodies persist for several months, and because not all patients have detectable IgM antibodies 6 to 10 days after onset, diagnosis based on a single IgM antibody MAC-ELISA result should be considered provisional.

Prevention and control Patients should be protected from mosquitoes and people should avoid mosquito bites in areas infested with *Ae. aegypti*. There are currently no licensed vaccines. Prevention and control can only be achieved by controlling *Ae. aegypti* in the large urban centres of the tropics. The most effective way to achieve this is via larval mosquito control by elimination of breeding sites in open stagnant water around communities where transmission is endemic/ epidemic.

Treatment Supportive care includes intensive monitoring of vital signs and haematocrit. If signs of shock appear, prompt replacement of plasma volume and correction of metabolic acidosis, electrolyte imbalance, and hypoglycaemia are essential. After 1 or 2 days, the capillary leakage ceases and resorption of extravasated fluid begins. Care must then be taken not to induce pulmonary oedema by excessive intravenous fluids. Treatment with corticosteroids does not reduce mortality in children with dengue shock syndrome. Aspirin (salicylic acid) should be avoided.

Japanese encephalitis

Aetiology and epidemiology

Japanese encephalitis virus is the type species of the Japanese encephalitis serocomplex which includes several antigenically related viruses, including St Louis encephalitis, Rocio, West Nile, Koutango, Usuto, Murray Valley encephalitis, Kunjin, Alfuy, Stratford, and Kokobera viruses. Sequence analysis of the structural proteins suggests there are several genotypes of Japanese encephalitis, in distinct geographical areas.

Japanese encephalitis has a widespread distribution throughout Asia which has expanded in the past 20 years, with outbreaks in the Pacific, Australia, Nepal, and Western India (Fig. 2). It is the most important cause of arboviral encephalitis, with about 45 000 cases reported annually. The highest incidence is in temperate and subtropical regions of China, northern Thailand, Nepal, and India. The virus is maintained in a cycle involving culicine mosquitoes and water birds and is transmitted to humans by *Culex* mosquitoes, primarily species of the *Cx. tritaeniorhynchus* complex, which breed in rice fields. Pigs are the primary amplifying host in the peridomestic environment. Epidemics occur in late summer in temperate regions and throughout the year in some tropical areas of Asia. Children have the highest attack rates, because of cumulative herd immunity with age.

Clinical characteristics (see also Chapter 24.14.2)

Only about one in 250 infections result in symptomatic infection, which ranges from a febrile illness with headache, to aseptic meningitis, to encephalitis, and death. After an incubation period of 6 to 16 days, illness usually begins with a prodrome lasting several days followed by abrupt onset of high fever, change in mental status, nausea and vomiting, headache, and seizures, which occur in more than three-quarters of all paediatric patients. Generalized weakness and changes in tone, especially hypertonia and hyper-reflexia are common, but focal motor deficits, including cranial nerve palsies, paresis, hemiplegia, or tetraplegia, may also

occur. Respiratory dysregulation, coma, abnormal plantar reflexes, and prolonged convulsions are associated with a poor prognosis.

Laboratory examination often reveals a moderate, peripheral leucocytosis and mild anaemia. Hyponatraemia, reflecting inappropriate antidiuretic hormone secretion, is common. Cerebrospinal fluid pressure is usually normal, pleocytosis ranges from a few to several hundred cells per mm³, and cerebrospinal fluid protein is moderately elevated in about half the cases.

Five to 30 per cent of cases are fatal; young children are more likely to die, and if they survive, are more likely to have residual neurological defects. Overall, up to 70 per cent of survivors have residual neurological abnormalities including parkinsonism, paralysis, behavioural changes, and psychological deficits. Evidence suggests that infection fails to clear in some patients, with clinical relapse several months after resolution of the acute illness. The clinical effects of congenital infection are unknown. Spontaneous abortions of women infected in the first and second trimesters have been reported.

Diagnosis

The differential diagnosis includes other viral encephalitides including arboviruses, herpes, and enteroviral infections, cerebral malaria, and bacterial infections. Epidemiological features such as place of residence or travel, season, and occurrence of other cases in the community provide clues to the diagnosis. Patients with encephalitis are rarely viraemic. Specific IgM can be detected in cerebrospinal fluid, serum, or both in nearly all patients by the seventh day after onset. Confirmation can be obtained by demonstrating four-fold or greater changes in specific IgM or neutralizing antibody titre.

Prevention and control

A formalin-inactivated mouse brain vaccine is used widely in Japan, Korea, Taiwan, Thailand, and other countries in Asia for childhood immunization and is licensed in Britain, the United States, and other developed countries to protect travellers. Hypersensitivity reactions to this vaccine, including generalized urticaria and angioedema, have occurred within minutes to as long as 2 weeks following vaccination at a rate of 1 to 104 per 10 000. Tissue culture based-vaccines (inactivated and live-attenuated) have been used in China. The risk to travellers to endemic areas during the transmission season can reach 1 per 5000 per month of exposure; risk for most short-term travellers may be less than 1 per million. In general, vaccine should be offered to people spending a month or more in endemic areas during the transmission season, especially if travel includes rural areas. Water and crop management and animal husbandry have been used to decrease human exposure to mosquito bites in the peridomestic environment.

Treatment

No specific therapy is available, but supportive treatment can reduce morbidity and mortality. One uncontrolled study showed a beneficial effect of α-interferon. Dexamethasone did not prevent death caused by oedema-induced increases in intracranial pressure in patients with severe encephalitis.

St Louis encephalitis

Aetiology and epidemiology

St Louis encephalitis virus is prevalent throughout the western hemisphere from Canada to Argentina (Fig. 1). The natural transmission cycle involves wild birds and *Culex* mosquitoes. Although clinical illness has been sporadically reported throughout much of this region, the highest incidence occurs in North America during epidemics. Fewer than 100 human cases are generally reported annually; epidemics with hundreds of cases have occurred in North America every 10 to 20 years.

Clinical characteristics

The ratio of infection to clinical illness is high, ranging from 800:1 in children under 10 years to 85:1 in persons over 60 years. Illness ranges from fever with headache, to aseptic meningitis, to encephalitis, and death. Advanced age is the strongest risk factor for both symptomatic disease and severity of encephalitis. After an incubation period of 4 to 21 days, the typical presentation of encephalitis is fever, headache, chills, nausea, and dysuria. Within 1 to 4 days, central nervous system signs appear and may include meningism, tremor, abnormal reflexes, ataxia, cranial nerve palsies, convulsions (especially in children), stupor, and coma. Complications include bronchopneumonia, sepsis, stress ulcer, and pulmonary embolism. Recovery is usually complete, except that 10 to 25 per cent of very young infants have residual mental deficits, personality changes, muscle weakness, and paralysis. Underlying diseases such as hypertension, diabetes, and alcoholism affect the outcome. The case fatality rate is about 6 per cent overall, but is only 1 per cent of those under 5 years, as the disease is generally milder in children. Short-lived sequalae of nervousness, memory impairment, and headache occur uncommonly in older children and adults.

The peripheral leucocyte count, serum transaminases, and creatine phosphokinase may be elevated. Hyponatraemia due to the syndrome of inappropriate antidiuretic hormone secretion may be noted in up to one-third of patients. The cerebrospinal fluid contains fewer than 500 cells/mm^3, principally leucocytes.

Diagnosis

The differential diagnosis includes other viral encephalitides such as arboviruses, herpes, and enterovirus, as well as other bacterial and fungal infections of the central nervous system. Epidemiological features (residence, season of the year, and occurrence of other cases in the community) provide diagnostic clues. Because of serological cross-reactivity with other flaviviruses, positive serum samples should be subjected to cross-neutralization tests. From fatal cases, virus may be isolated from brain tissue or demonstrated by immunofluorescence. Virus has not been isolated from the blood during the acute phase of illness.

Prevention and control

No vaccine is available. Prevention is aimed at personal protection from mosquito bites and mosquito abatement.

Treatment

Treatment is supportive; no specific therapy is available.

West Nile encephalitis (see also Chapter 24.14.2)

Aetiology and epidemiology

West Nile virus is enzootic in Africa, the Middle East, and western Asia, and has caused periodic outbreaks in humans and horses in southern and central Europe (Fig. 2). In 1999, the virus was first detected in the New World during an outbreak in New York City. By 2001 the virus' distribution expanded to the entire eastern half of the United States and southern Ontario. Continued geographic expansion throughout the Americas is likely.

Phylogenic studies indicate two viral lineages: lineage one includes most strains isolated in recent outbreaks in Europe, the Middle East, and North America; lineage two includes many of the strains enzootic in Africa. Kunjin virus (see below) is a variant of West Nile virus and fits within lineage one. West Nile virus is maintained in a cycle involving culicine mosquitoes and wild birds. Bird migration may be important for transporting the virus geographically, particularly to temperate areas.

From the 1950s to the 1970s, epidemics, rarely associated with severe neurological disease and death, occurred in Israel, France, and Africa. No epidemic activity was then reported until the mid-1990s when epidemics associated with severe neurological disease and death in humans and/or equines were recorded in Algeria, Morocco, Tunisia, Italy, Romania, Israel, southern Russia, France, and the United States. Several of these epidemics have included hundreds of cases. Outbreaks typically occur in late summer and early autumn in temperate regions.

Clinical characteristics

Illness ranges from fever with headache, to aseptic meningitis, to encephalitis, and death; but most infections are asymptomatic. Investigations in Romania and the United States showed that less than one per cent of those infected developed meningitis or encephalitis requiring hospitalization. Approximately 20 per cent of those infected developed a systemic febrile illness. Advanced age was the most important risk factor for developing both encephalitis and death. The incubation period is 3 to 7 days (range 3–15 days). Mild illness presents as a dengue-like illness with fever, headache, backache, myalgia, and anorexia that lasts 3 to 6 days. A roseolar or

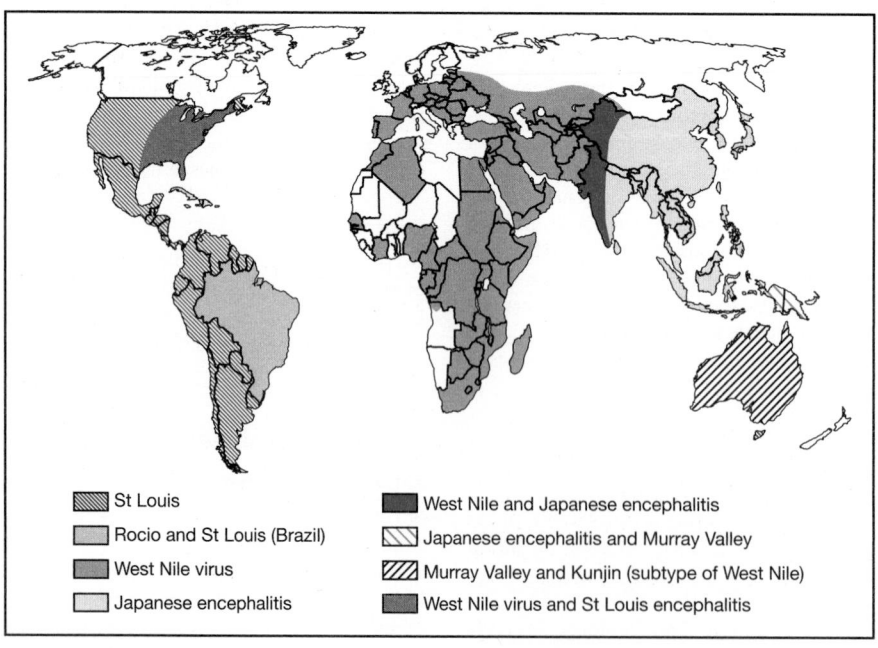

Fig. 2 The geographical distribution of the Japanese encephalitis serocomplex of the family Flaviviridae.

maculopapular rash occurs in about half the patients and lasts up to a week without scaling. Generalized lymphadenopathy has also been reported as a common finding. In recent outbreaks, however, only about one in five patients had a rash and lymphadenopathy was uncommon. Disorientation, disturbed consciousness, and generalized weakness are predominant signs in persons with encephalitis. Ataxia, extrapyramidal signs, hypotonia, hyper-reflexia, coma, and seizures may be present. Motor weakness may be profound, suggesting Guillain–Barré syndrome. Other serious, non-neurological, rare complications include myocarditis, pancreatitis, and fulminant hepatitis.

Recovery is usually complete, but among those with severe encephalitis, up to half of survivors have residual neurological deficits. Case fatality rates in recent large outbreaks have ranged from 5 to 14 per cent. The peripheral leucocyte count, serum transaminases, and alkaline phosphatase may be elevated. Thrombocytopenia and anaemia may be present. Hyponatraemia can occur in up to three-quarters of patients. The cerebrospinal fluid usually contains up to 2000 cells/mm³, mostly leucocytes, and moderately elevated protein.

Diagnosis

The differential diagnosis includes other viral encephalitides including arboviruses, herpes, and enterovirus, as well as other bacterial and fungal infections of the central nervous system. Guillain–Barré syndrome should be considered in patients with profound muscle weakness. Epidemiological features (residence, season of the year, and occurrence of other cases in the community) provide diagnostic clues. Because of serological cross-reactivity with other flaviviruses, positive samples should be tested by cross-neutralization. Virus isolation or nucleic acid amplification tests of acute-phase blood, cerebrospinal fluid, or brain biopsy samples may provide a definitive diagnosis, but will not detect virus in all patients.

Prevention and control

No vaccine is available. Prevention is aimed at surveillance, mosquito abatement, and taking personal precautions to avoid mosquito bites.

Treatment

Treatment is supportive; no specific therapy is available.

Yellow fever

Aetiology and epidemiology

Yellow fever was first described in the seventeenth century and was one of the great plagues of mankind for over 400 years. In 1900, mosquito transmission and the viral aetiology were proven. The virus was isolated in 1927 and a vaccine developed in 1937. The virus is present in tropical America and Africa, but does not occur in Asia. Epidemics still occur, especially in West Africa. Between 1986 and 1991, a series of outbreaks in Nigeria caused an estimated 100 000 cases (although only about 5000 were officially reported), with attack rates in affected areas of 30/1000 and case-fatality rates exceeding 20 per cent. In South America, the disease affects up to 300 people annually, principally young men working in forest areas exposed to *Haemagogus* mosquitoes breeding in tree holes (jungle yellow fever). Disease in unvaccinated travellers is rare; however, since 1996 four travellers died in the US and Europe of infection acquired in South America and Africa.

Yellow fever virus has two cycles of transmission: jungle yellow fever and urban yellow fever. The forest or jungle transmission cycle involves canopy-dwelling mosquitoes and monkeys. The urban cycle involves humans as the vertebrate host and *Ae. aegypti* as the principal vector. In the past 30 years, *Ae. aegypti* has reinvaded Central and South America and a small outbreak of urban yellow fever occurred in Bolivia in 1998. The American tropics currently have the highest risk of urban epidemics of yellow fever in over 50 years. Epidemics in Africa often occur in moist savannah regions, involving forest (sylvatic) or peridomestic *Aedes* mosquitoes and humans as viraemic hosts. In dry areas and urban centres, epidemic transmission occurs where water-storage practices breed domestic *Ae. aegypti*. Several hundred thousand people are infected annually; outbreaks are frequent.

Clinical features

Approximately 1 in 20 infections results in clinical disease with jaundice. In its classical form, disease occurs abruptly after an incubation period of 3 to 6 days. The initial phase ('period of infection') is characterized by viraemia, fever, chills, headache, lumbosacral pain, myalgia, nausea, and prostration. On examination, the patient may have a relative bradycardia, and conjunctival injection. Within several days, the patient may recover transiently ('period of remission'), only to relapse ('period of intoxication') with jaundice, albuminuria, oliguria, haemorrhagic manifestations (especially 'black vomit' haematemesis), delirium, stupor, metabolic acidosis, and shock. The prognosis in such cases is poor; 20 to 50 per cent die during the second week of illness.

Clinical laboratory tests reveal leucopenia, thrombocytopenia, hepatic dysfunction, and renal failure. The bleeding diathesis is caused by decreased synthesis of clotting factors and may be complicated by disseminated intravascular coagulation. Pathological findings include midzonal hepatic necrosis and eosinophilic degeneration of hepatocytes (Councilman bodies), possibly representing apoptosis, and acute renal tubular necrosis. Focal myocarditis, and brain swelling and petechial haemorrhages contribute to pathogenesis. Recovery is complete, without postnecrotic hepatic cirrhosis.

Diagnosis

Exposure and travel history provide important clues to aetiology. The differential diagnosis includes viral hepatitis, leptospirosis, rickettsial infections, dengue haemorrhagic fever, Rift Valley fever, Ebola, and Crimean–Congo haemorrhagic fever. Serological cross reactions with other flaviviruses may complicate serology. Postmortem histopathological examination of the liver is diagnostic, with or without immunocytochemical staining for viral antigen. Liver biopsy should never be performed on living patients, as it may precipitate haemorrhage.

Treatment

Treatment is symptomatic. Intensive care requires prompt awareness and treatment of acidosis, shock, and metabolic imbalance. Patients with renal failure may require dialysis.

Prevention and control

The live, attenuated 17D vaccine, delivered as a single 0.5-ml subcutaneous dose, is highly effective, and has minimal side-effects. Immunity is probably life long, but for travel certification, revaccination is recommended every 10 years. People with documented egg allergy should not be immunized or should be skin tested with the vaccine. The vaccine must not be given to children under 6 months of age, in whom there is a risk of postvaccinal encephalitis, and it is best to delay vaccination until 9 months of age. On theoretical grounds, immunosuppressed patients (including those with clinical AIDS) should not be immunized. The immune response in HIV infected persons is impaired. No evidence of clinical congenital infection has been found. Immunization during pregnancy is contraindicated, but, if inadvertently performed, recipients should be reassured and followed. The immune response in pregnancy was found to be impaired. Fatal infection following vaccination with the 17D strain has been rarely reported. Effective control has been achieved by controlling the principal urban mosquito vector, *Ae. aegypti*. This approach would also prevent epidemic dengue fever/dengue haemorrhagic fever in tropical urban centres.

Other mosquito-borne infections

Kunjin

Genomic sequencing indicates that Kunjin virus is a variant of West Nile virus. It is found over most of tropical Australia and Queensland and has a similar transmission cycle involving birds and *Culex* mosquitoes. Infection is usually asymptomatic, but occasional cases of encephalitis have been reported. Infections are generally milder than with Murray Valley encephalitis and are not life threatening. Kunjin virus infections that are non-encephalopathic usually present with fever, often with polyarthralgia. Cases occur sporadically, with only nine reported from 1990 to 1998. Treatment is supportive; there is no vaccine.

Murray Valley encephalitis

Murray Valley encephalitis is enzootic in New Guinea, in northern Western Australia, and in the Northern Territory, and possibly in northern Queensland (Fig. 1). The virus has a transmission cycle involving birds and *Culex* mosquitoes and is transmitted to man by *Cx. annulirostris* mosquitoes from the end of March to early June. Only one in 1000 to 2000 infections results in clinical illness; of those that have neurological disease, approximately one-third are fatal and a quarter have residual neurological deficits. Clinical illness resembles Japanese encephalitis. Children and the elderly are at the highest risk. In 1974, the largest recorded epidemic involved 58 cases and 10 deaths; since then, sporadic cases have been identified. Serological diagnosis is complicated by the presence of the closely related Kunjin virus, which also causes encephalitis. Treatment is supportive; there is no vaccine.

Rocio encephalitis

Rocio virus is antigenically related to St Louis encephalitis virus and is known only in Brazil. Epidemics in 1975 to 1976 caused 871 cases, principally among young adult, male, agricultural workers and fisherman. Since then, only sporadic illness has been reported. The probable vector is *Aedes scapularis* and wild birds are amplifying hosts. The clinical disease is typical viral encephalitis, with a 4 per cent mortality and 20 per cent of patients have neuropsychiatric sequealae. Virus is not recoverable from blood, but post-mortem diagnosis may be made by virus isolation from brain tissue. Treatment is supportive; there is no vaccine.

Tick-borne infections of the central nervous system

Tick-borne encephalitis

Aetiology and epidemiology

There are two subtypes of tick-borne encephalitis virus, eastern and western, which differ only slightly in viral protein structure. These viruses, along with the louping ill, Powassan, Kyasanur Forest disease, and Omsk haemorrhagic fever viruses, belong to the tick-borne encephalitis antigenic complex. The disease caused by the eastern subtype is also known as Russian spring/summer encephalitis and Russian epidemic encephalitis; and the western subtype as FSME (Fruehsommer-Meningo-Enzephalitis), early-summer encephalitis, and Kumlinge's disease. The geographic distribution of disease is determined by that of their tick vectors: *Ixodes persulcatus* for the eastern subtype causing human disease principally in the Far East, the Urals, and western Siberia; and *Ixodes ricinus* for the western subtype which occurs at highest incidence in eastern and central Europe, Moldavia, the Ukraine, and Byelorus, with smaller numbers of cases from western Europe, the Balkans, and Scandinavia.

Infections occur during the period of tick activity from April to November. Tick-borne encephalitis is largely a rural infection; occupational and vocational pursuits favouring tick exposure are risk factors. Human infection and outbreaks following consumption of raw milk or cheese from asymptomatic goats, or more rarely, sheep or cows, have been described. Hundreds to thousands of cases occur annually, with reported attack rates up to 200/100 000 residents in Latvia, the Urals, and Western Siberia. Aerosolized virus has caused laboratory infections.

Clinical features

Most human infections are subclinical. The illness produced by each subtype is generally similar but that produced by the eastern subtype carries a worse prognosis. The incubation period is 7 to 14 days, with a range of 2 to 28 days. Incubation periods of 3 to 4 days follow milk-borne exposure. The Western subtype typically produces a biphasic illness. The first phase is a non-specific, influenza-like, febrile illness lasting 2 to 7 days followed by an afebrile and relatively asymptomatic period lasting 2 to 10 days. Flushing, conjunctival haemorrhage, nausea, vomiting, dizziness, and myalgia are common findings. Approximately one-third of patients then develop higher fevers with aseptic meningitis or meningoencephalitis. The eastern subtype usually progresses without an asymptomatic phase. Signs and symptoms of meningoencephalitis or meningoencephaloymelitis include somnolence, coma, asymmetrical parasesis of the cranial nerves, tremors of the extremities, nystagmus, severe pain in the extremities, and flaccid paralysis of the neck and upper extremities.

Permanent paralysis develops in 2 to 10 per cent of patients with the western subtype, 10 to 25 per cent with the eastern. Corresponding case fatality rates are 0.5 to 2.0 per cent and 5 to 20 per cent for the western and eastern subtypes, respectively.

Laboratory findings include neutrophilia, although neutropenia, thrombocytopenia, and elevated liver enzyme levels may occur early. The cerebrospinal fluid white blood count is usually below 500/mm^3, primarily of mononuclear cells.

Diagnosis

The differential diagnosis is similar to Japanese encephalitis; the pattern of flaccid paralysis may be confused with poliomyelitis. A history of bite by small ixodid ticks is elicited in fewer than half the cases. Specific diagnosis is made by virus isolation from blood or cerebrospinal fluid during the first week of illness, or by serological tests, including IgM enzyme immunoassay and neutralization test.

Treatment

Treatment is supportive.

Prevention and control

Effective inactivated vaccines are available in Europe in formulations for adults and children. Mass vaccination in Austria produced a dramatic decline in disease incidence. Vaccines appear to produce equal protection against the eastern and western strains. Use of a vaccine, available in the United Kingdom, should be seriously considered for tourists planning camping or extensive outdoor activities during the tick transmission season in enzootic areas, particularly in Russia and Central Europe. Commercial hyperimmune globulin preparations are available for use after tick exposure or to provide short-term pre-exposure prophylaxis.

Louping ill

This is a disease of veterinary importance, causing neurological illness in sheep and to a lesser extent in cows, horses, farmed deer, sheep-dogs, and pigs. The virus, isolated in 1931, is a member of the tick-borne encephalitis complex, and is transmitted by *Ixodes ricinus*. Louping ill occurs in the hill country along the western coast of Scotland and northern England, Ireland, and Norway. Natural infections resulting in human disease have been rare, but laboratory infections are not uncommon. Ten naturally occurring cases have been documented, including a veterinarian, abattoir workers, and farmers. Some of these cases were attributable to contact with sheep blood. The human disease is typically aseptic meningitis or encephalitis; no fatal infections have occurred. Avoidance of tick bite in enzootic areas is recommended. The licensed tick-borne encephalitis vaccine may be protective.

Powassan encephalitis

The virus was first isolated from the brain of a fatal case in Powassan, Ontario in 1958. Since then, approximately 20 human cases have been recognized in eastern Canada and the eastern United States, primarily in children, with a case-fatality rate of 10 per cent and a high incidence of residual neurological dysfunction. Serological surveys indicate an antibody prevalence of 1 to 4 per cent. The distribution of the virus in North America is considerably wider than indicated by human cases, and the diagnosis should be suspected in any case of summer–autumn encephalitis. The virus is transmitted between *Ixodes scapularis* (ricinus complex) ticks and rodents. The clinical features are those of viral encephalitis, with localizing neurological signs and convulsions. There is no specific treatment or vaccine.

Tick-borne haemorrhagic fever

Kyasunur Forest disease

Aetiology and epidemiology

This virus is a member of the tick-borne encephalitis antigenic complex. The virus has been isolated from humans, monkeys, and ticks since it was first recognized in 1957 during an outbreak of haemorrhagic fever affecting wild monkeys in Karnataka (then Mysore) State, India. Several hundred cases are reported annually, principally among people working in the forest in Karnataka State. In 1983, 1555 cases, including 150 deaths, occurred. The peak seasonal incidence is between February and May. The virus is transmitted between immature ixodid ticks (*Haemaphysalis spinigera*) and small mammals (rodents, porcupines), passes to the adult stage during moulting, and is spread to man and wild monkeys by adult ticks.

In 1995, a subtype of Kyasanur Forest disease virus was isolated from patients in Jeddah, Saudi Arabia, with clinical symptoms ranging from febrile illness to fatal haemorrhagic disease. Human infections were associated with handling meat or drinking unpasturized camel's milk. The virus seems to be associated with sheep and camels, and to be transmitted by ticks.

Clinical characteristics

After an incubation period of 2 to 7 days, there is abrupt onset of fever, chills, headache, myalgia, abdominal pain, nausea, vomiting, and diarrhoea. Physical signs include bradycardia, lymphadenopathy, and haemorrhagic manifestations. Hypotension is frequently noted during the end of the acute stage. Fatal cases develop shock and pulmonary oedema. A biphasic illness is not uncommon, with resolution of the first phase in 5 to 12 days, and return of the fever and signs of meningoencephalitis after an interval of 1 to 3 weeks. Localizing neurological signs are infrequent, and residual defects are rare. Convalescence is prolonged. Laboratory abnormalities include leucopenia, thrombocytopenia, and elevated serum transaminases during the acute phase.

Diagnosis

Diagnosis is by virus isolation from blood collected during the first week after onset or by serological tests. Virus isolation should be conducted under biosafety level four conditions.

Prevention and control

Tick bites should be avoided in endemic areas. Proper care should be taken when handling raw meat, and camel's milk should be pasteurized. A formalin-inactivated virus is available in India.

Treatment

Treatment is supportive; specific therapy is not available.

Omsk haemorrhagic fever

This disease was first recognized in 1945 in western Siberia. Cases were frequent between 1945 and 1949, with morbidity rates of 500 to 1400/100 000, but subsequently have been rare, mainly occurring among residents of rural areas working in the fields. The virus is a member of the tick-borne encephalitis complex. Human infections are acquired by tick bite or contact with infected muskrats. The disease is characterized by abrupt onset of fever, headache, myalgia, facial flushing, conjunctival suffusion, minor haemorrhagic manifestations, and leucopenia. Recovery occurs in the second week, and the case fatality rate is low (0.5–3 per cent). The differential diagnosis includes tularaemia, rickettsial infection, and leptospirosis. Specific diagnosis is made by virus isolation from blood during the acute phase or by serological tests. Only a few laboratories outside Russia with biocontainment level 4 facilities are capable of providing laboratory assistance. Tick-borne encephalitis vaccines may cross-protect against Omsk haemorrhagic fever.

Further reading

Centers for Disease Control and Prevention (1993). Inactivated Japanese encephalitis virus vaccine. Recommendations of the Advisory Committee on Immunization Practices (ACIP). *Morbidity and Mortality Weekly Reports* **42**, 1–15.

Dumpis U, Crook D, Oski (1999). Tick-borne encephalitis. *Clinical Infectious Diseases* **28**, 882–90.

Gubler DJ (1998). Dengue and dengue hemorrhagic fever. *Clinical Microbiology Reviews* **11**, 480–96.

Gubler DJ, Roehrig JT (1998). Arboviruses (Togaviridae and Flaviviridae). In: Collier L, *et al. Topley and Wilson's microbiology and microbial infections*, 9th edn, Vol. 1, Virology, ch. 29, pp. 579–600. Arnold, London

Monath TP, Heinz FX (1996). Flaviviruses. In: Fields BN, Knipe DM, Howley PM, eds. *Fields virology*, pp. 961–1034. Lippincott-Raven, Philadelphia.

Solomon T, Dung NM, Kneen R, Gainsborough M, Vaughn DW, Khanh VT (2000). Japanese encephalitis. *Journal of Neurology, Neurosurgery and Psychiatry* **68**, 405–15.

7.10.14 Bunyaviridae

J. W. LeDuc and J. S. Porterfield

The family Bunyaviridae currently contains around 300 viruses, and is divided into five genera (see Table 1). The family name, and that of the genus *Bunyavirus*, is derived from the type species, Bunyamwera virus, which was isolated in Uganda from *Aedes* mosquitoes. The other genera are also named after viruses: the genus *Hantavirus* after Hantaan virus, the causative agent of Korean haemorrhagic fever; the genus *Nairovirus* after Nairobi sheep disease virus; the genus *Phlebovirus* after phlebotomus or sandfly fever virus; and the genus *Tospovirus* after tomato spotted-wilt virus. All members of the family share certain structural, biochemical, and genetic properties, such as a spherical, enveloped virion 80 to 120 nm in diameter (see Fig. 1), and a genome of single-stranded, negative-sense RNA divided into three segments. Members of different genera vary substantially in their biological and biochemical properties and in the details of their mechanisms of replication. Bunyaviruses, nairoviruses, and phleboviruses, which together make up the greater part of the family, are all arthropod-borne animal viruses, or arboviruses; these circulate in nature in a wide variety of different vertebrate hosts and are biologically transmitted between vertebrates and to humans by the bites of blood-sucking arthropods, principally mosquitoes for bunyaviruses, sandflies for phleboviruses, and ticks for nairoviruses. By contrast, hantaviruses are not arboviruses, but are zoonotic agents infecting rodents and other small mammals, which may spread to humans if they are in close contact with their infected excreta, and tospo-viruses are arthropod-transmitted plant viruses of no known medical importance.

Viruses within the larger genera are further subdivided into serogroups of more closely related members, there being at least 18 serogroups within the bunyaviruses, and seven within the nairoviruses (see Table 1). Of over 60 Bunyaviridae that are known to infect man, the type species and those that cause major human diseases are shown in bold type in Table 1 and are described in more detail in the following sections. Table 2 lists the continental distribution of the remaining viruses that cause only minor human infections and also indicates the principal arthropod vector of each virus. The habitats in which the different viruses and their vectors occur range from arctic to tropical, with every intermediate form. The enzootic cycles by which arboviruses are maintained in nature are very imperfectly understood; most viruses undergo alternate cycles of replication in vertebrate and invertebrate hosts, but transovarial and trans-stadial transmission within some mosquitoes, ticks, and phlebotomine flies, and venereal transmission from vertically infected male mosquitoes to uninfected females are also known to occur. Most arboviruses have a narrow host range, occur within a limited area, and are transmitted by specific vectors to a limited number of vertebrate hosts, but some viruses infect a wider host range, are transmitted by more than one type of vector, and may occur in more than a single continent. It is of interest that, for different members of the family, tick transmission predominates in Asia, but is unknown in South or Central America, and although some Bunyaviridae have been isolated in Australia, none is known to infect man in that continent. Further epidemiological details can be found in more specialized publications.

Following viral entry, whether through the skin after the bite of an infected arthropod or by another route, virus replicates in draining lymph nodes, which are frequently enlarged, and a viraemia follows. Symptoms develop when virus lodges in other sites and undergoes further replication cycles. Appropriate virucidal agents and methods include bleach, phenolic disinfectants and detergents, autoclaving or boiling, and the use of γ-irradiation. Various enzymes such as nucleases will also inactivate these viruses. For human pathogens with the ability to spread by the aerosol route, biosafety level 3 (hantaviruses, Oropouche virus, others) or 4 (Crimean–Congo haemorrhagic fever virus only) is recommended. Added precautions are necessary when handling hantavirus-infected animals and virus concentrates.

Genus *Bunyavirus*

Much of our knowledge about the family as a whole derives from intensive studies on the type species, Bunyamwera virus, and a few other members of this large genus. The three-segmented genome permits reassortment when two closely related viruses infect the same cell, either in nature or under controlled laboratory conditions. Such studies have been used to establish the genomic control of viral proteins, and to analyse the basis of virulence

Table 1 The family Bunyaviridae: its genera, serogroups, vectors, and viruses infecting man

Genus	Serogroup	Vector	Viruses infecting man
Bunyavirus (over 150)	Anopheles A (12)	Mosquito	Tacaiuma
	Anopheles B (2)	Mosquito	
	Bakau (5)	Mosquito	
	Bunyamwera (33)	Mosquito	**Bunyamwera**[1], Calovo, Gorissa, Germiston, Ilesha, Maguari, Shokwe, Tensaw, Wyeomyia
	Bwamba (2)	Mosquito	**Bwamba**, Pongola
	C group (14)	Mosquito	Apeu, Caraparu, Itaqui, Madrid, Marituba, Murutucu, Nepuyo, Oriboca, Ossa, Restan
	California (14)	Mosquito	**California encephalitis**, Guaroa, **La Crosse**, **Inkoo**, **Jamestown Canyon**, **snowshoe hare**, **Tahyna**, trivittatus
	Capim (10)	Mosquito	
	Gamboa (8)	Mosquito	
	Guama (12)	Mosquito	Catu, Guama
	Koongol (2)	Mosquito	
	Minatitlan (2)	Mosquito	
	Nyando (2)	Mosquito	Nyando
	Olifanstsvlei (5)	Mosquito	
	Patois (7)	Mosquito	
	Simbu (24)	Mosquito	**Oropouche**, Shuni
	Tete (5)	Mosquito	
	Turlock (5)	Mosquito	
	Unassigned (3)	Mosquito	
Hantavirus (8)	Hantaan (26)	None	**Andes, Bayou, Black Creek Canal, Dobrava, Hantaan, Juquitiba, Laguna Negra, Lechiguanas, Monongahela, Oran**, Prospect Hill, **Puumala, Seoul, Sin Nombre**
Nairovirus (32)	Crimean–Congo (3)	Tick	**Crimean–Congo haemorrhagic fever**, Hazara
	Dera Ghazi Khan (6)	Tick	
	Hughes (10)	Tick	Soldado
	Nairobi S.D. (3)	Tick	Dugbe, Ganjam, Nairobi sheep disease
	Qalyub (3)	Tick	
	Sakhalin (7)	Tick	Avalon
	Thiafora (2)	Tick	
Phlebovirus (57)	Phlebotomus (44)	Sandfly[2]	Alenquer, Candiru, **Chagres**, Corfu, **Punta Toro**, **Rift Valley fever**[2], **Naples**, **Sandfly Fever, and Sicilian, Toscana**
	Uukuniemi (13)	Tick	Uukuniemi, Zalev-Terpeniya
Unassigned (53)		Mosquito	Bangui, Kasokero, Tataguine
		Tick	Bhanja, Keterah, Tamdy, Wanowrie
Tospovirus (1)		Thrips	

Numbers in parentheses indicate the approximate number of viruses in the genus or serogroup.
[1] Bold type indicates the type species and viruses causing major disease in man.
[2] Mosquito vector for Rift Valley fever virus.

for both vertebrate and invertebrate hosts. Two bunyaviruses, Akabane and Aino viruses in the Simbu serogroup, are notable for their ability to produce congenital deformities in sheep, goats, and cattle in Japan, Australia, Africa, and in the Middle East. However, there is as yet no evidence that any member of the genus or family produces teratogenic effects in man, although there is concern that Oropouche virus, an important Simbu serogroup pathogen of northern South America, may be a threat to pregnant women.

Bunyamwera virus

Symptoms

A mild, febrile illness, usually with headache, joint and back pains, sometimes associated with a rash, and occasionally with mild involvement of the central nervous system. Serological surveys indicated that infection of man is widespread in sub-Saharan Africa but most infections are unrecognized. Laboratory infections have been recorded. Garissa virus, recently isolated from haemorrhagic fever patients during outbreak investigations in Kenya and Somalia, contains L and S genome segments virtually identical to Bunyamwera virus, but with the M segment coming from a virus most closely related to Cache Valley virus. Neither Bunyamwera nor Cache Valley virus is known to cause haemorrhagic disease in humans.

Fig. 1 Electron micrograph of Crimean–Congo haemorrhagic fever virus (× 400 000) (by courtesy of Dr D.S. Ellis).

Treatment and prognosis
No treatment is necessary and the prognosis is excellent.

California encephalitis virus, Inkoo, Jamestown Canyon, La Crosse, Tahyna, and snowshoe hare viruses

The viruses named above, and perhaps others currently unrecognized, are responsible for the clinical condition known as California encephalitis. The viruses are widely distributed in nature throughout many parts of North America, Europe, and Eurasia. Most recognized human infections in the United States are due to La Crosse virus and are reported from Ohio, Wisconsin, Minnesota, and West Virginia; in 1999 a total of 70 cases was reported from nine states. The great majority of these occur in children, more often males than females, although Jamestown Canyon virus is unusual in that more adults are involved. There is nearly always a history of outdoor exposure in areas where woodland mosquitoes are prevalent. The incubation period is 5 to 10 days. Most cases of La Crosse encephalitis are relatively mild with headache, fever, and vomiting, progressing to lethargy, behavioural changes, and occasional brief seizures, followed by improvement. Severe cases (10 to 20 per cent) have an abrupt onset of fever and headache, disorientation, and seizures during the first 24 h of illness, sometimes progressing to coma and requiring intensive supportive care. Overall, symptomatic children suffer seizures in about 50 per cent of cases, status epilepticus in 10 to 15 per cent, and mortality approaches 1 per cent. Residual seizures occur in 6 to 13 per cent, persistent hemiparesis in about 1 per cent, and cognitive dysfunction in a small but poorly defined percentage of cases.

In Europe, Tahyna virus is widely distributed in Austria, the former Czechoslovakia, France, Germany, Italy, Norway, Romania, the former Yugoslavia, and the former USSR. Antibody rates can exceed 95 per cent in certain parts of the former Czechoslovakia, and are around 50 per cent in the Rhone valley in France and the Danube basin near Vienna; however, overt disease is seldom recognized. Inkoo virus is prevalent in Finland and in neighbouring regions of Russia, with the great majority of adult Lapps having antibodies; emerging information suggests that small children may have signs of central nervous involvement during acute infection. Antibodies reactive with California serogroup viruses have also been found in human sera collected in Sri Lanka, China, and in the far northern latitudes of Eurasia where a number of California serogroup viruses have been isolated from mosquitoes, some related to Inkoo and Tahyna viruses, but others to snowshoe hare virus. In another Russian study of some 50 persons, mainly 14 to 30 years of age, with infections caused by California serogroup viruses, about two-thirds had an influenza-like illness without

Table 2 Bunyaviridae causing only mild or trivial infections in man, arranged on a geographical basis

Africa	North America	Central America	South America	Europe	Asia
Bangui (M)[1]	Avalon (T)[2]	Fort Sherman	Alenquer (P)[3]	Bhanja (T)	Batai (M)
Bhanja (T)	Keystone (M)	Madrid (M)	Apeu (M)	Calovo (M)	Bhanja (T)
Bwamba (M)	Tensaw (M)	Ossa (M)	Candiru (P)	Corfou (P)	Issyk-Kul (T)
Dugbe (T)	Trivittatus (M)	Restan (M)	Caraparu (M)	Inkoo (M)	Ganjam (T)
Germiston (M)		Trivittatus (M)	Catu (M)	Tahyna (M)	Hazara (T)
Ilesha (M)			Guama (M, P)	Tamdy (T)	Keterah (T)
Kasokero (M)			Guaroa (M)	Uukuniemi (T)	Wanowrie (T)
Nyando (M)			Maguari (M)		Zaliv Terpeniya (M, T)
Pongola (M)			Marituba (M)		
Shokwe (M)			Murutucu (M)		
Shuni (M)			Restan (M)		
Tataguine (M)			Tacaiuma (M)		
Thiafora			Wyeomyia (M)		
Wanowrie (T)					

[1] M indicates that the virus is transmitted by mosquitoes.

[2] T indicates that the virus is transmitted by ticks.

[3] P indicates that the virus is transmitted by phlebotomine flies.

central nervous involvement, while the remaining third had aseptic meningitis.

Control, treatment, and prognosis

Measures to limit mosquito breeding, particularly of *Aedes triseriatus*, are useful in endemic regions. No vaccines are available, and there is no specific treatment, although the fluid and electrolyte balance must be maintained, and anticonvulsive drugs may be required to control seizures. Intravenous ribavirin has been used to treat severe La Crosse encephalitis; however, more comprehensive clinical trials are needed.

Oropouche virus

Symptoms

Prior to 1961, Oropouche virus was known to have caused only a mild fever in a single forest worker in Trinidad, but that year it was responsible for a substantial epidemic in the Belem area of northern Brazil, with some 7000 individuals affected. Over the ensuing 40 years, massive epidemics of febrile illness have been recorded throughout the Amazon Basin, with perhaps as many as 200 000 persons infected. Symptoms include headache, generalized body pains, back pains, prostration, and moderately high fever (40°C). Rash occasionally accompanies infection, as does meningitis or meningismus. Illness lasts from 2 to 5 days, occasionally with protracted convalescence. No fatalities have been reported.

Control, treatment, and prognosis

No vaccine is available. Transmission is probably by the biting midge *Culicoides paraensis* and outbreaks appear to be a long-term consequence of agricultural development of the Amazon Basin. Accumulated organic waste from cacao and banana production provide ideal breeding sites for *Culicoides*, leading to massive populations and subsequent epidemic Oropouche disease. Thus, measures to reduce *Culicoides* breeding may be of benefit. Treatment is supportive, and the prognosis is good, although convalescence may be protracted.

Genus *Hantavirus*

Haemorrhagic fever with renal syndrome

The genus *Hantavirus* takes its name from Hantaan virus, the cause of Korean haemorrhagic fever in Korea. The name Hantaan in turn is from the Hantaan River near the demilitarized zone between North and South Korea, where the virus was first recovered from its rodent host, *Apodemus agrarius*. Hantaan virus was only isolated in 1976, although the clinical diseases it and related hantaviruses cause in the Eurasian continent have been known much longer under many different synonyms: epidemic haemorrhagic fever, Korean haemorrhagic fever, nephropathia epidemica, with haemorrhagic fever with renal syndrome preferred. Four distinct viruses are responsible for most recognized haemorrhagic fever with renal syndrome: Hantaan virus, found primarily in Asia; Dobrava virus, found in an enclave of disease in the Balkan region and sparsely elsewhere in Europe; Puumala virus, found in Scandinavia, western Russia, and much of Europe; and Seoul virus, probably globally distributed wherever *Rattus norvegicus* populations exist uncontrolled. Hantaan and Dobrava viruses cause severe, life-threatening disease with mortality of about 5 per cent, reaching as high as 30 per cent in select populations. Puumala virus infections are less severe, although patients still require admission to hospital, with death in less than 1 per cent of admitted cases. Seoul virus is thought to be the least severe of the pathogenic strains of hantaviruses, although it too has been associated with human deaths.

Each hantavirus is specifically associated with a particular rodent host in nature: Hantaan virus with the striped field mouse, *Apodemus agrarius*; Dobrava virus suspected with the yellow-necked mouse, *Apodemus flavicollis*; Puumala virus with the bank vole, *Clethrionomys glareolus*; and Seoul virus with the Norway rat, *Rattus norvegicus*. Human infection is from aerosols of infectious rodent excreta, or rarely by rodent bite, and is occupationally associated. Most disease is seen among adult men in rural environments. Those with occupations at greatest risk include farmers, woodcutters, shepherds, and especially the military in the field. Most hantavirus disease is markedly seasonal, with peak incidence seen in the late autumn and early winter, although the Balkan form is found most commonly during summer months in Greece and adjacent countries.

Symptoms

Incubation period for hantaviruses is rather variable, and may approach 2 months in some cases, but is generally 12 to 16 days. Severe disease, as typically associated with Hantaan or Dobrava virus infections in Asia or the Balkans, is characterized by five phases:

(1) febrile, of 3- to 7-day duration;

(2) hypotensive, lasting from a few hours to 3 days;

(3) oliguric, from 3 to 7 days;

(4) diuretic, from a few days to weeks;

(5) a prolonged convalescence.

Characteristic signs and symptoms of the febrile phase include fever, malaise, headache, myalgia, back pain, abdominal pain, nausea and vomiting, facial flushing, petechias, and conjunctival haemorrhage (Fig. 2). The hypotensive phase is characterized by nausea, vomiting, tachycardia, hypotension, blurred vision, haemorrhagic signs, and shock, with approximately one-third of the deaths occurring during this phase. In the oliguric phase, nausea and vomiting may persist, and blood pressure may rise; kidney failure presents, which may include frank anuria; and about one-third of the cases may experience severe haemorrhage as epistaxis, gastrointestinal, cutaneous, or bleeding at other sites. Nearly one-half of deaths occur during the oliguric phase. In the diuretic phase, urine output increases to several litres per day. Convalescence is protracted and may require months before full strength and function are regained.

Less severe forms of the disease may skip phases, or spend less time in each phase. The milder forms of haemorrhagic fever with renal syndrome, such as nephropathia epidemica due to Puumala virus, follow a similar, but less severe course, with abrupt onset of fever of 38 to 40 °C, headache, malaise, backache, and generalized abdominal pain. Back or loin pain is especially common. Signs of renal failure are usually not as pronounced, and the need for renal dialysis varies. Transient blurred vision occurs in about 10 per cent of cases. Infection due to Seoul virus follows a similar course, but may present with more evidence of liver involvement. There is no evidence of person-to-person transmission.

Fig. 2 Patient with acute Korean haemorrhagic fever, showing extensive conjunctival haemorrhages (by courtesy of Professor H.W. Lee).

Treatment and prognosis

Admission to hospital, avoidance of trauma and unnecessary movement, close observation, and careful supportive care are essential to patient survival. Treatment is phase specific, with special attention to fluid balance and volume, and control of hypotension and shock. Dialysis may be required in cases of acute renal failure. Specific antiviral therapy using ribavirin has been shown to be efficacious if started early in disease. Recovery is protracted, but until now considered complete and without permanent complications. Recent evidence, however, suggests that persons previously infected with Seoul virus may be at increased risk of chronic renal disease, hypertension, or stroke.

Hantavirus pulmonary syndrome

Recently, a new hantavirus disease, Hantavirus pulmonary syndrome, was reported from the United States and soon recognized in several South American countries as well. More than half the originally identified cases died in 1993, but mortality rates have declined to 20 to 40 per cent as clinical experience is gained. Cases were reported predominantly from the western United States and Canada, and more recently from Argentina, Chile, Brazil, and other South American countries. Sin Nombre virus was first associated with hantavirus pulmonary syndrome, but many additional hantaviruses have now been recognized as likely causes of this syndrome (Table 1). As Old World hantaviruses are generally associated with specific microtine rodents, so each American hantavirus appears to be associated with a specific sigmodontine host. A chain of apparent human-to-human transmission of Andes virus occurred during an outbreak in southern Argentina, including transmission to medical staff, suggesting that application of universal precautions when treating suspected cases of Hantavirus pulmonary syndrome may be warranted.

Symptoms

Hantavirus pulmonary syndrome is unusual in that symptoms are primarily those of acute unexplained adult respiratory distress syndrome, rather than renal disease. A nondescript prodrome of fever, myalgia, and malaise may last 4 to 6 days, with nausea, vomiting, and abdominal pain, often accompanied by dizziness. On admission, physical examination of patients with confirmed cases reveals fever (> 38 °C), tachycardia (> 100/min), tachypnoea (> 20/min), and often hypotension (systolic < 100 mmHg), and rales. Laboratory findings include hypoxia, leucocytosis, haemoconcentration, thrombocytopenia, atypical lymphocytosis, elevated serum lactate dehydrogenase and glutamic pyruvic transaminase, and prolonged prothrombin time (> 14 s). Chest radiography is helpful in diagnosis, noting progression from subtle interstitial findings to frank bilateral alveolar oedema; pleural effusions are usually present (Fig. 3). Thrombocytopenia and haemoconcentration are independent statistical predictors of Hanta-

virus pulmonary syndrome, although not present in every patient. Disease progresses rapidly once the lungs begin to fill, with death commonly seen in 24 to 48 h after admission, or sooner, due to hypoxia and/or circulatory failure. Hypotension and shock may occur independently in patients whose hypoxaemia is medically controlled.

Treatment and prognosis

Treatment is supportive, with careful management of hypoxia, fluid balance, and shock. About two-thirds of patients will require intubation and mechanical ventilation. Fluid loss into the lungs leads to haemoconcentration, but infusion of fluids exacerbates pulmonary oedema; consequently fluids should be administered with caution and careful monitoring. Limited experience in open label trials suggests that intravenous ribavirin does not have a marked effect on the course of Hantavirus pulmonary syndrome, perhaps because of the speed with which the disease progresses.

Control

Prevention involves avoidance of infected rodents, either through efficient rodent control programmes in urban settings for Seoul virus, or maintenance of clean campsites so that waste food is not allowed to accumulate and attract rodents. Vaccine development is under way, and nationally approved inactivated vaccines reported to be safe and efficacious against Hantaviruses are available for use in Asia.

Genus *Nairovirus*

The genus *Nairovirus* is named after Nairobi sheep disease, an acute, haemorrhagic gastroenteritis affecting sheep and goats in East Africa, with transmission by the sheep tick, *Rhipicephalus appendiculatus*. In addition to the type species, which has caused laboratory infections, the genus also includes several other viruses known to infect man, of which the most important is Crimean-Congo haemorrhagic fever virus. Other nairoviruses causing less important human infections are Ganjam virus, almost indistinguishable from Nairobi sheep disease virus but first isolated in India from *Haemaphysalis intermedia* ticks collected from healthy goats; Hazara virus, recovered from *Ixodes redkorzevi* ticks collected from the vole *Alticola roylei*, in a subarctic habitat at an altitude of 3660 m in the Khaghan valley of Hazara district, Pakistan; Dugbe virus, isolated in Nigeria from *Amblyomma variegatum* ticks collected from healthy cattle; and Soldado virus, repeatedly isolated from a variety of bird ticks but recently linked to a mild illness in man.

Crimean–Congo haemorrhagic fever virus

Crimean haemorrhagic fever was first recognized as a cause of an acute, febrile, haemorrhagic disease affecting man in the Crimean region of the

Fig. 3 Chest radiograph of patient with early Hantavirus pulmonary syndrome (L), and same patient 24 h later (R) showing development of bilateral perihilar alveolar oedema (by courtesy of Dr Loren Ketai).

former USSR, transmitted by ticks and carrying a mortality of 15 to 30 per cent. In Africa, Congo virus was first isolated in the then Belgian Congo (now Democratic Republic of the Congo) from the blood of a local 13-year-old boy, and it caused a moderately severe laboratory infection; related viruses were isolated in Uganda, where more laboratory infections occurred, one of which ended fatally after a severe haematemesis. In Asia, a virus indistinguishable from Congo virus was isolated from pools of ticks collected from a variety of wild and domestic animals in Western Pakistan. It was later demonstrated that Crimean haemorrhagic fever virus was serologically indistinguishable from Congo virus, hence the use of the term Crimean–Congo haemorrhagic fever virus. Different strains of this virus have been associated with outbreaks of severe and sometimes fatal disease in the Crimea, Rostov, and Astrakhan regions of the former USSR, in Albania, Bulgaria, and Yugoslavia, in East, West, and South Africa, in Iran, Iraq, and in Western Pakistan, and in China. Most infections are acquired by tick bites, but infections have occurred in both hospital and laboratory environments. In South Africa an association with wild birds has been reported.

The incubation period is about 1 week. The onset of fever is usually sudden, and fever is usually continuous, although occasionally remittent or biphasic. Signs and symptoms include fever, headache, nausea, vomiting, joint pains, backache, photophobia, together with circulatory disorders, thrombocytopenia, and leucopenia. Haemorrhagic manifestations are common, with bleeding from nasal, gastric, intestinal, uterine, and renal membranes (Fig. 4). Patients may present with acute abdominal pain, mimicking an acute surgical emergency, and operating-theatre staff have become infected and have died through contact with infected blood or secretions exposed at operation. The mortality is about 15 to 30 per cent, but may be as high as 40 to 80 per cent in hospital or nosocomial outbreaks. Transient hair loss has been reported.

Control, treatment, and prognosis

No vaccine is available. Avoidance of tick bites may reduce the risk of infection. In hospital outbreaks, meticulous attention to the containment of infected secretions is essential and barrier nursing should be used. There

Fig. 4 Patient with Crimean–Congo haemorrhagic fever showing extensive ecchymoses on the arms and thorax (by courtesy of Professor D.I.H. Simpson).

may be neurological involvement, which usually indicates a poor prognosis. Those patients who recover may be left with a polyneuritis that persists for months, but eventual recovery is to be expected.

Genus *Phlebovirus*

At least nine different phleboviruses are known to infect man (see Table 1). Pappataci fever, sandfly fever, or Phlebotomus fever was recognized as a clinical entity in the Mediterranean area during the nineteenth century, and the association with *Phlebotomus papatasi* sandflies was clearly demonstrated by showing that filtrates of human blood would reproduce the disease in human volunteers. For many years it was thought that man was the only vertebrate host, but antibody studies indicate that gerbils, cattle, and sheep may also be infected. Naples virus was isolated by American investigators from human serum collected during an outbreak of sandfly fever in Naples, and the Sicilian virus was isolated by the same workers from American troops with a similar fever in Palermo, Sicily. The two viruses have many common properties, but they are serologically quite distinct. Sandfly fever is widespread throughout the Mediterranean area, and also occurs in Egypt, Greece, Iran, Turkey, the former Yugoslavia, Bangladesh, India, Pakistan, and the southern states of the former USSR. Toscana virus, serologically related to the Naples virus, is found in countries bordering the Mediterranean; it is notable for its ability to infect the central nervous system, especially in central Italy where it is thought to be responsible for at least 80 per cent of acute summertime infections of the central nervous system in children. The viruses that cause classic sandfly fever do not occur in the New World, but in South and Central America a similar clinical condition follows infection with Alenquer, Candiru, Chagres, and Punta Toro viruses.

Rift Valley fever has long been known as a disease of domestic animals, mainly sheep, in East Africa, which occasionally spreads to farm workers and others handling infected animals. The infection is endemic, but seldom recognized, in many wild game animals in Africa. Molecular studies have established that Rift Valley fever virus is very similar to sandfly fever viruses and Punta Toro virus in having an ambisense replication mechanism; this property distinguishes the genus *Phlebovirus* from other genera within the family. In its biological properties, Rift Valley fever virus differs from the sandfly fever viruses, Punta Toro viruses, and most other members of the genus, in being normally transmitted by mosquitoes rather than sandflies. When it was recognized that the tick-transmitted Uukuniemi and Zaliv-Terpeniya viruses also shared an ambisense replication strategy, these viruses were removed from their earlier classification in the genus Uukuvirus and were redesignated to the genus *Phlebovirus*. The only evidence that Uukuniemi virus can infect man is the finding of specific antibodies in some human sera collected in Estonia and in the former Czechoslovakia. Zaliv-Terpeniya virus was isolated from bird ticks collected on an island in the Sea of Okhotsk, Sakhalin region, and there is some evidence that it may be pathogenic to man.

Sandfly fever, Naples, and Sicilian viruses

Symptoms

After an incubation period of 2 to 6 days, there is an abrupt onset of fever, chills, nausea and vomiting, epigastric pain, and often severe, generalized headache leading to incapacitating prostration. Fever of 38 to 40 °C usually resolves after 2 to 3 days, but may be biphasic and persist for a week. There is no rash, but small haemorrhages into the skin and mucous membranes may be seen. Photophobia and eye pain are not uncommon, lymphadenopathy is often seen, and the liver may be tender, although jaundice is rare. The disease is self-limiting, with complete recovery. No deaths have been attributed to either sandfly fever, Naples, or Sicilian viruses.

Rift Valley fever virus

Following its initial isolation in 1930 as the agent of enzootic hepatitis of domestic animals in Kenya, Rift Valley fever virus was recognized as the cause of sporadic human infections in East, Central, and West Africa, with a particular capacity to infect those handling the virus in the laboratory. In East and Central Africa the virus has been isolated from a variety of mosquito species and recent studies have shown that the virus is capable of persisting in mosquito eggs during the dry season, emerging when larvae hatch in the rainy season. From 1951 to 1956 there were severe epizootics in lambs in southern Africa, and many human cases occurred. Further human cases with several deaths were seen in South Africa in 1975, and a major outbreak occurred in East Africa following El Niño flooding in 1997 to 1998, apparently seeding a 'virgin soil' outbreak in Saudi Arabia and Yemen in 2000.

.In the Central African Republic in 1969 a virus isolated from *Mansonia africana* mosquitoes and named Zinga virus was associated with several cases of haemorrhagic fever; Zinga virus was later shown to be a strain of Rift Valley fever virus. In West Africa, Rift Valley fever virus was isolated from mosquitoes in Nigeria and from bats in Guinea, but despite the presence of antibodies in human sera collected in Nigeria and Senegal, human disease was unrecognized until 1987 when a substantial epidemic occurred in Mauritania, with further epidemics in following years. In 1977 the virus spread, apparently for the first time, into Egypt, producing a major epizootic in domestic animals, principally sheep and goats, but also cattle, and causing some 600 human deaths within a period of 3 months. The virus has been detected periodically since then in Egypt, and the principal vector seems to be the mosquito, *Culex pipiens*. It is of interest that both the Egyptian and the Mauritanian epidemics appear to be linked to major ecological changes following the construction of the Aswan Dam on the Nile and dams on the Senegal River.

Symptoms

After an incubation period of 3 to 6 days there is an abrupt onset of fever, shivering, nausea and vomiting, epigastric pain, and often severe, generalized headache. The fever may be biphasic, with temperatures between 38 and 40 °C, and may remain elevated for at least a week. There is no rash, but small haemorrhages into the skin and mucous membranes may be seen. Photophobia and eye pains are not uncommon; there may be conjunctival inflammation, and a central serous retinitis, leading to central scotoma and sometimes to retinal detachment. The fundus may show macular exudates that are slow to disappear. There is often a lymphadenopathy, and although the liver is frequently involved and may be tender, jaundice is rare, but appears to have been more common during the recent outbreaks in Mauritania. Convalescence may be protracted, but is usually uncomplicated; however, a small percentage of patients may suffer severe complications such as haemorrhagic fever, encephalitis, or eye lesions. Haemorrhagic disease presents as above, but progresses with petechial, mucous membrane, and gastrointestinal haemorrhagic, jaundice with severe liver and renal dysfunction often progressing to disseminated intravascular coagulation, hepatorenal syndrome, and may end in death. Patients with encephalitis typically recover from acute febrile disease only to present within a few days to 2 weeks later with headache, meningismus, confusion, and fever, often leading to residua or ending in death. Ocular complications are characterized by rapid onset of decreased visual acuity due to retinal haemorrhage, exudates, and macular oedema. These are also seen after apparent recovery from the initial disease. About half of these patients suffer some degree of permanent vision loss. Deaths from Rift Valley fever were rare before the 1977 outbreak in Egypt, but the Mauritanian epidemics in which at least 25 persons died with jaundice and haemorrhagic manifestations, and the recent East African and Arabian Peninsula outbreaks with several hundred suspect fatalities clearly establishes it as a life-threatening infection.

Control, treatment, and prognosis

Veterinary vaccines have been used for a number of years, and formalin-inactivated vaccines have also had limited use for the prevention of disease in laboratory workers and others exposed to high risk of infection. Improved vaccines based on molecular techniques are under development. Although there are no reports of nosocomial transmission, barrier nursing would be a sensible precaution.

Unassigned viruses and viruses causing only minor disease in man

The great majority of the viruses listed in Table 2 cause only a mild, febrile illness, but the following show certain additional features.

Bhanja virus (unassigned)

This virus was first isolated from *Haemaphysalis intermedia* ticks collected from healthy goats in India, but has since been isolated in Sri Lanka, in Africa, and in Europe. Infection of goats is widespread in Italy and in the former Yugoslavia, where there have been several reported human cases, including some with severe neurological disease, and at least two deaths. Laboratory infections have also occurred.

Bwamba virus (*Bunyavirus*)

This was first isolated in Uganda in 1941 and is very widespread throughout sub-Saharan Africa. More than 75 per cent of adult human sera collected in Nigeria and over 95 per cent of human sera collected in Uganda and Tanzania have antibodies against Bwamba virus. The original cases showed fever, headache, generalized body pains, and conjunctivitis, but no rash, although a rash has been described in the Central African Republic. No fatalities have been reported.

Nyando virus (*Bunyavirus*)

This virus was first isolated from mosquitoes in Kenya; it has since been isolated from man in the Central African Republic, where it caused fever, myalgia, and encephalitis.

Tataguine virus (unassigned)

This causes fever, rash, and joint pains in at least five African countries (Cameroon, Central African Republic, Ethiopia, Nigeria, and Senegal).

Wanowrie virus (unassigned)

This virus was first isolated in India from *Hyalomma marginatum* ticks collected from sheep. It has also been isolated in Egypt and Iran, and in Sri Lanka, where it was recovered from the brain of a 17-year-old girl who died following a 2-day fever with abdominal pain and vomiting.

Further reading

Bartelloni PJ, Tesh RB (1976). Clinical and serologic responses of volunteers infected with phlebotomus fever virus (Sicilian type). *American Journal of Tropical Medicine and Hygiene* 25, 456–62.

Calisher CH, Thompson WH, eds (1983). *California serogroup viruses. Progress in Clinical and Biological Research*, Vol 123. Alan R. Liss, New York.

Hooper JW, Li D (2001). Vaccines against hantaviruses. *Current Topics in Microbiology and Immunology* 256, 171–91.

LeDuc JW (1995). Hantavirus infections. In: Porterfield JS, ed. *Exotic viral infections*, pp 261–84. Chapman & Hall, London.

LeDuc JW, Pinheiro FP (1989). Oropouche fever. In: Monath TP, ed. *The arboviruses: epidemiology and ecology*, Vol 4, pp 1–14. CRC Press, Boca Raton, Florida.

Lee HW, Calisher C, Schmaljohn, CS (1999). *Manual of hemorrhagic fever with renal syndrome and hantavirus pulmonary syndrome*. WHO Collaborating Center for Virus Reference and Research (Hantaviruses), Seoul, Korea.

Monath TP, ed. (1989). *The arboviruses: epidemiology and ecology*. CRC Press, Boca Raton, Florida.

Peters CJ (1997). Emergence of Rift Valley fever. In: Saluzzo JF, Dodet B, eds. *Factors in the emergence of arbovirus diseases*, pp 253–64. Elsevier, Paris.

Peters CJ (1998). Hantavirus pulmonary syndrome in the Americas. *Emerging Infections* 2, 17–64.

Peters CJ, LeDuc JW (1991). Bunyaviridae: bunyaviruses, phleboviruses, and related viruses. In: Belshe RB, ed.. *Textbook of human virology*, 2nd edn, pp 571–614. Mosby Year Book, St. Louis.

Pinheiro FP *et al.* (1981). Oropouche virus. I. A review of clinical, epidemiological, and ecological findings. *American Journal of Tropical Medicine and Hygiene* 30, 149–60.

Saluzzo JF, Dodet B, eds (1999). *Factors in the emergence and control of rodent-borne viral disease (hantaviral and arenal diseases)*. Elsevier, Paris.

Swanepoel R (1995). Nairovirus infections. In: Porterfield JS, ed. *Exotic viral infections*, pp 285–93.Chapman & Hall, London.

Tesh RB (1989). Phlebotomus fevers. In: Monath TP, ed. *The arboviruses: epidemiology and ecology*, Vol 4, pp 15–27. CRC Press, Boca Raton, Florida.

7.10.15 Arenaviruses

Susan Fisher-Hoch and Joseph McCormick

General considerations

Ecology and epidemiology

Arenaviruses infect rodents in the New and Old Worlds. There are at least 15 arenaviruses but only five produce significant human disease (Fig. 1); Lassa, Junin, Machupo, Guanarito, Sabia and lymphocytic choriomeningitis virus (LCMV). Arenaviruses have coevolved over very long periods of time with their natural rodent host so that the distribution of a given virus is restricted to its host range. Further, division into Old World (LCMV, Lassa) and New World (Tacaribe complex) viruses based on geographic distribution and antigenic typing is endorsed by nucleocapsid sequencing data.

Rodents normally experience silent, lifelong infection, with perinatal transmission. Lifelong viruria is the primary source of contamination of the environment. Human infection results from intrusion into the rodents' ecological niche or infestation of poor housing. The virus infects through skin lesions and possibly mucosae or rodent-urine-contaminated dust aerosol. Human-to-human spread is common for Lassa fever both in community and hospital settings, but is apparently rare with the other pathogenic arenaviruses. Disease may be severe and haemorrhagic and all the pathogenic arenaviruses require Biosafety Level 4 (BSL4), except LCMV (BSL3).

Virology

By electron microscopy, host-cell ribosomes included in the virion resemble grains of sand ('arena' = sand in Latin) (Fig. 2). They are enveloped, pleomorphic, membrane viruses 50 to 300 nm (mean 110–130 nm) in diameter with a virion density in sucrose of 1.17 g/cm^3. They contain two segments of single-stranded RNA, tightly associated with a nucleocapsid protein of 65 000 to 72 000 molecular weight. The large strand of ambisense RNA, of molecular weight 2.0 to 3.2 × 10^6, codes for the viral polymerase and a zinc finger protein. The small single strand of ambisense RNA, molecular weight about 1.1 to 1.6 × 10^6, encodes the glycoprotein precursor and the nucleoprotein. The genome is enclosed in a membrane bearing two glycosylated proteins of molecular weights 34 000 to 44 000 (G1) and 54 000 to 72 000 (G2), derived from glycoprotein precursor by post-translational cleavage. Antigenic cross-reactivity is conserved at least at one epitope across all known arenaviruses.

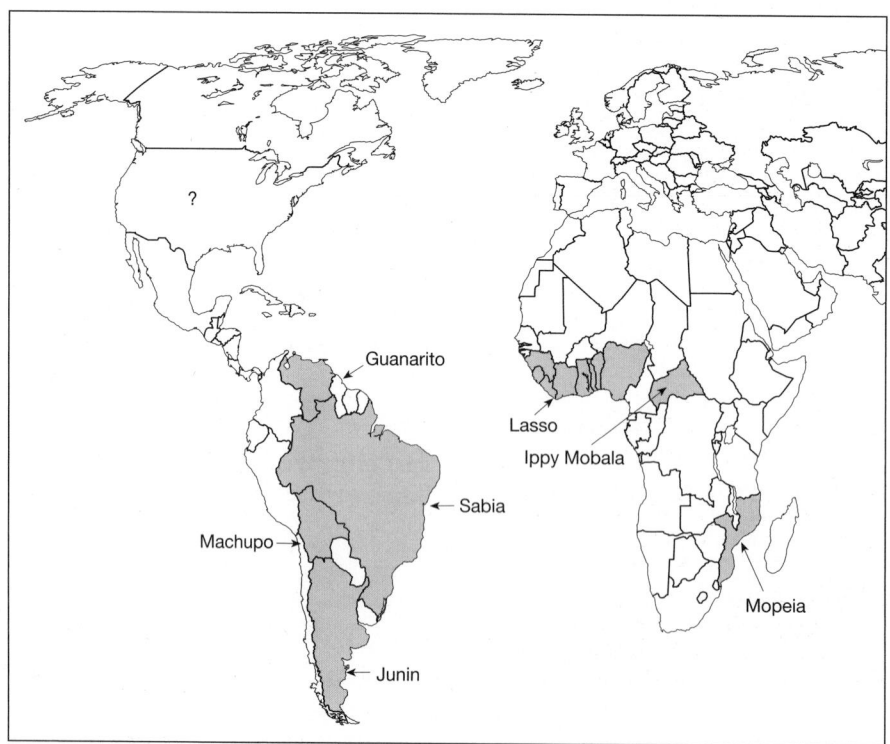

Fig. 1 World map showing the approximate distribution of arenaviruses.

Old World arenaviruses

Lassa fever

Epidemiology

Distribution and ecology

Lassa fever was first described in West Africa in the 1950s, but not isolated until 1969. It occurs from Northern Nigeria to Guinea, an area with a population of perhaps 180 million. Its only known reservoir is *Mastomys natalensis*, one of Africa's commonest rodents. In southern Africa, a related *Mastomys* carries the closely related Mopeia virus which can infect humans but is unable to cause significant clinical disease. *Mastomys* are highly commensal with man. In some areas, 50 per cent of domestic rodents may be *Mastomys*, averaging 2.4 animals per house, but they have limited movement within a village. Prevalence of Lassa virus infection is variable in *Mastomys* and tends to cluster in houses, so that infection is endemic but focal.

Lassa fever is the haemorrhagic fever most likely to occur in travellers returning to developed countries. In the year 2000, at least four cases were imported into Europe. Cases in foreigners in 2000 have been seen during peacekeeping efforts in Sierra Leone. The rebels' stronghold is at the centre of the Lassa fever endemic area.

(a)

(b)

Fig. 2 Electronmicrographs of arenaviruses. (a) Machupo virus in tissue culture. Arrow shows virus budding through cell membrane. (b) Lassa virus budding from cell membrane.

Epidemiology

Lassa fever is the arenavirus which affects the largest number of humans. Over 200 000 infections occur annually, and several thousand deaths. All age groups and sexes are affected. Antibody prevalence increases with age suggesting that most virus transmission to humans takes place in and around the home. Antibody prevalence ranges from 4 to 6 per cent in Guinea, 15 to 20 per cent in Nigeria, and up to 60 per cent in some villages in Sierra Leone. Seroconversion to Lassa virus positive ranged from 5 to 22 per cent/year among seronegative Sierra Leonean villagers. Disease to infection ratios range from 9 to 26 per cent in Sierra Leone, and the proportion of febrile illness associated with seroconversion to Lassa virus from 5 to 14 per cent. Five to 8 per cent of infected people may be hospitalized, of whom 17 per cent may die if untreated. However, the case fatality for all Lassa virus infections (hospitalized and non-hospitalized, symptomatic and asymptomatic) may be as low as 2 per cent. In endemic areas, Lassa fever may account for 10 to 16 per cent of all adult medical admissions and about 30 per cent of adult deaths among medical admissions.

Transmission

Direct contact between virus contaminated articles and surfaces and cuts and scratches on bare hands and feet may be the most important and consistent mode of transmission in endemic areas. The sporadic pattern of human infection in the community does not suggest aerosol transmission. Nosocomial spread in hospitals is associated with inadequate disinfection and direct contact with infected blood and contaminated needles. Increasing and indiscriminate use of routine intravenous therapy in West African hospitals, along with inadequate needle and syringe care, led to large-scale epidemics. A prospective study in a hospital in an endemic area showed that simple but rigorous barrier nursing techniques can reduce the frequency of infection in hospital personnel handling Lassa fever patients. In London, none of 159 unprotected hospital contacts of a severely ill Lassa fever patient was infected. In developed countries, (United Kingdom and United States) in 1990, there were no secondary infections among 907 documented hospital contacts of infected patients (188 classified as high risk).

Risk factors

Rodent-to-human infection is strongly associated with indiscriminate food storage, and practices such as catching, cooking, and eating rodents. Person-to-person spread is common in households. Risk of infection in villages is associated with direct contact, nursing care, or sexual contact with someone during the incubation, acute, or convalescent phases of illness.

Clinical features

Incubation period and prodrome

Following an incubation period of 7 to 18 days, symptoms begin insidiously with fever, weakness, malaise, severe, usually frontal, headache, and a painful sore throat (Fig. 3). More than 50 per cent of patients then develop joint and lumbar pain and 60 per cent or more develop a non-productive cough. Severe retrosternal chest pain, nausea with vomiting or diarrhoea, and abdominal pain are also common.

Respiratory and pulse rate and temperature are elevated and blood pressure may be low. There is no characteristic rash; petechiae and ecchymoses are not seen. About a third of patients will have conjunctivitis. More than two-thirds have pharyngitis, half with exudates, diffusely inflamed and swollen posterior pharynx and tonsils, but few ulcers or petechiae. The abdomen is tender in 50 per cent of patients. Neurological signs in the early stages are limited to a fine tremor, most marked in the lips and tongue.

Severe disease

Up to a third of hospitalized patients progress to a prostrating illness 6 to 8 days after onset of fever, usually with persistent vomiting and diarrhoea. Patients are often dehydrated with elevated haematocrit. Proteinuria occurs

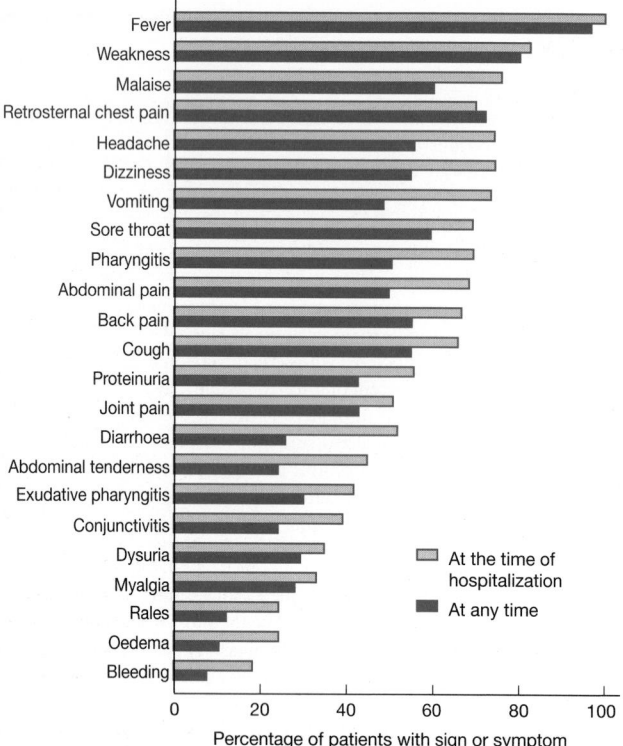

Fig. 3 Frequency of signs and symptoms of Lassa fever.

in two-thirds of patients, with moderately elevated blood urea nitrogen. About half of Lassa fever patients have diffuse abdominal tenderness without localizing signs or loss of bowel sounds. The severe retrosternal or epigastric pain seen in many patients may be due to pleural or pericardial involvement. Bleeding is seen in only 15 to 20 per cent of patients, restricted to mucosal surfaces, conjunctivitis, gastrointestinal, or genital tracts. Severe pulmonary oedema and adult respiratory distress syndrome is common in fatal cases with gross head and neck oedema, stridor, and hypovolaemic shock (Fig. 4).

Over 70 per cent of patients have abnormal electrocardiograms (nonspecific ST-segment and T-wave abnormalities, ST-segment elevation, generalized low voltage complexes, and changes reflecting electrolyte disturbance), but none correlates with clinical or other measures of disease

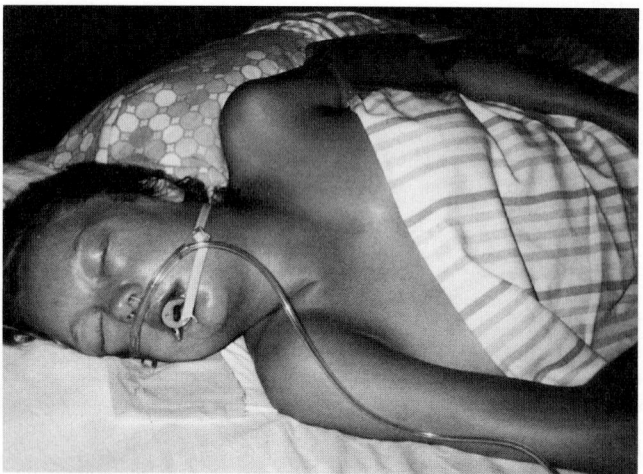

Fig. 4 Acute Lassa fever in a patient showing facial oedema, decerebrate posturing, and respiratory distress. This patient survived.

severity or outcome. There is no clinical evidence of myocarditis. Neurological signs are infrequent, but carry a poor prognosis, progressing from confusion to severe encephalopathy with or without general seizures, but without focal signs. Cerebrospinal fluid is usually normal, apart from a few lymphocytes, and low titres of virus relative to serum. Pneumonitis and pleural and pericardial rubs develop in early convalescence in about 20 per cent of hospitalized patients, sometimes associated with congestive cardiac failure.

Laboratory measurements

A normal mean white blood cell count on admission to hospital ($6 \times 10^9/1$) may mask early lymphopenia with relative or absolute neutrophilia, as high as $30 \times 10^9/l$. Thrombocytopenia is moderate, even in severely ill patients, but platelet function is markedly depressed. Serum aspartate aminotransferase levels greater than 150 U/l are associated with a case fatality of 50 per cent (Fig. 5). The ratio of aspartate aminotransferase to alanine aminotransferase is as high as 11:1. Prothrombin times, glucose, and bilirubin levels are nearly normal, excluding biochemical hepatic failure.

Viraemia of greater than 3 $\log_{10}$ TCID$_{50}$/ml is associated with increasing case fatality (Fig. 5). High virus titres occur in liver, ovary, pancreas, uterus, and placenta, but there is no histological evidence of organ failure. High viraemia and aspartate aminotransferase together carry a risk of death of nearly 80 per cent.

Mortality

The overall death rate for all infections may be as low as 2 per cent, but is about 16 per cent in hospitalized patients. In Nigeria, much higher death rates have been observed. The case fatality may be over 30 per cent in the third trimester of pregnancy, and 50 per cent in patients with haemorrhage.

Complications and sequelae

Nearly 30 per cent of patients develop uni- or bilateral-deafness beginning during convalescence. About half show a near or complete recovery after 3 to 4 months, but the other half remain permanently deaf. Many patients also exhibit transient cerebellar signs during convalescence, particularly tremors and ataxia. Infrequent complications are uveitis, pericarditis, orchitis, pleural effusion, ascites, and acute adrenal insufficiency. Renal and hepatic failure are not seen.

Lassa fever in pregnancy

Lassa fever is a common cause of maternal mortality in parts of West Africa. In the third trimester there is a two to three-fold risk of maternal death

Fig. 5 Cumulative survival in Lassa fever related to serum viraemia and aspartate aminotransferase (AST) levels.

from infection. Very high levels of virus replication have been found in placental tissue. Mortality was reduced four-fold in women spontaneously or therapeutically aborted (OR for fatality with pregnancy intact 5.5). Fetal loss is as much as 87 per cent, and does not seem to vary by trimester. Lassa virus is present in the breast milk of infected mothers, and neonates are therefore at risk of congenital, intrapartum, and puerperal infection.

Lassa fever in children

Lassa fever is common in children, but may be difficult to diagnose. In very young babies marked oedema has been reported. In older children the disease may manifest as diarrhoea, pneumonia, or an unexplained prolonged fever. In a hospital in Sierra Leone, 21 per cent of paediatric admissions had Lassa fever, with 12 per cent fatality. An outpatient study found 24/435 children (6 per cent) with evidence of previous Lassa infection and 68 who seroconverted (16 per cent).

Differential diagnosis

The diagnosis of Lassa fever must be considered if there is a history of potential exposure to rodents or patients in or from West Africa. Cerebral malaria or septicaemia must be excluded but double infections can occur, particularly with malaria. In West Africa, fever with pharyngitis, proteinuria, and retrosternal chest pain had a predictive value for Lassa fever of 81 per cent and a specificity of 89 per cent. Likewise a triad of pharyngitis, retrosternal chest pain, and proteinuria (in a febrile patient) correctly predicted Lassa fever 80 per cent of the time (sensitivity 50 per cent). Bleeding and sore throat had specificity for fatal outcome of 90 per cent (sensitivity only 36 per cent). In contrast, vomiting and sore throat had a specificity of only 47 per cent for fatal disease (sensitivity 89 per cent).

Pathogenic processes

Pathogenesis

Arenaviruses invade through broken skin to lymph nodes, progressing to generalized multiorgan infection, affecting especially the reticuloendothelial system. In Lassa fever, severe disease manifestations are intractable hypovolaemic shock, and/or severe central nervous system involvement, bleeding, and oedema of the face. There is endothelial and platelet dysfunction, despite adequate numbers of circulating platelets.

Pathology

There is focal necrosis of the liver, but damage is insufficient to cause fatal hepatic failure. A substantial macrophage response is seen with little, if any, lymphocytic inflammatory response. Moderate splenic necrosis primarily involves the marginal zone of the periarteriolar lymphocytic sheath. Diffuse focal adrenocortical cellular necrosis has been less frequently observed.

Immunology

The immunological response is complex. While neutralizing antibodies are associated with clearance of viraemia due to the South American arenaviruses, Lassa and lymphocytic choriomeningitis viruses appear to depend primarily on cytotoxic T-cell responses. There appears to be a brisk B-cell response with a classic primary IgG and IgM antibody response to Lassa virus early in the illness. By the sixth day of illness IgG antibodies are found in 46 per cent of patients and IgM antibody in 59 per cent. By the sixteenth day of illness both are found in 100 per cent of patients, but this does not coincide with virus clearance. A high viraemia and high IgG and IgM titres often coexist in both humans and primates, and virus may persist in the serum and urine of humans for several months after infection, and probably in occult sites, such as renal tissue, for years.

In a minority of patients, some low titre serum neutralizing activity may be observed several months after resolution of the disease. Controlled clinical trials with human convalescent plasma containing high titred antibodies have shown no protective effect. Thus the clearance of Lassa virus appears to be independent of antibody formation. In non-human primates, killed vaccine and vaccinia-vectored vaccines expressing the nucleoprotein elicited high level antibodies to Lassa virus but no protection, while vaccinia-vectored glycoprotein vaccine elicited little antibody, but nevertheless

provided protection. Reinfection following natural Lassa infection may occur in humans, apparently without clinical disease.

Laboratory procedures

Diagnosis

Laboratory diagnosis is by isolation of virus from serum, demonstration of a four-fold rise in antibody titre, or high-titre IgG antibody with virus-specific IgM antibody in association with compatible clinical disease, or more recently by detection of viral sequences by reverse transcriptase polymerase chain reaction (RT-PCR), or by detection of viral proteins using an ELISA system.

Virus isolation may be accomplished easily from serum or tissues in cell cultures, but should be performed in BSL4 laboratory facilities . Specimens should be drawn into a vacuum tube to minimize risk of infection. Virus has also been isolated from breast milk, spinal fluid, pleural and pericardial transudate, and from autopsy material. Virus excretion in urine is intermittent but may persist. Antigen detection in conjunctival scrapings, buffy coat preparations, cells from pharyngeal aspirates, and urinary sediment have not been successful. ELISA tests have been notoriously difficult to calibrate in the field, particularly in West Africa. Newer serological tests include recombinant immunoblot techniques. Because of its superior sensitivity and specificity, where possible the ELISA should be used. Specific IgM, if detected early in disease, indicates acute infection. Antigen detection by ELISA and ELISA for IgM have recently been shown to have a specificity of 90 per cent and a sensitivity of 88 per cent compared with RT-PCR, but IgG was only detected in 16 per cent of the cases. A rising titre, with or without IgM, can be very useful in acute diagnosis. The RT-PCR or hybridization is much more rapid, and is as sensitive as virus isolation, and more sensitive than antigen detection by ELISA, and is the assay of choice for reference laboratories when a rapid diagnosis is needed. No commercial diagnostic reagents are currently available. BSL4 reference laboratories do not produce non-infectious reagents for use by other laboratories.

Containment and disinfection

Lassa virus is robust, and withstands drying. Blood from severely ill patients may contain 10^9 infectious units per ml, and rodent urine may contain 10^4 infectious units/ml. However, it can be inactivated by heat, detergents, chlorine, formalin, and UV radiation (including sunshine). Antigenic properties are best conserved by inactivation with gamma irradiation. Disinfection by washing with 0.5 per cent phenol in detergent (for example Lysol), 0.5 per cent hypochlorite solution, formaldehyde, or paracetic acid is recommended.

Patient management

Supportive care

Fluid, electrolyte, respiratory, and osmotic imbalances should be corrected, and full intensive care support, including mechanical ventilation offered if required. However, even vigorous support may be insufficient to prevent fatal progression of advanced disease. Pregnant patients often present with absent fetal movements, and survival may depend on aggressive obstetric intervention.

Antiviral therapy

Ribavirin (tribavarin) is effective but must be given early in disease. Ribavirin is given by intravenous infusion as a 2-g loading dose followed by 1 g every 6 h for 4 days then 0.5 g every 8 h for 6 more days. Toxicity is confined to mild reversible anaemia. A five to ten-fold decrease in the case–fatality ratio was demonstrated in patients treated with ribavirin compared with untreated patients when therapy was given within the first 6 days of illness. Patients with high aspartate aminotransferase and viraemia, risk factors for unfavourable outcome (Fig. 5), who were treated within the first 6 days of illness suffered a 5 to 9 per cent case fatality. Those with the same risk factors receiving treatment more than 6 days after the onset of illness had a 26 to 47 per cent fatality, compared with 52 to 78 per cent untreated. Ribavirin is contraindicated in early pregnancy because of potential teratogenicity, but the fetus rarely survives the infection. It has been used in late pregnancy (>24 weeks) but its efficacy has not yet been determined.

Prevention

Hospital containment

The key to prevention of human-to-human transmission is isolation of febrile patients and rigorous use of gloves and disinfection. Complete support, including intensive care, or surgery, should be provided. Patient isolators should not be used since they induce loss of manual dexterity and inhibit intensive care and communication. Recommendations issued for patient management and handling of clinical specimens from AIDS patients are adequate for containment of Lassa fever.

Contacts

High risk is associated with percutaneous or mucosal contact with blood or body fluids. Medium risk contacts (unprotected contact with blood or body fluids) may safely be observed for development of persistent high fever for 3 weeks from the last date of contact by daily temperature measurement and telephone reporting. The practice of following up airline passengers and other low risk contacts (no unprotected physical contact with patient or body fluids) is unnecessary.

Prophylaxis

Oral ribavirin should be offered to high-risk contacts as soon as possible after exposure to Lassa virus (600 mg orally, four times a day for 10 days).

Vaccine

A vaccinia virus recombinant expressing Lassa glycoprotein (G) protected primates from infection, but a nucleoprotein expressing recombinant did not. Immunization of primates with inactivated (gamma irradiated) whole Lassa virus resulted in brisk antibody responses to both proteins, but all animals died with serum virus titres equal to unvaccinated controls. In humans, the presence of antibody to neither glycoprotein nor nucleoprotein at the time of hospital admission was associated with survival, or even severity of disease.

Following Lassa virus challenge, high survival rates are seen after vaccination with vaccines expressing G, despite low or undetectable antibody levels preinfection. The duration of the interval between vaccination and challenge, and the challenge dose, affected the efficacy of vaccines. Almost all surviving, asymptomatic animals experienced viraemia, even those vaccinated with Mopeia virus (essentially a live, attenuated Lassa virus), consistent with the hypothesis that virus replication is controlled by CTL responses and not antibody responses. These data show that the G gene is necessary and sufficient to protect primates against a large parenteral challenge dose (Table 1).

Persistence

Lassa virus may persist at low titre for a limited time in primates, but virus is sequestered, and transmission is unlikely. Viraemia in patients is quickly controlled. However, virus may be detected intermittently in human urine for up to 60 days.

Control

Control of rodents would prevent Lassa fever in West Africa. Improvement of housing and food storage might reduce the domestic rodent population, but such changes are not easily made without massive improvement in the local economy.

Lymphocytic choriomeningitis virus

Epidemiology

Distribution and ecology

Lymphocytic choriomeningitis (LCMV) virus was isolated in 1933 from the cerebrospinal fluid of a patient with suspected St Louis encephalitis. It is widely distributed in its natural host, *Mus musculus*. Transmission from feral rodents to humans rarely results in clusters of disease, and person-to-person spread has not been demonstrated. The virus has acquired scientific importance in laboratory studies of immunological tolerance and virus-induced immunopathological disease.

Epidemiology

The prevalence of antibody to LCMV virus in the general population is between 1 and 5 per cent. Sporadic disease in rural areas occurs during the colder months but in urban areas with large rodent populations the epidemiology may be different. In Baltimore, 4.7 per cent of those attending a sexually transmitted disease clinic had antibodies to LCMV.

Risk factors and transmission

Although feral mice cause sporadic infection, the most common sources of human infection are pet or laboratory rodents particularly hamsters, white mice, or nude mice. Laboratory outbreaks of human disease have followed contact with infected animals or virus, and aerosol transmission may have occurred.

Clinical features

Incubation period and disease

The incubation period is about 1 to 3 weeks. About 35 per cent of infections are asymptomatic, and a further 50 per cent have a febrile illnesses without significant central nervous system manifestations. About 15 per cent have lymphocytic choriomeningitis (disease to infection ratio 1:3). Illness begins with fever, malaise, weakness, myalgia, and headache, often severe, retro-orbital, and associated with photophobia. Anorexia, nausea,

Table 1 Results of vaccination with vaccines expressing different components of Lassa virus

Virion protein expression	Protection (%)	Vaccine	N	Survivors	Median day of death (range)	Mean viraemia at death (log₁₀)
None	0	NTBH Vaccinia	3	0	15 (15–19)	5.7
		None	7	0	12 (10–15)	
Single glycoproteins	0	V-LSG1	2	0	15 (14–16)	6.8
		V-LSG2	2	0	12.5 (12–13)	
Nucleoprotein	27	V-LSN	11	3	11.5 (9–13)	6.7
Full glycoprotein	88	V-LSG	7	6	21 (21)	2.5
		V-LSG1 + V-LSG2	2	2		
Full S-segment	90	Mopeia virus	2	2		
		V-LSG + V-LSN	6	5	11 (11)	7.0
		V-LSG/N	2	2		
Total			44	20		

dizziness, and myalgia are common. Only two deaths have been reported, but there is prolonged convalescence.

Laboratory findings

Leucopenia and mild thrombocytopenia are common, and cerebrospinal fluid from patients with meningeal signs contains several hundred white cells, predominantly lymphocytes (>80 per cent), with slightly increased protein and occasionally low sugar levels. Virus is found in spinal fluid during acute disease.

Complications and sequelae

About one-third of patients with central nervous system manifestations will develop encephalopathy while the rest exhibit aseptic meningitis. An interstitial pneumonia, alopecia, orchitis, and transient arthritis of the hands have been described. Convalescence is prolonged with persistent fatigue, somnolence, and dizziness, and deafness. Neurological sequelae are unusual.

Differential diagnosis

LCMV should be considered in patients with fever with persistent meningeal signs, particularly if a history of rodent contact is elicited.

Pathogenic processes

Pathology

There are no published descriptions of the pathology of LCMV infection in humans. In one report of a fatal case there was perivascular macrophage infiltration in multiple areas of the brain. Antigen was observed in the meninges and cortical cells by IFA. In animal studies, the leptomeninges show dense infiltration with lymphocytic cells, with little involvement of the brain parenchyma.

Immunology

Antibody to LCMV appears in the first week of illness, with titres peaking at 40 to 60 days. In the natural host, the mouse, the immunology of natural and experimental infection has been extensively studied, but extrapolation to human disease needs to be made with caution.

Laboratory diagnosis

Virus may be cultured from cerebrospinal fluid or detected using RT-PCR during the acute phase of disease. IgG and IgM antibody may be detected in serum.

Patient management

There is no standard treatment for LCMV infection. Ribavirin is effective *in vitro*, but penetration into the cerebrospinal fluid is poor, however as the disease is severely debilitating its use should be considered.

Prevention

Laboratory outbreaks continue to occur, particularly through handling of persistently infected mice. The virus is a major laboratory hazard, and care must be taken to avoid infection. Exposure is too infrequent for there to be a market for a vaccine.

New World arenaviruses

The New World arenaviruses causing human disease are Junin (Argentine haemorrhagic fever), Machupo (Bolivian haemorrhagic fever), Guanarito (Venezuelan haemorrhagic fever), and Sabia (Brazilian haemorrhagic fever). The most important rodent hosts are the South American genera *Calomys*, *Sigmodon*, and *Oryzomys*. Together these are known as the South American haemorrhagic fevers. All are endemic in geographically limited areas, but new, related viruses are emerging in other yet unaffected areas. Between June 1999 and May 2000 three patients, two from southern California and a third from the San Francisco Bay area, died of an acute febrile illness with lymphopenia, thrombocytopenia, and acute respiratory distress syndrome. Two had liver failure and haemorrhagic manifestations. RNA fragments detected by PCR from all three patients shared 87 per cent identity with a recently described arenavirus from New Mexico, Whitewater Arroyo virus.

Argentine haemorrhagic fever

Epidemiology

Distribution and ecology

Argentine haemorrhagic fever was first recognized in the 1950s in the fertile farmland of north-western Buenos Aires Province in Argentina, and Junin virus was first isolated in 1958. The major rodent hosts are *Calomys musculinus* and *Calomys laucha* which, unlike *Mastomys* or *Mus*, are affected by the virus, with up to 50 per cent fatality in infected suckling animals, and stunted growth in many others. These are agrarian rodents, and most human cases are male agricultural workers, particularly harvesters of sugar cane.

Virology

Monoclonal antibody studies show Junin to be most closely related to Machupo and Tacaribe viruses, otherwise cross-reactivity with other New World arenaviruses is restricted to the nucleoprotein. Junin viruses comprise three clades depending on geographical origin, with the live attenuated Argentine haemorrhagic fever vaccine strain, Candid 1, a fourth, separate clade. No particular viral epitopes have been associated with varying severity or clinical forms of the human disease.

Epidemiology

About 21 000 cases have been reported since the early 1960s, averaging about 360 a year with wide annual fluctuations. Peak incidence is during summer and early autumn. The disease appeared to spread to new areas as incidence in the earlier affected areas decreased, possibly because of the virus' effect on rodent populations. Overall human antibody prevalence is about 12 per cent, with predominance in male agriculture workers, and about 30 per cent had no history of typical illness, (disease to infection ratio 2:3). The recent introduction of a live attenuated vaccine has dramatically reduced the incidence.

Transmission

The major routes of virus transmission to humans is probably through virus-infected dust, and mechanical harvesters are traditionally cited. Whether infection is through contamination of cuts and abrasions or mucosae or by aerosol is unclear. There is no recorded person-to-person spread. Recent studies have shown that the major host species, *Calomys musculinus*, is most frequently captured from roadsides and fence lines.

Clinical features

Incubation period and prodrome

After an incubation period of about 12 days, there is insidious onset of malaise, high fever, severe myalgia, anorexia, lumbar pain, epigastric pain and abdominal tenderness, conjunctivitis and retro-orbital pain, often with photophobia, and constipation. Nausea and vomiting frequently occur after 2 or 3 days of illness. There is no lymphadenopathy or splenomegaly, sore throat or cough, but there is high fever, marked erythema of the face, neck, and thorax, and conjunctivitis. Respiratory symptoms are uncommon. Petechiae appear by the forth or fifth days of the illness. There may be a pharyngeal enanthem, but pharyngitis is uncommon.

Severe disease

The infection either resolves after about 6 days or progresses to severe disease. In contrast to Lassa fever, South American haemorrhagic fevers are associated with haemorrhagic manifestations in nearly half of the patients (gingival haemorrhages, epistaxis, metrorrhagia, petechiae, ecchymoses, purpura, melaena, and haematuria). Severe cases have nausea, vomiting, intense proteinuria, microscopic haematuria, oliguria, and uraemia. Fatal cases develop hypotensive shock, hypothermia, and pulmonary oedema.

Renal failure has been reported but glomerular filtration rates, renal plasma flow, and creatinine clearance are usually normal. There is some electro-cardiographic evidence of myocarditis. Fifty per cent of Argentine haemorrhagic fever and Bolivian haemorrhagic fever patients also have neurological symptoms during the second stage of illness, such as tremors of the hands and tongue, progressing in some patients to delirium, oculo-gyrus, and strabismus. Meningeal signs and cerebrospinal fluid abnormalities are rare.

Laboratory findings

A low white blood cell count and a platelet count are invariable. Bleeding and clot retraction times are concomitantly prolonged. Though reductions of levels of Factors II, V, VII, VIII, and X and of fibrinogen are observed, alterations in clotting functions are usually minor. Disseminated intravascular coagulation is not a significant feature, despite some reports of the presence of fibrinogen degradation products and absence of fibrinolysis. Proteinuria is common and microscopic haematuria also occurs. Liver and renal function tests are only mildly abnormal. Virus titres in serum are not as high as in Lassa fever, but the infection is also apparently pantropic.

In a febrile patient, the combination of a platelet count of less than $100\,000/mm^2$ and a white blood cell count of less than $2500/mm^2$ has a sensitivity and specificity of 87 per cent and 88 per cent respectively. The combination of a platelet count of less than $100\,000/mm^2$ and a white cell count of less than $4000/mm^2$ has a sensitivity of 100 per cent and a specificity of 71 per cent. These criteria are now recommended for use in screening patients for potential therapy with immune plasma or ribavirin.

Mortality

Mortality is about 16 per cent in laboratory-confirmed, hospitalized patients with untreated Argentine haemorrhagic fever. There are no estimates of overall mortality in populations.

Complications and sequelae

A late neurological syndrome in about 10 per cent of cases, consisting mainly of cerebellar signs, is associated with treatment using high titre antiserum. It begins between 4 and 6 weeks after onset of acute illness and lasts less than a week. It is characterized by fever, headache, ataxia, and intention tremors, and a mild cerebrospinal fluid pleocytosis with anti-Junin virus antibody in the cerebrospinal fluid. Most patients recover within 3 months. Mild permanent damage to acoustic centres has been detected in a small group of patients. Argentine haemorrhagic fever is reported to be severe in pregnancy.

Pathogenic processes

Pathogenesis

Despite the different degrees of bleeding , there are sufficient similarities between the course of disease in Argentine haemorrhagic fever, Bolivian haemorrhagic fever, and Lassa fever to speculate that they share pathophysiological pathways. Organ function, other than the endothelial system, appears to remain intact, and the critical period of shock is brief, lasting only 24 to 48 h. Hepatitis is mild and renal function is well maintained. Bleeding is more pronounced but is not the cause of shock and death. Capillary leakage is significant, but the dramatic head and neck oedema characteristic of severe Lassa fever is absent. Proteinuria is significant, and dehydration important. Though petechiae suggest endothelial damage, no clear evidence of virus replication in endothelium has been demonstrated. Persistent hypovolaemic shock despite intravascular volume expanders suggest that this is due to leakage of fluid into extravascular spaces. Adult respiratory distress syndrome is not described, but tissue oedema is frequent and pulmonary oedema may follow vigorous intravenous fluid replacement.

Other observations include high levels of interferon in severely ill patients, and a decrease in complement. More recently, proinflammatory cytokines, namely interferon-α and tumour necrosis factor-α (TNF-α) and interleukins, IL6, IL8, and IL10, have been variably reported. A platelet inhibitor, which may be interferon-α, similar to that described in Lassa fever, has inhibitory effects on thrombin-induced aggregation and ^{14}C serotonin release. Raised G-CSF levels correlated with TNF-α and disease severity.

Pathology

There are large areas of intra-alveolar or bronchial haemorrhage, petechiae on organ surfaces, and ulcerations of the digestive tract, although bleeding is not massive. Large areas of intra-alveolar or bronchial haemorrhage are often seen with no evidence of inflammatory process. Pneumonia with necrotizing bronchitis or pulmonary emboli is observed in half of the cases. Haemorrhage and a lymphocytic infiltrate have been observed in the pericardium, occasionally with interstitial myocarditis. Lymph nodes are enlarged and congested with reticular cell hyperplasia. Splenic haemorrhage is common, and medullary congestion with pericapsular and pelvic haemorrhages are frequently seen. Adrenal necrosis has not been reported. Renal damage occurs in about half of the fatal cases, and consists of severe structural damage in the distal tubular cells and collecting ducts with relative sparing of the glomeruli and proximal tubules. There is no evidence of direct viral central nervous system infection. Microscopically, there is mild oedema of the vascular walls, with capillary swelling and perivascular haemorrhage associated with viral antigen but no immunoglobulins. Electronmicroscopy shows intracytoplasmic and intranuclear inclusions and marked, non-specific cellular damage in all organs examined.

Immunology

In striking contrast to Lassa fever, the antibody response to Junin virus is effective in clearing virus during acute disease, and may also be sufficient to protect against infection. Neutralizing antibody may be detectable at the time the patient begins to recover from the acute illness, and the therapeutic efficacy of immune plasma in patients with Junin infection is directly associated with the titre of neutralizing antibody in the plasma given. This neutralizing antibody is directed towards the surface glycoproteins. Nevertheless, like Lassa, Junin virus may persist. In vaccine studies in Argentina, some people do not produce measurable neutralizing antibodies but do mount a Junin-virus-specific lymphocytic proliferative response. It is probable that both humoral and cellular immunity are important in limiting virus replication and thus in recovery and protection.

Differential diagnosis

Argentine haemorrhagic fever should be considered in patients in the endemic area, particularly male agricultural workers, who present with fever of unknown origin and a bleeding diathesis. No cases have been reported outside Argentina.

Laboratory diagnosis

Antibodies measured by IFA may be positive by the end of the second week of illness. Neutralizing and complement fixing antibody to Junin are usually detectable 3 to 4 weeks after onset. ELISA systems for antibody and antigen are described with sensitivity and specificity of 99.2 per cent and 98.8 per cent, respectively, but reagents are not generally available. Virus may also be cultured from serum, but this must be performed in BSL4 conditions. For acute diagnosis, RT-PCR on whole blood samples is now the method of choice with sensitivity of 98 per cent and specificity 76 per cent.

Patient management

Specific treatment

In contrast to Lassa fever, convalescent-phase plasma has been shown to be highly successful in Argentine haemorrhagic fever, reducing the mortality from 16 per cent to 1 per cent in patients treated in the first 8 days of illness. Viraemia is reduced within 24 h of treatment, and clinical symptoms and haematological alterations are less severe than in control cases receiving non-immune plasma. Efficacy is directly related to the concentration of neutralizing antibodies. Delayed treatment is less successful. Availability of appropriately screened plasma may be a problem. Ribavirin is effective in experimentally infected primates, and its therapeutic use late in disease is being explored. The late neurological syndrome of Argentine haemorrhagic fever may be associated with therapy, particularly very high titre immune plasma.

Prevention

The human–rodent encounter resulting in Argentine haemorrhagic fever occurs during crop harvests, and there are no means of controlling feral rodents. A successful live attenuated vaccine, Candid 1, for Argentine haemorrhagic fever has now undergone Phase III studies, and is in use in the endemic area of Argentina, where is has almost eliminated the disease. The vaccine has proved safe in large-scale trials, and has a protective efficacy of 84 per cent.

Bolivian haemorrhagic fever

Epidemiology

Bolivian haemorrhagic fever is caused by Machupo virus, first isolated in 1965, and is limited to a portion of the department of Beni in Bolivia. The only known reservoir is *Callomys callosus*, found in the highest density at the borders of tropical grassland and forest, in the eastern Bolivian plains, northern Paraguay, and adjacent areas of western Brazil. Infected rodents develop haemolytic anaemia and splenomegaly, with up to 50 per cent fatality among infected suckling animals, and stunted growth in many others. The virus renders *Callomys callosus* essentially sterile with the young dying *in utero*. Transmission from rodent to rodent is horizontal, not vertical, and is believed to occur through contaminated saliva and urine.

By 1962, more than 1000 cases had been identified in a confined area of two provinces. The largest known epidemic of Bolivian haemorrhagic fever, involving several hundred cases, followed a marked and unusual increase in the *Calomys* population in homes in the town of San Joaquin in 1963 and 1964. This seems to have been a unique event, and there have been virtually no cases until 1994, when there was an outbreak in north-eastern Bolivia. Since all ages and both sexes are affected, it can be assumed that most patients were infected in their homes. Person-to-person spread is rarely reported.

Virology

The sequence of the nucleocapsid protein of Machupo virus shows close relatedness to Junin and Tacaribe viruses. This, together with previous demonstrations of antigenic similarity and cross-protection, suggest that vaccines developed against Argentine haemorrhagic fever might also be effective against the Bolivian disease.

Clinical features

The incubation period, clinical disease, and pathology of Bolivian haemorrhagic fever closely resemble Argentine haemorrhagic fever. Initial symptoms include headache, fever, arthralgia, and myalgia. In the later stages of this illness, patients may develop haemorrhagic manifestations including subconjunctival haemorrhage, epistaxis, haematemesis, melena, and haematuria, as well as neurological signs including tremor, seizures, and coma. Case fatality in the 1960s was 22 per cent. Neurological sequelae are observed in experimentally infected primates. Diagnosis is made in the same way as for Argentine haemorrhagic fever. Machupo virus also induces a humoral immune response, which may include neutralizing antibody.

Treatment

During the 1960s, convalescent-phase immune plasma from survivors of Bolivian haemorrhagic fever was used. However, there is now a paucity of survivors of Bolivian haemorrhagic fever who can donate immune plasma, and there is no active program for collection and storage of Bolivian haemorrhagic fever immune plasma. In 1994, intravenous ribavirin was offered to two patients who both recovered without sequelae, but Machupo virus infection was only confirmed in one.

Prevention

The ideal method of prevention for these rodent-borne diseases is to prevent contact between rodents and humans. The effectiveness of this was admirably shown in the outbreaks of Bolivian haemorrhagic fever in the 1960s when rodent control programmes in the villages were highly successful in eliminating the epidemic situation. The Candid 1 vaccine used in Argentina has been proposed for use against infection with this virus.

Venezuelan haemorrhagic fever

Epidemiology

Guanarito virus, the aetiological agent of Venezuelan haemorrhagic fever, was first isolated in 1991. Person-to-person transmission is not reported, and is unlikely since there is low frequency of infection in family contacts and none in exposed hospital workers. That all ages and sexes are infected suggests transmission occurs in and around houses. Disease is endemic, without seasonal variation. There are no data on prevalence and risk factors for infection have not been identified. The cotton rat, *Sigmodon alstoni*, is now thought to be the principal rodent reservoir of Guanarito virus. Despite intensive surveillance, Venezuelan haemorrhagic fever has been detected in only the small region of western Venezuela where the first outbreak was seen.

Virology

Morphology and antigenic properties of Guanarito show it to be a new member of the Tacaribe complex with which it cross reacts broadly. Phylogenetic analysis of the nucleocapsid gene open reading frame showed that Guanarito virus is a genetically distinct arenavirus, with 32 per cent nucleotide sequence divergence ranging from 30 per cent (Junin) to 45 per cent (LCMV). This sequence region is a probable antigenic domain (amino acids 55–63) shared among all arenaviruses. Phylogenetic trees of rodent isolates delineate nine distinct Guanarito genotypes, most of which are restricted to discrete geographical regions. Human disease is not associated with a particular genotype or host rodent.

Clinical features

Little information is available but hospitalized patients with severe disease are described as febrile with prostration, headache, arthralgia, cough, sore throat, nausea/vomiting, and diarrhoea. Haemorrhage is manifest as epistaxis, bleeding gums, menorrhagia, and melaena. On physical examination, patients are toxic and usually dehydrated, with pharyngitis, conjunctivitis, cervical lymphadenopathy, facial oedema, or petechiae. Thrombocytopenia and neutropenia are common. The case fatality in 15 patients was over 60 per cent, but surveys suggest that overall mortality to infection ratio is much lower. Post mortem pathology included: pulmonary oedema with diffuse haemorrhages in the parenchyma and sub pleura; focal hepatic haemorrhages; cardiomegaly epicardial haemorrhages, splenic and renal swelling; and widespread bleeding into cavities. Like Argentine haemorrhagic fever and Bolivian haemorrhagic fever, antibodies to Guanarito virus appear later in the illness. The infection is likely to respond to ribavirin therapy, although no data are available.

Sabia virus

Sabia virus emerged in 1990 when it was isolated from a fatal case in São Paulo, Brazil. Subsequently, it caused two laboratory-acquired infections. Its natural distribution and host are still unknown. One incident involving a human exposure occurred in the Yale Arbovirus Research Unit on August 8, 1994 when a senior scientist was exposed to Sabia virus while purifying the virus from a large volume of tissue culture fluid. The patient treated himself immediately with ribavirin, and made a rapid and full recovery.

Molecular studies confirm that Sabia virus is distinct from all other members of the arenaviridae and shares a progenitor with Junin, Machupo, Tacaribe, and Guanarito viruses. It has a unique, predicted, three stem–loop structure in the S RNA intergenic region.

Further reading

Bowen MD, Peters CJ, Nichol ST (1997). Phylogenetic analysis of the Arenaviridae: patterns of virus evolution and evidence for cospeciation between arenaviruses and their rodent hosts. Molecular and Phylogenetic Evolution 8, 301–16.

Enria DA, Briggiler AM, Fernandez NJ, Levis SC, Maiztegui JI (1984). Importance of dose of neutralising antibodies in treatment of Argentine haemorrhagic fever with immune plasma. Lancet 2, 255–6.

Fisher-Hoch SP, Hutwagner L, Brown B, McCormick JB (2000). Effective vaccine for Lassa fever. Journal of Virology 74, 6777–83.

Holmes GP, McCormick JB, Trock SC, et al. (1990). Lassa fever in the United States. Investigation of a case and new guidelines for management [see comments]. New England Journal of Medicine 323, 1120–3.

Jahrling PB, Hesse RA, Eddy GA, Johnson KM, Callis RT, Stephen E (1980). Lassa virus infection of rhesus monkeys: pathogenesis and treatment with ribavirin. Journal of Infectious Diseases 141, 580–9.

Johnson KM, McCormick JB, Webb PA, Smith ES, Elliott LH, King IJ (1987). Clinical virology of Lassa fever in hospitalized patients. Journal of Infectious Diseases 155, 456–64.

Maiztegui JI, McKee KT Jr, Barrera Oro JG, et al. (1998). Protective efficacy of a live attenuated vaccine against Argentine hemorrhagic fever. AHF Study Group. Journal of Infectious Diseases 177, 277–83.

McCormick JB, King IJ, Webb PA, et al. (1987). A case-control study of the clinical diagnosis and course of Lassa fever. Journal of Infectious Diseases 155, 445–55.

McCormick JB, King IJ, Webb PA, et al. (1986). Lassa fever. Effective therapy with ribavirin. New England Journal of Medicine 314, 20–6.

McCormick JB, Webb PA, Krebs JW, Johnson KM, Smith ES (1987). A prospective study of the epidemiology and ecology of Lassa fever. Journal of Infectious Diseases 155, 437–44.

7.10.16 Filoviruses

Susan Fisher-Hoch and Joseph McCormick

Primary human infections with filoviruses are exceedingly rare. The first appearance of these viruses was in Marburg in 1967 when laboratory, medical, and animal care personnel exposed to tissues and blood from African Green monkeys were infected. A unique virus isolated from these patients had a strange, looped and branched filamentous form, hence filovirus. In 1976 and 1979, epidemics of a haemorrhagic disease with very high mortality in northern Zaire and in southern Sudan were found to be due to two strains of a related, yet distinct filovirus, named Ebola virus. Over the next 10 years rare, sporadic cases of filovirus infections in Africa were the only continuing evidence of the existence of these viruses. Their natural host and ecology remained elusive. In 1989, a filovirus was isolated near Washington, DC, from dying cynomolgus monkeys shipped to the United States from the Philippines. Since 1990, both Ebola and Marburg viruses have re-emerged in Central Africa causing several devastating epidemics.

Virology

Nucleotide sequence analyses now places the filovirus family in the order Mononegavirales. Filoviruses are among the largest known viruses, with highly variable length (up to 14 000 nm). They undergo rapid, lytic replication in the cytoplasm of a wide range of host cells. The virions are of uniform 80-nm diameter, with a helical nucleocapsid, consisting of a central axis, 20 to 30 nm in diameter, surrounded by a helical capsid, 40 to 50 nm in diameter, with 5-nm cross-striations. A host-cell membrane-derived layer with 10-nm projections in regular array surrounds the nucleocapsid.

The virions contain a single negative-strand RNA genome ranging from 4 to 4.5×10^6 daltons. The RNA is a template for at least seven polypeptides, a nucleoprotein (N), a glycoprotein (G), a polymerase (L), and four other undesignated proteins (VP40, VP35, VP30, and VP24), two of which are associated with the nucleocapsid. The surface glycoprotein is heavily glycosylated. An abundant, but poorly glycosylated protein, VP40, and the nucleoprotein (N) are associated with the nucleocapsid. There is apparently close identity at the glycoprotein level among Asian filoviruses, but not African filoviruses.

Epidemiology

In 1967, epidemiological investigations revealed that 20/29 persons with blood contact with Marburg infected monkeys became infected, and four of 13 exposed to tissue culture. Five of the secondary cases resulted from person-to-person contact at home or in hospital. About 400 to 600 animals originating from four shipments reached Europe from Uganda over a 3-week period. Data on concurrent Belgrade enzootics showed an unusually high mortality characterized by ongoing transmission during 6 weeks quarantine; 46/99 animals died from a first shipment, and 20 and 30 from another two. No evidence could be found of epizootics in Uganda, but later some indirect, controversial information emerged that there had at that time of the outbreak been excess deaths in monkey colonies in islands near Lake Kyoga, north of Lake Victoria. Since then there were three isolated, primary human Marburg infections and two secondary cases in tourists or expatriate residents; one a traveller in Zimbabwe and two others from the Mount Elgon region of western Kenya, not far from the shores of Lake Victoria. Extensive epidemiological investigations in Zimbabwe and on Mount Elgon revealed no clues of the origin of these infections. In May 1999, an outbreak of Marburg virus disease occurred in Watsa and Durba in eastern Democratic Republic of Congo. There were an estimated 76 cases with 52 deaths in miners and their families. The common risk factor in miners was illegally entering and working in an officially closed gold mine in an area with major rebel fighting and in which investigations proved difficult and dangerous. Since then, sporadic reports suggest that the suspect outbreak may be ongoing.

Nearly a decade after the Marburg outbreak, simultaneous outbreaks of another lethal haemorrhagic fever struck in northern Zaire (Republic of Congo) and Sudan in 1976. Two more filoviruses were isolated, Ebola (Zaire) and Ebola (Sudan); 280 deaths among 318 probable or confirmed cases were identified in Zaire (case fatality 88 per cent). The index case may have been a recent traveller in the northern Equateur region of Zaire who visited the clinic of a mission hospital in Yambuku. The subsequent nine cases, however, had all received treatment for other diseases at the hospital. The major risk factor was receiving an injection at this hospital. Eleven of the 17 staff members of the hospital died, and the outbreak only terminated when the hospital was closed . There was subsequent dissemination in surrounding villages to people caring for sick relatives, attending childbirth, or through sexual intercourse. The following year, 1977, a single fatal case was identified in Tandala, also in northern Zaire. Also in 1976, an outbreak of a similar disease occurred in southern Sudan, with the index case in a single cotton weaving factory. There were 151 deaths among 284 cases identified (case fatality about 53 per cent). The focus of the infection was in the town of Nzara where the factory was located, and spread was to close relatives. The epidemic was augmented by high levels of transmission at nearby Maridi hospital following transfer of one of the Nzara patients, and further cases transferred to Juba and Khartoum. There were 203 cases in Maridi, 93 of which were probably infected in the hospital and 105 in the community. Forty one staff members died, and at the height of the epidemic all wards contained patients with overt haemorrhage. In 1979, there was a similar outbreak in Sudan when 22 of 34 infections (65 per cent) were fatal. Though closely related, the viruses from Zaire and Sudan were found to be distinct. The two virus strains isolated in Sudan in 1976 and 1979, however, are identical.

A large outbreak of Ebola virus disease caused by the Zaire strain occurred in 1995 in Kikwit, Democratic Republic of Congo, resulting in 315 cases with 81 per cent case fatality. Eighty cases (25 per cent) occurred among health-care workers, and the epidemic centred again around the hospital with secondary spread in the community. The outbreak was terminated by the initiation of barrier-nursing techniques, health education efforts, and rapid identification of cases

In 1994 and 1995, 49 patients with haemorrhagic symptoms were hospitalized in north-eastern Gabon. Two other epidemics (spring and fall 1996) occurred in the same province, one of which was the result of contact of a number of young people with the carcass of a dead chimpanzee. This chimpanzee was later cooked and eaten. Infection was associated with handling the carcass or meat of the dead animal, but was not associated with eating cooked meat. A single case, infected with a closely related strain, occurred in a veterinarian working in Côte d'Ivoire. In 2001 further outbreaks occurred in Gabon.

Sudan virus Ebola haemorrhagic fever re-emerged in Uganda in August 2000 in a widespread epidemic which only terminated in January 2001; 425 presumptive cases were recorded from three districts in an estimated population of 1.8 million. The first cases came apparently from rebel areas, and no information is available on the source of this outbreak. There were 224 deaths (case fatality 53 per cent); 29 health-care workers were infected. Infection of 14/22 health-care workers after establishing isolation wards required reinforcement of infection control measures. Two distant focal outbreaks in Uganda were initiated by movement of infected contacts.

In 1989 and early 1990, a filovirus closely related to Ebola virus was isolated from cynomolgus monkeys recently imported from the Philippines (in quarantine facilities in Reston, Virginia, in Texas and in Pennsylvania) into the United States. No link with Africa or African animals could be identified and this must be considered at present an Asian filovirus. Pathogenicity for cynomolgus monkeys was uncertain because of a high rate of concurrent infection with Simian haemorrhagic fever virus (SHFV), a DNA virus which is a known, severe simian pathogen unrelated to the Filoviridae. Evidence for ongoing epizootics and transmission was found in the Philippine export facilities which had provided the monkeys. Further importations of infected monkeys into Italy and the United States have occurred since 1990.

In the Philippines, there was no illness in any individuals associated with infected monkeys, and no association between seropositivity and other risk factors, such as bites, scratches, or eating monkey meat. In the facility at Reston, Virginia, five animal handlers had a high level of daily exposure to infected and dying animals, and four of these developed antibodies. One cut his finger while performing a necropsy on an infected animal. Daily monitoring of this individual revealed transient viraemia and seroconversion, but neither he nor his colleagues had any illness attributable to filovirus infection.

Ecology

Transmission from the unknown natural reservoir to humans is rare. Searches for evidence of virus infection in many species of animals captured in central African countries have failed to provide any clues. Bats remain highly suspect, since they were indirectly implicated in the Kitum cave cases of Marburg disease and were also present in the sugar cane-processing factory where the index cases of both 1970s Sudan outbreaks worked.

Transmission and risk factors

Person-to-person spread has been the major mode of transmission in epidemics, with contact with patients ill with Ebola is the most important factor. Other risk factors are contaminated needles, blood or secretions, preparation of a body for burial, or, occasionally, sexual contact. Epidemiological studies do not suggest spread through casual contact or by aerosol transmission. The mode of acquisition of primary infection is totally unknown.

The most significant risk factor for the monkeys infected in the epizootic in the Philippines was being an occupant of a gang cage (six-fold increase of risk, p < 0.001, OR 5.96, 95 per cent CI 2.87–12.38). Ebola (Reston) has been identified at high titre in respiratory secretions in monkeys, and respiratory transmission at close quarters may be a factor in epizootics with this virus.

Laboratory infections and bioterrorism

The outbreak of Marburg virus in 1967 was in individuals handling fresh monkey tissues or contaminated equipment without gloves or other protective clothing. Otherwise there has only been one reported laboratory-acquired infection (needlestick) with Ebola virus in 1976. Because of its lethal potential, Ebola has been a candidate for biological warfare. Little information is available, but it has been handled extensively in biological research, and further accidental infections are said to have occurred with the death of one scientist in a laboratory in the former Soviet bloc. The key to safe laboratory handling of this virus is extreme care in avoiding accidental inoculation. Ebola has been named as a candidate for biowarfare or bioterrorism, but without extensive biological modification it is unsuitable for dissemination in this way.

Disease

Marburg and Ebola diseases are clinically indistinguishable. The incubation period is 3 to 10 days, shorter with needle transmission. The illness-to-infection ratio is high, though it is clear that asymptomatic infections occur. In contrast Ebola (Reston) virus is uniformly asymptomatic.

Onset is abrupt with fever, severe headache, myalgia, arthragia, conjunctivitis, and extreme malaise. Sore throat is often associated with severe swelling and dysphagia, but no exudative pharyngitis. A papular, eventually desquamating rash may occur. In non-human primates, petechiae are striking. Abdominal pain and cramping followed by diarrhoea and vomiting develop on the second or third day of illness. Jaundice is not a feature. There is invariably biochemical evidence of hepatic disease with elevated aspartate transaminase (AST) levels maximal by day seven of illness. Bilirubin is not elevated, and alanine transaminase (ALT) is disproportionately low. Bleeding begins about the fifth day of illness, most commonly from the mucous membranes. Death is associated with hypovolaemic shock and severe bleeding. Infection in pregnancy results in high maternal fatality and virtually 100 per cent fetal death. Central nervous system involvement has led to hemiplegia and disorientation, and sometimes frank psychosis. Even in convalescence, patients show prolonged weakness, severe weight loss, and in a few survivors serious but reversible personality changes are recorded, namely confusion, anxiety, and aggressive behaviour. Blindness has been recorded as a sequel.

Ten of the 29 known primary Marburg infections died (35 per cent). No fatalities occurred among the 10 secondary cases, overall mortality was 10/39 (25.6 per cent). The mortality ratios during the two epidemics of Ebola disease in Sudan were 55 and 65 per cent, while that during the Zaire epidemic in 1976 was 88 per cent. In the Kikwit epidemic of 1995, mortality was 81 per cent, and in Uganda in 2000, 53 per cent, though it was much higher in children (80 per cent).

Animal models

The monkey has been the most successful animal used for the study of Marburg and Ebola viruses, and has been used extensively for the study of pathogenesis of filovirus infection.. The ability of any of the viruses to kill guinea pigs is variable. Ebola (Zaire) kills guinea pigs consistently after several adaptive passages, the Sudan variant and Marburg virus do not. Only the Zaire virus is lethal for suckling mice.

Pathogenesis and immunopathogenesis

High titres of virus are found in serum and tissues taken at autopsy, and particles may be seen in large numbers with some obvious tropism for reticuloendotheial cells. The most profound physiological alteration, invariably associated with death, is hypotensive shock. Fatal infection is marked by absent specific IgG and barely detectable IgM, whereas in survivors early and increasing levels of Ebola-specific IgG against viral nucleoprotein (NP) and 40-kDa viral protein (VP40) is followed by activation of cytotoxic T cells. In fatal cases, DNA fragmentation in blood leucocytes and levels of 41/7 nuclear matrix protein in plasma indicate that massive intravascular apoptosis proceeds during the 5 last days of life. In survivors, upregulation of FasL, perforin, CD28, and IFNγ messenger (m)RNA in peripheral blood mononuclear cells coincide with clearance of circulating viral antigen. In survivors there is also early activation of T cells, evidenced by mRNA patterns in peripheral blood mononuclear cells and marked release of IFNγ in plasma. It is clear that events very early in Ebola virus infection determine control of viral replication, apoptosis of immune cells and possibly other cells, and recovery or death.

Bleeding is prominent, manifest as petechiae, uncontrolled bleeding from venepuncture sites and haemorrhagic effusions. Thrombocytopenia is invariable but bleeding is not usually of sufficient volume to account for the shock, nor is it associated with solid evidence of disseminated intravascular coagulation (DIC) in the small number of animals or humans studied so far, although much has been written about DIC in Ebola and Marburg disease. As in Lassa fever, platelet dysfunction has been described in experimentally infected primates, in which there is a decline in *in vitro* platelet aggregation beginning 1 to 3 days prior to the onset of bleeding and shock and progressing to virtually no aggregation at death. Liver enzymes (AST and ALT) are raised, but the rise in AST is disproportionately higher than ALT, as was described in the early Marburg cases.

At autopsy both Marburg and Ebola infected humans and primates show widespread haemorrhagic diathesis into skin, membranes, and soft tissue. There is focal necrosis in liver, lymph nodes, ovaries, and testis. Most prominent are eosinophilic inclusion bodies in hepatocytes (Councilman-like), without significant inflammatory response.

Several individuals in direct contact with blood or infectious secretions during two outbreaks in Gabon did not develop symptoms, but seroconverted with IgM and IgG between 2 and 4 weeks following exposure. Acute Ebola infection was confirmed by detection of viral genomic (negative-stranded) RNA in peripheral blood mononuclear cells for 2 weeks after exposure, together with positive-stranded viral RNA, indicating viral replication. These individuals mounted an early, strong inflammatory response, with high levels of IL-1α, IL-6, TNFα, MCP-1, and MIP-1α/β, but without evidence of an immediate T-cell response. This unexpected observation suggests that the early inflammatory response is able, in some individuals, to control viral replication and disease.

Diagnosis

Care should be taken in both drawing and handling blood specimens since virus titre may be extremely high, and the virus is stable for long periods even at room temperature. Sera may be safely handled for immunological tests by inactivating with gamma irradiation, or, if this is unavailable, heating for 60°C for 30 min. High or rising titre filovirus-specific IgG is diagnostic as is the presence of IgM by IFA. An antigen detection ELISA system has been found to be of considerable use in monitoring epidemics and epizootics. Virus may be isolated and identified within 2 to 3 days if suitable containment facilities are available. Polymerase chain reaction (PCR) assays are available for acute diagnosis.

Immunofluorescent antibody tests (IFA) used for serological studies is unreliable at low-titre or in the absence of a history of clinical disease. Antibody, sometimes with high prevalence, has been reported in monkeys and humans from many geographic locations, including unlikely populations such as Cona Indians from Central America and Alaskans. Newer generation tests using recombinant antigens appear to have reduced the number of non-specific reactions whilst retaining sensitivity.

Patient management

Fluid, electrolyte, respiratory and osmotic imbalances should be managed carefully. Patients may require full intensive care support, including mechanical ventilation, along with blood, plasma, or platelet replacement. The maintenance of intravascular volume is a particular challenge but every effort is justified since the crisis is short lived, and complete recovery can be expected in survivors. There is no specific therapy, and the value of immune plasma is unproven.

Control

Since the reservoir(s) of the viruses are not known, no specific precautions can be identified which would avoid infections from the natural source of the viruses. Interruption of person-to-person spread of the virus is essential to control. Early institution of safe and orderly care of the ill should be set up with effective surveillance of high-risk contacts and prompt isolation of further cases.

Vaccine

Recent vaccine candidates have been described in animal studies, including a DNA vaccine which protected guinea pigs and monkeys. Human vaccines are not available at the time of writing, but may become so shortly.

Further reading

Baize S, Leroy EM, Georges-Courbot MC, *et al.* (1999). Defective humoral responses and extensive intravascular apoptosis are associated with fatal outcome in Ebola virus-infected patients [In Process Citation]. *Nature Medicine* **5**, 423–6.

Baron RC, McCormick JB, Zubeir OA (1983). Ebola virus disease in southern Sudan: hospital dissemination and intrafamilial spread. *Bulletin of the World Health Organanization* **61**, 997–1003.

Ebola hemorrhagic fever: lessons from Kikwit, Democratic Republic of the Congo (1999). *Journal of Infectious Diseases* **179** (Suppl. 1).

Leroy EM, Baize S, Volchkov VE, *et al.* (2000). Human asymptomatic Ebola infection and strong inflammatory response. *Lancet* **355**, 2210–5.

MacDonald R (2000). Ebola virus claims more lives in Uganda. *British Medical Journal* **321**, 1037.

Report of a WHO/ International Study Team (1978). Ebola haemorrhagic fever in Sudan, 1976. *Bulletin of the World Health Organanization* **56**, 247–70.

Report of a WHO/ International Study Team (1978). Ebola haemorrhagic fever in Zaire, 1976. *Bulletin of the World Health Organanization* **56**, 271–93.

Sullivan NJ, Sanchez A, Rollin PE, Yang ZY, Nabel GJ (2000). Development of a preventive vaccine for Ebola virus infection in primates. *Nature* **408**, 605–9.

7.10.17 Papovaviruses

K. V. Shah

General description

Papovaviruses are small, spherical, non-enveloped, doubled-stranded DNA viruses that multiply in the nucleus. Viruses of the papovavirus family infect a wide variety of species including man and are largely host specific. They fall naturally into two subfamilies, papillomaviruses (wart viruses) and polyomaviruses. Papillomaviruses and polyomaviruses differ in many significant ways. The genetic information of papillomaviruses is carried on only one DNA strand but that of polyomaviruses is distributed over both strands. Papillomaviruses infect surface epithelia and produce disease at these sites. Polyomaviruses are carried by viraemia, after initial multiplication at the site of entry, to affect internal organs such as the kidney and the brain. Viruses of both subfamilies produce experimental tumours in laboratory animals but only papillomaviruses are related to naturally occurring cancers. Within each subfamily the viruses are immunologically related and share nucleotide sequences but the two subfamilies are distinct.

More than 100 human papillomaviruses have been recognized, 35 types infecting mucous membranes (genital and respiratory tracts, and the oral cavity). Human papillomaviruses are the aetiological agents of skin warts, genital warts, respiratory papillomatosis, and papillomas at other mucosal sites (e.g. mouth, eye). Infection with some genital tract human papillomaviruses causes cervical cancer, one of the most common female malignancies in the world. Human papillomaviruses contribute to cancers at other sites.

Two polyomaviruses, BK virus and JC virus, infect man. JC virus is the aetiological agent of progressive multifocal leucoencephalopathy, a fatal demyelinating disease of immunodeficient people. Because of the emergence of AIDS, it is now more frequent and is found in younger people. BK virus is associated with haemorrhagic cystitis in bone marrow transplant recipients, and with renal failure in renal transplant recipients.

Human papillomaviruses (HPVs)

Human papillomaviruses cannot be propagated in tissue culture and require nucleic acid hybridization assays for their identification. Their double-stranded circular genome contains about 8000 base pairs, divided into an early region, necessary for transformation, a late region, encoding for capsid proteins, and a regulatory region, containing control elements (Fig. 1). Open reading frames of the viral genome are located on one

Table 1 Functions of human papillomavirus open reading frames (modified from Shah and Howley (1996))

Function	ORF
Replication of viral DNA	E1, E2
Regulation of transcription	E2
Coding for late cytoplasmic protein	E4
Cellular proliferation	E5*
Transformation	E6, E7
Not known	E3, E8

ORF, open reading frame.

* In bovine papillomavirus, the major transforming activity is in E5.

strand: E1 to E8 in the early region and L1 and L2 in the late region. The functions assigned to the different open reading frames are listed in Table 1.

Human papillomaviruses only infect humans. They show a marked degree of cellular tropism. Mucosal human papillomaviruses do not readily infect cutaneous epithelia and cutaneous human papillomaviruses are rarely present on mucous membranes. Infection is initiated when, after minor trauma (e.g. during sexual intercourse or after minor skin abrasions), the basal cells of the epithelium come in contact with infectious virus particles. The virus stimulates the proliferation of basal cells. The early-region open reading frames are expressed in all layers of the infected epithelium, but expression of the late-region open reading frames and synthesis of viral particles occur only in the upper differentiating and keratinizing layers.

Important disease associations and characteristics of mucosal HPVs are listed in Table 2; the genital tract is the reservoir for all but a few mucosal human papillomaviruses and genital human papillomavirus infections constitute the most common viral sexually transmitted disease. Genital human papillomaviruses may sometimes infect non-genital mucosal sites, for example, the respiratory tract, the mouth, and the conjunctiva. Transmission of genital tract HPV types 6 and 11 from an infected mother to the baby at birth results in juvenile onset recurrent respiratory papillomatosis. Infection with two types, HPV-13 and HPV-32, appears to be confined to the mouth.

Table 3 lists disease associations of cutaneous HPVs, transmitted by direct contact with infected tissue or by contact with a contaminated object.

Anogenital warts*

Anogenital warts (condylomas) are the most commonly recognized clinical manifestations of genital HPV infections. More than 90 per cent of condlyomas result from infections with HPV-6 and HPV-11. It is estimated that in the United States there are more than a million annual consultations with private physicians for anogenital warts.

Table 2 Mucosal human papillomaviruses: chief clinical associations (modified from Shah and Howley (1996))

Clinical association	Viral type(s)
Exophytic condyloma; respiratory papillomas; oral and conjunctival papillomas	HPV-6, -11
Cervical cancer:	
'High-risk' infections	HPV-16, -18, -31, -45
'Intermediate-risk' infections	HPV-31, -33, -35, -39, -51, -52, -56, -58, -59, -68
'Low-risk' infections	HPV-6, -11, -42, -43, -44
Focal epithelial hyperplasia of the oral cavity	HPV-13, -32

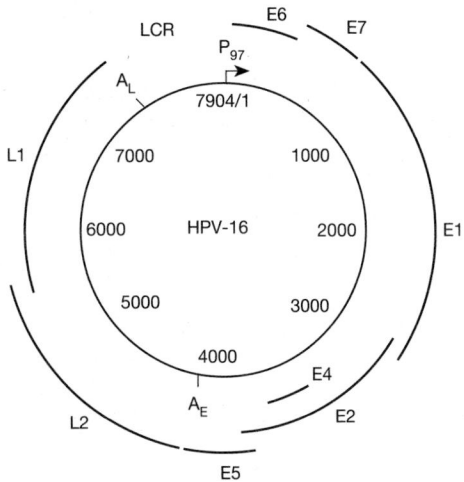

Fig. 1 Genomic map of HPV-16. On the inner circle, P97 represents the transcriptional promoter and A$_E$ and A$_L$ designate early and late polyadenylation sites. The location of the early-region open reading frames (E1–E8), the late-region open reading frames (L1, L2), and of the long control or regulatory region (LCR) are shown. (Reproduced from Shah and Howley (1990), with permission.)

* Includes material from *The Oxford Textbook of Medicine*, 3rd edn, pp 3366–9 (Chapter 21.7, Genital warts, J. D. Oriel).

Table 3 Cutaneous human papillomaviruses: chief clinical associations. (Modified from Shah and Howley (1996))

Clinical association	Viral type
Deep plantar wart	HPV-1
Common wart	HPV-2, -4
Mosaic wart (superficial spreading wart)	HPV-2
Flat warts	HPV-3, -10, -28, -41
Macular plaques of epidermodysplasia verruciformis	HPV-5, -8, -9, -12, -14, -15, -17, -19, -20, -21, -22, -23, -24, -25, -36, -47, -50

Epidemiology

Genital and anal warts are most common between the ages of 16 and 24 years. They are transmitted by direct sexual contact to 60 per cent of sexual partners of people with genital warts. Rarely, genital lesions are secondary to common warts on non-genital areas. Both anogenital warts and laryngeal papillomatosis may occur in children whose mothers had vulval warts at the time of delivery. Anogenital warts in children can also be due to close but non-sexual contact within a family or can be secondary to common skin warts, but in many cases sexual abuse by an infected adult is responsible.

Clinical features

The incubation period is between 3 weeks and 8 months (mean 2.8 months). In men, condylomata acuminata (exophytic condylomas) most often appear on areas exposed to coital trauma—the glans penis, coronal sulcus, prepuce, and terminal urethra. The soft fleshy vascular tumours are usually multiple and may coalesce into large masses (Fig. 2). Sessile or papular warts are more likely to occur on dry areas such as the shaft of the penis (Fig. 3). The raised pink or grey lesions, 0.5 to 3 mm in diameter, may occur alone or with exophytic condylomas. Subclinical HPV lesions (flat condylomas) are identiified by examining the genitalia with magnification after the application of 5 per cent aqueous acetic acid solution. The affected areas are slightly raised and shiny white (acetowhite), with a rough surface (Fig. 4). Flat condylomas affect the same areas as exophytic condylomas.

Perianal warts are usually exophytic and in moist conditions around the anus may reach a large size. In 50 per cent of cases, condylomas also appear in the anal canal (Fig. 5). Areas of acetowhite epithelium indicative of subclinical HPV infection may be associated with perianal warts or occur alone.

In women, exophytic condylomas are the most common HPV lesions (Fig. 6). They appear at the fourchette and adjacent areas, and may spread to the rest of the vulva, the perineum, anus, vagina, and cervix. Multiple

Fig. 3 Sessile (papular) warts of the penis.

Fig. 2 Condylomata acuminata (exophtic condylomas) of the penis.

Fig. 4 Subclinical HPV lesions (flat condylomas) of the penis after application of 5 per cent aqueous acetic acid.

Fig. 7 Subclinical HPV infection of the cervix.

Intraepithelial neoplasia comprises Bowen's disease, bowenoid papulois, and carcinoma *in situ*. They may be associated with genital warts but contain sequences of HPV-16 or HPV-18 and may become malignant.

Diagnosis and management
Genital warts must be distinguished from Fordyce's spots, fibroepithelial polyps, molluscum contagiosum, and the papillar lesions of secondary syphilis. Intraepithelial neoplasia may be difficult to distinguish; lesions that appear atypical or respond poorly to treatment must be biopsied early.

Associated sexually transmitted diseases must be excluded. Sexual partners should be examined. Intraepithelial neoplasia must be excluded. Cervical cytological examination should always be done on women with vulval warts and on female partners of men with penile warts.

No specific antiviral treatment is available. The application of podophyllin or other cytotoxic agents, such as 5-fluorouracil and tricloracetic acid, is often unsuccessful. Warts may be destroyed with cryotherapy by liquid nitrogen or a nitrous oxide cryoprobe, electrocautery, electrodessication, and scissor excision. Interferons have been used in the treatment of persistent anogenital warts. A topical cream, which can be self-administered and is immunomodulatory, has become available recently for the treatment of genital warts.

Cervical cancer (see Chapter 21.5)
Human papillomavirus DNAs are recovered from more than 90 per cent of cases of invasive cervical cancer and squamous intraepithelial lesions of the cervix, which precede invasive cancer. The viral genome is present in the tumour cells of primary as well as metastatic cervical cancer. The progression from low-grade squamous intraepithelial lesions to invasive cancer may take more than 10 years; human papillomaviruses are found throughout this disease process. The viruses are recovered much less frequently from cytologically normal women of comparable age. In prospective studies of women with normal cervical cytology, the presence of HPV is a strong risk factor for the subsequent development of squamous intraepithelial lesions.

Certain HPV types are preferentially associated with invasive cancers. From their distribution in normal individuals and in preinvasive and invasive cervical disease, genital tract HPVs have been categorized as 'high-risk', 'intermediate-risk', and 'low-risk' types (Fig. 8; Table 2). HPV-16 and HPV-18 are the predominant viruses in invasive cancers and account for 40 to 60 per cent and 5 to 20 per cent, respectively, of HPV-positive cancers in different studies. About a dozen additional types of HPV are found in small proportions of invasive cancers. The 'low-risk' HPVs are almost never detected in invasive cervical cancers.

Comparisons of different HPV types for their ability to transform human keratinocytes *in vitro* show that HPV-16 and HPV-18, those most

Fig. 5 Condylomata acynubate of the anal canal in an anoreceptive homosexual man.

sessile warts may affect the labia and perineum. Subclinical HPV infection presents as slightly raised acetowhite lesions: the fissuring of these may cause dyspareunia. About 15 per cent of women with vulval warts have exophytic condylomas on the cervix. Subclinial infection is more common, and consists of acetowhite lesions with punctation due to capillary loops, which can be identified by colposcopy (Fig. 7). Large, exophytic vulval condylomas may develop during pregnancy and may become so large that they compromise delivery. Most regress postpartum.

Fig. 6 Condylomata acuminata of the vulva.

clearly associated with naturally occurring cervical cancers, also have the greatest oncogenic potential in laboratory studies. The transforming functions of HPVs are localized to open reading frames E6 and E7; these are the frames consistently expressed in naturally occurring HPV-positive cancers. The viral genome is integrated into the cellular DNA in most cervical cancers. The break in the circular viral genome that is required for integration occurs most frequently in the E1/E2 region and results in an enhanced expression of the transforming E6 and E7 open reading frames. The transforming HPV proteins E6 and E7 interact with cellular tumour-suppressor proteins p53 and Rb, respectively. It is likely that the oncogenic effect of HPVs is mediated partly by their ability to inactivate the tumour-suppressor proteins which normally regulate the cell cycle.

Epidemiology

Human papillomavirus infections of the genital tract are extremely common in sexually active populations. In young sexually active women, prevalence of HPV infection as measured by the detection of HPV DNA in genital tract specimens by the sensitive polymerase chain reaction may be greater than 40 per cent. The prevalence decreases with increasing age. Most of these infections are found in women with normal cervical cytology and undoubtedly resolve without leaving a trace. Only a small proportion of infections progress to squamous intraepithelial lesions and then to invasive cancer. The cofactors that might be required for this progression are not conclusively identified, but smoking, use of oral contraceptives, parity, presence of other sexually transmitted diseases, and diet are incriminated to some degree, in some studies. Human immunodeficiency virus infection, and associated immunosuppression, leads to a much higher prevalence, and longer persistence, of HPV infections and to greater incidence of squamous intraepithelial lesions.

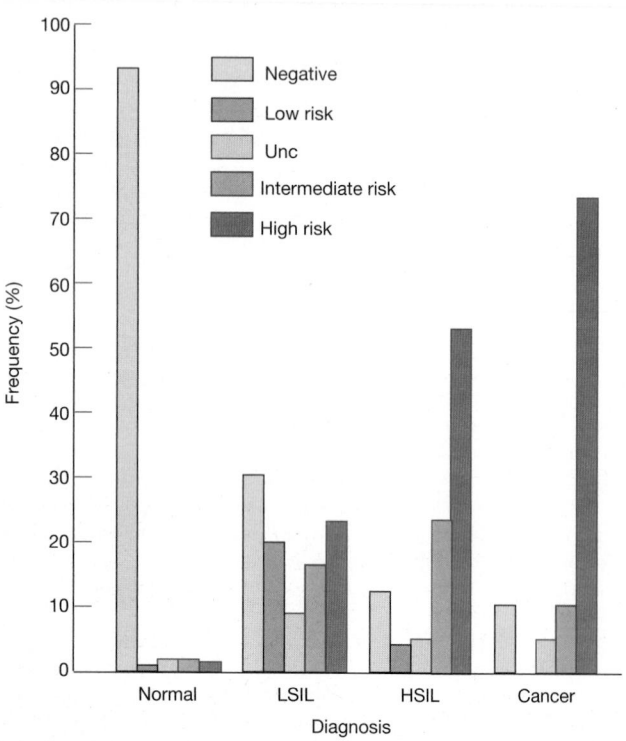

Fig. 8 Distribution of HPV types in normal women and in preinvasive (low-grade and high-grade squamous intraepithelial lesions (SILs)) and invasive cancer. In each diagnostic category, specimens are grouped as containing high-risk, intermediate-risk, and low-risk HPV types (see Table 2), or as containing unclassified HPVs (Unc), or as negative (Neg). (Modified and reproduced from Lörincz *et al.* (1992), with permission.)

Prevention and control of cervical cancer

Screening for cervical cytological abnormalities by Pap smear and treatment of preinvasive and invasive cancers identified by screening have been credited with the decrease in incidence of cervical cancer and mortality due to the disease that has been observed in many developed countries over the last 40 to 50 years. The recognition that HPVs are linked aetiologically to cervical cancers has led to the exploration of HPV-based strategies for prevention and control of cervical cancer.

Clinical management

Women who have cytological abnormalities which are low grade or of uncertain significance may benefit from an HPV diagnosis. The presence of cancer-associated HPVs (high risk plus intermediate risk) would indicate a need for closer monitoring and colposcopy; HPV-negative women would be monitored routinely.

Prophylactic vaccines

Tests in rabbits, cattle, and dogs show that immunization of these animals with conformationally correct L1 capsid protein of their respective papillomaviruses protects them against papillomavirus-induced disease. Vaccines based on HPV L1 proteins have been formulated and tested in human volunteers to evaluate their safety. It is anticipated that the efficacy of these vaccines will soon be tested in clinical trials.

Therapeutic vaccines

Human papillomavirus-associated cancers express HPV E6 and E7 proteins in their tumour cells. Candidate therapeutic vaccines targeted to these proteins are being developed for the treatment of high-grade squamous intraepithelial lesions and invasive cancer.

Cancers at other lower anogenital tract sites

Human papillomavirus infections are very common on the vulva, vagina, penis, perineum, and anus. Synchronous neoplasia at multiple sites in the female lower genital tract is almost always associated with HPVs, especially HPV-16. Carcinoma of the vulva is aetiologically heterogeneous. Vulval cancers occurring in younger women are associated with HPVs but the typical squamous cell carcinoma of the vulva in older women is not. Neoplasia of the anal canal, seen frequently in HIV-seropositive homosexual men, is strongly associated with HPVs.

Cancer of the oropharynx

Some pharyngeal cancers, especially tonsillar cancers, appear to be associated with high-risk HPVs, most often HPV-16. The HPV-positive cancers are characterized by more frequent basaloid pathology, less frequent p53 mutations, and better prognosis, than HPV-negative cancers.

Respiratory papillomatosis

This rare disease is most common in children under the age of 5 years. It may become life threatening if it obstructs the airways. Papillomatosis usually involves the vocal cords and presents with hoarseness or voice change. Papillomas may recur after surgical removal.

HPV-6 and HPV-11, genital tract HPVs that are responsible for most of the exophytic genital warts also cause respiratory papillomatosis. Infants are infected during passage through the birth canal. In adults, transmission may occur by sexual contact. Respiratory papillomas very rarely progress to invasive cancer. Irradiation of papillomas with X-rays (a practice now discontinued) increases the risk of malignancy.

Caesarean delivery for mothers who are found to have genital warts or are infected with HPV-6 or HPV-11 would reduce the risk of juvenile onset respiratory papillomatosis, but it is not generally recommended because of the small risk of disease following perinatal infection. Interferon therapy is not very effective in the treatment of respiratory papillomas.

Human papillomaviruses in the oral cavity

The genital tract HPVs, especially HPV-6 and HPV-11, may infect the oral cavity (Table 2) and are readily recovered from oral lesions diagnosed histologically as condylomas or warty lesions. Focal epithelial hyperplasia of the mouth is distributed worldwide but is highly prevalent in indigenous populations of Central and South America and of Alaska and Greenland; it is aetiologically associated with HPV-13 and HPV-32. These two types are found exclusively in the oral cavity.

Skin warts (see Chapter 23.1)

Skin warts and verrucas may occur anywhere on the skin and are morphologically diverse. They are most common in older children and young adults. Except in the rare condition known as epidermodysplasia verruciformis (see below), they almost never become malignant. Most regress within 2 years. Specific HPV types are strongly associated with specific types of warts (Table 3).

Epidermodysplasia verruciformis

This is a rare, lifelong disease in which a patient has extensive warty involvement of the skin that cannot be resolved. It generally begins in infancy or childhood with multiple, disseminated, polymorphic wart-like lesions on the face, trunk and extremities that tend to become confluent. The warts are either flat or reddish-brown macular plaques that resemble pityriasis versicolor. In about a third of the cases, foci of malignant transformation occur in macular plaques in areas of the skin exposed to sunlight. The tumours are slow growing and rarely metastasize.

Epidermodysplasia verruciformis is often familial. Patients sometimes have a history of parental consanguinity. The pattern of inheritance is suggestive of an X-linked recessive disease resulting in an immunological inability to resolve the infection. The flat warts yield the same HPV types as those of normal individuals but a very large number of HPVs that are seldom encountered in normal individuals are recovered from the macular plaques (Table 3). It is unclear how patients with epidermodysplasia verruciformis become infected with these particular papillomaviruses. The factors that contribute to the occurrence of carcinoma in these patients therefore include a genetic defect, infection with specific HPVs, for example, HPV-5 and HPV-8, and exposure of the affected area to sunlight.

Non-melanoma skin cancers

HPV sequences have been recovered frequently from normal skin, from psoriatic lesions, and from non-melanoma skin cancers of normal and immunosuppressed populations. The sequences represent cutaneous HPV types, epidermodysplasia verruciformis (EV)-associated HPVs and many novel HPV sequences. It appears that the normal skin is seeded with many HPV types but it is not clear to what extent they contribute to the development of non-melanoma skin cancers.

Human polyomaviruses

In 1971 BK virus was isolated from the urine of a renal transplant recipient and JC virus was recovered from the brain of a patient with progressive multifocal leucoencephalopathy. The viruses have a double-stranded DNA genome of about 5000 base pairs, which is divided into an early region encoding viral T proteins, a late region encoding viral capsid proteins, and a non-coding regulatory region. The early and late regions are transcribed from different strands of the viral DNA. Although BK and JC viruses are homologous for 75 per cent of their nucleotide sequence, the infections are readily distinguishable by conventional tests.

Infection occurs in childhood and is largely subclinical. Most children acquire antibodies to BK virus by the age of 10; infection with JC virus occurs at a later age. Early acquisition of antibodies suggests that infection occurs by the respiratory route. Both viruses establish latent, often lifelong, infection in the kidney and are occasionally excreted in the urine of normal people. Reactivation in immunodeficient people is responsible for most associated illnesses. The viruses are reactivated in pregnancy but without any apparent harm to the mother or the newborn.

BK virus-associated illnesses

Reactivation of BK virus in renal transplant recipients may cause ureteric obstruction, a late and uncommon complication of transplantation. Reactivated BK virus infection in patients with renal transplants has recently been linked and renal dysfunction and graft rejection . In bone-marrow transplant recipients receiving allogeneic marrow, late onset haemorrhagic cystitis and BK viruria are strongly correlated. Primary BK virus infection may be responsible for an occasional case of cystitis in normal children. A case of fatal tubulointerstitial nephritis in an immunodeficient child was ascribed to primary BK virus infection. Reports of the virus in pancreatic islet cell tumours and in brain tumours are unconfirmed.

Progressive multifocal leucoencephalopathy (see also Chapter 24.14.2)

JC virus causes progressive multifocal leucoencephalopathy, a subacute demyelinating disease of the central nervous system occurring in individuals with impaired cell-mediated immunity. Until recently, it was a rare disease found mainly in older patients with lymphoproliferative disorders or chronic diseases. In the past decade, it has been seen much more frequently and the majority of cases are in younger patients, as a complication in 1 to 2 per cent of AIDS cases. It has also been recognized in children who have inherited immunodeficiency diseases or have AIDS.

The key pathogenetic event in the leucoencephalopathy is the cytocidal JC virus infection of oligodendrocytes, which are responsible for the production and maintenance of myelin. This leads to foci of demyelination that tend to coalesce and eventually involve large areas of the brain. Infected oligodendrocytes, containing large inclusion-bearing nuclei filled with abundant virus particles, surround the foci of demyelination (Fig. 9). Enlarged astrocytes often show bizarre nuclear changes but are mostly virus negative. They are found within the foci of demyelination. JC virus is disseminated haematogenously to the central nervous system, probably through virus-infected B lymphocytes. The brain may be seeded with JC virus either at the time of primary infection or when the virus is reactivated in times of immunological impairment.

Progressive multifocal leucoencephalopathy starts insidiously. Early signs and symptoms indicate the presence of multifocal asymmetrical lesions in the brain and involve impairment of vision and speech, and mental deterioration. The disease is usually relentlessly progressive and fatal within 3 to 6 months but rarely it can become stabilized with survival for many years. Computed tomography and magnetic resonance imaging have

Fig. 9 A lesion of progressive multifocal leucoencephalopathy showing oligodendrocytes with enlarged, deeply staining nuclei (arrow) and giant astrocytes (left). A crystalloid array of JC virus particles in an infected oligodendrocyte nucleus (right). (Reproduced from Shah (1992), with permission.)

been successfully used for diagnosis. Treatment with cytosine arabinoside and the presence of an inflammatory response in the brain have been associated with the few relatively successful outcomes.

Further reading

Binet I *et al.* (1999). Polyomavirus disease under new immunosuppressive drugs. A cause of renal graft dysfunction and graft loss. *Transplantation* **67**, 918–22. Describes BK virus nephrology in renal transplant recipients.

Cuzick J *et al.* (1999). HPV testing in primary screening of older women. *British Journal of Cancer* **81**, 554–8.

Greenlee JE (1998). Progressive multifocal leukoencephalopathy—progress made and lessons relearned. *New England Journal of Medicine* **338**, 1378–80.

IARC (International Agency for Research on Cancer) (1995). *Monograph on the evaluation of carcinogenic risks to humans volume 64, Human papillomaviruses.* IARC, Lyon. Systematic literature review of HPV–cancer link.

Koutsky L (1997). Epidemiology of genital human papillomavirus infection. *American Journal of Medicine* **102**, 3–8.

Lörincz AT *et al.* (1992). Human papillomavirus infection of the cervix: relative risk associations of 15 common anogenital types. *Obstetrics and Gynecology* **79**, 328–7.

Shah KV (1992). Polyomavirus, infection and immunity. In: Roitt IM, ed. *Encyclopedia of immunology*, pp 1256–8. Academic Press, New York.

Shah KV, Howley PM (1996). Papillomaviruses. In: Fields BN *et al.*, eds. *Virology*, 3rd edn, pp 2077–109. Lippincott-Raven, Philadelphia.

Tindle RW, ed (1999). *Vaccines for human papillomavirus infection and anogenital disease.* RG Landes, Austin, TX. Multiauthored book discussing HPV vaccine candidates and strategies.

Weber T, Major EO (1997). Progressive multifocal leukoencephalopathy: molecular biology, pathogenesis and clinical impact. *Intervirology* **40**, 98–111.

7.10.18 Parvovirus B19

*B. J. Cohen**

Viruses of the subfamily Parvovirinae infect vertebrates

Introduction

Parvoviruses (family *Parvoviridae*) are widespread in nature causing disease in many animal species. They are small (23 nm), icosahederal, non-enveloped viruses (Fig. 1) containing a single-stranded DNA genome. The *erythrovirus* genus, which replicates only in nucleated red blood cell precursors includes human parvovirus B19 (B19 virus), the only member of the family *Parvoviridae* known to cause disease in humans. B19 virus was discovered in 1975 by chance as an asymptomatic infection in blood donors being screened for hepatitis B antigen.

Epidemiology

B19 infection is usually spread by respiratory droplets. Contamination of hands and surfaces may also contribute. More rarely, it is bloodborne, either across the placenta or by transfusion of contaminated blood com-

* Professor J.R. Pattison kindly wrote on Parvoviruses in the third edition of the *Oxford Textbook of Medicine*. Some of his text and Figures have been incorporated in this chapter and we are pleased to acknowledge his contribution.

Fig. 1 Immune electron micrograph of parvovirus particles in serum from a case of aplastic crisis. Some particles are penetrated by the negative stain and appear 'empty'; other particles resist the stain and appear 'full'.

ponents. Infection is most common in children between 6 and 10 years. By 20 years of age, 60 to 70 per cent of the population have been infected. Susceptible adults remain at risk of infection, often following exposure to B19 virus in their own children. Epidemics occur every 4 or 5 years with peaks of infection in winter and spring.

Clinical features of parvovirus B19 infection

At least a third of B19 infections in children and adults are asymptomatic or present as non-specific febrile illness.

Erythema infectiosum

The most common specific clinical manifestation is erythema infectiosum, an erythematous rash illness (fifth disease) of childhood. The rash has an incubation period of 17 to 22 days (Fig. 2 and Plate 1) and classically the illness begins with mild fever and lassitude followed by the facial erythema referred to as 'slapped cheek disease' (Fig. 3). Subsequently the rash spreads to the trunk and limbs where it has a lacy or reticular appearance and tends to fade and recrudesce for a week or so after its initial appearance. School outbreaks are common during epidemic periods. Sporadic cases in children and adults may be misdiagnosed as rubella, streptococcal infection, or allergy. Occasionally, B19 infection presents as a purpuric rash.

Acute arthropathy

More than 80 per cent of adults with B19 infection (especially women) present with painful or swollen joints. An acute-onset, symmetrical polyarthritis specifically affects the small joints of the hands and feet. It usually resolves within a few weeks. In about 20 per cent of adult females with B19 infection, joint symptoms persist for more than 2 months and may resemble rheumatoid arthritis. Rheumatoid factor is usually absent and there is no erosive joint disease. No association with rheumatoid arthritis has been confirmed.

Infection in pregnant women

About 10 per cent of B19 infections in the first 20 weeks of gestation end in spontaneous abortion, a rate of fetal loss about 10 times greater than that in unaffected pregnancies. Embryopathy usually presents as hydrops fetalis 4 to 6 weeks after a maternal infection, which may be symptomatic or clinically silent. In epidemic years, 10 to 20 per cent of cases of non-immunological hydrops fetalis are associated with B19 infection. Fetal anaemia due to B19 infection may be treated with *in utero* blood transfusions. Surviving infants have no evidence of congenital disease or malformation.

Fig. 2 Slapped cheek' rash of erythema infectiosum: note circumoral pallor. (By courtesy of Dr Ken Mutton.) (See also Plate 1.)

Transient aplastic crisis

Interruption of erythropoiesis caused by B19 is transient and insufficient to cause clinically significant anaemia in individuals with normal red cell life-span and function. In those with a shortened red cell lifespan, such as

Fig. 3 Sequence of events following intranasal inoculation of volunteers with parvovirus B19.

patients with sickle cell anaemia, B19 infection can rapidly lead to a more profound anaemia termed an aplastic crisis. In the acute phase there is erythroid aplasia and the absence of reticulocytes in peripheral blood and, in recovery, reticulocytosis and the appearance of giant pronormoblasts in the bone marrow. B19-induced aplastic crisis has also been recorded in patients with hereditary spherocytosis, β-thalassaemia intermedia, pyruvate kinase deficiency, and other red cell disorders.

Chronic anaemia in immunocompromised patients

Patients with congenital immunodeficiency, HIV infection, acute lymphatic leukaemia, or immunocompromise following organ transplantation fail to produce neutralizing antibody to B19 virus and infection becomes chronic. This results in persistent anaemia and patients may become transfusion dependent.

Prevention and therapy

A recombinant DNA-derived vaccine is being developed. To minimize spread by infected blood components, blood donor screening has been proposed, but its cost-effectiveness is unknown. The testing of plasma pools, however, is likely to become mandatory and should result in the reduction of viral load, if not the complete removal, of B19 virus from blood products. Early recognition of B19 infection in hospital patients is important for prevention of nosocomial transmission. Severe infections in immunocompromised patients are treated with high-dose intravenous normal immunoglobulin (400 mg/kg body weight for 5 or 10 days).

Laboratory diagnosis

Detection of B19 virus, by polymerase chain reaction (PCR) for example, is important for diagnosis in patients presenting in the viraemic phase of infection, including those with aplastic crisis, immunocompromise, and fetal infection. In most cases, however, the presenting symptoms of rash and arthropathy are postviraemic phenomena (Fig. 3) and the diagnosis is most commonly confirmed by detecting B19-specific IgM. The IgM response persists for 2 to 3 months after acute infection. Thereafter, B19-specific IgG remains as the sole marker of infection in the past and indicates immunity. Reinfection occurs only in the immunocompromised patient.

Further reading

Brown KE, Young NS, Liu JM (1994). Molecular, cellular and clinical aspects of parvovirus B19 infection. *Critical Reviews in Oncology/Hematology* **16**, 1–31.

Hall SM (1990). Parvovirus B19 and pregnancy. *Reviews in Medical Microbiology* **1**, 160–7.

Prowse C, Ludlam CA, Yap PL (1997). Human parvovirus B19 and blood products. *Vox Sanguinis* **72**, 1–10.

7.10.19 Hepatitis viruses (including TTV)

N. V. Naoumov

Viral hepatitis is an ancient disease which remains an important health problem worldwide. The archetypal viral hepatitis, yellow fever (Chapter 7.10.13), is not included within this group. Over the last 30 years five major hepatitis viruses have been identified—A, B, C, D, and E (Table 1). These unrelated human viruses, different in their genome organization, biology, and epidemiology, are similar in their hepatotropism. Ten to fifteen per cent of cases of viral hepatitis are considered as non-A to E hepatitis: their aetiology remains unknown. The search for new hepatitis agents led to the identification of hepatitis G virus (HGV or GB virus-C) and TT virus. Both have been detected in a high proportion of the general population, but their pathogenic role is uncertain. The search for new agents responsible for the small proportion of patients with cryptogenic hepatitis continues. Details of symptomatology, management, and prevention of viral hepatitis are given in Section 14.20.

Hepatitis A virus (HAV)

HAV particles were detected by immune electron microscopy in 1973 in stool samples of patients with hepatitis A. The virus is classified in the genus *Hepatovirus* within the Picornaviridae family. The genome of HAV is a single-stranded, linear RNA of approximately 7500 nucleotides (Table 1). This includes a 5′ non-translated region (5′NTR) of approximately 740 nucleotides, followed by a single long open reading frame (ORF) encoding a polyprotein of 2200 amino acids and a short 3′ non-translated segment. After translation, the HAV polyprotein undergoes multiple cleavages by a virally encoded enzyme—3C protease. The polyprotein is considered to contain three functionally separate domains. At the aminoterminal end is domain P1 that includes the major structural polypeptides of HAV in the following sequence—VP2, VP3, and VP1. A fourth very small polypeptide, VP4, presumed to be involved in the HAV capsid formation, is located at the extreme aminoterminal end of the polyprotein. These four structural polypeptides assemble into a viral capsid containing 60 copies of each. How the viral RNA is incorporated into the virion is unknown, but both empty and RNA-containing capsids have been observed in most virus preparations. The other P2 and P3 domains of the viral polyprotein include at least six separate proteins involved in viral replication. These include 2B and 2C helicase, 3A and 3B proteins, 3C (the viral protease), and 3D (an RNA-dependent RNA polymerase).

Hepatocytes are the predominant site of HAV replication *in vivo*. Recent data indicate that HAV may also replicate within the epithelial cells of the gastrointestinal tract. However, the mechanism by which HAV reaches the liver remains unknown. Maximal HAV replication in hepatocytes occurs before serum aminotransferases increase. The virus is excreted via the biliary system into the faeces where it can be found in high concentrations around 1 to 2 weeks before the start of clinical symptoms. Viraemia is present from the earliest phase of infection. It results from HAV replication within hepatocytes. HAV differs from other picornaviruses in its non-cytolytic replication. Liver injury is immune mediated by natural killer cells, virus-specific CD8+ cytotoxic T lymphocytes, and non-specific inflammatory cells recruited to the liver. When clinical symptoms appear there is a humoral immune response and antibodies to structural HAV proteins (anti-HAV) are detectable in the serum. Initially these are mainly IgM antibodies (IgM anti-HAV) that usually persist for approximately 6 months. During convalescence, anti-HAV of IgG class become the predominant antibodies. They remain detectable indefinitely, representing protective immunity to HAV.

Hepatitis B virus (HBV)

In 1965, Blumberg and colleagues identified the surface antigen (HBsAg) of HBV, initially termed 'Australia antigen', and in 1970 the complete virion (a 42 nm particle) was detected by Dane and colleagues, using electron microscopy. The genome of HBV, the smallest DNA virus, contains only 3200 nucleotides (Table 1). One of the DNA strands, the 'minus' strand, is an almost complete circle containing four overlapping reading frames: pre-core/core, polymerase, envelope, and X genes (Fig. 1). The other ('plus') strand is shorter and varies in length. HBV belongs to the hepadnavirus family that includes similar hepatotropic DNA viruses specific for woodchucks, ground squirrels, and Pekin ducks.

Genome organization

The envelope ORF contains three start codons separating the pre-S1, pre-S2 , and S sequences. The surface gene encodes the major envelope protein (HBsAg) of 226 amino acids. The translation product of the pre-S2 and S gene is the middle envelope protein and the product of pre-S1, pre-S2, and S gene is the large envelope protein. In addition to the complete virion, many more non-infectious, 22 nm, spherical and filamentous subviral particles are produced in infected hepatocytes. HBsAg and the middle envelope protein are present in all viral and subviral particles, while the large protein is present in the virions and in some subviral filaments. The domain which binds to a specific HBV receptor (still not defined) on the plasma membrane of hepatocytes resides within the pre-S1 region.

The precore/core ORF has two start codons encoding two closely related proteins. Translation from the preC-start codon produces a precursor molecule, designated precore protein. In the endoplasmic reticulum, this protein undergoes two proteolytic steps at the amino- and carboxy-terminal ends. The resultant polypeptide is secreted from hepatocytes as hepatitis B e antigen (HBeAg). This is a non-structural protein, which is not essential for viral replication. However, detection of HBeAg in serum is a good marker of HBV replication. Translation from the C-start codon yields the nucleocapsid protein (HBcAg) of 183 amino acids. In the cytoplasm of hepatocytes HBcAg assembles spontaneously into nucleocapsid particles. HBeAg and HBcAg share about 90 per cent of the amino acids but differ substantially in their conformation. The polymerase ORF encodes the HBV polymerase protein with 832 amino acids. It has three functional domains—terminal protein, reverse transcriptase, and RNAase H activity. The X ORF encodes a protein with 154 amino acids. The X protein is not essential for the replication of hepadnaviruses, but is believed to contribute to HBV-related hepatocarcinogenesis. It functions as a transactivator of cellular and other viral genes.

Seven different genotypes of HBV (A, B, C, D, E, F, and G) have been determined. The variations involve approximately 10 per cent of the genome. Genotype A is predominant in Central and Northern Europe, genotype D in the Mediterannean basin, genotypes B and C in Asia, and genotype E in Africa.

Viral replication

Following HBV entry into hepatocytes, the nucleocapsid is transported to the nucleus (Fig. 2). Cellular enzymes repair the open circular HBV DNA into covalently closed circular DNA (cccDNA), which serves as a template for synthesis of pregenomic and messenger RNAs. Viral DNA does not integrate into the host genome as part of the normal replication cycle. The pregenomic RNA is transported to the cytoplasm and serves as mRNA for translation of new core and polymerase proteins. When these three components (pregenomic RNA, core and polymerase proteins) reach sufficient quantities, they assemble into nucleocapsid particles. The polymerase protein is directly involved in the pregenomic RNA encapsidation. Inside the particles the pregenomic RNA is reverse transcribed into DNA 'minus' strand, while the RNA template is simultaneously degraded by RNAaseH. Finally, the 'plus' strand is produced, which completes a new partially double-stranded HBV DNA. Some of the newly synthesized nucleocapsids

Table 1 Main characteristics of hepatitis viruses

Virus	Family	Morphology	Genome	Proteins	Antibodies	Pathogenesis	Specific features
HAV	Picornaviridae	27–28 nm non-enveloped spherical particles	Single-stranded linear RNA, 7500 nt	Four capsid proteins, viral polymerase, and proteases	Anti-HAV	Non-cytopathic virus Immune-mediated acute hepatitis	No chronic infection Effective vaccines available
HBV	Hepadnaviridae	42 nm particle with nucleocapsid (core) and outer envelope (surface)	Partially double-stranded, circular DNA, 3200 nt	*Envelope* Major protein (HBsAg) Middle protein (PreS2+S) Large protein (PreS1+S2+S) *Nucleocapsid* (HBcAg) HBeAg non-structural, soluble protein	Anti-HBs Anti-HBc Anti-HBe	Non-cytopathic virus Immune-mediated acute and chronic hepatitis Weak T-cell reactivity—a dominant cause for persistent viral replication	In chronic infection spontaneous evolution from HBeAg(+) to anti-HBe(+) phase Mutant strains (surface, precore, polymerase) evolve under selection pressure DNA integration into host genome Trans-activation of cellular genes Effective vaccines available
		22 nm spherical and filamentous subviral particles		Envelope proteins only	Anti-HBs		
HCV	Flaviviridae	50–60 nm enveloped spherical particles	Single-stranded linear RNA, approx. 9500 nt	*Structural* Envelope 1 (E1) Envelope 2 (E2) Nucleocapsid (core)	Anti-E1 Anti-E2 Anti-core	Usually non-cytopathic virus Neutralizing antibodies (?)	High degree of virus heterogeneity (genotypes and quasispecies) High propensity to chronic infection No integration in host genome
		Six major genotypes		*Non-structural* NS2 NS3 NS4 NS5	Anti-NS3 Anti-NS4 Anti-NS5	T-cell reactivity—major role for resolution of acute infection	
HDV	Resembles viroids and plant viruses	35–37 nm enveloped particles	Single-stranded circular RNA, 1700 nt	HD-Ag (nucleocapsid) HBsAg (envelope)	Anti-HD Anti-HBs	Direct cytopathic and/or immune-mediated liver injury	Defective RNA virus Requires help from HBV for providing HBsAg
HEV	Caliciviridae	32–34 nm non-enveloped spherical particles	Single-stranded linear RNA, 7500 nt	ORF1—non-structural proteins ORF2—structural proteins ORF3—unknown function	Anti-HEV	Probably immune mediated (?)	Enterically transmitted hepatitis mainly in Asia, Middle East, and Central America No chronic infection
HGV/ GBV-C	Flaviviridae	?	Single-stranded linear RNA, 9400 nt	Conserved E2 No core protein	Anti-E2	Primary site of replication unknown Does not cause hepatitis	Can establish chronic infection No clear pathogenic role
TTV	Circinoviridae (?)	?	Single-stranded, circular DNA, approx. 3850 nt	?	?	Does not cause hepatitis	Can establish chronic infection High degree of virus heterogeneity No clear pathogenic role

NS, non-structural; nt, nucleotides; ORF, open reading frame.

Fig. 1 Schematic representation of hepatitis B virus genome. CP, core promoter; S1P, preS1 promoter; S2P, pre-S2 promoter; XP, X gene promoter; EnhI, enhancer I; Enh II, enhancer II; DR1 and DR2, direct repeat 1 and 2; EcoRI, restriction site for EcoRI enzyme used as a starting point for numbering.

with HBV DNA are transported back to the nucleus, which maintains a stable pool of cccDNA. Others are enveloped and leave the cell as new virions. Hepadnavirus replication differs from that of retroviruses. Integration into the host genome is not obligatory during replication and functional mRNAs are produced from several internal promoters of the circular DNA genome.

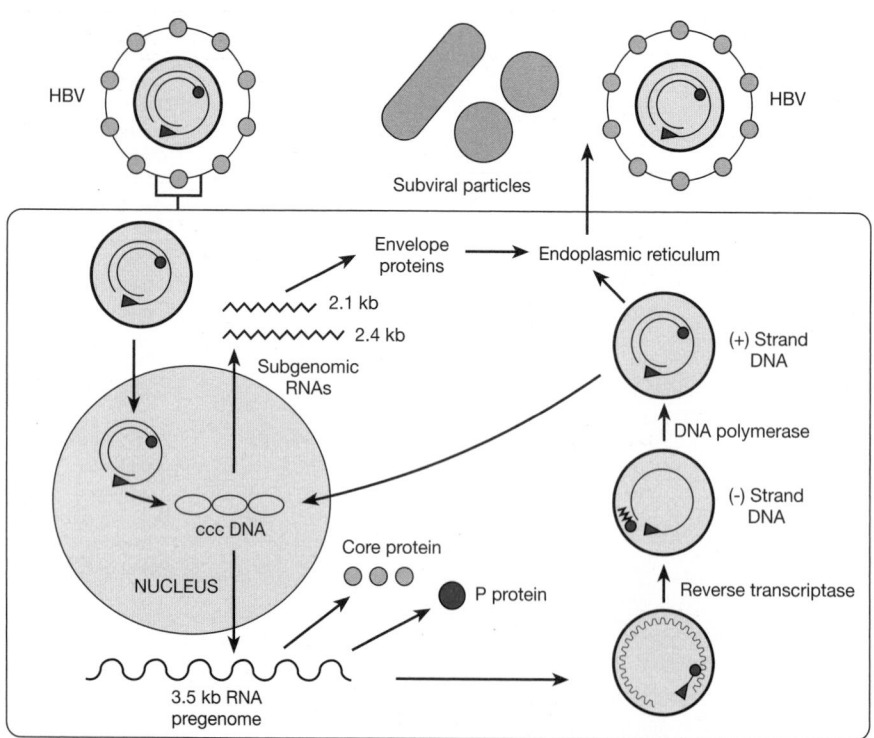

Fig. 2 Replicative cycle of hepatitis B virus.

Host immune response and pathogenesis

HBV is a non-cytopathic virus. The virus-specific cellular immune response is the main determinant of the outcome of infection. Both HLA class I- and class II-restricted T-cell responses are strong, polyclonal, and directed to multiple viral antigens in patients with acute self-limiting hepatitis B. Despite clearance of serum HBsAg, HBV DNA remains detectable by polymerase chain reaction (**PCR**) in most cases, and HBV-specific CD4+ and CD8+ T-cell reactivity has been demonstrated 10 to 20 years after acute infection. Cytokines released from these cells, especially interferon-γ, exert non-cytolytic control on HBV replication without causing cell death. Thus, eradication of HBV may be rare, but the effective immune response controls HBV DNA expression and there is no liver disease. Patients with chronic HBV infection (seropositive for HBsAg) show weak virus-specific T-cell reactivity, which is the dominant cause for HBV persistence. This ineffective response, together with antigen non-specific inflammatory cells, recruited at the site of inflammation, results in progressive liver damage. During the course of chronic HBV infection, spontaneous reactivation of hepatitis may occur, associated with enhanced immune reactivity.

The humoral immune response involves antibodies directed to different HBV antigens (Table 1). It is clinically significant for: (i) diagnosis—the antibody profile in the serum, together with the result of HBsAg and HBeAg, is used to define the phase of HBV infection; (ii) prophylaxis—the development and the level of the protective antibody (anti-HBs) is used to monitor the response to vaccination; (iii) pathogenesis—the humoral immune response contributes to viral elimination from the circulation by forming immune complexes. In some cases, tissue deposition of antigen–antibody complexes is responsible for extrahepatic pathology such as glomerulonephritis, polyarteritis nodosa, arthritis, and skin changes.

Evolution of chronic HBV infection

The changes in HBV–host interactions over time and associated liver disease define three consecutive phases, particularly after vertical transmission of HBV. The early 'immunotolerant' phase is characterized by high levels of virus replication. HBeAg and HBV DNA are readily detectable in serum, while there is minimal liver inflammation. Over the years this is followed by a phase with enhanced immune reactivity to the virus, as reflected by hepatic inflammation and elevated serum aminotransferases. Serum HBeAg is still positive and serum HBV DNA level is usually lower. Some patients will progress spontaneously to the next 'non-replicative' phase, manifested by seroconversion to anti-HBe, undetectable HBV DNA (by conventional techniques), and resolution of hepatic inflammation. Persistent virus replication leads to the emergence of mutations in the HBV genome. Three groups of HBV mutants have direct clinical significance. First, surface escape HBV mutants can emerge in recipients of active and passive immunization. They contain mutations within the immunodominant 'a' determinant of the HBsAg, which abrogate the neutralizing effect of anti-HBs. The second group includes HBV mutants with impaired translation of HBeAg—HBe minus mutants. The most frequent is a G to A mutation at position 1896, which results in a precore stop codon. The third group includes mutations in the polymerase gene that may emerge during treatment with nucleoside analogues, such as lamivudine or famciclovir. The most typical is a lamivudine-associated mutation in the conserved YMDD (tyrosine–methionine–aspartate–aspartate) region of the polymerase, leading to substition of methionine with valine or isoleucine.

Hepatitis C virus (HCV, see also Chapter 7.10.20)

HCV was identified in 1989 and was shown to be the main aetiological agent of parenterally transmitted non-A, non-B hepatitis. For the first time a virus was discovered and characterized by molecular techniques without being seen or grown in culture. The virus has been placed in a separate genus of the Flaviviridae family (Table 1). The lack of an *in vitro* system supporting HCV replication has been a major limitation to the understanding of its biology and the development of antiviral compounds. Synthesis of a full-length cDNA clone, capable of generating infectious RNA transcripts, is an important step to establish a tissue culture system.

Genome organization

The HCV genome is a single-stranded RNA containing a single ORF encoding a polyprotein of 3010 to 3033 amino acids (Fig. 3). Both at the 5′ and the 3′ ends, it has a non-translated region (NTR). The 5′NTR consists of 341 nucleotides and is the most conserved region of the genome. It forms multiple stem–loop structures, important for ribosome entry and presumably for viral RNA replication. The 3′NTR comprises several regions, including a highly conserved sequence of 98 nucleotides at the 3′ terminus, thought to be required for initiation of replication. Because HCV RNA does not replicate via a DNA intermediate, it does not integrate into the host genome. The HCV polyprotein undergoes proteolytic processing in the cytoplasm of infected cells resulting in 10 mature proteins from core to NS5B (Fig. 3). The putative nucleocapsid or core protein is conserved and highly immunogenic, containing several B- and T-cell epitopes. The envelope glycoproteins (E1 and E2) are believed to form the outer spikes of the viral envelope. The HCV E2 protein binds to the major extracellular loop of human CD81 molecule. CD81 is a cell surface protein, expressed on various cells including hepatocytes. It may act as a receptor for HCV. The first 27 amino acids at the N-terminus of the E2 region (between amino acids 384 and 410 of the polyprotein), which show a very high degree of variation, is termed hypervariable region I (**HVRI**). E2 is part of the virus envelope; it contains neutralizing epitopes, one of which appears to be in the HVRI; the immune pressure on this protein leads the selection of escape mutants. The NS3 serine protease domain and the NS4A protein form a complex that is essential for efficient polyprotein cleavage. Specific inhibition of the proteolytic activities of virally encoded proteases is regarded as a promising strategy for inhibiting HCV replication. The non-

Protein	Aminoacids	Function
Core	1–191	Structural, nucleocapsid
E1	192–383	Structural, envelope
E2	384–746	Structural, envelope (including HVRI)
p7	747–809	Unknown
NS2	810–1026	Auto-protease (?)
NS3	1027–1657	Serine protease, RNA helicase
NS4A	1658–1711	Co–factor for NS serine protease
NS4B	1712–1972	Unknown
NS5A	1973–2420	Interferon-α resistance (?)
NS5B	2421–3011	RNA-dependent RNA polymerase

Fig. 3 Hepatitis C virus genome and proteins.

structural protein NS5B possesses RNA polymerase activity. This enzyme is also essential for HCV replication and is another important target for antiviral drug development.

Genome variation and quasispecies

HCV is exceptionally heterogeneous. The NS5B replicase is an error-prone enzyme with no proof-reading activity. During HCV replication this generates many mutant strains which are selected on the basis of their fitness. Based on a phylogenetic analysis of the HCV core, E1, and NS5 regions, six major HCV genotypes (from 1 to 6) have been defined, with a further division into subtypes (1a, 1b, 2a, 2b, etc.). Isolates of type 1 are widely present throughout the world. Genotype 1a and 1b are predominant in North and South America and Europe. Genotypes 2 and 3 are widely distributed in many countries, but are rare in Africa. Genotype 4 is predominant in north and central Africa, especially Egypt, while genotype 5 is most frequent in southern Africa. Genotype 6 is responsible for many HCV infections in Hong Kong and Vietnam. HCV genotypes 7, 8, and 9 have been identified only in Vietnam where they represent almost 20 per cent of all HCV infections. Despite the substantial genomic variations between different HCV genotypes, both clinical and virological data show no significant phenotypic differences in the severity of liver damage or the potential to cause hepatocellular carcinoma. Genotype 1b responds less well than genotypes 2 or 3 to antiviral treatment.

In an individual host, the HCV population is a mixture of closely related, but heterogeneous, RNA sequences centred around one dominant viral sequence. The heterogeneous isolates in a single patient are termed 'quasispecies'. This is commonly based on the genomic variability within the HVRI region. Viral diversity increases during chronic HCV infection as a result of immune escape from antibodies directed to this hypervariable region.

Host immune response and pathogenesis

Clinical evidence suggests that HCV is not cytopathic for infected cells. A most striking feature of HCV is the high rate of chronic infection. The immune response is believed to play a central role in viral clearance and pathogenesis. Neutralizing antibodies are produced during HCV infection. However, they are isolate specific and are usually effective only against HCV strains present before the appearance of the corresponding antibodies. Although antibodies to core and non-structural proteins are detectable in the serum, no specific antibody profile has been established as a predictor of outcome. The titre of antibodies to E1 and E2 proteins correlate with viraemia. The presence of strong and multispecific T-helper cell responses to HCV results in viral clearance. In patients with chronic HCV infection both the CD4+ T-helper cell and the cytotoxic T-lymphocyte responses are much weaker than during acute, resolving infection. Although HCV-specific cytotoxic T lymphocytes have been detected in peripheral and intrahepatic lymphocytes, they seem functionally impaired as they are unable to clear the virus. HCV may escape immune elimination through peripheral tolerance, exhaustion of T-cell response by a high viral load, viral inhibition of antigen presentation, and viral mutations abrogating or antagonizing antigen recognition by virus-specific T cells. Further studies are needed to clarify these possibilities and to provide a scientific basis for new therapeutic concepts and the development of effective vaccine.

Hepatitis D virus (HDV)

HDV is a defective virus that causes acute and chronic liver disease only in association with hepatitis B virus. This unique pathogen was discovered in 1977 by M. Rizzetto in liver biopsies from patients with hepatitis B. HDV particles contain the viral RNA nucleocapsid, which is hepatitis δ-antigen (**HDAg**) and an outer envelope (HBsAg) provided by the helper virus HBV. The HDV genome is a single-stranded, circular RNA (Table 1). It is the smallest known animal virus genome. Because of a high degree of internal complementarity, 70 per cent of the nucleotides are base-paired. This gives it an unusual, rod-like structure. HDV RNA replicates via RNA-directed RNA synthesis by transcription of genomic RNA to a complementary antigenomic δ-RNA that serves as a template for subsequent genomic RNA synthesis. HDV produces a single protein, HDAg, which is encoded by the antigenomic RNA. RNA editing of the antigenomic RNA allows the virus to make two forms of HDAg—'small (S)' (195 amino acids) and 'large (L)' (214 amino acids). Both forms are present in the virions and have different functions in the HDV replicative cycle. HDAg-S facilitates HDV RNA replication, while HDAg-L inhibits replication and is required for assembly of the virion. Although the formation of δ-virions requires the helper fuction of HBV, the replication of HDV RNA within the cell can occur without HBV.

Three distinct HDV genotypes have been recognized. Genotype I, the most widespread, has been identified in North America, Europe, Africa, and Asia. It is associated with a broad spectrum of chronic liver disease. Genotype II is found only in east Asia and seems to cause mild hepatitis-δ. Genotype III is found exclusively in northern parts of South America and is associated with particularly severe hepatitis.

Host immune response and pathogenesis

HDV can infect either simultaneously with HBV (coinfection) or as a superinfection of a chronic carrier of HBsAg. Because HDV requires the helper function of HBV, the duration of δ-infection is determined by the duration of HBsAg positivity. Like antibodies to HBV nucleocapsid (anti-HBc), antibodies to HDAg are not protective. Chronic HDV infection is accompanied by high titres of IgG anti-HD. High serum levels of IgM anti-HD indicate acute δ-infection or exacerbation of chronic hepatitis D. The roles of cellular immune responses to HDAg, HBV antigens, or both in the immunopathogenesis of hepatitis D is uncertain. The lack of liver pathology in transgenic mice expressing HDV and data from experimental infections suggest that HDV is not cytopathic. This is supported by the experience with patients undergoing liver transplantation for HDV cirrhosis. Although HDV always recurs in the graft, necroinflammation is absent unless HBV recurs as well. The presence of microvesicular steatosis in severe hepatitis D indicates a possible direct cytopathic effect in some circumstances.

Hepatitis E virus (HEV)

HEV was first identified in 1983 by immune electron microscopy of the faeces of patients and is now recognized as the agent responsible for enterically transmitted non-A, non-B hepatitis. The virus is classified in the Caliciviridae family. Without a cell culture system, studies on HEV have required experimental transmission to susceptible non-human primates, such as cynomolgous macaques. The HEV genome is a single-stranded, polyadenylated RNA of approximately 7500 nucleotides containing three open reading frames (Table 1). ORF1 encodes non-structural proteins involved in virus replication—helicase and RNA-dependent RNA polymerase. ORF2, comprising approximately 2000 nucleotides, codes for the major structural proteins. ORF3 has 328 nucleotides and also appears to code for a structural protein. The genomic organization of HEV is different from HAV and HCV because the structural and non-structural proteins are coded by discontinuous, partially overlapping ORFs. Non-structural proteins are encoded at the 5′ rather than at the 3′ end of the genome. Unlike HAV, HEV infection may be zoonotic. HEV RNA has been found in the faeces of wild pigs. Serological evidence of infection has been found in pigs, cattle, and sheep in endemic regions. Sequence analyses have identified two major genotypes of HEV (isolates from Burma and Mexico), which show 25 per cent nucleotide variability. The amino acid variability ranges from 1 to 5 per cent among different HEV isolates from Asia to 14 per cent between the Mexican and Asian isolates. A new genotype was recently isolated from a patient in the United States.

The primary site of HEV replication is not fully understood. Following intravenous HEV inoculation in experimental models, the elevation of serum aminotransferases occurs after 24 to 38 days. Expression of HEV antigens has been detected in the cytoplasm of hepatocytes as early as 7 to 10 days after inoculation. Experimental data indicate that during an initial phase with high HEV replication, the virus may be released from hepatocytes into bile before serum 'liver' enzymes increase and there are morphological changes in the liver. Virus shedding ceases when serum aminotransferases return to normal. HEV RNA is detectable by reverse transcriptase polymerase chain reaction (**RT-PCR**) in the serum of virtually all patients within 2 weeks of the start of hepatitis. Prolonged viraemia (4 to 16 weeks) has also been reported. Detection of anti-HEV by enzyme immunoassay involving recombinant HEV antigens or synthetic peptides is the most frequently used method for diagnosis and for epidemiological studies.

The humoral immune response develops gradually in parallel with the rise in serum alanine aminotransferase. The serum level of anti-HEV IgM peaks around the time of peak enzyme levels and is detectable for 5 to 6 months. Although the IgG anti-HEV response persists for several years after the acute hepatitis, the natural history of protective immunity to HEV is not fully established. In contrast to HAV, hepatitis E shows an unusually high attack rate among adults, suggesting that immunity to HEV, if acquired in childhood, may wane.

GB virus-C (GBV-C) or hepatitis G virus (HGV)

The genome of GBV-C was identified in 1995 by molecular hybridization in the serum of a patient with the initials GB. Separately, another group of investigators identified the genome of a new RNA virus, named hepatitis G virus. The comparison of HGV and GBV-C genomes revealed high homology, both at nucleotide (86 per cent) and amino acid level (100 per cent). In is now accepted that they represent two isolates of the same virus. GBV-C/HGV is an RNA virus with a single ORF encoding a polyprotein of approximately 3000 amino acids (Table 1). Together with another two RNA viruses, GBV-A and GBV-B, it belongs to the Flaviviridae family. These three viruses show various similarities with HCV. Specific features of the GBV-C/HGV genome include absence of core gene (nucleocapsid); long 5'- and 3'NTR and lack of poly(A) tail. Unlike HCV, this virus has a very conserved E2 region. Longitudinal studies have shown that GBV-C/HGV can establish chronic infection with RNA persistence in serum for up to 15 years. Some patients clear the virus spontaneously and develop anti-E2 reactivity, which is used as a marker of past infection. Anti-E2 also seems to confer protective immunity. A large body of evidence suggests that GBV-C/HGV does not cause liver disease.

TT virus (TTV)

TTV was identified in 1997 by investigators in Japan. By applying the methodology used for the identification of GBV-C, they detected the genome of a new DNA virus in the serum of a patient with cryptogenic post-transfusion hepatitis. The patient's initials (TT) prompted the name of this new virus and a causative role for acute and chronic hepatitis was suggested. Subsequent studies revealed that the TTV genome is circular, single-stranded DNA of approximately 3850 nucleotides (Table 1). Two partial ORFs have been predicted, but TTV proteins have not been expressed so far. It is suggested that TTV belongs to a new family—Circinoviridae. TTV DNA has been detected in non-human primates and farm animals. The primary site of TTV replication is unknown. TTV DNA is present in the liver and in all fractions of peripheral blood mononuclear cells, although TTV RNA transcripts are detectable only in liver tissue. Unlike other DNA viruses, TTV shows remarkable genomic variability. The phylogenetic analysis demonstrates the presence of many genotypes although there is no internationally agreed classification yet. The TTV population in one patient could comprise several genotypes.

TTV infection is highly prevalent worldwide (for instance up to 92 per cent of healthy subjects in Japan). Initially, the virus was thought to be transmitted parenterally, although its prevalence in the general population indicates the importance of non-parenteral routes as well. Prevalence increases with age in paediatric and adult age groups.

It is uncertain whether TTV is pathogenic. Analysis of liver histology in patients with TTV infection and longitudinal studies, as well as experimental TTV inoculation in chimpanzees, demonstrate that this virus does not cause hepatitis. So far, TTV is an example of a human virus with no clear disease association.

Further reading

Cerny A, Chisari FV (1999). Pathogenesis of chronic hepatitis C: immunological features of hepatic injury and viral persistence. *Hepatology* **30**, 595–601.

Hadziyannis SJ (1997). Epidemiology of G/GBV-C infection. In: Boyer JL, Ockner RK, eds. *Progress in liver diseases*, Vol XIV, pp 219–45. WB Saunders, Philadelphia.

Lau JYN, Wright TL (1993). Molecular virology and pathogenesis of hepatitis B. *Lancet* **342**, 1335–40.

Major ME, Feinstone SM (1997). The molecular virology of hepatitis C. *Hepatology* **25**, 1527–38.

Rizzetto M (1983). The delta agent. *Hepatology* **3**, 729–37.

Torre F, Naoumov NV (1998). Clinical implications of mutations in the hepatitis B virus genome. *European Journal of Clinical Investigation* **28**, 604–14.

Wilson RA, ed. (1997). *Viral hepatitis. diagnosis, treatment, prevention*. Marcel Dekker, New York.

Zuckerman AJ, Thomas HC, eds (1998). *Viral hepatitis. Scientific basis and clinical management*, 2nd edn. Churchill Livingstone, Edinburgh.

7.10.20 Hepatitis C virus

D. L. Thomas

Introduction

By the mid 1970s, it was apparent that both acute and chronic hepatitis could be caused by something other than hepatitis A virus (**HAV**) or hepatitis B virus (**HBV**). This condition, called non-A, non-B hepatitis, was assumed to be a viral infection since it was reproduced in chimpanzees inoculated with blood from affected persons, even after passage through 90 nm filters. However, hepatitis C virus (**HCV**) was not discovered until the late 1980s when a portion of viral RNA was cloned, and the resulting antigen shown to react with sera from persons with non-A, non-B hepatitis. It is now clear that HCV causes most cases of bloodborne non-A, non-B hepatitis.

Aetiology (see Chapter 7.10.19)

Epidemiology

Prevalence of infection

An estimated 170 million people are infected with HCV worldwide. In economically developed nations, HCV infection is found typically in 1 to 2 per cent of the general population. A 10-fold higher HCV prevalence has been found in Egypt and in some regions of Japan, Taiwan, and Italy. In these highly-endemic regions a sharp decrease in prevalence is often found in those less than 30 to 40 years of age, a cohort effect that probably reflects discontinuation of a practice that once contributed to widespread infection. HCV infection occurs in 50 to 90 per cent of persons injecting illicit drugs, more than 90 per cent of patients with haemophilia transfused with clotting factors before they were inactivated, 10 to 50 per cent of patients on haemodialysis, 5 to 20 per cent of patients attending sexually transmitted disease clinics, and 1 to 3 per cent of health care workers. HCV infection is common in people with other bloodborne infections, such as HBV and HIV.

Transmission

Biological basis

Studies with molecular clones demonstrate that infection will occur if sufficient numbers of complete HCV RNA transcripts reach the liver. HCV RNA has been detected in blood, saliva, seminal fluid, and tears, and intravenously injected blood is clearly infectious. In addition, in one instance, a chimpanzee was infected by intravenous injection of saliva. It is not known if other body fluids contain enough intact virions to be infectious when administered percutaneously or if infection can be sustained when virions contact cells present in mucous membranes.

Percutaneous transmission

Nosocomial transmission

The principal route of HCV transmission worldwide is percutaneous exposure to HCV-containing blood. Transfusion of contaminated blood once accounted for 20 per cent of HCV infection in the United States. HCV has also been transmitted by intravenous administration of contaminated immunoglobulin and clotting factors, including several well publicized outbreaks in the United States and Europe. However, the incidence of HCV transmission through administration of blood and blood components has decreased dramatically in regions of the world where donors are screened for HCV antibody and viral deactivation procedures are now used for immunoglobulin and clotting factor products.

Although the incidence in economically developed nations is now very low, patient-to-patient HCV transmission has been documented following percutaneous medical procedures such as colonoscopy with biopsy and use of intravenous infusion devices. In such instances, a common source of transmission can be detected by higher than expected identity in RNA sequences from various persons, as has repeatedly been shown in haemodialysis centres. Nosocomial HCV transmission probably requires a breach in infection control policies, although this may be difficult to recognize retrospectively.

In economically developing nations, most HCV transmission occurs through medical treatments, both by modern and folk practices. In Egypt, where 50 per cent of persons more than 40 years of age are infected, HCV was transmitted through a widespread national campaign of injections to eradicate schistosomiasis. When this practice was discontinued, there was a sharp decrease in HCV prevalence in persons born thereafter. Elsewhere in the world, HCV transmission occurs where education and resources are insufficient to ensure sterilization of devices used for medical injections, scarification rituals, and other percutaneous practices. Misperceptions regarding the benefit of injections appear to be especially important.

Drug use

In some regions of the world, percutaneous exposure to contaminated needles and other drug-use implements is the dominant mode of HCV transmission. HCV infection, which often occurs within months of starting to abuse drugs by injection, is found in 50 to 90 per cent of people admitting drug use worldwide. There are conflicting data as to whether HCV can be transmitted by intranasal use of cocaine.

Sexual transmission

Transmission of HCV by intercourse has not been proven, but some data suggest that it occurs, albeit uncommonly. In some HCV-infected individuals, the only potential exposure that can be detected is sex with another infected person, and HCV infection occurs more often than expected in persons with multiple sexual partners. In the families of HCV-infected people, sexual partners are the only members whose risk of infection is increased. The viral nucleotide sequences often suggest a common source. However, most long-term sexual partners of people with hepatitis C are not infected, and in those who are infected, it is impossible to exclude exposures other than intercourse. In the few studies in which direct comparisons are possible, the prevalences of HBV and HIV in sexual partners are 5- to 10-fold higher than for HCV.

Most authorities do not recommend that people in monogamous relationships use condoms to prevent HCV transmission. However, many encourage HCV-infected people to discuss the risk of transmission with their sexual partners and encourage them to be screened.

Mother-to-infant transmission

HCV infection occurs in 2 to 8 per cent of infants born to HIV-infected mothers. This risk increases if the mother is also HIV infected or if the maternal level of HCV RNA is high. Because of passive transfer of maternal antibodies, the diagnosis of HCV infection in the child must be based on detection of HCV RNA or persistence of antibodies 18 months or more after birth. There is no conclusive evidence that HCV is transmitted by breast feeding, and only a single study that suggests the risk of perinatal infection is reduced by elective caesarian delivery.

Natural history and pathogenesis

Viral persistence

HCV RNA can be detected in blood within weeks of exposure and, for approximately 85 per cent of individuals, remains detectable indefinitely (Fig. 1). Most persistently-infected people have intermittent elevations in serum liver enzymes such as alanine aminotransferase (**ALT**) and after 10 to 20 years, 2 to 20 per cent develop cirrhosis. Within 5 years, approximately 20 per cent of those who develop cirrhosis will have a life-threatening complication, such as ascites, variceal bleeding, hepatic encephalopathy, or hepatocellular carcinoma.

The incidence of cirrhosis is higher in persons infected at older ages and those who ingest alcohol, especially more than 50 g/day (or the equivalent of three alcoholic drinks). The effect of smaller amounts of alcohol is not known. HIV and HBV infections also appear to increase the incidence of HCV-related cirrhosis. Neither HCV genotype nor HCB RNA level are strong determinants of disease progression.

The pathogenesis of cirrhosis is poorly understood. A few HLA alleles have been associated with cirrhosis and more vigorous cytotoxic

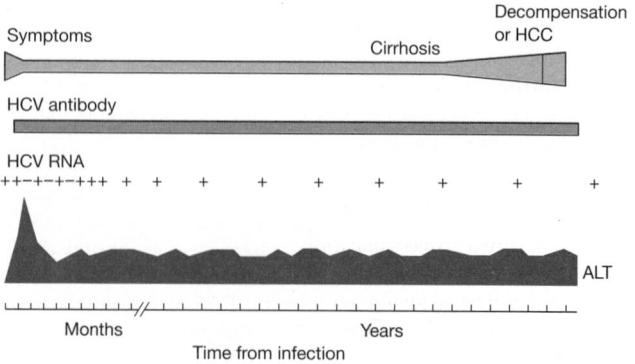

Fig. 1 Natural history of HCV infection.

T-lymphocyte responses have been associated with severe liver disease. Conversely, immunosuppression from sources as diverse as HIV infection, agammaglobulinaemia, and steroid use appears to increase the incidence of cirrhosis.

Viral clearance

In approximately 15 per cent of people, HCV RNA can no longer be detected in blood one or more years after exposure, although HCV antibody and T-lymphocyte responses may remain. Long-term sequelae like cirrhosis and hepatocellular cancer do not appear to occur in those with viral clearance.

The mechanisms of viral clearance are not known. Both humoral and cellular immune responses are detectable to multiple HCV antigens within months of exposure, but occur even in those with persistent infection. Over time, individual variants may be eliminated from the HCV quasispecies only to be replaced by others that are sufficiently different to escape immune effectors. Those who clear HCV infection also tend to have strong T-cell proliferation responses to HCV antigens and a T_{H1} cytokine phenotype. The importance of these findings in viral clearance remains to be shown.

Clinical features

Acute infection

Acute HCV infection is indistinguishable from other forms of acute viral hepatitis, causing malaise, nausea, and right upper quadrant pain, followed by dark urine and jaundice. These symptoms occur in approximately 20 per cent of acutely infected adults, less frequently and typically with less severity than for hepatitis A or hepatitis B. Fulminant hepatic failure is rare.

HCV RNA is detectable before symptoms occur, but the level of viraemia varies in the first 6 months and can be transiently undetectable even in those who ultimately have persistent infection. Serum levels of liver enzymes such as ALT rise more than 10 times normal, then decline and, for those with persistent HCV infection, fluctuate indefinitely. The serum bilirubin may also be elevated for weeks after symptoms are first noted, but ultimately returns to a normal level. HCV antibody can usually be detected within a month of symptoms and within 8 weeks of exposure.

Chronic infection

The 85 per cent of people who develop persistent infection can be differentiated from those with viral clearance by repeated testing for HCV RNA in blood for 12 or more months. Other tests, such as serum ALT levels and the quantity of serum HCV RNA, do not reliably predict the outcome.

Fatigue and malaise may herald the onset of cirrhosis, which is suggested by thrombocytopenia, neutropenia, hypoprothrombinaemia, and hypoalbuminaemia. These haematological indicators of cirrhosis develop as late findings and imply a bad prognosis. Liver enzymes fluctuate throughout the course of HCV infection with little correlation to symptoms or the long-term outcome. Cirrhosis can occur even in the 20 to 40 per cent of patients who have repeatedly normal ALT levels. The levels of HCV RNA and HCV genotype likewise are poor predictors of disease. Probably the only reliable marker of disease progression is the liver biopsy (see below).

Extrahepatic manifestations

These include mixed cryoglobulinaemic vasculitis and membranoproliferative glomerulonephritis (see Chapter 20.7.8). Diagnosis of cryoglobulin-related vasculitis is based on the clinical syndrome as HCV-infected people commonly have cryoglobulins detectable in their serum. HCV infection is commonly associated with sporadic porphyria cutanea tarda, and less commonly, with Sjögren's syndrome, lichen planus, idiopathic pulmonary fibrosis, and Mooren's corneal ulcers.

Pathology

The histopathological features of acute HCV infection are less severe than with the other hepatitis viruses. Mononuclear (mostly lymphocytic) inflammation is present throughout the lobule. Sinusoidal lining cells are activated and fat can be seen. Over time, the level of inflammation varies and fibrosis can occur, beginning in the portal areas and, in some cases, extending as septae beteween portal zones. Fibrous bands that bridge portal triads and formation of nodules denotes cirrhosis. The Knodell system quantifies the degree of periportal necrosis (0 to 10), intralobular necrosis (0 to 4), and portal inflammation (0 to 4) along with the stage of disease or fibrosis score (0 to 4). Although the histological findings fluctuate, this information remains the most important predictor of disease outcome and is often used to ascertain which individuals would benefit from treatment.

Liver cancer

Each year, an estimated 1 to 4 per cent of people with HCV-associated cirrhosis will develop hepatocellular cancer. The pathogenesis is unknown. The highest incidences are reported in Japan and Italy. In China and Korea, HBV infection is a more common cause of hepatocellular carcinoma. Serum α-fetoprotein levels and hepatic ultrasound are used for screening in persons with cirrhosis.

Diagnosis

Serological testing

HCV infection is usually diagnosed by testing for HCV antibodies in serum with an enzyme immunoassay that includes recombinant HCV proteins. Second and later generations of these antibody assays are highly sensitive screening tools (Table 1). Problems arise in acute infection as antibody development can be delayed for several months after exposure and in those with compromised antibody production (e.g. haemodialysis and agammaglobulinaemia). Uncommonly, false-negative enzyme results have been reported in persons on haemodialysis and, less commonly, HIV-positive people.

A positive HCV antibody test needs further evaluation. In low-risk screening (e.g. volunteer blood donation) an immunoblot assay can be used to detect antibodies to a variety of recombinant antigens. Reactions to more than one antigen strongly suggests infection. Where HCV infection is expected, HCV RNA testing is a more expedient confirmation approach, providing both an independent assessment of infection and indication of whether the infection has cleared or is ongoing.

HCV RNA testing

HCV RNA can be detected and quantified by a number of amplification techniques including reverse transcription polymerase chain reaction (**RT-PCR**). The reliability of HCV RNA assays has been questioned and the values of different quantitative tests are difficult to compare, although an international standard has been advanced. HCV genotype can be assessed by phylogenetic analysis of nucleotide sequences or detection of subtype-specific point mutations in RT-PCR amplified RNA.

Treatment

Interferon-α

Interferon-α induces expression of multiple genes that have antiviral and antiproliferative activity including those encoding RNAase L, 2′-5′ oligoadenylate synthase, M protein, and protein kinase R.

Almost half of the patients receiving interferon-α-2b (3 million units subcutaneously three times a week for 6 months) have a normal serum ALT

Table 1 Laboratory tests for HCV infection

Test	Comment
Diagnosis	
HCV antibody by EIA	High sensitivity, used to screen for infection
HCV antibody by RIBA	High specificity, used in low-prevalence settings (e.g. blood donations) to detect false-positive EIA results
HCV RNA	Used when EIA is positive in high-prevalence setting (e.g. persons with elevated ALT or HCV risk factor) or to identify acute infection before antibody is detectable. When detected, provides independent confirmation of EIA and indication of ongoing infection. RNA tests can be unreliable.
Pretreatment evaluation	
Liver biopsy	Best reflection of stage of disease, prognosis, and need for therapy
HCV genotype	Important predictor of treatment response and duration
HCV RNA level	Possible predictor of treatment response and duration

ALT, serum alanine aminotransferase; EIA, enzyme immunoassay; RIBA, recombinant immunoblot assay. See text for details.

and undetectable HCV RNA by the end of treatment (end of treatment response). However, many relapse and 6 months after completion of therapy, fewer than 20 per cent still have a normal ALT level and undetectable HCV RNA (sustained response). Longer treatment reduces the number of relapses, but overall sustained (6 months after treatment) response rates remain low. Higher interferon doses and daily administration accelerate the pace of viral clearance but do not consistently improve sustained virological response rates.

Interferon-α therapy causes a number of adverse reactions. Flu-like symptoms occur within 6 h of the first dose but generally diminish in 1 to 2 weeks. Fatigue, depression, and other mood disturbances may be severe, especially if there is a history of such problems in the past. Hair thinning and thyroid abnormalities may occur. Bone marrow suppression is common including neutropenia, thrombocytopenia, and anaemia. Interferon-α cannot be used safely in pregnancy.

Interferon-α therapy has been associated with improvements in quality-of-life indices and reductions in the incidence of hepatocellular cancer and cirrhosis. Although uncommon, sustained virological responses are durable; 5 years later more than 90 per cent of sustained responders still have normal serum ALT levels and no HCV RNA in blood or liver.

Other interferon formulations, including a recombinant consensus interferon, interferon-α-2a, and interferon-α-2b-n₁ (lymphoblastoid interferon) have similar efficacy and adverse effects. Interferon-α has been cova-lently linked to polyethylene glycol (pegylated interferon), resulting in a longer half-life (weekly dosing), higher sustained serum levels, and improved HCV clearance.

Interferon and ribavirin

Ribavirin is a guanosine analogue that has broad antiviral activity but may affect HCV by inducing a shift toward a T_{H1} immune response. Used orally alone, ribavirin returns the level of serum ALT to normal in some individuals but does not substantially change HCV RNA levels. However, in combination with interferon-α-2b, 1000 to 1200 mg of oral ribavirin daily improves the sustained virological response rates both for people who have never been treated and those who initially responded to interferon but then relapsed (but not those who never responded). As initial treatment, approximately one-third of patients treated with interferon and ribavirin have a sustained virological response. Responses to interferon-α and ribavirin vary according to pretreatment characteristics, especially HCV genotype (Fig. 2). It is likely that pegylated interferon-α and ribavirin will be the most effective therapy available in 2001.

Adverse reactions to ribavirin and interferon-α are similar to those with interferon-α alone, but ribavirin causes haemolytic anaemia in many patients. Ribavirin is teratogenic; pregnancy must be prevented during and for up to 1 year after administration, whichever sex is being treated.

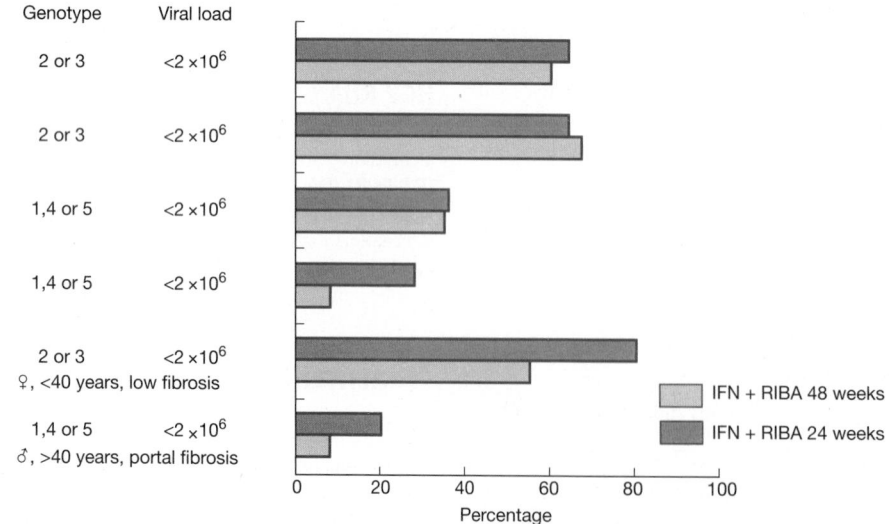

Fig. 2 Sustained virological response rates according to regimen and pretreatment factors.

Other therapies

Oral amantadine and herbal products such as milk thistle have been used to treat HCV infection. New drugs are expected that interfere with the viral protease, helicase, or replicase, or with viral translation.

Prevention

Primary prevention

HCV transmission is preventable by reducing percutaneous exposures, while ensuring the safety of those that are medically or culturally necessary. HCV-infected people should not allow others to come into contact with their blood, especially by sharing razors or dental devices. HCV is not transmitted by typical household exposures (hugging, kissing, sharing eating utensils or food). Counselling may be needed to prevent unwarranted ostracism.

No vaccination has been licensed to prevent HCV transmission. Since HCV reinfection has been demonstrated even with an autologous inoculum, it is difficult to induce immunity that protects against infection. However, it may be possible to reduce viral persistence by vaccination.

Secondary prevention

Once infection occurs, the incidence of cirrhosis and hepatocellular cancer can be reduced by medical treatment and elimination (or reduction) of alcohol ingestion. Because of drug toxicity and expense, interferon-α use is rare except among selected residents of economically developed nations. More accessible treatments are needed to prevent development of disease worldwide.

Postexposure prevention

Although administration of HCV antibody-containing immunoglobulin may increase the time to development of infection, infection is not usually prevented, and immunoglobulin preparations available in many countries no longer contain HCV antibodies. Therefore, most authorities recommend that persons exposed to HCV do not receive immunoglobulin. Exposed persons should be monitored (for example, at 2 and 6 months) for development of HCV antibodies and possibly HCV RNA, since treatment may be more effective if provided within the first year of infection. There are no interventions available to prevent HCV transmission from a mother to her infant; in particular, current medical treatments (interferon and ribavirin) are contraindicated in pregnancy, immunoglobulin administration is not advised, caesarian section is not routinely indicated, and breast feeding should not be discouraged.

Further reading

Alter MJ et al. (1998). Hepatitis C. Infectious Disease Clinics of North America 12, 13–26. [A review of the epidemiology of hepatitis C infection from an international expert.]

Bukh J, Miller RH Purcell RH (1995) Genetic heterogeneity of hepatitis C virus: quasispecies and genotypes. Seminars in Liver Disease 15, 41–63. [A comprehensive evalution of the genetic complexity of hepatitis C by the pioneers in the field.]

Centers for Disease Control and Prevention (1998). Recommendations for prevention and control of hepatitis C virus (HCV) infection and HCV-related chronic disease. Morbidity and Mortality Weekly Report 47 (No. RR-19), 1–39. [A thorough review of the epidemiology and management of hepatitis C infection.]

Chang K-M, Rehermann B, Chisari HV (1997). Immunopathology of hepatitis C. Springer Seminars in Immunopathology 19, 57–68. [A review of the immunology of hepatitis C infection by a group that has contributed substantially to the field.]

Davis GL, Nelson DR, Royes GR (1999). Future options for the management of hepatitis C. Seminars in Liver Disease 19(Suppl. 1), 103–12. [A review of the manamgent of hepatitis C infection by leading experts.]

Pawlotsky JM et al. (1998). What strategy should be used for diagnosis of hepatitis C virus infection in clinical laboratories? Hepatology 27, 1700–2. [A review of the approach to diagnosis of hepatitis C infection by an international expert.]

Seef LB (1997). Natural history of hepatitis C. Hepatology 26, 21S–28S. [A review of the natural history of hepatitis C by an international expert.]

Thomas DL, Lemon SM (2000). Hepatitis C. In: Mandell GL, Bennett JE, Dolin R, eds. Principles and practices of infectious diseases, 5th edn, pp 1736–60. [A well-referenced review of hepatitis C.]

7.10.21 HIV and AIDS

G. A. Luzzi, T. E. A. Peto, R. A. Weiss, and C. P. Conlon

Introduction

The acquired immunodeficiency syndrome (**AIDS**) was first recognized in 1981 in the United States, when several cases of *Pneumocystis carinii* pneumonia and Kaposi's sarcoma were reported in homosexual men in New York and California. The variety of unusual infections and other conditions declared a new form of cellular immunodeficiency. Soon after, the syndrome was reported in injecting drug users, haemophiliacs, and recipients of blood transfusions. Early epidemiological data suggested that the cause was a sexually transmissible bloodborne infective agent. During 1983, in France, a new retrovirus was isolated from a patient with persistent generalized lymphadenopathy. Initially referred to as 'lymphadenopathy-associated virus' (**LAV**) or 'human T-lymphotropic virus III' (**HTLV-III**), it was renamed 'human immunodeficiency virus' (**HIV**) in 1986.

At the time of its discovery, HIV was already widespread, the earliest infections probably having occurred before the 1950s. The recognition of heterosexual intercourse as the most common means of HIV transmission worldwide followed the investigation of epidemics in Africa and the Caribbean. Infected mothers could pass the virus on to their fetus or neonate, establishing vertical transmission as another important route of HIV infection.

In 1986 a second retrovirus causing AIDS, HIV-2, was identified in West Africa. It is largely confined to this region, while HIV-1 is the cause of the world pandemic of AIDS. Over the past 5 years there have been advances in the understanding of the pathogenesis of HIV, in clinical monitoring, and in therapy. Table 1 lists the milestones in the history of HIV and AIDS (acquired immunodeficiency syndrome).

Epidemiology

The global HIV-1 pandemic has affected developing countries in particular. Despite under-reporting, the World Health Organization (**WHO**) estimated that by the end of 1998 over 10 million people had died of HIV, and over 30 million people were alive and infected worldwide, of whom 90 per cent were living in sub-Saharan Africa, South and South-East Asia, and Central and South America (Fig. 1).

The numbers of people infected with HIV must be distinguished from cases of AIDS, which follows an asymptomatic period of about 10 years and may be influenced by interventions such as antiretroviral therapy. Worldwide, the WHO estimated a 9 per cent increase in new infections in 1997 compared with 1996.

In North America, western Europe, and Australasia the epidemic began in the late 1970s and early 1980s among homosexual men and injecting drug users. However, in these regions the proportion attributable to heterosexual transmission has increased. The estimated incidence of AIDS in western Europe rose every year between 1985 and 1994, stabilized in 1995, and fell by 10 per cent in 1996 and by over 20 per cent in 1997. A similar trend has been observed in North America. Cases attributed to injecting drug use form the largest proportion of diagnosed cases of AIDS in Europe. Large epidemics of HIV have been reported in injecting drug users in several countries of the former Soviet Union.

Some two-thirds of all cases are found in sub-Saharan Africa, where HIV transmission is predominantly heterosexual and perinatal. The estimated overall prevalence there is 7 to 8 per cent, rising to 20 to 30 per cent in some countries such as Zambia and Zimbabwe, where AIDS has curtailed population growth. Because of the predominant heterosexual transmission, the overall male-to-female ratio in Africa is approximately 1:1 compared with 9:1 in North America and western Europe.

In Africa, predicted rates of AIDS and new HIV infection were expected to plateau by 2000 and then to fall gradually, whereas trends suggest a continuing rise in South and South-East Asia, where the emergence of epidemic HIV occurred later. A rapid rise in incidence occurred in Thailand and India in the late 1980s, initially among intravenous drug users and prostitutes and then through heterosexual spread; the WHO estimates that 3 to 5 million people have been infected in India alone. Rapid spread and major epidemics of HIV have also been reported in China, Cambodia, Burma (Myanmar), and Vietnam.

High rates of transmission of HIV continue in developing countries because of the lack of awareness, poverty, high rates of other sexually transmitted infections, and higher risk behaviour such as the use of prostitutes and injecting drug use.

HIV-2 is endemic in parts of West Africa and is increasingly prevalent in Angola, Mozambique, France, and Portugal. In other parts of the world the prevalence is very low, although it is present in India. The clinical features of HIV-2 are similar to those of HIV-1, but some patients with HIV-2, for unknown reasons, appear to progress much more slowly.

HIVs may be regarded as zoonoses: HIV-1 is derived from a simian immunodeficiency virus in the chimpanzee (*Pan troglodytes troglodytes*), and the animal reservoir for HIV-2 is the sooty mangabey monkey (*Cercocebus atys*). Variation of HIV-1 RNA sequences has been identified, leading to a classification of 11 sequence subtypes (or clades), A to K, of the main group M, and N (new) and O (outlier) as two quite distinct groups in west central Africa. The subtypes have varying geographical distributions. For instance, subtypes A and D are found in central Africa, B in North America and Europe, and E in Thailand. Study of the genetic and geographical divergence of subtypes has shed light on the emergence and global spread of HIV.

Table 1 Milestones in the history of HIV and AIDS

pre-1970s	HIV-1 transmitted to humans in Africa, probably from chimpanzee source
1970s	Unrecognized global spread of HIV
1981	Epidemic pneumocystis pneumonia and Kaposi's sarcoma reported in New York, Los Angeles, and San Francisco
1983	New human retrovirus isolated from a patient in France
1984	Retrovirus confirmed as cause of AIDS; CD4 shown to be its binding receptor
	Screening for HIV antibodies in donated blood introduced in industrialized countries
1986	HTLV-III/LAV renamed human immunodeficiency virus (HIV) by the International Committee for Taxonomy of Viruses
	Effective prevention of pneumocystis pneumonia by co-trimoxazole and other drugs
	HIV-2 isolated from West African patients
1987	Zidovudine improves survival in AIDS
1990	Antigenic variation warns that development of HIV vaccines will not be easy
1993	Concorde trial demonstrates that survival benefit from zidovudine monotherapy is not sustained
1994	Zidovudine shown to reduce vertical transmission of HIV by two-thirds
	HHV-8 discovered: the cause of Kaposi's sarcoma
1995	High HIV and immune-cell turnover demonstrated during asymptomatic phase of HIV infection
	Dual combinations of nucleosides shown to be superior to monotherapy
1996	Prognostic value of plasma HIV RNA estimation (viral load) demonstrated
	Protease inhibitors in triple regimens show marked reduction in progression to AIDS and death over the short to medium term
	Chemokine co-receptors for HIV demonstrated; mutant receptors confer resistance to HIV infection in some exposed uninfected subjects
1997	Non-nucleoside reverse transcriptase inhibitors introduced
1998	Epidemiological studies show major reduction in death rates in patients with AIDS on triple therapy
	Vertical transmission of HIV shown to be reduced by elective caesarean section
2001	Inexpensive antiretroviral treatment available in resource-poor countries

Cellular biology of HIV

The viral replication cycle

HIV-1 (Fig. 2) and HIV-2 belong to the lentivirus subfamily of retroviruses. Retrovirus implies a 'backwards' step in biological information during viral replication attributable to its enzyme, reverse transcriptase. As with all retroviruses, the viral genes in infectious particles are carried as RNA, but upon infection of the host cell, reverse transcriptase catalyses the synthesis of a double-stranded DNA viral genome (Fig. 3). Insertion of the DNA genome into the chromosomal DNA of the infected cell is effected by viral integrase. The integrated provirus may remain latent, particularly in resting lymphocytes. In actively infected cells, however, RNA transcripts and proteins are synthesized, leading to the formation of new virus particles.

The core proteins derived from the *gag* and *pol* genes are made as large polypeptides that are then cleaved into smaller components representing the enzymes and building blocks of the virus. This cleavage is achieved by the viral protease. The unique reverse transcriptase and protease are targets of antiretroviral therapy (see Antiretroviral therapy below). Reverse transcriptase inhibitors such as zidovudine and lamivudine affect an early step in HIV replication, whereas the protease inhibitors, such as saquinavir or indinavir, block a late stage of virus assembly (Fig. 3). Compounds that inhibit any stage of HIV replication, without being too toxic to the infected person, are potential antiviral drugs. Agents have been developed to block viral entry (fusion inhibitors); in future, the integrase and viral RNA processing may become therapeutic targets.

HIV genes and proteins

Although regarded as a complex retrovirus, HIV has only nine genes (Fig. 4). The three structural genes are *gag*, *pol*, and *env*, encoding the core proteins p19, p24, and p17, the enzymes (protease, reverse transcriptase,

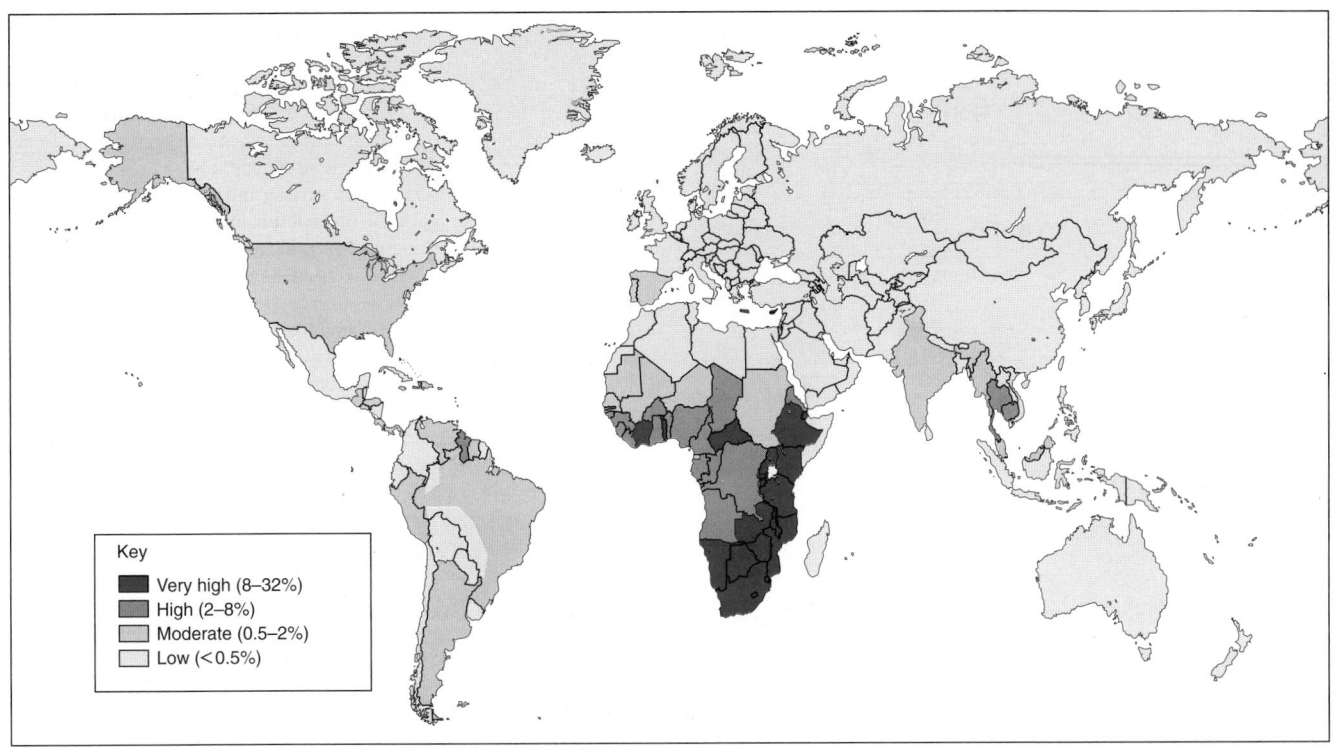

Fig. 1 World distribution of HIV (UNAIDS/WHO, 1998). (Reproduced from *Report on the global HIV/AIDS epidemic*, June 1998. (1998). UNAIDS/WHO, with permission.)

and integrase), and the envelope glycoproteins (gp120 and gp41), respectively. The major regulatory genes *tat* and *rev* encode proteins that are not assembled into the virus but are essential for replication in the cell. The Tat protein acts in positive feedback to enhance transcription of viral RNA from the DNA provirus, while the Rev protein helps the efficient transport of viral RNA from the nucleus to the cytoplasm. Either of these proteins could be a suitable target for antiviral therapy, particularly Tat, because the synthesis of all the other viral proteins depends on its activity.

The functions of the four accessory genes of HIV are less well understood. *Vif* encodes a protein assembled in virus particles that appears necessary for the infectivity at a stage soon after entry, possibly by facilitating disassembly of the virion to allow reverse transcription. Nef also effects an early postentry function; it is not needed by laboratory-adapted HIV strains or if virus enters via endosomal vesicles rather than fusing with the

outer cell membrane. It also downregulates surface expression of the primary cell-surface receptor for HIV, the CD4 antigen, by drawing CD4 into clathrin-coated pits. Vpu similarly interacts with CD4, promoting its degradation by directing it to the ubiquitin–proteasome pathway. Vpr has dual functions; first, it directs the preintegration complex of the virus, containing the newly synthesized DNA, into the nucleus so that it can integrate into chromosomal DNA; second, it blocks cell proliferation in the G2 phase of the cell cycle, thereby enhancing the amount of viral progeny released per cell.

Unlike HIV-1, HIV-2 and the simian immunodeficiency virus (**SIV**) lack *vpu*, but have an alternative gene, *vpx*. HIV-2 Vpr leads the viral genome into the cell nucleus but does not arrest the cell cycle. These proteins presumably recognize cellular proteins and some of these interactions are species-specific. Thus the Vpr and Vif proteins in SIV of African green

Fig. 2 Electron micrograph of HIV-1. (Reproduced by courtesy of H. Gelderblom.)

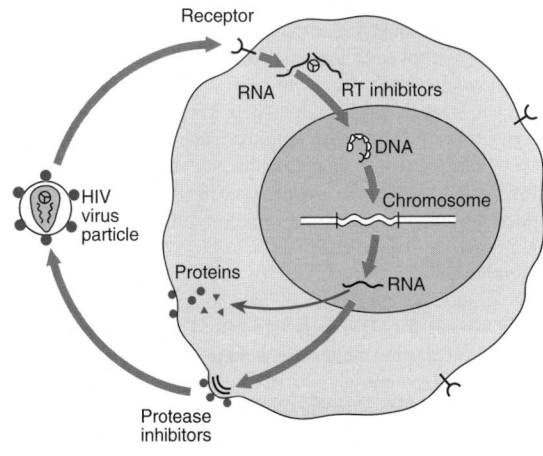

Fig. 3 Replicative cycle of HIV.

Fig. 4 HIV genome map.

monkeys do not function in human cells, while the equivalent proteins of SIV from sooty mangabey monkeys work well in human cells. This could explain why sooty mangabey SIV was able to infect humans and become HIV-2, whereas the more widespread African green monkey SIV has not led to a zoonosis. Another difference is that HIV-1 incorporates the cellular protein cyclophylin A (the target of the drug ciclosporin A) into virus particles, where it may co-operate with Vif and is required for steps early in the infection. In contrast, HIV-2 does not contain cyclophylin A and replicates well without it.

HIV receptors and cellular tropism

CD4 is the cell-surface receptor for HIV; it is expressed on T-helper lymphocytes, the cells that become depleted in AIDS. CD4 is also expressed (to a lesser extent but sufficient to permit infection) on macrophages, Langerhans dendritic cells in mucous membranes, and brain microglial cells. These are the other target cells for HIV infection. CD4 is necessary to initiate HIV infection but is not sufficient to allow the virus to fuse with host-cell membranes: another cellular component or co-receptor is required.

Different substrains of HIV, even those isolated from the same patient, exhibit specific tropisms for different cell types in culture. All isolates can infect primary CD4 lymphocytes, but only some infect macrophages while others can infect cell lines established from CD4+ leukaemic cells. Macrophage-tropic strains predominate early in the course of HIV infection, and may be more transmissible from person to person. They do not cause CD4 lymphocytes to fuse together in culture and hence are referred to as non-syncytium inducing (**NSI**) strains. In contrast, many HIV isolates established from late-stage infection rapidly adapt in culture to infect T-cell lines and are syncytium-inducing (**SI**). Approximately 50 per cent of patients with AIDS develop SI strains in addition to NSI strains. The differences in cellular tropism and SI/NSI phenotype occur in all HIV subtypes or clades, which appear to reflect geographical variation of HIV rather than specific biological properties of the virus.

The complex cellular tropism of HIV has been explained by the discovery that different members of the chemokine receptor family act as co-receptors to CD4 for HIV entry into cells. Chemokines are chemoattractant, locally acting hormones or cytokines that bind to one or more receptors which are structurally related to olfactory and neurotransmitter receptors. Following binding to the CD4 receptor, primary NSI strains use CCR5, the chemokine receptor for macrophage-inhibitory proteins (**MIP-1α, MIP-1β**) and RANTES. In contrast, the SI strains of HIV use the CXCR4 co-receptor, the receptor for another chemokine, stromal-derived

factor-1 (**SDF-1**). Other receptors such as CCR3 (the receptor of eotaxin) can be used by some NSI strains.

High levels of MIP-1α or -β in the blood correlate with relative resistance to HIV infection. Some exposed yet uninfected individuals are homozygous for an inherited defect of the CCR5 receptor involving a 32 base-pair deletion in the *CCR5* gene. This mutation has a high frequency in Caucasian people but is not found in African and Asian populations. Individuals who are homozygous for the deletion are healthy, indicating that the CCR5 receptor is not essential for the development of immune competence, probably because MIP-1 and RANTES can also bind to alternative receptors. However, homozygotes are genetically resistant to infection by NSI strains of HIV and the few homozygotes with A32 deletions who are HIV-positive appear to have been infected with SI strains that utilize CXCR4 instead. Other, more subtle, mutations in the promoter region of the *CCR5* gene allowing only low levels of co-receptor expression may confer relative resistance to HIV infection and also, if infection occurs, slower progression to AIDS.

The outer envelope glycoprotein, gp120, is the molecule on HIV that binds to CD4 and subsequently to the co-receptor. Gp120 is anchored to the viral envelope via gp41, the viral protein that is thought to effect membrane fusion. The gp120–gp41 is present in the viral envelope as a trimeric complex. SI strains have a gp120–gp41 structure that is less stable than NSI strains, readily undergoing conformational change on binding to CD4. This property makes SI strains more sensitive to neutralization by gp120 antibodies and also to inactivation by soluble forms of recombinant CD4, which were once seen as promising therapeutic agents. NSI strains, however, are more resistant. Mutations in the V3 loop of gp120 can convert NSI strains to SI strains. These mutations arise naturally during progression to AIDS and may allow HIV to switch to infect different cell types via new co-receptors.

The natural chemokines act as competitive inhibitors of HIV entry; certain chemically modified chemokines and chemical analogues act as strong HIV inhibitors without triggering the downstream signalling of the receptor. This has led to a new class of potential anti-HIV drugs, called 'co-receptor inhibitors'.

Diagnosis of HIV infection

Acute infection is accompanied by the development of serum antibodies to the core and surface proteins of the virus, usually within 2 to 6 weeks. Most seroconversions occur within 3 months of infection, and very rarely up to 6 months. Routine diagnostic tests, if negative, should be repeated 3 months after any possible exposure. Where there has been a high risk of transmission, additional tests that detect HIV directly (detection of viral RNA or DNA by polymerase chain reaction, **PCR**) should be used, and may confirm HIV infection before antibodies become detectable.

Following seroconversion, antibody to envelope protein persists indefinitely in the serum and forms a highly specific test for HIV infection. In general, one or more sensitive enzyme immunoassay tests that detect HIV-1 and HIV-2 antibodies are used as the initial screening tests. Positive screening tests are confirmed by additional tests to confirm the presence of HIV antibodies.

Pretest discussion and counselling

Where possible, patients should understand the implications of being tested for HIV and should give informed consent before the test is done. This is especially important for asymptomatic people. Awareness of being HIV-positive allows the use of effective prophylaxis against the major opportunistic infections, and highly active antiretroviral drugs. It should also encourage behavioural change to reduce the risk of transmission to sexual partners, and may benefit children exposed to perinatal infection. However, early diagnosis may cause distress and disruption of domestic, social, and professional lives, although the infected person may be free from symptoms for many years. HIV-positive people may find it difficult to obtain life or medical insurance, obtain work, buy a house, and travel abroad.

Where HIV is relevant to the investigation of a patient's symptoms, it is in their interest to be tested so that appropriate treatment for an opportunistic condition, antiretroviral therapy, and prophylaxis can be provided. Where the patient is too ill to give consent, testing may be justifiable on these grounds. A high level of confidentiality must be maintained; disclosure of HIV-positive status should generally be allowed only in the medical interests of the patient and with their knowledge and consent.

Clinical presentation and features

Acute HIV syndrome

Between 2 and 6 weeks after exposure to HIV, 50 to 70 per cent of those infected develop a transient, often mild, non-specific illness (sometimes called primary infection or seroconversion illness) similar to infectious mononucleosis, with fever, malaise, myalgia, lymphadenopathy, and pharyngitis. However, unlike infectious mononucleosis over 50 per cent of people develop a rash, typically erythematous, maculopapular, and affecting the face and trunk. Other rashes and patterns of distribution, and oral and genital ulcers have also been reported. The illness begins abruptly and usually lasts for 1 to 2 weeks, but may be more protracted. Neurological complications include acute encephalitis, lymphocytic meningitis, and peripheral neuropathy. Severe or long-lasting illness and neurological involvement are associated with accelerated progression to AIDS and a bad prognosis, which may be influenced by early antiretroviral therapy.

Diagnosis requires a high index of suspicion. Acute HIV infection is a time of high viraemia (typically 10^5 to 10^6 viral particles/ml) during which antibodies to HIV may initially be absent (Fig. 5). Serological tests often need to be repeated at intervals to establish the diagnosis. Rapid diagnosis during the early stages of acute infection may be provided by detecting HIV viraemia using tests for HIV RNA or proviral cDNA (by PCR). A transient decrease in CD4 lymphocytes is usual during primary illness. Occasionally this may be substantial and associated with opportunistic infections such as oral or oesophageal candidiasis, and rarely pneumocystis pneumonia.

Aggressive therapy of acute HIV infection with antiretroviral drugs does not eradicate the infection but, on theoretical grounds, may alter the natural history. After acute infection, the viral load becomes relatively stable after 6 to 9 months (Fig. 5). The plasma HIV RNA level at this virological steady state or 'set point' is of prognostic importance; therefore, treatment of the initial viraemic illness may lower the risk of progression. A placebo-controlled trial of zidovudine monotherapy during acute HIV infection showed a short-term benefit, but whether long-term outcomes are better compared with deferred treatment is not known. There are also concerns about the long-term toxicity of antiretroviral drugs. Current guidelines generally recommend considering treatment with highly active antiretroviral therapy, ideally within a clinical trial. The optimal duration of therapy for acute HIV infection is unknown.

Early HIV infection

Following the acute syndrome or subclinical seroconversion, there usually follows an asymptomatic period lasting an average of 10 years without antiretroviral therapy. Although a time of clinical latency, there is intense viral turnover: 10^9 to 10^{10} viral particles are replaced daily and the half-life of circulating CD4 lymphocytes is substantially reduced.

During the asymptomatic period, physical examination may be normal, but about one-third of patients have persistent generalized lymphadenopathy. The enlarged nodes, caused by a non-specific follicular hyperplasia, are usually symmetrical, mobile, and non-tender. The cervical and axillary nodes are most commonly affected. Nodes that are markedly asymmetrical, painful, or rapidly enlarging should be biopsied to exclude tumours such as lymphoma and opportunistic infections such as tuberculosis.

Symptoms of progressive HIV infection can be prevented by highly active antiretroviral treatment (see Management of HIV and prevention of complications, below). In the absence of treatment, patients often develop minor opportunistic conditions affecting the skin and mucous membranes. These are also common throughout the later stages of HIV disease. They include a range of infections: fungal (e.g. tinea, *Pityrosporum*), viral (e.g. warts, molluscum contagiosum, herpes simplex, herpes zoster), and bacterial (e.g. folliculitis, impetigo); and also eczema, seborrhoeic dermatitis, and psoriasis.

Drug rashes may occur at all stages of HIV, and particularly in late disease. Reactions to co-trimoxazole occur in up to 30 per cent of patients. They are most common when high doses are used in the treatment of pneumocystis pneumonia. Dapsone, clindamycin, β-lactam antibiotics, pentamidine, and nevirapine are commonly associated with drug rash.

Oral hairy leucoplakia usually appears as corrugated greyish-white lesions on the lateral borders of the tongue in homosexual men (Fig. 6). The condition is symptomless and non-progressive, but acts as a useful clue to HIV seropositivity. Epstein–Barr virus DNA has been demonstrated in these lesions.

One of the characteristic clinical presentations of HIV disease is a sore mouth and throat due to oropharyngeal candidiasis (oral thrush) (Fig. 7). This sign of worsening immunodeficiency may be recurrent. Topical antifungals (amphotericin lozenges or nystatin suspension) are usually effective in the early stages, but later oral azole antifungals (ketoconazole, fluconazole, or itraconazole) are needed. *Candida albicans* is usually responsible, but other species (e.g. *C. glabrata*) may be implicated.

There is an increased incidence of periodontal disease in those with HIV. Necrotizing (ulcerative) gingivitis and periodontitis may require extensive debridement and antimicrobials. Recurrent oropharyngeal aphthous ulceration is common and may be painful. Recurrent ulcers may occur in the oesophagus and other parts of the gastrointestinal tract. They usually respond to local or systemic corticosteroid therapy. Resistant cases may respond to thalidomide.

Later in the course of infection, intermittent or persistent non-specific constitutional symptoms may develop, which include lethargy, anorexia, diarrhoea, weight loss, fever, and night sweats. These symptoms may presage severe opportunistic infections or tumours.

Progression to AIDS

Various staging systems for HIV infection and case definitions of AIDS have been used since 1982 and modified by increased understanding of the pathogenesis and natural history. The 1987 Centers for Disease Control (**CDC**) definition listed a range of specific diseases indicative of AIDS. In

Fig. 5 Schematic representation of typical changes in CD4 lymphocyte count (left axis, per mm³) and plasma HIV-1 RNA (right axis, copies/ml) with time, during the natural history of HIV infection.

Fig. 6 Oral hairy leucoplakia.

1993, an expanded definition was introduced in the United States that included additional AIDS indicator diseases, people with proven HIV infection, and a CD4 lymphocyte count of less than 200/mm³ (0.2 × 10⁹/l), irrespective of clinical manifestations. This last criterion has not been adopted in Europe.

The value of making a distinction between AIDS (as defined) and HIV infection at other stages is questionable, especially in industrialized countries. AIDS-defining illnesses were essential for surveillance when HIV status was frequently unknown, the natural history of HIV infection was poorly understood (the proportion developing opportunistic complications was uncertain), and disease-modifying drugs were not available. However, effective prevention of many of the opportunistic infections has led to an increase in the proportion of symptomatic patients who do not fulfil the criteria for AIDS. Highly active antiretroviral therapy often improves the clinical condition and survival even when started after progression to AIDS. These factors have undermined the epidemiological value and prognostic importance of a strict AIDS case definition. It is probably more useful to consider progressive HIV disease as a continuous spectrum.

However, clinical criteria to identify symptomatic HIV disease and AIDS are needed in developing countries, where laboratory confirmation of HIV seropositivity and AIDS-defining diseases is not possible. The WHO has, therefore, adopted clinical case definitions for AIDS surveillance in

Fig. 7 Oral candidiasis.

resource-poor countries, based on clinical manifestations with or without laboratory confirmation of HIV infection.

Non-progression

While the average time between infection with HIV and the development of AIDS is about 10 years, approximately 20 per cent of patients progress rapidly to AIDS within 5 years and 10 to 15 per cent remain clinically well for 15 to 20 years. Long-term healthy survivors are often called non-progressors, and to an extent this subgroup represents simply the tail end of a normal distribution of progression rates. Cohort studies have demonstrated that most apparent non-progressors are slow progressors, in whom a gradual decline in the CD4 lymphocyte count and increments in HIV viral load can be demonstrated. Although several investigators have reported virological, genetic, and cellular and humoral immunological factors that may be associated with non-progression, limitations in study design have made it difficult to identify what was responsible. A mutation in the gene for the macrophage chemokine receptor CCR5 is associated with non-progression in the heterozygous state; homozygotes have high-level resistance to HIV infection (see Cellular biology, above).

Management of HIV and prevention of complications

Impact of highly active antiretroviral therapy

Although a decline in the number of cases of AIDS and mortality from HIV was reported from the United States and Europe before the advent of protease inhibitors in 1996, the subsequent marked reductions in morbidity and mortality are mostly attributable to antiretroviral regimens that include the newer potent agents (protease inhibitors or non-nucleoside reverse transcriptase inhibitors) in combination with nucleoside drugs. Among 1255 HIV-positive patients attending HIV clinics in eight cities in the United States, mortality declined from 29.4 per 100 person-years in 1995 to 8.8 per 100 person-years in the second quarter of 1997. The incidence of pneumocystis pneumonia, disseminated *M. avium* complex (**MAC**) infection, and cytomegalovirus (**CMV**) retinitis declined dramatically. The mortality of patients with CD4 counts below 100/mm³ fell for the first time in 1996, at a time when protease inhibitors were increasingly being included in treatment regimens. A decline in the incidence of opportunistic infections, notably oral candidiasis, toxoplasmosis, cryptosporidiosis, and cryptococcal meningitis, was reported from the United States and Europe.

In Europe, the expected survival 10 to 15 years after seroconversion was shown to have risen substantially after the introduction of highly active antiretroviral treatment (Fig. 8). For instance, in the 35 to 44 years' age group, survival 10 years after acquiring HIV in the era of highly active antiretroviral treatment (1997–98) was estimated to be 83 per cent, compared with 43 per cent for those infected between 1986 and 1996.

Whether antiretroviral drugs will ever eradicate HIV and bring about a 'cure' is regarded as unlikely. Although HIV may be undetectable in plasma for many months, a long-lived reservoir of infectious virus can be recovered from latently infected (resting) memory CD4 lymphocytes. Since the half-life of this cell population is about 6 months, many years of effective antiretroviral treatment would be needed to clear virus from this reservoir. Other compartments exist that are relatively inaccessible to drugs—for instance, in the central nervous system, retina and testes—and unless viral replication can be successfully prevented at such sites there is also the risk of reinfection of compartments previously cleared by therapy.

General management

Ideally, HIV infection should be identified at the asymptomatic stage. Clinical and laboratory monitoring can detect waning immunity and the risk of disease progression, prompting antiretroviral therapy and prophylaxis

Fig. 8 Estimated proportions of individuals surviving from HIV-1 seroconversion in 1986–96 (pre-HAART* period) and 1997-98 (HAART* period). *HAART, highly active antiretroviral therapy. (CASCADE collaboration, *Lancet* (2000), **355**, 1158.)

against infections such as pneumocystis pneumonia. Serological screening detects past or current infections such as toxoplasma, CMV, hepatitis B and C, and syphilis, which may be reactivated or progress during immunosuppression. Clinic visits provide an opportunity for discussion of such issues as safer sex. Many problems can be managed by a primary care physician. Routine dental care is needed. Clinical and laboratory monitoring, the management of late complications, and the prescription and monitoring of antiretroviral drugs require specialist supervision.

Monitoring

Monitoring involves regular clinical assessment and prognostic laboratory tests. Oral candidiasis, or physical signs such as asymptomatic cutaneous Kaposi's sarcoma are of prognostic importance. CD4 lymphocyte count and quantitative estimation of HIV RNA in the blood plasma (viral load) are the two laboratory markers that have the best prognostic value.

The CD4 lymphocyte (T-helper cell) count is a reliable indicator of HIV-related immune impairment. CD4 counts, normal at or above 600/mm^3, vary considerably, even in the absence of HIV infection. A fall in the CD4 lymphocyte count to below 200/mm^3 is associated with a risk of opportunistic infections of about 80 per cent over 3 years without antiretroviral treatment. However, progression is variable and a minority remain well for several years with stable low CD4 counts. This variability is explained partly by differences in HIV viral load. The level of CD4 lymphopenia generally determines the spectrum potential of infections (Table 2). For instance, whereas oral and oesophageal candidiasis and pneumocystis pneumonia are frequent at CD4 counts of 100 to 200/mm^3, disseminated MAC infection and CMV retinitis are rarely seen until the CD4 count is below 50/mm^3.

The prognostic value of measuring HIV RNA in plasma was reported from the United States in 1996. In HIV-positive men in a subgroup of the Multicenter AIDS Cohort Study, only 8 per cent with less than 5000 copies of HIV RNA/ml progressed to AIDS over 5 years, whereas 62 per cent with viral loads above 35 000 developed AIDS. For a given level of CD4 lymphocytes, variations in viral load predict the risk of progression. The most useful prognostic information is therefore derived from the CD4 count and viral load taken together (Fig. 9).

In industrialized countries, HIV viral load measurements have become widely available. Techniques include reverse transcription followed by amplification by the polymerase chain reaction (**RT-PCR**), branched DNA

Table 2 Principal complications of HIV infection

Infections	Neoplasms	Direct HIV effects
Early/intermediate HIV infection (CD4 >200/mm^3)		
Herpes zoster	Non-Hodgkin's lymphoma[*]	Persistent generalized lymphadenopathy
Oral hairy leucoplakia	Cervical intraepithelial neoplasia	Atopy; eczema
Oral candidiasis; candidal vaginitis	Anal intraepithelial neoplasia	Recurrent aphthous ulcers (oral and gastrointestinal tract)
Pulmonary tuberculosis[*]		Immune thrombocytopenia
Bacterial pneumonia, especially pneumococcal		Neutropenia
Bacteraemia, especially pneumococcal and salmonella		Neuropathy (mononeuritis multiplex; Guillian–Barré syndrome)
Bacillary angiomatosis		
Late HIV infection (CD4 <200/mm^3)		
Pneumocystis pneumonia[*]	Kaposi's sarcoma[*]	HIV enteropathy
Candidal oesophagitis[*]	Primary cerebral lymphoma[*]	Peripheral neuropathy (distal, axonal)
Cerebral toxoplasmosis[*]	[?]Hodgkin's lymphoma	Autonomic neuropathy
Cryptococcal meningitis[*]	[?]Cervical carcinoma[*]	Myelopathy
Chronic cryptosporidial diarrhoea[*]	[?]Anal carcinoma	HIV dementia[*]
Chronic isosporiasis[*], microsporidiosis		Wasting syndrome[*]
Chronic HSV[*] ulceration		HIV-associated nephropathy
Extrapulmonary tuberculosis[*]		Cardiomyopathy
Disseminated *M. avium* complex (MAC)[*]		
CMV (retinitis and disseminated)[*]		
Progressive multifocal leucoencephalopathy[*]		
Recurrent bacterial pneumonia[*]		
Recurrent bacteraemia, especially salmonella[*]		
Disseminated histoplasmosis[*], and *P. marneffei*		

[*] AIDS-defining conditions; incomplete list.

[?] Signifies suspected but unproven association. Many of the early/intermediate manifestations also occur in late-stage HIV disease; non-Hodgkin's lymphoma is more common during the later stages.

Fig. 9 Curves showing AIDS-free survival with time among groups with different baseline CD4 lymphocyte counts, according to HIV-1 RNA category. The five categories were (copies/ml): I, 500 or less; II, 501 to 3000; III, 3001 to 10 000; IV, 10 001 to 30 000; and V, above 30 000. (Sample sizes are shown in brackets).

(**bDNA**) signal amplification, and nucleic acid sequence-based amplification (**NASBA**). Highly sensitive tests with very low detection limits (about 20 copies/ml) are increasingly used.

Antiretroviral therapy

Nucleoside analogues

Knowledge of the viral lifecycle (Fig. 3) led to the development of a number of antiretroviral compounds with clinically useful activity against HIV

(Table 3). The forerunner of these was zidovudine (AZT or ZDV), first shown to be active against HIV *in vitro* in 1985. Zidovudine, a nucleoside analogue that inhibits HIV reverse transcriptase, slowed down the rate of disease progression over a 12-month period in patients with AIDS and improved short-term survival, well being, body weight, and neurological features. However, clinical progression associated with viral resistance to the drug was observed after a year or two of therapy. When early treatment with zidovudine was compared to deferred zidovudine, there was no difference in survival or disease progression after 3 years.

The clinical failure of monotherapy prompted combination therapy in an attempt to reduce the development of drug resistance. Double nucleoside combinations proved superior to zidovudine monotherapy, especially in patients without prior exposure to zidovudine. Treatment with at least three drugs is more effective and has become the standard of care. In general, two nucleoside drugs are used with either a non-nucleoside reverse transcriptase inhibitor or a protease inhibitor. A combination of three nucleoside analogues (zidovudine, lamivudine, and abacavir) can also be used, and is available as a single tablet taken twice daily (Table 4).

Non-nucleoside reverse transcriptase inhibitors

The prototype of the class is nevirapine, a potent and selective inhibitor of HIV reverse transcriptase. When nevirapine is given alone, resistance develops rapidly and this drug is of limited effectiveness in double therapy or when added to failing regimens. However, in antiretroviral-naive patients without AIDS (CD4 200 to 600/mm³), over a half of patients treated with nevirapine plus two nucleosides (zidovudine and didanosine) had undetectable plasma HIV RNA after 1 year of therapy, compared with 12 per cent for zidovudine/didanosine only. Efavirenz and delavirdine

Table 3 Principal antiretroviral agents

Nucleoside reverse transcriptase inhibitors	Non-nucleoside reverse transcriptase inhibitors	Protease inhibitors	Fusion inhibitors[a]
Zidovudine (AZT/ZDV)	Nevirapine	Saquinavir[b]	*Fusion inhibitors:*[a]
Didanosine (ddI)	Delavirdine[c]	Ritonavir	T-20
Zalcitabine (ddC)	Efavirenz	Indinavir[b]	T-1249
Lamivudine (3TC)		Nelfinavir	
Stavudine (d4T)	*Nucleotide reverse*	Amprenavir[b]	*Other*[d]
Abacavir (ABC)	*transcriptase inhibitor*	Lopinavir[b]	Hydroxyurea
	Tenofovir		Interleukin-2

Numerous other compounds are at earlier phases of development and evaluation.

[a] Undergoing clinical trials.

[b] Can be given with low-dose ritonavir for pharmacokinetic enhancement.

[c] Not licensed in Europe.

[d] Indirect activity; used as adjuvants.

Table 4 Initial antiretroviral regimens

Regimen	Examples	Comment
2 NRTIs + NNRTI	AZT/3TC + nevirapine OR efavirenz ddI/d4T + nevirapine OR efavirenz 3TC/d4T + nevirapine OR efavirenz	Preferred initial regimen; efficacy and ease of adherence
2 NRTIs + PI	AZT/3TC + nelfinavir OR other PI ddI/d4T + nelfinavir OR other PI 3TC/d4T + nelfinavir OR other PI	High pill burden; toxicity relatively common
2 NRTI + 2PIs*	AZT/3TC + ritonavir/other PI* ddI/d4T + ritonavir/other PI* 3TC/d4T + ritonavir/other PI*	Possible increase in toxicity and drug interactions
3 NRTIs	AZT/3TC/abacavir	Spares other drug classes; possibly less effective at high viral loads.

NRTI, nucleoside reverse transcriptase inhibitor; NNRTI, non-nucleoside reverse transcriptase inhibitor; PI, protease inhibitor; AZT, zidovudine; 3TC, lamivudine; ddI, didanosine; d4T, stavudine.

* Low-dose ritonavir (to improve pharmacokinetics) plus saquinavir, indinavir, or lopinavir.

(which is not licensed for use in the United Kingdom) are other non-nucleoside reverse transcriptase inhibitors with similar properties to nevirapine.

Protease inhibitors

The HIV-encoded protease (or proteinase) is required for the production of mature infectious viral particles. This enzyme cleaves a number of structural proteins and enzymes from the polyprotein precursors produced by translation of the *gag* and *gag–pol* genes. Inhibitors of HIV protease act synergistically with nucleoside drugs and are potent inhibitors of HIV replication.

Protease inhibitors have a greater effect on HIV viral load and CD4 counts than nucleoside reverse transcriptase inhibitors, especially when used in triple therapy.

Indinavir, in combination with two nucleoside analogues (zidovudine/lamivudine or stavudine/lamivudine) produced good results in a large controlled trial with clinical endpoints (ACTG 320). Compared to double therapy (two nucleosides), the triple combination reduced the proportion of patients who progressed to AIDS or death from 11 to 6 per cent over about 38 weeks. The responses of CD4 cells and plasma HIV RNA paralleled the clinical results. Similar results were reported for combinations that involved other protease inhibitors, saquinavir, ritonavir, and nelfinavir. Ritonavir, in low dosage, may be included to boost blood levels of other protease inhibitors (especially saquinavir, indinavir, and a newer drug, lopinavir) by competitive inhibition of their hepatic metabolism. Combinations of non-nucleoside drugs and protease inhibitors are also being evaluated.

Other drugs

Fusion inhibitors, such as T-20, stop the HIV glycoprotein gp41 from effecting fusion of the viral and cellular membranes, and thereby prevent HIV entry into host cells. Compounds that inhibit HIV integrase and prevent proviral DNA integration into the host cell genome are also being identified. Hydroxyurea, not in itself an antiviral compound, is sometimes used in combination with nucleoside reverse transcriptase inhibitors; *in vitro* studies suggest that it acts synergistically by reducing the intracellular substrate for making DNA and thereby increasing the efficiency of chain termination. Another adjunctive agent under investigation is interleukin-2 (given subcutaneously), which raises CD4 lymphocyte counts substantially when used in combination with antiretrovirals. Influenza-like side-effects are prominent and therapy is very expensive. Its long-term efficacy is currently unknown and being studied in a large trial (ESPRIT).

General points on HIV therapy

There is a plethora of results from clinical trials of antiretroviral drugs, but several large, randomized controlled trials have made the greatest impact. Comparison between trials may be difficult because of differences in the clinical stage of HIV disease in those enrolled, CD4 counts at entry, previous antiretroviral experience, duration of treatment, and in the drug regimens used. Many trials measure surrogate endpoints, especially HIV viral load reduction and changes in CD4 lymphocyte count. It is assumed that these reflect clinical effectiveness. However, trials conducted over periods of less than 1 year may not predict longer term results. The value of such short-term studies based on surrogate markers is to identify treatments that should be evaluated in large, well-designed controlled trials that measure clinical endpoints (progression of HIV disease or death) ideally over several years. HIV trials may be stopped prematurely when significant differences in clinical outcomes are demonstrable between study arms, but before longer term benefits can be assessed. In fact, the long-term efficacy of currently recommended anti-HIV treatment regimens remains unknown.

When to start treatment

The optimum time to start antiretroviral therapy is not known, and no trials have adequately addressed this question. Data from several clinical cohorts suggest that patients who start treatment when the CD4 count is below 200/mm³ have an increased mortality when compared with those starting at higher CD4 levels. Currently, there is no clear evidence for an advantage in starting treatment at any given range of CD4 count above 200/mm³. Therefore, recent guidelines generally recommend starting before the CD4 count drops to below 200/mm³, or if the patient develops symptomatic HIV disease. Asymptomatic patients with CD4 counts in the range of 200 to 350/mm³ whose CD4 counts are falling rapidly or who have a high viral load should be monitored more intensively, and earlier intervention may be considered.

What to start with

Highly active antiretroviral regimens consist of at least three drugs, usually a backbone of two nucleosides with either a non-nucleoside reverse transcriptase inhibitor or a protease inhibitor (see Table 4). As discussed above, for pharmacokinetic reasons, two protease inhibitors (one of which is low-dose ritonavir) may be used, and a triple nucleoside regimen is also available. The best starting regimen(s), and how treatment should subsequently be sequenced, have not been determined. No regimen or sequencing strategy has been shown to be clinically superior in controlled trials. Several factors should be taken into consideration when selecting initial therapy, including potential drug interactions, toxicity, and the likelihood of adherence. HIV viral load and CD4 count should be checked after 2 to 3 months. The aim of initial treatment is to achieve a reduction in viral load to undetectable levels (ideally <50 copies/ml) within 6 to 9 months of starting treatment. Whether initial regimens that include more than three drugs are clinically superior in the longer term is being studied in ongoing trials such as Initio.

Changing therapy

Recommendations for changing the treatment regimen are based on theoretical considerations. The principal reasons are treatment failure, toxicity, and poor adherence. There is no agreed definition for treatment failure. Patients whose viraemia was initially suppressed, and whose viral load subsequently rises, should be considered for changing to a completely new regimen of at least three drugs. This may be guided by a resistance test (see Drug resistance, below). However the optimal point at which the switch should be made remains to be defined. Poor absorption of protease inhibitors may sometimes cause treatment failure related to low blood levels, without development of resistance; measurement of blood levels may be useful in selected cases. In cases of drug toxicity (for instance, a severe rash), if the responsible agent is identified then a single drug substitution can be made. If adherence is poor or likely to be the cause of treatment failure, changing to a combination that is simpler to take should be considered, for instance based on once or twice daily dosage and low pill burden (see Patient adherence, below).

'Salvage' therapy

Salvage therapy is generally defined as treatment following exposure to multiple antiretroviral drugs. In this situation, numerous drug-resistance mutations are usually present and the likelihood of achieving sustained viral suppression below the detection level is much lower than for patients who have limited or no previous antiretroviral exposure. This is especially true if drugs from all three major classes have previously been used. Studies using clinical endpoints suggest that declines in viral load correlate with improvements in clinical outcome, even if suppression to below the detection limit is not achieved. Several factors may be considered when selecting a treatment regimen in these circumstances, including drugs or drug classes to which the patient has not been exposed, drugs with a lower likelihood of resistance that can be recycled, inclusion of new drugs or a new class of drug such as nucleotides, and results of tests for viral resistance. Whether 'mega' antiretroviral treatment using five or more drugs for salvage is superior to standard triple therapy is being examined in the OPTIMA trial in the United Kingdom, the United States, and Canada.

Patient adherence

A substantial proportion of HIV patients do not follow treatment recommendations. Reasons for non-adherence include poor communication, the complexity of drug regimens and number of tablets, disruption of life (including timing and food restrictions), side-effects, concerns about long-term effects, and lack of confidence in non-curative treatments of indefinite duration. Adherence to treatment requires a high level of understanding and motivation in the patient. This is of particular concern in HIV therapy because of the risk of developing drug-resistance mutations during sub-optimal therapy. The recent development of simplified regimens (for example, once or twice daily dosage; reduced pill burden) has helped.

Drug resistance

Viral resistance is a major factor in treatment failure. There is evidence that resistant mutants arise spontaneously even in the absence of antiretroviral therapy. This tendency is greatest when HIV viraemia is high, and lowest when HIV replication is completely suppressed by a potent drug combination.

Extensive genotypic variation of HIV occurs because of very high viral turnover and transcription errors by the reverse transcriptase enzyme, so that all possible single-point mutations are likely to occur frequently. While mutations causing resistance to single agents may be present before antiretroviral treatment, on statistical grounds it is unlikely that specific combinations of multiple mutations will be present. However, multiple mutations do develop during antiretroviral therapy with more than one drug when viral replication is at a high level. Therefore, controlling viral replication with a highly potent treatment regimen limits the appearance of resistant HIV mutants.

Genotypic and phenotypic assays have been developed to test for drug resistance in HIV isolates. Genotypic assays that identify codon mutations correlating with *in vivo* resistance to antiretrovirals are relatively easy to perform and inexpensive. Phenotypic assays that measure the ability of the virus to grow in increasing concentrations of drugs are time consuming and expensive, but provide more direct evidence of resistance to a particular drug. The clinical and prognostic value of resistance assays is being evaluated, and, increasingly, they are used in the selection of drug regimens and investigation of treatment failure. Interpretation of resistance patterns is increasingly difficult as the number of drugs and mutations involved increases.

Resistance mutations to antiretroviral agents are identifiable in up to 15 per cent of recent seroconverters in the United States, and transmitted drug resistance is increasing in Europe. Resistance mutations may be lost in the absence of therapy, so the clinical significance of the transmission of a virus carrying resistance mutations to one or multiple drugs is currently uncertain.

Drug toxicity and interactions

Adverse reactions to antiretroviral agents are relatively common; treatment may have to be stopped. Minor gastrointestinal disturbances (nausea, vomiting, diarrhoea), rashes, and headache are common, but some adverse reactions are serious. Drug interactions must be considered when prescribing antiretroviral drugs, especially in late HIV disease. Antiretroviral agents may interact with each other and with other drugs. Ritonavir, a potent inhibitor of cytochrome P-450, is especially prone to raising blood levels of other drugs and should not be given with most antiarrhythmics, anxiolytics, and antihistamines. Caution is required with several analgesics, anticonvulsants, and other categories of medication.

Metabolic complications, especially mitochondrial toxicity and disturbances of lipid and glucose metabolism, have emerged as important adverse effects of antiretroviral therapy. Mitochondrial toxicity is especially associated with nucleoside drugs (such as didanosine and stavudine) and may result in neuropathy, myopathy, pancreatitis, hepatic steatosis, and lactic acidaemia. Mild degrees of lactic acidaemia cause non-specific symptoms including malaise and gastrointestinal disturbance of gradual onset; pro-gression can lead to fatal lactic acidosis. Nucleoside drugs are thought to cause mitochondrial dysfunction by inhibiting mitochondrial DNA polymerase-γ.

A syndrome of lipodystrophy (loss of fat from face and limbs), truncal fat accumulation, hyperlipidaemia, and insulin resistance has been associated with protease inhibitors but has also been described with other antiretroviral drugs, and may not respond to changing the drug regimen. Whether the effects on lipid metabolism increase the risk of ischaemic vascular diseases is currently uncertain.

Considerable immune restoration seems to occur after treatment with potent antiretroviral regimens in patients with low CD4 lymphocyte counts. New disease manifestations have been reported. Disseminated MAC may cause widespread lymphadenopathy when antiretroviral therapy is started. Several new manifestations of CMV ocular disease have been reported, including vitritis, cystoid macular oedema (previously seen in HIV-negative patients following withdrawal of iatrogenic immunosuppression), and epiretinal membrane formation. These new disease manifestations are likely to be immune recovery phenomena.

Treatment interruptions

In general, once treatment is started it is continued indefinitely. There has been recent interest in whether interrupting treatment (in supervised or structured treatment interruptions) can be beneficial. In theory, such interruptions might enhance immune responses, reduce long-term toxicity, or reduce resistant virus by allowing repopulation with wild-type virus. The effect of treatment interruptions on clinical outcomes is being studied in clinical trials.

Late complications and their management

Pneumocystis carinii pneumonia

P. carinii pneumonia, one of the hallmarks of AIDS, is now less common because of primary prophylaxis and antiretroviral therapy. Some 85 per cent of cases occur in patients with CD4 lymphocyte counts below 200/mm³, and mostly at counts below 100/mm³. Symptoms—typically: increasing shortness of breath, dry cough, and fever—usually develop subacutely over a few weeks. Malaise, fatigue, weight loss, and chest pains or tightness may occur. Chest signs are usually minor (crackles) or absent. The characteristic chest radiograph shows bilateral perihilar interstitial shadowing (Fig. 10), but may be normal. Other appearances include localized infiltrates or consolidation, upper lobe shadows resembling tuberculosis,

Fig. 10 Chest radiograph: *Pneumocystis carinii* pneumonia.

Fig. 11 *Pneumocystis carinii* cysts in bronchoalveolar lavage aspirate.

nodular lesions, and pneumothorax; effusions are very rare. The arterial oxygen saturation is less than 95 per cent at rest or falls after exercise.

A foamy intra-alveolar exudate containing abundant *P. carinii* develops, which is associated with an interstitial inflammatory infiltrate and progressive impairment of lung function. The diagnosis can sometimes be confirmed by microscopy of sputum, which is induced by nebulized saline in isolated, properly ventilated rooms to reduce the risk of tuberculosis transmission (see Multidrug-resistant tuberculosis, below). *P. carinii* cysts and trophozoites are visualized by the use of special stains. If the result is negative, fibreoptic bronchoscopy with bronchial lavage may be indicated (Fig. 11); other causes of lung disease or coexistent infection may also be diagnosed by this technique, including tuberculosis, fungal infections, and Kaposi's sarcoma. Immunofluorescence using monoclonal antibodies, or DNA amplification by PCR, may improve diagnostic sensitivity when compared with conventional staining techniques, but these methods are not yet used routinely. In a minority of patients with *P. carinii* pneumonia the diagnosis is not confirmed.

High-dose co-trimoxazole (120 mg/kg daily in divided doses) for 3 weeks is the first-line treatment for pneumocystis pneumonia. Oral therapy is often adequate, but in moderate and severe cases the drug should be given intravenously. The drug can be given orally if fever, symptoms, and oxygenation have improved after 10 days. Adverse reactions to co-trimoxazole—especially neutropenia, anaemia, rash, and fever—occur in up to 40 per cent of patients, usually after 6 to 14 days. Intravenous pentamidine (4 mg/kg per day) is the second-line choice for patients who do not tolerate co-trimoxazole.

Patients intolerant of co-trimoxazole and pentamidine may be treated with clindamycin plus primaquine or dapsone plus trimethoprim. These regimens have only been evaluated in patients with mild to moderate pneumocystis pneumonia, as has atovaquone, an antiprotozoal drug that is active against *P. carinii*. Although slightly less effective than co-trimoxazole, atovaquone causes fewer adverse effects.

In patients with moderate or severe pneumocystis pneumonia, high-dose corticosteroids reduce morbidity and mortality. If the arterial oxygen tension (Pao_2) is less than 9.3 kPa or the alveolar–arterial oxygen gradient is greater than 4.7 kPa, oxygen and intravenous methylprednisolone or oral prednisolone should be given for 5 to 10 days. Patients who develop respiratory failure may require ventilatory support. After treatment for pneumocystis pneumonia has been completed, secondary prophylaxis should be given to prevent recurrence. This can be discontinued if there is a good response to antiretroviral treatment, with a rise in the CD4 count sustained above 200/mm³.

Bacterial pneumonia

The risk of bacterial pneumonia is increased in HIV, especially if the CD4 lymphocyte count is below 200/mm³. The most common cause is *Strepto-coccus pneumoniae*; *Haemophilus influenzae* and *Moraxella catarrhalis* are relatively common, and *Staphylococcus aureus*, *Klebsiella* spp., and other Gram-negative rods are important causes in advanced HIV disease. Rarer causes include *Nocardia* spp. and *Rhodococcus equi*. The presentation may be atypical, and radiological appearances frequently include diffuse infiltrates that resemble pneumocystis pneumonia, as well as more typical segmental or lobar patterns. Cavitation with abscess formation, pleural effusion, and empyema may occur. HIV predisposes to recurrent invasive pneumococcal infections with bacteraemia; recurrent bacterial pneumonia in a 12-month period is an AIDS-defining condition. Chronic lung damage with bronchiectasis and colonization by *Pseudomonas aeruginosa* have been reported.

Other pulmonary complications

Disseminated fungal infections, including *Cryptococcus* spp., may involve the lungs. In endemic areas histoplasmosis, coccidioidomycosis, and disseminated *Penicillium marneffei* infection need to be considered (see Other disseminated infections, below). Invasive *Aspergillus fumigatus* infections may occur in patients with advanced HIV disease who have additional risk factors such as severe neutropenia. Patients usually have severe systemic illness. The radiographic appearances in all these fungal infections are usually non-specific. Bronchoalveolar lavage may be needed for diagnosis. HIV-associated lymphocytic interstitial pneumonitis causes diffuse abnormalities, usually in children but occasionally in adults. Bronchiolitis obliterans-organizing pneumonia is a steroid-responsive cause of lung infiltrates, probably a tissue response to various underlying conditions, which has also been reported in HIV and may be confused with pneumocystis pneumonia.

Tuberculosis

The interaction between HIV and tuberculosis was recognized early in the HIV epidemic. Studies in Central Africa in the mid-1980s showed that more than 60 per cent of newly diagnosed tuberculosis patients were HIV-positive at a time when the background seroprevalence of HIV in the population was much lower. Intravenous drug users were shown to have an increased risk of developing active tuberculosis if they were HIV-positive. After decades of progressive decline in the incidence of tuberculosis in the United States, notifications increased during the mid-1980s, soon after the emergence of the HIV epidemic. A similar trend was subsequently observed in western Europe. Globally, tuberculosis remains the most frequent life-threatening opportunistic infection in AIDS.

Most cases of tuberculosis in HIV-positive individuals represent reactivation of dormant bacilli. However, molecular typing of isolates of *Mycobacterium tuberculosis* by restriction fragment length polymorphism (**RFLP**) analysis suggests that up to 40 per cent are new infections. The WHO estimates that one-third of the world's HIV-positive population is co-infected with tuberculosis. In communities where *M. tuberculosis* is a common endemic organism, those who are immunosuppressed by HIV have an increased risk of relapsing or contracting new infections. Where the background prevalence of tuberculosis is low, the disease is uncommon in HIV-positive patients unless they become exposed, for instance through travel. Testing for HIV should be considered in patients presenting with active tuberculosis, and tuberculosis should be considered as a cause of unexplained symptoms in patients with HIV.

Active tuberculosis may occur at any time during the course of HIV infection. In early-stage HIV, it is more likely to present with the typical clinical features: subacute history of cough, fever, and weight loss, upper lobe cavitary disease and/or pleural disease on chest radiographs, and a positive skin test to tuberculin. In late-stage HIV, infected patients are more likely to present atypically with unusual chest findings, extrapulmonary involvement, and cutaneous anergy. The chest radiograph may be normal in up to 40 per cent of cases. Sputum smears should be examined for acid-fast bacilli. Blood cultures may be positive for *M. tuberculosis*.

Studies in Zambia have shown that, compared with HIV-negative patients, HIV-positive individuals with tuberculosis are less likely to be sputum-positive on microscopy, show less cavitation and more involvement of the lower lobes, and are more likely to relapse after completion of therapy and to die prematurely. Patients with advanced HIV infection are more likely to develop extrapulmonary tuberculosis involving lymph nodes, pericardium, liver, bone marrow, or meninges.

The standard 6-month regimen of three or four antituberculosis drugs (isoniazid, rifampicin, pyrazinamide, and ethambutol) is generally effective in patients with HIV, unless there is resistance to one or more of these first-line drugs. The drug regimen may need to be adjusted when *in vitro* sensitivity results are known. For fully sensitive organisms, after 2 months on three or four drugs, isoniazid and rifampicin should be continued for a further 4 months. Patients with pulmonary tuberculosis should be isolated initially. Contact tracing is important; HIV-positive contacts are at particular risk. Tuberculin testing is used to determine whether contacts should take isoniazid chemoprophylaxis.

Up to 20 per cent of patients with HIV experience adverse reactions to antituberculosis drugs. In HIV-positive patients with tuberculosis in Africa, the sulpha-based drug thiacetazone has been associated with serious skin reactions, including toxic epidermal necrolysis and fatal cases of Stevens–Johnson syndrome. Whereas response rates for conventional short-course tuberculosis treatment in industrialized countries are similar to those achieved in HIV-negative patients, in resource-poor countries and where compliance is less easily achieved, cure rates are lower and there is a risk that resistance will develop. Several countries have adopted 'directly observed therapy' to address this problem.

Multidrug-resistant tuberculosis

Over 15 outbreaks of multidrug-resistant tuberculosis (**MDRTB**) have been reported since the late 1980s. MDRTB isolates are resistant to at least two first-line antituberculosis drugs, most commonly isoniazid and rifampicin, and are often resistant to several agents. Most have occurred in HIV units in hospitals, but there have been outbreaks in prisons, drug treatment centres, and nursing homes. Most documented outbreaks have been in the United States. Elsewhere, over 200 people were involved in Buenos Aires, Argentina, and another outbreak affected over 100 people in Lisbon, Portugal. In MDRTB outbreaks, healthcare workers may become infected. Initially, the mortality among HIV-positive patients was very high (up to 93 per cent), but more recently the outcome has improved because of more rapid diagnosis and treatment with at least four drugs to which the *M. tuberculosis* isolate is sensitive *in vitro*. To prevent outbreaks of MDRTB, special precautions are required when HIV-positive patients with possible tuberculosis are admitted to hospitals. Diagnosis must not be delayed, appropriate treatment must be started without delay, and drug resistance identified. Precautions include the isolation of patients in negative-pressure rooms, use of respiratory protection for staff, and special care during certain procedures such as bronchoscopy or nebulized pentamidine administration. With effective treatment, patients rapidly become non-infectious, but precautions need to be continued until the sputum is repeatedly smear-negative.

Mycobacterium avium complex

Patients with advanced HIV infection and CD4 lymphocyte counts below $50/mm^3$ are at high risk of disseminated *M. avium* complex (**MAC**) infection, particularly in industrialized countries where it is reported to develop in up to 40 per cent of patients with AIDS. *M. avium* is a ubiquitous environmental organism of low pathogenicity that can be isolated from domestic water supplies. Infection is likely to be through the gastrointestinal tract. MAC infection becomes widely disseminated in those with advanced HIV and causes fever, night sweats, weight loss, diarrhoea, abdominal pain, anaemia, disturbed liver function, and reduced overall survival. The organism can usually be cultured from blood or bone marrow, or may be recognized as acid-fast bacilli in tissue biopsies (for example from lymph node,

small bowel, or liver). It is unclear why the diagnosis is uncommon in underdeveloped countries; high mortality from other opportunistic infections at earlier stages of immunosuppression may be partly responsible.

MAC infection is intrinsically resistant to most first-line antituberculosis drugs. The optimal regimen has not been determined, and although clinical benefit and microbiological response is often achieved, survival benefit has been difficult to prove. Comparative trials suggest that initial therapy should be with two or three drugs: clarithromycin or azithromycin and ethambutol should be used, and additional rifabutin or a quinolone (e.g. ciprofloxacin) considered. In severely ill patients intravenous amikacin may be useful as the third agent. Lifelong treatment may be required to prevent relapse; but if immunity is restored by highly active antiretroviral therapy it may prove possible to cure MAC infection.

Other non-tuberculosis mycobacteria

Other mycobacteria, notably *M. kansasii*, *M. genavense*, and *M. celatum*, may cause opportunistic infections in those with HIV. *M. genavense*, which colonizes pet birds, was discovered in European patients with HIV and causes fever, diarrhoea, and severe weight loss. HIV does not seem to affect the incidence or natural history of leprosy (*M. leprae*).

Oesophageal candidiasis

Oesophagitis presents with retrosternal pain on swallowing, and in patients with HIV is most commonly caused by *Candida albicans*. Oesophageal candidiasis indicates advanced immunosuppression and is an AIDS-defining condition. The diagnosis should be suspected in a patient with oral candida and dysphagia, and may be supported by barium swallow or confirmed by endoscopy and biopsy. Treatment is with oral azole antifungal agents. Fluconazole may be more effective than ketoconazole. It may recur and in patients with severe immunosuppression, candida may become resistant to prolonged azole treatment. Resistance tends to develop gradually and can be monitored by *in vitro* testing. Such patients require treatment or continuous suppression with high doses of fluconazole (which is better tolerated than high doses of ketoconazole or itraconazole) or intermittent treatment with intravenous amphotericin. Azole-resistant oro-oesophageal candidiasis has become much less common since the advent of highly active antiretroviral therapy.

The differential diagnosis of oesophageal candidiasis includes oesophagitis caused by cytomegalovirus (**CMV**) or herpes simplex virus (**HSV**), which require specific antiviral therapy, and aphthous ulceration, which may respond to oral prednisolone or thalidomide.

HIV and the nervous system

The nervous system is a major site of involvement for direct and indirect complications of HIV at all stages of infection. All parts of the nervous system may be affected. In advanced HIV, opportunistic infections and tumours (lymphoma), and tissue damage caused by HIV replication in the brain and spinal cord, are important and relatively common during progressive HIV disease.

Cerebral toxoplasmosis

Cerebral infection with the intracellular protozoan *Toxoplasma gondii* is the most frequent infection of the central nervous system in AIDS when the CD4 lymphocyte count is below $200/mm^3$. It usually results from reactivation of toxoplasma cysts in the brain, leading to the formation of focal lesions that are typically multiple but may be single. Symptoms develop subacutely and include focal neurological disturbance, headache, confusion, fever, and convulsions. On CT scanning the lesions appear as ring-enhancing masses with surrounding oedema (Fig. 12). Magnetic resonance imaging (**MRI**) is more sensitive and frequently detects lesions not visible on the computed tomography (**CT**) scan. Serum antibodies to *Toxoplasma* spp. are usually detectable; their absence makes the diagnosis unlikely but

Fig. 12 Cerebral toxoplasmosis: ring enhancement and surrounding cerebral oedema (CT scan with contrast).

does not exclude it. Detection of toxoplasma DNA in cerebrospinal fluid by PCR is being evaluated as a diagnostic test. The principal differential diagnosis is cerebral lymphoma; other causes of focal brain lesions in AIDS include cryptococcoma, cerebral abscess (including infection with *Nocardia* spp.), tuberculoma, progressive multifocal leucoencephalopathy, and neurosyphilis. Brain biopsy is required for a definitive diagnosis, but is rarely performed. As toxoplasmosis is by far the most common treatable cause of focal cerebral lesions in HIV, it is standard practice to treat for this and only consider biopsy if there is no clinical improvement in 7 to 10 days.

The condition responds well if treatment is started early; a combination of sulfadiazine at 4 to 6 g/day and pyrimethamine at 50 to 75 mg/day is the treatment of choice. More than 40 per cent of patients experience adverse effects, especially rash and nephrotoxicity caused by sulfadiazine. The haematological toxicity of pyrimethamine may be reduced by adding folinic acid (10 mg/day). If sulpha drugs are not tolerated, clindamycin with pyrimethamine is an effective alternative. Highly active retroviral treatment should also be started. Corticosteroids may be used to reduce cerebral oedema in patients with large lesions and serious mass effects, but this is controversial.

Treatment is usually given for 3 to 6 weeks, and in the absence of effective antiretroviral treatment relapse is common after stopping. In these circumstances, lifelong maintenance treatment is usually required using pyrimethamine (25–50 mg/day) with a sulpha drug or clindamycin. However, these can be discontinued if antiretroviral treatment leads to sustained immunological recovery.

Cryptococcal meningitis

Although infection of the central nervous system with *Cryptococcus neoformans* can occur in the absence of immunodeficiency, it most commonly arises in association with HIV infection. Before the widespread use of azole antifungals for mucosal candidiasis it accounted for 5 to 10 per cent of opportunistic infections in patients with AIDS. The presentation is usually subacute and may be subtle and non-specific with headache, vomiting, and mild fever, and few neurological signs. Less frequently, psychiatric disturbance, convulsions, cranial nerve palsies, truncal ataxia, or focal intracerebral lesions may occur. Neck stiffness is unusual. The diagnosis is made by identifying cryptococci in the cerebrospinal fluid by India ink staining, detection of cryptococcal antigen in the cerebrospinal fluid (uniformly positive), and culture. Cryptococcal antigen is also usually detectable in serum. *C. neoformans* in patients with AIDS causes minimal inflammation so the white cell count of the cerebrospinal fluid is often only mildly raised and the protein and glucose levels of the cerebrospinal fluid may be normal.

A randomized, controlled trial showed that the combination of amphotericin B and 5-flucytosine was superior to amphotericin B alone or fluconazole alone for the treatment of cryptococcal meningitis. Amphotericin B and 5-flucytosine together lead to more rapid sterilization of the cerebrospinal fluid but are not as well tolerated as fluconazole. Most patients should be given the combination, but milder cases may be treated with fluconazole alone. Resistance of cryptococcus to fluconazole is very rare. Itraconazole can be effective, but is not generally recommended. Adverse reactions to amphotericin are frequent, especially fever, myalgia, renal impairment, and electrolyte disturbances. Close monitoring is required. Lipid formulations of amphotericin are reserved for patients intolerant of conventional formulation. Raised intracranial pressure is associated with clinical deterioration and the risk of blindness: repeated lumbar punctures, ventricular shunting, or acetazolamide therapy may be required.

Without secondary prophylaxis, cryptococcal meningitis relapses in 50 to 80 per cent of patients with HIV in the absence of antiretroviral treatment. Oral fluconazole (200 mg/day) is effective for lifelong maintenance. This can be discontinued if antiretroviral treatment leads to sustained immunological recovery.

Progressive multifocal leucoencephalopathy

Progressive multifocal leucoencephalopathy is a progressive demyelinating condition of advanced HIV disease caused by JC virus, a polyomavirus cytopathic for oligodendroglia. It presents with focal neurological deficits, personality changes, or ataxia; headache and mass effects are absent. Brain MRI, the investigation of choice, usually shows multiple white-matter lesions. JC virus is detectable in cerebrospinal fluid by PCR, but this is not usually necessary for diagnosis. There is no specific treatment. Survival of less than 6 months is usual, but progression may sometimes be halted or reversed by highly active antiretroviral therapy. Cidofovir is active against JC virus and is being evaluated in patients. The other human polyomavirus, BK virus, is a very rare cause of encephalitis and interstitial nephropathy in AIDS.

HIV encephalopathy

HIV can infect the nervous system directly, leading to a variety of clinical problems. Most patients dying of AIDS show histological evidence of brain involvement including neurone loss. A smaller number (up to 10 per cent) develop the cognitive, behavioural, and motor abnormalities of dementia. In the early stages, there is impairment of concentration and memory and mood changes mimicking depression; gradual progression leads to intellectual incapacity and motor disability so that patients cannot care for themselves. Neurological signs include slow movement, incoordination, motor weakness, hyperreflexia, and extensor plantar responses; brain imaging shows reduced grey matter volume in the cortex and basal ganglia. Ultimately, a nearly vegetative condition develops with virtual mutism, inability to walk, and incontinence. These patients die within 2 years. Antiretroviral treatment can prevent, and in the earlier stages reverse, AIDS dementia.

Other psychological/psychiatric problems include anxiety, panic attacks, and depression. Psychotherapy may be helpful. Antidepressants may be needed in severe cases. Acute psychosis is rare. Dystonic reactions to various drugs, such as metoclopramide, are more common in patients with HIV.

In the late stages of HIV disease, the differential diagnosis of HIV dementia includes cytomegalovirus (CMV) encephalitis. This usually presents with rapidly progressive confusion and dementia, impaired consciousness, fever, cranial nerve lesions, and convulsions. MRI shows necrotizing periventriculitis; protein levels in cerebrospinal fluid may be elevated and CMV DNA is detectable in the cerebrospinal fluid by PCR. Ganciclovir and other anti-CMV agents may reduce progression.

Peripheral neuropathy and myelopathy

Peripheral neuropathy can occur at any stage of HIV infection, even at seroconversion, but is most common in advanced disease, when 10 to 15 per cent of patients have a distal symmetrical sensorimotor neuropathy of axonal type causing pain and paraesthesias that may limit walking and, less often, distal weakness and atrophy. Mononeuritis multiplex and acute inflammatory demyelinating polyneuropathy resembling the Guillain–Barré syndrome are also described, generally at an earlier stage. Drugs used in patients with HIV, including stavudine, didanosine, and vincristine, may cause or exacerbate peripheral neuropathy. HIV-related autonomic neuropathy may cause postural hypotension, diarrhoea, impotence, impaired sweating, and bladder symptoms. CMV infection in patients with AIDS presents with a lumbosacral polyradiculopathy causing sacral paraesthesias and numbness, lower limb weakness, and urinary retention that may progress to flaccid paraparesis if untreated.

HIV may involve the spinal cord directly causing a vacuolar myelopathy. This usually presents with bilateral leg weakness and sensory symptoms, usually paraesthesias, and may progress to spastic paraparesis, ataxia, and incontinence.

Ocular disease

Cytomegalovirus retinitis (see also Section 25)

Without antiretroviral therapy, up to 30 per cent of patients with AIDS (and CD4 lymphocyte count below 50/mm³) develop reactivation of CMV in the form of a destructive and blinding retinitis. This is rare in other types of immunosuppression. It usually presents with blurring of vision, scotomas, floaters, or flashing lights. The characteristic retinal changes are patches of irregular retinal pallor, caused by oedema and necrosis, and haemorrhages in a perivascular distribution (Fig. 13). The retinitis usually starts peripherally and progresses rapidly to involve the macula and whole retina, leading to blindness. Complications include retinal detachment, branch retinal artery occlusion, persistent iritis, and cataract. CMV retinitis should not be confused with cotton-wool spots (HIV retinopathy)—small, pale retinal lesions without haemorrhages that commonly occur in patients with HIV. These are benign and often come and go.

The diagnosis of CMV retinitis is clinical, based on the characteristic retinal appearance (see Section 25). CMV viraemia may be detectable by PCR and high or rising CMV viral load is associated with an increased risk of developing retinitis and other CMV disease. Anti-CMV drugs (ganciclovir, foscarnet, cidofovir) are virustatic; before the availability of highly active antiretroviral drug combinations, the aim of treatment was to stop progression rather than to cure disease. First-line treatment is with intravenous ganciclovir, which may cause severe neutropenia and thrombocyto-

Fig. 13 Cytomegalovirus retinitis.

penia that are dose-limiting in about 10 per cent of patients. Foscarnet (phosphonoformate) is a relatively toxic second-line agent that causes dose-limiting reversible renal impairment and symptoms of hypocalcaemia in about 20 per cent of patients. Ganciclovir can also be given as a slow-release intraocular implant, but this may allow CMV to develop at other sites including the other eye.

For maintenance therapy, oral ganciclovir may be adequate, convenient, and well tolerated, although there is a greater risk of disease progression than with daily intravenous infusions of ganciclovir or foscarnet, and the eyes must be examined frequently. Cidofovir is more active against CMV than the other anti-CMV drugs. It can be given by intermittent intravenous infusion, initially weekly and then every 2 weeks. Whereas ganciclovir and foscarnet require a central venous catheter, cidofovir may be given in short infusions through a peripheral vein because of its prolonged antiviral effect. However, cidofovir is relatively toxic, causing irreversible nephrotoxicity, neutropenia, and peripheral neuropathy in over one-third of patients.

With the advent of highly active antiretroviral therapy, CMV retinitis is much less common in developed countries. Sustained suppression of HIV viral load and improvement in immune status can allow discontinuation of maintenance treatment. New manifestations of ocular CMV, such as vitritis, have been reported in patients treated with highly active antiretroviral therapy (see Impact of highly active antiretroviral therapy, below).

Other ocular syndromes

Acute retinal necrosis is a rare condition originally reported in reactivation of varicella zoster virus in otherwise healthy adults. In patients with advanced HIV infection it is usually preceded by dermatomal herpes zoster and typically presents with blurring of vision and pain in the affected eye. Progressive necrotizing retinitis leads to visual deterioration that may be associated with uveitis. An outer retinal necrosis syndrome with little ocular inflammation also occurs in patients with AIDS. There is a high risk of visual loss and retinal detachment. Both eyes may be affected. Suspected acute retinal necrosis should be treated with intravenous aciclovir.

Acute toxoplasma choroidoretinitis may resemble CMV retinitis, but the retinal scarring that follows treatment is distinctive. The disease is more common in countries such as Brazil and France where the background prevalence of toxoplasmosis is much higher than in the United Kingdom. Choroidoretinitis is also a rare complication of histoplasmosis and cryptococcosis.

HIV-related tumours

Kaposi's sarcoma

Kaposi's sarcoma characteristically presents as multiple, purplish nodular skin lesions (Fig. 14). Lesions start as small, pink, deep purple, or brown macules, and develop into nodules or plaques that may ulcerate. They also occur on mucosal surfaces, most commonly on the hard palate. Local or regional oedema and lymph node enlargement may occur. Mucocutaneous lesions are cosmetically and psychologically important but are rarely of clinical importance (Fig. 15). However, visceral disease, which most commonly affects the lungs and gastrointestinal tract, is an important cause of morbidity and even mortality. Lung lesions cause dyspnoea, cough, or haemoptysis, and gut involvement may cause abdominal pain, bleeding, or a rare protein-losing enteropathy. Extensive visceral involvement can cause constitutional symptoms such as fevers, night sweats, and weight loss. Kaposi's sarcoma rarely affects the central nervous system.

In industrialized countries, Kaposi's sarcoma is over 2000 times more common in HIV-infected individuals than in the general population. Classic Kaposi's sarcoma in HIV-negative individuals occurs in middle-aged and elderly men of Eastern European or Mediterranean origin. Endemic Kaposi's sarcoma in Africa has been known for decades. It is predominantly

Fig. 14 Cutaneous Kaposi's sarcoma.

a disease of older men that has a fairly indolent course. HIV-related Kaposi's sarcoma, on the other hand, is a more aggressive disease and occurs mostly in those people who have acquired HIV via a sexual route, namely homosexual and bisexual men and in younger African men and women. The epidemic of Kaposi's sarcoma in Central and East Africa exactly mirrors the HIV epidemic in these regions. Kaposi's sarcoma is rare in intravenous drug users and very rare in recipients of blood products, including those with haemophilia. These epidemiological features suggested a sexually transmissible aetiological agent.

In 1994, a new herpesvirus, human herpesvirus-8 (**HHV-8**), was found in HIV-related Kaposi's sarcoma and was soon detected in the lesions of all forms of Kaposi's sarcoma. Seroepidemiological studies show that HHV-8 is common only in certain geographical regions, corresponding to where Kaposi's sarcoma was endemic before the era of HIV. HHV-8 is detectable in saliva but less often in semen. This may explain why both sexual and other routes of transmission occur. For instance in Africa, where HHV-8 infection is common, it is transmitted perinatally from mother to child.

Kaposi's sarcoma lesions are characterized by proliferating spindle cells, possibly of endothelial origin, thin-walled slit-like vascular spaces, infiltration by lymphocytes and plasma cells, and extravasated red cells. Multiple lesions appear synchronously in widely dispersed areas. Recent work has suggested a monoclonal origin for Kaposi's sarcoma lesions, but they may be reactive proliferative rather than truly cancerous. HHV-8 is detectable in spindle cells and flat endothelial cells lining the vascular spaces of Kaposi's sarcoma lesions. It is likely that the virus triggers the release of cellular and virus-encoded cytokines that promote the proliferation of spindle cells.

Fig. 15 Kaposi's sarcoma of the palate in a patient with HIV infection (copyright D. A. Warrell).

Highly active antiretroviral therapy has led to a dramatic reduction in the frequency and mortality of Kaposi's sarcoma in developed countries. In early Kaposi's sarcoma the progression is often halted or reversed by starting antiretroviral treatment alone. Otherwise, cutaneous lesions may be left untreated or treated with local radiotherapy, cryotherapy, or intralesional vinblastine. Widespread skin or visceral disease is usually treated by systemic chemotherapy, with single or multiple-agent regimens of vincristine, vinblastine, bleomycin, etoposide, and anthracyclines. The combination of vincristine and bleomycin is effective in 50 per cent of patients and well tolerated, but responses are usually short-lived. Liposomal preparations of anthracyclines (such as daunorubicin) are more effective and better tolerated, and are now the treatment of choice. Treatment of disseminated Kaposi's sarcoma has not been considered to be curative, but remissions may be induced by a combination of highly active antiretroviral treatment and systemic chemotherapy.

Non-Hodgkin's lymphoma

Non-Hodgkin's lymphoma develops in 3 to 10 per cent of HIV-positive patients, an incidence 60 to 100 times higher than in the general population. Most tumours are extranodal and, histologically, 60 per cent are large-cell B-cell lymphomas; 30 per cent are Burkitt's type and the rest are of T-cell or non-B-, non-T-cell origin. Some 50 per cent are associated with Epstein–Barr virus (**EBV**) infection and are more aggressive with a shorter survival. A minority of HIV-related lymphomas are associated with HHV-8. They present as body-cavity lymphomas, causing pleural or peritoneal effusions (primary effusion lymphoma). Patients on highly active antiretroviral therapy have a reduced risk of developing Non-Hodgkin's lymphoma, and consequently the incidence of HIV-related lymphomas in developed countries has declined in recent years.

HIV-associated lymphoma outside the central nervous system may respond well to standard lymphoma chemotherapy regimens, in addition to highly active antiretroviral treatment. Response is better in those who are less immunosuppressed (CD4 above 200/mm^3 and no previous AIDS diagnosis). Opportunistic infections cause many deaths during chemotherapy. Lower dose or less toxic chemotherapy protocols are sometimes advocated for patients with more advanced HIV disease.

The central nervous system is a common site of HIV-associated non-Hodgkin's lymphoma, which is nearly always associated with EBV and sometimes with HHV-8 as well. Patients usually present with the symptoms and signs of a space-occupying cerebral tumour. Detection of EBV DNA in the cerebrospinal fluid may help to distinguish these lymphomas from cerebral toxoplasmosis. In the absence of antiretroviral therapy, neither chemotherapy nor radiotherapy have much impact, and the median survival after diagnosis is very poor, at about 3 months. However, this may be substantially prolonged in patients on highly active antiretroviral treatment.

Other tumours in AIDS

Some studies have reported an increased frequency of Hodgkin's disease in patients with HIV, particularly of the mixed cellularity type. Disseminated disease with a poor prognosis seems to be more frequent than for HIV-negative Hodgkin's disease. Castleman's disease (angiofollicular lymph node hyperplasia) is a lymphoproliferative condition that may be HHV-8 related and, in the multicentric form, is also associated with HIV. There is an increased incidence of squamous-cell carcinoma of the conjunctiva in patients with HIV infection, especially in Africa. HIV-infected women suffer a higher incidence of cervical intraepithelial neoplasia (**CIN**) and predisposition to cervical carcinoma; cervical cancer has been designated an AIDS-defining condition. The incidence of vulval intraepithelial neoplasia (**VIN**) is also increased by HIV infection. The incidence of squamous-cell anal carcinoma is increased in homosexual men, but the risk does not seem to be greatly magnified by HIV while the risk of anal intraepithelial neoplasia (**AIN**), a precursor of anal carcinoma, is significantly increased. The development of CIN, VIN and AIN may be related to co-infection with oncogenic types of human papillomavirus, especially type 16.

Common syndromes

Fever of unknown cause

Fever is rarely attributable to HIV infection *per se*, and patients should be fully investigated for other causes. There is increased susceptibility to pyogenic infections as well as opportunistic infections and tumours. Unlike fever of unknown origin (FUO) in other patients, however, most cases of FUO in HIV-positive patients are caused by an infection. Cultures of blood, urine, and faeces should be obtained, and chest radiography done. If sputum is available it should be stained and cultured for tuberculosis. In patients with intravenous lines and devices, catheter-related bacteraemia is an important cause. Occult infections (including sinusitis and dental sepsis) and drug-related fever should always be considered. Rarely, infection with *Pneumocystis* spp. and *Cryptococcus* spp. can present as fever without their typical focal signs, and dissemination to other sites (such as skin, fundi) may occur. Disseminated leishmaniasis is an important cause in those who have visited an endemic area (see Other disseminated infections, below).

In advanced disease, the most common causes of persistent high-swinging fevers are disseminated MAC infection (see *Mycobacterium avium* complex, above) and non-Hodgkin's lymphoma (see Non-Hodgkin's lymphoma, above). Imaging techniques, in particular CT scanning of the abdomen, are essential to find a suitable site for biopsy to diagnose lymphoma.

In some cases, the cause of fever is not found; in early disease the fever may resolve spontaneously. In advanced disease, fever and sweats may continue intermittently for many months. Symptomatic treatment includes non-steroidal anti-inflammatory drugs and low-dose prednisolone; therapeutic trials of anti-MAC treatment may be justified.

Breathlessness

Appropriate management of breathlessness is important because the most common cause, pneumocystis pneumonia, can be rapidly progressive. The differential diagnosis is broad, and includes bacterial pneumonia, pneumothorax, pulmonary Kaposi's sarcoma, other tumours, fungal infections, asthma, and heart failure. Routine investigations should include chest radiography, blood oxygen saturation, and peak flow measurement. Blood from febrile patients should be sent for culture. Sputum should be obtained, if necessary by induction with nebulized saline, and stained for the presence of *Pneumocystis* spp., mycobacteria, and fungi. Bronchoalveolar lavage should be considered early as patients sometimes progress quickly and become too ill for bronchoscopy without the support of mechanical ventilation.

Empirical treatment should cover *Pneumocystis* spp., *S. pneumoniae*, and *H. influenzae* by combining high-dose co-trimoxazole with a suitable broad-spectrum antimicrobial such as cefotaxime. A macrolide such as erythromycin or clarithromycin may be added if atypical pneumonia (such as mycoplasma) is suspected. If the clinical suspicion of pneumocystis is high, corticosteroids should be included if the patient is hypoxaemic (see *Pneumocystis carinii* pneumonia, above). Continuous positive airway pressure (**CPAP**) or mechanical ventilation may be needed in severe cases to allow diagnosis and time for patients to respond to treatment. If the chest radiograph shows diffuse bilateral infiltration and bronchoalveolar lavage fails to reveal any pathogen, presumptive treatment for pneumocystis pneumonia should be continued. If no diagnosis is made and deterioration occurs despite empirical treatment, open-lung biopsy should be considered to establish the diagnosis, but the prognosis is generally poor.

Diarrhoea

Chronic diarrhoea is a common problem in patients with advanced HIV infection, particularly in the tropics, and may be associated with weight loss and malabsorption. No cause other than HIV can be identified in at least half of cases; an HIV enteropathy characterized by partial villous atrophy has been described. The most common opportunistic cause is infection by the protozoan *Cryptosporidium parvum*, which causes a self-limiting gastroenteritis in those who are non-immunosuppressed. In HIV-positive patients diarrhoea may be protracted and severe, with marked fluid and electrolyte losses. The diagnosis is made by finding cryptosporidial oocysts in the stool using a modified acid-fast stain. Symptoms of cryptosporidiosis are often intermittent, as is excretion of the oocysts, so multiple stool specimens may need to be examined. Therapy with highly active antiretroviral drugs is the most important step in treatment. Symptomatic treatment with antidiarrhoeal drugs (such as loperamide), fluid and electrolyte replacement, and nutritional support are required. Octreotide may be useful in the most severe cases.

The coccidian protozoa *Isospora belli* and *Cyclospora cayetanensis* are important but less common causes of HIV-related chronic diarrhoea, diagnosed by the presence of sporocysts in the stool. Isosporiasis may respond to treatment with co-trimoxazole but the relapse rate after stopping treatment is 50 per cent, and similar experience is reported for cyclosporiasis. Microsporidia such as *Enterocytozoon bieneusi* and *Encephalitozoon intestinalis* are intracellular pathogens that may cause diarrhoea in advanced HIV disease. Special diagnostic staining methods applied to stool samples or electron microscopy of a rectal biopsy are needed to make the diagnosis. Albendazole may be effective, and treatment with highly active antiretroviral therapy may induce remission of intestinal microsporidiosis.

Giardia duodenalis and *Entamoeba histolytica* cysts are more commonly found in the faeces of homosexual men than heterosexual men, but these protozoa usually do not cause special problems in those with HIV. Bacterial infections with enteric pathogens such as salmonella, shigella, campylobacter, and *Clostridium difficile* do not lead to chronic diarrhoea but may take longer to clear. Salmonella infections may cause disseminated infection with recurrent bacteraemia that recurs even after prolonged antimicrobial therapy.

With advanced disease, MAC infection may cause diarrhoea among other symptoms. CMV causes a colitis that typically presents with abdominal pain and tenderness, fever, and bloody diarrhoea. Rectal or colonic biopsy may confirm the diagnosis by identifying the characteristic nuclear inclusion bodies. HIV-related autonomic neuropathy is a rare cause of diarrhoea that is often most troublesome at night; anticholinergic drugs may help in addition to antidiarrhoeal agents. Diarrhoea in HIV-positive patients is a frequent side-effect of medications such as antibiotics and antiretroviral drugs.

HIV wasting syndrome

Weight loss is one of the most distressing features of progressive HIV infection. Its course fluctuates even in advanced disease; frequently it is attributable to specific complications such as diarrhoeal diseases, lymphoma, or disseminated MAC infection. It may also progress with no cause identified other than advanced HIV infection. In developing countries, such as those in sub-Saharan Africa, the wasting syndrome is characteristic evidence of AIDS and has been called 'slim disease'. Despite severe weight loss, patients may remain well for many months or even years. Numerous therapeutic approaches have been tried, mostly with disappointing results, including oral nutritional support, enteral feeding, total parenteral nutrition, and trials of growth hormone and thalidomide. Anabolic steroids such as nandrolone and stanozolol may reverse HIV-related wasting, but they may cause serious side-effects and their use has not been widely adopted. Highly active antiretroviral therapy is important in the prevention and reversal of HIV-related weight loss, but the fat redistribution associated with some antiretroviral agents may cause face and limb wasting (see Drug toxicity and interactions, below).

Miscellaneous conditions

Bacillary angiomatosis

Disseminated infection with *Bartonella henselae*, the principal agent of cat-scratch disease, is the cause of bacillary angiomatosis, an HIV-associated condition that typically causes multiple subcutaneous vascular lesions, fever, liver lesions (bacillary peliosis hepatis), and osteolytic bone lesions. The skin lesions are usually purplish nodules that may be mistaken for Kaposi's sarcoma, but the histology is distinct, acute neutrophilic inflammation and capillary proliferation, and clusters of bacilli revealed by modified silver staining. The organism may be cultured from blood. A similar syndrome in HIV-positive patients can be caused by the agent of trench fever, *Bartonella quintana*. Bacillary angiomatosis usually responds to treatment with a macrolide antibiotic. Cats and cat fleas form a reservoir for *B. henselae*, and patients who develop bacillary angiomatosis frequently have a history of contact with cats.

Other disseminated infections

In regions where invasive fungal infections are endemic (such as *Histoplasma capsulatum* in the Mississippi river region, *Coccidioides immitis* in the southern United States, and *Penicillium marneffei* in South-East Asia) or where there is a relevant travel history, disseminated fungal infection should be considered in HIV-positive patients presenting with fever, weight loss, anaemia, pulmonary infiltrates, lymphadenopathy, and hepatosplenomegaly. Papular skin lesions may be seen in disseminated histoplasmosis and *P. marneffei* infection. Similar lesions resembling giant molluscum (see Skin conditions in advanced HIV, below) may occur with disseminated cryptococcosis. Blood or bone marrow cultures or direct identification by the use of special stains on tissue obtained from skin lesions, bone marrow, or liver are required for diagnosis. Initial therapy is generally with intravenous amphotericin; itraconazole (for histoplasmosis and *P. marneffei*) or fluconazole (for coccidioidomycosis) may be adequate for subsequent maintenance treatment.

HIV-associated disseminated leishmaniasis is mostly reported from the Mediterranean littoral, South America, and Africa. It is caused by dissemination of *Leishmania* spp., protozoan parasites transmitted by sandflies. A high index of clinical suspicion is required because although the classic features are fever, weight loss, anaemia, and hepatosplenomegaly, a high proportion of patients have fever alone. Most cases can be diagnosed by bone marrow examination. Treatment is usually with the organic antimonial compound sodium stibogluconate, given parenterally.

Other visceral disease

Cryptosporidium (see Diarrhoea, above) and CMV may cause a sclerosing cholangitis-like syndrome with irregular dilatations and stenoses of the biliary tree (demonstrable by endoscopic retrograde cholangiography), abnormal liver blood tests, and occasionally jaundice. CMV is frequently identified histologically in the pancreas at autopsy, but its role in the development of clinical pancreatitis is unproved. A characteristic nephropathy (HIV-related glomerulosclerosis), primary pulmonary hypertension, and cardiomyopathy (see Section 15.16) are well described in patients with AIDS.

Haematological conditions

Thrombocytopenia is relatively common (5 to 15 per cent) in HIV infection and is associated with antiplatelet antibodies; symptomatic thrombocytopenia is uncommon but more likely in the later stages of HIV infection. Life-threatening bleeding is rare. Thrombocytopenia is not a marker for HIV progression and spontaneous remissions are frequent. When treatment is required, the principles and response are similar to those that apply in the treatment of HIV-negative immune thrombocytopenia, and include the use of prednisolone, intravenous immunoglobulin, and splenectomy. Thrombocytopenia also frequently responds to antiretroviral therapy using combinations that include zidovudine, which improves platelet production.

Anaemia is common in patients with advanced HIV infection, and is frequently related to medications (such as zidovudine). Human (B19) parvovirus infection is an important reversible cause of chronic anaemia in HIV infection. Bone marrow biopsy typically shows an absence of erythroid development with occasional giant pronormoblasts, and B19 parvovirus is detected by PCR. The anaemia may respond to treatment with intravenous immunoglobulin.

Mild neutropenia is common in HIV-positive patients at all stages of infection, and may be partly responsible for the increased risk of pyogenic bacterial infections; however, profound neutropenia (below $0.5 \times 10^9/l$) is rare. Antineutrophil antibodies may be present. Drugs (such as co-trimoxazole, ganciclovir, antiretrovirals) may increase the incidence and severity of neutropenia. In selected HIV-positive patients with refractory or life-threatening bacterial or fungal infection and severe neutropenia, the addition of recombinant human granulocyte colony-stimulating factor to the treatment regimen may improve the outcome.

Skin conditions in advanced HIV

In the later stages of HIV infection a number of infections have atypical cutaneous manifestations. These include giant molluscum contagiosum, characterized by large flesh-coloured non-tender umbilicated lesions often affecting the face in homosexual men. In advanced HIV disease, genital herpes simplex infection may cause painful chronic genital or anal ulcers that can become resistant to aciclovir and related compounds; intravenous foscarnet or cidofovir are effective. Aciclovir-resistant varicella zoster virus also occurs in AIDS; and reactivation of varicella zoster virus can take an unusual form, with a subacute course and dissemination causing scattered vesicular lesions in the absence of dermatomal zoster. CMV is a cause of chronic perianal ulceration that can be treated with ganciclovir. Atypical cutaneous presentations of syphilis may occur at any stage of HIV infection. In Asia, the varied skin manifestations of *P. marneffei* infection are familiar.

Children and HIV

Most paediatric infections result from the vertical transmission of HIV, although some children may be infected by blood products. The risk of vertical transmission is increased during advanced maternal HIV disease, if delivery is by the vaginal route, and if the baby is breast fed (see Vertical transmission, below). Diagnosis is important during the first year of life because about 20 per cent of HIV-infected children progress rapidly to AIDS during that time; however, a special diagnostic approach is needed before 18 months of age, because over this period uninfected children may have maternal HIV antibody. Techniques for virus detection (for example, HIV DNA by PCR) allow confirmation of HIV infection in 95 per cent of infected infants by 1 month of age. The sensitivity of these virological assays increases over the first few months, so if negative at 3 to 6 weeks, the tests should be repeated at 3 to 6 months; if HIV is not detected at this time, loss of HIV antibody should be confirmed at 15 to 18 months before the child is assumed to be HIV-negative.

HIV-infected children should be managed by paediatricians with experience in HIV care, usually in specialized units. About 10 per cent die in infancy, and progression to AIDS subsequently occurs at the rate of about 5 per cent per year. In recent European series, 40 per cent of children had developed AIDS before the age of 5 years and 25 per cent had died. The commonest AIDS diagnosis in infancy is pneumocystis pneumonia. The CD4 lymphocyte count is less valuable for monitoring than in adults, particularly in very young children; consequently prophylaxis against *Pneumocystis* spp. is usually given regardless of the CD4 count during the first year. In older children, the principles of monitoring are similar to those in adults, using clinical status, CD4 counts, and viral load estimation by plasma HIV-1 RNA measurement. The CD4 percentage (percentage of total lymphocytes) and CD4:CD8 cell ratio vary less with age and are more useful than absolute CD4 counts in children under the age of 5 years.

In children, clinical conditions reasonably predictive of HIV infection include persistent oral candida, parotid swelling, and recurrent or frequent serious bacterial infections including pneumonia. Failure to thrive, diarrhoea, fever, lymphadenopathy, and hepatosplenomegaly are more common in HIV-infected infants but are non-specific and less predictive. HIV dementia, and other neurological and developmental problems are associated with a poor prognosis. HIV-related lymphocytic interstitial pneumonitis (**LIP**) is almost confined to children and characterized by progressive widespread reticulonodular shadowing on chest radiography. LIP develops gradually and may be asymptomatic; cough, breathlessness, clubbing, secondary bacterial infections, and bronchiectasis occur in severe cases and may be treated with oral prednisolone.

Principles of antiretroviral treatment are similar in children and adults. Clinical trials are in progress to determine optimal antiretroviral combinations, when to start treatment, and the tolerability of the newer drugs in all the major categories. Triple-therapy regimens are well tolerated in children and may produce sustained elevations in CD4 lymphocyte counts, but adherence is particularly difficult. As HIV-infected children grow older, the number of adolescents with perinatally acquired HIV is increasing, raising the need for advice on reducing the risk of sexual transmission.

Prevention of opportunistic infections (see Table 5)

The risk of developing an opportunistic infection rises greatly once the peripheral CD4 lymphocyte count falls consistently below 200/mm^3. It is standard practice to introduce low-dose co-trimoxazole prophylaxis for pneumocystis pneumonia at this stage. This also reduces the risk of cerebral toxoplasmosis and may prevent bacterial pneumonia.

The risk of developing active tuberculosis in HIV-positive American intravenous drug users with positive tuberculin skin tests has been shown

Table 5 Prophylaxis of major opportunistic infections in HIV

Infection	Indications	Regimens		Comments
		First line	**Alternatives**	
Pneumococcal pneumonia	All HIV-positive patients	Pneumococcal vaccine	None	Clinical effectiveness unproved; antibody response greater if CD4 >350/mm^3
P. carinii pneumonia	CD4 <200/mm^3; or symptomatic HIV; or following *P. carinii* pneumonia	Co-trimoxazole 480–960 mg daily (or 960 mg, 3 times per week)	Dapsone; dapsone with pyrimethamine; monthly nebulized pentamidine; atovaquone	May be stopped if CD4 rises to >200/mm^3 and very low viral load on anti-HIV treatment
Cerebral toxoplasmosis	CD4 <100/mm^3 plus toxoplasma IgG-positive	As above	Dapsone with pyrimethamine	Primary prophylaxis usually incidental to that for *P. carinii* prophylaxis; pentamidine not protective
	Following treatment of cerebral toxoplasmosis	Sulfadiazine 0.5–1 g, 4 times daily with pyrimethamine 25–75 mg/day, and folinic acid	Clindamycin with pyrimethamine, and folinic acid	See Cerebral toxoplasmosis section. Only sulfadiazine/pyrimethamine protects against *P. carinii* as well
Tuberculosis	Tuberculin reaction >5 mm induration with no previous BCG; or high-risk exposure to tuberculosis	Isoniazid 300 mg/day with pyridoxine 50 mg/day for 6–9 months (if isoniazid-sensitive)	Rifampicin with pyrazinamide for 2 months (if isoniazid-sensitive)	Rifampicin should not be given with protease inhibitors or non-nucleoside reverse transcriptase inhibitors
M. avium complex (MAC)	CD4 <50/mm^3	Clarithromycin 500 mg, twice daily, or azithromycin 1200 mg/week	Rifabutin; rifabutin with azithromycin	Adoption of primary prophylaxis varies
	Following treatment of disseminated MAC	Clarithromycin 500 mg, twice daily, with ethambutol 15 mg/kg per day with or without rifabutin 300 mg/day	Azithromycin with ethambutol with or without rifabutin	See *M. avium* complex section
Cytomegalovirus (CMV)	CD4 <50/mm^3 and CMV antibody-positive	Oral ganciclovir 1 g, 3 times daily	None	Primary prophylaxis not generally recommended because of lack of survival benefit, limited efficacy, toxicity, and cost
	Following CMV retinitis or other CMV disease	Ganciclovir 5–6 mg/kg IV on 5–7 day/week; or oral ganciclovir 1 g, 3 times daily	Foscarnet IV; cidofovir IV; ganciclovir intraocular implant; oral valganciclovir	
Cryptococcal meningitis	CD4 <50/mm^3	Fluconazole 100–200 mg/day orally	Itraconazole orally	Primary prophylaxis not generally recommended because cryptococcal disease uncommon
	Following treatment of cryptococcal meningitis	Fluconazole 200 mg/day orally	Amphotericin B IV weekly or 3 times/week; itraconazole orally	Fluconazole superior to itraconazole for secondary prophylaxis

IV, intravenous.

to be about 8 per cent per year and can be reduced by taking isoniazid for a year. In developing countries, in particular, the risk of active tuberculosis in HIV-positive individuals is high and isoniazid alone or in combination with rifampicin can reduce the risk, but the feasibility and cost-effectiveness of this approach in resource-poor countries require further evaluation. BCG vaccination does not appear to be protective in HIV.

Primary prophylaxis may prevent other conditions, such as CMV retinitis, cryptococcal meningitis, and histoplasmosis, but because of the relatively low incidence and lack of predictors of risk for these conditions, it is not cost-effective. Before the advent of highly active antiretroviral therapy, after treatment of an opportunistic infection the underlying tendency to the infection usually remained. Thus in early studies, following an episode of pneumocystis pneumonia, patients had a 50 per cent chance of a further episode within a year. Secondary prophylaxis with co-trimoxazole proved effective. Secondary prophylaxis for *Pneumocystis* spp. and other opportunistic infections, including MAC and CMV, can now usually be discontinued if there is a good response to antiretroviral treatment, with CD4 counts sustained above 200/mm^3 and low plasma levels of HIV RNA.

Simple measures, other than drugs, may reduce the risk of some infections. Avoiding undercooked eggs and poultry may reduce the risk of disseminated salmonella infection and adequate boiling of drinking water can prevent cryptosporidiosis. Stopping cigarette smoking may reduce the risk of bacterial chest infections

Prevention of HIV transmission

Sexual transmission

Sexual transmission accounts for most new cases of HIV infection. Education to alter behaviour and reduce the risk of HIV infection is an important part of HIV control programmes. The benefits of 'safer sex' should be publicized; condom promotion in Thailand has made an impact on HIV transmission rates. The presence of other sexually transmitted infections, especially those causing genital ulcers, facilitates HIV transmission. Accordingly, studies in Tanzania and elsewhere have demonstrated that programmes to prevent and treat sexually transmitted infections can reduce the incidence of new HIV infections.

Vertical transmission

As the number of women infected with HIV increases, the problem of vertical transmission of the virus assumes greater importance. In developed countries, the risk of transmission of HIV from a seropositive pregnant woman to her child is about 15 per cent, but this figure may be as high as 30 per cent in sub-Saharan Africa and other parts of the tropics. Although infection of the fetus can occur at any time during pregnancy and has been associated with breast feeding, most infections occur during labour. Zidovudine reduced the risk from 25 to 8 per cent, when given to women during late pregnancy and labour and to the neonate for 6 weeks. Simpler, cheaper regimens have been shown to be effective. During vaginal delivery, intrapartum interventions such as fetal blood sampling and use of fetal scalp clips should be avoided. Elective caesarean section further reduces vertical transmission (see British HIV Association guidelines in the Further reading list). Breast feeding should be avoided, if possible, but is still generally recommended in developing countries where the risks of bottle feeding probably outweigh the risks of breast feeding. Increasingly, the routine offer of HIV testing is being incorporated into antenatal care in developed countries where antiretroviral treatment is available.

Blood products

Screening of blood products began as soon as testing for HIV became available, and heat treatment for factor VIII concentrate was also introduced. These measures dramatically reduced the risk of virus transmission by blood and blood products in industrialized countries. However, there may still be a problem in developing countries where screening is not efficient, or where the background seroprevalence of potential donors is so high that HIV-infected blood may be screened as negative when donated by an individual in the 'window period' immediately after initial infection (see Diagnosis of HIV infection, above).

Injecting drug use

Needle-exchange programmes and the prescription of controlled drugs to registered addicts may reduce the incidence of new HIV infections in injecting drug users. Major problems still exist in countries such as India and Russia, where injecting drug use is becoming more common and education about the risk and the availability of clean needles is very limited.

Occupational exposure and postexposure prophylaxis

Based on data from more than 3000 occupational exposures to HIV, the average risk of HIV infection after needlestick injury or other percutaneous exposure was calculated to be 0.3 per cent (about 1 in 325). The risk following mucous membrane exposure has been estimated to be around 0.1 per cent. The risk of transmission is greatest for deep injuries; if there is visible blood on the device; during procedures involving direct cannulation of blood vessels; or if the source patient has advanced HIV disease. A small retrospective case-control study demonstrated an 80 per cent reduction in the likelihood of seroconversion in healthcare workers who took zidovudine soon after percutaneous exposure to HIV. In view of the greater activity of antiretroviral drug combinations but without direct evidence, it is currently recommended that high-risk occupational exposures to HIV are treated as soon as possible with two nucleoside inhibitors and a protease inhibitor (such as zidovudine, lamivudine, and nelfinavir) for 1 month. Nevirapine is not currently recommended in postexposure prophylaxis regimens because of a relatively high rate of adverse reactions. In the management of occupational exposure to HIV, a careful risk assessment should be done and information provided. If the risk of HIV transmission is identified, antiretroviral therapy should be offered and started promptly to maximize the chance of success. There is a theoretical argument for taking antiretroviral drugs after high-risk sexual exposure to HIV; at present there is no consensus on the appropriateness of postexposure treatment in this context, and no clinical or cost-effectiveness data are available.

Vaccine development

The high degree of viral variation and immune escape present difficulties for the development of an effective HIV vaccine. None the less, group-specific neutralizing antibodies and cross-reacting T-cell clones have been identified, and there is evidence from female prostitutes repeatedly exposed to HIV that certain individuals can develop specific T-cell responses without persistent infection. These individuals may be protected from infection when exposed to live virus.

To date, non-infectious killed whole virus or recombinant subunit vaccines have not been successful to date in protecting chimpanzees from HIV infection, or macaques from SIV infection and disease. Certain live attenuated strains of SIV, with deletion mutations in *nef* and other regulatory genes, initially appeared to protect adult monkeys from challenge with virulent SIV strains, but more recently were reported to cause AIDS.

Human testing of candidate HIV vaccines, including a vaccine made from tiny recombinant fragments of gp120, the surface glycoprotein of HIV that binds to host-cell CD4 receptors, has so far not been successful. Several new approaches are being examined, which may prove more effective in inducing protective humoral and killer T-cell-mediated immunity. These include DNA vaccines, consisting of pieces of HIV DNA incorporated into harmless plasmid DNA from bacteria, and the use of live vectors (for example, poxviruses such as canary pox and modified vaccinia) to deliver portions of the HIV envelope. Researchers in Oxford are investigating a strategy ('prime–boost') using a DNA vaccine followed by boosting with a modified vaccinia vector vaccine. This approach is also being evaluated for therapeutic vaccination in HIV-positive patients with suppressed viraemia who are being treated with antiretroviral agents, to determine if vaccination will allow interruption of treatment without loss of virological control. Effective vaccination is likely to hold the greatest promise for controlling HIV infection in the future.

Further reading

Basic science

Clapham PR, Weiss RA (1997). Immunodeficiency viruses: spoilt for choice of co-receptors. *Nature* **388**, 230–1.

Emerman M, Malim MH (1998). HIV-1 regulatory/accessory genes: keys to unravelling viral and host cell biology. *Science* **280**, 1880–4.

Esparza J (2001). An HIV vaccine: how and when? *Bulletin of the World Health Organization* **79**, 1133–7.

Ho DD, *et al.* (1995). Rapid turnover of plasma virions and CD4 lymphocytes in HIV-1 infection. *Nature* **373**, 123–6.

Levy JA (1998). *HIV and the pathogenesis of AIDS*, 2nd edn. ASM Press, Washington DC.

Wyatt R, Sodroski J (1998). The HIV-1 envelope glycoproteins: fusogens, antigens and immunogens. *Science* **280**, 1884–8.

Clinical trials

Concorde Coordinating Committee (1994). Concorde: MRC/ANRS randomised double-blind controlled trial of immediate and deferred zidovudine in symptom-free HIV infection. *Lancet* **343**, 871–81.

Delta Coordinating Committee (1996). Delta: a randomised double-blind controlled trial comparing combinations of zidovudine plus didanosine or zalcitabine with zidovudine alone in HIV-infected individuals. *Lancet* **348**, 283–91.

Hammer SM, *et al.* (1997). A controlled trial of two nucleoside analogues plus indinavir in persons with human immunodeficiency virus infection and CD4 cell counts of 200 per cubic millimeter or less. *New England Journal of Medicine* **337**, 725–33.

Epidemiology

Cascade collaboration (2000). Survival after introduction of HAART in people with known duration of HIV-1 infection. *Lancet* **355**, 1158–9.

Collaborative Group on AIDS Incubation and HIV Survival (2000). Time from HIV-1 seroconversion to AIDS and death before widespread use of highly-active antiretroviral therapy: a collaborative re-analysis. *Lancet* **355**, 1131–7.

Palella FJ Jr, *et al.* (1998). Declining morbidity and mortality among patients with advanced human immunodeficiency virus infection. *New England Journal of Medicine* **338**, 853–60.

Treatment

Carr A, Cooper DA (2000). Adverse effects of antiretroviral therapy. *Lancet* **356**, 1423–30.

Flexner C (1998). Drug therapy: HIV-protease inhibitors. *New England Journal of Medicine* **338**, 1281–92.

Perrin L, Telenti A (1998). HIV treatment failure: testing for HIV resistance in clinical practice. *Science* **280**, 1871–3.

On-line resources

www.aidsmap.com [UK national guidelines (British HIV Association, regularly updated)]

www.hivatis.org [US HIV Treatment Guidelines Library (regularly updated), includes: 2001 USPHS/IDSA Guidelines for the prevention of opportunistic infections in persons infected with human immunodeficiency virus]

hivinsite.ucsf.edu/cochrane [Cochrane Collaborative Review Group on HIV Infection and AIDS]

www.unaids.org [Joint United Nations programme on HIV/AIDS]

7.10.22 HIV in the developing world

Charles F. Gilks

Introduction

The first definite evidence of human infection with HIV dates from a blood sample taken from an unidentified African man in Leopoldville (now Kinshasa) in the Congo in 1959. What happened before then is conjecture but it seems clear that HIV was originally an African primate virus, and that by the time it had spread to North America in the mid- to late 1970s the epidemic in sub-Saharan Africa was already well established. Public health surveillance is poor across Africa, and the disease went essentially unrecognized until AIDS had been identified as a new clinical entity in the United States. It is an uncomfortable truth that the main impetus to discover the cause of AIDS and produce reliable diagnostic tests, and the subsequent search for effective therapies and vaccines, has been the size and scale of the HIV epidemic in the West rather than the developing world.

Unfortunately, massive Western involvement with the disease has not always been directly beneficial. It has taken far too long to appreciate that HIV/AIDS is not the same disease in resource-poor countries as it is in rich North American or European cities; and that different clinical interventions and preventive approaches are necessary. Few textbooks deal with HIV/AIDS as anything but a disease of affluent communities which have access to high-technology medicine and expensive, state-of-the-art therapy. Many policy makers view the epidemic, and possible responses, in the impossible-to-replicate context of the costs to an industrialized health service—rather than what is necessary and can be achieved even with limited resources.

Aetiology

HIV has two variants, type 1 and type 2; each has different groups and subtypes or clades. HIV-1 group M is the cause of the pandemic: in industrialized countries subtype B predominates. In Africa two rare groups N and O have recently been identified; and whilst within group M the whole alphabet of subtypes A to J exist, subtype B is uncommon. In other parts of the developing world, because of founder effects, there is less HIV-1 heterogeneity. HIV-2 is largely restricted to West Africa although localized foci exist elsewhere. Dual infection can occur and prior infection with one type does not appear to generate useful protection against the other.

Most commercial diagnostic kits identify all types and variants of HIV. Typing and subtyping requires special resources and is not routinely carried out. HIV-2 appears to have important biological differences from HIV-1: it is less efficiently transmitted both sexually and vertically; disease progression is slower but it results in the same spectrum of related diseases. Less is known about the biological attributes of HIV-1 subtypes, although disease progression may be faster with some types (for instance subtype A compared with D in Uganda). Immune responses to infection may be both type subtype-specific, which has considerably complicated vaccine development. This chapter deals only with HIV-1 infection.

Epidemiology

Distribution

All parts of the world have reported HIV infection (Table 1). Current estimates (end 1999) suggest that 50 million people have been infected, of whom over 16 million have already died. Sub-Saharan Africa has borne the brunt of the epidemic: although constituting about 10 per cent of global population, 70 per cent of people living with HIV and 85 per cent of deaths

Table 1 Regional HIV/AIDS statistics and features, December 1999

Region	Epidemic started	Adults and children living with HIV/AIDS	Adults and children newly infected with HIV	Adult prevalence rate (%)*	% HIV-positive women	Main mode(s) of transmission for those living with HIV/AIDS**
Sub-Saharan Africa	Late 1970s–early 1980s	23.3 million	3.8 million	8.0	55	Hetero
North Africa and Middle East	Late 1980s	220 000	19 000	0.13	20	IDU, Hetero
South and South-East Asia	Late 1980s	6 million	1.3 million	0.69	30	Hetero
East Asia and Pacific	Late 1980s	530 000	120 000	0.068	15	IDU, Hetero, MSM
Latin America	Late 1970s–early 1980s	1.3 million	150 000	0.57	20	MSM, IDU, Hetero
Caribbean	Late 1970s–early 1980s	360 000	57 000	1.96	35	Hetero, MSM
Eastern Europe and Central Asia	Early 1990s	360 000	95 000	0.14	20	IDU, MSM
Western Europe	Late 1970s–early 1980s	520 000	30 000	0.25	20	MSM, IDU
North America	Late 1970s–early 1980s	920 000	44 000	0.56	20	MSM, IDU, Hetero
Australia and New Zealand	Late 1970s–early 1980s	12 000	500	0.1	10	MSM, IDU
Total		33.6 million	5.6 million	1.1	46	

* The proportion of adults (15 to 49 years of age) living with HIV/AIDS in 1998, using 1997 population numbers.

** Hetero, heterosexual transmission; IDU, transmission through injecting drug use; MSM, sexual transmission among men who have sex with men.

come from the region. Ominously, the virus is continuing to spread rapidly in highly populous regions of India and South-East Asia. India has recorded 4 million cases, the largest number. In parts of east and central Africa, prevalence is stabilizing, sometimes at rates in excess of 30 per cent, and the 'HIV endemic' is emerging. In Uganda and Thailand, recent declines in HIV prevalence have been ascribed to behavioural change and successful control programmes. However, there is no developing country where the epidemic is in steady state. The burden of HIV/AIDS disease will continue to grow and the full impact of the epidemic on development and civil society will not be felt for many years.

Transmission

In developing countries, HIV is spread predominantly through heterosexual intercourse. Women become infected an average of 5 to 10 years earlier than men and in Africa more women than men are now infected. Several socio-economic and biological cofactors enhance transmission. In many cities there are large pools of migrant labour, women have few marketable skills, and there is often a preponderance of single men—all of which encourages the sex trade. Poor people have limited resources to devote to safer sex. Early sexual debut and frequent partner changes are common in some communities. Sexually transmitted infections facilitate transmission; in resource-poor societies treatment may often be delayed, incorrect, or inadequate.

Mother-to-child transmission is a direct result of the adult heterosexual epidemic. Infants can be infected transplacentally, during the birth process, or through breast feeding. Without intervention, overall risks are about 30 per cent. In high-prevalence regions up to 10 per cent of young children may be HIV infected. Those who escape infection may become orphans. The problem of AIDS orphans, particularly in urban centres, is a growing crisis. No simple solutions are emerging.

Intravenous drug use is widespread in certain areas and can be the vehicle for explosive transmission—as has occurred in Thailand, Vietnam, north-east India, and the Russian Federation. Needles and syringes may be shared by many individuals and tragically the epidemic may only be recognized when HIV is already well-established. Transmission through infected blood is important where transfusion is used indiscriminately, where inadequate provision is made for screening and quality control, where contaminated equipment is reused, and where professional donors and commercial blood banks resist supervision and regulation. China in particular is facing up to the consequence of poorly supervised and regulated blood transfusion practices.

Surveillance and disease burden

Accurate surveillance is essential to monitor the evolution of the HIV epidemic. Surveillance is often inadequate because of budgetary constraints, limited public health capacity, and occasionally lack of political will. Few countries can measure HIV incidence rates reliably. Antenatal clinic attenders have been the main focus for recording prevalence. At-risk or core transmission groups such as attenders of sexually transmitted disease (STD) clinics, and prostitutes are also important groups to monitor. Many countries have only limited and incomplete national prevalence data. The absence of such basic information has hindered the effectiveness of AIDS control programmes across the developing world.

Surveillance for clinical disease has focused on AIDS, using a clinical case definition and monitoring HIV prevalence in patients with tuberculosis. Given the importance of non-AIDS disease and death and very poor AIDS case reporting across the developing world, the continued promotion of AIDS surveillance must be questioned. Assessing HIV prevalence in specific patient groups, such as those admitted to hospital with acute conditions, will generate more accurate and useful information for health planners.

In high-prevalence countries the burden of disease caused by HIV/AIDS is far broader than appreciated—consequences of fear and denial in the community and inadequate disease surveillance (Fig. 1). Failure to recognize the true impact of HIV has led to fragmented care responses, which serve inadequately the needs of communities affected by HIV. Stigmatization is maintained and potential benefits of enhancing prevention, by linking it with effective care packages, are not realized.

Prevention and control

Control strategies relate to mode of transmission. All require appropriate health information and education, to inform rather than scare and to promote behaviour change. Unfortunately, the background in many developing countries continues to be one of hostility, fear, and denial, in which those infected are discriminated against and stigmatized. Until there is a more rational and accepting attitude to HIV/AIDS, it is difficult to see how interventions can be fully effective. The United Nations Programme on HIV/AIDS (UNAIDS) addresses this by advocating the view that people with HIV/AIDS are not the problem but are part of the solution.

Strategies to reduce sexual transmission concentrate on the universal message of safer sex, condom usage, and improved treatment of sexually transmitted diseases. When properly used, condoms are effective barriers to all sexually transmitted pathogens—not just HIV. Condoms can be distributed free, or sold by local traders who buy at discounted wholesale prices, a process known as social marketing. This encourages the condom market and accepts than clients are more likely to use condoms that have been bought rather than given away. In some countries this has greatly expanded the use of condoms. In other countries, male reluctance is an impediment to widespread usage.

The rationale for improving STD treatment to control HIV is based on the increased risks that any STD, inflammatory or ulcerative, generates for person-to-person transmission of HIV. Initial enthusiasm for this was based on a single, randomized, controlled trial in East Africa (Mwanza, Tanzania) which documented a 42 per cent (95 per cent confidence interval 21–58) reduction in transmission. A larger study in Rakai, Uganda, showed no effect of mass community-wide STD treatment. One further randomized clinical trial is still underway in Uganda. It may be that differences relate to the stage of the epidemic. Improved STD treatment may have most impact where the virus is still epidemic rather than endemic, and where sexual contact with high-risk core transmitter groups is more important that transmission from spouse or regular partner.

In the West, mother-to-child transmission can be virtually eliminated with comprehensive antenatal counselling and HIV testing, antiretroviral therapy, elective caesarian section, and avoidance of breast feeding. In high-prevalence developing countries, where need is greatest, the financial resources and capacity to implement such interventions are woefully lack-

ing. The promise of simple, cheap therapy with nevirapine reduces the cost barrier and has created a wide-ranging international debate with calls for charitable donations or concerted bilateral aid. However, reducing mother-to-child transmission may not be considered a leading public health priority in developing countries, particularly without robust policies addressing the care of AIDS orphans.

With intravenous drug users, education programmes promoting risk reduction, particularly avoiding the sharing of needles or syringes, have been effective in cities such as Bangkok. Implementing needle exchange programmes is usually a political, not public health, issue. Spread through infected blood has been the easiest route to control. Widespread provision of facilities and equipment for screening and, more recently, the advent of rapid single-use HIV tests have minimized the number of infected units transfused. Quality control remains the biggest single issue in maintaining the integrity of the blood supply. Establishing clear and appropriate guidelines for transfusion has reduced dramatically the numbers of units given, especially to anaemic children with malaria.

Clinical features
Natural history
Most people in the developing world who are immunosuppressed through HIV are poor. They are usually forced to live in unhygienic environments

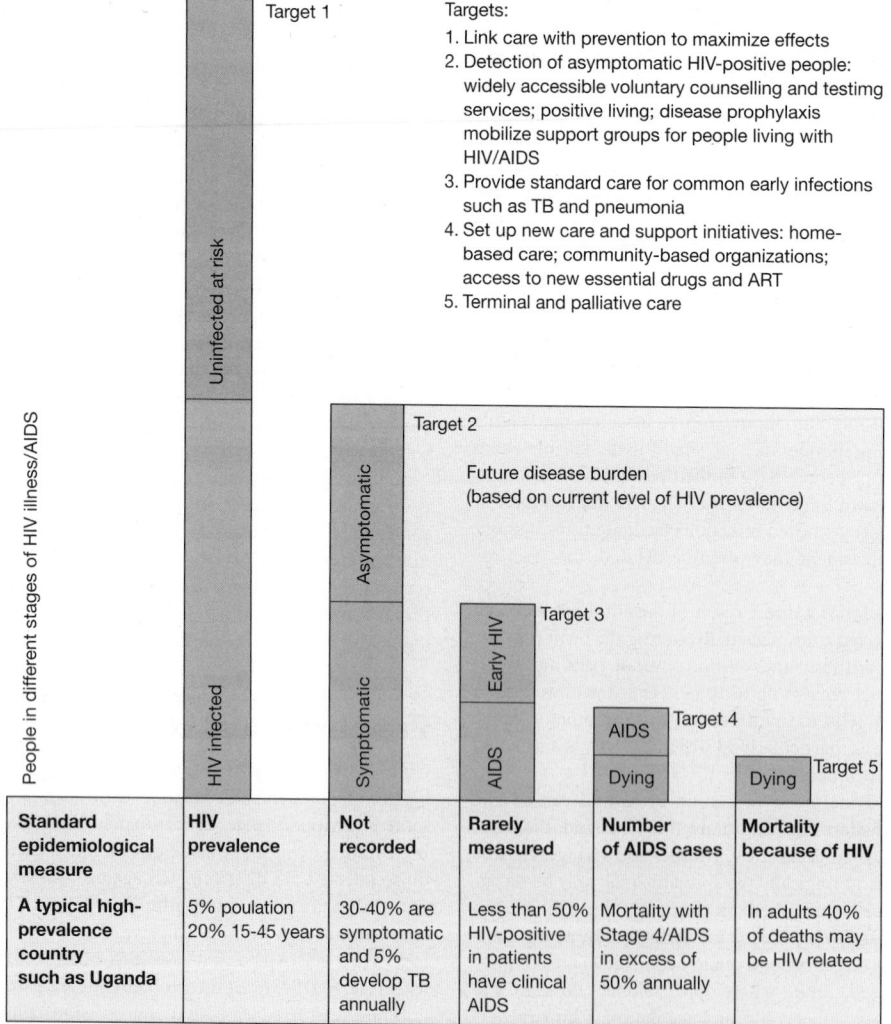

Fig. 1 The HIV/AIDS care burden in a community.

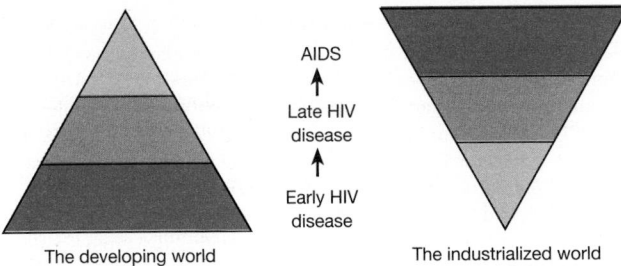

Fig. 2 The burden of disease caused by HIV infection in the developing world and the industralized world.

with inadequate sewerage and limited clean water, in overcrowded dwellings in close proximity to other sick and healthy people. There is substantial exposure to airborne and water-borne pathogens ensuring that rates of tuberculosis, pneumococcal disease, salmonellosis, and cryptosporidium are higher than in industrialized countries. With intense pathogen exposure, disease early on in the natural history of HIV is far more common (Fig. 2).

Poverty also limits the ability to maintain a healthy lifestyle and markedly reduces access to health care. Health-seeking behaviour is delayed and presentation with advanced disease is common. The quality of care available is often substandard. Health centres and hospitals may be rundown, poorly staffed, and lacking in even the most basic of drugs. Diagnostic capacity can be limited with few or no laboratory services provided. It seems obvious that survival will be severely compromised by such disadvantages.

Surprisingly, despite the scale of the HIV/AIDS epidemic in the tropics, there are few cohort studies in which the natural history of disease has been well characterized. In one seroincident cohort in rural Uganda, initial disease progression was similar to that in Western pretherapy cohorts, and suggested median survival of about 9 years. Several studies document poor survival, a year or less, following the onset of a major AIDS-defining illness. There are no data to suggest that reduced survival with HIV/AIDS in Africa relates overall to more rapid disease progression. Rather, early death from readily preventable or treatable infections shortens survival. Perhaps, once severe intercurrent disease has developed, viral replication may be enhanced causing more rapid disease progression. To date this has not been documented.

Clinical staging

A clinical staging classification has been developed by the World Health Organization for use in clinics without access to CD4 counts or viral load measurement. Patients with asymptomatic disease or minor clinical problems are classified as stage 1 and 2, respectively. The importance of high-grade virulent pathogens early on in the disease process is encompassed; pulmonary tuberculosis (now classified as an AIDS-defining disease in the United States) and severe bacterial infections are stage 3 problems. Opportunistic infections characteristic of AIDS are classified as stage 4 events. The staging system has recently been validated against CD4 counts in Uganda and is useful for predicting survival.

Specific clinical problems

Tuberculosis

HIV-related tuberculosis is of supreme importance. HIV renders the individual highly susceptible to primary infection or reinfection and is a potent reactivator of latent tuberculosis. About 75 per cent of patients have thoracic disease. Classic pulmonary tuberculosis with positive sputum smears is seen in the early stages of HIV, pleural effusions are common, and hilar or paratracheal glands are frequently enlarged. With more advanced immunosuppression, extensive pulmonary disease with negative sputum smears

develops. Extrapulmonary disease is common and dissemination with mycobacteraemia is increasingly recognized. Clinical features suggest both acute primary disease and reactivation are occurring.

Diagnosis can be difficult when only radiology and microscopy are available, particularly in smear-negative, disseminated, or extrapulmonary disease. Patients with early HIV disease usually respond well to standard therapy. National treatment guidelines should be followed and all cases notified to the tuberculosis control services. Thiacetazone is associated with high rates of hypersensitivity and should be avoided. In Africa, 25 to 30 per cent of patients may die during or soon after completing appropriate therapy, from community-acquired bacterial infections rather than poor therapeutic response. Treatment failure because of drug resistance is not yet a major problem in Africa but will be elsewhere. Tuberculosis frequently recurs through relapse and reinfection; rifampicin-based therapy may reduce relapse rates.

HIV-associated tuberculosis is preventable. The challenge is how to implement chemoprophylaxis without compromising existing tuberculosis control programmes or promoting drug resistance. One study in Abidjan showed that cotrimoxazole prophylaxis significantly improved survival of patients with tuberculosis/HIV, largely by reducing intercurrent bacterial infections. Studies are underway elsewhere to see how universally valid such an approach may be, given high rates of cotrimoxazole resistance across the developing world.

Pneumococcal infection

Streptococcus pneumoniae infection frequently develops with HIV. Lobar pneumonia accounts for about two-thirds of cases; acute sinusitis; occult bacteraemia, meningitis, pericarditis, skin sepsis, and pyomyositis also occur. Recurrent disease, primarily reinfection, is extremely common with rates of 25 to 30 per cent documented in East Africa.

Most patients with pneumonia are bacteraemic and Gram-positive diplococci are abundant in sputum. Patients respond well to standard penicillin therapy; ampicillin, chloramphenicol, and erythromycin are also effective. Lack of response suggests a second pathogen, often tuberculosis. Mortality rates are consistently higher in seropositive than seronegative patients. In Nairobi, penicillin resistance appears more frequent in pneumococci isolated from HIV-infected patients. Penicillin-resistant pneumococci are widespread; the worry is that HIV will facilitate further spread and evolution.

Polysaccharide pneumococcal vaccine is recommended (without efficacy data) in the United States and Europe. A randomized controlled trial in Uganda showed no efficacy but significantly higher rates of pneumonia in vaccine recipients. It should not be recommended in developing countries. The role of the new conjugate vaccines remains to be established. Studies in Abidjan showed reduced rates of pneumonia as well as other HIV-related problems with cotrimoxazole prophylaxis. Compliance remains a problem with long-term chemoprophylaxis.

Non-typhi salmonellas

Systemic salmonellosis is highly associated with HIV. *S. typhimurium* and *S. enteritidis* are most frequent; other non-typhi salmonellas are less important and HIV does not significantly predispose to *S. typhi* infection. Most patients present with bacteraemia and an enteric fever-like illness clinically indistinguishable from classical typhoid fever. Non-typhi salmonella coinfection also develops in patients with tuberculosis or pneumonia. Diagnosis requires blood culture. With inadequate microbiology facilities, few cases are identified and there is poor recognition of the general importance of non-typhi salmonellas or indeed other Gram-negative bacteraemic infections.

Patients with bacteraemia respond poorly if therapy is delayed, the diagnosis missed, or the organism is resistant. Antimicrobial resistance is common, especially to the widely used broad-spectrum antibiotics. Chloramphenicol, ampicillin and gentamycin, quinolones or third-generation cephalosporins are appropriate; use depends on cost and availability. Most centres treat for 2 to 3 weeks although optimal duration is not established. Relapse and reinfection both occur. Relapse usually develops within 6 to 8 weeks of stopping therapy and close follow-up is indicated. Quinolone maintenance therapy is effective but too costly for most patients. There are many environmental sources and no obvious ways to prevent exposure. Cotrimoxazole prophylaxis may prevent bacteraemia caused by non-typhi salmonellas.

Disseminated fungal infections

Cryptococcus neoformans is the most common disseminated fungal infection associated with HIV. There can be wide regional variations in incidence. In Abidjan evidence of infection was seen in only 2.5 per cent of autopsies. One cohort in Uganda diagnosed cryptococcosis at or around death in 25 per cent of patients. Most patients have subacute or chronic meningitis; some present with fever, non-specific pulmonary symptoms, and fungaemia; and cutaneous nodules occasionally develop. Diagnosis can be made by culture, antigen detection, or cerebrospinal fluid microscopy using Indian ink. Both fluconazole and amphotericin B are effective but lifelong maintenance therapy is required. Antifungal drugs are expensive and not usually considered essential drugs in low-income countries. Most poor families cannot afford therapy. Significant price reductions have recently been announced. Whether fluconazole prophylaxis is effective and implementable remains to be established.

Penicillium marneffei is an important HIV-related systemic mycosis in parts of South-East Asia. *Histoplasma duboisii* has been reported in HIV-positive patients in Central Africa and *H. capsulatum* in Central America and the Caribbean. Coccidioidomycosis and paracoccidioidomycosis have been associated with HIV infection in South America. Several other fungal diseases ecologically or geographically restricted to parts of the tropics may yet emerge as HIV-associated pathogens.

Chronic diarrhoea

Chronic diarrhoea with wasting, called 'slim' across Africa, is the most recognizable and obvious manifestation of AIDS in developing countries. Around 20 per cent of patients in a Ugandan cohort had slim at death. Rates elsewhere are not established.

Many potential pathogens have been associated. Cryptosporidium is probably the most important; prevalence of cyst excretion in African case series ranges from 5 to 48 per cent. In some areas *Isospora belli* is common; with improved diagnosis microsporidia are increasingly recognized. Other protozoan and helminth parasites are not important. Enteric bacteria can be isolated in perhaps 15 per cent of cases but their pathogenic role is uncertain; enteric viruses are not thought important. Disseminated tuberculosis is probably an agonal endstage infection. As in the West, only about 50 per cent of patients with slim fully investigated will have a putative pathogen identified.

There is no effective therapy for cryptosporidium. Isosporiasis clears with cotrimoxazole but maintenance therapy is necessary. Some microsporidia may respond to albendazole. Imodium or codeine phosphate can initially relieve symptoms; whether benefits are maintained with long-term treatment is not known. Enteric pathogens are ubiquitous and it is difficult to avoid exposure. Hygiene is important but, in practice, is not always easy to implement or affordable. Cryptosporidium cysts can withstand chlorination and it is necessary to bring water to the boil.

The endemic tropical parasitic diseases

For years it has been unclear whether HIV interacts significantly with malaria. As with other intercurrent infections, HIV viral load rises with acute malaria. There is now mounting evidence from pregnant women and adults that HIV-related immunosuppression reduces protective antimalaria responses. The prevalence of placental parasitaemia is twice as high in HIV-positive compared to HIV-negative multigravidas, and this significantly increases the risks of mother-to-child HIV transmission. In endemic malaria areas, adults with HIV infection experience increased rates of clinical malaria with higher parasite densities. Whether severe complicated disease is more common and response to therapy is compromised as malaria-specific immune responses are lost remains to be established. In adults who have no background immunity to malaria, it also appears that HIV is a significant risk factor for severe and complicated disease and death with epidemic *P.falciparum* infection. There are very few data on malaria in HIV-infected children or on the interactions of HIV with *P.vivax*.

Leishmaniasis is well described in patients with AIDS from southern Europe following acute exposure or reactivation of latent infection. There are few case reports from endemic tropical areas. HIV prevalence is low in many remote rural foci, the disease is difficult to diagnose, and patients may die before being immunosuppressed enough to develop disseminated leishmaniasis. Any significant interaction would be of great importance in the kala-azar belt of India.

Unusual manifestations of Chagas' disease have been linked with HIV. There is no clear association with African trypanosomiasis and neither pathogenic amoebas nor giardia are exacerbated by HIV infection. A few cases of *Strongyloides stercoralis* hyperinfection have been described; despite being AIDS defining, it is very uncommon. To date, there are no data suggesting important interactions between HIV and schistosomiasis (except perhaps to reduce egg excretion), other flukes, hookworm, ascaris, filariasis, or any of the cestode/tapeworm infections.

Malignancies

Kaposi's sarcoma and HHV8 are endemic in sub-Saharan Africa. However, Kaposi's sarcoma develops in less than 5 per cent of African patients with AIDS, perhaps related to different patterns of HHV8 exposure. HIV has markedly altered Kaposi's sarcoma epidemiology. Women are more likely to be affected although there is still a male preponderance. Lesions are more extensive, frequently involve the mucosa, and often the viscera. Disease is more aggressive and can progress rapidly. Cytotoxic therapy is expensive and not widely available in developing countries. A relatively cheap regimen using actinomycin D and vincristine has proved effective in Zambia. There are few data on Kaposi's sarcoma and HIV from other regions.

Conjunctival squamous cell carcinoma has been recorderd in East Africa. Lymphomas are uncommon and occur much less frequently than in industrialized countries. No impact on cervical carcinoma has been reported from the tropics.

Opportunistic infections

Many African studies have looked carefully for the classic Western AIDS-defining opportunistic infections. *Pneumocystis carinii* is diagnosed by bronchoscopy or at autopsy in perhaps 2 per cent of patients with chronic lung disease. *Mycobacterium avium* has been isolated from the environment but mycobacteraemic disease is rare; disseminated tuberculosis is far more common. Toxoplasmosis or active cytomegalovirus infections are rarely diagnosed or clinically manifest, although they may be seen at autopsy. The most likely explanation for their rarity is that few poor patients survive long enough to develop profound immunosuppression. In developing countries only the urban elites have such a 'Western' pattern of HIV/AIDS disease.

Future challenges

The critical issue remains to reduce the number of new infections, currently over 16 000 per day. More effective linkage of prevention with care and more attention to adolescent groups are priority areas for action. AIDS orphans are a growing and highly emotive problem. In high-prevalence countries strategies for coping with the profound change in the burden of disease are needed urgently. A growing threat is the increasing toll that HIV/AIDS is having on trained health-care personnel, who themselves are having to cope with the rising tide of HIV/AIDS disease. Continued advances in antiretroviral therapy highlight the inequity in access to care and poor survival in most developing countries. It is difficult to see how any of these challenges can be addressed without substantial increases in health care budgets and commitments from Western industrialized countries to reduce the global inequity in HIV/AIDS care. The new Global Fund may have a huge impact, if health systems are improved along with financing drug purchase..

Further reading

Gilks CF *et al.*, eds (1998). *Care and support for people with HIV/AIDS in resource-poor settings*. Health and Population Occasional Paper. Department for International Development, London.

Harries AD, Maher D (1996). *TB/HIV, a clinical manual*. WHO/TB/96.200. World Health Organization, Geneva.

Kaldor JM, ed. (1998). *AIDS in Asia and the Pacific*, 2nd edn. Rapid Science Publishers, London.

Laga M, ed. (1997). *AIDS in Africa*, 2nd edn. Rapid Science Publishers, London.

World Bank Policy Research Report (1997). *Confronting AIDS: public priorities in a global epidemic*. Oxford University Press, New York.

UNAIDS (Joint United Nations Programme on HIV/AIDS) and WHO (World Health Organization) (1999). *Global summary of the HIV/AIDS epidemic*. UNAIDS/99.53E—WHO/CDS/CSR/EDC/99.9. World Health Organization, Geneva.

7.10.23 HTLV-I and II and associated diseases

C. R. M. Bangham, M. Osame, and S. Nightingale

HTLV-I

Originally isolated from a patient with a cutaneous lymphoma, the human T-cell lymphotropic virus type I (**HTLV-I**) was the first pathogenic retrovirus to be discovered in humans. In contrast to the human immunodeficiency virus (**HIV**), HTLV-I causes disease in only about 5 per cent of infected people. However, the virus is of special interest and importance because it is associated with two different types of disease: adult T-cell leukaemia/lymphoma (**ATL**) and a range of chronic inflammatory conditions, of which the most commonly diagnosed is HTLV-I-associated myelopathy, also known as tropical spastic paraparesis (**HAM/TSP**). A suggested association with multiple sclerosis has been refuted.

HTLV-I is estimated to infect between 10 and 20 million people worldwide. There are large endemic areas in Central and West Africa, southern Japan, the Caribbean and South America, and smaller foci in the aboriginal populations of Australia, Papua New Guinea, and northern Japan. In Europe and North America the virus is found chiefly in immigrants from these endemic areas and in some communities of intravenous drug users. Within the endemic areas, the distribution of HTLV-I is characteristically uneven; the seroprevalence can vary between 1 and 20 per cent of adults in neighbouring towns.

There are three important modes of transmission: parental and neonatal infection from a seropositive mother, in which breast feeding is a significant factor; sexual transmission, particularly from males to females; and transmission by infected blood, either by transfusion or by sharing of needles among drug users. Transmission of the virus depends on transfer of cells from infected people, because there is little free virus in the serum. Blood for transfusion is now routinely screened for HTLV-I in several countries, including Japan, the United States, and Brazil.

HTLV-I is known as a complex retrovirus: in addition to the three genes present in other typical replication-competent exogenous retroviruses (*gag*, *pol*, and *env*) it encodes at least two further proteins—Tax, which stimulates transcription of the proviral genome, and Rex, which controls the splicing of HTLV-I mRNA. There are closely related leukaemia viruses in monkeys and cattle.

Although it can infect a wide variety of cell types *in vitro*, HTLV-I appears to replicate efficiently only in CD4+ (helper) T cells; these are the cells that are transformed in adult T-cell leukaemia/lymphoma. The cellular receptor for HTLV-I has not been identified, although the gene is known to lie on chromosome 17. Certain cell-surface adhesion molecules (ICAM-1, ICAM-3, and VCAM) also facilitate entry of HTLV-I into the cell.

Antibodies against the Gag protein are the first to appear after infection, and they predominate in the first 2 months. Thereafter, anti-envelope antibodies predominate, and about half of infected individuals subsequently produce antibodies to the Tax protein. Diagnosis of HTLV-I infection depends on the detection of specific antibodies by particle agglutination or enzyme-linked immunosorbent assay (ELISA), and confirmation by polymerase chain reaction (PCR) or western blot assay.

Most people infected with HTLV-I mount a vigorous, chronically activated, cytotoxic T-lymphocyte response to the virus, mostly directed against the viral Tax protein. This cellular response appears to play an important part in reducing the viral burden and the risk of the associated inflammatory diseases such as HAM/TSP.

HTLV-I associated myelopathy (HAM/TSP) and other inflammatory diseases associated with HTLV-I

The association between HTLV-I and HAM/TSP, formerly known as Jamaican neuropathy, was discovered in the Caribbean and in Japan in the mid-1980s. HTLV-I has since shown to be associated with uveitis, and a lymphocytic alveolitis (usually subclinical). There are also less certain associations with chronic infective dermatitis, polymyositis, arthritis, sicca syndrome, and a motor neurone disease-like disorder.

The prevalence of HAM/TSP is between 0.1 and 2 per cent of individuals infected with HTLV-I: about two-thirds of patients are female. Other known risk factors for HAM/TSP include a high proviral load of HTLV-I (Fig. 1) and the *HLA DRB1*0101* gene ('*HLA DR1*'). Possession of the *HLA A*02* gene is associated with a reduced proviral load and a reduced risk of HAM/TSP in Japan.

Clinical features

HAM/TSP is characterized by a spastic paraparesis that is slowly progressive, or in some cases static after initial progression, and anti-HTLV-I antibody positivity in serum and cerebrospinal fluid. Almost all patients show spasticity and/or hyperreflexia of the lower extremities, initially presenting as gait and urinary disturbances. Presentation is commonly with low back pain, weakness of the lower extremities and a poorly defined (mild) sensory affectation, and rarely, with cerebellar ataxia.

Patients with a younger age of onset (less than 15 years) tend to have short stature and slow progression of the disease, while patients with an older age of onset (more than 61 years) show faster progression regardless of the mode of transmission.

Aside from HTLV-I antibody positivity, other essential laboratory findings in the cerebrospinal fluid include lymphocytic pleocytosis and increased neopterin levels. In more than two-thirds of patients, magnetic resonance imaging shows high signals of T_2-weighted spin echo in the white matter of the brain indicating atrophy of the spinal cord.

Autopsy reveals severe involvement of the thoracic spinal cord with mononuclear infiltration, marked myelin and axonal destruction, and astrocytic gliosis.

Several clinical trials have shown transient beneficial effects from corticosteroids, α-interferon, azathioprine, high-dose vitamin C, pentoxifyllene, danazol, and plasmapheresis. The nucleoside analogues zidovudine and lamivudine can reduce the provirus load of HTLV-I, but the clinical benefit is unknown.

Adult T-cell leukaemia/lymphoma (ATL)

HTLV-I infection carries a 5 per cent lifetime risk of ATL; the interval between infection and disease is frequently over 20 years. The disease is slightly commoner in males (1.2:1), and there is evidence of familial clustering of cases. In highly endemic areas it is an important cause of malig-

nant disease: in Kyushu, Japan, ATL accounts for 75 per cent of non-Hodgkin's lymphomas.

The mean age at onset of ATL is about 60 years in Japan, and 40 years in the Caribbean and Brazil; the reason for this difference is not known.

The clinical features of ATL are those of a non-Hodgkin's lymphoma: malaise, fever, lymphadenopathy, hepatosplenomegaly, jaundice, drowsiness, weight loss, and opportunistic infections. Features particularly associated with ATL are skin involvement (nodules, plaques, or a generalized papular rash) and thirst. Laboratory findings include hypercalcaemia and high serum concentrations of lactate dehydrogenase and the soluble interleukin 2 (**IL-2**) receptor. The leukaemic cells are almost invariably CD4+, and are usually CD25+ (IL-2 receptor+). The transformed T cell has a characteristic appearance: the nucleus has several lobules, giving rise to the epithet 'flower cell'. Morphologically similar cells are found in small numbers in the peripheral blood in some asymptomatic carriers of the virus. When the proportion of abnormal cells is high, and there is a lymphocytosis, there is a greatly increased risk of development of ATL. However, in some cases the atypical cells regress spontaneously.

Southern blot analysis indicates the presence of oligoclonal or monoclonal proliferation of CD4+ cells carrying the HTLV-I provirus in their cellular DNA. Typically there is a progression from polyclonal to oligoclonal to monoclonal proliferation in the CD4+ population, accompanied by a progression to increasing IL-2-independence of cellular growth.

ATL is classified into clinical subtypes with different courses and prognoses. Intermediate states between lymphocytosis and frank ATL are called 'smouldering' or 'pre-' ATL. Initially response to standard chemotherapeutic regimes is commonly followed by early relapse with refractoriness to further chemotherapy after 2 to 6 months. Combination of interferon-α and zidovudine can prolong life expectancy by between 6 months and 2 years. The mean survival times (untreated) for acute, lymphomatous, and chronic ('smouldering') ATL in Japan are 6.2, 10.2, and 24.3 months, respectively.

HTLV-II

HTLV-II, a retrovirus closely related to HTLV-I, was first isolated from the tissue of a patient with an atypical form of hairy cell leukaemia. The virus occurs sporadically in West Africa. Among intravenous drug abusers in Europe and North America, infection with HTLV-II is as common as HTLV-I. HTLV-II is common in several native groups throughout the Americas.

HTLV-II is not associated with the typical B-cell form of hairy cell leukaemia, or with other haematological malignancies. A paralytic syndrome similar to HAM/TSP has been reported in individuals seropositive for HTLV-II. Paralysis may be flaccid rather than spastic. However, HTLV-II aetiology is not certain.

Further reading

Bangham CRM *et al.* (1999). Genetic control and dynamics of the cellular immune response to the human T-cell leukaemia virus HTLV-I. *Philosophical Transactions of the Royal Society of London Series B* **354**, 691–700.

Bangham CRM (2000). HTLV-I infections. *Journal of Clinical Pathology* **53**, 581–6.

Fields BN *et al.* (1996). *Fields virology*, 3rd edn. Lippincott-Raven, Philadelphia.

Nakagawa M *et al.* (1995). HTLV-I-associated myelopathy: analysis of 213 patients based on clinical features and laboratory findings. *Journal of Neurovirology* **1**, 50–61.

Uchiyama T (1997). Human T cell leukaemia virus type 1 (HTLV-I) and HTLV-I-associated diseases. *Annual Review of Immunology* **15**, 15–37.

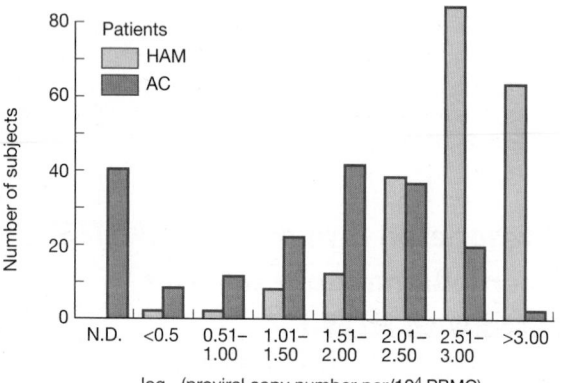

Fig. 1 Upper panel: distribution of HTLV-I provirus load in 202 patients with HAM/TSP (HAM) and 200 asymptomatic HTLV-I carriers (AC) in Japan. The median proviral load in HAM/TSP patients was 16 times greater than asymptomatic carriers. N.D., not detected. Lower panel: the risk of HAM/TSP in people infected with HTLV-I rises rapidly when the proviral load exceeds one copy per 100 peripheral blood mononuclear cells (PBMC). (Adapted from Figs 2 and 3 in Bangham *et al.* (1999).)

7.10.24 Viruses and cancer

R. A. Weiss

Introduction

Viruses are important in cancer for three main reasons: first, as a cause for about 15 per cent of the worldwide cancer burden; second, for the discovery and characterization of oncogenes and tumour suppressor genes; and third, as vectors for the delivery of gene therapy and immunotherapy.

Viruses as aetiological agents of cancer

Table 1 lists the viruses implicated in human cancer. In most but not all cases the viral genome is present in the malignant cells; the exceptions appear to be those that promote cancer indirectly, such as human immuno-deficiency virus (**HIV**) and hepatitis C virus (**HCV**).

Oncogenic viruses establish persistent, lifelong infections, so that the event of infection may be far removed from the event of malignancy. Moreover, cancer is often a rare outcome of virus infection, and other cofactors play a part in viral carcinogenesis. For example, Epstein–Barr virus (**EBV**) is a ubiquitous infection yet children's Burkitt's lymphoma occurs only in areas of holoendemic malarial infection, whereas undifferentiated naso-pharyngeal carcinoma occurs mainly in southern Chinese populations. Aflatoxin may act with hepatitis B virus (**HBV**) to cause liver cancer, and in hereditary epidermodysplasia verruciformis the ultraviolet radiation acts with human papillomavirus (**HPV**) strains to cause skin cancer.

Kaposi's sarcoma is a tumour that occurs much more frequently in immunodeficient patients. Its relative risk in recipients of organ transplants is about 400, and in persons with AIDS about 20 000. HIV probably contributes to Kaposi's sarcoma indirectly through immune suppression, although the Tat protein of HIV may also play a role. The primary cause of all forms of Kaposi's sarcoma is the recently discovered human herpes virus 8 (**HHV-8** or KSHV). This virus is also causally linked to primary effusion lymphoma and plasmablastic multicentric Castleman's disease.

Oncogenic viruses belong to many virus families, which have different routes of transmission. Some, like hepatitis B virus, are frequently acquired perinatally or through subsequent exposure to blood. With human T-cell lymphotropic virus type I (**HTLV-I**) the main route of transmission is vertical through infected cells in breast milk. Sexual transmission is common to HIV, HTLV-I (with a male to female bias), HBV, and HPV. Oncogenic viruses do not appear to be transmitted by the respiratory route, except adenoviruses, or via arthropod vectors, except some veterinary cases, such as bovine leucosis virus. Whereas EBV (transmitted through saliva) occurs worldwide, HBV, HTLV-I, and HHV-8 have a high prevalence mainly in those population groups in which the associated cancers occur.

Certain common human viruses are highly oncogenic in experimental animals but are not linked to human cancer, namely the polyomaviruses BK and JC, and the adenoviruses. Human adenovirus types 2 and 12 readily cause sarcomas and carcinomas in hamsters and other rodents. The viral genomes persist non-productively in the animal tumours and express early genes. It is surprising, then, that there is no epidemiological evidence linking adenovirus or BK infection with human cancer. There is some concern that a simian relative of BK virus, SV40, may be linked with mesothelioma, osteosarcoma, and ependymoma in humans, but these findings remain controversial.

Mechanisms of viral carcinogenesis

Physical and chemical carcinogens are usually mutagens. They cause DNA mutations in specific genes that contribute to the eventual malignant phenotype of the cancer. Oncogenes were first discovered in animal retro-viruses, such as the Rous sarcoma virus of chickens, and are now known to originate from cellular genes. Most retroviruses do not carry oncogenes but the DNA provirus integrates into chromosomal DNA and can activate adjacent cellular oncogenes. Oncogene activation by retroviruses is comparable with activation by chromosomal translocation.

The mechanism of cell transformation by HTLV-I is different from that of the majority of animal retroviruses. HTLV-I encodes a viral protein, Tax, which is essential to promote full viral gene transcription. Tax acts as a transcriptional activator by associating with host nuclear proteins which activate expression of the viral genome. However, Tax also up-regulates certain cellular genes such as the interleukin-2 receptor. HTLV-I 'immortalizes' CD4+ T lymphocytes in culture, rather as EBV immortalizes B lymphocytes, but this is only one step in the pathway to malignancy. HTLV-I leukaemia does not become manifest until 40 or more years after infection, and in only 5 per cent of infected people.

Cell transformation by DNA viruses is best understood for polyoma-viruses and adenoviruses. The transforming genes of these viruses are expressed early in the infection cycle and prevent tumour suppressor protein function. Adenovirus proteins E1A and E1B and BK T-antigen bind to p53 and Rb and block their normal interaction in the cell cycle. Thus instead of mutating these cellular tumour suppressor genes, the DNA tumour viruses block the normal function of their proteins, which similarly results in unregulated cell proliferation. The HHV-8 genome carries several oncogenes including a homologue of cyclin D2, which inactivates Rb by a different mechanism, phosphorylation.

To cause tumours, most oncogenic viruses persist in the tumour cells, often by integrating into chromosomal DNA. Oncogenic herpesviruses do not integrate but are maintained episomally. EBNA-1 is required for episomal replication of EBV (and LANA for HHV-8), while other nuclear and latent membrane proteins are responsible for the transformed cell phenotype. With HBV, integrated copies are found in many liver carcinoma lines, but a requirement for integration has not been unequivocally shown. HBV expresses transactivating functions from the *X* gene so its transformation may resemble that of HTLV-I. Some viruses might exert an oncogenic effect without persisting in the cells destined to become the malignant clone, by causing mutations in host DNA, thus acting in a 'hit-and-run' manner like other mutagens.

Indirect carcinogenic effects are those in which damage to tissues by viruses may allow clones of premalignant cells to proliferate that would not

Table 1 Viruses implicated in human cancer

Virus	Malignancy	Non-malignant disease
DNA viruses		
HPVs	Cervical cancer	Warts
	Skin cancer	
HBV	Primary liver cancer	Hepatitis
EBV	Nasopharyngeal carcinoma	
	Burkitt's lymphoma	
	Immunoblastic lymphoma	
	Hodgkin's disease	Infectious mononucleosis
	Leiomyosarcoma	
HHV-8	Kaposi's sarcoma	
	Primary effusion lymphoma	
	Multicentric Castleman's disease	
RNA viruses		
HTLV-I	Adult T-cell leukaemia	Tropical spastic paraparesis
HIV-1	Non-Hodgkin's lymphoma	AIDS
	Kaposi's sarcoma	
HCV	Primary liver cancer	Hepatitis

Abbreviations of virus names are explained in the text.

otherwise do so. HCV and possibly HBV might do this by destroying normal liver cells, resulting in a much greater rate of liver cell regeneration. HIV could be regarded as a special case of indirect viral carcinogenesis, promoting tumour development by destroying helper T-cell immunity to other viruses. The cancers elevated in AIDS are also seen in immunosuppressed transplant recipients, for example non-Hodgkin's lymphoma and Kaposi's sarcoma, and themselves have a viral aetiology.

Treatment and prevention

Oncogenesis is multifactorial, requiring several sequential events before a patient presents with a fully malignant tumour. Yet if a virus plays a crucial role in oncogenesis, its elimination should prevent that type of cancer. Currently, there is no special approach to the treatment of cancers that have a viral aetiology. Among the lymphoid malignancies, some respond well to radiotherapy or chemotherapy, such as Hodgkin's disease, whereas others seldom show remission, such as adult T-cell leukaemia. Cancers that express viral antigens should be responsive to immunotherapy. If immunosuppression promotes their presentation, they should be susceptible to immune attack. For tumours in which viral proteins are required for the maintenance of the malignant state, those proteins are potential molecular targets, as drugs that block them might spare normal cellular functions.

Prevention is preferable to cure and offers the greatest promise of reducing cancer mortality due to viruses. Prevention can be accomplished by three strategies: (i) early screening for tumours, (ii) screening for the virus with prevention of transmission, and (iii) immunization. Early screening is exemplified by cervical smears and, in China, for elevated serum IgA levels to EBV antigens for incipient nasopharyngeal carcinoma. Screening to prevent iatrogenic transmission via blood and blood products is routinely employed in many countries for potentially oncogenic viruses such as HBV, HCV, HIV, and HTLV-I. In Kyushu, Japan, where infection was endemic, HTLV-I is being steadily eradicated through a policy of antenatal screening to prevent milk transmission.

Prevention of cancer by immunization against oncogenic viruses is likely to have a major impact on world cancer mortality in the twenty-first century. Currently, the only proven, mass-produced vaccine against a human oncogenic virus is the HBV vaccine based on surface antigen. Indeed, it is the first efficacious recombinant subunit vaccine against any virus. Other vaccines under development that are likely to be successful within the next decade are for EBV, HPV, and HTLV-I. Intensive research is also being undertaken on vaccines for HIV and HCV. There are likely to be some obstacles on the route to successful immunization, as HIV is extraordinarily variable, and even the relatively stable HBV shows evidence of immune-escape mutants in the face of vaccination programmes. Nevertheless, immunization against oncogenic viruses is likely to become a most effective cancer prevention strategy.

Viruses as therapeutic agents

Viruses may be put to use in the fight against cancer. First, some cytopathic viruses preferentially replicate in proliferating cells and destroy them, such as parvoviruses and mutant adenoviruses. Second, viruses as foreign antigens may aid the recognition of cancer cells by the host's immune system. Although the mechanism is ill understood, 'xenogenization' of tumour cells by virus infection can, in some cases, enhance immune control of noninfected cells of the same tumour. Third, viruses are favoured vectors for immunization and for gene therapy, by restoring tumour suppressor functions, by enhancing immune responses through the expression of antigens or cytokines, and by locally delivering genes for enzymes that convert inert prodrugs into active, chemotherapeutic agents.

Further reading

Arrand JR, Harper DR, eds (1998). *Viruses and human cancer.* BIOS, Oxford.

Boshoff CH, Weiss RA, eds (1999). Human herpes virus 8. *Seminars in Cancer Biology* 9.

Dalgleish AG, Weiss RA, eds (1999). *HIV and the new viruses.* Academic Press, London.

Goedert JJ, ed. (2000). *Infectious causes of cancer. Targets for intervention.* Humana Press, Paterson, New Jersey.

Newton R, Beral V, Weiss RA, eds (1999). Infections and human cancer. *Cancer Surveys* 33.

7.10.25 Orf

N. Jones

Aetiology

Orf virus, a member of the *Parapox* genus, normally causes ecthyma contagiosum or 'scabby mouth' (contagious pustular dermatitis) in sheep and goats. Orf virions are ovoid (approximate size, 260 × 160 nm), with tubular threadlike structures criss-crossing the surface of the virions, visible by negatively stained electron microscopy. The orf virus genome is double stranded DNA of 135 kbp. The viral genome encodes a polypeptide homologous to IL-10, inhibitors of interferon, IL-2 and GM-CSF, and a vascular endothelial growth factor. These contribute to the dermal lesions characterized by capillary proliferation and dilatation.

Other Parapox viruses infect cattle, deer, and seals.

Epidemiology

The disease affects mainly young lambs, who contract the infection from one to another, or possibly from persistence of the virus in the pastures (the virus can remain viable for long periods in dried scabs from lesions). Human disease is usually occupational, following contact with infected sheep. It is not uncommon in shepherds, veterinary surgeons, and farmers (Fig. 1). One attack normally confers immunity and human to human spread has not been recorded.

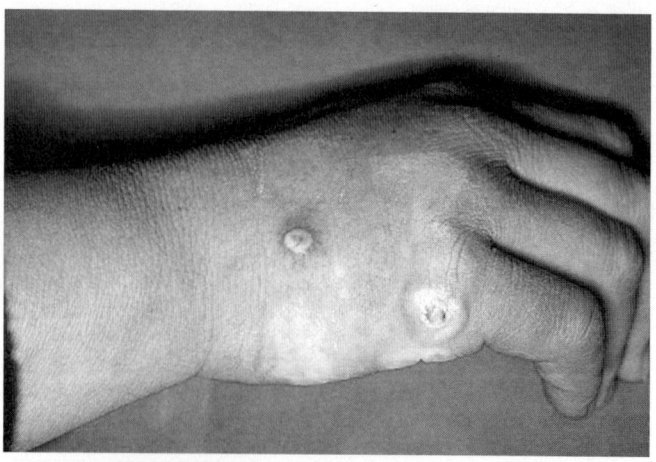

Fig. 1 Orf, typical lesions on a farmer's hand.

Fig. 2 Contagious pustular dermatitis ('orf') in a lamb.

Clinical features

In sheep, papules and vesicles appear on the lips (Fig. 2) and gradually heal with no scarring over 4 weeks. In humans, after an incubation period of 5 to 6 days, a small, red, firm papule enlarges to form a flat-topped haemorrhagic pustule or bulla; the centre may be crusted. The lesion is usually 2 to 3 cm in diameter, but may be as large as 5 cm. Lesions are solitary or few in number and commonly occur on the hands and forearms, occasionally the face. Lymphangitis or regional lymphadenopathy are not uncommon. Slight fever and malaise can occur. Recovery is usually complete in 6 weeks and is spontaneous.

Large fungating granuloma or tumour-like lesions have been reported, especially in association with haematological malignancy.

Erythema multiforme occasionally develops, typically 10 to14 days after the onset of orf (Fig. 3). Rarely, bullous pemphigoid has been reported in association with orf.

Diagnosis

The characteristic lesion in a person exposed to sheep and lambs allows a clinical diagnosis. This can be confirmed in the laboratory by electron microscopy of a biopsy of the orf lesion or by PCR. The virus can also be isolated in cell culture, but this is rarely performed. Histopathological examination of biopsy specimens shows a proliferation of keratinocytes with cellular swelling and balloon degeneration and B type cytoplasmic inclusion bodies.

Fig. 3 Erythema multiforme complicating orf of the left middle finger in a veterinary student.

Treatment

Secondary infection should be treated if it occurs. Large lesions can be removed surgically, but recurrence can occur in the immunocompromised. Cidofovir cream has been used successfuly to treat giant or persistent lesions in immunosuppressed patients.

Further reading

Gill, M.J., Arlette, J., Buchan, K.A., *et al.* (1990). Human orf. *Archives of Dermatology,* **126**, 356–8.

Groves, R.W., Wilson-Jones, E., and MacDonald, D.M. (1991). Human orf and milkers nodule: a clinicopathological study. *Journal of the American Academy of Dermatology,* **25**, 706–11.

Imlach W, *et al.* (2002). Orf virus-encoded interleukin-10 stimulates the proliferation of murine mast cells and inhibits cytokine synthesis in murine peritoneal macrophages. *Journal of General Virology* **83**, 1049–58.

Torfason EG, Gunadottir S (2002). Polymerase chain reaction for laboratory diagnosis of orf virus infections. *Journal of Clinical Virology* **24**, 29–84.

7.10.26 Molluscum contagiosum

N. Jones

Molluscum contagiosum is a benign skin tumour, caused by a poxvirus, which mostly affects children and young adults. It is exclusively a human disease.

Aetiology

Molluscum contagiosum virus (MCV), a large double-stranded DNA virus, is a member of the Poxviridae, genus *Molluscipox.* MCV has not been transmitted to laboratory animals and there is no *in vitro* cultivation system currently available. Restriction endonuclease analysis of the genome has identified three types, MCV I, MCV II, and MCV III. The majority of infections seem to be due to MCV 1. The virus encodes MC 159L protein which causes abnormal proliferation of epithelium by inhibiting TNF and apoptosis-inducing factors.

Epidemiology

Molluscum contagiosum is common and disease usually follows contact with an infected individual or contaminated object. In tropical countries, the infection tends to occur in younger children (1–4 years) than in temperate climates (10–12 years). Sexual transmission accounts for a second incidence peak in young adults. Unusually widespread lesions have been reported in HIV disease, sarcoidosis, and those taking immunosuppressive therapy.

Clinical features

The incubation varies from 14 days to 6 months. The individual lesion is a shining, pearly, hemispherical, firm, umbilicated papule with a central depression. Lesions can occur singly (Fig. 1) but are commonly multiple (Fig. 2). The lesions gradually grow to a diameter of 5 to 10 mm over 6 to 12 weeks. Occasionally one very large lesion can develop (> 10 mm), or a

Fig. 1 Single lesion on eyelid.

plaque of very small lesions (agimate form). Most cases persist for 6 to 9 months, occasionally as long as 5 years, following which spontaneous resolution occurs.

Lesions are commonly seen on the neck, trunk, or axilla, although any part of the skin can be affected. Lesions are rare on the palms, soles, and mucous membranes. Sexually acquired infections normally result in anogenital lesions. In about 10 per cent of cases, especially where there is a history of atopy, a patchy dermatitis develops around the lesions. In the HIV patient molluscum can be widespread, but particularly involves the face,

Fig. 2 Molluscum contagiosum: groups of papules characterized by a central punctum.

neck, and around and inside the mouth in male homosexuals. Lesions may become large and atypical, and are mistaken for basal cell carcinomas or other skin tumours. The disease is often unremitting with increasing severity, especially when HIV is advanced.

Diagnosis

The diagnosis is usually clinical, but histological and electron microscopic examination of a curetted lesion establishes the diagnosis. The differential diagnosis can include lepromatous leprosy and, in HIV-seropositive patients, disseminated cutaneous histoplasmosis or cryptococcosis.

Treatment (see also Chapter 23.1)

Advice on prevention of spread of the infection to others should be given, such as avoidance of swimming pools, contact sports, or shared towels, until the lesions have resolved. Treatment may not be necessary, and depends on the site and number of the lesions and the age of the patient.

Cryotherapy (with liquid nitrogen) is effective and should be repeated at 3–4-weekly intervals. Other techniques include diathermy or curettage. In children the application of local anaesthetic cream prior to the procedure may be necessary.

Topical agents such as phenol (10–20 per cent solution), salicylic acid (15–20 per cent), silver nitrate, trichloroacetic acid, lactic acid, tretinoin, and cantharidin are used. The agent can be delivered to the inside of the lesion using the sharpened end of a wooden applicator stick.

In severe cases associated with HIV, 5 per cent imiquimod cream has proved effective. Recently, the antiviral agent, cidofovir (intravenously or topically), has been successfully used to treat molluscum contagiosum.

Further reading

Birthistle, K. and Carrington, D. (1997). Molluscum contagiosum virus. *Journal of Infection*, **34**, 21–8.

Garvey TL, *et al.*(2002). Binding of FADD and Caspase-8 to *Molluscum contagiosum* virus MC 159v-FLIP is not sufficient for its antiapoptotic function. *Journal of Virology* **76**, 697–706.

Husar K, Skerlev M (2002). *Molluscum contagiosum* from infancy to maturity. *Clinics in Dermatology* **20**, 170–2.

Meadows, K.P., Tyring, S.K., Pavia, A.T., and Rallis, T.M. (1997). Resolution of recalcitrant molluscum contagiosum virus lesions in human immunodeficiency virus infected patients treated with cidofovir. *Archives of Dermatology*, **133** (8), 987–90.

Schwartz, J.J. and Myskowski, P.L. (1992). Molluscum contagiosum in patients with human immunodeficiency virus infection. A review of twenty seven patients. *Journal of the American Academy of Dermatology*, **27**, 583–8.

7.11 Bacteria

7.11.1 Diphtheria

Delia B. Bethell and Tran Tinh Hien

Introduction

Diphtheria is an acute infection of the upper respiratory tract, and occasionally of other mucous membranes or skin, usually caused by *Corynebacterium diphtheriae*. The disease was probably known to the Greeks and Romans. While virtually eliminated from most developed countries by mass immunization, diphtheria remains a threat in poorer countries. In the last decade there has been a resurgence in parts of the former Soviet Union.

Bacteriology

Morphology

C. diphtheriae are pleomorphic, Gram-positive rods or clubs. Adjacent cells lie at different angles to each other—'Chinese letters'. The presence of metachromatic granules, usually two or three per cell, is characteristic but not exclusive; these stain deep blue with Neisser's methylene blue or greyish-black with Albert's stain. Virulent and non-virulent *C. diphtheriae* cannot be distinguished by their morphological appearances.

Culture

C. diphtheriae does not grow well on ordinary agar, but prefers media containing blood or serum. Selective media, such as Loeffler's serum medium and blood tellurite agar, are necessary for its isolation from other respiratory flora, although other corynebacteria can also grow on these media. Biochemical tests are used to identify *C. diphtheriae*. There are three colonial types of *C. diphtheriae*: *gravis*, *intermedius*, and *mitis*. There is no good association between colonial appearance and disease severity.

Toxin production

The clinical manifestations of diphtheria are caused by an exotoxin produced by virulent corynebacteria. The structural gene of the toxin, *tox*, is carried by a lysogenic corynebacteriophage. The phage can pass from toxigenic to non-toxigenic strains; this may be important in outbreaks when harmless strains in carriers' throats may become toxigenic. TOX gene expression is regulated by the *C. diphtheria*-encoded, iron-activated, repressor DtxR; hence iron starvation leads to increased toxin production.

Production of toxin may be assessed using gel precipitation (Elek's test) or guinea-pig inoculation. More recently enzyme immunoassays have been developed.

Pathogenesis

Pseudomembrane formation

This results from an inflammatory reaction to the presence of multiplying toxigenic *C. diphtheriae*. Fluid and leucocytes move from dilated blood vessels to surround necrotic epithelial cells. The fluid clots to enmesh these dead cells, as well as leucocytes, diphtheria bacilli, cellular debris, and occasionally small blood vessels. The latter explains why the pseudomembrane is adherent to underlying tissues and often bleeds when it is pulled away.

Action of toxin

C. diphtheriae does not usually pass beyond the pseudomembrane site; it is the toxin that causes the severe complications of diphtheria. Diphtheria toxin is a 535-residue, 62-kDa exotoxin. It consists of two factors: spreading factor B attaches via its receptor (heparin-binding, epidermal growth factor-like precursor (**HB-EGF-LP**)) to the cell membrane allowing lethal factor A to enter the cell. Factor A catalyses the NAD+-dependent ADP-ribosylation of eukaryotic elongation factor 2, preventing protein synthesis. Locally the toxin causes tissue necrosis, leading to formation of the typical pseudomembrane and, when absorbed into the bloodstream, systemic complications. Diphtheria toxin affects all human cells, but the most profound effects are seen in the myocardium, peripheral nerves, and kidneys. Delivery of a single molecule of factor A to the cytosol of a eukaryotic cell will kill it.

Effects on the heart

Common changes are fatty degeneration of cardiac muscle (myocarditis) and infiltration of the interstitium with leucocytes, which may affect the conduction fibres. Parenchymal necrosis is rare. Generally the heart can recover completely from these effects, although severe fibrosis and scarring may lead to death in late convalescence. Mural endocarditis may cause embolism leading to cerebral infarction and hemiplegia. Valvular endocarditis is extremely uncommon. Neuritic changes may be seen in the nerves to the heart during the late paralytic stage of the disease.

Effects on nerves

Diphtheria toxin causes demyelination and degeneration of both sensory and motor nerves. It affects the nerves to the eye, palate, pharynx, larynx, heart, and limb muscles. It is unclear whether the toxin can cross the blood–brain barrier and cause central lesions.

Effects on other organs

Non-specific changes in the kidneys, adrenals, liver, and spleen may be seen.

Epidemiology

Man is the only known reservoir for *C. diphtheriae*. Spread is usually via respiratory droplets or direct contact with respiratory secretions or exudate from skin lesions. Cutaneous diphtheria is more contagious than respiratory diphtheria: skin infections are the main reservoir of *C. diphtheriae* in environments of poverty, overcrowding, poor hygiene, frequent and slowly healing traumatization of unprotected skin, and insect bites. Fomites and dust are not important means of transmission, although *C. diphtheriae* may resist drying and has been isolated from dust on the floor of a ward. Diphtheria has been spread by contaminated milk. *C. diphtheriae* is killed by pasteurization and by most common disinfectants. Patients may become carriers of the infection and continue to harbour the organism for weeks or months, or even for a lifetime.

There is no given level of circulating antibody indicating protection or susceptibility to infection. The Schick test is used to assess the antibody response to diphtheria toxin. A measured amount of toxin is injected into the forearm causing a red reaction (positive) unless the patient has a sufficient antibody response to prevent it (negative). A Schick-negative person is very unlikely to have clinically significant diphtheria, while a Schick-positive person may have an attack of any severity. Neonates are very often Schick-negative, protected by maternal antibody, but become Schick-positive around 6 months of age. *C. diphtheriae* tends to die out in a highly immunized population, and children may grow to adult life without encountering the bacillus. In areas of the world that lack an effective immunization programme children generally meet *C. diphtheriae* early, maybe becoming a faucial, nasal, or aural carrier, and young children may suffer severe or fatal attacks of diphtheria.

In the 1990s a diphtheria epidemic gripped parts of the former Soviet Union. Economic hardship, crowding due to large urban migration, low vaccination coverage, and poor primary vaccination practices due to failing health systems have contributed. This has led to large numbers of susceptible children as well as an increase in susceptible adults as immunity was not maintained by periodic boosters. Prior to the vaccine era, most people acquired natural lifelong immunity during childhood through their exposure to *C. diphtheriae*. Serological studies in several countries indicate that 20 to 50 per cent of adults over the age of 20 years are susceptible to diphtheria, with a significant trend of decreasing immunity with increasing age. This potential risk assumes a particular significance in today's international travel.

Clinical features

After an incubation period of 2 to 5 days, diphtheria presents in a variety of forms depending upon the location of the pseudomembrane—anterior nasal, faucial, tracheolaryngeal, malignant, and cutaneous.

Anterior nasal

This is usually unilateral and relatively mild unless it coexists with other forms. It is relatively common in infancy. There is a nasal discharge, initially watery, then purulent and blood-stained. The nostril may be sore or crusted and a thin pseudomembrane can sometimes be seen within the nostril itself.

Faucial

This is the commonest form of diphtheria. Malaise, sore throat, and moderate fever develop gradually. At the onset of symptoms only a small, yellow-grey spot of pseudomembrane may be present on one or both tonsils, easily mistaken for other types of tonsillitis. The surrounding areas are dull and inflamed. Over the next few days the pseudomembrane enlarges and may extend to cover the uvula, soft palate, oropharynx, nasopharynx, or larynx. There is tender cervical lymphadenopathy, nausea, vomiting, and painful dysphagia. The pseudomembrane becomes greenish-black and eventually sloughs off.

Tracheolaryngeal

Some 85 per cent of tracheolaryngeal presentations are secondary to faucial diphtheria, but occasionally there may be no pharyngeal pseudomembrane. Initial symptoms include moderate fever, hoarseness, and a non-productive cough. Over the next day, as the pseudomembrane and associated oedema spread, the child becomes increasingly dyspnoeic with severe chest recession and cyanosis and asphyxiation unless the obstruction is relieved. Tracheostomy brings instant relief if the obstruction is confined to the larynx and upper trachea. In a minority of cases the pseudomembrane also involves the bronchi and bronchioles and tracheostomy has little effect.

Malignant

The onset is rapid, with high fever, tachycardia, hypotension, and cyanosis. Pseudomembrane spreads from the tonsils to cover much of the nasopharynx. It has a thick edge and as this advances the earlier parts become necrotic and foul smelling. There is gross cervical lymphadenopathy. Individual lymph nodes are difficult to feel because of surrounding oedema; this is the characteristic 'bull neck' of malignant diphtheria. The patient may bleed from the mouth, nose, or skin. Cardiac involvement with heart block occurs within a few days. Acute renal failure may ensue. Survival is unlikely.

Cutaneous

In contrast to many faucial infections, cutaneous diphtheria is usually chronic but mild. The morphological features of individual lesions can be extremely variable as *C. diphtheriae* can colonize any pre-existing skin lesion (such as impetigo, scabies, surgical wounds, or insect bites) without altering their picture. However, the ulcerative form is the most frequent and typical. Initially vesicular or pustular, filled with straw-coloured fluid, it soon breaks down to leave a punched-out ulcer several millimetres to a few centimetres across. Common sites are the lower legs, feet, and hands. During the first 1 to 2 weeks it is painful and may be covered with a dark pseudomembrane. After this separates a haemorrhagic base is seen, sometimes with a serous or serosanguinous exudate. The surrounding tissue is oedematous and pink or purple in colour. Spontaneous healing to leave a depressed scar usually takes 2 to 3 months, sometimes much longer.

Systemic complications, such as myocarditis, are rare. Occasionally, the affected limb becomes paralysed.

Other sites

A mild conjunctivitis may accompany faucial diphtheria. Occasionally, pseudomembrane forms in the lower conjunctiva and spreads over the cornea causing considerable damage. Dysphagia may indicate that pseudomembrane has spread from the tonsils to the oesophagus. Other parts of the gastrointestinal tract are not usually affected, but melaena with colicky abdominal pain is described. Diphtheria may spread by fingers from the throat to vulva or penis causing localized sores. *C. diphtheriae* occasionally invades the vagina and cervix, allowing the absorption of toxin. In one patient, pseudomembrane was found on the wall of the bladder at operation; peripheral neuritis and fatal heart failure ensued. Endocarditis is rare, but at least one reported case recovered following antimicrobial treatment.

Other corynebacteria

C. ulcerans produces two toxins, one of which seems to be the same as diphtheria toxin. It may cause membranous tonsillitis but toxic manifestations are rare. However, at least one fatality due to *C. ulcerans* has been reported. *C. ulcerans* has been spread to humans in cows' milk.

C. pseudodiphtheriticum is commonly present in the flora of the upper respiratory tract. It is non-toxigenic, but can cause exudative pharyngitis with a pseudomembrane identical to that produced by *C. diphtheriae*. More commonly it causes endocarditis in patients with anatomical abnormalities or infections of the lungs, trachea, or bronchi in immunosuppressed patients or those with pre-existing respiratory disease.

C. xerosis has been isolated from the blood of patients with endocarditis and from prosthetic valves at operation. *C. haemolyticum* has caused outbreaks of tonsillitis with or without a maculopapular rash.

Complications

Patients surviving acute diphtheria may develop one or more complication. These result from delayed effects of the toxin following haematogenous spread. The risk and severity of complications correlates directly with the extent of the pseudomembrane and the delay in administration of antitoxin.

Cardiovascular

Approximately 10 per cent of patients with diphtheria will develop myocarditis. Some two-thirds of patients with severe infection will have some evidence of cardiac involvement. The frequency of cardiac involvement in laryngeal and malignant diphtheria is three- to eightfold higher compared with faucial diphtheria, and two- to threefold higher if antitoxin is given more than 48 h after onset of the disease.

Cardiac toxicity usually appears after the first week of illness, but in malignant forms can occur after just a few days. Patients complain of upper abdominal pain and may vomit. They become very lethargic and tired. Examination reveals a rapid thready pulse with hypotension. At this stage profound shock may lead to death. In less severe cases, congestive cardiac failure may develop, with a displaced apex beat, gallop rhythm, and murmurs audible over all areas of the heart. Profound bradycardia may result from heart block. The liver enlarges and oliguria develops. Most deaths from diphtheria occur at this stage. If the patient survives myocarditis, complete recovery is likely.

Electrocardiography (**ECG**) is the best way to demonstrate cardiac involvement. The most common abnormalities are T-wave inversion in one or more chest leads and prolonged QTc intervals. There may be right or left axis deviation, bundle-branch block, or heart block. Very occasionally, atrial fibrillation or tachyarrhythmias are seen. Many more bursts of arrhythmias can be demonstrated if 24-hour ECG monitoring is performed. Numerous ectopic beats have been recorded in patients who lacked other manifestations of cardiac involvement.

Neurological

Neurological complications usually appear weeks after the onset of the disease, when the patient appears to be recovering. Palatal paralysis is common and may be seen from the third week onwards. The patient develops a nasal voice and regurgitates fluids through the nose. This usually resolves within a week or so. A little later there may be blurred vision from paralysis of accommodation, or a transient squint from external rectus paralysis. About the sixth or seventh week more sinister paralyses may develop affecting muscles to the pharynx, larynx, chest and limbs. The nerves to the heart may be affected causing tachycardia and dysrhythmias. Patients may become profoundly hypotonic over a few hours and die from respiratory arrest. However, if intensive-care facilities and skilled staff are available, the patient should be able to make a complete recovery over the following weeks or months.

Diagnosis

In areas where diphtheria is relatively common it should be suspected in any child with exudate in the throat. If the exudate is thick and discoloured the child should be given antitoxin. Clinical diagnosis is much more difficult where diphtheria is rare. The differential diagnosis includes infectious mononucleosis, streptococcal or viral tonsillitis, peritonsillar abscess, oral thrush, and leukaemia and other blood dyscrasias. The bull-neck of malig-

nant diphtheria may be mistaken for mumps. In adults, secondary syphilis can sometimes cause a glairy (resembling egg-white) exudate on the tonsils, and may be accompanied by rash and laryngitis.

Direct smears of infected areas of the throat are often used for diagnostic purposes, but are only of value in experienced hands. Confirmation of the diagnosis depends on culture and identification of *C. diphtheriae* from infected sites. Atypical corynebacteria can be classified only in a reference laboratory.

Treatment

Antitoxin is the mainstay of treatment, but to be effective it must be given before the toxin has reached tissues such as the heart and kidneys, preferably within 48 h of the onset of symptoms. This means that it must be given before bacteriological confirmation. Dosage depends on the site of primary infection, the extent of pseudomembrane, and the delay between the onset of symptoms and antitoxin administration. Between 20 000 and 40 000 units are given for faucial diphtheria of less than 48 h duration or for cutaneous infection; 40 000 to 80 000 units for faucial in excess of 48 h or for laryngeal infection; 80 000 to 100 000 units for malignant diphtheria. For doses over 40 000 units a portion is given intramuscularly followed by the bulk of the dose intravenously after an interval of 30 min to 2 h. Anaphylaxis can occur following antitoxin administration, and adrenaline (epinephrine) should always be available.

Antibiotics are given to eradicate the organism and prevent further toxin production. Benzylpenicillin (penicillin G) 150 000 to 250 000 units/kg per day (90–150 mg/kg/day) is given intravenously in four to six divided doses in children aged 1 month to 12 years. In adults the dose of benzylpenicillin is 12 million to 20 million units/day (7.2–12 g/day) in four to six divided doses. Oral penicillin V is substituted when the patient is able to swallow. Erythromycin may be used for penicillin-sensitive individuals, but a recent study suggests it may not be as effective in eradicating carriage. Antibiotic therapy should continue for 10 to 14 days.

Facilities for urgent tracheostomy should always be available in case of respiratory obstruction. Indications include increasingly laboured breathing and agitation. This procedure will be life-saving in many cases. Most tracheostomies can be closed after just a few days. Steroids may be used in conjunction with tracheostomy to reduce airway swelling, but there have been no controlled trials to support their use. Steroids are of no benefit in preventing myocarditis or neuritis.

Patients with signs or symptoms of cardiac involvement need to be managed in intensive-care units. Oxygen should be given. Temporary cardiac pacing is useful in patients with heart block, but is of doubtful value in cases of malignant diphtheria. An isoprenaline infusion may buy valuable time while the patient is transferred to a centre with facilities for pacing. Digoxin has been used in congestive cardiac failure. It has been suggested that carnitine may prevent some cases of myocarditis.

There is no specific treatment for neuritis. The severest cases will need mechanical ventilation and intragastric or intravenous feeding. With skilled nursing care full recovery can be expected.

Prevention

Diphtheria is a devastating but preventable disease. Its resurgence in Eastern Europe has highlighted the importance of vaccination. Experience to date suggests that a large gap in the immunity of adults poses an outbreak risk, but is probably not sufficient to sustain a large diphtheria epidemic. However, an immunity gap in adults coupled with the presence of large numbers of susceptible children and adolescents creates the potential for an extensive epidemic. Population migration may lead to massive introduction and spread of toxigenic strains of *C. diphtheriae*.

In industrialized countries, infants, children, and adolescents can be effectively immunized using a six-dose schedule: three primary doses of **DTP** (adsorbed diphtheria–tetanus–pertussis) are given in infancy (in the

United Kingdom at 2, 3, and 4 months); a first booster dose with DTP vaccine at the end of the second year; a second booster dose with **DT** (adsorbed diphtheria-tetanus) (or DTP) at school entry; and a third booster dose with **Td** (adsorbed tetanus/low-dose diphtheria for adults) at school leaving. Protection against diphtheria may be inadequate if only a single booster of TD or Td vaccine is given at 4 to 10 years of age following the primary doses.

In developing countries, the immunization of infants with a primary series of three doses of DTP was introduced in the late 1970s. By 1995 the coverage of infants was 81 per cent. Where diphtheria is endemic this should be sufficient to prevent an epidemic of diphtheria, as natural mechanisms such as frequent skin infections caused by *C. diphtheriae* probably contribute to maintaining immunity. One or two DT or DTP booster doses may need to be added to the routine schedule in areas at increased risk of diphtheria.

Reduction in the *C. diphtheriae* reservoir due to the large-scale immunization of children means that adults in industrialized countries are no longer immune through natural exposure. Repeated doses of diphtheria toxoid are needed to maintain immunity in the adult population. A lower dose of toxoid is used in older children and adults because of a tendency for more severe adverse effects. Some industrialized countries schedule routine booster doses of Td for every 10 years, but this strategy is difficult to monitor. Adults in developing countries do not require routine immunization.

Aggressive action is needed in the event of a diphtheria outbreak. Groups at risk should be immunized, there should be prompt diagnosis and management of cases, and identification of close contacts should be made so that the spread of infection can be halted. A single dose of DTP should be used for children under 3 years of age, DT for children aged 3 to 7 years, and Td vaccine for all persons aged over 7 years. Additional doses of vaccine will be needed in non-immunized individuals.

Further reading

Bonnet JM, Begg NT (1999). Control of diphtheria: guidance for consultants in communicable disease control. *Communicable Disease and Public Health* **2**, 242–9.

Eskola J, Lumio J, Vuopio-Varkila J (1998). Resurgent diphtheria—are we safe? *British Medical Bulletin* **54**, 635–45.

Galazka AM, Robertson SE (1996). Immunization against diphtheria with special emphasis on immunization of adults. *Vaccine* **14**, 845–57.

Hofler W (1991). Cutaneous diphtheria. *International Journal of Dermatology* **30**, 845–7.

Public Health Laboratory Service website. www.phls.co.uk/facts/diphtheria/dip.htm [Information on UK notifications and vaccine uptake.]

Rakhmanova G, *et al.* (1996). Diphtheria outbreak in St. Petersburg: clinical characteristics of 1,860 adult patients. *Scandinavian Journal of Infectious Diseases* **28**, 37–40.

Vitek CR, Wharton M (1998). Diphtheria in the former Soviet Union: reemergence of a pandemic disease. *Emerging Infectious Diseases* **4**, 539–50.

WHO (1998). Diphtheria. *Bulletin of the World Health Organization* **78**(Suppl 2), 129–30. [A concise summary of the global problem.]

7.11.2 Streptococci and enterococci

S. J. Eykyn

The term *Streptococcus* was first used by Billroth in 1874 to describe chain-forming cocci seen in infected wounds. They were also seen in the blood in puerperal sepsis by Pasteur (1879). In 1884, Rosenbach defined these streptococci as *Streptococcus pyogenes*. This organism remains one of the most important human pathogens. The genus *Streptococcus* contains numerous other species of varying degrees of pathogenicity for humans and animals. *Streptococcus faecalis* and *S. faecium* were split from the genus *Streptococcus* in 1984 and became *Enterococcus* spp. and numerous other species have since been included in this genus. The nutritionally-exacting streptococci *S. adjacens* and *S. defectivus* have also been assigned to a new genus, *Abiotrophia*, to which the newly described species *A. elegans* has been added.

Classification

Traditionally, classification of streptococci has relied on serological reactions, particularly Lancefield grouping based on cell wall carbohydrates, and haemolytic activity on blood agar, which has led to rather unsatisfactory streptococcal taxonomy. Genetic analysis has now enabled the subdivision of the species of *Streptococcus* into six clusters or groups as follows: pyogenic streptococci, milleri or anginosus group, mitis group, salivarius group, mutans group, and bovis group. Since the medically important members of the mitis, salivarius, and mutans groups are all oral streptococci, and of clinical relevance predominantly in endocarditis, they will be considered together.

The pyogenic streptococci

The pyogenic streptococci include the major human pathogen *S. pyogenes* (Lancefield group A), group B streptococci (*S. agalactiae*), and groups C and G streptococci. These organisms are β-haemolytic on blood agar.

Streptococcus pyogenes (β-haemolytic group A)

Since the beginning of the last century, and long before the introduction of antibiotics, infections with *S. pyogenes* declined in incidence and severity until, in the 1980s, highly virulent streptococci appeared causing very severe infections often in otherwise healthy people. Such cases occurred not only in the United Kingdom but in most of the developed world. *S. pyogenes* infection is usually community-acquired but may be acquired in hospital, where the most serious infections are postoperative.

Carriage

Although *S. pyogenes* is an invasive organism, it lives on epithelial surfaces (asymptomatic carriage) usually in the nose and throat; carriage can also be anal, vaginal, and on the scalp. Pharyngeal carriage rates are usually much higher in healthy children (5 to 20 per cent) than in adults (0.5 per cent) and also vary with season, year, and geographical location; they are also higher in crowded living conditions. *S. pyogenes* can persist for months after acute pharyngitis, though in decreased numbers. Survival in the environment is poor and *S. pyogenes* can only survive on skin squames and dust for a limited period and in low numbers.

Pathogenicity, virulence, and typing

S. pyogenes is an extracellular pathogen and produces virulence factors that enable it to avoid host defences and spread in tissues. The main virulence factor is the M protein; streptococci rich in M protein resist phagocytosis by polymorphs. Immunity to *S. pyogenes* infection is associated with the development of opsonic antibodies to antiphagocytic epitopes of M protein; it is usually type specific and lasts for many years, perhaps indefinitely. M protein was first described in the 1920s by Rebecca Lancefield; over 100 M types have now been differentiated. Lancefield also developed the supplementary T typing system which distinguishes 26 serotypes of a trypsin-resistant surface protein (T antigen), most of which can be expressed by several different M types. Certain M types also produce a serum opacity factor (OF+). These typing systems are still widely used in epidemiological studies to distinguish between strains of *S. pyogenes*. Recent studies have shown considerable genetic diversity in *S. pyogenes*, and horizontal transfer and recombination of virulent genes have played a major role. This finding is likely to be relevant to the emergence of new, unusually virulent clones of the organism.

In addition to M protein, lipoteichoic acid, important in the host–bacterial interaction, is expressed on the surface of the organism and is the adhesin that binds the organism to fibronectin on the surface of the oral epithelial cell membranes and initiates the colonization that precedes infection. *S. pyogenes* has a hyaluronate capsule which, like M protein, is also antiphagocytic, and is an additional virulence factor. The extent of encapsulation varies and colonies with prominent capsules are very mucoid on blood agar. Strains of *S. pyogenes* that are both rich in M protein and heavily encapsulated are readily transmitted from person to person, and tend to produce severe infections.

S. pyogenes produces many extracellular substances, several of which are important in the pathogenesis of infection. The most familiar are streptolysin O, deoxyribonuclease (DNAase) B, and hyaluronidase as serum antibodies to these provide retrospective confirmation of recent streptococcal infection. Other extracellular products include DNAases A, C, and D, streptolysin S, proteinase, streptokinase, and the substances previously known as erythrogenic toxins. These toxins have now been designated streptococcal pyrogenic exotoxins (**SPE**) -A, -B, -C, and possibly -D. SPE-A, and possibly others, is coded by a phage gene. These toxins, known as superantigens, have diverse effects on the host. In addition to the rash of scarlet fever, they cause fever, changes in the blood–brain barrier, organ damage, and lethal shock in animals. They have profound effects on the immune system including increasing susceptibility to endotoxic shock, blockade of the reticuloendothelial system, and alterations in T-cell function.

When *S. pyogenes* enters the body, either through the upper respiratory tract mucosa or a break in the skin, a local lesion may occur or there may be spread along tissue planes or lymphatics. The M protein is not toxic in itself but protects the streptococcus from phagocytosis and antibodies to the M protein are opsonic. In some two-thirds of patients with serious invasive disease, who may present with fever, shock, and renal impairment, the portal of entry is the skin, and infection of soft tissue is apparent, but in others the site of infection may not be evident.

Infections caused by *S. pyogenes*

S. pyogenes causes a variety of illnesses ranging from very common, usually mild, conditions such as pharyngitis and impetigo, through common, temporarily disabling cellulitis, to less common, puerperal sepsis and very severe infections such as type II necrotizing fasciitis, bacteraemia, and toxic shock. It is also associated with the non-suppurative sequelae of acute rheumatic fever and acute glomerulonephritis.

Streptococcal pharyngitis

Streptococcal pharyngitis or tonsillitis is one of the commonest bacterial infections in children from 5 to 15 years, but all ages are susceptible. The incubation period, at least in outbreaks, is short (1 to 3 days) and the onset of the infection marked by the abrupt onset of sore throat and pain on swallowing with malaise, fever, and headache. The signs are redness and oedema of the pharynx, enlarged red tonsils with spots of white exudate, and enlarged tender anterior cervical lymph glands. Nausea, vomiting, and abdominal pain are common in children, and in infants and preschool children there may be few definite signs of pharyngitis but fever, nasal discharge, enlarged cervical lymph glands, and otitis media occur.

Suppurative complications

Direct extension of streptococcal pharyngitis can give rise to acute sinusitis or otitis media and other suppurative complications include peritonsillar abscess (quinsy) and retropharyngeal abscess, which often contain oral flora including anaerobes with or without *S. pyogenes*, and suppurative cervical lymphadenitis.

Scarlet fever

Scarlet fever results from infection with a strain of *S. pyogenes* that produces SPE (erythrogenic toxin). It is usually associated with streptococcal pharyngitis but may follow streptococcal infections at other sites and occurs with invasive disease. Scarlet fever rarely follows streptococcal pyoderma. Most cases occur in school-age children and the rash must be distinguished from viral exanthems, Kawasaki disease, and staphylococcal toxic shock syndrome. The rash, which generally appears on the second day of clinical illness, is usually a diffuse erythema, symmetrical, and blanches on pressure. It is seen most often on the neck, chest, folds of the axilla, and groin. Occlusion of sweat glands gives the skin a 'sandpaper' texture, a useful sign in dark-skinned patients. The face appears flushed with circumoral pallor. There are small red haemorrhagic spots on the palate and the tongue is initially covered with a white fur through which red papillas appear ('strawberry tongue') and then, usually after the rash develops, the white fur peels off leaving a raw red papillate surface ('raspberry tongue'). The rash persists for several days and later (up to 3 weeks) peeling may occur, usually on the tips of the fingers, toes, or ears and less often over the trunk and limbs. A similar rash may develop as a reaction to streptokinase thrombolytic therapy.

Streptococcal perianal infection (cellulitis)

This is a superficial, well-demarcated rash spreading out from the anus in young children, usually boys, associated with itching, rectal pain on defaecation, and blood-stained stools. *S. pyogenes* is isolated from perianal cultures and usually also from pretreatment throat swabs.

Streptococcal vulvovaginitis

Vulvovaginitis in prepubertal girls is often caused by *S. pyogenes* and presents with serosanguinous discharge and erythema of the labia and vaginal orifice. As with perianal infections, *S. pyogenes* is usually also found in the throat. In both streptococcal perianal infection and vulvovaginitis, more than one child in the family may be affected and nasopharyngeal carriage is likely in both infected and uninfected children.

Streptococcal skin and soft tissue infections

Pyoderma/impetigo

Almost any purulent lesion of the skin can yield *S. pyogenes*, sometimes with *Staphylococcus aureus*. Such lesions include impetigo, infected cuts and lacerations, insect bites, scabies, intertrigo, and ecthyma. *S. pyogenes* also often causes secondary infection in varicella, occasionally with resultant bacteraemia. The term pyoderma is used synonymously with impetigo for discrete, purulent, apparently primary infections of the skin that are prevalent in many parts of the world, especially in children. These lesions are initially papules, then vesicular with surrounding erythema, and finally pustules with crusting exudate; they may be localized to one part of the body or generalized. Outbreaks of impetigo can occur among adults subject to skin trauma, such as rugby football players (scrumpox), and streptococcal infection of cuts on the hands and forearms are an occupational hazard for workers in the meat trade. Ecthyma is an ulcerated form of impetigo in which ulceration extends into the dermis.

Invasive streptococcal infections of skin and soft tissues

Erysipelas

This is an acute inflammation of the skin with lymphatic involvement. The streptococci are localized in the dermis and hypodermis. It usually affects the face, particularly in the elderly, but may occur elsewhere. It may be bilateral (Plate 1) and is sometimes recurrent. There is usually a history of sore throat, but the mode of spread to the skin is unknown. It is usually accompanied by fever, rigors, and toxicity. The cutaneous lesion begins as a localized area of erythema and swelling and then spreads with rapidly advancing raised red margins that are well demarcated from adjacent normal tissue. Facial erysipelas begins over the bridge of the nose and spreads over the cheeks. Vesicles and bullas appear, which become crusted when they rupture. There is marked oedema and the eyes are often closed. When the infection resolves it is often followed by desquamation. Intense local allergic reactions to topical agents, such as cosmetics, may cause confusion.

Cellulitis (Plate 2)

Cellulitis is commonly caused by streptococci and *Staphylococcus aureus*. This is an acute spreading inflammation of the skin and subcutaneous tissues with local pain swelling and erythema. Fever, rigors, and malaise may precede by a few hours the appearance of the skin lesion and associated lymphangitis and tender lymphodenopathy. Streptococcal cellulitis differs from erysipelas in that the lesion is not raised and the demarcation between affected and unaffected skin is indistinct. It may result from infection of burns, mild trauma, or surgical wounds. When this involves the leg, fungal infection of the feet is often present and predisposes to streptococcal invasion. After the first episode, there is a tendency for recurrence in the same area. Intravenous drug users are also at risk of streptococcal cellulitis associated with skin and tissue infection and septic thrombophlebitis.

(Type II) necrotizing fasciitis (streptococcal gangrene)

This infection, described by Meleney in 1924, involves the deep subcutaneous tissues and fascia (and occasionally muscle as well) with extensive, rapidly spreading necrosis and gangrene of the skin and underlying structures. It is generally community-acquired, usually involving the arm or leg, but may also occur after surgery, even quite minor. Some victims are diabetic, but the majority were previously healthy. Risk factors, providing a portal of entry, include surgery, trauma, childbirth, intravenous drug abuse, and chickenpox. Blunt trauma and muscle strain which may generate a haematoma and use of non-steroidal anti-inflammatory agents are also implicated. The infection begins at the site of trivial or even inapparent trauma with redness, swelling, fever, and rapidly escalating focal pain followed by purple discoloration and the development of bullae, often haemorrhagic. Bacteraemia is often present and within days skin necrosis occurs followed by extensive sloughing. The patient is profoundly ill and the disease has a high case fatality of 30 to 70 per cent. Features of streptococcal toxic shock syndrome are associated in many cases. The United Kingdom media memorably dubbed *S. pyogenes* the 'flesh-eater' in reports of a cluster of cases of necrotizing fasciitis in 1994. Treatment involves early intravenous antibiotics (clindamycin has several theoretical advantages over penicillin), urgent surgical débridement of necrotic tissue, and intensive care to support failing organs and systems (e.g. cardiovascular and renal). Benefits of immunoglobulin are anecdotal.

Streptococcal toxic shock syndrome

This syndrome was described in 1987 in patients with severe *S. pyogenes* infection and clinical features remarkably similar to those of the staphylococcal toxic shock syndrome described a decade earlier. Neither are likely to be new diseases. Definitions of streptococcal toxic shock syndrome vary. Some limit the definition to cases of shock and multiorgan failure where there is a rash or desquamation, whilst others include all cases of shock and its non-specific sequelae such as coagulopathy, uraemia, or jaundice, irrespective of skin lesions. Streptococcal toxic shock syndrome is usually associated with necrotizing fasciitis or myositis. It can occur at all ages and many of those affected are young and previously healthy. Most cases have been community-acquired, though it can be acquired in hospital. M1 has been the predominant serotype in many countries, though others, especially 2, 3, 12, and 28, have also been implicated. Most strains produce SPE-A. Interestingly there is an amino acid homology of 50 per cent and immunological cross-reactivity between SPE-A and staphylococcal enterotoxins B and C, which together with staphylococcal TSS toxin-1 are relevant in non-menstrual staphylococcal toxic shock syndrome.

Streptococcal bacteraemia

In parallel with the increase in serious *S. pyogenes* infections there has been an increase in bacteraemic infections, both community- and hospital-

acquired (usually postoperative) (Plate 3). While many patients have an underlying disease, most often malignancy, immunosuppression, or diabetes, others are previously healthy adults between 20 and 50 years old. The portal of entry is usually the skin. The mortality is higher in patients with underlying disease.

Puerperal and neonatal infection

Historically *S. pyogenes* has always been an important cause of puerperal sepsis ('childbed fever'), but in the postantibiotic era it was rarely encountered in obstetric practice until the 1980s when sporadic cases occurred, some with streptococcal toxic shock syndrome, and some women have died. These infections follow abortion or delivery when streptococci (usually colonizing the patient herself) invade the endometrium, lymphatics, and bloodstream. They can be devastatingly severe and present with non-specific signs such as restlessness and gastrointestinal upset that may not immediately suggest sepsis. Fever may be absent resulting in further diagnostic confusion. The streptococcal infection not only involves the uterus and adnexa but sometimes distant sites such as joints as well. It can also affect the baby causing serious neonatal infection including meningitis. Instrumentation in the presence of asymptomatic vaginal or anorectal carriage of *S. pyogenes* can result in severe infection.

Other infections

S. pyogenes can, though rarely does, cause pneumonia (usually associated with viral infection or pulmonary disease), osteomyelitis, septic arthritis, meningitis, pericarditis (Plate 4), endophthalmitis, and endocarditis.

Laboratory diagnosis of S. pyogenes infection

S. pyogenes is easy to culture in the laboratory and usually grows on blood agar in 24 hours. Throat swabs must be taken before antibiotics are given or the chance of recovery is slim. Kits for the detection of the group A antigen directly from throat swabs are available and give few false-positive reactions, but they are seldom used in the United Kingdom. Even trivial skin lesions are worth swabbing (if necessary with a moistened swab) and a search for such lesions often pays dividends. Swabs from the surface of cellulitis and erysipelas rarely yield streptococci and although they may be recovered from specimens obtained by aspiration, in practice this is seldom done. Blood cultures should be done in any patient who is ill whether febrile or not. Serological confirmation of infection with *S. pyogenes* when the organism has not been isolated can be obtained by the detection of raised antibodies to its extracellular products. Most laboratories tend to use two or more tests. Interpretation requires knowledge of the level of titres in the community for those without a history of recent streptococcal infection. In the United Kingdom the upper limit of titres in teenagers and young adults without such a history is antistreptolysin O (ASO) 200, anti-deoxyribonuclease B (ADB) 240, and antihyaluronidase (AHT) 128.

Management and antibiotic treatment of S. pyogenes infection

Remarkably, *S. pyogenes* remains exquisitely sensitive to penicillin and this is the antibiotic of choice for treatment, parenterally for severe infections and orally otherwise. Conventionally, 10 days treatment is recommended for pharyngeal infections to eradicate the organism and prevent acute rheumatic fever. In practice, compliance with this regimen is poor as once the symptoms abate there is a natural reluctance to continue the antibiotic. Treatment of patients allergic to penicillin is most often with erythromycin or the newer macrolides (azithromycin and clarithromycin), but some 3 to 5 per cent of strains are erythromycin resistant. *S. pyogenes* is also sensitive to cephalosporins. Topical agents such as mupirocin and fusidic acid are useful in addition to systemic antibiotic treatment in impetigo and other skin lesions. Patients with streptococcal toxic shock syndrome will need intensive care and many require inotropic support, ventilation, and haemodialysis. Urgent surgical intervention is needed for necrotizing fasciitis and myositis. Clindamycin (in addition to penicillin) has been recommended for patients with established invasive streptococcal infections since this drug stops the metabolic activity of the streptococci and thus halts further production of toxin. This is specially relevant in type II necrotizing fasciitis/myositis and streptococcal toxic shock syndrome. Intravenous immunoglobulin has also been used in an attempt to neutralize the streptococcal toxins, but reports of its effects are inconclusive. Prevention of recurrent cellulitis of the lower legs involves meticulous foot hygiene with treatment of 'athlete's foot' fungi and reduction in skin carriage using topical mupirocin. Oedematous limbs can benefit from elastic stockings. Antibiotic prophylaxis may be required in cases of frequent recurrence refractory to these measures. Lastly it should be remembered that *S. pyogenes* is readily transmitted from person to person and thus appropriate infection control precautions should be taken until swabs show the organism has been eradicated.

β-Haemolytic groups C and G streptococci

These streptococci are sometimes referred to as 'large colony-forming group C and G streptococci' to distinguish them from the small colony-forming strains of streptococci with the same Lancefield antigens that belong to the anginosus or milleri group (see below). Groups C and G streptococci are closely related genetically. They are most conveniently regarded as 'pyogenes-like' as the infections they cause are similar to those caused by *S. pyogenes* though these streptococci tend to be less virulent than *S. pyogenes*. Infections with these streptococci are less common than *S. pyogenes* infections. Although post-streptococcal glomerulonephritis has been associated with pharyngitis caused by both groups C and G streptococci, acute rheumatic fever has not. Group C streptococci are less frequently encountered in human infections than group G and most group C infections are caused by *S. equisimilis*; those caused by *S. zooepidemicus* have an animal source. Group G streptococci are frequently isolated from leg ulcers and pressure sores, usually with other bacteria. In such patients cellulitis and systemic upset are rare and the organisms are just colonizing the lesions. They, like *S. pyogenes*, can cause cellulitis in lymphoedematous limbs.

β-Haemolytic group B streptococci (*S. agalactiae*)

The group B streptococcus has been known for over a century as a cause of bovine mastitis and in the 1930s it was recognized as a vaginal commensal, an occasional cause of puerperal fever, and an uncommon cause of invasive disease in adults. Not until the 1960s was it realized that the group B streptococcus was an important neonatal pathogen, and some 20 years later it had replaced *Escherichia coli* as the predominant neonatal pathogen.

Carriage

Group B streptococci can be recovered from various sites in healthy adults but vaginal carriage has been most extensively investigated. Swabs from the lower vagina are more often positive than cervical swabs and carriage rates of 3 to over 40 per cent have been reported. Higher rates have been obtained with selective media and enrichment techniques. Carriage also increases with sexual activity and is highest in women attending genitourinary clinics. The urethra, vagina, perineum, and anorectal region have all been suggested as the prime site of carriage. Some 5 to 10 per cent of normal adults carry group B streptococci in the throat, independent of urogenital and anorectal carriage.

Pathogenicity, virulence, and typing

The chief determinant of virulence appears to be the capsular polysaccharide, and most human strains carry one of six sialic acid-containing polysaccharides that surround the cell wall. In addition, a protein antigen (c, X, or R) may be carried. Certain combinations are common; serotypes III or III/R form one-quarter of all isolates from superficial sites on women, but three-quarters of all group B streptococci causing meningitis in infants. They are also the commonest serotypes found in adult (non-pregnant) infections. The type polysaccharide, like the M protein of *S. pyogenes*, inhibits phagocytosis. Colonization of the mucous membranes of the neonate results from vertical transmission of the organism from the mother either *in utero* by the ascending route or at delivery. The rate of vertical transmission in neonates born to mothers colonized with group B streptococci is about 50 per cent, but the incidence of symptomatic infection in neonates born to colonized mothers is only about 1 to 2 per cent. It is much higher in preterm infants. Nosocomial colonization of neonates can also occur. In most cases of adult infections (other than in pregnant women) the source of the infection is unknown.

Infections caused by group B streptococci

These are commonly neonatal or puerperal infections, but group B streptococci also cause infection in the non-pregnant adult.

Neonatal infection

The frequency of neonatal infection (bacteraemia, meningitis, or both) has been variously quoted as between 0.3 and 5.4 cases/1000 live births, but these figures have wide confidence limits. Two fairly distinct clinical patterns of disease predominate, but the spectrum is wide and includes impetigo neonatorum, septic arthritis, osteomyelitis, pneumonitis, peritonitis, pyelonephritis, facial cellulitis, conjunctivitis, and endophthalmitis.

Early-onset disease

Symptoms develop within the first 5 days of life with a mean of 20 h, though they can present at birth suggesting an intrauterine onset of infection. Early-onset disease is most often a bacteraemia with no identifiable focus of infection, but can also be pneumonia or, infrequently, meningitis. The presenting signs include lethargy, poor feeding, jaundice, grunting respirations, pallor, and hypotension and they are common to all types of disease. Respiratory symptoms are nearly always present. The only reliable way of detecting meningitis is by lumbar puncture. Mortality rates are high in low birth-weight babies. In addition to positive blood cultures, the infecting strain can be found in the mother's vagina and cultured from 'screening' sites on the baby; these include ear, throat, and nasogastric aspirate.

Late-onset disease

This usually presents between 7 days and 3 months after birth, often in previously healthy babies born after a normal labour who are admitted unwell from home. The pathogenesis is less clear than in cases of early-onset disease and only about half the cases are associated with mucosal colonization during delivery. Most babies have meningitis and concomitant bacteraemia and present with non-specific symptoms such as lethargy, poor feeding, irritability, and fever. Neurological sequelae are common among survivors.

Puerperal infection

Puerperal infection with Group B streptococci usually occurs within 24 to 48 h of delivery or abortion. The source of the organism is always the vagina and infection is more likely when there has been premature rupture of the membranes and chorioamnionitis. Most infections are endometritis with fever and uterine tenderness sometimes associated with retained products of conception, but group B streptococci can also cause wound infection after caesarean section. Bacteraemia is common. Other bacteria, both aerobes and anaerobes, are sometimes isolated from the genital tract and wounds in addition to the group B streptococcus. Very rarely the streptococcus may spread to other sites in puerperal women.

Infection in non-pregnant adults

The prominence given to group B streptococci as neonatal and puerperal pathogens has tended to overshadow their importance in non-pregnant women and men in whom they cause significant morbidity and mortality. Most infections are community-acquired, occur in the middle aged and elderly, and are as common in males as females. Many, though by no means all, patients with group B streptococcal infection have underlying diseases, particularly diabetes and myeloma. Skin and soft tissue infections are especially common in patients with diabetes. Occasional urinary tract infections occur, in men as well as women. Bacteraemic infections serve to emphasize the virulence of group B streptococci, and they have increased in incidence, or perhaps have been increasingly recognized, since the early 1990s. Community-acquired group B streptococcal bacteraemia is similar in many respects to that caused by *Staphylococcus aureus* since common clinical manifestations include endocarditis, vertebral osteomyelitis, septic arthritis, endophthalmitis, and meningitis. As with staphylococcal infections, some bacteraemic patients have more than one metastatic focus of infection, which can lead to diagnostic confusion.

Laboratory diagnosis of group B streptococcal infection

Group B streptococci are readily isolated from any clinical specimen in the laboratory and easily identified by Lancefield grouping. The group B antigen is not shared by any other streptococcus. Importantly the antigen can be reliably detected in fluids such as blood, urine, or cerebrospinal fluid by latex particle agglutination enabling a rapid diagnosis.

Treatment of group B streptococcal infection

Group B streptococci are sensitive to penicillin and this is the antibiotic of choice for treatment. They are rather less sensitive to penicillin than *S. pyogenes* with minimum inhibitory concentrations some four- to 10-fold higher. For this reason penicillin is sometimes combined with gentamicin for meningitis and other serious infections, though this is not of proven benefit. Certainly, the maximum recommended dose of parenteral penicillin should be given whether combined with gentamicin or not. Penicillin allergy is not likely to be an issue in neonates; adults with meningitis can be treated with chloramphenicol. Most group B streptococci are sensitive to erythromycin and they are sensitive to cephalosporins.

Prevention of neonatal infection with group B streptococci

During the 1990s the incidence of disease caused by mother-to-child transmission of group B streptococci in the United States fell by two-thirds as a result of the increased use of intrapartum penicillin in women at high risk of transmitting the infection, an intervention largely brought about by parental pressure. The American authorities recommend either prenatal screening or a risk-based strategy to identify women to receive intrapartum antibiotics. Similar recommendations are to be introduced in the United Kingdom. Any protocol for prophylactic penicillin based on the isolation of group B streptococci in late pregnancy would present difficulties in a busy obstetric unit and culture methods may also fail to detect the organism unless vaginal and rectal swabs are cultured in selective broth media. Maternal colonization with group B streptococci can be identified rapidly and reliably by polymerase chain reaction assay, but this is unlikely to be adopted as a routine round-the-clock service. An effective vaccine is an alternative approach, as yet unavailable.

Streptococci of the anginosus or milleri group

This group of streptococci has been a source of considerable taxonomic confusion, partly the result of a lack of international consensus on nomenclature, but also because of a lack of reliable phenotypic differences between taxa within the group. Most clinicians are familiar with the organism they know as 'Streptococcus milleri'. There are three species of milleri streptococci, S. anginosus, S. constellatus, and S. intermedius, but despite increasing awareness of the clinical significance of the *milleri* group little is known about the association between individual species and specific sites of isolation and diseases. These streptococci are found in large numbers in the normal flora of the upper respiratory tract, gastrointestinal tract, and genital tract, and are commonly isolated from a range of pyogenic infections, sometimes in pure culture, but often with other organisms, particularly anaerobes. These infections include dental abscesses, intra-abdominal abscesses (especially of the liver), subphrenic abscesses, lung abscesses and empyema, and brain abscesses. Such is the propensity of these organisms to cause deep-seated abscesses that isolation of a milleri streptococcus from a blood culture should prompt investigations to detect such a focus. Milleri streptococci are also commonly isolated from inflamed appendices and postappendicectomy wound infection. Unlike other viridans and non-haemolytic streptococci, milleri streptococci seldom cause endocarditis. They form minute colonies on blood agar and are preferentially anaerobic on primary isolation. They may be α-, β-, or non-haemolytic. Some have the Lancefield antigens A, C, G, or F. All group F streptococci are milleri group whereas not all milleri streptococci are group F. Another useful clue to their identity in the laboratory is the distinct caramel smell of many strains on blood agar, the result of the diacetyl metabolite. Most strains are very sensitive to penicillin.

The mitis, salivarius, and mutans groups of streptococci (oral/viridans streptococci)

This group of usually α-haemolytic (viridans) streptococci includes *S. pneumoniae* and those oral streptococci (*S. mitis, S. oralis, S. sanguis, S. gordonii*, and rarely, *S. salivarius*) that are the commonest cause of infective endocarditis of oral or dental origin. These streptococci occasionally cause bacteraemia in neutropenic patients who sometimes have detectable mouth lesions and neonatal infection as they are found as part of the normal vaginal flora.

The bovis group of streptococci

Although this group comprises at least three species, S .bovis is the main species of medical importance. S. bovis is similar to the enterococci in that it bears the Lancefield group D antigen and is a gastrointestinal commensal, but unlike the enterococci, it is sensitive to penicillin. It can be misidentified in the laboratory either as an oral streptococcus or as an enterococcus. Most patients with *S. bovis* bacteraemia will have endocarditis and it is seldom isolated from other sites. It is important to recognize *S. bovis* in a blood culture as the organism is associated with colonic pathology, and patients should be specifically investigated for this.

Nutritionally variant organisms previously classified as streptococci, now *Abiotrophia* spp.

These organisms, which occasionally cause endocarditis, require pyridoxal or thiol group supplementation for growth in the laboratory and tend to form satellite colonies round *Staphylococcus aureus*. Although most blood culture media will support their growth, successful subculture requires supplementation or cross-streaking of the plates with *S. aureus* to provide the necessary growth factors. The *Abiotrophia* include three species, *S. adjacens*, *S. defectivus*, and the recently described *A. elegans*. They are less susceptible to penicillin than other streptococci.

Streptococcus suis

This streptococcus, which can be misidentified in the laboratory as *S. bovis* or an enterococcus as it reacts with group D antiserum, is an important pathogen of young pigs causing meningitis, septicaemia, arthritis, pneumonia, and endocarditis and is also carried in the pharynx of healthy pigs. *S .suis* type II (also referred to as group R streptococci) is not only the most invasive type in pigs, it can cause serious infection—mainly septicaemia and meningitis, but also septic arthritis, pneumonia, and endophthalmitis—in humans, in whom it is an occupational disease of pig farmers, abattoir workers, and factory workers handling pig meat (see Chapter 24.14.1). The streptococcus probably enters the bloodstream via skin abrasions that are common in the above occupations. *S. suis* type II meningitis results in deafness in about half of those affected.

Enterococci

Enterococci are Lancefield group D, Gram-positive cocci that can grow and survive in extreme cultural conditions, and are also more resistant to antibiotics than streptococci. They form part of the normal gut flora of humans and animals. Overall, the commonest clinical isolates of enterococci are *Enterococcus faecalis*, but the more antibiotic-resistant species *E. faecium* is increasingly encountered in hospitals. Nosocomial isolates of enterococci have dramatically increased in the 1990s. Other species, including *E. casseliflavus*, *E. durans*, and *E. avium*, are occasionally isolated. In most cases it is unnecessary to determine the species of enterococci in a clinical laboratory but sometimes differentiation between *E. faecalis* and *E. faecium* is helpful, for instance in epidemiological studies and in endocarditis because of their different antibiotic susceptibilities.

Infections caused by enterococci

Enterococci are an increasingly important cause of nosocomial infection and colonization, possibly the result of the large-scale use of antibiotics such as cephalosporins and quinolones to which they are inherently resistant. They occasionally cause community-acquired urinary tract infections but the most important community-acquired infection is endocarditis, which is increasing in incidence. This infection is almost always caused by *E. faecalis*. Any patient admitted from the community with *E. faecalis* in blood cultures should be assumed to have endocarditis until proved otherwise. Enterococci are predominantly hospital pathogens and cause urinary infection, particularly after instrumentation, intra-abdominal infections, wound infections (usually with other organisms), infections associated with intravascular devices and dialysis, and occasionally endocarditis.

Antibiotic sensitivity and treatment

Enterococci are not only intrinsically resistant to many antibiotics, they show a remarkable ability to acquire new mechanisms of resistance. This allows them to survive in environments in which large amounts of antibiotics are used and also has important therapeutic consequences, particularly for the treatment of endocarditis and other serious infections. Fortunately many patients from whom enterococci are isolated do not require antibiotic treatment. Sensitive enterococci cannot be killed by ampicillin/amoxycillin alone, though combination with an aminoglycoside is bactericidal (synergy); but many strains now exhibit high-level gentamicin resistance and for them the combination is not bactericidal. *E. faecium* is almost always resistant to ampicillin/amoxycillin and *E. faecalis* is occasionally. The first published report of vancomycin-resistant enterococci (**VRE**) was in 1988 from a London hospital outbreak, though such strains had been recognized a year before in Paris. Most strains of VRE in the

London outbreak were *E. faecium* and overall most VRE are *E. faecium*. There are four recognized phenotypes of vancomycin resistance; the first isolates of VRE were highly resistant to vancomycin and teicoplanin and exhibit what is known as the VanA resistance phenotype. Since then, levels of resistance to teicoplanin in this phenotype have been more varied. Most VanA enterococci are *E. faecium*, but this phenotype also occurs in *E. faecalis* and occasionally in other species. The VanB phenotype is associated with low-level vancomycin resistance and sensitivity to teicoplanin and is found in both *E. faecalis* and *E. faecium*. Both VanA and VanB are acquired traits. The VanC phenotype is an intrinsic property of *E. casseliflavus* and *E. gallinarum* and these species have low-level resistance to vancomycin but are sensitive to teicoplanin. A fourth phenotype, VanD, has been described in a single strain of *E. faecium*. Vancomycin-resistant *E. faecium*, though not vancomycin-resistant *E. faecalis*, are sensitive to quinupristin/dalfopristin (Synercid) and all VRE are sensitive to the oxazolidinone Linezolid.

The antibiotic susceptibilities of the enterococci outlined above serve to emphasize that these bacteria are the most antibiotic-resistant Gram-positive bacteria now encountered in hospital practice. Fortunately many, perhaps most, of the patients from whom they are isolated do not require antibiotic treatment at all, but for those who do, the effective treatment of serious infection caused by enterococci and particularly antibiotic-resistant strains requires microbiological expertise.

Further reading

Bisno AL, Stevens DL (2000). *Streptococcus pyogenes* (including streptococcal toxic shock syndrome and necrotizing fasciitis). In: Mandell GL, Bennett JE, Dolin R, eds. *Principles and practice of infectious diseases*, pp 2101–17. Churchill Livingstone, New York.

Colman G *et al.* (1993). The serotypes of *Streptococcus pyogenes* present in Britain during 1980 to 1990 and their association with disease. *Journal of Medical Microbiology* **39**, 165–78.

Edwards MS, Baker CJ (2000). *Streptococcus agalactiae* (Group B streptococcus). In: Mandell GL, Bennett JE, Dolin R, eds. *Principles and practice of infectious diseases*, pp 2156–67. Churchill Livingstone, New York.

Jacobs JA (1997). The 'Streptococcus milleri' group: *Streptococcus anginosus*, *Streptococcus constellatus* and *Streptococcus intermedius*. *Reviews in Medical Microbiology* **8**, 73–80.

Katz AR, Morens D (1992). Severe streptococcal infections in historical perspective. *Clinical Infectious Diseases* **14**, 298–307.

Murray BE (1990). The life and times of the *Enterococcus*. *Clinical Microbiological Reviews* **3**, 46–65.

Stevens DL (1992). Invasive Group A streptococcus infections. *Clinical Infectious Diseases* **14**, 2–13.

Stevens D (1995). Streptococcal toxic shock syndrome: spectrum of disease, pathogenesis and new concepts of treatment. *Emergencies in Infectious Disease* **1**, 69–78.

Woodford N (1998). Glycopeptide-resistant enterococci: a decade of experience. *Journal of Medical Microbiology* **47**, 849–62.

7.11.3 Pneumococcal diseases

Keith P. Klugman and Brian M. Greenwood

Streptococcus pneumoniae (the pneumococcus) causes a considerable burden of vaccine-preventable disease. It is a leading cause of bacterial meningitis, pneumonia, otitis media, and sinusitis. The global HIV pandemic has greatly increased the burden of pneumococcal disease in both children and adults and the dissemination of a number of multiresistant pneumococcal clones has complicated the management of this disease. In the first decade of the twenty-first century it is likely that the introduction of pneumococcal conjugate vaccines will reduce the burden of pneumococcal disease in children and may also contribute to interrupting the transmission of antibiotic-resistant strains.

History and biology of the pathogen

Streptococcus pneumoniae is a Gram-positive, lanceolate-shaped diplococcus that was isolated independently by Sternberg and Pasteur in 1881. They had inoculated human sputum into rabbits. The first demonstration of the pathogen as a cause of pneumonia was made by Friedlander in 1883. The sensitivity of the pathogen to ethylhydrocupreine (optochin) was noted in the early 1900s and the use of this agent to treat experimental pneumococcal disease was one of the first examples of antibacterial chemotherapy. The emergence of resistance following treatment was noted in that study in humans and its use was abandoned due to side-effects, including temporary blindness. The multiple serotypes of the pneumococcus are due to 90 distinct capsular polysaccharides. The pneumococcus has played a role in biology beyond that of the description of its virulence factors. The discovery of DNA as the transforming principle was based on the transformation of pneumococcal serotypes.

Adherence and pathogenesis

Newborn infants are free of pneumococcal colonization, and infections follow colonization. Colonization occurs rapidly in developing countries and, in such communities, most infants are nasopharyngeal carriers before the age of 6 months. Early colonization is associated with an increased incidence of otitis media. It is probable that multiple serotypes of pneumococci are carried simultaneously and that current methods of detection fail to identify subdominant strains. The duration of carriage varies by serotype and there is some evidence that the risk of invasive disease is greatest at the time of acquisition of a new serotype.

Pneumococci bind to specific galactose receptors on nasopharyngeal epithelial cells and pneumocytes. The bacteria undergo phase variation into transparent and opaque phenotypes. The transparent phenotype is better able to adhere to epithelial cells in the nasopharynx and adherence is enhanced by interleukin-1 (IL-1) and by tumour necrosis factor-α(TNF-α). The basis for the invasion of colonizing pneumococci is not clearly understood although preceding viral infections, such as influenza or respiratory syncytial virus infection, may be important. Influenza virus enhances the adhesion of pneumococci to respiratory cells and the binding of pneumococci to platelet activating factor is associated with invasion of activated cells. The binding of transparent phenotype pneumococci to the PAF receptor is mediated by a phosphorylcholine ligand. Other surface receptors such as pneumococcal surface adhesin A (PsaA), pneumococcal surface protein C (PspC), and choline-binding protein A (CbpA) also play a role in adhesion.

Once invasion has occurred, other components of the bacterium such as the phosphorylcholine moiety of techoeic acid C polysaccharide in the cell wall contribute to the induction of a marked acute inflammatory response. Cytokines, such as tumour necrosis factor and interleukin 1, play an important part in the pathogenesis of this inflammatory process. Reduction of the inflammatory response of animals with experimentally induced pneumococcal meningitis with drugs such as corticosteroids increases their survival, but it is not known whether this is also the case in humans (see below). Virulence may also be enhanced by pneumococcal surface protein A (PspA), and by the production of bacterial enzymes such as hyaluronidase, neuraminidase, and pneumolysin. The direct neurotoxicity of nitrous oxide may also be important in the neurological damage of pneumococcal meningitis. The pathway of pneumococcal infection is illustrated in Fig. 1 and the pathogenesis of infection is summarized in Fig. 2.

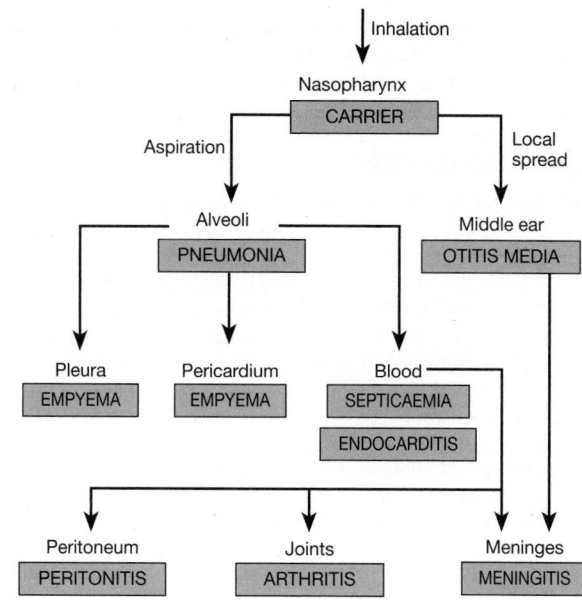

Fig. 1 The pathway of pneumococcal infection.

Antibiotic resistance

There was the emergence of a global pandemic of antibiotic resistance in the pneumococcus during the 1990s. The use of antibiotics selects resistant pneumococci at the national, provincial, hospital, and individual level. The identification of penicillin resistance in the pneumococcus was first made by Hansman and Bullen in 1967, although resistance to macrolides and tetracycline had already been described. Multiresistant pneumococci were found first in South Africa in 1978. These strains were also fully resistant to penicillin (minimum inhibitory concentration greater than 1 μg/ml). The

Fig. 2 The pathogenesis of pneumococcal infection.

selection of multiresistant strains is complex in that the differential ability of each of the antibiotic classes to select the multiresistant pathogen is not clearly understood. There are data to suggest that trimethoprim sulphamethoxazole may select for multiresistant strains more successfully than β-lactams, and reduction in the use of macrolides and trimethoprim sulphamethoxazole has been associated with a reduction in the prevalence of multiresistant pneumococci.

The nasopharyngeal carriage rate of antibiotic-resistant strains has been shown to predict closely the susceptibility of strains isolated from blood and cerebrospinal fluid. Pneumococcal nasopharyngeal carriage is seasonal with increased rates in winter. There is evidence that HIV infection increases the carriage rate of pneumococci in adults. Carriage can be reduced by the administration of conjugate pneumococcal vaccine. There is some evidence that the same total dose of antibiotic given in low daily doses for a longer period of time may increase the risk of selection of resistant strains, compared to a shorter course in a higher dose.

While β-lactam and multiple resistance in the pneumococcus now have a global distribution, recent emerging problems include very high levels of macrolide resistance in China and fluoroquinolone resistance in Canada and Hong Kong.

Mechanisms of antibiotic resistance

The molecular basis of penicillin resistance in the pneumococcus is the creation of mosaic genes of the penicillin-binding proteins (PBPs) 2X, 2B, and 1A by the transformation and horizontal transfer of DNA from related streptococcal species. The interaction of these altered gene products in the construction of the pneumococcal cell wall is not yet understood but resistant pneumococci make altered cell walls. In certain genetic backgrounds, alterations in the MurM protein may contribute to very high penicillin MICs of 8 to 16 μg/ml. Tetracycline resistance is caused by the acquisition of the tetracycline resistance determinant *tet*M or rarely *tet*O. Macrolide resistance is due to the acquisition of the methylating enzyme encoded by *erm*AM, by the acquisition of an efflux mechanism encoded by the *mef*E gene, by mutations in 23S RNA, or by mutations in the L4 riboprotein. Chloramphenicol resistance is due to the acquisition of the *cat* gene encoding chloramphenicol acetyltranferase. The acquisition of this gene has been shown to be associated with the integration and linearization of a plasmid into the pneumococcal genome. Rifampicin resistance is due to mutations in the *rpo*B gene, which may occur in one of two domains. Additional mechanisms of rifampicin resistance remain to be described. Trimethoprim resistance is caused by an altered *dhfr* chromosomal gene and is mediated by a single base mutation at position 100. Sulphonamide resistance is due to expansions in a small area of the *dhps* gene. While pneumococcal tolerance to vancomycin and other antibiotics has been described to be due to a deletion in the DNA encoding a two-component signalling system, resistance to vancomycin has not yet been described in this pathogen. Fluoroquinolone resistance is mediated by single base mutations in the *par*C gene and high levels of resistance may be obtained by a combination of mutations in the *par*C and *gyr*A genes. Mutations in the *par*E and *gyr*B genes may also contribute to pneumococcal resistance to the fluoroquinolones. The expression of a multidrug inhibitor protein *pmr*A can also confer low levels of fluoroquinolone resistance in the pneumococcus.

Serotype distribution

The distribution of pneumococcal serotypes causing invasive disease differs between children and adults. The so-called paediatric serotypes are serotypes 6A, 6B, 9V, 14, 19A, 19F, and 23F. All these serotypes commonly colonize young infants and most strains multiresistant to antibiotics belong to these serotypes. Serotypes 1 and 5, which are important invasive serotypes in developing countries, are rarely carried in the nasopharynx and thus are less commonly resistant to antibiotics—it is hypothesized that most selection for antibiotic resistance takes place in the nasopharynx. Serotype 1 is a relatively uncommon cause of invasive disease in adults in the United States but remains important in the adult population in most other parts of the world. The serotype 3 capsule is distinguished by its mucoid appearance and encapsulated type 3 pneumococci can often be distinguished from other pneumococci by visual inspection of an agar plate. There is evidence that the serotype distribution of pneumococci causing invasive disease in HIV-infected adults is different to that in adults with no HIV infection. The paediatric serotypes are more common in HIV-infected adults suggesting that these patients may have lost immunity to paediatric serotypes. Antimicrobial resistance has contributed to an increase in the proportion of paediatric serotypes causing invasive disease in both children and adults.

The capsular type is determined by a set of capsular genes. There are common genes in the regions of DNA flanking the capsular genes allowing homologous recombination to occur, and capsular switching of pneumococcal clones has been documented. In some parts of the world (especially Papua New Guinea) children are colonized at a young age with adult serotypes. The reason for the unusual distribution of serotypes in these children is not known. The distribution of serotypes in pneumococci isolated from the nasopharynx cannot be used to predict accurately the serotypes causing invasive disease because some of the most important invasive strains (notably serotypes 1 and 5) are, as mentioned above, rarely carried.

The global burden of pneumococcal disease

The global burden of pneumococcal disease is not known with certainty. However, the World Health Organization estimates that 1 million of the estimated 5 million deaths from pneumonia that occur in young children each year are caused by the pneumococcus. The incidence of pneumococcal bacteraemia in adults over 65 years of age is about 50/100 000 persons per year. The incidence of invasive pneumococcal disease is greatly increased in both adults and children by HIV infection. In South Africa, the incidence of invasive pneumococcal disease in children under the age of 2 years is 1844/100 000 per year.

Risk factors

Predisposing factors to invasive pneumococcal disease are listed in Table 1.

Diagnosis

The mainstay of the diagnosis of invasive pneumococcal disease is the isolation of the organism from a sterile site. Ten to 30 per cent of patients with pneumococcal pneumonia have a positive blood culture. Patients with suspected pneumococcal pneumonia should have an adequate volume of blood cultured because an association has been found in clinical practice between the isolation rate and the volume of blood cultured. Culture of cerebrospinal fluid remains the gold standard for the identification of *Streptococcus pneumoniae* as a cause of meningitis. Gram stain of cerebrospinal fluid and detection of capsular antigen are both useful diagnostic tests, especially when antibiotics have already been given. The definitive identification of a pneumococcal aetiology of otitis media or sinusitis requires the culture of the organism from the middle ear following tympanocentesis or the sinus following sinus puncture.

While a negative pneumococcal culture from the nasopharynx reduces the likelihood of a pneumococcal aetiology of otitis media, there is little clinical use associated with a positive nasopharyngeal culture. Nasopharyngeal cultures can be used to predict the susceptibility of invasive isolates, but they are not of much diagnostic use in individual patients. The identification of Gram-positive, lanceolate-shaped diplococci in a sputum sample

Table 1 Some important risk factors for pneumococcal pneumonia and septicaemia

Damage to the respiratory tract epithelium
Adverse climatic conditions
　　Low absolute humidity
　　Cold
Air pollution
　　Respirable particles
　　Toxic gases
Chemical
　　Anaesthetics
　　Inhaled poisons
　　Cigarette smoke
Infectious
　　Viral infections
　　Mycoplasma infections
Mechanical
　　Bronchial obstruction
Impaired systemic immunity
Hypogammaglobulinaemia
　　Congenital
　　Acquired
Splenic hypofunction
　　Traumatic
　　Sickle-cell disease
Alcoholism and drug addiction
Systemic lupus erythematosus
HIV infection

of good quality remains a useful diagnostic aid for pneumococcal pneumonia. In children the most sensitive method of diagnosing pneumococcal pneumonia is lung puncture. While this procedure carries a minimal morbidity in experienced hands, it is not widely used in clinical practice. Some promising data have recently been reported for the direct urinary detection of pneumococcal capsular polysaccharide antigens in adults. The polymerase chain reaction has not yielded a useful clinical advantage when used on blood, compared with blood culture as the gold standard. However, PCR can be used on cerebrospinal fluid to make a rapid diagnosis and can even be used directly to identify penicillin-resistant pneumococcal meningitis.

The microbiological identification of pneumococci rests on the demonstration of typical draftsman colonies producing an α-haemolytic reaction on blood agar. Pneumococci are generally optochin sensitive and are always bile soluble. Agglutination with polyvalent serum can be used to confirm their identity.

Susceptibility testing

Disc susceptibility to a 1µg oxacillin disc is the best predictor of penicillin susceptibility of the pneumococcus. Pneumococci are defined as susceptible to penicillin when they are inhibited by a minimum inhibitory concentration (**MIC**) of less than 0.1 µg/ml. A MIC of 0.1 to 1 µg/ml defines intermediate susceptibility and greater than 1 µg/ml resistance to penicillin. Resistance to amoxicillin is defined as an MIC greater than 2 µg/ml. Susceptibility to the third-generation cephalosporins, cefotaxime or ceftriaxone is defined by a MIC less than 1 ug/ml. Intermediate susceptibility and resistance to these agents are defined by MICs of 1 µg/ml and more than 1 µg/ml, respectively. The differentiation of fully resistant from intermediately penicillin-resistant pneumococci and the identification of cephalosporin-resistant pneumococci cannot be done by disc testing. The definitive method for susceptibility testing of pneumococci is by an agar dilution or micro-broth dilution method. However, many laboratories use the E test to identify penicillin- and cephalosporin-resistant pneumococci. Susceptibility testing to trimethoprim sulphamethoxazole requires the use of lysed blood. Susceptibility to most other agents is predicted by routine

disc methods, although there are currently no phenotypic methods available to detect first-step mutants that lead to fluoroquinolone resistance.

Clinical features

The clinical features of pneumococcal infection are described most conveniently in relation to the main clinical syndromes that can be caused by pneumococci. However, these syndromes are not mutually exclusive and many patients with pneumococcal disease have more than one clinical manifestation of the infection, for example pneumonia and meningitis.

Pneumonia

Pneumonia is one of the most common manifestations of pneumococcal disease.

Symptoms

In a typical case of pneumococcal pneumonia, the onset of illness is sudden, although there may be a history of a recent upper respiratory tract infection. Fever is usually the first symptom and it is frequently accompanied by rigors. The patient feels ill, anorexic, and weak. Headache and myalgia may be severe.

Chest pain usually appears during the course of illness although it may not be present on initial presentation. The pain, which results from involvement of the parietal pleura, is sharp and stabbing and is aggravated by deep inspiration or coughing. The patient may try to obtain relief by splinting the affected side of his chest with his hands or lying on the affected side. If the diaphragmatic pleura is involved, pain may be referred to the shoulder or to the abdomen.

Cough may be absent at the onset of the illness but, in most patients, it becomes a prominent symptom. Cough is initially non-productive and painful. Subsequently it becomes productive of a blood-tinged, 'rusty' sputum. Finally, the sputum becomes frankly purulent.

Among young children and elderly people, pneumococcal pneumonia may present less dramatically. The mothers of young children with pneumonia usually give a history of fever and cough and the mother may have noticed that the child has rapid respiration. Elderly patients and those who are immunocompromised may have little or no fever and few respiratory symptoms. In such patients, general malaise and confusion may be the presenting symptoms. The classic features of pneumococcal pneumonia may also be modified by prior antibiotic treatment.

Physical signs

Adult patients with lobar pneumonia are usually febrile and toxaemic. The rectal temperature may be as high as 40°C. Oral temperature may be lower because of hyperventilation. When the patient is first examined, no abnormal physical signs may be detected in the respiratory system. Later the classic signs of lobar consolidation may appear. The patient's breathing becomes rapid and distressed, and the nostrils may dilate on inspiration. Cyanosis may be present as a result of diminished alveolar ventilation or shunting of desaturated blood through the consolidated lung. Chest movement is diminished on the affected side. A dull note is obtained on percussion over the affected lobe. On auscultation, bronchial breathing is sometimes detected, fine crepitations are frequent, and a pleural rub may be heard.

General examination usually shows tachycardia and an atypical systolic murmur may be detected, as in any patient with a high fever. Examination of the abdomen may show some distension or, when the diaphragmatic pleura has been involved, upper abdominal tenderness and guarding. Jaundice may be present. The patient, especially if elderly, may be confused.

The classic signs of lobar consolidation are found infrequently in infants with pneumococcal pneumonia, although some auscultatory abnormalities, such as crepitations, can usually be detected. In young children, the most prominent features of pneumococcal pneumonia are usually a raised respiratory rate, chest-wall indrawing (Fig. 3), and nasal flaring.

Fig. 3 Severe lower-chest indrawing in a child with pneumococcal pneumonia (by courtesy of Dr Alice Greenwood).

Investigations

A polymorphonuclear neutrophil leucocytosis is usually present; a white-cell count of 15×10^9/l or more is found in about three-quarters of cases and counts as high as 40×10^9/1 may occur. A low white-cell count is associated with a poor prognosis. There may be a reticulocytosis. Both conjugated and unconjugated bilirubin levels are raised in jaundiced patients, and serum transaminases may be elevated. The Po_2 is often diminished, and measurement of the degree of hypoxaemia gives an important indication of the severity of the infection, but the Pco_2 is normal unless terminal respiratory failure occurs.

The sputum of untreated patients usually shows large numbers of Gram-positive diplococci, together with polymorphonuclear neutrophils, and culture is frequently positive for pneumococci. However, in industrialized countries, where many patients have received partial treatment before presentation at hospital, sputum microscopy is positive in only about one-quarter of patients and culture positive in only about a half. Blood culture is positive in 10 to 30 per cent of patients.

Radiographs of the chest usually show homogeneous opacification of the affected part of the lung, but may appear normal on first presentation. Posteroanterior and lateral views are required to make an accurate diagnosis of the site of the infection. A small pleural effusion can be seen in some patients. Pneumococci can cause either segmental or lobar consolidation, or patchy shadowing. The latter is encountered more frequently in children. The lower lobes are affected more frequently than the upper. In about one-third of patients, more than one lobe is involved.

Differential diagnosis

The initial febrile phase of acute pneumococcal pneumonia cannot be differentiated from that of any other acute febrile illness. Once the characteristic respiratory symptoms and signs have appeared, a diagnosis of acute pneumonia can usually be made on clinical grounds, but chest signs may be absent when the patient is first seen. In developing countries, most cases of pneumococcal pneumonia in young children are diagnosed and treated by paramedical primary health-care workers, who may have only limited diagnostic skills. For this reason the World Health Organization (**WHO**) has devised a simple diagnostic scheme, based predominantly on measurement of the respiratory rate and on observation of lower chest-wall indrawing, to help primary health-care workers determine which children with acute respiratory-tract infections probably have pneumonia and require antibiotic treatment (Table 2). This scheme has played an important part in the rationalization of the management of acute respiratory infections in developing countries, but other severe infections, including malaria, can give rise to cough and a raised respiratory rate in young children, thus fulfilling the diagnostic criteria for pneumonia. For this reason an integrated approach

Table 2 WHO criteria for the diagnosis of pneumonia in young children who present with cough or difficulty in breathing

Cough or difficulty with breathing
plus
Rapid respiration/indrawing
< 2 months > 60/min
2–11 months > 50/min
12–59 months > 40/min
Pneumonia is considered to be severe, requiring admission, if there is chest-wall indrawing and very severe if the child has cyanosis or stops feeding

to the management of childhood illness by primary health-care workers is now advocated by WHO and UNICEF. An algorithm has been developed which gives guidance on diagnosis and management; it is now being used in many developing countries.

Two important pulmonary conditions that may be confused with acute bacterial pneumonia in adult patients are infarction and atelectasis. Rigors and a high fever favour a diagnosis of pneumonia as opposed to one of infarction; a very sudden onset of symptoms and frank haemoptysis favour a diagnosis of infarction. Pulmonary atelectasis, resulting from the aspiration of mucus, may give rise to symptoms and signs that are very similar to those of pneumonia. Fever and signs of toxaemia are usually less marked in patients with atelectasis than in those with pneumonia unless the collapsed area of lung has become infected. In elderly patients, heart failure with atypical pulmonary oedema may sometimes mimic pneumococcal pneumonia.

Occasionally, subdiaphragmatic lesions such as cholecystitis, a subphrenic abscess, or an amoebic liver abscess cause a clinical picture that mimics that of lower-lobe pneumonia. Conversely, lower-lobe pneumonia, by producing abdominal pain and guarding, may suggest the diagnosis of an acute abdominal condition such as a perforated peptic ulcer, acute cholecystitis, or appendicitis.

Pneumococcal pneumonia can usually be differentiated from viral pneumonias or pneumonia caused by *Mycoplasma pneumoniae* because of its sudden onset, associated severe toxaemia, and accompanying polymorphonuclear neutrophil leucocytosis, but differentiation from other forms of acute bacterial pneumonia cannot be made without the aid of microbiological investigations. Klebsiella pneumonia, staphylococcal pneumonia, and legionnaires' disease may all produce a similar clinical picture. Confusion, signs of multisystem damage, lymphopenia, or a low serum sodium should raise the possibility of legionnaires' disease. In HIV infected patients the differential diagnosis also includes patients infected with *Pneumocystis carinii* and mycobacterial species.

Course and prognosis

Untreated patients who survive long enough to make specific anticapsular polysaccharide antibody recover spontaneously by crisis, or by a more gradual lysis, 7 to 10 days after the onset of their illness. Without treatment the mortality of acute pneumococcal pneumonia is high, especially when bacteraemia is present. Among patients treated promptly with antibiotics, overall mortality is about 5 per cent, but mortality remains as high as 30 per cent in patients with bacteraemia despite antibiotic treatment. Mortality is highest among the elderly and the very young, and among those with an associated underlying illness, such as cirrhosis, alcoholism, or heart disease. HIV infection probably increases mortality in children but this has not been found in all studies. Infection with certain pneumococcal serotypes, involvement of more than one lobe of the lung, bacteraemia, leucopenia, and jaundice are all bad prognostic signs. Most deaths from treated pneumococcal pneumonia occur within the first few days of admission to hospital. It is often difficult to establish an exact cause of death in such patients —peripheral circulatory collapse, cardiac arrhythmias, and respiratory failure are some of the contributory factors.

Complications of pneumococcal lobar pneumonia result from local or lymphatic spread of bacteria to adjacent pleura or pericardium, producing pleural or pericardial effusions, or from bacteraemic spread to meninges and other distant foci. The likelihood of one of these infective complications developing is reduced, but not completely abolished, by prompt treatment with antibiotics. Pneumococcal pneumonia may precipitate congestive cardiac failure in elderly patients and can precipitate acute dilatation of the stomach or paralytic ileus. Herpes labialis is a common accompaniment of the infection.

Pleural effusion and empyema

A large pleural effusion or an empyema develops during treatment in a small percentage (2 to 5 per cent) of patients with established pneumococcal pneumonia. Other patients present with the clinical features of pleural effusion without any preceding symptoms of pneumonia.

Symptoms

Some patients give a history suggestive of a previous parenchymatous lung infection. A history of days or weeks of fever, malaise, anorexia, and marked weight loss is often obtained. Fever may be hectic and accompanied by rigors and episodes of profuse sweating. Patients with a large pleural effusion are breathless and they may complain of dull pain on the affected side. A productive cough is unusual unless a bronchopleural fistula is present.

Physical signs

General examination shows persistent fever and tachycardia. The patient may look toxaemic and there may be signs of recent weight loss. Examination of the chest usually shows the characteristic signs of a pleural effusion—diminished chest movement, dullness of percussion, and diminished breath sounds over the accumulated fluid. The chest wall overlying an empyema may be tender.

Investigations

A persistent polymorphonuclear neutrophil leucocytosis is nearly always present. Radiographs or ultrasonography may be very helpful in localizing a loculated effusion. On aspiration, turbid fluid or thick pus is obtained, which contains pneumococci and degenerate white cells. If antibiotics have been given it may not be possible to culture pneumococci, but pneumococcal antigen can usually be detected by immunological assays.

Differential diagnosis

Association of persistent pyrexia and leucocytosis with abnormal chest signs indicates a chronic pulmonary infection. Absence of copious, purulent sputum differentiates the condition from a lung abscess. Differentiation from tuberculosis may be difficult on clinical grounds alone. Diagnosis of an empyema is confirmed by the aspiration of pus from the pleural cavity. Repeated needling with a wide-bored needle, preferably under ultrasound control, may be needed to find a loculated empyema. Pleural biopsy may provide diagnostic histology.

Course and prognosis

Untreated, an empyema may rupture through the chest wall (empyema necessitas) or rupture into a bronchus causing a bronchopleural fistula. Even when pus is aspirated and healing achieved, subsequent fibrosis and calcification may seriously restrict expansion of the underlying lung.

Pericardial effusion and empyema

Pneumococci may spread from an infected lower lobe to produce pericarditis. Pericarditis is clinically silent in some patients; in other patients it is manifest only as a transient pericardial rub or as an abnormal electrocardiogram. However, occasionally pericardial involvement is the dominant feature of a pneumococcal infection. Only a proportion of such patients give a history suggestive of an initial acute respiratory-tract infection.

Symptoms

Patients with a pneumococcal pericardial empyema usually give a history of several days, or even weeks, of persistent fever, malaise, anorexia, and weight loss. They may complain of dull or pleuritic central chest pain and they may have noted swelling of the ankles or of the abdomen.

Physical signs

Many patients with a pneumococcal pericardial empyema are critically ill by the time that they reach hospital. They are febrile and toxaemic. There may be signs of severe pericardial tamponade—a rapid, small-volume pulse, pulsus paradoxus, a low blood pressure, elevation of the jugular venous pressure with a further increase during inspiration, and peripheral oedema and ascites. Percussion of the chest may show some enlargement of the area of cardiac dullness but this is an unreliable clinical sign. The heart sounds are usually faint and, in some patients, a pericardial rub is heard.

Investigations

A peripheral blood polymorphonuclear neutrophil leucocytosis is present and blood culture may be positive for pneumococci. A chest radiograph may show globular enlargement of the heart and there may be radiological evidence of an associated lung infection. An ultrasonographic examination may help to define the best site for drainage. The electrocardiogram shows low-voltage potentials and S-T elevation or depression may be present. On aspiration of the pericardium, turbid fluid or thick pus is obtained from which pneumococci can be isolated or in which pneumococcal antigen can be detected.

Differential diagnosis

Detection of the signs of pericardial tamponade in a patient who is febrile and toxaemic should suggest a diagnosis of pericardial empyema. The condition may be confused with tuberculous constrictive pericarditis, but patients with the latter condition usually have a longer history than patients with a pneumococcal pericardial empyema and are less toxic. Staphylococci and, rarely, other pyogenic bacteria can produce a similar clinical picture to that of pneumococcal pericardial empyema. Diagnosis of a pericardial empyema is confirmed by ultrasound and by pericardial aspiration. A pneumococcal pericardial empyema is a medical emergency and, following ultrasonographic examination if this is available, pericardial aspiration should be undertaken, if necessary at more than one site, as soon as this diagnosis is seriously suspected.

Course and prognosis

Pneumococcal pericardial empyema is a serious condition with a high mortality, even in treated patients. Patients who survive the initial episode may develop constrictive pericarditis within weeks or months of their acute illness.

Otitis media

Otitis media is probably the most common form of pneumococcal infection. The condition is seen most frequently in young children but it may also affect adults.

Symptoms

The onset of an attack of acute otitis media is sudden, although there may be a history of a recent upper respiratory-tract infection. Fever and severe pain in the ear are the usual presenting complaints in adults and older children, and patients may complain of deafness and tinnitus. Fever, crying, and extreme irritability are the usual features of the condition in young children, in whom febrile convulsions may occur.

Physical signs

On examination of the affected ear, the tympanic membrane is seen to be red and swollen, and it may bulge outwards into the external ear. If perforation has occurred, the external ear may be full of pus and a ragged hole may be seen in the tympanic membrane. The affected ear is usually partially deaf. In children, meningism may be present; this must be differentiated from meningitis by lumbar puncture.

Laboratory findings

A polymorphonuclear neutrophil leucocytosis is usually found. If the drum has ruptured, pneumococci may be found in the purulent discharge present in the external ear but contaminants are likely to be present also.

Differential diagnosis

A clinical diagnosis of otitis media is rarely difficult provided that the ears of all febrile and irritable children are examined carefully. A tympanogram usually shows a characteristic pattern. The aetiology of the condition can be established by examination of fluid obtained from the middle ear with a fine needle. This technique, widely practised in some countries but not in others, may become increasingly useful as determination of the antibiotic sensitivity pattern of pneumococci becomes an essential requirement for optimum treatment of pneumococcal infections.

Course and prognosis

Prompt treatment is usually followed by a rapid and complete resolution of the infection. However, some patients, especially those in whom rupture of the drum has occurred, are left with partial conductive deafness. When untreated, pneumococcal otitis media can give rise to a chronic discharging ear requiring prolonged and complicated treatment. Spread of the infection posteriorly may result in acute mastoiditis, and spread of the infection upwards can cause pneumococcal meningitis and/or a cerebral abscess.

Pneumococcal meningitis (see also Chapter 24.14.1)

Pneumococcal meningitis may follow damage to the base of the skull, and it can occur as a complication of pneumococcal otitis media or pneumococcal pneumonia. However, many patients with this condition, the proportion varying from series to series, present with the clinical features of acute pyogenic meningitis and have no features to suggest a primary focus of pneumococcal infection.

Symptoms

Fever and headache are the usual presenting symptoms of pneumococcal meningitis. Headache usually comes on gradually over a few hours; it is generalized and may be very severe. Nausea, backache, and photophobia may develop, and convulsions may occur. Confusion may be the most prominent symptom in elderly patients, and failure to feed the first symptom in infants.

Physical signs

Patients with pneumococcal meningitis are febrile and toxaemic. Neck stiffness and a positive Kernig's sign are usually found in adults and in older children. Impairment of consciousness is often present, which varies in severity from drowsiness and confusion to deep coma. Bradycardia and hypertension may indicate the presence of raised intracranial pressure, but papilloedema is rarely seen. Bulging of the anterior fontanelle may be present in infants. Cranial nerve palsies, most frequently of the VIth or of the IIIrd cranial nerve, may be found on presentation and, occasionally, other peripheral localizing neurological signs are present.

An associated pneumococcal lesion, such as otitis media or pneumonia, may be detected. Petechiae are rarely seen. Herpes labialis may be present.

Laboratory findings

A peripheral blood polymorphonuclear neutrophil leucocytosis is usually found and a positive blood culture may be obtained.

Examination of the cerebrospinal fluid shows a turbid fluid, which usually contains an increased number of cells and many bacteria. Most of the leucocytes are polymorphonuclear neutrophils. Cerebrospinal fluid bacterial counts are often very high in patients with pneumococcal meningitis, on average 10 times higher than in patients with meningococcal meningitis. Leucocytes are present in only small numbers in the cerebrospinal fluid of some patients; in such instances the fluid may still be turbid because of the presence of numerous bacteria. The protein level in cerebrospinal fluid is increased and its glucose level decreased below that of blood. Gram stain and culture are usually positive for pneumococci.

Differential diagnosis

It is not usually difficult to establish a clinical diagnosis of pyogenic meningitis in adults and older children. However, problems may arise in the very young and in the very old; signs of meningeal irritation may be absent in both these groups of patients. Fever and irritability may be the only clinical signs of pneumococcal meningitis in an infant. The appearance of confusion may be the only sign indicating involvement of the meninges in an elderly patient with pneumococcal pneumonia. An adverse change in the psychological or neurological state of an elderly patient with pneumonia is an indication for lumbar puncture.

On clinical grounds, pneumococcal meningitis cannot be differentiated with certainty from other forms of pyogenic meningitis. An associated ear infection or pneumonia favours the diagnosis of pneumococcal infection but is not diagnostic. If petechiae are found, meningococcal meningitis is more likely. Bacteriological diagnosis of pneumococcal meningitis is confirmed by examination of the cerebrospinal fluid.

Course and prognosis

The prognosis of patients with pneumococcal meningitis is poor. Many patients make no response to treatment, their conscious level deteriorates progressively, and they die within the first 24 to 48 h after their admission to hospital. Other patients make some initial response to treatment but then relapse, their conscious level deteriorates, and new neurological signs appear. This deterioration may be due to the collection of pus in the extradural space or brain but, more usually, follows a vascular occlusion. Patients who deteriorate after an initial clinical improvement must be fully investigated to exclude the presence of a space-occupying lesion. The clinical course of survivors of the early phase of pneumococcal meningitis is often stormy, being complicated by conditions such as bedsores, pneumonia, and venous thrombosis. It has been estimated that over one-half of survivors from pneumococcal meninigitis are left with some intellectual impairment or residual neurological disability such as deafness or partial hemiplegia. Small children who survive may develop hydrocephalus. Relapses may occur when treatment is stopped. Mortality figures for pneumococcal meningitis vary from series to series but in industrialized countries the true mortality from pneumococcal meningitis is probably around 30 per cent. In developing countries, mortality figures of around 50 per cent have been found consistently. Impairment of consciousness on admission to hospital, associated pneumonia, a low white-cell count, and a high bacterial count in the cerebrospinal fluid are all poor prognostic features. Death is almost inevitable in patients who are in deep coma at the time they are admitted to hospital.

Why the prognosis of pneumococcal meningitis is so poor is uncertain. Although there is little difference in the clinical features of patients with pneumococcal or meningococcal meningitis on presentation at hospital, death is at least five times more likely in a patient with pneumococcal meningitis than in a patient with meningococcal meningitis regardless of the level of patient care available. Vascular damage, rapid multiplication of bacteria, and defective leucocyte function have all been suggested as possible causes for the poor outcome of patients with pneumococcal meningitis, but the reasons for the very poor prognosis of patients with this condition remain a mystery.

Other clinical syndromes

The pneumococcus is an important cause of bacterial sinusitis. The likelihood of a bacterial aetiology of acute sinusitis is increased if the duration of symptoms exceeds 7 days.

Acute, fulminating septicaemia is a rare form of pneumococcal infection and is encountered most frequently in patients without a spleen or in those who are immunocompromised in some way. A sudden onset of fever, peripheral circulatory collapse, and bleeding (purpura fulminans) are the usual presenting features of this condition, which is indistinguishable from other forms of overwhelming bacterial septicaemia. Leucopenia is usually found. Bleeding is due to disseminated intravascular coagulation. The mortality of this condition is very high, even when treatment is started promptly. A milder form of bacteraemia is sometimes encountered in children who present with fever or febrile convulsions without any obvious focus of pneumococcal infection (occult bacteraemia).

Acute endocarditis may complicate pneumococcal septicaemia but this condition is now encountered only rarely. Healthy heart valves, especially the aortic valve, may be attacked and rupture of the aortic valve may occur, producing severe aortic incompetence. Emboli derived from cardiac vegetations may reach the brain and other organs. Progressions of the cardiac lesions may be very rapid and the prognosis of this condition is poor. Valve replacement may be necessary for patients who survive the initial episode.

During the course of pneumococcal septicaemia, with or without endocarditis, bacteria may reach many sites where they can multiply to produce a purulent lesion. Pneumococcal arthritis, verterbral osteomyelitis, ophthalmitis, and orchitis may be produced in this way. The pneumococcus has been rarely associated with the toxic shock syndrome and with the haemolytic–uraemic syndrome.

Pneumococcal peritonitis is an uncommon condition that is encountered most frequently in patients with the nephrotic syndrome or cirrhosis of the liver, conditions frequently resulting in ascites and generalized impairment in immunity. The condition has been described also in healthy young girls, perhaps as a complication of pelvic infection, and occasionally in neonates. The condition is characterized by a sudden onset of fever, and abdominal pain and tenderness. The ascitic fluid is turbid and contains polymorphonuclear neutrophils and pneumococci. The general features of an acute infection may not be so obvious in patients with cirrhosis, and peritonitis must be considered as a possible diagnosis in any patient with this condition whose clinical state shows a sudden deterioration. The prognosis of pneumococcal peritonitis is poor in patients with a serious underlying illness.

Treatment

In the era of the antibiotic-resistant pneumococcus, the appropriate treatment of pneumococcal disease is determined by pharmocodynamic principles. These suggest that successful β-lactam therapy of invasive pneumococcal disease requires drug levels at the site of infection that exceed the MIC of the organism for at least 50 per cent of the dosing interval. The same principle applies to therapy with macrolides. Fluoroquinolones, azalides, and aminoglycosides exert a concentration-dependent killing effect on pneumococci. The best predictor of an appropriate outcome is a measure that includes both the peak concentration and time above the MIC. This is best described by the area under the drug concentration curve over 24 h ($AUC24$). The ratio of the AUC_{24} to the MIC (AUIC) predicts optimal efficacy at a value of ≥ 125. The application of these principles probably applies to all invasive diseases caused by pneumococci. Their application to the treatment of otitis media has, however, been best studied to date.

Pneumonia

Clinical studies have shown that the drug level most predictive of outcome in pneumonia is the serum concentration. Measurement of these concentrations suggests that β-lactam therapy of pneumonia will successfully treat penicillin-resistant pneumococcal pneumonia. When the drug is given in high dose intravenously is it likely that pneumonia caused by pneumococci with MICs up to 4 μg/ml will respond. A number of studies in both adults and children have shown that the most important predictors of outcome in the management of pneumococcal pneumonia are severity of disease and the presence of underlying disease. β-Lactam susceptibility does not affect outcome when adequate doses of intravenous β-lactam drugs are used to treat the infection. The optimal drugs for treating pneumococcal pneumonia are penicillin or amoxycillin. When there is a high index of suspicion of a pneumococcal aetiology in a patient with pneumonia, intravenous management with penicillin, ampicillin, or amoxycillin is appropriate (amoxycillin has higher antipneumococcal activity than ampicillin). When the aetiology of pneumonia is unclear, empirical management requires broader-spectrum cephalosporin therapy such as treatment with cefuroxime. Cefotaxime or ceftriaxone are more active against pneumococci and ought to be effective against cephalosporin-resistant pneumococcal pneumonia caused by pneumococci with cephalosporin MICs of 1 to 2 μg/ml. The clinical relevance of macrolide resistance remains unclear, but it is likely that macrolide treatment of pneumonia caused by pneumococci with MICs in a range of 1 to 2 μg/ml (*mef*E-mediated resistance) will respond to intravenous macrolide therapy. Pharmocodynamic principles suggest that higher levels of macrolide resistance are likely to result in clinical failure. Newer fluoroquinolones are under development for the management of pneumococcal pneumonia. This class of agent has, until recently, had marginal activity against the pneumococcus, but newer agents with enhanced antipneumococcal activity may be useful for the management of highly penicillin-resistant pneumococcal pneumonia in adults. There is currently no indication for the addition of vancomycin to the management of patients with pneumococcal pneumonia. There are few data on the appropriate antibiotic for oral management of antibiotic-resistant pneumococcal pneumonia and it is in this situation that very high doses of amoxycillin or the new fluoroquinolones may have their most important role.

Otitis media

While the use of antibiotics for the treatment of otitis media remains controversial, pneumococcal otitis media will resolve in a minority of cases only with appropriate antibiotic therapy. Bacterial eradication from middle ear fluid correlates well with clinical response in the management of otitis media. Oral cephalosporins with poor antipneumococcal activity are inferior to amoxycillin in their ability to eradicate bacteria from the middle ear. The choice of appropriate antibiotic therapy for the management of otitis media requires evaluation of local studies in which initial and follow-up tympanocentesis has been performed. Studies with clinical endpoints lack the ability to differentiate between highly active and poorly active agents. Current guidelines suggest that high doses of amoxycillin (90 mg/kg.day) represent the best available oral therapy for pneumococcal otitis media. Patients in whom this therapy has failed require tympanocentesis to document the cause of the failure. Should a highly penicillin-resistant pneumococcus be isolated, the appropriate therapy is intravenous or intramuscular ceftriaxone for 3 days.

Meningitis

The mainstays of therapy of pneumococcal meningitis in developing countries, namely penicillin and/or chloramphenicol, can no longer be relied upon to treat this disease, given the global epidemic of β-lactam-resistant strains. In a study from South Africa in which the usefulness of this combination was tested against penicillin-resistant, but chloramphenicol-susceptible, strains there was a poorer outcome in patients with penicillin-resistant disease compared with those with penicillin-susceptible pneumococcal meningitis. Pharmocodynamic principles suggest that penicillin and chloramphenicol are an inadequate form of therapy for even intermediately penicillin-resistant pneumococcal meningitis. The drugs of choice for the management of pneumococcal meningitis are thus cefotaxime

(300 mg/kg.day divided into 3 or 4 doses) or ceftriaxone (100 mg/kg.day divided into 2 doses). Adults should receive full doses of antibiotic. In communities where, for financial reasons, only limited amounts of cephalosporins are available, patients with pneumococcal meningitis should be given a high priority for treatment with these drugs because of the severity of this condition. In some parts of the world, strains with intermediate or full resistance to cefotaxime or ceftriaxone have emerged. In these countries the appropriate initial empiric management of meningitis includes the addition of vancomycin (60 mg/kg.day divided into 4 doses). Amongst the other available cephalosporins, ceftazidime should not be used for the management of pneumococcal meningitis. Cefepime has activity similar to that of cefotaxime and ceftriaxone, and may be used. Cefpirome has enhanced antipneumococcal activity but there are no clinical studies of the efficacy of this agent in the management of meningitis. Amongst the carbapenems, imipenem when used for meningitis is associated with an increased incidence of seizures. Two studies have demonstrated that patients treated with meropenem were not at increased risk of seizures on therapy compared with patients treated with cefotaxime. While newer fluoroquinolones are under clinical trial for the management of meningitis, there are insufficient data to recommend their use at this time.

The use of dexamethasone immediately prior to or simultaneously with the administration of cefotaxime, or ceftriaxone, appears to improve the outcome of pneumococcal meningitis in children. The use of this agent in adult pneumococcal meningitis is unproven and its use in conjunction with penicillin and/or chloramphenicol is controversial.

Other infections

There is little published information on the clinical impact of antibiotic resistance on the management of pneumococcal infections other than pneumonia, meningitis, and otitis media. The pharmocodynamic principles outlined above may be useful in guiding empiric therapy for these conditions.The principles of treatment for pneumococcal sinusitis are the same as those of otitis media. While pneumococci are intrinsically less susceptible than viridans streptococci to aminoglycosides, the addition of an aminoglycoside may have a synergistic effect on the bacterial killing rate in the treatment of pneumococcal endocarditis.

The minimum duration of therapy for invasive pneumococcal infections is under review, but the current usual duration is shown in Table 3.

Chemoprophylaxis

Children at particularly high risk of pneumococcal disease (such as those with sickle cell disease or nephrotic syndrome, or post-splenectomy) should receive regular oral penicillin prophylaxis for the first 5 years of life. The value of prophylaxis after this age is unproven, but should be considered in those who may not have responded to vaccine (such as patients with recurrent bacteraemia). Vaccination of high-risk children should be given at 2 years of age with the 23 valent vaccine. Conjugate vaccine is recommended in infancy, followed by a booter with the 23 valent vaccine at 2 years of age.

Patients who have undergone splenectomy should be educated about the risks of bacteraemia, and have prompt initiation of antibiotic therapy for febrile episodes.

Table 3 The duration of antibiotic treatment required in different forms of pnemococcal disease

5–7 days	10–14 days	4–6 weeks
Otitis media	Meningitis	Endocarditis
Pneumonia	Septicaemia	Empyema
	Sinusitis	Septic arthritis

Immunity and vaccines

The basis of immunity to invasive pneumococcal disease is thought to be the development of serotype-specific capsular antibodies of the IgG_2 subclass. These antibodies stimulate opsonophagocytosis, a process that is facilitated by the binding of complement. Previous studies of specific capsular polysaccharide antibody levels in adults have used a radioimmunoassay which detected both specific antibody and antibody to C polysaccharide. The use of C polysaccharide absorption in ELISA assays has helped to make these antibody assays more specific. The IgG response to capsular polysaccharide is poorly developed in young infants and the affinity and opsononophagocytic activity of these antibodies is reduced in older patients and patients infected with HIV.

The first attempt to develop a multivalent pneumococcal vaccine was made by Sir Spencer Lister at the South African Institute for Medical Research in 1917. Robert Austrian pioneered the development of multivalent capsular polysaccharide vaccines in the 1970s when these vaccines were shown to be effective in reducing the incidence of invasive pneumococcal disease in otherwise healthy adult gold miners. The vaccine also reduced the incidence of lobar pneumonia in miners. There is indirect evidence of the efficacy of pneumococcal polysaccharide vaccine against bacteraemia in high-risk groups of adults who have received this vaccine. The most compelling evidence comes from indirect cohort studies. There is less evidence of the efficacy of the vaccine in immunocompromised patients. Protection against pneumonia in the elderly has not been demonstrated in prospective randomized trials. Current indications for the use of the vaccine in the United States are listed in Table 4. Use of pneumococcal polysaccharide vaccines has generally been low in adults in industrialized countries, although in some there has been a recent improvement. Following the results of a trial in Uganda, which showed an increased incidence of invasive pneumococcal disease in HIV-positive subjects who had received polysaccharide vaccine, no firm recommendation about the use of this vaccine in patients who are not on antiretroviral therapy can be made before further studies are performed.

Protein vaccines are an attractive option for developing vaccines that are not serotype specific. The most promising vaccines are based on PspA and PsaA proteins which are conserved among pneumococci of various serotypes. These vaccines are in early clinical trial in humans.

In contrast to polysaccharide or protein vaccines, pneumococcal conjugate vaccines contain polysaccharide chemically linked to protein. These conjugate vaccines are immunogenic in young infants and induce immunological memory. They also reduce nasopharyngeal carriage of pneumococci of vaccine serotype, although in some studies this has been accompanied by an increase in the carriage rate of pneumococci of non-vaccine serotype. This replacement may be a function either of exogenous

Table 4 Indications for immunization with pneumococcal capsular polysaccharide vaccine recommended in the United States

Children over 2 years old
Hyposplenia including sickle-cell disease
Nephrotic syndrome
Cerebrospinal fluid leak
Immunosuppressive disorders including HIV
Other at-risk groups such as Eskimos
Adults
Those over the age of 65 years
Immunocompetent adults with an increased risk of pneumococcal disease such as those with chronic cardiovascular or pulmonary disease, diabetes, alcoholism, and cirrhosis
Immunocompromised subjects with hyposplenia, lymphoma, chronic renal failure, or nephrotic syndrome, and those on immunosuppressive drugs
Subjects with HIV infection

infection with non-vaccine strains or simply the eradication of the domin-ant strain by the vaccine thus unmasking subdominant strains. Pneumo-coccal conjugate vaccines have been shown to reduce the carriage of antibiotic-resistant pneumococci.

A number of efficacy trials of these vaccines are under way. Results from a trial conducted in California recently became available; over 90 per cent efficacy against invasive pneumococcal disease was found and significant protection, although less marked, was obtained against radiographic pneu-monia and recurrent otitis media. Because of serotype replacement the overall impact on pneumococcal otitis media was reduced further. In another study, undertaken in Finland, a conjugate vaccine reduced by 57 per cent the incidence of serotype-specific otitis media. These vaccines thus have the potential greatly to reduce mortality and morbidity from invasive pneumococcal disease and pneumonia in young infants and their availability in the first decade of the new millennium may be one of the most important public health interventions of this decade.

Further reading

Arason VA *et al.* (1996). Do antimicrobials increase the carriage rate of penicillin resistant pnuemococci in children? Cross-sectional prevalence study. *British Medical Journal* **313**, 387–91.

Chen DK *et al.* (1999). Decreased susceptibility of *Streptococcus pneumoniae* to fluoroquinolones in Canada. *New England Journal of Medicine* **341**, 233–9.

Dowson CG *et al.* (1989). Horizontal transfer of penicillin-binding protein genes in penicillin-resistant clinical isolates of *Streptococcus pneumoniae*. *Proceedings of the National Academy of Sciences, USA* **86**, 8842–6.

Friedland IR, Klugman KP (1992). Failure of chloramphenicol therapy and penicillin-resistant pneumococcal meningitis. *Lancet* **339**, 405–8.

Gillespie SH, Balakrishnan I (2000). Pathogenesis of pneumococcal infection. *Journal of Medical Microbiology* **49**, 1057 – 67.

Greenwood BM (1999). The epidemiology of pneumococcal infection in children in the developing world. *Proceedings of the Royal Society of London, Series B* **354**, 777–85.

Musher DM (1992). Infections caused by *Streptococcus pneumoniae*: the clinical spectrum pathogenesis, immunity and treatment. *Clinical Infectious Diseases* **14**, 801–9.

Pallares T *et al.* (1995). Resistance to penicillin and cephalosporin and mortality from severe pneumococcal pneumoniae in Barcelona, Spain. *New England Journal of Medicine* **333**, 474–80.

Watson DA *et al.* (1993). A brief history of the pneumococcus in biomedical research: a panoply of scientific discovery. *Clinical Infectious Diseases* **17**, 913–24.

7.11.4 Staphylococci

S. J. Eykyn

Although both Koch and Pasteur made observations on coccal organisms, the polyglot Scottish surgeon Alexander Ogston first associated cluster-forming cocci with abscesses. He presented his findings in German to the Surgical Congress in Berlin in 1880 and his classic paper *Über Abscesse* was published the same year. The Professor of Greek at Aberdeen University suggested the name 'staphylococcus' for the organism (*staphyle*—bunch of grapes; *kokkos*—berry) to distinguish it from the chain-forming strepto-cocci. Rosenbach divided the genus *Staphylococcus* into *Staphylococcus aur-eus* and *S. albus*. Ogston's coccus was of course *S. aureus*.

Table 1 Classification of *Staphylococcus* spp. associated with human infection

Family	Genus	Species
	Staphylococcus	
	Coagulase-positive	*S. aureus*
	Coagulase-negative	*S. auricularis*
		S. capitis
		S. cohnii
		S. epidermidis
		S. haemolyticus
Micrococcaceae		*S. hominis*
Catalase-positive		*S. lugdunensis*
Gram-positive		*S. saccharolyticus*
cocci in clusters		*S. saprophyticus*
		S. schleiferi
		S. simulans
		S. warneri
	Micrococcus	
	Stomatococcus	
	Planococcus	

Taxonomy

Staphylococci are Gram-positive cluster-forming cocci. There are some 32 recognized species of the genus *Staphylococcus* but only about half are of human origin (Table 1). Staphylococci are skin commensals of mammals and birds and some species, particularly *S. aureus*, are important human pathogens. In the clinical laboratory *S. aureus* is distinguished from other staphylococci by its ability to coagulate plasma. The slide coagulase test detects cell-associated clumping factor (bound coagulase), which reacts with fibrinogen to cause aggregation of the organisms. Commercial kits are used for this test and some also detect protein A, present in most strains of *S. aureus*. Occasional strains do not produce clumping factor or protein A, and certain other species of staphylococci produce clumping factor, hence the gold standard for the identification of *S. aureus* in the laboratory is the tube coagulase test in which staphylococci are mixed with plasma in a test tube. This detects extracellular coagulase (free coagulase), which activates prothrombin and initiates clot formation. The slide coagulase test is used to screen organisms, whereas the tube test is confirmatory and of more taxo-nomic significance. Other useful screening tests for *S. aureus* are the detec-tion of DNAase activity and fermentation of mannitol, but neither is as reliable as the tube coagulase test.

Many clinical laboratories report any coagulase-negative staphylococcus other than *S. saprophyticus* as *S. epidermidis* without formal speciation and some still refer to these bacteria as '*Staph. albus*'. Availability of commercial identification kits has enabled speciation of coagulase-negative staphylo-cocci in the routine laboratory though this is seldom undertaken routinely. Most clinical isolates are *S. epidermidis* (*sensu stricto*) or *S. saprophyticus* but several other species such as *S. lugdunensis* can occasionally be import-ant pathogens.

Typing

Epidemiological studies of *S. aureus* infection, and increasingly these con-cern methicillin-resistant strains (**MRSAs**), require typing methods to dis-tinguish between epidemic and endemic strains. Typing can also confirm the correlation between specific staphylococcal infections and a particular type of the organism. In many countries including the United Kingdom such studies still rely on bacteriophage typing. Phage typing has been organized internationally since 1953. The basic international set of phages consists of 23 phages (Table 2). There are four major phage groups—I, II, III, and V—and staphylococci may be lysed by a single phage from one group, more than one phage from a single group, or by phages from more

Table 2 International phage typing scheme for *S. aureus*

Phage group	Individual phages
I	29, 52, 52A, 79, 80
II	3A, 3C, 55, 71
III	6, 42E, 47, 53, 54, 75, 77, 83A, 84, 85
V	94, 96
Unclassified	81, 95

than one group. The internationally recognized gold standard for discriminating between strains of *S. aureus* is pulse field gel electrophoresis (**PFGE**), a DNA finger printing technique. It is neither necessary nor feasible to use PFGE for typing all strains of *S. aureus* as most can be satisfactorily differentiated by phage typing. Epidemic MRSAs are designated specific numerical types (1 to 17) as well as phage types. Phage typing is much less satisfactory for coagulase-negative staphylococci and has largely been abandoned. Epidemiological studies on these bacteria are seldom required in clinical practice but could be done by PFGE.

Staphylococcus aureus

Pathogenicity

S. aureus produces a remarkable variety of extracellular substances that include: general toxic agents such as catalase, hyaluronidase, lipase, and membrane-damaging toxins that may be involved in the pathogenesis of local or systemic inflammation; and specific toxins such as enterotoxins and epidermolytic toxins that mediate particular non-suppurative diseases.

Membrane-damaging toxins

S. aureus produces five toxins that disrupt cell membranes—α-, β-, γ-, and δ- toxins and leucocidin. Many of these toxins disrupt red cell membranes producing haemolysis. The most extensively studied is α-toxin, which is formed by most strains and produces impressive biological effects; it is cytotoxic and necrotizing, kills leucocytes, lyses platelets, releases catecholamines, and causes renal cortical necrosis yet remarkably its specific role in staphylococcal infection in humans has yet to be defined.

Enterotoxins

There are now 11 staphylococcal enterotoxins—types A, B, D, E, G, H, I, and J which show major antigenic differences and type C which is subdivided into C1, C2, and C3 on the basis of minor antigenic differences. Enterotoxins G, H, I, and J were only described recently and have not yet been confirmed as emetic in humans. Enterotoxin F is identical to toxic shock syndrome toxin 1 and is now known as TSST-1. About 40 per cent of *S. aureus* produce enterotoxin, sometimes of more than one type. Staphylococcal food poisoning results from the ingestion of foods containing preformed enterotoxin. Most outbreaks in the United Kingdom are caused by enterotoxin A with or without D (see Table 3). Staphylococcal enterotoxins have a range of biological activities in addition to their ability to induce vomiting; they are pyrogenic, mitogenic, and can produce thrombocytopenia and hypotension.

Epidermolytic toxins

These toxins cause intraepidermal splitting and are responsible for the scalded skin syndrome and the blistering of impetigo. The production of epidermolytic toxin is particularly associated with (though not confined to) *S. aureus* of phage group II. There are two epidermolytic toxins, ETA which is heat stable and under chromosomal control, and ETB which is heat labile and plasmid-mediated, and most phage group II staphylococci produce ETA or both ETA and ETB.

Table 3 Enterotoxin production by strains of *S. aureus* implicated in 359 outbreaks of food poisoning in the United Kingdom (1969 to 1990)[*]

Enterotoxin produced	Strains positive
A	205 (57%)
B	6
C	5
D	15
E	3
A and B	12
A and C	9
A and D	55 (15%)
A, B and D	4
B and D	1
C and D	28 (8%)
None (not A–E)	16

[*] From Wieneke AA, Roberts D, Gilbert RJ (1993). Staphylococcal food poisoning in the United Kingdom. *Epidemiology and Infection* **110**, 519–31.

Toxic shock syndrome toxin (TSST-1)

This toxin is responsible for the toxic shock syndrome (**TSS**). Most cases of menstrually associated TSS are mediated by TSST-1 produced by *S. aureus* of phage group I, usually phage 29 or 52; TSS not associated with menstruation can occur with strains producing TSST-1, but also with phage group V strains that produce enterotoxin B.

Carriage

S. aureus is part of the normal flora in some individuals; about 25 per cent of people 'carry' the organism permanently, a similar proportion never do, and the rest do so intermittently. Common carriage sites are the nose, axilla, perineum, and toe webs. Nasal carriage rates vary from 10 to 40 per cent in normal adults outside hospital, but higher rates are often found in patients in hospital, particularly those who have been in hospital for several weeks. High carriage rates are also found in those with skin diseases such as eczema, those with insulin-dependent diabetes, patients on chronic haemodialysis or chronic ambulatory peritoneal dialysis, intravenous drug users, and HIV-positive patients. Some carriers, designated 'shedders', disperse large numbers of staphylococci into the environment on skin squamas. The carrier state is highly relevant to the epidemiology of *S. aureus* infection as to whether or not this complicates surgery or trauma and the source of the *S. aureus* in most patients who develop staphylococcal infection is endogenous.

Host factors in *S. aureus* infection

Intact skin and mucous membranes are important defences against staphylococcal infection. Wounds, whether traumatic or surgical, frequently become colonized with *S. aureus*, which may result in localized infection or in dissemination via the bloodstream to distant sites. Sometimes trivial, even unrecognized, skin trauma precedes such haematogenous spread. Burns and skin diseases are also important portals of entry for staphylococci. Certain viral infections such as influenza damage the respiratory epithelium and allow secondary staphylococcal invasion. Foreign material including intravascular devices, arteriovenous shunts, and vascular and orthopaedic prostheses is also relevant to the pathogenesis and perpetuation of staphylococcal infection.

Once *S. aureus* gains access to the tissues, polymorphs are the most important line of defence. Phagocytosis involves chemotaxis, opsonization, and intracellular killing. Chemotactic defects occur, for example, in Job syndrome (in which patients with recurrent eczema suffer from repeated skin infections and cold abscesses with *S. aureus*) and also in certain other rare syndromes. Opsonic defects tend to predispose to a variety of pyogenic infections, including, but not specifically, *S. aureus* infection, but *S. aureus* is a major pathogen in chronic granulomatous disease producing local and metastatic abscesses. In this disease, intracellular killing by the polymorphs is defective.

Susceptibility of *S. aureus* to antibiotics and antiseptics

Resistance to antibiotics is not a marker for virulence in *S. aureus* and strains that are sensitive to all antistaphylococcal antibiotics, including penicillin, can cause severe community-acquired infections. However, *S. aureus* has a record of rapid and successful development of resistance to antibiotics. Most isolates, whether acquired in the community or in hospital, produce penicillinase (β-lactamase) and are thus resistant to penicillin itself and related compounds including ampicillin and amoxycillin. Staphylococcal β-lactamase has a negligible effect on methicillin, cloxacillin, and flucloxacillin, which were sequentially introduced specifically for the treatment of staphylococcal infection. Methicillin-resistant strains of *S. aureus* (MRSAs) were detected soon after the introduction of methicillin in 1960, and reports of their isolation increased until 1971 when they accounted for some 5 per cent of strains submitted to the Staphylococcus Reference Laboratory of the Central Public Health Laboratory in the United Kingdom. MRSAs then diminished in frequency in the United Kingdom, possibly as a result of increased prescribing of aminoglycosides, but there was a resurgence in the early 1980s and for some years now virtually all hospitals have patients who are colonized or infected with MRSAs. MRSAs are usually, but not always, resistant to a variety of other antibiotics in addition to methicillin, and are resistant to all cephalosporins. *S. aureus* other than MRSA, whether penicillinase producing or not, are sensitive to many cephalosporins, though the newer third-generation cephalosporins, such as ceftazidime, are much less active than cefuroxime and cefotaxime. The incidence of erythromycin resistance relates to its use and varies from about 5 to 20 per cent. Gentamicin resistance is unusual, except in MRSA. Resistance of *S. aureus* to fusidic acid is uncommon, but most cultures contain a few resistant mutants and a fully resistant population can emerge, particularly after topical use. Since 1996 MRSAs of reduced sensitivity to vancomycin have been reported from Europe, Asia, and the United States. Such strains are referred to by the acronyms 'VISA' (vancomycin-intermediate *S. aureus*) and 'GISA' (glycopeptide-intermediate *S. aureus*); GISA is the more appropriate as these strains are of intermediate resistance to both the glycopeptide drugs vancomycin and teicoplanin, but the term glycopeptide is less familiar to clinicians. The emergence of such resistance is of concern as glycopeptides are extensively used for MRSA infections. However VISA/GISA and other MRSAs are sensitive to quinupristin/dalfopristin (Synercid) and the oxazolidinone Linezolid Rifampicin is highly active against *S. aureus*, but as with fusidic acid, minority populations of resistant cells are found and resistance may emerge during treatment.

The topical antibiotic mupirocin (Bactroban) is active against many *S. aureus* although unfortunately in some hospitals mupirocin resistance is common thus limiting the use of mupirocin to eradicate MRSA from the nose and other superficial sites. Most disinfectants and antiseptics inhibit or kill *S. aureus*. Chlorhexidine, hexachlorophane, triclosan, and iodine-containing compounds such as povidone iodine are all used for skin disinfection and when used correctly are highly effective in removing staphylococci from the skin.

Prevention of spread of *S. aureus*

Although any strain of *S. aureus* can spread between people whether patients or staff, measures to control spread are now largely directed at the nosocomial spread of MRSAs. MRSAs have caused innumerable hospital outbreaks in many countries; sometimes these outbreaks have involved colonization rather than infection, but severe infection is increasingly encountered and the MRSA has become the scourge of elective surgery in some hospitals. Several distinct strains have caused epidemics and the prevalent type varies: in the United Kingdom overall type 15 is most common, but in London the incidence of types 15 and 16 is equal. Epidemic strains not only spread readily but can cause severe invasive infection. Colonization with MRSA is a notoriously recalcitrant problem in hospitals, particularly on elderly care units, and is also an increasing problem in nursing and residential homes. Eradication of MRSA from the nose and from some surface lesions is readily achieved with topical agents such as mupirocin, but it is virtually impossible to eradicate MRSA from the throat, sputum, or from sites associated with a foreign body such as an indwelling catheter or tracheostomy unless these are removed. Repeated careful handwashing by all staff in contact with patients is the single most effective measure in preventing spread of staphylococci.

Clinical manifestations

S. aureus usually causes localized infection, sometimes with local spread, but this may result in bacteraemia and dissemination of the infection. Certain staphylococcal syndromes are produced by extracellular toxins rather than local invasion and will be considered separately.

Localized infections

Infection of the skin and its appendages
These infections often arise in association with hair follicles, and minor trauma, maceration, and skin diseases also predispose to them. Folliculitis is a superficial infection of the hair follicle commonly caused by *S. aureus*. Boils (furuncles) are deep-seated infections around a hair follicle usually on the neck, axilla, buttock, or thigh, often recurrent, and sometimes involving more than one member of a family. When several adjacent hair follicles are involved a carbuncle develops, usually on the back of the neck, with multiple draining sinuses and systemic disturbance. Although boils are very common, carbuncles are now rarely seen. Impetigo is a blistering skin lesion with crusting exudate affecting exposed areas (often the face) usually in children. Epidermolytic toxin is associated with these infections. Most acute paronychias are caused by *S. aureus*. Mastitis and breast abscess in the puerperium are caused by *S. aureus* as are many non-puerperal breast abscesses. Newborn babies commonly suffer from staphylococcal infection, with septic spots, 'sticky umbilicus', 'sticky eye', and occasionally breast abscess, as well as the much rarer toxin-mediated staphylococcal diseases. Styes, purulent infections of the glands of the eyelid, are caused by *S. aureus*.

Wound infection
S. aureus is the commonest cause of wound infection after surgery or trauma that does not involve the mucous membranes with their rich anaerobic commensal flora. Staphylococcal wound infection varies from minimal erythema and serous discharge, through small abscesses often in relation to sutures, to marked cellulitis, deep pus, and wound dehiscence with pain and systemic disturbance. It is of particular concern after operations involving prosthetic material such as joint or vascular prostheses or heart valves as the infection can extend from the wound to infect the prosthesis with disastrous results.

Ear, nose, and throat infection
Staphylococcal infection of the hair follicles or sebaceous glands in the outer external auditory canal causes acute localized otitis externa with severe pain and itching. Acute otitis media and sinusitis are seldom caused by *S. aureus*. Although *S. aureus* is commonly grown from throat swabs, it behaves as a commensal at this site, and such patients have usually been taking antibiotics.

Pleuropulmonary infection
Staphylococcal pneumonia arises either from aspiration or by haematogenous spread with metastatic seeding of the lung. Aspiration pneumonia generally complicates pre-existing lung disease or viral respiratory disease, usually influenza. In children, other viral infections of the respiratory tract, including severe measles in developing countries, may be followed by secondary bacterial infection with staphylococci. *S. aureus* from carriage sites

presumably reaches the damaged lung tissue via the trachea and bronchi. In contrast to aspiration pneumonia, haematogenous staphylococcal pneumonia characteristically affects a previously normal lung. There may sometimes be an identifiable local infection, often of the skin and usually trivial, that has resulted in haematogenous seeding or there may be evidence of release of infected thrombi via the venous system as in tricuspid endocarditis or occasionally when there is an infected intravascular device. Staphylococci can usually be isolated from the blood in haematogenous pneumonia, though seldom in aspiration pneumonia. Whatever its pathogenesis, *S. aureus* pneumonia is a severe disease. When secondary to influenza, it may occur without an obvious influenza-like prodromal illness and with alarming suddenness (Fig. 1(a and b)). It is usually complicated by abscess formation, empyema, and in children, by pneumatoceles and pyopneumothorax, but the radiological findings at initial presentation vary from local

Fig. 1 Chest radiograph of a 24-year-old man with severe staphylococcal pneumonia. (a) on admission and (b) 13 days later. The patient was also suffering from influenza B.

consolidation, to multiple patchy infiltrates, and abscess formation may or may not be detected.

Urinary tract infection

S. aureus urinary tract infection is uncommon and unlikely to occur in patients with a normal urinary tract except in staphylococcal bacteraemia with microabscesses in the kidney as may occur in staphylococcal endocarditis. *S. aureus* urinary infection sometimes occurs in patients with abnormal bladder function but in association with instrumentation or catheterization, presumably from previous urethral colonization with the strain.

Bacteraemia, septicaemia, and metastatic (haematogenous) infection

Bacteraemia in the strict sense means bacteria in the blood, that is, a positive blood culture. This may or may not be symptomatic in the patient. A symptomatic bacteraemia is referred to as a septicaemia. In fact, *S. aureus* in the blood is almost always symptomatic and thus strictly a septicaemia, but the terms tend to be used interchangeably adding to the confusion. Bacteraemia will be used here.

Community-acquired bacteraemia

In most patients who acquire *S. aureus* bacteraemia in the community the staphylococcus has entered the bloodstream from a carrier site or from a trivial unnoticed abrasion and seldom from a defined local lesion. Such bacteraemia then results in serious deep-seated infection. Such bacteraemias have been called 'primary' and are usually much more severe than those secondary to a defined focus of infection. Primary bacteraemia can occur at any age, and often in a previously healthy individual. Such patients may, but often do not, present with initial infection at a specific site. An ill patient with a community-acquired *S. aureus* bacteraemia and no detectable focus of infection will generally have endocarditis (see below).

Hospital-acquired bacteraemia

Nosocomial *S. aureus* bacteraemia usually results from an infected intravascular access site and this is as likely to be a peripheral cannula as a central catheter. There will often be obvious infection at the insertion site, but sometimes only minimal local signs with severe systemic disturbance. Such bacteraemias can result in metastatic infection involving bone, joint, lung, or heart valve. These disastrous iatrogenic sequelae of intravenous access are increasing. Nosocomial bacteraemia also sometimes occurs with severe wound sepsis.

Endocarditis

S. aureus endocarditis is a devastating illness often occurring in a previously healthy individual, but an asymptomatic left-sided valvular abnormality such as a bicuspid aortic valve or mitral leaflet prolapse is sometimes present. The infection typically presents as an influenza-like illness, often with gastrointestinal disturbance. Meningism is seen in about 25 per cent of cases and polymorphs, though seldom organisms, are detected in the cerebrospinal fluid. There may be systemic emboli. Valvular insufficiency can develop within days, sometimes hours, of admission. Staphylococcal endocarditis is a rapidly destructive disease, justifiably called malignant endocarditis by Osler.

The skin manifestations can be mistaken for meningococcal infection (Fig. 2(a and b)). Figure 3(a) and (b) show another fatal staphylococcal infection in a previously healthy 54-year-old man who was febrile and confused at presentation and hemiplegic within 48 h. Blood and CSF (which contained 5000 polymorphs) grew *S. aureus*.

Staphylococcal endocarditis is occasionally complicated by splenic abscess (Fig. 4). Intravenous drug users are at particular risk of staphylococcal endocarditis, but unless the affected individual has a previous valvular abnormality, the infection is likely to involve the tricuspid valve and present with fever, malaise, and respiratory signs that result from septic pulmonary emboli.

Bone and joint infections

S. aureus is the commonest cause of acute bone and joint infection. These infections can result from a 'primary' bacteraemia, but also from a contiguous focus of infection after trauma or surgery, especially that involving prosthetic implants. The overall incidence of acute haematogenous osteomyelitis has decreased but there has also been a change in its localization. Osteomyelitis of the long bones seen primarily in children, particularly boys, is now uncommon, but vertebral osteomyelitis has increased or is increasingly recognized. Patients with staphylococcal vertebral osteomyelitis are usually middle aged or elderly. This shift in the localization of the infection has not been explained. Vertebral osteomyelitis can be a notoriously difficult diagnosis, repeatedly referred to in the literature as a 'diagnostic pitfall'. Pain, not always localized to the spine is the only consistent feature. Fever is sometimes absent but at least if present should initiate a blood culture, which is likely to be positive whatever the temperature. Any patient with backache, a high C-reactive protein and erythrocyte sedimen-

(a)

(b)

Fig. 3 Meningococcaemic-like disease. (a) Hand and (b) foot of a man with primary staphylococcal bacteraemia and meningitis who had disseminated intravascular coagulation.

Fig. 2 Meningococcaemic-like infection in a 22-year-old man who died from an aortic root abscess from *S. aureus* endocarditis on a bicuspid aortic value. A false-positive meningococccaemic latex agglutination test on the cerebrospinal fluid (which contained 1500 polymorphs, but no organisms) taken on admission further increased the clinical confusion.

Fig. 4 Splenic abscess complicating staphylococcal endocarditis.

tation rate, and *S. aureus* in the blood should be assumed to have vertebral infection.

Staphylococcal septic arthritis may occur in previously normal or abnormal joints and at any age. It may involve one or more joints and multiple infection can occur in patients with previous joint pathology such as rheumatoid arthritis, when it may be difficult to diagnose.

Renal cortical abscess (carbuncle) and perinephric abscess

These metastatic staphylococcal infections are rare and usually cause diagnostic confusion. A renal cortical abscess, also known as a carbuncle, is a multilocular abscess involving the renal parenchyma, the result of the coalescence of cortical microabscesses from haematogenous seeding of the kidney from a previous infection, typically a boil, with *S. aureus*. The patient complains of fevers and loin pain but urinary symptoms are usually absent and unless the abscess communicates with the excretory system, the urine contains neither pus cells nor *S. aureus*. Although *S. aureus* is the commonest pathogen in renal carbuncle, perinephric abscesses—those external to the renal capsule but within the perinephric fascia—are more commonly caused by Gram-negative aerobes such as *Escherichia coli* or *Proteus* spp. than staphylococci. A renal carbuncle may rupture into the perinephric space producing a perinephric abscess. Again, urine cultures are unlikely to be positive and the signs are similar to those of a renal carbuncle.

Pyomyositis

See Chapter 24.22.6 for discussion.

Infections mediated by toxins of *S. aureus*

Staphylococcal food poisoning

This syndrome, characterized by vomiting, nausea, abdominal cramps, and diarrhoea, is caused by the ingestion of staphylococcal enterotoxin preformed in the food. The onset occurs within hours of ingestion of food contaminated during its preparation by an individual infected with, or shedding, an enterotoxin-producing staphylococcus. Unrefrigerated protein-rich foods containing meat or milk are likely to support the growth of staphylococci and the subsequent production of heat-stable enterotoxin. Only about 5 per cent of outbreaks of bacterial food poisoning reported to the Communicable Disease Surveillance Centre for which an aetiological agent is identified are caused by *S. aureus*. The diagnosis can be confirmed by culturing incriminated food, any skin lesions, the nose of food handlers, and the stools of the victims. In most outbreaks, both the organism and its toxin can be defined, but occasionally, enterotoxin alone is demonstrated in the food.

Staphylococcal scalded skin syndrome

This rare disease, originally known as Ritter's disease when it was first seen in infants in the late nineteenth century, is more commonly seen in children (Fig. 5) than adults (Fig. 6). It is characterized by the sudden onset of extensive erythema followed by bullous desquamation of large areas of skin. It is caused by the epidermolytic toxins of *S. aureus*. The disease of scalded skin syndrome must be distinguished from a similar clinical entity unassociated with *S. aureus*, that of toxic epidermal necrolysis (Lyell's syndrome) which occurs in older children and adults and results from drug hypersensitivity. Histologically the two diseases can be readily distinguished as in scalded skin syndrome there is intraepithelial splitting at the level of the stratum granulosum and in toxic epidermal necrolysis there is total epidermal loss with separation at the dermal–epidermal junction.

Staphylococcal toxic shock syndrome (TSS)

This syndrome (Fig. 7) of high fever, mental confusion, erythroderma, diarrhoea, hypotension, and renal failure was first defined in children in 1978, but had been described 50 years earlier and thought to be staphylococcal scarlet fever. In the late 1970s there was an epidemic of toxic shock syndrome in women associated with menstruation and tampon use, initially, and predominantly, in the United States, but later, though in far fewer

Fig. 5 Staphylococcal scalded skin syndrome in a child. (Reproduced by courtesy of Professor W.C. Noble.)

numbers, in other countries. Toxic shock syndrome has also been described in women who were not menstruating and in men in association with a wide variety of conditions and operations including burns in children. Toxic shock syndrome may be fatal and a mortality rate of around 5 per cent was reported during the 'tampon epidemic'. Since the syndrome is mediated by toxin, the mainstay of treatment is supportive. Antistaphylococcal antibiotics should be given to eradicate *S. aureus* from the local site. Bacteraemia has rarely been reported in toxic shock syndrome. The staphylococci isolated are usually resistant only to penicillin.

Laboratory diagnosis of *S. aureus* infection

S. aureus is readily isolated in the laboratory. A Gram-stained film may enable a rapid diagnosis of a staphylococcal aetiology; the characteristic clumps of Gram-positive cocci, often intracellular as well as extracellular and sometimes of variable size, are readily identifiable. The diagnosis can

Fig. 6 Staphylococcal scalded skin syndrome in an adult.

be confirmed by culture within 18 to 24 h. Staphylococcal bacteraemia is readily detected by routine blood culture methods. The isolation of *S. aureus* from blood is almost always indicative of a genuine bacteraemia and the organism should only be dismissed as a contaminant if the patient has extensive skin disease such as eczema, rarely otherwise.

Treatment

Drainage of any pus is an essential prerequisite of the management of *S. aureus* infection. This may occur spontaneously or with only minor surgical intervention in most superficial infections such as boils, paronychias, styes, and stitch abscesses. Deep abscesses in wounds or organs and osteomyelitis that has progressed to the point of pus formation require definitive surgical drainage. Infections associated with intravascular devices or other prosthetic material seldom resolve with antibiotics and removal of the foreign material is usually required.

Antibiotics are indicated if the patient is systemically unwell or the infection is spreading and sometimes when given early in the course of a potentially localizing pyogenic infection may arrest its progress. They are of no benefit in staphylococcal food poisoning but should be given in scalded skin syndrome and toxic shock syndrome to eradicate toxin-producing *S. aureus*. The initial choice of agent for staphylococcal infection before sensitivities become available depends on whether the staphylococcus was acquired in the community or in hospital. For community-acquired infections a β-lactamase-resistant penicillin such as flucloxacillin or cephalosporin such as cefuroxime will be appropriate initial treatment and

Fig. 7 Toxic shock syndrome. Desquamation of (a) hand and (b) feet in a girl with tampon-associated disease. (Reproduced by courtesy of Dr D.C. Shanson.)

probably also definitive therapy. Penicillin is suitable only if the strain does not produce β-lactamase, and should never be used for the initial 'blind' treatment. Similar constraints apply to ampicillin and amoxicillin. Alternative agents to β-lactams for community-acquired infection when the patient is hypersensitive to penicillin include the macrolides erythromycin, clarithromycin, and azithromycin. Fusidic acid is an excellent antistaphylococcal agent although resistance may arise during treatment, especially when the organism cannot readily be eradicated. When the infection is acquired in hospital and the patient is unwell, in most hospitals it should be assumed to be an MRSA until cultures prove otherwise. The only agents with reliable activity against MRSA are vancomycin, teicoplanin, the combination drug quinupristin/dalfopristin (Synercid), and the oxazolidinone Linezolid. Most staphylococcal infection is satisfactorily treated with a single antibiotic. Combination therapy is often used for serious infections such as endocarditis and bone or joint infection but there is minimal evidence of any advantage over a single agent.

The length of the antibiotic course to treat staphylococcal infection is unknown, but for serious infections such as endocarditis, bone and joint infections, and pneumonia several weeks' treatment may be needed. For most other infections, antibiotics should be given until there is clinical improvement or for about 48 h after fever has resolved. Most patients are treated for too long inviting side-effects. Blood cultures that are persistently positive for *S. aureus* despite appropriate antibiotic therapy are seldom an indication for changing the antibiotics, but rather for an assessment of the need for intervention, for example to remove an infected intravascular device, excise an infected heart valve, or aspirate and wash out an infected joint. Topical antibiotics and antiseptics are useful for the treatment of staphylococcal skin infections.

Coagulase-negative staphylococci

Coagulase-negative staphylococci are the commonest contaminants in the laboratory, particularly, though not exclusively, in blood cultures, but they can also be important pathogens whose incidence continues to increase. The availability of commercial kits for their speciation has served to emphasize that they cannot be regarded as a homogeneous entity; the different species vary not only in their incidence in clinical infections but also in the type and severity of disease produced. Most infections with coagulase-negative staphylococci are hospital acquired, but certain species cause severe community-acquired infection.

Pathogenicity

Coagulase-negative staphylococci (usually *S. epidermidis*) that cause infections associated with prosthetic devices and intravascular catheters produce an exopolysaccharide ('slime') which is important in enabling these organisms to adhere to plastic material and probably also in their resistance to phagocytosis, other host defences, and to antimicrobial action. Coagulase-negative staphylococci from clinical infections produce a variety of potential toxins including haemolysins, cytotoxins, deoxyribonuclease, fibrinolysin, proteinase, and lipase-esterase, similar to those produced by *S. aureus*, and infection caused by some species, especially *S. lugdunensis* and *S. simulans*, mimics that caused by *S. aureus*.

Carriage

Coagulase-negative staphylococci, together with coryneforms, comprise most of the human skin flora. Many different species are found on the skin but the commonest is *S. epidermidis*; *S. hominis* and *S. haemolyticus* are also common. Distribution of species varies on different skin areas: the predominant species on the head and trunk is *S. epidermidis*, on the arms and legs it is *S .hominis*, and as its name suggests *S. capitis* is found mainly on the head. There are also geographical variations.

Host factors in coagulase-negative staphylococcal infection

Most infection with coagulase-negative staphylococci is associated with prosthetic material both in immunocompromised and non-immunocompromised patients. Infection of intravascular catheters arises via the catheter access site or the catheter hub from frequent disconnections. Prosthetic material can also become infected at implantation.

Antibiotic susceptibility

Hospital-acquired coagulase-negative staphylococci, particularly *S. epidermidis* and *S. haemolyticus*, are usually multiply resistant. Most are resistant to methicillin (and thus to cephalosporins), and many to gentamicin and erythromycin. Thus the usual nosocomial strain of coagulase-negative staphylococcus has an antibiotic susceptibility pattern akin to many MRSAs. Rare resistance to vancomycin and teicoplanin has been reported, initially in *S. haemolyticus*. In marked contrast to hospital-acquired infections those acquired in the community are usually caused by very sensitive strains; many are sensitive to penicillin.

Infections caused by coagulase-negative staphylococci

Most infections caused by coagulase-negative staphylococci are acquired in hospital and are increasingly common. They usually arise in association with an intravascular or prosthetic device or implant. Infection with more than one strain may occur in nosocomial infections.

Community-acquired infections though rare are probably increasing or increasingly recognized and are usually severe. In most community-acquired infections, repeated isolation of the same coagulase-negative staphylococcus from the blood is essential for the diagnosis, and true bacteraemia must be distinguished from contamination.

Intravascular devices

There has been a marked increase in infection of intravascular devices with coagulase-negative staphylococci, particularly in neonates and immunocompromised patients, and they are the commonest bacteria in such infections. The degree of systemic disturbance varies, and this should determine the approach to treatment. In contrast to infections of intravascular devices caused by *S. aureus* for which it is usually necessary to remove the device to control the infection, with those caused by coagulase-negative staphylococci the catheter can often be left *in situ* and the infections controlled with antibiotics. If this fails, the device must be removed. Very occasionally, as with *S. aureus*, persistent bacteraemia can result in metastatic seeding of a heart valve or vertebral body.

Cerebrospinal fluid shunts

Coagulase-negative staphylococci, predominantly *S. epidermidis*, are the commonest cause of infection of cerebrospinal fluid shunts and these infections can present weeks, months, or years after the shunt insertion. They also cause infection of cerebrospinal fluid reservoirs used for chemotherapy. Signs of meningitis may be absent and usual findings include low-grade fever, malaise, and shunt malfunction. Serum antibodies to *S. epidermidis* can be used to monitor treatment and detect relapse. Treatment may require removal of the shunt and antibiotics, usually vancomycin with rifampicin, are best given intraventricularly. Occasionally, glomerulonephritis ('shunt nephritis') occurs in patients with colonized shunts as a result of deposition of immune complexes on the basement membranes of the glomeruli.

Peritonitis associated with continuous ambulatory peritoneal dialysis

Coagulase-negative staphylococci, predominantly *S. epidermidis*, are the commonest cause of peritonitis associated with continuous ambulatory peritoneal dialysis. The bacteria probably gain access to the peritoneum as a result of manipulation of the catheter connections. Patients have abdominal pain, occasionally nausea, diarrhoea, and fever, and abundant polymorphs in the dialysate in which Gram-positive cocci, usually scanty and intracellular, may be detected on a Gram-stained smear. The antibiotic sensitivities of infecting strains vary and since treatment must always be started before this information is available, vancomycin (preferably intraperitoneally) is the drug of choice.

Endocarditis

Coagulase-negative staphylococci can infect native or prosthetic heart valves. Nosocomial native valve infections with coagulase-negative staphylococci (usually *S. epidermidis*) generally result from infected intravascular devices; the affected valve may or may not have been previously abnormal. Nosocomial prosthetic valve endocarditis can be acquired in the theatre at the time of valve replacement surgery or shortly thereafter and presents within weeks or more often months of surgery ('early-onset'). In many series, coagulase-negative staphylococci are the commonest cause of early-onset prosthetic valve endocarditis. Prosthetic infection can also be acquired from an infected intravascular device. Community-acquired coagulase-negative staphylococcal endocarditis, which usually involves native valves, is increasingly recognized and most patients will have a pre-existing cardiac abnormality. The organisms must derive from the patient's skin, but predisposing skin lesions are seldom detected. The infection often mimics *S. aureus* endocarditis with rapidly destructive valvular disease, neurological manifestations, and concomitant vertebral osteomyelitis. The commonest pathogen is *S. epidermidis*, but there are increasing reports of other species, particularly *S. lugdunensis*, which seems to be especially virulent. These community-acquired strains are frequently penicillin sensitive.

Urinary tract infection

Coagulase-negative staphylococci are urinary pathogens both in the community and in hospital but different species are involved. In the community the curiously named *S. saprophyticus* is an important urinary pathogen in sexually active women, second only to *Escherichia coli*. It commonly produces cystitis, but may cause upper urinary tract infection and has been isolated from infected calculi. *S. saprophyticus* is a skin commensal but is not normally found colonizing the urethra, though it has been isolated from the rectal flora of women. Most strains are readily recognized in the laboratory by their resistance to novobiocin. They are sensitive to a wide range of antibiotics. Some nosocomial urinary tract infections are also caused by coagulase-negative staphylococci, predominantly *S. epidermidis*. These infections, usually after urological surgery, are seldom accompanied by pyuria, and may clear spontaneously on removal of the catheter. Nosocomial urinary isolates of coagulase-negative staphylococci are often multiply resistant.

Other infections

Coagulase-negative staphylococci are increasingly isolated from the blood of neonates and immunocompromised, neutropenic patients. Distinguishing true bacteraemia from contamination can be difficult. In many cases bacteraemia is related to the presence of an intravascular catheter (see above). In premature neonates, colonization of the respiratory tract occurs and respiratory infection can result. Infection of prosthetic joints and vascular prostheses is sometimes caused by coagulase-negative staphylococci. The organisms are introduced at the time of the surgery, although the clinical signs of infection may not become evident for weeks or months. Attempts to treat such infections with antibiotics generally fail and removal of the prosthesis is required. Coagulase-negative staphylococci are also the commonest cause of postoperative endophthalmitis after intraocular surgery.

Laboratory diagnosis

The laboratory diagnosis of much infection with coagulase-negative staphylococci poses greater difficulties than the diagnosis of *S. aureus* infection. The clinician is advised to enlist the help of a competent microbiologist when assessing the validity of culture results of invasive specimens growing coagulase-negative staphylococci. A further problem with these organisms occurs with the use of broth enrichment cultures for specimens of excised tissue; a single contaminating staphylococcus will multiply in liquid medium, thereby misleading unwary clinicians.

Treatment

As well as the prescribing of antibiotics, an integral part of the successful treatment of infections with coagulase-negative staphylococci is a critical clinical assessment of the need for removal of any prosthetic material with which so many infections are associated. So many nosocomial infections are caused by resistant strains that the only reliable initial therapy is vancomycin or teicoplanin. The length of treatment in most instances is somewhat arbitrary and the same principles apply to infections with these organisms as to those with *S. aureus*. Community-acquired infections, usually endocarditis, can often be treated with β-lactam antibiotics, sometimes with penicillin. As with serious *S. aureus* infections, combination therapy is often used.

Further reading

Archer GL (2000). *Staphylococcus epidermidis* and other coagulase-negative staphylococci. In: Mandell GL, Bennett JE, Dolin R, eds. *Principles and practice of infectious diseases*, pp 2092–100. Churchill Livingstone, New York. [Comprehensive chapter with large number of references.]

Chesney PJ *et al.* (1984). The disease spectrum, epidemiology, and etiology of toxic-shock syndrome. *Annual Review of Microbiology* **38**, 315–38.

Espersen F *et al.* (1991). Changing pattern of bone and joint infections due to *Staphylococcus aureus*: study of cases of bacteraemia in Denmark, 1959 to 1988. *Reviews of Infectious Diseases* **13**, 347–58.

Etienne J, Eykyn SJ (1990). Increase in native valve endocarditis caused by coagulase negative staphylococci: an Anglo-French clinical and microbiological study. *British Heart Journal* **64**, 381–4.

Vandenesch F *et al.* (1993). Endocarditis due to *Staphylococcus lugdunensis*: report of 11 cases and review. *Clinical Infectious Diseases* **17**, 871–6.

Waldvogel FA (2000). *Staphylococcus aureus* (including staphylcoccal toxic shock). In: Mandell GL, Bennett JE, Dolin R, eds. *Principles and practice of infectious diseases*, pp 2069–92. Churchill Livingstone, New York. [Very comprehensive chapter with large number of references.]

7.11.5 Meningococcal infections

P. Brandtzaeg

Neisseria meningitidis infection remains a major public health problem worldwide by causing clusters or epidemics of meningitis and acute lethal sepsis. Case fatality has gradually declined from 80 to 90 per cent to approximately 10 per cent but has remained at this level since the introduction of antimicrobial chemotherapy in 1937.

Bacterium

Neisseria meningitidis is an obligate human Gram-negative diplococcus normally located in the mucous membrane of the upper respiratory tract. Invasive isolates from blood or cerebrospinal fluid are encapsulated and express pili. Capsular polysaccharides that inhibit phagocytosis and bacterial adhesion are divided into 12 different serogroups (A, B, C, 29-E, H, I, K, L, W-135, X, Y, and Z). Serogroups A, B, and C account for more than 90 per cent of all invasive isolates. Less than 10 per cent of clinical isolates are from serogroups W-135 and Y.

The bacterial cell wall consists of an outer lipid bilayer containing lipopolysaccharides (endotoxin) and outer membrane proteins, a thin peptidoglycan layer, and the cytoplasmic membrane. Lipid A is a glycolipid that anchors the lipopolysaccharide to the lipid membrane. It is the major inflammatory (toxic) component of *N. meningitidis*. It can activate a variety of cells via CD14–toll-like receptor-4 interaction or indirectly through activation of blood coagulation, fibrinolysis, kallikrein–kinin, and complement systems. During growth, meningococci release outer membrane vesicles containing large amounts of lipopolysaccharides.

Outer membrane proteins are classified according to electrophoretic mobility into five major classes. Por A (class 1 protein) and Por B (class 2 or 3 proteins) are cation- and anion-selective porins, respectively. Surface exposed loops of Por B and Por A define serotype and serosubtype, respectively. Loops 1 and 4 in Por A are major epitopes inducing bactericidal and opsonophagocytic antibodies when exposed to the human immune system.

Meningococci are fastidious bacteria that readily autolyse. They grow well on blood agar, supplemented chocolate agar, trypticar soy base, Mueller–Hinton agar, and selective GC-medium. Optimal growth occurs at 35 to 37°C in a humid atmosphere with 5 to 10 per cent carbon dioxide. The convex colonies (diameter: 1 to 4 mm) are transparent, non-pigmented, and non-haemolytic. They produce cytochrome oxidase and ferment glucose and maltose, but not lactose and sucrose, to acid without gas formation.

Practical handling of clinical specimens

Blood culture (10 ml for adults, 2 to 4 ml for infants/children) and swabs from the nasopharynx and the tonsils are collected immediately. Media for blood culture and transportation of swabs should be optimal for recovery of meningococci. Cerebrospinal fluid is best cultured by direct plating of 0.1 ml on supplemented chocolate agar or a similar medium, incubated at 35 to 37°C in 5 to10 per cent carbon dioxide. If direct plating is impossible or delayed, the sample should be stored at +4°C to +20°C, preferably at refrigerator temperature. Recovery of live meningococci may increase if some drops of the cerebrospinal fluid are stored on a sterile swab in transport medium or injected into blood culture medium and incubated at 35 to 37°C.

Direct visualization of *N. meningitidis* in clinical specimens

Intra- and extracellular diplococci can be observed in the cerebrospinal fluid, peripheral blood buffy coat (fulminant septicaemia), and biopsies of haemorrhagic skin lesions using Gram or acridine orange stains.

Polymerase chain reaction

Using primers that recognize various DNA sequences coding for different genes in *N. meningitidis*, it is possible to detect and classify meningococci in cerebrospinal fluid and blood without positive cultures.

Epidemiology

Industrialized countries

Infection presents as single cases or in small clusters. The incidence is usually 1 to 3 per 100 000 inhabitants per year. Strains belonging to specific clonal complexes may cause a hyperendemic situation characterized by a much higher incidence than usually observed (4 to 30 per 100 000 per year). This epidemiological situation may last for more than a decade in defined geographical areas before slowly declining. Serogroup A has disappeared as a cause of significant epidemics. Outbreaks in Finland in the 1970s and in New Zealand in the 1980s were exceptions.

Developing countries

Large-scale epidemics are confined to developing countries, primarily in sub-Saharan Africa. The incidence approaches 10 to 25 per 100 000 inhabitants per year. During epidemic peaks in Africa, as many as 500 to 1000 per 100 000 inhabitants may contract meningococcal infections. Serogroup A and to lesser extent serogroup C dominate the isolates of large epidemics.

The meningitis belt in sub-Saharan Africa

The area stretches from the Gambia in the west to Ethiopia in the east including Senegal, Guinea, Mali, Burkina Faso, Ghana, Togo, Benin, Nigeria, Niger, Chad, Cameroon, The Central African Republic, and Sudan. Mainly serogroup A strains belonging to a few clonal complexes cause the increased attack rate. In some of these countries large-scale epidemics occur every 8 to 12 years.

Season

In temperate climates most cases occur during the winter and early spring. In the sub-Saharan African meningitis belt the incidence increases from the middle and reaches its maximum at the end of the dry season (harmattan). New cases decline rapidly after the start of the rainy season.

Preceding infections

Influenza A predisposes to invasive meningococcal infections. Mycoplasma infections and rubella have been associated with outbreaks.

Age distribution

Cases are seen in all age groups. However, most occur from 0 to 4 years with a smaller peak from 13 to 20 years. During epidemics the median age appears to increase. Complement-deficient patients may contract the infection when they are older than others.

Genetic diversity

N. meningitidis can exchange and incorporate DNA from other Neisseria or closely related species. It reveals more genetic diversity than many other human pathogens. However, strains from certain clonal complexes may persist for many decades over wide areas, retaining their pathogenicity. Strains from seven clonal complexes have predominated since the late 1960s.

Predisposing factors for invasive disease (Table 1)

Lack of protective antibodies

Antibodies against serogroups A, C, W-135, and Y capsule polysaccharides are bactericidal and confer protection at concentrations of 1 to 2 µg/ml of serum. Serogroup B polysaccharide induces a weak, transient IgM response that is not protective. Bactericidal and opsonophagocytic antibodies recognizing surface-exposed epitopes of the outer membrane protein, in particular Por A, developing after infection, are important for protection. Antilipopolysaccharide antibodies, recognizing commonly shared epitopes among virulent and non-pathogenic Neisseria and closely related species, presumably play a role in protection.

Table 1 Factors predisposing for meningococcal infections

Lack of bactericidal and/or opsonizing antibodies
Lack of properdin or late complement components
Polymorphism of the Fcγ-receptor II (Fcγ-RIIa, CD32) and Fcγ-receptor III (Fcγ-RIIIb, CD16).
Low levels of mannan-binding lectin

Defects in the complement system

Defects in the complement system can increase susceptibility to meningococcal infections up to 6000 times. The commonest are absent or malfunctioning properdin or late complement components C5 to C9. Properdin defects predispose to rapidly progressing, overwhelming septicaemia. Defects in C5 to C9 are associated with recurrent meningococcal infections. Previous studies suggested that the case fatality rate was reduced in those with late complement defects. However, a recent Dutch study found case fatality rates of 16 per cent and 32 per cent among patients with late complement defects and properdin defects, respectively—a difference that was not statistically significant, compared with 7.7 per cent in the general population. Defects in the classical pathway do not predispose to meningococcal infection. Complement defects are rare. They play a minor role in the development of serogroup A, B, and C systemic meningococcal disease, but are over-represented in patients with the uncommon serogroups W-135, X, Y, and Z.

Defects in the mannan-binding lectin

Mannan-binding lectin is a calcium-dependent, opsonizing, acute-phase protein. Mutations in codons 54, 57, and 52 in the mannan-binding lectin gene result in low serum levels. Defects in this protein have been associated with 1/3 of all meningococcal cases in England and Ireland.

Polymorphism of Fcγ-receptor II and Fcγ-receptor III

Polymorphisms of Fcγ-receptor II (Fcγ-RIIa, CD32) and Fcγ-receptor III (Fcγ-RIIIb, CD16) on phagocytic cells are associated with reduced binding of antibodies. They are over-represented in patients with defects in the late complement components and in children with fulminant meningococcal sepsis. Fcγ-RIIa receptors where arginine has replaced histidine at position 131 are associated with reduced binding of IgG2 subclass (antipolysaccharide) antibodies.

Nasopharyngeal colonization

Upper respiratory tract mucosa is the natural habitat of N. meningitidis. It is spread from person to person by droplets and direct mucosal contact. Most colonizing meningococci are non-pathogenic, genetically and phenotypically different from virulent invasive strains. Only a small minority of those colonized with virulent strains will develop invasive disease. Colonization is asymptomatic. It induces local and systemic immune responses within 1 to 2 weeks.

Carriage

Cross-sectional studies in England and Norway in the 1980s and 1990s indicated that approximately 10 per cent of the population harboured meningococci in the upper respiratory tract. However, only 1 per cent of the healthy normal population carried strains from typical virulent clones

Table 2 The levels of lipopolysaccharides and inflammatory mediators related to the clinical presentation

	Shock No meningitis	No shock Meningitis	Shock Meningitis	No shock No meningitis
Circulation	++++	(+)	++	(+)
Subarachnoid space	(+)	+++++	+++	(+)

Shock denotes persistent hypotension requiring treatment with volume and pressor for 24 h.

Meningitis denotes 100×10^6/l or more leucocytes in the cerebrospinal fluid or clinically distinct signs of meningism.

prevalent at the time. The acquisition rate leading to carriage appears to be independent of season, whereas invasive meningococcal infections peak in the winter and early spring in temperate countries.

The carriage rate in England is low (2 to 3 per cent) in the first 4 years of life, rising in children 10 to 14 years of age (9 to 10 per cent), reaching a maximum among young adults of 15 to 19 years (20 to 25 per cent), and than gradually declining to less than 15 per cent in persons above 25 years. It increases in closed or semi-closed communities and is particularly high in military camps where strains change frequently. In university communities with bar and catering facilities the carriage rate is high. Smoking increases the carriage rate.

Reservoir of virulent meningococci

Healthy adults carrying virulent strains of *N. meningitidis* are the main reservoir. Household members and kissing contacts of a patient harbour virulent strains more often than the average population. In industrialized countries, infants and children are usually infected by a local adult carrier. Spread from patients to medical staff is very uncommon. In Africa, children may more commonly infect each other with serogroup A strains.

Invasive infection

Most patients appear to develop invasive disease 2 to 4 days after acquiring the virulent strain in the upper respiratory tract, but some are carriers for up to 7 weeks before invasive infection develops. *N. meningitidis* adheres to specific structures on the epithelial cells in the nasopharynx and on the tonsils. During a period of adaptation and proliferation, meningococci presumably alter various surface structures (lipopolysaccharides, pili, outer membrane proteins) by phase variation before starting transepithelial migration. They reach submucosal tissue and via capillaries gain access to the circulation.

The initial bacteraemic phase

Bacteraemia is a prerequisite for systemic meningococcal infection. Meningococci may be eliminated from the blood by phagocytosis of opsonized bacteria and lysis induced by bactericidal antibodies and complement. Persistent bacteraemia allows meningeal invasion.

Bacterial proliferation and an inflammatory response may occur predominantly in either the subarachnoid space, causing meningitis, or in the circulation, causing meningococcaemia with or without shock.

The rash

Haemorrhagic skin lesions are the hallmark of systemic meningococcal disease, occurring in 70 to 80 per cent of all cases in industrialized countries. They appear as red or bluish petechiae. These lesions are larger and more irregular in size than the petechiae of thrombocytopenic purpura. Each lesion represents a local nidus of meningococci within the endothelial cells, thrombus formation, and extravasation of erythrocytes. The petechial rash indicates meningococcaemia, not necessarily severe sepsis. However, in fulminant meningococcal septicaemia the haemorrhagic lesions are larger (ecchymoses) with a propensity to locate on extremities (Plate 1). Some patients develop relatively large, non-specific, maculopapular lesions, with or without haemorrhagic lesions, at an early stage (Plates 2, 3). The petech-

ial lesions are difficult to discover on dark skin but may be observed in the conjunctivae.

Clinical presentations

Initial symptoms of systemic meningococcal infection are attributable to meningococcaemia. This may persist as a low-grade bacteraemia or develop into septic shock and multiple organ failure in a few hours. Most commonly the patient develops meningococcaemia without circulatory impairment which gradually evolves to meningitis within 12 to 72 hours. Occasionally, patients develop meningitis and persistent shock simultaneously. Based on easily recognizable clinical symptoms, meningococcal infections can be classified as (i) meningitis without shock, (ii) shock without meningitis, (iii) meningitis and shock, and (iv) meningococcaemia without shock or meningitis. Each clinical presentation is associated with a distinct pathophysiological background and prognosis (Table 2).

Distinct meningitis without persistent shock

Meningism dominates the clinical presentation. The onset is often insidious. The patients, particularly children, may complain of general malaise, nausea, and headache. They vomit and become febrile. The temperature may fluctuate and can be normal at times. Many patients are initially diagnosed as 'gastric flu', gastroenteritis, or upper respiratory tract infection. Gradually, the symptoms of meningitis dominate the clinical picture. The patient complains of headache, vomits, develops nuchal and back rigidity, photophobia, and in more advanced cases altered consciousness. Kernig's and Brudinski's signs become positive. Many patients are lethargic, some are agitated. The blood pressure is normal or slightly elevated by stress. Occasionally it is low but can be restored to normal by infusion of a limited volume of fluid. In untreated cases brain oedema develops, the intracranial pressure rises, and the central circulation is increasingly compromised. Finally, herniation of the cerebellum occurs with arrest of the brain circulation. The case fatality rate is usually less than 5 per cent.

Meningococcal meningitis without persistent shock accounts for more than 50 per cent of all cases of systemic meningococcal infections in industrialized countries and an even higher proportion of cases reaching hospitals in developing countries. The combination of multiple petechiae and symptoms of meningitis supports a diagnosis of meningococcal meningitis.

Pathophysiological background

In untreated patients, *N. meningitidis* can be cultivated from cerebrospinal fluid and blood. The concentration of lipopolysaccharides, reflecting the microbial proliferation, is 100 to 1000 times higher in cerebrospinal fluid than plasma. Levels of bioactive inflammatory mediators such as tumour necrosis factor-α, interleukins 1β, 6, 8, 10, and 12, and soluble receptors of these interleukins are much higher in cerebrospinal fluid than plasma. Plasma proteins, mainly albumin, leak into the cerebrospinal fluid. The influx of mainly neutrophils causes the pleocytosis. The glucose level of the cerebrospinal fluid is reduced mainly as a result of increased central glucose consumption rather than the pleocytosis.

Laboratory findings

The erythrocyte sedimentation rate, C-reactive protein, and leucocyte count in the peripheral blood are markedly elevated with increased numbers of band forms. Sodium, potassium, calcium, and magnesium ions, pH, renal, hepatic, and coagulation parameters are usually within normal range. Cerebrospinal fluid shows a marked pleocytosis (more than 100×10^6 leucocytes/l), with increased levels of protein and decreased level of glucose. Intra- and extracellular Gram-negative diplococci can be detected by direct microscopy.

Persistent septic shock without distinct meningitis

Fulminant meningococcal septicaemia (Waterhouse–Friderichsen syndrome) is characterized by persistent circulatory failure and severe coagulopathy leading to thrombosis and extensive haemorrhage of the skin, thrombosis and gangrene of the extremities, and impaired renal, adrenal, and pulmonary function.

Symptoms develop very rapidly. Six to 12 hours after recognizing their first symptoms the patients are often desperately ill. Initially, they complain of 'flu-like' symptoms, such as fever, aching muscle, prostration, abdominal pain, and nausea. The temperature rises rapidly, commonly to between 39.0 and 41.5°C, but occasionally lower. Diarrhoea is quite common during the first few hours. The patient appears worryingly sick to relatives. Before the appearance of petechiae and ecchymoses the symptoms are often misinterpreted as influenza or acute gastroenteritis.

The haemorrhagic skin lesions are first seen as bluish petechiae, which rapidly increase in size and number. They are distributed all over the body but are often more pronounced and detected earliest on the extremities. Occasionally they are seen on the conjunctivae and other mucous membranes.

The circulation is severely impaired. The extremities are often cold and cyanotic. The blood pressure is low despite tachycardia. The tissue perfusion remains inadequate despite extensive fluid and pressor therapy. Initially, the circulation is hyperdynamic, but gradually becomes hypodynamic from persistent vasodilatation and gradually reduced myocardial performance. The heart becomes dilated with a reduced ejection fraction.

Patients usually lack nuchal and back rigidity. Kernig's sign is negative. Despite impaired circulation, many patients remain awake and alert on hospital admission, being able to communicate their complaints. They hyperventilate to compensate for the pronounced metabolic acidosis. Urine output gradually dwindles. They may develop acute respiratory distress syndrome (ARDS), i.e. pulmonary oedema after fluid volume repletion.

Circulatory collapse dominates the clinical picture during the first 48 to 96 h. Death is usually within 48 h. Later, ARDS, renal failure, and the consequences of the diffuse thrombosis of the extremities and the skin dominate the picture. The case fatality rate ranges from 29 to 53 per cent.

Rapidly evolving symptoms with fever, circulatory shock, and extensive skin haemorrhages in a person without a history of splenectomy makes the diagnosis of fulminant meningococcal septicaemia likely. The same clinical picture is, however, observed in cases of overwhelming *Streptococcus pneumoniae*, *Haemophilus influenzae*, *Streptococcus pyogenes*, and *Capnocytophaga canimorsus* infections and with viral haemorrhagic fevers (Plate 4).

Pathophysiological background

There is very rapid microbial proliferation in the circulation, generating large amounts of bacterial lipopolysaccharides in a few hours, but with limited or no bacterial growth in the subarachnoid space. The levels of lipopolysaccharides in the plasma predict the development of persistent septic shock, multiple organ failure, and death. Among 100 Norwegian patients with systemic meningococcal disease, admission levels of lipopoly-

Fig. 1 The relationship between the levels of bacterial lipopolysaccharides in plasma and case fatality rate related to the development of septic shock and multiple organ failure in 100 Norwegian patients with systemic meningococcal disease.

saccharides in the plasma of less than 1000 pg/ml (10 endotoxin units/ml) were associated with no mortality caused by septic shock, rising to 100 per cent mortality in patients with more than 15 000 pg/ml (150 endotoxin units/ml), that is, 1.2 log higher (Fig. 1).

Coagulopathy

Coagulation is activated primarily via the extrinsic (tissue factor–FVIIa) pathway. In patients with fulminant meningococcal septicaemia, there are increased levels of tissue factor in monocytes and on microparticles released from monocytes. The platelets disappear rapidly and remain at a low level for many days due to extensive consumption and a presumably altered endothelial surface. The activation of the coagulation system, as measured by formation of fibrin, is gradually reduced after antibiotic and fluid therapy is initiated (Table 3).

Inhibited fibrinolysis

Concurrent with activation of coagulation, fibrinolysis is inhibited by high levels of plasminogen activator inhibitor 1 (**PAI-1**), released from activated endothelial cells and platelets. High levels of PAI-1 are associated with development of persistent septic shock and a fatal outcome. Allelic variations in the promoter region of the PAI-1 gene enhance production and are associated with an increased risk of dying.

Thrombus formation

Thrombosis occurs particularly in the skin, kidneys, adrenals, muscles, peripheral extremities, and to some extent in the lungs. Levels of the natural coagulation inhibitors antithrombin III and protein C decline due to consumption, whereas tissue factor pathway inhibitor rises. Low levels of protein C are associated with diffuse thrombosis and necrosis of the skin even in non-septic patients.

Table 3 Factors contributing to the coagulopathy in fulminant meningococcal septicaemia

Procoagulant factor	Tissue factor in monocytes ↑
Anticoagulant factors	Antithrombin III ↓
	Protein C ↓
	Tissue factor pathway inhibitor ↑
Profibrinolytic factor	Tissue plasminogen activator ↑ ↓
Antifibrinolytic factor	Plasminogen activator inhibitor 1 ↑

Pro- and anti-inflammatory mediators

A multitude of bioactive pro- and anti-inflammatory mediators are released into the plasma. The complement and the kallikrein–kinin systems generate anaphylatoxins (C3a, C4a, C5a) and bradykinin, which are potent vasodilators. Proinflammatory cytokines, notably tumour necrosis factor-α, IL-1β, IL-6, and IL-8, are all massively upregulated. Concomitantly, high levels of soluble receptors of the same cytokines are released. The anti-inflammatory cytokines IL-10 and IL-1 receptor antagonist are present in high levels and suppress the cell-activating effect of the bacterial lipopolysaccharides and the many proinflammatory cytokines. It is uncertain whether inducible nitric oxide synthase, augmenting the production of nitric oxide in the endothelial cells, plays a role in meningococcal septic shock.

The subarachnoid space

Microbial proliferation is limited or absent although meningococci may be cultured from cerebrospinal fluid in as many as 50 per cent of untreated cases. The inflammatory response is very limited with a leucocyte count usually in the range of 10 to 100×10^6/l and normal contents of protein and glucose.

Laboratory findings

The erythrocyte sedimentation rate and C-reactive protein are only moderately elevated on admission, rising to high levels within 48 h. The leucocyte count is usually low with a marked shift to young band forms of neutrophils. There is evidence of a partly compensated metabolic acidosis with decreased levels of pH and $P\text{CO}_2$. Creatinine and urea are elevated, serum glucose is variable (high, normal, or low), potassium, calcium, and magnesium are low. Potassium rises with the renal failure. Serum aspartate aminotransferase and alanine aminotransferase are slightly elevated, whereas γ-glutamyl transferase remains normal. Creatine kinase rises within 1 to 3 days, indicating rhabdomyolysis. Prothrombin, activated partial thromboplastin, and thrombin times are prolonged. The levels of platelets, fibrinogen, coagulation factors VII, X, and V, and prothrombin are low. Antithrombin III and protein C are low whereas tissue factor pathway inhibitor is elevated. Fibrin(ogen) degradation products, thrombin–antithrombin complexes, and PAI-1 are elevated. Lumbar puncture should be avoided in view of the bleeding diathesis.

Distinct meningitis and persistent shock

There are meningeal and circulatory symptoms. Usually the symptoms from the inflamed meninges dominate the picture. On admission there are classic signs and symptoms of meningitis such as headache and nausea, nuchal and back rigidity, and a positive Kernig's sign. The blood pressure remains low despite fluid volume repletion.

Circulating levels of bacterial lipopolysaccharide and inflammatory mediators are lower than in patients with fulminant septicaemia, and case fatality is lower. However, it is higher than in patients with meningitis without compromised circulation.

Meningococcaemia without distinct meningitis and persistent shock

The patient is febrile and usually presents with a rash but without symptoms of persistent septic shock or meningitis. It is a composite group of patients. Many of these patients have been admitted to hospital early, 12 to 24 h after their first symptoms. The case fatality rate is zero. Left untreated they might have developed symptoms of meningitis or fulminant shock.

Transient benign meningococcaemia

These patients develop fever and often an uncharacteristic rash, but no meningism. They are diagnosed as most likely having a viral infection and receive no antibiotic. When the blood culture results are known, the symptoms have disappeared spontaneously, usually within 1 to 3 days. This syndrome may occur in infants and young children.

Subacute meningococcaemia

A few patients develop fever, an uncharacteristic maculopapular rash, general malaise, and arthralgia but no signs of meningitis or shock. They feel uncomfortable but are not severely ill. Meningococci are isolated from blood cultures. Untreated the symptoms may last for days to several weeks but disappear within 1 to 2 days after penicillin therapy is initiated.

Chronic meningococcaemia

The patient develops undulating fever, arthralgia, and maculopapular rash. At times the symptoms may disappear completely. The symptoms may last for months. Blood cultures are sometimes repeatedly negative. Patients are often treated with corticosteroids because an underlying autoimmune disease is suspected. The fever disappears temporarily before reappearing. At this stage meningococci may well be isolated from blood cultures. Antibiotic treatment clears the symptoms within a few days.

Other organ manifestations

Pericarditis

The pericardium is seeded during meningococcaemia. Subsequent inflammation and exudate may lead to cardiac tamponade if left untreated. The patient is febrile, nauseated, and may complain of epigastric pain. The condition is often misdiagnosed as an acute abdominal condition. Blood cultures may be negative. *N. meningitidis* can be cultured and seen in aspirated pus by direct microscopy. Treatment consists of evacuating the pus and benzylpenicillin. The condition should be followed daily by ultrasound examination. Serogroup C organisms have been particularly implicated in these cases.

Arthritis

Acute meningococcal arthritis is an uncommon clinical manifestation of a preceding, often low-grade, meningococcaemia. It is usually located to one, or more rarely, several large joints. If the characteristic petechial rash is absent, isolation of meningococci from blood or joint cultures is necessary for a correct diagnosis. Arthritis caused by *Neisseria gonorrhoeae* is considerably more common than primary meningococcal arthritis. The symptoms disappear rapidly after penicillin treatment without long-term complications.

Arthritis induced by immune complexes

This is more common than the meningococcal arthritis. One or several large joints become swollen and painful. The symptoms usually develop at the end of the first week of treatment. Blood and joint cultures are negative. The temperature and inflammatory markers may rise after an initial decline. The symptoms disappear gradually after some days of treatment with non-steroidal anti-inflammatory drugs. Extended antibiotic therapy is not necessary.

Cutaneous vasculitis and episcleritis

This appears simultaneously with the immune complex arthritis and is commonly observed in sub-Saharan Africa. The vasculitis causes multiple blisters that readily rupture leading to multiple superficial skin ulcers.

Table 4 Doses of prehospital antibiotic to be administered in suspected cases of meningococcal infection

< 2 years	300 mg (0.5×10^6 IU) benzylpenicillin intramuscularly
2–7 years	600 mg (1×10^6 IU) benzylpenicillin intramuscularly
> 7 years	1.2 g (2×10^6 IU) benzylpenicillin intravenously or intramuscularly

Ocular infections

Conjunctivitis or panophthalmitis may precede other symptoms of invasive meningococcal infection. They are primarily observed in infants and children. The patient develops a red eye which in the case of panophthalmitis becomes painful with impaired vision. Local formation of microthrombi may complicate the infection.

Pneumonia

Strains belonging to serogroup Y and W-135 or more rarely other serogroups may cause pneumonia in adults and children. The diagnosis depends on detecting meningococci in a representative specimen from the low respiratory tract. It cannot be differentiated from pneumonia caused by other agents on the clinical symptoms alone.

Treatment

Prehospital antibiotic treatment

Health authorities in many countries advise general practitioners to start prehospital antibiotic treatment (i.e. benzylpenicillin) in suspected cases of meningococcal infection. The doses in Table 4 rapidly lead to bactericidal concentrations in plasma.

The penicillin is injected laterally in one or both thighs in infants and children. The primary goal is to stop rapid growth of meningococci in the circulation before the intravascular inflammation becomes irreversible or causes grave sequelae. The patients most likely to benefit from this strategy, if applied early enough, are those who are distant from the hospital and have rapidly evolving symptoms leading to a compromised circulation and extensive haemorrhagic skin lesions. Retrospective studies in England suggest that prehospital penicillin treatment reduces case fatality.

Initial evaluation in hospital

The patients should be regarded as emergency cases. The main clinical presentation and severity should be evaluated immediately. A variety of prognostic scores have been developed. The Glasgow Meningococcal Septicaemia Prognostic Score is the one most commonly used. Scores can be used to select patients for intensive care treatment. They should never be used to justify withholding treatment as they often overestimate case fatality.

Antibiotic treatment

Adequate doses of benzylpenicillin, cefotaxime, ceftriaxone, or chloramphenicol effectively stop further proliferation of *N. meningitidis* in the circulation, cerebrospinal fluid, and other extravascular sites. Induction of an explosive release of bacterial lipopolysaccharides leading to a Jarisch–Herxheimer reaction has never been documented in patients receiving antibiotics for meningococcal infection. Plasma levels of lipopolysaccharides and the levels of important inflammatory mediators decline immediately after treatment with antibiotics is initiated in these patients (Table 5).

Benzylpenicillin, chloramphenicol, cefotaxime, ceftriaxone, and meropenem are bactericidal to *N. meningitidis*. Benzylpenicillin remains the drug of choice in most countries. It is effective, cheap, and non-toxic in high doses as long as renal function is normal. High doses are necessary since it penetrates the cerebrospinal fluid relatively poorly. In patients with fulminant septicaemia and severe renal dysfunction the doses should be reduced after 24 to 48 h.

Strains whose sensitivity to penicillin is reduced because of altered penicillin-binding protein 2 are an increasing problem. In most industrialized countries they account for less than 5 per cent of all meningococcal isolates, but the frequency is higher in Mediterranean countries, particularly Spain. Patients infected with these strains have been adequately treated with benzylpenicillin as long as dosage is adequate. Penicillinase-producing meningococci remain extremely rare.

Chloramphenicol is a good alternative in patients hypersensitive to β-lactam antibiotics. In developing countries it is the best and cheapest alternative to benzylpenicillin. Meningococcal strains resistant to chloramphenicol have recently emerged in France.

In many industrialized countries cefotaxime or ceftriaxone is combined with vancomycin as empirical treatment of bacterial meningitis until the aetiological agent has been identified. Cefotaxime and ceftriaxone are highly effective antibiotics that penetrate the blood–brain barrier better than benzylpenicillin. Meningococci remain fully sensitive to both drugs. Meropenem is a carbapenem highly active against *N. meningitidis*, *H. influenzae*, and *S. pneumoniae*. It does not induce seizures as observed with the imipenem–cilastatin combination.

In each country the health authorities and microbiological laboratories should recommend the optimal and affordable drug regimen.

Antibiotic treatment should be initiated promptly. Immediately after the first clinical evaluation and collection of the necessary samples for microbiological diagnosis, therapy should start. If there are contraindications to lumbar puncture or if it is delayed until after brain imaging, antibiotic treatment should be started immediately. Five days of treatment is adequate to eradicate sensitive meningococci.

Supportive treatment

Patients with persistent shock should be given extensive volume replacement, whereas patients with meningitis should receive a moderate amount of fluid. All patients should be monitored closely to detect early signs of a deteriorating circulation, renal and pulmonary failure, or increasing intracranial pressure.

Volume treatment

Patients with persistent hypotension and signs of inadequate peripheral circulation require massive fluid volume repletion. The extensive capillary leak syndrome increases the volume required. Children and adults may require an infused volume that is one to several times their circulating blood volume in the first 24 h. The optimal solution has not yet been defined. Colloids are often combined with crystalloid. Albumin and fresh frozen plasma were previously extensively used. However, the use of albumin in septic shock is controversial, expensive, and was not supported in a recently published meta-analysis. In many countries the use of fresh frozen plasma is no longer recommended because of the risk of transmitting pathogens, especially HIV.

Patients presenting with distinct signs of meningitis without shock should receive the basic daily requirement of fluid supplemented with extra volume for dehydration and loss due to vomiting and fever. Excessive hydration should be avoided since it may precipitate irreversible brain oedema and cerebellar herniation. In patients with persistent shock and meningitis, treatment of shock is the priority.

Inotropic support

If initial volume repletion fails to improve the circulation, inotropic support should be added. Dopamine, dobutamine, noradrenaline, and adrenaline are used. Most physicians start with dopamine at 2 to 10 μg/kg.min, or dobutamine at 1 to 10μg/kg.min. Ideally, patients should be infused through a central line.

Table 5 Antibiotics in meningococcal meningitis or sepsis

Antibiotics	Dose per 24 h		Dose interval (h)
	Adult (g)	Child (mg/kg)	
Benzylpenicillin	14.4	180	6
	24×10^6 IU	300 000 IU/kg	6
Cefotaxim	9	200	8
Ceftriaxone	4	80	24
Chloramphenicol	3	100	6
Meropenem	6	120	8

Corticosteroid therapy

The use of corticosteroids in meningococcal septic shock is controversial. Methylprednisolone in pharmacological doses did not increase 28-day survival in two large series of patients with septic shock of various causes. Adrenal haemorrhage is common in patients with fulminant meningococcal septicaemia. It is also present in surviving patients. In most fatal cases of meningococcal infection, plasma cortisol levels are normal or high. Few patients have low levels. However, serial measurements of plasma cortisol and adrenal stimulation tests suggest a relative deficiency. Corticosteroids are not recommended routinely unless a deficiency is documented.

The benefit of dexamethasone in meningococcal meningitis is controversial. Efficacy has never been evaluated in double-blind, randomized, controlled clinical trials involving enough patients with meningococcal meningitis to allow a firm conclusion. In an open randomized study in Egypt involving 267 patients, dexamethasone injected every 12 h for 3 days did not improve the outcome. Corticosteroid treatment has been associated with relapse of the meningitis in patients who had otherwise been adequately treated. At present, dexamethasone is not recommended for routine use in patients with meningococcal meningitis.

Ventilatory support

Patients receiving volume treatment for profound shock are in danger of developing ARDS from capillary leak syndrome and volume overload. Increasing oxygen demand, decreased pulmonary compliance, and the appearance of diffuse infiltrates on chest radiograph indicate the development of ARDS. Some paediatricians advocate elective intubation and mechanical ventilation if more than 40 ml/kg per 24 h resuscitation fluid is needed to combat the septic shock, even if the oxygenation is normal.

Renal support

Patients with persistent septic shock and coagulopathy develop renal dysfunction from acute proximal tubular necrosis. Thrombosis in the small peritubular vessels, in glomeruli, and myoglobinaemia may contribute to the renal dysfunction. Serum creatinine and urea are elevated on admission and continue to increase for many days without adequate treatment. Hyperkalaemia, which may develop during the first 24 to 48 h, is an immediate threat. If possible, continuous haemofiltration should be used. Peritoneal dialysis, although less effective, is an alternative to continuous haemofiltration.

Treatment of disseminated intravascular coagulation

The first priority is to stop further bacterial proliferation with antibiotics. In the 1970s heparin was extensively used. Two small controlled trials did not document any survival benefit in patients receiving heparin. Infusion of a continuous low-dose unfractionated heparin (10 to 15 IU/kg.h) has recently been advocated as supplement to treatment with concentrated protein C. The antithrombin III levels should be kept above 35 to 40 IU/ml.

Infusion of the natural anticoagulant protein C (loading dose: 100 IU/kg, followed by 15 IU/kg.h for days to keep the plasma concentration between 0.8 and 1.2 IU/ml) may possibly limit thrombus formation, skin necrosis, and the need for amputation. If used it should be started early. In the few uncontrolled studies that have been published, several patients treated with protein C concentrate still needed amputation. Randomized controlled trials have not been carried out.

Routine transfusion of platelets is controversial. In patients with life-threatening bleeding, massive platelet transfusion may be life saving. However, it may also aggravate thrombus formation by increasing levels of PAI-1 released from the platelets.

Fibrinolysis

To overcome inhibition by PAI-1, recombinant human tissue plasminogen activator (0.25 to 0.5 mg/kg in 1.5 to 4 h) has been infused to enhance fibrinolysis. Dramatic improvement was observed in some children. Recombinant human tissue plasminogen activator increases the risk of an intracerebral haemorrhage. If used, it should be started early. Efficacy has never been evaluated in a randomized controlled trial.

Plasmapheresis and blood exchange

Plasmapheresis or exchange blood transfusion have been tried, to remove pathologically activated plasma and leucocytes; 50 ml plasma/kg body weight has been exchanged with fresh plasma. These techniques do not increase the clearance of bacterial lipopolysaccharide substantially. Results suggest improved survival but adequate control groups are lacking. Even desperately ill patients have tolerated the procedures.

Extracorporal membrane oxygenation

A limited number of children have been treated with extracorporal membrane oxygenation in a few centres with apparently good results. However, equally good results have been achieved in another paediatric intensive care unit without using the procedure, suggesting that the experience of the intensive care unit is more important than the procedure per se.

Neutralization of bacterial lipopolysaccharides

Three different antiendotoxin principles, the anti-J5 serum, the human monoclonal IgM (HA-1A) antibody, and the recombinant bactericidal/permeability increasing protein (BPI_{21}) have been evaluated in randomized, double-blind, controlled clinical trials. None increased survival significantly. However, fewer patients treated with BPI_{21} required multiple severe amputations and more patients had a functional outcome similar to that before illness 60 days after treatment. None of the principles are presently commerically available.

Antimediator therapy

Strategies to neutralize tumour necrosis factor-α, IL-1, bradykinin, platelet-activating factor, and prostaglandins in patients with septic shock have not increased the 28-day survival rate. They have not been specifically evaluated in meningococcal septic shock.

Sequelae

Meningitis

Neurogenic deafness occurs in 1 to 10 per cent of the patients. It develops at an early stage and is usually irreversible. Reversible paresis of brain nerves IV, VI, or VII is occasionally observed. Epilepsy, hydrocephalus, and diffuse brain damage are at present rare complications in industrialized countries.

Persistent headache, altered sleep pattern, concentration difficulties, irritability, and neurasthenia may persist in 5 to 8 per cent of all patients.

Shock and coagulopathy

Most long-term complications are related to development of gangrene of the extremities requiring amputation and necrotic skin lesions requiring extensive grafting. The renal failure is usually reversible. Permanent adrenal insufficiency develops very rarely in survivors. Acute respiratory distress syndrome may lead to permanent pulmonary fibrosis and reduced function.

Vaccination

Capsule polysaccharide vaccine (A, C, Y, and W)

The serogroup A polysaccharide vaccine is immunogenic from 6 months of age. Infants vaccinated at 3 and 7 months develop higher antibody levels than do infants vaccinated only at 7 months, suggesting a booster effect. The serogroup C polysaccharide vaccine induces a short-lived immune response at 3 months but normal immune response in children above 18 months. No booster response is present. Revaccination may reduce the antibody level. When vaccination is required for serogroup A infection, infants of less than 24 months should receive two doses with at least a 1-month interval, whereas those above 2 years should receive one dose. For serogroup C infection, one dose should be given from 18 months. In children with malaria, the immune response is reduced. An antibody level of 1 to 2 µg/ml appears to be necessary for protection.

Indications for vaccination

Routine immunization with the A, C, Y, and W polysaccharide vaccine is advocated for people with documented deficiencies in the late complement components and properdin.

Non-outbreak situation

Indications for vaccination with A or C polysaccharide vaccine are, according to Peltola: close contacts of an index case, travellers to high-risk areas, military recruits, persons with asplenia, and alcoholics.

Outbreak situation

Vaccination has been recommended if two or more are attacked by the same strain in a school class or day-care centre, the attack rate exceeds 10 cases/100 000 population per 3 months, or the attack exceeds 1/1000 with 3 or more cases in a closed group setting.

Epidemic situation

An advocated threshold for mass vaccination is 15 cases/100 000 population per week for 2 consecutive weeks caused by the same strain. A steadily increasing number of cases and an increase in the median age of the patients indicate an epidemic.

Conjungate polysaccharide protein vaccine

Serogroup C polysaccharide conjugated to a protein carrier induces a significant booster response in infants vaccinated at 2, 3, and 4 months of age. The same has been shown for toddlers. The United Kingdom is the first country to start mass vaccination with serogroup C conjugate vaccine of infants, children, and adolescents owing to the increasing number of serogroup C cases.

Outer membrane vesicle vaccine

Since the capsule polysaccharide of serogroup B strains induces a short-lived IgM but no lasting IgG response, several groups have developed an outer membrane vesicle vaccine. The protection rate after two doses is lower (57 to 80 per cent) than for the polysaccharide A, C, Y, and W vaccines and is relatively strain specific. The protection rate in children below 4 years of age is much lower than for adults. Three doses induce a significantly better immune response than two doses given with a 6-week interval. Only one vaccine is available for sale.

Secondary prophylaxis

Antibiotic prophylaxis

Household contacts of an index case have a 100 to 1000 times increased relative risk for developing meningococcal infections. Usually the second case occurs within 2 weeks of the index case if no eradication treatment is given. However, there is doubt about the effectiveness of eradication treatment when the causative strain belongs to serogroup B.

Health authorities in most countries advise that close contacts have eradication treatment with rifampicin at 10 mg/kg, maximum dose 600 mg every 12 h for 48 h. Recently, 500 mg of ciprofloxacin or 400 mg of ofloxacin as a single dose has replaced rifampicin for adults in many countries. Pregnant women should receive 250 mg, and children of less than 12 years 125 mg, of ceftriaxone as one intramuscular injection.

Future prospects

The development of effective and affordable conjugate vaccines covering serogroups A and C will be a major step forward. They will cover the age group 2 months to 2 years where protection is most required and pave the way for routine vaccination. Development of a serogroup B vaccine with documented effect for infants and children is urgently needed.

Further reading

Brandtzaeg P (1996). Systemic meningococcal disease: clinical pictures and pathophysiological background. *Reviews in Medical Microbiology* 7, 63–72.

Cartwright K, ed. (1995). *Meningococcal disease.* Wiley, Chichester.

Caugant DA (1998). Population genetics and molecular epidemiology of *Neisseria meningitidis. Acta Pathologica, Microbiologica et Immunologica Scandinavica* 106, 505–25.

Girgis NI *et al.* (1989). Dexamethasone treatment for bacterial meningitis in children and adults. *Pediatric Infectious Disease Journal* 8, 848–51.

Oppenheim BA (1997). Antibiotic resistance in *Neisseria meningitidis. Clinical Infectious Diseases* 24 (Suppl. 1), 98–101.

Peltola H (1998). Meningococcal vaccines. Current status and future possibilities. *Drugs* 55, 347–66.

Pollard AJ *et al.* (1999). Emergency management of meningococcal disease. *Archives of Disease in Childhood* 80, 290–6.

Van Deuren M, Brandtzaeg P, van der Meer JWM (2000). Update on meningococcal disease, with special emphasis on pathogenesis and clinical management. *Clinical Microbiology Review* 13, 144–66.

7.11.6 *Neisseria gonorrhoeae*

D. Barlow and C. Ison

Neisseria gonorrhoeae, the gonococcus, has changed in three important ways since the advent of effective treatment: sensitivity to antibiotics has decreased (and continues to do so); its symptom-producing capabilities have lessened; and its incubation period has lengthened. A study from the United Kingdom in the early nineties gave a mean incubation period of 5.6 days and a median of 8.6 days in men.

Pathogenesis

N. gonorrhoeae is a particularly successful pathogen, with mechanisms that evade host defences and cause repeated infection. The major antigens of the outer membrane (**OM**) of the gonococcus that are exposed to the immune response are pili, lipo-oligosaccharide (**LOS**), and three major OM proteins, Por, Opa, and Rmp. *N. gonorrhoeae* primarily colonizes columnar epithelium of the lower genital tract and only occasionally progresses to the upper genital tract or invades to cause systemic disease. Successful colonization requires attachment and invasion of the epithelial layer to avoid being swept away by cervical secretions in women or urine in men. *N. gonorrhoeae* expresses receptors on the cell surface for transferrin or lactoferrin from which iron is released, unlike many other bacteria that produce soluble sideropores. Lack of iron can be a growth-limiting factor. For invasion to occur, gonococci must resist the bactericidal activity of serum. *In vivo* gonococci are serum resistant as a result of sialylation of LOS. *In vitro* most strains revert to serum sensitive, although a few remain resistant suggesting an additional unidentified mechanism.

Pili, Opa, and LOS have the ability to alter the surface-exposed part of the molecule and hence present a new antigen to the immune system. In the gonococcus this alteration occurs at a frequency higher than the normal mutation rate and is known as antigenic variation. On each encounter between the organism and the host, the gonococcus presents a range of immunologically distinct proteins which are not recognized by the host. The interaction of these bacterial receptors with the host cell is complex and the host-cell receptors are currently being unravelled, ranging from complex carbohydrates and glycosamines to lipoproteins and glycoproteins.

Epidemiology

Gonorrhoea is almost exclusively transmitted by sexual activity and, like HIV infection, is not evenly distributed amongst the sexually active population. The highest incidence is found in young (teenaged women, men in their twenties), urban, socio-economically deprived persons and ethnic minorities. Figure 1 shows the number of cases in England up to 2000, the

Fig. 1 Reported cases of gonorrhoea in England between 1918 and 2000 (Department of Health).

drop in reported cases since 1974 being reversed in the early nineties. Use of antimicrobials has less effect on endemic levels than might be expected, although it reduces the incidence of complications. Gonorrhoea facilitates HIV transmission, producing an increase in detectable virus in urethral secretions when infection is present; this is reversed following antibiotic treatment.

The incidence and prevalence of gonorrhoea serve as useful surrogates for unsafe sexual behaviour since diagnosis is swift and accurate and the infection can be treated and reacquired repeatedly. The incidence of neonatal gonococcal ophthalmia and the prevalence of antenatal infection measure the success, or otherwise, of a control programme. By both criteria, gonorrhoea is not a serious problem in the United Kingdom.

The infectivity of the gonococcus is probably higher from male to female and may reach 80 per cent. Condoms, when used invariably and throughout sexual contact, prevent transmission of gonorrhoea.

Symptoms, signs, and complications

Gonorrhoea in women

Because of the lack of specific symptoms there is no meaningful incubation period for uncomplicated gonorrhoea in women. The sites most commonly affected are cervix (90 per cent), urethra (75 per cent), rectum (40 per cent), and oropharynx (5 to 15 per cent). Signs at all these sites are unhelpful—the 'cervicitis' ascribed to gonorrhoea being found in other conditions and in healthy individuals. Symptoms likewise are absent or non-specific, including alteration in vaginal discharge or, rarely, mild dysuria. Women with gonorrhoea depend on notification by a partner or development of complications to alert them to the possibility of infection. Spread of the gonococcus to infect the endometrium, fallopian tubes, and pelvic adnexas is the most common complication (5 per cent of infections) and occurs at or soon after the menstrual period, probably resulting from retrograde flow of menses. Coincidental infection with *Chlamydia trachomatis* is common enough to warrant treatment of both organisms. Gonococcal infection of Bartholin's, Skene's, or periurethral glands is rare in the United Kingdom.

Disseminated gonococcal infection is four or five times more common in women than men, a reflection of women's lack of genital symptoms. Almost always caused by penicillin-sensitive organisms, disseminated gonococcal infection is a comparatively benign bacteraemia affecting joints and skin. The shoulder and knee are most commonly affected followed by the wrist, elbow, and small joints of the hands and feet, often with an associated tenosynovitis. The pathognomonic, painless, skin lesions, usually 4 to 10 in number, evolve through vesicular, pustular, and haemorrhagic stages before healing (Plates 1, 2). Erythema nodosum-like lesions have been described. The constitutional upset tends to be minimal and the white cell count and erythrocyte sedimentation rate are not greatly raised. Response to antibiotic treatment is rapid but joints may need to be aspirated. Blood or joint fluid culture may yield gonococci but the quickest diagnosis comes from anogenital and throat culture.

Perihepatitis, the FitzHugh–Curtis syndrome, more frequently appears with *C. trachomatis* than *N. gonorrhoeae*. Right hypochondrial pain, referred to the shoulder, occasionally with pleural effusion and rub, results in referral to a surgeon or a general, rather than geniturinary, physician.

Gonorrhoea in men

Affected sites are the urethra and oropharynx, and the rectum in homosexual men. Rectal and throat infections tend to be silent while discharge is the commonest urethral symptom. When the infection is fully developed, the discharge is white/yellow/green and profuse, staining the underwear. Differential diagnosis includes foreign body and, unusually, non-gonococcal urethritis. Scanty mucoid or mucopurulent discharge is seen in early infection. Discomfort on urination no longer seems to be severe or as common as before, with one large United Kingdom study eliciting dysuria as a presenting symptom in only 50 per cent of men. Asymptomatic patients (less than 10 per cent) include presymptomatic, post-symptomatic, and unobservant men. Urethral gonorrhoea acquired following fellatio is increasingly seen in gay men practising 'safe' sex and may be passed on as rectal gonorrhoea to a regular partner. Infection spreading to the epididymis and testis is more often due to *C. trachomatis* than the gonococcus, and other complications—tysonitis, prostatitis, periurethral abscess, or infection of the median raphe—constitute very few cases in the United Kingdom.

Diagnosis

Microscopy

Even in genitourinary medicine departments, the majority of patients will not have gonorrhoea. Much time and effort is spent excluding rather than diagnosing the disease. Investigations therefore need high sensitivity. The diagnosis of gonococcal infection is easier in men than in women.

Microscopy of a suitably stained specimen is the first line in diagnosis. The organisms must be Gram-negative, intracellular (within the cytoplasm of a leucocyte), and diplococci (GNID) (Plate 3). In samples from the male urethra, microscopy is highly sensitive (identifying 98 per cent of positives) and highly specific (less than 1 per cent will be found on culture to be *Neisseria meningitidis* or other species).

Microscopy of stained samples from rectum, cervix, and female urethra although much less sensitive, with identification of only 55 per cent or less of true positives, should still be performed since it has the advantage, where positive, of enabling immediate diagnosis and treatment. Because of the preponderance of other neisserias in the oropharynx, microscopy of samples from this site is not helpful.

Routine culture of samples from the male urethra provides an important means of quality control of the laboratory service, so crucial for diagnosis in women. It also enables assessment of antibiotic sensitivities and other characteristics of the organism for epidemiological and management purposes.

Laboratory detection of *N. gonorrhoeae*

Isolation of the causative organism, *N. gonorrhoeae*, has been regarded as the gold standard for the diagnosis of gonorrhoea for many years. However, the application of molecular techniques, such as polymerase chain reaction or the ligase chain reaction, are being more widely used.

Isolation and identification of *N. gonorrhoeae*

N. gonorrhoeae is fastidious in its growth requirements. It needs an enriched medium, such as Thayer–Martin or Modified New York City, which consist of GC agar base supplemented with a source of iron (lysed horse blood) and essential amino acids and glucose (IsoVitaleX or Vitox), and incubation in moist conditions with 5 to 7 per cent carbon dioxide at 37°C. Good specimen collection and efficient transport to the laboratory are crucial to successful isolation.

Specimens are taken using disposable loops or swabs and inoculated in the clinic or sent to the laboratory in transport medium. The isolation rates vary little if the specimen is dealt with rapidly. Isolation is enhanced by the addition of antibiotics to the medium to suppress other organisms that colonize the anogenital tract. While occasional problems can arise due to antibiotic-sensitive strains, a selective medium is essential and non-selective media should only be used as an adjunct not as a replacement.

After incubation, colonies that are oxidase positive (presence of cytochrome c oxidase), Gram negative, and cocci are considered to be *Neisseria* spp. In many parts of the world this would be considered presumptive identification of *N. gonorrhoeae*. However, in the industrialized world confirmation of identity as *N. gonorrhoeae* is usual. Historically, this has been achieved using carbohydrate utilization tests; *N. gonorrhoeae* differs from other species in that it alone produces acid from glucose. Identification kits

combining carbohydrate utilization and enzyme profiles are commonly used. An alternative approach is to use immunological reagents; two reagents are available which contain antibodies raised to epitopes on the two types of the major outer membrane protein, Por or PI, linked to fluorescein (GC Microtrak, Syva Company, USA) and to staphylococcal Protein A (Phadebact Monoclonal GC OMNI test, Boule AB Sweden). These sensitive and specific reagents can identify colonies direct from the primary isolation medium and a result can be obtained on the same day as the organism is isolated. Correct identification of *N. gonorrhoeae* is most important in cases of sexual or child abuse. In such instances it is sensible to use more than one of the identification tests available to confirm an isolate as *N. gonorrhoeae*.

Molecular detection of *N. gonorrhoeae*

Antigen detection assays for *N. gonorrhoeae*, both immunological and molecular, have been largely unsuccessful because they offer little advantage over the Gram stain and culture and they cannot provide an organism for susceptibility testing. However, the sensitivity and specificity of detection assays by DNA amplification, polymerase chain reaction (**PCR**) and ligase chain reaction (**LCR**), now appear to be equal or superior to conventional techniques and may be less affected by suboptimal handling or transport. These assays may also be useful on non-invasive specimens such as urine or self-taken swabs. Currently there are no molecular tests available for determining antibiotic susceptibility, but the sequence of the appropriate resistance genes or mutations is known and could be detected using PCR or LCR. Assays that offer the combination of detection of *N. gonorrhoeae* and susceptibility to antibiotics are likely to be available in the near future.

Typing

Typing is useful for studying reinfection, treatment failure, coinfection, and to show correlations with pathogenicity and antimicrobial susceptibility patterns. Auxotyping is the determination of nutritional requirement. A large number of auxotypes have been described but in most studies three or four types predominate: non-requiring (NR) or prototrophic (Proto), proline-requiring (Pro), arginine-requiring (Arg), and those requiring arginine, hypoxanthine, and uracil (AHU). Serotyping, using a panel of monoclonal antibodies, divides strains into 24 IA serovars and 32 IB serovars. Auxotyping and serotyping are often used in combination to produce auxotype/serovar (A/S) classes giving greater discrimination. A variety of genotypic methods have also been used, from plasmid analysis, which is poorly discriminatory, to pulse-field gel electrophoresis or DNA sequencing, which are highly discriminatory.

Antibiotic resistance

Penicillin has been used as first-line therapy for gonorrhoea for many years. *N. gonorrhoeae* is inherently sensitive to most antibiotics such as penicillin, but with increased usage both chromosomally-mediated and plasmid-mediated resistance has developed. Resistance is most prevalent in the developing world where the incidence of gonorrhoea is high and appropriate antibiotics are often unavailable or misused. However, in the industrialized world these strains are often imported and then spread by the indigenous population. In 1989 the World Health Organization issued new guidelines for the treatment of gonorrhoea stating that penicillin should only be used as first-line treatment if the gonococcal population is known to be sensitive. If resistance is high or the susceptibility of the gonococcal population is unknown, alternative treatment is recommended: ciprofloxacin (a quinolone), ceftriaxone (a third-generation cephalosporin), or spectinomycin (a macrolide). Of these antibiotics, ciprofloxacin is used increasingly is the United Kingdom because it is administered orally and is highly effective and inexpensive.

Chromosomally-mediated resistance

Decreased susceptibility to penicillin was detected as early as 1958, but this could be overcome by increasing the dose of penicillin and by adding probenecid. It was not until the 1970s that strains begun to appear with minimum inhibitory concentrations (**MICs**) to penicillin of greater than 1.0 mg/l and posed a therapeutic problem. Chromosomal resistance to penicillin in *N. gonorrhoeae* is the result of the additive effects of mutations at multiple loci, *penA*, *mtr*, and *penB*, the products of which reduce the permeability of the cell wall to penicillin.

Resistance to the alternative therapies—ceftriaxone, spectinomycin, and ciprofloxacin—has begun to emerge. Therapeutic failure to ceftriaxone has not yet been documented, but the loci responsible for chromosomal resistance to penicillin also confer decreased susceptibility to the earlier cephalosporins. If this type of resistance to penicillin continues to increase and is treated inappropriately, resistance to cephalosporins could emerge. Therapeutic resistance to spectinomycin has been reported sporadically, is high level, and due to a mutation on the chromosome that affects ribosomal binding. Spectinomycin has been an extremely useful antibiotic in treating resistant gonorrhoea and may be important in the future if mechanisms of resistance continue to evolve to newer antibiotics. Ciprofloxacin is now a popular alternative for the treatment of gonorrhoea because it is highly effective in a single oral dose of 500 mg. However, high-level resistance, resulting in therapeutic failure, has emerged in strains primarily originating from the western Pacific with mutations in the DNA gyrase gene, *gyrA*, and the topoisomerase IV gene, *parC*. The level of resistance may be enhanced by additional mutations in the *gyrB* gene or in changes in cell wall permeability, possibly due to efflux mechanisms. Surveillance of gonococcal isolates in the Western world should prolong the life of this useful antimicrobial agent.

Plasmid-mediated resistance

N. gonorrhoeae exhibiting plasmid-mediated resistance to penicillin were first described in 1976. Simultaneous reports appeared of two strains, one from Africa carrying a plasmid of 3.2 megadaltons (MDa) and the second from the Far East carrying a plasmid of 4.4 MDa. Both plasmids encode for the TEM-1 type β-lactamase (penicillinase). The smaller plasmid of 3.2 MDa has a deletion from the 4.4 MDa plasmid in a non-functional region. Penicillinase-producing *N. gonorrhoeae* carrying the 3.2 MDa and 4.4 MDa plasmids have now disseminated worldwide, although their prevalence is greatest in countries of the developing world. Penicillinase-producing *N. gonorrhoeae* carrying plasmids of differing size (2.9, 3.0, and 4.8 MDa) have been described more recently but have not spread in the same manner.

In 1985 plasmid-mediated resistance to tetracycline was first detected. It is high-level (MIC ≥ 16 mg/l) and is due to the acquisition of the *tetM* determinant by the conjugative plasmid of *N. gonorrhoeae* resulting in a plasmid of 25.2 MDa. Strains carrying this plasmid are known as tetracycline-resistant *N. gonorrhoeae*. Tetracycline is not the treatment of choice for gonorrhoea but is commonly used, particularly in African countries, because it is inexpensive and available.

Susceptibility testing

The primary aim of susceptibility testing of *N. gonorrhoeae* is to predict therapeutic failure. However, it is also important to monitor drifts in susceptibility and to detect the emergence of resistant strains to the main first-line therapies. There is much controversy over the correct method for achieving this for gonococci. Determination of zones of inhibition around antibiotic-containing discs has been the method chosen by most clinical laboratories, but gonococci vary in their growth patterns and this method can be difficult to control and interpret. In recent years the breakpoint agar dilution technique, which uses one or two concentrations of antibiotic to estimate the MIC and categorize strains into susceptible, reduced susceptibility, and resistant, has been used increasingly. Determination of the full MIC is not necessary for most laboratories and is best performed by reference centres.

Plasmid-mediated resistance to penicillin can be easily detected using the chromogenic cephalosporin (nitrocefin) test, which can be performed direct from the primary isolation plate. Plasmid-mediated resistance to tetracycline can be detected using either the absence of a zone of inhibition around a 10 μg tetracycline disc or presence of growth on GC agar containing 10 mg/l of tetracycline. In a similar manner, high-level resistance to ciprofloxacin can be detected by screening for isolates that can grow on agar containing 1 mg/l ciprofloxacin.

Treatment

Treatment of uncomplicated gonorrhoea in both sexes is ideally by a single dose of antibiotics, the choice of which will depend on where the infection was acquired and from whom. In the Far East and Africa, a high percentage of strains will have chromosomal and/or plasmid-associated resistance, whereas organisms in the United Kingdom, unless imported, are still largely sensitive to penicillin, and with doses less than those required, say, in America. Standard treatment should cure at least 95 per cent of presenting cases of gonorrhoea and, in the United Kingdom, 2 or 3 g of amoxycillin or ampicillin, with 1 g of probenecid achieves this aim. Alternatively, 500 mg of ciprofloxacin has the advantage of higher cure rates in oropharyngeal infection. Treatment with 250 mg of ceftriaxone, 500 mg of spectinomycin, or 500 mg of cefotaxime, all intramuscularly, is suitable for infections acquired outside the United Kingdom, cefotaxime being particularly useful for organisms with both plasmid and high chromosomal resistance such as those found in the Philippines.

Many physicians add 1 g of azithromycin, or 100 mg of doxycycline twice daily for 1 week, for possible coincidental chlamydial infection.

American and British guidelines suggest that gonococcal pelvic infection or perihepatitis be treated with parenteral antibiotics although the evidence for this is not strong. All are agreed that antichlamydial therapy should be included. A single intramuscular dose of 250 mg of ceftriaxone or 2 g of cefoxitin, followed by 100 mg of doxycycline and 400 mg of metronidazole, both twice daily for 2 weeks, is recommended. For infection acquired in the United Kingdom, with no foreign connections, cure should occur with any of the standard single-dose treatments followed by doxycycline with metronidazole for 2 weeks, as above.

Gonococcal epididymo-orchitis can be treated with 500 mg of ciprofloxacin followed by 100 mg of doxycycline twice daily (or 2 g of erythromycin stearate daily in divided doses) for at least 2 weeks. A scrotal support eases symptoms.

Tracing of contacts of all cases of gonorrhoea and exclusion of other sexually transmitted infections must be undertaken.

Further reading

Bignell C (2000). European guidelines for the management of gonorrhoea. *International Journal of Sexually Transmitted Diseases and AIDS* **12** (Suppl 3), 27–9 and www.mssvd.org.uk.

Centers for Disease Control (1998). Sexually transmitted disease treatment guidelines 1988. *Morbidity and Mortality Weekly Report* **47**, 1–111.

Hook EW, Handsfield HH (1999). Gonococcal infections in the adult. In: Holmes KK *et al.*, eds. *Sexually transmitted diseases*, 3rd edn, pp. 451–6. McGraw-Hill, New York.

Ison CA (1996). Antimicrobial agents and gonorrhoea: therapeutic choice, resistance and susceptibility testing. *Genitourinary Medicine* **72**, 253–7.

Ison CA (1998). Gonorrhoea. In: Woodford N, Johnson AP, eds. *Methods in molecular medicine*, Vol 15. *Molecular bacteriology: protocols and clinical applications*, pp 293–308. Humana Press, New Jersey.

Nassif X *et al.* (1999). Interactions of pathogenic neisseria with host cells. Is it possible to assemble the puzzle? *Molecular Biology* **32**, 1124–32.

Taylor-Robinson D, Thomas B, Ison C (1999). Diagnostic procedures in genitourinary medicine: practical laboratory aspects. In: Barton SE, Hay PE, eds. *Handbook of genitourinary medicine*, pp. 19–48. Arnold, London.

7.11.7 Enterobacteria, campylobacter, and miscellaneous food-poisoning bacteria

G. T. Keusch and M. B. Skirrow

Humans are colonized by a huge number of micro-organisms, prominent among which are the Enterobacteriaceae, a large grouping of small, facultatively anaerobic, Gram-negative bacilli capable of residence in the gastrointestinal tract, and therefore often grouped together as the enterobacteria. However, Enterobacteriaceae are not just commensals in the intestinal flora; they may also be important causes of disease, both locally in the gut and at times invasively in the blood and elsewhere in the body. This chapter begins with a short general description of enterobacteria and the infections they cause outside the intestinal tract. It then focuses on these organisms as enteric pathogens. In the latter role the enterobacteria most often cause diarrhoea, which remains a major cause of morbidity in advanced industrial economies and mortality in developing countries, especially among children.

Although *Salmonella typhi* and *S. paratyphi*, the causes of typhoid and paratyphoid fever, are enterobacteria, their special attributes are described in detail in Chapter 7.11.8. Likewise, *Yersinia* infections are described in Chapter 7.11.17. However, enteritis due to Gram-negative non-Enterobacteriaceae, namely *Campylobacter, Aeromonas, Plesiomonas* spp., *Vibrio parahaemolyticus*, and other non-cholera vibrios are included here. Descriptions of food poisoning due to the Gram-positive bacteria *Clostridium botulinum* and *C. perfringens* are provided in Chapter 7.11.21. *Bacillus cereus*, and *Staphylococcus aureus* food poisoning are presented here. An overview of infections of the intestinal tract is given in Chapter 14.17.

The enterobacteria

Definition and general description

Strictly speaking, the term 'enterobacteria' applies to members of the large family Enterobacteriaceae that are found in the intestinal tract of humans and animals, or are associated with plants and soil. Classical taxonomy based on biochemical and immunological criteria has resulted in a family that includes a number of major tribes with widely varying properties, including 30 genera and at least 120 species. Within these various tribes, the genera most likely to be encountered in medical practice are *Salmonella, Shigella, Escherichia, Klebsiella, Enterobacter, Citrobacter, Serratia, Hafnia, Edwardsiella, Erwinia, Kluyvera, Proteus, Providencia, Morganella,* and *Yersinia*. However, this classical schema is likely to be altered as DNA homology becomes the basis of microbial classification. *Escherichia coli, Salmonella* spp., and *Shigella* spp. are the principal enteric pathogens among these groups. The others may cause enteric disease but are more commonly the cause of systemic infection, usually through a specific portal of entry, especially in immunologically compromised hosts.

Enterobacteriaceae are Gram-negative, oxidase-negative, non-spore-forming straight rods, most of which are motile by means of peritrichous flagella. Although they are aerobes, many are capable of growth under anaerobic conditions. Microbiologists divide the group into those capable of mixed-acid fermentation resulting in the production of acetate from pyruvate (such as *Escherichia coli, Salmonella,* and *Shigella*) and those that produce butanediol as the end-product of fermentation (*Serratia, Enterobacter,* and *Erwinia*). They are easy to cultivate in the laboratory on simple bacteriological media (most can grow using D-glucose as the sole source of carbon, producing acid), indeed they often outgrow and mask the presence of more fastidious bacteria. However, they are vulnerable to environmental stress, such as heating to 60 °C for 20 min, and desiccation. Many are acid-sensitive, but some are resistant to acid pH, which may serve as a virulence factor in the gastrointestinal tract.

The clinical microbiology laboratory takes advantage of the inability of *Salmonella* and *Shigella* spp. to ferment lactose by screening cultures for the presence of non-lactose-fermenting organisms. This is a useful initial and simple distinguishing feature, because virtually all other enterobacteria—with the exception of *Proteus, Providencia,* and *Morganella*—ferment lactose freely. By including lactose and a pH indicator in a culture medium, the colonies of non-lactose fermenters stand out from the lactose fermenters, which produce acid and change the colour of the included pH-sensitive indicator dye. This makes it simple to pick the pale non-lactose-fermenting colonies for further study. The lactose-fermenting enterobacteria are commonly grouped together as 'coliforms', a clinically convenient term that has little logic to commend it. It is particularly unfortunate that this rubric may serve to hide significant pathogens, as the notation is often interpreted to mean harmless organisms resembling ordinary *E. coli*.

Microbial structure and antigenicity

The Enterobacteriaceae are typical Gram-negative rods, in that they possess a complex cell wall containing three major layers: (1) the inner cytoplasmic membrane; (2) an intermediate region made up of peptidoglycan; and (3) an outer cell membrane, which is itself composed of an inner phospholipid–protein layer and an outer covering of lipopolysaccharide (**LPS**). In addition, some members of the group possess an outermost antigenic carbohydrate capsule, while others possess one or more flagella and hence are motile. The cytoplasmic membrane functions, as it does for all micro-organisms, to regulate the transport of metabolites, sugars, amino acids, small peptides, and ions into and out of the microbial cell. Peptidoglycan, a long-chain linear polymer and structural element common to Gram-positive and Gram-negative bacteria, covers this membrane. It is composed of alternating *N*-acetylmuramic acid and *N*-acetylglucosamine residues with a pentapeptide side chain terminating in a D-alanyl-D-alanine dipeptide. This dipeptide is the site for the formation of cross-linking peptide bonds between adjacent linear aminosugar chains, providing structural stability to the bacterial cell. Crosslinking is catalysed by transpeptidase enzymes, which are the targets of action of the β-lactam antibiotics, such as the penicillins and cephalosporins.

A major difference in the peptidoglycan layer between Gram-positive and Gram-negative bacteria is the greater thickness of the structure in Gram-positive bacteria. The region between the peptidoglycan layer and the outer cell membrane is known as the periplasmic space. Critical cell functions also take place within this space, for example the assembly and modification of microbial proteins and antigens that are inserted in, or excreted through, the outer layer. The latter is a complex structure commonly referred to as endotoxin because it contains lipid A, the endotoxic moiety of LPS, linked to a common-core carbohydrate structure. A highly variable polymer of sugar residues, the O-specific oligosaccharide chain, is displayed on the outermost microbial surface, and contains critical, specific, heat-stable antigenic carbohydrate determinants designated O-antigens. Oligosaccharides, even when composed of just a few sugar residues, are well suited to express immunologically specific and recognizable antigens, because they permit a large number of small stereospecific changes that can be distinguished by antigen-specific antibodies. It is this structural feature of the O-specific oligosaccharides that permits the separation of many different O-antigen serotypes within a species—160 in *E. coli* alone. In the case of motile strains, flagellar proteins are also expressed well, so additional heat-labile protein (H) antigens are identifiable. Finally, some Enterobacteriaceae produce an outer capsular layer possessing yet more (carbohydrate) antigens designated K antigens. K antigens may cover and mask the underlying O-antigens and obscure the identity of the organism unless first removed by boiling the culture.

Taken together, these three types of antigen form the basis of a useful system for the identification and differentiation of enterobacteria in the laboratory, originally devised by Kaufmann and White. Because these antigens induce the formation of specific antibodies, which may be employed as immunoreagents that are specific for particular microbial structures, they turn out to be highly useful for the serological diagnosis of specific infections. When there is a rise in antibody to the O, H, and, if present, K antigens, which represent the 'signature' of particular members of the group, a serological diagnosis can be made. However, adding to the complexity, a single organism can express multiple O, H, and K antigens and individual antigens; moreover, O-specific oligosaccharides may be shared by two or more specific organisms within a genus or across species. Therefore immunological identification of individual organisms and serological diagnosis of an infection is based on the pattern of antigens detected, or on a significant rise in antibody titre to a particular battery of antigens. This serological 'fingerprint' is often supplemented by biological and biochemical information for the purposes of identification. Capsular antigens, when present, can add additional information, for example the Vi antigen of *Salmonella typhi*, which is shared with just one organism, *Citrobacter freundii*. Serological identification of specific strains of enterobacteria is of enormous utility for epidemiological investigations.

Extraintestinal infections caused by enterobacteria and related organisms

Before proceeding to specific diarrhoeal diseases caused by enterobacteria, a brief account of their infective role elsewhere in the body is provided. It is convenient to include other non-fastidious Gram-negative bacilli that behave clinically in a similar manner to enterobacteria and which are often found in mixed infections with them. Chief among these is *Pseudomonas aeruginosa*, which is notorious as a 'hospital' organism and as a cause of opportunistic and sometimes fatal systemic infection in debilitated or immunosuppressed patients. *Ps. aeruginosa* is naturally resistant to most of the commonly used antimicrobials and also to many antiseptics. Indeed certain pseudomonads, notably *Ps. cepacia*, are capable of growth in antiseptic solutions stored at dilute working strengths in hospital wards. Other common opportunistic Gram-negative bacilli are found in the genera *Alcaligenes*, *Acinetobacter*, *Aeromonas*, *Flavobacterium*, and *Chromobacterium*.

Gram-negative sepsis occurs when these organisms reach the bloodstream and result in clinical symptoms. The incidence of Gram-negative sepsis steadily increased from the 1970s to the 1990s, particularly in hospital patients. The widespread use (and abuse) of broad-spectrum antibiotics, which were generally more active against Gram-positive bacteria, is one reason, but another is the increasing proportion of susceptible patients being treated: more elderly patients; more receiving immunosuppressive or cytotoxic therapy; more with catheters, pacemakers, and prostheses that provide favourable sites for infection; and more undergoing more complex and adventurous surgery. Enterobacteria, pseudomonads, and similar Gram-negative bacilli easily acquire resistance to antimicrobials, which helps them to colonize the hospital environment. Such organisms quickly replace the normal sensitive bowel flora of patients admitted to hospital, particularly if antibiotics are being given. In this way the patient's anus becomes the gateway to colonization and infection elsewhere in the body. Interestingly, during the past decade Gram-negative bacteraemia diminished relative to Gram-positive bacteraemia. Today, almost 50 per cent of bloodstream isolates are Gram-positive (Table 1). This reflects acquired resistance among the Gram-positives and the use of newer broad-spectrum drugs with better coverage of the Gram-negative bacteria, which are often given empirically for the treatment of presumptive infection without a specific known aetiology.

Table 1 Causes of bloodstream infection in patients in Intensive Care Units, United States, 1987–2000

Isolate	Percentage of total isolates
Coagulase-negative staphylococci*	35.5
*Staph. aureus**	13.7
Enterococci*	13.3
Candida albicans	5.4
Enterobacter†	4.8
Ps. aeruginosa†	3.9
K. pneumoniae†	3.2
E. coli†	2.4
Acinetobacter†	2.2
Serratia†	1.7
Others	13.9

Source: National Nosocomial Infections Surveillance System, National Center for Infectious Diseases, Centers for Disease Control and Prevention, Atlanta, GA, USA.
* Gram-positive; †Gram-negative.

It is against this background that one must consider Gram-negative sepsis, and it is not surprising that these organisms turn up in a wide variety of clinical material. They are frequently found colonizing wounds, sinuses, ulcers, burns, and chronically discharging ears—in fact wherever the body integument is broken. In many cases they are probably of little consequence, but their presence deep in a wound may cause harm by consuming oxygen and enhancing the growth of anaerobes. This is a common finding in foot infections in diabetic patients, for example. Distinguishing between simple colonization and infections of consequence can be challenging. This is one reason why practice of the specialty of infectious diseases requires both knowledge and thoughtful analysis—reflex administration of antimicrobials can be harmful to the health of the patient.

Specific types of infection

Urinary tract infection (Chapter 20.12)

The urinary tract is the most common site for genuine infection as opposed to simple colonization. Such infections range from a simple cystitis to pyelonephritis and pyonephrosis. Most infections are caused by *E. coli*, but resistant strains of *Klebsiella*, *Enterobacter*, *Proteus*, and *Ps. aeruginosa* are more likely to be the infecting agents in patients with complications: those with indwelling catheters; those who have undergone genitourinary surgery; and those with recurrent episodes of urinary tract infection treated with many courses of antimicrobial therapy. Septicaemia may arise from such infections, particularly after surgery (Chapter 7.5); even the simple removal of a urethral catheter from an infected individual may cause bacteraemia. *E. coli* strains causing parenteral infection usually belong to one of only 12 or so serogroups. Proteus infections in male children should alert a clinician to the possibility of a congenital abnormality of, for example, a urethral valve.

Sepsis linked to the intestinal tract

In these infections coliform bacteria are usually found with other bowel flora such as *Bacteroides* spp. and microaerophilic streptococci. Peritonitis secondary to a perforated bowel, intraperitoneal abscess (for example, pelvic, subphrenic, retrocaecal), cholecystitis, cholangitis, and liver abscess are examples of such infections. Coliforms and other bowel flora may also cause remote focal infections such as endocarditis or cerebral abscess.

Respiratory tract infections (Chapter 17.5.2)

Coliform bacteria seldom cause significant respiratory tract infections, but they are often isolated from sputum samples due to a tendency to colonize the mouths and upper respiratory tract of ill patients, particularly babies, the elderly, and debilitated patients in the intensive-care unit. Such colonization is significantly encouraged by antimicrobial chemotherapy, but this is not essential. The presence of colonizing coliforms in sputum is therefore commonly of no immediate clinical consequence, although true pneumonia may result. A classical example is caused by *Klebsiella pneumoniae* subspecies *pneumoniae* (Friedlander's bacillus), which has a characteristic morphology in the Gram stain of sputum (a fat Gram-negative rod with a large capsule) and a particular radiological appearance in the lung (sagging fissure, presumably due to the weight of capsular polysaccharide present). However, this organism accounts for only a tiny proportion of all bacterial pneumonias; most of the klebsiellae isolated from sputum are of the common aerogenes type and are not endowed with the thick capsule that characterizes *K. pneumoniae*. Patients with bronchiectasis or cystic fibrosis are especially prone to chronic bronchial superinfection, notably with capsulated 'mucoid' variants of *Ps. aeruginosa*.

K. ozaenae and *K. rhinoscleromatis* are associated with the uncommon nasal diseases ozaena and rhinoscleroma (Chapter 7.11.9). In the tropics, *Chromobacterium violaceum* occasionally causes a potentially fatal, rapidly progressive, septicaemic illness, with pneumonia and multiple abscess formation.

Neonatal infections

Newborn babies are especially liable to suffer from serious Gram-negative infections. This may be partially due to the immaturity of some host defence mechanisms, for example the complement system. Gram-negative septicaemia, which usually arises from an infected umbilicus, invariably involves the meninges as an incipient, if not overt, meningitis (Chapter 24.15.1). Fortunately such events are rare, but coliforms are the most common cause of neonatal meningitis, a fact that contrasts sharply with the scarcity of coliform meningitis after the age of 1 month. *E. coli* is usually responsible, but any of the enterobacteria may be involved. *Proteus mirabilis* infections, which take the form of a meningoencephalitis, are particularly severe, and occasionally this common organism, for reasons that are not understood, has caused disastrous outbreaks in hospital nurseries.

Specific enterobacterial infections of the gut

Escherichia coli infections

We begin with *E. coli* because the genus illustrates the vast range of pathogenic mechanisms available to the enterobacteria, together with the varied pathophysiology and clinical manifestations that ensue from infection. Most *E. coli* do not cause human illness, but are merely commensals that colonize the lower intestine from the terminal ileum to the anus. It is this property that has given rise to the term 'coliforms'. However, some have acquired virulence factors that have placed them among the leading causes of diarrhoea, particularly in the developing world. The concept that *E. coli*

might be capable of causing enteritis is not a recent one. In 1895 the German paediatrician, Escherich, suspected that certain strains of '*Bacterium coli*' caused infantile diarrhoea, but attempts to differentiate pathogenic from non-pathogenic strains were unsuccessful, mainly because adequate serological classification was not then available. In the past 25 years, the combined approach using epidemiology, clinical research, and molecular biology has identified at least five distinct groups of *E. coli* that cause disease when they colonize the intestine of non-immune subjects, typically young children, or less commonly adults with no prior contact with these organisms (Table 2).

Enterovirulent *E. coli* possess a number of specific virulence genes, in addition to sharing the general properties of *E. coli* encoded in the genome of K-12 strains (the minimal genome necessary to be classified as an *E. coli* species). These are often concentrated in islands of DNA known as 'pathogenicity islands', which are segments of DNA that differ significantly in base composition from the backbone *E. coli* K-12 genome, signifying that they have most likely been imported from other bacteria by DNA transfer, infecting phage, or via plasmids. It is the cluster of virulence genes present in strains of *E. coli* that give each the capacity to cause specific types of intestinal disease. These clusters of virulence genes are often associated with specific O and H serotypes, which thus may serve as surrogate and putative markers for pathogenic strains; although as discussed below, this is not always sufficient to define which *E. coli* are the pathogens (see Table 2). The five groups of enterovirulent *E. coli* are now described.

Enteropathogenic E. coli (**EPEC**)

EPEC strains are most important as a cause of endemic diarrhoea in developing countries, where they primarily infect children between the ages of 6 and 18 months. In developed countries, EPEC infection has declined to low levels over the last several decades. Some EPEC can infect adults, often in the context of traveller's diarrhoea. Their discovery goes back to the early 1940s when certain *E. coli*, recognized by the production of a distinct odour when grown on agar plates, were associated with severe outbreaks of diarrhoea in neonatal nurseries. When the Kaufmann–White scheme for serotyping *E. coli* was subsequently developed, these original strains, designated EPEC, were found to be from serogroups O111 and O55. Over the years, additional serotypes have been added to the EPEC group (see Table 2), and the epidemiology has changed from that of a strong association with neonatal units to that of a watery diarrhoea in young infants and children between 6 months and 3 years of age. Hospital microbiology units were capable of serotyping the 12 most frequent O-antigen types associated with these infections using commercial kits. Hospital clinical laboratories

Table 2 The major groups of *Escherichia coli* causing diarrhoea in humans

Pathogenicity group	Pathogenicity factor or marker	Commonly found serogroups	Associated disease
Enteropathogenic *E. coli* (EPEC) and other enteroadherent *E. coli* (EAEC)	Locally adherent*	O55, O86, O111, O114, O119, O125, O126, O127, O128, O142, O158	Watery diarrhoea, mainly in children but also adults
	Diffusely adherent*	O15, O75, O126 and various others	Not clearly established
	Aggregatively adherent*	O3, O15, O44, O51, O77, O78, O86, 091, 092, O111, O113, O126, O141, O146	Acute and persistent diarrhoea in children
Enterotoxigenic *E. coli* (ETEC)	Heat-labile toxin (LT), or heat-stable toxin (ST), or both	O6, O8, O15, O25, O27, O63, O78, O115, O148, O153, O159, O167, and various others	Watery diarrhoea in children in developing world; travellers' diarrhoea
Enteroinvasive *E. coli* (EIEC)	Cell invasion like shigellae	O28ac, O112ac, O124, O136, O143, O144, O152, O164	Most commonly watery diarrhoea. Also causes a shigella-like bloody diarrhoea or, on occasion. dysentery
Enterohaemorrhagic *E. coli* (EHEC) or shiga- toxin-producing *E. coli* (STEC)	Shiga-like toxins: Stx-1, Stx-2 and variants	O157, O26, O103, O104, O111 and many others	Haemorrhagic colitis; haemolytic-uraemic syndrome

* See text.

could then report back that a potentially enteropathogenic serotype of *E. coli* was isolated.

The modern era in the study and definition of EPEC was ushered in by the first successful human experimental infections with EPEC strains in 1978. In this experiment, two of three EPEC strains (an O127 and an O142) previously isolated from neonatal diarrhoea outbreaks caused clinical illness in adult United States volunteers, whereas the third (an O128) as well as a classical 'normal flora' strain (HS) were clinically benign. This indicated that it was possible to distinguish between virulent and avirulent EPEC and explain the finding that had puzzled clinical investigators and microbiologists for quite some time, namely that EPEC serotypes were frequently isolated from clinically well individuals. The use of animal models and *in vitro* experiments with cultured human cells soon demonstrated that virulent EPEC caused a unique pathological lesion. This consisted of the close attachment of organisms to the host intestinal-cell membrane and a change in the structure of the microvillus, which effaced and mounded up to form a platform-like pedestal upon which the attached organism was found. This characteristic change was therefore designated the 'attaching and effacing' (A/E) lesion, and was soon shown to occur *in situ* in human patients from whom biopsy tissue was available.

Clinical features After an incubation period of a few days, the duration being inversely related to the inoculum size, the onset of diarrhoea is abrupt or gradual, with a tendency for cases with an abrupt onset to be more ill than the others. The stools become loose and green, then orange-coloured, and eventually watery. Vomiting is common in more severely affected children and it may even be projectile. The combination of watery diarrhoea and vomiting quickly leads to dehydration. The child is at first irritable, may have convulsions, and the temperature rises to 39 to 40 °C. In the absence of prompt fluid replacement, dehydration and metabolic disturbances may become irreversible, with the result that the child becomes apathetic, hypotensive, hypoglycaemic, and dies. Yet the disease may be mild, and marked only by the passage of a few loose stools without vomiting or general illness; this is the usual pattern in healthy children in developed countries. Occasionally, especially in poorly nourished infants in developing countries, the loose stools persist for days or even weeks, but beyond this time it becomes increasingly likely that other factors are involved, and in these subjects enteroaggregative *E. coli* may be identified.

Enteroaggregative E. coli (**EaggEC**)

EaggEC are typically associated with infantile diarrhoea, and seem to be more commonly present in cases of persistent diarrhoea lasting more than 14 days. It is not clear whether these organisms are the cause of these persistent episodes, or whether they are simply able to colonize the intestine damaged by another cause of diarrhoea. Persistent episodes are associated with significant nutritional deficits, and in developing countries EaggEC are a major cause of diarrhoeal mortality in young infants. When investigators first began to classify isolates of *E. coli* associated with diarrhoea by determining the pattern of adherence to certain cells in tissue culture, three distinct types were identified: those attaching in discrete packets; those adhering diffusely to the whole perimeter of the cell; and those that appeared to autoaggregate, stacking upon one another like bricks in a wall. Initially, this phenotypic characteristic, and then molecular methods that were used to identify associated and putative virulence genes, helped to define the epidemiology of EaggEC. The precise pathogenesis of EaggEC infection remains to be defined. A heat-stable toxin designated **EAST** (enteroaggregative stable toxin) has been identified in many isolates and appears to be a marker of virulence.

Enterotoxigenic E. coli (**ETEC**)

ETEC are common causes of diarrhoeal disease at any age. Because they produce toxins related to cholera toxin, ETEC can result in a clinical illness that resembles cholera. For most of these infections, the source is usually contaminated food or water. The inoculum size is generally high, and therefore contaminated unrefrigerated food can be an excellent vehicle in which a small inoculum can multiply to sufficient numbers to cause disease.

In studying patients with clinical cholera from whom *Vibrio cholerae* could not be isolated, investigators working in Calcutta in the mid-1960s found certain *E. coli* serotypes which, to their great surprise, caused fluid secretion in animal diarrhoea models. Two major classes of enterotoxins have since been identified: heat-labile proteins called labile toxin (**LT**), of which several subtypes have been identified; and small heat-stable peptide toxins (**ST**), which possess multiple disulphide bonds that enhance their resistance to heat inactivation, of which several subtypes have also been identified. LT acts in a manner similar to cholera toxin, catalysing the ADP-ribosylation of adenylate cyclase, the host enzyme involved in the production of cyclic-AMP. This product is an intracellular signal which, in intestinal epithelial cells, leads to a reduction in sodium absorption and increase in chloride secretion. The accumulation of excess NaCl in the intestinal lumen results in the movement of water into the lumen to maintain isosmolarity, which results in diarrhoea when the volume exceeds the absorptive capacity of the gut. It was a surprise, however, when ST was found to activate the particulate guanylate cyclase of intestinal epithelial cells and to increase intracellular cyclic-GMP, which also increased the lumenal accumulation of NaCl to cause diarrhoea, because in most other systems the effects of cAMP and cGMP tend to offset one another, providing the basis for an effective feedback control system.

ETEC also colonize the small intestine by means of adherence factors termed 'colonization-factor antigens' (**CFAs**). These are plasmid-encoded proteins expressed on the surface of the bacterium, either on a pilus or as a surface-displayed antigen. Some *E. coli* express more than one CFA antigen. These adhesins are used by the organism to attach to host cells via specific binding-to-host-cell receptors. These events are essential for virulence, for without the adherence mechanism, ETEC would just pass through the small bowel instead of intensely colonizing the proximal small bowel, a feature essential to the production of enterotoxins such as LT and ST.

The main features of ETEC infection are diarrhoea and vomiting, but proportionally more older children are affected compared with EPEC infection, and the fluid losses usually result in mild to severe dehydration. There is nothing particularly distinctive about this presentation, and it is difficult to distinguish between ETEC and rotavirus diarrhoea in these young children.

Enteroinvasive E. coli (**EIEC**)

Enteroinvasive *E. coli* were first identified as a cause of bloody diarrhoea in an outbreak in the United States that was traced to contaminated imported French Camembert cheese. In subsequent studies, these organisms have been identified in a low percentage of diarrhoeal illnesses in children under the age of 5 years in developing countries. These infections are rarely bloody or dysenteric, although some serotypes have been associated with a shigella-like illness. These serotypes have been shown to possess genes similar to those of *Shigella*, conferring the property of invasion of epithelial cells (this is described more fully below in the section on *Shigella*). Suffice it here to say that the products of these genes induce normally non-phagocytic cells, such as intestinal epithelial cells, to ingest the organisms within a phagocytic vacuole. Intracellular multiplication of the organisms is associated with cell damage, possibly by an apoptotic mechanism, and altered host physiology leading to diarrhoea.

In some geographical locations, EIEC are identified in about 5 per cent of watery diarrhoea episodes. They may cause disease in adults as well as children. Foodborne outbreaks have also occurred in industrialized nations, sometimes due to the importation of food from other industrialized nations tainted with the pathogenic organisms. EIEC are not as well adapted as pathogens as are *Shigella* spp., which require fewer bacteria to cause illness and generally result in more severe symptoms and complications. Clinically, EIEC infection is indistinguishable from most other causes of watery diarrhoea.

*Enterohaemorrhagic E. coli (**EHEC**)*

These organisms appear to be an evolutionary development of EPEC, as they possess the genetic determinants for the A/E lesion, engage the same signal-transduction pathways, and produce the characteristic pathological changes in the gut mucosa as EPEC. They were first identified in the United States during 1982 associated with outbreaks of bloody diarrhoea traced to contaminated hamburgers from fast-food restaurants. A serotype of *E. coli*, O157:H7, previously unknown as a cause of human illness, was isolated from these patients, who had a distinctive haemorrhagic colitis. This haemorrhagic colitis represents the most severe end of the spectrum of *E. coli* infections. It has taken the better part of the past two decades to determine that the colitis is not the only manifestation of infection with EHEC, that a number of different *E. coli* serotypes other than O157:H7 can be implicated, and that a common characteristic of the group is their ability to produce shiga toxins. Hence these organisms are now more commonly designated 'shiga-toxin-producing *E. coli*' or **STEC**. (It should be noted that in some parts of Canada, the United Kingdom, and Europe, shiga toxin from *E. coli* is known as verotoxin (**VT**), because Vero cells were used to characterize its properties. Those who use the VT terminology refer to the group as 'verotoxin-producing *E. coli*' or **VTEC**. (However, the term 'STEC' is more correct, as it is named for the gene designation for the prototype shiga toxin from *Shigella dysenteriae* type 1.) There is an important epidemiological distinction between the terms 'EHEC' and 'STEC'. The former refers to STEC associated with a distinctive clinical syndrome, haemorrhagic colitis, most commonly due to serotype O157:H7. Yet, other STEC can produce a range of diarrhoeal illnesses that do not fit this description. Thus, all EHEC are STEC, but only some STEC are EHEC, and STEC is a more comprehensive term.

Epidemiology STEC are found in cattle, and occasionally in other farm animals, in which they appear to be part of the normal flora. Ground hamburger meat prepared in large lots at slaughterhouses, then quick-frozen for distribution and later cooking, have been implicated in outbreaks of human infection. Under these conditions, one carcass contaminated with STEC from its faeces can contaminate meat prepared from a number of carcasses. Freezing preserves the organisms, and cooking the meat rare allows bacteria in the interior of a hamburger patty to survive. Disease results because the required inoculum size is only between 50 and 100 organisms. Hamburgers prepared in supermarkets have become a major source for sporadic cases or small outbreaks associated with picnics, school meals, church barbecues, and other similar small gatherings. Salami, sausage, and raw milk have also been implicated in outbreaks. A huge outbreak affecting over 10 000 school-age children occurred in Japan during 1996 caused by contaminated prepared school lunches.

Organisms can also be disseminated from farm animals to ground water and adjacent crops; lettuce, alfalfa sprouts, apple cider, and unpasteurized apple juice have been vehicles of infection. In fact, non-beef foods have become increasingly important sources of STEC, accounting for approximately 50 per cent of all cases in the United States. Direct infection from contact with animals, notably in children on school visits to farms, is another form of transmission. Person-to-person transmission is also well documented, which reflects the small inoculum size needed to cause infection.

Clinical features Perhaps as a consequence of the small inocula of STEC, the incubation period is often as long as 5 to 7 days. The initial watery stools become blood-tinged and then grossly bloody over the course of a day or two, and there are abdominal cramps and tenderness. This is due to a diffuse inflammatory colitis with vascular leaks, rather than ulceration as in shigellosis. Lesser degrees of colon involvement lead to milder symptoms with less blood in the stool, with mild infections remaining as a watery diarrhoea. Patients usually improve clinically in 5 to 7 days. However, at about this time, particularly in infections with O157:H7, microangiopathic haemolytic anaemia, thrombocytopenia, and oliguric renal failure—the haemolytic-uraemic syndrome (**HUS**)—develop in 5 to 10 per cent of patients. In some patients, these manifestations are mild and self-limited; in others, rapidly developing hypertension may lead to haemorrhagic strokes and death in the acute phase. In still others, management of renal failure becomes a major clinical problem, requiring peritoneal or even haemodialysis before improvement occurs. In a small, but unknown, proportion of patients, manifestations of chronic renal damage occur a decade or more after the initial episode. Because HUS is also associated with shiga-toxin-producing *Shigella dysenteriae* type 1, it is apparent that this toxin is a significant pathogenetic factor.

Laboratory diagnosis of pathogenic E. coli

Although identifying an organism as an *E. coli* is simple, diagnosis of the different *E. coli* strains causing intestinal disease is both hard and easy. It is hard because, with the exception of O157:H7 STEC strains (see below), there are no simple screening tests for their identification. It is easy because the virulence genes that characterize the different groups can be readily identified by polymerase chain reaction (**PCR**) and other genotyping methods; the problem is that PCR is not yet suitable for routine use in the clinical laboratory. Serotyping, as noted previously, is not specific enough, even for the EPEC strains that have classically been identified by this method. There are tissue culture methods that detect some virulence properties, such as cell-adherence patterns, or the ability to polymerize actin and reorganize cytoskeletal microfilaments and the microvillus surface, but routine clinical laboratories do not perform these tests. Modernization of the laboratory is imperative to enable the full diagnosis of *E. coli* infections, but fiscal and other considerations are likely to limit the rapidity with which this can be achieved.

The identification of O157:H7 STEC is more straightforward. Most *E. coli* O157:H7 do not ferment sorbitol and can therefore be detected on sorbitol–MacConkey (SMAC) agar. Other STEC can be detected by commercially available enzyme-linked immunosorbent assay (**ELISA**) tests for toxin production; however, most clinical laboratories do not seek these organisms.

The detection of systemically invading *E. coli*, for example as the cause of sepsis and circulatory shock, is not a problem for the laboratory as *E. coli* are not 'normal flora' except in the colon. Sampling normally sterile sites, such as the bloodstream, readily yields the organisms, unless the patients have been given antibiotics in advance. The organisms are not fastidious, they grow rapidly, and are easily identified and tested for antimicrobial sensitivity within 48 h.

Treatment and prevention of pathogenic E. coli

With the exception of STEC infection, the main danger to an infant with *E. coli* gastroenteritis is dehydration; thus, the most urgent need is to replace fluid and electrolyte losses. Infants may require parenteral fluids, particularly with ETEC infection, but oral rehydration fluids are generally sufficient.

With STEC infection, dehydration is not the prime concern as the fluid losses are typically not severe. It is the systemic complications—the microangiopathic haemolytic anaemia and renal failure (HUS)—that are the clinical challenge. The use of antimicrobial therapy, even in STEC infection, is neither generally necessary nor advocated. While some believe the early use of antimicrobials to treat STEC will prevent the late complications, there is sufficient evidence to the contrary to pause for consideration. Certain antimicrobials induce shiga-toxin production and may predispose to HUS or increase its severity, and many believe antibiotic treatment to be contraindicated. There is no definitive, controlled clinical-trial evidence to resolve this controversy. Antimotility agents do not diminish fluid losses, so much as they prolong the interval between stooling. There is some evidence that antimotility agents can exacerbate illness and increase its severity by prolonging the contact between the pathogen and the gut mucosa, particularly in young children, and therefore they are generally considered both ineffective and potentially harmful. Measures taken to prevent infection are the same as those for shigellosis, notably good personal hygiene, especially among medical staff caring for these patients; the risk among neonatal infants is particularly high.

Shigella infections

But for history, the genus *Shigella* would be another type of *E. coli*. This is because the identification of the prototype organism of the genus occurred in 1896 rather than in 1996 when it became known that *Shigella* and *Escherichia* could not be distinguished by DNA hybridization. This bacterium, ultimately named *Shigella dysenteriae* type 1, honours the Japanese microbiologist, Kiyoshi Shiga, who isolated it from patients with dysentery during a particularly severe epidemic in Japan. Shiga proved its aetiological significance by demonstrating a rise in agglutinating antibodies during convalescence. The epidemic affected at least 100 000 individuals, with a mortality rate close to 25 per cent. After World War I, this species declined in prevalence, and was only rarely isolated. However, in 1968 it re-emerged as the cause of a widespread epidemic of dysentery in Central America and Mexico. Early in the epidemic, mortality rates reached levels similar to those in Japan 60 years before, partly because the organism was initially not grown from stool and partly because the presence of amoebic cysts was interpreted to mean that the disease was amoebic dysentery. As a result, the use of emetine (a highly toxic drug) to treat victims contributed to the high mortality. Once better media for the isolation of this organism were employed, the true cause of the outbreak was identified, proper antibiotic treatment was given, and deaths were reduced. With time, strains with multiple antibiotic resistance emerged, but the epidemic had already waned.

Soon after the publication of Shiga's work, Flexner, Sonne, and Boyd described related groups of organisms. By 1938, four groups of dysentery bacilli could be differentiated according to their biochemical reactions and antigenic structure (Table 3). Shigellae, like the salmonellae, are non-lactose fermenters (albeit, *S. sonnei* does ferment lactose after 24 h in culture), but they are unusual among the enterobacteria in lacking flagella (non-motile) and, with one minor exception, they are anaerogenic—they do not produce gas from sugars. *S. sonnei* and *S. boydii* are the least pathogenic species and usually cause minor illness. *S. flexneri* is of intermediate pathogenicity.

Epidemiology

S. dysenteriae type 1 remains the most virulent of the shigellae. It is the principal species involved in major epidemics. It thrives under conditions of poverty, overcrowding, and squalor, particularly where there are no proper means of sewage disposal. However, the same can be said for the more frequently encountered *S. flexneri* and *S. sonnei*. It is not clear, therefore, why *S. dysenteriae* disappeared after the First World War, to be replaced by *S. flexneri*, or why *S. flexneri* diminished in prevalence in industrialized nations after the Second World War, where it was replaced by *S. sonnei*. Nor is it clear why *S. dysenteriae* type 1 reappeared in Mexico and Central America during 1968, in the Indian subcontinent during 1975, or in Central Africa during 1985, where it is now an endemic cause of dysentery. Shigellosis differs from other common diarrhoeal diseases of the developing world in that it affects older children and adults rather than targeting young infants.

Sources and transmission Unlike salmonellae, shigellae are only found naturally in humans and occasionally certain non-human primates, which probably acquire infection from humans. Shigellosis is the most communicable of all bacterial infections of the gut; in adult human-volunteer challenge studies, dysentery has been produced by as few as 10 to 100 bacteria. This is partly because it resists acid pH and is able to survive passage through the stomach. Not surprisingly, the principal route of transmission is person to person by the direct faecal–oral spread of bacteria, mainly via the fingers. Apart from the obvious contaminating action of finger-to-mouth contact after touching or scratching the anal area, or not washing one's hands after defaecation, infective doses of bacteria can also be transferred to food or water. These can be ideal vehicles for transmission because shigellae do not have to multiply in food to cause infection. Thus the greatest risk is from foods that are most handled during preparation, such as salads, sandwiches, and fruit.

The global market in foods has resulted in many new ways of transporting and transferring shigellae. For example, an outbreak in Europe was caused by injecting watermelons with contaminated water in North Africa in order to increase their market weight. Lettuce fertilized with human faeces ('night-soil') in Mexico has transmitted shigellosis in the United States, facilitated in some instances by the shredding of lettuce for distribution to fast-food restaurants. It is not clear how much shigellosis is transmitted by contact with fomites, such as lavatory seats, flushing handles, taps, door knobs, roller towels, and other objects in the toilet. Cool, dark, damp conditions favour the prolonged survival of shigellae deposited on hard surfaces in this way, and under such conditions organisms have been shown to survive for at least 17 days on wooden lavatory seats.

Occasionally, large outbreaks have arisen through the faecal pollution of municipal water supplies. In countries lacking flushing toilets and sewerage systems, flooding has coincided with simultaneous increases in dysentery as flood waters wash infected human faeces deposited in fields into well water or other sources of drinking water. Flies can also transmit infection from exposed human faeces to food, and in such settings fly control reduces the incidence of infection.

Pathogenesis

The cardinal pathogenic feature of shigellae is their ability to invade and multiply in epithelial cells. Invasion occurs by a process analogous to phagocytosis, mediated by a set of genes present in a large-virulence plasmid. A number of different mutations in these genes will impair or eliminate this property and result in attenuation of virulence. *S. dysenteriae* type 1 also produces a powerful exotoxin (shiga toxin), which is associated with the haemolytic-uraemic syndrome (HUS). As described above, certain *E. coli* (STEC) that are also associated with HUS produce structurally and functionally related toxins. In experimentally infected rhesus monkeys, colonization initially takes place in the jejunum and upper ileum, giving rise to secretory diarrhoea. This may be due to the action of one of two shigella enterotoxins (Shet-1 and Shet-2), distinct from shiga toxin, but not all diarrhoea-causing shigellae produce these proteins. Because a huge dose of organisms (>10^{10} bacteria) is required to cause symptomatic infection in these animals, this finding may not be representative of human infection.

Table 3 The four *Shigella* spp.

Serological Group	Organism	Number of strains	Comments
A	*Shigella dysenteriae*	10 types	Types 1 and 2 are human pathogens. Type 1 responsible for the most severe forms of shigellosis
B	*Shigella flexneri*	13 serotypes and subtypes	Most common isolate in developing countries. Usually causes severe bloody diarrhoea or dysentery
C	*Shigella boydii*	15 serotypes	Prevalent in the Indian subcontinent but not elsewhere. Usually mild disease
D	*Shigella sonnei*	1 serotype but many phage or colicin types	Most common isolate in developed countries. Typically causes a mild watery diarrhoea

The characteristic pathology produced by shigellae is an acute, locally invasive colitis. This ranges in severity from mild inflammation of the mucous membrane of the rectum and sigmoid colon, typical of *S. sonnei* infections, to severe, necrotizing lesions affecting the whole colon and sometimes the terminal ileum, such as are seen in the worst forms of *S. dysenteriae* type 1 infection. Shigellae penetrate and multiply in the submucosa and within the epithelial cells of the colon, close to the enteric vasculature, and yet bacteraemia is rare, though less rare in patients with malnutrition. In severe cases the colon may be so damaged that it is confused with a global ulcerative colitis.

Local mucosal changes consist of oedema, capillary engorgement, and neutrophil infiltration. Small haemorrhages are common and the submucous veins may be engorged or thrombosed. The mucous membrane becomes intensely red and blood-stained mucus may be present. In the most severe forms of the disease, areas of mucosa undergo coagulation necrosis, which appear as thickened, semi-rigid, greyish patches. These eventually separate to leave raw, ulcerated areas. Haemorrhage and perforation may also result from such lesions. Extensive lesions lead to considerable protein loss, which adds to the severe debility that accompanies these infections. Extensive production of inflammatory cytokines is responsible for these mucosal responses.

Clinical features

The incubation period is usually between 2 and 3 days, but exceptionally it may be as long as a week. The illness usually starts with fever, abdominal colic, and watery diarrhoea. In many *S. sonnei* infections these are the only features and there is spontaneous resolution. In the more severe forms of shigellosis, diarrhoea and fever is accompanied by headache, anorexia, myalgia, and malaise. After 1 to 3 days the diarrhoea becomes bloody, and in some cases it may progress further to dysentery, characterized by the very frequent passage of small amounts of blood-stained mucus ('red-currant jelly') and pus, with abdominal cramps and tenesmus—the classic dysenteric syndrome. In severe forms of the disease this sequence is telescoped so that bloody, mucoid stools are passed virtually from the outset. The patient becomes toxic and restless, the pulse rapid and feeble, and there is a risk of death from hyponatraemia, hypoglycaemia (Fig. 1), septic shock due to polymicrobial bacteraemia with other coliforms, or renal failure and hypertension associated with acute HUS. Recovery in such cases is invariably slow, and occasionally patients continue with chronic or relapsing infection resembling ulcerative colitis. Indeed, 50 years ago some experts believed shigellae were the cause of ulcerative colitis. Exacerbation of haemorrhoids and rectal prolapse may result from rectal oedema and straining at stool. Shigellae are usually excreted in the faeces for a few weeks after the illness.

Fig. 1 Bangladeshi child with pouting and upward deviation of the eyes associated with profound hypoglycaemia complicating shigellosis. (Courtesy of RE Phillips)

Malnourished individuals, particularly young children, may excrete the organisms for months.

Children may show striking meningism, which, in the presence of fever and headache, can be misleading if it occurs before the onset of diarrhoea. Shigellosis in children may also be associated with appendicitis and occasionally with intussusception in infants. The catabolic response, protein-losing enteropathy, and anorexia that occur and persist in shigella infections in children in developing countries can lead to acute protein-energy malnutrition (kwashiorkor). This is associated with frequent intercurrent infections and high mortality rates. Shigellae are rare causes of vaginitis in children and, as this focal infection can develop without any obvious history of diarrhoea, it can easily pass unrecognized.

Reactive arthritis or full Reiter's syndrome, associated with the HLA-B27 haplotype, purulent keratoconjunctivitis, and neuritis are uncommon late complications of infection with any of the shigellae.

Laboratory diagnosis

Isolation in culture remains the standard method for detecting shigellae. Faecal samples rather than rectal swabs should be submitted. Shigellae are delicate bacteria, so it is necessary to plate samples rapidly or inoculate a buffered transport medium if there is to be any delay before a stool can be delivered to the laboratory and processed. Some bacteriological media are more inhibitory to shigellae than others. For example, Salmonella–Shigella (**SS**) agar is moderately inhibitory, whereas Hektoen enteric and xylose–lysine–deoxycholate agar are less so. Multiple agars should be used to maximize the chance of isolation.

Antimicrobial chemotherapy

Although antimicrobial therapy is seldom needed for *S. sonnei* and other mild self-limited forms of shigellosis, it is the mainstay of treatment for severe shigellosis, especially for *S. dysenteriae* type 1 and *S. flexneri* infections. Laboratory identification should always be sought, as well as antimicrobial susceptibility data. Strains showing multiple antimicrobial resistances are common, especially in developing countries. Suppression of the normal microbial flora by inappropriate antimicrobial therapy exacerbates infection.

Co-trimoxazole and ampicillin have for many years been the drugs of choice for shigellosis, but most strains are now resistant; many are also resistant to tetracycline and chloramphenicol. Nalidixic acid is effective and cheap, but high resistance rates have arisen where the drug has been used intensively. Resistance to ciprofloxacin, which is 100 times more active against shigellae than nalidixic acid, is currently uncommon. A single dose of 1 g is effective in adults infected with shigellae other than *S. dysenteriae* type 1, but 3 to 5 days of treatment is usually required for the latter species. The treatment of children with antibiotic-resistant shigella infection is difficult, as quinolones are potentially toxic for the young. A short course of a fluoroquinolone may be necessary to treat severely affected children, but parenteral ceftriaxone (50 mg/kg per day for 5 days) and pivmecillinam are alternatives that have been used successfully.

Prevention and control

The safe disposal of excreta, provision of purified water, and control of flies are fundamental to the control of shigellosis. Where these are lacking, the incidence can still be reduced by the promotion of personal and domestic hygiene, notably hand washing after defaecation and before handling food. Unpurified water can be made safe by boiling or by the addition of hypochlorite tablets; salads and fruit can be disinfected by soaking in water containing 80 parts per million of free chlorine from household bleach. Breast feeding substantially increases resistance to infection in children. Oral vaccines for use in developing countries are being developed.

Outbreaks of *S. sonnei* dysentery in schools are difficult to control, but measures should be aimed at preventing spread by the hands. Supervised washing and disinfection of hands after defaecation, and frequent disinfection of lavatory seats, taps, and door knobs are effective if rigorously applied. Only disposable hand towels should be provided in this setting. It is impracticable to detect and exclude all children excreting shigellae, and therefore children suffering from diarrhoea, regardless of whether or not *S. sonnei* is isolated from stool, should be restricted from school until recovered.

Food handlers suffering from diarrhoea or dysentery should be excluded from work until they have produced at least three consecutive negative stool samples taken not less than 24 h apart, and at least 2 days after the cessation of any antimicrobial chemotherapy.

Salmonella infections

The genus *Salmonella* is a large complex group of organisms that continues to challenge the ability of taxonomists to classify them. After many years, and many schemes, the genus *Salmonella* is now considered to comprise a single species designated *S. enterica*. All of the more than 2400 individually distinguishable strains (based on their possession of sets of microbiological, biochemical, and serological properties), such as *S. choleraesuis, S. typhi, S. paratyphi* A or B, *S. typhimurium, S. dublin,* and *S. enteritidis,* are now considered to be serovars of *S. enterica.* This leads to a complex nomenclature in which the particular strain previously known as *S. enteritidis* is now called *S. enterica* serovar enteritidis. While this is now taxonomically correct, it is clinically awkward and clinicians will no doubt continue to use the old nomenclature. *S. enterica* is divided into seven subspecies, which largely correspond to the old 'subgenera'. Members of subspecies I are predominantly parasites of warm-blooded animals and include almost all the salmonellae pathogenic for humans. The other subspecies include organisms found mainly in cold-blooded animals or the environment. Subspecies IIIa and IIIb (the 'Arizona' group) are a group of organisms that, in contrast to subspecies-I organisms, ferment lactose. This makes their recognition in the laboratory more difficult because they initially resemble normal flora coliforms.

Salmonella in subspecies I fall into three epidemiological groups:

(1) those highly host-adapted to humans, such as *S. typhi* and *paratyphi* A, which cause the distinctive clinical syndromes typhoid and paratyphoid fever;

(2) those that are highly host-adapted to animals but which cause no human illness (e.g. *S. pullorum* in chickens);

(3) a large group that are not particularly host-adapted, such as *S. typhimurium, S. dublin, S. heidelberg.*

It is in the third group that the food-poisoning salmonellae are found. Many of them are named after the city or place where they were first identified. While there are a huge number of distinguishable strains included in this group, only a few are commonly found causing human illness. Identification of uncommon serovars can be extremely useful in determining their source and mode of transmission.

Epidemiology

Salmonellae are one of the major causes of foodborne illness throughout the world, but particularly in industrialized countries. This is because many processed foods contain animal products likely to be contaminated with salmonellae, such as poultry and egg products. The latter have been particularly effective vehicles for spreading *S. enteritidis* originating in egg-laying hens (see below). It is remarkable how many processed foods contain potential sources of *Salmonella.* The socioeconomic cost of salmonella infection is enormous. In the United States it is estimated to be $1.4 billion per annum. The cost of mounting an outbreak investigation may seem high, but it is trivial in relation to the savings that can be made in medical and social costs by rapid interventions.

Animal and food sources The food-poisoning salmonellae are enzootic in a wide range of vertebrates, unlike the typhoid and paratyphoid bacilli, which are highly host-adapted to humans. Infection may be acquired from direct contact with infected animals. On the farm, the source is often scouring calves; and in the home, family pets—even terrapins and turtles. But in general, animals are more important as a source of infection through the food chain. In developed countries, intensive animal husbandry and mass production methods encourage the spread of salmonellae. In the example

of poultry, modern mechanized plucking and eviscerating methods, which are capable of processing 5000 birds an hour, can readily lead to gross cross-contamination.

Animal feeds are often the portal of entry for new *Salmonella* serotypes. The appearance and spread of *S. agona* in Britain and the United States in the early 1970s was traced to its introduction via Peruvian fish meal used in poultry and pig feed. Similarly, in the late 1970s, *S. hadar,* formerly unknown in Britain, became well established in turkey stocks after its introduction in feedstuffs from abroad. The prevalence of serotypes is constantly changing. Since 1985, the incidence of *S. enteritidis* infection has risen to unprecedented heights in Europe (mainly phage type 4) and North America (mainly phage types 8 and 13a), and probably elsewhere. The main source is poultry, for which these strains are more than usually invasive, causing oviduct infection and contamination of fresh eggs through vertical transmission, a new epidemiological dimension that had far-reaching political consequences.

The net result of the enzootic state is that raw meat and animal products, especially poultry and eggs, are commonly contaminated with salmonellae of one or another serovar. The consequences are not always as serious as they might appear, for healthy adults are able to deal with small inocula and, in general, clinical symptoms are unlikely unless multiplication of the inoculum is allowed to occur in the food before consumption. Thus correct handling, preparation, and storage of food can prevent clinical infection. Unfortunately, this ideal is not always attained. Failure to handle raw meats separately from cooked foods leads to cross-contamination, and incomplete thawing of large frozen carcasses, such as turkeys, results in inadequate cooking and the multiplication of surviving bacteria. Raw milk is often contaminated at source and is a regular cause of infection in those unwise enough to drink it. Faults in food processing plants can lead to widespread outbreaks corresponding to the distribution of the product. Major incidents have been caused by failure of heat treatment, or contamination of a food after heat treatment. The list of foods implicated is long, but a few examples are liquid egg, dried egg, dried-milk infant food, desiccated coconut, bean sprouts, chocolate, and meat pies topped up after cooking with jelly from contaminated dispensing machines.

Human sources Infection is not readily transmitted from person to person because of the relatively high inoculum required, a consequence of the acid susceptibility of these organisms. Infants, old people, and patients living in closed communities such as nursing homes and institutions for retarded or mentally ill individuals, in whom it may be difficult to maintain high levels of sanitation, are at particular risk. Salmonellae can be especially troublesome in hospital maternity units.

The importance of a *Salmonella*-excreting food handler as a source of infection has been exaggerated. These individuals are more likely to be the victim of handling contaminated animal products at work than a source of infection. It is rarely necessary to suspend an otherwise healthy food handler from duty until clear of salmonellae, providing the stools are formed and good standards of hygiene are maintained. However, it is mandatory to suspend food handlers with diarrhoea, whatever the apparent cause.

Pathogenesis

The infective dose is governed by many factors. As noted above, the inoculum required to cause infection is several hundred thousand organisms, as determined in experimental infections in human volunteers, even when the organism is administered in buffered solutions. There are important exceptions. The inoculum is lowered when taken in a food meal, which buffers gastric acidity and protects the organisms in their journey through the stomach to the small bowel. In fact, as few as 50 bacteria contained in certain high-fat foods, notably chocolate, cheese, and salami, can cause illness. Anything that reduces gastric acidity, such as atrophic gastritis, treatment with H_2-receptor blocking agents, and previous gastric surgery, also lowers the infective dose. Broad-spectrum antibiotics increase susceptibility by suppressing the normal competitive microflora of the gut. The newborn are especially susceptible before the gut becomes colonized with the normal intestinal flora.

The distal small intestine is the main site of infection, but the colon can also be affected. Salmonellae provide chemical signals to intestinal epithelial cells, leading to bacterial uptake within vesicles and translocation across the cytoplasm to the lamina propria where the organisms multiply and invade the bloodstream. Whereas circulating bacteria are generally contained and quickly eliminated, bacteria in the mucosa result in an acute inflammatory response with polymorphonuclear leucocytic infiltration of the submucosa. Flattening or loss of secretory epithelium occurs adjacent to these inflamed areas. Inflammatory cells are usually present in the stools, which provides a diagnostic clue to the invasive process. The mechanism by which salmonellae cause tissue damage and fluid secretion is not well understood. Production of inflammatory products that alter electrolyte and fluid transport (for example, prostaglandins and enterotoxins), and described in some strains, are considered to be responsible.

Although bacteraemia probably occurs in most infections at the outset, positive cultures are obtained in only a few per cent of all laboratory diagnosed infections. Yet, certain strains are associated with high rates of bacteraemia, for example *S. cholerae-suis* (75 per cent), *S. dublin* (25 per cent), and *S. virchow* phage-type 19 (5.5 per cent). Some of these so infected patients suffer a typhoidal illness, or even the severe manifestations of septic shock, and focal infection may arise in almost any organ of the body. *S. cholerae-suis* has a particular predilection for the aorta, where it can cause life-threatening mycotic aneurysms.

Clinical features

There are broadly six major clinical manifestations of salmonella infection, the first of which is asymptomatic infection (Table 4). Most people ingesting salmonellae never become ill. In every food-poisoning outbreak, despite the likelihood of a high inoculum in the suspect food, there are unaffected persons who excrete the organism in their faeces. Others suffer a typical attack of acute febrile enteritis lasting 2 or 3 days, and there are usually a few who suffer a more severe, prolonged attack. The proportion of people who become ill is determined by the extent of contamination of the food and the characteristics of the infecting strain.

The incubation period is usually 24 h, but it may range from 6 to 48 h, depending on the size of the infecting dose. The onset is abrupt, with malaise, nausea, headache, abdominal pain, and diarrhoea. Some patients vomit, but seldom more than once or twice. Shivering and fever is common in those who are more than mildly affected. Occasionally there is severe diarrhoea, with fluid, green, offensive stools that may contain mucus and blood. Dehydration, with cramps, oliguria, and uraemia may occur, most likely among those at the extremes of age who are at risk of a fatal outcome. Patients whose distal colon and rectum are severely affected occasionally develop tenesmus with the passage of small, bloody dysenteric stools, and there may be tenderness over the sigmoid colon. Salmonella enterocolitis may trigger off an attack of non-specific colitis, acute appendicitis in the young, or mesenteric thrombosis in the elderly. Bacteraemia early in the course of infection can lead to focal infection in certain organ systems (see below).

Reactive arthritis is an occasional late sequel of infection. Estimates of its incidence range from 1.2 to 7.3 per cent of all infections. Patients with the HLA-B27 haplotype have a strong predisposition for this complication, in whom it sometimes becomes a chronic, destructive arthritis.

Convalescent excretion Most patients continue to excrete small numbers of salmonellae in their faeces for a few weeks after infection—about 4 to 8 weeks for adults, and 8 to 24 weeks for infants. The number of organisms present is usually low, but excretors have been found with 10^5 to 10^7 organisms per gram of faeces. Carriage of salmonellae, other than typhoid or paratyphoid bacilli, for more than 6 months is rare.

Focal infection Focal infections are often difficult to diagnose because they may first manifest themselves long after an episode of enteritis—or the original bowel infection may even have been silent. Focal infections have a tendency to chronicity and can mimic tuberculosis, particularly in cases of osteomyelitis of a vertebra or paravertebral abscess. Salmonella osteomyelitis and arthritis are strongly associated with sickle-cell disease, where bony infarcts can be infected during the asymptomatic bacteraemic phase of salmonella enteritis. Salmonella abscesses may develop in virtually any site: the liver, gallbladder, spleen, psoas muscle, uterus (after septic abortion), and the peritoneal cavity (for example, subphrenic, pelvic) are the most common. Patients with a deep-seated salmonella infection who remain untreated suffer high mortality.

Laboratory diagnosis

Definitive diagnosis depends on the isolation of the infecting organism, for salmonella enteritis cannot be distinguished from other forms of enteritis on clinical grounds alone. The isolation methods for salmonellae allow the detection of small numbers of organisms, even when greatly outnumbered by other bacteria. While most specific serovars can only be identified in reference laboratories possessing a full set of serotyping antisera, most clinical laboratories are able to narrow identification down to a short-list by the use of restricted sets of commercially available antisera. Some reference laboratories offer strain identification of *S. typhimurium*, *S. enteritidis*, and other common serovars by phage-typing techniques. Patients produce antibody to their infecting strain during convalescence, but this is seldom of diagnostic value.

Antimicrobial chemotherapy

The mainstay for the treatment of salmonella gastroenteritis is fluid replacement. This can usually be accomplished by the use of oral rehydration solutions, which are discussed more fully in Chapter 14.17. In the past, antimicrobials were not recommended for treating this infection since there was no apparent shortening of the clinical illness and there was a tendency for carriage to persist longer. None the less, more aggressive treatment should be considered for certain severely affected patients or in particular situations. Examples are patients with bloody diarrhoea and those with an underlying illness such as sickle-cell disease or AIDS, which predispose patients to more severe, focally invasive, and sometimes fatal infections.

The ever-increasing rates of antimicrobial resistance among salmonellae to chloramphenicol, co-trimoxazole, tetracyclines, and ampicillin mean that ciprofloxacin and other related 4-quinolones are now the agents of choice. At times, because the 4-quinolones rapidly sterilize the stool and stop transmission, treatment may be warranted during an institutional outbreak in order to reduce the excretion and spread of salmonellae. Ciprofloxacin has also been used with remarkable success to eradicate salmonellae from chronic carriers (including those with *S. typhi*) after other treatments have failed, probably because it is concentrated in bile and mucus. Treatment is essential for invasive and focal disease, which requires full dosage of the drug for several weeks, as the serovars causing invasive infection may be more virulent than the run-of-the-mill serovars causing diarrhoea. Resistance to ciprofloxacin (and other quinolones) developing during treatment has been reported, thus emphasizing the need for close laboratory control. The drug is not recommended for use in children because of a concern that it may cause cartilage damage, although there is little evidence for this from human studies.

Prevention and control

The correct hygienic preparation, handling, and storage of food dramatically reduces the transmission of salmonella infection, but lapses are inevitable at home and in restaurants. The most common fault is the failure to appreciate that even the briefest contact between a raw animal product and

Table 4 Human disease syndromes due to *Salmonella* spp.

Asymptomatic infection (or persistent carrier state)
Fever and bacteraemia
Non-specific watery diarrhoea
Bloody diarrhoea, enterocolitis, and dysentery
Focal infections (hepatitis, cholecystitis, nephritis)
Typhoid fever syndrome

other foods can transfer an inoculum to the latter and initiate a salmonella outbreak; strict separation of the two is a fundamental food-safety pre-requisite. Ideally, animal products should be salmonella-free, but this is far from the case. Methods of animal husbandry, slaughtering, processing, marketing, and policies for the safe disposal of animal and human waste are all reflected in the incidence of human infection.

Examples of control measures in animals are the compulsory heat treatment of imported and recycled animal feeds, and the competitive exclusion of salmonellae from chicks by dosing with normal gut flora. There should be severe restriction on the use of antimicrobial agents in animal rearing, particularly those drugs that are especially valuable for treating human disease, such as the fluoroquinolones. Unfortunately, economic considerations of animal husbandry seem to count more than human health, and it has proven difficult to restrict the use of antibiotics in animal feed. Because of market globalization, restrictions in one country may not affect the movement of drug-resistant organisms elsewhere. Terminal disinfection of poultry carcasses by irradiation would eliminate all pathogens including salmonellae, but irradiation has gained a bad public image and it may be a while before this will change. However, just as there was initial opposition to the pasteurization of milk (a measure of unquestioned public health value and of no risk), irradiation may be more widely used in the future to reduce foodborne infections.

Campylobacter infections

The name Campylobacter (Greek, curved rod) was coined by French workers in 1963 for a group of small, curved or spiral, Gram-negative bacteria formerly classified as vibrios. They now form part of a unique superfamily of mainly spiral bacteria that includes *Campylobacter*, *Arcobacter*, and *Helicobacter*. Campylobacters have a single flagellum at one or both poles of the bacterial cell, giving them a characteristic, rapid darting motility (Fig. 2). The type species, *Campylobacter fetus* (originally *Vibrio fetus*), was first isolated in England in 1906 from aborted sheep fetuses. In the ensuing years it became clear that this species was a major cause of infectious abortion in cattle and sheep, but it was not until the 1970s that *C. jejuni* and *C. coli* were recognized as a common cause of enteritis in humans. The reason they escaped detection for so long was that special methods are required for their isolation from faeces. *C. fetus* occasionally infects humans, but only as an uncommon opportunist causing systemic infection, sometimes with diarrhoea, in patients with immune deficiency or a serious underlying disease. Exceptionally, *C. fetus*, as well as *C. jejuni* and *C. coli*, cause human fetal infection and septic abortion.

Campylobacter enteritis

In industrialized countries almost all campylobacter enteritis is caused by *C. jejuni* and *C. coli*. These differ from most other *Campylobacter* species in having the high optimum growth temperature of 42 °C, in keeping with their adaptation to birds and other animals. In most regions about 90 per cent of infections are caused by *C. jejuni*. Many hundreds of strains exist, which are primarily defined serologically according to two classes of antigen: heat-stable O (lipopolysaccharide) antigens, and heat-labile surface and flagellar protein antigens. Serotypes can be further subdivided into phage types, and even finer discrimination can be attained by DNA analy-

Fig. 2 Electron micrograph of a campylobacter (6650 ×). (By courtesy of Mr DR Purdham.)

sis. In the United Kingdom, 473 serophage types were found among 9600 routine human isolates.

Several other campylobacters and related bacteria are associated with infection of the human intestinal tract. *C. lari* accounts for about 0.1 per cent of all cases of campylobacter enteritis. A subgroup of *C. jejuni* (*C. jejuni* subsp. *doylei*) and *C. upsaliensis*, *C. hyointestinalis*, and *Arcobacter butzleri* are scarce in industrialized countries, but more frequent in children in developing countries; although *A. butzleri* was implicated in an outbreak of abdominal pain, without diarrhoea, in an Italian school. *Helicobacter cinaedi* and *H. fennelliae* are associated with proctitis in homosexual men.

Epidemiology

Campylobacter enteritis is the most common bacterial infection of the gut in industrialized countries. Some 55 000 laboratory isolations per annum are currently reported in the United Kingdom, representing an annual incidence of 100/100 000, but the true incidence is likely to be at least ten times this figure. Incidences are similar in the United States, where the total number of cases is estimated to be 2.4 million per year, with 50 to 150 deaths. The economic burden of the disease runs to millions of dollars annually. In temperate zones there is a remarkably consistent and unexplained peak of incidence in early summer. In developed countries campylobacter enteritis affects people of all ages, especially young adults, but in developing countries it is almost entirely confined to children below the age of 2 to 3 years, after which they are immune through repeated exposure to infection.

Like salmonellosis, campylobacter enteritis is a zoonosis. Campylobacters are found in a wide variety of warm-blooded animals, especially birds, in which they form part of the normal intestinal flora. Pigs are the main host of *C. coli*. A few infections are acquired by direct contact with infected animals, either occupationally (farmers, slaughtermen, poultry processors) or domestically (typically contact with a puppy or kitten with campylobacter diarrhoea), but most are acquired indirectly via contaminated meat, milk, or water. Normal cooking destroys campylobacters, but the consumption of raw or barbecued meats, especially poultry, carries a distinct risk of infection.

Broiler chickens are the most prolific source of campylobacters. Retailed chickens are almost universally contaminated (frozen ones less so than fresh ones), so self-infection when handling them in the kitchen, or cross-contamination to other foods, readily occurs if good hygienic practice is not observed. Campylobacters do not multiply in food like salmonellae, but the infective dose is small enough for food to act as a passive vehicle, just as it does for shigellae. Foodborne infection therefore tends to be sporadic, or in small family outbreaks, rather than in the form of explosive outbreaks. Yet, major outbreaks of campylobacter enteritis affecting 3000 people at a time have been caused by the consumption of raw milk or contaminated municipally supplied water. The ubiquitous nature of campylobacters makes it difficult to pinpoint the sources of sporadic infections. There are probably many routes of infection yet to be discovered. For example, in certain areas of Britain during early summer, infections are caused by the consumption of milk contaminated by wild birds (magpies and jackdaws) pecking the foil caps of doorstep-delivered milk bottles.

Campylobacters do not survive well on inanimate objects, which is probably why person-to-person infectivity is low. Secondary cases are unusual in common-source outbreaks. Food handlers who are healthy excreters with formed stools are a negligible risk to others. The only human sources of consequence are toddlers with campylobacter diarrhoea and infected mothers at term, who may infect their babies during labour.

Pathology

Infection starts in the upper ileum and progresses distally to affect the terminal ileum and colon. The spiral configuration and motility of campylobacters enables them to penetrate, migrate, and colonize the mucus covering the intestinal epithelium in a way that conventional bacteria cannot. Histology shows an acute inflammatory response, with crypt abscess formation in the mucosa indistinguishable from that caused by salmonellae or shigellae. This, and the presence of mesenteric adenitis, suggest that campylobacters invade the mucosa. Bacteraemia is detected in only 0.1 to 0.2 per cent of infections; however, this figure probably underestimates the true incidence, as blood cultures are seldom taken from patients with diarrhoea early in the disease. Many strains produce a cholera-like enterotoxin and/or cytotoxins *in vitro*, but their role in the pathogenesis of the disease is unclear.

Specific antibodies to the infecting strain appear in patients' blood from about the fifth day of illness and remain detectable for several months.

Clinical features

After an incubation period of between 2 and 7 days (mean 3 days) the illness starts either with abdominal pain and diarrhoea, or with a prodromal period of fever, headache, and other influenza-like symptoms that precedes the diarrhoea by a few hours to a few days. A fever of 40 °C or more is not unusual and may be associated with convulsions in children and delirium in adults. Vomiting is not a conspicuous feature of the disease, except in infants, but nausea is common. Abdominal pain tends to be particularly severe and can be of a type and severity that suggests acute appendicitis (see below). Inflammatory cellular exudate can usually be detected microscopically in the stools and frank blood may appear after a day or two. Severe diarrhoea seldom lasts for more than 2 or 3 days, but loose stools and abdominal pain may persist for a while and patients feel 'washed out' and wretched. A brief relapse occurs in 10 to 15 per cent of patients. Death is rare and usually due to some associated disorder. Chronic disease or long-term carriage of campylobacters has not been recorded in normal subjects, but it has in patients with immune deficiency, such as hypogammaglobulinaemia or AIDS. The stools of most patients are culture-negative after about 5 weeks.

Misleading presentations and complications

Suspected appendicitis, particularly in older children and young adults, is the main reason for the referral of patients with campylobacter enteritis to hospital. If laparotomy is performed, the usual findings are an inflamed, oedematous ileum and enlarged, fleshy, mesenteric lymph nodes. Occasionally there is genuine appendicitis. In uncomplicated infection, abdominal tenderness may be present, but not the true signs of acute peritonitis.

Some patients present with the symptoms and sigmoidoscopic appearances of acute ulcerative colitis. The danger here is that they might be given steroids rather than antibiotics. On the other hand, campylobacter infection can exacerbate pre-existing ulcerative colitis and treatment must be given for both conditions.

Campylobacter biliary tract infection and cholecystitis are uncommon complications of infection and there are a few reports of pancreatitis and hepatitis. Other rare acute-stage complications are gastrointestinal haemorrhage, haemolytic-uraemic syndrome, glomerulonephritis, and rashes in the form of urticaria or erythema nodosum. Maternal infection and septic abortion is another rare complication that may arise without the mother having had obvious diarrhoea. Another consequence of maternal infection is neonatal infection occurring during labour. Infants may pass blood-stained stools and have symptoms that mimic intussusception. Outbreaks within neonatal units have been described, and some neonates have developed campylobacter meningitis, albeit of a relatively benign nature.

Reactive arthritis is a late complication arising 1 to 3 weeks after the onset of illness. It affects about 1 per cent of patients, or more if the frequency of the HLA-B27 haplotype in the population is high. Clinically, it is no different from the reactive arthritis following salmonella or other bacterial diarrhoeas.

Guillain-Barré syndrome The link between campylobacter infection and Guillain-Barré syndrome (**GBS**), or postinfective polyneuropathy, was not recognized for several years. In fact, campylobacter enteritis is now the most frequently identified antecedent event in GBS (26–41 per cent of cases); moreover, patients with campylobacter-associated GBS have a worse prognosis than others. It is certainly the most distressing and dangerous of the regular complications of campylobacter enteritis. Like reactive arthritis, it arises 1 to 3 weeks after the onset of diarrhoea. Campylobacter infection is also associated with the Miller–Fisher variant of GBS, in which cranial nerves are affected, and the so-called Chinese paralytic syndrome. The demyelination of nerve sheaths that occurs in GBS is thought to be caused by an immunological crossreaction between parts of the lipopolysaccharide in the cell wall of certain *C. jejuni* strains, which initiates an autoimmune reaction. GBS and related diseases are described in Chapter 24.19.

Laboratory diagnosis

Diagnosis depends on the isolation of campylobacters from faeces, as the disease cannot be distinguished clinically from other forms of bacterial diarrhoea. The isolation of campylobacters is not difficult, but it does require special selective media and microaerobic atmospheric conditions. Campylobacters are labile bacteria, so faecal samples held for more than a few hours should be refrigerated. Faeces should be placed in transport medium if delays of more than a day are anticipated. A laboratory result is normally available in 48 h. It is conventional for laboratories to report the presence (or absence) of campylobacters without specifying whether the species is *C. jejuni* or *C. coli*, as the distinction is immaterial for clinical purposes. However, it could be important if an outbreak is suspected.

Methods for detecting campylobacters by DNA probes with PCR amplification work well, but they are currently too complex for use in routine clinical laboratories. In circumstances where a quick answer is required, such as a patient with suspected appendicitis or ulcerative colitis, the direct microscopy of faeces can be helpful—campylobacters are usually abundant in the acute stages of infection and their typical morphology and motility make them easily recognizable by a trained eye.

A retrospective serological diagnosis can be made in patients who have a late complication, such as reactive arthritis or Guillain-Barré syndrome, and in whom cultures are negative or were not performed.

Treatment

Oral rehydration and electrolyte replacement is all that is required for most patients with campylobacter enteritis. Antimicrobial therapy is of limited value because patients are usually recovering by the time a bacteriological diagnosis is made, yet it is effective if given early in the disease. Antimicrobials should be reserved for patients who are acutely ill or have complications. The choice is then between erythromycin (or another macrolide) if campylobacters are known or suspected to be the cause of illness, or ciprofloxacin given empirically if the cause of enteritis is unknown. Resistance to erythromycin rarely exceeds 5 per cent of strains in most countries (there are notable exceptions) and this figure has not changed substantially in years. Suitable dosage regimens are erythromycin stearate 500 mg twice daily for 5 days for adults, and erythromycin ethyl succinate 40 mg/kg per day for children. By contrast, resistance to ciprofloxacin and other fluoroquinolones has risen sharply in recent years; examples of current recent resistance rates are: United Kingdom, 20 per cent; United States, 24 per cent; Spain, 70 per cent. A major factor in the acquisition of quinolone resistance in *C. jejuni* is believed to be the extensive use of enrofloxacin in poultry. The traditional dosage of ciprofloxacin is 500 mg taken orally twice daily for 5 days, but shorter courses are probably effective.

For patients with life-threatening septicaemic infections, gentamicin or imipenem are the agents of choice. They are highly active against campylobacters and resistance is almost unknown. It should be noted that campylobacters are naturally resistant to most cephalosporins, and so must be considered as possible infecting agents in febrile patients who do not respond to these broad-spectrum antibiotics.

Prevention and control

As with any infection transmitted by the faecal–oral route, the safe disposal of sewage and the purification of water supplies are fundamental control measures. However, because campylobacter enteritis is a zoonosis, there is much more to its control. Prevention must be aimed at minimizing infection in food-producing animals and preventing their arrival and survival in food. Many of the measures taken to prevent salmonellosis, such as the pasteurization of milk, apply to campylobacters. Much could be done to reduce infection in broiler chickens, which are a major source of infection, but this is a complex matter that will cost money and require changes in attitude in the industry and the public. Good hygienic practice in the preparation and handling of chickens and other raw meats removes the risk of infection, but the public is largely ignorant of this and needs to be educated.

Miscellaneous food-poisoning bacteria

Although most infections of the intestinal tract are transmitted via food or water, only a limited number are typically classified under the heading of food poisoning. Of these, the minority are in fact due to microbial 'poisons' (or toxins) present in the food or water source. This convention is odd, as it groups both infections and toxin ingestions as a subset of foodborne infections. Yet the use of the term 'food poisoning' seems to be firmly fixed in the literature. For example, a Medline search for 'food poisoning' in February 2002 reveals 9086 citations, the vast majority of which refer to non-typhoidal *Salmonella* spp., enterotoxin-producing *Staphylococcus aureus*, *Clostridium* spp., *Bacillus* spp., or *Listeria monocytogenes*, as well as 1046 papers on mushroom and 588 papers on fish toxin (ciguatera) poisoning.

'Food poisoning' is most often recognized in the context of an outbreak involving a number of individuals exposed to the same food or water source. It is the number of cases that calls attention to the event and leads to the investigation that establishes a confirmed or probable aetiology. Because individual and sporadic cases are seldom investigated, particularly when symptoms are transient and insufficiently severe to lead to hospitalization or death, they are neither classified nor tabulated and remain epidemiologically invisible. However, the total number of such individuals affected in a given year probably greatly exceeds the total number of individuals involved in outbreaks.

Classification and differential diagnosis of food poisoning

Food poisoning episodes can be classified into three principal syndrome groups:

(1) watery diarrhoea;

(2) primarily vomiting and/or cramps; and

(3) neurological symptoms.

A limited differential diagnosis (a listing of the possible causes of a clinical presentation) of food poisoning episodes can be constructed in this manner. Alternatively, a presumptive differential diagnosis can be developed by classifying the episode according to a critical epidemiological feature, for example the time elapsed between the ingestion of the presumed causative food or water and the appearance of symptoms, whatever nature they may take. In general, symptoms of food poisoning episodes occur in three time periods: within 4 h; between 8 and 16 h; 24 h or more. These periods correspond to distinct sets of common aetiologies. Therefore, simple outbreak epidemiology to determine when the suspect meal occurred in relation to the onset of symptoms can itself limit the differential diagnosis (Table 5). A third way to organize thinking about food poisoning agents is to separate them according to microbiological and taxonomic considerations, such as their Gram-stain reaction. There are certain advantages to each approach, but in clinical practice the most accurate diagnosis results from the integration of all three sources of information.

Non-cholera vibrios and vibrio-like organisms

Vibrio parahaemolyticus

This marine organism was first associated with human illness in Japan in 1963, since when it has come to be recognized as the most common cause of food poisoning in that country. Seafood is the main source of the organism, and the high incidence of infection in the Far East is doubtless due to the popularity of eating raw fish in the region. *V. parahaemolyticus* is most plentiful in warm waters, but it has been isolated from North Atlantic and Pacific coastlines, and cases of food poisoning have been reported from most continents, usually after the consumption of crabs, prawns, or raw oysters. Cooked shellfish may become contaminated after cooking, for a few bacteria picked up from a working surface contaminated with the raw product can multiply at atmospheric temperatures. This is one reason why the incidence in temperate regions is highest in summer.

After ingestion, *V. parahaemolyticus* multiplies in the gut to produce an enterotoxin, which causes watery diarrhoea and sometimes vomiting lasting for 1 or 2 days. The incubation period is usually 10 to 20 h (range 4–96 h). Despite excretion of the bacteria in enormous numbers in diarrhoeal stools, victims are not a significant source of infection. Tetracycline shortens the period of excretion (seldom more than 10 days), but antibiotics are not justified for such a short illness.

As marine vibrios fail to grow properly on routine media that are not supplemented with extra salt, it is essential for clinicians to notify the laboratory if *V. parahaemolyticus* is suspected. A positive Kanagawa test

Table 5 Classification of food poisoning by incubation period*

Duration of incubation period	Usual causes	Main symptoms	Mechanisms
Short (1–4 h)	*Staphylococcus aureus* enterotoxins	Vomiting	Preformed toxins; activation of emetic centres of brain
	B. cereus cereulide toxin		
Intermediate (8–16 h)	*Clostridium perfringens* enterotoxins	Abdominal pain and to a lesser extent watery diarrhoea	Production of toxin *in situ* in the intestine
	B. cereus enterotoxins	Watery diarrhoea and to a lesser extent abdominal pain	
Long (1 to 7 days)	Non-typhoidal *Salmonella*; *Shigella sonnei*; ETEC; *Campylobacter*; *Vibrio parahaemolyticus*;	Febrile watery diarrhoeal illness	Replicating infection in the small or large bowel, with adherence, invasion, production of enterotoxins, or other signalling mechanism for the activation of ion-secretory pathways
	Listeria monocytogenes (Chapter 7.11.34) Norwalk and small, round-structured viruses (Chapter 7.10.8)	Mainly vomiting but also diarrhoea	
Variable (a few hours to several days)	*Clostridium botulinum* (Chapter 7.11.21)	Neurological	Toxin, preformed in food

* This table does not include marine or mushroom toxin-mediated syndromes (see Chapters 8.2 and 8.3)

(β-haemolysis on medium containing human blood) is an indication of pathogenicity of the isolated strain.

Other non-cholera vibrios

Several other aquatic vibrios are capable of causing human gastroenteritis. A study in the southern United States showed that over half of the cases were linked to the consumption of raw oysters. Apart from *V. parahaemolyticus*, the species isolated were *V. mimicus*, *V. fluvialis*, *V. hollisae*, *V. vulnificus*, and *V. alginolyticus*. Half of the patients had fever and one-quarter had bloody stools. *V. vulnificus* is better known as a cause of severe, often fatal, septicaemic wound infection, which may arise from eating raw oysters or through damaged skin. *V. alginolyticus* also causes wound infection, but more typically otitis externa in swimmers. *Photobacterium damsela* (formerly *V. damsela*) causes a septicaemic infection like *V. vulnificus*. Again, as most of these bacteria are halophilic, it is essential to notify the laboratory of their possible presence so that high salt-containing media can be inoculated.

Aeromonas and Plesiomonas spp.

Aeromonads are ubiquitous in water, soil, and cold-blooded animals; some are major pathogens of fish. Their status as human pathogens is unclear, but it seems that some strains, mainly *Aeromonas hydrophila* (others are *A. sobria* and *A. caviae*) are capable of causing diarrhoea. Aeromonads are more frequent in hot climates, so most aeromonas infections are encountered in travellers visiting tropical and subtropical regions. Persistent aeromonas-associated diarrhoea with blood and mucus mimicking ulcerative colitis has been described in patients in Western Australia. These patients were treated successfully with trimethoprim. Most aeromonas infections are thought to be waterborne, but the absence of common-source outbreaks suggests their status as enteric pathogens is low.

Plesiomonas shigelloides is another aquatic vibrio-like organism that is occasionally associated with diarrhoea, usually of a mild nature. It has been implicated in outbreaks of diarrhoea in the Far East and has been isolated from sporadic cases throughout the world. Fewer than 100 cases a year are reported in the United Kingdom.

Gram-positive bacterial food poisoning

A limited number of Gram-positive bacteria are frequent causes of food poisoning in the strict sense of the term, namely the ingestion of preformed toxins in a meal that results in clinical illness. Gram-negative organisms do not cause 'food poisoning' in this manner even though they may produce toxins that are involved in the pathogenesis of clinical disease. The major Gram-positive causes are several species of rod-shaped bacilli (*Clostridium* spp., *Bacillus* spp.) and certain *Staphylococcus aureus* strains.

Clostridium botulinum

See Chapter 7.11.21 for further discussion.

Clostridium perfringens

See Chapter 7.11.21 for further discussion.

Bacillus cereus

This is another Gram-positive spore-forming bacillus like the clostridia, but it exhibits aerobic rather than anaerobic metabolism. It is normally and widely present in soil, hay, trees, and other plants and is frequently present in both raw and processed foods. As a spore former it is resistant to heat, chlorine, and other chemicals used to eliminate microbial contamination, and humans are constantly exposed to this organism. While this provides an epidemiological edge for the organism, it is not a common cause of human disease, accounting for just 1 per cent of foodborne illness in Europe.

The virulence properties of *B. cereus* are not well studied. Some strains produce a chemically unique cyclic toxin, cereulide, and one or more enterotoxins acting on the intestinal mucosa by uncertain mechanisms. Cer-

eulide is elaborated in food sources and thus causes a true food poisoning when preformed toxin is ingested in a food meal. Cereulide consists of three repeats of four different amino acids that have been modified so that every other residue and half the amino acids are α-hydroxy acid derivatives in ester, rather than amide, linkage. The cyclic structure provides heat stability, so that once elaborated by the organism the toxin is neither denatured nor detoxified by cooking. Systemically administered cereulide is a mitochondrial toxin that uncouples oxidative phosphorylation. While this may explain rare fatal cases of *B. cereus* food poisoning associated with liver failure, it does not offer any ready explanation for the self-limited emetic syndrome typical of human cases.

B. cereus also produces several distinctive enterotoxins that are suspected to cause watery diarrhoea by uncertain mechanisms. Spores induced to germinate in food by heating then develop into the replicating vegetative bacillary form in the intestinal tract where the enterotoxins are synthesized. These toxins are heterotrimers comprising three distinct polypeptides of an aggregate molecular weight greater than 100 000. A 41-kDa single peptide chain enterotoxin is present in some strains.

Food poisoning with the emetic toxin results in the rapid onset of profuse vomiting within hours of ingesting contaminated food. Most commonly this is boiled or fried rice prepared in Chinese restaurants in large amounts, stored at room temperature, and reheated before serving. Diarrhoea and abdominal pain due to enterotoxin production in the gastrointestinal tract is a longer 8- to 16-h incubation illness resembling *C. perfringens* food poisoning. It is transmitted by a number of food vehicles, including meats, stews, sauces, and dairy products. In some more recent outbreaks, the related organism *B. thuringensis*, producing similar enterotoxins, has been identified. This species is more commonly associated with its ability to produce a different toxin that kills insect larvae and is used for pest control in agriculture. However, were these strains of *B. thuringensis* to acquire the genes for enterotoxicity in nature, its use to control pest insects would be seriously compromised. The gene for this protein has been cloned into some genetically modified crops to endow them with insect-resistance properties, which, although a controversial strategy for pest control, would not carry the same risk.

Specific diagnosis depends on the isolation of high numbers of organisms from food, diarrhoea, or vomitus. Typically, however, the high temperature that induces germination and cereulide production kills the bacteria in the emetic form. Cell culture and ELISA tests for toxin are available in reference laboratories. Management of clinical cases is supportive, as symptoms are short-lived.

Listeria monocytogenes

See Chapter 7.11.34 for further discussion.

Staphylococcus aureus (see also Chapter 7.11.4)

Enterotoxin-producing strains of *Staph. aureus* are a classical cause of another true food poisoning, which results from the ingestion of preformed staphylococcal toxins produced in contaminated foods. The source of the bacteria is usually a food handler or preparer, as these organisms are ubiquitous colonizers of the skin, nasal, oral, and rectal mucous membranes. Fingers then readily transmit the bacteria from these sites to food in preparation. Such food handlers often have minor skin infections, such as boils, paronychia, impetigo, or an infected cut or skin abrasion, which facilitates the contamination of the food. The clinical illness is predominantly a short-incubation vomiting syndrome, with watery diarrhoea and abdominal cramps as less prominent symptoms. It is very common and is undoubtedly underdiagnosed.

Many foods can serve as a vehicle for the growth of *Staph. aureus*, including sliced meats, custards and cream pastries, potato and salads containing mayonnaise, and various dairy products. Organisms grow and elaborate toxins if the food is stored unrefrigerated or kept warm for serving.

Staphylococcal food poisoning is not more common as relatively few isolates are toxin producers and because the ubiquitous coagulase-negative staphylococci are toxin-negative. There are eight serologically identifiable, small, structurally related, 22- to 28-kDa linear polypeptide toxins, designated staphylotoxin enterotoxins (**SE**) A to E and G to I (SEA, SEB, etc.). Another distinctive toxin, formerly identified as staphylococcal enterotoxin F, is uniquely able to translocate across mucosal surfaces and is now known as toxic-shock syndrome toxin-1 (**TSST-1**). The enterotoxin terminology is engrained in use, however inappropriate this now seems as these peptides are not prominent causes of diarrhoea. Rather they appear to target the stomach where they activate gastric emetic responses by, as yet, uncertain mechanisms. For example, it is not known what the gastric mucosal receptors for staphylococcal enterotoxins are, or even whether small quantities are absorbed to act centrally in the brain. Ultimately, however, it is the activation of medullary emetic centres in the brainstem via vagal or sympathetic-nerve transmitted signals that causes symptoms. Pathology in primates reveals inflammatory changes of the gastric mucosa, and to a lesser extent in the proximal jejunum. Brush-border alterations and mucopurulent exudates are also present. Some investigators theorize that the toxins induce mast-cell degranulation via direct binding to these cells, whereas others suggest that neuropeptides are first released from sensory nerves and secondarily stimulate mast cells to release inflammatory mediators.

Diagnosis is dependent on the isolation of high numbers of toxin-producing *Staph. aureus* from the suspect food. Stool culture is not diagnostic because *Staph. aureus* can often be found in stool in small numbers. None the less, stool culture can be useful epidemiologically if the same phage type of toxin-producing *Staph. aureus* is recovered from the food and the patient and other possible aetiologies are not found. If a food handler is suspected of being the source, culture of skin lesions for enterotoxin-producing *Staph. aureus* is also epidemiologically helpful. Treatment is supportive, as the symptoms are short-lived, generally just a matter of hours.

Summary

It is clear that Enterobacteriaceae constitute a clinically important group of organisms, primarily involved in intestinal infection, with a number of systemic syndromes due to microbial penetration of the intestinal mucosa. In addition, there are a number of foodborne illnesses due to Gram-positive organisms that overlap the spectrum of enteric disease caused by the Enterobacteriaceae. There has been considerable progress in understanding basic microbiology, epidemiology, clinical manifestations, and treatment and prevention strategies of all these organisms. Beyond the scope of this chapter, and therefore not discussed, are the general measures that are or could be taken to reduce the contamination of food and water sources of infection. These range from basic sanitation and safe food handling—for example, Hazard Analysis Critical Control Point (**HACCP**) systems to control microbial contamination of food in processing plants, or proper cooking and refrigeration of food in the home—to the use of large-scale, gamma-irradiation of food to diminish microbial counts, or other potential innovative methods to reduce the contamination of food and water sources with disease-causing micro-organisms. However, the physician must be familiar with all of these aspects of Enterobacteriaceae infections in order to properly diagnose and treat disease when prevention fails.

Further reading

Acheson DW, Kane AV, Keusch GT (2000). Shiga toxins. *Methods in Molecular Biology* **145**, 41–63.

Altekruse SF, *et al.* (2000). Vibrio gastroenteritis in the US Gulf of Mexico region: the role of raw oysters. *Epidemiology and Infection* **124**, 489–95.

Bennish ML, *et al.* (1990). Hypoglycemia during diarrhea in childhood. Prevalence, pathophysiology and outcome. *New England Journal of Medicine* **322**, 1357–63.

Blaser MJ, *et al.*, eds. (2002). *Infections of the gastrointestinal tract.* Lippincott, Williams and Wilkins, Philadelphia.

Brunder W, Karch H (2000). Genome plasticity in Enterobacteriaceae. *International Journal of Medical Microbiology* **290**, 153–65.

Crane JK (1999). Preformed bacterial toxins. *Clinics in Laboratory Medicine* **3**, 583–99.

Dinges MM, Orwin PM, Schlievert PM (2000). Exotoxins of *Staphylococcus aureus. Clinical Microbiology Reviews* **13**, 16–34.

Donnenberg MS (2000). Pathogenic strategies of enteric bacteria. *Nature* **406**, 768–74.

Donnenberg MS, Whittam TS (2001). Pathogenesis and evolution of virulence in enteropathogenic and enterohemorrhagic Escherichia coli. *Journal of Clinical Investigation* **107**, 539–48.

Dooley JSG, Roberts TA (2000). Control of vegetative micro-organisms in foods. *British Medical Bulletin* **56**, 142–57.

Farkas J (1998). Irradiation as a method for decontaminating food. *International Journal of Food Microbiology* **44**, 189–204.

Fierer J, Swancutt M (2000). Non-typhoid Salmonella: a review. *Current Clinical Topics in Infectious Diseases* **20**, 134–57.

Fleckenstein JM, Kopecko DJ (2001). Breaching the mucosal barrier by stealth: an emerging pathogenic mechanism for enteroadherent bacterial pathogens. *Journal of Clinical Investigation* **107**, 27–30.

Godaly G, *et al.* (2000). Innate defences and resistance to Gram negative mucosal infection. *Advances in Experimental Medical Biology* **485**, 9–24.

Granum PE, Lund T (1997). *Bacillus cereus* and its food poisoning toxins. *FEMS Microbiology Letters* **157**, 223–8.

Janda JM, Abbott SL (1999). Unusual food-borne pathogens. *Listeria monocytogenes, Aeromonas, Plesiomonas,* and *Edwardsiella* species. *Clinical and Laboratory Medicine* **19**, 553–82.

Keusch GT, Bennish ML (1998). Shigellosis. In: Evans AS, Brachman, PS, eds. *Bacterial infections of humans,* pp 631–56. Plenum Press, New York.

Nachamkin I, Blaser MJ, eds. (2000). Campylobacter, 2nd edn. ASM Press, Washington DC.

O'Hara CM, Brenner FW, Miller JM (2000). Classification, identification, and clinical significance of Proteus, Providencia, and Morganella. *Clinical Microbiology Reviews* **13**, 534–46.

Roberts JA (2000). Economic aspects of food-borne outbreaks and their control. *British Medical Bulletin* **56**, 133–41.

Sahly H, Podschun R, Ullmann U (2000). Klebsiella infections in the immunocompromised host. *Advances in Experimental Medicine and Biology* **479**, 237–49.

Sansonetti PJ (2001). Rupture, invasion and inflammatory destruction of the intestinal barrier by Shigella, making sense of prokaryote-eukaryote cross-talks. *FEMS Microbiology Reviews* **1**, 3–14.

Schimpff SC (1993). Gram-negative bacteremia. *Support Care Cancer* **1**, 5–18.

Skirrow MB, Blaser MJ (2002). *Campylobacter jejuni.* In: Blaser MJ, *et al.*, eds. *Infections of the gastrointestinal tract.* Lippincott, Williams and Wilkins, Philadelphia.

Tauxe R (1997). Emerging foodborne diseases: an evolving public health challenge. *Emerging Infectious Diseases* **3**, 425–34.

Thorpe CM, *et al.* (1999). Shiga toxins stimulate secretion of IL-8 from intestinal epithelial cells by altering regulation of cell processes. *Infection and Immunity* **67**, 5985–93.

Threlfall EJ, *et al.* (2000). The emergence and spread of antibiotic resistance in food-borne bacteria. *International Journal of Food Microbiology* **62**, 1–5.

Vallance BA, Finlay BB (2000). Exploitation of host cells by enteropathogenic Escherichia coli. *Proceedings of the National Academy of Sciences, USA* **97**, 8799–806.

7.11.8 Typhoid and paratyphoid fevers

J. Richens and C. Parry

Typhoid

Typhoid and paratyphoid, types A, B, and C (collectively known as enteric fevers) make up the group of salmonelloses whose main host is human. Their clinical features resemble other salmonelloses, ranging from gastroenteritis (more common with paratyphoid) to the septicaemic illness of severe typhoid.

Epidemiology

Worldwide, 15 to 30 million cases of typhoid occur each year with half a million deaths. In affluent countries, typhoid is seen in travellers or when food or water safety measures fail; with antibiotic treatment death is rare. High rates of transmission are seen in sub-Saharan Africa, the Indian subcontinent, central Asia, Vietnam, and Indonesia where annual incidence reaches 100 to 1000 cases per 100 000 population and up to 1 per cent of the population may carry *S. typhi*. In these countries, transmission has been exacerbated by antibiotic resistance. Peaks of transmission occur in dry weather or at the onset of rains. Case-fatality rates have exceeded 10 per cent in hospitalized patients in Indonesia and Papua New Guinea.

Pathogenesis

Aetiology

Salmonella enterica serovar *typhi* (*S. typhi*) is a Gram-negative bacillus capable of surviving in hostile environments and proliferating dangerously within dairy products, processed meats, and shellfish. Three antigens have been exploited for serodiagnosis; the somatic oligosaccharide O antigen (9 and 12), the protein flagellar H-d antigen, and the polysaccharide envelope Vi antigen which confers virulence by masking the O antigen from immunological attack. Antibiotic resistance is conferred by R plasmids, usually of the incompatibility group IncH-1 (chloramphenicol, amoxicillin, co-trimoxazole), and mutations in the chromosomal *gyrA* gene (fluoroquinolones). Many of the genes that give *S. typhi* its ability to survive in hostile extracellular and intracellular environments have been identified. The genome of *S. typhi* has a remarkable plasticity compared to other bacteria, which allows recombination of homologous rRNA operons as well as insertion of non-homologous DNA. The recent sequencing of an isolate of *S. typhi* will shed further light on the pathogenicity of this organism.

Transmission

Sources of typhoid transmission are excreting chronic or convalescent carriers and the acutely infected. Transmission occurs through contamination by carriers of food or water by effluents containing infected urine or faeces. 'Typhoid Mary' was a cook who infected 53 people early last century. The Aberdeen outbreak in 1964 was traced to a leaking corned beef tin which had been cooled with contaminated river water. Transmission of typhoid has also been attributed to flies, laboratory mishaps, unsterile instruments, and anal intercourse.

Infective dose

Hornick demonstrated that 10^7 organisms of Quailes strain of *S. typhi* infected 50 per cent of experimental subjects. Susceptibility is increased by antacids or vagotomy. The virulence of *S. typhi* varies. Infection may lead to acute disease, transient symptoms, or to a symptomless carrier state.

Multiplication and dissemination

Bacteria pass from the gut through the cytoplasm of enterocytes and M cells overlying lymphoid tissue (Peyer's patches) of the small intestine to reach the lamina propria from which they are conveyed to the mesenteric nodes, before reaching the blood stream via the thoracic duct. During a transient primary bacteraemia the organism is seeded to reticuloendothelial sites where intracellular multiplication occurs throughout a 7 to 14-day incubation period. A second bacteraemia follows, accompanied by symptoms as the infection spreads throughout liver, gallbladder, spleen, Peyer's patches, and bone marrow. Multiplication of *S. typhi* occurs mainly in macrophages. Concentrated sites of infection in reticuloendothelial tissues, known as typhoid nodules, are characterized by infiltrates of lymphocytes and macrophages. At post mortem, hypertrophy of lymphoid tissue is often visible within liver, spleen, mesenteric nodes, and Peyer's patches. Ulceration of Peyer's patches is seen where the inflammatory process has resulted in ischaemia and necrosis (Fig. 1).

Endotoxin plays a central role in stimulating the release of cytokines such as tumour necrosis factor and interleukins 1 and 6 from macrophages and neutrophils, by activating the complement cascade and upregulating the adhesive capacity of neutrophils and endothelial cells. These processes inflict inflammatory damage through the release of neutrophil proteases, free oxygen radicals, and arachidonic acid metabolites. Unlike in meningitis and malaria, no correlation between levels of tumour necrosis factor and clinical outcome has been demonstrated in typhoid. Levels of circulating tumour necrosis factor receptors are increased and the capacity of whole blood to produce proinflammatory cytokines following stimulation is reduced in patients with severe typhoid.

Immune response

In patients there is a cell-mediated immune response lasting about 16 weeks, a mucosal immune response lasting for up to 48 weeks, and persistent circulating anti-O and -H agglutinins for up to 2 years. The predominance of clinical typhoid among children and young adults in endemic areas suggests a degree of acquired immunity. Only 25 per cent of volunteers given a standard inoculum of *S. typhi* 20 months after an initial infection developed clinical illness. Prolonged elevation of Vi antibody occurs in typhoid carriers. Immunodeficiency reduces the ability to clear *Salmonella* infections.

Clinical features

Typhoid is predominantly an infection of children and young adults, affecting both sexes equally. The incubation period ranges from 3 to 60 days, but most infections occur 7 to 14 days after exposure.

Fig. 1 Typhoid at autopsy, showing transmural ulceration of Peyer's patches in the distal ileum.

The main focus of typhoid is in the small bowel, but systemic symptoms often overshadow abdominal symptoms. The predominant symptom is the fever which rises gradually to a high plateau of 39 to 40°C, and shows little diurnal variation. Rigors are uncommon, except in late or complicated typhoid or in patients treated with antipyretics.

Most patients complain of headache and malaise. Constipation is a frequent early symptom. Most patients will experience diarrhoea and typhoid can present as an acute gastroenteritis. Severe diarrhoea or colitis has been reported in HIV-infected patients. Bloody diarrhoea may be seen. The abdominal pain is usually diffuse and poorly localized but occasionally sufficiently intense in the right iliac fossa to suggest appendicitis. Nausea and vomiting are infrequent in uncomplicated typhoid but are seen with abdominal distension in severe cases. Other early symptoms include cough, sore throat, and epistaxes.

In developing countries, patients with typhoid in its second to fourth week present with accelerating weight loss, weakness, altered mental state, intestinal haemorrhage and perforation, refractory hypotension, pneumonia, nephritis, and acute psychosis. Those infected with multidrug resistant *S. typhi* may suffer more severe disease.

Physical examination is often unremarkable apart from fever. Careful examination may reveal splenomegaly, hepatomegaly, or rose spots. Tachycardia is common although temperature pulse-dissociation (relative bradycardia) is considered characteristic. Hypotension has important implications (see below, Severe typhoid). A coated tongue is often observed. The lenticular rose spots, appear at the end of the first week. They form a sparse collection of maculopapular lesions on the abdominal skin, which blanch with pressure and fade after 2 or 3 days. Osler found them in 90 per cent of whites and 20 per cent of black skins. The rash may extend on to the trunk and arms. Melanesian typhoid patients develop purpuric macules that do not blanch (Plate 1).

Adventitious lung sounds, especially scattered wheezes, are common and may suggest pneumonia. These findings with a normal chest radiograph and high fever should prompt consideration of typhoid.

Abdominal examination may reveal the typhoid rash, distension, or a diffuse tenderness, occasionally localized to the area of the terminal ileum. Intra-abdominal inflammation sometimes provokes retention of urine. A moderate, soft, tender hepatosplenomegaly eventually develops in most patients but it less likely to be found early.

Patients with advanced illness may display the 'typhoid' facies (Fig. 2), a thin, flushed face with a staring, apathetic expression. Mental apathy may progress to an agitated delirium, frequently accompanied by tremor of the hands, tremulous speech, and gait ataxia. If the patient's condition deteriorates further the features described in the writings of Louis and Osler make their appearance—muttering delirium, twitchings of the fingers and

Fig. 2 Typhoid facies: 18-year-old male with severe typhoid.

wrists (subsultus tendinum), agitated plucking at the bedclothes (carphology), and a staring, unrousable stupor (coma vigil).

Typhoid in children

Typhoid can develop in neonates born to infected mothers. The disease tends to take a milder course in children but case-fatality rates are higher in under-fives. The main differences, compared to adults, are a greater frequency of diarrhoea and vomiting, jaundice, febrile convulsions, nephritis (3 per cent in one series), or typhoid meningitis. Community-based studies in Chile and India have shown that unrecognized *S. typhi* and *paratyphi* bacteraemia can behave like a mild respiratory illness in very young children. Relative bradycardia is of greater diagnostic significance for typhoid in febrile children.

Diagnosis

A secure diagnosis of typhoid rests on the isolation of *S. typhi*. Many viral, bacterial, and protozoal infections as well as non-infectious conditions characterized by fever, such as lymphoproliferative disorders and vasculitides, resemble typhoid. Typhoid should always be considered when suspected malaria has not been confirmed or has not responded to antimalarial therapy.

Culture

S. typhi can be isolated from blood, bone marrow, stool, urine, bile, cerebrospinal fluid, and rose spots. Bone marrow gives the highest yield, including those exposed to antibiotics, but yields only marginally more than blood. For bone marrow culture the fine needle technique described by Hedley can be recommended (Hedley *et al.* (1982). *Lancet* **ii,** 415–16). Most clinicians culture blood, stool, and sometimes urine.

The median number of bacteria present in the blood of children are higher than adults and decline with increasing duration of illness. In mild typhoid, the number of bacteria may be as low as one colony forming unit per ml. Successful culture from blood can be achieved in 80 per cent of patients but depends on taking a generous volume of blood and using the correct volume of blood to broth (1:10). Automated continuously monitored culture systems (e.g. Bactec and Bact/Alert systems) can accelerate the culture from blood. Culture of bile obtained from an overnight duodenal string capsule gives a similar yield to blood and offers additional means to isolate *S. typhi* from children or from carriers. Rose spots, when present, can give a positive culture in 70 per cent of patients.

The number of organisms recoverable from faeces increases through the illness. Rectal swabs are less satisfactory than faecal samples. The results must be interpreted with caution in areas with many carriers. Isolation from urine is more common in areas endemic for schistosomiasis.

Serology

The use of a tube or slide agglutination test (the Widal test) to diagnose typhoid is cheaper and simpler than culture but fraught with pitfalls. The demonstration of a four-fold rise in titre of antibodies to *S. typhi* suggests typhoid but is too slow to help clinical decision-making and is not observed in all patients. Single measurements of antibody titres has been found useful in populations where accurate, up-to-date information about the predictive value of the test at specific cut-off points is available. False positive serological tests are obtained from persons with previous infection, infection with cross-reacting organisms, or following vaccination.

Other tests for typhoid

Many other tests for the detection of antibodies, *S. typhi* antigens, and salmonella DNA in body fluids have been described: these include passive haemagglutination, latex agglutination, counterimmune electrophoresis, radioimmunoassay, enzyme immunoassay, indirect fluorescent antibody tests, monoclonal antibodies, IgM capture, DNA probes, and PCR. Few have so far been adopted for routine use.

Other laboratory findings in typhoid

A mild normochromic anaemia, mild thrombocytopenia, and an increased erythrocyte sedimentation rate are common. The frequency of true leucopenia has been overstated in the past; most patients have a total white-cell count within the normal range. Leucocytosis suggests either perforation or another diagnosis. Laboratory evidence of mild disseminated intravascular coagulation is common but rarely of clinical significance. Common biochemical findings include hyponatraemia, hypokalaemia, and elevation of liver enzymes. The urine often contains some protein and white cells.

Management

The aims of management are to eliminate the infection swiftly with antibiotics, to restore fluid and nutritional deficits, and to monitor the patient for dangerous complications.

Antibiotics (see Table 1 for doses)

Effective antibiotic therapy in typhoid reduces mortality and complications and shortens the illness. Chloramphenicol was the first antibiotic found to be effective and the standard against which subsequent antibiotics have been measured. Ampicillin, amoxicillin, and co-trimoxazole have been shown to have comparable efficacy to chloramphenicol while having less toxicity. In many areas these drugs are no longer used because of the spread of multidrug resistant (MDR) strains of *S. typhi*. New antibiotics active against MDR *S. typhi* have emerged. Most active are the fluoroquinolones but resistance is again emerging. Other useful antibiotics are the extended-spectrum cephalosporins and azithromycin.

Most physicians start with a fluoroquinolone—ofloxacin, ciprofloxacin, fleroxacin, or pefloxacin. Treatment can be completed in a week or less with minimal toxicity In an analysis of 19 randomized trials of fluoroquinolones in the treatment of 788 patients with culture-confirmed enteric fever (>95 per cent *S. typhi* infection), the fever clearance was 2.5 to 5.2 days with a pooled cure rate of 97.3 (95 per cent CI, 96–98 per cent). Over half the studies reported no relapses and only one carrier (0.2 per cent) was detected among 591 patients followed up. Response rates in endemic areas may be better than those of non-immune travellers. For immunocompromised patients treatment may need to be extended for weeks or months. Questions remain about the safety of fluoroquinolones in children and during pregnancy. Careful follow-up studies of children in Vietnam following fluoroquinolone therapy have shown no toxicity and there is a growing consensus that the advantages of therapy outweigh the dangers. Ampicillin or amoxicillin is considered to be the safest drug to use in pregnancy with typhoid but should not be used in preference to a fluoroquinolone in patients likely to have MDR typhoid.

Strains of *S. typhi* with reduced susceptibility to fluoroquinolones are common in Asia and can be identified by being resistant to nalidixic acid. Patients infected with these strains may require longer courses of fluoroquinolones at the maximum dose or they may be treated with extended spectrum cephalosporins (ceftriaxone or cefixime). Azithromycin has recently shown to be effective in mild to moderate typhoid but currently cannot be recommended for severe disease.

Supportive care

Cooling is preferred to antipyretics for relief of fever. Simple analgesics may be used to relieve headache but note that paracetamol has been reported to lengthen the half-life of chloramphenicol five-fold. Most patients can eat and drink normally. Special diets do not protect the bowel from perforation. Daily assessment of the patient's mental and circulatory status are required plus examination of the abdomen for signs of impending perforation. Severely ill patients require intensive care with parenteral fluids, intravenous steroids (see below), inotropic support, and sedation.

Complications

Table 2 lists complications of typhoid. Most are rare and only likely to be encountered in patients who present with untreated disease lasting 2 or more weeks. Occasionally, a complication dominates the clinical picture and deflects attention from the underlying diagnosis of typhoid.

Severe typhoid

Studies from Indonesia and Papua New Guinea have revealed an important subgroup of patients with mental confusion or shock (defined as a systolic blood pressure of less than 90 mmHg in adults or less than 80 mmHg in children), with evidence of decreased skin, cerebral, or renal perfusion, who have a 50 per cent fatality and account for most typhoid deaths. In one study in Jakarta, high doses of dexamethasone substantially reduced the mortality of such severe cases. The criteria for severe typhoid were marked mental confusion or shock. In adults, dexamethasone, 3 mg/kg infused intravenously over half an hour, followed by eight doses of 1 mg/kg 6-hourly, resulted in a 10 per cent case-fatality compared to 55.6 per cent in controls.

Intestinal haemorrhage and perforation

Perforation of ileal ulcers occurs in less than 5 per cent of typhoid patients. The development of acute abdominal signs is often gradual, making diagnosis difficult. Severely ill patients display only restlessness, hypotension,

Table 1 Guidelines for drug dosages in typhoid

Antibiotic	Daily dose	Route[a]	Doses/day	Duration
Chloramphenicol	50–75 mg/kg	O/IM/IV[b]	4	14 days
Co-trimoxazole	6.5–10 mg/kg trimethoprim; 40 mg/kg sulfamethoxazole	O/IM/IV	2–3	14 days
Amoxicillin	75–100 mg/kg	O/IM/IV	3	14 days
Furazolidone	7.5 mg/kg	O	4	14 days
Ceftriaxone	50–60 mg/kg	IM/IV	2	7–14 days
Cefixime	20 mg/kg	O	2	7–14 days
Ciprofloxacin	0.5–1 g	O/IV	2	7–14 days
Ofloxacin	800 mg	O/IV	2	7–14 days
Pefloxacin	800 mg	O/IV	2	7–14 days
Fleroxacin	400 mg	O/IV	1	7–14 days
Azithromycin	500 mg	O	1	7 days
Treatment of carriers				
Ampicillin or amoxicillin with probenecid	100 mg/kg	30 mg/kg	3–4	3 months[c]
Co-trimoxazole	6.5–10 mg trimethoprim	O	2	3 months
Ciprofloxacin	1500 mg	O	2	28 days

[a] Oral therapy is satisfactory for most patients. Parenteral therapy is generally reserved for severely ill patients.

[b] The oral route is preferred; there are reports of lower blood levels of chloramphenicol in patients given parenteral therapy.

[c] The duration of treatment can be shortened if parenteral therapy is given, e.g. 8-hourly intravenous ampicillin for 2 weeks.

O, oral; IM, intramuscular; IV, intravenous.

Table 2 Complications of typhoid

Abdominal
Intestinal perforation
Intestinal haemorrhage
Hepatitis
Cholecystitis (usually subclinical)
Spontaneous splenic rupture
Rupture and haemorrhage from mesenteric nodes
Pancreatitis

Genitourinary
Retention of urine
Glomerulonephritis
Pyelonephritis
Cystitis
Orchitis

Cardiovascular
Asymptomatic ECG changes
Myocarditis
Pericarditis
Endocarditis
Phlebitis and arteritis
Deep venous thrombosis
Gangrene
Shock
Sudden death

Respiratory
Bronchitis
Laryngeal ulceration
Glottal oedema
Pneumonia (*S. typhi*, *Strep. pneumoniae*)

Neuropsychiatric
Delirium
Psychotic states
Depression
Deafness
Meningitis
Encephalomyelitis
Transverse myelitis
Signs of upper motor-neurone lesions
Signs of extrapyramidal disorder
Impairment of co-ordination
Optic neuritis
Peripheral and cranial neuropathy
Guillain–Barré syndrome
Pseudotumour cerebri

Haematological
Disseminated intravascular coagulation (usually subclinical)
Anaemia
Haemolysis
Haemolytic uraemic syndrome

Focal infections
Abscesses of brain, liver, spleen, breast, thyroid, muscles, lymph nodes
Parotitis
Pharyngitis
Osteitis, especially tibia, ribs, spine
Arthritis

Other
Myopathy
Hypercalcaemia
Decubitus ulceration
Abortion
Relapse

and tachycardia. A chest radiograph may show free gas under the diaphragm. Ultrasonography is useful for demonstrating and aspirating faeculent fluid in the peritoneal cavity. To manage perforation start nasogastric suction, administer fluids to correct hypotension, and proceed to surgery promptly. Simple closure of perforations is adequate but experienced surgeons use procedures to bypass the worst-affected sections of the ileum in order to reduce postoperative morbidity. Closure of perforations should be accompanied by vigorous peritoneal toilet. Metronidazole or clindamycin should be added to the therapy of fluoroquinolone-treated patients. Metronidazole and aminoglycosides are recommended for patients receiving chloramphenicol, ampicillin, or co-trimoxazole. The survival of patients undergoing surgery for perforation is generally 70 to 75 per cent, but reaches 97 per cent in the best series. This compares with survival rates of around 30 per cent in conservatively managed patients.

Silent bleeding may be signalled by sudden collapse of a patient or a steadily falling haematocrit. Severe bleeding is sometimes seen in advanced typhoid. It is rarely fatal. Most bleeding episodes are self-limiting. A few require transfusion. In exceptional circumstances, surgery or intra-arterial vasopressin have been to halt haemorrhage.

Relapse

Relapse in typhoid is a second episode of fever, usually milder than the first, occurring a week or two after the recovery from the first episode. Isolates from relapsing patients usually have identical antibiotic susceptibility to those identified during the first episode. Relapse rates of 10 per cent have been described in untreated typhoid and chloramphenicol-treated patients. Relapse is managed with a similar or abbreviated course of the same therapy used in the initial episode.

Carriers

Many patients excrete *S. typhi* in their stools or urine for some days after starting antibiotic treatment. Convalescent carriers excrete for periods up to 3 months. Patients still excreting at 3 months are unlikely to cease and at 1 year meet the formal definition of 'chronic carrier'. Amongst carriers detected by screening, 25 per cent give no history of acute typhoid. Faecal carriage is more frequent in individuals with gallbladder disease and is most common in women over 40; in the Far East there is an association with opisthorchiasis. Urinary carriage is associated with schistosomiasis and nephrolithiasis. Acute typhoid in carriers has been reported. There is an increased risk of carcinoma of the gallbladder.

Patients discharged after treatment for typhoid with six negative stool and three negative urine specimens and negative Vi serology are considered free of infection. Most patients with positive stools at the completion of treatment excrete temporarily and can be safely followed up. Antibiotic eradication of carriage is advised in those still excreting at 3 months, or earlier in those at particular risk of communicating infection to others. The patient with a persistently elevated or rising Vi antibody titre is likely to be a carrier. Repeated checks of urine and faeces should be made and consideration given to obtaining bile cultures if these are negative. In Egypt, demonstration of H antibody in urine has been useful in identifying carriers.

Eradication of carriage requires prolonged, high-dose antibiotics (Table 1). Ampicillin, amoxicillin, and co-trimoxazole have been used with some success. More recently, good results have been reported with fluoroquinolones. Cholecystectomy and nephrectomy, once used to eliminate carriage (and not without operative mortality), are hard to justify on public health grounds alone, but can be considered if antibiotic methods fail and there are additional indications for operation. The success rates of surgery are increased by giving antibiotics as well.

Prevention

The elimination of typhoid from industrialized countries can be attributed to the provision of safe drinking water, safe disposal of sewage, legal enforcement of high standards of food hygiene, programmes to detect, monitor, and treat chronic carriers, and prompt investigation and intervention when these safeguards are breached. The tools of outbreak investigation are phage typing of isolates, DNA fingerprinting using pulse field gel electrophoresis or ribotyping, registers of known carriers and their phage types, and sewer swabs used to trace isolates back to their source.

Measures for individual protection are to kill *S. typhi* in water by heating to 57°C, iodination or chlorination, care with uncooked or reheated food, and immunization. Patients and convalescents with typhoid should be advised to wash their hands after using the toilet and before preparing food and to use separate towels.

Vaccines

The greatest need for typhoid vaccination is among children in endemic areas, especially where antibiotic resistance is increasing, and among laboratory workers handling *S. typhi*. In practice, vaccines are given mostly to travellers to endemic areas. A recent meta-analysis has suggested that whole cell vaccines (which are no longer widely available) are the most effective although side-effects are prominent. The most convenient is the Vi vaccine, as a single 25-µg intramuscular dose, giving 70 to 80 per cent protection for 3 years. An alternative is the live attenuated oral Ty21a vaccine which gives 65 to 70 per cent protection for 3 to 7 years. This vaccine can cause abdominal symptoms. Effectiveness can be reduced by mefloquine and antibiotics and it should not be given to immunosuppressed persons. Typhoid vaccines do not protect against paratyphoid infection and the protection afforded by vaccination can be overcome by large inocula of bacteria. Efficacy figures derive largely from trials conducted in partly immune populations and overestimate benefit in persons without prior exposure. The risks of typhoid among travellers are low (105–118 cases per million travellers to India) and the precise efficacy of currently recommended doses in previously unexposed adults remains unknown. A number of new vaccines are currently being evaluated, notably a Vi conjugate vaccine undergoing phase III clinical trials in Asia. For full details of typhoid vaccination readers should consult specialist texts.

Paratyphoid fever

Paratyphoid, type B has the widest distribution and resembles typhoid most closely. Paratyphoid A occurs chiefly in Asia and Africa and paratyphoid C in Asia and the Middle East. Paratyphoid A and C are more likely to present with a gastroenteritic than a typhoidal type of illness. *S. Paratyphi* causes more asymptomatic infections than *S. typhi*. Outbreaks of paratyphoid are much more often food-borne than water-borne, probably because larger inocula are needed to establish infection. Paratyphoid has a shorter incubation period (4–5 days), shorter duration, and lower incidence of complications, including relapse and long-term carriage. Deaths are rare. The skin lesions of paratyphoid are larger, more numerous, and more extensive than those of typhoid. The management of paratyphoid is the same as that of typhoid. Paratyphoid organisms may display multidrug resistance as in *S. typhi*. Eradication of carriage with quinolones has been less successful in paratyphoid than in typhoid.

Further reading

Butler T, Knight J, Nath SK, Speelman P, Roy SK, Azad MAK (1985). Typhoid fever complicated by intestinal perforation: a persisting fatal disease requiring surgical management. *Reviews of Infectious Diseases* 7, 244–56.

Christie AB (1987). Typhoid and paratyphoid fevers. In: Christie AB, ed. *Infectious diseases: epidemiology and clinical practice*, 4th edn, Vol. 1, pp. 100–64. Churchill Livingstone, Edinburgh. [An outstanding, detailed, and generously referenced monograph on typhoid.]

Engels EA *et al.* (1998). Typhoid fever vaccines: a meta-analysis of studies on efficacy and toxicity. *British Medical Journal* 316, 110–16.

Forsyth JRL (1998). Typhoid and paratyphoid. In: Smith GR, Easmon CSF, eds. *Topley and Wilson's principles of bacteriology, virology and immunity*, 9th edn, Vol. 3, pp. 459–78. Arnold, London. [A useful chapter covering microbiological aspects of typhoid in depth.]

Hoffman SL *et al.* (1984). Reduction of mortality in chloramphenicol-treated severe typhoid fever by high-dose dexamethasone. *New England Journal of Medicine* 310, 82–8.

Information concerning the *S. typhi* genome sequence can be accessed through the Sanger Centre web site, http://www.sanger.uk/Projects/Microbes

7.11.9 Intracellular Klebsiella infections

J. Richens

Rhinoscleroma

Rhinoscleroma or scleroma in an infection of the upper airways characterized by inflammatory growths and caused by *Klebsiella pneumoniae*, subspecies *rhinoscleromatis*. Small endemic foci have been described in Africa (especially Egypt and Uganda), Siberia, Turkestan, the Middle East, the Indian subcontinent, China, the Philippines, Indonesia, and Papua New Guinea. There are many foci in South and Central America; it remains common in Guatemala where it has been identified in terracotta Maya heads of AD 300 to 600. The disease has retreated in Eastern and Central Europe where it was first described by Hebra and Kaposi in 1870.

Aetiology

K. rhinoscleromatis can be isolated from about 60 per cent of patients and is seen as intracellular inclusions in material taken from lesions. Patients show high titres of antibody which react with this organism and with the inclusions seen in sections.

Pathogenesis

Transmission is believed to occur from person to person in endemic areas. No incubation period has been defined. Initially patients infected with this organism may develop an atrophic rhinitis with squamous metaplasia, hyperkeratosis, and atrophy. The most characteristic phase of the disease is the nodular stage during which a granulomatous reaction to the organisms within macrophages leads to the development of bulky masses within any part of the respiratory tract from nares to tracheal bifurcation. The process can extend into and destroy neighbouring soft tissues, cartilage, bone, and skin. Histology shows a dense infiltrate of plasma cells among which are seen large foamy histiocytes (Mikulicz cells) containing Gram-negative bacteria and Russell bodies which are thought to be effete plasma cells. Patients with late-stage disease are liable to develop fibrosis and strictures.

Clinical features

Rhinoscleroma runs a slow, fluctuating course over several years, progressing through atrophic, nodular, and fibrotic stages. Systemic symptoms are not seen. The usual presentations are with nasal obstruction and bleeding and nasal deformity (splaying of the lower nose, often with a visible growth extending down to the upper lip known as Hebra nose) (Fig. 1). Some patients present with ozaena, which is an atrophic rhinitis accompanied by a foul smell and formation of crusts within the nose. Patients with tracheal involvement may present with stridor. With the help of sinus endoscopy and newer imaging techniques it is not unusual to find evidence of spread into the sinuses, orbits, cranial cavity, middle ear, and regional lymph nodes.

Fig. 1 Rhinoscleroma in a 30-year-old man from Papua New Guinea causing characteristic nasal splaying (Hebra nose) and obstruction of the left nostril. (Reproduced from Cooke R (1987). *Colour atlas of anatomical pathology*, p. 31. Churchill Livingstone, Edinburgh, with permission.)

Diagnosis

The diagnosis is usually made by demonstrating intracellular organisms in Giemsa or silver-stained sections taken from typical lesions combined with culture. Haemagglutination tests for Klebsiella capsular antigen III have high sensitivity and specificity. CT scanning and endoscopic techniques provide useful ways to define the extent of the disease.

Treatment

Rhinoscleroma is usually managed by ear, nose, and throat specialists using a combination of antibiotic therapy and surgery for obstructing lesions. Atrophic rhinitis may benefit from nasal lavage with saline. Treatment with ciprofloxacin, 250 mg twice daily for 4 weeks, appears to be substantially superior to previously used antibiotic regimens (rifampicin, streptomycin, tetracyclines, ampicillin and co-trimoxazole). The efficacy of fluoroquinolones may derive from their excellent intracellular penetration. For the same reason, azithromycin would be a logical choice for rhinoscleroma, particularly in view of its excellent results in donovanosis, which is caused by a very closely related intracellular Klebsiella infection. Debulking operations may be needed if there is obstructing nasal and tracheal disease and tracheostomy may be required as a temporary measure. Reconstructive surgery may be needed to deal with late fibrotic stenosis.

Donovanosis (granuloma inguinale)

Donovanosis is a sexually transmitted infection characterized by ulcers of the anogenital and inguinal areas. The name of the causative organism has recently been changed from *Calymmatobacterium granulomatis* to *Klebsiella granulomatis*. The disease is also known by the names granuloma inguinale and granuloma venereum, but should not be confused with lymphogranuloma venereum. The intracellular Gram-negative bacteria found within lesions (Donovan bodies) were first described by the same Charles Donovan who found protozoal inclusions in visceral leishmaniasis (Leishman–Donovan bodies).

Aetiology

Recent research has indicated that it is possible to isolate an unusual Gram-negative bacillus in HEp-2 cells or human peripheral blood mononuclear cells from patients with characteristic lesions. This organism will not grow on conventional solid media. Previously named *Donovania* and subsequently *Calymmatobacterium*, it is now been classed as *Klebsiella granulomatis* on the basis of close DNA homology with other *Klebsiella* species.

Klebsiella granulomatis shows morphological identity with Donovan bodies observed within clinical lesions of donovanosis and patients with characteristic lesions have high levels of antibody that react equally with Donovan bodies and with *K. granulomatis*. *K. granulomatis* is pathogenic only to man. Experimental transmission has been reported with lesion material, but to date not with a pure culture of this organism. Donovanosis shows a close macroscopic and microscopic similarity to rhinoscleroma which produces granulomatous lesions of the upper airways containing intracellular clusters of the closely related organism, *Klebsiella rhinoscleromatis*.

Epidemiology

Donovanosis is found in small endemic foci. The best known of these are in Papua New Guinea, India, southern Africa, Brazil, and among Australian aborigines. Smaller foci have been described in the Caribbean region and China. Where endemicity is greatest it is unusual for donovanosis to account for more than 20 per cent of genital ulcers. In most parts of the world donovanosis seems to be retreating, raising hopes of eventual eradication. Where it occurs, donovanosis appears particularly linked to poverty, poor hygiene, and prostitution. Dark-skinned persons appear to have greater susceptibility. Infectivity is believed to be low and sexual partners often remain free of infection despite prolonged exposure. The highest rates reported in partners have been 50 per cent. In the past, epidemics of donovanosis have occurred in New Guinea where they were linked to ritual homosexual and heterosexual promiscuity. The predilection of lesions for the anogenital region of sexually active adults and the frequent association with other sexually transmitted infections point to most transmission being sexual. Goldberg has put forward arguments for non-sexual transmission of an opportunistic rectal pathogen based on a single questionable isolation of the causative organism from faeces. Perinatal transmission has been observed in a few cases.

Pathogenesis

Transmission requires direct contact with an infected lesion and is thought not to occur through intact skin. The organism has a special tropism for dermal macrophages, in which it is able to avoid damage by lysosomal enzymes and toxic oxygen metabolites. The response to infection is characterized by vigorous granulomatous inflammation that damages the skin and subcutaneous tissues. Extension of the infection is predominantly a local process of spreading ulceration. The frequent inguinal lesions are probably seeded by lymphatic spread but, in general, involvement of lymphatics and lymph nodes in donovanosis is much less prominent than in lymphogranuloma venereum. Haematogenous dissemination and spread to the upper genital tract of women occur exceptionally and demonstrate the organism's ability to survive in deeper tissues. Lesions in women tend to be more extensive and may progress rapidly during pregnancy.

Clinical features

The best estimates of the incubation period range from 3 to 40 days. The early lesion is most common on the distal penis in men and near the introitus in women. Starting as a non-specific papule, the early lesion soon becomes an ulcer displaying a deep red colour, contact bleeding, low levels of pain and tenderness unless secondary infection is present, and a well-defined, rolled edge. Frequently lesions take the form of hypertrophic masses that pout outwards from the surrounding skin. Lesions are often accompanied by local oedema, particularly in women. Atypical lesions include: dry, warty, hypertrophic lesions with a cobblestone appearance; painful, excavated ulcers; and lesions with an ill-defined edge showing diffuse subcutaneous infiltration. Chronic lesions tend to expand gradually along skin folds and across to apposed skin surfaces forming a large, continuous area of ulceration, with a characteristic serpiginous outline (Fig. 2). Inguinal lesions are common, especially in men. They start as firm, subcutaneous swellings and often go on to ulcerate. The term 'pseudobubo'

Fig. 2 Characteristic serpiginous ulcer in female patients with long-standing donovanosis.

Fig. 3 Donovan bodies: Giemsa-stained smear from donovanosis lesion demonstrating the characteristic 'closed safety pin' appearance of encapsulated organisms within a large histiocyte.

was originally coined to describe a subcutaneous inguinal abscess in donovanosis (rare) but tends to be used now to describe the more common ulcerating inguinal lesions. Primary lesions of the cervix are notorious for simulating carcinoma of the cervix. The uterus, fallopian tubes, ovaries, and adnexas may all be involved, simulating other forms of pelvic inflammatory disease with abscess formation or simulating malignancy with development of a frozen pelvis, large, hard masses, or hydronephrosis. Anal lesions in women commonly spread directly from the introitus; in men they are associated with anal intercourse. Involvement of the rectum very seldom occurs.

Extragenital lesions of donovanosis occur most often in and around the mouth and sometimes on the neck. Haematogenous dissemination of donovanosis is associated especially with the trauma to an infected uterine cervix during pregnancy. The manifestations include lytic bone lesions, psoas, and perinephric abscesses. Spread to liver, spleen, and lung occurs exceptionally. Lesions in infants tend to involve the ears and regional lymph nodes.

Complications of donovanosis include extensive scar formation, lymphoedema of the genitalia, penile autoamputation, and the development of squamous carcinoma in active or healed lesions. Secondary infection with fusospirochaetal organisms can cause rapid, extensive, and sometimes fatal tissue destruction.

Diagnosis

Donovanosis is traditionally diagnosed by demonstrating the presence of Donovan bodies lying within histiocytes in material taken from a typical lesion (Fig. 3). The number of Donovan bodies present varies considerably so that sometimes a swab or scraping is sufficient to make a diagnosis whilst at other times a careful search must be made of biopsy material. Donovan bodies show well with Giemsa, Leishman, and Wright stains but poorly with haematoxylin and eosin. Histology typically shows a heavy plasma cell infiltrate and epithelial hyperplasia in addition to histiocytes containing Donovan bodies. The use of tissue culture, serological tests, and polymerase chain reaction to diagnose donovanosis have all been described recently, but are not yet commercially available. All patients should be offered

screening for other sexually transmitted infections, especially syphilis and HIV. Donovanosis often causes diagnostic confusion when encountered outside endemic areas. Common misdiagnoses are squamous carcinoma of the cervix, vulva, or penis, secondary syphilis, and conditions that produce genital lymphoedema such as filariasis and lymphogranuloma venereum.

Treatment and prevention

Recently published guidelines for the management of donovanosis recommend the use of azithromycin, ceftriaxone, ciprofloxacin, doxycyline, erythromycin, or co-trimoxazole. No randomized comparative trials have been conducted. Antibiotics are given at standard dosage until lesions have re-epithelialized. Expert opinion suggests that azithromycin gives the best results at a daily dose of 500 mg or weekly doses of 1 g. Antibiotic susceptibility testing is not currently feasible. Treatment failure with older antibiotics, such as doxycyline and co-trimoxazole, is well documented in individual cases. Erythromycin is safe and gives good results in pregnant women. Women in labour found to have untreated lesions of the cervix should be delivered by caesarian section to reduce known risks of haematogenous dissemination and transmission to the neonate. Patients with genital deformity may benefit from plastic surgical procedures. Partners of patients should be examined and treated if infected. A week of epidemiological treatment may be offered to healthy contacts to abort incubating infections. The main hopes for the control of donovanosis lie in strengthening services for patients with sexually transmitted infections in endemic areas, the use of newer antibiotics such as azithromycin coupled with health education and condom promotion. Eradication is currently being attempted in Australia.

Further reading

Borgstein J, Sada E, Cortes R (1993). Ciprofloxacin for rhinoscleroma and ozena. *Lancet* **342**, 122.

Bowden F, Savage J (1998). Is the eradication of donovanosis possible in Australia. *Australia and New Zealand Journal of Public Health* **22**, 7–8.

Carter JS *et al.* (1999). Phylogenetic evidence for reclassification of *Calymmatobacterium granulomatis* as *Klebsiella granulomatis* comb. nov. *International Journal of Systematic Bacteriology* **49**, 1695–1700.

Gamea AM (1990). Role of endoscopy in diagnosing scleroma in its uncommon sites. *Journal of Laryngology and Otology* **104**, 619–21.

Maher AI *et al.* (1990). Rhinoscleroma management by carbon dioxide surgical laser. *Laryngoscope* **100**, 783–8.

Meyer PR *et al.* (1983). Scleroma (rhinoscleroma). A histologic immunohistochemical study with bacteriologic correlates. *Archives of Pathology and Laboratory Medicine* **107**, 377–83.

Paul C *et al.* (1993). Infection due to *Klebsiella rhinoscleromatis* in two patients infected with human immunodeficiency virus. *Clinical Infectious Disease* **16**, 441–20.

Richens J (1992). The diagnosis and treatment of donovanosis (granuloma inguinale). *Genitourinary Medicine* **32**, 441–52.

Sehgal VN, Prasad AL (1986). Donovanosis. Current concepts. *International Journal of Dermatology* **24**, 8–16.

Ssali CLK (1975). The management of rhinoscleroma. *Journal of Laryngology and Otology* **89**, 91–9.

7.11.10 Anaerobic bacteria

S. J. Eykyn

Definition of an anaerobe

The definition of an anaerobe is not entirely straightforward microbiologically. Anaerobes vary in their tolerance of oxygen and some strains will grow only in a very low concentration while others are relatively aerotolerant. In practice in the routine microbiology laboratory, bacteria that fail to grow on the surface of solid medium in 10 per cent CO_2 in air are classified as anaerobes. Confusion sometimes arises with organisms that while preferentially anaerobic (that is, they usually grow only on the anaerobic plate on primary isolation from a clinical specimen) are actually microaerophilic or capnophilic; these include *Actinomyces* which are often erroneously referred to as anaerobes. In this case the confusion is compounded as the clinical infection of actinomycosis (see Chapter 7.11.26) is usually caused by both *Actinomyces* and anaerobes. Preferentially anaerobic bacteria also include the 'milleri' group of streptococci which can readily be mistaken for anaerobic streptococci.

Incidence of anaerobic infection

Anaerobic infections are common, even if not always recognized as such, and may affect any tissue or organ and thus present to most clinicians regardless of specialty. Postoperative anaerobic sepsis was dramatically reduced when the prophylactic use of highly effective antianaerobic antibiotics was introduced in the 1970s. Although anaerobic bacteria were extensively studied in Europe in the late 19th and early 20th centuries, they were then largely ignored for many years. Anaerobes (with the exception of *Clostridium perfringens* and the occasional *Bacteroides fragilis*) were seldom isolated in clinical laboratories until the mid-1970s when an 'anaerobic renaissance' was initiated by American researchers and the anaerobes were 'rediscovered' as common and important human pathogens. This coincided with the advent of highly effective antianaerobic antimicrobials. Since then enormous advances have been made in the isolation, taxonomy, clinical diagnosis, management, and prevention of anaerobic infection.

Taxonomy

The classification and characterization of many anaerobic bacteria presents considerable difficulties and only dedicated anaerobists can hope (or need) to be abreast of current taxonomy. The many synonyms for some of these organisms bear witness to these difficulties; Finegold, for example, quoted over 50 for the organism now classified as *Fusobacterium necrophorum*. Such taxonomic confusion is further compounded by the many reports that refer to any Gram-negative anaerobic bacillus as a 'Bacteroides' and to those resistant to penicillin and ampicillin as *B. fragilis*. The use of genetic techniques has resulted in the reclassification of many anaerobes. The genus *Bacteroides* is limited to the *Bacteroides fragilis* group. The saccharolytic species previously included in the *B. melaninogenicus–oralis–ruminicola* group have been assigned to the new genus *Prevotella* which includes both pigmented and non-pigmented species. The asaccharolytic, pigmented, Gram-negative rods are now in the new genus *Porphyromonas*. Other taxonomic changes have affected the anaerobic Gram-positive cocci which have almost all become *Peptostreptococcus*. As these taxonomic changes affect some clinically important anaerobes, the new nomenclature will be used in this chapter. Table 1 lists some of the clinically important anaerobes and their old and new names where appropriate. Of the many hundreds of anaerobic species, only a small number are likely to be relevant to clinical practice and specifically reported by clinical microbiology laboratories.

Anaerobic commensal flora of man

The commensal flora of man is largely anaerobic; anaerobes are found on all the mucosal surfaces and on the skin.

Skin

It is surprising that although the skin is constantly exposed to the air, it still supports a considerable anaerobic microflora, predominantly 'anaerobic diphtheroids' that is the propionibacteria, including the lipolytic species *Propionibacterium acnes* associated with acne.

Mouth

Anaerobes are found in the tonsillar crypts, tongue crypts, gingival crevices, and dental plaque. Although some anaerobic species are found in young infants, the variety and number of anaerobes increases markedly with the eruption of the teeth. Predominant members of the oral anaerobic flora include *Prevotella*, *Fusobacterium*, *Peptostreptococcus*, *Veillonella*, and various anaerobic Gram-positive bacilli. The group *B. fragilis* group of anaerobes are rarely found in the mouth and *Porphyromonas* only in small numbers if at all.

Table 1 Some clinically important anaerobic bacteria including taxonomic changes where relevant

Anaerobic bacilli
Gram-positive bacilli
Spore forming:
Clostridium perfringens
Other *Clortridium* spp.
Non-spore-forming:
Actinomyces spp.
Bifidobacterium spp.
Eubacterium spp.
Probionibacterium spp.
Gram-negative bacilli
Bacteroides fragilis
Bacteroides spp. (*fragilis*-like)
Prevotella melaninogenica
Other *Prevotella* spp.
Porphyromonas asaccharolytica
Fusobacterium necrophorum
Other *Fusobacterium* spp.
Anaerobic cocci
Gram-positive cocci
Peptostreptococcus spp.
Gram-negative cocci
Veillonella spp.
Spirochaetes
Treponema vincenntii

Intestine

The stomach and upper small intestine are normally sterile or contain transient, small numbers of anaerobic organisms derived from food, saliva, and nasopharyngeal secretions. The terminal ileum resembles the colon with a vast and diverse anaerobic flora which is established by the second year of life. Anaerobes account for about 99 per cent of the bacterial faecal mass and *Bacteroides* spp. are the commonest species. *B. vulgatus* and *B. thetaiotaomicron* are more frequently encountered than *B. fragilis*. Clostridia are also found in large numbers. Many hundred different species of anaerobe are found in the colon.

Genitourinary tract

The normal flora of the vagina is predominantly anaerobic, mostly lactobacilli, but also small numbers of *Prevotella*, fusobacteria, and peptostreptococci are found. The urethral flora consists of similar anaerobes.

Pathogenesis

The anaerobic bacteria that cause human infection are almost always derived endogenously from the host's own commensal flora. Exceptions to this include: bite and punch injuries, in which the anaerobic oral flora of assailant or victim is involved; animal and human bites (animal oral flora has large numbers of anaerobes as well as aerobic bacteria specific to animals such as *Pasteurella*); and neonatal sepsis in which the maternal vaginal anaerobes cause infection in the new-born baby. Many clostridia are found not only as normal gastrointestinal flora in man and animals but also in the soil. Clostridia are sporing anaerobes and cause infection in man in two distinct ways: firstly certain species produce potent toxins and these cause specific toxin-mediated infections that will be considered elsewhere; secondly, Clostridia, including sometimes *Clostridium perfringens*, often occur with non-sporing anaerobes in a variety of anaerobic infections in which they do not exert their toxic potential, and their presence or absence has no effect on the course of the disease. Most anaerobic infections are polymicrobial with not only several anaerobic species involved but usually aerobic species as well. The anaerobic component of these mixed infections seems to be the more important. Predisposing factors include disruption of normally intact cutaneous or mucosal barriers, tissue injury and necrosis, impaired blood supply, and obstruction. Virulence factors are also involved and include adhesins, capsules, lipopolysaccharide, hydrolytic and other enzymes, soluble metabolites, and growth factors. Precise virulence determinants for most anaerobic infections have not been established.

Adhesins

Surface attachment structures such as fimbriae have been described in some strains of *B. fragilis* and in other anaerobic species and may enable adherence to epithelial cells, an important factor in the initiation of colonization and infection.

Capsules

Capsule formation has been described in *B. fragilis* and some other anaerobes. Capsules confer resistance to phagocytosis, inhibit the migration of macrophages, and potentiate abscess formation.

Lipopolysaccharide

The lipid A component of the *B. fragilis* lipopolysaccharide differs chemically in certain respects from lipid A and this may account for its low endotoxic activity. *F. necrophorum* and *F. nucleatum* interestingly have conventional endotoxic lipopolysaccharide.

Enzymes

Most anaerobic pathogens produce numerous enzymes, including immunoglobulin proteases, enzymes capable of inactivating plasma proteins important in the initiation and control of the inflammatory response, and enzymes that degrade tissue components.

Diagnosis of anaerobic infection

Clinical

A working knowledge of the nature and whereabouts of the normal human commensal anaerobic flora is invaluable to the clinician as anaerobic infection frequently arises in association with this. Putrid discharge characterizes some, though not all, anaerobic infections and this results from the metabolic products of the bacteria. No other group of organisms can produce pus with such a foul, nauseating smell. Anaerobic infections, particularly necrotizing infections, are sometimes associated with cellulitis and gas formation. The former may be mistaken for streptococcal cellulitis and the latter for clostridial gas gangrene but anaerobic gangrene with gas formation generally causes far less toxaemia and prostration than clostridial infection in which the patient is alarmingly ill. Nor is the formation of gas in tissues confined to anaerobes, as aerobes are occasionally also involved. Another useful clue to the presence of anaerobes in a specimen is a report from the laboratory of 'sterile pus' despite the presence of organisms on a Gram-stained film. Lastly, in any patient who is receiving antibiotics inactive against anaerobes such as aminoglycosides, and still remains septic, an anaerobic infection should be considered.

Collection and transport of specimens for anaerobic bacteriology

All anaerobic bacteria are sensitive to oxygen but they vary in their aerotolerance. *B. fragilis* and *C. perfringens* will tolerate 2 to 4 per cent oxygen but fusobacteria and some peptostreptococci are much more sensitive to oxygen, hence more difficult to grow in the laboratory, and less likely to survive the journey from patient to culture medium. Until the renewed interest in anaerobes in the 1970s few laboratories ever isolated the more fastidious species. The best specimens for the isolation of anaerobes are aspirates, pus (in a universal container), or excised tissue and, although rapid delivery of specimens to the laboratory is desirable, in practice, anaerobes (even fastidious species) survive well in pus and tissue. Swabs are less satisfactory but are often all that is available, and for them a transport medium should be used. Complex commercial systems for the collection and transport of specimens for anaerobic bacteriology have been devised but are expensive and unlikely to appeal to clinicians. Many clinical specimens will be routinely cultured for anaerobes and no specific directive from the clinician will be required. One exception is expectorated sputum and clinicians should be aware that the microbiological diagnosis of anaerobic pleuropulmonary infection is best made from an invasive specimen.

Laboratory

The putrid smell of the pus in many anaerobic infections has been mentioned, and even swabs in such cases will be noticeably foul when processed. The Gram-stained smear of anaerobic discharge is often diagnostic to the experienced microscopist as it characteristically contains a variety of different bacteria, Gram-negative and Gram-positive rods and cocci. Filamentous or spindle-shaped Gram-negative rods (often hard to see) confirm the presence of fusobacteria. Successful culture of anaerobes requires fresh media and a reliable anaerobic atmosphere with 10 per cent carbon dioxide. Most laboratories now have either special anaerobic cabinets or automated systems using anaerobic jars. Relatively aerotolerant species will often grow in 24 to 48 h but fastidious anaerobes require undisturbed anaerobiosis for much longer (3–5 days) and if inoculated anaerobic culture plates are left out on the bench in the laboratory, such anaerobes will die.

Even with the availability of commercial identification systems the definitive identification of many anaerobes is a technically demanding process and taxonomic exactitude has minimal appeal to clinicians. In clinical practice it is usually sufficient to recognize the *B. fragilis* group and Clostridia but it is clearly important that a limited number of laboratories (increasingly reference or research laboratories) retain sufficient skill to advise on the more unusual species and to define the patterns of infection associated with different sites.

Clinical spectrum of anaerobic infection

Infections of the head and neck

Acute necrotizing ulcerative gingivitis

This condition, also known as Vincent's disease, Vincent's angina, Vincent's gingivostomatitis, trench mouth, and fusospirochaetosis, affects the gingiva and buccal mucosa and was one of the earliest anaerobic infections described. The characteristic symptoms of painful bleeding gums, sometimes with a pseudomembrane, and foul breath readily suggest the diagnosis which can be confirmed with a Gram-stained smear in which large numbers of spirochaetes, fusiform, and other bacteria are seen.

Dental sepsis

The anaerobic oral commensal flora is found (with aerobic and microaerophilic bacteria) in periodontal infection, dental abscesses, and in postoperative infections associated with maxillofacial surgery.

Infections of the neck and jaw

These unusual necrotizing infections are frequently anaerobic and may be accompanied by marked cellulitis and oedema and cause respiratory embarrassment. Ludwig's angina is infection involving the main anterior compartment of the neck, the submandibular space. The source of the infection is usually the lower molar teeth, but it can arise from tonsillar infection as in the patient shown in Fig. 1. These infections spread via the fascial planes and may involve the chest with mediastinal abscess and empyema formation.

Ear, nose, and throat infections

Anaerobes are frequently isolated from tonsillar tissue in recurrent streptococcal tonsillitis and are also involved in peritonsillar abscesses (quinsy). They are commonly found in chronic infection of the sinuses, middle ear, and mastoid. Chronic sinus infection occasionally results in acute orbital cellulitis.

Fig. 1 Spreading cellulitis of the neck resulting from tonsillar sepsis (fatal)— 'anaerobic neck'.

Infections of the central nervous system

Anaerobic bacteria are the major pathogens in cerebral abscesses other than those that follow surgery or trauma. Otogenic cerebral abscesses are most common and involve the temporal lobe or cerebellum. *B. fragilis* is usually isolated and aerobes, particularly *Proteus* spp. are often present. Frontal lobe abscesses of sinusitic or dental origin are usually caused by *S. milleri* group although oral anaerobes may also be found.

Pleuropulmonary infection

Anaerobic pleuropulmonary infection usually results from oropharyngeal aspiration but also occasionally from haematogenous seeding, particularly by fusobacteria (see necrobacillosis). Anaerobic pleuropulmonary infections include aspiration pneumonia, necrotizing pneumonitis, lung abscess, and empyema, as well as infection secondary to bronchiectasis and bronchial carcinoma. The anaerobes involved in these infections are the oropharygeal commensals. Patients with an anaerobic lung abscess will usually admit to the revolting taste (as well as smell) of their sputum. Definitive bacteriological diagnosis of anaerobic pleuropulmonary infection usually requires culture of an invasive specimen obtained either by bronchoscopy or percutaneous transthoracic aspiration. Expectorated sputum is rarely suitable. Specimens should preferably be obtained before antibiotics are given.

Intra-abdominal infections

These infections are usually associated with intra-abdominal pathology such as perforated gastric or duodenal ulcers, appendicitis, diverticulitis, inflammatory bowel disease, or malignancy and produce peritonitis or abscesses. Most are polymicrobial and the predominant anaerobes are those of the *B. fragilis* group. Before the advent of effective antianaerobic prophylaxis for intestinal surgery, anaerobic postoperative wound infection, abscess formation, and even septicaemia were commonly seen on surgical wards.

Hepatic and biliary tract infection

Hepatic abscesses are rare but likely to be caused by anaerobic bacteria (usually fusobacteria and *B. fragilis*) as well as by *S. milleri* group. They result from biliary tract infection, haematogenous spread from an intestinal source or direct extension of contiguous infection. Anaerobes are found in the bile in obstructive disease with stasis, and may cause cholangitis in patients who have had previous enterobiliary anastomoses.

Infections of the female genital tract and neonatal infection

Anaerobic bacteria cause bacterial vaginosis, tubo-ovarian sepsis, Bartholin's abscess, endometritis, septic abortion, and infection associated with intrauterine contraceptive devices. Vaginal hysterectomy carries a high risk of postoperative anaerobic infection, but wound infection after abdominal hysterectomy is uncommon and likely to be caused by *S. aureus*. Prolonged rupture of the membranes is associated with anaerobic infection and foul smelling liquor is often noted. Anaerobes, of vaginal origin, can be cultured from the liquor, the placenta, and the nasogastric aspirate, ear, and other surface swabs of the baby, which may develop anaerobic pneumonitis.

Infections of the male genitalia and prostate

The commensal anaerobic flora of the urethra is found in balanoposthitis, whose foul odour is well known to genitourinary physicians. Anaerobes also cause secondary infection of penile lesions. Scrotal abscesses are usually caused by anaerobes unless they follow acute epididymo-orchitis. Anaerobic scrotal abscesses which are often recurrent arise either *de novo*, and probably result from secondary infection of blocked apocrine glands or after surgery to the genitalia or urethra.

The eponymous term Fournier's gangrene was originally used at the end of the 19th century to describe necrotizing infections involving the peno-scrotum and perineum that occurred in young, previously healthy men; these infections were almost certainly caused by *S. pyogenes*. Since then the term has been used for anaerobic (synergistic) necrotizing infections of the scrotum and perineum that sometimes also involve the thighs and abdominal wall. These infections are characterized by sudden intense pain and swelling with foul discharge and gas in the tissues as well as marked systemic disturbance and occur in middle aged or elderly men, particularly diabetics and alcoholics. There is a cutaneous, anorectal, or genitourinary source for the anaerobes.

Acute prostatic abscesses are rare but are sometimes caused by anaerobes. Anaerobes may also be relevant in chronic prostatitis, and can sometimes be cultured from prostatic secretions.

Infection of the urinary tract

Anaerobic urinary infection is very rare, so much so that urine is not routinely cultured anaerobically. Anaerobes can be recovered from the urine when there are abnormalities within the urinary tract such as vesicocolic fistulae, tumours, pyonephrosis, or perinephric abscess, and sometimes from ileal conduit specimens.

Bone and joint infection

Anaerobes are uncommon pathogens in acute haematogenous osteomyelitis and septic arthritis. Acute anaerobic osteomyelitis affecting long bones is likely to be caused by fusobacteria, whereas vertebral osteomyelitis, a infection occurring mainly in elderly patients, is likely to be caused by *B. fragilis*. Anaerobic septic arthritis usually occurs in patients with rheumatoid arthritis or other joint pathology and is also likely to be caused by *B. fragilis*. It can also result from bite and punch injuries to the hand in which the pathogens are oral bacteria, both anaerobic and aerobic. Anaerobes are sometimes isolated (with aerobes) in chronic osteomyelitis.

Skin and soft tissue infection

Diabetic foot ulcers

These often grow anaerobes, and the infections may be associated with underlying chronic osteomyelitis and sometimes with cellulitis, necrotizing fasciitis, and gas formation.

Venous ulcers

Anaerobes, particularly peptostreptococci, are often isolated from venous ulcers but are secondary invaders and are not relevant to the aetiology or perpetuation of the ulcer.

Decubitus ulcers

These are frequently infected with anaerobes, particularly *B. fragilis*, and anaerobic bacteraemia may occasionally result.

Sebaceous cysts

Anaerobes, especially peptostreptococci, are often isolated from infected sebaceous cysts.

Axillary abscess and hidradenitis suppurativa

Most axillary abscesses are caused by *S. aureus*, but some are anaerobic. Anaerobic abscesses are recurrent and more indolent than staphylococcal abscesses. Recurrences can result in hidradenitis suppurativa (Fig. 2). Anaerobic axillary abscesses and hidradenitis suppurativa result from apocrine blockage and infection is secondary. Hidradenitis suppurativa is not confined to the axilla but can affect the perineum, groins, buttocks, and back. Patients afflicted with this condition complain bitterly of the foul smell of their lesions.

Fig. 2 Hidradenitis suppurativa of axilla.

Perirectal abscess

These abscesses are frequently caused by anaerobes and when associated with an underlying fistula yield gut-specific anaerobes of the *B. fragilis* group and coliforms. Perirectal abscesses without a fistula are usually also caused by anaerobes but not gut-specific anaerobes; they may result from infection of blocked apocrine glands.

Breast abscess

Breast abscesses are usually assumed to be staphylococcal but in the non-puerperal woman are as likely to be anaerobic. Anaerobic breast abscesses are secondary infections of an underlying blocked duct, and are usually recurrent, subareolar, and associated with inverted nipples.

Human and animal bites

Human bites have been mentioned with reference to infection of the joints of the hand, but they may involve other parts of the body. Animal bites can also give rise to anaerobic infection but are more likely to become infected with *Pasteurella multocida* (see Chapter 7.11.17).

Paronychia

Paronychia can be caused by anaerobes, usually with aerobes. The anaerobes are oral commensals and are probably transferred to the fingers by licking or biting. Anaerobic paronychias are usually less acute than those caused by *S. aureus* or *Streptococcus pyogenes*.

Synergistic necrotizing infections

Anaerobic bacteria, usually with aerobes, cause a range of 'synergistic' infections. These infections can involve skin, fascia, and sometimes muscle and affect many areas of the body, occurring either spontaneously or after trauma or surgery (Fig. 3 and see Fournier's gangrene above).

Bacteraemia and endocarditis

Anaerobic infection at any site, but particularly intra-abdominal infection, can cause bacteraemia sometimes with shock but anaerobes only account for less than 5 per cent of positive blood cultures, with the *B. fragilis* group most common. Anaerobes are also found in polymicrobial bacteraemia. Anaerobic endocarditis is very rare.

Fusobacterial bacteraemia, necrobacillosis, and Lemierre's postanginal septicaemia

Although most anaerobic infections are polymicrobial with not only several anaerobic species but also several aerobic species frequently isolated, fusobacteria, that is *F. necrophorum*, *F. nucleatum* and possibly other species, can be sole pathogens and produce severe infections. Their virulence is

Fig. 3 Necrotizing fasciitis involving perineum, buttock, and thigh 3 weeks after gastrectomy for carcinoma.

Fig. 4 Chest radiograph taken on admission to hospital of a 21-year-old heating engineer who had developed rigors and severe shortness of breath about a week after a sore throat. He was thought to have possible Legionnaire's disease, hence given erythromycin (to which fusobacteria are usually resistant); *F. necrophorum* was isolated from blood cultures.

probably attributable to their lipopolysaccharide which is similar to that of Gram-negative aerobic bacteria. Although these serious infections are rare, they were well-described in the preantibiotic era. They are now being constantly 'rediscovered' by different clinicians and microbiologists, each convinced that they are describing a new disease. The species most often isolated from septicaemic disease is *F. necrophorum* and it is to this species that the term necrobacillosis refers.

Necrobacillosis

The earliest reports of necrobacillosis in man were of zoonotic skin infections acquired from animals with local infection with *F. necrophorum* usually in mixed culture, but in 1930 two fatal cases that presented 'hitherto undescribed clinical and pathological features of systemic infection' were described: a girl of 19 who died of lung abscesses, septic arthritis of the hip, and jaundice six days after a sore throat with rigors, and a man of 64 who died of a retropharyngeal abscess with gangrene and extension into the peritracheal and subcutaneous tissues. The former case is the 'postanginal septicaemia' later described by Lemierre (see below). The latter sounds like necrotizing fasciitis. Further clarification of the entity of necrobacillosis was provided in 1955 by Alston who recognized four different types of infection caused by *F. necrophorum*: those involving the skin and subcutaneous tissues, a large group where the infection started with a sore throat or otitis media, a third group associated with the female genital tract, the alimentary tract, or the urinary tract, and a fourth with empyema. Pyaemia and abscesses were very common in the last three groups. Alston's second group corresponds to Lemierre's postanginal septicaemia although Lemierre considered septicaemias arising from otitis media and mastoiditis to be a separate group. Since Alston's study, there have been numerous sporadic case reports of necrobacillosis but quite large series were published from the United Kingdom in 1989 and from Denmark in 1998. The term necrobacillosis is best used for any septicaemic infection with *F. necrophorum*, and postanginal septicaemic infection designated Lemierre's disease since this is a distinct clinical entity.

Lemierre's postanginal septicaemia (Lemierre's disease)

This unique manifestation of necrobacillosis occurs in previously healthy young people, usually adolescents or in their twenties. Lemierre suggested that it affected both sexes equally but recent series found a male predominance. There is an antecedent sore throat, often severe, and sometimes acute tonsillitis. Painful cervical lymphadenopathy is usual and septic jugular thrombophlebitis can occur. Within days, sometimes only hours, of the onset of sore throat, rigors develop with marked systemic upset and often impaired renal and hepatic function. Metastatic spread is characteristic, most commonly involving the lung, but also bone, joint, liver, brain, and heart valves. The 'pneumonia' is often severe and extensive, and cavitation

of the septic infarcts and empyema may occur. Unless the relevance of the antecedent sore throat is appreciated, the diagnosis will be missed. There are occasional reports of coincidental Epstein–Barr virus infection in Lemierre's disease and viral infection might act as a trigger for fusobacterial invasion. Figure 4 shows the chest radiograph taken on admission to hospital of a 21-year-old heating engineer with rigors and severe shortness of breath about a week after a sore throat. He was thought to have Legionnaire's disease hence given erythromycin (to which fusobacteria are usually resistant); *F. necrophorum* was isolated from blood cultures. Although *F. necrophorum* is very sensitive to both penicillin and metronidazole, the infection responds only very slowly to antibiotic treatment, a reflection of the innate virulence of the organism.

Sensitivity of anaerobic bacteria to antimicrobial agents

The susceptibility of most anaerobic bacteria to antimicrobial agents is remarkably uniform. Intrinsic resistance is often predictable and acquired resistance uncommon.

Metronidazole (and other nitroimidazoles)

Metronidazole is unique amongst the antimicrobial agents that are active against anaerobic bacteria as it is only active against anaerobes, with no activity against aerobes. Although it has been used to treat anaerobic infections for nearly 40 years, most clinically important anaerobes remain sensitive. There is little to choose between the activity of the different nitroimidazoles.

β-Lactam antibiotics

Contrary to popular belief, many anaerobes are still very sensitive to penicillin including many strains of *Prevotella*, *Porphyromonas*, and fusobacteria as well as clostridia, peptostreptococci, and spirochaetes. The *B. fragilis* group are almost uniformly resistant to penicillin, and resistance is also increasing amongst *Prevotella* and *Porphyromonas*. These penicillin-resistant anaerobes are also resistant to ampicillin, amoxycillin, piperacillin, ticarcillin, and most cephalosporins; cephamycins such as cefoxitin and carbapenems such as imipenem and meropenem have some useful activity.

The addition of the β-lactam inhibitor clavulanic acid to amoxicillin, ticarcillin, and piperacillin renders the *B. fragilis* group susceptible to these antibiotics.

Other agents

Most anaerobes are sensitive to clindamycin, and the antianaerobic activity of clindamycin is similar to that of metronidazole. Chloramphenicol is also highly active against anaerobes. Other agents with useful activity include erythromycin (though not against most fusobacteria), co-trimoxazole, and tetracyclines. The glycopeptides vancomycin and teicoplanin, whilst inactive against most Gram-negative anaerobes, possess useful activity against clostridia and peptostreptococci. Anaerobic bacteria are resistant to aminoglycosides and quinolones.

Treatment of anaerobic infections

Surgical intervention, particularly drainage of pus and excision of necrotic tissue, is of paramount importance in anaerobic infections and in many cases this will be all that is required to treat the infection. Indeed failure to carry out effective surgery will often result not only in the persistence of the infection but also in extension of this whatever antibiotic is given. Since most anaerobic infections are mixed with aerobes, it may be necessary to treat both groups of organisms. For anaerobic infections other than those of the *B. fragilis* group there is a wide choice of agent, but few clinicians think of anaerobes in distinct groups, and it is easier to recommend overall anaerobic cover which is best provided by metronidazole.

Prevention of anaerobic infection

Antibiotic prophylaxis for operations likely to be followed by postoperative anaerobic wound infection did not become routine until the mid 1970s but since then many trials bear witness to the efficacy of such prophylaxis in surgery involving sites with an anaerobic commensal flora and the putrid wound infections so familiar to gastrointestinal surgeons in the past are now rare. The patient in Fig. 5 featured in the trial of intravenous metronidazole versus placebo (saline) in elective colorectal surgery that took place at St Thomas' Hospital in 1976; he received saline! Such a trial would be

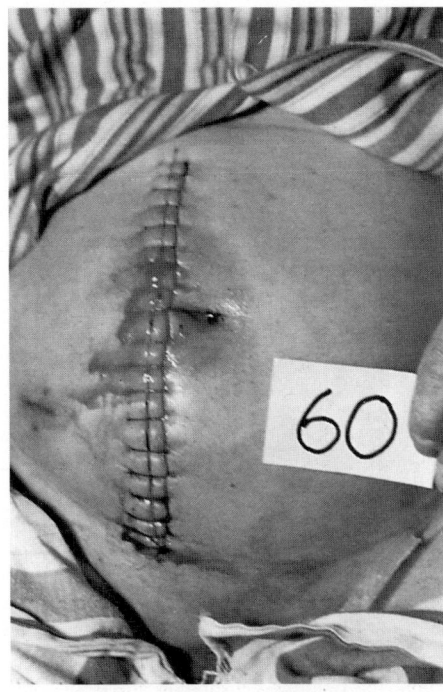

Fig. 5 Wound sepsis following elective colorectal surgery.

quite unethical today. Most prophylactic regimens include cover for both aerobes and anaerobes. Antianaerobic prophylaxis is given for many different types of surgery, but particularly for that involving the gastrointestinal tract, genital tract, and upper respiratory tract. Such prophylaxis should be perioperative, intravenous, and of short duration (1–3 doses). There are many possible regimens but cefuroxime and metronidazole are widely used in the United Kingdom.

Further reading

Alston JM (1955). Necrobacillosis in Great Britain. *British Medical Journal* **ii**,1524–28. Old paper providing insight into various clinical presentations of fusobacterial septicaemia.

Eykyn SJ (1989). Necrobacillosis. *Scandinavian Journal of Infectious Diseases* **62** (Suppl.), 41–6.

Finegold SM, George WL, eds (1989). *Anaerobic infections in humans*. Academic Press, New York.

Hagelskjær LH, Prag J, Malczynski J, Kristensen JH (1998). Incidence and clinical epidemiology of necrobacillosis, including Lemierre's syndrome, in Denmark 1990–1995. *European Journal of Clinical Microbiology and Infectious Diseases* **17**, 561–5.

Lemierre A (1936). On certain septicaemias due to anaerobic organisms. *Lancet* **i**, 701–3. This paper contains the classic description of postanginal septicaemia.

Unattributed (1984). International symposium on anaerobic bacteria and their role in disease. *Reviews of Infectious Diseases* **6** (Suppl.1).

7.11.11 Cholera
Michael L. Bennish

Introduction

Cholera has caused millions of deaths during seven pandemics affecting all six inhabited continents over the past 200 years. Cholera can cause massive diarrhoea, dehydration, and death in healthy persons within 12 h of the onset of illness. Epidemics only occur where hygiene and social conditions are poor. This has made cholera a metaphor for death and decay in both the public ('cholera zoll der treppen'—'may the cholera strike you' is the traditional Yiddish curse) and the literary (*Love in the time of cholera* by Gabriel Garcia Marquez) imaginations. Cholera continues to cause tens of thousands of death annually in poor countries, despite ample evidence that the provision of clean water prevents disease and that inexpensive and simple-to-administer fluid therapy prevents death in those infected. That this is so is an indictment of our continuing neglect of global public health.

Aetiology

Cholera is caused by infection with one of two serogroups of *Vibrio cholerae*—O1 or O139—having been identified as the causative agent of cholera by Robert Koch in 1883. *V. cholerae* O1 and O139 are facultatively anaerobic, motile, curved Gram-negative rods that contain polar flagella and grow best in media containing increased concentrations (5 to 15 mmol/l) of sodium chloride when compared to most pathogenic microorganisms. Hence their predilection for brackish environments—such as the Ganges Delta in the Indian subcontinent, the historic home of cholera. In addition to serogroup (determined by the somatic antigen type, of which more than 150 have been identified), *V. cholerae* serogroup O1 can be further divided into two biogroups, classical and El Tor (determined by their phenotypic characteristics) and three serotypes—Inaba, Ogawa, and Hikojima. Differences in virulence and epidemiological pattern have been described by biogroup (classical being more virulent than El Tor) but not for serotype.

Before 1992, all cholera was caused by infection with the O1 serogroup, the only serogroup then known to produce cholera toxin. In 1992, a new cholera toxin-producing serogroup—O139—was identified. This serogroup arose from the horizontal transfer of genes encoding the O139 lipopolysaccharide into a toxigenic El Tor *V. cholerae* strain. After explosive epidemics following its emergence (immunity to serogroup O1 did not protect against infection with O139) the new O139 serotype is now largely restricted to the Indian subcontinent. Despite fears that it would cause a new pandemic, it has not become endemic or epidemic elsewhere.

V. cholerae virulence genes have a number of recently defined mechanisms for horizontal transfer. The genes for cholera toxin are encoded on a filamentous phage, the receptor for which is the toxin co-regulated pilus. The latter is itself encoded by a lysogenic inovirus. In addition to being an example of evolutionary co-adaptation, the mobility of these virulence elements raises the concern of additional pathogenic strains arising.

Epidemiology

As convincingly demonstrated by the seminal epidemiologist John Snow in 1855, cholera occurs where clean drinking water is not available. *V. cholerae* resides in brackish surface water (perhaps in association with zooplankton), and initial infections during outbreaks most often stem from drinking such water. Once infection is established in a community, subsequent infections may occur by dissemination from infected individuals via contaminated food, or from drinking water newly contaminated by faecal pollution from a *V. cholerae*-infected individual. Since *V. cholerae* infections are more often asymptomatic than symptomatic, asymptomatic people may play a role in transmission. Chronic carriers are rare and do not play an important role in transmission. Because of the high inoculum required, infection rarely occurs directly from person-to-person without contaminated water or food as an intermediary vehicle. *V. cholerae* may remain viable on food (and multiply under favourable conditions) for days.

Although cholera has been present in the Indian subcontinent for centuries, the worldwide spread of cholera in modern times has been categorized as having occurred during seven pandemics. The first pandemic was recorded as starting in 1817, when Western observers became aware of the spread of cholera outside the Indian subcontinent. The current seventh pandemic, caused by an El Tor strain, started during 1961 in Sulawesi, Indonesia. Classical strains are now confined to Bangladesh.

Currently, cholera is periodically epidemic in many parts of Asia, Africa, and in Latin America, where it returned in 1991 after an absence of almost 100 years. Cholera is endemic and seasonally epidemic in the Ganges Delta, including most of Bangladesh and West Bengal, India. In 2000, 56 countries reported 137 071 cases of cholera and 4908 cholera deaths to the World Health Organization: 87 per cent of cases were in Africa. These figures are gross underestimates, both because of incomplete ascertainment and incomplete reporting. For instance, Bangladesh, where hundreds of thousands of cases of cholera occur annually, does not report cases to the World Heath Organization, presumably because of concerns about the effect on food exports.

Epidemics can be particularly severe in refugee camps, where crowding is common, and hygiene and clean water are often absent. Some 12 000 persons died in 3 weeks from a cholera outbreak in Rwandan refugee camps in Goma, Zaire.

Sporadic cases of cholera occur in the Gulf Coast region of the United States, Naples Bay in Italy, and other estuaries where *V. cholerae* lives. Infection in these areas is often linked to eating raw seafood. Because of good sanitation, epidemics no longer occur in industrialized countries following these sporadic cases. Because the infectious dose of *V. cholerae* is very high (10^9 or greater in normal hosts) infections in travellers with normal gastric acid secretion (*V. cholerae* are acid-labile—hypochlorhydria reduces the

infective dose 3- or more fold) are exceedingly rare, and occur only when there are gross errors in standard hygienic practices.

Where cholera is endemic it disproportionately affects children, as many adults are immune. During epidemics in non-endemic regions, adults and children share similar risks of disease. Patients with blood group O are also thought to be at a moderately (20–100 per cent) increased risk of contracting the disease.

Pathogenesis

Depending on the inoculum and the host response, ingestion of *V. cholerae* can fail to establish infection, cause infection but not illness, or can result in disease. The incubation period between the ingestion of *V. cholerae* and the emergence of symptoms ranges from 12 to 72 h.

V. cholerae O1 or O139 cause disease by colonizing the small bowel and producing an enterotoxin—cholera toxin—that causes a massive secretion of electrolytes and water into the gut lumen. This results in the profound diarrhoea that is the hallmark of cholera. The toxonosis is the only gut derangement during *V. cholerae* infection. *V. cholerae* organisms do not invade the gut epithelium (with the exception of the antigen-processing M cells), there is no histological change in the mucosa during infection, and no inflammatory response.

Two virulence factors have been demonstrated in all cholera causing *V. cholerae* O1 or O139: toxin co-regulated pilus and cholera toxin. Toxin co-regulated pili are essential for colonization of the intestinal epithelium brush border, an essential step for proliferation in the intestinal milieu. Cholera toxin is composed of two subunits, A and B. The monomeric A subunit is non-covalently linked to a pentameric B subunit. The B subunit binds to a glycolipid receptor present on enterocytes (and many other eukaryotic cells), ganglioside GM$_1$. This binding becomes rapidly irreversible at body temperature. The A subunit is the active moiety, being internalized in the cell following proteolytic cleavage into two polypeptide chains (A$_1$ and A$_2$).

The A$_1$ subunit alters concentrations of cyclic AMP, an important intracellular messenger. It does this by catalysing the ADP-ribosylation of a protein—G$_s$—that upregulates adenylate cyclase activity. The latter mediates the transformation of ATP to cyclic AMP. Cyclic AMP in turn activates a protein kinase that causes protein phosphorylation, which affects ion channels and ion movement. There is increased Cl$^-$ secretion from intestinal crypt cells into the gut lumen (which drags water with it by changing the osmotic gradient) and decreased NaCl-coupled water absorption in the villus cells.

Virulence genes in *V. cholerae* exist in two clusters—the CTX element, containing the toxin genes, and the TCP pathogenicity island, where genes coding for the toxin co-regulated pilus reside. Expression of these genes, and a number of other putative virulence factors in these gene clusters, are controlled by the transmembrane ToxR regulatory protein. ToxR directly affects transcription of the genes coding for toxin, and indirectly controls transcription of other virulence genes by initiating a cascading system of regulatory factors. Expression of ToxR occurs in response to environmental factors present in the gut lumen. This co-ordinated expression of virulence factors is required for pathogenesis, and also perhaps for survival of *V. cholerae* in the intestinal lumen, giving the *V. cholerae* that possess virulence factors a selective advantage.

An increased secretion of fluid and electrolytes in crypt cells, and decreased absorption in villus cells, results in isotonic fluid accumulation in the small-bowel lumen. The rate of fluid loss is greatest in the jejunum, where fluid losses of 11 ml/cm of jejunum per hour may occur. Diarrhoea results when the amount of fluid produced exceeds the colon's absorptive capacity (approximately 6 litres/day). Because water and ions are lost in equal proportion, the resulting dehydration affects all compartments—intracellular, extracellular, and intravascular—equally.

Clinical and laboratory features

Signs and symptoms

Cholera is one of the most distinctive of clinical illnesses, and its severe form is immediately recognizable. Dr William O'Shaugnessy's description of a patient with cholera in Sunderland in 1831, during the second pandemic of cholera, captures the clinical features of disease as well as any description in the ensuing 170 years:

> On the floor…lay a girl of slender make and juvenile height, but with the face of a superannuated hag. She uttered no moan, gave no expression of pain, but she languidly flung herself from side to side…her eyes were sunk deep into her sockets, as though they had been driven an inch behind their natural position; her mouth was squared; her features flattened; her eyelids black; her fingers shrunk, bent and inky in their hue. All pulse was gone at the wrist, and a tenacious sweat moistened her bosom.

Vomiting and watery diarrhoea are the initial signs of cholera. Diarrhoea may be modest at first—and consist of faecal matter and watery stool. In the majority of infected persons the illness will not advance beyond this stage, and the disease will not be distinguishable from other more common causes of diarrhoea, such as that caused by enterotoxigenic *Escherichia coli*.

In some patients, the diarrhoea becomes profound—exceeding 200 ml/kg body weight per day. In these patients the stool will become 'rice-watery' in character—in other words, it resembles the opaque white water discarded after rice has been washed—it will not contain fecal matter, and is not malodorous. Diarrhoea is painless and patients are often incontinent of stool. In the absence of antimicrobial treatment, the total stool volume during the illness can exceed total body weight.

Vomiting—following by retching as the stomach contents are emptied—almost always occurs in patients with severe diarrhoea. The vomiting tends to abate after the first 24 h of illness. The cause of the vomiting has not been well established—being attributed to both direct effects of *V. cholerae* on intestinal motility, and to acid–base disturbances.

In the absence of effective fluid replacement, dehydration and prostration occurs in those patients with high rates of fluid loss. The features of dehydration in cholera are unmistakable. They include markedly diminished skin turgor, reflecting diminished interstitial fluid. Alterations in skin turgor are demonstrated most graphically by pulling the abdominal subcutaneous tissues between the thumb and forefinger. In the dehydrated patient the tissues will tent (Fig. 1). Other signs of dehydration in patients with cholera include wrinkled fingers ('washerwoman's hands'), sunken eyes, dry mucous membranes, tachypnoea, altered consciousness (apprehensiveness, lethargy, stupor), diminished urine volume, and tachycardia with a diminished or absent radial pulse. Blood pressure is often not recordable.

For purposes of management, dehydration is divided into three categories—none or mild, moderate or some, and severe—based upon the presence and severity of clinical findings (Table 1).

Abdominal cramping can occur, presumably because of gut distension. Cramping of the extremities is a common symptom. Carpopedal spasm and tetany may occur because of alterations in calcium homeostasis resulting from rapid changes in the acid–base status. The presence of coma may indicate severe hypoglycaemia.

Laboratory features

Laboratory abnormalities in patients with cholera result from the intravascular volume contraction and resultant prerenal azotaemia. Creatinine and blood urea nitrogen values are elevated as a result of the prerenal failure, and the packed cell volume and serum protein concentration are elevated as a result of haemoconcentration. Patients are acidaemic because of bicarbonate loss in the stool and lactic acidosis from volume contraction

Fig. 1 Young girl with severe dehydration as fluid infusion is begun. In this picture the sunken eyes and lassitude of severe dehydration can be appreciated, as can the abdominal skin tenting following the assertive pinching of the abdominal subcutaneous tissues.

and hypoperfusion. There is no inflammatory response, although leucocyte numbers may be mildly increased because of the haemoconcentration.

Laboratory diagnosis

Cholera is a clinical diagnosis, especially because most cases of cholera occur in locations where laboratory facilities are not readily available. Because the treatment of any severely dehydrating diarrhoea is the same—fluid replacement—identification of the pathogen is not essential for patient management. As severe dehydration is rare in adults, in the right epidemiological setting the existence of adults with severe dehydration should alert the clinician and public health authorities to the presence of cholera.

A definitive diagnosis is made by isolating *V. cholerae* from stool or rectal swab samples on selective media, and then using sera to identify the pathogenic serogroups 01 and 0139 and Ogawa or Inaba serotypes using slide agglutination tests. Since routine enteric media are not appropriate for the identification of *V. cholerae*, a more-selective media such as thiosulphate–citrate–bile salts–sucrose agar (**TCBS**) should be used. Because TCBS is expensive, and not always available, some laboratories in developing countries rely on less selective and efficient media, such as gelatin, meat extract, or MacConkey agar.

Specimens for dispatch to a laboratory distant from the site of patient care should be placed in a transport media: Cary–Blair medium is the most effective because of its high pH and ready commercial availability. Alkaline peptone water can be used when the time required for transport to laboratory is 6 h or less. When patients are in the same facility as the laboratory, plating should be done at the bedside. Because *V. cholerae* are excreted in such high numbers in stool ($>10^7$ organisms/ml of stool) enrichment of samples before plating is not routinely required.

Serological tests (vibriocidal or antitoxin antibodies) are useful only for retrospective epidemiological studies.

Treatment

This section will focus on treatment under conditions in which most cholera patients present—clinics or hospitals in developing countries with few resources. Only 35 cases of cholera were reported in Europe during 2000, and 9 cases in North America, and so the chances of physicians caring for patients with cholera in industrialized countries are remote.

Initial intravenous therapy

Treatment of the severely dehydrated patient with cholera is a medical emergency. With appropriate therapy, no patient with cholera who reaches a treatment facility alive should die; without adequate therapy, the death rate may be as high as 50 per cent.

The cornerstone of the treatment of cholera patients is rapid replacement of the fluid deficit. Estimates of the degree of dehydration should be made using the categories listed in Table 1, and the corresponding fluid deficit replaced in 2 to 4 h. Patients with severe dehydration should have their fluid volume replaced using intravenous fluid. The composition of the fluid used should closely resemble that lost in the cholera stool (Table 2). Such fluids have been developed in areas where cholera is common (Dhaka solution and Peru polyelectrolyte solution). Ringer's lactate is the commercially available intravenous solution that most closely meets these require-ments. In the absence of an appropriate solution, the emphasis should still be on volume replacement. The maxim 'the dumbest kidney is smarter than the smartest intern' is appropriate here; if the intravascular volume (and renal perfusion) is restored, the kidney will achieve, albeit more slowly, electrolyte and acid–base homeostasis.

Deaths due to cholera usually occur because of the failure to realize the extent of fluid requirements in severely dehydrated patients (7 to 10 litres required during the first 2–4 h for a 75-kg severely dehydrated individual) and the need for close monitoring and continued high-volume fluid replacement after initial rehydration (Table 3). Patients who are not closely monitored can quickly again become dehydrated—and this time not in the high-visibility area of the triage or admission desk, but in the far corner of a rehydration tent set up for delivering care during an epidemic. Patients should be monitored every 1 to 2 h during the first 24 h of illness. Stool and urine volume should be collected and quantified. This can be most exped-itiously achieved using a cholera cot—a simple cot with a plastic sheet and a hole in the middle so that stools and urine drain into a calibrated bucket. Rectal catheters can also be used for stool collection. Fluid replacement should then be adjusted to match continued fluid losses.

Although large-volume intravenous replacements are best accomplished using large-bore needles, any fluid replacement is better than none: even small-calibre needles can be used to initiate therapy. If an intravenous line

Table 1 Categorization of dehydration and fluid deficit based on clinical findings

Feature	Sign, symptom, or laboratory finding with:		
	No or mild dehydration	Moderate or some dehydration	Severe dehydration
Elasticity of subcutaneous tissues as determined by skin pinch*	Normal	Pinch retracts slowly	Tissues remain tented and retract very slowly
Eyes	Normal	Sunken	Dramatically sunken
Respiratory rate and character	Normal	Tachypnoeic	Tachypnoeic, deep, laboured
Heart rate	Normal	Tachycardic	Tachycardic
Radial-pulse character	Normal	Normal	Feeble or non-detectable
Mentation	Alert	Restless or lethargic	Apprehensive, lethargic, stuporous, or comatose
Thirst	Present	Present	Marked
Urine flow	Normal	Scant and dark	Scant or absent
Serum specific gravity†	<1.027	1.028–1.034	>1.034
Approximate fluid deficit, mg/kg of body weight	<50	51–90	> 90
Preferred method of fluid replacement	Oral rehydration therapy	Oral or intravenous, depending on presence of vomiting and rate of continued stool loss	Intravenous

* Sign may be difficulty to distinguish from increased skin elasticity in children with malnutrition and the elderly.

† Patients with malnutrition may have a lower baseline specific gravity; thus the values listed may not be applicable to these patients.

Table 2 Electrolyte composition of cholera stool, and fluids used for rehydration

Fluid	Electrolyte and glucose concentration (mmol/l)					
	Na$^+$	Cl$^-$	K$^+$	HCO$_3^-$	Glucose or dextrose	Osmolality (mosmol/l)^a
Cholera stool						
Adults	130	100	20	44	0	300^b
Children	100	90	33	30	0	300^b
Rehydration solutions						
WHO oral rehydration solution	90	80	20	30^c	111	331
Intravenous solutions						
Lactated Ringer's	130	109	4	28^d	0^e	271
Dhaka	133	98	13	48	0	292
Peru—poly-electrolyte	90	80	20	30	111	331
Normal saline	154	154	0	0	0^e	308

^{a} For rehydration solutions, the value listed is the calculated osmolality. Actual osmolality is slightly less, as the salts do not completely disassociate.

^{b} Osmolality includes unmeasured osmotically active molecules (primarily organic acids) in addition to electrolytes.

^{c} Often replaced with 10 mmol/l of trisodium citrate which has a longer shelf-life.

^{d} As lactate.

^{e} Preparations of these solutions containing 5 per cent dextrose (277 mmol/l) are preferred, as they prevent hypoglycaemia from occurring, or treat it if present.

cannot be established, oral rehydration solutions should be given by mouth if the patient is alert, or otherwise using a nasogastric tube.

Antimicrobial therapy

Antimicrobial therapy can halve the duration and volume of diarrhoea. All patients requiring intravenous therapy, or admission to clinic or hospital, should receive an antimicrobial agent. Almost all patients given an effective antimicrobial drug can be discharged within 24 h of admission, in contrast to 72 h or more if they are left untreated. Especially during epidemics, this reduction in hospital stay, and the associated reduction in demand for intravenous and oral fluids, can be critical for an effective response by already strained healthcare services.

Single-dose therapy—of which there are a number of options—is the preferred regimen, especially in epidemic settings (Table 4). Resistance in *V. cholerae* is not predictable, and hence the need to obtain isolates for susceptibility testing during an outbreak. Since outbreak strains are usually clonal, empirical therapy can be based upon a limited number of isolates. Resistance to fluoroquinolones and azithromycin has not been reported,

and if these drugs are available at generic prices they, along with doxycycline (if the strain is susceptible), are the drugs of choice.

Oral rehydration

Oral rehydration fluids containing glucose and salts were developed following the observation that, although cholera toxin poisons the neutral sodium-chloride absorption channels in the intestinal mucosa, the glucose-mediated cotransport of sodium (and water) remains intact. Oral rehydration fluids should be given immediately after the onset of diarrhoea in an effort to prevent the development of dehydration. They should also be used in severely dehydrated patients following rehydration. Most patients can be managed with oral fluids alone within 12 to 24 h of admission. Provision of oral rehydration fluids is an inexact art, but the amount provided should be somewhat more than the volume of stool lost.

The most readily available oral rehydration salts are the sachets distributed by UNICEF and the WHO containing 90 mmol of sodium for reconstitution in water. Homemade solutions—using sucrose and salt, or cereal and salt—are also effective. Oral rehydration solution can be drunk from a cup by adults or fed to young children and infants using a spoon (Fig. 2).

Table 3 Changes in plasma electrolytes, creatinine, and protein following rapid 2–4 h rehydration

Time	Na$^+$ (mmol/l)	K$^+$ (mmol/l)	HCO$_3^-$ (mmol/l)	Creatinine (mmol/l)	Protein (g/l)
Admission	132	4.4	13.3	138	102
4 h	135	3.8	19.4	106	72
24 h	134	3.7	21.9	83	73

Based upon 32 children with severe dehydration who received a polyelectrolyte solution for initial rehydration, and then primarily received oral rehydration solution. (Taken with permission from Rahman O, *et al.* (1988). Rapid intravenous rehydration by means of a single polyelectrolyte solution with our without dextrose. *Journal of Pediatrics* **113**, 654–60.)

Table 4 Options for antimicrobial therapy of patients with cholera

Drug	Adults	Children
Azithromycin	Not evaluated in controlled trials; 1 g as a single dose likely to be effective	20 mg/kg body weight as a single dose; maximum dose 1 g
Ciprofloxacin	1 g as a single dose	Not evaluated; 20 mg/kg body weight as a single dose (maximum 1 g) likely to be effective and safe
Doxycycline	300 mg as a single dose	Not evaluated; 6 mg/kg body weight as a single dose likely to be effective
Erythromycin	500 mg four times daily for 3 days	12.5 mg/kg body weight four times daily for 3 days; maximum individual dose 500 mg
Furazolidone	100 mg four times daily for 4 days	1.25 mg/kg body weight per dose; four doses daily for 3 days; maximum individual dose 100 mg
Tetracycline	1 g as a single dose	12.5 mg/kg body weight four times daily for 3 days; maximum individual dose 500 mg
Cotrimoxazole	320 mg trimethoprim/1600 mg of sulfamethoxazole twice daily for 3 days	4 mg trimethoprim/20 mg of sulfamethoxazole/kg body weight twice daily for 3 days; maximum dose same as adult

Complications

Rapid correction of the acidosis in patients with cholera may reduce ionized calcium concentrations, resulting in tetany. If tetany occurs, the rehydration solution used should be changed to normal saline for a brief period. Rapid correction of the acidosis can also result in a drop in the serum potassium concentration, but this is rarely symptomatic.

Renal failure is rare. Most patients thought to have renal failure actually have inadequate fluid replacement. Even with rapid rehydration, most children and adults produce no urine during the first 4 h of treatment, and only a median of 1 ml/kg body weight in the next 24 h. Patients with diminished urine output should be followed, and their creatinine level measured if possible. Additional fluids should be given, and the patients followed closely for oedema and other signs of fluid overload.

Hypoglycaemia occurs because of a failure of gluconeogenesis in stressed children; in Bangladesh the rate of severe hypoglycaemia in children with dehydrating cholera was 0.5 per cent. Thus dextrose-containing solutions, such as Ringer's lactate with 5 per cent dextrose, are preferred for rehydrating patients with cholera. In the absence of such a solution, children should have their blood glucose measured with a glucometer, or be given a bolus of glucose if they are in a state of altered consciousness.

If the patient develops a fever, or appears septic, the most likely cause is contamination of the infusate and/or the intravenous apparatus. The treatment is to replace both. Adherence to infection-control techniques is an important part of the management of patients, especially in epidemic situations.

Prevention and future research

The provision of clean water is the primary means of preventing cholera. In the absence of potable water, chlorine or iodine can be added to drinking water. Alum potash has also been reported to be effective. All sterilizing agents are ineffectual in water that has a high turbidity from suspended organic material. Food is best eaten cooked, and not from street vendors.

There are currently three vaccines available for cholera: a parenterally administered vaccine containing whole cells killed by phenol; and two oral vaccines: a killed, whole-cell recombinant B-subunit toxin vaccine; and a live, attenuated, *V. cholerae* vaccine strain—CVD 103—that does not express the cholera-toxin A subunit. The parenteral vaccine is of uncertain efficacy and is toxic because of its lipopolysaccharide content; the two oral vaccines have minimal toxicity and provide limited protection for short periods to persons living in endemic areas. The oral vaccines are not widely available in developing countries, and are not licensed in the United States. These vaccines are of limited utility; travellers are at a miniscule risk of contracting cholera, and the limited long-term efficacy of these vaccines makes them inappropriate for routine use in developing countries. They may have more use during epidemics; but epidemics are likely to have run their course before supplies can be mobilized and immunity induced.

There is a need to develop a vaccine that provides long-duration, high-level protection against cholera. Perhaps the most pressing research need is for a better understanding of how resources can be mobilized to provide clean water and sanitation to the billions of persons who currently lack it.

Fig. 2 Mother providing oral rehydration solution to her reluctant child using the recommended method of a cup and spoon. In the background note the cholera cots and the buckets placed underneath the cutouts in the cot ('poop-chutes') that allow stool to be measured. Cots are covered with a plastic liner that is changed daily.

Further reading

Dhar U, *et al.* (1996). Clinical features, antimicrobial susceptibility and toxin production in *Vibrio cholerae* O139 infection: comparison with *V. cholerae*

O1 infection. *Transactions of the Royal Society of Tropical Medicine and Hygiene* **90**, 402–5.

Faruque SM, Albert MJ, Mekalanos JJ (1998). Epidemiology, genetics, and ecology of toxigenic *Vibrio cholerae*. *Microbiology and Molecular Biology Reviews* **62**(4), 1301–14.

Field M, *et al.* (1972). Effect of cholera enterotoxin on ion transport across isolated ileal mucosa. *Journal of Clinical Investigation* **51**, 796–804.

Heidelberg JF, *et al.* (2000). DNA sequence of both chromosomes of the cholera pathogen *Vibrio cholerae*. *Nature* **406**, 477–83.

Hirschhorn N, *et al.* (1968). Decrease in net stool output in cholera during intestinal perfusion with glucose-containing solutions. *New England Journal of Medicine* **279**, 176–81.

Khan WA, *et al.* (1996). Randomised controlled comparison of single-dose ciprofloxacin and doxycycline for cholera caused by *Vibrio cholerae* 01 or 0139. *Lancet* **348**, 296–300.

Ryan ET, Calderwood SB (2000). Cholera vaccines. *Clinical Infectious Diseases* **31**, 561–5.

Waldor MK, Mekalanos JJ (1996). Lysogenic conversion by a filamentous phage encoding cholera toxin. *Science* **272**, 1910–14.

7.11.12 *Haemophilus influenzae*

E. R. Moxon

General

Haemophilus influenzae, a Gram-negative bacterium, is a commensal and potential pathogen that resides in the nasopharynx, the conjunctivae, and occasionally the genital tract of humans. Carriage of one or more strains for periods of days to months is common and most carriers are, and remain, healthy. However, *H. influenzae* is pathogenic and can result in two distinct patterns of disease (Table 1). First, there are infections in which there is invasion of the bloodstream and dissemination to distant sites, for example the meninges or synovial joints. These are usually caused by encapsulated type b strains and occur typically in infants. Second, there are infections that occur as a result of contiguous spread of *H. influenzae* within the respiratory tract, for example otitis media, sinusitis, and pneumonia. These are usually, but not invariably, caused by unencapsulated or non-typeable

Table 1 Carriage and pathogenicity of *Haemophilus influenzae*

Strains	Common upper respiratory tract carriage rates (%)	Principal manifestations of pathogenicity
Non-encapsulated	50–80	Exacerbations of chronic bronchitis, otitis media, sinusitis, conjunctivitis; bacteraemic infections rare; patients commonly adults
Encapsulated, type b	2–4	Meningitis, epiglottitis, pneumonia and empyema, septic arthritis, cellulitis, osteomyelitis, pericarditis, bacteraemia; rare manifestations include glossitis, tenosynovitis, peritonitis, endocarditis, ventriculitis, associated with infected shunt tubing
Encapsulated types a, c–f	1–2	Rarely incriminated as pathogens

(NT) strains and are relatively common in children; however, they also occur in adults.

Epidemiology, pathogenesis, and immunology

Humans are the sole reservoir of *H. influenzae*; person-to-person spread is therefore crucial to the survival of the species. Transmission occurs by airborne droplets, or by direct contagion with secretions. The age of acquisition is extremely variable. In socio-economically deprived countries, most children are densely colonized with *H. influenzae* immediately after birth, whereas acquisition may be delayed for several weeks in infants living in, for example, Europe or the United States. Most of the colonizing strains are unencapsulated or so-called non-typeable (NT) organisms, but in 3 to 5 per cent of people, the *H. influenzae* express one of six, antigenically distinct polysaccharide capsules, designated a to f, the basis of the major typing system. Carriage of several different strains concurrently has been well described. Over time, phenotypic changes in major surface antigens, such as outer membrane proteins, occur in response to host immune selection pressures. The factors influencing acquisition and colonization of *H. influenzae* include a variety of surface adhesins, including pili, the production of IgA1 proteases, the inhibition of host clearance mechanisms by the inhibitory effect of cell wall glycopeptides, and the production of both local and serum antibodies. Colonization is a permissive event in the pathogenesis of disease and the importance of the type b capsule as a crucial factor in systemic, bacteraemic infections has been well established in animal models. Capsule impedes the clearance of organisms by phagocytes and complement-mediated killing. The core sugars of lipopolysaccharide also play an important role in promoting survival of *H. influenzae* and another key component, endotoxin (lipid A), is critical in mediating the damage to tissues, such as inflammation and breakdown of the blood–meningeal barrier. Prior viral infections such as influenza potentiate infection and appear to facilitate both contiguous spread within the respiratory tract—as in otitis media, sinusitis, or lower respiratory tract infection——and the probability of dissemination into the blood.

Serum antibodies to type b capsule mediate protective immunity against systemic infections in humans. The serum of newborn babies and young infants, up until the age of 3 months, generally has sufficient amounts of passively acquired maternal antibodies to afford protection. Thereafter, the natural decline of maternally derived antibodies is followed by a period lasting until the age of 2 to 4 years when the levels of antibody are absent, or inadequate to provide protection.

In contrast to systemic type b infections where deficiencies in opsonophagocytic mechanisms are paramount, impairment of non-specific host defence mechanisms (e.g. impaired ciliary clearance) is the most obvious feature of those who have disease caused by NT *H. influenzae*. Other predisposing factors include smoking, viral infections, immunodeficiency, or chronic lung disease such as cystic fibrosis.

Haemophilus influenzae type b

Meningitis

Despite the availability of antibiotics, and more recently the highly effective conjugate vaccines, type b meningitis remains the commonest cause of purulent meningitis in early childhood worldwide, and the cause of many deaths and permanent central nervous system damage in survivors. The majority of the cases occur in young children aged less than 5 years, the peak incidence being from about the age of 3 months to 2 years. Reported risk factors include male sex, black rather than white race, absence of breast feeding, socio-economic deprivation, winter months, siblings (often asymptomatic carriers), and attendance at day-care or preschool nurseries.

Typically, meningitis presents after a few hours or days of antecedent symptoms, most commonly those of an upper respiratory tract infection in a young child; an associated or preceding otitis media is common. The most common symptoms and signs are fever, lethargy, vomiting, neck stiffness, and altered nervous system function, ranging from irritability to coma, but young babies may be afebrile and have few symptoms or signs. Raised intracranial pressure produces headache and vomiting and may cause a bulging fontanelle in young infants. Seizures are common in children; subdural effusions are present in about 33 per cent of children and occur most frequently in young infants. The key to diagnosis is to perform a lumbar puncture and examine the cerebrospinal fluid. This typically reveals inflammatory cells, raised protein and lowered glucose concentrations, and there are often organisms that can be seen by microscopy after staining with Gram's stain or methylene blue.

If diagnosis and treatment are prompt, more than 95 per cent of patients with *H. influenzae* meningitis will survive, but about 8 per cent of survivors have serious central nervous system sequelae, the commonest being sensorineural deafness. Before the advent of effective vaccines, this was said to be the most important cause of acquired mental handicap in the United States.

Epiglottitis

Acute respiratory obstruction, caused by a cellulitis of the epiglottis and aryepiglottic folds, usually occurs as a fulminating, life-threatening infection. Sore throat, fever, and dyspnoea progress rapidly to dysphagia, pooling of oral secretions, and drooling of saliva from the mouth. The child is toxic, restless, anxious or lethargic, and adopts a sitting position with an extended neck and protruding chin in an effort to to minimize airway obstruction. The voice and cry are muffled and the child may be reluctant to talk. Stridor is often absent; if present it is soft and wheezy. Cough is unusual. In the absence of adequate treatment death commonly occurs within a few hours. The course may be less dramatic with a prodromal illness of sore throat and hoarseness from one to several days preceding the onset of acute symptoms. The characteristic findings are that the epiglottis is red and swollen, obstructing the pharynx at the base of the tongue. Lateral radiographs reveal the swollen 'thumb-shaped' epiglottis. Examination of the larynx should be attempted only where there are facilities for immediate intubation/tracheotomy, since fatal respiratory obstruction may occur abruptly. The most important aspect of management of acute epiglottitis is the provision of an adequate airway and ventilation in addition to antibiotic treatment.

Pneumonia and empyema

Lower respiratory tract infections occur most often in children aged less than 5 years and present as lobar pneumonia, often with pleural involvement. In many of the poorer countries of the world, such as New Guinea, *H. influenzae* type b pneumonia is second only to that caused by the pneumococcus and in these regions is a greater public health problem than *H. influenzae* meningitis. Type b pneumonia is also well recognized in adults as a primary cause of pneumonia, especially in alcoholics.

Cellulitis

This important infection occurs in young children who present with hectic fever and a raised, warm, tender area of distinctive reddish-blue hue, most often located on one cheek or in the periorbital region, that evolves over a few hours.

Septic arthritis

H. influenzae type b is one of the commonest causes of septic arthritis in children of less than 2 years of age. Typically, there is involvement of a single large, weight-bearing joint, usually without osteomyelitis. Response to drainage and appropriate systemic antibiotics is usually dramatic and apparently curative, but long-term follow-up is important since residual joint dysfunction occurs in a proportion of children.

Treatment of diseases caused by type b strains

Prior to the availability of antibiotic treatment, *H. influenzae* meningitis was invariably fatal. With the introduction of chloramphenicol in 1950, survival rates of 95 per cent or more have been possible. Overall, chloramphenicol remains an excellent drug for treating *H. influenzae* meningitis, but occasional isolates show resistance. Chloramphenicol carries a dose-related, reversible bone marrow toxicity, but this is rarely clinically a problem and can be completely avoided if blood levels are monitored. Idiosyncratic bone marrow aplasia has been reported but is extremely rare. Ampicillin, formerly considered an ideal treatment for *H. influenzae* meningitis, is no longer favoured because of the relatively high prevalence of resistant (β-lactamase producing) strains. The treatment of choice is parenteral third-generation cephalosporins such as ceftriaxone or cefotaxime; these have been shown to be highly effective as initial treatment of suspected bacterial meningitis. Cefuroxime is less effective.

Young children in the same household as a patient with invasive type b disease are at significantly increased risk of secondary invasive infection by *H. influenzae* type b. Rifampicin given orally once daily for 4 days is effective in eradicating nasopharyngeal carriage, and is recommended for all household contacts (children and adults).

Experimental and clinical studies support the administration of corticosteroids to reduce the incidence of neurological sequelae, especially sensorineural deafness. The presumed mechanism is the reduction of inflammation that results from release of bacterial cell wall fragments. Dexamethasone therapy (0.6. μg/kg.day) intravenously in four divided doses for 4 days is recommended for children older than 2 months of age.

Active immunization

In the 1940s, serum antibodies specific for the type b capsule were used as treatment of type b infection. Efforts to develop a vaccine for active immunization using purified type b capsule did not begin until the 1970s. However, by the 1980s, it was clear that this vaccine did not protect children aged less than 2 years old. Further research was directed towards developing conjugate vaccines in which type b capsule is covalently linked to a carrier protein, such as tetanus toxoid. Several commercially manufactured conjugate vaccines have been licensed and all have proved to be very safe and capable of affording high levels of protection to children immunized as early as 2 months of age. In the United Kingdom, conjugate vaccines have been given to infants as part of the routine immunization schedule since 1992 and their protective efficacy is more than 95 per cent.

Diseases caused by non-typeable *H. influenzae*

Pneumonia

Non-typeable strains are an important cause of pneumonia in children and adults, especially the elderly, and in those with established lung disease, such as chronic bronchitis. In many countries where adverse socio-economic circumstances are prevalent, acute lower respiratory tract infections in infants caused by NT *H. influenzae* represent an uncertain but probably major cause of morbidity and mortality.

It has been recognized for many years that exacerbations of chronic bronchitis correlate with an increase in the production of purulent sputum from which NT *H. influenzae* strains are cultured. Such episodes are often precipitated by prior viral infection. Progressive lung damage in conditions such as chronic bronchitis, cystic fibrosis, and hypogammaglobulinaemia is thought to result from heightened and protracted inflammatory response to a variety of bacteria, including NT *H. influenzae*, in people whose respiratory tract lacks the appropriate clearance mechanisms.

Maternal and neonatal sepsis

NT *H. influenzae* are a well-documented cause of tubo-ovarian abscess or chronic salpingitis. More ominously, the infants born to such mothers, often prematurely, may develop life-threatening neonatal septicaemia, meningitis, and a form of acute respiratory distress syndrome that is indistinguishable from that caused by group B streptococci.

Acute otitis media and sinusitis

H. influenzae accounts for about one-fifth of all cases of acute bacterial otitis media. More than 90 per cent of the organisms isolated from middle ear fluid are NT strains. Although such episodes occur at any age, they are most common in children aged 6 months to 5 years. Since more than two-thirds of children have one or more episodes of otitis media by the age of 3 years, a conservative estimate would indicate that more than 100 000 cases of *H. influenzae* otitis media occur each year in the United Kingdom. NT strains are also a common cause of sinusitis in both adults and children.

Conjunctivitis

H. influenzae is an important cause of purulent conjunctivitis. Most are NT strains that were formerly considered to be sufficiently distinctive to be referred to as *H. aegyptius*. Interest in these strains was heightened when, in 1984, an apparently new and serious disease was described in Brazilian children who developed a life-threatening infection known as Brazilian purpuric fever. Its peak age incidence is 1 to 4 years; purulent conjunctivitis, high fever, vomiting, purpura, vascular collapse, and a high mortality are characteristic.

Other infections

All of the diseases that are commonly caused by type b strains can, on rare occasions, be caused by strains of capsular serotypes a, c, d, e, and f as well as NT strains. A number of other unusual infections have been described including: endocarditis, pericarditis, peritonitis, and epididymo-orchitis. Two other closely related species, *H. parainfluenzae* and *H. aphrophilus*, are also causes of disease, such as endocarditis.

Treatment

Serious infections caused by NT strains such as meningitis, lower respiratory tract infections, tubal abscess, and neonatal sepsis require systemic treatment with third-generation β-lactams or co-trimoxazole. Chloramphenicol is highly effective but blood levels need to be monitored carefully, especially in young infants, because of potential toxicity. Sinusitis and otitis media are often treated effectively with oral amoxycillin, but augmentin would be preferable, given the relatively high incidence of strains producing β-lactamase. Oral co-trimoxazole would be an equally sound or alternative choice for trimethoprim-susceptible strains. The use of antibiotics as prophylaxis or treatment of exacerbations of chronic bronchitis is controversial, but many advocate their use either to reduce the number of haemophili in the lower respiratory tract or to eradicate them. Drugs of the tetracycline group are effective, but are contraindicated in pregnancy, patients with impaired renal function, or children less than 10 years of age; amoxycillin and co-trimoxazole have also proved useful.

Passive immunization

People with increased susceptibility to infection with *H. influenzae*, but particularly NT strains, may have a deficiency of antibody synthesis. They benefit from immunoglobulin preparations administered either intramuscularly or intravenously. This form of immunoglobulin replacement undoubtedly decreases the incidence of systemic infections and the number of episodes of both upper and lower respiratory tract infections caused by NT *H. influenzae*.

Further reading

Booy R *et al.* (1997). Surveillance of vaccine failures following primary immunisation of infants with Hib conjugate vaccine: Evidence for protection without boosting. *Lancet* **349**, 1197–1202.

Hoiseth SK (1991). The genus *Haemophilus*. In: Balows A *et al.*, eds. *The prokaryotes, a handbook on the biology of bacteria: ecophysiology, isolation, identification, applications*. Springer-Verlag, New York.

Moxon ER, Murphy TF (1999). *Haemophilus influenzae*. In: Mandell GL, Bennett JE, Dolin R, eds. *Mandell, Douglas, and Bennett's principles and practice of infectious diseases*, 5th edn, pp 2369–78. Churchill Livingstone, Philadelphia.

Murphy TF, Apicella MA (1987). Non-typeable *Haemophilus influenzae*: A review of clinical aspects, surface antigens, and the human immune response to infection. *Reviews of Infectious Diseases* **9**, 1–15

Turk DC (1982). Clinical importance of *Haemophilus influenzae*. In: Sell SH, Wright PF, eds, Haemophilus influenzae, *epidemiology, immunology and prevention of disease*, pp 30–3. Elsevier Biomedical, New York.

7.11.13 *Haemophilus ducreyi* and chancroid

Allan R. Ronald

Introduction

Genital ulcer disease is the presenting feature of sexually transmitted diseases in about 5 per cent of patients in Western societies; in the developing world, 10 to 50 per cent of patients with sexually transmitted diseases present with genital ulcer disease. In the West, genital herpes and primary syphilis are the commonest aetiological agents. In the developing world *Haemophilus ducreyi* accounts for most genital ulcer disease. Granuloma inguinale and lymphogranuloma venereum are occasionally imported from remaining foci in sub-Saharan Africa and Asia.

The epidemiological association between genital ulcer disease, particularly chancroid, and the risk of transmission of HIV-1 and HIV-2 has increased interest in its control.

Soft chancre was differentiated from the hard indurated chancre of syphilis by Ricord in 1838. In 1889, the Neapolitan physician Ducreyi identified short-chaining streptobacillary rods in exudate from ulcers following inoculation with chancroid pus.

Aetiology

Haemophilus ducreyi is a faintly bipolar staining Gram-negative rod. Due to extracellular linkage of the bacteria, the organism forms chains and demonstrates a 'school of fish' arrangement. *H. ducreyi* colonies appear after 48 h of incubation, are yellow-grey, dome-shaped, and variable in size and opacity. Colonies are cohesive and can be nudged intact with a straight wire.

Epidemiology

Chancroid is endemic in eastern and southern Africa, India, and the Caribbean where the annual incidence in adult males can exceed 1/1000. It occurs sporadically in industrialized countries, most frequently at major ports of entry. During the last two decades, there have been over 20 discrete outbreaks in North America. Prostitutes are the usual reservoir for dissemination of *H. ducreyi* and the male to female ratio usually is 5:1 or higher. Male circumcision decreases susceptibility to infection by about threefold.

Asymptomatic carriage has no proven role in the spread of *H. ducreyi*. In one study of men with culture-positive chancroid, all source contacts had genital ulcers. *H. ducreyi* is rarely transmitted non-sexually. Chancroid lesions on the fingers or breasts reflect direct contact from a genital lesion on the sexual partner or autoinoculation.

Pathogenesis and pathology

After an incubation period of 3 to 10 days, an inflammatory papule develops which ulcerates. Bacterial virulence factors include a haemolysin and a cytolethal distending toxin that interferes with intracellular signalling. Both humeral and cell-mediated responses to *H. ducreyi* occur, but their role in preventing or modifying infection is unknown. On histological examination, perivascular and interstitial mononuclear cell infiltrates predominate with occasional giant cell granulomas. Endothelial disruption with neutrophil invasion occurs superficially.

Clinical features

Chancroid begins as a tender papule which ulcerates. It is painful, rarely indurated, irregular, and sharply demarcated, usually with no surrounding inflammation. The ulcer base is uneven with a greyish-yellow exudate which bleeds readily. About 50 per cent of men and most women have multiple ulcers.

Numerous variants of chancroid occur including giant rapidly spreading ulcers, dwarf chancroid resembling herpes, follicular chancroid that mimics pyogenic infection, transient ulceration associated with lymphadenitis similar to lymphogranuloma venereum, a painless single ulcer similar to primary syphilis, and raised indurated 'beefy' lesions not unlike granuloma inguinale. In the absence of laboratory investigation, in men as many as 25 per cent and in women at least 50 per cent of ulcers could be attributed on clinical surmise to aetiological agents other than *H. ducreyi*. The index of suspicion for chancroid increases where the disease is highly prevalent.

Chancroid occurs anywhere on the genitalia. However, in uncircumcised men, over 50 per cent of ulcers are on the prepuce. The coronal sulcus is a common site with a circle of ulcers surrounding the entire sulcal circumference. Contact lesions are common on adjacent cutaneous surfaces. In women lesions occur in decreasing frequency on the fourchette, labia majora and labia minora, perianal area, and medial aspects of the thighs. Cervical and vaginal ulcers are uncommon.

Inguinal lymphadenopathy appears in about 40 per cent of men and 20 per cent of women within 7 to 10 days of ulceration. The lymph nodes are discrete, very tender, and often bilateral. If untreated, lymphadenitis progresses to a suppurative bubo which may form an inguinal abscess. Abscesses can penetrate deeply into the groin.

Laboratory diagnosis

Definitive diagnosis of chancroid requires culture of *H. ducreyi*. The Gram stain is not sufficiently sensitive or specific to diagnose *H. ducreyi* infection. No serological test is available. Diagnostic nucleic acid probes are under investigation. The sensitivity of *H. ducreyi* culture is in the range of 50 to 80 per cent. However, specificity is high as asymptomatic carriage of *H. ducreyi* is rare. Two or more sexually transmitted pathogens are present in 10 to 15 per cent of patients presenting with genital ulcers; *H. ducreyi* may be cultured concomitantly with either *Herpes simplex* or *Treponema pallidum*. Although the classic features of syphilis and chancroid appear to place them at opposite ends of a spectrum of genital ulceration, in about 20 per cent of patients the presentations are indistinguishable.

Whenever possible, exudate from the ulcer or bubo should be inoculated directly on to the primary selective media. Organisms will survive longer on a swab at 4°C than at room temperature. *H. ducreyi* grows well on gonococcal agar with added vancomycin (3 mg/l) to inhibit growth of Gram-positive bacteria, a vitamin supplement, and 0.25 per cent activated charcoal. Cultures for *H. ducreyi* should be incubated at 33°C in 5 per cent carbon dioxide and maximum humidity. A candle extinction jar with a moist paper towel is adequate. Distinct colonies appear within 72 h. *H. ducreyi* is identified by its Gram stain and its ability to use nitrate, a positive oxidase test, and a requirement for X factor.

Agar dilution tests with *H. ducreyi* correlate with the clinical response. Plasmid-mediated resistance, as in *Neisseria gonorrhoeae* and *Haemophilus influenzae*, encodes for β-lactamase production; other plasmids enable sulphonamide, tetracycline, and chloramphenicol, kanamycin, and streptomycin resistance. These plasmids have spread rapidly.

Fortunately, all isolates remain susceptible to the third-generation cephalosporins, the fluoroquinolones, and the macrolides.

Treatment

In the absence of specific treatment, chancroid is a prolonged illness with slow resolution and frequent recurrence. Genital ulcers and inguinal abscesses have been reported to persist for years.

Circumcision, cleanliness, and saline soaks were used prior to the sulphonamides. Ampicillin, streptomycin, and tetracycline were each shown to be equivalent treatment regimens with a mean time to complete healing of 10 days. Trimethoprim/sulphonamide combinations became standard therapy, but the emergence and rapid spread of trimethoprim resistance has thwarted its continuing use.

Other treatment regimens include ceftriaxone (a single dose of 250 mg intramuscularly), ciprofloxacin (a single oral dose of 500 mg), fleroxacin (a single dose of 400 mg), erythromycin (250 mg three times a day for 7 days), and azithromycin (a single oral dose of 1 g). All cure over 95 per cent of HIV-seronegative men with chancroid. Patients with chancroid concurrently infected with HIV are more likely to fail to respond to treatment with β-lactam antibiotics.

Epidemiological associations between HIV-1 and *Haemophilus ducreyi*

Chancroid is a risk factor for the heterosexual spread of HIV-1 and HIV-2. Chancroid in women increases the risk of acquisition of HIV-1 following heterosexual contact with HIV-1-infected men by four- to eightfold. The presence of chancroid in HIV-1-infected individuals increases the shedding of HIV-1 and the probability that partners will become HIV-1 infected.

Prevention and control

The control of chancroid can reduce heterosexual transmission of HIV substantially, perhaps by 30 per cent or more, in societies where both pathogens are being spread, particularly from prostitutes to their clients. Effective control of chancroid has been achieved on numerous occasions by treating men with ulcers and their sexual contacts. Most women who are source contacts of men with chancroid have few symptoms, despite the presence of ulcers, and so contact tracing is essential. The use of condoms by clients dramatically reduces the acquisition of chancroid from prostitutes.

Chancroid control is an essential cost-effective intervention to slow the transmission of HIV-1.

Further reading

Cameron DW *et al.* (1989). Female to male transmission of human immunodeficiency virus type 1: risk factors for seroconversion in men. *Lancet* **ii**, 403–7.

Coqtes-Bratti X *et al.* (1999). The cytolethal distending toxin from the chancroid bacteria *Haemophilus ducreyi* induces cell-cycle arrest in the G2 phase. *Journal of Clinical Investigation* **103**, 107–15.

Martin DH *et al.* (1995). Comparison of azithromycin and ceftriaxone for the treatment of chancroid. *Clinical Infectious Diseases* **21**, 409–14.

Ndinya-Achola JO *et al.* (1996). Presumptive specific clinical diagnosis of genital ulcer disease (GUD) in a primary health care setting in Nairobi. *International Journal of AIDS and STD* **7**, 201–5.

Trees DL, Morse SA (1995). Chancroid and *Haemophilus ducreyi*: an update. *Clinical Microbiology Reviews* **8**, 357–75.

7.11.14 Bordetella

Calvin C. Linnemann, Jr

Bacteria of the genus *Bordetella* are primarily pathogens of the respiratory tract of humans and animals because they can adhere to ciliated epithelial cells. The whooping cough syndrome or pertussis is characterized by paroxysmal coughing, an inspiratory whoop, and lymphocytosis. *B. pertussis*, *B. parapertussis*, and *B. bronchiseptica* can cause disease in man. *B. holmesii* has also been recovered from patients with whooping cough. Misattribution of pertussis to viral infection resulted from the difficulty in isolating *B. pertussis* and frequent coinfection with adenoviruses.

Bordetella infections should be suspected in patients with persistent lower respiratory tract infection and paroxysmal coughing, with or without an inspiratory whoop, or those with any respiratory symptoms after close contact with a documented infection. Most bordetella infections will go unrecognized because the symptoms are indistinguishable from other respiratory tract infections, and because appropriate diagnostic tests are usually done only in patients with typical pertussis. *B. bronchiseptica*, a common pathogen in animals, should be considered in animal handlers with respiratory tract infections.

The causative agent

Bordetella are small, aerobic, Gram-negative coccobacillary organisms. *B. pertussis* are slow growing and are inhibited by a variety of media constituents such as fatty acids that must be inactivated if culture is to be effective (see below). *B. parapertussis* and *B. bronchiseptica* are less fastidious and faster growing.

Bordetella pertussis adheres to ciliated epithelial cells in the respiratory tract. Attachment is followed by ciliostasis and subsequent loss of the ciliated cells. Biologically active components include filamentous haemagglutinin, fimbrias, pertactin, pertussis toxin (lymphocytosis-promoting factor), adenylate cyclase, and tracheal cytotoxin. Acellular vaccines, containing only selected components such as the filamentous haemagglutinin and pertussis toxin, protect against severe symptomatic infection. *B. pertussis* is non-invasive, usually remaining on the surface of the respiratory tract, but *B. parapertussis*, *B. bronchiseptica*, and *B. holmesii* bacteraemias have been reported.

Epidemiology

Humans are the only known reservoir of *B. pertussis* and *B. parapertussis*, whereas *B. bronchiseptica* is found in other mammals. *B. pertussis* is transmitted by droplets from symptomatic patients. Asymptomatic infections are not important in the spread of disease, and there are no chronic carriers. It is assumed that the transmission of *B. parapertussis* is similar to that of *B. pertussis*. Humans and other mammals may be reservoirs of *B. bronchiseptica*.

Before vaccine was available, epidemics of *B. pertussis* spread through schools, and were carried by the schoolchildren to their homes. Secondary attack rates in susceptible children were 25 to 50 per cent in schools, and 70 to 100 per cent in homes, reflecting the intense and prolonged exposure at home. Most children developed symptoms. Mild infections or reinfections in adults caring for sick children were known as 'grandmother's cough' or 'nurse's cough'.

In the vaccine era, major epidemics have disappeared in most developed countries. Mortality from *B. pertussis* was decreasing before the introduction of vaccine, but not the number of cases. In the United States and Canada, where effective vaccines have been widely used, the incidence of pertussis has decreased to 1 to 3/100 000 per year (Fig. 1). Results were less dramatic in the United Kingdom, related, perhaps, to early problems with vaccine efficacy and lower levels of vaccine usage. Pertussis did decrease in the United Kingdom, and the resurgence of *B. pertussis* in the late 1970s, following a decrease in vaccine usage, demonstrated the efficacy of vaccine.

In a highly vaccinated population, older children and adults make up a larger proportion of cases and may play a more important part in the transmission of disease. Before vaccine was available, the source of infection could be identified in most cases as another child. It is now more difficult to trace the source, but in very young infants an adult family member frequently appears to be the source. Hospital epidemics have also demonstrated the part adults play in transmission. Doctors and nurses may

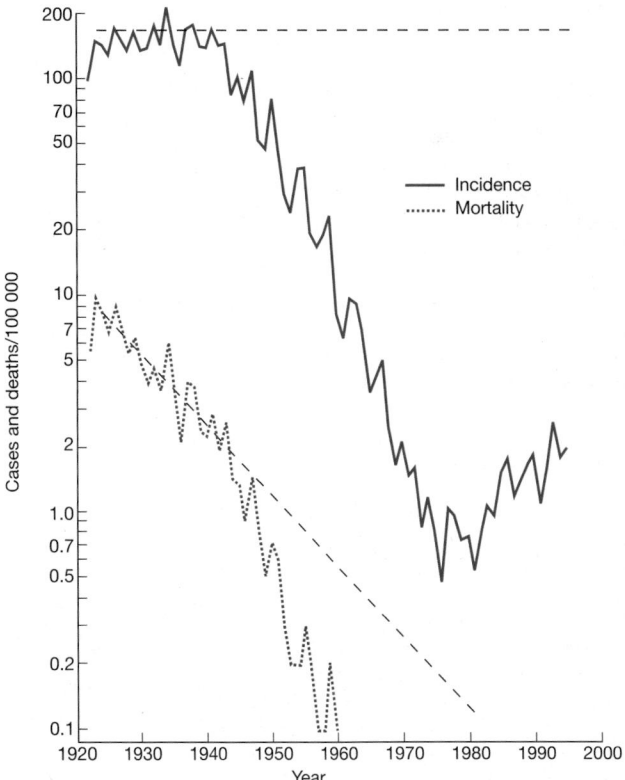

Fig. 1 The effect of pertussis vaccine on the incidence and mortality of pertussis in the United States. The lines superimposed on the graph indicate the trends prior to the vaccine and as projected if vaccine had not been introduced.

acquire infection from a patient and then transmit it to other hospital staff and to patients.

The epidemiology of *B. parapertussis* has not been modified by vaccine usage. It is widespread in many countries, but it is seldom recognized because of the mildness of the disease. In Denmark epidemics occur every 4 years, alternating with epidemics of *B. pertussis*.

Clinical manifestations

In *B. pertussis* infection, non-specific upper respiratory symptoms, malaise, anorexia, and sometimes a low-grade fever begin 7 to 10 days after infection. This 'catarrhal stage' is indistinguishable from other mild respiratory infections. Towards the end of this stage a dry, hacking cough appears and progresses. Older, presumed partially immune, patients may not progress further. After 1 to 2 weeks, the paroxysmal stage begins and continues for several weeks. The cough is now paroxysmal. Prolonged coughing episodes may be followed by the characteristic 'whoop', produced by forced inspiration through a partially closed glottis. In severe cases, paroxysms of coughing are followed by vomiting, and may be associated with epistaxis, petechias, conjunctival or scleral haemorrhages, haemorrhagic myringitis, or periorbital oedema. Young infants may not have the whoop. Their paroxysms of coughing may be followed by cyanosis and apnoea. Fever is uncommon at this stage in uncomplicated infections. The convalescent stage begins after 2 to 4 weeks, with gradually resolving paroxysms of coughing. Patients may cough for weeks to months. Their whooping may be exacerbated by subsequent viral respiratory infections.

Leucocytosis with lymphocytosis appears toward the end of the catarrhal stage and continues in the paroxysmal stage. Lymphocytosis is most marked when coughing is worst. There is a proportional increase in both T and B lymphocytes. Lymphocytosis may not occur in very young infants, older children, and adults.

Fever suggests a complicating bacterial infection. Otitis media and pneumonia are the most common. Atelectasis results from bronchial obstruction by the thick mucus. Bronchiectasis is uncommon. High pressures caused by paroxysmal coughing contribute to pulmonary, haemorrhagic, and gastrointestinal complications. These include mediastinal and subcutaneous emphysema, pneumothorax, inguinal hernias, and rectal prolapse. The extremely rare neurological complications include convulsions, paralysis, coma, blindness, deafness, and movement disorders.

B. parapertussis infections are clinically milder. Twenty per cent or less of children will develop the whooping cough syndrome. *B. bronchiseptica* rarely causes whooping cough. It is usually a non-pathogen in the respiratory tract but may cause bronchitis. In immunosuppressed patients, *B. bronchiseptica* can cause sinusitis, tracheobronchitis, and pneumonia. Bacteraemia, endocarditis, peritonitis, and meningitis have also been reported. *B. bronchiseptica* and *B. pertussis* have been reported in HIV-infected patients. *B. holmesii* septicaemia has been reported in compromised hosts.

Diagnosis

Definitive diagnosis is by isolation of the organism. Fluorescent antibody staining of material obtained by nasopharyngeal swabs from patients with *B. pertussis* infections provides only presumptive diagnosis. Polymerase chain reaction can be used for diagnosis, but assays are expensive and not standardized. Antibody responses can be measured in acute and convalescent sera by enzyme immunoassay.

The cough plate technique has been replaced by the nasopharyngeal culture technique. A wire calcium alginate swab is passed through the nose until it touches the posterior nasopharynx, allowed to remain for a few seconds, and removed. Cotton swabs may be used if the cotton has been shown to be non-bacteriostatic for *B. pertussis*. The swabs are streaked on

to Bordet–Gengou agar plates, both with and without an antibiotic such as cephalexin. Multiple cultures increase recovery of *B. pertussis*. The organism has not been recovered from blood or other sites. Cultures must be held for 6 days before being discarded.

B. parapertussis, *B. bronchiseptica*, and *B. holmesii* can also be recovered on Bordet–Gengou medium and they also grow on routine media used for recovery of Gram-negative bacteria. These three organisms have been recovered from blood cultures, and *B. bronchiseptica* has been cultured from urine.

Treatment

Most patients can be managed at home. Very young children may need good nursing care in hospital. Cough medicines are useless as is passive immunization with available immunoglobulin preparations. Salbutamol and steroids may be useful. Sedation of young children is potentially dangerous but is practised by some paediatricians.

B. pertussis, *B. parapertussis*, and *B. holmesii* are sensitive to erythromycin, tetracycline, chloramphenicol, and trimethoprim–sulphamethoxazole. Early treatment, during the catarrhal stage, shortens the clinical illness. Treatment started at the paroxysmal stage is much less effective. The best results are achieved by treating symptomatic contacts of patients with diagnosed infections. Despite limited clinical benefit, patients in the paroxysmal stage should be treated to render them non-infectious. Erythromycin is the drug of choice: 40 to 50 mg/kg per day for children, 1.5 to 2 g per day for adults, for 14 days. Nasopharyngeal cultures become negative in the first few days of treatment, but the erythromycin should be continued to prevent bacteriological relapses (Fig. 2). Trimethoprim–sulphamethoxazole has been used in children who do not tolerate erythromycin, although its efficacy has not been proved. The newer macrolides, clarithromycin and azithromycin, at 10 mg/kg per day for 5 to 7 days may be as effective as erythromycin.

B. bronchiseptica is sensitive to tetracycline and chloramphenicol but not to erythromycin. Antipseudomonal penicillins and aminoglycosides have been proved successful in serious infections.

Prevention

Patients with *B. pertussis* should avoid close contact with susceptible individuals to prevent droplet transmission. Untreated patients remain contagious for weeks. Communicability decreases rapidly after starting erythromycin. Nasopharyngeal cultures become negative within 48 to 72 h. Patients admitted to hospital are usually isolated for the first 5 days of treatment.

Chemoprophylaxis with erythromycin may be effective. Close contacts of patients with *B. pertussis* infection should be treated with erythromycin. Vaccination should continue according to routine schedules. Some recommend that, in addition to erythromycin, a booster dose of vaccine should be given to preschool children who have not received a booster within 6 months. Lower risk exposures, such as those occurring outside the home or day-care centre, require erythromycin only if respiratory symptoms develop.

Vaccination

Whole-cell pertussis vaccine prevents disease, but frequently causes local reactions, with or without fever, and rare neurological complications. Serious reactions occur less frequently after vaccination than with clinical disease. The killed whole-bacterial preparation is given with diphtheria and tetanus toxoids. An effective immunizing schedule includes three injections at 1- to 2-month intervals beginning at 6 to 12 weeks of age, and a fourth dose given 6 to 12 months after the third. A booster dose is given before

Fig. 2 Duration of excretion of *B. pertussis* as detected by fluorescent antibody staining and culture, and the effect of antimicrobial treatment. The graphs compare (group means) patients treated with antimicrobial agents with untreated control patients. (Reproduced from Bass JW *et al.* (1969), *Journal of Pediatrics* **75**, 768, with permission.)

entry to school. Acellular vaccines, containing three or four bacterial components—including pertussis toxoid, filamentous haemagglutinin, pertactin, and fimbriae—are replacing whole-cell vaccines, using the same immunization schedules.

Vaccination is usually restricted to children less than 7 years of age because of the local reactions, but immunity is neither complete nor life-long. Protection may last only 12 years. Duration of immunity after acellular vaccines is unknown. Re-exposure to *B. pertussis* may induce continuing immunity in previously vaccinated patients. In future, acellular vaccines may be deployed in older children and adults. There are no vaccines generally available for *B. parapertussis* or *B. bronchiseptica*.

Further reading

Hoppe JE (1999). Update on respiratory infection caused by *Bordetella parapertussis*. *Pediatric Infectious Disease Journal* **18**, 375–81.

Linnemann CC Jr (1979). Host–parasite interactions in pertussis. In: Manclark C, Hill J, eds. *International symposium on* pertussis, pp 3–18. US Government Printing Office, Washington, DC.

Muller FM, Hoppe JE, Wirsing von Konig CH (1997). Laboratory diagnosis of pertussis: state of the art in 1997. *Journal of Clinical Microbiology* **35**, 2435–43.

Thomas MG (1989). Epidemiology of pertussis. *Review of Infectious Diseases* **11**, 255–62.

Woolfrey BF, Moody JA (1991). Human infections associated with *Bordetella bronchiseptica*. *Clinical Microbiology Reviews* **4**, 243–55.

7.11.15 Melioidosis and glanders
D. A. B. Dance

Melioidosis

Definition and aetiology

Melioidosis is an infection of humans or animals caused by the saprophytic bacterium *Burkholderia* (previously *Pseudomonas*) *pseudomallei*. It is an ovoid, oxidase-positive, motile, Gram-negative bacillus that often exhibits 'safety-pin' bipolarity. It grows well on most standard culture media, producing wrinkled and smooth colony types and giving off a sweet, earthy smell. It has often been overlooked or discarded as a contaminant by bacteriologists unfamiliar with its characteristics. A pattern of resistance to aminoglycosides and polymyxins with susceptibility to co-amoxiclav is a useful clue to its identity.

Epidemiology

Distribution

Melioidosis is endemic throughout south and south-east Asia and northern Australia. Its incidence varies within these regions in both place and time, being particularly high in north-east Thailand during heavy monsoon years. It is likely to be underdiagnosed unless good laboratory facilities are available. Sporadic cases have been reported from sub-Saharan Africa, Central and South America, the Caribbean, and Iran. A unique outbreak occurred in France during the mid-1970s.

Reservoir and transmission

B. pseudomallei is an environmental saprophyte found in soil and surface water, particularly rice paddy, in endemic areas. A closely related, arabinose-assimilating, avirulent soil organism, *Burkholderia thailandensis*, has recently been recognized and may contribute to the high seropositivity rate in endemic areas (up to 80 per cent by the age of 4 years in north-east Thailand). Humans and animals are probably usually infected through contaminated scratches and abrasions or occasionally aspiration of fresh water, although a specific episode of exposure is rarely identified. Iatrogenic infections have also been described. Other possible modes of acquisition include inhalation and ingestion. Direct transmission from infected humans or animals is extremely rare.

Descriptive epidemiology and risk factors

Melioidosis is a disease of people in regular contact with soil and water, such as rice farmers. It has a bimodal age distribution, with a peak incidence between the ages of 40 and 60 years. Males outnumber females by 3:2 in Thailand but more in Australia and Singapore. The disease is markedly seasonal, some 80 per cent of cases presenting during the rainy season in north-east Thailand, when *B. pseudomallei* accounts for almost 20 per cent of cases of community-acquired septicaemia. Most such infections are probably recently acquired, although periods of latency as long as 29 years have been described, which is highly unusual for a bacterial infection. The proportion of seropositive people who are latently infected is unknown.

Pathogenesis

The outcome of contact with *B. pseudomallei* depends on the size of the inoculum, the virulence of the infecting strain, and the host response. Massive exposure will overwhelm a normal immune system, but most infections are self-limiting, resulting merely in asymptomatic seroconversion.

Host response

Clinically apparent melioidosis is an opportunistic disease, over 70 per cent of patients having underlying predisposition to infection. Diabetes mellitus is particularly strongly associated with melioidosis, but pre-existing renal disease and thalassaemia are also significant independent risk factors, and other reported associations include alcoholism and cirrhosis, malignant disease, immunosuppressive and steroid therapy, and pregnancy. In animal models, a T-helper type 1 immune response confers relative resistance to infection, and γ-interferon plays a crucial role in protecting against overwhelming sepsis. However, an overexuberant host response may also be damaging, as serum levels of several cytokines have been associated with a fatal outcome in human melioidosis. Humoral immunity may also play a role in defence, since animals may be passively protected by antibodies to lipopolysaccharide and flagellin, and levels of antilipopolysaccharide II correlate with survival in human melioidosis.

Virulence factors

Many putative virulence factors have been described in *B. pseudomallei* and transposon mutagenesis is proving useful in identifying their relative importance. For example, mutants deficient in one of the two forms of lipopolysaccharide produced by *B. pseudomallei*, lipopolysaccharide II, lose the natural resistance to complement-mediated bacteriolysis of the species and are 10 to 100 times less virulent in animal models than their parent strains. Other characteristics which may contribute to the pathogenicity of *B. pseudomallei* include: the ability to enter and survive in eukaryotic cells; the secretion of various extracellular enzymes (e.g. protease, lecithinase, and lipase); peptide, protein, and glycolipid toxins; extracellular polysaccharide; pili; a siderophore (malleobactin); and acid phosphatase.

Clinical features

B. pseudomallei may cause acute, chronic, localized, or disseminated infections. A 'flu-like' illness associated with seroconversion has been reported from Australia. Latent infections (see above) usually relapse at times of intercurrent stress ('Vietnam time bomb').

Septicaemic melioidosis

Sixty per cent of cases of culture-positive melioidosis have positive blood cultures. Most are clinically septicaemic; some have a more typhoid-like presentation. There is usually a short history (median 6 days; range 1 day to 2 months) of high fever and rigors. Approximately half the patients have evidence of a primary focus of infection, usually pulmonary or cutaneous. Confusion and stupor, jaundice, and diarrhoea may be prominent features. Initial investigations typically reveal anaemia, neutrophil leucocytosis, coagulopathy, and evidence of renal and hepatic impairment. Such patients often deteriorate rapidly, developing widespread metastatic abscesses, particularly in the lungs, liver, and spleen, and metabolic acidosis with Kussmaul's breathing. Once septic shock has supervened, case fatality approaches 95 per cent, many patients dying within 48 h of admission. Other poor prognostic features include absence of fever, leucopenia, azotaemia, and abnormal liver function tests.

If the patient survives this acute phase, multiple foci of dissemination become prominent. Cutaneous pustules or subcutaneous abscesses occur in approximately 10 per cent of cases and an abnormal chest radiograph is found in 80 per cent of patients, the most common pattern being widespread nodular shadowing ('bloodborne pneumonia'; Fig. 1). Other common sites for secondary lesions include the liver, spleen, kidneys, prostate, bones, and joints. Involvement of the central nervous system may also occur.

Fig. 1 Septicaemic melioidosis: widespread nodular shadowing—'bloodborne pneumonia' (by courtesy of Professor Sornchai Looareesuwan).

Localized melioidosis

The lung is the most frequent site. There is subacute, cavitating pneumonia accompanied by profound weight loss, often confused with tuberculosis (Fig. 2). Relative sparing of the apexes and infrequent hilar adenopathy may help to distinguish melioidosis from tuberculosis. There is a predilection

Fig. 2 Necrotizing *B. pseudomallei* pneumonia with central cavitation and fluid level in a rice farmer in north-east Thailand being treated with corticosteroids for nephrotic syndrome. Such patients are often misdiagnosed as having smear-negative tuberculosis, but fail to respond to antituberculous chemotherapy. (By courtesy of Professor Sornchai Looareesuwan.)

for the upper lobes. Complications include pneumothorax, empyema, purulent pericarditis, and progression to septicaemia.

Acute suppurative parotitis is a characteristic manifestation of melioidosis in children, accounting for approximately one-third of childhood cases in north-east Thailand (Fig. 3). The reason is unknown. Most cases are unilateral and result in parotid abscesses requiring surgical drainage. They may rupture spontaneously into the auditory canal. Facial nerve palsy and septicaemia are rare complications.

Other sites of localized infection include cutaneous and subcutaneous abscesses, lymphadenitis, osteomyelitis and septic arthritis, liver and/or splenic abscesses, cystitis, pyelonephritis, prostatic abscesses, epididymo-orchitis, keratitis, and rarely, brain abscesses.

(a)

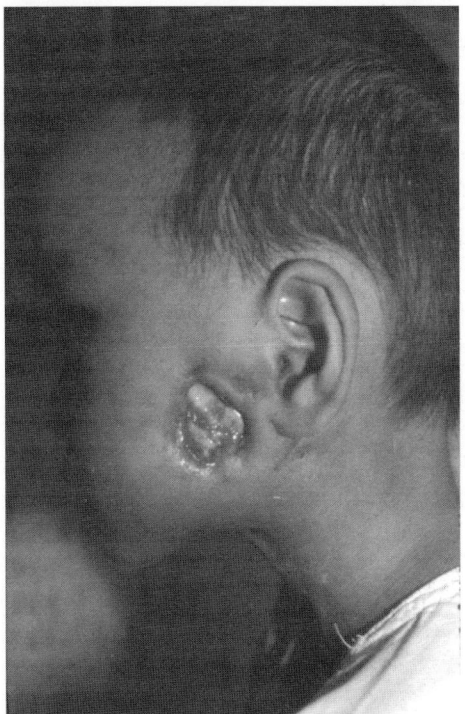

(b)

Fig. 3 (a) Acute suppurative parotitis—a common manifestation of childhood melioidosis in north-east Thailand. This child had parotid abscesses that required drainage despite having already ruptured into the auditory canal, extensive overlying ulceration, facial nerve palsy, and septicaemia. (b) Ulceration over healing parotid abscess.

Pathology

B. pseudomallei is pyogenic, causing localized abscesses or granulomas, depending on the duration of the lesion. The presence of 'globi' of Gram-negative bacilli within macrophages and giant cells may give a clue to the aetiology.

Laboratory diagnosis

The diagnosis should be considered in any patient who has ever visited an endemic area and presents with septicaemia, abscesses, or chronic suppuration, particularly if there is evidence of an underlying disease such as diabetes mellitus. Specific diagnosis depends on the detection of *B. pseudomallei* or of corresponding antibodies. The laboratory should always be warned if melioidosis is suspected, both to enable appropriate methods and media to be employed, and to alert staff to the risk of infection (containment level 3 organism).

Microscopy and culture

Gram staining of smears of pus or secretions may reveal bipolar or unevenly staining Gram-negative rods, but this is neither specific nor sensitive. The most useful rapid diagnostic technique is immunofluorescent microscopy of smears. The mainstay of diagnosis is isolation and identification of *B. pseudomallei* from blood, pus, urine, sputum, or other specimens. The organism is not difficult to grow, although special selective media will increase the isolation rate from sites with a normal flora.

Serodiagnosis

Several tests for antibodies to *B. pseudomallei* have been described. The indirect haemagglutination test remains the most widely available. Assays that detect IgG give similar results. These tests are useful in patients from non-endemic areas in whom a single indirect haemagglutination titre in excess of 1:40 is highly suggestive of melioidosis. In populations continually exposed to *B. pseudomallei*, the high background seropositivity reduces the predictive value of the tests, and in such patients only a rising or very high titre suggests active melioidosis. Assays that detect specific IgM correlate better with disease activity but are not widely available.

Antigen and nucleic acid detection

Numerous antigen detection and polymerase chain reaction systems have been described, but all have problems of specificity and sensitivity.

Treatment

Treatment—general

Patients with septicaemic melioidosis require intensive supportive treatment, ideally in an intensive care unit. Particular attention should be paid to correction of volume depletion and septic shock, respiratory and renal failure, and hyperglycaemia or ketoacidosis. Abscesses should be drained whenever possible.

Antibiotic susceptibility

B. pseudomallei is intrinsically resistant to many antibiotics, including aminoglycosides and early β-lactams. Failure to respond to these agents may suggest the diagnosis of melioidosis.

Antibiotic therapy—acute phase

Five, randomized, controlled studies of regimens for the treatment of acute severe melioidosis have now been published. Two showed that regimens containing β-lactam approximately halved the mortality compared with conventional chloramphenicol plus doxycycline plus co-trimoxazole. Imipenem/cilastatin had a lower treatment failure rate than ceftazidime, which itself had a lower failure rate than co-amoxiclav. β-Lactam/co-trimoxazole combinations may have lower mortality and relapse rates than β-lactams alone, but larger studies are needed to confirm this. Unfortunately, all these

Table 1 Treatment regimens used for the acute phase of therapy in acute severe melioidosis

Agent	Dose (mg/kg.day)	
Imipenem	50	(3 divided doses)
Ceftazidime	120	(3 divided doses)
Ceftazidime	100	(3 divided doses)
plus co-trimoxazole	8/40	(3 divided doses)
Cefoperazone/sulbactam	25	(3 divided doses)
plus co-trimoxazole	8/40	(3 divided doses)
Co-amoxiclav	160	(6 divided doses)
Chloramphenicol	100	(4 divided doses)
plus doxycycline	4	(2 divided doses)
plus co-trimoxazole	10/50	(2 divided doses)

All regimens should be given for at least 2 weeks and should be followed by maintenance therapy. Doses should be adjusted according to renal function.

β-lactams are too expensive to be practical in most endemic countries. The regimens used for acute treatment are listed in Table 1.

Antibiotic therapy—maintenance phase or mild disease

Long courses of oral antibiotics are needed to prevent relapse. Less than 12 weeks of treatment is inadequate, and the usual recommendation is 20 weeks. The conventional combination regimen was associated with a lower relapse rate than co-amoxiclav. The latter is preferable in children and pregnant women because of the risks of toxicity. Fluoroquinolones and doxycycline alone give unacceptable results, but co-trimoxazole alone warrants further evaluation. Regimens are given in Table 2.

Prognosis

In septicaemic melioidosis, the level of bacteraemia correlates with outcome. Even with optimal treatment, case fatality from acute severe melioidosis is high (25 to 40 per cent). Often survivors remain chronically ill both from the disease itself and the underlying conditions. At least 5 per cent of patients will still relapse despite long courses of antibiotics, particularly if compliance is poor. Antibiotic resistance may develop during treatment. Long-term follow-up should therefore be arranged. Monitoring of IgM titres or C-reactive protein may help early detection of relapse.

Prevention and control

No vaccines are available for human use. The only preventive measure is avoidance of exposure to the organism in soil for high-risk groups (e.g. people with diabetes). Both ciprofloxacin and doxycycline confer partial protection when given prophylactically to animals. Although person-to-person spread is rare, isolation of patients is recommended.

Glanders

Definition and aetiology

Glanders is a disease of horses caused by *Burkholderia mallei*, which may occasionally be transmitted to humans or other animals. Traditionally,

Table 2 Maintenance treatment regimens for melioidosis

Agent	Dose (mg/kg.day)
Co-amoxiclav	60/15 (4 divided doses)
Chloramphenicol	40 (4 divided doses for the first 4 weeks)
plus doxycycline	4 (2 divided doses)
plus co-trimoxazole	10/50 (2 divided doses)

These should be given following acute-phase treatment to complete at least 12 weeks, and preferably 20 weeks, of treatment in total. Doses should be adjusted according to renal function.

glanders, a systemic respiratory tract disease, has been distinguished from farcy, a cutaneous infection.

In the early 1900s, equine glanders occurred worldwide. Over 200 000 horses were destroyed because of glanders during the First World War. However, no naturally acquired case has been reported in the United States or the United Kingdom since 1938.

It is thought still to occur in the Middle East, Africa, and Asia. Human infection, always uncommon, is confined to those in close contact with horses.

B. mallei is closely related to *B. pseudomallei* both taxonomically and antigenically, but it grows less luxuriantly in culture and is non-motile.

Clinical features

Glanders resembles melioidosis. Manifestations include septicaemia, wound infection, ulceration, lymphangitis with abscesses along the course of lymphatic drainage ('farcy buds'), ulceration of the respiratory (especially nasal) mucosa, polyarthritis, pneumonia and lung abscesses, nodular abscesses in any site, particularly muscle and subcutaneous tissue, and a widespread pustular rash.

Laboratory diagnosis

Diagnosis hinges on a history of contact with horses in an endemic area or laboratory exposure, and either the isolation of *B. mallei* or detection of specific antibodies. Like *B. pseudomallei* it requires handling in a containment level 3 laboratory.

Treatment

In vitro susceptibility is similar to that of *B. pseudomallei*, and so glanders should respond to the regimens used for melioidosis.

Further reading

Melioidosis

Chaowagul W *et al.* (1999). A comparison of chloramphenicol, trimethoprim–sulfamethoxazole, and doxycycline with doxycycline alone as maintenance therapy for melioidosis. *Clinical Infectious Diseases* **29**, 375–80.

Chong VFH, Fan YF (1996). The radiology of melioidosis. *Australasian Radiology* **40**, 244–9.

Dance DAB (1991). Melioidosis: the tip of the iceberg? *Clinical Microbiology Reviews* **4**, 52–60.

Simpson AJ *et al.* (1999). Comparison of imipenem and ceftazidime as therapy for severe melioidosis. *Clinical Infectious Diseases* **29**, 381–7.

Woods DE *et al.* (1999). Current studies on the pathogenesis of melioidosis. *Microbes and Infection* **2**, 157–62.

Glanders

Howe C. (1950). Glanders. In: *Oxford system of medicine*, Vol. 5, pp. 185–202. Oxford University Press.

7.11.16 Plague

T. Butler

History

Plague may have caused more deaths than most other diseases and warfare combined; it was estimated to have killed a quarter of Europe's population in the Middle Ages. The present pandemic of plague began in China in the 1860s and was spread by rats transported on ships to California and to ports in South America, Africa, and Asia. The genus of the plague bacillus is called *Yersinia* because Alexandre Yersin (1863 to 1943) went to Hong Kong in 1894 and successfully isolated the causative organism in pure culture. Urban plague transmitted by rats was brought under control in most affected cities, but the infection was transferred to sylvatic rodents, allowing it to become entrenched in rural areas of these countries. In the 1960s and 1970s, Vietnam during its war became the leading country for plague, reporting more than 10 000 cases a year. In 1994 in Surat, India, an outbreak of primary pneumonic plague was reported. There were hundreds of suspected cases, with 50 deaths, and thousands fled the city. However, none of the cases were confirmed by sputum culture. In 1997, Madagascar experienced an epidemic of pneumonic plague in which 8 out of 18 infected persons died.

Bacteriology

Yersinia pestis (formerly *Pasteurella pestis*), the cause of plague, is an aerobic, Gram-negative bacillus of the family Enterobacteriaceae. It is readily identified by its failure to ferment lactose on MacConkey agar, an alkaline slant and acid butt in triple-sugar–iron agar, and negative reactions for citrate utilization, urease, and indole. *Y. pestis* is virulent because it carries a 45 MDa plasmid that encodes for V and W antigens, which confer a requirement for calcium to grow at 37°C. Additionally, it produces lipopolysaccharide endotoxin and a capsular envelope containing the antiphagocytic principle fraction I antigen.

Epidemiology

From 1990 to 1996, there were 16 000 cases of plague and 1214 deaths (7.6 per cent) reported to the World Health Organization. The countries that reported more than 100 cases were, in the order from greatest number to least: Tanzania, Madagascar, Vietnam, Congo, Peru, India, Myanmar, Zimbabwe, China, and Uganda. In the United States, all the 64 plague cases occurred in the south-western states of New Mexico, Arizona, Colorado, Utah, and California. Most of the American cases occur during the months of May to October, when people are outdoors coming into contact with rodents and their fleas. Each endemic region has a specific season when plague tends to occur.

Plague is a zoonotic infection transmitted among animal reservoirs by flea bites and ingestion of animal tissues. The major animal reservoirs are urban and domestic rats as well as rural field rodents including ground squirrels and prairie dogs. The oriental rat flea *Xenopsylla cheopis* is the most efficient vector. When bitten by a rodent flea humans become an accidental host and play no role in disease transmission except in rare epidemics of pneumonic plague. Epizootics usually accompany human cases and can cause large die-offs of susceptible rodent species. Human plague affects both sexes and children of all ages depending on their exposure to rodent fleas. Risk factors for acquiring plague include contact with rodents or carnivores and presence of refuges or food sources for wild rodents near the home.

Pathogenesis

Bacteria are inoculated into the skin by a flea bite and migrate to regional lymph nodes, where they multiply during an incubation period of 2 to 8 days. Inflamed lymph nodes called buboes show polymorphonuclear leucocytes, destruction of normal architecture, haemorrhagic necrosis, and dense concentrations of extracellular plague bacilli. Bacteraemia occurs and results in purulent, necrotic, and haemorrhagic lesions in many organs.

Table 1 Plague syndromes

Syndrome	Features
Bubonic	Fever, painful lymphadenopathy (bubo)
Septicaemic	Fever, hypotension without bubo
Pneumonic	Cough, haemoptysis, with or without bubo
Cutaneous	Pustule, eschar, carbuncle, or ecthyma gangrenosum, usually with bubo
Meningitis	Fever, nuchal rigidity, usually with bubo

Clinical manifestations

Bubonic plague

The most common presentation is acute lymphadenitis called bubonic plague (Table 1). The people of plague endemic regions know the disease and have local names, such as *dich hach* in Vietnamese, that conjure up the horror of recalled fatalities during previous seasons. Patients are affected by the sudden onset of fever, chills, weakness, and headache. Usually, at the same time, after a few hours, or on the next day, they notice the bubo, which is signalled by intense pain in one anatomical region of lymph nodes, usually the groin, axilla, or neck. A swelling evolves in this area, which is so tender that the patients typically avoid any motion that might provoke discomfort. For example, if the bubo is in the femoral area, the patient will characteristically flex, abduct, and externally rotate the hip to relieve pressure on the area and will walk with a limp. When the bubo is in an axilla, the patient will abduct the shoulder or hold the arm in a splint. When a bubo is in the neck, patients will tilt their head to the opposite side.

The buboes are oval swellings that vary from 1 to 10 cm in length and elevate the overlying skin, which may appear stretched or erythematous. They may appear either as a smooth, uniform, ovoid mass or as an irregular cluster of several nodes with intervening and surrounding oedema (Fig. 1). There is warmth of the overlying skin and an underlying tender, firm, nonfluctuant mass. Occasionally, there is a large area of oedema extending from the bubo into the region drained by the affected lymph nodes. Although infections other than plague can produce acute lymphadenitis, plague is virtually unique for the suddenness of onset of the disease and fulminant clinical course that can produce death in 2 to 4 days after the onset of symptoms. The bubo of plague is also distinctive for the usual absence of a detectable skin lesion or ascending lymphangitis in its anatomical region.

The patients are typically prostrate and lethargic, and often exhibit restlessness or agitation. Occasionally, they are delirious with high fever, and seizures are common in children. Temperature is usually elevated in the range 38.5 to 40.0°C, and the pulse rate is increased to 110 to 140/min.

Fig. 1 A right femoral bubo consists of an enlarged, tender lymph node with surrounding oedema.

Fig. 2 A right axillary bubo was accompanied by a purulent ulcer on the abdomen, which was the presumed site of the flea bite.

Fig. 3 Bubo aspirate shows bipolar bacilli stained with methylene blue (Wayson's stain).

Blood pressure is characteristically low, around 100/60 mmHg, and may be unobtainable if shock ensues. The liver and spleen are often palpable and tender.

About one-quarter of patients in Vietnam showed varied skin lesions including pustules, vesicles, eshars, or papules in the anatomical region that is lymphatically drained by the affected lymph nodes, and they presumably represent sites of the flea bites (Fig. 2). Purpuric lesions may develop and become necrotic, resulting in gangrene of distal extremities, the probable basis of the epithet 'Black Death' attributed to plague through the ages.

Other plague syndromes

Less common presentations may accompany the bubo or occur without a bubo. Septicaemic plague refers to bacteremia without a bubo. Pneumonic plague occurs as a secondary pneumonia due to bacteremic spread in about 10 per cent of patients with bubonic plague. Person-to-person spread of pneumonia by a coughing patient is less common, and a few cases of inhalation pneumonia have occurred in persons who handled sick cats. Bacterial meningitis is a rare complication of plague. Acute pharyngitis may occur.

Laboratory findings

The white blood-cell count is typically elevated in the range of 10 000 to 20 000 cells/mm³, with a predominance of immature and mature neutrophils. Occasionally, some patients, especially children, may develop myelocytic leukaemoid reactions with white cell counts as high as 100 000/mm³. Blood platelets may be normal or low in the early stages of bubonic plague. Although patients with plague rarely develop a generalized bleeding tendency from profound thrombocytopenia, disseminated intravascular coagulation is common in this infection. Liver function tests, including serum aminotransferases and bilirubin, are frequently abnormally high. Renal function tests may be abnormal in hypotensive patients.

Diagnosis

Plague should be suspected in febrile patients who have been exposed to rodents or other mammals in the known endemic areas of the world. A bacteriological diagnosis is readily made by Gram stain and culture of a bubo aspirate. The aspirate is obtained by inserting a 20-gauge needle on a 10-ml syringe containing 1 ml of sterile saline into the bubo and withdrawing it several times until the saline becomes blood tinged. Because the bubo does not contain liquid pus, it may be necessary to inject some of the saline and immediately reaspirate it. The Gram stain will reveal polymorphonu-

clear leucocytes and Gram-negative coccobacilli and bacilli ranging from 1 to 2 μm in length (Fig. 3). Smears of blood, sputum, or spinal fluid can be handled similarly (Fig. 4).

The aspirate, blood, and other appropriate fluids should be inoculated on to blood and MacConkey agar plates and into infusion broth for bacteriological identification. At some reference laboratories, a serological test, the passive hemagglutination test or an ELISA utilizing fraction I of *Y. pestis*, is available for testing acute- and convalescent-phase serum. A fourfold or greater increase in titre or a single titre of 1:16 or higher is presumptive evidence of plague.

Treatment and prevention
Antimicrobials

Untreated plague has an estimated mortality rate of more than 50 per cent. Therefore, the early institution of effective antimicrobial therapy is mandatory following appropriate cultures. In 1948, streptomycin was identified as the drug of choice for the treatment of plague by reducing the mortality rate to less than 5 per cent. Streptomycin should be given intramuscularly in two divided doses daily, totalling 30 mg/kg body weight per day for 10 days. Most patients improve rapidly and become afebrile in about 3 days. The 10-day course of streptomycin is recommended to prevent

Fig. 4 Gram stain of spinal fluid in plague meningitis shows numerous Gram-negative bacilli.

relapses because viable bacteria have been isolated from buboes of patients with plague during convalescence.

When an oral drug is preferred, tetracycline is a satisfactory alternative. It is given orally in a dose of 2 to 4 g/day in four divided doses for 10 days. Tetracycline is contraindicated in children younger than 7 years of age and in pregnant women because it stains developing teeth. It is also contraindicated in renal failure. As an alternative drug that is especially suitable for meningitis, chloramphenicol can be given intravenously as a loading dose of 25 mg/kg of body weight followed by 60 mg/kg of body weight per day in four divided doses. After clinical improvement, chloramphenicol can be continued orally in a dose of 30 mg/kg to complete a total course of 10 days. There is no rationale for using multiple antibiotics to treat plague.

Other antimicrobial drugs have been used in plague or in experimental animal infections with varying success. These include sulphonamides, trimethoprim–sulphamethoxazole, kanamycin, gentamicin, ampicillin, cephalosporins, and fluoroquinolones. These drugs either are less effective than streptomycin or have not been subjected to adequate clinical studies and, therefore, should not be routinely chosen. An isolate from a 16-year-old boy in Madagascar in 1995 was resistant to streptomycin, tetracycline, chloramphenicol, and sulphonamide but was susceptible to trimethoprim–sulphamethoxazole. He recovered after receiving trimethoprim–sulphamethoxazole. Other than this case, antibiotic resistance in *Y. pestis* from humans has never been reported, nor has resistance emerged during antibiotic therapy.

Supportive therapy

Intravenous 0.9 per cent saline solution should be given to most patients for the first few days of the illness or until improvement occurs. Patients in shock will require additional quantities of fluid, with haemodynamic monitoring and use of vasopressors. The buboes usually recede without local therapy. Occasionally, however, they may enlarge or become fluctuant during the first week of treatment, requiring incision and drainage.

Precautions and prevention

Patients with plague who are promptly treated present no health hazard to other people. Those with a cough or other signs of pneumonia must be placed in respiratory isolation for at least 48 h after starting therapy or until the sputum culture is negative. The bubo aspirate and blood must be handled with gloves and with care to avoid aerosolization. Vaccines have been developed but at present are not available. Health departments advise personal protection against rodents and fleas, including living in rat-proof houses, wearing shoes and garments to cover the legs, and dusting houses with insecticide. For persons who report close contact with a coughing patient, prophylaxis with oral doxycycline or trimethoprim–sulfamethoxazole is advised.

Further reading

Butler T (1994). *Yersinia infections*: Centennial of the discovery of the plague bacillus. *Clinical Infectious Diseases* 19, 655–63.

Byrne WR et al. (1998). Antibiotic treatment of experimental pneumonic plague in mice. *Antimicrobial Agents and Chemotherapy* 42, 675–81.

Campbell GL, Hughes JM (1995). Plague in India: a new warning from an old nemesis. *Annals of Internal Medicine* 122, 151–3.

Chanteau S et al. (1998). F1 antigenaemia in bubonic plague patients, a marker of gravity and efficacy of therapy. *Transactions of the Royal Society of Tropical Medicine and Hygiene* 92, 572–3.

Crook LD, Tempest B (1992). Plague. A clinical review of 27 cases. *Archives of Internal Medicine* 152, 1253–6.

Galimand M et al. (1997). Multidrug resistance in *Yersinia pestis* mediated by a transferable plasmid. *New England Journal of Medicine* 337, 677–80.

Ratsitorahina M et al. (2000). Epidemiological and diagnostic aspects of the outbreak of pneumonic plague in Madagascar. *Lancet* 355, 111–13.

7.11.17 Yersinia, Pasteurella, and Francisella

*David Lalloo**

Yersiniosis

Definition

Yersiniosis is a disease caused by two species of enteric bacteria, *Yersinia enterocolitica* and *Yersinia pseudotuberculosis*. They cause a wide spectrum of clinical manifestations, which includes acute watery diarrhoea, acute mesenteric adenitis, extraintestinal infection, and bacteraemia. Postinfectious sequelae such as arthritis or erythema nodosum are also common.

The organisms

Yersinia sp. belong to the family Enterobacteriaceae. They are aerobic facultative and anaerobic, Gram-negative coccobacilli which grow on bile-containing media. There are three human pathogens within the genus, *Y. pseudotuberculosis*, *Y. enterocolitica*, and *Y. pestis*. The last, the causative organism of plague, is considered elsewhere (Chapter 7.11.16). Yersinia are usually non-lactose fermenting, catalase positive, and oxidase negative. The recovery of yersinia from stool samples can be improved by use of cefsulodin–irgasan–novobiocin (**CIN**) agar, cold enrichment, or potassium hydroxide pretreatment, but such manoeuvres are only occasionally necessary for clinical specimens. *Y. enterocolitica* can be divided into five biovars on the basis of biochemical reactions. The clinical and epidemiological significance of these biovars remains uncertain. Over 50 serogroups of *Y. enterocolitica* have been described, on the basis of O (somatic lipopolysaccharide) and H (flagellar) antigens. Six serotypes of *Y. pseudotuberculosis* have been described.

Virulence and pathogenicity

There are clear differences in virulence between strains of *Y. enterocolitica*; human disease is caused by a limited number of serotypes. A number of important factors have been identified. The possession of a 40 to 50 MDa plasmid is associated with virulence *in vitro* and the VW antigen complex and plasmid-encoded yersinia outer membrane proteins (YOPs) appear to be important in pathogenesis. The ability of yersinia to utilize exogenous iron by a number of mechanisms, including binding of exogenous siderophores, also appears to be an important factor in virulence; serious yersinia infections are much more common in patients with iron-overload syndromes. The vast majority of isolates produce enterotoxin, which is related to the enterotoxin of *Escherichia coli*. However, the role of enterotoxin in the production of diarrhoea remains uncertain and enterotoxin production does not correlate with other tests of virulence.

Most yersinia infections result from invasion via the gastrointestinal tract. Organisms adhere to the surface of the ileum and may invade the intestinal mucosa, via a bacterial outer membrane protein, invasin, which binds to a ligand on the cell surface. Bacteria multiply within intestinal epithelial cells and may reach Peyer's patches, where further multiplication occurs, with the potential for systemic spread.

Epidemiology

Y. enterocolitica causes infection throughout the world, but appears most common in the temperate regions, particularly northern Europe and North

* This chapter is based on A. D. Pearson's account in the third edition of the *Oxford Textbook of Medicine* and the editors and author take pleasure in acknowledging his contribution.

America. Both sporadic infections and outbreaks occur. Infection with serotypes 03 and 09 predominate in Europe whereas 08 and 03 are more commonly responsible for infection in North America. Yersiniosis is a zoonotic infection but usually causes foodborne illnesses. Animal reservoirs of *Y. enterocolitica* include pigs, rabbits, goats, cattle, horses, rodents, dogs, and cats. Animals may carry the organism asymptomatically in the oropharynx or gastrointestinal tract. The most important source of infection for man is the pig, although contact with household pets has also been implicated. Humans are infected via the faecal–oral route, usually after eating or drinking contaminated food or water; incompletely cooked pork is a major risk factor. Infection may also occur by person-to-person or direct animal-to-person contact and transmission through contaminated blood products has been reported. Infants and young children appear to be more susceptible to infection with *Y. enterocolitica* than adults. Most infections are sporadic but a number of specific outbreaks have been identified, following ingestion of contaminated foods such as pork chitterlings (intestines), water, or dairy products.

Infection with *Y. pseudotuberculosis* is less common, although cases are increasingly reported from Japan. Infection results from contact with both sylvatic and domestic animals and a number of birds. It most commonly affects patients aged between 5 and 20 years.

Clinical features

The usual incubation period for the acute manifestations of yersiniosis is 3 to 7 days. Common clinical syndromes are shown in Table 1. The most common manifestation of infection with *Y. enterocolitica* is an acute gastroenteritis, which particularly affects young children. Diarrhoea, fever, and abdominal pain may all be prominent. Stools contain mucus, leucocytes, and red blood cells; the organism can usually be detected on stool cultures. Clinically, the syndrome is indistinguishable from salmonella or campylobacter infection. Symptoms may last for up to 3 weeks and patients remain infectious over this period with continuous shedding of organism in the faeces. Rare complications include diffuse ulceration of the small intestine and colon, perforation, intussusception, toxic megacolon, cholangitis, and mesenteric vein thrombosis.

Older children more often develop mesenteric adenitis and terminal ileitis with either *Y. enterocolitica* or *Y. pseudotuberculosis* infection; this is the most common manifestation of *Y. pseudotuberculosis* infection. The presentation mimics appendicitis with fever, abdominal pain, right lower quadrant pain, and leucocytosis. Diarrhoea is unusual. Ultrasound and/or computed tomography may be helpful in demonstrating a normal appendix and enlarged mesenteric nodes. The infection is usually self-limited. At laparotomy, enlarged mesenteric lymph nodes are found in the iliocaecal angle and there may be swelling of the terminal ileum or caecum. This presentation must be distinguished from acute appendicitis, or diseases causing terminal ileal disease such as Crohn's, tuberculosis, and rarely, neoplasia.

Y. enterocolitica may cause focal infection both in the absence of detectable bacteraemia and following bacteraemia. Isolated focal infection has been described in many sites, including the pharynx, skin and subcutaneous tissues, bones and joints, the conjunctiva, the renal tract, lungs, and

Table 1 Common clinical manifestations of Yersinia infection

Y. enterocolitica	Gastroenteritis
	Mesenteric adenitis
	Terminal ileitis
	Bacteraemia
	Pharyngitis
	Hepatic abscesses
	Erythema nodosum
	Reactive polyarthropathy
Y. pseudotuberculosis	Mesenteric adenitis
	Terminal ileitis
	Bacteraemia

peritoneum. *Y. enterocolitica* bacteraemia most often occurs in patients with chronic conditions such as diabetes, chronic liver disease, malignancy, and conditions causing immunosuppression. There is also a strong association with iron-overload syndromes or the treatment of iron overload (*Y. enterocolitica* is able to use exogenous iron chelators such as desferrioxamine to acquire iron itself). Over half of systemic bacteraemias are in patients with iron-overload syndromes; multiple hepatic abscesses may occur and the case fatality rate may reach 50 per cent in this population. Overall, the case fatality rates for *Y. enterocolitica* bacteraemia have ranged from 7.5 to 25 per cent over the last decade. Bacteraemia may lead to metastatic infections including endocarditis, intravenous line infection, meningitis, and septic arthritis.

Y. pseudotuberculosis bacteraemia is much less common, but is often associated with chronic illness. Case fatality rates are extremely high in the immunocompromised population. In Japan, *Y. pseudotuberculosis* infection has been associated with renal failure in young children.

Secondary, postinfective, complications are common following yersinia infection. In Scandinavia, they have been reported in up to 30 per cent of patients with *Y. enterocolitica* infection. A reactive polyarthropathy or erythema nodosum are the most common manifestations, classically occurring 1 to 2 weeks after an acute illness. Reiter's syndrome, glomerulonephritis, and myocarditis have also been described. The arthritis is polyarticular and asymmetrical, typically affecting the large joints of the lower limbs. There is a strong association with the possession of HLA B27. Synovial fluid culture is normally sterile although yersinia antigens can be found in the synovial tissue of patients. Symptoms of reactive polyarthritis may take several months to settle. The exact immunological mechanism of these postinfectious manifestations remains uncertain.

Diagnosis

Yersinia infection should be considered in anyone with fever and abdominal pain. A definitive diagnosis of yersiniosis may be made by culture of the organism from stool, lymph nodes, or blood depending upon the clinical presentation. However, isolation from stool may sometimes be slow because of the overgrowth of other faecal flora. Cold enrichment or CIN media may be used to optimize recovery from faecal samples.

A number of serological techniques, including tube agglutination assay, radioimmunoassays, and enzyme immunoassays, have been used to diagnose infection with yersinia. High titres in a previously healthy individual are suggestive of infection, but fourfold rises in titre are rarely found. Interpretation may be made difficult by cross-reactivity with *Brucella*, *Rickettsia*, and *Salmonella* spp. and possibly thyroid tissue antigens; some populations also have a high background prevalence of positive serology. Negative or minimal titres can occur following yersiniosis in infants or immunocompromised patients. Definitive diagnosis therefore depends upon the culture of the organism. However, serology is often the only way of diagnosing postinfectious complications as stool cultures may be negative by the time of appearance of symptoms such as arthritis. *Y. pseudotuberculosis* may be found in sterile site samples, but is rarely isolated from stool. Serology is often the only mode of diagnosis available; antigens cross-react with those of *Y. enterocolitica*.

Treatment

Antimicrobial therapy is not indicated in uncomplicated disease and treatment does not shorten the course or severity of enterocolitis. Localized infection, bacteraemia, and systemic disease, or enterocolitis in an immunocompromised patient, should be treated. *Y. enterocolitica* is resistant to most penicillins and first-generation cephalosporins due to the production of chromosomally encoded β-lactamases. Minimum inhibitory concentrations for amoxycillin/clavulanate combinations vary considerably; this drug should not be used for the treatment of infections. Aminoglycosides, chloramphenicol, tetracycline, and co-trimoxazole are all effective *in vitro* and have been used clinically with success. Third-generation cephalosporins are also effective, although in one recent study they were only successful in 85 per cent of cases, even when used in combination with other drugs. Fluoroquinolones have very good *in vitro* activity against yersinia and have been used successfully in clinical practice, but the optimal antibiotic therapy for the treatment of *Y. enterocolitica* has still to be determined. *Y. pseudotuberculosis* is sensitive to ampicillin and cephalosporins in addition to the drugs already discussed.

Pasteurella

Introduction

Pasteurella spp. are Gram-negative coccobacilli which cause a wide spectrum of disease in humans, ranging from local infection and abscesses to severe systemic infection. The majority of human infections are caused by *P. multocida*. They are most often acquired from contact with domestic animals.

The organism

Pasteurella spp. are small, non-motile, Gram-negative coccobacilli. They grow aerobically or as facultative anaerobes on standard media at 37°C; growth is enhanced by enrichment with carbon dioxide. They are oxidase and catalase positive and may stain bipolarly on Gram stain, sometimes being confused with *Haemophilus*, *Neisseria*, or *Acinetobacter* spp. *Pasteurella* spp. are a major veterinary pathogen, but only four species have been associated with human disease. The vast majority of human infections are caused by *P. multocida*, subspecies *septica* and subspecies *multocida*. Four capsular antigens and 15 somatic antigens of *P. multocida* have been identified. The capsule appears to be important in pathogenesis; heavily capsulate strains are resistant to phagocytosis.

Epidemiology

P. multocida is widely distributed as a nasopharyngeal or gastrointestinal commensal of animals and birds. The organism is carried by 70 to 90 per cent of cats and 50 to 70 per cent of dogs, but is also found in a large number of other domestic and wild animals. The organism can survive in water or soil for up to a month. *P. multocida* is a major animal pathogen, causing a number of different diseases, including fowl cholera and haemorrhagic septicaemia in wildstock.

Humans usually acquire infection with *P. multocida* from bites, scratches, or licks of dogs and cats, or close contact with these animals. However, in up to 15 per cent of cases, no known animal contact occurs. *Pasteurella* spp. can be isolated from 20 to 30 per cent of dog bite wounds and 50 per cent of cat bite wounds, although only a small proportion will become clinically infected. In clinically infected wounds, *Pasteurella* spp. are identified in 50 per cent of dog bites and 75 per cent of cat bites. Person-to-person spread has not been recorded, although *P. multocida* can occasionally be found in the nasopharynx of healthy humans exposed to animals.

Clinical features

P. multocida has been associated with a wide variety of different clinical presentations, outlined in Table 2. The vast majority of infections are due to animal bites which cause local soft tissue infection manifesting with remarkable rapidity. Symptoms and signs may develop within several hours of the bite. Local erythema, swelling, and purulent discharge are common; fever, lymphangitis, and local lymph node swelling may also occur. Soft tissue infections may also involve deeper tissues, causing abscesses, tenosynovitis, septic arthritis, or osteomyelitis.

The second most common site of isolation of *P. multocida* is the respiratory tract. Some of these patients have no history of animal contact, but over 90 per cent have chronic respiratory tract disease, particularly chronic obstructive pulmonary disease, bronchiectasis, or malignancy. Isolation of *Pasteurella* spp. may sometimes represent long-term colonization, but acute

Table 2 Infections caused by *Pasteurella multocida*

Skin and soft tissue infections
Cellulitis; subcutaneous abscess; infected ulcers; wound infection

Oral and respiratory infections
Tonsillitis or peritonsillar abscess; sinusitis, pharyngitis, and epiglottitis; otitis media, mastoiditis and submandibular abscess; pneumonia; tracheobronchitis, empyema, and lung abscess

Serious invasive infections
Cardiovascular: endocarditis; bacteraemia; mycotic aneurysm; purulent pericarditis; infected vascular graft
Bone and joint: septic arthritis; osteomyelitis; bursitis; prosthetic joint infection
Central nervous system: meningitis; brain abscess; subdural empyema
Gastrointestinal tract: Liver abscess; spontaneous bacterial peritonitis; omental or appendiceal abscess; peritonitis and gastroenteritis
Genitourinary tract: cystitis or pyelonephritis; infected ileal loop and renal abscess; uterine infection; vaginitis, cervicitis; Bartholin's gland abscess; chorioamnionitis; epididymitis
Eyes: conjunctivitis; corneal ulcer; endophthalmitis

upper and lower respiratory tract infection does occur. Acute pneumonia, tracheobronchitis, empyema, and occasionally, lung abscess are the most commonly reported clinical syndromes. Most patients with pneumonia are elderly and bacteraemia occurs in 25 to 55 per cent of cases of respiratory infection with a reported case fatality rate of 29 per cent. There are no specific diagnostic features of *P. multocida* pneumonia; although lobar consolidation is the commonest chest radiograph appearance, multilobar and diffuse infiltrates also occur. Spread of Pasteurella infection from the upper respiratory tract may occasionally cause tonsillitis, sinusitis, pharyngitis, and epiglottitis.

Bacteraemia occurs in association with localized infections in many different sites. It is more common in patients with liver dysfunction. Bacteraemia is most often associated with meningitis (53 per cent of cases), respiratory disease, and septic arthritis (24 per cent). Endocarditis has been reported but appears to be relatively rare. Pasteurella meningitis affects mainly infants or the elderly. Septic arthritis normally affects already damaged joints. It is sometimes associated with bites distal to the joint, but also occurs in patients with no trauma or even in some who have no pets. A number of different intra-abdominal infections have been reported; bacterial peritonitis is a particular problem in patients with liver disease.

Diagnosis

A history of animal exposure should always suggest the possibility of Pasteurella infection. *Pasteurella* spp. can be identified as small Gram-negative rods which may stain bipolarly and can be isolated from sputum, pus, blood, or cerebrospinal fluid. Differentiation from *Haemophilus*, *Acinetobacter*, and *Neisseria* spp. is important.

Prevention and treatment

The most important factor in avoiding Pasteurella infections is the adequate treatment of bites. Thorough cleaning and debridement of wounds is crucial. The role of prophylactic antibiotics is controversial; approximately 5 to 15 per cent of dog bites and up to 50 per cent of cat bites become infected. Most clinicians advocate prophylactic antibiotics for 'high-risk' bites, crush injuries, deep puncture wounds, and wounds to the hands. Patients who are immunosuppressed, who have asplenism, or have alcoholic liver disease should certainly be treated. One recent meta-analysis suggested that routine antibiotics reduced the incidence of infection with a number needed to treat (NNT) of 14 to prevent one infection. In view of the strong association of Pasteurella infection with domestic animal contact, some clinicians have suggested that patients who are immunocompromised or who have chronic disease such as cirrhosis should try to avoid contact with dogs or cats.

Penicillin is the treatment of choice for established infections, although occasional clinical isolates that produce β-lactamase have been reported. Oral agents with good *in vitro* activity include tetracyclines, amoxicillin, amoxicillin/clavulanate, co-trimoxazole, and most fluoroquinolones. Azithromycin appears to be the most effective macrolide. Erythromycin has poor activity and *P. multocida* is resistant to clindamycin and many first-generation cephalosporins. Penicillin, third-generation cephalosporins, particularly cefotaxime, and chloramphenicol have all been used successfully in severely ill patients admitted to hospital.

Although penicillin has good activity against *Pasteurella* spp., prophylactic antibiotics for bites need to cover other organisms commonly found in the oral flora of dogs and cats, for instance *Staphylococcus aureus*, other staphylococcal species, anaerobes, and *Capnocytophaga canimorsus*. Amoxycillin/clavulanate is the prophylactic drug of choice. Treatment options in penicillin-hypersensitive patients include tetracycline or a combination of clindamycin and a fluoroquinolone.

Tularaemia

Introduction

Tularaemia is a zoonotic, arthropod-, and water-borne disease caused by *Francisella tularensis*, a small Gram-negative bacterium that has a natural lifecycle in mammalian hosts and may be transmitted by ticks and biting flies. Human infections occur predominantly in the northern hemisphere causing several different clinical syndromes, ranging from the combination of a fever, cutaneous ulcer, and lymphadenopathy to severe systemic disease and pneumonia. Three biogroups of *F. tularensis* can be distinguished by their geographical distribution, epidemiology, and virulence.

Bacteriology

Francisella spp. are small, non-motile, pleomorphic, Gram-negative coccobacilli. The organism has a thin capsule and may stain only faintly or exhibit bipolar staining with Gram or Giemsa stains. *Francisella* spp. grow only on media that contains cystine or cysteine and are strict aerobes. Optimal growth occurs at 35°C with carbon dioxide enrichment. They are oxidase negative and weakly catalase positive. Several species exist within the genus, but the major human pathogen is *F. tularensis*. Several biogroups of *F. tularensis* can be distinguished by biochemical characteristics; these biogroups vary markedly in their geographical distribution, epidemiology, and virulence for humans. *F. tularensis* biogroup *tularensis* and *F. tularensis* biogroup *palearctica* cause the vast majority of human disease. *F. tularensis*

biogroup *novicida* causes milder forms of tularaemia and *F. philmiragia* has occasionally been reported to cause infection in specific host groups.

Epidemiology

Although foci of disease occur throughout the world, the vast majority of cases have occurred in the northern hemisphere. The distribution of *F. tularensis* throughout Europe is shown in Fig. 1. A significant number of cases have also been reported from Japan. In North America, tularaemia has been reported from all states of the United States, Canada, and Mexico. However, the disease is now particularly associated with the Midwest in summer owing to transmission by tick bites and east of the Mississippi in winter from rabbit hunting. Transmission of the disease does not occur in the United Kingdom. Although tularaemia was extremely common in the United States, former Union of Soviet Socialist Republics, and Scandinavia in the middle of the last century, the recognition of occupational hazards and vaccination campaigns have reduced the incidence considerably. In the United States, the number of cases has declined from around 2000 per year in the post-war era to an average of 146 cases per year from 1990 to 1994, the last year for which tularaemia was a notifiable disease. Hundreds of thousands of cases occurred in the Union of Soviet Socialist Republics around the time of the Second World War, but the Russian Federation only reported 2019 cases in the 10 years from 1987 to 1997.

Infection in humans is predominantly caused by two biogroups; *F. tularensis* biogroup *tularensis* (synonymous with type A or *nearctica*) and *F. tularensis* biogroup *palearctica* (synonymous with type B or *palearctica*). Ninety-five per cent of North American human infections are due to biogroup *tularensis*. In Europe, infection is by the less virulent biogroup *palearctica*, which has a greater variety of reservoirs and vectors than the North American biogroup.

In the United States, biogroup *tularensis* particularly infects ground squirrels, cottontail rabbits, hares, and jackrabbits, but also occurs in other wild and domestic animals. Human infections usually arise from contact with affected animals or following tick or fly bites. Hunting, skinning, or eating infected animals is a particular risk factor. Inoculation through the skin or airborne transmission may occur during preparation of carcasses and infection can also be acquired by ingestion of infected meat or contaminated water and through mammal bites. *F tularensis* biogroup *tularensis* may be transmitted by a wide range of arthropod vectors, including ticks of the genera *Dermacentor* and *Amblyomma*.

Biogroup *palearctica* is less common in the United States; strains of this type have been isolated from muskrats, in which they cause epizootics. In northern Europe, biogroup *palearctica* infects a wide variety of mammals,

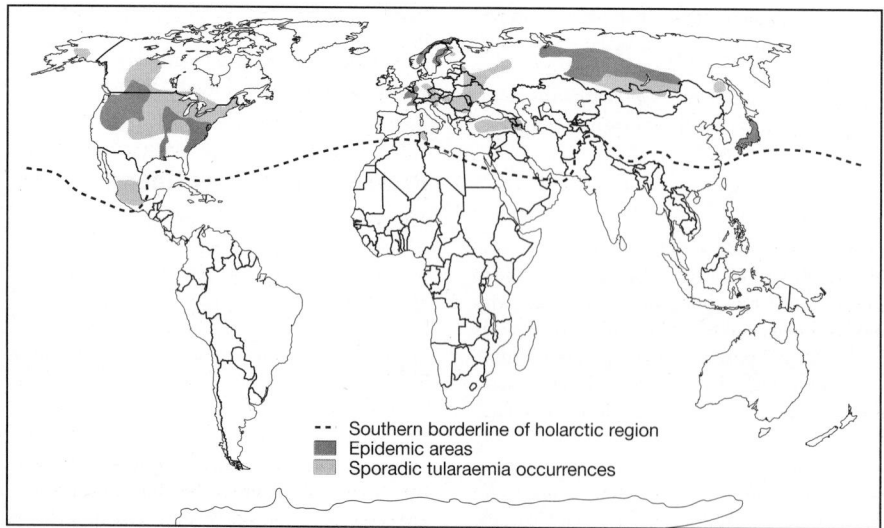

Fig. 1 Tularaemia foci in Europe.

mainly rodents, as well as hares. The main insect vectors are mosquitoes of the genus *Aëdes*, but ticks and biting flies also transmit the disease. Outbreaks of disease have often been reported. Human infections arise by a number of different mechanisms, apart from hunting and arthropod bites. Outbreaks have occurred from exposure to water contaminated by dead bodies or excreta of infected animals and from airborne dissemination of infection acquired by the inhalation of contaminated particles, such as dust from rodent-infested hay.

Pathogenicity

F. tularensis is primarily an intracellular pathogen that can multiply within mononuclear cells. Experimentally, as few as 50 organisms may cause infection through inoculation or inhalation; higher numbers are need to cause infection following ingestion. The organism spreads to regional lymph nodes from where it may be disseminated. Immunity is primarily cell mediated; focal necrosis and granulomas may be found in affected tissue. Little is known of the molecular basis of virulence, but loss of the capsule is associated with decreased virulence.

Clinical presentations of tularaemia (rabbit fever, deerfly fever, Ohara disease)

The clinical presentation of tularaemia depends on the route of transmission and virulence of the organism. Although clinical disease traditionally has been classified differently in the United States and Europe, manifestations of infection by *F. tularensis* biogroups *tularensis* and *palearctica* are essentially similar, except that biogroup *palaearctica* in Europe is clearly less virulent. The incubation period for tularaemia is usually between 3 and 5 days, but may be as long as 3 weeks. Most patients describe fever, chills, and prostration, and have a relapsing, protracted illness unless treated or vaccinated. A number of different discrete clinical syndromes (Table 3) have been described but there is considerable overlap between them.

Ulceroglandular tularaemia (Plates 1, 2, 3)

This is the most common presentation, particularly in North America. Patients present with sudden chills, fever, and often severe headache. An indurated and ragged ulcer evolves at the site of the initial entry of the organism; this is usually small and causes little pain. The ulcers are occasionally multiple and their site is related to the mode of contact. Local lymph nodes are tender, steadily increase in size, and frequently suppurate. If untreated, the ulcer may heal over several weeks leaving a scar.

Glandular tularaemia

Tularaemia may also present with lymphadenopathy without an obvious skin ulcer. Small lesions may be missed or have healed before presentation. Nodes may sometimes persist for weeks before the diagnosis is made. The differential diagnosis of glandular and ulceroglandular tularaemia includes pyogenic bacterial disease, cat-scratch disease, syphilis, mycobacterial infection, plague, and toxoplasmosis.

Oropharyngeal tularaemia (Plate 4)

This may occur due to oral contact with infected material and causes a pharyngitis, sometimes with ulceration, and enlargement of local lymph nodes. It may be more common in children than in adults. Pharyngitis and enlarged nodes may also occur in other forms of tularaemia. Pharyngeal tularaemia must be distinguished from other bacterial and viral causes of pharyngitis.

Oculoglandular tularaemia

This is a relatively rare form of tularaemia. The primary lesion is in the conjunctiva or cornea; infection usually occurs from splashing the face while cleaning infected animals, swimming in contaminated water, or from laboratory accidents. Conjunctivitis occurs along with chemosis and lid oedema. Unilateral preauricular lymphadenopathy is commonly observed. The differential diagnosis includes viral and bacterial causes of conjunctivitis including herpes simplex and syphilis.

Typhoidal tularaemia

This form of tularaemia occurs following any mode of acquisition of infection. Lymphadenopathy is not a feature. It appears to be more common in patients with pre-existing chronic illness. A febrile illness is associated with systemic symptoms which include fevers, chills, pharyngitis, myalgia, and gastrointestinal symptoms including watery diarrhoea. Meningism may occur. Patients may become severely ill and secondary pneumonic involvement occurs in over 40 per cent of patients.

Pulmonary tularaemia

Pulmonary disease may be primary, resulting from the inhalation of infected aerosols, or secondary from haematogenous spread. Pneumonia is commonly associated with typhoidal disease and also occurs in around a third of patients with ulceroglandular disease. Some patients have respiratory symptoms and signs of pneumonia, but a significant number of patients with tularaemia have asymptomatic radiological abnormalities. The commonest radiological finding is multiple parenchymal infiltrates in one lobe, but bilateral infiltrates and pleural effusions also occur. Hilar lymphadenopathy may be present. Examination of the sputum is rarely helpful. Most infiltrates clear rapidly on therapy. Tularaemia should be considered in any patient in an endemic area who presents with a community-acquired pneumonia which is resistant to standard therapy. The disease needs to be distinguished from all other causes of atypical pneumonia.

Secondary rashes have been reported following acute infection in all forms of tularaemia. Erythema nodosum has particularly been associated with pneumonic forms. *F. tularensis* biogroup *novicida* has low virulence for humans but may cause mild forms of tularaemia. *F. philmiragia* has been reported to cause severe infection in patients with chronic granulomatous disease or myeloproliferative disease and victims of near drowning.

Complications

Suppuration of lymph nodes is common in glandular forms, even after antibiotic treatment. Some patients may be unwell with malaise and fatigue for several months. In severe disease, impaired renal and hepatic function, elevated creatine kinase levels, and disseminated intravascular coagulation may occur. Severe disease is more common in patients with pre-existing illness and the elderly. Bacteraemia, renal impairment, pulmonary involvement, and elevated creatine kinase levels are all associated with a poorer prognosis. Overall case fatality rates for tularaemia in North America are approximately 2 to 3 per cent in patients treated with appropriate antibiotics. Deaths are rare in biogroup *palearctica* infections.

Diagnosis

In regions where *F. tularensis* is endemic, a provisional clinical diagnosis can often be made from the patient's exposure history and clinical signs. However, if there is no local ulcer, and if the patient has left the area in which the infection was acquired, patients who present with a persistent fever, lymphadenopathy, pneumonitis, or tonsillitis may be more difficult

Table 3 Clinical syndromes of human tularaemia

Syndrome	Frequency (%)
Ulceroglandular	40–80
Glandular	10–20
Typhoidal	5–15
Pneumonic	5–20
Oropharyngeal	< 5
Oculoglandular	< 5

to diagnose. A detailed travel and epidemiological history may help. Routine laboratory investigations are rarely helpful, although sterile pyuria has been noted in up to 20 per cent of cases.

A definitive diagnosis can be made by isolation of the organism, but *F. tularensis* will not grow on routine plating and samples require inoculation on to supportive media. The organism can be isolated from blood, lymph nodes, wounds, and occasionally sputum, but even in optimum conditions, the organism grows slowly and prolonged culture may be needed. Clinicians should inform the laboratory if tularaemia is suspected; laboratory aerosols cause serious, occasionally fatal, laboratory-acquired infection. Swabs or aspirates from local lesions and lymph glands should be transported in approved containers. Immunofluorescence methods may be more sensitive for identification of organisms in smears and tissues, and reduce the risk to laboratory staff.

Traditionally, most diagnoses have been made serologically using various agglutination assays. A fourfold rise in titre, or a titre of 1:160 in a single sample by the end of the third week of illness, is considered to be diagnostic of tularaemia. Antibody may persist for years after infection. Cross-reactivity with *Brucella* and *Yersinia* antibodies occurs. Enzyme-linked immunosorbent assay (**ELISA**) techniques are more sensitive for the early detection of tularaemia and can detect class-specific immunoglobulins. Delayed hypersensitivity skin testing has been used for diagnosis, but antigens have not been standardized. The polymerase chain reaction (**PCR**) has been used for the detection of *F. tularensis* DNA in animal tissues and initial studies on clinical wound specimens suggest that the technique may be more sensitive than culture. *F. tularensis* DNA has also been detected in patients who are serologically negative but have other evidence of infection with *F. tularensis*. Further study is need to determine the role of PCR and improved ELISA techniques in the diagnosis of tularaemia.

Treatment

Aminoglycosides have been used most widely for the treatment of tularaemia because of their bactericidal activity against *F. tularensis*. Streptomycin is the drug of choice and usually produces a dramatic clinical response. Gentamicin is an effective alternative, although relapses are more common than with streptomycin, occurring in 6 per cent of patients. Treatment is normally given for 10 to 14 days; shorter courses are associated with relapse. Tetracycline and chloramphenicol have been used successfully for the treatment of tularaemia, although relapse rates of 12 and 21 per cent, respectively, have been reported. Tetracyclines may be adequate for mild infections with biogroup *palaearctica* when given in high oral doses for 2 weeks.

Francisella spp. are resistant *in vitro* to most β-lactam antibiotics with the exception of third-generation cephalosporins. However, clinical experience with ceftriaxone has been disappointing. Quinolones have good *in vitro* activity against *F. tularensis* and successful clinical outcomes have been reported in a number of patients who have been treated with ciprofloxacin. Further study is required to define the role of these drugs in the treatment of tularaemia.

Prevention

Most important is reduction in human contact with infected animals and vectors in endemic areas. Protective clothing and insect repellent should be used when walking in endemic areas. Ticks should be sought out regularly and removed. Gloves should be worn when skinning or preparing rabbits; meat should be thoroughly cooked and sick animals should not be handled or eaten. Care should be taken in the laboratory to prevent transmission from potentially infective samples; *Francisella* spp. are category 3 pathogens and should be handled accordingly. Vaccines developed from live attenuated strains of biogroup *palaearctica* are effective and should be considered for laboratory workers who regularly handle *F. tularensis* or for others with repeated occupational exposure. There is no evidence of efficacy of chemoprophylaxis for exposed individuals.

Further reading

Adlam C, Rutter JM (1989). Pasteurella *and pasteurellosis*. Academic Press, London.

Cover TL, Aber RC (1989). *Yersinia enterocolitica. New England Journal of Medicine* **321**, 16–24.

Enderlin G et al. (1994). Streptomycin and alternative agents for the treatment of tularaemia. *Clinical Infectious Diseases* **19**, 42–7.

Evans ME et al. (1985). Tularaemia: a 30-year experience with 88 cases. *Medicine (Baltimore)* **64**, 251–69.

Gayraud M et al. (1993). Antibiotic treatment of *Yersinia enterocolitica* septicemia: a retrospective review of 43 cases. *Clinical Infectious Diseases* **17**, 405–10.

Gill V, Cunha BA (1997). Tularaemia pneumonia. *Seminars in Respiratory Infection* **12**, 61–7.

Koornhof HJ, Smego RA Jr, Nicol M (1999). Yersiniosis. II: The pathogenesis of *Yersinia* infections. *European Journal of Clinical Microbiology and Infectious Diseases* **18**, 87–112.

Larson JH (1979). The spectrum of clinical manifestations of infections with *Yersinia enterocolitica* and their pathogenesis. *Contributions to Microbiology and Immunology* **5**, 257–69.

Limaye AP, Hooper CJ (1999). Treatment of tularaemia with fluoroquinolones: two cases and review. *Clinical Infectious Diseases* **29**, 922–4.

Naktin J, Beavis KG (1999). *Yersinia enterocolitica* and *Yersinia pseudotuberculosis*. Clinics in Laboratory Medicine **19**, 523–36.

Smego RA, Frean J, Koornhof HJ (1999). Yersiniosis I: microbiological and clinicoepidemiological aspects of plague and non-plague *Yersinia* infections. *European Journal of Clinical Microbiology and Infectious Diseases* **18**, 1–15.

Talan DA et al. (1999). Bacteriologic analysis of infected dog and cat bites. *New England Journal of Medicine* **340**, 85–92.

Weber DJ et al. (1984). *Pasteurella multocida* infections. *Medicine* **63**, 133–56.

7.11.18 Anthrax

Thira Sirisanthana

Introduction

Anthrax is an acute bacterial infection caused by *Bacillus anthracis*. Herbivores are particularly susceptible to anthrax. They acquire the infection after coming into contact with soil-borne spores. Humans are infected when spores of *B. anthracis* enter the body through contact with infected animals or animal products, ingestion, or inhalation. The disease occurs in three clinical forms: cutaneous, gastrointestinal, and inhalation. Septicaemia and meningitis may occur from any of these primary foci. Other names for anthrax include malignant pustule, Siberian ulcer, charbon, malignant oedema, Milzbrand, and woolsorter's disease.

Anthrax has been known since antiquity. The fifth and sixth plagues described in the Bible are most likely outbreaks of anthrax in cattle and humans. Several distinguished scientists in the nineteenth century characterized the pathogenesis of the disease. In 1877, Robert Koch grew the organism in pure culture. He defined the stringent criteria needed to prove that the organism caused anthrax (Koch's postulates), then met them experimentally. Koch also discovered the spore stage that allows persistence of the organism in the soil. Louis Pasteur, in 1881, made a convincing field demonstration at Pouilly-le-Fort to show that vaccination of sheep, goats, and cows with heat-attenuated strain of *B. anthracis* prevented anthrax. In 1939, Sterne developed an animal vaccine that is a spore suspension of an avirulent, non-capsulated live strain. This is the animal vaccine still in use today.

Anthrax practically disappeared from North America, Western Europe, and Australia after the disease was eradicated in livestock following extensive vaccination programmes. However, it is still prevalent in developing countries, especially in Asia and Africa, where livestock are only poorly subjected to veterinary control, and where environmental conditions are favourable for an animal–soil–animal cycle to be established.

Recent interest in anthrax has been excited by fear of the use of anthrax spores as a biological weapon both in the battlefield and in a terrorist strike. An accident involving aerosolized anthrax spores at a Soviet military compound in 1979 (see below), and the revelation that Iraq had produced weapons containing anthrax spores during the 1991 Gulf War, confirm this fear.

Aetiology

B. anthracis is a large, non-motile, encapsulated, Gram-positive, aerobic, spore-forming bacillus that grows well in most nutrient media at 35°C. Spores are not produced in living animals. In the clinical laboratory, *B. anthracis* is recognized by its tendency to form very long chains of rods with elliptical central spores. The rectangular shape of the individual bacteria gives chains of *B. anthracis* a 'joint bamboo rod' appearance (Fig. 1 and Plate 1). On blood agar, *B. anthracis* forms non-haemolytic or weakly haemolytic greyish-white, rough colonies. In the presence of excess carbon dioxide, the organisms form capsules, and colonies are smooth and mucoid. The colonies produce a typical 'medusa head' or 'curled hair' appearance caused by chains of bacilli growing out from the edge of colonies. *B. anthracis* are pathogenic for small rodents. White mice, rabbits, and guinea pigs develop fatal infections after subcutaneous inoculation of very small numbers of the virulent organisms. The virulence factors of *B. anthracis* include a capsule that inhibits phagocytosis and three proteins collectively called anthrax toxin. The organism can be further identified by determination of susceptibility to bacillus phage γ and by demonstration of species-specific antigens (including the capsule and the anthrax toxin). The spores of *B. anthracis* are very resistant and will resist dry heat at 140°C for 1 to 3 h or moist heat at 100°C for 5 min. They can persist in nature for many years. Boiling for 10 min, treatment with oxidizing agents such as potassium permanganate, or with formaldehyde will kill the spores. Most strains of *B. anthracis* are susceptible to penicillin. During growth inhibition by penicillin, the cell cylinders of *B. anthracis* tend to bulge, resulting in the classic 'string of pearls' reaction.

Epidemiology

Anthrax is usually acquired through unrecognized breaks in skin or mucous membranes to which spores of *B. anthracis* gain access. The spores germinate to yield vegetative cells, which multiply and produce either localized or severe systemic infection depending on the animal species infected.

Fig. 1 Large Gram-positive bacilli in chains are typical of *B. anthracis*. An individual bacillus is 3 to 5 μm long and 1 to 1.25 μm wide with a flattened end. (See also Plate 1.)

Different species of animals are susceptible to varying degrees. Herbivores such as horses, sheep, goats, and cattle are most susceptible and develop fatal systemic disease. Dying herbivores have overwhelming bacteraemia and often bleed from the nose, mouth, and bowel, thereby contaminating soil with vegetative *B. anthracis*, which can sporulate and persist in the soil for a long time. The carcasses of infected animals provide additional potential foci of contamination. *B. anthracis* spores become part of the normal soil flora and can undergo bursts of local multiplication that increase the number of organisms in the soil. The cause of this local multiplication of anthrax bacilli is not known, but it is usually associated with major changes in the soil microenvironment such as those seen after abundant rainfall or a drought.

Human cases may occur in agriculture or industry. Agricultural cases result from direct contact with infected animals (herders, butchers, and slaughterhouse workers) and those who consume contaminated meat. Industrial cases involve those in contact with infected animal product such as hides, wool, goat's hair, or bone. All human cases are zoonotic in origin. No human-to-human transmission has been reported. The worldwide incidence of human anthrax is not known because many cases, especially in developing countries, do not receive medical attention and are not reported. However, one estimate puts the incidence at between 20 000 and 100 000 cases annually. Cutaneous anthrax typically follows skin exposure to infected animals or animal products. It is the most common form of the disease. Gastrointestinal anthrax follows ingestion of *B. anthracis*-contaminated food. Although rarely reported, gastrointestinal anthrax may not be uncommon in parts of Asia and Africa. Inhalation anthrax is a result of spore deposition in the lungs. Historically, woolsorters at industrial mills were at highest risk. Naturally occurring inhalation anthrax is now a rare disease.

Recent important epidemics of human anthrax include those from Zimbabwe between 1978 and 1982, from Switzerland in 1991, and from Sverdlovsk in the former Soviet Union in 1979. The outbreak in Zimbabwe is the largest reported agricultural outbreak. There were more than 10 000 cases. Most patients had cutaneous infections, but some gastrointestinal cases were also reported. This happened after a cattle outbreak during the Rhodesian civil war that caused disruption to veterinary anthrax vaccination programmes. In the Swiss outbreak, 25 workers in one textile factory contracted the disease. Twenty-four cases had cutaneous and one inhalation anthrax. The factory had imported *B. anthracis*-contaminated goat hair from Pakistan. This outbreak shows that the potential for industrial transmission of *B. anthracis* still exists in the Western world. In the former Soviet Union, the health authorities initially attributed the outbreak in Sverdlovsk to meat from infected animals. It is now known that deaths were in fact due to inhalation anthrax, the result of an accidental aerosolized release of anthrax spores from a microbiology laboratory in the local military facility. There were at least 77 cases of anthrax and 66 deaths.

Pathogenesis

Pathological changes result from tissue invasion by *B. anthracis* and effects of its exotoxin. The organism is an extracellular pathogen that multiplies rapidly, invades the bloodstream and kills quickly. Virulent strains of *B. anthracis* possess two virulence factors: a capsule and a three-component protein exotoxin (anthrax toxin) that is made up of protective antigen (**PA**), oedema factor (**EF**), and lethal factor (**LF**). The capsule, which is composed of D-glutamic acid polypeptide, enhances virulence by making the organism resistant to phagocytosis. The genes encoding the anthrax capsule are carried on an extrachromosomal plasmid. A second plasmid carries the gene for the three proteins: PA, EF, and LF. PA is so named because it is the main protective constituent of anthrax vaccines. PA binds to a cell-surface receptor on the target cell and is cleaved by a protease into two fragments. After the cleavage, the larger membrane-bound fragment displays a binding site for EF and LF and mediates their entry into the target cell. EF, a calmodulin-dependent adenylate cyclase, increases intracellular cyclic adenosine monophosphate levels. The biological effects of EF include the formation of oedema characteristic of the disease. A mixture of EF and PA, known together as oedema toxin, also inhibits phagocytosis by polymorphonuclear leucocytes. The action of LF, believed to be a metalloproteinase, is less understood. Its exact intracellular target is not known. One recent study showed that LF inactivates an enzyme responsible for activating mitogen-activated protein kinase (**MAPK**). Thus, LF blocks the MAPK signal transduction pathway, an evolutionarily conserved pathway that controls cell proliferation and differentiation. Injection of a mixture of PA and LF, known together as lethal toxin, causes death in many species of experimental animals. Lethal toxin has been shown at high concentration to kill macrophages and at low concentration to cause macrophages to release tumour necrosis factor and interleukin 1.

When spores of *B. anthracis* are introduced subcutaneously, they germinate and multiply. The antiphagocytic capsule facilitates local spread. The oedema and lethal toxins impair leucocyte function and contribute to tissue necrosis, oedema, and relative absence of leucocytes in the skin lesion. The bacilli spread to the draining lymph node resulting in the typical findings of haemorrhagic, oedematous, and necrotic lymphadenitis. Gastrointestinal anthrax follows ingestion of contaminated and undercooked meat. Multiplication of the bacilli in the oropharynx and the draining lymph nodes causes the oropharyngeal ulcer and neck swelling. When the organisms are deposited in the duodenum, ileum, or caecum, they cause mucosal inflammation and ulcers. Transport of the bacteria to the mesenteric lymph nodes results in the development of haemorrhagic adenitis and ascites. Inhalation anthrax follows deposition of spore-bearing particles of 1 to 5 μm into alveolar spaces. They are phagocytosed by alveolar macrophages and transported to the tracheobronchial and mediastinal lymph nodes, where they germinate. Production of toxins leads to haemorrhagic, oedematous, and necrotic lymphadenitis and mediastinitis.

In all primary forms of anthrax, especially inhalation anthrax, the bacilli can spread through the blood causing septicaemia and at times haemorrhagic meningitis. Autopsies show numerous bacteria in blood vessels, lymph nodes, and other organs.

Clinical features

Cutaneous anthrax

The cutaneous lesion in anthrax is most often found on exposed areas of skin such as the face, neck, arms, or hands. The incubation period is 1 to 7 days, usually 2 to 5 days. Initially a small papule develops at the site of infection. During the next week, the lesion typically progresses through vesicular and pustular stages to the formation of an ulcer with a depressed black eschar (Fig. 2 and Plate 2). A striking degree of non-pitting oedema surrounding the lesion is typical. The early lesion may be pruritic. The fully developed lesion is painless. Small satellite vesicles may surround the original lesion. Lymphangitis and painful regional lymphadenitis is common. Associated systemic symptoms are usually mild, and the lesion heals after the eschar separates. In about 10 to 20 per cent of the patients, the disease progresses with massive local oedema, toxaemia, and bacteraemia, and a fatal outcome if untreated. Cutaneous anthrax should be considered when patients have painless ulcers associated with vesicles, oedema out of proportion to the size of the lesion, and have had contact with animals or animal products. The differential diagnosis includes staphylococcal skin infections, tularaemia, plague, cutaneous diphtheria, orf, rickettsial pox, and scrub typhus.

Gastrointestinal anthrax

Because gastrointestinal anthrax develops following consumption of contaminated meat, it can occur as familial clusters. The disease has been described in two forms. The incubation period is 2 to 5 days. Oropharyngeal anthrax follows deposition of the bacteria in the oropharynx. Patients present with fever, neck swelling, sore throat, and dysphagia. The neck swelling is caused by enlargement of the lymph nodes together with subcutaneous oedema as in diphtheria. The lymph node enlargement commonly involves the upper group of the jugular chain. There is an inflammatory lesion in the oral cavity or oropharynx. The lesion starts as an inflamed mucosa, progressing through necrosis and ulceration to the formation of a pseudomembrane covering the ulcer (Fig. 3 and Plate 3). In severe cases, the subcutaneous oedema extends to the anterior chest wall and axilla, with the overlying skin showing signs of inflammation. Toxaemia and death may follow. Oropharygeal anthrax should be considered in patients who present with fever, neck swelling, sore throat, and oropharyngeal ulcer and who give a history of eating raw or undercooked meat. The differential diagnosis includes diphtheria and peritonsillar abscess.

In another form of gastrointestinal anthrax, the organisms are deposited in the duodenum, terminal ileum, or caecum. The onset is with fever, nausea, vomiting, and abdominal pain, followed by rapidly developing ascites and bloody diarrhoea. Haematemesis, melaena, haematochezia, and/or profuse watery diarrhoea may occur in some patients. In severe cases, toxaemia, shock, and death follow. It is difficult to make a diagnosis in the early stage, except in an epidemic setting.

Inhalation anthrax

Inhalation anthrax (woolsorter's disease) has been described as a two-stage illness. The incubation period is 1 to 5 days. It starts with malaise, myalgia, fever, and non-productive cough, symptoms similar to those of viral respiratory diseases. Signs of illness and laboratory results are non-specific. In some patients there is a transient improvement after 2 to 4 days. The second stage begins with severe respiratory distress, cyanosis, stridor, and

Fig. 2 Cutaneous anthrax lesion on the forearm on day 10 showing an ulcer with a depressed black eschar. (See also Plate 2.)

Fig. 3 Oropharyngeal anthrax on day 9 showing a pseudomembrane covering an ulcer. (See also Plate 3.)

profuse sweating. Subcutaneous oedema of the chest and neck may develop. A characteristic radiographic finding is symmetric mediastinal widening with or without pleural effusion. Blood culture will grow *B. anthracis*. Up to half of patients develop anthrax meningitis. Shock and death typically follow in less than 24 h. The initial phase of the disease is very difficult to diagnose in the absence of a known outbreak. Advanced disease may be suspected in the presence of a characteristically widened mediastinum despite otherwise normal chest radiographic findings. Inhalation anthrax must be distinguished from pneumonic plague.

Meningeal anthrax

Anthrax meningitis, frequently a consequence of overwhelming *B. anthracis* bacteraemia, may complicate any primary form of anthrax. Rarely, a case of anthrax meningitis has been reported in which the primary site was not identified. Within a few days of the primary lesion, the patient develops sudden onset of confusion, loss of consciousness, and focal neurological signs. The cerebrospinal fluid is haemorrhagic, purulent, or both. The disease is almost always fatal.

Laboratory diagnosis

Clinical specimens taken before antibiotic therapy is instituted will grow *B. anthracis* in culture. Gram stain of these specimens may show Gram-positive rods. These specimens include vesicular fluid (cutaneous anthrax), swabs from oropharyngeal lesions, ascitic fluid (gastrointestinal anthrax), and cerebrospinal fluid (meningeal anthrax). Severe cases of anthrax, especially the inhalation form, may have bacteraemia, but by the time blood cultures become positive many patients will have died. Because *Bacillus* species are frequent laboratory contaminants, most laboratories do not identify them further unless specifically asked to do so. Thus, it is important to notify the laboratory when *B. anthracis* infection is suspected. Laboratory confirmation can also be made by demonstration of *B. anthracis* in the clinical specimens by direct fluorescent antibody staining.

Serological tests are helpful in making a diagnosis, especially when prior antibiotics have eradicated the bacteria before cultures or smears were obtained. However, patients with severe disease, especially inhalation anthrax, die so quickly that these tests may not be helpful to the clinician. Useful tests include an enzyme-linked immunosorbent assay (ELISA), which detects antibodies to the capsular antigen and/or PA, and an electrophoretic immunotransblot test (Western blot), which detects antibodies to PA and/or LF. These tests are only available at national reference laboratories.

Treatment

Most strains of *B. anthracis* are susceptible to penicillin, which should be started as soon as possible. Mild cases of cutaneous anthrax may be treated with oral penicillin at the dose of 250 mg 6-hourly for 5 to 7 days. For extensive lesions, parenteral penicillin G, 2 million units 6-hourly, should be given until systemic toxicity subsides. The patient may then take oral penicillin for a total treatment period of 7 to 10 days. Ciprofloxacin, erythromycin, doxycycline, or chloramphenicol can be used in penicillin-sensitive patients. Antibiotics decrease systemic toxicity, but the skin lesions will continue to progress to the eschar phase. The skin lesion should be covered with a sterile dressing. Used dressings should be decontaminated. In gastrointestinal or inhalation anthrax or in anthrax meningitis, intravenous penicillin G, 4 million units 4-hourly, should be administered. Other drugs are intravenous ciprofloxacin (800 mg/day) or intravenous doxycycline (200 mg/day). Many patients will require intensive supportive care including vigilant monitoring and correction of electrolyte and acid–base disturbance, mechanical ventilation, and vasopressor administration.

Prognosis

A case fatality rate of 10 to 20 per cent has been reported for untreated cases of cutaneous anthrax. With appropriate antibiotic treatment, fatalities are rare. Almost all cases of inhalation anthrax and anthrax meningitis are fatal. Oropharyngeal anthrax causes death in about 15 per cent of the patients. The case fatality rate of the other form of gastrointestinal anthrax is not known.

Prevention and control

Control of anthrax in animals is essential to control of the disease in humans. Routine immunization of animals should be instituted in areas with continuing cases of animal anthrax. All cases of animal or human anthrax should be reported to the appropriate authorities. During an outbreak, suspected animals should be quarantined and infected herds sacrificed. Carcasses of animals that have succumbed to anthrax are buried intact or cremated to avoid sporulation and further contamination of the environment. Gastrointestinal anthrax can be prevented by public education about consumption of contaminated meat. Anthrax vaccines should be given to those at risk of acquiring the disease such as agricultural workers or veterinarians who have contact with potentially infected animals, laboratory workers who work with *B. anthracis*, and workers involved in the industrial processing of animal products. The incidence of industrial anthrax has been further decreased by educating workers about how anthrax is transmitted, improvement in industrial hygiene, better manufacturing equipment and environmental control, as well as the decline in using fibres of animal origin as raw material.

Current anthrax vaccines for human use include cell-free preparations consisting of alum-precipitated and aluminum hydroxide-adsorbed extracellular components (primarily PA) of uncapsulated *B. anthracis*, available in the United Kingdom and the United States, respectively. A live attenuated anthrax spore vaccine is available in countries of the former Soviet Union, but is not used elsewhere because of safety concerns. The current cell-free vaccines are manufactured from an undefined crude culture supernatant. They must be given several times to ensure protection and local reactions have been reported. These drawbacks and the potential use of *B. anthracis* as a biological weapon have stimulated efforts to develop improved vaccines. A minimally reactogenic, recombinant PA vaccine has been investigated. Other approaches, made possible by modern molecular biology technology, include cloning the PA gene into other bacteria or viruses and development of mutant avirulent strains of *B. anthracis*.

Further reading

Hanna P (1998). Anthrax pathogenesis and host response. *Current Topics in Microbiology and Immunology* 225, 13–35. [A review on the pathogenesis of *Bacillus anthracis*.]

LaForce FM (1994). Anthrax. *Clinical Infectious Diseases* 19, 1009–13. [A good review article on anthrax.]

Meselson M *et al.* (1994). The Sverdlovsk anthrax outbreak of 1979. *Science* 266, 1202–8. [Description of the outbreak at a military facility at Sverdlovsk in the former Soviet Union.]

Pile JC *et al.* (1998). Anthrax as a potential biological warfare agent. *Archives of Internal Medicine* 158, 429–34. [A good review article on anthrax in general and as a potential biological weapon.]

Sirisanthana T *et al.* (1988). Serological studies of patients with cutaneous and oral-oropharyngeal anthrax from northern Thailand. *American Journal of Tropical Medicine and Hygiene* 39, 575–81. [Studies of serological diagnosis in patients with oropharyngeal and cutaneous anthrax.]

7.11.19 Brucellosis

M. Monir Madkour

Brucellosis is a common, classic zoonotic disease of worldwide distribution. It is transmitted to man from infected animal reservoirs. Human brucellosis may be caused by one of four species: *Brucella melitensis* (the most common cause) from goats, sheep, and camels; *B. abortus* from cattle; *B. suis* from pigs; and *B. canis* from dogs. Brucella organisms are small, non-encapsulated, non-motile, non-sporing, Gram-negative, aerobic bacilli, which are facultative intracellular parasites. They can survive for up to 8 weeks in unpasteurized, white, soft goat's cheese. They tend to die within 60 to 90 days in cheese that has undergone lactic acid fermentation during the period of maturing. Freezing milk or its products does not destroy the organism, but they are killed by boiling or pasteurization. Brucella organisms are shed in urine, stools, vaginal discharge, and products of conception. They remain viable in dried soil for up to 40 days and for longer if the soil is damp.

Epidemiology

There are only 17 countries in the world that are brucellosis free: Norway, Sweden, Finland, Denmark, Switzerland, the former Czechoslovakia, Romania, the United Kingdom including the Channel Islands, the Netherlands, Japan, Luxembourg, Cyprus, Bulgaria, Iceland, and the Virgin Islands of the United States. Canada and New Zealand are about to be declared brucellosis-free countries. However, the overall incidence of brucellosis in the world is increasing. With the ease of modern travel, patients may contract the disease while visiting endemic countries. The true global incidence of human brucellosis is difficult to determine because of the lack of essential statistics, disease reporting, and notification systems in many countries. Even in developed countries there are reports indicating that the incidence of human brucellosis is estimated to be 3 to 26 times higher than official figures.

The risk to public health

In endemic areas of developing countries, brucellosis affects predominantly males and younger age groups. Farm animals such as goats, sheep, camels, and cattle are kept in the backyards of houses and considered as pets. Childhood brucellosis indicates endemicity of the disease in that area. Serious human maternal morbidity and fetal loss through abortion, intrauterine death, and premature delivery, or active disease in neonates, are public health risks in endemic areas of developing countries. Where brucellosis is controlled in animals, human brucellosis is mostly an occupational disease, particularly among workers in meat-processing industries and in farmers, veterinarians, and laboratory workers.

Modes of transmission

In endemic areas, animal contact through inhalation of organisms is the most frequent cause of infection, and affects herdsmen, dairy-farm workers, and laboratory workers. *Brucella melitensis* is included among 10 types of biological warfare or bioterroristic agents which can be released as aerosols. Ingestion of untreated milk or its products, or raw meat, liver, or bone marrow, is a common route of infection through the gastrointestinal tract, particularly among those taking antacids. Penetration of intact or abraded skin is a common route of infection among abattoir workers in developing and developed countries. Accidental autoinoculation or conjunctival splashing of live brucella vaccine during animal vaccination are well-recognized routes of infection among veterinarians. Laboratory infections have been described. Transplacental transmission of infection from mother to fetus may occur. Brucella organisms have been isolated from human breast milk and nursing mothers may infect their infants through breast feeding.

Sexual transmission in man is similar to that in animals, and has recently been reported, with isolation of the organisms from human semen. Other uncommon routes of transmission include blood transfusion and bone marrow transplants.

Pathogenesis

Polymorphonuclear cells and activated macrophages migrate to the site of entry of brucella organisms. During the early phase of invasion, extracellular killing is carried out by IgM and complement-mediated mechanisms.

However, brucella organisms can resist such killing. During invasion and phagocytosis, the organisms are killed inside macrophages by oxidative burst or oxygen-based killing using the myeloperoxide–hydrogen peroxide–halide system. The interaction between the organisms and macrophages will determine the severity and outcome of infection. Organisms surviving within or escaping from phagocytic cells multiply and reach the bloodstream via the lymphatics to enter body organs rich in reticuloendothelial cells. Other organs and tissues are also invaded through the bloodstream. Inflammatory responses with or without granulomas and caseation or even abscess formation may occur. The cytotoxic activity of natural killer cells, with decrease in the CD4+ and increase in the CD8+ lymphocyte subpopulations, is depressed in patients with active brucellosis. Cytokines including interleukin12 and tumour necrosis factor-α appear to play an important role in host defence against brucella infection.

Clinical features

The incubation period is about 1 to 3 weeks but may extend up to several months. Brucellosis is a disease of protean manifestations that may simulate other febrile illnesses. Its clinical features are not specific. In endemic areas, diagnosis is relatively easy. However, in non-endemic areas of developed countries, clinicians should remember brucellosis in the differential diagnosis of a febrile illness. A history of travel to endemic areas should be obtained, as well as the patient's occupational history. The clinical features of brucellosis largely depend on the species of the organism and may vary widely. *B. melitensis* has a high pathogenicity, producing more intense symptoms. The onset may be sudden (1 to 2 days) or gradual (1 week or more). It presents as a febrile illness, with or without localization to particular organs. Brucellosis is classified according to whether or not the disease is active (i.e. history, clinical features, and significantly raised brucella agglutinins with or without positive blood cultures) and whether or not there is localized infection. Evidence of active disease and the presence of localization have a significant impact on recommended treatment. Classification of brucellosis as acute, subacute, chronic, serological, bacteraemic, or mixed types serves no purpose in diagnosis and management. The term 'active brucellosis with/without localization' is recommended. The most frequent symptoms are given in Table 1. The fever has no distinctive pattern that could differentiate it from other febrile illnesses, despite the old name 'undulant fever'. It usually shows diurnal variation, being normal in the morning and high in the afternoon and evening. Chills or rigors with profuse sweating may simulate malaria. Patients with brucellosis commonly look deceptively well and, less frequently, may look acutely ill. Physical signs may be lacking despite the multiplicity of symptoms, which may be labelled as psychological. The frequency of physical signs is shown in Table 2.

Localizations

Bones and joints

Reactive arthritis may occur in brucellosis. Septic arthritis may result from bloodborne spread to the synovium or from extension of brucellar osteomyelitis in a neighbouring long bone. Brucella spondylitis starts in the superior end-plate, an area of rich blood supply. The infection may either

Table 1 History and symptoms in 500 patients with brucellosis due to *B. melitensis*

History/symptoms	No.	%
Animal contact	368	73.6
Raw milk/cheese	350	70
Raw liver ingestion	147	29.4
Family history	188	37.6
Fever	464	92.8
Chills	410	82.0
Sweating	437	87.4
Body aches	457	91.4
Lack of energy	473	94.6
Joint pain	431	86.2
Back pain	431	86.2
Headaches	403	80.6
Loss of appetite	388	77.6
Weight loss	326	65.2
Constipation	234	46.9
Abdominal pain	225	45.0
Diarrhoea	34	6.8
Cough	122	24.4
Testicular pain (of 290 males)	62	21.3
Skin rash	72	14.4
Sleep disturbances	185	37.0

regress and heal or progress to involve the entire vertebra, disc space, and adjacent vertebrae. Early lesions are localized in the anterior aspect of the superior end-plate at the disc–vertebral junction, leading to a small area of bone destruction. Bone healing takes place at the same time, leading to sclerosis.

Arthritis is commonly polyarticular and migratory, affecting mainly the large joints including the knee, hip, sacroiliac, shoulder, sternoclavicular, wrist, ankle, and interphalangeal joints in decreasing order of frequency. Septic monoarthritis may lead to destruction of the affected joint if undiagnosed. Joints affected include the knee, hip, sternoclavicular, and sacroiliac joints and the shoulder. Spondylitis may involve single or, less frequently, multiple sites. The lumbar spine, particularly L4, is the most frequent site. The average age of onset of brucella spondylitis is 40 years; it is extremely rare during childhood.

Extraspinal brucella osteomyelitis is rare. Long bones, particularly the femur, tibia, humerus, or manubrium sterni, may be affected. Bursitis, tenosynovitis, and subcutaneous nodules may also occur. Unlike with septic arthritis and osteomyelitis due to other organisms, the peripheral white-cell count is normal and the erythrocyte sedimentation rate is normal or accelerated. The total white-cell count in synovial fluid ranges from 4000 to 40 000/mm³ with 60 per cent polymorphonuclear cells. Glucose in synovial

Table 2 Signs in 500 patients with brucellosis due to *B. melitensis*

Signs	No.	%
Ill looking	127	25.4
Pallor	110	22.0
Lymphadenopathy	160	32.0
Splenomegaly	125	25.0
Hepatomegaly	97	19.4
Arthritis	202	40.4
Spinal tenderness	241	48.0
Epididymo-orchitis (of 290 males)	62	21.3
Skin rash	72	14.4
Jaundice	6	1.2
CNS abnormalities	20	4.0
Cardiac murmur	17	3.4
Pneumonia	7	1.4

fluid may be reduced, but protein is usually raised and culture is positive in about 50 per cent of the cases.

Cardiovascular

These localizations may include endocarditis, myocarditis, pericarditis, aortic-root abscess, mycotic aneurysms, thrombophlebitis, and pulmonary embolism. The most frequent of these is endocarditis, which used to be the leading cause of death. The outcome is now more favourable with recent advances in diagnosis, cardiac surgery, and treatment. Brucella endocarditis usually occurs on a previously damaged valve or a congenital malformation, but can occur even on normal valves. The clinical features are similar to those caused by other organisms. Patients who live in endemic areas and have what has been labelled as 'sterile infective endocarditis' should have their blood culture extended for a period of up to 6 weeks.

Respiratory

Respiratory symptoms are common but, because they are usually mild, clinicians tend to overlook them. A flu-like illness with sore throat and mild dry cough is a common feature. Other rare foci of infection include hilar and paratracheal lymphadenopathy; pneumonia, with solitary or multiple nodular lung shadowing or even with abscess formation; soft-tissue miliary shadowing; pleural effusion; empyema; or mediastinitis.

Gastrointestinal

Gastrointestinal infections are usually mild and are rarely a presenting feature of the disease. They include tonsillitis, and hepatitis with mild jaundice (either non-specific or granulomatous with suppuration and abscess formation). Actual cirrhosis is rare. Deep jaundice is not a feature of brucellosis. Splenic enlargement with abscess formation is rarely reported. Mesenteric lymphadenopathy with abscess formation, cholecystitis, peritonitis, pancreatitis, and ulcerative colitis are described. The liver transaminases, alkaline phosphatase, and serum bilirubin may be mildly raised. The clinical and biochemical evidence of liver involvement is far less frequent than liver biopsies have indicated. The diagnostic significance of splenomegaly becomes doubtful in countries where malaria and bilharzia are also common.

Genitourinary

Genitourinary localizations may be the presenting feature of brucellosis. They include unilateral or bilateral epididymo-orchitis in children and in adults, prostatitis, seminal vesiculitis, dysmenorrhoea, amenorrhoea, tubo-ovarian abscesses, chronic salpingitis, and cervicitis. Acute nephritis or acute pyelonephritis-like features, renal calcifications, and calyceal deformities may occur. Renal granulomatous lesions with abscess formation, with caseation and necrosis may occur, as may cystitis and posterior urethritis.

Urine culture may be positive in about 50 per cent of patients with brucellosis. Brucella organisms have recently been isolated from human semen during investigation of possible sexual transmission.

Neurobrucellosis

Neurobrucellosis is uncommon but serious. Despite the multiplicity of symptoms, abnormal neurological findings may be lacking. They include meningoencephalitis, multiple cerebral or cerebellar abscesses, ruptured mycotic aneurysm, cranial nerve lesions, transient ischaemic attacks, hemiplegia, myelitis, radiculoneuropathy and neuritis, Guillain–Barré syndrome, a multiple sclerosis-like picture, paraplegia, sciatica, granulomatous myositis, and rhabdomyolysis.

The psychiatric features of brucellosis are no more severe than those caused by other infections. Neurobrucellosis may be caused by direct bloodborne invasion by brucella organisms, pressure from destructive spinal lesions, vasculitis, or an immune-related process. In meningoencephalitis the cerebrospinal fluid pressure is usually elevated and the fluid may look clear, turbid, or rarely, haemorrhagic; the protein, cells (predominantly lymphocytes), and oligoclonal immunoglobulin are raised, while glucose may be reduced or normal. Brucella organisms may be cultured from cerebrospinal fluid.

Pregnancy

In endemic areas the outcome of pregnancy in humans is similar to that in animals: normal delivery, abortion, intrauterine fetal death, premature delivery, or retention of the placenta and other products of conception.

Skin

Skin manifestations are uncommon. They include maculopapular eruptions and contact dermatitis, particularly among veterinarians and farmers assisting animal parturition. Other dermatological manifestations include erythema nodosum, purpura and petechias, chronic ulcerations, multiple cutaneous and subcutaneous abscesses, vasculitis, superficial thrombophlebitis, discharging sinuses, and rarely, pemphigus.

Ocular

Direct splashing of live brucella vaccine into the eyes may cause conjunctivitis. Keratitis, corneal ulcers, uveitis, retinopathies, subconjunctival and retinal haemorrhages, retinal detachment, and endogenous endophthalmitis with positive vitreous cultures are well documented. Neuro-ophthalmic complications of brucella meningitis may lead to papilloedema, papillitis, retrobulbar neuritis, optic atrophy, and ophthalmoplegia due to lesions on the IIIrd, IVth, and VIth cranial nerves.

Endocrine

Localization of brucella infection with or without abscess formation in the endocrine glands is commonly reported in the testicle and epididymis. Other endocrine gland localizations with or without abscess formation are well documented but rare. These include the thyroid, ovaries, mammary glands, the adrenals, and the prostate. Reported cases of endocrine gland localizations are commonly not associated with disturbed hormonal secretions, perhaps with the exception of the adrenals. The syndrome of inappropriate secretion of antidiuretic hormone as well as raised serum calcium are reported in patients with active brucellosis.

Diagnosis

The diagnosis of brucellosis depends on the presence of clinical features and brucella agglutinins in a significantly raised titre. A positive blood or tissue culture is not always present. The organism's identity is confirmed by phage typing, DNA characterization, or metabolic profiling. Use of a carbon dioxide detection system (such as BACTEC; Becton Dickinson, Sparks, MD) for blood culture provides a more sensitive and rapid culture result than standard methods, with positivity usually apparent after only 2 to 5 days of incubation. Alternatively, extended incubation of blood cultures for up to 6 weeks (incubated at 37°C with and without an atmosphere of 10 per cent carbon dioxide) should be requested. Most authorities will consider an agglutination titre of 1/160 or higher to be significant in a symptomatic patient living in a non-endemic area. However, in endemic areas only titres of 1/320 to 1/640 or higher are considered significant. In endemic areas, otherwise asymptomatic individuals offering to donate blood may be found to have high brucella titres and should not be considered to be suffering from active brucellosis. Follow-up 2 to 4 weeks later is necessary in such individuals to exclude subclinical infection.

The presence of brucella antibodies in the patient's serum can be detected by the standard tube test, rose bengal plate test, 2-mercaptoethanol test, antihuman globulin test (Coomb's), radioimmunoassay, enzyme immunoassay, and polymerase chain reaction (**PCR**). The PCR is specific and highly sensitive for the detection of brucella agglutinins (the

DNA used for the amplification is either phenol purified or comes directly from a suspension of brucella organisms). The antigens commonly used for serological screening are prepared from *B. abortus*, which cross-reacts with *B. melitensis* and *B. suis* antibodies as well. However, they do not cross-react with *B. canis* antibodies. To detect these antibodies, antigen prepared from *B. canis* organisms is needed, but they are not available commercially. A cross-reaction with tularaemia and cholera may occur. This can be distinguished by testing simultaneously for brucella, tularaemia, and cholera antibodies. Occasionally, brucella agglutination tests are negative in patients with positive tissue cultures. The prozone phenomenon is a false-negtive standard tube test caused by the presence of blocking antibodies in the α-globulin (IgG) and in the α_2-globulin (IgA) fractions. This phenomenon can be avoided by screening sera at low and high titres. An elevated IgM antibody indicates recent infection, while low titres indicate previous contact with the organism. An elevated IgG indicates active disease.

Haematological changes

The total white-cell count is usually normal and leucopenia with relative lymphocytosis does not always occur. Thrombocytopenia is less common and haematological features of disseminated intravascular coagulation are rare. The erythrocyte sedimentation rate is of no diagnostic value. Liver function tests, liver biopsies, and cerebrospinal and synovial fluid changes have been discussed under pathogenesis and localizations.

Treatment

Control and prevention of brucellosis should be directed primarily towards eradication of the disease in animals. The brucella organism is intracellular and therefore relatively inaccessible to antimicrobials. A combination of a tetracycline and an aminoglycoside remains the most effective regimen because of its synergistic effect. Oral doxycycline (100 mg, twice daily) is preferred to other tetracyclines (500 mg, 6-hourly) because of its rapid and complete absorption from the duodenum, longer half-life (18 h), and more efficient tissue penetration (it is more lipid soluble). Suitable aminoglycosides are streptomycin, netilmicin, or gentamicin. Streptomycin is given intramuscularly in a dose of 1 g/day for patients under 45 years of age and 0.5 to 0.75 g/day for older patients. The plasma trough concentration should be 1 to 2 µg/ml. Netilmicin, 4 to 6 mg/kg a day intramuscularly in two divided doses, can be used for outpatient treatment. The plasma trough concentration should be 2 to 4 µg/ml. Gentamicin is only used for patients in hospital as it is usually given as an intravenous infusion of 2 to 5 mg/kg daily, in divided doses, 8-hourly. The plasma trough should be 1 to 2 µg/ml. Combined therapy with a tetracycline and an aminoglycoside should be given for 1 month, followed by a tetracycline and rifampicin (600 to 900 mg/day as a single oral dose) or a tetracycline and co-trimoxazole (two tablets, 480 mg each, twice daily) for a further 1 to 2 months. This regimen has a relapse rate of 7 per cent. A three-drug regimen in combination with urgent surgical intervention is required in those with endocarditis, aortic root abscess, spondylitis, osteomyelitis, and abscesses in organs or other tissues. Neurobrucellosis without abscesses formation will require a three-drug regimen. The combination of doxycycline–netilmicin/gentamicin–rifampicin should be given for 4 weeks. A doxycycline–rifampicin combination should be continued for a further 4 to 8 weeks. Single daily dosing of netilmicin or gentamicin has been successfully used for other infections. Such dosing is being assessed at present for treatment of brucellosis and results are not yet available. Shorter periods of treatment have a higher relapse rate. Most patients with brucellosis are treated as outpatients and only those with localizations (e.g. endocarditis, neurobrucellosis, osteomyelitis, septic arthritis, and renal impairment), or who are pregnant or are infants, require admission to hospital.

Ciprofloxacin (750 mg, 12-hourly, orally) and other fluoroquinolones are synthetic broad-spectrum antibiotics with intracellular penetration used by some for treatment of brucellosis. There are reports of the development of resistance and cross-resistance with other quinolones and high relapse rates. Quinolones showed no synergism with other agents.

Children

Infants and children under 7 years of ages should be treated with a combination of rifampicin and co-trimoxazole for 2 to 3 months. However, in those with serious localizations in endemic areas where some discoloration of the teeth is of secondary importance, doxycycline can be used, in combination, as described above—doxycycline, 50 to 100 mg/day orally; gentamicin: infants aged up to 2 weeks, 3 mg/kg every 12 h; aged 2 weeks to 12 years, 2 mg/kg every 8 h intramuscularly or by slow intravenous injection or intravenous infusion; netilmicin: infants aged up to 1 week, 3 mg/kg every 12 h; aged over 1 week, 2.5 to 3 mg/kg every 8 h intramuscularly or by intravenous injections or infusions; rifampicin, 10 to 20 mg/kg a day, either orally or by slow intravenous injection as a single daily dose; co-trimoxazole paediatric suspension (240 mg/ml) is given 12-hourly orally as follows: 6 weeks to 5 months of age, 120 mg; 6 months to 5 years, 240 mg; 6 to 12 years, 480 mg. Intravenous infusion: 54 mg/kg daily in two divided doses.

Renal impairment and pregnancy

Patients with renal impairment should be carefully monitored for serum concentration of aminoglycoside. If such monitoring is not available, then a doxycycline–rifampicin regimen should be administered. In pregnancy, co-trimoxazole–rifampicin for 8 to 12 weeks is the most suitable regimen.

Response to treatment

Patients become afebrile and other constitutional symptoms greatly improve within 4 to 14 days. The liver and spleen become impalpable within 2 to 4 weeks. Patients may experience an acute, intense flare-up of symptoms—the Jarisch–Herxheimer reaction—shortly after starting treatment, particularly with tetracyclines. This reaction is only transient and does not necessitate discontinuation of therapy. Follow-up of clinical, blood culture, and serological tests should be done every 3 to 6 months for 1 to 2 years.

Human vaccine

Human vaccine for brucellosis, used in the former Soviet Union, China, and France, was found to be effective in reducing markedly the rate of infection. Two injections, each of 1 mg of phenol-insoluble fraction, were given 2 weeks apart. It provides effective but short-lived immunity and should be repeated every 2 years. Vaccination is indicated in workers with an occupational risk of developing brucellosis. The outer membrane proteins (OMPs) are showing promise in experimental work on the development of a new vaccine.

Further reading

Banntyne RM *et al.* (1997). Rapid diagnosis of brucellar bacteraemia by using the BACTEC 9240 system. *Journal of Clinical Microbiology* **35**, 2673–4.

Berkowsky PB *et al.* (1997). Why should we be concerned about biological warfare? *Journal of the American Medical Association* **278**, 431–2.

Madkour MM (1989). *Brucellosis*, 1st edn. Butterworths, London.

Madkour MM (2001). *Madkour's brucellosis*, 2nd edn. Springer-Verlag, Heidelberg. [A complete monograph on brucellosis, enhanced by 216 figures of plain radiography, CT, and MRI modalities.]

Sharif HS *et al.* (1989). Brucellar and tuberculous spondylitis: comparative imaging features. *Radiology* **171**, 419–25.

Solera J *et al.* (1996). Treatment of human brucellosis with netilmicin and doxycycline. *Clinical Infectious Diseases* **22**, 441–5.

7.11.20 Tetanus

F. E. Udwadia

Tetanus is an acute, often fatal disease, resulting from the contamination of a wound by *Clostridium tetani*, a spore-forming, Gram-positive, motile, rod-shaped, obligate anaerobic organism. Under anaerobic conditions the vegetative form of the organism produces a powerful exotoxin, which on reaching the central nervous system causes the increased muscle tone and spasms that characterize the disease.

Epidemiology

The spores of *Cl. tetani* are ubiquitous, but the natural environment is soil, particularly cultivated soil rich in manure. Spores are commonly found in animal faeces, may also be detected in human faeces, and can occasionally be recovered from house dust or from the air of occupied buildings, slums, and even hospitals and operating theatres.

Tetanus is a killer disease chiefly afflicting the poor, uneducated, and underprivileged people of the world. It is thus widely prevalent in India, Bangladesh, Pakistan, parts of South-East Asia, Africa, the eastern Mediterranean region, and South America. In these countries where immunization programmes are inadequate, the disease is most common in the young and newborn and is more frequent in males than in females. In the 1980s, 1 million newborn babies died of tetanus every year. The annual worldwide mortality had declined to 480 000 by 1994 and to 277 400 in 1997. However, neonatal tetanus still accounts for 23 to 73 per cent of neonatal deaths in developing countries. An estimated 70 000 cases continue to occur in India every year. The decline in incidence of the disease in the nineties is largely due to the substantial increase in immunization coverage of pregnant women with a protective dose of tetanus toxoid. It is estimated that effective vaccination programmes have prevented 500 000 deaths in the South-East Asia region out of the 700 000 deaths prevented globally. Ninety per cent of the deaths prevented in South-East Asia are in India, Bangladesh, and Indonesia. In the West the disease is increasingly rare, fewer than 60 cases being reported annually from the United States between 1991 and 1994. The disease in the West is more frequent in people older than 60 years, in whom effects of immunization have worn off, in the unimmunized, impoverished, and in drug addicts.

Physiopathology

Under anaerobic conditions (e.g. presence of necrotic tissue, active infection, foreign body), the tetanus bacillus within a wound produces two toxins—tetanospasmin and tetanolysin. Only tetanospasmin has clinical effects. Tetanospasmin is a 150 kDa protein consisting of a heavy (100 kDa) chain and a light (50 kDa) chain joined by a single disulphide bond. The mechanism of spread of tetanospasmin is illustrated in Fig. 1. The released toxin spreads to underlying muscles and is bound by its heavy chain to receptors containing gangliosides on the neuronal membranes of presynaptic nerve terminals. The toxin is then internalized and transported intra-axonally and retrogradely within the peripheral nerves to cells of motor neurones of that segment of the cord supplying those muscles. The toxin almost always also enters and circulates in the bloodstream. It does not cross the blood–brain barrier, but by haematogenous spread binds to nerve terminals in muscles throughout the body. It is then transported retrogradely within numerous axonal pathways of all peripheral nerves to reach the α motor-neurone cell bodies of the whole spinal cord and brainstem. It thereby also reaches the sympathetic chain, the preganglionic sympathetic neurones in the lateral horns of the spinal cord, and the parasympathetic centres.

After reaching the cell bodies in the spinal cord and brainstem, the toxin, by an unknown mechanism, passes retrogradely across the presynaptic cleft to bind to ganglioside receptors on presynaptic nerve terminals of inhibitory interneurones. The light chain of the toxin now acts to block the release of the inhibitory neurotransmitters, chiefly glycine and γ-aminobutyric acid (**GABA**), from synaptic vesicles within nerve terminals of inhibiting neurones. This blockage releases motor and autonomic neurones from inhibitory control. The molecular mechanism behind this action is unknown. The toxin may well alter a calcium-dependant process necessary for neurotransmitter release. The uncontrolled excessive, disinhibited efferent discharge from motor neurones in the cord and brainstem to both agonist and antagonist muscles leads to widespread muscle rigidity and to reflex spasms characteristic of generalized tetanus. Muscles of the jaw, face, and head are involved first because the toxin has to travel along shorter axonal pathways to reach their controlling motor neurones in the brainstem. Muscles of the trunk and limbs are involved a little later because the toxin travels along longer axonal pathways to their controlling motor cells in the cord. Disinhibited autonomic discharge leads to disturbances in autonomic control, particularly to sympathetic overactivity with excessive catecholamines in the blood. Medullary centres and hypothalamic centres may also be affected by tetanus toxin. Myocardial dysfunction and disturbances in impulse conduction may occur.

When, rarely, tetanus toxin does not reach the bloodstream but spreads from the site of the wound along regional axonal pathways to motor neurones in a localized segment of the cord; local tetanus results. Rigidity and spasms are restricted to a group of muscles.

Tetanus toxin can also produce a peripheral neuromuscular blockade by preventing release of acetylcholine, similar to the effect of botulinum toxin. This peripheral paralytic effect is observed in cephalic tetanus.

Fig. 1 Retrograde intra-axonal transport of tetanospasmin and its main site of action in the central nervous system.

Altered haemodynamics

Severe tetanus without complications is characterized by a high-output, hyperkinetic circulatory state with marked tachycardia, increased stroke-volume index, increased cardiac index, and a normal, left ventricular stroke-work index (Fig. 2). There is also an increase in the compliance of the vascular system due to arteriolar, capillary, and venous dilation, chiefly in skeletal muscle. These changes have been attributed to increased muscle contraction, increased sympathetic tone, and a rise in core temperature.

Disturbances in the autonomic nervous system lead to marked cardiovascular instability with wide fluctuation in heart rate, systemic vascular resistance, and blood pressure.

Clinical features

Some 15 to 25 per cent of patients with tetanus have no evidence of recent wounds, for the disease can result from the most trivial of wounds. Contamination of the wound with garden soil or manure, or injury by rusty metals, are particularly dangerous. Tetanus can complicate burns, ulcers, gangrene, necrotic snake bites, frostbite, discharging middle-ear infections, septic abortions, childbirth, ritual scarification, and female circumcision. It can occur after intramuscular injections, particularly of drugs producing tissue necrosis (such as quinine), and after surgery. Tetanus neonatorum is most often due to non-sterile obstetric techniques, and in India to the dreadful practice of applying cow dung to the cut surface of the umbilical cord.

The clinical features of tetanus are rigidity, muscle spasms, and seizures. Severe tetanus is invariably associated with autonomic disturbances.

Muscle stiffness or rigidity

Stiffness of the masseters is often the first manifestation of the disease, resulting in difficulty in opening the mouth—trismus or lockjaw. Typically, stiffness extends to the muscles of the face, all skeletal muscles, and often involves muscles of swallowing, causing dysphagia. The facial expression in tetanus is diagnostic. The eyes appear partially closed, the forehead is furrowed, the corrugator muscle contracted, the nostrils flared, nasolabial folds prominent, and the lips pursed, thinned, and stretched, with the angles of the mouth extending outwards and often turned slightly down, producing a 'risus sardonicus' (Fig. 3 and Plate 1). This smile is perhaps more pathetic than sardonic. The expression is one of pain, anguish, and fear. Stiffness of the neck muscles results in retraction of the head. The muscles of the chest are stiff and the breathing movements are restricted. The abdomen often shows board-like rigidity. The arms and legs are often ramrod stiff and in children marked stiffness in the muscle of the back can lead to opisthotonos similar to that observed in meningitis (Fig. 4 and Plate 2).

Muscle spasms

Mild cases of tetanus exhibit only stiffness without spasms. Spasms or seizures are characterized by a marked reflex exaggeration of the underlying rigidity, producing tonic contraction of the stiff muscles. They are frequently brought on by touch but may also be triggered by visual, auditory, or emotional stimuli. Seizures vary in severity and frequency. They may be mild, infrequent, and brief (lasting a few seconds) or severe, protracted, painful, and spontaneous, the patient appearing to be in a state of perpetual convulsion. Severe protracted spasms render breathing impossible or shallow, irregular, and ineffective, so that the patient becomes very hypoxic and even cyanosed. Spasm of pharyngeal muscles prevents swallowing of saliva, so that pharyngeal secretions accumulate and are often aspirated into the lungs, causing atelectasis and aspiration pneumonia. Laryngeal spasm may occur by itself; it may accompany generalized spasms and can produce unexpected sudden death from asphyxia.

Patients with severe tetanus have fever, tachycardia, and often, an unstable cardiovascular system. Unless expertly managed, they usually die of respiratory complications, circulatory failure, or cardiac arrest.

Autonomic nervous system disturbances

In severe tetanus there is invariably involvement of the sympathetic and parasympathetic nervous systems. Features include tachycardia exceeding 150 beats/min, drenching sweats, frequent modest elevation in systolic and/or diastolic arterial blood pressure, increase in salivary and tracheobronchial secretions, and evidence of increased reflex vagal tone and activity.

Severity of tetanus

Grading the severity of tetanus is not just an academic exercise; it is useful both in prognosis and in the management of the disease. The criteria listed below are subjective and arbitrary but have stood the test of time in our unit.

Grade I (mild)

There is mild to moderate trismus, general spasticity, no respiratory embarrassment, no spasms, and little or no dysphagia.

Grade II (moderate)

There is moderate trismus, well-marked rigidity, mild to moderate short-lasting spasms, moderate respiratory embarrassment with tachypnoea in excess of 30 to 35/min, and mild dysphagia.

Grade III (severe)

There is severe trismus, generalized spasticity, reflex and often spontaneous prolonged spasms, respiratory embarrassment with tachypnoea in excess of 40/min, apnoeic spells, severe dysphagia, and tachycardia in excess of 120/min.

Grade IV (very severe)

The features are the same as grade III plus violent autonomic disturbances involving the cardiovascular system.

Cephalic tetanus

This occurs after an injury to the head and is confined to muscles innervated by the cranial nerves. It is characterized by unilateral facial palsy (Fig. 5 and Plate 3), trismus, facial stiffness of the unparalysed half, nuchal rigidity, pharyngeal spasms causing dysphagia, and frequent laryngeal spasms with danger of death from asphyxia. Rarely, facial palsy is bilateral. Paresis of the glossopharyngeal, vagus, and rarely of the oculomotor nerves may also occur. Cephalic tetanus may graduate to generalized tetanus.

Tetanus neonatorum

The earliest symptom is a difficulty or inability to suckle and swallow owing to stiffness of muscles of the jaw and pharynx. There is increasing stiffness, with the classic tetanus facies (Fig. 6 and Plate 4), flexion at the elbows with the fists clenched and drawn to the thorax, extension of the knees with plantar flexion of the ankles and toes, and opisthotonos. Muscle spasms make breathing difficult; autonomic disturbances are frequent and death results from cardiorespiratory failure.

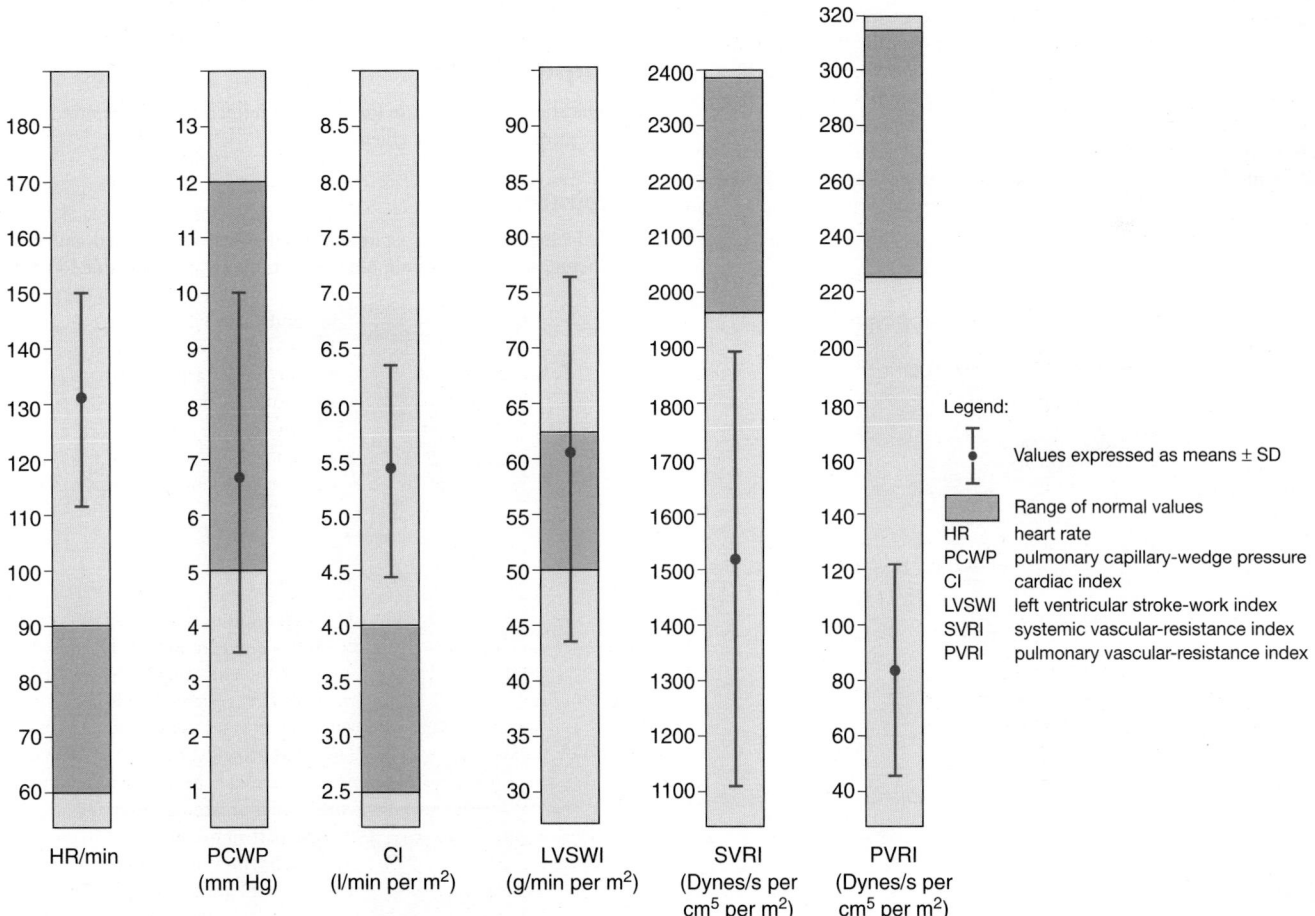

Fig. 2 Haemodynamic observations in 19 patients with severe uncomplicated tetanus.

Fig. 3 Facies in tetanus. (See also Plate 1.)

Local tetanus

Rarely, rigidity and spasms may be localized to muscles adjacent to the wound or confined to a limb.

Natural history

The incubation period of tetanus (time between the injury and the first symptom) averages 7 to 10 days, but may range from 1 to 2 days to 2 months. The period of onset is the time between the first symptom and onset of spasms, and ranges from 1 to 7 days. The shorter the incubation period and the period of onset, the greater the severity of the disease. The disease peaks over 7 to 10 days, plateaus over the next 3 weeks, and then subsides over the next 2 weeks. Muscle stiffness and ankle clonus may persist for months after recovery. Severe tetanus is a markedly catabolic disease and significant weight loss is always observed even in patients who recover.

Fig. 5 Brazilian patient with local tetanus confined to muscles innervated by the left VIIth cranial nerve and with trismus, showing the wound causing the infection. (By courtesy of Dr Pedro Pardal, Belém, Brazil.) (See also Plate 3.)

Complications

Complications in tetanus are frequent and numerous. The respiratory and cardiovascular systems are chiefly involved.

Respiratory

These include atelectasis, aspiration pneumonia, pneumonia, and bronchopneumonia. Bronchopulmonary infections are generally due to Gram-

Fig. 4 Opisthotonos in severe tetanus during seizures. (See also Plate 2.)

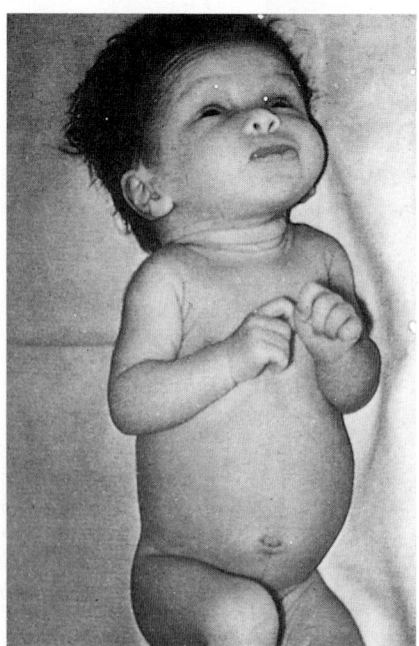

Fig. 6 Characteristic facies in neonatal tetanus. (See also Plate 4.)

negative organisms—chiefly *Klebsiella* spp.and *Pseudomonas aeruginosa*. Prolonged laryngeal spasms if unrelieved can cause death. Severe hypoxia and respiratory failure due to incessant spasms are a certainty if these patients are not given curare-like drugs and ventilated. Episodes of severe unexplained tachypnoea and respiratory distress are probably central in origin. The acute respiratory distress syndrome can be caused by tetanus *per se* or may be due to complicating sepsis. Complications related to tracheostomy and ventilator support are also observed.

Cardiovascular and autonomic

Sustained tachycardia (more than 160/min), persistent hypotension, labile or sustained hypertension, and 'autonomic storms' complicate severe tetanus. Autonomic storms are due to wild fluctuations in sympathetic activity causing episodes of hypertension and tachycardia alternating within minutes or hours with hypotension and bradycardia. Such cardiovascular instability may be a forewarning of cardiac arrest and death. Increased vagal tone can cause bradycardia and sudden death, particularly during suctioning of tracheal secretions. Supraventricular arrhythmias, ventricular tachycardia, and infranodal conduction defects can also occur. Hyperthermia and rarely hypothermia suggest hypothalamic involvement.

Sudden death

Sudden cardiac arrest causing death remains the single most dreaded complication of moderate and severe tetanus. It may be related to cardiovascular instability due to fluctuating autonomic tone, excessive vagal activity, severe hypoxia, sudden hyperpyrexia, impaired infranodal conduction, massive pulmonary embolism, or no obvious reason.

Other complications

These are generally incidental to prolonged management of critically ill patients on ventilator support. They include: iatrogenic sepsis with multiple organ failure; gastrointestinal bleeds, ileus, or diarrhoea; renal insufficiency; fluid, electrolyte, and acid–base disturbances; fractures generally of one or more thoracic vertebrae during severe spasms; miscellaneous complications—bedsores, thrombophlebitis, rhabdomyolysis, peripheral neuropathy, corneal ulcers, anaemia, hypoproteinaemia, and deep vein thrombosis which may cause pulmonary embolism.

Diagnosis

Diagnosis is based solely on clinical features. Absence of a wound does not exclude tetanus. Trismus produced by tetanus should be distinguished from masseter spasm due to an alveolar or peritonsillar abscess. Dystonic reactions caused by phenothiazines and metoclopramide, spasms due to hypocalcaemic tetany, and seizures due to strychnine poisoning may superficially mimic tetanus. Meningitis and meningoencephalitis can also produce trismus, rigidity, seizures, and opisthotonus, but can be differentiated by a cerebrospinal examination, which is normal in tetanus. Cephalic tetanus can be mistaken for rabies because of severe dysphagia—however, hydrophobia never occurs in tetanus.

Mortality

Tetanus neonatorum carries a mortality of 60 to 80 per cent. Mortality in adult tetanus ranges from 20 to 60 per cent. It is higher in the older age group and in those with a short incubation period (under 4 days). A short period of onset (under 2 days) more reliably prognosticates severe disease. The introduction of critical care and ventilator support in severe tetanus has led to a drop in overall mortality from 30 to 12 per cent, and the mortality in fulminant tetanus from near 100 to 23 per cent, in our unit. In a good, well-equipped, critical care unit in Bombay, the mortality in severe tetanus in adults remains as low as 6 per cent.

Management

Mild tetanus (grade I) poses no serious problems. However, grade I (mild) tetanus can over a period of days graduate to grade II (moderate) or even grade III and grade IV (severe) tetanus. Such patients merit close observation. Wherever possible, all patients with tetanus should be admitted to an intensive care unit. Unfortunately this is not always feasible in poor developing countries. However, motivation and training for better patient care coupled with basic equipment for respiratory care and support can work wonders in reducing mortality even in the absence of full intensive care facilities.

The use of antiserum

Equine antiserum is generally available in poor countries; 10 000 units are given intravenously on admission after first doing a sensitivity test. However, fatal anaphylaxis can occur even when skin sensitivity is not observed. Human tetanus immunoglobulin is superior to equine antiserum, produces no hypersensitivity reactions, and if available should be given in preference to the equine antiserum in a dose of 5000 units intravenously. The intrathecal use of tetanus antiserum is best avoided as claims of its efficacy remain unproven. Local infiltration of 3000 units of antitoxin around an obvious wound is practised in some units, but its value is uncertain. Antitoxin has no action on the toxin that has already been fixed to the nervous tissue; at best, it serves to neutralize newly liberated tetanus toxin. Antitoxin should be given before local manipulation of the wound, which is treated according to usual surgical principles with debridement of necrotic tissue and delayed primary suturing.

Antibiotics

Two mega-units of penicillin are given intravenously four times a day for 8 days. Though effective against *C. tetani in vitro*, its use in this disease is disappointing. Clindamycin or erythromycin are alternatives for penicillin-sensitive patients. Metronidazole at a dosage of 500 mg four times a day for 10 days is currently preferred. Other appropriate antibiotics may be necessary to counter secondary complicating infections.

Management strategies

Mild or grade I tetanus should be treated conservatively with the use of sedatives and muscle relaxants. Patients with grade II or moderate tetanus should, in addition to sedatives and relaxants, have a tracheostomy. Patients with grade III or IV (severe) tetanus require sedation, tracheostomy, and continuous ventilatory support after they have been paralysed with curare-like drugs, until spasms relent and recovery ensues.

Use of sedatives and muscle relaxants

The use of sedatives and muscle relaxants remains the cornerstone of management in grade I and grade II tetanus. The aim is to reduce rigidity and control spasms without significantly depressing respiration. Diazepam, a benzodiazepine and a GABA antagonist, is the drug of choice in most units. The dosage is 5 to 20 mg thrice daily in children and adults, and 2 mg thrice daily in neonates. In mild tetanus it is given orally; in moderately severe tetanus it is given in a slow intravenous infusion over 24 h. It is best not to exceed 120 to 150 mg/24 h in adults even in the presence of marked rigidity. Higher doses will inevitably depress respiration. Lorazepam with a longer duration of action and midazolam with a shorter half-life may also be used, but offer no advantage over diazepam. Chlorpromazine and phenobarbitone are second-line drugs that can be used in combination with diazepam when there is no alternative. The ideal sedative and muscle relaxant dosage schedule for each patient should be tailored to ensure continuous sedation at a level that ensures sleep, but that allows the patient to be aroused to obey commands. An objective guide, particularly in moderately severe tetanus, is relaxation of the abdominal muscles, which feel much less stiff to palpation.

Tracheostomy

Tracheostomy is mandatory for severe (grade III, IV) tetanus. Preferably, it should also be done in moderate tetanus simply because, even in an intensive care unit setting, the most important preventable cause of death is a sudden prolonged laryngeal spasm leading to asphyxia. The patient's inability to handle upper respiratory secretions in the presence of dysphagia, and the use of heavy sedation in many cases of moderately severe tetanus are both indications for elective tracheostomy.

Induced paralysis with ventilator support

Severe tetanus has a forbiddingly high mortality if management is conservative and confined to the use of high doses of sedatives and muscle relaxants. These patients require a tracheostomy, induced paralysis by curare-like drugs (pancuronium or vecuronium), and ventilatory support in an intensive care unit. In poor countries, this management strategy can also be implemented in the absence of good monitoring facilities provided the unit or ward has basic equipment for respiratory care and a trained medical and nursing staff. Results in such units may not be as good as in well-staffed and -equipped intensive care units but are still far superior to those observed with conservative management. Pancuronium is used in a dose of 2 to 4 mg intravenously every 30 min to 2 h; the dose of vecuronium is 0.1 mg/kg intravenously. Alternatively, either of these drugs may be given in a slow intravenous infusion, the dose being titrated to produce a degree of neuromuscular blockade and paralysis that allows efficient ventilator support. As the patient improves, pancuronium or vecuronium are given at longer intervals or the infusion rate is reduced. In fulminant tetanus with continuous spasms it may be almost impossible to induce complete paralysis. Twitches invariably break through within 30 min of the use of the drug, but these do not interfere with efficient ventilatory support. The average period of ventilatory support in severe tetanus is around 3 to 4 weeks, but may vary from 10 days to 6 weeks. Once spasms cease, the neuroparalytic drug is stopped; ventilator support is continued until such time as the patient is deemed fit to be weaned.

It is unnecessary, unwise, and probably dangerous in our opinion to use large doses of intravenous diazepam (a frequent practice in many units) in paralysed patients on ventilator support. A dose of 40 to 60 mg of diazepam intravenously over 24 h suffices to counter anxiety without dangerously depressing vital centres.

In poor countries the correct mode of management in severe tetanus is often constrained by a paucity of trained staff and material resources (particularly ventilators). Ethical considerations then restrict the use of ventilator support to: (i) patients with grade IV tetanus; (ii) patients with grade III tetanus whose spasms are uncontrolled on a conservative regime and whose $P(a)o_2$ is less than 55 mmHg on 6 to 8 litre/min of oxygen; and (iii) patients who develop any serious complication that in itself merits ventilatory support.

Treatment of autonomic circulatory disturbances

Intravenous β-blockers, heavy sedation, intravenous morphine sulphate, intravenous labetalol, intravenous infusion of magnesium sulphate, and intravenous clonidine have all been used to control autonomic storms in severe tetanus. These drugs do not alter the high mortality. It is best to rely on good overall critical care and efficient cardiorespiratory support and avoid drugs that strongly depress the central and autonomic nervous systems. Hypotensive spells are treated by a volume load and if this is ineffective or contraindicated, by inotropic support with dopamine or dobutamine to maintain a systolic pressure just above 100 mmHg. Hypertensive episodes with a systolic blood pressure in excess of 200 mmHg or a diastolic in excess of 100 mmHg are treated with a small oral dose of propranolol (10 mg) or 5 mg of sublingual nifedipine. Intravenous propranolol is dan-

gerous and can cause sudden death, but a titrated infusion of esmolol (a β-blocker with a very short half-life) is useful in a hypertensive crisis. Bradyarrhythmias are treated with intravenous atropine, and persistent sinus tachycardia of more than 170/min with 40 mg of verapamil orally twice or thrice daily. In this situation it is best not to use more than 50 mg of diazepam intravenously per day. Sedatives and drugs used at a dosage that strongly depresses the central or autonomic nervous system probably contribute to a high mortality by predisposing to cardiac arrest (particularly after sudden hypotensive spells and sudden bradyarrhythmias) and by preventing successful resuscitation. These management principles have achieved a very low mortality (6 per cent) in severe tetanus.

Treatment of other complications

Complications may involve almost every system in the body. These should be promptly recognized and treated.

Critical care and nursing

Good critical care and expert nursing play a vital role in reducing complications and preventing death. The following are of particular importance:

(1) ensuring patency of the airway and care of the tracheostomy in scrupulous detail;

(2) ensuring an adequate arterial oxygen saturation and oxygen transport to tissues through efficient cardiorespiratory support;

(3) expert physiotherapy to the chest timed specifically during periods of drug-induced muscle relaxation;

(4) maintaining fluid, electrolyte, and acid–base balance;

(5) prevention, early detection, and prompt control of infection and sepsis with appropriate antibiotics;

(6) supporting nutrition, if necessary by intravenous alimentation;

(7) detection (by frequent monitoring) and treatment (by physical methods and by paracetamol) of hyperpyrexia—a surreptitious killer in tetanus.

Use of tetanus toxoid

Tetanus does not confer immunity. Active immunization is necessary and is achieved by giving the first dose of tetanus toxoid during convalescence and the next two doses at the recommended intervals.

Prevention

Tetanus is a preventable disease through active immunization with adsorbed tetanus toxoid (**ATT**) and by proper management of wounds.

Active immunization

The following regime is advocated. In infancy and childhood, three doses of triple vaccine (tetanus, diphtheria, pertussis) are given at monthly intervals, and a booster dose is given at 4 to 6 years of age. Unimmunized individuals older than 7 years should be given triple vaccine in three doses: the first and second 6 weeks apart, and the third dose 6 months after the second. Booster doses of ATT are advocated every 10 years, but this remains a practical impossibility in poor countries.

Immunization after minor, uninfected wounds

Passive immunization with equine or human tetanus antitoxin is not indicated for minor, clean wounds. Active immunization (with 0.5 ml ATT) is indicated if immunization status is unknown or more than 10 years have elapsed after the last dose of ATT. Under the above circumstances, especially in poor countries, ATT is also administered prior to emergency surgery, deliveries, and obstetric procedures.

Immunization after infected or major wounds

Passive immunization (250 to 500 units of human tetanus immunoglobulin or 5000 units of equine antitoxin, intramuscularly) is recommended in all individuals who are not immunized, partially immunized, or whose immunization status is unknown. Indication for administration of ATT is the same as for minor, uninfected wounds. However, it would be safer to use a booster dose of ATT even in a well-immunized individual if more than 5 years have elapsed since the last dose of ATT.

Prevention of tetanus neonatorum

Primary immunization of pregnant patients with two injections of ATT a month apart, preferably during the last two trimesters, together with education of nurses and midwives on sterile obstetric techniques, would further reduce the incidence of tetanus neonatorum in developing countries.

Further reading

Gupta SD, Keyl PM (1998). Effectiveness of prenatal tetanus toxoid immunization against neonatal tetanus in a rural area in India. *Pediatric Infectious Diseases Journal* **17**, 316–21.

Park K (1997). Tetanus. In: Banarsidas Bhanot, ed. *Park's textbook of preventive and social medicine*, 15th edn, pp 237–40. Jabalpur, India.

Sutton DN *et al.* (1990). Management of autonomic dysfunction in severe tetanus: the use of magnesium sulphate and clonidine. *Intensive Care Medicine* **16**, 75–80.

Udwadia FE (1994). *Tetanus.* Oxford University Press, Bombay.

Udwadia FE *et al.* (1987). Tetanus and its complications: intensive care and management experience in 150 Indian patients. *Epidemiology and Infection* **99**, 675–84.

7.11.21 Botulism, gas gangrene, and clostridial gastrointestinal infections

H. E. Larson

Botulism

Definition

Botulism is an acute, symmetrical, descending paralysis caused by a neurotoxin produced by *Clostridium botulinum*. Food contaminated by *C. botulinum* spores and elaborated toxin produces illness when ingested. Wound infections with *C. botulinum* or intestinal tract colonization in infants and adults occasionally cause botulism.

Occurrence

C. botulinum is ubiquitously distributed in soil and mud. The surfaces of potatoes, vegetables, and other foods are easily contaminated with spores, which survive brief heating at 100°C. The anaerobic conditions characteristic of canning, smoking, or fermentation facilitate clostridial growth and toxin release. Spores germinate in sausage or cheese if they are kept for extended periods at room temperature. An eighteenth century report asso-

ciated paralytic illness with eating sausages, hence *botulus*, Latin for a sausage. Cases have been associated with fermented milk in Africa, cheese sauce on baked potatoes in North America, fermented stew in Japan, and imported fish in the United Kingdom.

Although past outbreaks typically involved small groups of people, home-canned peppers served in a restaurant caused two large outbreaks in the United States. Outbreaks caused by commercially processed foods are infrequent, but contamination of hazelnut purée added to commercially produced yoghurt caused 27 cases of botulism in Wales and north-west England in 1989, the largest recorded outbreak in the United Kingdom. Most of the contaminated cartons could not be accounted for, suggesting that the attack rate varied or that mild symptoms were not diagnosed as botulism. Commercially prepared, chopped garlic in soybean oil caused 36 cases dispersed over eight provinces and states in North America.

Some outbreaks involved only single contaminated items, such as in the Loch Maree episode in 1922 where eight people died after eating duck paste, the 1978 outbreak in Birmingham involving four people who ate tinned Alaskan salmon, and one case in 1989 following a meal on a commercial airliner. Uneviscerated fresh fish have been associated with botulism, usually where there have been deficiencies in refrigeration.

Purified botulinum toxin has recently come into therapeutic use. Toxin injections produce temporary muscle weakness in the treatment of strabismus, blepharospasm, torticollis, and for cosmetic purposes. Treatment doses are considered too small to account for systemic symptoms. Under experimental conditions aerosolized botulinum toxin causes illness in monkeys and the toxin has been mooted as an effective agent for biological warfare or terrorist activity. Botulinum toxin was loaded into SCUD missile warheads by Iraq during the Gulf War and stockpiled by the Aum Shinrikyo cult in Japan.

The toxin

There are seven serological types of botulinum toxin (A–G). Types A, B, and E account for nearly all human cases. Serotypes implicated in outbreaks of botulism parallel the geographical distribution of soil spores. Type E is nearly always associated with fish, but outbreaks caused by fish products involve types A and B. Spores of *C. botulinum* can survive up to 2 h of boiling (100°C), but are killed rapidly at autoclave temperatures (120°C).

C. botulinum toxin is heat labile and rapidly inactivated at ordinary cooking temperatures. It is a protein neurotoxin, and a dose as small as 0.1 µg has been estimated to cause death in a human being. The 150-kDa molecule is composed of two peptide chains connected by disulphide bonds. One chain binds to and penetrates the neurone, the other cleaves a protein essential for neurotransmitter release, reducing acetylcholine availability for impulse transmission. Toxin types A, C, and E hydrolyze a protein in the presynaptic membrane while types B, D, F, and G hydrolyze a protein in the synaptic vesicle.

Pathogenesis

Botulinum toxin is absorbed directly across mucous membranes. Locally acting toxin may produce some symptoms but cranial nerve paralysis results from blood stream distribution. Cranial nerves are preferentially affected because botulinum toxin binds more rapidly to sites where the cycles of depolarization and repolarization are frequent. Binding is irreversible and the toxin cannot thereafter be neutralized by antitoxin. Recovery occurs when nerve terminals sprout from the axon to form new motor endplates.

Botulinum toxin blocks impulse transmission mediated by acetylcholine at myoneural junctions, at autonomic ganglia, and at parasympathetic nerve terminals. Transmission is blocked because the toxin prevents release of acetylcholine from the presynaptic membrane. Impulse conduction within peripheral nerves and muscle contraction are not affected. Synthesis of acetylcholine and impulse transmission within terminal nerve fibrils remain intact. On the other hand, the miniature end-plate potentials spontaneously generated by release of acetylcholine in a resting nerve decrease and eventually disappear in the presence of toxin. If a poisoned nerve is stimulated repetitively, temporary summation of acetylcholine release occurs, producing an augmented response.

History

The symptoms of botulism vary from mild fatigue to severe weakness and collapse leading to death within a day. Initially, nausea, vomiting, abdominal bloating, and dryness in the mouth and throat may suggest gastrointestinal tract illness. Diplopia, blurred vision, dizziness, unsteadiness on standing, and difficulty with speech or swallowing are common early neurological symptoms. Subsequently, there is progression to weakness or paralysis in the limbs, and generalized weakness and lassitude. The dryness of the mouth and throat may become so severe as to cause pain. Eventually there may be difficulty holding up the head, constipation, urinary hesitancy, and problems in breathing. The incubation period is between 12 and 72 h. Patients with short incubation periods are likely to have ingested large amounts of toxin. However, individuals are known to have ingested large amounts of contaminated food without developing symptoms.

Physical examination

Negative findings in botulism are pertinent. Higher mental functions are preserved, although sometimes patients are drowsy. Sensation is intact. Fever is unusual. The mouth is dry and the tongue is furrowed. Lateral rectus weakness in the eyes produces internal strabismus. Failure of accommodation is common and the pupils may be fixed in mid position or dilated and unresponsive to light. Ptosis, weakness of other extraocular muscles, and inability to protrude the tongue or to raise the shoulders are other early findings. Weakness in the limbs is of the flaccid, lower motor neurone type and deep tendon reflexes are initially preserved. Facial muscles may be spared; gag and corneal reflexes are not lost.

Weakness of the respiratory muscles develops early in relation to other findings and deterioration can be rapid. Paralysis descends symmetrically from cranial nerves to upper extremities to respiratory muscles to the lower extremities in a proximal to distal pattern. Hypotension without compensatory tachycardia, intestinal ileus, and urinary retention are evidence of the widespread autonomic paralysis. Symptoms and signs can be confined to the autonomic nervous system.

Diagnosis

The diagnosis in the first case of an outbreak can be missed because cranial nerve symptoms and signs are ignored in what is apparently a gastrointestinal disturbance. The differential diagnosis usually lies between botulism and the descending form of acute inflammatory polyneuropathy or Guillain–Barré syndrome. There can be similarities in the clinical presentation and progression of symptoms in the two diseases. Patients with botulism have normal cerebrospinal fluid findings and respiratory weakness and failure develop early, prior to the presence of severe limb weakness. Patients with the Guillain–Barré syndrome have marked limb weakness prior to the development of respiratory failure. Sensation and mental status are preserved in botulism.

Other diagnoses that may be considered include diphtheria, intoxication with atropine or organophosphorus compounds, myasthenia gravis, cerebrovascular disease involving the brainstem and producing bulbar palsy, paralytic rabies, tick paralysis, and neurotoxic snake bite. Botulism is distinguished from polymyositis and periodic paralysis by its rapid progression and cranial nerve abnormalities. Sometimes patients with other types of poisoning are thought to have botulism, most often with an outbreak of staphylococcal food poisoning. Individuals with carbon monoxide poisoning have been mistakenly been thought to be poisoned by food, but they invariably have headaches and altered consciousness. Poisoning from chemicals or fish produces rapid onset of symptoms. Mushroom poisoning is characterized by severe abdominal pain.

The diagnosis of botulism can be confirmed by testing for botulinum toxin in the patient's serum, urine, stomach contents, or in the suspect food. Mice are inoculated intraperitoneally with 0.5 ml of sample, with and without mixing with polyvalent botulinum antitoxin, and observed for signs of botulism. Electromyography can be helpful in confirming a diagnosis of botulism. Single or low-frequency stimuli evoke muscle action potentials that are reduced in amplitude; tetanic or rapid stimuli produce an enhanced response. Nerve conduction velocities are normal. This result readily differentiates botulism from the Guillain–Barré syndrome. Patients with myasthenia gravis usually have muscle action potentials of normal or minimally decreased amplitude.

Treatment

The priorities in management are assessment of respiratory function followed by administration of antitoxin. Respiration should be monitored closely with a view to elective intubation since deterioration can occur rapidly. Prolonged respiratory support may be required. Profound hypotension can be secondary to hypoxaemia, acidosis, and accumulated fluid deficits or be a feature of the autonomic paralysis. Treat autonomic paralysis by expanding the intravascular volume using whole blood, protein, and/or saline while monitoring central venous pressure or by infusing low dose dopamine.

Trivalent (types A, B, and E) antitoxin has been shown to reduce case fatality and shorten the course of the illness. To be useful it must be given early, before free circulating toxin has bound to its peripheral targets and before the diagnosis can be confirmed by animal tests. Multivalent equine antitoxin is available from designated regional hospitals in the United Kingdom; half the dose is given intramuscularly and half intravenously. An intradermal 0.1-ml test dose is given, but most serum reactions are not predicted by this test. Human botulism immune plasma can be obtained from the Centers for Disease Control, Atlanta, Georgia, United States.

Many years ago it was shown that patients dying of botulism carried bacilli in their intestine. The discovery that clinical disease can result from toxin formed within the gastrointestinal tract of infants and adults makes antimicrobial treatment theoretically appealing. Gastric lavage, repeated high enemas, and cathartics have been given to attempt to remove unabsorbed toxin. Drugs capable of reversing neuromuscular blockade have been used to treat patients with botulism, but without any noticeable effect on respiratory muscle weakness or tidal volume.

The mortality from botulism in the early part of the twentieth century was 60 to 70 per cent, but this improved to 23 per cent for cases reported between 1960 and 1970 since the use of respiratory support. In a single, large outbreak in 1977 there were no deaths among 59 cases. Recovery from botulism depends upon the formation of new neuromuscular junctions; clinical improvement thus takes weeks to months. One severe case required respiratory support for 173 days with eventual recovery. Very prolonged fatigue and dyspnoea on exertion can be due to factors other than the neuromuscular blockade.

Wound botulism

Symptoms and signs of botulism can develop in people with injuries. Recognition may be complicated by the presence of fever from wound infection or gas gangrene, or by the absence of gastrointestinal symptoms. The diagnosis is confirmed by electromyography; botulinum toxin is detected in serum in only about half of the reported cases. The incubation period averages 7 days with a range of 4 to 17 days. Clinical findings and management are the same as for patients with food-borne botulism. Since 1991, wound botulism has increasingly become a complication of injection drug abuse; small abscesses at injection sites yield *C. botulinum*. An epidemic of wound botulism in the United States has been associated with the injection of black tar heroin. *C. botulinum* can be recovered from wounds in the absence of clinical botulism.

Infant botulism

Sporadically, cases of botulism are recognized in infants under 6 months of age. Previously healthy babies develop constipation, which progresses over 3 to 10 days to poor feeding, irritability, a hoarse cry, and weakness in head control. Examination shows a generally weak, hypotonic, afebrile infant. Abnormalities in eye movements and pupillary reactions are sometimes present and deep tendon reflexes are reduced or absent. There is considerable range in severity; respiratory failure can develop but most recover completely.

The diagnosis can be confirmed by finding *C. botulinum* and toxin in the faeces, and by electromyography. Botulinum toxin is not present in the serum. The disease is thought to follow ingestion of *C. botulinum* spores, which multiply in the infant's gastrointestinal tract and produce toxin. Excretion of *C. botulinum* and toxin may continue for as long as 3 months. Honey has been a source of spores for some cases. Other than supportive measures, no consistent pattern in treatment using antitoxin, antibiotics, cathartics, or enemas has been established.

Gas gangrene

Definition

Gas gangrene is a rapidly developing and spreading infection of muscle by toxin-producing clostridial species, especially *C. perfringens* (formerly known as *C. welchii*). It is accompanied by profound constitutional toxicity and is invariably fatal if untreated.

Aetiology

Although gas gangrene conjures up visions of battlefield injury, cases occur after civilian and iatrogenic trauma. Disease occurrence depends upon a conjunction of factors. Viable forms of clostridia must be present and the wound environment must be conducive to their growth. Proximity to faecal sources of bacteria is a risk factor, as in hip surgery, adrenaline injections into the buttock, and amputation of the leg for ischaemic vascular disease. Wound contamination with dirt, shrapnel, or bits of clothing reduces local oxygen concentrations. Similarly, wounds involving large muscle masses in the shoulder, hip, thigh, and calf, damage to major arteries, crush injuries, open fractures, and burns carry a higher risk. High-velocity missiles and impacts are regular features of modern injuries in both wartime and civilian life and such injuries produce extensive tissue damage.

The incidence of gas gangrene after trauma reflects the speed at which injured people can be evacuated and receive appropriate treatment. During the Vietnam and Falklands conflicts there were very few cases of gas gangrene among American and British wounded cared for by highly organized surgical teams. In comparison, when a jet airliner crashed in the Florida everglades, eight of the 77 injured survivors developed the disease.

Gas gangrene is caused by anaerobic, Gram-positive, spore-forming bacilli capable of producing potent exotoxins. Most cases are caused by *C. perfringens* type A, but some are due to *C. novyi* and a few to *C. septicum. C. histolyticum, C. sordellii*, and *C. fallax* cause few cases and not uncommonly more that one species is isolated. Clostridia are mainly saprophytes, occurring naturally in soil and in the gastrointestinal tracts of man and animals. Oxygen inhibits their growth and prevents toxin production. Possession of superoxide dismutase can permit the organisms to survive in the presence of small amounts of oxygen. Necrotic tissue, foreign bodies, and ischaemia in a wound reduce the locally available oxygen. Infrequently, gas gangrene occurs without preceding trauma. It can be a primary infection of the perineum or scrotum, or present in a limb, secondary to seeding from clostridial colonization of a colonic neoplasm. *C. septicum* is found in a higher percentage of these cases than where there is a history of trauma.

C. novyi and other clostridia cause soft tissue infections at injection sites in drug addicts. An epidemic of these infections was reported in Scotland, Ireland, England, and the United States in 2000 associated with hypotension, severe constitutional toxicity, and a high case fatality rate.

Toxins

The clostridia responsible for gas gangrene elaborate a wide range of toxin activities, with from four to more than 12 separate toxins described for *C. septicum, C. novyi*, and *C. perfringens*. The principal toxin of *C. perfringens* is α toxin; the toxic action has been shown to be due to an ability of the molecule to insert into and interact with a phospholipid membrane. Electron microscopy shows gaps of 7.5 to 18 nm appearing in the plasma membrane as early as 1 h. These plasma membrane defects increase with time and can be visualized adjacent to toxin molecules that have been labelled with ferritin. Toxin is not detected in the tissues or serum of patients with gas gangrene, possibly because the toxin binds rapidly and irreversibly.

History

The incubation period of gas gangrene is usually less than 4 days, often less than 24 h, and occasionally as short as 1 to 6 h. Pain is the most characteristic symptom. Patients describe this as severe or excruciating and sudden in onset. Evolution of symptoms and signs can be very rapid. Toxicity may prevent the patient from giving an adequate history.

Physical examination

Early on it may be difficult to account for the patient's pain by objective physical findings. Swelling, bluish discoloration, or darkening of the skin occurs at the affected site. The traumatic or surgical wound becomes oedematous and a thin, serous ooze emerges. Pain steadily increases in severity: the overlying skin becomes stretched and develops a brown or 'bronzed' discoloration. Haemorrhagic vesicles and finally areas of frank necrosis appear. A sweet odour from the wound has been described. In spite of the name, gas is not invariably present, especially early. Later, crepitus and exquisite tenderness are present in the wound.

Profound constitutional changes occur. Patients become sweaty and febrile, and though alert and oriented, are very distressed. The pulse is elevated out of proportion to the fever. Death may occur within 48 h. At operation, infected muscle appears dark red with purple discoloration; frank gangrene and liquefaction may be seen. Involved muscle does not contract after direct stimulation.

Clostridial myonecrosis must be distinguished from anaerobic cellulitis and from anaerobic streptococcal myositis. Anaerobic cellulitis occurs where putrefying anaerobic clostridia produce a purulent infection in traumatized muscle and other tissues. Streptococcal myositis is a spreading muscle infection with anaerobic streptococci and either *Streptococcus pyogenes* or *Staphylococcus aureus*. Neither is associated with the constitutional toxicity characteristic of gas gangrene and neither requires as radical excision. Diabetic patients develop gas gangrene due to ischaemic vascular disease. Numerous micro-organisms, both aerobic and anaerobic, produce gas in tissues.

Diagnosis

The diagnosis of gas gangrene has to be made on clinical grounds. Prompt recognition and treatment improves the prognosis. Sudden deterioration in a postoperative patient or following trauma requires examination of the wound and surrounding tissue. Cases of primary gas gangrene and cases following elective surgery may have a higher fatality because recognition is delayed. Gram stain of the wound discharge, of an aspirate, or of a needle biopsy may aid diagnosis. In gas gangrene there are many large, plump, Gram-positive bacilli, usually without spores. Few, if any, polymorphonuclear leucocytes are present. On the other hand, both anaerobic streptococcal myositis and anaerobic cellulitis show many leucocytes and the former is characterized by long chains of Gram-positive cocci.

CT scanning can detect gas deep in muscle, but the absence of gas does not exclude the diagnosis. Culture of clostridia does not confirm a diagnosis of gas gangrene, as simple colonization without clinical disease occurs in up to 30 per cent of wounds. Efforts to establish a portal of entry for cases of spontaneous, non-traumatic gas gangrene may improve the prognosis.

Treatment

Surgical removal of all affected muscle is essential. Although not substitutes for surgery, antimicrobials, hyperbaric oxygen, and administration of antitoxin have been thought to be helpful adjunctive therapies. Penicillin has been the drug of choice, but there is experimental evidence that clindamycin and metronidazole might be superior to penicillin, perhaps by inhibiting toxin production. This has led to the use of penicillin and clindamycin as combination therapy. Ceftriaxone or erythromycin are alternative choices for severely penicillin-allergic patients.

Hyperbaric oxygen is used to treat gas gangrene. An effect on mortality has never been shown by controlled trials, and comparable mortality rates have been achieved without using it. One hundred per cent oxygen is given at 303 kPa for 60 to 120 min, two to three times daily. Therapeutic administration of gas-gangrene antitoxin made from horse serum is controversial. Use during the Second World War reduced mortality but serum sickness and other allergic reactions occur. It is no longer produced in the United States. Shock, blood loss, dehydration, and septicaemia with micro-organisms such as *Escherichia coli* should be treated appropriately. *C. perfringens* septicaemia in association with gas gangrene is not common.

Prevention

The mortality of established disease still ranges between 11 and 31 percent. Prophylactic antibiotic treatment effectively eliminates this risk. A first generation cephalosporin is given intravenously before surgery and for three doses postoperatively. Metronidazole may be useful in patients who are hypersensitive to β-lactam antibiotics. Antibiotic levels can be detected in ischaemic tissues.

Traumatic wounds are treated to eliminate the conditions that allow gas-gangrene bacilli to grow. High-velocity missiles distribute energy radially from their path, producing more extensive tissue damage than missiles at low speeds or with a small mass. Wounds should be excised widely by resection back to healthy, viable muscle and skin. Closure is delayed for 5 to 6 days until it is certain that the wound is free of infection. Military surgeons usually give penicillin in high dosage over this period. Experimentally, active immunization protects, but in man this requires the clear definition of risk categories.

Clostridial infections of the gastrointestinal tract

Pseudomembranous colitis

Definition

Pseudomembranous colitis is an acute exudative infection of the colon caused by *C. difficile*. The name derives from plaques of necrotic membrane that adhere to the mucosal surface in the clinically most severe form of the disease.

Aetiology

Pseudomembranous colitis was described as a clinical and pathological entity in 1893 with its clostridial aetiology becoming known in 1977. *C. difficile* is an anaerobic, spore-forming, bacillus found in the environment. Healthy adults are only rarely colonized with *C. difficile*. Antimicrobial treatment reduces resistance to intestinal colonization. Colonization and toxin production produce colitis. Because colonization and antimicrobial treatment may occur at different times, antibiotic-susceptible strains of *C. difficile* are able to produce disease. Resistance to colonization requires viable intestinal bacteria, but it is not known which species or combination of species determines this resistance. Usually resistance to colonization will spontaneously reconstitute itself unless an antimicrobial effect persists

within the gut. Infants and young children can be asymptomatically colonized even in the absence of antimicrobial treatment.

Clinical history

The single most pertinent detail of the medical history is previous antimicrobial treatment. Direct questioning may be needed to elicit this history; antimicrobials may have been self-administered, taken for trivial complaints, or used as long as 3 or 4 weeks before the start of diarrhoea. Pseudomembranous colitis has been reported to follow the use of every antimicrobial in common medical practice, but its association with lincomycin, clindamycin, ampicillin, amoxacillin, and cephalosporins is strongest. It occasionally occurs in individuals with no history of antimicrobial treatment or as a complication of chronic colonic obstruction, carcinoma, leukaemia, or uraemia. Pseudomembranous colitis was identified as a pathological entity before any clinical use of antimicrobials. Community-acquired cases occur sporadically but case clustering in hospitals or nursing homes is not uncommon. The disease is more common in older patients but the typical syndrome has been described in people of all ages including infants.

Initial symptoms vary from mild, self-limiting diarrhoea to acute fulminating toxic megacolon. Illness can begin surreptitiously where persistent diarrhoea resists all efforts at symptomatic relief. Community-acquired cases tend to have a week or more of diarrhoea before seeking medical attention. Stools are described as watery or porridge-like, or patients may be obstipated. Other initial symptoms are sudden chills, fever, and signs of an abdominal catastrophe. Elderly patients may have diarrhoea that resolves and then recurs at intervals of one to several days. Severe abdominal pain is not common and a history of frank blood in the stools suggests a different type of colitis.

Physical examination

Elderly patients appear tired, toxic, and ill. Low fever, a dry furred tongue, and abdominal tenderness, sometimes with peritonism, are the most common clinical signs. Signs of dehydration may be present, but hypotension attributable to hypovolaemia is not common. Spiking temperatures may also be seen and a distended, tense, abdomen can suggest colonic obstruction. Reactive arthritis, IgA nephropathy, and hypoproteinaemia are potential complications of *C. difficile* colitis.

Diagnosis

Many patients show polymorphonuclear leucocytosis, sometimes with counts of 30 000/ul or more. Leucocytes are present in the faeces. Chemical findings in patients with prolonged diarrhoea include azotaemia and hypoalbuminaemia; the azotaemia may appear to be out of proportion to the dehydration. The presence of *C. difficile* toxin establishes a mechanism for the diarrhoea.

Sigmoidoscopy can be helpful in making an early diagnosis because the raised, mucoid to opaque yellow plaques (0.2–2 mm across) are diagnostic. If the mucosa appears normal, biopsy and multiple sectioning may reveal microscopic lesions. Some patients with *C. difficile* colitis do not have pseudomembranes, either because lesions are distributed unevenly in the colon or because the illness is mild. In these cases the diagnosis can only be confirmed by testing for toxin and *C. difficile*. Rarely, patients with pseudomembranes on sigmoidoscopy or rectal biopsy may fail to yield *C. difficile*. Usually confluent rather than focal mucosal necrosis is found. This appears to be the end result of several types of colonic mucosal injury, not specific to *C. difficile* infection.

The differential diagnosis of pseudomembranous colitis includes other forms of antimicrobial-associated colitis, diarrhoea due to *Salmonella*, *Shigella*, and *Campylobacter* species, intestinal amoebiasis, Crohn's disease, and non-specific ulcerative colitis. These can be differentiated by sigmoidoscopy and rectal biopsy, or by microscopy and culture of the faeces. Two-thirds or more of patients with simple antimicrobial-associated diarrhoea do not have infection with *C. difficile*. Often they complain of sudden abdominal pain and bloody diarrhoea that subsides within a day or two of stopping antimicrobial treatment. Occasionally, patients may be infected with *C. difficile* in addition to another micro-organism capable of causing diarrhoea. Infection with *C. difficile* may exacerbate symptoms in some patients with inflammatory bowel disease.

Treatment

Stopping the associated antimicrobial may allow *C. difficile* colitis to resolve spontaneously. If clinical circumstances dictate active treatment, the antimicrobial of choice is one to which *C. difficile* is susceptible and which is not absorbed following oral administration. Vancomycin is used in a dose of 125 mg every 6 h. Metronidazole, 250 mg four times a day, also appears to be effective, although it is absorbed. Some physicians regard it as less effective than vancomycin. Bacitracin may also be useful. Severe cases usually show improvement after 48 h of treatment and signs and symptoms rapidly return to normal. Failure to respond to vancomycin suggests that the diagnosis is incorrect or that an additional condition or complication may be present.

Patients who are dehydrated need fluid resuscitation. Cholestyramine resins bind *C. difficile* toxin *in vitro*, but have no effect on the clinical course of the colitis. Pseudomembranous colitis has been successfully treated by colectomy. However, the disease is completely reversible by appropriate antimicrobial treatment. In patients who are unable to take vancomycin orally, some physicians have attempted to instil it into the colon via a caecostomy tube; others combine intragastric vancomycin, intermittent clamping of the nasogastric tube, and parenteral metronidazole. *C. difficile* antitoxin is not available in the United Kingdom.

Any of the suggested antimicrobial treatment regimens for pseudomembranous colitis may be followed by relapse. The relapse illness can be clinically more severe than the original. There has never been any evidence that relapse is due to antimicrobial resistance and patients continue to respond to treatment with the original or an alternative drug. Patients relapse both because antimicrobial treatment may not completely clear them of *C. difficile* or because a new exposure to environmental strains has occurred. There is evidence that vancomycin and metronidazole themselves can reduce resistance to the infection; prolonged treatment may produce prolonged susceptibility. On the other hand, patients whose *C. difficile* colitis resolves without antimicrobial treatment usually do not relapse.

Occasional patients may have multiple relapses and many regimens have been suggested for their management. These include tapering doses of vancomycin, a *Lactobacillus* preparation three times a day, or cholestyramine three times a day after a therapeutic course of vancomycin. Cholestyramine can not be combined with vancomycin. In a patient recovering from multiple relapses, tapering vancomycin doses to once daily when diarrhoea stops, then to alternate days, then to progressively longer intervals, can prevent early relapse. Some patients with severe colitis or multiple relapses may continue to have diarrhoea without toxin in their stools. This resembles postdysenteric colitis where continued diarrhoea is due to lingering mucosal injury. Bowel rest with total parenteral nutrition can allow healing and recovery; continued treatment against *C. difficile* is not required. Normal flora may be reconstituted by giving a suspension of normal faeces as an enema.

It may be necessary under certain circumstances to continue an antimicrobial when a patient has developed pseudomembranous colitis. There is no evidence to suggest that concurrent therapy with vancomycin will not be successful, although clinical improvement occurs more slowly. It is reasonable to replace a drug commonly associated with pseudomembranous colitis by one which is not, such as a quinolone, aminoglycoside, tetracycline, or sulphonamide. Repeat treatment with an inducing antimicrobial at some later time is not contraindicated in a patient who has recovered from pseudomembranous colitis.

Prevention

Clusters of cases of pseudomembranous colitis were reported before its infectious aetiology was understood. Now it is known that *C. difficile* may contaminate the environment of a patient, that patients acquire the organism, and that cross-infection is confirmed by strain typing. The chain of infection for isolated cases may be difficult to trace because spores can persist for months. Since patients receiving antimicrobial treatments are at risk, those with colitis ought to be nursed in barrier isolation. Patients with diarrhoea, especially those who are incontinent, are more important sources of cross-contamination than those with formed stools. Physical cleanliness, enteric precautions, confinement to a single room, and reduced use of the most frequent inducing antimicrobials are the approaches most often used to reduce institutional cross-infection. There is no proven value in retesting patients until they are free of toxin nor in treating asymptomatic toxin excretors.

Necrotizing enterocolitis

Definition

Necrotizing enterocolitis is a fulminating clinical illness characterized by extensive necrosis of the intestinal mucosa and wall. Terms such as darmbrand (Germany), enteritis necroticans, pig bel (Papua New Guinea), or gas gangrene of the bowel describe geographical variants. Cases occur sporadically in adults or as epidemics in all ages. Necrotizing enterocolitis occurs in infants, sometimes in clusters, but is not proven to be due to clostridial infection.

Aetiology

C. perfringens (*C. welchii*) is considered to be the cause. Sporadic cases usually yield *C. perfringens* type A. Gram stain of the necrotic mucosa and the bowel wall shows many Gram-positive bacilli. However, in the German and especially in the Papua New Guinea outbreaks, there is substantial evidence implicating *C. perfringens* type C. Type C produces large amounts of β-toxin, which has lethal and necrotizing effects. Papua New Guinea highlanders have a high prevalence of antibodies to β-toxin; antibodies are rare in people who live where the disease is uncommon. Patients with pig bel have rising levels of antibodies to β-toxin, and specific passive or active immunization has been shown to prevent disease. It is not clear whether exogenous human infection with these organisms occurs or whether the lesions are produced by the overgrowth of endogenous clostridia. Sweet potato, a local dietary staple, contains an inhibitor of trypsin. Combined with a low-protein diet this may impair the ability of the intestine to inactivate endogenously produced β-toxin. However, the methods used for roasting the pigs offer many opportunities for clostridial contamination.

History and physical examination

Sporadic cases, over 50 years of age or recovering from gastric surgery, are regularly reported from Scandinavia, Europe, the United States, Australia, and the Middle East. Alternatively, epidemic outbreaks as described in post-war Germany and among the highlanders of Papua New Guinea follow ingestion of contaminated food or a dramatic change in eating habits. Symptoms develop suddenly in someone who was previously well. There is severe abdominal pain, which is colicky at first and afterwards becomes continuous. Bloody diarrhoea and vomiting may occur. The patient may be extremely toxic and go into shock. On examination there is fever, with abdominal distension, localized or diffuse tenderness, and reduced bowel sounds. A tender mass may be palpated. Later, malabsorption or chronic partial obstruction may develop because of intestinal scarring.

Treatment and prevention

Patients with suspected pig bel should be treated with nasogastric suction and intravenous fluids. Pyrantel is given by mouth and the bowel rested by fasting. One megaunit of benzylpenicillin is given intravenously every 4 h and the patient observed for surgical complications. Mild cases recover without surgical intervention, but if surgical indications are present, the mortality ranges from 35 to 100 per cent. As pig bel continues to be a common disease in Papua New Guinea, consideration should be given to the use of a *C. perfringens* type C toxoid vaccine in local areas. Two doses spaced 3 to 4 months apart have been shown to prevent the disease.

Clostridium perfringens food poisoning

Occurrence and clinical findings

In the United Kingdom and the United States, food poisoning caused by *C. perfringens* is the third most common type of food-borne illness. Meat and poultry are responsible for at least 90 per cent of the outbreaks, which occur where food is prepared in large quantities. Two-thirds of the reported outbreaks are in schools, hospitals, factories, restaurants, or catering establishments, and in a typical outbreak 35 to 40 people are affected. An estimated 12 000 cases were associated with a single out-break in 1969.

The circumstances surrounding an outbreak repeat themselves with monotonous regularity. A meat dish is prepared by stewing, braising, boiling, or steaming and this is allowed to stand at ambient temperatures for a period of 4 to 24 h. The food is served cold or after desultory rewarming. Six to 12 h after eating the meal, the victims complain of crampy abdominal pain and then diarrhoea. Vomiting is unusual and fever inconsequential. Twelve to 24 h later the diarrhoea and pain have subsided. Fatal cases occur rarely; at autopsy they show severe enterocolitis.

Undoubtedly many cases of *C. perfringens* food poisoning occur at home but are not reported. Antibodies to the toxin mediating the symptoms are very common and it is likely that nearly everyone has experienced this disease once or more in their lifetime.

Aetiology

C. perfringens is an ubiquitous, sporulating anaerobe with an unparalleled virtuosity for production of biologically significant toxins. The clinical effects of infection with any particular strain may depend largely on its toxin-producing capacity. Strains associated with food poisoning have a number of special characteristics. They are type A, although their production of α-toxin is variable; they are often heat resistant. Eighty-six per cent of food-poisoning strains produce a specific, heat-labile enterotoxin. Toxin production *in vitro* is closely associated with sporulation rather than with the multiplication of vegetative cells. *In vivo*, toxin probably acts by damaging enterocyte membranes. Free enterotoxin has been detected in diarrhoeal stool after *C. perfringens* food poisoning, antibody to enterotoxin increases after such episodes, and ingestion of 8 to 12 mg of enterotoxin by volunteers produces abdominal pain and diarrhoea.

C. perfringens is a normal human faecal organism, is regularly found in the intestinal tract of domestic animals, often contaminates raw meat, and can be carried by flies. The distribution of enterotoxin-producing strains may be more restricted. However, surface contamination of meat with *C. perfringens* is common and subsequent rolling or grinding will distribute these organisms throughout. Heat-resistant strains survive at maximum temperatures of 100°C. Spores then germinate and multiply to 10^6 to 10^7 cells/g in the highly advantageous, anaerobic environment created when meat cools slowly or stands at ambient temperature. Reheating may not kill these cells; when ingested they multiply still further, sporulate, and release their toxin.

Enterotoxin-producing strains of *C. perfringens* may sometimes cause diarrhoea by means of overgrowth in the gut. Patients, usually elderly, begin to experience diarrhoea without known contact with contaminated food. The diarrhoea may be short lived or persist intermittently for several months. Colony counts of 10^8 to 10^{10}/g of faeces are associated with the presence of high titres of free toxin. Previous antimicrobial treatment may encourage the overgrowth and the same strain has been found to cross infect patients.

Further reading

Botulism

Cherington M (1998). Clinical spectrum of botulism. *Muscle and Nerve* 21, 701–10.

Maselli RA (1998). Pathogenesis of human botulism. *Annals of the New York Academy of Sciences* 841, 122–39.

Schreiner MS, Field B, Ruddy R (1991). Infant botulism: a review of 12 years' experience at the Children's Hospital of Philadelphia. *Pediatrics* 87, 159–65.

Hayes MT, Seto O, Ruoff KL (1997). Weekly clinicopathological exercises: Case 22-1997: A 58-year-old woman with multiple cranial neuropathies. *New England Journal of Medicine* 337, 184–90.

Gas gangrene

Centers for Disease Control (2000). Update: *Clostridium novyi* and unexplained illness among injecting-drug users. *Morbidity and Mortality Weekly Report* 49, 543–5.

Darke SG, King AM, Slack WK (1977). Gas gangrene and related infection: classification, clinical features and aetiology, management and mortality. A report of 88 cases. *British Journal of Surgery* 64, 104–12.

Maclennan JD (1962). The histotoxic clostridial infections of man. *Bacteriology Reviews* 26, 177–276.

Naylor CE, Eaton JT, Howells A, *et al.* (1998). Structure of the key toxin in gas gangrene. *Nature Structural Biology* 5, 738–46.

Rood JI (1998). Virulence genes of *Clostridium perfringens*. *Annual Review of Microbiology* 52, 333–60.

Shouler PJ (1983). The management of missile injuries. *Journal of the Royal Navy Medical Service* 69, 80–4.

Gastrointestinal infections

Bartlett JG (1992). The 10 most common questions about *Clostridium difficile* and diarrhea/contis. *Infectious Diseases in Clinical Practice* 1, 254–9.

Hobbs BC (1974). Clostridium welchii and Bacillus cereus infection and intoxication. *Postgraduate Medical Journal* 50, 597–602.

Larson HE, Price AB, Honour P, Borriello SP (1978). *Clostridium difficile* and the aetiology of pseudomembranous colitis. *Lancet* i, 1063–6.

Lawrence GW, Murrell TGC, Walker PD (1979). Pigbel. *Papua New Guinea Medical Journal* 22, 1–86.

7.11.22 Tuberculosis

Richard E. Chaisson and Jean Nachega

Introduction

Tuberculosis is one of the most important diseases in the history of humanity, and remains an extraordinary burden on human health today. Archaeological evidence demonstrates that tuberculosis was present in antiquity, and large epidemics of the disease emerged in Europe in the Middle Ages. While contemporary physicians consider tuberculosis to be one of the classical infectious diseases, recognition of the clinical manifestations of the disease has evolved over the past two millenia. The Greek term *phthisis* was used by Hippocrates to describe the wasting disease later known as tuberculosis. While the Greeks recognized various clinical manifestations of tuberculosis, understanding of the connection between the forms was limited. In the Middle Ages, the study of anatomy and the correlation of pathological findings with clinical syndromes led to a better understanding of the disease. The term 'tuberculosis' was introduced in the early nineteenth century, derived from the tubercles characterized in the study of pathological features of the disease.

The impact of tuberculosis on mankind cannot be overstated, as the disease has killed hundreds of millions of people over the centuries and has had economic and social effects perhaps unparalleled in the history of medicine. Between 1700 and 1950, tuberculosis was a great killer in the developed world, earning the sobriquet 'the captain of the men of death ...' from John Bunyan, and 'the White Plague' from René and Jean Dubos. The inspiration that artists have drawn from tuberculosis, portrayed in literature, opera, and art, testifies not only to the importance of the disease within their contemporary societies, but also to the extent to which tuberculosis affected artists themselves. The annals of art are rife with those who succumbed to tuberculosis, including Keats, Chopin, the Brontë sisters, Robert Louis Stevenson, Poe, and many others.

The conquest of tuberculosis through the development of vaccines, drugs, and diagnostics was a principal goal of biomedical research in the nineteenth and twentieth centuries. The first description of the tubercle bacillus as the cause of tuberculosis by Robert Koch in 1882 was a scientific landmark. The postulates established by Koch for determining the microbial aetiology of disease have continuing influence today, and molecular correlates of those derived by Koch further strengthen the ingenuity of his thesis. The discovery of streptomycin by Schatz and Waksman in 1943 was a major triumph; both Koch and Waksman received the Nobel prize for their efforts. The development of additional antimicrobial agents against tuberculosis in the 1950s, 1960s, and 1970s and the evaluation of chemotherapy in elegant studies conducted by the British Medical Research Council, the United States Public Health Service, and the United States Veterans Administration led to a marked apathy about tuberculosis in the closing decades of the twentieth century.

Despite the availability of curative chemotherapy for more than half a century, however, tuberculosis continues to cause an enormous amount of suffering, disability, and mortality. In 1994, the World Health Assembly declared that tuberculosis was a global health crisis, and the situation has only grown more grave since then. Epidemics of HIV-related tuberculosis and multidrug-resistant disease have expanded in the past 5 years, and global control of tuberculosis is a remote possibility at present.

The unique biological properties of the causative organism, *Mycobacterium tuberculosis* complex, allow for a long incubation period between the time of infection and the development of symptoms. Latent tuberculosis infection can persist for decades prior to causing disease, or can persist for the lifetime of an infected person without ever causing clinically evident illness. Because latent infection creates a large reservoir of carriers of the infection, disease elimination is difficult to contemplate.

Aetiology

Tuberculosis is a granulomatous disease caused by organisms of the *M. tuberculosis* complex, including *M. tuberculosis*, *M. bovis*, and *M. africanum*, with *M. tuberculosis* greatly predominating. *M. tuberculosis* and the other mycobacteria are small, rod-shaped or curved bacilli in the Order Actinomycetales, Family Mycobacteriaceae, with a unique, thick cell wall composed of glycolipids and lipids. The lipid-rich coat of the mycobacteria renders these organisms resistant to acid decolorization following carbolfuschin staining, hence the term 'acid-fast bacilli.' Classification of the mycobacteria was based for many years on the staining and growth properties described by Runyon, but this unwieldy system has been largely replaced with modern techniques that identify mycobacteria by specific DNA sequences and, to a lesser extent, biochemical assays. Mycobacteria are frequently considered according to the diseases they cause rather than their behaviour in the laboratory: *M. tuberculosis* complex causing tuberculosis; *M. leprae* the cause of leprosy; and the non-tuberculous mycobacteria, including rapid growers, associated with a wide range of manifestations, particularly in immunocompromised hosts.

The organisms of the *M. tuberculosis* complex are remarkably slow growing, with a generation time of between 20 and 24 h. The exceedingly slow intrinsic reproductive rate of *M. tuberculosis* contributes both to its behaviour as a pathogen and to difficulties in recovering the organism in culture. Moreover, *M. tuberculosis* is able to persist in a latent form within cells and granulomas for many years, and can reactivate to cause disease decades after infection is acquired. Tubercle bacilli are not known to form spores, but both typical bacilli and non-staining forms of the bacteria persist in cells and tissues, as evidenced by detection of DNA, years after infection is

acquired and retain the capacity to replicate and produce clinical illness. These unique biological characteristics make the tubercle bacillus exceedingly difficult to combat and control.

Epidemiology

Despite the widely held belief that tuberculosis was waning during the 1980s, global tuberculosis incidence has been steady or increasing for several decades. In Western Europe and North America, the incidence of tuberculosis peaked in the 1700s and 1800s, then declined over a period of years prior to the development of chemotherapy. Improvements in hygiene and nutrition, along with reductions in household crowding, were credited with these trends. Following the introduction of curative treatment for tuberculosis in the era following Second World War, the incidence of disease fell even further, and tuberculosis deaths were greatly decreased. The success in controlling tuberculosis experienced in the Western nations was not replicated in developing countries, and increasing epidemics of the disease have been occurring in these areas. Ironically, progress in tuberculosis control in the Western nations led to neglect of public health programmes that were responsible for reductions in morbidity. As a consequence of inattention to control, the United States experienced a resurgence of tuberculosis between 1985 and 1992, with a 21 per cent increase in the annual number of reported cases during that time. In the United Kingdom, tuberculosis incidence has plateaued over the past decade, with an annual incidence of 11 cases per 100 000 population since 1991. Worldwide, tuberculosis continues to kill more than 2 million people per year, making it the second leading infectious cause of death after HIV infection. In fact, tuberculosis is a leading cause of death in AIDS, and HIV-related tuberculosis deaths are attributed to AIDS, not tuberculosis. If these deaths were attributed to tuberculosis, it would remain the leading infectious cause of death worldwide.

The World Health Organization estimates that 2 billion people, or one-third of the world's population, are infected with *M. tuberculosis*. From this seedbed of latent infection, about 8 million new cases of active disease arise each year, with a global incidence of approximately 160 cases per 100 000 population. The global distribution of tuberculosis case rates is shown in Fig. 1. Disease due to *M. tuberculosis* is most common in developing nations, both in absolute numbers and incidence of new cases. Twenty-two countries account for 80 per cent of all tuberculosis, with India and China responsible for 23 and 17 per cent of cases, respectively. In general, the highest incidence of disease is found in the countries of sub-Saharan Africa, where HIV infection has contributed to extraordinary increases in case rates, while the greatest number of cases arise in the populous nations of Asia, which have moderately high rates of disease per capita. The global incidence of tuberculosis is increasing slightly, although population growth is resulting in higher numbers of cases each year. Declines in incidence in the developed world have been offset by increasing rates in the HIV-ravaged countries of Africa and by escalating incidence in Eastern Europe in the aftermath of the collapse of communism and its public health infrastructure.

Typically tuberculosis affects young adults, with peak incidence in those aged 25 to 44. The dynamics of tuberculosis within a particular country or region, however, reflects both historical trends in tuberculosis transmission and current risk factors and practices of disease control. In Western Europe, for example, tuberculosis is seen in two demographic groups: elderly native Europeans who were presumably infected many years ago and who experience reactivation of latent infections as they age or become immunocompromised, and younger immigrants from high-incidence countries in the developing world. In the United States, tuberculosis is seen in young adults who have immigrated from endemic areas and in those with HIV infection, whereas reactivation tuberculosis in the elderly is increasingly uncommon. In the developing world, tuberculosis most commonly occurs in young adults, with rapidly escalating rates in those with HIV infection. In all countries where tuberculosis is prevalent, young children who acquire

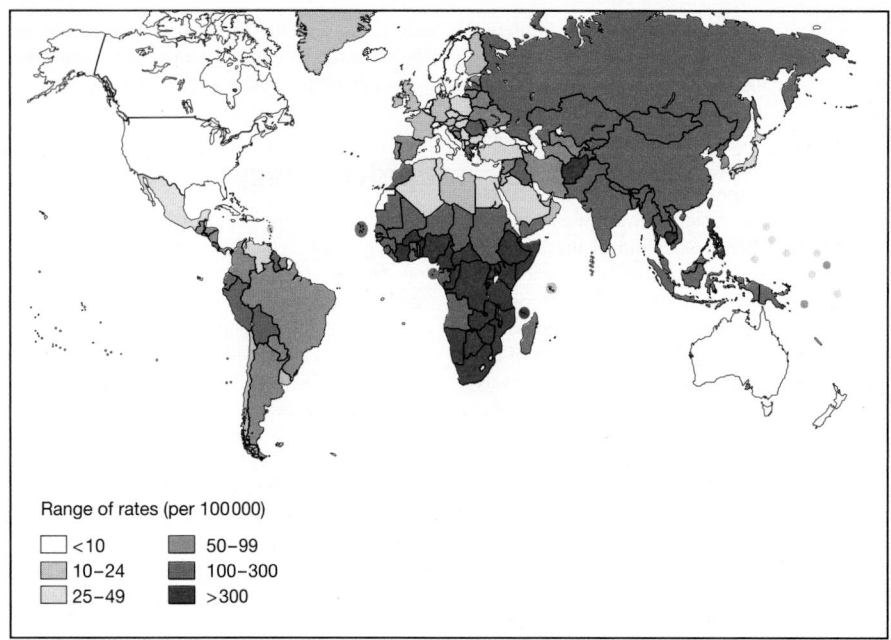

Fig. 1 Global tuberculosis incidence 1999.

tuberculosis from adults account for a small proportion of all cases. It is interesting that children between the ages of 5 and 15 have extremely low rates of tuberculosis, even in areas with a high disease burden.

The epidemiology of tuberculosis is a function of two distinct but related phenomena: the likelihood of becoming infected with *M. tuberculosis* and the probability of developing disease once infection has occurred. Risk factors for becoming infected relate to exposure to infectious individuals. Throughout the world, living with someone who has infectious tuberculosis is the most important risk factor for acquiring infection. The longer the duration of undiagnosed tuberculosis, the greater the severity of disease and probability of transmitting infection. The more intimate the contact, the greater the chance of becoming infected. Exposure to infectious individuals in other environments, including hospitals, prisons, and the workplace, is another important route of infection. In areas of the world where tuberculosis is frequent, exposure in the community is probably unavoidable. In low-prevalence countries community exposure is most likely to occur in distinct pockets of increased incidence, such as poorer areas of large cities or neighbourhoods with high HIV prevalence.

After *M. tuberculosis* infection is acquired, the risk of developing disease is dependent on host immunity. As discussed below, a number of conditions have been identified that increase the risk of active disease in a person with latent tuberculosis infection, most notably HIV infection. Strain differences in *M. tuberculosis* have not been associated with the risk of disease, although inoculum size is associated with the probability of becoming ill. Household contacts who are infected by patients with high sputum levels of acid-fast bacilli have a higher incidence of active disease than contacts of patients who have sputum smears negative for acid-fast bacilli. On the other hand, while there is some evidence that specific strains of *M. tuberculosis* may infect contacts more successfully than other strains, the risk of disease in those infected with these transmissable strains is not elevated.

Tuberculosis is a disease traditionally associated with specific population groups, notably the poor, alcohol and drug abusers, and more recently, those with HIV infection. The increased incidence of tuberculosis in impoverished populations is probably multifactorial, involving increased risk of infection (for example due to crowded living conditions and a higher background prevalence of disease in the community) and increased risk of developing disease after infection (for example due to malnutrition).

Similar reasons may explain the higher rates of tuberculosis seen in alcohol and drug abusers, with suppression of host cellular immunity either directly or indirectly from substance abuse. The more recent association of tuberculosis and HIV infection is clearly related to development of cellular immunodeficiency in those with HIV, but in many settings those at highest risk for HIV infection are also more likely to be latently infected with *M. tuberculosis* than others.

The impact of HIV infection on the epidemiology of tuberculosis is striking. As will be discussed below, HIV infection is the most potent known biological risk factor for tuberculosis. The relative risk of tuberculosis in an HIV-infected person is 200- to 1000-fold greater than in someone without HIV infection. As a result of the extraordinary risk conferred by HIV infection, the majority of patients with tuberculosis in many sub-Saharan countries are HIV seropositive. In the United States and the United Kingdom, HIV infection accounts for a substantial proportion of tuberculosis cases in many cities. HIV infection is the unifying theme in many nosocomial outbreaks of tuberculosis, as infection is spread among immunocompromised patients receiving medical care at the same facility. It is increasingly apparent that control of tuberculosis will not be possible globally without control of HIV infection.

Another very important trend in tuberculosis epidemiology is the growing problem of drug-resistant tuberculosis. There are two categories: primary resistance, which is the presence of drug resistance in someone who has never had treatment for tuberculosis, and secondary resistance, the presence of resistance in a patient who has previously been treated for tuberculosis. Primary resistance results from acquiring an infection that is already drug resistant, while acquired resistance is the result of inappropriate therapy that selects for resistant mutants of *M. tuberculosis*. A global survey of resistance performed by the World Health Organization and the International Union Against Tuberculosis and Lung Disease found that the median prevalence of primary drug resistance was 10 per cent, and the median prevalence of acquired resistance was 36 per cent. Moreover, 'hot spots' of drug-resistant tuberculosis were identified on all continents, most notably in the former Soviet nations, where multidrug-resistant tuberculosis is identified in 10 to 20 per cent of all cases. Multidrug-resistant tuberculosis is exceedingly difficult to cure, and so failure to control its spread has ominous implications.

Pathogenesis

The development of active tuberculosis, like all infectious diseases, is a function of the quantity and virulence of the invading organism and the relative resistance or susceptibility of the host to the pathogen. Tubercle bacilli are transmitted between people by aerosols generated by coughing or otherwise expelling infectious pulmonary or laryngeal secretions into the air. *M. tuberculosis* bacilli excreted by this action are contained within droplet nuclei, extremely small particles (less than 1 μm) that remain airborne for long periods and are disseminated by diffusion and convection until they are deposited on surfaces, diluted, or inactivated by ultraviolet radiation. People breathing air into which droplet nuclei have been excreted are at risk of becoming infected if inhaled nuclei are deposited in their alveoli. Transmission of tuberculous infection by other routes, such as inoculation in laboratories and aerosolization of bacilli from tissues in hospitals, has been documented, but these are an insignificant means of spread. *M. bovis* can be acquired from contaminated milk from tuberculous cows, but modern animal husbandry practices and pasteurization of milk have virtually eliminated this mode of infection throughout most of the world.

The natural history of tuberculosis in humans is illustrated in Fig. 2. People who are in contact with someone with infectious tuberculosis may acquire infection, as described above. Factors that affect the likelihood of infection being transmitted include the severity of the disease in the index case (such as extent of radiographic abnormalities, cavitation, frequency of cough), the duration and closeness of exposure, and environmental factors such as humidity, ventilation, and ambient ultraviolet light. A number of studies in diverse locations and circumstances have shown that approximately 20 to 30 per cent of close contacts of a patient with untreated tuberculosis become infected with *M. tuberculosis*, as demonstrated by the development of a reactive tuberculin skin test.

Deposition of tubercle bacilli in the alveoli results in a series of protective responses by the cellular immune system that forestall the development of disease in the majority of infected people. Alveolar macrophages ingest tubercle bacilli, which then multiply intracellularly and eventually cause cell lysis with release of organisms. Killing of *M. tuberculosis* within macrophages is prevented by inhibition of phagolysosome formation by the tubercle bacilli through a process that is not understood. Additional alveolar macrophages engulf progeny bacilli, resulting in further intracellular growth and cell death. Over a period of weeks, as tubercle bacilli proliferate within macrophages and are released, infection spreads to regional lymph nodes, elsewhere in the lungs, and systemically. Foci of tubercle bacilli can be established in multiple organs, including the lymph nodes, brain, kidneys, and bones. In most people, after several weeks, specific immunity is developed, with activated T lymphocytes mediating a T_{H1}-type response. Macrophages act as antigen-presenting cells, interacting with CD4 lympho-cytes primed for *M. tuberculosis* antigens. Activated CD4 lymphocytes produce both IL-2, which promotes activation of additional T lymphocytes, and interferon-γ, which binds with receptors on macrophages and promotes intracellular killing of organisms. Tumour necrosis factor-α production is induced in macrophages, and this too promotes killing of intracellular bacilli. The specific role of CD8 cells in the control of tuberculosis has not been fully elaborated, although there is evidence that cytotoxic T lymphocytes may play a role in containing a tuberculous infection. In addition, CD8 lymphocytes also produce interferon-γ and participate in granuloma formation.

The classic immunological response to infection with tubercle bacilli is the walling off of viable bacilli in granulomas, collections of cells surrounding a focus of *M. tuberculosis*, usually within macrophages but sometimes extracellular organisms, that serve to contain the infection. Granulomas consist of macrophages, CD4 and CD8 lymphocytes, fibroblasts, giant cells, and epithelioid cells that produce an extracellular matrix of collagenous and fibrotic materials that are continually remodelled and can become calcified. A calcified granuloma at the initial site of infection in the lung is referred to as a Ghon complex, while the combination of a Ghon complex and a calcified regional lymph node is called a Ranke's complex.

The development of the cellular immune response to *M. tuberculosis* is accompanied by the development of delayed-type hypersensitivity to specific antigens from tubercle bacilli. While delayed-type hypersensitivity is distinct from the cell-mediated immunity that provides protection from disease, this sensitivity to tubercle-derived proteins has proved enormously useful for diagnosing tuberculosis infection. Use of purified protein derivatives (**PPD**) of tuberculin is the basis for estimating the prevalence of latent tuberculosis infection in populations. This is essential in studying the natural history of tuberculosis infection, and is frequently helpful in evaluating patients with suspected tuberculosis disease. The difference between delayed-type hypersensitivity and immunity to tuberculosis is illustrated by the observation that 80 to 90 per cent of patients with active disease, and therefore clearly not immune, have positive tuberculin tests.

For the majority of people acquiring a new tuberculous infection, the development of cell-mediated immunity to the organism is protective and holds the bacilli in check, although viability is usually maintained. A small minority will be unable to contain the infection and progress to active tuberculosis disease, often referred to as primary tuberculosis. Early progression of infection to disease is associated with immunosuppression, particularly with HIV infection, a higher inoculum of organisms, malnutrition, and perhaps, concomitant illness. While rates of active disease in young children who are contacts of infected individuals are no higher than for older contacts, young children with primary tuberculosis do develop more severe forms of tuberculosis than adults, including disseminated disease and tuberculous meningitis.

Those who successfully contain the organisms have a latent tuberculosis infection that may reactivate later in life. Studies of latent tuberculosis infection acquired in childhood or adolescence suggest a lifetime risk of reactivation of *M. tuberculosis* of about 10 per cent. Table 1 lists risk factors for reactivation of latent tuberculosis infection. The most potent is HIV infection, which increases the rate of reactivation by as much as 1000-fold. Immunosuppression from malignancy, cytotoxic therapy, corticosteroids, and other agents that alter cellular immune responses can also reactivate latent tuberculosis infection. Other potentiating factors include diabetes, endstage renal disease, injection drug use (independent of HIV infection), low body weight, gastrointestinal surgery, and silicosis. Cigarette smoking is associated with increased tuberculosis incidence (notably in India), as is alcohol abuse. Inhibitors of tumour necrosis factor-α used to treat rheumatoid arthritis or inflammatory bowel disease increase the risk of tuberculosis. Tuberculosis rates are usually higher in the elderly than in younger adults in developed countries, but this may represent a higher prevalence of latent infection in older cohorts, rather than immunological senescence.

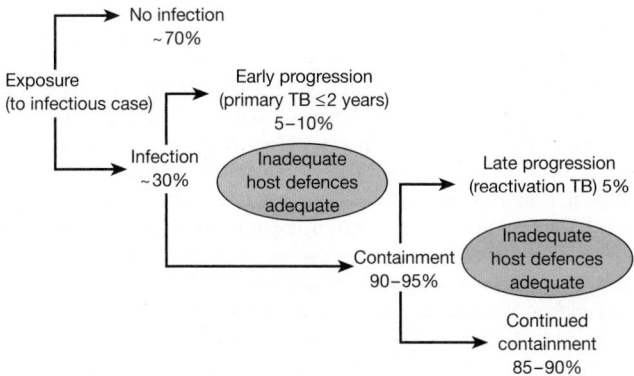

Fig. 2 Natural history of tuberculosis.

Table 1 Incidence of active tuberculosis in persons with a positive tuberculin skin test, by selected risk factors

Risk factor	Tuberculosis cases/ 100 persons-years
Recent tuberculosis infection:	
Infection less than 1 year previously	2–8
Infection 1 to 7 years previously	0.2
HIV infection	3.5–14
Injection drug use:	
HIV seropositive	4–10
HIV seronegative	1
Silicosis	3–7
Radiographic findings consistent with prior tuberculosis	0.2–0.4
Weight deviation from standard:	
Underweight by 15% or more	0.26
Underweight by 10 to 14%	0.20
Underweight by 5 to 9%	0.22
Weight within 5% of standard	0.11
Overweight by 5% or more	0.07
Diabetes mellitus	0.3
Renal failure	0.4–0.9
None of the above factors	0.01–0.1

Clinical features

Classification of tuberculosis infection and disease

Infection with *M. tuberculosis* can result in clinical manifestations ranging from asymptomatic carriage of latent bacilli to life-threatening pneumonia. Classification of the different stages of *M. tuberculosis* in humans by the American Thoracic Society (**ATS**) is shown in Table 2. This system is used more for public health purposes than for clinical management, but is useful because it reflects the natural history of *M. tuberculosis* and categorizes patients according to the type of evaluation and treatment they may need.

ATS Category 0 describes people with no history of tuberculosis exposure and a negative tuberculin skin test (if performed). Category 1 includes those people exposed to an infected individual but in whom no evidence of infection is found. This is a temporary category used during the evaluation of contacts of tuberculosis cases; repeat tuberculin testing several months after the exposure would result in these individuals being reclassified to another category. Category 2 is defined as latent tuberculosis infection without evidence of disease, and is based on a positive tuberculin skin test without clinical or radiographic signs of illness. Category 3 is confirmed, active tuberculosis disease requiring treatment. As discussed below, this category is further divided according to the site of disease and laboratory features, including results of acid-fast bacilli smears. Category 4 is defined as inactive tuberculosis. Patients in this category do not have clinical or laboratory evidence of active disease, but are known to have suffered previously from tuberculosis. This category includes those who have been

Table 2 American Thoracic Society classification system for tuberculosis

Classification	Description
TB0	No exposure, no infection
TB1	Exposed to tuberculosis, infection status unknown
TB2	Latent infection, no disease (positive PPD tuberculin test)
TB3	Active tuberculosis
TB4	Inactive tuberculosis, healed or adequately treated
TB5	Possible tuberculosis, status unknown ('rule out' tuberculosis)

treated and cured of active tuberculosis, as well as individuals who have spontaneously recovered from tuberculosis without treatment. Finally, category 5 refers to patients in whom tuberculosis is suspected, but who are still undergoing evaluation. Depending on the degree of suspicion of the diagnosis, such people might be started on presumptive therapy for tuberculosis pending the outcome of cultures and other laboratory assessments. Like category 1, it is a temporary category for patients undergoing evaluation. All are subsequently reclassified on the basis of diagnostic studies.

The clinical presentation of active tuberculosis is highly variable, depending on the site and extent of disease and the immune status of the host. Historically, active tuberculosis has been classified as 'primary' or 'post-primary' on the basis of both the presumed duration of infection and the clinical features of the disease. However, molecular epidemiological studies suggest that this classification may be unreliable. For example, the 'classic' presentation of reactivation tuberculosis has been seen in patients whose infection is clearly newly acquired, such as in nosocomial outbreaks where DNA fingerprinting confirms recent transmission. For practical purposes, tuberculosis is generally divided into pulmonary and extrapulmonary forms, with considerable clinical heterogeneity within these categories.

Pulmonary tuberculosis

Pulmonary tuberculosis is usually a subacute respiratory infection with prominent constitutional symptoms. The most frequent symptoms of pulmonary tuberculosis are cough, fever, night sweats, and malaise. Cough in pulmonary tuberculosis is initially dry, but often progresses to become productive of sputum and, in some instances, haemoptysis. The sputum is generally yellow in colour, and is neither malodorous nor thick. Haemoptysis may occur acutely in patients with untreated tuberculosis, but is also a feature of treated tuberculosis; damage from prior tuberculosis may result in bronchiectasis or residual cavities that can either become superinfected or erode into blood vessels or airways, producing haemoptysis. Advanced tuberculosis may also present with bloody sputum. Rarely, the bleeding is massive leading to shock, asphyxia, and death.

Chest pain is not a prominent symptom in pulmonary tuberculosis, although coughing may cause musculoskeletal pain. Patients with tuberculous pleurisy may experience pleuritic pain. Radicular chest pain may be associated with spinal tuberculosis. Dyspnoea alone may be a sign of extensive parenchymal destruction, large pleural effusions, endobronchial obstruction, or pneumothorax.

Patients with tuberculosis also experience loss of appetite and weight loss or cachexia, often out of proportion to their diminished intake of food. Elevations in tumour necrosis factor-α may be responsible. Mild symptoms include emotional lability, irritability, depression, and headache.

Most patients present after feeling unwell for weeks or months. In surveys of populations with high rates of disease and poor access to medical care, a history of cough for more than 3 weeks was strongly associated with a diagnosis of active tuberculosis. Untreated tuberculosis is associated with high mortality, but many patients may have persistent symptoms for years. A study of untreated pulmonary tuberculosis in the pre-therapy era found that after 5 years 50 per cent of patients had died, 25 per cent had spontaneously healed, and 25 per cent were chronically ill with pulmonary disease. A subset of patients have rapidly progressive disease, the so-called 'galloping consumption' of old. This is now most often seen in patients with HIV infection or other forms of severe immunosuppression. These patients have progressively severe pulmonary symptoms over a period of several weeks, often in the setting of disseminated disease. Failure to diagnose and treat these patients promptly may result in death.

Physical findings in pulmonary tuberculosis may be of limited usefulness in making a diagnosis. Fever is an irregular and unreliable feature in tuberculosis. While most patients complain of fevers prior to presentation, only one-half to three-quarters of patients with confirmed tuberculosis have a documented fever. Examination of the chest may reveal dullness to percussion and rales, although these findings are highly variable and non-specific. Signs of consolidation are usually absent. The classic post-tussive rales described in the last century are not often present and are not specific to tuberculosis. Patients with disseminated tuberculosis may have lymphadenopathy, hepatomegaly, or evidence of central nervous system involvement, but these are not generally seen in typical pulmonary tuberculosis. Clubbing and cyanosis are findings associated with prolonged and advanced pulmonary disease. Thus, the diagnosis of tuberculosis almost always rests on the patient's history and epidemiological characteristics, in conjunction with laboratory studies described below. The most important step in making a timely diagnosis of tuberculosis is to think of it in the first place.

Radiological evaluations play a critical role in the diagnosis of pulmonary tuberculosis. Disease due to *M. tuberculosis* can involve any portion of the lungs, and radiographic findings are usually only suggestive, not diagnostic, of tuberculosis. The typical radiological manifestations of pulmonary tuberculosis are upper lobe infiltrates that may show cavitation. *M. tuberculosis* exhibits a unique predilection for the upper zones of the lungs for reasons that are not well understood. Latent infection characteristically reactivates in the apical segments of the upper lobes, or the superior segments of the lower lobes. The infiltrates are often fibronodular and irregular, and may be diffuse and associated with volume loss. Cavities, when present, are rarely symmetrical and do not usually have air–fluid levels, such as those seen in pyogenic lung abscesses. Examples of the radiographic appearance of pulmonary tuberculosis are seen in Fig. 3.

The classic radiographic presentation described above is neither pathognomonic nor highly sensitive for pulmonary tuberculosis. A number of other lung infections, notably the pulmonary mycoses, can present with similar findings. More important, one-third to one-half of patients with

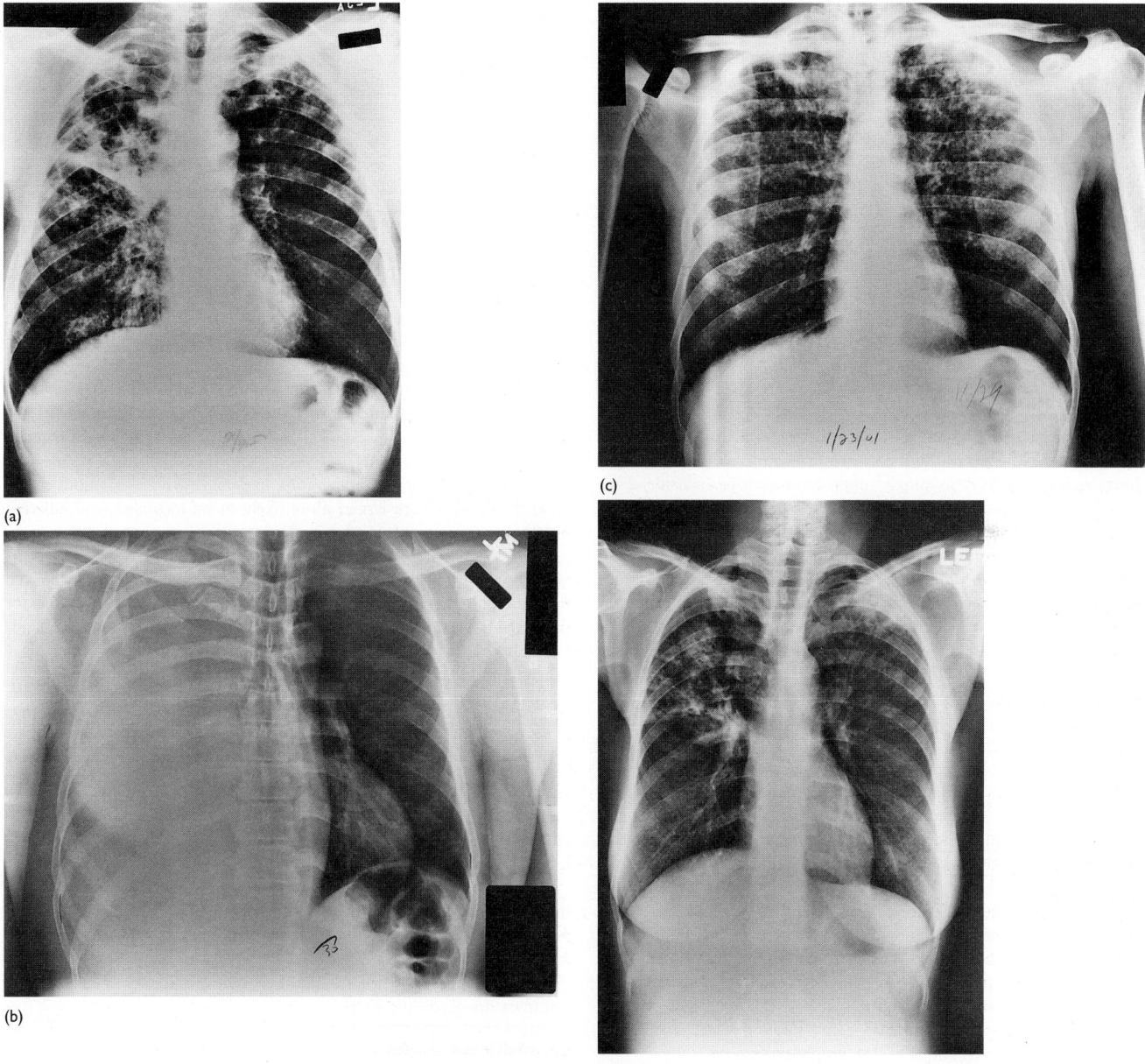

Fig. 3 Radiographic appearance of pulmonary tuberculosis. (a) Extensive tuberculosis with right upper lobe volume loss and multiple small cavities. This patient was the source of at least 14 secondary cases in contacts. (b) A 69-year-old man with right pleural tuberculosis. (c) Diffuse pulmonary nodules in an HIV-infected man with pulmonary tuberculosis. (d) Cavitary upper lobe disease in an HIV-infected woman.

pulmonary tuberculosis lack these classic radiographic findings. Lower lung zone infiltrates, mid-lung focal infiltrates, pulmonary nodules, and infiltrates with mediastinal or hilar adenopathy are also seen. In particular, HIV-infected patients with tuberculosis tend to present with 'atypical' findings, and up to 5 per cent of them may have a normal chest radiograph but sputum cultures that yield *M. tuberculosis*. The lack of typical radiographic features is not, therefore, grounds for rejecting the diagnosis in a patient with a history and symptoms compatible with tuberculosis.

Computed tomography (CT) is increasingly used to evaluate radiographic findings that are not readily explained after an initial assessment. They may reveal more extensive involvement than conventional radiographs, including multiple nodules, small cavities, and multilobar infiltrates.

The laboratory diagnosis of pulmonary tuberculosis relies on examination and culture of sputum or other respiratory tract specimens. Definitive diagnosis requires growth of *M. tuberculosis* from respiratory secretions, while a probable diagnosis can be based on typical clinical and radiographic findings with either sputum positive for acid-fast bacilli or other specimens, or typical histopathological findings on biopsy material. The specificity of these latter approaches depends on the prevalence of disease due to non-tuberculosis mycobacteria in the population.

Throughout most of the world, acid-fast staining of sputum is the sole test available to confirm the diagnosis of pulmonary tuberculosis. In developing countries, the positive predictive value of the sputum acid-fast smear is very high, as the likelihood of non-tuberculous mycobacterial disease is quite low. In industrialized countries, disease due to the non-tuberculous mycobacteria is relatively more common and reliance on smears without cultures is potentially misleading. Despite the best efforts of clinicians, a confirmed diagnosis of tuberculosis cannot be established in some patients who have the disease, and a response to presumptive therapy forms the basis for establishing the diagnosis.

Extrapulmonary tuberculosis

In the United States, extrapulmonary tuberculosis is defined as disease outside the lung parenchyma, and in the United Kingdom, as disease outside the lungs and pleura. This seemingly subtle distinction has considerable epidemiological significance, however, as pleural tuberculosis is the most common extrapulmonary site of disease in the United States.

During the initial seeding of infection with *M. tuberculosis*, described earlier, haematogenous dissemination of bacilli to a number of organs can occur. These localized infections, as in the lung, can progress into primary tuberculosis or become walled off in small granulomas where bacteria may remain dormant if they are not killed by cell-mediated immune responses. Extrapulmonary tuberculosis, therefore, can either be a presentation of primary or reactivation tuberculosis.

Extrapulmonary tuberculosis may be generalized or confined to a single organ. In otherwise immunocompetent adults, extrapulmonary tuberculosis is found in 15 to 20 per cent of all tuberculosis cases. In young children and immunosuppressed adults, rates of extrapulmonary disease are substantially higher. It is seen in more than half of patients with HIV-related tuberculosis and one-quarter of patients with tuberculosis under 15 years of age. Children less than 2 years old have high rates of miliary and meningeal disease.

The organs most frequently involved are listed in Table 3. To some extent the frequency with which specific organs are involved reflects the pathophysiology of the disease. Infection spreads from the lungs, the primary site of inoculation, by lymphatic and haematogenous routes, to the pleura, lymph nodes, kidneys and other genitourinary organs, bone, and central nervous system. Bacteraemia is transient and rarely detected except in patients with HIV infection and low CD4 lymphocyte counts.

Both pulmonary and extrapulmonary disease are found in up to 50 per cent of patients with HIV-related tuberculosis, so it is important to consider the possibility of extrapulmonary pathology when pulmonary tuberculosis is diagnosed in an HIV-infected patient (and vice versa). Pulmonary

Table 3 Common sites of extrapulmonary tuberculosis

Site	Percentage of extrapulmonary cases
Pleura	20–25
Lymphatics	20–40
Genitourinary	5–18
Bone/joint	10
Central nervous system	5–7
Abdominal	4
Disseminated	7–11

involvement is seen in up to one-quarter of patients with tuberculous meningitis and less frequently with other sites of disease.

Pleural tuberculosis

This is the result of two distinct pathophysiological sequences, which present in strikingly different manners. Most pleural tuberculosis is associated with primary infection, and is the result of seeding of the visceral pleura with relatively small numbers of tubercle bacilli via direct extension from adjacent lung tissue. A large proportion of patients with this form of tuberculous pleurisy will have evident pulmonary disease, although findings may be subtle. The duration of symptoms is generally brief, usually several weeks. Patients complain of fever, chest pain, and non-productive cough. Other constitutional and respiratory symptoms may be present. Unlike pneumococcal pneumonia, which presents abruptly, tuberculous pleurisy has a more insidious onset.

The second form of pleural tuberculosis occurs when larger numbers of bacilli invade the pleural space and multiply, producing frank empyema. Tuberculous empyema is seen in older patients, almost all of whom have extensive pulmonary disease. Patients present with prolonged cough, chest pain, fever, cachexia, and night sweats. Pneumothorax is a common complication that may be associated with a more rapid disease course.

The radiographic picture in tuberculous pleurisy reflects the underlying pathophysiology of the disease. Patients with the primary type of pleurisy tend to have small, unilateral effusions, and up to half have visible parenchymal lesions on plain radiographs. In patients with tuberculous empyema, the effusions are larger, more likely to be loculated, and adjacent pulmonary involvement is often evident.

When pulmonary parenchymal involvement is manifest, sputum smears and cultures are likely to be diagnostic and pleural disease can be inferred from the pulmonary findings. When pulmonary findings are minimal, or the initial test results unrevealing, analysis of pleural fluid is essential. Acid-fast stains of pleural fluid are most often negative in patients with primary tuberculous pleurisy, as few organisms are present. Repeated sampling will show organisms in less than half of cases. Similarly, cultures may be negative. The pleural fluid is usually serous and exudative, with a protein concentration that is more than 50 per cent of the serum level, normal or low glucose, and a slightly acidic pH. The white blood cell count of the pleural fluid is usually in the range of 1000 to 10 000/μl, with a lymphocytic predominance. Lactate dehydrogenase and adenosine deaminase levels are generally elevated. These tests are non-specific and cannot reliably distinguish tuberculous pleurisy from other pleural diseases.

Percutaneous biopsy of the pleura reveals granulomatous inflammation in up to 80 per cent of cases, and cultures obtained at the time of biopsy are positive in over half of patients. If a first attempt fails to provide a diagnosis, a second biopsy may be successful. Compared with blind sampling with a percutaneous pleural needle, viewing biopsy targets by thorascopy improves the diagnostic yield.

Lymphatic tuberculosis

This can occur in any location, but classic scrofula, involving the cervical or supraclavicular chains, is the most common presentation. Mediastinal and hilar lymphatic tuberculosis is a feature both of primary and disseminated disease, but discovery of these lesions is usually incidental. Lymphatic tuberculosis is thought to result from drainage of bacilli in the lungs into supraclavicular and posterior cervical lymph node chains. In contrast, lymphatic disease caused by non-tuberculous mycobacteria more often involves anterior cervical, preauricular, or submandibular lymph nodes, suggesting acquisition through the oropharynx. In patients with HIV infection, many groups of lymph nodes may be involved, including axillary, inguinal, mesenteric, and retroperitoneal.

Symptoms in lymphatic tuberculosis are generally limited, unless the disease is disseminated. Painless swelling of a lymph node is the most common presentation. Constitutional symptoms are not prominent in most cases. Examination of the area may reveal several enlarged lymph nodes, as only about 20 per cent of patients have disease of a solitary node.

The diagnosis of lymphatic tuberculosis usually depends on cultures from affected nodes. Biopsies may show granulomatous changes and acid-fast bacilli. Such findings are non-specific, however, and cannot distinguish tuberculous from non-tuberculous lymphadenitis. As discussed elsewhere, the presence of a positive tuberculin skin test with typical biopsy findings is strongly suggestive of tuberculosis. If lymphatic tuberculosis is suspected, these findings warrant presumptive therapy.

Genitourinary tuberculosis

This encompasses a broad array of clinical entities, ranging from disease of the kidneys to endometrial, prostatic, and epididymal disease. The most common of these is renal tuberculosis, which results from haematogenous seeding of the renal cortex during the primary infection. The pathogenesis of other genitourinary sites is either from downstream extension of renal infection over time or from haematogenous seeding at the time of the initial acquisition of *M. tuberculosis*.

Renal tuberculosis is probably underdiagnosed because it is frequently asymptomatic. Many cases are diagnosed as a result of routine detection of sterile pyuria. The development of symptoms reflects a more advanced stage of disease, associated with considerable tissue destruction. When genitourinary tuberculosis is symptomatic, the most common complaints are localized, including urinary symptoms and flank pain. In men, tuberculosis can cause prostatitis and epididymitis, both of which can present with pain resulting from swelling. In women, genital tract tuberculosis may be symptomatic when it involves the ovaries and fallopian tubes; pelvic pain is also a feature of endometrial tuberculosis. However, menstrual abnormalities and infertility may be the only signs of genital disease.

The diagnosis of genitourinary tuberculosis depends on the anatomical site of the disease. Renal tuberculosis, suggested by sterile pyuria, is diagnosed by isolation of organisms in the urine. Early morning urine is more likely to grow *M. tuberculosis* than spot samples obtained at other times. In patients with symptoms of upper urinary tract illness, radiological studies are often helpful. The kidneys may appear calcified on abdominal radiographs. Intravenous pyelography may show distorted or dilated calyces or renal pelvis, papillary necrosis, cavitation or abscesses of the renal parenchyma, or intrarenal or ureteric obstructions. Use of renal ultrasound or CT scanning may be more sensitive for identifying the abnormalities of renal tuberculosis, but there is the greatest experience with contrast radiography. When tuberculosis of the bladder is suspected, cystoscopy with biopsy may lead to the identification of granulomas prior to identification of organisms by culture. Diagnosis of prostatic, testicular, or epididymal tuberculosis is usually accomplished with cultures obtained by fine needle aspiration or transurethral resection of the prostate. Cervical and endometrial tuberculosis can be diagnosed by biopsy with culture.

Tuberculous meningitis (see also Chapter 24.14.1)

This is the most common central nervous system manifestation of tuberculosis. It is much more likely to occur in children under the age of 5 and HIV-infected patients than in immunocompetent adults. Although meningitis accounts for only a small fraction of all cases of tuberculosis, it is a devastating form of the disease that is uniformly fatal if left untreated.

The pathogenesis of meningeal tuberculosis varies with the age and immunological status of the patient. Reactivation of microscopic granulomas in the meninges was found by Rich to cause diffuse meningeal infection. These foci of infection are probably implanted at the time of primary bacillaemia. When they rupture into the subarachnoid space they invoke an inflammatory response leading to tuberculous meningitis. Meningeal disease can also occur in conjunction with miliary disease, especially in children. Adults can acquire meningeal disease during bacillaemia of miliary disease, but this is not the usual pathogenesis of meningeal infection. Rarely, invasion into the spinal canal from a paraspinous or vertebral focus can be the source of central nervous system involvement.

Historically, the clinical spectrum of tuberculous meningitis has been categorized in three stages, defined by the British Medical Research Council in 1948. Stage 1 consists of a prodrome lasting for 1 to 3 months. Nonspecific symptoms such as fever, malaise, and headache predominate. In this stage, patients are conscious and rational, but may have meningism. Focal neurological signs are absent and there are no signs of hydrocephalus. In stage 2 disease, single cranial nerve abnormalities, such as ptosis or facial paralysis appear, and paresis and focal seizures may occur. Kernig's and Brudzinski's signs and hyperactive deep tendon reflexes may be found. Prominent signs include altered cerebration, behavioural change, impaired cognitive ability, and increasing stupor. Headache and fever are common.

In stage 3, patients are comatose (Glasgow coma scale less than 8) or stuporous and often have multiple cranial nerve palsies and hemiplegia or paraplegia. By this stage, hydrocephalus is common and chronic inflammation in the enclosed space of the skull may result in intracranial hypertension. Seizures may be a prominent feature.

Fever, headache, changes in cerebration, and meningism are present in the majority of patients in most large studies, although no one single sign or symptom is reliably sensitive or specific. Children can be especially difficult to diagnose as symptoms such as fever, vomiting, drowsiness, or irritablity are commonly seen in many minor viral illnesses.

Transient tuberculous meningitis that presents as an aseptic meningitis and resolves without treatment has been described. Benign presentations of meningeal tuberculosis are exceedingly uncommon in clinical practice, and when the diagnosis is made, treatment is mandatory, even in the patient with seemingly trivial symptoms.

Diagnosis is often difficult and requires a high degree of suspicion. In disseminated disease, signs of tuberculosis in other organs, particularly the lungs, are often present. Between 25 and 50 per cent of patients with meningitis in most series also have radiographic evidence of pulmonary tuberculosis, either active or healed. The critical features of tuberculous meningitis, however, are found in the cerebrospinal fluid. Patients with tuberculous meningitis usually have elevated cerebrospinal fluid pressure. An exudative fluid with a mononuclear cell pleocytosis is characteristic. Cerebrospinal fluid is usually clear and the protein is generally in the range of 100 to 500 mg/dl. Hypoglycorrhachia is typical, with cerebrospinal fluid glucose less than 50 per cent of the serum value. The white blood cell count is rarely above 1000/µl, and cell counts of below 500/µl are typical. In early meningitis the cells may be predominantly neutrophils, but mononuclear cells predominate in most instances. Acid-fast stains of concentrated cerebrospinal fluid are only positive in one-third or fewer of patients, and cultures are positive in only one-half, although repeated sampling increases the yield.

The disastrous consequences of failing to diagnose tuberculous meningitis, coupled with the low yield of acid-fast stains and cultures from cerebrospinal fluid, has prompted the development of additional tests for establishing a diagnosis. Adenosine deaminase was initially reported to be exceptionally accurate for tuberculous meningitis. Subsequent experience, however, has found it to be insufficiently specific to distinguish tuberculosis from a variety of other acute and chronic meningitides. A number of other tests based on identification of mycobacterial antigens or specific antibodies have been evaluated, but none has been found to be reliable. Nucleic acid amplification tests such as the polymerase chain reaction (**PCR**) have great appeal, but the sensitivity and specificity of available assays are only moderately good. Thus, the diagnosis of tuberculous meningitis often rests upon the astute judgment of a clinician with a high degree of suspicion based on epidemiological and clinical clues. Presumptive therapy is frequently necessary.

Central nervous system tuberculomas are an unusual manifestation and are seen in a small proportion of patients with tuberculous meningitis. Tuberculomas are the result of enlarging tubercles that extend into brain parenchyma rather than into the subarachnoid space. Patients with HIV infection appear to have an increased risk of tuberculomas of the central nervous system, but the disease is far less common than toxoplasmosis, even in areas where tuberculosis is highly prevalent. Tuberculomas of the central nervous system may appear with clinical features of meningitis or of intracranial mass lesions. In the absence of meningeal involvement, seizures or headaches may be the only symptoms. The diagnosis is suggested by brain imaging; MRI is more sensitive than CT scanning. Biopsy of the lesion is required for diagnosis, and material should be submitted for histopathological staining and culture.

Bone and joint tuberculosis

This may affect a number of areas, but vertebral tuberculosis (Pott's disease) is the most common form, accounting for almost one-half of cases. Haematogenous seeding of the anterior portion of vertebral bone during initial infection sets the stage for later development of Pott's disease. Infection grows initially within the anterior vertebral body, then may spread to the disc space and to paraspinous tissues. Destruction of the vertebral body causes wedging and eventual collapse. Patients usually complain of back pain, with constitutional symptoms less prominent. Neurological impairment is a late complication, but delays in diagnosis are common and many patients experience neurological sequelae. Imaging studies of the spine most often reveal anterior wedging, collapse of vertebrae, and paraspinous abscesses. The diagnosis is established with bone biopsy or curettage, or by culture of the drainage from a paraspinous abscess.

Miliary tuberculosis and disseminated tuberculosis

These terms are used interchangeably to describe widespread infection and absent or minimal host immune responses. The term 'miliary tuberculosis' is derived from the classic radiographic appearance of haematogenous tuberculosis, in which tiny pulmonary infiltrates with the appearance of millet seeds are distributed throughout the lungs. Miliary tuberculosis is a more common consequence of primary tuberculosis infection than reactivation, and is seen more frequently in children and immunocompromised adults. Primary miliary tuberculosis presents with fever and other constitutional symptoms over a period of several weeks. Clinical evaluation may reveal lymphadenopathy or splenomegaly, and laboratory tests may show only anaemia. The chest radiograph is initially normal but later develops the typical miliary pattern. Involvement of multiple organ systems is the rule, most often the liver, spleen, lymph nodes, central nervous system, and urinary tract. Patients with reactivation of latent infection who present with miliary disease may have a more fulminant course although, without treatment, progression to severe disease is the rule in all patients. The diagnosis is made on tissue biopsy and culture, as sputum smears are often negative, reflecting the small numbers of bacilli typically present in respiratory secretions.

Other forms of extrapulmonary tuberculosis

These less common sites of infection are diagnosed by a combination of clinical suspicion and the results of biopsies and cultures. Abdominal, ocular, adrenal, and cutaneous tuberculosis are rarely encountered in the modern era, even in immunocompromised patients.

Laboratory diagnosis

Evaluation of patients for *M. tuberculosis* infection or disease relies on both non-specific and specific tests. Imaging studies, body fluid chemistry and cell counts, and histochemical staining, as described above, are useful and important tests for the diagnosis of tuberculosis. Specific studies for identifying mycobacterial infections include the tuberculin skin test, acid-fast microscopy, and mycobacterial culture.

Tuberculin skin testing

Tuberculin skin testing involves the intradermal injection of purified proteins of *M. tuberculosis* (purified protein derivative, or PPD tuberculin) that provokes a cell-mediated delayed-type hypersensitivity reaction, which produces a zone of induration. Tuberculin originated with Robert Koch, who prepared a tubercle sensitin that he thought would cure tuberculosis. Administration of Koch's tuberculin, of course, did not cure the disease, and hypersensitivity reactions to the agent were sometimes severe or fatal, bringing Koch great discredit.

Fortunately, it was recognized that because tuberculin induced reactions in people who were infected with tuberculosis, the substance might prove a better diagnostic test than treatment. Over a period of years, refinements were made in the preparation of tuberculins, and in 1939 Seibert and Glenn produced the reference lot of tuberculin, called PPD-S, which has served as the international standard. Current tuberculin preparations are composed of a variety of small tuberculous proteins derived from culture filtrates and stabilized with a detergent (Tween) to prevent precipitation. The standard dose of tuberculin is 5 tuberculin units (**TU**) of PPD-S, equivalent to 0.1 mg of tuberculin in a volume of 0.1 ml. Commercial and other tuberculin products are standarized against PPD-S to ensure bioequivalence.

Tuberculin testing is used to identify individuals with *M. tuberculosis* infection, and the test cannot distinguish those who have disease from those with latent infection. Intradermal injection of tuberculin into an infected individual invokes a delayed-type hypersensitivity response. Specific T lymphocytes sensitized to tuberculous antigens from prior *M. tuberculosis* infection cause a local reaction at the site of injection. Inflammation, vasodilatation, and fibrin deposition at the site result in both erythema and induration of the skin, the key feature of a tuberculin response. The result of tuberculin testing is categorized according to the amount of induration measured.

Tuberculin skin testing should be done by the Mantoux method, as this is the only technique that has been standardized and extensively validated. An injection of 0.1 ml of PPD-S is given intradermally in the volar surface of the forearm using a tuberculin syringe and small-gauge needle, causing a small wheal. Injection subcutaneously will result in uninterpretable results. Multipuncture devices should not be used. The amount of induration should be measured 2 to 5 days after the injection; measurements performed precisely 48 to 72 h later are not essential. The transverse diameter of induration should be measured in millimetres using a ruler. The edge of the induration can be seen and marked, or the margins can be detected using the ballpoint pen method, in which the pen is rolled over the skin with light pressure and its progress is stopped at the demarcation of the indurated area.

Criteria for the interpretation of tuberculin skin tests vary according to clinical and epidemiological circumstances. Cut-offs for positive tests developed by the American Thoracic Society and the Centers for Disease Control and Prevention are listed in Table 4. A cut-off of 5-mm induration is used for those at high risk of tuberculosis infection, or at high risk of disease if infected. This category includes close contacts of infectious individuals and patients with radiographic abnormalities consistent with tuberculosis. The rationale for the 5-mm cut-off in these patients is their high pretest probability of being infected. A 5-mm cut-off is also used for HIV-infected patients and those immunocompromised by corticosteroids or other agents. Failure to diagnose tuberculosis infection in these people could be calamitous, so a lower threshhold is used to maximize sensitivity. The use of control antigens such as *Candida* or tetanus toxoid to aid the interpretation of tuberculin tests in HIV-infected patients has been shown to be of no value and is not recommended.

A cut-off of 10-mm induration is used for people from populations with a high prevalence of tuberculosis or for people with conditions that increase the risk of developing active disease if infected. This would include

Table 4 Criteria for tuberculin positivity, by risk group

Reaction ≥ 5 mm of induration	Reaction ≥ 10 mm of induration	Reaction ≥ 15 mm of induration
HIV-positive persons	Recent immigrants (i.e. within the last 5 years) from high-prevalence countries or regions	Persons with no risk factors for tuberculosis
Recent contacts of patients with infectious tuberculosis	Injection drug users	
Persons with fibrotic changes on chest radiograph consistent with prior tuberculosis	Residents and employees of the following high-risk settings: prisons and jails, nursing homes and other long-term facilities for the elderly, hospitals and other health care facilities, residential facilities for patients with AIDS, and homeless shelters	
Patients with organ transplants and other immunosuppressed patients (receiving the equivalent of ≥ 15 mg/day of prednisone for 1 month or more)	Mycobacteriology laboratory personnel Persons with the following clinical conditions that place them at high risk: silicosis, diabetes mellitus, chronic renal failure, some haematological disorders (e.g. leukaemias and lymphomas), other specific malignancies (e.g. carcinoma of the head or neck and lung), weight loss of ≥ 10% of ideal body weight, gastrectomy, and jejunoileal bypass Children younger than 4 years of age, or infants, children, and adolescents exposed to adults at high risk	

immigrants from endemic areas, residents of some inner cities, and health care workers, as well as patients with diabetes, renal disease, silicosis, and other medical conditions associated with an elevated risk of reactivation of latent tuberculosis. Finally, a cut-off of 15 mm is used in people who have no risk factors for tuberculosis infection or disease. These people are unlikely to be tested.

Tuberculin skin testing is frustratingly crude and somewhat cumbersome, but has proved superior to numerous more 'modern' assays, including antibody tests, quantitative interferon-γ detection assays, and other *in vitro* immunodiagnostics. Recently, the use of Elispot assays to detect antigen-recognizing T cells has shown promise as an alternative to tuberculin testing, although further validation is required.

The test does suffer, however, from limitations in both sensitivity and specificity. The 5-TU dose of tuberculin used diagnostically is based on studies in the 1940s that showed that 99 per cent of patients with chronic tuberculosis responded to this dose, while less than 20 per cent of persons without disease and no history of tuberculosis exposure had a response. Subsequent research suggested that the lack of specificity of tuberculin testing may be the result of cross-reactions due to exposure to non-tuberculous mycobacteria. Use of tuberculin derived from *M. avium intracellulare* (PPD-B), for example, induces larger reactions than PPD-S in healthy people from areas where this organism is widespread in the environment. Another important cause of non-specific reactions to tuberculin is vaccination with BCG (bacille Calmette–Guérin). While the reactogenicity of BCG vaccine differs according to the strain, immunization with BCG can produce falsely positive skin test results. Reactions induced by BCG tend to be smaller than true positive reactions, and wane over a period of several years. Studies in populations with high rates of BCG coverage indicate that tuberculin testing can still be used to predict those who are most likely to be infected with *M. tuberculosis*, even though precision is reduced because of cross-reactions.

False-negative tuberculin tests result from both errors in applying and interpreting the test and from anergy. Errors in injection of tuberculin are common, and inter-reader variability in measuring results is high. Fortunately, if there is doubt about the interpretation of a skin test, multiple readers can measure the result over a period of days, or the test can be repeated and reinterpreted. Specific anergy to tuberculin is seen in several situations. Approximately 10 to 20 per cent of patients with culture-confirmed pulmonary tuberculosis fail to respond to tuberculin as a result of anergy. These patients will often mount a response after their disease has been treated. HIV-infected patients have a high prevalence of anergy, both

to tuberculin and other antigens. Only 10 to 40 per cent of patients with low CD4 counts and confirmed tuberculosis respond to tuberculin. Transient anergy is associated with acute viral infections such as measles, or live virus vaccinations, and other acute medical illnesses.

Microscopic staining

Microscopic staining of acid-fast bacilli is the method most widely used to diagnose tuberculosis throughout the world. Acid-fast staining is inexpensive, rapid, and technologically undemanding, making it an attractive technique for identifying mycobacterial infections. The waxy glycolipid matrix of the mycobacterial cell wall is resistant to acid-alcohol decolorization after staining with carbolfuchsin dyes, and red bacilli are visible after counterstaining. Both the Ziehl–Neelsen method (which requires heat fixation) and the Kinyoun method utilize methylene blue or malachite green counterstains, and have similar sensitivities for identifying acid-fast bacilli in clinical specimens.

The major limitation of acid-fast staining is that a relatively large number of bacilli must be present to be seen microscopically. Acid-fast smears are generally negative when there are fewer than 10 000 bacilli/ml of sputum, and many microscope fields need to be examined to identify bacilli even when there are 10 000 to 50 000 bacilli/ml. Thus, up to 50 per cent of patients with sputum cultures positive for *M. tuberculosis* have negative acid-fast smears. Where the sputum smear is the only test performed to confirm tuberculosis, a large number of smear-negative cases go undetected. This is a serious problem for patients without cavitary tuberculosis, who tend to have fewer bacilli in their sputum, including many HIV-infected patients with tuberculosis in developing countries.

Several techniques can be used to improve the yield of sputum smears. The most important method is enrichment of the specimen through concentration of the sputum. Centrifugation of sputum allows examination of the bacilli-rich pellet, which improves the sensitivity of smears substantially. Treatment of sputum with mucolytic agents is also helpful in identifying organisms by both smear and culture. Use of fluorochrome procedures to identify mycobacteria is more sensitive, but less specific, than acid-fast stains. Auramine O or auramine-rhodamine dyes are used on concentrated smears and examined under a fluorescence microscope. This technique allows much more rapid screening of slides that the traditional methods, but confirmation of positive results with Ziehl–Neelsen or Kinyoun staining is essential, as false-positive fluorochrome results are not uncommon.

The proper collection of specimens is also important for optimizing the results of microscopy and culture. Early morning sputum specimens tend to have a higher yield than specimens collected at other times, and overnight sputum collections provide even greater sensitivity. Morning gastric aspirates have a moderate yield for acid-fast bacilli in children, who generally have a difficult time producing sputum. Sputum induction with hypertonic saline is useful in evaluating patients with minimal or no sputum production, and the use of fibreptic bronchoscopy is often advocated for patients with negative sputum smears. In several series, however, the yield of post-bronchoscopy spontaneous sputum samples was higher than the bronchoalveolar lavage fluid. While the goal of sputum collection is to collect a pure lower respiratory tract sample, specimens that appear to consist primarily of upper respiratory tract or oral secretions often are smear or culture positive in patients with pulmonary tuberculosis.

Examination of multiple specimens increases the sensitivity of sputum microscopy for acid-fast bacilli. The first smear identifies 70 to 80 per cent of patients, the second another 10 to 15 per cent, and the third another 5 to 10 per cent. Review of additional specimens has little value.

In addition to the modest sensitivity of acid-fast staining, the specificity of this technique can also present problems. The morphological properties of the mycobacteria are sufficiently similar to make distinguishing M. tuberculosis from non-tuberculous mycobacteria impossible on the basis of acid-fast smears. This is not a serious concern where tuberculosis is common and non-tuberculous mycobacterial infections are unusual. However, in many industrialized countries, disease due to the non-tuberculous mycobacteria is relatively common compared with tuberculosis, and distinguishing these types of infections has important therapeutic and public health implications. Thus, while sputum microscopy is useful because of its rapidity and low cost, it should be supplemented with culture or other more sensitive and specific tests whenever feasible.

Culture, nucleic acid amplification, and susceptibility testing

Cultivation of M. tuberculosis in the laboratory is the gold standard for confirming the diagnosis of tuberculosis. A variety of media are available that support the growth of mycobacteria, including egg- and potato-based solid media and several broth-based media. The intrinsic growth rate of M. tuberculosis makes the recovery of the organism in culture a slow process. In traditional egg-based media such as Lowenstein–Jensen, growth of colonies of M. tuberculosis takes between 3 and 6 weeks, and 7H11 agar requires an average of 3 to 4 weeks to show colonies. Obviously, the glacial pace of these traditional culture systems interferes with optimal patient management, and more rapid techniques are required.

Several faster (not rapid) systems for detection of mycobacteria in culture have been commercially developed. The radiometric BACTEC system (BD Biosciences) utilizes ^{14}C palmitate in 7H12 broth to detect mycobacterial growth more quickly. Uptake and metabolism of the palmitate by mycobacteria releases $^{14}CO_2$ which is detected radiometrically. The relative amount of $^{14}CO_2$ produced is used to calculate a growth index, which is considerably more sensitive than visual inspection of colonies on agar. The average time to positive culture by BACTEC is 8 to 12 days, rather than the 3 to 4 weeks required with conventional media. The technology is automated so that regular visual inspection of culture bottles is not required, but BACTEC systems are expensive and require radioisotopes.

The Septi-Chek system combines solid and broth media. The Mycobacterial Growth Indicator Tube (MGIT) is a broth-based system that uses automated fluorescence detection to monitor growth. Both systems are more rapid than conventional culture.

Many clinical laboratories use more than one culture system for mycobacteria, both to increase the overall recovery rate and to provide quality control. In addition, if one culture becomes contaminated, alternative cultures can still be utilized.

Preparation of specimens for mycobacterial culture follows the same steps as outlined for acid-fast smears. In addition, specimens being submit-

ted for culture also require decontamination to prevent overgrowth by more rapidly multiplying bacteria. Sodium hydroxide and N-acetyl-L-cysteine are commonly used together for mucolysis and decontamination. By necessity, decontamination also inactivates more than 50 per cent of mycobacteria in a specimen, thereby reducing the potential yield of the culture. Failure to decontaminate, however, leads to bacterial overgrowth and uninterpretable results. Lack of growth as a result of over-decontamination and bacterial overgrowth resulting from under-decontamination emphasize the importance and utility of obtaining multiple specimens for culture, when possible. As with sputum smears, the yield of mycobacterial culture increases with evaluation of additional specimens.

After mycobacterial growth has been identified, speciation of the organism is required. Conventional techniques for identification involve characterization of colony morphology, pigmentation, rate of growth, and biochemical tests. Niacin reduction, nitrate reduction, and lack of catalase activity at elevated temperatures are all characteristic of M. tuberculosis. Species identification using these methods is time consuming and tedious, and further delays the diagnosis of tuberculosis.

The use of nucleic acid probes has dramatically simplified species identification of mycobacteria over the past decade. DNA probes that react with specific mycobacterial rRNA sequences to form DNA–RNA hybrids that can readily be detected by chemoluminescence are commercially available for M. tuberculosis, M. avium complex, M. kansasii, and M. gordonae. These tests can be performed within hours of detection of mycobacterial growth, and accelerate the diagnosis of specific pathogens. The sensitivity of these probes is approximately 90 to 95 per cent, depending on the species, with specificities approaching 100 per cent. Cultures that fail to respond to any of the DNA–RNA probes are almost always due to another mycobacterial species, but final identification depends on the traditional laborious biochemical techniques.

The difficulties of identifying mycobacteria in patient specimens accentuate the need for rapid and sensitive diagnostic methods for tuberculosis. If any infection seems suited to diagnosis by nucleic acid amplification assays, it would appear to be tuberculosis. Multiple studies of 'in-house' PCR assays for M. tuberculosis have shown modest sensitivity and specificity. PCR inhibitors in sputum have been a knotty problem in the molecular diagnosis of pulmonary tuberculosis, although the sensitivity has been lower than that of culture in non-respiratory specimens as well. Recently, several commercial nucleic acid amplification tests have been introduced or are nearing approval, including assays based on RT-PCR, transcription-mediated amplification, ligase chain reaction, and strand displacement amplification. All of these techniques use specific M. tuberculosis DNA sequences (most use the M. tuberculosis transposon IS6110) as targets for nucleic acid amplification. The great advantage of these assays is that they can provide results within 1 day of the collection of specimens. Their disadvantage is that they are uniformly less sensitive than culture, particularly in patients who have negative sputum smears. Early studies of these techniques have suggested that specificity was excellent overall but was reduced in smear-positive samples; further refinement in these assays has resulted in improved sensitivity and specificity.

Evaluation of nucleic acid amplification assays under field conditions has generally shown favourable results. When using these tests, however, clinicians must not forget fundamental clinical and epidemiological principles governing the diagnosis of tuberculosis: a negative test in a patient suspected of having tuberculosis should not exclude the diagnosis, nor should a positive test confirm it if clinical circumstances do not support the diagnosis. While both the positive and negative predictive values of nucleic acid amplification tests are high (70 to 90 per cent and over 90 per cent, respectively), misclassification of patients does occur, and it is important to use mycobacterial culture to validate the results of these rapid assays.

Drug susceptibility testing of M. tuberculosis isolates is essential for both clinical management and public health purposes. Susceptibility tests for the first-line antituberculosis drugs should be performed on at least one culture at the time of diagnosis for all patients. If the initial isolate is susceptible to the first-line agents, and treatment proceeds without incident, additional susceptibility tests are not required. Susceptibility testing should be performed for patients who relapse with tuberculosis and for patients whose treatment is a failure after 3 to 4 months of therapy.

Susceptibility testing for *M. tuberculosis* uses standard concentrations of antituberculosis drugs to measure inhibition of bacterial growth in culture. Drugs tested routinely include isoniazid, rifampicin, pyrazinamide, ethambutol and streptomycin. Testing of second-line antituberculosis drugs is only done when resistance to the first-line agents is documented or strongly suspected.

Susceptibility testing is generally performed on subcultures of the primary isolate, although direct inoculation of sputum or other specimens can be performed in the case of a strongly positive acid-fast bacilli smear. The standard method for measuring susceptibility to antituberculosis drugs is the proportions method. The organism is grown on agar plates in the presence of known concentrations of specific drugs. Growth on the plates is then compared with growth on control plates. By convention, if the test plate shows a colony count that is more than 1 per cent of the control value, the isolate is resistant. Laboratories will report the isolate as being susceptible or resistant to the concentration of the drug used in the assay.

An alternative method for susceptibility testing is the BACTEC system, in which culture bottles contain antituberculosis drugs. Growth indices are compared with control cultures to determine susceptibility. The BACTEC system provides results more quickly than the proportions method, is automated, but is more expensive. Other automated commercial culture systems have also been developed for determining drug susceptiblity.

The use of molecular methods to determine drug susceptibility is promising but not currently in routine use. Specific mutations in *M. tuberculosis* have been identified which confer resistance to antituberculosis drugs. For example, mutations in a small region of the *rpo*B gene of *M. tuberculosis* are responsible for more than 90 per cent of all rifampicin resistance. Sequencing of this portion of the genome using a variety of techniques has been shown to be feasible in research laboratories. Rapid identification of rifamicin resistance would be of enormous clinical benefit, as almost all rifampicin-resistant *M. tuberculosis* isolates are also resistant to isoniazid and, by definition, multidrug resistant. Molecular diagnosis of other types of resistance is more difficult, as the genetic basis of resistance to other drugs is either heterogenous or not completely understood.

Treatment of active tuberculosis

The treatment of tuberculosis requires the use of a combination of antimycobacterial drugs active against the strain of *M. tuberculosis* causing the patient's disease. The use of multiple agents is necessitated by the emergence of drug resistance when single agents are used. Mutations that confer resistance to antimycobacterial drugs arise spontaneously in wild-type populations of *M. tuberculosis* in frequencies ranging from 1 in 10^5 to 1 in 10^8 bacilli. When there are large numbers of organisms, such as are present during active pulmonary disease, a single agent will kill susceptible bacilli, but naturally drug-resistant mutants will survive and eventually emerge to cause drug-resistant disease. Since the mechanisms of resistance are genetically distinct and arise independently, multiple drug resistance within a single organism is exceedingly rare in nature. The use of two or more agents with different mechanisms of action assures that populations of drug-resistant bacilli are not selected for during therapy.

Drugs for tuberculosis are divided into first-line and second-line agents. First-line agents are widely available and used routinely in the treatment of tuberculosis, while second-line agents are generally less potent, more toxic, and less readily available. An exception to this is the fluoroquinolones, which appear to have moderately good antituberculosis activity and are widely available; their utility in tuberculosis, however, remains unstudied. Second-line drugs are reserved for the treatment of drug-resistant tuberculosis. Table 5 lists the first-line antituberculosis drugs, their activity in the treatment of tuberculosis, and common toxicities.

Table 5 Drugs for the treatment of tuberculosis

Agent	Activity	Toxicity
Isoniazid	Bactericidal	Liver, peripheral nerves, hypersensitivity
Rifampicin	Bactericidal	Liver, gastrointestinal, discoloration of body fluids, nausea, haematological
Pyrazinamide	Sterilizing	Liver, hyperuricaemia, gout, malaise, gastrointestinal
Ethambutol	Bacteriostatic (dose-dependent)	Liver, optic neuritis, skin
Streptomycin	Bactericidal	Ototoxicity, kidneys

Regimens currently used for the treatment of tuberculosis are based in part on trials conducted by the British Medical Research Council over the past 30 years. By combining drugs that target both rapidly growing bacillary populations and slow-growing or semi-dormant organisms within cells, modern short-course chemotherapy can successfully cure drug-susceptible pulmonary tuberculosis in 6 months. The regimens recommended for treatment of drug-susceptible tuberculosis are shown in Table 6. Treatment of extrapulmonary tuberculosis is generally for the same duration as for pulmonary disease, with the exceptions of bone and joint and central nervous system tuberculosis, which are treated for 12 months. HIV-related tuberculosis is also treated for 6 months.

The dynamics of mycobacterial growth are such that treatment needs to be administered only once daily, and can be given as infrequently as twice per week. The long generation time of *M. tuberculosis* and a postantibiotic effect of antituberculosis drugs renders more frequent drug dosing unnecessary. The dosages for drugs are listed in Table 7 according to the frequency with which they are administered.

Isoniazid is a key component of treatment because of its high bactericidal activity. Rifampicin is essential for short-course therapy because it is active against all populations of bacilli, both within and outside cells. Pyrazinamide is uniquely active during the first 2 months of therapy, but appears to have no activity thereafter. The addition of pyrazinamide to the treatment regimen allows the duration of therapy to be reduced from 9 to 6 months, however. Streptomycin has bactericidal activity against *M. tuberculosis*, and ethambutol has bacteriostatic activity at lower doses and bactericidal activity at high doses. These latter agents are given primarily to prevent the emergence of drug resistance, as they appear to add little activity to combination regimens against drug-susceptible tuberculosis.

Although antituberculosis therapy is remarkably well tolerated and almost always given to ambulant patients, important drug toxicities do exist. The most serious adverse drug reaction during tuberculosis treatment is liver toxicity, which may occur in up to 5 to 10 per cent of treated patients. Isoniazid, rifampicin, and pyrazinamide are all associated with liver toxicity. Use of these agents together increases the risk of a reaction. Isoniazid causes more hepatotoxicity than rifampicin or pyrazinamide, and is the agent most frequently implicated when reactions occur. Isoniazid can produce an idiosyncratic hepatocellular injury, manifested by elevated liver enzymes and clinical hepatitis. Elevation of transaminases does not always portend the development of hepatitis, but may serve as an important signal to anticipate clinical toxicity. The development of signs and symptoms of hepatitis, such as abdominal pain, nausea, vomiting, or jaundice, requires immediate discontinuation of isoniazid, as continuing treatment may result in death from hepatic failure. Risk factors for developing isoniazid hepatotoxicity include increasing age, chronic liver disease, alcohol abuse, daily dosing of isoniazid, and use of other hepatotoxic drugs, including rifampicin. In addition, people with a slow isoniazid-acetylation genotype are significantly more likely to develop hepatoxicity from the drug than intermediate or rapid acetylators.

Isoniazid interferes with metabolism of pyridoxine (vitamin B₆), which can result in a sensory neuropathy. Co-administration of pyridoxine with

Table 6 Treatment regimens for tuberculosis in children and adults

	Frequency	Drugs
Option 1	Intensive phase, daily	Isoniazid, rifampicin, pyrazinamide, and ethambutol or streptomycin[a] for 8 weeks
	Continuation phase, daily or 2 to 3 times weekly[a]	Isoniazid and rifampicin for 16 weeks
Option 2	Intensive phase, daily	Isoniazid, rifampicin, pyrazinamide, and ethambutol or streptomycin[a] for 2 weeks
	Intensive phase, twice weekly	Same drugs for 6 weeks[a]
	Continuation phase, twice weekly[b]	Isoniazid and rifampicin for 16 weeks
Option 3	Entire course of therapy, three times weekly[b]	Isoniazid, rifampicin, pyrazinamide, and ethambutol or streptomycin for 24 weeks

[a] In areas where drug resistance is <4%, omit fourth drug.

[b] Intermittent dosing should be directly observed.

isoniazid abrogates this effect without compromising the antimicrobial activity.

Rifampicin also causes hepatotoxicity, although the characteristic picture of liver disturbances due to rifampicin is cholestasis. However, the incidence of hepatotoxicity when rifampicin is given with isoniazid is substantially greater than when isoniazid is given alone. Rifampicin predictably causes a discoloration of body fluids, resulting in orange-tinted tears, sweat, and urine. Haematological toxicity from rifampicin includes thrombocytopenia and anaemia. Higher doses of rifampicin may produce a hypersensitivity reaction, with fever, rash, and joint swelling. For this reason, doses of rifampicin are not escalated during intermittent therapy, whereas the intermittent dosages of the other drugs are increased to deliver weekly doses that are equivalent to daily dosing.

Pyrazinamide is often associated with arthralgias, and may precipitate gout. Pyrazinamide inhibits renal tubular excretion of uric acid, resulting in increased serum levels of uric acid. Frank gouty arthritis is relatively uncommon with pyrazinamide use, and its frequency is reduced with intermittent dosing. Routine use of allopurinol to prevent gout is not recommended.

The major toxicity of ethambutol is optic neuritis, which is common at doses above 30 mg/kg daily and unusual at doses below 25 mg/kg daily. Patients receiving ethambutol should have baseline tests of visual acuity and colour discrimination, with monthly monitoring while on treatment. Ethambutol use is discouraged in children under 7 years old because of their inability to report visual disturbances reliably. The incidence of optic neuritis with the doses of ethambutol typically used is so low that use in young children is only relatively contraindicated.

Streptomycin was a staple of antituberculosis therapy for many years, but its use has been greatly curbed in recent years. A number of studies have demonstrated that regimens containing isoniazid, rifampicin, and pyrazinamide are equally efficacious with or without streptomycin. Streptomycin is given by intramuscular injection, causing discomfort to patients and creating an infection risk for patients and health care workers. In addition, streptomycin can be ototoxic and nephrotoxic. Consequently, ethambutol has replaced streptomycin in many parts of the world.

Patients receiving therapy for tuberculosis require regular monitoring to assess compliance, clinical response, and adverse reactions. In the initial phase of therapy, monitoring by a nurse or other trained clinician at least weekly is recommended, and supervision of every dose of medication is suggested by the World Health Organization and other authorities (see below). Patients should be observed for clinical responses, including defervescence, improvement in cough and appetite, and weight gain. Improvement in these symptoms and signs may take several weeks, but usually occurs within 3 weeks after starting treatment. Failure to improve suggests that the patient is not adhering to treatment, has drug-resistant tuberculosis, or has another illness in addition to or instead of tuberculosis.

Treatment response should also be documented with repeated sputum smears and cultures and a follow-up chest radiograph after 2 to 3 months (for pulmonary tuberculosis). All patients should have a repeat sputum smear and culture after 2 months of therapy; those who are smear or culture positive at 2 months should have another at 3 months. Failure to convert sputum smears and cultures to negative with 3 months of therapy is associated with a high risk of treatment failure; patients who are still smear or culture positive at 4 months of treatment are considered to have experienced treatment failure and should be evaluated for drug-resistant disease. A culture at the end of therapy is recommended to document cure, while a radiograph at this time is not necessary.

Monitoring for drug toxicity is also required throughout therapy. At least monthly monitoring for symptoms and signs of liver toxicity is essential, and patients should be advised to stop therapy and seek care if evidence of hepatitis is noted. Routine liver enzyme monitoring is recommended primarily for patients with underlying liver disease or baseline abnormalities in liver enzymes. Patients with symptoms of hepatitis, of course, should have liver studies obtained. As noted above, monthly visual assessment is also recommended when ethambutol is given.

For more than 40 years, experts in tuberculosis have noted that the success of treatment depends largely on adherence to therapy. Poor adherence to therapy is responsible for treatment failures, early relapses, and the emergence of drug-resistant disease. Two major interventions to improve adherence and prevent bad outcomes are directly observed therapy (**DOT**) and the use of fixed-dose combination tablets. DOT was first promoted in

Table 7 Dosage recommendation for the initial treatment of tuberculosis in children and adults

Drugs (mg/kg)	Daily dose		Twice-weekly dose		Thrice-weekly dose	
	Children	Adults	Children	Adults	Children	Adults
Isoniazid	10–20	5	20–40	15 max	20–40	15 max
	Max 300 mg	Max 300 mg	Max 900 mg	Max 900 mg	Max 900 mg	Max 900 mg
Rifampicin	10–20	10	10–20	10	10–20	10
	Max 600 mg	Max 600 mg	Max 600 mg	Max 600 mg	Max 600 mg	Max 600 mg
Pyrazinamide,	15–30	15–30	50–70	50–70	50–60	50–60
	Max 2 g	Max 2 g	Max 4 g	Max 3.5 g	Max 3.5 g	Max 3.5 g
Ethambutol[a]	15–25	15–25	50	50	25–30	25–30
	Max 1.5 g	Max 1.5 g	Max 4 g	Max 4 g		
Streptomycin	20–40	15	25–30	25–30	25–30	25–30
	Max 1.0 g	Max 1.0 g	Max 1.5 g	Max 1.5 g	Max 1.5 g	Max 1.5 g

[a] Ethambutol is not recommended for children or other patients whose visual acuity cannot be monitored.

the 1950s in India, and experience with DOT grew over the ensuing years. Intermittent dosing of tuberculosis therapy, along with the relatively short course of treatment, make supervision of treatment feasible in many situations. Ecological and programmatic studies of DOT programmes have shown that their introduction improves cure rates for tuberculosis, reduces non-compliance, and reduces the emergence of drug-resistant disease. Two observational studies have shown better survival of HIV-infected patients with tuberculosis who receive DOT.

On the other hand, two randomized trials of DOT in developing countries have not found improved treatment completion rates compared with self-administered treatment. These trials have been criticized for demonstrating only that even DOT can be carried out badly, but the lack of randomized studies documenting that DOT *per se* leads to improved outcomes is of some concern. The data from observational studies are compelling, however, and DOT is strongly encouraged by many experts and professional organizations.

The use of fixed-dose combination tablets is intended to reduce the risk of selecting for drug resistance, as opposed to improving adherence generally. By combining two, three, or four medications in the same tablet, depending on the regimen being used, the opportunity for patients to receive partial treatment that would select for drug resistance is avoided. The bioequivalence of fixed-dose combinations to individual medications has been established for some, but not all, of the combination products on the market.

The catastrophic state of global tuberculosis control led the World Health Organization (**WHO**) to develop the **DOTS** strategy (or directly observed therapy, short-course). This strategy is a series of policies related to national tuberculosis control practices. The five elements of the DOTS strategy are:

(1) governmental commitment to tuberculosis control;

(2) a reliable supply of tuberculosis drugs;

(3) diagnosis of tuberculosis cases microscopically;

(4) a registration system for tracking the outcomes of treatment; and

(5) supervision (DOT) of at least the first 8 weeks of treatment.

The DOTS strategy has been extremely successful in focusing attention on serious problems in tuberculosis treatment and control, and implementation of the programme in a number of countries has produced remarkable improvements in clinical outcomes for patients with tuberculosis. There is strong evidence that the use of the DOTS strategy results in lower rates of drug-resistant tuberculosis. None the less, the WHO estimates that in 2000 only 25 per cent of patients with tuberculosis in the world were treated within a DOTS programme. Further expansion of the DOTS strategy and improvements in tuberculosis treatment programmes are clearly needed.

The treatment of drug-resistant tuberculosis is beyond the scope of this chapter. Patients with drug-resistant tuberculosis should be managed by a physician who is a tuberculosis expert. Supervised therapy is considered mandatory for patients with resistant tuberculosis. Physician mistakes remain one of the leading causes of the emergence of drug resistance, and the identification of a drug-resistant isolate of *M. tuberculosis* should result in immediate expert consultation.

Treatment of latent tuberculosis infection

Prevention of tuberculosis with isoniazid therapy was first documented in children in the mid-1950s. Subsequently, a number of controlled trials of isoniazid chemoprophylaxis were undertaken, and its efficacy firmly established. A meta-analysis of 11 placebo-controlled trials of isoniazid, involving more than 70 000 persons, found that treatment reduced tuberculosis incidence by 63 per cent. Among patients who adhered to more than 80 per cent of the isoniazid regimen, protection was 81 per cent. These studies also showed that isoniazid chemoprophylaxis reduced tuberculosis deaths by

72 per cent. The efficacy of isoniazid therapy in preventing tuberculosis in high-risk persons is incontrovertible.

Enthusiasm for isoniazid chemoprophylaxis was considerably dampened in the late 1960s and early 1970s when drug-related hepatotoxicity, including deaths, was observed. A number of studies based on decision analysis or modelling suggested that the risks of chemoprophylaxis might outweigh the benefits, and use of preventive therapy was curtailed or ignored in many settings. Because the risk of isoniazid-related hepatotoxicity increases with age, use of chemoprophylaxis in people over 35 years old was particularly discouraged. The resurgence of tuberculosis in the developed world, particularly HIV-related tuberculosis, and the uncontrolled global epidemic have renewed interest in the use of preventive therapy in high-risk individuals.

The use of preventive therapy for tuberculosis now focuses on high-risk groups of individuals who are either known or strongly suspected to be latently infected with *M. tuberuclosis*. The term 'treatment of latent tuberculosis infection' is now preferred, emphasizing that preventive treatment is really targeted at an established infection. The American Thoracic Society and the Centers for Disease Control and Prevention published guidelines in 2000 on screening for latent tuberculosis that stress the importance of targeting efforts on populations and patients who would benefit from treatment to prevent active disease. In the past, screening for tuberculosis infection has been unfocused and often directed at patients who, if found to be infected, would have little risk of progressing to active disease. The new guidelines propose that only people with a high risk of disease or high prior probability of latent tuberculosis be tested, and that treatment be offered to infected individuals regardless of age. Individuals who should be targeted for tuberculin testing are those listed in the first two columns of Table 4, that is, those in whom a positive test is considered as 5- or 10-mm or more induration. People without risk factors for tuberculosis (those in whom a positive test is 15 mm or more) should not be tested.

Treatment regimens for latent tuberculosis are listed in Table 8, along with the rating given to the regimen by the American Thoracic Society (ATS) and Centers for Disease Control and Prevention (CDC). Isoniazid remains a favoured drug for tuberculosis preventive therapy because of its well-documented efficacy, low cost, and relatively low toxicity. The optimal duration of isoniazid therapy for latent tuberculosis has been the subject of extensive debate in the past 20 years. The International Union Against Tuberculosis and Lung Disease conducted a landmark trial in Eastern Europe in the 1970s and 1980s that compared no treatment with 3, 6, or 12 months of isoniazid in adults with fibrotic changes on radiography. The results showed that, compared with placebo, 12 months of isoniazid reduced the incidence of tuberculosis by 75 per cent, compared with 66 per cent for 6 months and 20 per cent for 3 months. In addition, patients who completed the 12 months of therapy and were judged to be compliant experienced a 92 per cent reduction in tuberculosis risk, compared with a 69 per cent decrease for compliant patients completing a 6-month regimen.

Table 8 Treatment regimens for latent tuberculosis

Drug regimen	Duration (months)	Interval	Rating HIV -ve	HIV +ve
Isoniazid	9	Daily	A II	A II
Isoniazid	9	Twice weekly	B II	B II
Isoniazid	6	Daily	B I	C I
Isoniazid	6	Twice weekly	B II	C I
Rifampicin and pyrazinamide	2	Daily	B II	A I
Rifampicin and pyrazinamide	2–3	Twice weekly	C II	C I
Rifampicin	4	Daily	B II	B III

Ratings: A, strongly recommended; B, recommended; C, optional; I, randomized trials; II, data from other scientific studies; III, expert opinion.

A meta-analysis by the Cochrane Collaborative found that 12 months of isoniazid was more effective than 6 months for prevention of tuberculosis. A recent analysis of varying durations of isoniazid therapy in Alaskan natives revealed that the effectiveness of isoniazid therapy was optimal after 9 months, and that further treatment conferred no additional benefit. The new ATS/CDC statement, therefore, recommends 9 months of isoniazid as the preferred regimen, with 6 months considered an alternative, but less effective, course of treatment.

Although isoniazid is a well tolerated drug, serious hepatotoxicity can occur in a small proportion of patients. Isoniazid may result in asymptomatic elevations in hepatic transaminase levels, but this does not always signal impending clinical toxicity. Hepatotoxicity is of concern when symptoms of hepatitis, including pain, nausea, vomiting, and jaundice, develop. Continuing isoniazid in the presence of symptoms may lead to death from fulminant hepatic necrosis and liver failure, with a case–fatality rate of 10 to15 per cent. Studies in the 1960s and 1970s found evidence of hepatotoxicity in 1 to 5 per cent of isoniazid recipients, with higher rates among older patients. More recent experience with isoniazid therapy that is closely monitored shows a risk of hepatotoxicity in the range of 0.1 to 0.3 per cent. Thus, appropriate patient screening and follow-up makes the use of isoniazid for treating latent infection markedly safer.

One of the most important new developments in the treatment of latent tuberculosis is the development of alternative regimens that shorten the duration of treatment. Based on studies in animal models of latent tuberculosis, rifampicin alone given for 3 to 4 months, or rifampicin and pyrazinamide given for 2 to 3 months, were felt to be potentially active regimens and were tested in clinical trials. A 3-month regimen of rifampicin alone was found to reduce the incidence of tuberculosis by about 65 per cent in men with silicosis, and was more effective than 6 months of isoniazid. Three studies of rifampicin and pyrazinamide for latent tuberculosis in HIV-infected, tuberculin-positive patients have been carried out. In each of these studies, the combination of rifampicin and pyrazinamide was as effective as 6 or 12 months of isoniazid. A meta-analysis of the studies found rifampicin with pyrazinamide was equivalent to isoniazid for preventing active tuberculosis, with an odds ratio of 1.0.

Rifampicin with pyrazinamide is generally well tolerated, but can be associated with serious hepatotoxicity. However, the use of rifampicin does pose the risk of important drug interactions. For example, reduction in methadone concentrations caused by rifampicin can precipitate narcotic withdrawal. Moreover, rifampicin can lower levels of protease inhibitors and non-nucleoside reverse transcriptase inhibitors used to treat HIV infection. Substitution of rifabutin for rifampicin in patients receiving anti-HIV drugs is based on the observation that rifabutin is equally as efficacious as rifampicin in the treatment of active tuberculosis.

Candidates for treatment of latent tuberculosis are listed in Table 4. Criteria for treatment include a positive tuberculin test according to the categories in Table 4, elevated risk for developing active tuberculosis if untreated, and exclusion of active tuberculosis by clinical evaluation and chest radiography. In addition, HIV-infected and other severely immunocompromised persons who are contacts of a patient with infectious tuberculosis should be treated for latent tuberculosis regardless of tuberculin skin test results.

Patients receiving treatment for latent tuberculosis should be monitored for drug toxicity, as well as to promote adherence to therapy. As in the treatment of active tuberculosis, patients receiving isoniazid should be warned about signs and symptoms of hepatotoxicity and advised to discontinue therapy and seek care if any of these occur. Patients with or at risk for chronic liver disease should have baseline liver enzymes obtained, with monthly monitoring if the results are abnormal. All patients should be clinically evaluated at least monthly to assess toxicity and those receiving rifampicin and pyrazinamide more often. Treatment of patients with mild transaminase elevations (3 times upper limits of normal or less) can proceed with regular clinical and laboratory monitoring. Higher elevations of transaminases, or the development of symptoms or signs of hepatitis, should be managed with discontinuation of therapy at least temporarily.

Patients who complete therapy for latent tuberculosis do not require any periodic monitoring for tuberculosis subsequently.

Prevention of tuberculosis

Strategies to control tuberculosis are aimed at the prevention of the spread of *M. tuberculosis* infection and the development of clinical tuberculosis. The principal approaches employed toward this end are:

(1) identification and treatment of infectious tuberculosis cases;

(2) treatment of latent tuberculosis infection;

(3) prevention of exposure to infectious particles in air, especially in hospitals and other institutions; and

(4) vaccination.

Case identification and treatment reduces transmission by rendering patients with communicable tuberculosis non-infectious. Patients with pulmonary tuberculosis produce infectious aerosols that may transmit tubercle bacilli to contacts breathing the same air. When cases are identified and treated, infectiousness is rapidly eliminated. The duration of treatment required to prevent further transmission of infection is not known precisely, but experimental, clinical, and microbiological data suggest that the level of infectiousness is reduced enormously within several days of beginning effective treatment. The number of secondary infections generated by a patient with infectious tuberculosis varies greatly, depending on the duration of illness, the extent of pulmonary pathology, the amount of patient coughing, and the environment into which the patient expels infectious aerosols. Early diagnosis and treatment reduces the number of secondary infections, while delays can result in ongoing transmission to large numbers of contacts. Failure to retain patients in treatment until they are cured also contributes to spread of infection.

Treatment of latent tuberculosis infection has been discussed above (Table 8). The benefit of treating latent infection is not only to the individual patient, who does not fall ill with tuberculosis, but also accrues to the potential contacts of that patient, who might become secondarily infected were disease to develop. Targeting of high-risk groups for screening and treatment of latent tuberculosis thereby reduces tuberculosis incidence within communities. Groups that should be targeted for screening are listed in the first two columns of Table 4.

Control of exposure to infectious aerosols can have a major impact on the spread of tuberculosis. In the late 1980s and early 1990s, transmission of tuberculosis, including multidrug-resistant tuberculosis, was widespread in hospitals, shelters for the homeless, and correctional facilities in New York City. The congregation of large numbers of highly susceptible people, especially HIV-infected persons, in closed environments with individuals with untreated tuberculosis resulted in numerous microepidemics of both drug-susceptible and drug-resistant tuberculosis. Reversal of the resurgence of tuberculosis in New York at that time was attributable in large part to strengthening of infection control practices.

Tuberculosis infection control involves prompt identification and isolation of patients with suspected tuberculosis. The decision to isolate a patient in a hospital setting is a function of epidemiological and clinical factors. Patients with known risk factors for tuberculosis who present with symptoms and signs characteristic of pulmonary tuberculosis should be placed in respiratory isolation. Local epidemiological data should influence isolation practices. Where tuberculosis is prevalent, all HIV-infected patients with pneumonia may require isolation, whereas isolation is more selective and based on individual patient features in low-prevalence settings.

Respiratory isolation requires nursing the patient in a room with negative air pressure relative to adjoining areas. Ventilation to the room should provide at least six complete air changes per hour, and air should not be recirculated without filtering or irradiation. Patients should be instructed always to cover their mouths when coughing, and should wear surgical face

Table 9 Criteria for discontinuing respiratory isolation for tuberculosis in hospital inpatients

Alternative diagnosis established
Infectious tuberculosis ruled out
Tuberculosis diagnosed and:
    treatment given for at least 14 days and
    clinical response to therapy documented, including improvement in
        fever and cough, and
    acid-fast smears of sputum negative, or
        patient discharged to home

masks when outside the room to reduce aerosol generation. Anyone entering the patient's room should wear an appropriate face mask or respirator to prevent inhalation of droplet nuclei with tubercle bacilli. Much debate has occurred in recent years in the United States about what constitutes appropriate protection for health care workers exposed to infectious tuberculosis. This debate is influenced as much by philosophy as by science, and will not be detailed here. Use of surgical masks for protection against tuberculosis is clearly inappropriate, even though these masks are useful when placed on patients to prevent creation of infectious aerosols. Tightly fitting face masks that filter out more than 99.7 per cent of particles greater than 0.5 µm in size (high efficiency particle air—HEPA—filters) are effective. Other devices, including positive air pressure respirators (PAPRs), are also effective.

Ultraviolet germicidal irradiation can be useful for reducing the number of infectious particles in ambient air in settings where ventilation alone is not sufficient. Ultraviolet light must be concentrated in areas of rooms where exposure to people will not occur, such as upper air zones, in order to prevent skin and ocular toxicity. Areas where ultraviolet lights are often used include bronchoscopy suites, inside air circulation ducts, in emergency rooms, and in shelters for the homeless.

Criteria for discontinuation of respiratory isolation are listed in Table 9. Guidelines for taking patients out of isolation in the hospital are strict and are intended to protect other vulnerable patients and hospital staff from any exposure to the disease. Respiratory isolation is not usually required or practical in the home setting, and patients with infectious tuberculosis do not need to be admitted to hospital solely for respiratory isolation. It is assumed that contacts in the home environment will already have significant exposure to tuberculosis by the time a diagnosis is made, and isolation of the patient affords no measurable benefit. Exceptions to this may include patients living in congregate living facilities or other special situations. The primary protective measures for contacts of infected individuals are a clinical evaluation to identify and evaluate symptoms of tuberculosis and tuberculin skin testing, with treatment of latent infection if present.

Vaccination against tuberculosis with BCG vaccine is widely administered throughout the world, but remains controversial. BCG is an attenuated live bacterial vaccine developed in the early twentieth century by Calmette and Guérin at the Institut Pasteur. After a series of uncontrolled and anecdotal assessments of the vaccine, a series of controlled trials of BCG was begun in the 1930s and continued through the 1990s. The efficacy of BCG has varied greatly in these studies, ranging from more than 80 per cent protection to complete lack of protection, with possibly increased risk in vaccine recipients. A meta-analysis of BCG trials performed in the early 1990s found that the weighted protective benefit of BCG was about 50 per cent for both the prevention of active tuberculosis disease and death.

In addition to the protective efficacy observed in trials of BCG, there is evidence that BCG diminishes haematogenous dissemination of primary tuberculosis infection and thereby reduces the incidence of miliary tuberculosis and tuberculous meningitis in children. It is primarily for this reason that BCG is included in the Expanded Program on Immunization of the WHO.

The current efficacy of BCG for preventing pulmonary tuberculosis is debated on the basis of several recent trials which have failed to show pro-

tection. A number of hypotheses have been proposed for the variation in efficacy reported in various studies, including differences in susceptibility within populations, environmental exposure to mycobacteria which masks vaccine effect, and attenuation of vaccine immunogenicity. The last explanation is very compelling and fits well with clinical trials data. Unlike most vaccines, BCG is not standardized and there is no seedlot of vaccine from which new batches are derived. BCG is grown in a number of laboratories around the world and has not been re-passaged in animals since it was derived from cattle a century ago. Multiple commercial and non-commercial BCG products are in use at present, and comparative genomic analysis demonstrates considerable genetic heterogeneity in these strains, with many gene deletions and polymorphisms. One analysis of BCG trials found that protective efficacy was reduced in studies using multiply-passaged vaccine strains. The evidence supports the hypothesis that BCG has become further attenuated over time and no longer promotes immunity to *M. tuberculosis* infection and disease in adults. This position has not been universally accepted, however, and BCG remains one of the most widely administered vaccines in the world, largely for its perceived effects on paediatric tuberculosis.

Areas for further research

Effective global tuberculosis control will require a co-ordinated set of clinical and public health strategies based on a thorough understanding of the epidemiology, pathogenesis, and therapy of infection with *M. tuberculosis*. It appears that the WHO DOTS strategy, which focuses on finding and effectively treating cases, is not sufficient to control or eliminate tuberculosis, particularly in countries with large HIV epidemics. Improved methods for the diagnosis and treatment of tuberculosis infection and disease, particularly drug-resistant tuberculosis, are urgently needed. Effective regimens for the treatment of multidrug-resistant tuberculosis, with both existing and new agents, need to be developed. A better understanding of the pathogenesis of and natural immunity to tuberculosis may contribute to the development of a more effective vaccine. The sequencing of the genome of *M. tuberculosis* promises to open the door to a new generation of research on tuberculosis and its control. Scientific progress alone, however, will be insufficient to combat tuberculosis worldwide. The willingness of societies and nations to pay for the deployment of the fruits of biomedical research, both past and future, to combat the disease where it is prevalent will be required for the conquest of tuberculosis.

Further reading

American Thoracic Society (1994). Treatment of tuberculosis and tuberculosis infection in adults and children. *American Journal of Respiratory and Critical Care Medicine* **149**, 1359–74.

American Thoracic Society/CDC (2000). Targeted tuberculin testing and treatment of latent tuberculosis infection. *American Journal of Respiratory and Critical Care Medicine* **161**, S221–47.

American Thoracic Society (2000). Diagnostic standards and classification of tuberculosis in adults and children. *American Journal of Respiratory and Critical Care Medicine* **161**, 1376–95.

Brudney K, Dobkin J (1991). Resurgent tuberculosis in New York City. Human immunodeficiency virus, homelessness, and the decline of tuberculosis control programs. *American Review of Respiratory Diseases* **144**, 745–9.

Chin DP *et al.* (1996). Reliability of anergy skin testing in persons with HIV infection. *American Journal of Respiratory and Critical Care Medicine* **153**, 1982–4.

Colditz GA *et al.* (1995). Efficacy of BCG vaccine in the prevention of tuberculosis. *Clinical Infectious Diseases* **20**, 126–35.

Comstock GW (1994). Field trials of tuberculosis vaccines: how could we have done them better? *Controlled Clinical Trials* **15**, 247–76.

Davies PDO, ed. (1998). *Clinical tuberculosis*, 2nd edn. Oxford University Press.

Dye C *et al.* (1999). Global burden of tuberculosis: estimated incidence, prevalence, and mortality by country. WHO Global Surveillance and Monitoring Project. *Journal of the American Medical Association* **282**, 67–86.

Ellner JJ (1997). Review: The immune response in human tuberculosis: implications for tuberculosis control. *Journal of Infectious Diseases* **176**, 1351–9.

El-Sadr WM *et al.* (1998). Evaluation of an intensive intermittent-induction regimen and duration of short-course treatment for human immunodeficiency virus-related pulmonary tuberculosis. *Clinical Infectious Diseases* **26**, 1148–58.

Ferebee SH (1970). Controlled chemoprophylaxis trials in tuberculosis: a general review. *Advances in Tuberculosis Research* **17**, 28–106.

Frieden TB *et al.* (1995). Tuberculosis in New York City—turning the tide. *New England Journal of Medicine* **333**, 229–33.

Fine PEM (1995). Variation in protection by BCG: implications of and for heterologous immunity. *Lancet* **346**, 1339–45.

Fox W, Ellard GA, Mitchison DA (1999). Studies on the treatment of tuberculosis undertaken by the British Medical Research Council tuberculosis units, 1946–1986, with relevant subsequent publications. *International Journal of Tuberculosis and Lung Diseases* **3**(Suppl 2), S231–79.

Graham NMH *et al.* (1992). Prevalence of tuberculin positivity and skin test anergy in HIV-1-seropositive and HIV-1-seronegative intravenous drug users. *Journal of the American Medical Association* **267**, 369–73.

Grzybowski S, Burnett G, Stybblo K (1975). Contacts of cases of active pulmonary tuberculosis. *Bulletin of the International Union Against Tuberculosis* **60**, 90–106.

Iseman MD (1993). Treatment of multidrug-resistant tuberculosis. *New England Journal of Medicine* **329**, 784–91.

Iseman MD (2000). *A clinician's guide to tuberculosis*. Lippincott Williams & Wilkins, Philadelphia.

Lalvani A, *et al.* (2001). Rapid detection of *Mycobacterium tuberculosis* infection by enumeration of antigen-specific T cells. *American Journal of Respiratory and Critical Care Medicine* **163**, 824–9.

Mahmoudi A, Iseman MD (1993). Pitfalls in the care of patients with tuberculosis: common errors and their association with the acquisition of drug resistance. *Journal of the American Medical Association* **270**, 65–8.

McKenna MT, McCray E, Onorato I (1995). The epidemiology of tuberculosis among foreign-born persons in the United States, 1986–93. *New England Journal of Medicine* **332**, 1071–6.

Murray CJL, Stybblo K, Rouillon A (1990). Tuberculosis in developing countries: burden, intervention and cost. *Bulletin of the International Union Against Tuberculosis* **65**, 1–20.

Reichman LB, Hershfield ES, eds (2000). *Tuberculosis: a comprehensive international approach*, 2nd edn. Marcel Dekker, New York.

Reider HL, Snider DE, Cauthen GM (1990). Extrapulmonary tuberculosis in the United States. *American Review of Respiratory Diseases* **141**, 347–51.

Rom WN, Gary S, eds (1996). *Tuberculosis*. Little Brown, Boston.

Ryan F (1992). *The forgotten plague: how the battle against tuberculosis was won—and lost*. Little Brown, Boston.

Small PM *et al.* (1991). Treatment of tuberculosis in patients with advanced human immunodeficiency virus infection. *New England Journal of Medicine* **324**, 289–94.

World Health Organization (1997). *Anti-tuberculosis drug resistance in the world. The WHO/IUATLD global project on drug resistance surveillance, 1994–1997*. World Health Organization, Geneva.

World Health Organization (2001). *Global tuberculosis control, WHO Report 2001*. World Health Organization, Geneva.

7.11.23 Disease caused by environmental mycobacteria

J. M. Grange and P. D. O. Davies

Introduction

In addition to the tubercle and leprosy bacilli, the genus *Mycobacterium* contains at least 60 species that exist naturally as environmental saprophytes and some of these occasionally cause opportunist disease in humans and animals. The environmental mycobacteria are divisible into two main groups, the slow and rapid growers, according to their rate of growth on subculture. Originally allocated to broad groups according to pigmentation and other cultural characteristics, almost all environmental mycobacteria are now readily identifiable at species level.

Most of the slow growers are able to cause human disease and the commonest pathogens are the closely related species *M. avium* and *M. intracellulare*, which are usually grouped together as the *M. avium* complex. With rare exceptions, the only pathogenic rapid growers are *M. chelonae* (including *M. abscessus*) and *M. fortuitum*. The principal pathogenic environmental mycobacteria are listed in Table 1.

The environmental mycobacteria cause two named diseases with characteristic features: swimming pool granuloma caused by *M. marinum* and Buruli ulcer caused by *M. ulcerans*. The other mycobacterioses are much less specific, often resembling tuberculosis, and require identification of the causative organism for diagnosis.

Ecology and epidemiology

The environmental mycobacteria are particularly associated with water and are found in swamps, ponds, rivers, and also colonize piped water supplies. They are readily transmissible to humans by drinking water, by inhalation of aerosols, or by traumatic inoculation. Infection of humans by environmental mycobacteria is widespread and common but overt disease is rare. In some regions such infection may be sufficient to cause cross-reactions on tuberculin testing and to modify the protective efficacy of subsequent

Table 1 The principal environmental mycobacteria causing opportunistic disease in humans

Slow growers	
M. avium[a]	Pulmonary disease
M. intracellulare[a]	
M. scrofulaceum	
M. kansasii	Pulmonary disease
M. xenopi	Pulmonary disease
M. malmoense	Pulmonary disease
M. szulgai	Pulmonary disease
M. simiae	
M. marinum	Cause of swimming pool granuloma
M. ulcerans	Cause of Buruli ulcer
M. haemophilum	Rare cause of disease, usually skin granulomas in transplant recipients
M. gordonae	Common in the environment but rare cause of disease
M. terrae	Rare cause of infection of wounds contaminated by soil
Rapid growers	
M. chelonae[b]	
M. fortuitum	

[a] These are usually grouped together as the *M. avium* complex (MAC).

[b] Some workers divide this species into *M. chelonae* and *M. abscessus*.

BCG vaccination, thereby possibly explaining the diversity of protection seen in major BCG trials.

The incidence of overt disease due to environmental mycobacteria is related to the species and numbers of mycobacteria in the environment, the opportunities for infection, and the susceptibility of the human population. Person-to-person transmission of overt disease very rarely, if ever, occurs and the prevalence of such disease is unaffected by tuberculosis control measures designed to break the cycle of person-to-person transmission. In recent years there has been an increase in the incidence of disease due to environmental mycobacteria in many countries because of immunosuppression, notably due to HIV infection.

The types of environmental mycobacterial disease in humans

The environmental mycobacteria cause four main types of disease: chronic pulmonary, lymphadenitis, postinoculation, and disseminated.

Chronic pulmonary disease

This form of environmental mycobacterial disease usually occurs in patients with predisposing local lung lesions, including industrial dust disease, old tuberculous cavities, chronic obstructive pulmonary disease, cancer, cystic fibrosis, and bronchiectasis, or generalized autoimmune or immunosuppressive disorders. However, a substantial minority of cases occur in people who otherwise appear healthy. Most patients are middle aged or elderly and men are usually more frequently affected than women. Environmental mycobacterial infection is also commoner in people who smoke. In some areas of the United Kingdom the incidence of environmental mycobacterial disease in the middle aged and elderly white population exceeds that of tuberculosis.

The most frequent causes worldwide are the *M. avium* complex and *M. kansasii*. *M. xenopi* is more restricted geographically but frequently occurs in southern England while, for unknown reasons, *M. malmoense* is encountered as a pathogen with increasing frequency in many parts of Europe including northern England. Rarer causes include *M. scrofulaceum*, *M. szulgai*, and *M. chelonae*.

Clinical presentation

Symptoms develop insidiously over weeks or months and include cough, malaise, weight loss, and sweats, in a pattern similar to tuberculosis but more chronic.

There are no diagnostically reliable clinical and radiological differences between pulmonary environmental mycobacterial disease and tuberculosis and diagnosis therefore depends on the isolation and identification of the causative organism. In contrast to *M. tuberculosis*, environmental mycobacteria isolated from sputum may not be the primary cause of disease; they may be transitory contaminants of the pharynx or secondary saprophytes of diseased tissue. There are no absolute criteria for distinguishing between these possibilities, but at least two pure cultures from specimens taken at least 1 week apart from patients with compatible symptoms and radiological signs in whom other causes, including tuberculosis, have been rigorously excluded render the diagnosis very likely. In some cases, a diagnosis is made or confirmed by microbiological examination of washings, brushings, or biopsies obtained by fibre-optic bronchoscopy.

Lymphadenitis

This is principally a disease of young children, occurring most frequently in the second year of life and then declining in frequency up to the fifth year, after which it is seldom encountered. The risk is reduced by neonatal BCG vaccination. The disease usually affects the cervical lymph nodes but other nodes, such as axillary and inguinal, may be involved, especially in older patients. Lymphadenitis is caused by many mycobacterial species, the commonest cause being the *M. avium* complex and *M. scrofulaceum*. Most cases occur in otherwise healthy children with no obvious predisposing cause but some cases, particularly in older age groups, are associated with human immunodeficiency virus (**HIV**) infection.

In most cases without predisposing causes, a single node is involved and surgical excision, if technically possible, is curative. More limited treatment, such as incision and drainage, may lead to sinus formation and should be avoided. Disseminated disease may develop in a few children, particularly those with some form of congenital immune deficiency, and in HIV-positive people.

Postinoculation mycobacterioses

Buruli ulcer is thought to result from inoculation of the causative organism, *M. ulcerans*, into the skin, principally by spiky vegetation. This disease is described elsewhere.

The natural habitat of *M. marinum*, the cause of swimming pool granuloma or fish tank granuloma, is water: it enters cuts and abrasions acquired whilst indulging in aquatic activities such as swimming and tending to tropical fish-tanks. The cutaneous lesions are usually warty, although pustules and ulcers may develop. There may be 'sporotrichoid' spread of lesions along the draining lymphatics (Fig. 1). The lesions usually heal spontaneously after a few months, but chemotherapy (see below) accelerates resolution. There have been occasional reports of tenosynovitis, carpal tunnel syndrome, osteomyelitis, and disseminated disease due to *M. marinum*.

Most other cases of postinoculation disease are caused by the rapid growers *M. chelonae* and *M. fortuitum*. The most common lesions are post-injection abscesses, which may occur sporadically or in mini-epidemics due to the use of contaminated multidose vaccines or other injectable materials. Abscesses develop from 1 to 12 months after injection and may enlarge to 7 cm or more in diameter. They tend to be chronic and localized, but multiple abscesses with spreading cellulitis may develop in people with insulin-dependent diabetes. Localized abscesses usually respond well to excision or curretage, but chemotherapy (see below) may be required for multiple or spreading lesions.

Trauma to the cornea predisposes to infection by rapid growers *M. chelonae* and *M. fortuitum*. Treatment with topical amikacin and eythromycin may lead to temporary resolution but relapse is common, especially in cases due to *M. chelonae*, and corneal grafting is usually required.

More serious infections have followed accidental inoculation during surgical operations, especially when contaminated materials, including heart valve xenografts, have been inserted. Contamination during cardiac valve surgery has resulted in mycobacterial endocarditis with septicaemia and osteomyelitis of the sternum requiring extensive debridement.

Fig. 1 *Mycobacterium marinum* infection. A small lesion at the base of the thumb (arrowed) and secondary lesions on the wrist and forearm due to 'sporotrichoid' spread (by courtesy of Dr G. Haase).

Fig. 2 Ulcers of the lower lip as the initial manifestation of disseminated *Mycobacterium chelonae* infection in a 4-year-old girl with autosomal IgA deficiency (by courtesy of Dr K. Schopfer).

Disseminated disease

Before HIV, disseminated disease due to environmental mycobacteria was very rare. Some cases, usually due to the *M. avium* complex or *M. chelonae*, occur in young people with congenital immune deficiencies (Fig. 2) and others, due principally to *M. chelonae*, occur in renal transplant recipients. *M. haemophilum* is a cause of multiple skin lesions in transplant recipients. As suggested by the name, this mycobacterium requires the addition of blood or other sources of iron in the medium for its *in vitro* cultivation.

The situation changed dramatically after the advent of the HIV pandemic and disseminated environmental mycobacterial disease was reported in 30 to 50 per cent of patients with AIDS, particularly in the United States. For reasons that are not clear, the great majority of such cases, 90 per cent or more, are caused by the *M. avium* complex, usually those identifiable by DNA homology as *M. avium* rather than *M. intracellulare*. Some cases are due to *M. genevense*, a very slowly growing species which, like *M. avium*, has been isolated from diseased birds. The number of cases of disseminated AIDS-related environmental mycobacterial disease has declined in the wealthier nations following the introduction of highly active antiretroviral therapy (HAART). Although HIV infection is common in Africa, and *M. avium* is present in the environment, AIDS-related disease due to this species is, for unknown reasons, rare in that continent.

The mechanism of the establishment of this disease in humans is poorly understood. Some workers consider it to be the result of recent infection while others postulate that the disease emerges from dormant foci of infection in the lymphatic tissues of the alimentary or respiratory tracts acquired many years previously.

The symptoms—fever, night sweats, weight loss, those of anaemia and general malaise—are rather non-specific and may be caused by other AIDS-related infections. Involvement of the intestine may lead to malabsorption and chronic diarrhoea. The diagnosis of AIDS-related *M. avium* complex disease is made by culture of blood or of biopsies of liver, lymph nodes, or bone marrow. The bacilli may be isolated from faeces in disseminated disease, but they may also be present in the intestinal tract of healthy persons.

Treatment of established disease improves the quality of the remainder of the patient's life. Opinions differ as to the place for prophylactic therapy, but the introduction of highly active antiretroviral therapy makes this less relevant.

Therapy

This depends on the site and severity of the infection, the presence of predisposing conditions such as congenital or acquired immunosuppression, the species of mycobacterium, and the result of *in vitro* drug-susceptibility tests.

As indicated above, skin lesions may be cured by excision, curettage, or drainage. Surgical excision, when technically possible, is used to treat lymphadenitis and should be considered in cases of localized pulmonary lesions.

Most cases of pulmonary disease due to the *M. avium* complex and other slow-growing environmental mycobacteria respond to regimens containing rifampicin, ethambutol, and isoniazid. In contrast to tuberculosis, ethambutol appears to be more effective than isoniazid and should be continued for the full duration of therapy, provided that ocular toxicity does not occur. Treatment for 18 or 24 months produces up to 80 per cent cure rate in disease due to the *M. avium* complex, *M. xenopi*, and *M. malmoense*. Shorter regimens are effective for treatment of *M. kansasii* infections. Recommended regimens are summarized in Table 2. Surgery may be considered in certain cases where chemotherapy is ineffective.

There is evidence that the regimens based on the newer macrolides, as used to treat disseminated AIDS-related *M. avium* disease (see below), are effective in the treatment of pulmonary disease due to this complex in HIV-negative patients, but their suitability for the treatment of such diseases caused by other slow-growing species has not been established.

There have been no comparative trials of drug regimens for disease due to the rapidly growing species *M. chelonae* and *M. fortuitum*. Therapy is therefore based on anecdotal experience and the results of *in vitro* susceptibility tests. The duration of therapy depends on clinical response. Localized disease often responds to erythromycin with trimethoprim, while spreading or disseminated disease may require the addition of amikacin or a cephalosporin such as ceftriaxone. Limited experience indicates that the fluoroquinolones are effective against *M. fortuitum* and imipenem or meropenem against *M. chelonae*.

Skin lesions due to *M. marinum* respond to doxycycline or minocycline, or a combination of rifampicin and ethambutol.

The newer macrolides, clarithromycin and azithromycin, form the basis of therapy of disseminated infection, usually due to the *M. avium* complex in patients with AIDS. Commonly used regimens contain one of these together with rifabutin and ethambutol, but revision on the basis of *in vitro* drug susceptibility testing may be required. The duration of therapy depends on clinical and bacteriological response. At one time merely palliative, such regimens may be curative when combined with antiretroviral therapy. The place for prophylaxis, usually clarithromycin, is controversial and rendered less relevant by the advent of antiretroviral therapy.

Table 2 Recommended regimens for treatment of pulmonary infections due to the more usually encountered slow-growing environmental mycobacteria

---

M. avium complex, *M. xenopi*, *M. malmoense* in HIV-
  negative patients:
  24 months' rifampicin, ethambutol, and isoniazid
Or
  24 months' rifampicin, ethambutol, clarithromycin,
  and/or ciprofloxacin
M. kansasii in HIV-negative patients:
  9 months' rifampicin and ethambutol
M. avium complex in patients with AIDS:
  A macrolide (clarithromycin or azithromycin) and
  ethambutol with, depending on response, the addition
  of rifabutin and/or ciprofloxacin.

Further reading

Banks J, Campbell IA (1998). Environmental mycobacteria. In: Davies PDO, ed. *Clinical tuberculosis*, 2nd edn, pp 521–33. Chapman & Hall Medical, London.

Collins CH *et al.* (1985). *Mycobacterium marinum* infections in man. *Journal of Hygiene (Cambridge)* **94**, 135–49.

Davies PDO, Ormerod LP (1999). Environmental mycobacteria. *Case presentations in clinical tuberculosis*, 259–75. Arnold Publishers, London.

Grange JM (1996). *Mycobacteria and human disease*, 2nd edn. Arnold Publishers, London.

Grange JM *et al.*. (1988). Inoculation mycobacterioses. *Clinical and Experimental Dermatology* **13**, 211–20.

Official Statement of the American Thoracic Society (1997). Diagnosis and treatment of disease caused by nontuberculous mycobacteria. *American Journal of Respiratory and Critical Care Medicine* **156**, S1–S25.

Subcommittee of the Joint Tuberculosis Committee of the British Thoracic Society (2000). Management of opportunist mycobacterial infections: Joint Tuberculosis Committee guidelines 1999. *Thorax* **55**, 210–18.

Wansborough-Jones MH, Banerjee D (1999). Non-tuberculous or atypical mycobacteria. In: James DG, Zumla A, eds. *The granulomatous disorders*, pp 189–204. Cambridge University Press, Cambridge.

7.11.24 Leprosy (Hansen's disease)

Diana N. J. Lockwood

Definition

Leprosy is a chronic granulomatous disease caused by *Mycobacterium leprae*. Its principal manifestations are anaesthetic skin lesions and peripheral neuropathy with peripheral nerve thickening. The clinical form is determined by the degree of cell-mediated immunity towards *M. leprae*. High levels of cell-mediated immunity with elimination of leprosy bacilli produces tuberculoid leprosy, whereas absent cell-mediated immunity results in lepromatous leprosy. Complications of leprosy result from nerve damage, immunological reactions, and bacillary infiltration. Nerve damage accompanying leprosy is a serious complication because it causes lifelong morbidity. Current antileprosy drugs are highly effective in killing bacilli but may not halt nerve damage. Patients with leprosy the world over are frequently stigmatized. Words such as 'leper' should be avoided and the disease should be referred to as Hansen's disease.

Aetiology

Leprosy is caused by *M. leprae*, an acid-fast intracellular organism not yet cultivated *in vitro*. It was first identified in the nodules of patients with lepromatous leprosy by Hansen in 1873. *M. leprae* preferentially parasitizes skin macrophages and peripheral nerve Schwann cells.

In vivo cultivation of *M. leprae*

M. leprae can be grown in the mouse footpad, but growth is slow, taking over 6 months to produce significant yields. The nine-banded armadillo is susceptible to *M. leprae* infection, and develops lepromatous disease. The armadillo and mouse models of *M. leprae* infection have been useful for producing *M. leprae* for biological studies and studying drug sensitivity patterns, respectively.

Biological characteristics

M. leprae is a stable, hardy organism, withstanding drying for up to 5 months. It has a doubling time of 12 days (compared with 20 min for *Escherichia coli*). The optimum growth temperature is 27°C to 30°C, consistent with the clinical observation of maximal *M. leprae* growth at cool superficial sites (skin, nasal mucosa, and peripheral nerves). *M. leprae* is a single species with isolates having similar biological characteristics and identical genotypes (using restriction fragment polymorphism analysis) irrespective of the type of leprosy, race, or geographical origin of the isolate.

Mycobacterial structure and metabolism

M. leprae possesses a complex cell wall comprising lipids and carbohydrates. It synthesizes a species-specific phenolic glycolipid and lipoarabinomannan. Antibody and T-cell screening has identified numerous protein antigens that are important immune targets.

M. leprae genome

M. leprae has a 3.27 Mb genome that displays extreme reductive evolution. Less than half the genome contains functional genes and many pseudogenes are present. One hundred and sixty-five genes are unique to *M. leprae* and functions can be attributed to 29 of them. Analysis of these unique proteins will be critical for developing new diagnostic tests. Comparison of biosynthetic pathways with *M. tuberculosis* is giving new insights into *M. leprae* metabolism. For lipolysis *M. leprae* has only two genes (*M. tuberculosis* has 22); *M. leprae* has also lost many genes for carbon catabolism and many carbon sources (e.g. acetate and galactose) are unavailable to it. This gene loss leaves *M. leprae* unable to respond to different environments and underlies the impossibility of growing the organism *in vitro*.

Epidemiology

Today, about 4 million people are disabled by leprosy. The much quoted figures of a fall in registered patients on treatment from 12 million in 1988 to 0.82 million in 1999 are misleading. Prevalence has fallen by means of effective antibiotic therapy and altered case definition. However, incidence remains stable at around 800 000 new cases annually with high rates of childhood cases. Intensive leprosy elimination campaigns held in 1998 and 1999 detected large numbers of new cases. A week-long campaign in Nepal found 11 696 new cases, doubling the national case load.

Geographical distribution

Seventy-seven per cent of patients with leprosy live in South-East Asia, 8.3 per cent in Africa, and 10 per cent in the Americas. India dominates the picture with 70 per cent of the world's leprosy cases; 86 per cent reside in six countries (India, Brazil, Indonesia, Myanmar, Madagascar, and Nepal). Leprosy has not always been a tropical disease; it was widespread in medieval Europe and was endemic in Norway until the early twentieth century. In North America, small foci of infection are still found in Texas and Louisiana. Nearly all new patients now seen in Europe and North America have acquired their infection abroad.

Risk factors

Leprosy is a chronic disease with a long incubation period. An average incubation time of 2 to 5 years has been calculated for tuberculoid cases and 8 to 12 years for lepromatous cases. American servicemen who developed leprosy after serving in the tropics presented up to 20 years after their presumed exposure. Age, sex, and household contact are important determinants of leprosy risk; incidence reaches a peak at 10 to 14 years; the excess of male cases is attributed to women's reluctance to present to health workers with skin lesions. Poor nutritional status is cited as predisposing to leprosy but no good evidence substantiates this. Improved socio-economic conditions, extended schooling, and good housing conditions reduce the risk of leprosy. Subclinical infection with *M. leprae* is probably common but the development of established disease is rare. Little work has been done on the early events in infection with *M. leprae* because there is no simple test that can establish whether an individual has encountered *M. leprae* and mounted a protective immune response.

HIV and leprosy

Studies from Malawi, Uganda, Mali, and South India have not found HIV infection to be a risk factor for leprosy. HIV/leprosy coinfected patients have typical skin lesions and typical leprosy histology and granuloma formation despite low circulating CD4 counts.

Transmission

The transmission of *M. leprae* is only partially understood. Untreated lepromatous patients discharge abundant organisms from their nasal mucosa into the environment. Studies in Indonesia and Ethiopia using polymerase chain reaction (PCR) primers to detect *M. leprae* DNA in nasal swabs have shown that up to 5 per cent of the population in leprosy endemic areas carry *M. leprae* DNA in their noses. The organism is then inhaled, multiplies on the inferior turbinates, and has a brief bacteraemic phase before binding to and entering Schwann cells and macrophages. The combination of an environmentally well-adapted organism, high carriage rates, and a long incubation period means that, even with effective antibiotics, transmission will continue for a long time.

Pathogenesis

Leprosy is a bacterial infection in which clinical features are determined by the host's immune response (Table 1).

The immune response to *M. leprae* and the leprosy spectrum

The Ridley–Jopling classification (Fig. 1) places patients on a spectrum of disease according to their clinical features, bacterial load, and histological and immunological responses. The two poles of the spectrum are tuberculoid (**TT**; paucibacillary) and lepromatous leprosy (**LL**; multibacillary). At the tuberculoid pole, well-expressed cell-mediated immunity effectively controls bacillary multiplication with the formation of organized epithelioid-cell granulomas; at the lepromatous pole there is cellular anergy towards *M. leprae* with abundant bacillary multiplication. Between these two poles is a continuum, varying from the patient with moderate cell-mediated immunity (borderline tuberculoid, **BT**) through borderline (**BB**) to the patient with little cellular response, borderline lepromatous (**BL**). The polar groups (TT, LL) are stable, but within the central groups (BT, BB, BL) the disease tends to downgrade to the lepromatous pole in the absence of treatment and upgrading towards the tuberculoid pole may occur during or after treatment.

Both T cells and macrophages play important roles in the processing, recognition, and response to *M. leprae* antigens. In tuberculoid leprosy, *in vitro* tests of T-cell function such as lymphocyte transformation tests show a strong response to *M. leprae* protein antigens with the production of T_{H1}-type cytokines (interferon-γ and interleukin 2, **IL-2**). Skin tests with lepromin, a heat-killed *M. leprae* preparation, are strongly positive. Staining of skin biopsies from tuberculoid lesions with T-cell markers shows highly organized granulomas composed predominantly of CD4 cells and macrophages with a peripheral mantle of CD8 cells. This strong cell-mediated immune response clears bacilli but with concomitant local tissue destruction, especially in nerves.

Patients with lepromatous leprosy have no cell-mediated immunity to *M. leprae* with a failure of the T-cell and macrophage response. Tests for lepromin are negative. This anergy is specific for *M. leprae*. Patients with LL disease respond to other mycobacteria such as *M. tuberculosis*, both *in vitro* and in skin tests. Identification of cell types in LL granulomas shows a disorganized mixture of macrophages and T cells, mainly CD8 cells. The T-cell failure may be due to clonal anergy or active suppression. Defects in cytokine production have been demonstrated; intralesional injections of recombinant IL-2 reconstitute the local immune response with elimination of *M. leprae* from macrophages. The T-cell cytokines that are produced are of the T_{H2} type. Macrophage defects described in LL disease include: defective antigen presentation and recognition, defective IL-1 production, a failure of macrophages to kill *M. leprae*, and a macrophage suppression of the T-cell response. Patients with lepromatous leprosy produce a range of autoantibodies that are both organ specific (against thyroid, nerve, testis, and gastric mucosa) and non-specific, such as rheumatoid factors, anti-DNA, cryoglobulins, and cardiolipin.

Table 1 Major clinical features of the disease spectrum in leprosy

Clinical features	Classification				
	Tuberculous—paucibacillary (TT)	Borderline tuberculoid (BT)	Borderline (BB)	Borderline lepromatous (BL)	Lepromatous—multibacillary (LL)
Skin					
Infiltrated lesions	Defined plaques, healing centres	Irregular plaques with partially raised edges	Polymorphic, 'punched out centres'	Papules, nodules	Diffuse thickening
Macular lesions	Single, small	Several, any size, 'geographical'	Multiple, all sizes, bizarre	Innumerable, small	Innumerable, confluent
Nerve					
Peripheral nerve	Solitary enlarged nerves	Several nerves, asymmetrical	Many nerves, asymmetrical pattern	Late neural thickening, asymmetrical, anaesthesia and paresis	Slow symmetrical loss, glove and stocking anaesthesia
Microbiology					
Bacterial index	0–1	0–2	2–3	1–4	4–6
Histology					
Lymphocytes	+	++	+/–	++	+/–
Macrophages	–	–	+/–	–	–
Epithelioid cells	++	+/–	–	–	–
Antibody, anti-*M. leprae*	–/+	–/++	+	++	++

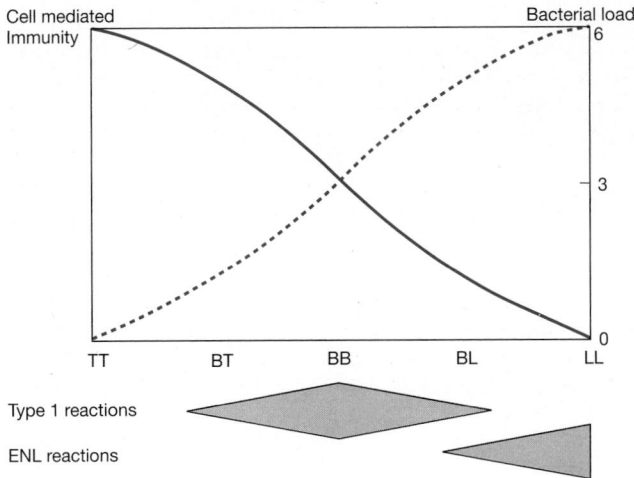

Fig. 1 The Ridley–Jopling spectrum of bacterial load, cell-mediated immunity, and reactions.

Bacterial load

In lepromatous leprosy, bacilli spread haematogenously to cool, superficial sites including eyes, upper respiratory mucosa, testes, small muscles, and bones of the hands, feet, and face as well as to peripheral nerves and skin. The heavy bacterial load causes structural damage at all these sites. In tuberculoid leprosy, bacilli are not readily found.

Leprosy reactions

Leprosy reactions are events superimposed on the Ridley–Jopling spectrum. Type 1 (reversal reactions) occur in borderline patients (BT, BB, BL) and are delayed hypersensitivity reactions caused by increased recognition of *M. leprae* antigens in skin and nerve sites. They are characterized by an increase in lymphocytes (CD4 and IL-2-producing cells) within lesions, severe oedema with disruption of the granuloma, and giant cell formation. There is local production of cytokines such as interferon-γ and tumour necrosis factor-α. Type 1 reactions are probably associated with a switch from production of T$_{H1}$- to T$_{H2}$-type cytokines.

Type 2 reactions, erythema nodosum leprosum (**ENL**), are partly due to immune complex deposition and occur in BL and LL patients who produce antibodies and have a large antigen load. There is vasculitis with lesional immunoglobulin, complement, and polymorphs and circulating immune complexes. There is also enhanced T-cell activity with increased CD8 cells, increased circulating IL-2 receptors, and high levels of circulating tumour necrosis factor-α. After reaction, lepromatous patients revert to a state of immunological unresponsiveness.

Nerve damage

Nerve damage occurs in skin lesions and in peripheral nerve trunks. Myelinated and unmyelinated sensory fibres are affected early. In tuberculoid disease, epithelioid granulomas and perineural inflammation occur. In established lepromatous infection, almost all the cutaneous nerves and peripheral nerve trunks are involved. Bacilli are found in Schwann, perineurial, and endothelial cells. Extensive demyelination occurs and later wallerian degeneration. Despite large numbers of organisms in the nerve there is only a small inflammatory response, but ultimately the nerve becomes fibrotic and is hyalinized. The formation of small granulomas is characteristic of borderline leprosy; granulomatous regions may abut strands of normal looking but heavily bacillated Schwann cells. The combination of lepromatous bacillation and cell-mediated immunity produces widespread nerve damage in borderline leprosy.

Clinical features of leprosy

Patients commonly present with skin lesions, weakness or numbness due to a peripheral nerve lesion, or a burn or ulcer in an anaesthetic hand or foot. Borderline patients may present in reaction with nerve pain, sudden palsy, multiple new skin lesions, pain in the eye, or a systemic febrile illness.

The cardinal signs are:

(1) typical skin lesions, anaesthetic at the tuberculoid end of the spectrum;

(2) thickened peripheral nerves; and

(3) acid-fast bacilli on skin smears or biopsy.

Presenting symptoms

Early lesions

The commonest early lesion is an area of numbness on the skin or a visible skin lesion. The classic early skin lesion, especially in surveys, is indeterminate leprosy, which is commonly found on the face, extensor surface of the limbs, buttocks, or trunk. Indeterminate lesions consist of one or more slightly hypopigmented or erythematous macules, a few centimetres in diameter, with poorly defined margins. Hair growth and nerve function are unimpaired. A biopsy may show the perineurovascular infiltrate and only scanty acid-fast bacilli. The indeterminate phase may last for months or years before resolving or developing into one of the determinate types of leprosy.

Skin

The commonest skin lesions are macules or plaques; papules and nodules are more rare. In lepromatous leprosy a diffuse infiltration of the skin often occurs. Lesions may be found anywhere although rarely in the axillas, perineum, or hairy scalp. Tuberculoid patients have few, hypopigmented lesions while lepromatous patients have numerous, sometimes confluent lesions. The few tuberculoid lesions are usually asymmetrical, more numerous lesions are likely to be distributed symmetrically.

Anaesthesia

Anaesthesia may occur in skin lesions when dermal nerves are involved or in the distribution of a large peripheral nerve. In skin lesions the small dermal sensory and autonomic nerve fibres supplying dermal and subcutaneous structures are damaged causing local sensory loss and loss of sweating within that area.

Peripheral neuropathy

Peripheral nerve trunks are vulnerable at sites where they are superficial or are in fibro-osseous tunnels. At these points a small increase in nerve diameter raises intraneural pressure causing neural compression and ischaemia. Damage to peripheral nerve trunks produces characteristic signs with dermatomal sensory loss and dysfunction of muscles supplied by that peripheral nerve. The sites of predilection for peripheral nerve involvement are ulnar (at the elbow), median (at the wrist), radial, radial cutaneous (at the wrist), common peroneal (at the knee), posterior tibial and sural nerves at the ankle, facial nerve as it crosses the zygomatic arch, and great auricular in the posterior triangle of the neck. All these nerves should be examined for enlargement and tenderness.

Tuberculoid leprosy (TT)

Infection is localized and asymmetrical. A typical tuberculoid skin lesion is a macule or plaque, single, erythematous or purple with raised and clear-cut edges sloping towards a flattened hypopigmented centre. The surface is anaesthetized, dry, and hairless. Sensory impairment may be difficult to demonstrate on the face, where there are abundant nerve endings. If one palpates the edge of the lesions, a thickened cutaneous nerve may be found. If peripheral nerve trunk involvement is present, only one nerve trunk is

Fig. 2 Active tuberculoid annular lesions showing the sharp outer edge, thin, raised, erythematous, dry rim, and the broad, hypopigmented, dry centre with slight hair loss. The 'satellite' lesion at the lower outer edge indicates that this is borderline tuberculoid leprosy. As shown, biopsies and smears should be taken from the raised, active rim.

enlarged. No *M. leprae* are found in skin smears. True tuberculoid leprosy has a good prognosis, many infections resolve without treatment and peripheral nerve trunk damage is limited.

Borderline tuberculoid (BT) (Plate 1)

The skin lesions are similar to TT leprosy and there may be few or many lesions (Fig. 2). The margins are less well defined and there may be satellite lesions. Damage to peripheral nerves is widespread and severe, usually with several thickened nerve trunks. It is important to recognize BT leprosy because these patients are at risk of reversal reactions leading to rapid deterioration in nerve function with consequent deformities.

Borderline leprosy (BB)

BB disease is the most unstable part of the spectrum and patients usually downgrade towards lepromatous leprosy if they are not treated or upgrade towards tuberculoid leprosy as part of a reversal reaction. There are numerous skin lesions which may be macules, papules, or plaques and vary in size, shape, and distribution. The edges of the lesions may have streaming, irregular borders. Annular lesions with a broad, irregular edge and a sharply defined punched-out centre are characteristic of BB disease (Fig. 3). Nerve damage is variable.

Borderline lepromatous leprosy (BL)

This is characterized by widespread, variable, asymmetrical skin lesions. There may be erythematous or hyperpigmented papules, succulent nodules or plaques, and sensation in the lesions may be normal. Peripheral nerve involvement is widespread. While patients with BL leprosy do not suffer the extreme consequences of bacillary multiplication that are seen in LL disease, they may experience either or both reversal and ENL reactions.

Lepromatous leprosy (LL) (Plate 2)

The patient with untreated polar lepromatous leprosy may be carrying 10^{11} leprosy bacilli. The onset of disease is frequently insidious, the earliest lesions being ill defined, shiny, hypopigmented or erythematous macules. Gradually the skin becomes infiltrated and thickened and nodules develop (Fig. 4); facial skin thickening causes the characteristic leonine facies

Fig. 3 Borderline annular lesions on the shoulder and back: the rim is broad, the edge irregular, and the 'punched-out' centre is hypopigmented and anaesthetized.

(Fig. 5). Hair is lost, especially the lateral third of the eye brows (madarosis). Dermal nerves are destroyed leading to a progressive glove and stocking anaesthesia and sensory loss (light touch, pain, and temperature) which begins at the hands and feet and gradually extends to the whole body except for the axillas, groins, and scalp. Position sense is preserved. Sweating is lost, which is uncomfortable in the tropics as compensatory sweating occurs in the remaining intact areas. Damage to peripheral nerves is symmetrical and occurs late in disease. Infiltration of the corneal nerves causes anaesthesia, which predisposes to injury, secondary infection, and blindness.

Nasal symptoms can often be elicited early in the disease, and 80 per cent of patients with newly diagnosed lepromatous leprosy have hyperaemic or ulcerated nasal mucosa. Septal perforation may occur. There may be papules on the lips and nodules on the palate, uvula, tongue, and gums. Bone involvement is common, with absorption of the terminal phalanges and pencilling of the heads and shafts of the metatarsals. Testicular atrophy results from diffuse infiltration and the acute orchitis that occurs during ENL reactions. The consequent loss of testosterone leads to azoospermia

Fig. 4 Active, untreated lepromatous leprosy, showing generalized infiltration of the skin, swelling of fingers and lips, and thinning of eyebrows and eyelashes. The residual annular lesions visible in both pectoral regions indicate that this patient has 'downgraded' from borderline.

Fig. 5 Leonine facies in advanced untreated lepromatous leprosy, with gross thickening of the ear lobes. The skin of the trunk and limbs is infiltrated and mildly erythematous, and small papules are present on some knuckles.

Fig. 6 Type 1 (reversal) reaction: this BL patient developed new, sharp-edged, well-defined, erythematous plaques with desquamating surfaces about 6 months after starting chemotherapy.

and gynaecomastia. The extremities become oedematous. The skin of the legs becomes icthyotic and ulcerates easily.

Other forms of leprosy

There are several variant forms of leprosy. Pure neural leprosy occurs principally in India, where it is the presenting form for 10 per cent of patients. There is asymmetrical involvement of peripheral nerve trunks and no visible skin lesions. On nerve biopsy all types of leprosy have been found.

Histoid lesions are distinctive nodules occurring in lepromatous cases which have relapsed due to dapsone resistance or non-compliance with chemotherapy.

Lucio's leprosy is a form of lepromatous leprosy found only in Latin Americans, with a uniform, diffuse, shiny skin infiltration.

Eye disease in leprosy

Blindness due to leprosy, which occurs in at least 2.5 per cent of patients, is a devastating complication for a patient with anaesthesia of the hands and feet. Eye damage results from both nerve damage and bacillary invasion. Lagophthalmos results from paresis of the orbicularis oculi due to involvement of the zygomatic and temporal branches of the facial (VIIth) nerve. These superficial branches are frequently involved in borderline tuberculoid cases, particularly if there are facial skin lesions. In lepromatous disease, lagophthalmos occurs later and is usually bilateral. Damage to the ophthalmic branch of the trigeminal (Vth) nerve causes anaesthesia of the cornea and conjunctiva resulting in drying of the cornea and makes the cornea susceptible to trauma and ulceration. Lepromatous infiltration in corneal nerves produces punctate keratitis and corneal lepromas. Invasion of the iris and ciliary body makes them extremely susceptible to reactions.

Leprosy reactions

Type 1 (reversal reactions) (Plates 3, 4)

These are characterized by acute neuritis and/or acutely inflamed skin lesions (Fig. 6). Nerves become tender with new loss of sensation or motor weakness. Existing skin lesions become erythematous or oedematous; new

lesions may appear (Fig. 7). Occasionally oedema of the hands, face, or feet is the presenting symptom, but constitutional symptoms are unusual. Type 1 reactions occur in borderline patients—35 per cent of BL patients will experience a type 1 reaction. The commonest time for reactions is in the first 2 months after starting treatment and in the puerperium.

Type 2 (ENL reactions)

These occur in LL and BL patients. Before multidrug therapy some 50 per cent of LL patients experienced erythema nodosum leprosum (ENL) reactions, the clofazimine component of multidrug therapy has reduced this to 15 per cent. Attacks are acute and may recur over several years. ENL manifests most commonly as painful red nodules on the face and extensor surfaces of limbs (Fig. 8). The lesions may be superficial or deep, with suppuration or brawny induration when chronic. Acute lesions crop and desquamate, fading over several days. ENL is a systemic disorder producing

Fig. 7 Reversal-reaction plaque on the left cheek and ear: the edge of this BT lesion has become very sharply defined, more raised, and erythematous, dry, and scaly. Treatment with corticosteroids is imperative, as the patient is at grave risk of rapidly developing lagophthalmos due to associated involvement of branches of the facial nerve.

Fig. 8 Erythema nodosum leprosum (ENL) on the forehead of a patient with early lepromatous leprosy. The papules (and nodules) are firm and tender, with rather indefinite edges. In dark-skinned patients the ENL lesions are often easier to feel than to see, especially over the extensor surfaces of the arms and thighs.

fever and malaise and may be accompanied by uveitis, dactylitis, arthritis, neuritis, lymphadenitis, and orchitis.

Neuritis (Plates 5, 6)

Silent neuropathy is an important form of nerve damage and presents as a functional neural deficit without a manifest acute or subacute neuritis. An Indian study following a cohort of 2608 patients found that 75 per cent of those developing deformity had no history of reactions. In Ethiopian and Bangladeshi cohort studies, silent neuritis accounted for most neuritis. This emphasizes the importance of regular nerve function testing so that new deficits can be detected.

Diagnosis

The diagnosis is made on the clinical findings of one or more of the cardinal signs of leprosy and supported by the finding of acid-fast bacilli on slit skin smears. The whole body should be inspected in a good light otherwise lesions may be missed, particularly on the buttocks. Skin lesions should be tested for anaesthesia to light touch, pin prick, and temperature. The peripheral nerves should be palpated systematically examining for thickening and tenderness. Wherever possible the diagnosis should be supported by a skin biopsy, which is essential for accurate classification. Serology is not usually helpful diagnostically because antibodies to the species-specific glycolipid PGL-1 are present in 90 per cent of untreated lepromatous patients but only 40 to 50 per cent of paucibacillary patients and 5 to 10 per cent of healthy controls. Polymerase chain reaction for detecting *M.leprae* DNA has not proved sensitive or specific enough for diagnosis.

Outside leprosy endemic areas doctors frequently fail to consider the diagnosis of leprosy. Of new patients seen from 1995 to 1999 at The Hospital for Tropical Diseases, London, diagnosis had been delayed in over 80 per cent of cases. Patients had been misdiagnosed by dermatologists, neurologists, orthopaedic surgeons, and rheumatologists. A common problem was failure to consider leprosy as a cause of peripheral neuropathy in patients from leprosy endemic countries. These delays had serious consequences for patients; over half of them had nerve damage and disability.

Slit skin smears

The bacterial load is assessed by making a small incision through the epidermis, scraping dermal material, and smearing evenly on to a glass slide. At least six sites should be sampled (earlobes, eyebrows, edges of active lesions). The smears are then stained and acid-fast bacilli are counted. Scoring is done on a logarithmic scale per high-power field. A score of 1+ indi-

cates 1 to 10 bacilli in 100 fields, 6+ over 1000 per field. Smears are useful for confirming the diagnosis and should be done annually to monitor response to treatment.

Differential diagnosis

Doctors should be aware of the normal range of skin colour and texture in their local population, and also of the common endemic skin diseases, such as onchocerciasis, that may coexist or mimic leprosy.

Skin

The variety of leprosy skin lesions means that a potentially wide range of skin conditions are in the differential diagnosis. At the tuberculoid end of the spectrum, anaesthesia differentiates leprosy from fungal infections, vitiligo, and eczema. At the lepromatous end the presence of acid-fast bacilli in smears differentiates leprosy nodules from onchocerciasis, Kaposi's sarcoma, and post-kala-azar dermal leishmaniasis.

Nerves

Peripheral nerve thickening is rarely seen except in leprosy. Hereditary sensory motor neuropathy type III is associated with palpable peripheral nerve hypertrophy. Amyloidosis, which can also complicate leprosy, causes thickening of peripheral nerves. Charcot–Marie–Tooth disease is an inherited neuropathy that causes distal atrophy and weakness. The causes of other polyneuropathies such as HIV, diabetes, alcoholism, vasculitides, and heavy metal poisoning should all be considered where appropriate.

Treatment

There are five main principles of treatment:

(1) stop the infection with chemotherapy;

(2) treat reactions;

(3) educate the patient about leprosy;

(4) prevent disability; and

(5) support the patient socially and psychologically.

These objectives need the patient's co-operation and confidence. In endemic countries, this will usually be achieved through the leprosy outpatient clinic. In countries where leprosy is uncommon, or when the clinical or social situation is complicated, it is often best to admit the patient to an experienced unit. This permits careful assessment together with accurate evaluation of nerve and eye involvement, patient education, and initiation of treatment.

Chemotherapy

All patients with leprosy should be given an appropriate multidrug combination. In the hospital setting, where skin smears and skin biopsies can be combined with clinical data, patients can be classified into paucibacillary (skin smear-negative tuberculoid and BT) and multibacillary (skin smear-positive BT, all BB, BL, and LL). The first-line antileprosy drugs are rifampicin, clofazimine, and dapsone. Table 2 gives the drug combinations, doses, and duration of treatment. Patients with multibacillary disease and an initial bacterial index greater than 4 will need longer treatment and the duration should be guided by their clinical status and bacterial index.

Rifampicin is a potent bactericide for *M. leprae*. Four days after a single 600 mg dose, bacilli from a previously untreated patient with multibacillary disease were no longer viable in a mouse foot-pad test. It acts by inhibiting DNA-dependent RNA polymerase. Because *M. leprae* can develop resistance to rifampicin as a one-step process, this drug should always be given in combination with other antileprotics.

Plates for Section 5
Chapter 5.4 Complement

(a)

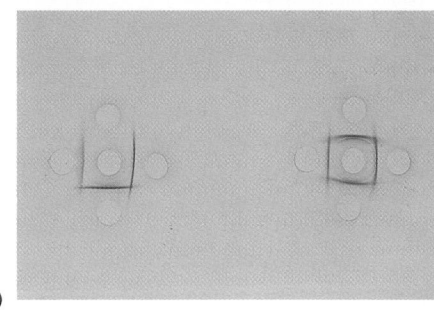

(b)

Plate 1 Patient with hereditary deficiency of C6 who presented with meningococcal septicaemia. (a) A subconjunctival haemorrhage. (b) The deficiency of C6. Serum from the patient was placed in the central well of an agarose-coated plate. In each of the outer wells was placed anti-serum to, respectively, C5, C6, C7, and C8. The antibody and antigen were allowed to diffuse in the gel and where the antibody encountered its antigen a precipitate formed, which was stained blue. No precipitate formed between the anti-C6 antibody and the patient's serum, indicating the presence of C6 deficiency.

Plates for Section 6
Chapter 6.2 The nature and development of cancer

(a)

(b)

Plate 1 In a spectral karyotype (SKY), each normal chromosome stains homogeneously with a single distinct colour, making translocations evident by the presence of more than one colour in a single chromosome. (a) Forty-five chromosomes are visible in this karyotype (left) from a patient with Turner's syndrome. Despite the loss of the X chromosome, the spectral karyotype (right) clearly shows the homogeneous chromosomal staining pattern typical of normal chromosomes. (b) In contrast, SKY analysis of a metaphase spread prepared from a breast cancer cell line displays both numerical and structural chromosomal aberrations. (By courtesy of Dr Bassem Haddad, Department of Oncology, Georgetown University Medical Center.)

Plates for Section 7
Chapter 7.10.2 Herpesviruses (excluding Epstein-Barr virus)

Plate 1 Primary herpetic gingivostomatitis.

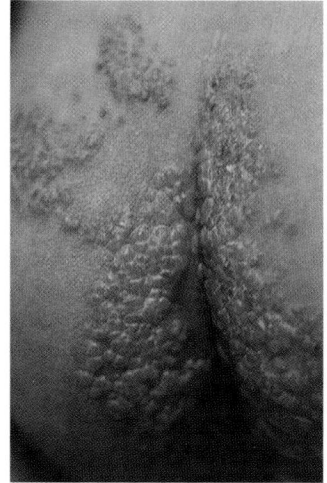

Plate 2 Primary HSV-2 of the buttocks.

(a)

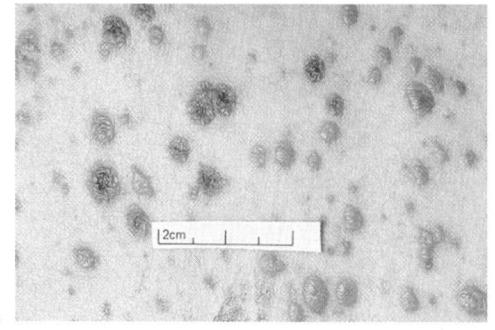

(b)

Plate 3 (a) Severe chickenpox also involving the lungs. (b) Details of the rash.

Plate 4 Herpes zoster affecting the ophthalmic division of the Vth nerve.

Plate 5 Human cytomegalovirus.

Plate 6 Kaposi's sarcoma affecting the palate and producing symmetrical skin lesions in association with HIV infection.

Chapter 7.10.4 Poxviruses

Plate 1 Ethiopian patient, in 1968, showing classical centrifugal distribution of lesions. (Copyright D.A. Warrell.)

Plate 2 Tanapox lesion on the leg of a Kenyan patient (by courtesy of the late P.E.C. Manson-Bahr).

Chapter 7.10.6 Measles

Plate 1 Measles rash on the legs of an English teenager. (Copyright D.A. Warrell.)

Plate 2 Measles rash (African).

Plate 3 Stomatitis with Herpes simplex ulcers in an African child with severe measles. (Copyright D.A. Warrell.)

Plate 4 Herpes simplex keratoconjunctivitis in an African child with severe measles. (Copyright D.A. Warrell.)

Plate 5 Measles rash (African).

Chapter 7.10.6.1 Nipah and Hendra viruses

Plate 1 Pteropid fruit bat (flying fox), the natural reservoir of Nipah, Hendra, and Menangle paramyxoviruses and Australian bat lyssavirus. (From the painting by John Gould.)

Chapter 7.10.9 Rhabdoviruses

Plate 1 Street rabies virus in human cerebellar Purkinje cells as seen with the light microscope. Several Negri bodies can be seen (one is arrowed). (By courtesy of the Armed Forces Institute of Pathology 73–12330.)

Chapter 7.10.18 Parvovirus B19

Plate 1 'Slapped cheek' rash of erythema infectiosum: note circumoral pallor. (By courtesy of Dr Ken Mutton.)

Chapter 7.11.2 Streptococci and enterococci

Plate 1 Bilateral facial erysipelas. (Copyright S. Eykyn.)

Plate 2 Cellulitis. (Copyright S. Eykyn.)

Plate 3 *Streptococcus pyogenes* bacteraemia 3 days after a skin graft. (Copyright S. Eykyn.)

Plate 4 Peeling of the skin of the soles of the feet in a patient with *Streptococcus pyogenes* pericarditis. (Copyright S. Eykyn.)

Chapter 7.11.5 Meningococcal infections

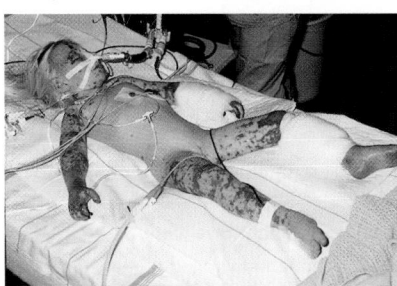

Plate 1 Massive skin haemorrhage on the extremities of a 4-year-old girl with fulminant meningococcal septicaemia. The infection was caused by *Neisseria meningitidis* group B. The left leg had to be amputated below the knee. She needed extensive skin transplantation and several fingers had to be amputated.

Plate 2 Macular lesions on the legs, some with a central haemorrhagic spot in a 17-year-old girl with mild meningococcaemia caused by *Neisseria meningitidis* group C. She recovered completely after 5 days treatment with benzylpenicillin.

Plate 3 Macular and haemorrhagic lesions on the legs of a 21-year-old man with mild meningococcaemia caused by *Neisseria meningitidis* group B. He recovered completely after 5 days of penicillin treatment.

Plate 4 The 'glass test' used to differentiate haemorrhagic skin lesions from viral or drug rash in an infant with meningococcal meningitis caused by *Neisseria meningitidis* group B. There was complete recovery after 5 days treatment with benzylpenicillin.

Chapter 7.11.6 *Neisseria gonorrhoeae*

Plate 1 Disseminated gonococcal infection, haemorrhagic vesiculopustule.

Plate 2 Disseminated gonococcal infection: healing lesions with desquamation and deposition of haemosiderin.

Plate 3 Gram-stained urethral discharge showing Gram-negative intracellular diplococci.

Chapter 7.11.8 Typhoid and paratyphoid fevers

Plate 1 Typhoid rash in a Melanesian child – sparse, purpuric (non-blanching) macules.

Chapter 7.11.17 Yersinia, Pasteurella, and Francisella

Plate 1 Hands in a case of ulcero-(cutano)-glandular tularaemia (by courtesy of A. Berglund, Fallund, Sweden).

Plate 2 Inguinal lymphadenopathy in ulceroglandular tularaemia (by courtesy of A. Berglund, Fallund, Sweden).

Plate 3 Hypersensitivity reaction in infection with *Francisella tularensis* subsp. *holarctica* (type B) in Scandinavia (by courtesy of A. Berglund, Fallund, Sweden).

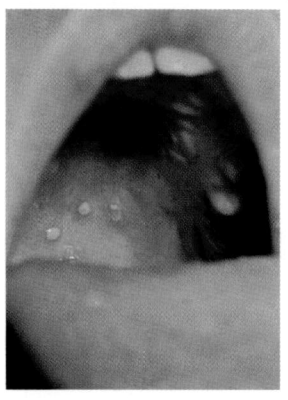

Plate 4 Oral tularaemia in a case from northern Sweden (by courtesy of A. Berglund, Fallund, Sweden).

Chapter 7.11.18 Anthrax

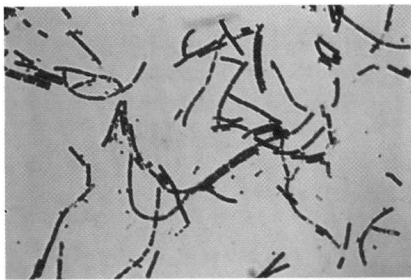

Plate 1 Large Gram-positive bacilli in chains are typical of *Bacillus anthracis*. An individual bacillus is 3 to 5 µm long and 1 to 1.25 µm wide with a flattened end.

Plate 2 Cutaneous anthrax lesion on the forearm on day 10 showing an ulcer with a depressed black eschar.

Plate 3 Oropharyngeal anthrax on day 9 showing a pseudomembrane covering an ulcer.

Chapter 7.11.20 Tetanus

Plate 1 Facies in tetanus.

Plate 2 Opisthotonos in severe tetanus during seizures.

Plate 3 Brazilian patient with local tetanus confined to muscles innervated by the left VIIth cranial nerve and with trismus, showing the wound causing the infection. (By courtesy of Dr Pedro Pardal, Belém, Brazil.)

Plate 4 Characteristic facies in neonatal tetanus.

Chapter 7.11.24 Leprosy (Hansen's disease)

Plate 1 BT leprosy. This Ethiopian woman has several hypopigmented patches. Testing for anaesthesia will confirm the diagnosis of BT leprosy.

Plate 2 Advanced nodular lepromatous leprosy. This Indian patient presented with ulcerating nodules all over his body.

Plate 3 Reversal (Type 1) reaction. This Ethiopian woman had a postpartum reaction presenting with numerous erythematous raised lesions 8 weeks after delivery.

Plate 4 Severe reversal (Type 1) reaction. This Indian woman has erythematous, oedematous, and desquamating reactional lesions.

Plate 5 Peripheral nerve thickening in leprosy. This young man had marked thickening of his great auricular nerve.

Plate 6 Nerve damage in leprosy. This patient with BT leprosy has damage to the ulnar and median nerves on both sides. This has resulted in hands which are wasted, clawed, and lack finger and thumb opposition.

Plate 7 Complications of lepromatous leprosy. Gynaecomastia is visible in this man, secondary to testicular involvement in lepromatous leprosy. Multiple nodules are present, many dark brown, due to clofazimine pigmentation. He also has new erythematous lesions of ENL.

Chapter 7.11.25 Buruli ulcer: *Mycobacterium ulcerans*; infection

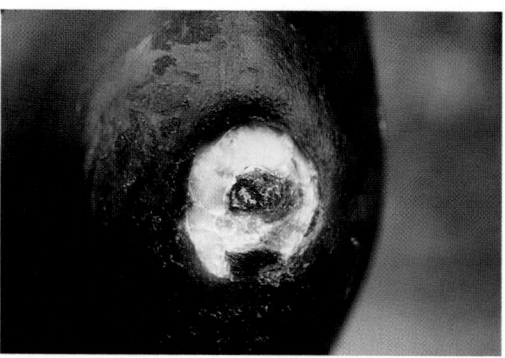

Plate 1 Buruli ulcer on the left deltoid area in a 12-year-old Congolese boy who had received a hypodermic injection at this site 3 months previously. Note central necrotic slough in the base of the ulcer, and undermined edges.

Chapter 7.11.29 Lyme borreliosis

Plate 1 Adult female (right) and nymphal (left) – ticks of the *Ixodes scapularis* species.

(a)

(b)

Plate 2 Erythema migrans rashes from patients who were culture positive for borrelia. (a) A rash with typical central clearing appearance. (b) A rash with more homogenous appearance.

Chapter 7.11.30 Other borrelia infections

Plate 1 *Borrelia recurrentis* spirochaetes in a Giemsa-stained thin blood film from a patient with louse-borne relapsing fever. (Copyright D.A. Warrell.)

Plate 2 Spleen in louse-borne relapsing fever. Warthin Starry stain showing *Borrelia recurrentis* (arrows). (By courtesy of Dr Ken Fleming.)

Plate 3 Cerebral haemorrhage in a patient with louse-borne relapsing fever. (Copyright D.A. Warrell.)

Plate 4 Petechial haemorrhages on the surface of the kidney in a victim of louse-borne relapsing fever. (Copyright D.A. Warrell.)

Plate 5 Ethiopian patient with severe louse-borne relapsing fever. Note emaciation and petechial rash. (Copyright D.A. Warrell.)

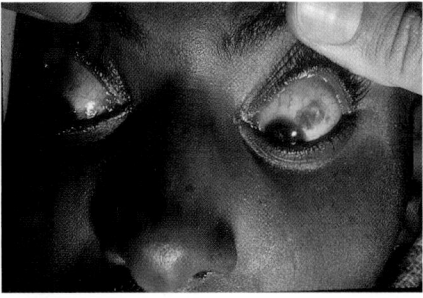

Plate 6 Subconjunctival haemorrhages in louse-borne relapsing fever. (Copyright D.A. Warrell.)

Chapter 7.11.31 Leptospirosis

Plate 1 Jaundice, haemorrhage, and conjunctival suffusion in acute leptospirosis.

Chapter 7.11.36 Rickettsial diseases including ehrlichiosis

Plate 1 Boutonneuse fever (South African tick typhus). Eschar with lymphangitic lines spreading towards the femoral lymph nodes in a patient who had visited the Kruger National Park, South Africa, 7 days earlier. (Copyright D.A. Warrell.)

Plates 2 and 3 Boutonneuse fever (South African tick typhus) in a British traveller. (Copyright E. Dunbar.)

Chapter 7.11.37 Scrub typhus

(a)

(b)

(c)

Plate 1 Typical eschars (a, b) and one less typical (c) on the distal foreskin. Lesions in locations such as these can be easily missed during a cursory examination of a febrile patient presenting to a busy outpatient clinic.

Plate 2 Diagnosis by rapid immunoblot dipstick. The test strip above indicates active scrub typhus, with clearly visible staining within several circles. The test strip below was read as non-reactive, because only the reagent control (last dot on the right) contains staining.

Chapter 7.11.39 Bartonellosis

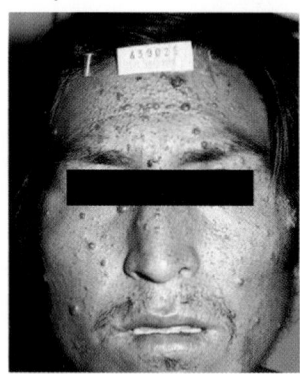

Plate 1 Miliary haemangioma-like of 'verruga peruana'.

(a)

(b)

Plate 2 (a, b) Nodular lesions of 'verruga peruana'.

Chapter 7.11.40 Chlamydial infections including lymphogranuloma venerum

Plate 1 Everted upper eyelid showing follicular trachoma (TF).

Plate 2 Everted upper eyelid showing intense inflammatory trachoma (TI).

Plate 3 Extensive neovascularization of the cornea (pannus) due to trachoma.

Plate 4 Everted upper eyelid showing trachomatous scarring (TS).

Plate 5 Trachomatous trichiasis (TT).

(a)

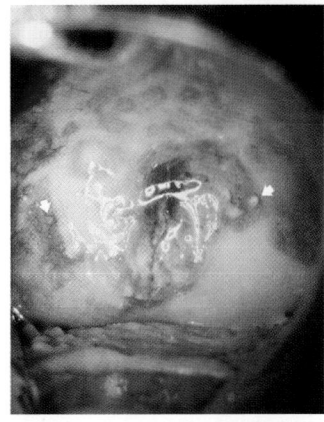

(b)

Plate 6 (a) Mucopurulent cervicitis; (b) follicular cervicitis.

Plate 7 Laparoscopic view of inflamed fallopian tube due to *C. trachomatis*. (By courtesy of P. Greenhouse.)

Plate 8 Adhesions in perihepatitis (Curtis Fitz-Hugh syndrome) due to *C. trachomatis*. (By courtesy of P. Greenhouse.)

Plate 9 Mucopurulent neonatal conjunctival discharge due to *C. trachomatis*.

Plate 10 Germinal centre formation in lymphoid follicle of cervicitis due to *C. trachomatis*.

Chapter 7.12.1 Fungal infections

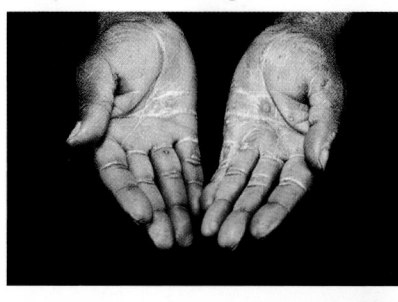

Plate 1 Palmar scaling due to *Trichophyton rubrum*.

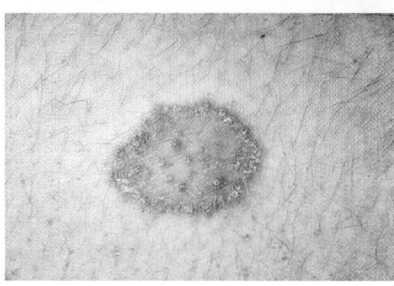

Plate 2 Tinea corporis due to *Microsporum gypseum*.

Plate 3 Oral candidosis in a patient with chronic mucocutaneous candidosis.

Plate 4 Grains in abscess in actinomycetoma (*Nocardia brasiliensis*) (H & E).

Plate 5 A mycetoma caused by *Madurella grisea*.

Plate 6 *Nocardia brasiliensis* actinomycetoma draining sinus.

Plate 7 Lobo's disease in a Brazilian man. (Copyright D.A. Warrell.)

Plate 8 Nodular subcutaneous lesions of African histoplasmosis in a Nigerian man. (Copyright D.A. Warrell.)

Plate 9 Candidosis disseminated to skin (methenamine silver × 516).

Chapter 7.13.1 Amoebic infections

Plate 1 Amoebic colitis. Crypt abscess. PAS stains amoebae red. (Copyright Viqar Zaman.)

Plate 2 Amoebic colitis. Superficial ulcer breaching the muscularis mucosae. (Copyright Viqar Zaman.)

Plate 3 'Anchovy sauce' pus drained from an amoebic liver abscess. (Copyright Viqar Zaman.)

(a)

(b)

Plate 4 Sixteen-year-old Peruvian boy with a chronic facial lesion that had been present for 3 years and intracranial space-occupying lesions cuased by *Balamuthia mandrillaris* (a). Perforating lesion of the palate (b). (Copyright D.A. Warrell.)

Plate 2 Section of frontal cortex from a Vietnamese patient who died of cerebral malaria, showing sequestration of parasitized red blood corpuscles in blood vessels (N=neurone, V=vessel). (By courtesy of Dr Gareth Turner, Oxford.)

Plate 3 Retinal haemorrhages close to the macula in a Thai patient with cerebral malaria. (Copyright D.A. Warrell.)

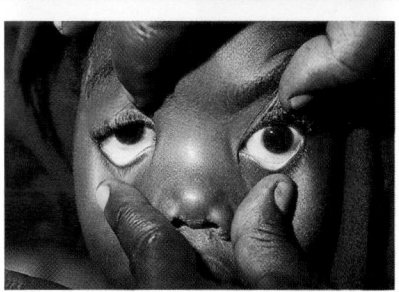

Plate 4 Profound anaemia (haemoglobin 1.2 g/dl) in a Kenyan child with *P. falciparum* parasitaemia. (Copyright D.A. Warrell.)

Chapter 7.13.2 Malaria

	Gametocytes		Schizonts		Trophozoites		
	Female	Male	Mature	Immature	Old	Young	
							P. falciparum
							P. vivax
							P. malariae
							P. ovale

Plate 1 Malaria parasites developing in erythrocytes. (By courtesy of The Wellcome Trust.)

Plate 5 Cerebral malaria. Spontaneous systemic bleeding in a Thai patient with disseminated intravascular coagulation. (Copyright D.A. Warrell.)

Plate 2 Modified Ziehl-Neelsen-stained faecal smear showing oocysts of *C. parvum* examined with × 100 oil-immersion objective lens. The uniformity of size (4.5-5 μm) but variability of staining of oocysts can be seen.

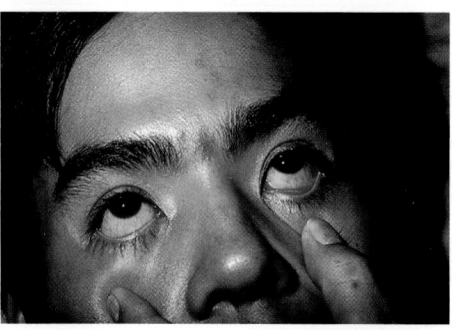

Plate 3 Modified Ziehl-Neelsen-stained faecal smear showing oocysts of *C. parvum*. The uniformity of size (4.5-5 μm) is apparent but the oocysts in this preparation show a definite increase in refractility and marked failure to take up the stain (identity confirmed by immunofluorescence and electron microscopy).

Plate 6 Deep jaundice in a Vietnamese man with severe falciparum malaria. (Copyright D.A. Warrell.)

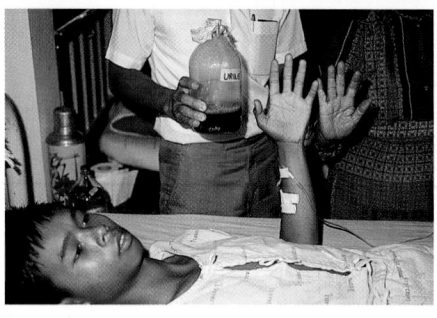

Plate 7 Intravascular haemolysis in a Karen patient with glucose 6-phosphate dehydrogenase deficiency in whom treatment with an oxidant drug resulted in haemoglobinuria and anaemia (normal hand in comparison). (Copyright D.A. Warrell.)

Plate 4 Modified Ziehl-Neelsen-stained faecal smear showing oocyst-like bodies (mushroom spores) examined with × 100 oil-immersion objective lens (from specimen submitted to Reference Unit for identification).

Plate 5 Modified Ziehl-Neelsen-stained faecal smear showing oocyst-like bodies (mould spores) examined with × 100 oil-immersion objective lens. The spores are uniform in size but a little smaller (4.0 μm) than oocysts of *C. parvum*. They are generally more uniform in their acid-fast staining (identity confirmed by mycological culture and electron microscopy).

Chapter 7.13.3 Babesia

Plate 1 *Babesia divergens* infection in a 29-year-old French man, infected in Normandy. He had been splenectomized 4 months previously for idiopathic thrombocytopenia. Parasitaemia reached 30 per cent. He was successfully treated with exchange transfusion, clindamycin, and quinine. (Copyright P. Brasseur.)

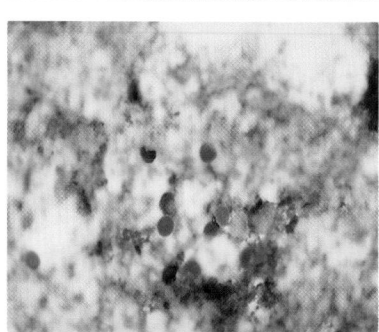

Chapter 7.13.5 Cryptosporidium and cryptosporidiosis

Plate 1 Modified Giemsa-stained faecal smear showing oocysts of *C. parvum*, examined with × 100 oil-immersion objective lens. The uniformity of size (4.5-5 μm) but variability of staining of oocysts can be seen. The eosinophilic nuclei and basophilic bodies of the sporozoites can be clearly seen within the oocysts that have taken up the stain.

Plate 6 Phenol-auramine/carbol fuchsin-stained faecal smear showing oocysts of *C. parvum*, examined with × 20 dry objective lens (screening magnification) on a fluorescence microscope.

Plate 7 Phenol-auramine/carbol fuchsin-stained faecal smear showing oocysts of *C. parvum*, examined with × 100 oil-immersion objective lens on a fluorescence microscope.

Plate 8 Fluorescent dye-tagged monoclonal antibody-stained faecal smear showing oocysts of *C. parvum*, examined with × 50 oil-immersion objective lens (screening magnification) on a fluorescence microscope. The suture or associated surface cleft or fold, through which the sporozoites are released, can be seen.

Plate 3 Jejunal biopsy from a patient with cyclosporiasis showing jejunitis with blunting of villi (low power H & E stain). (By courtesy of Dr Sebastian Lucus, London.)

Chapter 7.13.10 Human African trypanosomiasis

Plate 1 Adult tsetse fly (*Glossina morsitans*).

Plate 9 Modified Ziehl-Neelsen-stained sputum smear from an AIDS patient with respiratory involvement (examined with × 100 oil-immersion objective lens). The *C. parvum* bodies present may include endogenous (tissue) stages attached to exfoliated cells. For this reason, oocyst wall-specific indirect immunofluorescence may show a poor reaction. There may also be less uniformity of size and differences in the staining appearance of the internal structures.

Plate 10 Toluidine blue-stained semithin section of human rectal biopsy tissue of an AIDS patient with cryptosporidiosis. The apparent pseudo-external location of the parasite can be seen, the true location being intracellular but extracytoplasmic.
Plates for this chapter were kindly provided from photographs by A. Curry and D.P. Casemore.

Chapter 7.13.6 Cyclospora

Plate 1 Unstained wet preparation of human faecal material showing oocysts of *Cyclospora* sp., examined with × 100 water-immersion objective lens by phase-contrast microscopy. The uniformity of size (8-10 µm) and the morular (mulberry) internal structure of the oocysts can be seen.

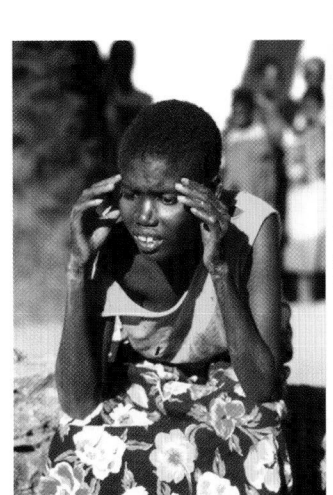

Plate 3 Patient with late-stage trypanosomiasis.

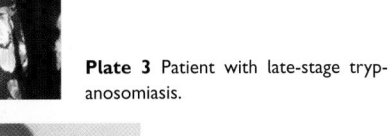

Plate 2 Trypanosomal chancre on the shank of a missionary returning from the Congo.

Plate 2 Modified Ziehl-Neelsen-stained faecal smear showing oocysts of *Cyclospora* sp. examined with × 50 oil-immersion objective lens. The uniformity of size (8-10 µm) but variability of staining of the oocysts can be seen. Apart from the greater size, the oocysts can be distinguished from those of *Cryptosporidium parvum* by the different pattern of acid-fast staining. Unstained oocysts within the smear sometimes show the morular structure apparent in wet preparations.

Plate 4 Trypanosomes in thin human blood film (Giemsa stain, × 1000 magnification).

Plate 4 Romaña's sign in acute Chagas' disease.

Plate 5 Morular cell of Mott in a histological brain section of a stage II HAT patient (H & E stain, × 1000 magnification).

Chapter 7.13.11 Chagas' disease

Plate 1 Adult female triatomine bug (*Panstrongylus megistus*), with a single egg shown adjacent to the tip of the abdomen. (By courtesy of Dr T.V. Barrett.)

Plate 5 Apical aneurysm of the left ventricle in chronic Chagas' disease. (By courtesy of Dr J.S. de Oliveira.)

(a)

(b)

Plate 6 Mural thrombus filling the right atrial appendage. (Copyright D.A. Warrell.)

Plate 2 (a) Pseudocyst of *Trypanosoma cruzi* in heart muscle. (By courtesy of J.E. Williams.) (b) Pseudocyst of *Trypanosoma cruzi* in umbilical cord, from a congenital case of Chagas' disease. (By courtesy of Dr Hipolito de Almeida.)

Plate 7 Mega-oesophagus seen by radiography in chronic Chagas' disease. (By courtesy of Dr J.S. de Oliveira.)

Plate 3 *Trypanosoma cruzi* C-shaped trypomastigote in blood, note large posterior kinetoplast.

Plate 8 Megacolon postmortem in chronic Chagas' disease. (By courtesy of Dr J.S. de Oliveira.)

Chapter 7.13.12 Leishmaniasis

Plate 1 Shallow ulcer with raised edge due to *L. brasiliensis* (copyright A.D.M. Bryceson).

Plate 2 Lupoid or recidivans leishmaniasis in a citizen of Baghdad. (By courtesy of Dr Ahmed.)

Plate 3 Swollen upper lip and nose due to mucosal leishmaniasis in Peru (copyright A.D.M. Bryceson).

Plate 4 Infiltration of lip and palate due to mucosal leishmaniasis in Peru (copyright A.D.M. Bryceson).

Chapter 7.13.13 Trichomoniasis

Plate 1 Trichomonads, Giemsa stain, in vaginal secretions. (Copyright J.P. Ackers.)

Chapter 7.14.1 Cutaneous filariasis

Plate 1 A 3-cm subcutaneous nodule.

Plate 2 Excoriated papular lesions of onchocerciasis with hyperpigmentation.

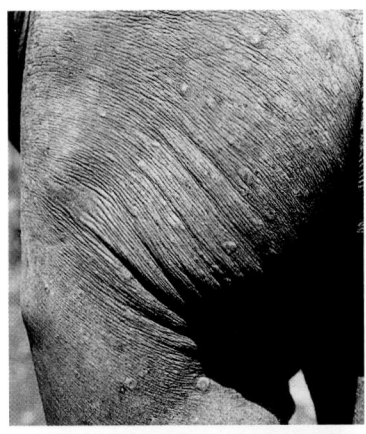

Plate 3 Lichenified skin lesions with atrophy.

Plate 4 Depigmented 'leopard skin'.

Plate 5 Migrating *Loa loa*.

Chapter 7.14.2 Lymphatic filariasis

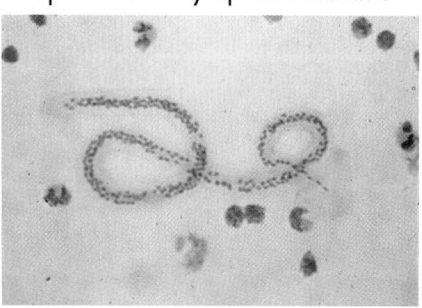

Plate 1 Microfilaria of *Wuchereria bancrofti* in a blood film from a patient in Samoa. (By courtesy of the Wellcome Museum of Medical Science.)

Chapter 7.14.3 Guinea-worm disease: dracunculiasis

Plate 1 Blister at site of imminent emergence of the female worm. (By courtesy of the late P.E.C. Manson-Bahr.)

Plate 2 Emergent female worm being wound out on a stick. (Copyright D.A. Warrell.)

Plate 3 Guinea worm in the scrotum. (Copyright D.A. Warrell.)

Chapter 7.14.4 Strongyloidiasis, hookworm, and other gut strongyloid nematodes

Plate 1 *Strongyloides stercoralis* in the intestinal mucosa. (Copyright Viqar Zaman.)

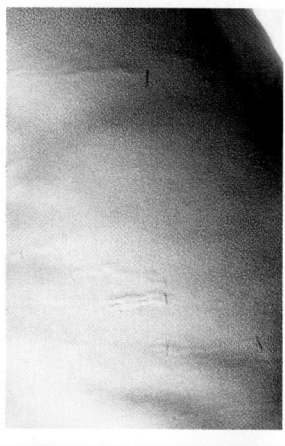

Plate 2 Larva currens rash on the back of a Nigerian patient resulting from autoinfection with *Strongyloides stercoralis*. (Copyright D.A. Warrell.)

Plate 3 Adult *Ancylostoma duodenale* – scale in millimetres. (Copyright Viqar Zaman.)

Plate 4 Cutaneous larva migrans of the hand in a Thai patient. (Copyright Sornchai Looareesuwan.)

Chapter 7.14.6 Other gut nematodes

Plate 1 Ascaris – scale in millimetres.

Plate 2 Ascaris in the lungs. (Copyright Viqar Zaman.)

Plate 3 Enterobius – scale in millimetres.

Chapter 7.14.8 Angiostrongyliasis

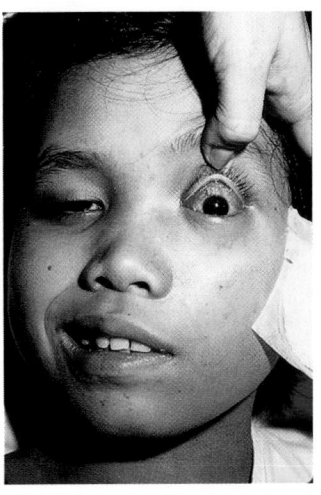

Plate 1 *Angiostrongylus cantonensis* under the conjunctiva in a Thai girl with a left facial nerve palsy. (Copyright D.A. Warrell.)

Chapter 7.15.1 Cystic hydatid disease (*Echinococcus granulosus*)

Plate 1 Hydatid cyst in muscles excised from around the femoral head (same case as shown in Fig, 3).

Chapter 7.16.1 Schistosomiasis

Plate 1 Giant urticarial rash in a patient with Katayama fever (*Schistosoma mansoni* infection). (Copyright R.N. Davidson.)

Plate 2 Schistosomal granuloma in the appendix. (Copyright Gareth Turner.)

(a)

(b)

Plate 3 The liver in *Schistosoma mansoni* infection in South Africa. Clay pipestem fibrosis. (Copyright Gareth Turner.) (a) Macrosopic view. (b) Masson trichrome stain.

Plate 4 Schistosomal granuloma in the lung. (Copyright Gareth Turner.)

Chapter 7.16.3 Lung flukes (paragonimiasis)

(a)

(b)

Plate 1 Adult lung fluke. (a) *Paragonimus heterotremus* (1.5 cm). (b) *P. westermani* (1.5 cm). (Copyright Sanan Yaemput.)

(a)

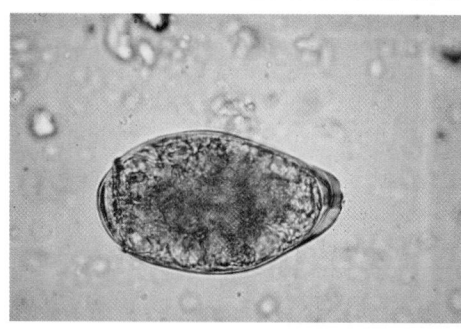

(b)

Plate 2 Ova of lung flukes. (a) *Paragonimus heterotremus*. (b) *P. westermani*. (Copyright Sanan Yaemput.)

(a)

(b)

Plate 3 Metacercariae of lung fluke in crabs, the second intermediate host. (a) *Paragonimus heterotremus*. (b) *P. westermani*. (Copyright Sanan Yaemput.)

Plate 4 Freshwater crab *Larnaudia beusekomae* (*Tawaripotamon beusekomae*), the second intermediate host. (Copyright Sanan Yaemput.)

Chapter 7.17 Non-venomous arthropods

Plate 1 Bedbugs, *Cimex lectularius*.

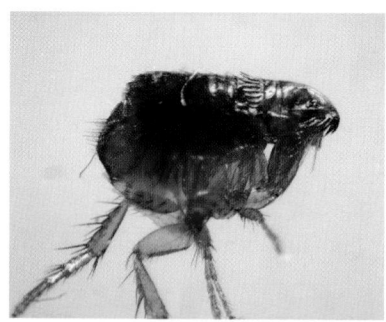

Plate 2 Catflea, *Ctenocephalides felis*: a common cause of flea bites in humans.

Plate 3 Underside of hedgehog tick, *Ixodes hexagonus* to show sucking mouthparts (hypostome).

Plate 4 Louse, *Pediculus humanus*: head lice and body lice are morphologically similar.

Plate 5 An Asian carabid beetle, *Sciates sulcatus*, from a patient complaining of vaginal discharge: a rare example of genital canthariasis.

Plate 6 Larvae of African tumbu fly, *Cordylobia anthropophaga*: a common agent of dermal myiasis.

Plates for Section 8
Chapter 8.2 Injuries, envenoming, poisoning, and allergic reactions caused by animals

Plate 1 Shark attack: wounds inflicted on the thigh by a tiger shark (*Galeocerdo cuvier*), Madang, Papua New Guinea. (Copyright S. Allen.)

Plate 2 Farmer swallowed by a reticulated python (*Python reticulatus*), Palu, Sulawesi. (Copyright Excel Sawuwu.)

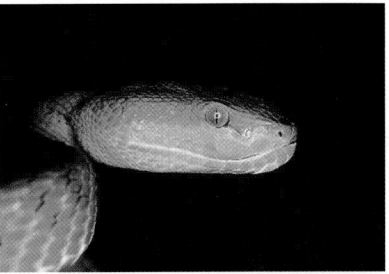

Plate 3 White-lipped pit viper from south-east Asia (*Trimeresurus albolabris*) showing the heat-sensitive pit organ between eye and nostril. (Copyright D.A. Warrell.)

Plate 4 Bleeding from gingival sulci in a victim of the West African saw-scaled or carpet viper (*Echis ocellatus*). (Copyright D.A. Warrell.)

Plate 5 The two species of venomous lizards: left, Mexican beaded lizard (*Heloderma horridum*); right, gila monster (*H. suspectum*). (By courtesy of the Zoological Society of London.)

Plate 6 Poison frog – *Dendrobates histrionicus* (Dendrobatidae) from Bahia Solauo, Colombia. Its skin secretion contains potent nicotinic receptor antagonists, histrionicotoxins. (Copyright D.A. Warrell.)

Plate 7 Poison dart frogs – *Phyllobates terribilis* (Dendrobatidae) from the Chocó region of Colombia, where their skin secretions, containing potent batrachotoxins, are used to coat blow gun darts. (Copyright D.A. Warrell.)

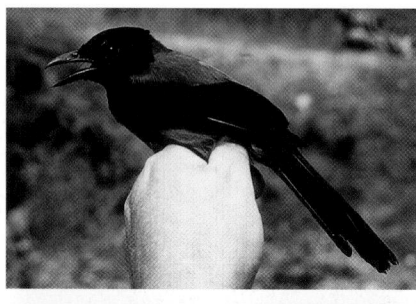

Plate 8 Hooded Pitohui (*Pitohui dichrous*), Vararata National Park, near Port Moresby, Papua New Guinea. (By courtesy of Dr Ian Burrows, Port Moresby.)

Plate 9 Venomous lion fish or butterfly cod (*Brachirus* or *Dendrochirus zebra*), from Madang, Papua New Guinea. (Copyright D.A. Warrell.)

Plate 10 Necrotic and secondarily infected wound at the site of a sting by a freshwater ray (*Potamotrygon hystrix*) in a Brazilian patient. (By courtesy of Dr João Luiz Costa Cardoso, São Paulo, Brazil.)

Plate 11 Extensive weals from contact with the stinging tentacles of the box jellyfish (*Chironex fleckeri*) in an Australian patient stung in Darwin. (By courtesy of Drs B. Currie and P. Nitschke, Darwin.)

Plate 12 Geography coneshell (*Conus geographus*) 10 cm long, responsible for killing a nine-year-old boy at Samarai, Papua New Guinea. (Copyright D.A. Warrell.)

Plate 13 Northern blue-ringed or spotted octopus (*Hapalochlaena lunulatus*) from Madang, Papua New Guinea. (Copyright D.A. Warrell.)

Plate 14 Fourteen-year-old Brazilian boy severely envenomed after more than 1000 stings by Africanized honey bees (*Apis mellifera scutellata*). (Copyright D.A. Warrell.)

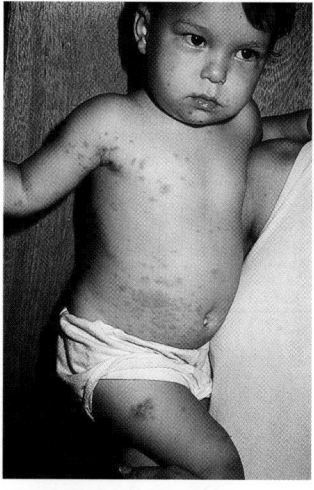

Plate 15 Lepidopterism. Lesions caused by urticating abdominal hairs of female moths (*Hylesia* sp.) during an epidemic on the Brazilian coast near São Paulo. (Copyright D.A. Warrell.)

Plate 16 Caterpillar of *Lonomia achelous* whose bristle venom can cause a fatal bleeding diathesis. (By courtesy of Dr Habib Fraiha, Belém, Brazil.)

Plate 17 Beetle (*Paederus crebripunctatus*, Staphylinidae) responsible for causing 'Nairobi eye'. (By courtesy of Dr John Paul, Brighton.)

Plate 22 Australian red back spider (*Latrodectus hasseltii*). (Copyright D.A. Warrell.)

Plate 18 Scorpion (*Tityus serrulatus*) from Brazil. (Copyright D.A. Warrell.)

(a)

Plate 19 Local blistering and necrosis caused by the sting of the scorpion *Hemiscorpius lepturus* (Scorpionidae) found in Iran and Iraq. (By courtesy of Dr M. Radmanesh, Shiraz, Iran.)

(b)

Plate 20 Threatening posture of a female Brazilian 'banana spider' (*Phoneutria nigriventer*). Note multiple eyes and large chelicerae. (Copyright D.A. Warrell.)

(c)

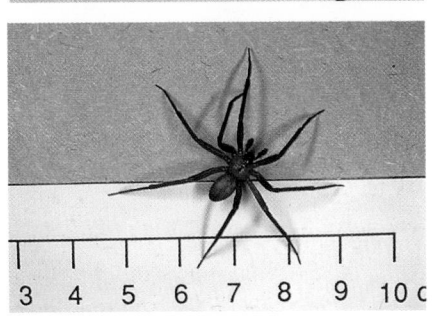

Plate 21 Female *Loxosceles laeta*. (Copyright D.A. Warrell.)

Plate 23 Necrotic araneism. Evolution of the typical lesion following bites by *Loxosceles gaucho* in Brazil. (a) Early ischaemic lesion showing the 'red, white, and blue' sign. (b) 2 weeks later. (c) Necrotic eschar 6 weeks later. (Copyright D.A. Warrell.)

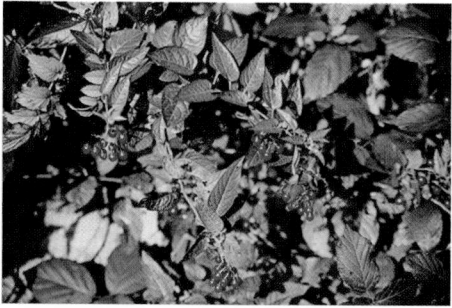

Plate 24 Local sweating and piloerection at the site of a bite by the banana spider *Phoneutria nigriventer*. (Copyright D.A. Warrell.)

Plate 5 Woody night-shade, *Solanum dulca-mara* (GTC).

Chapter 8.3 Poisonous plants and fungi

Plate 1 Dumb cane, *Dieffenbachia* sp. (GTC).

Plate 2 Laburnum, *Laburnum anagyr-oides* (GTC).

Plate 6 Foxglove, *Digitalis purpurea* (GTC).

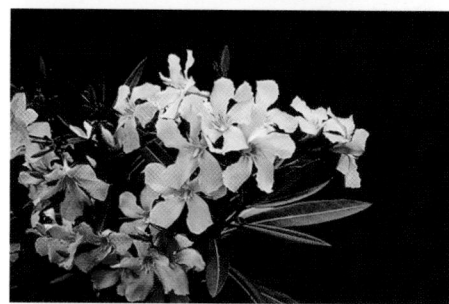

Plate 3 Jequirity beans, *Abrus precatorius* (RBG, Kew).

Plate 7 Oleander, *Nerium oleander* (GTC).

Plate 4 Castor beans, *Ricinus communis* (GTC).

Plate 8 Monkshood, *Aconitum* sp. (GTC).

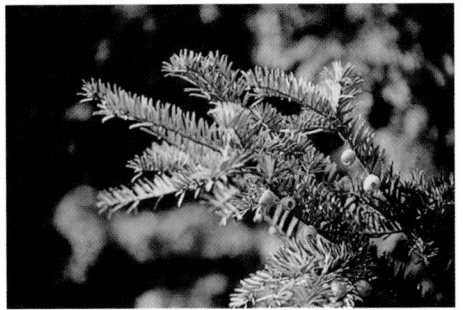

Plate 9 Yew, *Taxus baccata* (GTC).

Plate 10 Khat, *Catha edulis* (RBG, Kew).

Plate 13 Giant hogweed, *Heracleum mantegazzianum* (GTC).

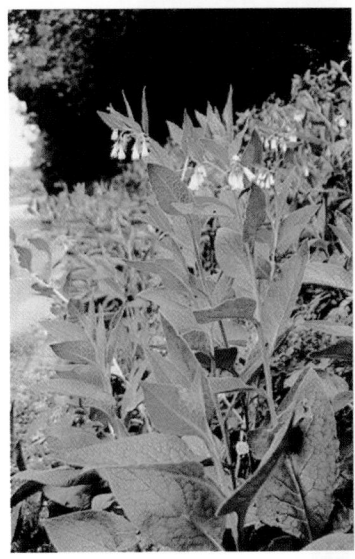

Plate 11 Comfrey, *Symphytum officinale* (GTC).

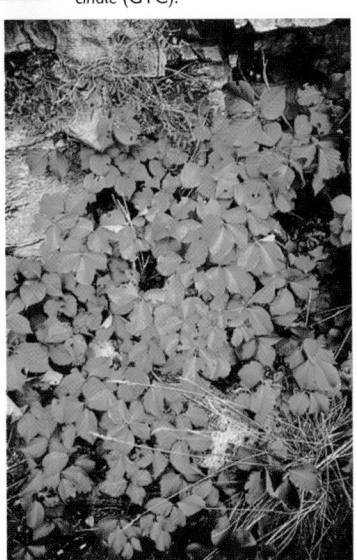

Plate 12 Poison ivy, *Rhus radicans* (MCC).

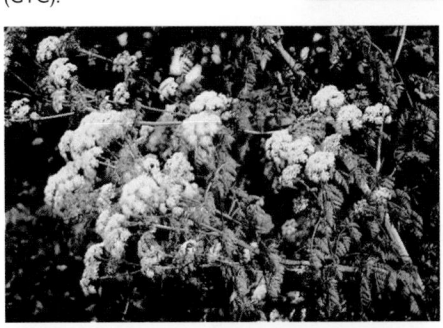

Plate 14 Rue, *Ruta graveolens* (GTC).

Plate 15 Hemlock, *Conium maculatum* (GTC).

Plate 16 Deadly nightshade, *Atropa belladonna* (GTC).

Plate 17 Angel's trumpets, *Brugmansia* sp. (GTC).

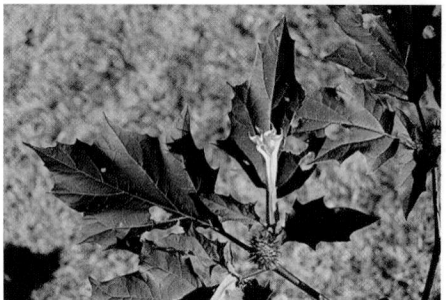

Plate 18 Thorn apple, *Datura stramonium* (GTC).

Plate 19 Cycad, *Zamia* sp. (GTC).

Plate 20 Fly agaric, *Amanita muscaria* (GTC).

Plate 21 Death cap, *Amanita phalloides* (GTC).

Plate 22 Roll-rim cap, *Paxillus involutus* (GTC).

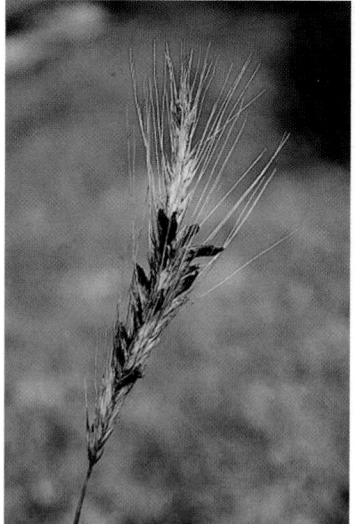

Plate 23 Ergot, *Claviceps purpurea* (JW).

We thank the following for permission to reproduce their photographs: The Trustees, The Royal Botanic Gardens, Kew (RBG, Kew), G.T. Cooper (GTC), M.C. Cooper (MCC), and Professor J. Webster (JW).

Table 2 Modified WHO recommended multidrug therapy regimens

Type of leprosy	Drug treatment		
	Monthly supervised	Daily self-administered	Duration of treatment
Paucibacillary	Rifampicin 600 mg	Dapsone 100 mg	6 months
Multibacillary	Rifampicin 600 mg	Clofazimine 50 mg	24 months
	Clofazimine 300 mg	Dapsone 100 mg	
Paucibacillary single-lesion	Rifampicin 600 mg, ofloxacin 400 mg, minocycline 100 mg		Single dose

WHO Classification for field use when slit skin smears are not available.

Multibacillary—more than five skin lesions; paucibacillary—two to five skin lesions; paucibacillary single-lesion leprosy—one skin lesion.

In this field classification WHO recommends treatment of multibacillary patients for 12 months only.

Dapsone (**DDS**, 4,4-diaminodiphenylsulphone) is weakly bactericidal. Oral absorption is good and it has a long half-life, averaging 28 h. It commonly causes mild haemolysis, but rarely anaemia. Glucose-6-phosphate dehydrogenase deficiency is seldom a problem. The 'DDS syndrome', which is occasionally seen in leprosy, begins 6 weeks after starting dapsone and manifests as exfoliative dermatitis associated with lymphadenopathy, hepatosplenomegaly, fever, and hepatitis.

Clofazimine is a red, fat-soluble, crystalline dye. The mechanism of its weakly bactericidal action against *M. leprae* remains unknown. The most troublesome side-effect is skin discoloration, ranging from red to purple-black, the degree depending on the drug dose and extent of leprous infiltration. The pigmentation usually fades within 6 to 12 months of stopping clofazimine, although traces of discoloration may remain for up to 4 years. Urine, sputum, and sweat may become pink. Clofazimine also produces a characteristic icthyosis on the shins and forearms.

New drugs bactericidal for *M. leprae* have been identified, notably the fluoroquinolones pefloxacin and ofloxacin, minocycline, and clarithromycin. These agents are now established second-line drugs and may replace dapsone and clofazimine. Minocycline causes a black pigmentation of skin lesions and so may not be an appropriate substitute for clofazimine if pigmentation is to be avoided.

Since the introduction of multidrug therapy more than 10 million patients have been treated successfully. Clinical improvement has been rapid and toxicity rare. The treatment duration has been shortened. Monthly supervision of the rifampicin component has been crucial to success. Other benefits are reduced deformity rates, increased compliance in control schemes, a halving of the annual case load, and reduction of the long-term (though not short-term) cost of control schemes. At the end of a 6-month treatment of borderline disease there may still be signs of inflammation, which should not be mistaken for active infection. The distinction between relapse and reaction may be difficult. World Health Organization (**WHO**) studies have reported a cumulative relapse rate of 1.07 per cent for paucibacillary leprosy and 0.77 per cent for multibacillary leprosy at 9 years after completion of multidrug therapy. *M. leprae* is such a slow-growing organism that relapse only occurs after many years. *M. leprae* isolates from relapsed patients who have received multidrug therapy are fully drug sensitive and patients can be retreated with the same regimen.

A single-dose triple-drug combination (rifampicin, ofloxacin, and minocycline) has been tested in India for patients with single skin lesions and improved 98 per cent of patients. Although the study had major flaws and single-dose treatment is less effective than the conventional 6-month treatment for paucibacillary leprosy, it is an operationally attractive field regimen and has been recommended for use by the WHO.

Reactions may develop months or years after stopping chemotherapy, especially in BL or LL patients. It is therefore vital when discharging patients to warn them to return should new symptoms appear, especially in hands, feet, or eyes. Patients with reactions or physical or psychological complications will need long-term care.

Management of reactions

Awareness of the early symptoms of reversal reactions by both patient and physician is important because, if left untreated, severe nerve damage may develop. The peak time for reversal reactions is in the first 2 months of treatment. Patients should be warned about reactions because the sudden appearance of reactional lesions after starting treatment is distressing and undermines confidence. The treatment of reactions is aimed at controlling acute inflammation, easing pain, reversing nerve and eye damage, and reassuring the patient. Multidrug therapy should be continued.

Type 1 (reversal) reactions

Simple anti-inflammatory drugs are rarely sufficient to control symptoms. If there is any evidence of neuritis (nerve tenderness, new anaesthesia, and/or motor loss), corticosteroid treatment should be started. Prednisolone should be given, starting at 40 to 60 mg daily, reducing to 40 mg after a few days, and then by 5 mg every 2 to 4 weeks. Patients with BT leprosy in reaction commonly need 2 to 4 months of steroids while BL reactions may need 6 months.

Type 2 (ENL) reactions (Plate 7)

This is a difficult condition to treat and frequently requires treatment with high-dose steroids (80 mg daily, tapered down rapidly) or thalidomide. Since ENL frequently recurs, steroid dependency can easily develop. Thalidomide (400 mg daily) is superior to steroids in controlling ENL and is the drug of choice for young men with severe ENL. Women with severe ENL may benefit from thalidomide treatment. This is a difficult decision for the woman and her physician and needs careful discussion of the benefits and risks (phocomelia when thalidomide is taken in the first trimester). Women should use double contraception and report immediately if menstruation is delayed. Unfortunately, the problems with thalidomide mean that it is unavailable in several leprosy endemic countries despite its undoubted value. Clofazimine has a useful anti-inflammatory effect in ENL and can be used at 300 mg per day for several months. Low-grade chronic erythema nodosum, with iritis or neuritis, will require long-term suppression, preferably with thalidomide or clofazimine. Acute iridocyclitis is treated with 4-hourly instillation of 1 per cent hydrocortisone eye drops and 1 per cent atropine drops twice daily.

Neuritis

Silent neuritis should be treated similarly to reversal reactions—prednisolone in a dose of 40 mg daily and reducing slowly over a period of months.

Education of the patient

Stigmatization due to leprosy occurs worldwide. Patients are frightened of social ostracization, physical rejection, and the development of deformities. It is often useful to ask them about their fears so that these can be addressed. They should be reassured that having started treatment they are not infectious to family or friends. The importance of compliance with antibiotic therapy needs to be emphasized. The patient needs a careful explanation of the diagnosis, aetiology, and prognosis.

Prevention of disability

The morbidity and disability associated with leprosy is secondary to nerve damage. A major goal in prevention of disability is to create patient self-awareness so that damage is minimized. Monitoring sensation and muscle power in patient's hands, feet, and eyes should be part of the routine follow-up so that new nerve damage is detected early. The patient with an anaesthetized hand or foot needs to understand the importance of daily self-care, especially protection when doing potentially dangerous tasks and inspection for trauma. It is helpful to identify for each patient potentially dangerous situations, such as cooking, car repairs, or smoking. Soaking dry hands and feet followed by rubbing with oil keeps the skin moist and supple.

An anaesthetized foot needs the protection of an appropriate shoe. For anaesthesia alone, a well-fitting 'trainer' with firm soles and shock-absorbing inners will provide adequate protection. Once there is deformity, such as clawing, shoes must be made specially to ensure protection of pressure points and even weight distribution.

The patient should be taught to question the cause of an injury so that the risk can be avoided in the future. Plantar ulceration occurs secondary to increased pressure over bony prominences. Ulceration is treated by rest. Unlike ulcers in the feet of patients with diabetes or ischaemia, ulcers in leprosy heal if they are protected from weight-bearing. No weight-bearing is permitted until the ulcer has healed. Appropriate footwear should be provided to prevent recurrence.

Physiotherapy exercises should be taught to maximize function of weak muscles and prevent contracture. Contractures of hands and feet, foot drop, lagophthalmos, entropion, and ectropion are amenable to surgery.

Social, psychological, and economic rehabilitation

The social and cultural background of the patient determine the nature of many of the problems that may be encountered. The patient may have difficulty in coming to terms with leprosy. The community may reject the patient. Education, gainful employment, confidence from family, friends, and doctor, and plastic surgery to correct stigmatizing deformity all have a role to play.

Prognosis

The majority of patients—especially those who have no nerve damage at the time of diagnosis—do well on multidrug treatment with resolution of skin lesions. Left untreated, borderline patients will downgrade towards the lepromatous end of the spectrum and lepromatous patients will suffer the consequences of bacillary invasion. Borderline patients are at risk of developing type 1 reactions, which may result in devastating nerve damage. Treatment of the neuritis is currently unsatisfactory and patients with neuritis may develop permanent nerve damage despite corticosteroid treatment. It is not possible to predict which patients will develop reactions or nerve damage. Nerve damage and its complications may be severely disabling, especially when all four limbs and both eyes are affected.

Leprosy in women

Women with leprosy are in double jeopardy, not only may they develop postpartum nerve damage but they are at particular risk of social ostracization with rejection by spouses and family.

Pregnancy and leprosy

There is little good evidence that pregnancy causes new disease or relapse. However, there is a clear temporal association between parturition and the development of type 1 reactions and neuritis when cell-mediated immunity returns to prepregnancy levels. In an Ethiopian study, 42 per cent of pregnancies in BL patients were complicated by a type 1 reaction in the postpartum period. In the same cohort, LL patients experienced ENL reactions throughout pregnancy and lactation. ENL in pregnancy is associated with early loss of nerve function compared with non-pregnant individuals.

Pregnant and newly delivered women should have regular neurological examination and steroid treatment instituted for neuritis. Rifampicin, dapsone, and clofazimine are safe during pregnancy. Clofazimine crosses the placenta and babies may be born with mild clofazimine pigmentation. Lepra reactions can be managed with the steroid regimens given above but with a more rapid reduction in dose. Women should be warned before becoming pregnant of the risk that their condition will deteriorate after delivery. Ideally pregnancies should be planned when leprosy is well controlled.

Prevention and control

The current strategy of leprosy control in endemic countries through vertical programmes providing case detection, treatment with WHO multidrug therapy, and contact examination and supported by case-finding campaigns, especially in schools, has been very successful. Effective treatment is not merely restricted to chemotherapy but also involves good case management with effective monitoring and supervision. An important secondary role of leprosy control programmes is the prevention of disabilities.

Vaccines against leprosy

The substantial cross-reactivity between bacille Calmette–Guérin (**BCG**) and *M. leprae* has been exploited in attempts to develop a vaccine against leprosy. Trials of BCG as a vaccine against leprosy in Uganda, New Guinea, Burma, and South India showed it to confer statistically significant but variable protection, ranging from 80 per cent in Uganda to 20 per cent in Burma. A case–control study in Venezuela showed BCG vaccination to give 56 per cent protection to the household contacts of patients with leprosy. Combining BCG and killed *M. leprae* has been tried, but in both a large population-based trial in Malawi and an immunoprophylactic trial in Venezuela there was no advantage for BCG plus *M. leprae* over BCG alone.

Areas of uncertainty/controversy

The optimum duration of treatment is a controversial area. The last WHO expert committee recommended that treatment for multibacillary cases could be reduced from 24 to 12 months. The classification of leprosy cases has been simplified. Cases are now classified by the number of lesions; slit skin smears are not mandatory. The decision to stop recommending slit skin smears was made because of the poor standard of smears in the field. A WHO sponsored trial comparing 12 months with 24 months treatment is in progress, but intake only started in 1992 and a 10-year follow-up is needed to assess relapse rates. Data from India show that patients with a high initial bacterial load (bacterial index greater than 4) treated with 2 years of rifampicin, clofazimine, and dapsone had a relapse rate of 8/100 person years, whereas patients treated to smear negativity had a relapse rate of 2/100 person years. The dilemma is that if skin smears are abandoned then those patients in need of longer treatment courses cannot be identified. These arguments illustrate the difficulty in providing sound evidence for policy decisions when a decade-long wait is needed.

The shortening of drug treatment for leprosy means that the vertical leprosy programmes are now treating far fewer patients. There is considerable discussion about how best to detect, treat, and prevent leprosy disability in the future. There are several possibilities—integration with tuberculosis programmes, dermatology programmes, or at health centre level. Whichever model is chosen as being locally appropriate, it should be remembered that treating patients with leprosy is a long-term enterprise involving patients, their families, and health workers.

Areas where further research is needed

The epidemiology of leprosy still poses unanswered questions. Why are 70 per cent of all patients with leprosy in India? Is this due to living conditions, genetic susceptibilty, or particular environmental conditions in India?

Early detection of cases is vital both at an individual and population level. It is now recognized that substantial nerve damage occurs before diagnosis. A test for early infection might help detect individual cases before nerve damage is established and before the spread of infection. Leprosy-specific peptides for skin tests have been generated and are being evaluated.

The medical management of reactions and nerve damage is currently limited to steroids. These are not effective for about 30 per cent cases. Thus trials of new immunosuppressants are urgently needed.

The WHO started the 1990s with the bold slogan of 'Eliminating leprosy as a public health problem by 2000'. This initiative galvanized leprosy control programmes worldwide, but the unique biology of *M. leprae* and its interaction with the human host meant that the target was unattainable. As the millennium approached the slogan was quietly dropped to the disappointment of many leprosy workers and governments. Leprosy is a bacterial disease with challenging immunological complications and will be a global and individual problem for many decades. It is unlikely to be eradicated until there is considerable improvement in general health, wealth, living conditions, and education.

Further reading

Britton WJ (1998). The management of leprosy reversal reactions. *Leprosy Review* **69**, 225–34. [A comprehensive review.]

Khanolkar-Young S *et al.* (1995). Tumour necrosis factor-α synthesis is associated with the skin and peripheral nerve pathology of leprosy reversal reactions. *Clinical and Experimental Immunology* **99**, 196–202. [Key paper demonstrating a tissue-damaging cytokine in leprosy nerves.]

Lockwood DNJ (1996). The management of erythema nodosum leprosum: current and future options. *Leprosy Review* **67**, 253–9.

Lockwood DNJ (1997). Rifampicin, ofloxacin, and minocycline (ROM) for single lesions in leprosy. What is the evidence? *Leprosy Review* **68**, 299–300. [A critical analysis of the trial report for single-dose treatment.]

Ponnighaus JM *et al.* (1992). Efficacy of BCG vaccine against leprosy and tuberculosis in northern Malawi. *Lancet* **339**, 636–9. [Demonstrates that adding killed *M. leprae* to BCG vaccine does not enhance protection against leprosy. This study also shows that BCG protects better against leprosy than tuberculosis in Africa.]

Sampaio EP *et al.* (1995). Cellular immune response to *Mycobacterium leprae* infection in human immunodeficiency virus infected individuals. *Infection and Immunity* **63**, 18848–54. [Key paper showing normal granuloma formation in patients coinfected with leprosy and HIV.]

Waters M (1998). Is it safe to shorten multidrug therapy for lepromatous (LL and BL) leprosy to 12 months? *Leprosy Review* **69**, 110–11. [Succinct review of the problems and uncertain data for short-course chemotherapy in leprosy.]

WHO expert committee on leprosy (1998). *WHO Technical Report Series.* World Health Organization, Geneva. [Summary of current recommendations for the management of leprosy in the field.]

Yamamura M *et al.* (1992). Cytokine patterns of immunologically mediated tissue damage. *Journal of Immunology* **149**, 1470–5. [Paper showing that lepromatous disease is associated with a T_{H2} pattern of cytokine production and TT with a T_{H1} pattern.]

7.11.25 Buruli ulcer: *Mycobacterium ulcerans* infection

Wayne M. Meyers and Françoise Portaels

Introduction

Buruli ulcer, also known as Bairnsdale or Searles' ulcer (Australia), and Kakerifu or Toro ulcer (Congo), is an indolent, necrotizing infection of the skin, subcutaneous tissue, and bone, caused by *Mycobacterium ulcerans*. After tuberculosis and leprosy, Buruli ulcer is the third most common mycobacterial disease, and is recognized by the WHO as a re-emerging infection.

Aetiology

In 1948 MacCallum and colleagues first isolated the causative agent from patients in Australia. *M. ulcerans* is a slow-growing, acid-fast bacillus which grows optimally at 32°C, and elaborates mycolactone, a cytotoxic and immunosuppressive polyketide. Putatively, this toxin is the primary virulence factor of *M. ulcerans*. Data from 16S rRNA sequences define four groups of *M. ulcerans*: African, American, Asian, and Australian strains.

Epidemiology and transmission

All endemic foci of Buruli ulcer are near rural freshwater wetlands, especially still or slow-moving water (ponds and swamps). All foci except those in southern Australia and northern Asia are tropical. Major endemic areas are Benin, Ghana, Ivory Coast, Nigeria, Congo, Gabon, Uganda, and adjacent countries. There are minor foci in South and Central America and south-east and northern Asia.

Documented environmental sources of *M. ulcerans* include water in irrigation systems and water bugs that dwell in the roots of aquatic plants in the bottom mud of swamps. In Australia, koala, possum, and naturalized alpaca contract the infection naturally.

Outbreaks of disease often follow environmental changes that promote flooding or alter water courses, such as deforestation or construction of dams and irrigation systems. Increases in farming populations near wetlands may contribute to the rapid re-emergence of Buruli ulcer in Africa. Approximately 75 per cent of all new infections are in children, who often play semi-naked in swampy terrain.

We postulate that humans become infected by traumatic introduction of the bacillus into the dermis or subcutis from the overlying *M. ulcerans*-contaminated skin surface. The trauma may be as slight as a hypodermic injection or as severe as a land-mine wound or snakebite. Biting insects (e.g. water bugs) may serve as mechanical vectors. Aerosols arising from the surface of ponds and swamps may disseminate *M. ulcerans*. Patient-to-patient transmission is rare.

Pathogenesis

No predisposing host factors are known. Once introduced, the small amount of mycolactone produced by a few *M. ulcerans* bacilli causes tissue necrosis and suppresses local immune responses ensuring survival of the bacillus in a nidus of nutrient necrotic tissue. The toxin targets subcutaneous fat cells so that necrosis can spread in and just superficial to fascial planes. *M. ulcerans* invades lymphatics and probably blood vessels, causing metastatic spread.

Clinical features

Clinical effects may be localized or disseminated. Except for those with massive lesions, patients are usually surprisingly well without specific systemic symptoms or abnormal laboratory findings.

Localized disease

Typically the initial cutaneous lesion is a single, firm, painless, non-tender, movable subcutaneous nodule up to 3 cm in diameter. Limbs are most frequently affected, often around joints. There is marked variation in the natural history of the disease, but nodules usually ulcerate within 1 to 3 months of inoculation. A whitish necrotic slough develops in the base of the ulcer and the surrounding skin is indurated and hyperpigmented. Ulcer borders are undermined, sometimes extending 15 to 20 cm or more (major ulcerative disease) (Fig. 1 and Plate 1). Some small (1 to 2 cm in diameter) ulcerated lesions with shallow undermining self-heal early without sequelae (minor ulcerative disease). Without treatment, major ulcerative lesions tend to become inactive, usually after months or years, and heal by scarring. Typically the scars are depressed and stellate, often causing disfiguring and crippling cicatricial contractions.

Disseminated disease

Disseminated disease may pass only through the nodular stage or arise from localized major ulcerative lesions; however, following inoculation, the disease sometimes disseminates directly and rapidly. These patients present with indurated plaques of varying size, sometimes covering an entire limb or vast areas of the trunk. Without treatment, such lesions will eventually slough, leaving a large ulcer with continuing extension of disease at the borders. Structures such as eyes, breasts, and genitalia may be damaged or lost.

While metastatic spread may arise from localized disease, patients with the highly bacilliferous disseminated cutaneous form are more prone to develop metastatic lesions. Spread may be to distant skin sites or to bone. Bones of the limbs are affected most frequently. *M. ulcerans* osteomyelitis is an increasing problem in many endemic areas, and often leads to amputations and other disabilities.

Differential clinical diagnosis

Diagnosis of the nodular stage is often perplexing. Differential diagnoses include bacterial, mycotic, and parasitic infections, inflammatory lesions, and tumours. Ulcers resembling Buruli ulcer include tropical phagedenic

Fig. 1 Buruli ulcer on the left deltoid area in a 12-year-old Congolese boy who had received a hypodermic injection at this site 3 months previously. Note central necrotic slough in the base of the ulcer, and undermined edges. (See also Plate 1.)

ulcer (malodorous and not undermined), venous stasis ulcer (not undermined), and bites by venomous snakes or spiders (history helpful).

Pathology

Optimal biopsy specimens contain the necrotic base of ulcers and undermined edge of lesions and subcutaneous tissue and fascia. Histopathological sections reveal a contiguous coagulation necrosis (non-caseating) of the deep dermis, panniculus, and fascia. Vasculitis and mineralization in these areas are common. Clumps of extracellular acid-fast bacilli are most plentiful in the base of the ulcer. Necrosis extends well beyond the location of the bacilli. Local and regional lymph nodes are often invaded and sometimes necrotic. In bone, the marrow is necrotic and contains acid-fast bacilli, and trabeculas are eroded. Development of delayed-type hypersensitivity granulomas heralds healing and eventual fibrosis.

Laboratory diagnosis

Smears stained by the Ziehl–Neelsen method from the ulcer base often reveal acid-fast bacilli in clumps. Cultures for *M. ulcerans* are often positive. Polymerase chain reaction is available for specific identification of *M. ulcerans*. Histopathological changes are characteristic.

Treatment

Wide surgical excision and skin grafting is the recommended treatment. Antimicrobial agents (e.g. rifampin and clarithromycin) should be administered before and after surgery to limit bacterial dissemination. Heating the lesion to 40°C is a useful adjunct. Oral antimycobacterial therapy without surgery may heal nodules and minor ulcerative lesions, but controlled trials are needed to establish efficacy. Physiotherapy is essential to prevent contraction deformities.

Prevention and control

Bacille Calmette-Guérin (BCG) vaccination provides short-lived protection. There are no practicable effective control measures for inhabitants of endemic areas. Tourists can avoid the wetlands in endemic countries.

Socio-economic impact

Patients are often disabled for life and require welfare services, often locally limited or unavailable. They require hospital stays of many months, taxing overburdened services.

Further reading

Asiedu K, Etuaful S (1998). Socioeconomic implications of Buruli ulcer in Ghana: a three-year review. *American Journal of Tropical Medicine and Hygiene* **59**, 1015–22. [Stresses the burden of Buruli ulcer as a chronic disease on the health-care delivery system of developing countries.]

George KM *et al.* (1999). Mycolactone: a polyketide toxin from *Mycobacterium ulcerans* required for virulence. *Science* **283**, 854–7. [Describes purification and characterization of the toxin of *M. ulcerans*, potentially opening new approaches to the treatment and prevention of Buruli ulcer.]

Meyers WM (1995). Mycobacterial infections of the skin. In: Doerr W, Seifert G, eds. *Tropical pathology*, pp 291–377. Springer-Verlag, Berlin. [Extensive coverage of the clinical and pathological features of Buruli ulcer.]

Van der Werf TS *et al.* (1999). *Mycobacterium ulcerans* infection. *Lancet* **354**, 1013–18. [A review of the current status of the epidemiology, diagnosis, and treatment of *M. ulcerans* infection in the world.]

7.11.26 Actinomycoses

K. P. Schaal

Definition

Actinomycoses are subacute to chronic, granulomatous as well as suppurative inflammatory diseases that tend to progress slowly and usually give rise to multiple abscesses and draining sinus tracts. Various fermentative (facultatively anaerobic or capnophilic) actinomycetes of the genera *Actinomyces* and *Propionibacterium*, but rarely also *Bifidobacterium*, may act as the principal causative agents of the disease. Because the term 'actinomycoses' denotes a polyaetiological inflammatory syndrome rather than a condition attributable to a single pathogenic actinomycete species, it should only be used in the plural.

Aetiology of human actinomycoses

Actinomyces israelii and *A. gerencseriae* are by far the most frequent and most characteristic pathogens aetiologically involved in the human form of the disease. *Propionibacterium propionicum*, *Actinomyces naeslundii*, *A. odontolyticus*, *A. viscosus*, *A. meyeri*, and *Bifidobacterium dentium* (formerly '*Actinomyces eriksonii*') are further potential but less common causes of actinomycotic infections, while *Actinomyces bovis* has been recovered solely from animals (Table 1).

Pathogenesis and pathology

Most of the fermentative actinomycetes pathogenic to man are found regularly and abundantly in the mouths of healthy adults. However, these microbes occur only sporadically or in low numbers in the digestive, respiratory, and genital tracts, as well as in the mouths of babies before teething and of adults without any natural teeth or tooth implants. Therefore, these actinomycetes may be considered facultatively pathogenic commensals of the human mucous membranes, which, apart from the very rare actinomycotic wound infections after human bites or fist fights, produce disease exclusively as endogenous pathogens.

For active invasion of the tissue, the classical pathogenic fermentative actinomycetes apparently require a negative redox potential, which may result either from insufficient blood supply (caused by circulatory or vascular diseases, crush injuries, or foreign bodies) or from the reducing and necrotizing capacity of other microbes in the lesion. Defective functions of the immune system do not specifically predispose to actinomycotic infections.

Synergistic polymicrobial infection

True actinomycoses are essentially always synergistic mixed infections, in which the actinomycetes act as the specific component, the so-called 'guiding organisms', which decide on the characteristic course and the late symptoms of the disease. The so-called concomitant microbes (Table 2), which may vary considerably in composition (about 100 aerobic and anaerobic species) and number (up to 10 per case) of species from case to case, are often responsible for the clinical picture at the beginning of the infection and for certain complications; they are also part of the resident or transient surface microflora of the mucous membranes of man.

Particularly pronounced synergistic interactions appear to exist between pathogenic fermentative actinomycetes, especially *Actinomyces israelii* and *A. gerencseriae*, and *Actinobacillus actinomycetemcomitans*. The latter organism, the name of which refers to its characteristic association with actinomycetes, may even sustain the inflammatory process under similar clinical symptoms after chemotherapeutic elimination of the causative actinomycete.

Histopathology

Initially, an inflammatory granulation tissue develops, which usually breaks down to form either an acute abscess or chronic multiple abscesses with proliferation of connective tissue. The pathognomonic sulphur granules are formed primarily in the infected tissue, but may also appear as free structures in abscess content or sinus discharge. They are then of the highest diagnostic importance.

Sulphur granules, which were originally designated 'Drusen' in Harz's first description of *Actinomyces bovis* in 1877, are macroscopically visible (up to 1 mm in diameter), yellowish, reddish to brownish particles, which

Table 1 Fermentative actinomycetes isolated from human abscess or empyema content or sinus discharge at the Institute of Hygiene, University of Cologne, between 1969 and 1984 and at the Institute for Medical Microbiology and Immunology, University of Bonn, between 1984 and 1991 (modified from Schaal and Lee (1992))

Species identified	No.	Percentage of cases
Actinomyces israelii	588	56.4
Actinomyces gerencseriae	259	24.9
Actinomyces naeslundii	79	7.6
Actinomyces odontolyticus	12	1.2
Actinomyces viscosus	43	4.1
Actinomyces meyeri	3	0.3
Bifidobacterium dentium	5	0.5
Propionibacterium propionicum	36	3.5
Corynebacterium matruchotii	12	1.6
Rothia dentocariosa	5	0.5
Total number of isolates	1042	100.0

Table 2 Concomitant actinomycotic flora (predominantly cervicofacial infections) (modified from Schaal and Lee (1992))

Species/group identified	No.	Percentage of cases
Aerobically growing organisms		
Coagulase-negative staphylococci	891	27.9
Staphylococcus aureus	405	12.7
α-haemolytic streptococci	357	11.2
β-haemolytic streptococci	157	4.0
Haemophilus influenzae/parainfluenzae	3	0.1
Enterobacteriaceae	81	2.5
Neisseria spp.	47	1.5
Non-fermenters	6	0.2
Yeasts	3	0.1
No aerobic growth	1509	47.2
Anaerobes and capnophils		
Actinobacillus actinomycetemcomitans	731	22.9
'Microaerophilic' streptococci	937	29.3
Peptostreptococcus spp.	583	18.2
Black-pigmented bacteroidaceae	1204	37.7
Non-pigmented Bacteroides/Prevotella spp.	446	14.0
Fusobacterium spp.	1040	32.5
Leptotrichia buccalis	653	20.4
Eikenella corrodens	527	16.5
Capnocytophaga spp.	14	0.4
Propionibacterium spp.*	974	30.5
Lactobacillus spp.	17	0.5
Total number of cases examined	3197	100.0

*Other than P. propionicum.

Fig. 1 Actinomycotic sulphur granule. Micrograph of a particle embedded in 1 per cent methylene-blue solution, original diameter 0.8 mm. Note the cauliflower-like structure in the centre of the particle and the partially dark-stained granulocytes in the periphery.

exhibit a cauliflower-like appearance under the microscope at low magnifications (Fig. 1). They consist of a conglomerate of filamentous actinomycete microcolonies formed *in vivo* and surrounded by tissue reaction material, especially polymorphonuclear granulocytes. At high magnification, a Gram-stained smear of the completely crushed granule reveals the presence of clusters of Gram-positive interwoven branching filaments with radially arranged peripheral hyphae and of a variety of other Gram-positive and Gram-negative rods and cocci, which represent the concomitant flora. A club-shaped layer of hyaline material may be seen on the tips of peripheral filaments, which can aid in the differentiation of actinomycotic sulphur granules from macroscopically similar particles of various other microbial and non-microbial origins.

Clinical manifestations

The primary actinomycotic lesion usually develops in tissue adjacent to a mucous membrane at sites such as the cervicofacial, thoracic, and abdominal areas. The infection tends to progress slowly and to penetrate without regard to natural organ borders, or to spread haematogenously even to distant sites. Remission and exacerbation of symptoms with and without antimicrobial treatment is characteristic. As in other endogenous microbial diseases, the incubation period of actinomycoses is not defined.

Cervicofacial actinomycoses

In the vast majority of cases, actinomycotic lesions primarily involve the face or neck. Conditions predisposing to these cervicofacial infections include tooth extractions, fractures of the jaw, periodontal abscesses, foreign bodies penetrating the mucosal barrier (bone splinters, fish bones, awns of cereals), or suppurating tonsillar crypts.

Initially, the cervicofacial actinomycoses present either as an acute, usually odontogenic, abscess or cellulitis of the floor of the mouth, or as a slowly developing, chronic, hard, painless, reddish or livid swelling. Small acute actinomycotic abscesses may heal after surgical drainage alone. More often, however, the acute initial stage is followed by a subacute to chronic course if no specific antimicrobial treatment is given, thereby imitating the primarily chronic form, which is characterized by regression and cicatrization of central suppurative foci while the infection progresses peripherally producing hard, painless, livid infiltrations. These may lead to multiple, new areas of liquefaction, fistulae (Fig. 2), which often discharge pus containing sulphur granules, and multilocular cavities with poor healing and a tendency to recur after temporary regressions of the inflammatory symptoms.

Fig. 2 Primarily chronic cervicofacial actinomycosis with several draining sinus tracts and livid discoloration of the skin in a 42-year-old man.

With inappropriate or no treatment, cervicofacial actinomycoses extend slowly, even across organ borders, and may become life-threatening by invasion of the cranial cavity, the mediastinum, or the bloodstream.

Thoracic actinomycoses

Thoracic manifestations, which are much less common than the cervicofacial form (Table 3), usually develop after aspiration or inhalation of material from the mouth (dental plaque or calculus, tonsillar crypt contents) or a foreign body that contains or is contaminated with the causative agents. Occasionally, this form of disease may result from extension of an actinomycotic process of the neck, from an abdominal infection perforating the diaphragm, or from a distant focus by haematogenous spread.

Primary pulmonary actinomycoses present as bronchopneumonic infiltrations that may imitate tuberculosis or bronchial carcinoma radiographically, appearing as single dense or multiple spotted shadows in which cavitations may develop (Fig. 3). If not diagnosed and treated properly, pulmonary infections may extend through to the pleural cavity producing empyema, to the pericardium, or to the chest wall; they may even appear as a paravertebral (psoas) abscess tracking down to the groin.

Abdominal actinomycoses

Actinomycoses of the abdomen and pelvis are rare (Table 3). They originate either from acute perforating gastrointestinal diseases (appendicitis, diverticulitis, various ulcerative diseases), from surgical or accidental trauma including injuries caused by ingested bone splinters or fish bones, or from inflammations of the female internal genital organs.

Women who wear intrauterine contraceptive devices or vaginal pessaries for long periods often show a characteristic colonization of the cervical canal and the uterine cavity by various fermentative actinomycetes and other anaerobes resembling the synergistic actinomycotic flora. However, this colonization only rarely results in an invasive actinomycotic process.

Table 3 Localization of human actinomycotic infections (modified from Schaal KP and Pulverer G (1984))

Body site involved	Number	Percentage of cases
Cervicofacial area	3197	97.9
Thoracic organs	41	1.3
Abdominal organs including small pelvis	20	0.6
Extremities	4	0.1
Central nervous system	4	0.1
Total number of cases	3266	100.0

Fig. 3 Chest radiograph of pulmonary actinomycosis of the right upper lobe in a 62-year-old man. The disease was only diagnosed after a huge subcutaneous abscess had developed covering the whole right shoulder blade.

Most abdominal actinomycoses present as slowly growing tumours, which, in the absence of sinus tracts discharging pus with sulphur granules, are difficult to differentiate from malignant neoplasms such as colonic, rectal, ovarian, or cervical carcinomas. By direct extension, any abdominal tissue or organ may be involved including muscle, liver, spleen, kidney, fallopian tubes, ovaries, testes, bladder, or rectum. Haematogenous liver abscesses have been seen, especially associated with genital actinomycoses.

Actinomycotic infections of the central nervous system

Actinomycoses of the brain and the spinal cord are very rare. They may arise from direct extension of cervicofacial infections. Haematogenous spread is also possible, particularly from primary lesions in the lungs or abdomen. The spinal canal may be directly involved from these sites. Brain abscess is much more common than meningitis.

Actinomycoses of the bone

Bone involvement is also very rare. It usually develops by direct extension from soft tissue infection resulting in a periostitis with new bone formation visible by radiography. If the bone itself is invaded, localized areas of bone destruction surrounded by increased bone density usually develop. Mandible, ribs, and spine are most frequently involved.

Cutaneous actinomycoses

Actinomycotic lesions of the skin are extremely rare. Usually, they originate from wounds that were contaminated with saliva or dental plaque following human bites or fist fights, but they may also result from haematogenous spread. Symptoms are similar to those of cervicofacial actinomycoses.

Diagnosis

Clinical symptoms are often misleading, especially in the early stages of the disease, histopathological appearances are unreliable, and diagnosis chiefly rests on bacteriological methods.

Radiography

In cervicofacial cases, radiography is useful only for detecting bone involvement. A pulmonary infiltrate associated with a proliferative lesion or destruction of ribs is highly suggestive of either actinomycosis or a tumour. Radiography may also help to locate the abdominal processes and to identify the involvement of organs such as liver, kidney, urinary bladder, or ureter. In general, however, radiographic changes are not diagnostic.

Laboratory diagnosis

Clinical chemistry and haematology

Small, localized actinomycotic lesions are not usually associated with abnormalities. In advanced cases, however, especially those in the thoracic or the abdominal area, a raised erythrocyte sedimentation rate and pronounced leucocytosis may be found. When the central nervous system is involved, a polymorphonuclear or mononuclear pleocytosis is commonly found. The protein content of the cerebrospinal fluid is frequently elevated and the sugar content moderately depressed.

Bacteriology

Pus specimens containing sulphur granules and occasionally looking like semolina should prompt the clinician to ask and the bacteriologist to look specifically for actinomycetes using suitable cultural techniques and other methods.

Pus, sinus discharge, bronchial secretions, granulation tissue, or biopsy materials are suitable specimens. Precautions must be taken to prevent contamination of the specimen by the indigenous mucosal flora. In cases of cervicofacial actinomycoses, pus should therefore be obtained only by transcutaneous puncture of the abscesses or by transcutaneous needle biopsy. When abscesses have already been incised, a sufficient amount of pus should be collected instead of using only a swab. Because sputum always contains oral actinomycetes, bronchial secretions should be obtained by transtracheal aspiration, or material should be collected by transthoracic percutaneous needle biopsy. Percutaneous puncture of suspected abscesses is often the only way of obtaining suitable specimens for diagnosing abdominal actinomycoses.

The transport of specimens to the bacteriological laboratory should be as fast as possible, preferably by messenger. Alternatively, a reducing transport medium such as one of the modifications of Stuart's medium should be used. The specimen should arrive in the laboratory within 24 h, although it has occasionally proved possible to isolate actinomycetes from samples that took 7 days or more to get to the diagnostic laboratory by post.

A quick and comparatively reliable tentative diagnosis is possible microscopically when sulphur granules are present (Fig. 1). The demonstration of concomitant bacteria in Gram-stained smears prepared from crushed granule material allows the differentiation of actinomycotic granules from similar particles produced by *Nocardia*, *Actinomadura*, or *Streptomyces* species.

Use of transparent culture media and careful microscopic examination of the cultures, preferably on Fortner plates, after at least 2, 7, and 14 days of incubation, enables a specialized laboratory to detect possible actinomycete colonies and to subculture them for identification. Isolation and definite identification to the species level may require a further 1 to 2 weeks. Techniques such as the application of gene probes or the polymerase chain reaction for detecting and identifying fermentative actinomycetes are not yet widely used.

Serological diagnosis

None of the routine serological methods has yet provided satisfactory results because sensitivity and specificity have been found to be too low.

Treatment

As the aetiology of human actinomycoses is always polymicrobial, the antibacterial drugs used for treatment should in principle cover both the causative actinomycetes and all of the concomitant bacteria. This usually requires the administration of drug combinations, in which aminopenicillins currently represent the therapeutic basis because they are slightly more active against the pathogenic actinomycetes than is penicillin G and because they are able to inhibit *Actinobacillus actinomycetemcomitans* which is usually resistant to narrow-spectrum penicillins. However, the presence of concomitant β-lactamase producers such as *Bacteroides fragilis*, *B. thetaiotaomicron*, or *Staphylococcus aureus* (β-lactamase producing) may impair the therapeutic efficacy of aminopenicillins and that of many other β-lactams so that the combination with a β-lactamase inhibitor is advisable or even necessary.

For cervicofacial actinomycoses, amoxicillin plus clavulanic acid has proved to be the treatment of choice. Three doses of 2.0 g amoxicillin plus 0.2 g clavulanic acid per day for 1 week and three doses of 1.1 g of the combination for an additional 7 days usually result in complete cure. Thoracic actinomycoses mostly respond to the same regimen. However, it is advisable to maintain doses of 2.2 g, three times per day, for 2 weeks, and to continue treatment for 3 to 4 weeks. Advanced pulmonary cases may require the addition of 2 g ampicillin, three times a day, in order to increase the tissue concentration of aminopenicillin and, depending on the composition of the concomitant flora, the use of an antimicrobial specifically active against resistant enterobacteriaceae; the application of drugs such as metronidazole or clindamycin against strict anaerobes is only necessary, as an adjunct to the aminopenicillins, in chronic cases with reduced blood supply.

Since in abdominal actinomycoses enterobacteriaceae and β-lactamase producing *Bacteroides* species are usually present and the correct diagnosis is mostly established late, suitable antimicrobial combinations for these cases are amoxicillin plus clavulanic acid plus metronidazole plus tobramycin (gentamicin) or ampicillin plus clindamycin plus an aminoglycoside. Imipenem might also be a good choice, but this drug has not yet been widely used for treating actinomycotic infections.

Neither clindamycin nor metronidazole should be used alone. Clindamycin is almost completely ineffective against *Actinobacillus actinomycetemcomitans* and metronidazole shows no activity at all against pathogenic actinomycetes. The use of further combinations, including additional aminoglycosides, cephalosporins, or β-lactamase-stable penicillins, may be necessary depending on the presence of unusual aerobic organisms. In patients allergic to penicillins, tetracyclines or possibly cephalosporins may be tried instead of aminopenicillins. Incision of abscesses and drainage of pus may still be necessary as an adjunct to the antimicrobial chemotherapy and may help to accelerate recovery and to decrease the risk of relapses.

Prognosis

The prognosis of cervicofacial and cutaneous actinomycotic infections is good provided that the diagnosis is established early and antimicrobial treatment is adequate. However, thoracic, abdominal, and systemic manifestations remain serious conditions that require all possible diagnostic and therapeutic efforts. Without proper treatment, the prognosis is grave.

Epidemiology

Actinomycoses are not transmissible and cannot be brought under control by vaccination or by measures that prevent spread. Sporadically, they occur worldwide. In Germany, the incidence of the disease was estimated to range from 1 in 40 000 (acute and chronic cases together) to 1 in 80 000 (chronic cases alone) per year, but appears to be decreasing in recent years.

Adult males are affected two to four times more frequently than are females by cervicofacial actinomycoses. Although actinomycoses may be found in patients of any age, men are predominantly affected between their 20th and 40th years and women in the second and third decade of their lives. Before puberty and in old age, actinomycoses occur sporadically in patients of both sexes.

Other diseases caused by fermentative actinomycetes

Fermentative actinomycetes play some part in dental caries and periodontal disease, but are clearly not the most important microbes contributing to these important health problems. Lacrimal canaliculitis with and without conjunctivitis is commonly caused by fermentative actinomycetes, in particular *Propionibacterium propionicum*, *Actinomyces viscosus*, or *A. israelii* and rarely by other actinomycete species. The concomitant flora, when present, is usually less complex than that of typical actinomycoses. Removal of the lacrimal concretions that are usually present and local application of antimicrobials always result in prompt cure.

Arcanobacterium pyogenes and *A. haemolyticum* (formerly 'Corynebacterium (Actinomyces) pyogenes' and 'C. haemolyticum') cause acute pharyngitis, urethritis, or cutaneous or subcutaneous suppurations. The recently described species *Actinomyces neuii* subspecies *neuii* and subspecies *anitratus*, *A. graevenitzii*, *A. europaeus*, *A. radingae*, *A. turicensis*, *A. funkei*, *A. radicidentis*, and *A. urogenitalis*, as well as *Arcanobacterium (Actinomyces) bernardiae* and *Actinobaculum schaalii* have been isolated from various clinical sources including abscesses and blood cultures, and may also be associated with mixed bacterial flora. *A. turicensis* and possibly *A. urogenitalis* seem to be particularly common in genital infections while *A. radingae* was found only in patients with skin-related pathologies, *A. europaeus* was detected in patients with urinary tract infections, and *A. radicidentis* was isolated from infected root canals of teeth.

Further reading

McNeil MM, Schaal KP (1998). Actinomycoses. In: Yu VL, Merigan TC Jr, Barriere SL, eds. *Antimicrobial therapy and vaccines*, pp 14–22. Williams and Wilkins, Baltimore.

Schaal KP (1986). Genus *Arachnia* Pine and Georg 1969, 269. In: Sneath PHA, Mair NS, Sharpe ME, Holt JG, eds. *Bergey's manual of systematic bacteriology*, Vol. 2, pp 1332–42. Williams and Wilkins, Baltimore.

Schaal KP (1986). Genus *Actinomyces* Harz 1877, 133. In: Sneath PHA, Mair NS, Sharpe ME, Holt JG, eds. *Bergey's manual of systematic bacteriology*, Vol. 2, pp 1383–418. Williams and Wilkins, Baltimore.

Schaal KP (1992). The genera *Actinomyces*, *Arcanobacterium*, and *Rothia*. In: Balows A, Trüper HG, Dworkin M, Harder W, Schleifer KH, eds. *The prokaryotes. A handbook on the biology of bacteria: ecophysiology, isolation, identification, applications*, 2nd edn, Vol. 1, pp 850–905. Springer, Berlin.

Schaal KP, Lee HJ (1992). Actinomycete infections in humans – a review. *Gene* **115**, 201–11.

Schaal KP, Pulverer G (1984). Epidemiologic, etiologic, diagnostic, and therapeutic aspects of endogenous actinomycete infections. In: Ortiz-Ortiz L, Bojalil LF, Yakoleff V, eds. *Biological, biochemical, and biomedical aspects of actinomycetes*, pp 13–32. Academic Press, Orlando.

7.11.27 Nocardiosis

R. J. Hay

Nocardiosis (nocardiasis) is the infection caused by *Nocardia* species, usually *Nocardia asteroides* but, less commonly, *N. brasiliensis*, *N. otitidiscaviarum*, and *N. transvaliensis*. The term is most commonly applied to systemic infection due to these organisms but can also be used to describe cutaneous disease that follows the implantation of infection. These organisms are also important causes of actinomycetoma, particularly in Mexico and Central America.

The nocardias are Gram-positive, filamentous, branching bacteria that ramify in infected tissues. They can also break up into bacillary forms and, in some conditions, aggregate into grains typical of mycetomas. These organisms are aerobic and partially acid fast. They grow readily on ordinary laboratory media.

Pathogenesis

Nocardia species are found in soil, particularly where there is decaying vegetation. They can also be isolated from the air and, in most cases, systemic infection is by the airborne route; rarely nocardiosis can be acquired after inoculation into the skin. The characteristic histopathological response to infection is the production of polymorphonuclear leucocyte abscesses without extensive fibrosis. Caseation and palisading granulomas are not generally seen. Metastases can occur in other organs. Dissemination of infection to the skin can occur in such systemic infections. By contrast, in primary cutaneous infections the lesion is usually localized to an abscess containing filaments at the site of inoculation and is accompanied by local lymphadenopathy. Mycetoma grain formation may occur in some of these infections that follow inoculation. It is not known why, in some patients, transcutaneous infection with nocardia results in the development of a mycetoma whereas in others a subcutaneous abscess containing filaments is formed. The tendency to develop into mycetomas appears to be more common with *N. brasiliensis* infections.

Epidemiology

Otherwise healthy patients may be infected by nocardia, although the frequency of subclinical exposure and sensitization in normal populations is unknown. However, the majority of patients with systemic nocardiosis are immunocompromised, most commonly with a condition that affects the expression of T-lymphocyte-mediated immune responses. The list of underlying conditions includes:

(1) malignancies, including cancer and lymphoma;

(2) AIDS and other immunodeficiency states such as chronic granulomatous disease;

(3) solid-organ transplantation;

(4) other conditions that require high doses of corticosteroids, such as collagen-vascular disease and rheumatoid arthritis; and

(5) pre-existing pulmonary disease—alveolar proteinosis, in particular, seems to predispose to nocardiosis.

The usual site of primary infection is the lung and the disease may remain restricted to this site. It may also be disseminated to other organs, particularly to the brain and skin. Nocardiosis can occur at any age, although it is rare, particularly in childhood.

Clinical features

Primary cutaneous nocardiosis

This is an uncommon infection that appears to follow traumatic inoculation of organisms in a superficial abrasion. The usual primary lesion is a small nodule, ulcer, or abscess at the site of inoculation. There may be a small chain of secondary nodules (cf. sporotrichosis) along the course of a lymphatic and local lymphadenopathy is common. Some such cases resolve spontaneously. This form of disease is usually caused by *N. asteroides*.

Nocardia mycetoma

This is discussed in Chapter 7.12.1. *N. brasiliensis* is the usual cause.

Pulmonary nocardiosis

Pulmonary infection is seen in about 75 per cent of cases of systemic nocardiosis, even where there are disseminated lesions elsewhere. Symptoms of pulmonary nocardiosis are variable, with cough, fever, and leucocytosis. In otherwise healthy individuals the changes and signs may be very similar to pulmonary tuberculosis, whereas in the immunocompromised patient the lesions present as rapidly developing, single or multiple lung lesions. In patients with AIDS, symptoms are often minimal, even in the presence of extensive disease. These changes are reflected by the course of the disease. In some patients, progression is rapid, in others chronic.

Chest radiographs may show segmental or lobar infiltrates, cavitation, nodules, or diffuse miliary infiltrates. Calcification is not common. The infection may spread locally to involve adjacent structures such as the pleural space and diaphragm or may spread to other sites. Very occasionally, nocardias can be isolated from sputum of otherwise healthy patients. Whether this reflects the process of asymptomatic sensitization is not known. Most cases of pulmonary nocardiosis are caused by *N. asteroides*.

Disseminated nocardiosis

Haematogenous spread is common in the immunocompromised patient and may occur without evidence of pulmonary infection. The most common site for dissemination is the brain, where it presents with localized abscesses without meningeal involvement. The signs are those due to an intracerebral space-occupying lesion. Spread to other sites is less common, although dissemination to skin, liver, kidneys, and bone may occur.

The acute disseminated forms and those with involvement of the central nervous system have the worst prognosis. Continued therapy with corticosteroids also appears to have bad prognostic significance. Infection in patients with AIDS may not be recognized before death. Rapid diagnosis is therefore a key to successful management. By contrast, pulmonary infection in otherwise healthy patients is usually a chronic process and has to be distinguished from tuberculosis.

Laboratory diagnosis

The infection is often recognized initially by direct microscopy of pus, bronchial washings, or tissue. In Gram stains the organisms can be shown as fine, branching filaments, although distinction from other bacteria may be difficult if short, rod-like forms predominate. A modified acid-fast stain using weak acid can be used to demonstrate filaments.

Nocardia species grow on ordinary media aerobically. Colonies may take 2 to 3 weeks to appear and cultures need prolonged incubation. Growth is generally more rapid on Lowenstein–Jensen medium.

Histopathological examination is useful in some cases. Filaments stain with modified acid-fast stains using an aqueous solution of a weak acid for decolorization, but can also be highlighted with the methenamine–silver stain (Grocott modification). The branching nature of the organism is best appreciated in histopathological material. Other pathogens such as *Pneumocystis* species may also be present in histopathological material.

Serological tests (usually counterimmunoelectrophoresis or enzyme immunoassay) can be obtained in reference centres and are generally used to monitor the progress of therapy rather than establish the diagnosis.

Therapy

The mainstays of therapy are sulphonamides such as sulphadiazine and sulphafurazole, given in doses of 4 to 6 g daily. Co-trimoxazole is also effective, particularly in pulmonary forms, although the ratio of the trimethoprim to sulphonamide components is not ideal for intracerebral infections. In many cases, drainage of abscesses may hasten recovery. Unfortunately, there have been no multicentre clinical studies aimed at reaching a consensus on the most appropriate therapy for this uncommon infection. Thus, much of the recommended drug therapy is derived from the personal experiences of few cases. It is, for instance, the general practice to use two antibiotics.

Other drugs that have been used include amikacin, ampicillin, and minocycline—although testing is necessary before using these. Experience of other drugs is similarly limited. For instance, ciprofloxacin, cefotaxime, and imipenem are all active *in vitro* but clinical experience with them is limited at present.

Clustering of cases may occur occasionally, suggesting exposure to a common source of infection. In two such episodes there had been extensive construction work in the vicinity of the hospital involved. At present, no methods of prevention are known, although the existence of more than two cases in a single or adjacent wards should alert clinicians to the possibility of environmentally acquired infection.

Further reading

Boiron P *et al.* (1992). Review of nocardial infections in France, 1987–1990. *European Journal of Clinical Microbiology and Infectious Diseases* **11**, 709–14.

Curry WA (1980). Human nocardiosis. *Archives of Internal Medicine* **140**, 818–24.

Georghiou PR, Blacklock ZM (1992). Infection with *Nocardia* species in Queensland. A review of 102 clinical isolates. *Medical Journal of Australia* **156**, 692–7.

Hay RJ (1983). Nocardial infections of the skin. *Journal of Hygiene* **91**, 385–91.

Houang ET *et al.* (1980). *Nocardia asteroides* infection—a transmissible disease. *Journal of Hospital Infection* **1**, 31–6.

Javaly K, Horowitz HW, Wormser GP (1992). Nocardiosis in patients with human immunodeficiency virus infection. Report of two cases and review of the literature. *Medicine* **71**, 128–38.

Sakai C, Takagi T, Satoh Y (1999). *Nocardia asteroides* pneumonia, subcutaneous abscess and meningitis in a patient with advanced malignant lymphoma: successful treatment based on *in vitro* antimicrobial susceptibility. *Internal Medicine* **38**, 683–6.

7.11.28 Rat-bite fevers

D. A. Warrell

Introduction

Rat bites are not uncommon, even in cities. Young children are often bitten while asleep. Patients with diabetic or leprous neuropathy are particularly vulnerable. Rodent bites can transmit lymphocytic choriomeningitis and other arenaviruses, rabies, leptospirosis, melioidosis, tularaemia, plague, murine typhus, trench fever, *Pasteurella multocida*, and the two rat-bite fevers caused by *Streptobacillus moniliformis* and *Spirillum minus*.

Streptobacillus moniliformis infection (streptobacillary rat-bite fever and Haverhill fever)

This organism is part of the normal pharyngeal flora of up to 50 per cent of wild and laboratory rats and can be recovered from the nasopharynx, middle ear, saliva, and urine. It can also cause severe disease in rodents: septicaemia, pneumonia, conjunctivitis, polyarthritis, and abortion. It has been isolated from rats, mice, guinea-pigs, gerbils, squirrels, and turkeys as well as animals that feed on rodents such as cats, dogs, pigs, ferrets, and weasels.

S. moniliformis derives its name from the filaments and chains with yeast-like swellings seen in mature cultures on solid media. It is a non-motile, pleomorphic, filamentous, Gram-negative rod, 1 to 5 μm long, and is microaerophilic. It can be grown in ordinary blood culture media, but thrives only when blood, serum, or ascitic fluid are added (for example, trypticase soy agar with 20 per cent horse or rabbit serum added under 8 per cent CO_2). In liquid media, 'puff ball' colonies appear in 1 to 6 days. In concentrations exceeding 0.0125 per cent, sodium polyanethol sulphonate ('Liquoid'), a laboratory anticoagulant often added to blood culture broths for isolating aerobic bacteria, inhibits the growth of *S. moniliformis*. In culture, L-phase variants occur spontaneously. These lack a cell wall and are therefore resistant to penicillin. The organism has been cultured from patients' bite wounds, blood, synovial and pericardial fluid, and from abscesses.

Epidemiology

The infection occurs worldwide in two forms. Rat-bite fever is caused by bites or scratches by rodents or their predators or mere contact with these mammals whether living or dead. In some countries, 10 per cent of those bitten by wild rats will be infected. Most rat-bite victims are children of poor families living in urban areas. The bite may not be suspected since many are inflicted while the patient is asleep. Laboratory staff who work with rats are also at special risk. Haverhill fever, named after a town in Massachusetts, follows ingestion of raw milk, food, or water contaminated by rats. An outbreak in a boarding school in England in 1983 affected 304 people, 43 per cent of the school's population, and was attributed to contamination of the water supply by rats.

Clinical features

After an incubation period, which is usually less than 10 days and often as short as 1 to 3 days, there is a sudden high fever with rigors, vomiting, severe headache, myalgia, and muscle tenderness. Evidence of the bite has usually disappeared by this stage. About 75 per cent of patients develop a rash between 1 and 8 days later. Discrete erythematous macules, 1 to 4 mm in diameter, appear symmetrically on the lateral and extensor surfaces and over the joints. They are often most marked on the hands and feet (palms and soles) with associated petechiae, but they also occur on the face. Papules, vesicles, and pustules with scabs have also been described. About half the patients develop an asymmetrical migratory polyarthralgia or arthritis, usually involving the knees, ankles, elbows, shoulders, and hips and often associated with effusions. Joint pains may be the dominant symptom in patients with rat-bite fever. Diarrhoea and loss of weight are described in young children. Fever and other symptoms subside in a few days in treated cases, but fever may persist for 1 to 2 weeks (or relapse over several months) and arthritis for many months in those untreated. Severe infections can lead to bronchitis, pneumonia, metastatic abscess formation (including cerebral abscess), myocarditis, pericarditis with effusion, subacute glomerulonephritis, interstitial nephritis, splenitis or splenic abscess, amnionitis, and anaemia. Infective endocarditis, usually with underlying rheumatic or other valve disease, has been described in 18 cases, one with human immunodeficiency virus (HIV) infection.

Haverhill fever (erythema arthriticum epidemicum) follows a similar clinical course after the patient has drunk unpasteurized milk or contaminated water. Vomiting, stomatitis, and upper respiratory tract symptoms such as sore throat are said to be more prominent than in rat-bite fever.

Diagnosis

Unlike *Spirillum minus* infection (sodoku), the incubation period is short, the bite wound heals permanently with little local lymphadenopathy, the rash is morbilliform or petechial, and arthritis is common.

The diagnosis can be confirmed by culturing the organism from blood, joint fluid, or pus. In patients with infective endocarditis the differential diagnosis of the slow-growing, microaerophilic organism will include *Haemophilus aphrophilus*, *Cardiobacterium hominis*, *Actinomyces actinomycetencomitans*, and *Eikenella corrodens*. A high or rising titre of agglutinins, complement-fixing or fluorescent antibodies, may be detected between 2 and 3 weeks. A peripheral leucocytosis of 10 000 to 30 000/µl is usual and false-positive serological tests for syphilis are found in 15 to 25 per cent of cases.

Treatment

Streptobacillus moniliformis is sensitive to penicillin and can be treated with procaine benzylpenicillin (adult dose 600 mg or 600 000 units) by intramuscular injection every 12 hours for 7 to 14 days, or by penicillin-V 2 g a day by mouth. Penicillin-resistant L-variants are susceptible to streptomycin, tetracycline, and probably erythromycin. For patients hypersensitive to penicillin, erythromycin, chloramphenicol, tetracycline, or cephalosporins can be used. Erythromycin was used successfully in the boarding-school outbreak of Haverhill fever in England in 1983.

Patients with endocarditis should be treated with intravenous benzylpenicillin, 4.8 to 14.4 g (8–24 000 000 units) each day for between 4 and 6 weeks, or 4.8 mega units of procaine benzylpenicillin daily by intramuscular injection for 4 weeks if the cultured organism has a sensitivity of 0.1 µg/ml. The addition of streptomycin improves bactericidal activity and eliminates L-forms.

Prognosis

The untreated case fatality was reported to be 10 to 13 per cent. However, the overall mortality in patients with endocarditis is about 50 per cent. Residual arthralgia, persisting for as long as 10 years, has been described.

Spirillum minus infection (sodoku, sokosha)

Spirillum minus may be found in the blood of up to 25 per cent of apparently healthy rodents and in the eye discharge and mouths of rats with interstitial keratitis and conjunctivitis. *S. minus* is a relatively thick, tightly coiled, Gram-negative spirillum (**not** a spirochaete), between 2.5 and 5.0 µm long, with 2 to 6 (commonly 3) spirals, resembling campylobacters. It darts about under the power of its terminal flagella. Continuous culture on artificial media has not been achieved, but the organism can be demonstrated by inoculating material from the bite wound, regional lymph nodes, or blood intraperitoneally into mice or guinea-pigs. Organisms usually appear in the rodent's blood within 5 to 15 days of inoculation.

Epidemiology

Sodoku is found worldwide but is particularly common in Japan. It results from bites, scratches, or mere contact with rodents or their predators including dogs, cats, and pigs.

Clinical features

The initial bite wound usually heals without signs of local inflammation. After an incubation period of between 5 and 30 days, usually 7 days or more, there is sudden fever which, in untreated cases, reaches its height in 3 days and resolves by crisis after a further 3 days. Other acute symptoms include rigors, myalgia, and prostration. At the start of the illness the healed bite wound becomes inflamed and swollen; it may break down to become necrotic or suppurative. Regional lymph nodes are usually enlarged and tender. The exanthem often starts at the site of the bite and spreads from there. It consists of angry purplish or reddish-brown indurated papules, plaques, or macules with urticarial lesions. Arthralgia may be severe but there are no joint effusions. Severe manifestations including meningitis, cerebral abscess, encephalitis, endocarditis, myocarditis, myocardial abscess, pleural effusion, chorioamnionitis, subcutaneous abscesses, and involvement of liver, kidney, and other organs are seen in about 10 per cent of cases. Relapses of fever, rash, and other symptoms lasting 3 to 6 days may occur between remissions of a week or so for 2 to months and occasionally up to a year in untreated patients.

Diagnosis

Clinically, sodoku is distinguishable from streptobacillary rat-bite fever by its longer incubation period, by the marked reaction at the bite site with local lymphadenopathy at the start of symptoms, by the different rash (dark papular rather than morbilliform and petechial), and by the rarity of arthritis. The diagnosis can be confirmed by examining an aspirate from the bite wound, lymph nodes, exanthem, or blood (thick and thin films) by dark-field microscopy or by staining with Wright's or Giemsa stain. Spirochaetes can be detected in the blood, peritoneal fluid, or heart muscle of inoculated rodents but cannot be cultured on artificial media. No specific serological tests are available. False-positive serological tests for syphilis are found in 50 to 60 per cent of cases, and reactions with Proteus OXK are also common.

Differential diagnosis of rat-bite fevers

An acute, severe, febrile illness following a rat bite, or other contact with rodents or their predators, should raise the possibility of other rodent-related infections. These include: *Pasteurella multocida*, which produces local pain and erythema within a few hours of the bite; plague; tularaemia; leptospirosis; murine typhus; and arenaviruses such as lymphocytic choriomeningitis, Lassa fever (Africa), or Argentine, Bolivian, or Venezuelan haemorrhagic fevers (South America). Ingestion of raw milk should also raise the possibility of brucellosis.

Treatment

Penicillin is the drug of choice. For adults, procaine benzylpenicillin 600 mg (600 000 units) should be given every 12 hours for 7 to 14 days. Penicillin-V, 2 g/day by mouth, is also said to be effective. A Jarisch–Herxheimer reaction may complicate penicillin treatment.

Prognosis

Untreated case fatality is about 2 to 10 per cent.

Prevention of rat-bite fevers

These infections can be prevented by rodent control, by encouraging laboratory workers to wear gloves and use correct techniques when handling rodents, to clean all rodent bite wounds, and to take prophylactic penicillin when bitten. Haverhill fever is prevented by avoiding the consumption of raw milk, by monitoring water supplies (especially those not derived from the mains), and by controlling rat populations.

Further reading

McEvoy MB, Noah ND, Pilsworth R (1987). Outbreak of fever caused by *Streptobacillus moniliformis*. *Lancet* **ii**, 1361–3.

Raffin BJ, Freemark M (1979). Streptobacillary rat bite fever: a pediatric problem. *Pediatrics* **64**, 214–17.

Roughgarden JW (1965). Antimicrobial therapy of rat bite fever. A review. *Archives of Internal Medicine* **116**, 39–54.

Rupp ME (1992). *Streptobacillus moniliformis* endocarditis: case report and review. *Clinical Infectious Diseases* **14**, 769–72.

7.12.29 Lyme borreliosis

John Nowakowski, Robert B. Nadelman, and Gary P. Wormser

Lyme borreliosis (also called Lyme disease) is an infection caused by the spirochaete, *Borrelia burgdorferi*, which is transmitted to humans by the usually asymptomatic bite of certain ticks of the genus *Ixodes* (Plate 1). The entire chromosome of *Borrelia burgdorferi* and 11 of its plasmids have been sequenced. Ticks acquire this borrelial infection in a complex tick–vertebrate transmission cycle. The white-footed mouse is the most important reservoir for *B. burgdorferi* in North America, but in Europe a variety of small mammals and birds are involved, possibly reflecting the much more varied and complex ecology of the *Ixodes* ticks in Eurasia. White-tailed deer, an important host for adult *Ixodes* ticks, are not a reservoir for *B. burgdorferi*.

Lyme borreliosis occurs in north-eastern, mid-Atlantic, north-central, and far western regions of the United States, limited foci in Canada (mainly in eastern Ontario), and much of Europe and northern Asia. Migrating birds may play a role in the spread of ticks and *B. burgdorferi* to new geographical locations.

Lyme borreliosis occurs equally in males and females, and affects people of all ages. There is a bimodal age distribution with the highest rates in children 5 to 9 years old and adults more than 30 years old.

Clinical manifestations

The somewhat different manifestations of Lyme borreliosis in Eurasia compared with North America (Table 1) may be explained by the wider variety of genospecies of *B. burgdorferi*. Clinical features are similar in adults and children.

Erythema migrans (Plate 2)

Erythema migrans, the clinical hallmark of Lyme borreliosis, is recognized in approximately 90 per cent of patients with objective evidence of *B. burgdorferi* infection. Typically, erythema migrans begins as a red macule or papule at the site of a tick bite that occurred 7 to 10 days earlier. The rash expands over days to weeks. Central clearing may or may not be present. Secondary cutaneous lesions may develop after haematogenous spread of spirochaetes. Erythema migrans must be distinguished from local tick bite reactions, tinea, insect and spider bites, bacterial cellulitis, and plant dermatitis.

Systemic complaints in patients with erythema migrans are more common in the United States than in Europe, perhaps as a result of illness caused by a more virulent genospecies (*B. burgdorferi sensu stricto* rather than *B. afzelii*) or more frequent coinfection with other tickborne pathogens. Symptoms include fatigue, myalgia, arthralgia, headache, fever and/ or chills, and stiff neck. Prominent respiratory and/or gastrointestinal complaints are so infrequent that their presence should suggest an alternative diagnosis or coinfection. The most common objective physical findings are regional lymphadenopathy and fever. Occasional cases of febrile viral-like illness without erythema migrans have been attributed to Lyme borreliosis.

Carditis

Typically cardiac disease develops within weeks to months after infection. It is usually manifested by fluctuating degrees of atrioventricular block which may cause the patient to complain of dizziness, palpitations, dyspnoea, chest pain, or syncope. Pericarditis with effusion is rarely observed. The incidence (as measured by ECG-confirmed heart block) has been observed to be low in both the United States (< 1 per cent) and Europe (< 4 per cent). *B. burgdorferi* has been recovered in culture from the myocardium of several European patients with congestive heart failure including two with acute myocarditis and one with chronic cardiomyopathy.

Table 1 Lyme borreliosis in North America compared with Eurasia

	North American Lyme borreliosis	Eurasian Lyme borreliosis
Vector	*Ixodes scapularis* or *Ixodes pacificus*	*Ixodes ricinus* or *Ixodes persulcatus*
Aetiological agent	*B. burgdorferi sensu stricto*	*B. burgdorferi sensu stricto* (in Europe), *B. afzelii*, or *B. garinii*
Erythema migrans	Recollection of tick bite infrequent (< 30%)	Recollection of tick bite common (64%)
	Short duration of rash at presentation (median 4 days)	Long duration of rash at presentation (median 14 days to 5–6 weeks)
	Central clearing uncommon (< 35%)	Central clearing common (> 65%)
	Systemic symptoms common (up to 80%)	Systemic symptoms uncommon (< 35%)
	Multiple lesions (about 13%)	Multiple lesions (≈ 7%)
	Seronegativity at presentation common (about 50%)	Seronegativity at presentation very common (up to 80%)
Borrelial lymphocytoma	Rare	Well documented
Acrodermatitis chronica atrophicans	Rare	Well documented
Neurological disease	Cranial nerve palsy (usually 7th) with or without meningitis most common (< 10%)	Painful meningoradiculoneuritis with or without cranial palsy most common (10–20%)
	Chronic neuroborreliosis rare	Chronic neuroborreliosis rare
Rheumatological disease	Arthritis common in untreated patients with erythema migrans (51%)	Arthritis uncommon in untreated patients with erythema migrans
	Chronic synovitis in 11% of untreated patients with erythema migrans	Chronic synovitis rare

Neurological disease

The incidence of neurological Lyme disease in Europe (20 per cent) may be higher than in the United States (< 10 per cent). One explanation may be the greater neurotropism of *B. garinii* (a genospecies which has not been isolated in North America). The principal early neurological manifestations are cranial neuropathy (typically 7th nerve palsy), radiculopathy, and meningitis, which may occur alone or together. Late neurological manifestations are uncommon and include peripheral neuropathy, encephalopathy, and encephalomyelitis.

Antibiotics appear to hasten the resolution of meningitis but most studies are uncontrolled. The rate of resolution of motor dysfunction, which is fully reversible in the vast majority of cases, is not enhanced by antimicrobial therapy. Symptoms of encephalopathy and peripheral neuropathy improve or do not progress after treatment with antibiotics.

Rheumatological disease

Lyme arthritis is more frequently diagnosed in North America than in Europe. In a study of 55 untreated patients with erythema migrans diagnosed in the United States between 1977 and 1979, followed for a mean duration of 6 years, objective arthritis developed in more than half, occurring within 1 year for 90 per cent of patients. Without antibiotic treatment, intermittent attacks of migratory monoarthritis or asymmetric oligoarthritis occur, lasting a mean of 3 months (range 3 days to 11.5 months). The knee is affected at some point in almost all patients, but other large and (less often) small joints may be affected. Temporomandibular joint involvement occurred in 11 (39 per cent) of 28 patients with arthritis in one series. Although large effusions may occur, joint pain and erythema are often minimal. Baker's cysts may develop. Typically, synovial fluid analysis reveals a modestly elevated protein and white cell count (median 24 250 white cells/mm^3; range 2100 to 72 250 white cells/mm^3) with a polymorphonuclear predominance and a normal glucose level. Synovitis lasting 1 year or more may ensue for a minority of American patients, sometimes associated with joint destruction. Although *B. burgdorferi* DNA can be detected by polymerase chain reaction (**PCR**) in the synovial fluid of up to 85 per cent of untreated patients with Lyme arthritis, *B. burgdorferi* has rarely been successfully cultured from joint fluid. In patients who receive antibiotics, the presence of *B. burgdorferi* can no longer be detected by PCR in repeat synovial fluid examinations.

Acrodermatitis chronica atrophicans

This develops insidiously on a distal extremity. It is a skin lesion that is swollen, bluish-red, and which ultimately atrophies. One-third of patients have an associated (usually sensory) polyneuropathy. *B. burgdorferi* has been recovered from skin biopsy specimens of acrodermatitis chronica atrophicans lesions of more than 10 years' duration. Since the usual causative agent, *B. afzelii*, does not occur in the United States, acrodermatitis chronica atrophicans is essentially a European disease.

Miscellaneous clinical manifestations

Borrelia lymphocytoma, principally caused by *B. afzelii* and *B. garinii*, is a tumour-like nodule which typically appears on the pinna of the earlobe or on the nipple or areola of the breast. Lesions resolve spontaneously but disappear within a few weeks after antibiotics. This lesion does not occur in North America.

Direct involvement of the eye (e.g. uveitis, keratitis, vitritis, or optic neuritis) has been attributed to *B. burgdorferi* infection. However, since ophthalmological disorders have almost never been associated with the isolation of *B. burgdorferi* in culture, the actual pathogenesis in these cases is uncertain. Conjunctivitis, originally described in 11 per cent of patients with erythema migrans, was rare (< 5 per cent) in recent studies of culture-positive patients.

Case reports have suggested that adverse outcomes may be associated with pregnancies complicated by maternal Lyme borreliosis. The risk of transplacental transmission of *B. burgdorferi*, however, is probably minimal when appropriate antibiotics (Table 2) are given to pregnant women with Lyme borreliosis. There are no published data to support a congenital Lyme borreliosis syndrome.

Laboratory tests

Where Lyme borreliosis is endemic, diagnosis of erythema migrans is purely clinical. Laboratory testing is neither necessary nor recommended. However, culture is virtually 100 per cent specific and appears to be more sensitive (57 to 86 per cent) than serology (50 per cent in the United States and less than 50 per cent in Europe).

In patients with suspected extracutaneous Lyme borreliosis, serological testing is essential to support the diagnosis. Culture of *B. burgdorferi* has been a highly insensitive diagnostic technique for this group of patients, presumably because of inaccessibility of tissues which contain the organism.

A two-step approach to serological diagnosis has recently been proposed in the United States (and is being studied in Europe) to increase the specificity of a positive test. A positive or equivocal first-stage test (usually an enzyme-linked immunosorbent assay [ELISA] or indirect immunofluorescence assay [IFA]) is followed on the same serum sample by a second-stage test (immunoblot). Two-step testing, however, is not indicated for those with little or no clinical evidence of Lyme borreliosis because of a low positive predictive value. Since IgM and IgG antibodies to *B. burgdorferi* may persist in serum for years after clinical recovery, serology has no role in measuring response to treatment.

Patients with extracutaneous Lyme borreliosis almost always have diagnostic serum antibodies to *B. burgdorferi*, except for some patients with early 7th nerve palsy or occasional patients in whom antibodies to *B. burgdorferi* are present in cerebrospinal fluid only.

Coinfection

Ixodes scapularis (Plate 1) ticks are the vectors for several other infections which may be transmitted separately or simultaneously with *B. burgdorferi* such as *Babesia microti*, and the rickettsial agent that causes human granulocytic ehrlichiosis. In Europe, species of *Babesia* and *Ehrlichia* are present in *Ixodes ricinus* ticks, which are also vectors for a flavivirus causing tick-borne encephalitis. Coinfection may alter the clinical presentation and response to treatment of Lyme borreliosis.

Treatment

Although most manifestations of Lyme borreliosis resolve spontaneously, antibiotics may speed the resolution of some manifestations and almost certainly will prevent the progression of disease. An approach to treatment is summarized in Table 2. Currently available quinolones, sulpha drugs, first-generation cephalosporins, rifampicin, and aminoglycosides have no appreciable activity against *B. burgdorferi* and should not be used. In addition, there is no evidence to support combination antimicrobial therapy, prolonged (> 1 month) or repeated courses of antibiotics, and 'pulse' or intermittent antibiotic therapy. Within 24 h after initiation of antibiotics, approximately 15 per cent of patients may develop transient intensified signs (e.g. rash and fever) and symptoms (e.g. arthralgias) consistent with a Jarisch–Herxheimer reaction. Treatment is symptomatic.

Most people treated for Lyme borreliosis have an excellent prognosis. Although some patients treated for erythema migrans in recent series continue to have a variety of mild non-specific complaints following antibiotic

Table 2 Treatment of Lyme borreliosis

Manifestation	Antibiotic[a, b]	Route/dose Adults	Route/dose Children[b, c]	Duration (days)	Comments
Cutaneous disease Erythema migrans					Amoxicillin, cefuroxime axetil, and doxycycline probably equally effective; treatment failure rate < 5% (objective findings); no evidence that intravenous ceftriaxone advantageous in 'disseminated' early disease
	Doxycycline[b]	Orally, 100 mg twice daily	2–4 mg/kg.day in 2 divided doses (max 200 mg/day)	14–21	Includes coverage of human granulocytic ehrlichiosis (HGE); ↑ risk of photosensitivity
	Amoxicillin	Orally, 500 mg thrice daily	40–50 mg/kg.day in 3 divided doses (max 1500 mg/day)	14–21	Not active against HGE
	Cefuroxime axetil	Orally, 500 mg twice daily	30 mg/kg.day in 2 divided doses (max 1000 mg/day)	14–21	Useful when cellulitis cannot be distinguished from EM (as is amoxicillin/ clavulanic acid); alternative for some penicillin-allergic patients; most expensive; not active against HGE
	Phenoxymethyl penicillin (penicillin V)	Orally, 500 mg four times daily	50 mg/kg.day in 4 divided doses (max 2000 mg/day)	14–21	Has been given at an oral dose of $1-1.5\times10^6$ units thrice daily in European studies. Not active against HGE
	Tetracycline[b]	Orally, 500 mg four times daily	25–50 mg/kg.day in 4 divided doses (max 2000 mg/day)	14–21	Includes coverage of HGE; ↑ risk of photosensitivity
	Azithromycin	Orally, 500 mg once daily	5–12 mg/kg once daily (max 500 mg/day)	7–10	Second-line choice; more objective failures compared with amoxicillin-treated patients (34); not active against HGE.
Borrelial lymphocytoma	First line oral EM regimen[b]			14–21	
Acrodermatitis chronica atrophicans	First line oral EM regimen[b]			21–28	Evaluation for concurrent neuropathy prudent; intravenous antibiotics (see below) may be effective, but regimen and advantages over oral therapy not established
Extracutaneous disease Carditis	First line oral EM regimen[b]			14–21	For primary or secondary heart block
	Ceftriaxone	Intravenously, 2 g once daily	75–100 mg/kg once daily (max 2000 mg/day)	14	For advanced (tertiary) heart block; no proof that intravenous treatment more effective than oral therapy
Facial nerve palsy	First line oral EM regimen[b]			14–21	No clinical trials; treatment does not shorten course; perform lumbar puncture if clinical signs of meningitis
Meningitis, radiculoneuritis	Ceftriaxone	Intravenously, 2 g once daily	75–100 mg/kg once daily (max 2000 mg/day)	14–28	
Peripheral neuropathy, encephalomyelitis, chronic encephalopathy	Cefotaxime	Intravenously, 2 g thrice daily	150–200 mg/kg.day in 3–4 divided doses (max 6000 mg/day)		
	Penicillin G	Intravenously, 18–24×10^6 units/day in 6 divided doses	3×10^5 units/kg.day in 6 divided doses (max 18–24×10^6U/day)	14–28	
	Doxycycline[b]	Orally, 100–200 mg twice daily	2–4 mg/kg.day in 2 divided doses (max 200 mg/day)	14–28	Effective in meningitis and radiculoneuritis in European studies; no data in chronic neurological disease
Arthritis					Some patients treated with oral agents develop subsequent neurological disease (see text); role of PCR of synovial fluid to determine treatment duration unclear; no comparison studies with shorter courses of therapy
	Doxycycline[b]	Orally, 100 mg twice daily	2–4 g/kg.day in 2 divided doses (max 200 mg/day)	28	

Table 2 Continued

Manifestation	Antibiotic[a, b]	Route/dose		Duration	Comments
		Adults	Children[b, c]	(days)	
	Amoxicillin	Orally, 500 mg thrice daily	40–50 mg/kg.day in 3 divided doses (max 1500 mg/day)	28	
	Ceftriaxone	Intravenously, 2 g once daily	75–100 mg/kg once daily (max 2000 mg/day)	14	
Asymptomatic tick bite	No treatment				Efficacy of prophylaxis has not been demonstrated; risk of adverse effects for the 10-day antibiotic regimens studied is comparable with risk of contracting Lyme borreliosis

EM, erythema migrans; HGE, human granulocytic ehrlichiosis.

[a] Few regimens studied in published trials in children; selection of amoxicillin in preference to penicillin V, or doxycycline to tetracycline is based upon convenience (decreased dosing) and theoretical concerns (higher attainable levels) and not upon comparison studies.

[b] Pregnant or lactating women, and children 9 years or younger should not receive tetracylines; tetracyclines are the only antimicrobial agents known to be effective against the agent of human granulocytic ehrlichiosis.

[c] Paediatric dose should not exceed maximum adult dose.

[d] Limited data are available on treatment duration; the only studies comparing treatment duration in erythema migrans showed no outcome differences; duration of treatment for erythema migrans ranging from 10 to 30 days has been recommended. In one study of patients with objective late Lyme disease (mostly arthritis), there was no difference in outcome for patients treated with either 14 or 28 days of ceftriaxone.

therapy, the development of objective extracutaneous disease after treatment is extremely rare. Lyme borreliosis may trigger a fibromyalgia syndrome that does not appear to respond to repeated courses of antibiotics, but may improve with symptomatic therapy. Patients with carditis and neurological disease also tend to do well, but may sometimes have residual deficits (e.g. mild 7th nerve palsy) after treatment. In patients with arthritis, clinical recovery typically occurs in conjunction with oral antibiotic therapy (often with a non-steroidal anti-inflammatory medication); occasionally such patients with subtle signs of neuroborreliosis who are treated with oral antibiotics may develop overt neuroborreliosis and require parenteral therapy. A small number of American patients with Lyme arthritis and the HLA DR4 haplotype, who continue to have synovial inflammation for months or even several years after the apparent eradication of *B. burgdorferi* from the joint following antibiotic therapy, have improved after synovectomy. An immunological mechanism rather than active infection may be responsible for the continued inflammatory response in these patients.

A sizeable number of American patients with a variety of complaints of uncertain aetiology, including pain and fatigue syndromes, have been labelled as having 'chronic Lyme disease' or 'post-Lyme syndrome'. This entity is controversial.

Prevention

This includes avoiding exposure by limiting outdoor activities in tick-infested locations, using tick repellents, tucking in clothing to decrease exposed skin surfaces, and frequent skin inspections for early detection and removal of ticks. Use of acaracides on property and construction of deer fences have also been proposed.

Antibiotic prophylaxis given after recognized *I. scapularis* tick bites has not been shown to be effective in reducing the low (< 5 per cent) risk of acquiring Lyme borreliosis after tick bites. Vaccination with a single recombinant outer surface protein A (**OspA**) preparation has been found to be safe and effective for preventing Lyme disease in the United States. The efficacy of this OspA vaccine may be related to the ability of OspA antibodies (ingested during the blood meal by the vector tick) to kill *B. burgdorferi* in the tick gut, thus preventing transmission of the spirochaete. A single antigen OspA vaccine is expected to be less effective in Eurasia where species of *Borrelia* are more heterogeneous and OspA is more variable.

Further reading

Aguero-Rosenfeld M *et al.* (1993). Serodiagnosis in early Lyme disease. *Journal of Clinical Microbiology* **31**, 390–5. [Serological response to *Borrelia burgdorferi* by ELISA and immunoblot in early Lyme disease.]

Barbour AG, Fish D (1993). The biological and social phenomenon of Lyme disease. *Science* **260**, 1610–16. [Description of the emergence of the disease in the United States and its importance to human and animal health.]

Dattwyler RJ *et al.* (1997). Ceftriaxone compared with doxycycline for the treatment of acute disseminated Lyme disease. *New England Journal of Medicine* **337**, 289–94. [Study demonstrating equivalent efficacy of oral doxycycline compared with intravenous ceftriaxone in patients with disseminated early Lyme disease.]

Nadelman RB, Wormser GP (1998). Lyme borreliosis. *Lancet* **352**, 557–65. [Comprehensive review of the disease.]

Steere AC, Schoen RT, Taylor E (1987). The clinical evolution of Lyme arthritis. *Annals of Internal Medicine* **107**, 725–31. [Description of the progression to Lyme arthritis in untreated patients with erythema chronicum migrans.]

Strle F *et al.* (1999). Comparison of culture-confirmed erythema migrans caused by *Borrelia burgdorferi sensu stricto* in New York State and by *Borrelia afzelii* in Slovenia. *Annals of Internal Medicine* **130**, 32–6. [Clinical comparison of the disease in the United States and Slovenia.]

7.11.30 Other borrelia infections

D. A. Warrell

The borreliae are large, loosely coiled, motile spirochaetes. *B. recurrentis* (Plate 1), first described by Obermeier in 1867, causes louse-borne relapsing fever; *B. duttonii* and a number of other species or groups of *Borrelia* cause tick-borne relapsing fever; and *B. burgdorferi* causes Lyme disease. *B. vincentii* (now renamed *Treponema vincentii*) was, with *Fusobacterium*

(*Bacteroides*) *nucleatum* (*fusiforme*), implicated in acute necrotizing ulcerative gingivitis and Vincent's angina but is now regarded as part of the normal oral flora.

Relapsing fevers

The borreliae that cause relapsing fevers are spirochaetes, 8 to 20 µm long and 0.2 to 0.6 µm thick with between 3 and 15 coils and, in some strains, 15 to 30 axial filaments or flagella. These motile organisms divide by transverse binary fission. Several species of *Borrelia* including *B. recurrentis* can be cultured in Kelly's BSKII artificial media. *Borrelia* spp. can also be cultured on chick chorioallantoic membrane and perpetuated in rodents and ticks. Plasmid DNA has been detected in at least three *Borrelia* species.

Epidemiology

Louse-borne (epidemic) relapsing fever (LBRF)

Humans are probably the only reservoir of LBRF. The vector is the human body louse, *Pediculus humanus* and, to a lesser extent, the head louse, *P. capitis*. *B. recurrentis*, ingested by the louse during a blood meal, multiplies in its body cavity. Under conditions of crowding and poor hygiene, lice move from person to person. When the host's body surface temperature deviates far from 37 °C, as a result of death, fever, or exposure, or if infested clothing is discarded, the louse is forced to find a new host. A new person is infected when the infected louse is crushed and its body haemolymph applied to mucous membranes, such as to the conjunctiva by rubbing the eye, or to abraded skin, or inoculated through intact skin by scratching. Transmission is possible by blood transfusion, needlestick injuries, or even, in medical personnel, by contamination of broken skin such as paronychia on the fingers, by infected patients' blood. Unlike the tick vectors or tick-borne relapsing fever, which are also reservoirs of the infection, lice cannot transmit the infection transovarially to their progeny.

Wars, famine, and other disasters and the resulting large numbers of refugees favour the spread of lice and epidemic louse-borne infections such as relapsing fever and typhus. The yellow plague in Europe in AD 550 and the famine fevers of the seventeenth and eighteenth centuries were probably LBRF. During the first half of the twentieth century there were an estimated 50 million cases worldwide with a 10 per cent mortality. Epidemics began in Europe, the Middle East, and northern Africa during 1903, 1923, and 1943. An endemic focus persists in the Horn of Africa. In Ethiopia there is an annual epidemic of thousands of cases coinciding with the cool, rainy season. Poor people with lice-infested clothes crowd together for shelter. Recent outbreaks have occurred in the Sudan, Somalia, West Africa, and Vietnam. Since there is no known animal reservoir, the infection must persist in humans between epidemics, in mild or asymptomatic form.

Tick-borne (endemic) relapsing fever (TBRF)

There is a close relationship between particular species of *Borrelia*, their soft tick vectors, and reservoirs (Argasidae genus *Ornithodoros*) and mammal reservoir species. In East and Central Africa, domestic ticks of the *O. moubata* complex transmit *B. duttonii* between humans, the only one of these infections that is not a zoonosis. In North, West, and East Africa and the Middle East small rodents have burrows in or near human dwellings, and borreliae of the *Crociduriae* group, may be transmitted to man by the rodent tick *O. sonrai* (formerly *O. erraticus sonrai*). In the Central and West United States and Mexico, *O. hermsi*, a parasite of chipmunks and other tree squirrels, transmits *B. hermsi* to humans especially to those individuals who sleep in tick-infested log cabins near the Grand Canyon, Arizona. Other important borreliae causing tick-borne relapsing fever (and their tick vectors) include: *B. hispanica* (*O. sonrai*) in Africa; *B. persica* (*O. tholozani* = *O. papillipes*) in the Middle East; *B. venezuelensis* (*O. venezuelensis*) in Central and South America; and *B. turicatae* (*O. turicatae*), *B. parkeri* (*O. parkeri*) and *B. mazzotti* (*O. mazzotti*) in North America. Tick-borne relapsing fever may result when night-feeding ticks have access to man.

TBRF has occurred in most continents except Australasia and the Pacific region. It is particularly common in West Africa, where a recent survey revealed a prevalence of 1 per cent among children (in western Senegal). Each year 1650 proven cases are treated at one health centre in Rwanda (6 per cent of all patients). Although cases are usually isolated and sporadic in North America, in 1968 a total of 11 out of a group of 42 boy scouts were infected while camping in rodent-infested cabins on Browne Mountain, Washington; and in 1973 there were 62 cases among people staying in the log cabins along the north rim of the Grand Canyon in Arizona. During the past 25 years, 280 cases of TBRF have been identified in the United States. In Colorado the incidence is increasing (23 confirmed cases since 1977). In Jordan between 1959 and 1969 there were 723 cases of TBRF with four deaths.

Spirochaetes enter the tick in its blood meal from infected humans or animals. Unlike *B. recurrentis*, they invade the tick's salivary and coccal glands and genital apparatus and so can be transmitted when the tick feeds on a new host and transovarially to the tick's progeny. Unlike lice, ticks are reservoirs of *Borrelia* spp. They infest the burrows, caves, tree stumps, and roughly built shacks that harbour their mammalian hosts—rodents, insectivores, lagomorphs, bats, and small carnivores. In western countries, TBRF is occasionally diagnosed in travellers, intravenous drug abusers, and recipients of blood transfusions.

Pathophysiology

The physiological changes during the spontaneous crisis and the Jarisch–Herxheimer reaction (**J-HR**) induced by antimicrobial treatment in LBRF are typical of an 'endotoxin reaction'. Endotoxin-like activity has been described for some spirochaetes: *B. burgdorferi*, *Treponema hyodysenteriae*, *B. vincentii* and *B. buccalis*, and *Leptospira canicola*, but not in *B. recurrentis*, *B. hispanica*, or *Treponema pallidum*. It is the outer-membrane, variable major lipoprotein (**VMP**) of *B. recurrentis* that stimulates monocytes to produce tumour necrosis factor (**TNF**) through NF-kappaB. In patients treated with antibiotics, symptoms of the severe J-HR are associated with a transient marked elevation in plasma concentrations of tumour necrosis factor-α (**TNF-α**), interleukin-6, interleukin-8, and interleukin-1β (Fig. 1). The stimulus for cytokine release is the phagocytosis of spirochaetes made susceptible by the action of penicillin. Benzylpenicillin attaches to penicillin-binding protein I in *B. hermsi* spirochaetes. Large surface blebs are produced and the damaged spirochaetes are phagocytosed rapidly by neutrophils in the blood and by the spleen. Complement may enhance phagocytosis of spirochaetes, especially in the non-immune host, but the complement system is not essential for elimination of spirochaetes whether or not specific immunoglobulins are present. *In vitro*, surface contact with spirochaetes induces mononuclear leucocytes to produce pyrogen and thromboplastin, which could be responsible for the fever and disseminated intravascular coagulation in LBRF. Kinins may be released during the J-HR of syphilis and LBRF. The marked peripheral leucopenia that develops during the reaction reflects sequestration, perhaps in the pulmonary blood vessels, rather than leucocyte destruction. Spirochaetes may be found in those organs that bear the brunt of the infection (liver, spleen (Plate 2), myocardium, and brain), but it is unclear how their pathological effects are produced. The petechial rash results from thrombocytopenia not vasculitis. The cardiorespiratory and metabolic disturbances in relapsing fever are principally the result of persistent high fever, accentuated by the J-HR or spontaneous crisis.

Immunological basis of the relapse phenomenon

Borrelia recurrentis exhibits antigenic variation of variable membrane proteins (**VMPs**), which are outer membrane lipoproteins. The organism has a repertoire of many VMPs but, at any one time, only one is expressed and is immunodominant. The expressed *VMP* gene is situated near the end of a linear plasmid and changes every 1 to 10 000 cell divisions. IgM is induced against the immunodominant VMP, leading to selection of borreliae of the next, emerging serotype. This explains the relapse phenomenon and the

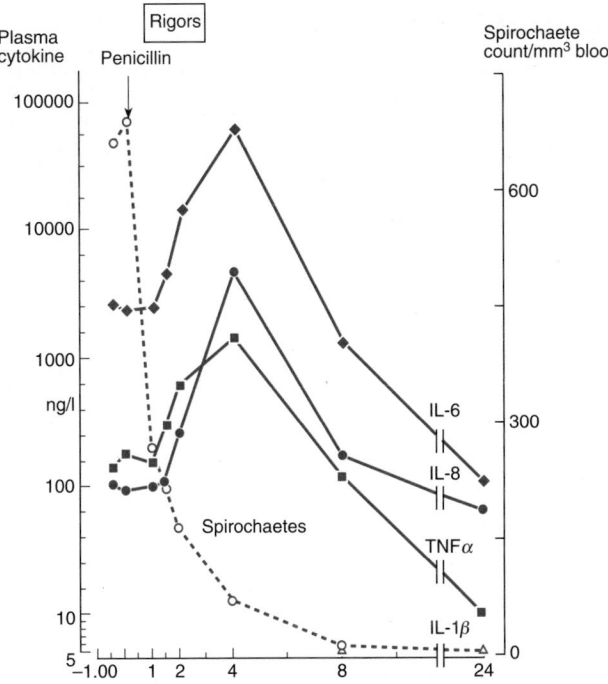

Fig. 1 Typical response in a patient treated with intravenous penicillin. Following penicillin, the number of spirochaetes fell abruptly; and circulating levels of TNF-α, IL-6, IL-8, and IL-1β started to rise after about 1 h, peaking at 4 h. This patient experienced sustained rigors as cytokine levels were increasing, which subsided before peak levels were achieved.

successive appearance of borreliae expressing different VMPs during the course of an untreated infection. These same VMPs are the principal TNF-α-inducing factors in LBRF. VMPs may differ in their potency as TNF inducers; they may also determine invasiveness of the borreliae (for example, into the central nervous system) and may affect virulence in other ways.

Pathology

The vast majority of spirochaetes are confined to the lumen of blood vessels, but tangled masses are also found in the characteristic splenic miliary abscesses (Fig. 2) (Plate 2) and infarcts as well as within the central nervous system adjacent to haemorrhages. Some strains of tick-borne borreliae can invade the CNS, aqueous humour, and other tissues. In LBRF, a perivascular histiocytic interstitial myocarditis, found in the majority of cases, may be responsible for conduction defects, arrhythmias, and myocardial failure resulting in sudden death. Splenic rupture with massive haemorrhage, cerebral haemorrhage (Plate 3), and hepatic failure are other causes of death. The liver shows hepatitis with patchy mid-zonal haemorrhages and necrosis (Fig. 3). There is meningitis and perisplenitis: most serosal cavities and surfaces of viscera are studded with petechial haemorrhages (Plate 4). Thrombi are occasionally found occluding small vessels, but the peripheral gangrene sometimes found in patients recovering from louse-borne typhus is not seen.

Clinical features

Poor, indigent, malnourished street-dwellers, beggars, and prisoners seem most likely to become infected, especially young men. Pregnant women appear to be specially susceptible to severe disease and abortions are frequent.

After an incubation period of 4 to 18 (average 7) days, the illness starts suddenly with rigors and a fever that mounts to nearly 40 °C in a few days. Early symptoms are headache, dizziness, nightmares, generalized aches and pains (especially affecting the lower back, knees, and elbows), anorexia, nausea, vomiting, and diarrhoea. Later there is upper abdominal pain, cough, and epistaxis. Patients are usually prostrated. Most are confused. Hepatic tenderness is the commonest sign (about 60 per cent). The liver is palpably enlarged in about 50 per cent of cases. Splenic tenderness and enlargement are slightly less common. Jaundice has been reported in between 10 and 80 per cent of cases. A petechial or ecchymotic rash is seen in between 10 and 60 per cent of cases: the lesions occur particularly on the trunk (Plate 5). Other sites of spontaneous bleeding include the nose in 25 per cent and less commonly the lungs, gastrointestinal tract, and conjunctivas (Plate 6) and retinas. Many patients have tender muscles. Meningism occurs in about 40 per cent of cases: other neurological features include cranial nerve lesions, monoplegias, flaccid paraplegia, and focal convulsions attributable, perhaps, to cerebral haemorrhages.

Time course and relapses

In untreated cases of the louse-borne disease, the first attack of fever resolves by crisis in 4 to 10 (average 5) days, whereas the initial fever in tick-borne disease lasts only about 3 days. There follows an afebrile remission of 5 to 9 days, and then a series of up to five relapses in louse-borne disease and up to 13 in tick-borne disease (Fig. 4). No petechial rash occurs during the relapses, which are generally less severe than the initial attack but may be associated with iritis or iridocyclitis and severe epistaxis.

Differences between louse-borne and tick-borne relapsing fever

The tick-borne disease is generally milder and less drawn out. The incidence of some symptoms and signs in the two diseases appears strikingly different. For example, in some series of cases, only 7 per cent of patients with tick-borne relapsing fever were jaundiced and neurological signs were more common than in the louse-borne disease.

Severe manifestations

These include myocarditis that presents as acute pulmonary oedema, liver failure, and severe bleeding attributable to thrombocytopenia, liver damage, and disseminated intravascular coagulation. Dysentery, salmonellosis, typhoid, typhus, malaria, and tuberculosis have been described in association with relapsing fever.

The spontaneous crisis and Jarisch–Herxheimer reaction

Whether or not treatment is given, an attack of relapsing fever usually ends dramatically. About 1 h after intravenous tetracycline, or on about the fifth day of the untreated illness, the patient becomes restless and apprehensive and suddenly begins to have distressingly intense rigors that last between 10 and 30 min. The ensuing phenomena have features of a classical endotoxin reaction. During the initial chill phase, temperature, respiratory and pulse rates, and blood pressure rise sharply. Delirium, gastrointestinal symptoms, cough, and limb pains are associated. Some patients die of hyperpyrexia at the peak of fever. The flush phase, which lasts several hours, is characterized by profuse sweating, a fall in blood pressure, and a slow decline in temperature. Deaths during this phase follow intractable hypotension or the development of acute pulmonary oedema and are attributable to myocarditis. The classical J-HR is in syphilis. Milder reactions have been described in Lyme disease and leptospirosis (treated with penicillin), sodoku (arsenicals), *Brucella melitensis* (tetracycline), and even in meningococcal infections.

Laboratory findings

Spirochaete densities may exceed 500 000/mm³ of blood. Other abnormalities include a moderate normochromic anaemia, neutrophil leucocytosis (with marked leucopenia during the spontaneous crisis or J-HR), thrombocytopenia, mild coagulopathy, biochemical evidence of hepatocellular damage (raised levels of aminotransferases, alkaline phosphatase, direct and total bilirubin, low albumin) and mild renal impairment. The cerebrospinal fluid shows a polymorph/lymphocyte pleocytosis without visible spirochaetes.

ECG evidence of myocarditis includes prolonged Q–Tc, T-wave abnormalities, and ST-segment depression with transient acute right heart strain after the J-HR. Chest radiographs show pulmonary oedema in some cases.

Diagnosis

In febrile patients, spirochaetes can usually be demonstrated in thin or thick blood films stained with Giemsa or Wright's stain and counterstained for 10 to 30 min with 1 per cent crystal violet (Plate 1), by dark-field examination or the quantitative buffy-coat technique. Towards the end of the attack, during remissions, and particularly in children with tick-borne disease, spirochaetaemia may not be detectable. In these cases, blood or CSF can be injected intraperitoneally into young mice which will develop spirochaetaemia within 14 days. Serological methods are not generally used, but LBRF has been diagnosed by the detection of antibodies to glycerophosphodiesterase from *B. recurrentis*. The serum of patients with relapsing fever may give positive reactions with *Proteus* OXK, OX19, and OX2 and false-positive serological responses for syphilis in 5 to 10 per cent of cases.

Differential diagnosis

In a febrile patient with jaundice, petechial rash, bleeding, and hepatosplenomegaly, the differential diagnosis will include falciparum malaria, yellow fever and other viral haemorrhagic fevers, viral hepatitis, rickettsial infections (especially louse-borne typhus), and leptospirosis. The diagnosis can be quickly confirmed by examining a blood smear, but the possibility of a complicating infection, particularly typhoid, should not be forgotten.

Prognosis

The mortality in treated cases is less than 5 per cent. During major LBRF epidemics, mortalities of 40 per cent or higher have been reported. Deaths during relapses are most unusual: they occur only in the tick-borne disease.

Treatment

Antimicrobials

Although TBRF is usually milder than the louse-borne variety, it is more difficult to treat because spirochaetes persist in tissues, such as the central nervous system and eye, and produce relapses. Oral tetracycline, 500 mg every 6 h for 10 days is, however, effective. Oral erythromycin can be given

(a)

(b)

(c)

(d)

Fig. 2 Splenic miliary abscesses in louse-borne relapsing fever. (a) Section of spleen at autopsy (copyright DA Warrell). (b) Biliary microabscesses as seen under the microscope; 71 × (Armed Forces Institute of Pathology photograph, negative number 75–8838). (c) Microabscesses involve both follicles and extrafollicular areas of the spleen, the pale area of extrafollicular necrosis is clearly demarcated from the surrounding pulp; 145 × (Armed Forces Institute of Pathology photograph, negative number 77326). (d) Warthin–Starry stain showing tangled masses of spirochaetes at the periphery of an abscess; 2280 × (Armed Forces Institute of Pathology photograph, negative number 77317).

to pregnant women (500 mg every 6 h for 10 days) and children (125–250 mg every 6 h for 10 days). In patients unable to swallow tablets, treatment can be initiated with 250 mg intravenous tetracycline hydrochloride or with 300 mg erythromycin lactobionate.

LBRF is readily cured with a single oral dose of 500 mg tetracycline or 500 mg erythromycin stearate. Few patients with severe louse-borne relapsing fever are able to swallow the tablets without vomiting them up: a more reliable treatment is a single intravenous dose of 250 mg tetracycline hydrochloride or, for pregnant women and children, a single intravenous dose of 300 mg erythromycin lactobionate (children 10 mg/kg body weight). In mixed epidemics of LBRF and louse-borne typhus a single oral dose of 100 mg doxycycline has been effective.

Benzylpenicillin (300 000 units), procaine penicillin with benzylpenicillin (600 000 units), and procaine penicillin with aluminium monostearate (600 000 units), all by intramuscular injection, have been used; but they may fail to prevent relapses, and the long-acting preparations produce only slow clearance of spirochaetaemia. Chloramphenicol is effective in TBRF in a dose of 500 mg every 6 h for 10 days in adults, and 250 mg every 6 h for

10 days in older children; and in louse-borne relapsing fever in a single dose of 500 mg by mouth or intravenous injection in adults.

Jarisch–Herxheimer reaction

Antimicrobials have reduced the mortality of relapsing fevers from between 30 and 70 per cent to less than 5 per cent; however, drugs such as tetracycline, which generally rapidly eliminate spirochaetes from the blood and prevent relapses, usually induce a severe J-HR that may occasionally prove fatal. Clearly, in a disease with such a high natural mortality, treatment cannot be withheld, especially as severe spontaneous crises, which may also prove fatal, occur in a large proportion of louse-borne cases after the fifth day of fever. There is no evidence, however, that the shorter and more intense reaction following tetracycline is more dangerous than the more prolonged but apparently milder reaction following slow-release penicillin. Treatment with hydrocortisone, in doses up to 20 mg/kg, and paracetamol does not prevent the reaction but reduces peak temperatures, hastens the fall in temperature, and lessens the fall in blood pressure during the flush phase. Pretreatment with oral prednisolone can prevent the J-HR of early syphilis; but in LBRF, neither an oral dose of 3 mg/kg prednisolone given 18 h beforehand nor an infusion of 3.75 mg/kg betamethasone prevented the reaction to tetracycline treatment. However, meptazinol, an opioid antagonist with agonist properties, diminishes the reaction when given in a dose of 100 mg by intravenous injection. The discovery of an explosive release of TNFα, IL-6, and IL-8 just before the start of the J-HR prompted the testing of a polyclonal ovine Fab anti-TNFα antibody. Infused for 30 min before treatment with intramuscular penicillin, this antibody suppressed the J-HR.

Supportive treatment

Patients must be nursed in bed for at least 24 h after treatment to prevent postural hypotensive collapse and the precipitation of fatal cardiac arrhythmias. Hyperpyrexia should be prevented with antipyretics and vigorous fanning with tepid sponging. Although patients with acute LBRF have an expanded plasma volume, most are dehydrated and relatively hypovolaemic. Adults may need 4 or more litres of isotonic saline intravenously during the first 24 h. Infusion should be controlled by monitoring jugular venous, central venous, or pulmonary artery wedge pressures. Acute myocardial failure may develop, particularly during the flush phase of the J-HR or spontaneous crisis. This is signalled by a rise in central venous pressure above 15 cm H_2O; 1 mg digoxin should be given intravenously over 5 to 10 min. Because of the intense vasodilatation, diuretics may accentuate the

Fig. 3 Liver in louse-borne relapsing fever. Congestion with prominent Kupffer cells and lymphocytic and neutrophil infiltrate predominantly in the central and mid-zonal areas; 500 × (Armed Forces Institute of Pathology photograph, negative number 75–6523)

Fig. 4 Temperature chart of J Everett Dutton who, with JL Todd, discovered the transmission of tick-borne relapsing fever in the Congo. Dutton contracted tick-borne relapsing fever at the beginning of November 1904. He had relapses of fever and spirochaetaemia on the 7 and 16 December and the 8 January 1905. His death on 27 February 1905 has been attributed by some, but not by Todd, to relapsing fever (Dutton JE, Todd JL (1905). The nature of human tick-fever in the eastern part of the Congo Free State with notes on the distribution and bionomics of the tick. *Liverpool School of Tropical Medicine Memoir XVII*).

circulatory failure by causing relative hypovolaemia. Oxygen should be given during the reaction, particularly in severe cases. Vitamin K should be given in all cases with prolonged prothrombin times. Heparin is not effective in controlling coagulopathy and should not be used. Complicating infections—typhoid, salmonellosis, bacillary dysentery, tuberculosis, typhus, and malaria—must be treated appropriately.

Control

No vaccines are available.

Delousing

Patients with LBRF are infectious until their louse-infested clothing is disinfected by heat, such as washing in water hotter than 60 °C, preferably followed by ironing. It is also recommended that infested people should wash their bodies with soap and a 1 per cent lysol (disinfectant) solution; however, most lice are attached to clothing not body hairs. These simple approaches are impracticable in epidemic situations and so insecticides are widely used for louse control. An insecticidal duster can be used to blow a 10 per cent DDT powder between the body and clothing. If DDT-resistant lice are present then dusts of 1 per cent malathion, 2 per cent temephos (Abate), 1 per cent propoxur, or 0.5 per cent permethrin can be used. Improved hygiene discourages lousiness, impregnation of clothing with a pyrethroid insecticide may give long-lasting protection against lice, and treated clothes may remain effective even after 6 to 8 washings. A study in Ethiopia demonstrated that treatment of cases of LBRF with antimicrobials was not effective in controlling an epidemic without the addition of vigorous delousing measures.

Tick control

Ticks should be searched for and removed. However, they usually feed for a short time and then detach and so are rarely found by the time the patient presents with tick-borne relapsing fever.

Ticks may be discouraged by insecticide-impregnated clothes or by applying repellents to the skin (for example, diethyltoluamide). Dwellings should be constructed with solid floors and walls to reduce tick infestation. Sleeping off the floor and under an insecticide-impregnated bed net can also reduce the risk of bites.

Tick control can be attempted by spraying buildings with insecticides such as pyrethroids, carbamates, and organophosphates and by reducing the numbers of rodent vectors.

Further reading

Bryceson ADM, *et al.* (1970). Louse-borne relapsing fever. A clinical and laboratory study of 62 cases in Ethiopia and a reconsideration of the literature. *Quarterly Journal of Medicine* **39**, 129–70.

Cutler SJ, *et al.* (1994). Successful *in-vitro* cultivation of *Borrelia duttonii* and its comparison with *Borrelia recurrentis*. *International Journal of Systematic Bacteriology* **49**, 1793–9.

Fekade D, *et al.* (1996). Prevention of the Jarisch–Herxheimer reactions by treatment with antibodies against tumor necrosis factor α. *New England Journal of Medicine* **335**, 311–15.

Felsenfeld O (1965). Borrelia, human relapsing fever and parasite–vector–host relationships. *Bacteriological Reviews* **29**, 46–74.

Felsenfeld O (1971). *Borrelia: strains, vectors, human and animal borreliosis.* WH Green, St Louis.

Negussie Y, *et al.* (1992). Detection of plasma tumor necrosis factor, interleukins-6 and -8 during the Jarisch–Herxheimer reaction of relapsing fever. *Journal of Experimental Medicine* **175**, 1207–12.

Scragg IG, Kwiatkowski D (2000). Structural characterization of the inflammatory moiety of a variable major lipoprotein of *Borrelis recurrentis*. *Journal of Biological Chemistry* **275**, 937–41.

Sundnes KO, Teklehaimanot A (1993). Epidemic of louse-borne relapsing fever in Ethiopia. *Lancet* **342**, 1213–15.

Trape JF, *et al.* (1991). Tick-borne borreliosis in West Africa. *Lancet* **337**, 473–5.

Udalova IA, *et al.* (2000). Direct evidence for involvement of NF-kappaB in transcriptional activation of tumor necrosis factor by a spirochetal lipoprotein. *Infection and Immunity* **68**, 5447–9.

Vidal V, *et al.* (1998). Variable major lipoprotein is a principal TNF-inducing factor of louse-borne relapsing fever. *Nature Medicine* **4**, 1416–20.

Warrell DA, *et al.* (1983). Pathophysiology and immunology of the Jarisch–Herxheimer like reaction in louse-borne relapsing fever: comparison of tetracycline and slow-release penicillin. *Journal of Infectious Diseases* **147**, 898–909.

Warrell DA, *et al.* (1970). Cardiorespiratory disturbance associated with infective fever in man: studies of Ethiopian louse-borne relapsing fever. *Clinical Science* **39**, 123–45.

7.11.31 Leptospirosis
George Watt

Leptospirosis is a worldwide zoonosis of the greatest public health importance in the tropics. Infection may be asymptomatic, but 5 to 15 per cent of cases are severe or fatal. Most cases go undiagnosed because symptoms and signs are often non-specific and serological confirmation is rarely available where most disease transmission occurs. Failure to diagnose leptospirosis is particularly unfortunate: severely ill patients often recover completely with prompt treatment but if therapy is delayed or not given, death or renal failure are likely to ensue.

Aetiology

The organism responsible is a tightly coiled spirochaete with an axial filament and hooked ends, 0.1 to 0.2 μm wide and 5 to 20 μm long. Leptospires are aerobic and travel with a corkscrew-like motion. Unstained organisms can be seen only by darkfield or phase-contrast microscopy. Silver staining is the method of choice for demonstrating leptospires in tissue specimens. The genus *Leptospira* contains two species: *Leptospira interrogans*, which is pathogenic, and *Leptospira biflexa*, which is saprophytic. Stable antigenic differences allow subclassification into serotypes, referred to in the literature as serovars (serovarieties). Antigens common to several serovars permit arrangement into broader serogroups. More than 200 serovars belonging to 23 serogroups have been identified for *L. interrogans*. Leptospirosis taxonomy is evolving and it has been proposed to establish five new species based on DNA relatedness.

Epidemiology

Measuring incidence by active surveillance confirms that leptospirosis is a surprisingly common disease. Antibody positivity rates of 37 per cent have been recorded in rural Belize and 23 per cent in Vietnam. More than 2527 human cases and 13 deaths were reported for the first 9 months of 1999 by the Ministry of Public Health in Thailand. Human leptospirosis is of significance in eastern and southern Europe, Australia, and New Zealand. In the United States, the disease is primarily of veterinary importance, with only 50 to 150 human cases reported annually.

Leptospires nest in the renal tubules of mammalian hosts and are shed in the urine. They can survive for several months in the environment under moist conditions, particularly in the presence of warmth (above 22 °C) and a neutral pH (pH 6.2 to 8.0). These conditions occur all year round in the tropics but only during the summer and autumn months in temperate climates. Roughly 160 animal species harbour organisms, but rodents are the most important reservoir. Carrier rates of over 50 per cent have been measured in Norway rats, which shed massive numbers of organisms for life without showing clinical illness. Some serovars appear to be preferentially adapted to select mammalian hosts. For example, the serovar icterohaemorrhagiae is primarily associated with the Norway rat, canicola with dogs, and pomona with swine and cattle. However, a particular host species may serve as a reservoir for one or more serovars and a particular serovar may be hosted by many different animal species.

The transmission of infection from animal to man usually occurs through contact with contaminated water or moist soil. Organisms enter man through abrasions of the skin or through the mucosal surface of the eye, mouth, nasopharynx, or oesophagus. Crowded Asian or Latin American cities that are flood-prone and have large rat populations provide ideal conditions for disease transmission. A outbreak in Nicaragua in 1995 and an urban epidemic in Salvador, Brazil in 1999 were associated with particularly heavy rains and flooding. Intense exposure to leptospires has been documented in rice, sugar cane, and rubber plantation workers. Less frequently, leptospirosis is acquired by direct contact with the blood, urine, or tissues of infected animals. Epidemiological patterns in the United States and United Kingdom have changed. Recreational exposure to fresh water (canoeing, sailing, water skiing) and animal contact at home have replaced occupational exposure as the chief source of disease.

Pathology and pathogenesis

Leptospires are disseminated by the blood and may be recovered from all organs within 48 h of entering the host. Leptospiraemia lasts from 4 to 7 days and ends when agglutinizing antibodies appear. Leptospires can persist for months in the kidneys and ocular tissue. Much of the pathogenesis of leptospirosis remains unexplained. There are only minor histopathological changes in the kidneys and livers of patients with marked functional impairment of these organs. Patients who survive severe leptospirosis have complete recovery of hepatic and renal function—consistent with the lack of structural damage to these organs.

Severely ill patients typically have marked leucocytosis but no leucocytic infiltrates in organs, a pattern produced by some toxins. Fatally infected animals and some human patients exhibit changes similar to those produced by the endotoxaemia of Gram-negative bacteraemia. An endotoxin-like substance is present in the cell wall of leptospires but lacks the ketodeoxyoctanoate of true endotoxin.

Kidney

Renal failure is the most common cause of death in leptospirosis. Leptospires are frequently found in human renal tissue, but their role in mediating kidney damage is unknown. Interstitial nephritis is found primarily in individuals who have survived until inflammation has had an opportunity to develop, but is frequently absent in patients with fulminant disease.

Impaired renal perfusion constitutes the fundamental nephropathic change. Oliguria is rapidly reversed by administration of intravenous fluid in many patients, suggesting that volume depletion is frequent. Hypovolaemia is multifactorial: insensible water loss, diarrhoea, vomiting, reduced fluid intake, and haemorrhage can all contribute. A defect in the kidney's ability to concentrate urine increases fluid loss while renal potassium wasting can lead to hypokalaemia. Widespread endothelial injury causes fluid to move from the intravascular to the extracellular space in some patients. Hypotension of cardiac origin is rare.

Liver

The pathogenesis of jaundice is unexplained; neither haemolytic anaemia nor hepatocellular necrosis are prominent features of leptospirosis. The most severe hepatic pathological changes are seen when organisms are difficult to demonstrate in tissue, suggesting subcellular toxic or metabolic insults.

Striated muscle

Myalgia is typical of early infection, and is presumably due to invasion of skeletal muscle by leptospires. Muscle biopsies in patients with early illness demonstrate vacuolation of the myofibrillar cytoplasm, loss of cellular detail, and fragmentation. Leptospiral antigen can be demonstrated by immunofluorescence within muscle tissue. Muscle pain resolves as antibody appears and organisms are cleared from the blood. Pathological changes are usually absent in muscle tissue from patients who have died, and myalgia is generally waning at the time of death.

Lungs

Localized or confluent haemorrhagic pneumonitis is the usual pulmonary finding, with petechial and ecchymotic haemorrhages noted throughout the lungs, pleura, and tracheobronchial tree. Early, life-threatening pulmonary haemorrhage has long been reported from Asia, and is now being increasingly recognized in Latin America. Necropsy findings include massive intra-alveolar haemorrhage with or without diffuse alveolar damage. Leptospires can be demonstrated in lung tissue.

Haemorrhage

A progressive severe haemorrhagic diathesis is a prominent feature of experimental leptospirosis. In humans, bleeding is generally restricted to the skin or mucosal surfaces, although occasionally massive gastrointestinal or pulmonary haemorrhage occurs. Coagulopathy and/or thrombocytopenia are common in leptospirosis but do not adequately explain bleeding. By exclusion, capillary damage is the postulated mechanism, and toxins have been suggested as the mediators of endothelial injury.

Meningitis

Organisms easily enter the cerebrospinal fluid during leptospiraemia, and this is thought to explain the high incidence of meningitis. However, signs of meningeal irritation are not due to the invasion of the meninges by leptospires, a process that elicits little reaction. Organisms are frequently isolated from cerebrospinal fluid that is otherwise normal and from individuals without clinically detectable involvement of the nervous system. Symptoms of meningitis coincide with the development of antibody and disappearance of leptospires from the blood and cerebrospinal fluid, suggesting an immunological mechanism. Pathological changes are minimal or absent, and the prognosis is excellent.

Heart

Focal haemorrhagic myocarditis has been reported, but hypovolaemia, electrolyte imbalance, and uraemia are more frequent causes of cardiac dysfunction. Minor electrocardiographic changes such as first-degree heart block are common and reversible.

Eye

The aqueous humour provides a protective environment for leptospires, which readily enter the anterior chamber of the eye during the leptospiraemic phase of the disease. There they can remain viable for months, despite the development of serum antibodies. Uveitis is common. Inflammation of the anterior uveal tract begins weeks or even months after the onset of disease and has been attributed to the persistence of organisms in the anterior chamber.

Clinical manifestations (see Table 1)

Subclinical infection is common and less than 10 per cent of symptomatic infections result in severe, icteric illness. Even relatively virulent serovars such as icterohaemorrhagiae lead more often to anicteric than to icteric disease. Old terms such as peapicker's disease, swineherd's disease, and

Table 1 The most common clinical manifestations of 208 leptospirosis patients in Puerto Rico. (Adapted from Diaz-Rivera RS *et al.* (1963). *Zoonosis Research* 2, 159)

Symptoms (% of cases)	Anicteric (106 cases)	Icteric (102 cases)
Fever	100	99
Myalgia	97	97
Headache	82	95
Chills	84	90
Sore throat	72	87
Nausea	71	81
Vomiting	65	75
Eye pain	54	38
Diarrhoea	23	30
Decreased urine	20	30
Cough	15	32
Haemoptysis	5	14
Signs (% of cases)		
Conjunctival injection	100	98
Muscle tenderness	70	79
Hepatomegaly	60	60
Pulmonary findings	11	36
Lymphadenopathy	35	12
Petechiae and ecchymoses	4	29

canicola fever, which linked specific serotypes with distinct disease manifestations, are misleading and should be abandoned. The median incubation period is 10 days, with a range of 2 to 26 days. The duration of the incubation period has no prognostic significance. Once symptoms develop, they are said to follow a biphasic course: After an initial febrile illness, there is defervescence of fever and symptomatic improvement, followed by a second period of disease. However, a clear demarcation between the first and second stages is atypical of icteric leptospirosis and in mild cases the distinction can be unclear, or the second stage may never occur. The diagnostic usefulness of a history of a biphasic illness has been overemphasized. HIV coinfection does not seem to affect the clinical presentation of leptospirosis in the few coinfected patients described thus far.

Anicteric leptospirosis

Symptoms and signs

The disease typically begins with the abrupt onset of intense headache, fever, chills, and myalgia. Fever often exceeds 40 °C (103 °F) and is preceded by rigors. Muscle pain can be excruciating and occurs most commonly in the thighs, calves, lumbosacral region, and abdomen. Abdominal wall pain accompanied by palpation tenderness can mimic an acute surgical abdomen. Nausea, vomiting, diarrhoea, and sore throat are other frequent symptoms. Cough and chest pain figure prominently in reports of patients from Korea and China.

Conjunctival suffusion is a helpful diagnostic clue which usually appears 2 or 3 days after the onset of fever and involves the bulbar conjunctiva. Pus and serous secretions are absent, and there is no matting of the eyelashes and eyelids. Mild suffusion can easily be overlooked. Less common and less distinctive signs include pharyngeal injection, splenomegaly, hepatomegaly, lymphadenopathy, and skin lesions.

Within a week most patients become asymptomatic. After several days of apparent recovery, the illness resumes in some individuals. Manifestations of the second stage are more variable and mild than those of the initial illness and usually last 2 to 4 days. Leptospires disappear from the blood, cerebrospinal fluid, and tissues but appear in the urine. Serum antibody titres rise—hence the term 'immune' phase. Meningitis is the hallmark of this stage of leptospirosis. Pleocytosis of the cerebrospinal fluid can be demonstrated in 80 to 90 per cent of all patients during the second week of illness, although only about 50 per cent will have clinical signs and symp-

toms of meningitis. Meningeal signs can last several weeks but usually resolve within a day or two. Uveitis is a late manifestation of leptospirosis, generally seen 4 to 8 months after the illness has begun. The anterior uveal tract is most frequently affected, and pain, photophobia, and blurring of vision are the usual symptoms.

Laboratory findings

The white blood cell count varies but neutrophilia is usually found. Urinalysis may show proteinuria, pyuria, and microscopic haematuria. Enzyme markers of skeletal muscle damage, such as creatine kinase and aldolase, are elevated in the sera of 50 per cent of patients during the first week of illness. Chest radiographs from patients with pulmonary manifestations show a variety of abnormalities, but none is pathognomonic of leptospirosis. The most common finding is small, patchy, snowflake-like lesions in the periphery of the lung fields.

Icteric leptospirosis (Weil's disease)

This dramatic, life-threatening illness is characterized by jaundice, renal dysfunction, haemorrhagic manifestations, and a high mortality rate. Though jaundice is the hallmark of severe leptospirosis, fatalities do not occur because of liver failure. The degree of jaundice has no prognostic significance, but its presence or absence does—virtually all leptospirosis deaths occur in icteric patients. Icterus first appears between the fifth and ninth days of illness, reaches maximum intensity 4 or 5 days later, and continues for an average of 1 month. Hepatomegaly is found in the majority of patients and hepatic percussion tenderness is a reliable clinical marker of continuing disease activity. There is no residual liver dysfunction in survivors of Weil's disease, consistent with the absence of structural damage seen on pathological examination of this organ.

Bleeding is occasionally seen in anicteric cases but is most prevalent in severe disease. Purpura, petechiae, epistaxis, bleeding of the gums, and minor haemoptysis are the most common haemorrhagic manifestations, but deaths occur from subarachnoid haemorrhage and exsanguination from gastrointestinal bleeding. Conjunctival haemorrhage is an extremely useful diagnostic finding, and when combined with scleral icterus and conjunctival suffusion, produces eye findings strongly suggestive of leptospirosis (see Fig. 1 and Plate 1). The frequency with which severe pulmonary haemorrhage complicates leptospirosis is variable, but is a cardinal feature of some outbreaks.

Life-threatening renal failure is a complication of icteric disease, though all forms of leptospirosis may be associated with mild kidney dysfunction. Oliguria or anuria usually develop during the second week of illness, but may appear earlier. Complete anuria is a grave prognostic sign, often seen in patients who present late in the course of illness with frank uraemia and

Fig. 1 Jaundice, haemorrhage, and conjunctival suffusion in acute leptospirosis. (See also Plate 1.)

irreversible disease. Because renal failure develops very quickly in leptospirosis, symptoms and signs of uraemia are frequently encountered. Anorexia, vomiting, drowsiness, disorientation, and confusion are seen early and progress rapidly to convulsions, stupor, and coma in severe cases. Disturbances of consciousness in a patient with severe leptospirosis are usually due to uraemic encephalopathy, whereas in anicteric cases aseptic encephalitis is the usual cause. Renal function eventually returns to normal in survivors of Weil's disease, through detectable abnormalities may persist for several months.

Laboratory features of Weil's disease

Hyperbilirubinaemia results from increases in both conjugated (direct) and unconjugated (indirect) bilirubin, but elevations of the direct fraction predominate. Prolongations of the prothrombin time occur commonly but are easily corrected by the administration of vitamin K; modest elevations of serum alkaline phosphatase are typical. There is mild hepatocellular necrosis; greater than fivefold increases of transaminase (aminotransferase) levels are exceptional.

Jaundiced patients usually have leucocytosis in the range of 15 000 to 30 000 per mm^3, and neutrophilia is constant. Anaemia is common and multifactorial; blood loss and azotaemia contribute frequently, intravascular haemolysis less often. Mild thrombocytopenia often occurs, but decreases in platelet count sufficient to be associated with bleeding are exceptional. The specific gravity of the urine is high. Hypokalaemia due to renal potassium wasting can occur.

Diagnosis

The diagnosis of leptospirosis is usually based on serology. The old commercially available microscopic slide agglutination test is being supplanted by a new generation of rapid serodiagnostic kits. Some enzyme-linked immunosorbent (EIA), agglutination, and immunofluorescent assays are very promising, although more data from prospective evaluations conducted in endemic areas are required. The need for practical, affordable diagnostic kits to be available in areas where leptospirosis is common cannot be overemphasized. The polymerase chain reaction and urine antigen detection are research tools which would be of greatest potential diagnostic value in patients who present early, before antibodies have reached detectable levels. The microscopic agglutination test is considered the serodiagnostic method of choice for leptospirosis, but its complexity limits its use to reference laboratories. Dilutions of patient sera are applied to a panel of live, pathogenic leptospires. The results are viewed under dark-field microscopy and expressed as the percentage of organisms cleared from the field by agglutination.

Isolation of leptospires from blood or cerebrospinal fluid is possible during the first 10 days of clinical illness, but specialized media are necessary. Serially diluted urine provides the highest yield. Unfortunately, culture results are only known 4 to 6 weeks later—too late to benefit hospitalized, severely ill patients.

Treatment

The approach to the patient with possible leptospirosis is summarized in Fig. 2. Placebo-controlled double-blind trials have proved that doxycycline benefits patients with early, mild leptospirosis, and that intravenous penicillin helps adults with severe, late disease. The outcome of severe, paediatric leptospirosis is also improved by penicillin therapy. Antibiotics should therefore be given to all patients with leptospirosis, regardless of age or when in their disease course they are seen. Doxycycline is given at doses of 100 mg orally twice a day for 1 week. Patients who are vomiting or are seriously ill require parenteral therapy. Intravenous penicillin G is administered as 1.5 million units every 6 h for 1 week. There is controversy regarding the occurrence of a Jarisch–Herxheimer reaction in leptospirosis. If present, it is much less prominent in leptospirosis than in other spiro-

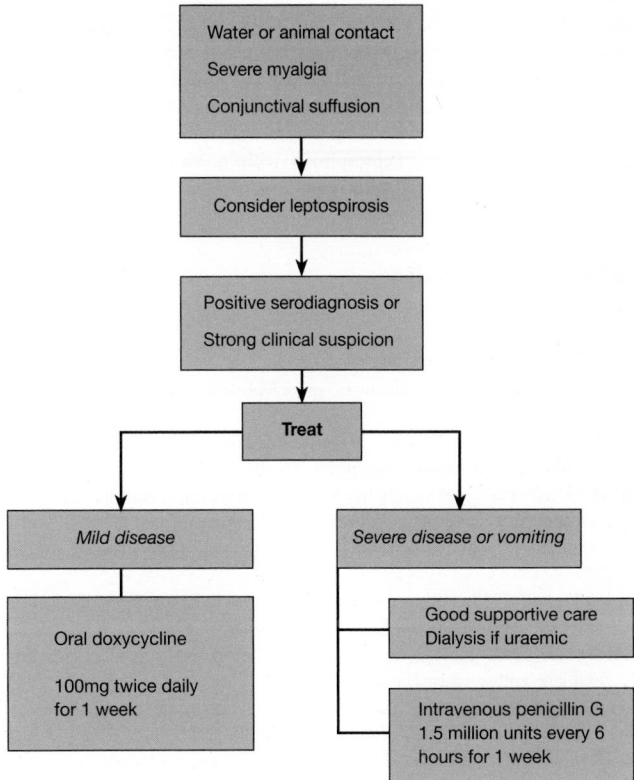

Fig. 2 Management of a febrile patient with possible leptospirosis.

chaetal illnesses. The important practical consideration is that antibiotics should not be withheld because of the fear of a possible Jarisch–Herxheimer reaction.

The management of pulmonary haemorrhage often requires prompt intubation and mechanical ventilation. Respiratory support to maintain adequate tissue oxygenation is essential because in non-fatal cases complete recovery of pulmonary function can be achieved. Ensuring adequate renal perfusion prevents renal failure in the vast majority of oliguric individuals. Peritoneal dialysis is preferred to haemodialysis; frequent dialyses may be necessary because renal failure in leptospirosis is hypercatabolic.

Prevention

Doxycycline, 200 mg taken once a week, prevents infection by *L. interrogans*. Widespread use of doxycycline prophylaxis is not indicated, but it can benefit those who are at high risk for a short time, such as military personnel and certain agricultural workers.

Infection by leptospires confers only serovar-specific immunity; second attacks due to different serovars can occur. The efficacy and safety of human leptospiral vaccines have yet to be conclusively demonstrated. Prevention of leptospirosis in the tropics is particularly difficult. The large animal reservoir of infection is impossible to eliminate, the occurrence of numerous serovars limits the usefulness of serovar-specific vaccine, and the wearing of protective clothing (e.g. rubber boots in rice fields) is both prohibitively expensive and impractical.

Prognosis

It is imperative to bring affordable tests to areas where leptospirosis is common because treatment (or lack of it) has a substantial impact on outcome. Atypical or mild cases are often confused with other entities such as aseptic meningitis, influenza, appendicitis, and gastroenteritis. Viral hepatitis is a common misdiagnosis in patients with Weil's disease. Leucocytosis, elevated serum bilirubin levels without marked transaminase elevations, and renal dysfunction are typical of leptospirosis but unusual in hepatitis. Malaria, typhoid fever, relapsing fever, scrub typhus, and Hantaan virus infection (haemorrhagic fever with renal syndrome) are important differential diagnoses in the tropics. Leptospirosis with prominent haemorrhagic manifestations is commonly misdiagnosed as dengue fever.

Further reading

Abdulkader RCRM *et al.* (1996). Peculiar electrolytic and hormonal abnormalities in acute renal failure due to leptospirosis. *American Journal of Tropical Medicine and Hygiene* **54**, 1–6.

Ko AI *et al.* (1999). Urban epidemic of severe leptospirosis in Brazil. *The Lancet* **354**, 820–5.

Marott PC *et al.* (1997). Outcome of leptospirosis in children. *American Journal of Tropical Medicine and Hygiene* **56**, 307–10.

Nicodemo AC *et al.* (1997). Lung lesions in human leptospirosis: microscopic, immunohistochemical, and ultrastructural features related to thrombocytopenia. *American Journal of Tropical Medicine and Hygiene* **56**, 181–7.

Sitprija V *et al.* (1980). Pathogenesis of renal disease in leptospirosis: clinical and experimental studies. *Kidney International* **17**, 827–36.

Watt G *et al.* (1988). Placebo controlled trial of intravenous penicillin for severe and late leptospirosis. *The Lancet* **1**, 433–5.

Zaki SR, Shieh WJ, the Epidemic Working Group. (1996). Leptospirosis associated with outbreak of acute febrile illness and pulmonary haemorrhage, Nicaragua. *The Lancet* **347**, 535–6.

7.11.32 Non-venereal endemic treponemoses: yaws, endemic syphilis (bejel), and pinta

P. L. Perine and D. A. Warrell

The endemic treponematoses are chronic, granulomatous diseases caused by spirochaetes belonging to the genus *Treponema*. Yaws occurs mainly in children living in rural areas in warm, humid climates in tropical countries. About 10 per cent of untreated cases develop late, disfiguring or crippling lesions of skin, bone, and cartilage.

Aetiology

Yaws is caused by *Treponema pallidum* ssp. *pertenue*, a spirochaete that is morphologically identical to *T. pallidum* ssp. *pallidum* (the cause of venereal syphilis) and *T. pallidum* spp. *endemicum* (the cause of non-venereal syphilis (bejel)), and to *T. carateum* (the cause of pinta). These treponemes share common antigens, so that infection by one species produces varying degrees of cross-immunity to the others. No serological test can differentiate the antibodies produced, and none of these organisms grows *in vitro*. The only means of differentiating yaws, syphilis, and non-venereal syphilis are their epidemiological characteristics and the pattern of infection produced in humans and experimentally infected laboratory animals (Table 1). Pathogenic treponemes can be differentiated at the molecular level by differences in the 5′- and 3′-flanking regions of their 15-kDa lipoprotein genes (*tpp*15).

The treponemes of yaws, syphilis, and pinta are fragile and readily killed by exposure to atmospheric oxygen, drying, mild detergents, or antiseptics. They prefer temperatures below 37 °C, which may explain their predilection for the skin and bones of the extremities. These organisms cannot penetrate intact skin, and gain entry to the body through small abrasions and lacerations.

Epidemiology (Table 1)

Yaws is transmitted by direct contact with an infectious lesion or by fingers contaminated with lesion exudate. It is enhanced by a crowded environment with poor sanitation and personal hygiene. The disease is usually acquired in childhood between the ages of 5 and 15. In endemic areas more than 80 per cent of the population are infected. In humid, warm environments the early lesion tends to proliferate and teems with spirochaetes, thus increasing the infectious reservoir; whereas in dry, arid climates or seasons the reverse is true.

There was a precipitous decrease in cases of yaws and other endemic treponematoses following mass penicillin-treatment campaigns during the 1950s and 1960s sponsored by the World Health Organization. An estimated 152 million people were examined and 46.1 million clinical cases, latent infections, and contacts were treated. The yaws reservoir was greatly reduced in West and Central Africa, Central and South America, and Oceania. However, over the past decade, yaws has been resurgent in the rural populations of Ecuador, the Ivory Coast, Ghana, Togo, Benin, Zaire, the Central African Republic, and Ethiopia in Africa, and in the island nations in the Pacific. Several nations initiated new campaigns of mass treatment during the 1980s.

Some African nations, such as Nigeria, previously rendered yaws-free by mass treatment campaigns, have also experienced a sharp rise in the incidence of venereal syphilis, perhaps representing a decline of herd immunity to yaws, and thereby to syphilis.

Endemic syphilis is transmitted by non-venereal contact among children. In contrast to yaws, transmission of infection by contaminated drinking vessels may be more common than by direct contact with infectious lesions. The disease tends to be familial, with spread of infection from children to adults rather than to the community in general. Endemic syphilis lesions are virtually indistinguishable from early yaws, and the two diseases may occur at different times in the same population but not in the same person. Venereal syphilis can be acquired by children through social contact with adults suffering from venereal syphilis, and then be spread by non-venereal, person-to-person contact if levels of sanitation and personal hygiene are low.

The Sahelian nations of Mauritania, Mali, Niger, Burkina Faso, and Senegal have reported dramatic increases in the number of cases of endemic syphilis. In Naimey (Niger), seroprevalence was 12 per cent among children under 5 years of age. The disease is also prevalent among the nomadic tribes of the Arabian peninsula, where late complications such as osteoperiostitis predominate.

Several variants of endemic syphilis are recognized by their geographical distribution: bejel of the Eastern Mediterranean, North Africa, and Niger; and njovera or dichuchwa of Africa; Bejel is the only type of endemic syphilis still prevalent. It is found in mainly seminomadic people such as the Tuareg living in the Saharan regions of Africa. Pinta is found only in remote parts of Central and South America, principally in the semiarid region of the Tepalcatepec Basin of southern Mexico and focal areas of Colombia, Peru, Ecuador, and Venezuela.

Pathogenesis

The lesion of yaws and the other treponematoses are due largely to the host's immune response to the treponeme. None of these treponemes carries or produces toxic substances. They have the ability to invade living cells without causing apparent injury. Cell destruction and tissue damage are

Table 1 Major features of the treponematoses

Feature	Venereal syphilis	Yaws	Endemic syphilis	Pinta
Organism*	T. pallidum, ssp. pallidum	T. pallidum, ssp. pertenue	T. pallidum, ssp. endemicum	T. carateum
Age of infection (years)	5–10	5–15	2–10	10–30
Occurrence	Worldwide	Africa, South America, Oceania, Asia	Africa, Middle East	Central, South America
Climate	All	Warm, humid	Dry, arid	Warm, rural
Transmission				
Direct:				
venereal	Common	No	Rare	No
non-venereal	Rare	Common	Rare	Common
congenital	Yes	No	Unproven	No
Indirect:				
contaminated utensils	Rare	Rare	Common	No
Insects	No	Rare	No	No
Reservoir of infection	Adults	Infectious and latent cases; ?non-human primates	Infectious and latent cases	
Infectious cases				
Ratio infectious: latent cases	1:3	1:3–5	1:2	?
Late complications:				
Skin	+	+	+	+
Bone, cartilage	+	+	+	No
Neurological	+	No	Unproven	No
Cardiovascular	+	No	Unproven	No

probably due to the action of immune cells that injure normal tissue in the process of killing treponemes.

Host immunity reaches its highest level after several months of infection, just before disseminated lesions heal and latency begins. Thereafter the host is immune to reinfection and is not contagious, but since not all treponemes are killed, infectious lesions may reappear as immunity wanes over time. Most patients with yaws experience two or three infectious relapses during the first 5 years of infection.

In venereal, and possibly endemic, syphilis, infection is systemic and late lesions may develop in any organ or tissue of the body. In yaws, *T. pertenue* produce lesions only in skin and osseous tissue, although it is certain that periodically the organism spreads systemically; *T carateum* resides only in the skin. This peculiar tissue tropism is unexplained. It is probably an inherent property of the treponeme, acting in contact with climatic factors.

Clinical features

Like venereal syphilis, the clinical course of yaws and endemic syphilis have primary, secondary, and tertiary or late stages, separated by quiescent or latent periods.

The initial lesion in yaws usually appears on the extremities after an incubation period of 3 to 5 weeks. Characteristically it is a papule; a painless lesion that appears at the site of infection, enlarges, forming a raspberry-like ('framboesia'), vegetative lesion called a papilloma. The papilloma is round to oval, elevated and not indurated, ranging in size from 1 to 3 cm in diameter. The surface teems with spirochaetes and is often covered by a thin yellow crust, which is easily removed. The papilloma may ulcerate as it enlarges and becomes secondarily infected with other micro-organisms. Lymph nodes draining the initial lesion may enlarge and become tender, but systemic symptoms are rare.

Secondary or disseminated papillomas appear after 2 to 6 months, often without an intervening latent period, on the skin of moist areas such as the axillas, joint flexures, genitalia, and the gluteal cleft (Fig. 1). They also occur on the soles and palms and, because they are tender, may interfere with gait and use of the hands. Papillomas in different stages of development persist for 6 to 8 months and heal without scars unless they become secondarily infected. Despite the size and number of lesions, children with generalized papillomas experience little discomfort or other constitutional symptoms.

Slightly raised, scaly, pigmented, macular yaws lesions measuring between 1 and 4 cm in diameter commonly occur when the climate is dry and arid. These lesions have the same distribution as papillomas and may appear together with lesions of different morphology in the same patient (maculopapular yaws).

The periosteum and osseous tissue of the bones of the extremities are frequently inflamed during early yaws, causing swelling, night-pain, and tenderness. There is dactylitis of the proximal phalanges. Painful osteoperiostitis of the legs, affecting mainly the tibias and fibulas, is especially common. Hypertrophic osteitis of the maxilla, either side of the bridge of the nose, can cause grotesque swellings ('goundo'). Scaly, tender, hyperkeratotic lesions of the palms and soles also occur and may be incapacitating. Hyperkeratotic and bone lesions are not contagious, and macular lesions are only minimally so.

Fig. 1 Early ulceropapillomatous yaws. (Copyright PL Perine.)

One or more relapses of secondary-type lesions usually occur during the first 5 years of infection, each separated by a period of latency. Late yaws' lesions occur thereafter in about 10 per cent of untreated cases.

Late yaws' lesions are not infectious because they contain few treponemes. Cutaneous plaques produce atrophic scars; subcutaneous, granulomatous nodules erode skin and produce deep ulcers that destroy underlying tissue and disfigure. Hyperkeratotic palmar and plantar yaws are incapacitating and often prevent use of the hands, or the ability to walk normally. The weight is placed on the sides of the feet, which produces a gait much like that of a crab ('crab' yaws; Fig. 2).

The granulomas of late yaws have a histological appearance like the gummas of syphilis. These proliferative lesions may involve the palate and destroy the soft tissues of the nose, causing a terrible disfiguration called gangosa (Fig. 3). Gummatous periostitis of the skull, fingers, and long

Fig. 2 Planter papillomas with hyperkeratotic, macular, early plantar yaws ('crab yaws'); these lesions are painful. (Copyright PL Perine.)

Fig. 3 Gangosa (rhinopharyngitis mutilans) of endemic syphilis and yaws in an adolescent child. (Copyright PL Perine.)

bones is erosive and often retards or stops growth. Active periostitis is occasionally found in young and middle-aged adults who had yaws in childhood.

The initial lesions of endemic syphilis usually appear at the mucocutaneous borders of the mouth or on the oral mucous membranes (mucous patches) as the result of transmission by contaminated drinking vessels. Late ulceronodules and osteoperiostitis are seen in late endemic syphilis, but cardiovascular and neurological complications are extremely rare.

In pinta, the initial papule appears on the skin of the extremities and enlarges slowly over a period of several weeks or months to form an erythematous plaque. Satellite papules form at the edge of the lesion and undergo a similar type of evolution. The plaques coalesce to form violaceous, pigmented plaques that, in several years, slowly depigment from lighter shades of blue to white, leaving atrophic depigmented scars.

Ulceronodular skin lesions of yaws and endemic syphilis resemble tropical ulcers. Yaws' lesions are not as painful, necrotic, nor as deep as tropical ulcers, which are usually singular and restricted to the lower one-third of the leg.

Plantar warts are frequently confused with plantar papillomas of yaws, and both conditions may occur in the same patient.

Diagnosis

The diagnosis of yaws is made by a combination of clinical assessment, of positive dark-ground examination of lesions, and of reactive serological tests for syphilis.

The diagnosis of early yaws, or endemic syphilis, is not difficult in endemic areas where the disease is familiar. The most difficult diagnostic problem arises when a person who had yaws as a child emigrates to an area of the world where the disease never existed. Such a person usually has reactive serological tests for syphilis and may have a few atrophic scars suggestive of earlier infection. What are the chances that this patient has or has had venereal syphilis? Should he be treated for latent yaws or syphilis?

The patient's social and medical history should be carefully reviewed. Clinical findings suggestive of old yaws (scars, inactive tibial periostitis), and the absence of signs of congenital and venereal syphilis support the diagnosis of inactive or treated yaws.

If the patient has a reagin titre of less than 1:8 dilutions, they probably do not have active latent yaws or syphilis. If they received at least one therapeutic dose of long-acting penicillin in their native country during a yaws campaign, they require no further treatment. On the other hand, if the patient is a contact of a case of infectious venereal syphilis, they should be treated as being potentially infected with syphilis, because *T.p. pallidum* occasionally superinfects people who had yaws as children. If treatment is given, the patient should receive a certificate stating the drug and dosage used and the results of their serological tests to prevent unnecessary future treatment.

Treatment and prevention

Long-acting benzylpenicillin given by intramuscular injection is the recommended treatment for all the endemic treponematoses. The preparation used in previous mass treatment campaigns was penicillin aluminium monostearate (**PAM**), but benzathine penicillin is currently recommended because it is longer acting and more readily available than is PAM. Active infections and non-infectious cases should be given 1.2 mega units in a single intramuscular injection; children under 10 years of age receive 0.6 mega units. Patients allergic to penicillin may be given tetracycline or erythromycin, 500 mg by mouth four-times daily for 2 weeks; children under 10 years of age should be given erythromycin in dosages adjusted for their age. Treatment failures have been reported in Papua New Guinea.

Prevention of yaws in a community requires elimination of the reservoir of infection, often by treating the entire population with penicillin.

Further reading

Centurion-Lara A, *et al.* (1998). The flanking region sequences of the 15-kDa lipoprotein gene differentiate pathogenic treponemes. *Journal of Infectious Diseases* **177**, 1036–40.

Engelkens HJ, Vuzevski VD, Stolz E (1999). Non-venereal treponematoses in tropical countries. *Clinics in Dermatology* **17**, 105–6, 143–52.

Guthe T (1969). Clinical, serological and epidemiological features of framboesia tropica (yaws) and its control in rural communities. *Acta Dermatologica-Venerologia*, Stockholm, **49**, 343–68.

Hackett CJ, Loewenthal LJA (1960). *Differential diagnosis of yaws*. World Health Organization, Geneva.

Paris JL (2000). Treponemal infections in the pediatric population. *Clinics in Dermatology* **18**, 687–700.

Perine PL, *et al.* (1984). *Handbook of endemic treponematoses*. World Health Organization, Geneva.

Walker SL, Hay RJ (2000). Yaws—a review of the last 50 years. *International Journal of Dermatology* **39**, 258–60.

7.11.33 Syphilis

D. J. M. Wright and S. E. Jones

Definition

Venereal syphilis is a systemic, contagious disease of great chronicity, caused by *Treponema pallidum*, and capable of congenital transmission. The natural host is man. The incubation period is around 3 weeks, at the end of which a primary sore develops at the site of inoculation, usually on the genitalia, associated with regional lymphadenitis. In most patients, this is followed by the secondary bacteraemic stage characterized by a symmetrical rash, generalized lymphadenopathy, and other lesions. After a latent period of many years, in 40 per cent of cases a destructive late stage develops involving the skin, mucous membranes, skeleton, central nervous system, eyes, hearing, and, especially, the aorta. Any of these stages may be absent or inapparent. Venereal syphilis, unlike non-venereal syphilis, is distributed world-wide.

Bacterial taxonomy

T. pallidum is a bacterium which causes venereal syphilis and the non-venereal, endemic childhood syphilis, bejel and njovera. Other pathogenic treponemes include *T. pertenue* (yaws) and *T. carateum* (pinta). Although these spirochaetes produce distinct diseases, molecular techniques have not yet been able to demonstrate consistent differences in their genomic DNA.

There are a number of non-pathogenic treponemes (*T. denticola* etc.) in the mouth which are difficult to distinguish from *T. pallidum*. For that reason dark-field examination of samples from mouth lesions should be avoided because of the danger of misdiagnosis. Other treponemes of low pathogenicity (e.g. *T. balanitides*) reside in the genital tract and, together with fusiform bacilli, can under anaerobic conditions superinfect genital lesions producing 'fusospirochaetosis'.

The completed sequence of the 1.14 Mb genome of *T. pallidum* (website 1) revealed that this parasitic spirochaete had few sets of enzymes for basic metabolic processes—as expected, since *T. pallidum* has remained unculturable *in vitro*. Transporter systems (for amino acids, carbohydrates, and cations) comprise 5 per cent of the genome, and the lack of genes coding for protection from oxygen-derived free radicals indicates that *T. pallidum* will only survive in oxygen-depleted conditions.

T. pallidum is a delicate, motile spiral organism, 6 to 15 μm long and 0. 15 μm wide which renders it below the level of resolution of light micro-

Table 1 *Borrelia* and *Treponema* compared

Characteristic	Borrelia	Treponema
Length (mm)	7–24	4–19
Width (mm)	0.2–0.5	0.15–0.3
Wavelength (mm)	1.7–3.3	0.5–1.8
Number of flagella	7–30[a]	1–9
Cytoplasmic tubules	–	–
Mode of division	septum	constriction
Romanowsky stain	+	–
Arthropod borne	+	–
Genome size	1.6 Mb	1.4 Mb
Open reading frames	1620[b]	1041[b]
Plasmids	+ (21)	

[a] Seven flagella have been found in isolates of *Borrelia burgdorferi*.

[b] 476 open reading frames(46 per cent) in *T. pallidum* have orthologues in *B. burgdorferi*, including 115 open reading frames which encode proteins of unknown function; 50 per cent of these (57 open reading frames) are unique to spirochaetes (by database analysis).

scopy and hence the need for dark-field or phase contrast illumination. It has an outer membrane, an electron-dense layer, and a cytoplasmic membrane. As with other bacteria, the cell wall has a trilaminar structure, the inner membrane constituting of a cytoplasmic membrane, while between the outer two layers there are axial filaments, structurally analogous to bacterial flagella, which wind around the axis of the organism and may be responsible for the motility of *T. pallidum*. All treponemes have not more than nine axial filaments, which distinguishes treponemes from borrelia (Table 1). *T. pallidum* has the unique ability of being able to bend in the middle to form a V-shape, if suspended in a medium of low viscosity. Motility does not necessarily indicate viability as mobile *T. pallidum* have been observed after they have been retained for 90 days in capillary tubes. *T. pallidum* may remain infective for up to a week in 'survival media' and, depending on the nature of the media, show limited multiplication; however, attempts at reproducible subculture of the microbe have to date been unsuccessful. Low concentrations of oxygen (between 3 and 5 per cent) may enhance survival. In practice, *T. pallidum* is propagated in rabbits.

Experimental inoculation of *T. pallidum* into man or animals shows that the organism divides every 30 to 32 h, suggesting approximate infective dose are between 10^6 and 10^7 organisms and an average incubation period of 3 weeks. Peptidoglycan in the inner layer of the bacterial membrane accounts for its susceptibility to penicillin. The phospholipids in the outer membrane, of which cardiolipin is the most prominent hapten, provides the antigenic basis for the synthetically substituted VDRL (Venereal Disease Reference Laboratory (test)) used as a serological test for syphilis. Flagella antigen reacts non-specifically with antibodies found in most known sera.

Origin of syphilis

Clinical differences between treponematoses have been explained as an adaptation of the organism to changing climatic factors, especially humidity and temperature, and with improvement in hygiene, the wearing of clothes, and less frequent intimate contacts between children. Yaws is found throughout the tropical belt, while pinta was forced to retreat into remote indigenous communities in South and Central America. Non-venereal childhood syphilis, such as bejel and similar conditions, was formerly found in more temperate climes including the Middle East, Yugoslavia, British Isles, Scandinavia, and South Africa. The lack of congenital transmission of these venereal treponematoses arose because they were essentially childhood infections and by the time these children were old enough to have their own offspring, the disease had become non-infectious. The treponeme causing venereal syphilis was perhaps an adaptation to people wearing clothes, when it was obliged to seek shelter in the protected, warm, and moist regions of the genitalia, so becoming sexually transmitted. It spread throughout the world as an adult disease and, because there appears to be no solid cross-immunity, may coexist with non-venereal treponematoses.

This adaptive theory fails to explain why *T. pallidum, sensu stricto*, unlike the other treponematoses, involves the central nervous system, aorta, and visceral organs and why, at the end of the fifteenth century, the virulent venereal form swept through Europe and Asia, eventually to become the milder modern syphilis. The alternative Columbian theory suggests that Columbus introduced this new disease from the Caribbean islands.

There are no definite descriptions of syphilis before this time. The finding of skeletons with long bone lesions compatible with syphilis, centuries before the fifteenth century epidemic of syphilis, remains speculative, though Boylston (reviewed by Morton (2001)) has reported syphilitic changes in the bones of pre-1450 skeletons found in Hull. The lack of such skeletons from America makes the relationship with the coincidental discovery of America and the advent of 'new world' syphilis even more doubtful.

The recognition of the contagious nature of the disease was recorded in 1530 by Fracastro. Klebs ultimately proved the infectivity of syphilis by reproducing syphilitic lesions by inoculating of syphilitic tissue into rabbits. The use of a prolonged Giemsa stain, allowed Schaudinn finally to identify the treponemes in 1905.

Epidemiology (see also Chapter 21.1)

Transmission

Sexual transmission is the rule in adult patients. The untreated patient remains infective for 4 years after acquiring the infection. Asexual transmission by close contact with an open lesion of early acquired or congenital syphilis is rare, as is direct blood transfusion with blood from an infectious individual or contact with infected fomites. Congenital syphilis still remains a problem, except in Northern Europe.

Incidence

There has been a steady decline in the incidence of syphilis in the West since the 1850s, interrupted only by major wars. Since 1940, there has been a 99 per cent drop in admissions of general paresis of the insane and congenital syphilis in the United States, with similar trends in the United Kingdom and Europe. There has also been a sharp reduction in all other forms of late syphilis. Gumma have almost disappeared. Early syphilis has not declined to the same degree since the Second World War. In the United States, syphilis reached a low in 1956, with 6576 reported cases but by 1992 had risen to 83 902 acquired cases. The introduction of health measures is reflected in the recent fall in the number of cases. A similar pattern is also found in most European countries. During the 1970s and 1980s, there was a steady increase in the number of cases of early syphilis. In the Russian Federation, where there has been a breakdown in public health, up to 1 per cent of the population has been affected by syphilis, especially around St Petersburg and Moscow. In 1980, 58 per cent of cases of syphilis in the United Kingdom were in homosexuals.

Since that time, the United Kingdom and American rates have diverged. The appearance of AIDS and the national programmes for 'safe sex' has resulted in the annual number of cases of infectious syphilis falling to 337 in the United Kingdom in 1993, most of the recent infections being acquired heterosexually abroad. In the United States, however, despite the fall in the number of homosexual males infected, the number of cases of syphilis has continued to rise, especially in the underprivileged Afro-American and Hispanic community and among HIV-infected drug abusers. In 1992, there were approximately 34 000 cases of primary and secondary syphilis, and 3850 cases of congenital syphilis in children under the age of 2 years, compared with 1986 when only 57 such cases were recorded in the United States. The failure of the Public Health Service in the United States to cope is reflected in the resurgence of congenital syphilis. Following the public health initiative in the United States, started in 1997,

the number of cases of primary and secondary syphilis reported for 2000 was 5979, while congenital syphilis had fallen to 529 cases. The comparative number of cases of syphilis seen in the genitourinary medicine clinics in England and Wales in 2000 was 328. In other parts of the world, notably in the Far East, infected prostitutes may play a central role in the spread of early syphilis. Estimates by the World Health Organization suggest that there are 10 to 20 million cases of syphilis each year.

The changing clinical presentation of syphilis

There is some clinical evidence that syphilis is becoming milder and less typical. This has been especially noted in neurosyphilis and the virtual disappearance of the gumma. The widespread use of antibiotics for unrelated conditions may be responsible. This is supported by finding that meningo-vascular syphilis has not shown the dramatic decrease of general paresis of the insane and tabes dorsalis, possibly because the last two conditions take many more years to develop, giving cumulative chances of antibiotics being given. It is also possible that the disease is tending to become milder and less typical as a result of 'natural' changes which appear to have started long before the antibiotic era. For whatever reasons, syphilis is apparently becoming clinically less clear-cut. Its exclusion by serology and other tests becomes more important in patients attending the dermatologist, neurologist, ophthalmologist, the ENT specialist, or cardiologist with conditions of uncertain pedigree.

The advent of AIDS has led to a re-examination of the progression and manifestations of concomitant syphilis. Although a variety of unusual syphilitic rashes, in particular more ulcerating multiple chancres and florid secondary rashes, have been described in association with HIV infections, all of them are recorded in the older literature. The suggestions that there might be an increase in syphilitic meningovascular relapse in patients with HIV infections, again may reflect the natural history of syphilis, since approximately 20 per cent of patients with early syphilis have a pleocytosis in the cerebrospinal fluid. If these patients are untreated, about one-fifth develop neurosyphilis. The high prevalence of syphilis in HIV patients leads to an apparent, rather than a real, increase in syphilis complications. Holtom, in California, found that in patients partially treated for syphilis with concomitant HIV infections, about 9 per cent developed a pleocytosis and 1 per cent then developed neurological disease. Unlike mycobacterial infections where unusual presentations of tuberculosis occur in patients with AIDS, the presentation of early neurosyphilis seems to be characteristic of the disease. This is possibly because the vasculitis of syphilis is not due to the cellular immune response but to the adherence of the spirochaete to the endothelial layer of the blood vessel. The blood vessel first becomes more permeable and subsequently there is proliferation of this layer. Simultaneously, the spirochaete induces a cellular infiltrate. These changes lead to endarteritis, which is the hallmark of the disease. What is true is that syphilitic relapses do not occur despite the potential for the persistence of spirochaetes (see below) and that benzathine penicillin G is less effective in eliminating spirochaetes (see below) in patients with altered immunity. Any persistence of cerebrospinal fluid pleocytosis in the neurosyphilitic patient with HIV after adequate penicillin treatment should lead to an investigation of causes of meningitis other than syphilis. However, doubt has been cast as to whether eradication of spirochaetes always occurs in the non-immunocompromised patient. Wilner and Brody found that one-third of the patients with a syphilitic encephalitis (general paresis of the insane) who had been followed for 30 years, developed neurological signs at the end of the period, despite having had 'adequate' penicillin therapy. Only 7 per cent of the non-syphilitic control group of demented patients, evinced new neurological signs. These were presumably due to cerebrovascular degenerative disease. Even in the pre-AIDS era, Rothenberg, when he reviewed the efficacy of penicillin in the treatment of neurosyphilis, found that it was not always effective. Lastly, laboratory experiments show that it is more likely that syphilis has a deleterious effect on the progression of AIDS rather than the reverse.

Sex and race

Early syphilis is less florid in women than men and is almost asymptomatic during pregnancy. Cardiovascular syphilis is at least twice as common in men than women, where it is more severe and appears earlier. Neurosyphilis is always more common in men than women. The reasons for these differences are not known.

Caucasians suffer more commonly from neurosyphilis than black Africans and they in turn are much more prone to develop cardiovascular syphilis than Caucasians.

Infectivity

The estimated figure for infectivity varies but is commonly assumed to be around 50 per cent for both homosexual and heterosexual patients. After a single exposure the figure is nearer 25 per cent.

Some control measures

The main reason for increased case identification is the more intensive use of serological tests for syphilis. Another valuable control measure is contact tracing, which varies greatly in different countries, but should be standard practice everywhere. Its use across international borders should be developed with proper safeguards to preserve confidentiality. This has proved especially useful in tracing networks of infection seen in the United Kingdom in recent years, such as the mini-outbreaks in Bristol (1999) and Manchester (2000). The application of social network analysis often traces more sexual contacts than direct partner notifications. Other measures which should prove valuable are the education of the young without inducing anxiety, information about sexually transmitted diseases on internet sex clubs, the education of doctors, and the encouragement of regular checkups of high-risk individuals, such as homosexual men and prostitutes. A more controversial suggestion is to treat contacts of infectious syphilis epidemiologically in certain situations, for example promiscuous individuals, known defaulters, and those who may infect their regular consort if not treated. In England and Wales, during the years 1995 to 2000, 425 such contacts were so treated in genitourinary (STD) clinics (PHLS and DHSS Report, 2001). These measures can be expected to uncover up to 75 per cent of all cases of syphilis.

Persistence of treponemal forms

Persistence of *T. pallidum*-like forms in the cerebrospinal fluid, aqueous humour, lymph nodes, and other tissues in penicillin-treated patients with late or late latent syphilis has been reported from several centres.

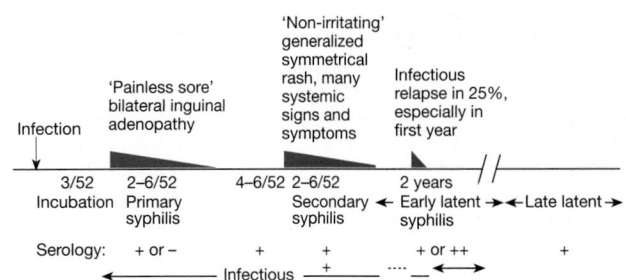

*Pregnant women may infect the fetus in early latency and during the early part of late latency

Fig. 1 The course of untreated, early-acquired syphilis.

The natural course of untreated syphilis

T. pallidum penetrates the abraded skin and intact mucous membrane. Within hours it has disseminated via the bloodstream and lymphatics and is beyond any effective local treatment. The incubation period is traditionally given as 9 to 90 days but in practice it is around 3 weeks (range, 2 to 6 weeks). The time depends on the size of the inoculum, sexual practice, and hygienic measures. A single treponeme leads to the longest incubation period. The primary lesion develops at the site of contact and heals in 2 to 6 weeks. In a proportion of patients, a secondary stage appears 6 weeks after the primary lesion has healed but there may be an overlap of the healing primary and the onset of the secondary stage. In some cases, the period between these stages can be prolonged to several months. The main characteristic of the secondary stage is a generalized, symmetrical, painless, and non-irritating rash. In about 20 per cent of cases, infectious relapses occur during the following year (range, 1 to 4 years). In the rest, the latent symptomatic period follows and may persist for life in at least 60 per cent. In 30 to 40 per cent, a third, late destructive stage develops. Its more benign form involves only the skin, mucous membranes, and bones. In the serious form, the central nervous system, aorta, and other internal organs are affected. The major events are shown in Figs 1 and 2.

Clinical features

Primary syphilis

The first sign is a small, painless papule which rapidly ulcerates. The ulcer (chancre) is usually solitary, round or oval, painless, and often indurated

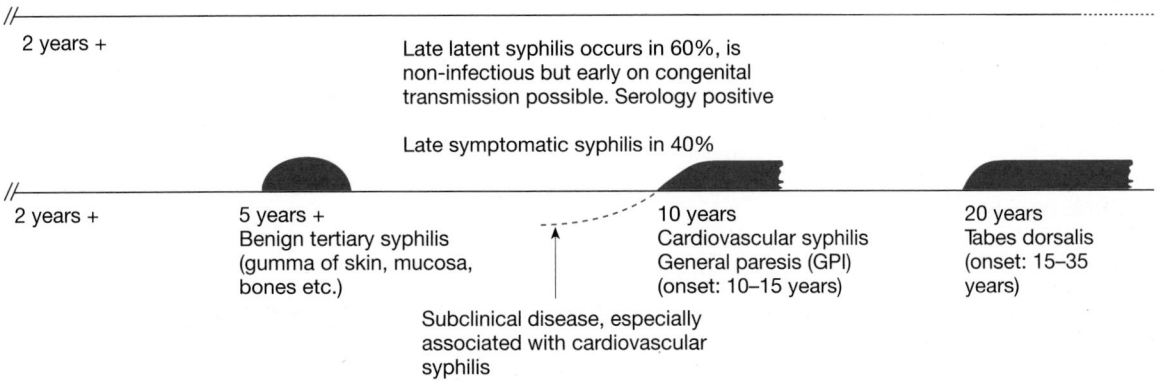

Fig. 2 The course of untreated, late-acquired syphilis. Asymptomatic neurosyphilis is present in 20 per cent and 20 per cent of these develop clinical neurosyphilis. Cardiovascular syphilis starts subclinically many years earlier and when clinically apparent, it is in fact in an advanced state. Prognosis: gumma heals spontaneously in a few years. Cardiovascular syphilis is usually fatal without treatment. Neurosyphilis: general paresis has a poor prognosis without treatment, meningovascular syphilis commonly responds well to penicillin, tabes progresses slowly but penicillin has no obvious influence. Overall mortality of untreated syphilis: 20 to 30 per cent.

Fig. 3 Large primary sore. Note the even shape and the absence of secondary infection.

(Fig. 3). It is surrounded by a bright red margin. It is not usually secondarily infected, a feature of all open syphilitic lesions of any stage. *T. pallidum* can be demonstrated in the serum from the sore which is easily obtained after slightly abrading the base. In heterosexual men, the common sites are the coronal sulcus, the glans, and inner surface of the prepuce but may be found on the shaft of the penis and beyond. In homosexual men, the ulcer is usually present in the anal canal, less commonly in the mouth and genitalia. In women, most chancres occur on the vulva, the labia, and, more rarely, the cervix where they are liable to be overlooked.

Extragenital chancres usually involve the lips, where they become large and associated with some oedema. Other sites are the mouth, buttocks, and fingers. The regional lymph nodes are invariably enlarged a few days after the appearance of the chancre and with genital sores the lymph nodes are bilaterally involved. They are painless, discrete, firm, and not fixed to surrounding tissues.

Atypical primary sores are not uncommon and depend on the size of the inoculum and the immunological status of the patient; thus a small inoculum usually produces a small, atypical ulcer or papule and looks trivial. This may also be the case in patients who had previously treated syphilis and the lesion may be dark-field negative.

Histologically, the chancre shows perivascular infiltration with plasma cells and histiocytes, capillary proliferation and obliterative endarteritis and periarteritis. The affected lymph nodes contain numerous treponemes, a depletion of lymphocytes, follicular hyperplasia, and histiocytic infiltration. If *T. pallidum* cannot be recovered from the primary sore, it may possibly be demonstrated from a needle aspirate of the regional lymph node.

Differential diagnosis (see also Chapter 23.1)

All genital sores must be regarded as syphilitic until proven otherwise, especially when solitary and painless. The following must be differentiated:

1. Genital herpes (see Chapter 7.10.2), which is much more common than syphilis in either sex, produces a crop of painful or irritating vesicles which develop into shallow erosions. In the first attack there is also painful inguinal adenitis.

2. Traumatic sores are painful, irregular erosions which may become secondarily infected.

3. Erosive balanitis causes inflammatory, irregular erosions which may become purulent in the uncircumcized.

4. Fixed drug eruptions are macules or occasionally ulcers following various drugs, especially tetracyclines.

5. Chancroid is mostly seen in the tropics, presenting as painful, superficial, 'soft chancre', often multiple, with painful suppurative regional adenitis.

Other conditions include scabies, Behçet's syndrome, donovanosis, and lymphogranuloma venereum.

Secondary syphilis

The lesions are numerous, variable, and affect many systems. Inevitably there is a symmetrical, non-irritating rash and generalized, painless lymphadenopathy. Constitutional symptoms are mild or absent; they include headaches, which are often nocturnal, malaise, slight fever, and aches in joints and muscles. The rash is commonly macular, pale red, and sometimes so faint as to be appreciated only in tangential light. It may be papular and sometimes squamous (Fig. 4). Pustular and necrotic rashes are rarely seen in temperate climates but still occur in tropical regions. The later the secondary rash develops, the more exuberant it becomes. The distribution of the rash can be of great diagnostic help. It usually covers the trunk and proximal limbs, but when it is seen on the palms, soles, and the face, syphilis should always be high on the list of probable causes (Figs 5 and 6). In warm and moist areas such as the perineum, female external genitalia, perianal region, axillae, and under pendulous breasts, the papules enlarge into pink or grey discs, the condylomata lata, which are highly infectious (Fig. 7). Mucous patches in the mouth and genitalia are painless greyish-white erosions forming circles and arcs ('snail-track ulcers'). They too are very infectious.

Meningism and headache, especially at night, are due to low-grade meningitis which can be confirmed by a raised cell count and raised protein in the cerebrospinal fluid. Less common lesions include alopecia and laryngitis. Syphilitic hepatitis is usually associated with a marked rise in serum alkaline phosphatase. The non-specific inflammatory changes in liver biopsy material are quite unlike those of viral hepatitis. Nephrotic syndrome may develop with glomerular immune-complex deposits. Pain in the bones, often worse at night, is attributable to periostitis. Uveitis occurs in secondary and tertiary syphilis. In about one-fifth of patients, recurrent infectious episodes occur especially during the first year after the secondary stage. All these lesions disappear spontaneously leaving no trace.

Latent syphilis

By definition the patient is asymptomatic with normal cerebrospinal fluid findings but positive serology for syphilis. It is arbitrarily divided into early (<2 years) and late latent (>2 years) syphilis. Infectiousness does not stop with the advent of latency, as women may continue to give birth to congenitally infected infants during the early latent stage and for at least 2 years into the late latent stage. Approximately 60 per cent of patients remain latent for the rest of their lives, the only evidence of syphilis being positive serology, usually with a low titre. The rest develop clinical late syphilis but autopsy studies indicate that a higher proportion has subclinical infection, especially of the cardiovascular system.

Late syphilis (tertiary syphilis)

This includes late latent syphilis already referred to, benign tertiary syphilis, involvement of viscera, the central nervous system, and the aorta.

Pathogenesis of late benign syphilis

The gumma is a chronic, granulomatous lesion which is an intense inflammatory response to a few treponemes. Histologically, there is central necrosis with peripheral cellular infiltration of lymphocytes, mononuclear cells, and occasional giant cells with perivasculitis and obliterating endarteritis. *T. pallidum* is present and can be demonstrated by rabbit inoculation.

(a)

(b)

(c)

Fig. 4 (a and b) Secondary maculo-papular syphilitic rashes. (c) Late secondary early/tertiary papulosquamous lesions.

Fig. 5 Secondary papulosquamous rash of the soles.

Clinical manifestations

Cutaneous gumma

Gummas are usually single but may be multiple or diffuse (Fig. 8). Clinically, it starts as a slowly progressive, painless nodule which becomes dull red and breaks down into one or several indolent punched-out ulcers. The base has a 'wash-leather' appearance, is remarkably free from secondary infection (Fig. 9), and often resembles other granulomatous conditions. It heals slowly from the centre which may become depigmented, whilst the periphery shows hyperpigmentation. Eventually, a paper-thin scar forms. Common sites are the face, legs, buttocks, upper trunk, and scalp.

Mucosal gumma

These are most commonly seen in the oropharynx, involving the palate, pharynx, and the nasal septum. They tend to be destructive, causing perforation of the hard palate and the nasal septum and severe scarring of the pharynx and larynx. The most serious lesion is the diffuse gummatous infiltration of the tongue, leading first to a general swelling of the organ, then due to loss of papillae to a smooth red surface. After a while, the poor blood supply produces necrotic white patches on the dorsum of the tongue

Fig. 6 Secondary rash of the palms.

Fig. 7 Condylomata lata.

Fig. 9 Single gumma. Note the punched-out ulcer and absence of secondary infection.

(Fig. 10). This leucoplakia has a strong tendency to become malignant. Penicillin has no effect on the progress of late syphilitic glossitis.

Late syphilis of bones

Osteoperiostitis of long bones such as the tibia and fibula causes thickening and irregularities which may be diffuse as in the 'sabre tibia' or localized as a circumscribed bony swelling. Unlike most other syphilitic lesions, those of the bone are often painful, especially at night. Very rarely the process breaks through the skin producing a chronic 'syphilitic osteomyelitis'. Lesions of the palate, nasal septum, and the skull are destructive, leading to

bone defects of the hard palate and nasal septum and multiple osteolytic lesions of the skull.

Differential diagnosis

Mucocutaneous gumma

Superficial skin lesions must be differentiated from fungal skin lesions, psoriasis, Kaposi's sarcoma, and iodide rashes. Deep gummas may resemble

Fig. 8 Multiple gummatous ulcers. This is a typical site.

Fig. 10 Late syphilitic glossitis, early stage.

Table 2 Interpretation of serological tests in syphilis

Diagnosis	VDRL	Titre	TPHA	FTA–ABS		Comment
				IgG	IgM	
Early untreated primary syphilis	+ or −	Rising	+ or −	+	+	FTA–ABS is the first test to become +. VDRL − in 30%
Untreated late primary or secondary syphilis or reinfection or untreated or recently treated late syphilis	+	High or rising	+	+	+	
Untreated latent syphilis	+ or −	Moderate	+	+	+	
Treated early syphilis	−		+ or −	−	−	
Treated latent syphilis	+ or −	Low	+ or −	−	−	
Neurosyphilis any type, treated or untreated or cardiovascular syphilis	+ or −	Varies	+ or −	+	+	CSF: FTA–ABS often +. VDRL − in 30%
Active gumma (skin, mucosa, bone)	+	Varies	+	+	+	
Early congenital syphilis	+	Rising	+	+	+	In some infants, tests may be negative for weeks until immunologically more mature
Passive transfer of maternal antibodies	+	Same or lower than mother	−	+	−	FTA–ABS IgM
Late congenital syphilis	+	Low or moderate	+	+	+	
Biological false-positive reaction	+	Low	−	−	−	FTA–ABS may be weakly positive

False positive reaction: VDRL will be of low titre. TPHA may give false positive results in 2 per cent. FTA–ABS may give borderline positive in pregnancy and systemic lupus. TPI negative in such problem sera.

deep mycoses, sarcoidosis, tuberculosis, leprosy, donovanosis, lymphogranuloma venereum, reticulosis, and epithelioma of the skin. Serological tests for syphilis, which must include specific reactions such as the FTA–ABS (fluorescent treponemal antibody-absorbed test), prompt response to penicillin, and evidence of syphilis elsewhere clarify the diagnosis.

Late syphilis of bones

Primary and secondary carcinoma, Paget's disease, chronic osteomyelitis, tuberculosis, and leprosy should be considered. All forms of non-venereal syphilis, except pinta, give rise to similar lesions.

Visceral syphilis

This is not common and response to treatment is variable.

Liver

Multiple gummas of the liver give rise to irregular hepatomegaly ('hepar lobatum'), which may be asymptomatic. Symptoms may result from pressure on bile ducts or blood vessels or destruction of liver parenchyma.

Eyes

Uveitis, choroidoretinitis, or optic atrophy may sometimes be the sole feature of late syphilis. Uveitis can also develop during early syphilis, particularly in association with HIV, where bilateral uveitis is more commonly seen. Response of the late form to penicillin is poor. Optic atrophy is further discussed under neurosyphilis. The cerebrospinal fluid should be examined in all patients.

Stomach

Single or diffuse gummatous infiltrations of the stomach may respond to antisyphilitic treatment.

Lungs

Single or multiple gummas are rare and respond to treatment.

Testis

Gummatous infiltration and dense fibrosis may produce smooth, painless enlargement of a testis. Testicular sensation is lost.

For discussion of paroxysmal cold haemoglobinuria and neurosyphilis see Chapter 24.14.4.

Laboratory diagnosis of syphilis

Dark-field microscopy

The organism is seen in the wet preparation by dark-field microscopy in fluid taken from open lesions in early syphilis or needle aspirate from affected lymph nodes. In late lesions, the organism is not readily demonstrable by microscopy. Treponemes causing syphilis, non-venereal syphilis, yaws, and pinta cannot be differentiated morphologically. They give rise to the same serological reactions and are susceptible to penicillin.

Immunostaining directly with monoclonal antibody or by indirect fluorescent antibody staining of air-dried smears or tissue specimen has recently been reported to show numerous *T. pallidum* in a cutaneous gumma but that were not observed by dark-field microscopy or silver staining. Immunoperoxidase staining is useful in archival material.

Serology

Two classes of antibody tests are available:

(a) those that measure non-specific antibodies (IgG and IgM) against lipoidal antigens (lipoidal antibody tests formerly called reagin tests);

(b) those that measure specific antibodies stimulated by antigenic components of the treponeme and further divided into those stimulated by antigens found in pathogenic treponemes only and those shared with non-pathogenic treponemes.,

The non-specific cardiolipin antibodies act on lipoidal antigen which results from the action of *T. pallidum* on host tissue; it mirrors disease activity. The specific antigen is derived from *T. pallidum* and does not differentiate between past or present infection and is therefore of no value in assessing current activity. None of the tests distinguishes syphilis from other treponematoses. The interpretation of the tests is given in Table 2.

Animal inoculation

Animal inoculation with material from late lesions or from cases of 'persistent *T. pallidum*-like forms' is usually reserved for research purposes. PCR detection of treponemal nucleotides in amniotic or cerebrospinal fluid has proved no more sensitive than the detection of live spirochaetes by animal inoculation of these fluids.

Current serological tests for syphilis

The basis of these tests is shown in Table 3.

Lipoidal antigen tests

Rapid plasma reagin (RPR) test This can be automated and is useful for screening purposes. It is the least technically demanding test (no microscope needed). It uses carbon-containing cardiolipin antigen and requires a minimal amount of blood. Filter paper or glass fibre discs can be used to post samples to laboratories; they are therefore mainly for use by primary health centres in outlying rural areas.

VDRL test This is the preferred test and as it is used world-wide there is a good chance of it becoming standardized. It is simple and inexpensive. It is, above all, a quantitative test and as the titres reflect activity, it is of great value for this purpose. It may, for example, be the only evidence of reinfection in a patient with previous syphilis whose VDRL was either negative or weakly positive after treatment. A sharp, sustained rise of the titre, four-fold or higher, even in the absence of clinical signs is good evidence of active infection. False-positive VDRL is usually of a low titre (1:8 or less). The VDRL test becomes positive during the primary stage and rises to its maximum during the secondary stage (1:32 or more). After successful treatment, the titre declines (1:4 or less) and if treatment was given early in the disease it often becomes negative. An occasional, small and transient rise in titre (two tubes) is of no significance. The immunofluorescent test which detects cardiolipin F levels tends to be positive only in active infections.

Specific antitreponemal tests

***T. pallidum* haemagglutination (TPHA) test or *T. pallidum* particle agglutination test (TPPA)** This is a very valuable and simple test using an indirect haemagglutination method with red cells or by gelatin particles attached to sonicate of *T. pallidum* extract. It is almost as specific as the near-obsolescent TPI (treponemal immobilization test) reaction but is less sensitive than the FTA–ABS test. False-positive reactions occur in up to 2 per cent. The micromethod is particularly suitable for screening purposes. This test together with the VDRL it is probably the best combination for routine use. In cases of doubt, the FTA–ABS test is added. TPHA can be adapted for automation. There is no standard 'cut off' for the TPHA in the cerebrospinal fluid.

The FTA–ABS test This uses the indirect fluorescent technique with killed *T. pallidum* as antigen. The organisms are fixed on a slide to which the serum is added. The antibody in the serum will unite with the treponemes and this can be made visible by adding antihuman globulin conjugated with a fluorescent stain which attaches itself and produces fluorescence of the treponemes seen by fluorescent microscopy. The test has been made more specific by absorbing the group antibodies with a sonicate derived from Reiter's treponemes. The test is then called FTA–ABS. The FTA–ABS is the most sensitive test available and is also specific. It becomes positive earlier during the primary stage of syphilis than other procedures. It is not

suitable for assessing activity, as it persists long after successful treatment. When the routine serology includes the VDRL and TPHA tests, the FTA–ABS test should be added in cases of problem sera.

The FTA–ABS–IGM test In the search for a specific test to differentiate active infection which has to be treated from adequately treated or 'burnt-out' inactive disease, the FTA–ABS–IGM is being evaluated to test for specific IgM which develops in the course of syphilis. This test sometimes gives false-positive reactions owing to the presence of anti-IgG globulins (e.g. rheumatoid factor) and false-negative reactions have also occurred; thus there are problems in the use of this test in the elderly. Its use in the rapid, early diagnosis of congenital syphilis was considered some years ago to be great advance. The basis for its use is that IgG is a small molecule and passes through the placenta; thus the baby may inherit maternal IgG but not necessarily the infection. Tests such as the VDRL may therefore be positive in the newborn by passive transfer and may take 3 months to disappear. IgM is a large molecule and does not pass through the placenta; thus if it is found in the neonate, it must be assumed that it has been produced by the infected infant.

Newer tests

Enzyme immunoassay (EIA) tests (e.g. CAPTIA IgG, IgM) have no practical advantage over current tests. Attempts with purified antigens from *T. pallidum* may be specific, although they tend to loose sensitivity, for example, those employing the TpN19 or Tp44.5 antigens. The problem is that early cases may not always have antibodies to a specific antigen. It would be better, therefore, to screen with as many antigens as possible. This is achieved by western blotting, which allows the separation by gel electrophoresis of all the major, stable antigens of the spirochaete, and enables a distinction to be made between the non-specific and specific antibody reactions with given bands. The major antigens are shown in Table 4.

This technique may have special application in seronegative syphilis (perhaps syphilis occurring with HIV infection) but not in primary syphilis, where up to half the cases show no reaction. The immunoblot may also be helpful in distinguishing false positive tests caused by borrelia infections.

Diagnosis of neurosyphilis by examination of the cerebrospinal fluid

The traditional tests include the VDRL, cell count, total protein globulin, and goldsol curve. The last two tests are now obsolete. The cerebrospinal fluid VDRL is unreliable as it can be negative in up to 50 per cent of samples from patients with active neurosyphilis. Cell counts exceeding 5/mm^2 (but usually not above 50/mm^2) and protein above 40 mg/ml (60 mg/ml in patients older than 65 years) are non-specific signs of inflammation. The specific FTA–ABS and TPHA tests in the cerebrospinal fluid may be positive due to passive transfer of serum IgG from adequately treated patients. If they are negative, active neurosyphilis can almost certainly be excluded.

Table 3 Basis of tests for syphilis (adapted from Egglestone *et al.* (2000)

Test	Antigen	Captive system
FTA-abs	Whole treponemes	Treponemes fixed on microscope slides (immunofluorescence)
TPHA	Treponemal sonicates	Attached to red blood cells (agglutination)
TPPA	Treponemal sonicates	Attached to gelatin particles (agglutination)
EIA (ELISA)	Treponemal sonicates	Attached to microtitre plates (conjugated antibody labelling)
Recombinant antigens	Recombinant products	As above
DNA probes	Extracted treponemal DNA	(Hybridization and amplification of product)
VDRL[1]	Cardiolipin	Liposome (flocculation)
RPR[1]	Cardiolipin	As above, but with trapping charcoal particles (flocculation)
EIA[1]	Cardiolipin	Cardiolipin attached to microtitre plates (conjugated labelled antibody)
SPEA[1] (solid phase erythrocyte adherence)	Cardiolipin	As above (agglutination with anti-immunoglobulin coated red cells)
Cardiolipin fluorescence	Tissue sections	Cardiolipin in tissue sections (immunofluorescence)

[1] Non-treponemal tests.

Biological false-positive tests for syphilis

These concern mainly the cardiolipin tests and are classified as acute, as in drug addicts, or chronic if they occur in autoimmune disease (when they may precede the symptoms by years), leprosy, and in a small proportion of people over 70. The concurrence of HIV and syphilis in drug abusers makes the investigation of these false-positive reactions particularly important. There is no evidence for an increase in false-positive tests in patients with HIV. Particular mention should be made of the thrombotic antiphospholipid syndrome since the condition is associated with early miscarriage and cerebral thrombosis, manifestations which might be confused with syphilis. The confirmatory TPHA and FTA–ABS tests are always negative. A biological false-positive test may occur acutely in the cerebrospinal fluid in aseptic meningitis or in a seropositive patient, when a traumatic tap may give a false impression of a positive cardiolipin test in the cerebrospinal fluid, following transfer of plasma antibody.

The management of syphilis

Suggestions for drug treatment of syphilis are given in Table 5. It has been found that adherence to clinical guidelines is better maintained when treatment and follow-up is performed by a sexually transmitted disease clinics than by a non-institutional practitioner. As soon as a diagnosis of infectious syphilis has been made, the patient should be interviewed by a social worker regarding all sexual contacts. In the case of primary syphilis, this should cover the previous 3 months; in patients with secondary syphilis this should be extended to 1 year; and in patients with early latent syphilis to 2 years because of the possibility of infectious relapses during that

Table 4 Major antigens of *Treponema pallidum*

Designation*	MW	Description and comments
TPO748	82 000	Cytoplasmic filament protein (CfpA)
TPO030	59 000	Homologue of Hsp60 or GroEL heat shock protein. Cross-reactive antigen
TPO971	45 000	Lipoprotein. The most abundant polypeptide and dominat antigen
TPO768	42 000	Lipoprotein. Also abundant. Recombinant form (TmpA) purified and experimental diagnostic reagent
TPO545	39 000	Lipoprotein. Homologue of the MglB periplasmic sugar binding protein of *Escherichia coli*
TPO249	37 000	FlA flagellin. Abundant, dominant antigen. Member of class of spirochaetal flagellar and ldquo; sheath and rdquo; proteins
TPO821	35 500	Lipoprotein. less abundant and dominant antigen
TPO868	34 500	FlaB flagellins, homologues
TPO792	33 000	of other bacterial flagellins
TPO870	32 000	Form flagellar core
TPO319	30–38 000	Lipoprotein, moderately antigenic
TPO993	24–29 000	Lipoprotein, moderately antigenic
TpN19 (4D)	19 000	Subunit of a large, heat labile complex which in recombinant *E. coli* is a ring structure
TPO435	17 000	Lipoprotein, strongly antigenic
TPO171	15 000	Lipoprotein, strongly antigenic

* TP designations are those given in Fraser et al. (1998) where applicable, otherwise the convention of Norris et al. (1993) is followed.

period. The patient is warned against intercourse during treatment and for a further 2 weeks. Experience suggests that advice for longer abstinence will be disregarded in many cases and is almost certainly unnecessary.

If the patient gives no history of penicillin allergy, it is the first choice for the treatment of all stages of the disease. Penicillin is as effective now as it was more than 40 years ago when it was first introduced. Resistance to penicillin has not been described, perhaps related to the novel penicillin binding of the T$_P$47 (TPO971) protein. If there is penicillin allergy, the alternative drugs are tetracycline/doxycycline and erythromycin. The recent finding of a wild strain of *T. pallidum* resistant to erythromycin has led to an extensive investigation into the use of newer cephalosporins. Cephalosporins are effective but there is cross-allergy with penicillin in 5 to 7 per cent of patients.

The optimal dose or duration of treatment with penicillin, or the other drugs, has not been established and therefore a great variety of treatment schemes have been put forward, although the results appear to be similar, suggesting that a fair degree of variation is permissible. The general tendency is to treat with larger doses and over a longer period of time in the later stages of syphilis; some prefer to repeat the course. There is no convincing evidence that large, much extended, or repeated courses give any added benefit.

There is good experimental evidence that serum concentrations of penicillin should be at least 0.003 µg/ml, should be maintained for 8 to 10 days, and that troughs in the concentration should not exceed 15 h. Some physicians prefer a single injection of the long-acting benzathine penicillin (2.4 million units) for simplicity, but the concentration reached is low and does not give a useful level in the cerebrospinal fluid; also the injection is quite painful. Others repeat this dose weekly, for 3 weeks. In patients with neurosyphilis and HIV infections, treponemes have been demonstrated in the cerebrospinal fluid after benzathine penicillin G treatments and in these patients the expected decline in VDRL cerebrospinal fluid titres after treatment occurred less often than in those without concurrent HIV infection. All treponemal infections are unaffected by sulphonamides, gentamicin, rifampicin, and quinolones in clinical dosage.

Procaine penicillin has several advantages over other penicillin preparations and is preferred by many. In some centres, the course is 1 million units/day for 10 days; in others it is given for 20 days though evidence that such a prolonged course gives better results is lacking. Procaine penicillin in 2 per cent aluminium monostearate (PAM) has a prolonged action and was used extensively by the World Health Organization in their mass campaign against non-venereal syphilis.

Penicillin reactions

All patients receiving penicillin injections should be kept in the clinic for 15 to 20 min as severe reactions needing immediate treatment will develop well within this period. An emergency tray to deal with anaphylactic penicillin reaction must be readily available wherever penicillin is given. It should contain ampoules of 1:1000 adrenaline (epinephrine) solution, syringes and needles, intravenous hydrocortisone, injectable antihistamine, aminophylline, an airway respirator (Ambu bag or Brooke's respirator), and oxygen with face mask or nasal catheter.

Prevention of penicillin reactions

Some 3 to 5 per cent of the population in the United Kingdom are allergic to penicillin and it is essential to enquire about this; if there is a history, penicillin must not be given. This fact should be displayed prominently on the cover of the medical notes and the patient told to inform any doctor who may wish to give this antibiotic. Careful history taking may, however, show that the 'allergy' to penicillin is doubtful, for example the rash antedated the giving of penicillin and may have been due to one of the childhood infections. It is quite common to be told that patients who apparently did have a penicillin reaction, had no problems when the antibiotic was inadvertently given subsequently as penicillin allergy is a transient phenomenon. In such cases we still prefer to avoid giving penicillin.

Clinical features

The most serious reaction is anaphylactic shock appearing immediately or within a minute or two after the injection. The more immediate the onset, the more severe the attack. The patient becomes unconscious, stops breathing, and becomes pulseless. Very rarely, the patient dies immediately. A fatal outcome is estimated to occur one or two times per 100 000 injections. In the more moderate reaction, the patient feels faint with acute anxiety and a feeling of impending death; there may be oedema of the face, possibly with an asthmatic attack, soon followed by urticaria. Arthralgia and some pyrexia may develop. The urticaria is liable to last 1 to 2 weeks.

The commonest form is the delayed reaction when urticaria appears days after injection or oral penicillin. Arthralgia and fever may develop. Sometimes a local reaction around the injection site is seen. It can be urticarial but is more commonly a painful red swelling and usually responds to rest. It is best to discontinue the course, as recurrences are otherwise common. In some patients a hysterical episode follows an injection and this may be due to procaine or possibly inadvertent intravenous injection. It passes off spontaneously.

Table 5 Treatment for syphilis based on WHO draft recommendations 1993, modified by Vader *et al.* (1998) and CDC (1998)

Type of syphilis	Treatment
Early syphilis (primary, secondary, early latent, early reinfection)	Aqueous procaine penicillin G[b] 1200 mg/day, single IM injection, 10 days *or* Benzathine penicillin 1800 mg (2.4 MU) for 1 day, IM
Late latent syphilis (more than 2 years) and late benign syphillis[a]	Aqueous procaine penicillin G 1200 mg/day, single IM injection, 15 days *or* Benzathine penicillin G Total 5400 m (7.2 MU)g, IM, weekly, for 3 weeks, at weekly intervals
Cardiovascular syphilis	Aqueous procaine penicillin G 1200 mg/day, single IM injection, 20 days Benzathine penicillin G not to be given
Neurosyphilis (and uveitis)	Aqueous procaine penicillin G 1200 mg/day, single IM injection + probenecid 500 mg by mouth, 4 times per day[c] both for 10—14 days *or* Aqueous crystalline penicillin G (12–24 megaunit) daily, given as 3–4 megaunits every 4 h, IV[d], for 14 days
Optic atrophy (congenital or acquired)	As for neurosyphilis
Eighth nerve deafness and vertigo	As for neurosyphilis *plus* corticosteroids
Syphilis of the tongue	As for late syphilis and consult ENT specialist for regular follow-up
Early congenital syphilis including suspected early congenital syphilis	Crystalline penicillin G 50 mg/kg IM in 2 divided doses, for 10 days *or* Aqueous procaine penicillin G 37.5 mg/kg IM, single daily dose, for 10 days
Late congenital syphilis (over 2 years duration)	As for late latent syphilis (dose adjusted for age)
Interstitial keratitis (2 years duration)	Procaine penicillin as for neurosyphilis *plus* 0.5% prednisolone eye drops hourly until controlled
Patients with HIV and syphilis	As for stage of syphilis but not benzathine penicillin
Patients allergic to penicillin—non-penicillin regimens	
Acquired syphilis of less than 2 years' duration	Tetracycline 500 mg by mouth, four times daily, for 15 days *or* Doxycycline 100 mg × 2, for 14 days *or* Ceftriaxone 1 × 250 mg IM, for 10 days *or* Azithromycin 500 mg daily by mouth, for 10 days[e] *If pregnant* Erythromycin, 500 mg by mouth four times daily, for 15 days
Acquired syphilis of more than 2 years' duration	Tetracycline 500 mg by mouth four times daily, for 30 days *or* Erythromycin 500 mg by mouth four times daily, for 30 days

[a] In patients with gumma of the larynx, late neurosyphilis, especially general paresis, and cardiovascular syphilis, especially with angina try to minimize any Herxheimer reaction by covering the first injection of penicillin with corticosteroid started the day before injection. In patients diagnosed as symptomatic cardiovascular syphilis consult cardiac surgeon from the start with a view to possible cardiac surgery (removal of coronary ostial stenosis, aortic valve replacement, repair or replacement of aneurysmal aortic segment). If there is congestive heart failure treat it before giving penicillin.

[b] The dosages of penicillin are usually expressed in terms of weight. Procaine penicillin G, 300 mg = 300 000 units; benzathine penicillin G, 900 mg = 1.2 megaunits; aqueous crystalline penicillin G = 0.5 megaunits ≅ 300 mg. Note that 1 mg Na penicillin = 1667 units, 1 mg K penicillin = 1599 units.

[c] It has been suggested that probenecid increases the CSF penicillin level at the expense of the tissue level. Probenecid should also be used with caution in AIDS patients since it increases the half-life of zidovudine.

[d] Doxycycline, 200 mg × 2 for 28 days, has been suggested for neurosyphilis.

[e] None of these alternative regimens has been rigorously tested in clinical trials with prolonged follow-up but these recommended regimens are based on small, uncontrolled series.

Treatment of the anaphylactic reaction

The patient is laid flat with feet up and head down. Blood pressure and pulse are monitored throughout. Adrenaline 1:1000 (adult dose 0.5–1.0 ml) is given intramuscularly without delay. If bronchospasm develops, 250 mg aminophylline in 10 ml water is administered by slow intravenous injection. Intravenous hydrocortisone (100 mg) may also be tried and may be repeated. Some prefer intravenous antihistamine (chlorpheniramine injection 10–20 mg). Adrenaline, nevertheless, is the mainstay of treatment. If there is no response, the cardiac arrest team is summoned. If recovery is slow, the patient should be admitted as recurrences may occasionally occur. In any case, the patient must be kept under observation for several hours. Later, urticaria develops in most patients and prophylactic antihistamines by mouth are indicated.

Treatment of the delayed reaction

The leading feature is urticaria, possibly with oedema of the face, arthralgia, and some fever. Such patients respond to oral antihistamines such as chlorpheniramine 4 mg four times daily or terfenadine 60 mg twice daily until the condition is controlled. If it is very severe, prednisolone 10 mg four times daily may be added for a few days, reducing it as soon as possible. Penicillinase is not recommended as it may produce reactions of its own.

Procaine reaction

Two types of reaction are recognized:

1. The patient shows extreme anxiety with a feeling of impending death. Sometimes there are hallucinations, disorientation, and depersonalization. The reaction is self-limiting. It may be due to reduced procaine esterase leading to high procaine blood levels. Patients should be restrained and reassured.

2. The reaction is similar but associated with hyperventilation, hypertension, tachycardia, and vomiting. Rarely cardiovascular collapse has been reported but without fatalities. The reaction is thought to follow accidental intravenous administration of procaine penicillin leading to microemboli of the lungs and brain. Supportive treatment is usually sufficient.

Vasovagal attacks

These occur most commonly in young men following intramuscular injection or after having blood taken. The patient looks very pale and may faint. He may slump to the floor and occasionally go stiff and have jerky movements. The most important diagnostic sign is a slow pulse. Recovery is rapid once he is laid flat on a couch. There is a tendency for recurrence in the same individual under similar circumstances and this can usually be prevented by giving injections or taking blood whilst the patient is lying down.

Jarisch–Herxheimer reaction (see also Chapter 7.11.30)

This systemic reaction is believed to be due to the release of endotoxin-like substances when large numbers of *T. pallidum* are killed by antibiotics. It is mainly associated with early syphilis. The incidence of the reaction appears to be related to the total number of the organism in the body. The mechanism may not be straightforward as it is not a feature of neonatal syphilis or non-venereal syphilis in childhood. The reaction can be expected in 50 per cent of primary syphilis, 90 per cent of secondary syphilis, and in 25 per cent of early latent infection, but is very rare in late syphilis. It has been suggested that it is more often seen in patients with HIV.

The reaction begins 4 to 12 h after the first injection, lasts for a few hours or up to a day, and is not seen with subsequent treatment. There is malaise, slight to moderate pyrexia, a flush due to vasodilation, tachycardia, and leucocytosis, and existing lesions become more prominent. In some patients with early syphilis, a secondary rash may become visible which was absent before treatment. Rarely, syphilis may be suspected by the appearance of the febrile reaction of the Jarisch–Herxheimer, perhaps with a fleeting rash, when treating another infection with a treponemocidal antibiotic (e.g. penicillin in gonorrhoea).

In early syphilis the reaction is only a minor nuisance. In late syphilis it can on very rare occasions be more serious. Thus in neurosyphilis it may lead to epilepsy or a rapid. irreversible progression, and in general paresis it can cause exacerbation amounting to temporary psychosis. Sudden death has been reported in cardiovascular syphilis. In laryngeal gumma, local oedema may necessitate tracheotomy. In the later stages of pregnancy, fetal monitoring is advised.

It is customary to give corticosteroids in late symptomatic syphilis starting a day before the first penicillin injection and tailing it off the day after the first injection. This does not prevent the Jarisch–Herxheimer reaction but is said to ameliorate it. The analogous reactions in relapsing fever have been modified by meptazinol or pretreatment with infusions of polyclonal anti-TNF-α Fab with concomitant reduction in the plasma concentration of interleukin 6 and 8.

Follow-up

It is generally sufficient to perform blood tests 1, 3, 6, and 12 months after treatment of early syphilis. In late symptomatic syphilis, surveillance is for life. Patients with leucoplakia of the tongue should be checked every 3 months. In symptomatic cardiovascular syphilis regular radiological and clinical examination is essential to determine any change which might suggest the need for cardiac surgery. In neurosyphilis an annual review might be adequate.

In latent syphilis, if there is a satisfactory serological response, 2 to 3-yearly follow-up seems reasonable. The cerebrospinal fluid need not be examined in the non-immunocompromised patient, except in the presence of neurological signs. In early congenital syphilis, the observation time should be similar to that of early acquired syphilis. In late latent congenital syphilis, no further attendance is necessary unless symptoms of interstitial keratitis or other lesions not prevented by penicillin develop.

In high-risk patients such as male homosexuals and prostitutes a regular check-up every 3 months is advised. If such patients have had syphilis, the VDRL should have become negative or of a low titre after treatment. If the titre suddenly rises four-fold or more, reinfection must be assumed and treatment is indicated.

Prophylaxis

Treatment of asymptomatic contacts of early syphilis is recommended in the United States as there is a 50 per cent chance of infection. Such pre-emptive treatment is likely to reduce the spread of infection in the promiscuous or in those likely to infect their spouses or regular sexual partners. Use of condoms should be recommended. Various vaginal chemical spermicidal creams give a small degree of protection but are unreliable.

Further reading

Borisenko KK, Tikhonova LL, Renton AM (1999). Syphilis and other sexually transmitted infections in the Russian Federation. *International Journal of STD and AIDS* **10**, 665–8.

Byrne RE, Laska S, Bell M, Larson D, Phillips J, Todd J (1992). Evaluation of a *Treponema pallidum* western immunoblot assay as a confirmatory test for syphilis. *Journal of Clinical Microbiology* **30**, 115–22.

CDC (1998). Guidelines for treatment of sexually transmitted diseases. *Syphilis* **47**, (RRI) 28–48.

Egglestone SI, Turner AJL (2000). Serological diagnosis of syphilis. *Communicable Disease and Public Health* **3**, 158–62.

Grimble AS (1971). Venereal disease in the young patient: a perspective. *Guy's Hospital Reports* **120**, 323–6.

Haake DA (2000). Spirochaetal lipoproteins and pathogenesis. *Microbiology* **146**, 1491–504.

Kell P, McMorrow S, Smith A (2000). Management of syphilis in pregnancy. *Bulletin of Sexually Transmitted Infections and HIV* **4**, 9–12.

Luger AF, Schmidt BL, Kaulich M (2000). Significance of laboratory findings for the diagnosis of neurosyphilis. *International Journal of STD and AIDS* **11**, 224–34.

Morton RS (2001). 'The syphilis enigma', the riddle resolved. *Sexually Transmitted Infections* **77**, 322–4.

Norris SJ (1993). Polypeptides of *Treponema pallidum*: progress towards understanding their structural, functional and immunologic roles. *Microbiology Reviews* **57**, 750–79.

Oriel JD (1994). *Scars of Venus: a history of venereology*, pp. 1–181. Springer Verlag, London.

PHLS, DHSS and PS and the Scottish ISD (D) 5 Collaborative Group. Sexually transmitted infections in the UK. new episodes seen at genito-urinary medicine clinics, 1995 to 2000. *Public Health Laboratory Service*, London.

Subramanian G, Koonin EV, Aravind A (2000). Comparative genome analysis of the pathogenic spirochetes *Borrelia burgdorferi* and *Treponema pallidum*. *Infection and Immunity* **68**, 1633–48.

US Department of Health and Human Services, Public Health Services: Centers for Disease Control (1 993) (1992). *Sexually transmitted disease surveillance*, pp. 6–11, 139–148, (definitions: 185–187). Atlanta, GA.

Van Vorst Vader PC (1998). Syphilis management and treatment. *Dermatology Clinics* **16**, 699–711.

White RM (2000). Unravelling the Tuskegee study of untreated syphilis. *Archives of Internal Medicine* **160**, 585–98.

Wilner E and Brody JA (1968). Prognosis of general paresis after treatment. *Lancet* **2**, 1370–1.

World Health Organization (1993). *Draft recommendations for the management of sexually transmitted diseases*. WHO advisory group meeting, WHO/GPA/STD/93. 1, pp. 24–31. WHO, Geneva.

Young H (2000). Guidelines for serological testing for syphilis. *Sexually Transmitted Infections* **76**, 403–5.

Website addresses

Website 1 http://www.tigr.org The Institute for Genomic Research

Website 2 download by anonymous ftp at ftp://ncbi.nlm.nih.gov/pub/Koonin/Spirochetes

7.11.34 Listeriosis

P. J. Wilkinson

Listeriosis has been recognized since the 1920s as a systemic infection of man, domestic and farm animals, and rodents. Because the disease in rabbits and guinea pigs was characterized by a marked mononuclear leucocytosis, the causative Gram-positive bacillus was named *Bacterium monocytogenes*, then (in honour of Lord Lister) *Listerella* and finally *Listeria*. Human listeriosis was a relatively obscure disease until the 1980s, when a series of food-borne outbreaks awakened interest. Listeriosis remains a rare infection but carries a significant morbidity and mortality.

Listeria monocytogenes

Listeria spp. are non-sporing, facultatively anaerobic, Gram-positive bacilli that are ubiquitous in the environment and distributed world-wide. *L. monocytogenes* is the major pathogen, although occasional human infections with *L. ivanovii* and *L. seeligeri* have been reported. *L. ivanovii* and *L. innocua* can infect animals. *L. welshimeri* and *L. grayii* are not known to cause disease. Enrichment and selective methods are now well established for the isolation of listeria from food or the environment; immunoassays and nucleic acid amplification techniques have also been used. The ability to multiply at temperatures of 0 to 40° C and tolerate preserving agents makes listeria of particular concern if present in refrigerated foods that are consumed without further cooking.

Several typing methods are used to trace food sources, distinguish relapses from reinfections, and investigate outbreaks. Thirteen serovars are currently recognized, of which three (1/2a, 1/2b, and 4b) cause more than 90 per cent of human and animal infections. Phenotypic subtyping systems, based on patterns of lytic reactions with bacteriophages, bacteriocin (monocin) production, and multilocus enzyme electrophoresis have been enhanced by genotypic analysis, particularly pulsed field gel electrophoresis (PFGE).

Epidemiological associations

L. monocytogenes has been isolated from many foods, and the consumption of contaminated meat, milk, seafood, or vegetables is the principal route of infection. Outbreaks have been associated with coleslaw, raw fish, raw hot dogs, undercooked chicken, meat paté, pork rillettes, turkey franks, smoked fish or shellfish, and cheese and dairy products, particularly when pasteurization has been ineffective. The United Kingdom Department of Health advises pregnant women and immunocompromised persons not to eat soft ripened cheese (e.g. Brie, Camembert, and blue-vein types), all types of paté, and cook-chill meals and poultry unless thoroughly reheated until piping hot.

Direct transmission through contact with infected animals can give rise to primary cutaneous listeriosis, an occupational disease of farmers and veterinarians. Laboratory workers have acquired eye and skin infections from direct exposure to culture material. Nosocomial infection has spread between neonates in association with poor hand hygiene, close contact between infected patients and their mothers, and fomites such as rectal thermometers. Hospital outbreaks, which may have been food-borne, have also occurred in adult immunosuppressed patients.

Pathogenesis

Although listeria displays many characteristics of saprophytes, specific adaptations allow *L. monocytogenes* to become an intracellular pathogen where invasion and multiplication in both phagocytic and non-phagocytic cells occurs. CR3 complement receptors may be involved in the adhesion to phagocytes. Internalin, a listerial surface protein similar to the M protein of group A streptococci, plays a part in the initial stages of invasion of all cell types, as may p60, another cell surface protein with murein hydrolase activity. After internalization, *L. monocytogenes* becomes encapsulated in a vacuole, the membrane of which is dissolved by a thiol-activated haemolysin (listeriolysin O) and possibly also by phospholipase C. Having entered the host cell cytoplasm, the organisms grow, polymerize actin, acquire intracellular mobility, and spread to adjacent cells.

Clinical features

Although listeriosis is generally an opportunistic infection of the elderly, patients with severe underlying illness, pregnant women, newborn babies, and individuals without these risk factors can also become infected. The clinical presentation varies from a mild, influenza-like illness to fatal septicaemia and meningoencephalitis. The syndromes recognized include maternofetal and neonatal listeriosis, septicaemia, meningoencephalitis, cerebritis, gastroenteritis, and localized infections.

- In maternofetal listeriosis, the mother may develop a fever, headache, myalgia, and low back pain, associated with the bacteraemic phase of the disease. Transplacental infection causes amnionitis and usually leads to spontaneous septic abortion or to premature labour with the delivery of a severely infected fetus or baby.

- Neonatal listeriosis of early onset results from intrauterine infection and has a high mortality. The liquor is meconium-stained and the baby septic and jaundiced, with signs of purulent conjunctivitis, bronchopneumonia, meningitis, or encephalitis. Granulomas affect many organs, hence the term 'granulomatosis infantisepticum'. Late-onset disease, which develops several days to weeks in a baby who was initially healthy but subsequently develops meningitis, which may be acquired from the mother's genital tract or through cross-infection from an early-onset case.

- Septicaemia occurs mainly in adult patients with malignancies, in transplant recipients, and in immunosuppressed and elderly people. Most present with fever, hypotension, and shock but a third to a half develop meningitis, which is often then the presenting feature.

- Meningoencephalitis may start abruptly but, in adults, can also develop insidiously, with progressive focal neurological signs even in the absence of a brain abscess. Most patients have meningism, but fever may not be marked, particularly in elderly or immunosuppressed people. This infection should be considered in any patient with an acute brain-stem disorder associated with fever, particularly if there are no risk factors for cerebrovascular disease.

- Cerebritis is increasingly recognized, particularly in the immunosuppressed patient. Headache, fever, and varying degrees of paralysis can resemble a cerebrovascular accident. Rhomboencephalitis begins with a headache, fever, nausea, and vomiting followed in several days by symmetrical, progressive cranial nerve palsies, decreased consciousness, and cerebellar signs. Areas of uptake without ring enhancement may be shown by MRI or CT scan, and the cerebrospinal fluid shows few, if any, cells, and normal protein and sugar concentrations.

- Gastroenteritis with arthromyalgia, fever, diarrhoea, nausea, vomiting, and an incubation period of 1 to 3 days has recently been described in outbreaks of infection in immunocompetent adults who have ingested contaminated food. Because diagnostic laboratories do not usually culture diarrhoeal stools selectively for listeria, *L. monocytogenes* may be missed. Recent outbreaks have come to light when blood cultures from hospitalized patients have yielded the organism, or when serological testing of the blood of recently affected patients has shown antibody to listeria.

- Localized infections are rare, occur mainly in immunosuppressed people, and include abscesses, cholecystitis, endocarditis, endophthalmitis, osteomyelitis, septic arthritis, and peritonitis. They usually result from seeding during an initial bacteraemic phase, but focal skin and eye infection can also result from direct, occupational exposure.

Diagnosis

The microbiological diagnosis of invasive listeriosis is made by culture of the organism from meconium, nose or eye swabs, urine, cerebrospinal fluid, blood, tracheal aspirate, placental tissue, and/or lochia. Gram-positive bacilli may be seen in a stained smear. In listeria meningoencephalitis, the cerebrospinal fluid exudate is predominantly mononuclear and, if no bacteria are seen in a Gram-stained film, may be confused with viral meningitis; however, unlike viral meningitis, the cerebrospinal fluid protein is high and the glucose concentration low in relation to that in the peripheral blood. Tests for listeria antibodies in maternal and cord blood samples do not contribute to the diagnosis of the acute infection. Selective culture techniques have considerably improved the isolation rate.

Antibiotic treatment

There are no controlled trials of antibiotic treatment for listeriosis. All strains are susceptible to ampicillin, which acts synergistically with aminoglycoside antibiotics, and high-dose intravenous ampicillin in combination with gentamicin remains the treatment of choice. Gentamicin is best avoided in pregnancy, when ampicillin may be used alone, or erythromycin if the patient is penicillin-allergic. Intravenous co-trimoxazole is the best second-line treatment for listeria meningoencephalitis. Vancomycin has been successfully used with gentamicin to treat bacteraemic illness, but does not cross the blood–brain barrier. Rifampicin and ciprofloxacin have not been evaluated in human listeriosis.

L. monocytogenes is inherently resistant to the cephalosporins and it is very important to be aware that treatment with this class of antibiotics is likely to fail. Since acute pyogenic meningitis is usually treated, until the pathogen is known, with ceftriaxone or cefotaxime, ampicillin should also be given with this initial treatment whenever listeriosis is a clinical possibility, unless the cerebrospinal fluid Gram-film shows good evidence of another bacterial cause, or the patient has unequivocal clinical features of meningococcal disease.

Intravenous ampicillin should be given in a daily dose of 200 to 300 mg/kg (neonates) or 6 to 12 g (adults) in three to four divided doses for 2 weeks (uncomplicated bacteraemia), 4 to 6 weeks (meningoencephalitis), or 6 to 8 weeks (endocarditis). Intravenous gentamicin should be given for the first 14 days in a dosage adjusted with the help of plasma concentration measurement. Focal listeriosis may be treated with ampicillin or amoxicillin, 3 to 6 g daily, until clinical resolution. In cases of genuine penicillin allergy, intravenous co-trimoxazole, 20 mg/kg per day (trimethoprim component) may be given in four divided doses. Alternatively, intravenous minocycline, which may have to be obtained specially from the manufacturer, can be used in a daily dose of 200 mg (adults) or 4 mg/kg (children), in combination with gentamicin.

Prognosis

Despite antibiotic therapy, the mortality of septicaemia and meningoencephalitis with *L. monocytogenes* remains high (20–50 per cent). There is significant long-term morbidity in the survivors. Efforts should therefore continue to be focused on the prevention of this infection by improvement in the microbiological safety of methods of food production and preparation and by the continued education of the public so that vulnerable people can avoid high-risk foods.

Further reading

Jones EM, MacGowan AP (1995). Antimicrobial chemotherapy of human infection due to *Listeria monocytogenes*. *European Journal of Clinical Microbiology and Infectious Diseases* **14**, 165–75.

McLauchlin J (1997). The pathogenicity of *Listeria monocytogenes*: a public health perspective. *Reviews in Medical Microbiology* **8**, 1–14.

McLauchlin J, Jones D (1998). Erysipelothrix and Listeria. In: Balows A and Duerden BI, eds. *Topley and Wilson's microbiology and microbial infections*, Vol. 2, pp. 683–703. Arnold, London.

McLauchlin J, Low JC (1994). Primary cutaneous listeriosis in adults: an occupational disease of veterinarians and farmers. *Veterinary Record* **135**, 615–17

Schlech WF III (1991). Listeriosis: epidemiology, virulence and the significance of contaminated foodstuffs. *Journal of Hospital Infection* **19**, 211–24.

Schlech WF III (1997). Listeria gastroenteritis—old syndrome, new pathogen. *New England Journal of Medicine* **336**, 130–2.

Salamina G *et al.* (1996). A foodborne outbreak of gastroenteritis involving *Listeria monocytogenes*. *Epidemiology and Infection* **117**, 429–36.

7.11.35 Legionellosis and legionnaires' disease

J. B. Kurtz and J. T. Macfarlane

In 1976 an outbreak of pneumonia occurred among American legionnaires who had attended a convention in a Philadelphia hotel. A total of 221 people developed pneumonia, 'legionnaires' disease', of whom 34 died. A newly identified organism, named after this outbreak, *Legionella pneumophila*, was responsible. Since then other outbreaks and sporadic cases have been recognized and 16 *L. pneumophila* serogroups, and other species of legionella besides *L. pneumophila* have been isolated from clinical and environmental samples. There are now at least 43 recognized species in the Legionellaceae family. Clinical illness caused by members of the family Legionellaceae is referred to as legionellosis. The pneumonia is called legionnaires' disease. Non-pneumonic legionellosis ('Pontiac fever') is a self-limiting, influenza-like illness, without radiographic changes in the lung, caused by many different legionella species. What determines the type of illness that will follow infection is unknown. Although, in a given outbreak, disease of both pneumonic and non-pneumonic types occurs, usually either one or other form predominates. *L. pneumophila* is responsible for over 80 per cent of legionellosis, and of the 16 serogroups serogroup 1 is the most frequently encountered in human infections. In some parts of Australia, however, *L. longbeachae* is the most frequently identified species causing legionnaires' disease. Other legionella species appear to be less pathogenic and are more frequently found as opportunist pathogens in immunocompromised people. Some have caused disease, others have only been isolated from the environment and have yet to be implicated as human pathogens.

The organism

The Legionellaceae are aerobic, non-sporing bacilli whose cell walls contain distinctive branched-chain fatty acids.

In the laboratory, legionellae are fastidious in their growth requirements and will not grow on standard bacteriological media. Aces buffered charcoal yeast-extract agar, pH 6.9, supplemented with L-cysteine, α-ketoglutarate, and iron, is a very satisfactory medium. On this medium, incubated at 35 to 37 °C, typical colonies usually appear in 3 to 5 days; occasional slow-growing strains require the plates to be incubated for 10 days. When isolates from a patient and a suspected environmental source (see below) have been obtained, an accurate comparison of the strains should be undertaken. Both genotypic (e.g. amplified fragment length polymorphism) and phenotypic (e.g. monoclonal antibody reaction pattern) methods of identification should be used in parallel to see whether the two isolates are indistinguishable or different.

Epidemiology

The natural habitat of legionellae is in freshwater streams, lakes, and thermal springs, moist soil, and mud. They have been found worldwide in waters with temperatures varying from 5 to 62 °C and pH values of 5.4 to 8.2. These organisms are inhibited by sodium chloride and are not found in sea water. In natural habitats they are found in only small numbers, forming part of the consortium of micro-organisms that makes up the biofilm. This includes amoebae and other protozoa, in certain of which legionellae multiply and later re-emerge. Inside these protozoa the bacteria form microcolonies, which are protected from adverse conditions (for example, in amoebic cysts from desiccation and up to 50 parts per million of free

chlorine). This association enables the bacteria to survive and to disseminate widely in the natural environment.

Legionellae have been found in small numbers in water distribution systems, through which they can colonize man-made habitats, again as part of the biofilm from which they are shed into the water. Factors that encourage colonization and multiplication are temperature (20–45 °C) and stagnation. The most common sites in buildings in which legionellae have been found are hot-water calorifiers and storage tanks. Piped water, especially hot water from the calorifiers in large buildings and industrial complexes with long runs of pipework, is a potential source of infection. Other well-recognized sources include:

- recirculating water in air-conditioning and cooling systems;
- whirlpool spas and other warm-water baths;
- decorative fountains;
- nebulizers and humidifier reservoirs of hospital ventilation machines if topped up with contaminated tap water;
- potting compost for *L. longbeachae* serogroup 1 in Australia.

Dissemination of infection is by contaminated water droplets (aerosol), which are inhaled. In order to cause infection the droplets must be of a size (less than 5 μm diameter) that can reach the alveoli of the lungs. Taps and shower heads produce very localized aerosols, whereas the water droplets (drift) contained in the airstream released from a cooling tower may be carried a considerable distance and expose a greater number of people to risk. For example, in the 1976 Philadelphia outbreak, those infected in the street developed 'Broad Street pneumonia' and passers-by were infected in both the Stafford District General Hospital outbreak in 1985 (101 cases, 28 deaths) and near the BBC building, London, in 1988 (79 cases, 2 deaths). Person-to-person spread of legionellosis has never been recorded. Aspiration of contaminated water as might occur in hospital following an anaesthetic is also a well-recognized route of infection.

Although most studies of legionnaires' disease have been of outbreaks, sporadic cases account for about three-quarters of those reported in England and Wales. A source is only exceptionally found for them. Some of these sporadic events become part of an outbreak when other cases can be linked to them epidemiologically, as when patients from different geographical areas give a history of visiting a common site within the incubation period of their illnesses. An association with overseas travel was found in one-third of the sporadic cases in England and Wales for the years 1979 to 1986. Apart from travel, an analysis of sporadic (better called non-travel, non-outbreak) cases in Glasgow between 1978 and 1986 supported the hypothesis that cooling towers were the source of the infections. The relative risk was three times greater for people living within 500 m of a cooling tower compared with those living more than 1000 m away.

In temperate countries legionellosis has a seasonal pattern, most cases occurring in the summer and autumn. A multicentre British Thoracic Society study of community-acquired pneumonia requiring hospital admission in 1982 to 1983 showed that 2 per cent had legionnaires' disease. This suggests that about 1500 cases occur per year in Britain.

The susceptibility to infection of exposed people varies. For non-pneumonic legionellosis the attack rate is very high. In contrast, the attack rate for legionnaires' disease is about 1 per cent, although subclinical or mild infections can follow exposure, as indicated by serological surveys. For example, of the staff at the Stafford District General Hospital who were tested following the outbreak in 1985, 42 per cent had an antibody titre of 1 in 16 or greater.

Hospital-acquired legionellosis has been a particular problem. This is because of the complexity of the buildings and the difficulty of keeping the hot water hot (storage at 60 °C and 50 °C at the taps), either because of the length of pipework or for fear of scalding patients. Hospital patients, too, are a highly susceptible population and species other than *L. pneumophila* more frequently cause infections in these circumstances. In intensive care units, inhalation of air passed through contaminated humidifiers or aspiration of contaminated water are other potential sources of infection.

Clinical manifestations

Legionella pneumonia

Large studies have suggested that legionella infection is the cause of around 2 to 5 per cent of cases of community-acquired pneumonia admitted to hospital, although there is wider geographical and seasonal variation. Infection tends to lead to moderate or severe infection rather than mild illness, and most patients require hospital admission within 5 to 7 days of the start of symptoms.

The incubation period is usually 2 to 10 days, with a mean of 7 days; males are two to three times more frequently affected than females. Infection at the extremes of age is rare and the highest incidence is in 40- to 70-year-old people, with a mean age of 53 years. People particularly at risk include cigarette smokers, alcoholics, diabetics, and those with chronic illness or who are receiving corticosteroids or immunosuppressive therapy. Consequently, the type of patient who requires admission to hospital is particularly at risk from a nosocomial source.

Clinical features (Table 1)

Typically, the illness starts fairly abruptly with high fever, shivers, bad headache, and muscle pains. Upper respiratory tract symptoms, herpes labialis, and skin rashes are uncommon. The cough is usually dry initially but dyspnoea is common and the illness often progresses quickly. Sometimes there may be a history of a recent hotel holiday abroad or a stay in hospital, which can alert the clinician to the possible diagnosis.

The patient commonly looks toxic and ill, with a high fever over 39 °C. Confusion and delirium or diarrhoea can dominate the clinical picture, masking the true diagnosis of pneumonia. Focal neurological signs, particularly of a cerebellar type, are well described. Amnesia on recovery is common.

Laboratory findings

The total white count is usually only moderately raised, to $15\,000 \times 10^6$/litre, often with a lymphopenia. Hyponatraemia, hypoalbuminaemia, and abnormality of liver function tests are detected in over half of the cases. Other non-specific features may include raised blood urea and muscle enzymes, hypoxaemia, haematuria, and proteinuria. Gram staining of sputum typically shows few pus cells and no predominant pathogen; initial blood and sputum cultures are negative unless dual infection is present.

Table 1 Clinical features of 739 patients with legionella pneumonia

Symptom	Percentage of patients showing symptom
Respiratory symptoms	
Cough	75
New sputum production	45
Dyspnoea	50
Chest pain	36
Haemoptysis	21
Bronchial breathing in lung	16
Crepitations in lung	74
General symptoms	
Rigors	59
Headaches	32
Confusion	45
Diarrhoea	33
Fever over 39 °C	70

(Data adapted with permission of the publishers from Table 3.2 in Bartlett CR, Macrae AD, Macfarlane JT (1986). *Legionella infections*. Edward Arnold, London)

Fig. 1 Chest radiograph of a 58-year-old man who returned from a Mediterranean hotel holiday with legionella pneumonia. There is extensive, bilateral, homogeneous consolidation. He required assisted ventilation for worsening respiratory failure.

Radiographic features

Radiographic shadowing is usually homogeneous. Characteristically, radiographic deterioration occurs with spread of shadows both within the same lung and to the opposite side. (Fig. 1).

Clearance of pulmonary shadows in survivors is particularly slow, with only two-thirds of radiographs being clear within 3 months and some taking more than 6 months to clear.

Complications

A wide variety of complications has been reported. The most important complication is acute respiratory failure requiring assisted ventilation, which occurs in up to 20 per cent of cases. Cardiac complications including pericardial and myocardial involvement are well recognized. A wide variety of neurological complications has been reported, leading to the suggestion of a specific neurotoxin. Acute, but usually reversible, renal failure may be seen in severe disease. There is anecdotal evidence that full clinical recovery may be very slow.

Pontiac fever

This is the acute non-pneumonic form of legionella infection and presents as a short-lived, self-limiting, influenza-like illness, dry cough, but no localizing signs in the chest (Fig. 2). The attack rate is extremely high, with an incubation period of usually 36 to 48 h. Investigations and chest radiograph are normal, and the illness improves spontaneously, usually within 5 days.

Laboratory diagnosis

There is a range of laboratory procedures that can be used to diagnose legionellosis:

(1) culture on a permissive medium, e.g. Aces buffered charcoal yeast-extract agar;

(2) direct detection of bacteria or their nucleic acid;

(3) urinary antigen detection;

(4) serological response.

Suitable specimens from which legionellae can be isolated are expectorated sputum, endotracheal aspirates, bronchoalveolar lavage fluid, pleural aspirates, and lung. Isolation provides definite proof of infection, as colonization without infection has not been demonstrated. In addition it allows

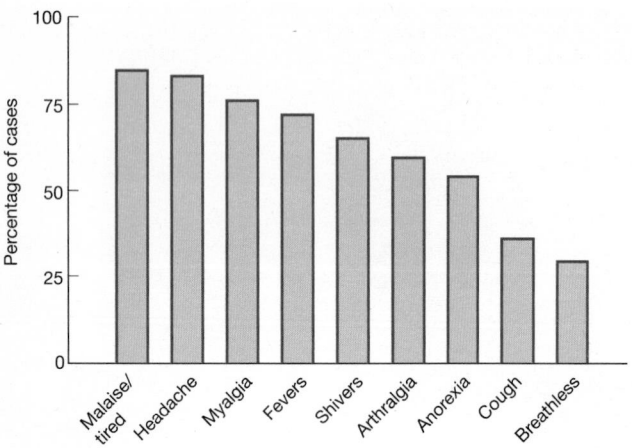

Fig. 2 Clinical features of 314 patients with non-pneumonic legionellosis (Pontiac fever). (Data adapted from Glick *et al.* (1978). *American Journal of Epidemiology* **107**, 149–60 and Goldberg *et al.* (1989). *Lancet* **i**, 316–18.)

the causative strain to be typed and compared with those from the environment. A quicker diagnosis can be made by examining these samples directly for evidence of legionellae. With specific monoclonal antisera the bacteria can be visualized by immunofluorescence or immunoperoxidase techniques. Alternatively the use of the polymerase chain reaction can detect the bacterial nucleic acid directly in a specimen.

Soluble antigen is excreted in the urine for 1 to 3 weeks during the acute pneumonia and longer in immunocompromised infected patients. Tests to detect *L. pneumophila* serogroup 1 urinary antigen have a high specificity and sensitivity, making this assay the most valuable for the prompt diagnosis of legionnaires' disease. Urine antigen testing for legionella should be undertaken for any patient with severe community-acquired pneumonia.

Serology is the most widely used diagnostic approach. The major problem with serodiagnosis is the delay due to the slow production of antibodies. Only 20 per cent of patients with legionnaires' disease have diagnostic titres of antibody within 3 days of hospital admission, although about 40 per cent will have lesser but suggestive antibody levels by that time. Approximately 20 per cent of those infected appear not to respond serologically.

Although some heterologous cross-reacting antibodies may be produced, infections with legionellae other than *L. pneumophila* serogroup 1 do not necessarily give rise to antibody to the latter. Reference laboratories therefore use a battery of antigens to increase their ability to diagnose legionellosis. In Denmark, for example, 13 antigens are used and, in 1990, of 171 serologically diagnosed cases, 93 were *L. pneumophila* serogroup 1 to 6 while 78 were non-*L. pneumophila* legionellosis caused by other species. Occasionally patients with Q fever, leptospirosis, *Citrobacter freundii*, and more commonly with campylobacter infections make antibodies that cross-react with *L. pneumophila* serogroup 1. As diarrhoea can be an early feature of legionnaires' disease as well as the major consequence of campylobacter enteritis, it is important to culture stool samples and interpret with caution the legionella serology from such patients.

Differential diagnosis

Unfortunately there is no distinctive pattern that allows the early clinical differentiation of legionella infection from other, more common, causes of pneumonia. Epidemiological clues such as recent foreign travel can be valuable pointers, as well, of course, as knowledge of a local epidemic. Important clues suggesting legionella pneumonia in this context include high fever, confusion, multisystem involvement, absence of a predominant bacterial pathogen on sputum examination, and lack of response to β-lactam antibiotics.

Therapy

There are no clinical trials, and recommendations are based on retrospective case studies as well as *in vitro* and animal experiments. The most relevant factor is the ability of the antibiotic to penetrate intracellularly into alveolar macrophages where the legionella organism hides and divides. A macrolide such as erythromycin or clarithromycin is at present recommended as the drug of first choice, in dosages of 500 to 1000 mg every 6 h for erythromycin and 500 mg twice daily for clarithromycin, being given intravenously if required.

In vitro and animal experiments and clinical experience support the efficacy of rifampicin and fluoroquinolones. Rifampicin is often recommended as additional therapy to erythromycin, in a dose of 600 mg once or twice daily in patients with severe infection or who are deteriorating. Fluoroquinolones are preferred by some experts in immunocompromised patients. Anecdotal reports also support the use of doxycycline.

General supportive measures are particularly important, with attention to adequate hydration and correction of hypoxaemia with the early use of assisted ventilation for advancing respiratory failure.

Prognosis and mortality

The two most important factors affecting outcome include the prior health of the patient and appropriate, early therapy. The fatality rate in previously fit patients is low, of the order of 5 to 15 per cent, but in immunosuppressed individuals it can approach 75 per cent. The mortality is about 30 per cent in those requiring assisted ventilation.

Pathology

Legionellae are intracellular pathogens, both in protozoa in the environment and in animal hosts. Following infection, the bacteria are taken up by macrophages and internalized in macrophage endosomes. Legionellae block the development of the endosome to a phagolysosome which prevents the normal cellular killing mechanism of the ingested bacteria. Instead, legionellae multiply within the cell with a generation time of 1 to 2 h. When an intracellular microcolony has formed , the legionellae produce a pore-forming toxin which damages the cell's membrane and allows the bacteria to escape from the cell.

The lungs are usually the only organs affected in fatal cases and reveal lobar consolidation. Affected lung tissue shows a severe inflammatory response, with alveoli and terminal bronchioles distended by fibrin-rich debris, mononuclear inflammatory cells, and neutrophils. Organisms can be demonstrated within alveolar spaces by silver or immunofluorescence stains. In survivors alveolar and interstitial fibrotic changes can result.

Prevention

There are three aspects to consider in reducing the risk of legionellosis:

(1) Measures to minimize colonization, growth, and release of legionellae into the atmosphere.

(2) Physical or chemical treatment of water to kill the bacteria.

(3) The protection of maintenance personnel who work on contaminated systems.

In Britain, particularly following the Stafford District General Hospital outbreak, a large number of publications aimed at minimizing the risk of legionellosis have appeared. In 1991 in Britain the Health and Safety Executive booklet HS(G)70 *The control of legionellosis including legionnaires' disease* was published, and it should be consulted for more details.

The most important principle to follow is to avoid holding water at temperatures between 20 and 45 °C, which is the range in which legionella multiplication occurs.

Further reading

Bhopal RS *et al.* (1991). Proximity of the home to a cooling tower and the risk of non-outbreak Legionnaires' disease. *British Medical Journal* **302**, 378–83.

Cunha BA (1998). Clinical features of legionnaires' disease. *Seminars in Respiratory Infections* **13**, 116–27.

Edelstein PH (1995). Antimicrobial chemotherapy for legionnaires' disease: a review. *Clinical Infectious Diseases* **21** (Suppl. 3), 5265–76.

Health and Safety Commission (2000). *Legionnaires' disease: the control of legionella bacteria in water systems. Approved code of practice and guidance L8.* HSE Books, Sudbury, Suffolk, UK.

Kwaik YA (1998). Fatal attraction of mammalian cells to *Legionella pneumophila. Molecular Microbiology* **30**, 689–95.

Ratcliffe RM *et al.* (1998). Sequence-based classification scheme for the genus Legionella targeting the *mip* gene. *Journal of Clinical Microbiology* **36**, 1560–7.

Woodhead MA, Macfarlane JT (1985). The protean manifestations of Legionnaires' disease. *Journal of the Royal College Physicians (London)* **19**, 224–30.

7.11.36 Rickettsial diseases including ehrlichioses

D. H. Walker

Introduction

Rickettsiae (Table 1) are obligate intracellular bacteria, which, during at least a part of their existence, occupy specific arthropods as their environmental niche. Rickettsiae are transmitted to man by their arthropod hosts and invade the endothelial cells of the blood vessel. In contrast, organisms of the genus *Ehrlichia* invade mainly phagocytes and do not cause primary vascular injury. Humans acquire *Coxiella burnetii* mainly by inhalation of aerosols from birth products of infected animals. The organisms proliferate within the acidic phagolysosome of host macrophages and cause an illness that ranges from acute atypical pneumonia to chronic endocarditis.

The public health importance of rickettsioses is underestimated because of difficulties with clinical diagnosis and lack of laboratory methods in many geographical areas. Active surveillance and serological surveys suggest that there is significant, unrecognized exposure to rickettsial organisms. It is particularly important to consider a rickettsial diagnosis when caring for the neglected poor of developing countries and travellers returning from areas endemic for murine typhus, scrub typhus, boutonneuse fever, African tick-bite fever, other spotted fevers, and Q fever. Rickettsiae infect previously healthy, active persons, and if undiagnosed, diagnosed late, or untreated, Rocky Mountain spotted fever, epidemic typhus, scrub typhus, Q fever endocarditis, boutonneuse fever (Plates 1, 2, 3), human ehrlichioses, and murine typhus are life threatening.

Many commonly prescribed antibiotics, including the penicillins, cephalosporins, and aminoglycosides, have no effect on the course of rickettsial diseases, but those antimicrobials active against rickettsial organisms can reduce morbidity and mortality.

Epidemics of louse-borne typhus fever have influenced the outcome of many wars between the 1500s and the 1920s. Wherever there are wars, famines, floods, and other massive disasters leading to widespread louse infestation of a population, the threat of epidemic typhus exists. Recent epidemics have occurred in Burundi, the economically devasted former USSR, and in extremely poor populations in the Andes.

Contemporary molecular analyses reveal that the spotted fever and typhus groups of the genus *Rickettsia* are very closely related to one another but not to *Orientia* (formerly *Rickettsia*) *tsutsugamushi*. They are relatively close relatives of *Ehrlichia* and the facultatively intracellular *Bartonella* and are evolutionarily distant from *Coxiella* and *Chlamydia*.

Vasculopathic rickettsial diseases of the spotted fever and typhus groups

Aetiological agents

These organisms measure approximately 0.3 by 1.0 μm and have a cell wall typical of Gram-negative bacteria.

Epidemiology

Seasonal incidence and geographical distribution are determined by the vector's activity. Spotted fever group rickettsiae are maintained in nature principally by transovarial and transstadial transmission in their tick or mite hosts. The most virulent rickettsiae are capable of killing their arthropod hosts (e.g. *R. prowazekii*) and require horizontal transmission to initiate epidemics of typhus fever. Reactivation of latent *R. prowazekii* infection in humans is the source for infection of lice that initiates epidemics of typhus fever.

Spotted fever group rickettsiae are transmitted to humans by secretion of infected tick saliva into the blood pooled in the site of the bite, and typhus group rickettsiae by infected louse or flea faeces deposited on human skin during arthropod feeding. Fluid or faeces of infected arthropods crushed between the fingers may enter a cutaneous wound or be rubbed into the conjunctiva.

Pathogenesis

Rickettsiae of some species of the spotted fever group frequently invade endothelial cells at the cutaneous portal of entry, proliferate, and cause a focus of dermal and epidermal necrosis, an eschar. Rickettsiae spread via the bloodstream to all parts of the body, where they infect endothelial cells lining the blood vessels. Typhus rickettsiae reach massive numbers intracellularly until the endothelial cell bursts. Spotted fever group rickettsiae are propelled through the cytosol by stimulating F-actin polymerization at one pole and spreading from cell to cell. Rickettsial lipopolysaccharides are non-endotoxic, and there is no evidence of any rickettsial exotoxin.

Host immune, inflammatory, and coagulation systems are activated with apparent overall benefit to the patient.

Progressive, disseminated infection and injury to endothelial cells cause increased vascular permeability, oedema, hypovolaemia, and signs and symptoms resulting from multifocal vascular injury in affected organs (Fig. 1). Infection of the pulmonary microcirculation and the resulting increased vascular permeability produce adult respiratory distress syndrome. Despite an interstitial myocarditis, myocardial function is usually preserved. Arrhythmias may result from vascular lesions affecting the conduction system. The vascular lesions in the brain are associated with coma and seizures in severe cases (Fig. 2). Multifocal infectious lesions in the dermis are the basis for the maculopapular, sometimes petechial, rash. Acute renal failure occurs in severe cases, usually as prerenal azotaemia or less frequently as acute tubular necrosis associated with severe hypotension.

Clinical manifestations

The incubation period averages 1 week (range: 4 days to 2 weeks) after cutaneous inoculation. It is related inversely to the dose of inoculum.

Symptoms start with non-specific malaise, chills, fever, myalgia, and headache that is often severe, followed by anorexia, nausea, vomiting, abdominal pain, photophobia, and cough. A rash usually appears after 3 to 5 days of illness. Initially, it consists of macular or maculopapular lesions, 1 to 5 mm in diameter, that blanch on pressure. Later petechiae appear.

Table 1 Aetiology, epidemiology, and ecology of rickettsial diseases

Disease	Agent	Geographical distribution	Natural history	Transmission to man
Spotted fevers				
Rocky Mountain spotted fever	R. rickettsii	North, Central, and South America	Transovarial maintenance in ticks; less extensive horizontal transmission from tick to mammal to tick	Tick bite
Boutonneuse fever	R. conorii	Mediterranean basin, Africa, Asia	Transovarial maintenance in ticks; role of horizontal transmission is not clear	Tick bite
African tick-bite fever	R. africae	Southern and eastern Africa	Presumably transovarian maintenance in ticks	Tick bite
North Asian tick typhus	R. sibirica	Russia, China, Mongolia, Pakistan, Kazakhstan, Kirgiziya, Tadzhikistan	Transovarial maintenance in ticks; horizontal transmission from tick to mammal to tick	Tick bite
Japanese spotted fever	R. japonica	Japan	Presumably a transovarial tick host; the role of horizontal transmission is not clear	Tick bite
Flinders Island spotted fever	R. honei	Southern Australian islands, Thailand	Unknown	Presumably tick bite
Queensland tick typhus	R. australis	Eastern Australia	Transovarial transmission in Ixodes ticks; the role of horizontal transmission is not clear	Tick bite
Rickettsialpox	R. akari	United States, Ukraine, Croatia, possibly worldwide	Transovarial transmission in Liponyssoides sanguineus mites; horizontal transmission from mite to mouse to mite	Mite bite
Cat flea typhus	R. felis	Presumably worldwide	Transovarial transmission in Ctenocephalides felis fleas	Unknown
Typhus fevers				
Epidemic typhus	R. prowazekii	South America, Africa, Asia, Central America, Mexico	Man to louse to man	Louse faeces scratched into skin
Sylvatic typhus	R. prowazekii	United States	Flying squirrel to louse and flea ectoparasites to flying squirrel	Presumably flea of flying squirrels to man
Recrudescent typhus	R. prowazekii	Worldwide	Reactivation of latent human infection years after acute illness	None
Murine typhus	R. typhi	Worldwide, predominantly tropical and subtropical	Rat to rat flea to rat; opossum to cat flea to opossum	Flea faeces scratched into skin, rubbed into conjunctiva, or inhaled
Scrub typhus	O. tsutsugamushi	Japan, southern and eastern Asia, northern Australia, islands of the western and south-western Pacific	Transovarial transmission in Leptotrombidium chiggers	Chigger bite
Ehrlichioses				
Human monocytotropic ehrlichiosis	E. chaffeensis	North America, Portugal, Spain, Mali, Thailand, Mexico	Horizontal transmission between mammals (e.g. deer, dogs) and ticks	Tick bite
Human granulocytotropic ehrlichoisis phagocytophila	A. phagocytophila	United States, Europe	Horizontal transmission between mammals (e.g. white footed mice, red deer, sheep, cattle, horses) and Ixodes ticks	Tick bite
Human granulocytotropic ehrlichosis ewingii	E. ewingii	United States	Horizontal transmission between mammals (e.g. dogs) and ticks	Tick bite
Sennetsu ehrlichiosis	E. sennetsu	Japan, Malaysia	Maintenance in fish or snail flukes	Suspected ingestion of raw fish infected with ehrlichia-infected flukes
Q fever	C. burnetii	Worldwide	Mammals including sheep, goats, cattle, rabbits, and cats; ticks	Aerosol of infected mammalian birth products
Bartonella infections				
Trench fever	B. quintana	Europe, North America	Louse to man to louse	Louse faeces
Cat-scratch disease	B. henselae / B. clarridgei	Worldwide	Cat-to-cat, flea-to-cat	Cat scratch or bite
Bacillary angiomatosis, peliosis	B. henselae / B. quintana	Worldwide	Cat-to-cat, flea-to-cat	Cat scratch or bite
Endocarditis	B. quintana / B. henselae / B. elizabethae	Worldwide	Cat-to-cat, flea-to-cat	Cat scratch or bite
Oroya fever, verruga peruana	B. bacilliformis	Peru, Ecuador, Colombia	Human to sandfly to human	Sandfly presumably via bite

Fig. 1 Immunoperoxidase-stained *Rickettsia rickettsii* appear as dark bacilli in endothelial cells of a cerebral blood vessel with perivascular oedema but no host immune-cell infiltration.

Pulmonary involvement causes cough, pulmonary oedema, radiographic infiltrates, hypoxaemia, dyspnoea, and pleural effusions in severe cases. Neurological manifestations consist of lethargy, progressing to confusion, delirium, stupor, ataxia, coma, focal neurological signs, and seizures. There may be a cerebrospinal fluid pleocytosis of 10 to 100 cells/µl with variable proportions of mononuclear and polymorphonuclear leucocytes, and/or an increased protein concentration.

Although serum aminotransferases and bilirubin may be elevated, jaundice is observed in fewer than 10 per cent of patients, and hepatic failure

Fig. 2 Epidemic typhus fever. The typical lesion of rickettsial encephalitis is exemplified by the typhus nodule in the brain of a patient (death about 12th day) showing perivascular infiltration by macrophages and lymphocytes. (Reproduced from *Medical Clinics of North America* (1959), **43**, 1512, with permission.)

does not occur. The white blood-cell count is usually normal. The acute-phase reaction occurs in many patients. Hypoalbuminaemia is the result of leakage of this plasma protein into the interstitial space because of increased permeability of the microcirculation. Hyponatraemia is most often the result of the appropriate secretion of antidiuretic hormone in response to the hypovolaemic state.

Diagnosis

Differential diagnosis

Early, before the rash appears, the differential diagnosis includes influenza, typhoid fever, enteroviral infection, and infectious diseases suggested by geographical exposure (e.g. malaria, Lassa fever, louse-borne relapsing fever). Nausea, vomiting, and abdominal pain may suggest infectious enterocolitis. Prominent abdominal tenderness has occasionally led to the differential diagnosis of acute surgical abdomen and to exploratory laparotomy. Cough and abnormalities of physical and radiographic examination of the chest may suggest bronchitis or pneumonia. Fever, seizures, coma, neurological signs, and abnormalities of the cerebrospinal fluid may lead to consideration of meningitis and arboviral or herpes viral encephalitis. If an eschar is detected, the differential diagnosis may include cutaneous anthrax, tularaemia, syphilis, and chancroid. Once a rash has developed, differential diagnosis includes meningococcaemia, toxic-shock syndrome, leptospirosis, disseminated gonococcal infection, secondary syphilis, measles, rubella, enteroviral exanthem, infectious mononucleosis, dengue, filoviral or arenaviral haemorrhagic fevers, idiopathic or thrombotic thrombocytopenic purpura, and immune-complex vasculitides (e.g. systemic lupus erythematosus). It is important to enquire about exposure to ticks, fleas, mites, and lice and to consider the seasonal occurrence and geographical exposure, but people are frequently unaware of their exposure to arthropods, and cases may occur outside of the seasonal peak.

Laboratory diagnosis

Serological tests are useful in confirming the diagnosis in the convalescent stage, but seldom detect specific antibodies during the first week of illness. At present, the generally available serological assays are an indirect immunofluorescent antibody test, indirect immunoperoxidase antibody test, and dot enzyme immunoassay. These tests detect antibodies that are cross-reactive within the spotted fever or typhus group. The Weil–Felix test should be replaced because of poor sensitivity and specificity unless, as in some underdeveloped areas, nothing else is available. Isolation of the aetiological rickettsia, the definitive diagnosis of an infectious disesae, is seldom attempted because of the biohazard and technical challenges.

Detection of rickettsiae by immunohistochemistry in skin requires the presence of a rash to determine the site for biopsy and has sensitivity of approximately 70 per cent and a specificity of 100 per cent in the hands of an experienced microscopist. An approach that can be employed even during the period of illness before the onset of rash is immunofluorescent staining of rickettsiae in circulating endothelial cells captured by a monoclonal antibody fixed to immunomagnetic beads. Polymerase chain reaction has not been very successful in diagnosing Rocky Mountain spotted fever early in the course of illness, but has proved useful in murine typhus, epidemic typhus, Japanese spotted fever, boutonneuse fever, *R. felis* infection, and scrub typhus. Treatment should never be withheld while awaiting the results of laboratory tests.

Treatment

Spotted-fever and typhus-group rickettsioses respond favourably to treatment with doxycycline (200 mg/day for adults and children heavier than 45 kg, and 4.4 mg/kg body weight per day for smaller children), tetracycline (2 g/day in four divided doses for adults, and 25 mg/kg body weight per day in four divided doses for children), or chloramphenicol (2 g/day in four divided doses for adults, and 50 mg/kg body weight per day in four divided doses for children). Ciprofloxacin (200 mg intravenously every 12 h, or

750 mg orally every 12 h), ofloxacin (200 mg orally every 12 h), and pefloxacin (400 mg intravenously or orally every 12 h) have been used successfully to treat boutonneuse fever. Epidemic typhus fever has been treated effectively under field conditions with a single, 200 mg dose of doxycycline. Treatment is generally continued for 2 or 3 days after defervescence to avoid relapse of the infection.

Intravenously administered doxycycline or chloramphenicol is employed when oral treatment cannot be used because of vomiting or coma. Chloramphenicol and josamycin (3 g/day for 8 days) have been used to treat rickettsioses during pregnancy when the tetracyclines are contraindicated.

Seizures should be treated with anticonvulsants. Renal failure is managed by haemodialysis, and hypoxaemia associated with interstitial pneumonitis and adult respiratory distress syndrome may require oxygen and mechanical ventilation.

Prevention

Immunization

Immunity to reinfection with spotted-fever or typhus-group rickettsiae is quite strong, although some patients with epidemic typhus fever will develop recrudescence of latent *R. prowazekii* infection many years after their acute infection.

Vaccines containing whole, killed organisms can reduce severity of illness and mortality, but a live, attenuated vaccine against *R. prowazekii* confers protection. However, some vaccine recipients develop mild typhus fever, and the vaccine strain may revert to a pathogenic state. Thus, there are at present no vaccines in general use against rickettsial diseases.

Vector control

Delousing reduces the spread of louse-borne epidemic typhus. Rodent control and insecticides decrease the incidence of murine typhus and rickettsialpox.

Regular daily or twice-daily inspection of the entire body, especially the scalp and groin, and prompt removal of ticks prevents inoculation of rickettsiae. Ticks are best removed by grasping their anterior parts firmly with pointed forceps flush with the skin and exerting steady traction until the intact tick is removed, frequently with a bit of attached skin. Care should be taken to avoid introduction of potentially infected tick fluids into the wound or mucous membranes.

Spotted fevers

Boutonneuse fever

Aetiology

The most prevalent spotted-fever rickettsiosis in Europe is boutonneuse fever, or Mediterranean spotted fever. *Rickettsia conorii* has been isolated in Spain, France, Italy, Croatia, Georgia, Russia, Ukraine, India, Pakistan, South Africa, Kenya, Somalia, and Ethiopia. *R. conorii* has more antigenic diversity than the other carefully analysed spotted-fever group rickettsia, *R. rickettsii*.

Epidemiology

The incidence of boutonneuse fever underwent a dramatic increase in Spain, France, Italy, and Portugal a decade or two ago. *R. conorii* is maintained transovarially in *Rhipicephalus sanguineus* and is transmitted to humans by tick bite. The peak incidence along the Mediterranean coast of southern Europe is in July and August when immature stages of the tick predominate.

Mortality rates of 1.4 to 5.6 per cent have been observed in patients admitted to hospital. In those who are elderly or have underlying diseases, suffer from alcoholism, or glucose-6-phosphate dehydrogenase deficiency, case fatality may be 33 per cent.

Pathogenesis

Reduction in the number of rickettsiae in the *tache noire* (black spot) or eschar at the site of the infective tick-bite eschar is associated with a perivascular influx of lymphocytes and macrophages. Autopsies of fatal cases of boutonneuse fever show systemic vascular infection and injury by *R. conorii*, with lesions in the brain, meninges, lungs, kidney, gastrointestinal tract, liver, pancreas, heart, spleen, and skin including sites of peripheral gangrene. Direct rickettsial injury of infected endothelial cells is the major pathogenic event. Hepatic biopsies show multifocal dead hepatocytes with a predominantly mononuclear cellular response.

Clinical manifestations

During the incubation period of boutonneuse fever, a red papule appears at the site of the tick bite and progresses to an eschar in approximately 70 per cent of cases, often associated with regional lymphadenopathy. The illness starts with fever, sometimes accompanied by headache and myalgias. The rash usually appears on the fourth day of illness as maculopapules, is petechial in 10 per cent of patients, and often involves the palms and soles. Other features include nausea, vomiting, cough, dyspnoea, conjunctivitis, stupor, meningismus, and hepatomegaly. Increased vascular permeability manifests as mild oedema, hypoalbuminaemia, and arterial hypotension. The white blood-cell count is usually normal. Platelet counts less than $100 \times 10^9/l$ are detected in 12.5 per cent of the patients. Hyponatraemia of less than 130 mmol/l occurs in 23 per cent, and hypoproteinaemia is observed in 23 per cent of patients.

Serum urea and creatinine concentrations are elevated in 25 and 17 per cent of patients, respectively. Serum concentrations of aspartate and alanine aminotransferases are increased in 39 and 37 per cent, respectively, and serum bilirubin is greater than 20 µmol/l in 9 per cent. Severe features (6 per cent of patients) include cutaneous purpura and other haemorrhagic phenomena, neurological signs, altered mental status, respiratory symptoms, hypoxaemia, and acute renal failure.

Diagnosis

In the acute stage, diagnosis can be established by immunohistological demonstration of *R. conorii* in a biopsy of the *tache noire* or rash, or in circulating endothelial cells (see above). *R. conorii* can be isolated in cell culture. Serological methods include immunofluorescent antibody assay, latex agglutination test, indirect immunoperoxidase assay, dot enzyme immunoassay, and complement fixation test.

Treatment

See above.

Prevention

There is no vaccine to protect against *R. conorii*.

Rocky Mountain spotted fever

R. rickettsii is pathogenic for *Dermacentor* ticks, perhaps explaining why fewer than 1 in 1000 ticks in endemic areas contains this organism. *R. rickettsii*, the most virulent rickettsia, is also more invasive than other rickettsial species, causing infection not only of endothelial cells but also vascular smooth-muscle cells. Host factors also play a part in severity of illness. Fatality rates are higher in older patients, males, and black people. Fulminant Rocky Mountain spotted fever with death occurring within 5 days after onset is associated with haemolysis, particularly in black males with glucose-6-phosphate dehydrogenase deficiency.

Untreated, Rocky Mountain spotted fever has a 20 per cent fatality rate. In recent series, the death rate has been 5 per cent, with respiratory failure in 12 per cent, acute renal failure in 14 per cent, and anaemia requiring red-cell transfusion in 11 per cent. Thrombocytopenia occurs in 32 to 52 per cent of patients. Coma is a grave prognostic sign.

Early in the illness, nausea or vomiting occurs in 38 to 56 per cent of cases and abdominal pain in 30 to 34 per cent. The rash usually appears on

Fig. 3 The early rash of Rocky Mountain spotted fever consists of pink macules in this 4-year-old boy on the fourth day of illness.

the third day of illness, but may be delayed to or after day 6 in 20 per cent (Fig. 3). In 10 per cent of patients, a rash never appears. Petechiae occur in only 41 to 59 per cent of cases and appear late in the course, often only on or after day 6. The palms and soles are affected by the rash in 36 to 82 per cent with involvement often occurring after day 5 (Fig. 4).

A history of tick exposure is obtained from only 60 per cent of patients. Reagents for indirect immunofluorescent antibody assay, latex agglutination test, and dot enzyme immunoassay for antibodies to *R. rickettsii* are commercially available.

Rickettsialpox

R. akari has been isolated in the United States, Ukraine, Croatia, and Korea. It is maintained by transovarian transmission in the gamasid mite *Liponyssoides sanguineus*, whose host is the domestic mouse, *Mus musculus*.

A cutaneous papule appears during the incubation period at the site where the mite has fed and evolves into an eschar over the next 2 to 7 days. About 10 days later, malaise, fever, chills, severe headache, and myalgia develop. A macular rash of discrete erythematous lesions, 2 to 3 mm in diameter, appears 2 to 6 days later and evolves into maculopapules, some of which develop central, deep-seated vesicles.

Other spotted-fever rickettsioses

R. sibirica, *R. australis*, *R. japonica*, *R. honei*, and *R. africae* differ antigenically in their surface proteins, DNA sequences, tick hosts, and known geographical distribution, but their clinical manifestations are similar to boutonneuse fever. The spotted-fever rickettsiosis of Flinders Island, Australia and Queensland tick typhus are clinically similar. Israeli spotted fever is a variant of boutonneuse fever in which eschar formation is usually lacking. *R. africae* is associated with a relatively less severe illness in which rash is less prevalent, but there are often multiple eschars. *Rickettsia slovaca*, previously considered as non-pathogenic, has recently been associated with clinical illness in Europe. *R. felis* is maintained in cat fleas and causes an emerging infectious disease.

In Sweden, *R. helvetica*, transmitted by *Ixodes ricinus* ticks, has been suggested to cause fatal chronic perimyocarditis. *R. conorii*, *R. typhi*, and *R.*

rickettsii are also known to affect the microcirculation of the myocardium.

Typhus fevers

Murine typhus

Endemic flea-borne typhus fever caused by *R. typhi* is more prevalent in warm, coastal ports. It is maintained in a commensal cycle involving rat fleas, *Xenopsylla cheopis*, and rats, *Rattus rattus* and *Rattus norvegicus*. Rats are infected by *R. typhi* in flea faeces deposited on the skin. Fleas become infected for life after a rickettsaemic blood meal. Other species of fleas and other mammals can also maintain an infectious cycle of *R. typhi* (see Table 1).

A rash is detected in 80 per cent of fair-skinned and 20 per cent of black people. Other features include nausea (48 per cent), vomiting (40 per cent), abdominal pain (23 per cent), diarrhoea (26 per cent), cough (35 per cent), abnormal chest radiographs (23 per cent), thrombocytopenia (48 per cent), elevated serum aminotransferases (90 per cent), and central nervous abnormalities (8 per cent) including confusion, stupor, and hallucinations. Nearly 10 per cent of patients admitted to hospital are severely ill with acute renal failure, respiratory failure, or severe neurological abnormalities including seizures. Older age, delayed treatment, and initial treatment with sulphonamides are risk factors for severe disease. Case fatality is 1 to 2 per cent.

Epidemic typhus, recrudescent typhus, and sylvatic typhus

R. prowazekii causes epidemic louse-borne typhus fever, recrudescence of latent infection years after acute epidemic typhus, and zoonotic infection acquired from the ectoparasites of infected flying squirrels in North America. There is intense headache, prostration, continuous high fever, a macular rash usually appearing on the fourth or fifth day of illness, myalgia, and neurological abnormalities. Within 24 to 48 h of its appearance, the rash becomes petechial and does not blanch on pressure (Fig. 5). Its development is centrifugal from the trunk to the extremities. Other symptoms include cough, rales (71 per cent), nausea (30 per cent), abdominal pain (30 per cent), mental dullness (14 per cent), delirium (48 per cent), coma (6 per cent), seizures (1 per cent), and gangrene (3 per cent).

The infection is now restricted to a few foci of sporadic occurrence in eastern Europe, central Africa, Ethiopia, southern Africa, Afghanistan, northern India, China, Mexico, Central America, and the Andes Mountains of South America. However, the danger of spread still exists as occurred recently during the war in Burundi where it is estimated that 100,000 cases occurred.

Recrudescent typhus (Brill–Zinsser disease) is the most important reservoir for initiation of epidemic louse-borne typhus in a susceptible population. Clinically it is milder than epidemic typhus (Fig. 6).

Ehrlichial diseases

Aetiological agents

Ehrlichiae are small, Gram-negative obligately intracellular bacteria that reside in a cytoplasmic vacuole and are transmitted by ticks. The four established human pathogens are *Ehrlichia chaffeensis*, *Anaplasma phagocytophila*, *E. ewingii*, and *Neorickettsia sennetsu*.

Ehrlichiae enter the host cell via phagocytosis, and they actively inhibit fusion of lysosomes with the phagosomes. They undergo binary fission to form clusters within a host vacuole. When stained by the Wright–Giemsa method, the cluster of organisms appears dark violet-blue and stippled and is called a morula from the Latin word for mulberry.

Epidemiology (see Table 1)

Ehrlichioses are maintained in cycles involving a mammalian host and a tick vector. *N. sennetsu* is a member of a genus which resides in flukes that parasitize fish and snails.

Most patients recall a recent tick bite. *E. chaffeensis* and *A. phagocytophila* infections peak between May and July in the United States, the season of greatest tick activity.

Human ehrlichioses

Haemopoietic cells are the primary targets of infection by *E. chaffeensis*, *A. phagocytophila*, and *E. ewingii*. Leucopenia and thrombocytopenia are probably caused by peripheral sequestration. Perivascular lymphohistiocytic infiltrations without vascular damage are observed in virtually any organ, including meninges. Hepatic involvement may include focal hepatocellular apoptosis and granulomas. Interstitial mononuclear pneumonitis has been observed, as well as diffuse alveolar damage.

Clinical severity ranges from asymptomatic seroconversion to fatal infection, very likely related to both host and microbial virulence factors. *E. chaffeensis* is the most pathogenic. Most patients have a fever, headache, chills, malaise, nausea, myalgias, and anorexia. Respiratory or renal insufficiency and abnormalities of the central nervous system have been reported. Pleocytosis, leucopenia, thrombocytopenia, and elevations in serum hepatic aminotransferases are the most often demonstrated clinical laboratory abnormalities. Overwhelming, often fatal, cases occur in immunosuppressed patients, particularly those with HIV-1 infection.

Differential diagnoses include Rocky Mountain spotted fever, meningococcaemia, bacterial sepsis, and infective endocarditis.

Human isolates of *E. chaffeensis* and *A. phagocytophila* have been obtained in cell culture of a dog histiocytoma cell line and a human promyelocytic leukemia cell line, respectively. Ehrlichiae, particularly *A. phagocytophila*, can sometimes be seen in peripheral white blood cells. The standard diagnostic test is indirect immunofluorescent antibody assay. A fourfold rise or fall in titre with a peak of 64 or greater is considered diagnostic. Human ehrlichiosis can also be diagnosed by detection of ehrlichial DNA amplified from the peripheral blood by polymerase chain reaction. Although these tick-borne human ehrlichioses were discovered only recently in the United States, human infections with *A. phagocytophila* have been reported in Europe.

Human ehrlichioses respond to treatment with doxycycline (200 mg/day in two divided doses) or tetracycline (25 mg/kg body weight per day in four divided doses).

Prevention is by avoiding tick bites.

Further reading

Bakken JS *et al.* (1996). Clinical and laboratory characteristics of human granulocytic ehrlichoisis. *Journal of the American Medical Association* **275**, 199–205.

Buller RS *et al.* (1999). *Ehrlichia ewingii*, a newly recognized agent of human ehrlichiosis. *New England Journal of Medicine* **341**, 148–55.

Fig. 4 Rocky Mountain spotted fever. Series showing haemorrhagic exanthem in a 4-year-old boy on about the eighth day of illness. Note oedema of face, hands, arms, and feet, and bleeding from mouth. Specific therapy with chloramphenicol resulted in complete recovery.

Fig. 5 Epidemic typhus fever. Typical truncal rash in louse-borne typhus on about the eighth day of illness showing many discrete haemorrhagic lesions.

Dumler JS, Taylor JP, Walker DH (1991). Clinical and laboratory features of murine typhus in South Texas, 1980 through 1987. *Journal of the American Medical Association* **266**, 1365–70.

Elghetany MT, Walker DH (1999). Hemostatic changes in Rocky Mountain spotted fever and Mediterranean spotted fever. *American Journal of Clinical Pathology* **112**, 159–68.

Kass EM *et al.* (1994). Rickettsialpox in a New York City hospital, 1980 to 1989. *New England Journal of Medicine* **331**, 1612–17.

LaScola B, Raoult D (1997). Laboratory diagnosis of rickettsioses: current approaches to diagnosis of old and new rickettsial diseases. *Journal of Clinical Microbiology* **35**, 2715–27.

Lotric-Furlan S *et al.* (1998). Human granulocytic ehrlichiosis in Europe: clinical and laboratory findings for four patients from Slovenia. *Clinical Infectious Diseases* **27**, 424–8.

McDade JE, Newhouse VF (1986). Natural history of *Rickettsia rickettsii*. *Annual Review of Microbiology* **40**, 287–309.

Nilsson K, Lindquist O, Pahlson C (1999). Association of *Rickettsia helvetica* with chronic perimyocarditis in sudden cardiac death. *Lancet* **354**, 1169–73.

Perine PL *et al.* (1992). A clinico-epidemiological study of epidemic typhus in Africa. *Clinical Infectious Diseases* **14**, 1149–58.

Fig. 6 Recrudescent typhus (Brill–Zinsser disease). Note the erythematous macular rash on the trunk. Illness is in an adult whose initial infection with typhus was 30 years earlier in Poland; the second attack was a week after appendicectomy and there was full recovery.

Raoult D, Brouqui P (1999). *Rickettsiae and rickettsial disease at the turn of the third millenium*. Elsevier, Paris.

Raoult D *et al.* (1986). Mediterranean spotted fever: clinical, laboratory and epidemiological features of 199 cases. *American Journal of Tropical Medicine and Hygiene* **35**, 845–50.

Rikihisa Y (1991). The tribe *Ehrlichieae* and ehrlichial diseases. *Clinical Microbiology Reviews* **4**, 286–308.

Walker DH, Dumler JS (1996). Emergence of ehrlichiosis as human health problems. *Emerging Infectious Diseases* **2**, 18–29

Walker DH, Dumler JS (1997). Human monocytic and granulocytic ehrlichioses. Discovery and diagnosis of emerging tick-borne infections and the critical role of the pathologist. *Archives of Pathology and Laboratory Medicine* **121**, 785–91.

Walker DH, Fishbein DB (1991). Epidemiology of rickettsial diseases. *European Journal of Epidemiology* **7**, 237–45.

7.11.37 Scrub typhus

George Watt

Scrub typhus, or tsutsugamushi fever, is a zoonosis of rural Asia and the western Pacific islands. The causative organism, *Orientia* (formerly *Rickettsia*) *tsutsugamushi*, is transmitted to humans by the bite of a larval *Leptotrombidium* mite (chigger). An eschar and regional lymphadenopathy often develop at the site of infection, and may by followed by a systemic illness ranging in severity from inapparent to fatal. Many cases go undiagnosed, particularly those in which an eschar cannot be found. Rapid non-microscopic diagnostic tests are available and should enable more *O. tsutsugamushi* infections to be diagnosed.

Aetiology and epidemiology

Orientia tsutsugamushi has a different cell wall structure and genetic makeup from rickettsiae but looks like a rickettsia under light microscopy. The organism is an obligately intracellular Gram-negative bacterium. There are multiple serotypes of *O. tsutsugamushi*, and infection with one type confers only transient cross-immunity to another. Scrub typhus is a zoonosis. Larval mites (of the *Leptotrombidium deliense* group) usually feed on small rodents, particularly wild rats of the subgenus *Rattus*. Man becomes infected when he accidentally encroaches in a zone where there are infected mites. These zones are often made up of secondary or 'scrub' growth, hence the term scrub typhus. However, mite habitats as diverse as seashores, rice fields, and semideserts have been described. Infected chiggers are generally found in only very circumscribed foci within these zones. Large numbers of cases can occur when humans enter these so-called 'mite islands.' Disease transmission occurs when infected mites burrow into the skin, take a meal of tissue fluid, and inoculate the infectious organisms. Human to human transmission of scrub typhus via contaminated blood has never been documented. The endemic area forms a triangle bounded by northern Japan and southeastern Siberia to the north, Queensland, Australia, to the south and Pakistan to the west (Fig. 1). Disease transmission occurs in rural and suburban areas as well as in villages, but inhabitants of city centres are not at risk.

Pathology and pathogenesis

Much remains unknown about the pathogenesis of scrub typhus, partly because most descriptions of severe cases pre-date advances made in immunohistology since the 1950s. Marked geographical variations in severity of the illness occur but determinants of severity are poorly characterized. Strains which differ in virulence, partial immunity, and regional differences in general health could affect disease presentation, but coinfection with the HIV-1 virus does not. Scrub typhus is a vasculitis, but clinical and pathological findings do not correlate closely. The host cell of *O. tsutsugamushi* in humans is thought to be the endothelial cell because of findings in experimental animals and by analogy with other rickettsial infections. However, in human liver infected with scrub typhus examined by electron microscopy, organisms predominate in Kupffer cells and hepatocytes rather than within endothelial cells (Fig. 2). *O. tsutsagamushi* is present in peripheral white blood cells of patients with scrub typhus. The HIV-1 viral load falls markedly in some AIDS patients who acquire acute *O. tsutsagamushi* infection. Some sera from HIV-seronegative patients with scrub typhus inhibit HIV replication *in vitro*.

Clinical features

The painless chigger bite can occur on any part of the body, but is often in difficult to see in locations such as under the axilla or in the genital area. An eschar (Plate 1) forms at the bite site in about half of primary infections, but in a minority of secondary infections. The eschar begins as a small, painless papule which develops during the 6- to 18-day (median 10 days) incubation period. It enlarges, undergoes central necrosis, and acquires a blackened scab to form a lesion resembling a cigarette burn. Regional lymph nodes are enlarged and tender. The eschar is usually well developed by the time fever appears and is often healing by the time the patient presents to hospital.

Fever, headache, myalgia, and non-specific malaise are common symptoms. Hearing loss concurrent with fever is reported by as many as one-third of patients and is a useful diagnostic clue. Conjunctival suffusion and generalized lymphadenopathy are common, helpful physical signs. A transient macular rash may appear at the end of the first week of illness but is often difficult to see. The rash first appears on the trunk and becomes maculopapular as it spreads peripherally. Cough sometimes accompanied by infiltrates on the chest radiograph is one of the commonest presentations of *O. tsutsugamushi* infection. In severe cases, tachypnoea progresses to dyspnoea, the patient becomes cyanotic and full-blown adult respiratory distress syndrome may ensue. Apathy, confusion, and personality changes frequently occur and only rarely progress to stupor, convulsions, and coma. Abnormalities resolve completely in non-fatal cases.

Diagnosis

The eschar is the single most useful diagnostic clue, and is pathognomonic when seen by a physician experienced in diagnosis of scrub typhus. Even typical eschars can be overlooked or misdiagnosed, however, and atypical presentations are common. Eschars in the genital area often lose their crust and can be confused with the ulcers of chancroid, syphilis, or lymphogranuloma venereum.

There is no constellation of laboratory test results which strongly suggests *O. tsutsugamushi* infection. Slight increases in the number of circulating white blood cells are common. Atypical lymphocytes and moderately elevated serum transaminase levels are not uncommon. Laboratory findings are chiefly useful to rule out other infections. A low white cell count and thrombocytopenia with a haemorrhagic rash suggest infection with dengue virus rather than *O. tsutsugamushi*. Raised serum creatinine and serum bilirubin levels with marked myalgia suggest leptospirosis rather

Fig. 1 Geographical distribution of scrub typhus.

than scrub typhus. Enteric fever rarely causes generalized lymphadenopathy or conjunctival suffusion.

The Weil–Felix test using the Proteus OX-K antigen is a commercially available serodiagnostic test which has been used for many years, but is insensitive. Immunofluorescent assay and the immunoperoxidase test are the confirmatory tests of choice but their complexity limits their use to a small number of reference centres. An accurate, rapid, dotblot immunoassay which does not require a microscope has been developed (Plate 2). Such kits would be of enormous benefit if they could be made affordable for use in rural tropical Asia where most scrub typhus cases occur.

Treatment

Prompt antibiotic therapy shortens the course of the disease and reduces mortality. Treatment must often be presumptive, but the benefits of avoiding severe scrub typhus by early antibiotic administration generally far outweigh the risks of a 1-week course of tetracycline—the treatment of choice. Either oral tetracycline 500 mg four times daily, or oral doxycycline 100 mg twice daily for 7 days are recommended. Oral chloramphenicol 500 mg four times a day is a cheaper alternative. Treatment for less than a week is

(a)

(b)

Fig. 2 *Orientia tsutsugamushi* in human liver visualized by electron microscopy (by courtesy of Dr Emsri Pongponratn). (a) Three hepatocytes (H) and a perinuclear scrub typhus organism (arrow) attached to the nuclear membrane. (b) *O. tsutsugamushi* piercing a hepatocyte nuclear membrane.

initially curative, but may be followed by relapse. Parenteral doxycycline should be administered to patients who cannot swallow tablets or who are severely ill. A 7-day course of parenteral chloramphenicol (50–75 mg/kg/day) is an effective alternative in areas where parenteral formulations of tetracyclines are unavailable. Good supportive care and early detection of complications is important in severe cases if a good outcome is to be obtained.

Scrub typhus cases from northern Thailand which respond poorly to conventional therapy have been described, but neither the mechanism of resistance nor its geographical distribution have been defined. A controlled, blinded study demonstrated that patients treated with rifampin in northern Thailand became afebrile twice as quickly as did patients who received doxycycline. However, the optimum therapeutic regimen for the treatment of drug-resistant scrub typhus has not yet been determined. Therapy for pregnant women and children poses several problems. Chloramphenicol is best avoided during pregnancy and cannot be given to neonates; tetracycline is contraindicated in pregnancy and long courses administered to young children cause staining of the permanent teeth. Newer macrolide antibiotics appear to be effective for scrub typhus. Cases of both drug-sensitive and drug-resistant scrub typhus have been cured by azithromycin and three Japanese patients were treated successfully with clarithromycin. If their efficacy is confirmed, macrolides would be particularly useful for the treatment of infection during pregnancy and early childhood.

Prevention and control

Weekly doses of 200 mg of doxycycline can prevent *O. tsutsugamushi* infection. Chemoprophylaxis should be considered for non-immunes sent to an enzootic area to perform work which places them at high risk of acquiring scrub typhus. Soldiers and road construction crews are typical examples, but chemoprophylaxis should also be considered in high-risk travellers such as trekkers. Contact with chiggers can be reduced by applying repellant to the tops of boots, socks, and on the lower trousers and by not sitting or lying directly on the ground. Unfortunately these measures are frequently not practicable in those exposed occupationally. There is no vaccine for scrub typhus.

Prognosis

Scrub typhus was a dreaded disease in the preantibiotic era; case fatality rates reached as high as 50 per cent. Prompt antibiotic therapy generally prevents death, but up to 15 per cent of patients still die in northern Thailand. Deaths are attributable to a variety of factors including late presentation, delayed diagnosis, and drug resistance.

Further reading

Chayakul P, Panich V, Silpapojakul K (1988). Scrub typhus pneumonitis:an entity which is frequently missed. *Quarterly Journal of Medicine* **256**, 595–602.

Kantipong P *et al.* (1996). HIV infection does not influence the clinical severity of scrub typhus. *Clinical Infectious Diseases* **23**, 1168.

Olson JG *et al.* (1980). Prevention of scrub typhus. Prophylactic administration of doxycycline in a randomized double blind trial. *American Journal of Tropical Medicine and Hygiene* **29**, 989.

Pongponratn E *et al.* (1998). Electron microscopic examination of *Rickettsia tsutsugamushi*-infected human liver. *Tropical Medicine and International Health* **3**, 242–8.

Silpapojakul K *et al.* (1991). Scrub and murine typhus is children with obscure fever in the tropics. *International Journal of Systematic Bacteriology* **10**, 200–3.

Silpapojakul K *et al.* (1991). Rickettsial meningitis and encephalitis. *Archives of Internal Medicine* **151**, 1753–7.

Watt G *et al.* (1996). Scrub typhus infections poorly responsive to antibiotics in Northern Thailand. *Lancet* **348**, 86–9.

7.11.38 *Coxiella burnetii infections (Q fever)*

T. J. Marrie

History

In August 1935, Dr Edward Holbrook Derrick, Director of the Laboratory of Microbiology and Pathology of the Queensland Health Department in Brisbane, Australia, was asked to investigate an outbreak of undiagnosed febrile illness among workers at the Cannon Hill abattoir. Derrick realized that he was dealing with a type of fever that had not been previously described—he named it Q (for query) fever. A couple of years later, Sir Frank Macfarlane Burnet in Australia and Herald Rea Cox in the United States isolated the micro-organism responsible for Q fever.

Coxiella burnetii (Fig. 1)

This micro-organism, the sole species of its genus, has a Gram-negative cell wall and measures $0.3 \times 0.7\ \mu m$. It is an obligate phagolysosomal parasite of eukaryotes that sporulates, stains well by the Gimenez stain, and multiplies by transverse binary fission. *C. burnetii* undergoes phase variation akin to the smooth to rough transition in some enteric Gram-negative bacilli. In nature and laboratory animals it exists in the phase-I state. Repeated passage of phase-I virulent organisms in embryonated chicken eggs lead to the conversion to phase-II avirulent forms. Antibodies to phase-I antigens predominate in chronic Q fever, while phase-II antibodies are higher than phase I in acute Q fever.

C. burnetii has survived for 586 days in tick faeces at room temperature, 160 days or more in water, in dried cheese made from contaminated milk for 30 to 40 days, and for up to 150 days in soil.

Epidemiology

Q fever is a zoonosis. There is an extensive wildlife and arthropod (mainly ticks) reservoir of *C. burnetii*. Domestic animals are infected through inhal-

Fig. 1 Transmission electron micrograph showing *Coxiella burnetii* cells within a macrophage in the heart valve of a patient with Q fever endocarditis. The dark material in the centre of each cell is condensed DNA. 15 000 ×.

ing contaminated aerosols or by ingesting infected material. These animals rarely become ill but abortion and stillbirths may occur. *C. burnetii* localizes in the uterus and mammary glands of infected animals. During pregnancy there is reactivation of *C. burnetii* and it multiplies in the placenta, reaching 10^9 hamster infective doses per gram of tissue. The organisms are shed into the environment at the time of parturition. Man becomes infected after inhaling organisms aerosolized at the time of parturition, or later when organisms in dust are stirred up on a windy day. Infected cattle, sheep, goats, and cats are the animals primarily responsible for transmitting *C. burnetii* to man. There have been several outbreaks of Q fever in hospitals and research institutes due to the transportation of infected sheep to research laboratories. Some studies have suggested that ingestion of contaminated milk is a risk factor for the acquisition of Q fever; volunteers seroconverted but did not become ill after ingesting such milk.

Percutaneous infection, such as when an infected tick is crushed between the fingers, may occur but is rare. Transmission via a contaminated blood transfusion has rarely occurred.

Vertical transmission from mother to child has been infrequently reported. A 1988 review documents 23 cases of Q fever in pregnant women. These authors found that Q fever was present in 1 per 540 pregnancies in an area of endemic Q fever in Southern France.

Person-to-person transmission has been documented on a few occasions. To date, 45 countries on five continents have reported cases of Q fever. Q fever is estimated to cost $A1 million in Australia each year and results in the loss of more than 1700 weeks of work.

Clinical features

Man is the only animal known consistently to develop illness following infection with *C. burnetii*. There is an incubation period of about 2 weeks (range 2 to 29 days) following inhalation of *C. burnetii*. A dose–response effect has been demonstrated experimentally and clinically. *C. burnetii* is one of the most infectious agents known to man; a single micro-organism is able to initiate infection. The resulting illness in man can be divided into acute and chronic varieties.

Acute Q fever

Self-limiting febrile illness

The most common manifestation of acute Q fever is a self-limiting febrile illness.

Q fever pneumonia (Figs 2 and 3)

This is the most commonly recognized manifestation of Q fever. There is often a seasonal distribution, most of the cases occurring between February and May. The onset is non-specific with fever, fatigue, and headache. The headache may be very severe, occasionally so severe that it prompts a lumbar puncture. A dry cough of mild to moderate intensity is present in 24 to 90 per cent of patients. About one-third have pleuritic chest pain. Nausea, vomiting, and diarrhoea occur in 10 to 30 per cent of patients. Most cases of *C. burnetii* pneumonia are mild; however, about 10 per cent are severe enough to require admission to hospital; rarely, assisted ventilation is necessary. Death is rare in Q fever pneumonia and is usually due to comorbid illness. The white blood-cell count is usually normal, but is elevated in one-third of patients. Liver enzyme levels may be mildly elevated, at two to three times normal. Alkaline phosphatase is raised in up to 70 per cent of cases and 28 per cent are hyponatraemic. Reactive thrombocytosis is surprisingly common. Microscopic haematuria is a common finding.

The chest radiographic manifestations of Q fever pneumonia are usually indistinguishable from those of other bacterial pneumonias (Fig. 3). However, rounded opacities are suggestive of this infection (Fig. 2). Some investigators have reported delayed clearing of the pneumonia; however, in our experience resolution is usually complete within 3 weeks.

Fig. 2 Serial chest radiographs of a 35-year-old patient with Q fever pneumonia. The first radiograph (1 August 1989) shows a round opacity in the right upper lobe, which increases in size over the next 6 days. The pneumonia has completely cleared by 19 September 1989.

Hepatitis

The liver is probably involved in all patients with acute Q fever. There are three clinical pictures:

(1) pyrexia of unknown origin with mild to moderate elevation of liver function tests;

(2) a hepatitis-like picture—liver biopsy shows distinctive doughnut granulomas consisting of a granuloma with a central lipid vacuole and fibrin deposits;

(3) 'incidental hepatitis'.

Neurological manifestations

Encephalitis, encephalomyelitis, toxic confusional states, optic neuritis, and demyelinating polyradiculoneuritis are uncommon manifestations of Q fever.

Fig. 3 Portable anteroposterior chest radiograph of a 72-year-old male with Q fever pneumonia. This radiographic picture is indistinguishable from pneumonia due to any other microbial agent.

Rare manifestations

These include myocarditis, pericarditis, bone marrow necrosis, rhabdomyolysis, glomerulonephritis, lymphadenopathy, pancreatitis, mesenteric paniculitis, erythema nodosum, epididymitis, orchitis, priapism, and erythema annulare centrifugum.

Chronic fatigue may be a sequel of Q fever in some patients.

Chronic Q fever

The usual manifestation of chronic Q fever is that of culture-negative endocarditis. Some 70 per cent of these patients have fever and nearly all have abnormal native or prosthetic heart valves. Hepatomegaly and or splenomegaly occur in about half of these patients and one-third have marked clubbing of the digits. A purpuric rash due to immune complex-induced leucocytoclastic vasculitis and arterial embolism occurs in about 20 per cent of patients. Hyperglobulinaemia (up to 60 g/l) is common and is a useful clue to chronic Q fever in a patient with the clinical picture of culture-negative endocarditis.

Other manifestations of chronic Q fever include osteomyelitis, infection of aortic aneurysm, and infection of vascular prosthetic grafts.

The strains of *C. burnetii* that cause chronic Q fever do not differ from those that cause acute Q fever. Peripheral blood lymphocytes from patients with Q fever endocarditis are unresponsive to *C. burnetii* antigens *in vitro*, while responding normally to other antigens.

Diagnosis

A strong clinical suspicion based on the epidemiology and clinical features as outlined above is the cornerstone of the diagnosis of Q fever. This suspicion is confirmed by determining a fourfold or greater increase in antibody titre between acute and 2- to 3-week convalescent serum samples. A variety of serological tests are available: complement fixation, microimmunofluorescence, and enzyme immunoassay. The immunofluorescence antibody test is easiest to use. In acute Q fever the antibody titre to phase-II antigen is higher than that to phase-I antigen, while the reverse occurs in chronic Q fever. In chronic Q fever, antibody phase-I titres are extremely high, in the order of 1:8192 and higher. In acute Q fever, antibody titres to phase-I antigen are rarely in excess of 1:512, while peak antibody titres to phase-II antigen are between 1:1024 and 1:2048. The micro-organism can be isolated in embryonated eggs or in tissue culture; however, a biosafety level-3 laboratory is required. The polymerase chain reaction can be used to amplify *C. burnetii* DNA from tissues or other biological specimens.

Treatment

Acute Q fever is treated with a 2-week course of tetracycline or doxycycline. Chronic Q fever should be treated with two antimicrobial agents for at least 2 years. Some authorities recommend lifelong therapy for chronic Q fever. We use rifampicin, 300 mg twice a day, and ciprofloxacin, 750 mg twice a day, as agents of first choice. Rifampicin and doxycycline or tetracycline and trimethoprim–sulfamethoxazole have also been used to treat chronic Q fever. Another regimen for the treatment of chronic Q fever is doxycycline 100 mg once daily and hydroxychloroquine 600 mg once daily to maintain a plasma level of between 0.8 and 1.2 µg/ml. This regimen is given for 18 months. Photosensitivity is a potential adverse reaction and patients should be warned to take preventive measures. In addition, an ophthalmologist must examine the optic fundus every 6 months for chloroquine accumulation. Antibody titres should be measured every 6 months for the first 2 years. A progressive decline in antibody titre reflects the successful treatment of chronic fever. Cardiac valve replacement may be necessary as part of the management of chronic Q fever.

Prevention

A formalin-inactivated *C. burnetii*, whole-cell vaccine is protective against infection and has a low rate of side-effects; 1 per cent of vaccinees developed an abscess at the inoculation site and another 1 per cent had a lump at this site 2 months after vaccination. The vaccine should be offered to those whose occupation places them at high risk for *C. burnetii* infection. Other measures to reduce Q fever infection are the use of only seronegative pregnant sheep in research facilities and the control of ectoparasites on livestock.

Further reading

Sawyer LA, Fishbein DB, McDade JE (1987). Q fever: current concepts. *Reviews of Infectious Diseases* 9, 935–46.

7.11.39 Bartonelloses, excluding *Bartonella bacilliformis* infections

James G. Olson

Background

Bacteria belonging to the genus *Bartonella* cause human diseases, including verruga peruana (discussed elsewhere), cat-scratch disease, trench fever, and bacillary angiomatosis–peliosis. During the last two decades, the aetiology of cat-scratch disease was discovered, bacillary angiomatosis was recognized, and the relationship of these diseases to trench fever, an epidemic scourge of soldiers in the First World War, was demonstrated. Because of recent microbiological and genetic evidence, the aetiological agents of these diseases have been included in the genus *Bartonella*. Recent progress has lead to an improved understanding of the aetiology, diagnosis, and epi-

demiology of infections with *Bartonella*, and some improvements in patient care and prevention.

Cat-scratch disease

Introduction

Cat-scratch disease, in most patients, is an acute, self-limiting infection characterized by development of a papule at the site of inoculation by a cat, followed by regional adenopathy that may persist for 1 to 4 months. In a small percentage of patients, serious systemic complications may arise, including involvement of the central nervous system, liver, spleen, lung, bone, eyes, and skin.

Epidemiology

Cat-scratch disease occurs world-wide in all races, more often in males than in females. Most cases of cat-scratch disease occur in children, but the disease is rare in infants. Estimates of the proportion of cases occurring before the age of 18 years range from 55 to 87 per cent. In the United States, the estimated incidence of cat-scratch disease in ambulatory patients is nine cases/100 000 population. Some 0.8 cases/100 000 population are discharged from hospital with a diagnosis of cat-scratch disease. These data support earlier estimates and suggest that cat scratch disease affects about 24 000 people each year in the United States, resulting in approximately 2000 hospital admissions. Incidence in the United States is highest in humid southern states and lowest in arid western states. Most reported cases occur in the fall and winter, but patients can be infected during any season. About 90 per cent of patients have a history of exposure to cats. Cat-scratch disease is strongly associated with owning a kitten, particularly one with fleas, and the presence of a scratch or bite by a kitten. Although they remain asymptomatic, domestic cats serve as major persistent reservoirs for *B. henselae*. Blood samples cultured from pet and impounded cats suggest that more than 40 per cent of cats are bacteraemic. *B. henselae* was also detected in fleas taken from an infected cats by both direct culture and PCR. Cat fleas from infected cats readily transmit *B. henselae* to uninfected cats. *B. henselae* is readily transmitted to uninfected cats by the subcutaneous inoculation of infectious flea faeces. The cat flea certainly plays an indirect role in human disease by increasing the size of the feline reservoir, and a direct role by producing infectious faeces that are inoculated into the human via the scratch of the cat.

Aetiology

Serological, epidemiological, and molecular findings indicate that *B. henselae* is responsible for cat-scratch disease. *B. henselae* is a small, curved, pleomorphic, fastidious, Gram-negative rod that is oxidase and catalase negative, and X-factor dependent. Colony morphology is varied, ranging from small, dry, grey-white colonies to smooth, creamy-yellow colonies. Its slow-growing sensitivity to a broad range of commonly used antimicrobials (including ampicillin, tetracycline, trimethoprim–sulfamethoxazole, and aminoglycosides) does not always correlate with *in vivo* efficacy. It is most closely related to *B. quintana*, the louse-borne agent of trench fever. There are many newly described species in the genus *Bartonella* that have been recovered from animals, but only four, *B. henselae*, *B. quintana*, *B. elizabethae* (which was isolated from a single patient with endocarditis), and *B. bacilliformis* have been associated with human disease. *Afipia felis* was claimed to be the aetiological agent of cat-scratch disease but was probably a soil contaminant.

Pathology

Examination of the primary inoculation lesion demonstrates dermal necrosis with variable numbers of histiocytes and occasional multinucleate giant cells accompanied by scattered microabscesses with mixed inflammatory cells, including neutrophils, eosinophils, lymphocytes, and plasma cells. The epidermal changes are non-specific with parakeratosis, hyperkeratosis, oedema, and exocytosis of inflammatory cells.

Adenopathy

Early in the course of infection lymph nodes show reactive lymphoid follicular hyperplasia with initial minute microabscesses adjacent to the subcapsular sinus. As the disease progresses, characteristic histopathology is necrotizing granulomas with central microabscesses and palisading histiocytes. Most of the necrotic centres have a stellate configuration. Multinucleated giant cells in lymph nodes are either rare or absent. A perivascular neutrophilic infiltrate may be present. The Warthin–Starry or Steiner silver impregnation stains may reveal pleomorphic bacilli in clusters or short chains within the areas of central necrosis or around small vessels (Fig. 1). Although these histopathological features are characteristic of cat-scratch disease, they are not diagnostic and must be correlated with clinical findings and serological studies. Other infections, such as tularaemia, lymphogranuloma venereum, and fungal and mycobacterial infections, may have a similar histology.

Clinical presentation

The typical course of cat-scratch disease begins with an erythematous papule or pustule at the inoculation site of a scratch or contact with a cat which usually persists for 1 to 3 weeks (Fig. 2). An inoculation site may be detected in over two-thirds of patients. Within 2 weeks, lymph nodes draining the site of inoculation become enlarged and tender. Lymphadenopathy occurs in more than 90 per cent of patients; it usually resolves spontaneously within a period of several months. In about 50 per cent, regional lymphadenitis is the only manifestation of the disease. Usually a single node or group of nodes is affected. The most common sites of lymphadenopathy are axillary, cervical, inguinal/femoral, and epitrochlear lymph nodes. Affected nodes are often tender and suppurate in about 10 per cent of the patients. Constitutional symptoms of fever, anorexia, malaise, and headache accompany the lymphadenitis in 75 per cent of patients, but in the vast majority these symptoms are mild. About one-third of patients complain of fever and one-quarter have malaise or fatigue. Other non-specific clinical features are headache, anorexia, weight loss, vomiting, sore throat, rashes (maculopapular and rarely erythema nodosum), and splenomegaly. Although considered to be a self-limiting illness, signs and symptoms of cat-scratch disease often persist for 2 to 4 months, and adenopathy for longer.

Atypical presentations occur in up to 15 per cent of patients. The most common, Parinaud's oculoglandular syndrome, was first described by Henri Parinaud in 1889. It is characterized by ocular granuloma or conjunctivitis with preauricular lymphadenopathy and fever. The affected eye is painless and non-pruritic and shows no evidence of discharge. Most patients recover spontaneously without any sequelae in 2 to 4 months. Other atypical manifestations include encephalopathy, aseptic meningitis, seizures, neuroretinitis, transverse myelitis, osteolytic lesions, hepatic and splenic granulomas, thrombocytopenic purpura, haemolytic anaemia, endocarditis, atypical pneumonia, pleural effusion, pulmonary nodules,

Fig. 1 Bacilli in tissue. Photomicrograph of Warthin–Starry silver impregnation stained section of an inguinal lymph node from a patient with a skin test positive for cat scratch disease. A vessel containing erythrocytes is cut in cross-section, bacilli are seen singly and in chains outlining the vessel (× 630). (Reproduced from Wear et al. (1983). *Science* **221**, 1403–5, Armed Forces Institute of Pathology negative 82–11271, with permission).

Fig. 2 Crusted erythematous papules at the site of a cat scratch above the umbilicus with bilateral inguinal lymphadenopathy, which developed 10 days later, in a 7-year-old boy (Copyright D.A. Warrell).

breast mass, multiple granulomatous skin lesions, and recurrent adenopathy. In patients with central nervous system involvement, encephalopathy is the most commonly reported manifestation, occurring in 2 to 3 per cent of patients. Typically, 1 to 6 weeks after onset of lymphadenopathy, patients become abruptly confused and disoriented, rapidly progressing to coma. Cranial computed tomography is generally normal, and cerebrospinal fluid shows minimal pleocytosis or elevation of protein. Electroencephalography is frequently abnormal. Neurological recovery is almost always complete over 1 week, but persistent deficits have been reported. There have also been reports of patients presenting with recurrent fever, malaise, fatigue, and weight loss without obvious focal infection. The symptoms may persist for weeks to months before the diagnosis is made. Hepatic granulomas, osteomyelitis, and pulmonary involvement have also been reported as rare complications. All parts of the respiratory tract may be affected; bilateral hilar lymphadenopathy and primary atypical pneumonia have been reported. Severe manifestations have been described in an immunocompromised patient. Fatalities are extremely rare.

Diagnosis

The diagnosis of cat-scratch disease has evolved from a diagnosis by exclusion to one based on the laboratory confirmation of infection with the aetiological agent, *B. henselae*. The current case definition includes lymphadenopathy, with a serum IgG antibody titre more than 64 when tested by indirect immunofluorescence using *B. henselae* antigen; or PCR product specific for *B. henselae* as determined by RFLP or sequence analyses. Isolation of *B. henselae* is not practicable as viable bacteria are seldom present when the patient seeks medical care.

Differential diagnoses include lymphogranuloma venereum, syphilis, typical or atypical tuberculosis, other forms of bacterial adenitis, sporotrichosis, tularaemia, brucellosis, histoplasmosis, sarcoidosis, toxoplasmosis, infectious mononucleosis, and benign or malignant tumours.

Treatment

In the majority of patients, cat-scratch disease resolves spontaneously in 1 to 2 months. Azithromycin, rifampin, ciprofloxacin, trimethoprim-sulfamethoxazole, and gentamicin may benefit some patients. Antimicrobials should be considered for severe cases of cat-scratch disease but for uncomplicated cases of classical cat-scratch disease, treatment should be directed toward relief of discomfort. Application of moist soaks, local heat, analgesics, limitation of activity, and aspiration of suppuration may help to relieve the pain and resolve the inflammation. Aspiration is preferred to surgical drainage, which may lead to fistula formation or scarring. Spontaneous resolution of the infected node is common, but aspiration or surgical removal may be necessary. Healing is usually rapid. Treatment with erythromycin or doxycycline—either alone or in combination with rifampin—at standard doses but for longer duration (4 to 6 weeks) have been reported as effective and safe in both immunocompetent and immunosuppressed patients. Currently, the role of systemic steroid therapy, including in patients with neuroretinitis, is not clear.

Complications are uncommon and the prognosis is excellent. Recurrent attacks are rare and systemic sequelae are unusual.

Prevention

Isolation of patients is unnecessary. No vaccines are available, however, cat vaccines to protect cats from infection are under development. Treatments that prevent flea infestations in cats may be an effective means of preventing human infections. Cat owners should be encouraged to take their pets to routine veterinary visits and prevent ectoparasite infections, and to avoid cat scratches and bites. Cats implicated in transmission need not be destroyed.

Trench fever

Introduction

Trench fever is a febrile illness first described among British soldiers in 1915. From 1915 to 1918 it was thought to account from 40 to 60 per cent of all illnesses among soldiers. There were no deaths but much morbidity. By 1918 it was concluded that trench fever was an infectious disease and that the aetiological agent was transmitted by the human body louse. In 1961, *B. quintana* was isolated from the blood of a patient with trench fever and Koch's postulates for the causation of trench fever by *B. quintana* were fulfilled in 1969. Since the end of the Second World War, reports of trench fever have been rare but recent data suggest that cases may have escaped recognition; clusters of cases in homeless alcoholic men have been identified in the United States and France.

Epidemiology

Endemic foci of trench fever have been identified in Poland, the former Soviet Republics, Mexico, Bolivia, North Africa, Ethiopia, and Burundi, but its true incidence and geographical distribution are unknown.

B. quintana is transmitted by inoculation of contaminated louse faeces through a break in the skin from a louse bite or other injury. The incubation period is 7 to 30 days. It is not transmitted directly from person-to-person. The human body louse becomes infected by ingesting infected human blood.

In the 1980s, *B. quintana* re-emerged as an opportunistic pathogen among HIV-infected people in whom it causes bacillary angiomatosis, endocarditis, and bacteraemia. It has been isolated from AIDS patients in France and the United States. *B. henselae* is probably a more common cause of bacillary angiomatosis and bacteraemia among HIV-infected people.

More recently, *B. quintana* has been identified as a cause of invasive infection among HIV-seronegative, inner-city, homeless, alcoholics in Seattle, Washington, and Marseilles, France. A seroprevalence study conducted one year after the *B. quintana* outbreak among patients at a downtown Seattle clinic serving a primarily indigent and homeless population found that 20 per cent of patients had microimmunofluorescence titres at or greater than 64. Interpretation of these results is limited by the high cross-reactivity of the assay to *B. henselae*. The results suggest, however, that exposure to the organism was common in that population and that many cases of infection may have been asymptomatic or minimally symptomatic.

The mode of transmission of *B. quintana* among homeless persons is not well defined. Lice were detected on one patient at the time of presentation and five patients were reported to have been previously diagnosed with scabies. Transmission via a louse or other ectoparasitic vector is therefore a plausible hypothesis. Currently, the human body louse is the only known vector of *B. quintana*. No non-human vertebrate reservoir is known.

Clinical presentation

High fever is the most common clinical feature. Headache and myalgia are common prodromal symptoms. Fever starts acutely or insidiously and is often associated with headache, dizziness, and pains in the back, eyes, and legs, especially in the shins. Splenomegaly is common and a red macular rash (lesions 2–4 mm in diameter) may appear transiently. Complete recovery usually occurs within 5 to 6 weeks without antimicrobial therapy. Trench fever is not fatal but about half of the patients will have relapse of illness with fever and myalgia. Endocarditis has been described.

Four clinical patterns have been recognized:

(1) asymptomatic or minimally symptomatic infection;

(2) a single, acute, febrile attack lasting 3 to 4 days;

(3) a periodic form, with multiple febrile paroxysms; and

(4) a continuous form with weeks of fever.

Studies involving inoculation of humans with *B. quintana* from infected louse faeces suggest that the incubation period ranges from 5 to 20 days depending on the size of the inoculum. *B. quintana* may circulate in the blood for weeks after resolution of symptoms and infection may last as long as a year.

The clinical spectrum of infection among HIV-negative, alcoholic and homeless people has varied. Of these 13 cases of 'urban trench fever', five developed left-sided endocarditis which required valve replacement in four despite antibiotic therapy. One patient died 4 months after valve replacement surgery and one patient who had a concurrent positive blood culture for *Streptococcus pneumoniae* also died, presumably due to pneumococcal sepsis. Many of the patients with *B. quintana* bacteraemia presented with a subacute course of chronic fever, fatigue, and weight loss. Two patients had splenomegaly; however, other symptoms associated with classical trench fever, such headache, rash, and bone pain, were not reported.

Diagnosis

Bartonella quintana are slow growing bacteria which require special culture methods for isolation. The use of Isolator (lysis–centrifugation) tubes improves the yield from blood cultures. Specimens should be plated on enriched media (blood or chocolate agar) incubated at 35 to 37°C in 5 per cent CO_2 and high humidity and held for at least 4 weeks. The organism can also be isolated from blood using Bac Tec or resin-containing culture media if the contents are stained with acridine orange after 1 week of incubation. All stain-positive bottles are then subcultured onto enriched media and processed as above. Cocultivation of blood samples with endothelial cells has also been used for isolation of *Bartonella* species. With more widespread use of culture methods appropriate for the isolation of *Bartonella* species in clinical laboratories, the spectrum and apparent extent of infections due to this organism may be expanded.

Enzyme-linked immunosorbent (ELISA) and immunofluorescence (IFA) assays are available for serological diagnosis. Both exhibit substantial cross-reactivity between *Bartonella* species. The use of paired sera obtained four or more weeks apart is recommended. PCR amplification from infected tissues of DNA specific to *Bartonella* species has also been used.

Treatment

Optimal treatment has not been established. Erythromycin has been the drug of choice, although doxycycline, tetracycline, or azithromycin appear to be acceptable alternatives. At least 14 days of oral therapy is recommended for uncomplicated infection and for bacteraemia at least 4 weeks of therapy is indicated. Most of the few patients identified with *B. quintana* endocarditis have required cardiac valve replacement. Parenteral therapy for 2 to 3 months should therefore be considered for cases of suspected or confirmed *B. quintana* endocarditis.

Relapsing disease is well described, especially if therapy is terminated prematurely. In the Seattle outbreak one patient who was non-compliant with therapy had documented bacteraemia over an 8-week period. It is not known whether extended therapy will prevent relapses.

In immunocompetent hosts, infection with *B. quintana* is usually self-limited unless complicated by endocarditis. The disease is more severe in immunocompromised hosts and may progress to death.

Prevention

Control of the human body louse will prevent transmission of trench fever.

Bacillary angiomatosis–peliosis

Introduction

Bacillary angiomatosis was described in 1983 in an HIV-infected patient with fever and skin nodules. Since then it has been seen in many other HIV-

infected patients and in a few apparently immunocompetent individuals. Bacillary angiomatosis represents one aspect of a spectrum of infections due to the fastidious organisms *Bartonella quintana* and *B. henselae*. A similar disorder known as verruga peruana, caused by *B. bacilliformis*, is restricted to Peru and several neighbouring countries. More reliable diagnostic and identification methods are providing a better understanding of the ubiquitous distribution of both organisms and of the expanding spectrum and overlap of disease they cause. Like *B. bacilliformis*, *B. quintana* and *B. henselae* cause acute febrile illnesses (trench fever, Oroya fever), recurrent asymptomatic bacteraemias, skin lesions, and aseptic meningitis, while ocular involvement (Leber's stellate neuroretinis) appears to be limited to *B. henselae* infections. *B. elizabethiae* has been associated with endocarditis.

Epidemiology

Most cases of bacillary angiomatosis–peliosis have been reported from the United States but its incidence and global distribution are unknown. Epidemiological information is based on case reports, small case series, and a single case–control study. In the largest reported series of cases ($n = 49$), 45 (92 per cent) were HIV infected, one was HIV negative and immunodeficient, and three (6 per cent) were HIV negative and apparently immunocompetent.

Patients infected with *B. henselae* but not *B. quintana* were more likely than controls to own cats, to have been bitten or scratched by cats, to have been exposed to a household cat with fleas, and to have been bitten by cat fleas. The cat flea serves as an arthropod vector for *B. henselae*. Patients with *B. quintana* infections were more likely than controls to be homeless, to have a low annual income, and to be infested with head or body lice. The human body louse is the most likely vector of *B. quintana*. Neither those infected with *B. henselae* or *B. quintana* were more likely than controls to be alcoholic or to use intravenous drugs.

Aetiology

B. quintana and *B. henselae* have recently been isolated from cutaneous lesions of bacillary angiomatosis. Their aetiological role is also supported by serological and molecular assay data. The morphological and staining characteristics, biochemical and antimicrobial sensitivity profiles, and phylogenetics of *B. quintana* are similar to those of *B. henselae* in cat-scratch disease.

Clinical presentation

Bacillary angiomatosis derives its name from the vascular proliferation and presence of numerous bacillary organisms in affected tissues. It has been reported to involve numerous tissues including skin, lymph node, muscle, bone, bone marrow, brain, liver, and spleen. Bacillary angiomatosis affecting the liver (also 'bacillary peliosis hepatis') and spleen has been referred to as 'bacillary peliosis'. Bacillary angiomatosis most commonly presents as single or clustered, reddish, papular lesions on the skin, but may also occur as brownish patches or subcutaneous nodules and may be confused with Kaposi's sarcoma or disseminated fungal infections, such as *Cryptococcus neoformans*, in the HIV-infected individual. Rarely, diffuse or isolated lymph node involvement can be seen without the characteristic rash. Systemic involvement may also occur, causing lytic bone lesions, peliosis hepatis, or disseminating to other visceral organ in more severe cases. Although descriptions of the disease were in patients with immune deregulation due to neoplastic processes, HIV-1 infection, or immunosuppressive therapy, bacillary angiomatosis has also been described in essentially immunocompetent individuals.

Diagnosis

Biopsy and histological examination of affected tissue is needed for diagnosis of bacillary angiomatosis. It is not possible to distinguish bacillary angiomatosis clinically from Kaposi's sarcoma or other diseases that may affect the skin, spleen, liver, and other tissues, especially in HIV-infected or other immunocompromised persons. Histological criteria for the diagnosis of bacillary angiomatosis include characteristic vascular proliferation on routine haematoxylin-and-eosin staining, and of demonstration of bacillary organisms by silver staining (Warthin–Starry, Steiner, or Dieterle) or electron microscopy.

B. henselae and *B. quintana* have been isolated from cutaneous lesions of bacillary angiomatosis after cultivation of tissue homogenates with endothelial cell monolayers, followed by plating of the supernatants on to solid agar. These organisms can also be isolated from the blood using a lysis–centrifugation method. Serological responses with an indirect immunofluorescence assay for antibodies to *B. quintana* and *B. henselae* may indicate recent infection and provide supporting evidence in a clinical syndrome compatible with diseases. While the duration of antibody responses is not known, IFA reactivity has been documented to last for over 1 year in several longitudinally followed cases. Tissue and blood for culture may also be useful—a positive culture is conclusive, but elusive. PCR of the 16s ribosomal subunit or the citrate synthase gene with restriction fragment length polymorphisms may also be employed.

Treatment

Most *Bartonella* infections are self limiting, particularly when associated with cat-scratch or isolated lymphadenopathy. However, with more disseminated disease such as bacillary angiomatosis, systemic antimicrobial therapy is necessary, particularly when it is an opportunistic infection in AIDS patients. Antimicrobial agents which achieve high intracellular concentrations, such as doxycycline, rifampin, erythromycin, and the macrolides, and possibly trimethoprim–sulfamethoxazol are the most effective in treating and clearing infection. In severe cases, combination therapy with doxycycline or a macrolide and rifampin have been used with success. Fluoroquinolones and cell-wall-active agents, including penicillins and cephalosporins, and aminoglycosides are ineffective. There is no clearly defined duration of therapy, although relapses have been seen when less than 4 weeks of antimicrobial treatment has been given both in HIV-infected and immunocompetent patients.

Prevention

Macrolide antibiotic (erythromycin, clarithromycin) prophylaxis is effective in preventing bacillary angiomatosis–peliosis. Both *B. henselae* and *B. quintana* can be transmitted by arthropod vectors to humans. Elimination of body louse infestations among human populations and cat flea infestations among domestic cats provide a potential means for preventing infections. The domestic cat is the zoonotic reservoir for *B. henselae*, and despite the fact that infected cats show no or mild clinical signs, effective clearance of infection may be achieved through the use of a variety of oral antibiotics.

Further reading

Bass JW, Freitas BC, Freitas AD, *et al.* (1998). Prospective randomized double blind placebo-controlled evaluation of azithromycin for treatment of cat-scratch disease. *Pediatric Infectious Disease Journal* 17, 447–55.

Broqui P, Lascola B, Roux V, Raoult D (1999). Chronic *Bartonella quintana* bacteremia in homeless patients. *New England Journal of Medicine* 340, 184–9.

Drancourt M, Mainardi JL, Brouqui P, *et al.* (1995). *Bartonella* (*Rochalimaea*) *quintana* endocarditis in three homeless men. *New England Journal of Medicine* 332, 419–23.

Koehler JE, Quinn FD, Berger TG, LeBoit PE, Tappero JW (1992). Isolation of *Rochalimaea* species from cutaneous and osseous lesions of bacillary angiomatosis. *New England Journal of Medicine* 327, 1625–31.

Margileth AM (1992). Antibiotic therapy for cat-scratch disease: clinical study of therapeutic outcome of 268 patients and a review of the literature. *Pediatric Infectious Disease Journal* 11, 474–8.

Spach DH, Kanter AS, Dougherty MJ, *et al.* (1995). *Bartonella* (*Rochalimaea*) *quintana* bacteremia in inner-city patients with chronic alcoholism. *New England Journal of Medicine* 332, 424–8.

Tappero JW, Koehler JE, Berger TG, *et al.* (1993). Bacillary angiomatosis and bacillary splenitis in immunocompetent adults. *Annals of Internal Medicine* 118, 363–5.

Zangwill KM, Hamilton DH, Perkins BA, *et al.* (1993). Cat scratch disease in Connecticut. Epidemiology, risk factors, and evaluation of a new diagnostic test. *New England Journal of Medicine* 329, 8–13.

7.11.39.1 *Bartonella bacilliformis* infection

A. Llanos Cuentas

Definition

Bartonellosis (Carrión's disease, verruga peruana, Oroya fever, Guaitará fever) is a non-contagious infectious disease that is endemic in the western Andes and inter-Andean valleys of Peru and occasionally has been reported in Colombia and Ecuador. The acute stage is characterized by infection of red blood cells leading to anaemia; in the late stage the patients develop dermal nodules, which are called 'verrugas'. This disease produces a temporary, reversible immunosuppression in the host, which explains why secondary opportunistic infections are common.

Aetiological agent

Barton, a Peruvian physician, described the causative organism in 1905. *Bartonella bacilliformis* is a small, motile, aerobic, Gram-negative bacillus that stains deep red or purple with Giemsa (Fig. 1). This facultative intracellular haemotrophic bacterium varies in morphology and quantity during various stages of the disease. In spite of being a pleomorphic organism, two essential types are distinguishable: bacilli or rod-shaped forms and coccoid forms. Rod-shaped forms predominate in the acute stage of the disease and coccoid in the convalescent stage. *B. bacillifomis* may infect red blood cells (Fig. 2), endothelial cells of capillaries, and sinusoidal lining cells. The organism is 2 to 3 μm long and 0.2 to 2.5 μm thick. In cultures, 1

Fig. 1 Smear of peripheral blood with red blood cells parasitized by coccoid forms of *B. bacillifomis* (Wright's stain, × 1048). (Reproduced by courtesy of Professor Juan Takano Moron.)

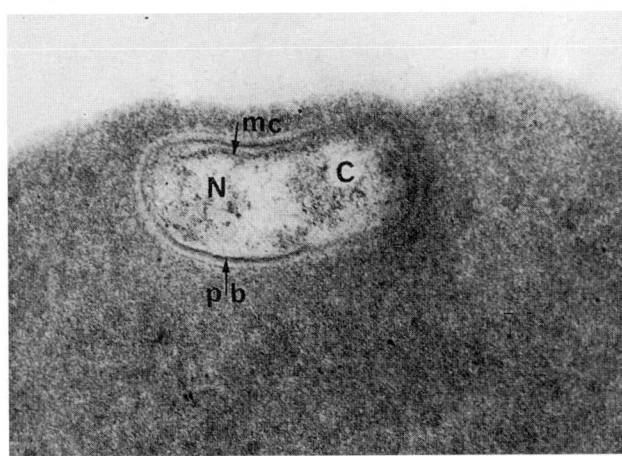

Fig. 2 Ultrastructure of coccobacillary form of *B. bacilliformis* in a red blood cell (× 31 915): mc, cell membrane; N, nucleus; C, cytoplasm; pb, bacterial cell wall. (Reproduced by courtesy of Professor Juan Takano Moron.)

Fig. 4 Geographical distribution of bartonellosis. Coloured spots represent endemic areas of bartonellosis.

to 10 flagella 3 to 10 μm long may originate from one end of the organism. Bartonella can be cultured in Columbia agar supplemented with 5 per cent defibrinated human blood or other supplemented media containing rabbit serum and haemoglobin at 28°C under aerobic conditions for up to 6 weeks.

Epidemiology

The disease has occurred since pre-Columbian times, as proved by artistic representations in pre-Inca potteries as well as lesions in a mummy. Bartonellosis is an endemic disease mainly in narrow river valleys and canyons usually in west Andean, and increasingly frequently in inter-Andean, valleys of the central and east Andes of Peru and high jungle areas (Fig. 3). Bartonellosis is a re-emergent disease that is extending its range in Peru. During the last two decades the disease has become endemic in new areas of Ayacucho, Huancavelica, Amazonas, Huanuco, Junín, and Cusco departments and important outbreaks have been reported in recent years. Outbreaks have been described in similar areas in Nariño, Colombia (in 1939) and in Loja and Chichipe areas, Ecuador (Fig. 4). It occurs between 500 and 3200 m above sea level. There are annual high and low transmission seasons and the transmission is greatest towards the end of the rainy season (March to May). Interepidemic periods occur every 10 to 15 years, influenced by climate, environmental, and ecological changes such as El Niño phenomenon.

In recent years, other human infections by haemotrophic bacteria have been included in the genus *Bartonella*: *B.* (formerly *Rochalimaea*) *quintana*, the agent of trench fever, *B. henselae*, the major cause of cat-scratch disease, *B. elizabethae*, an aetiological agent of infective endocarditis, and *B.* (formerly *Rochalimaea*) *vinsonii*, until recently not considered to be a pathogen. In immunocompromised people, especially those with AIDS, *B. henselae* and *B. quintana* cause opportunistic infections, frequently manifested as cutaneous bacillary angiomatosis, resembling verruga peruana.

In endemic areas the disease appears in childhood and usually produces few symptoms. Outsiders generally develop acute severe forms of the disease (Oroya fever). Large epidemics have occurred when large groups of non-residents have entered endemic areas. In 1870 an epidemic involved workers building the railroad from Lima to Oroya (Fig. 5); the estimated mortality was 7000. Infection results from the bite of female sandflies of the genus *Lutzomyia*, the most important species being *L. verrucarum*. The vectors are closely associated with human dwellings and, because they are active during twilight hours, people acquire bartonellosis in the hours around sunrise and sunset. Although the reservoir is unknown, there is increasing evidence that humans are the major host. Asymptomatic infection by *B. bacilliformis* has been demonstrated in people of endemic areas.

Fig. 3 Endemic area for bartonellosis, Rimac Valley, Peru. (By courtesy of Professor David H. Molyneux, Liverpool.)

Fig. 5 Puente verrugas' at an altitude of 1800 m above sea level near Lima, Peru. (By courtesy of Mr E. J. Perez.)

However, since bartonellosis can be acquired in several Andean areas uninhabited by humans, other reservoirs for the disease may exist. Some domestic animals, including horses, donkeys, mules, dogs, and cats, are susceptible and develop lesions similar to verrugas. *Bartonella*-like isolates have been obtained from a *Phyllotis* mouse.

Pathogenesis

After inoculation of *B. bacilliformis* through a sandfly bite, the bacteria multiply in endothelial cells of small vessels, and phagocytic cells near the skin. Systemic invasion and multiplication in endothelial cells and red blood cells follows. In the most serious cases, 95 to 100 per cent of red cells are infected with numerous bacteria. The hallmark of the disease is the severe anaemia caused by massive infection of red blood cells and subsequent erythrophagocytosis. Several mechanisms contribute to anaemia: increased fragility, form and size alteration, and reduced half-life of infected and non-infected red cells. Some inhibition of haemoglobin synthesis, probably induced by toxic factors, has also been invoked, since production of red cells increases dramatically with reduction of bacteraemia. Erythrophagocytosis contributes to lymphadenopathy and hepatosplenomegaly. Blockade of the mononuclear phagocytic system and the presence of the circulating iron leads to superinfection, usually by enterobacteria, during the anaemia stage or early recovery from it. Transient depression of cellular immunity has been reported. During the anaemic phase, mild lymphopenia with a reduction of OKT4, a mild increase of OKT8, and decrease of the polyclonal stimulation of the lymphocytes occurs.

A few weeks to months after the acute illness has subsided, the cutaneous form 'verruga peruana' may develop (Fig. 6). The vascular skin lesion shows endothelial proliferation and histiocytic hyperplasia (the cells contain degenerate organisms; Fig. 7), with later fibrosis and necrosis. Electron microscopy of verrucous tissue shows *B. bacilliformis* in the interstitial tissue, indicating that the presence of the bacteria is important for this unusual vascular response to occur. Verruga peruana results from persistent infection, a probably insufficient immune response, and a peculiar vascular reaction, which could be caused by bacterial products acting as an angiogenic factor. In 1885, D.A. Carrión, a Peruvian medical student, linked both phases of the disease by self-experimentation and died.

Clinical features

The disease has two stages, anaemic and eruptive, with an asymptomatic intermediate period. After an incubation period of around 60 days (range 10 to 210 days), non-specific prodromal symptoms appear: onset is usually gradual with malaise, mild chills, fever, and headache. Occasionally, high fever may develop rapidly or build up over a few days. It is accompanied by

Fig. 6 Histological section of miliary skin lesion of 'verruga peruana', a sessile or partly pedunculated molluscum-like lesion. (Armed Forces Institute of Pathology photograph negative no. 77355.)

Fig. 7 Electron micrograph of a vascular skin lesion (verruga peruana) showing six *B. bacilliformis* in the fibrillar intertitial matrix (FIM). The cell wall, cell membrane, and internal structure of the bacteria can be seen. The clear cytoplasm of a histiocyte (H) can also be seen. (Reproduced by courtesy of Professor Sixto Pecevarren, Department of Pathology, UPCH and HNCH.)

sweating and rigors. Common symptoms include weakness, aching of the head, back, and extremities, prostration, and depression. The clinical picture is dominated by severe (haemolytic) anaemia: the patient rapidly become pale, dyspnoeic, and jaundiced. There may be hepatosplenomegaly, generalized lymphadenopathy, myocarditis, pericardial effusion, exudates, and retinal haemorrhages in the fundus; sometimes there is generalized oedema, a fine vesicular or petechial rash, and exceptionally, meningoencephalomyelitis. The duration of this state is variable (generally 2 to 4 weeks). In pregnant women the disease in this phase may cause abortion, fetal death, and be transmitted transplacentally; maternal death is common.

In the intermediate period the patients are asymptomatic and recover from the anaemia through great bone marrow activity. This pre-eruptive period varies from weeks to months.

In the eruptive stage, many nodular lesions of varying size appear on the face, trunk, and limbs during a period of one or more months and usually persist for 3 or 4 months. There is accompanying mild arthralgia, myalgia, and sometimes fever. The red or purplish skin lesions vary from papules a few millimetres across. Most often the eruption is miliary (miliary form) with many haemangioma-like lesions of the dermis (Plate 1). Nodular lesions (modular form) are larger but fewer and more prominent on the extensor surfaces or arms and legs (Plate 2). They are painless and prone to bleeding, secondary infection, and ulceration. The appearance may resemble haemangioma, granulome pyogenicum Kaposi's or fibrosarcoma, leprosy (hystioid form), or yaws. Occasionally, one to a few, large, deep-seated lesions that often ulcerate (mular form) develop. These tend to appear near joints, where they may be painful and limit motion. Apart from skin, the mucous membranes of the mouth, conjunctiva, and nose, serous cavities, and the gastrointestinal and genitourinary tracts may be involved. The eruptive phase tends to heal spontaneously, although the course is often prolonged. Inhabitants of endemic areas usually develop the eruptive stage as the sole manifestation of the disease.

The principal complication is superinfection, leading to septicaemia, which occurs at different stages of the disease but generally in the later part of the anaemic stage and during the intermediate stage. Formerly, *Salmonella typhi*, *S. typhimurium*, *S. dublin*, *S. anatum*, *S. enteritidis*, *Mycobacterium tuberculosis*, and *Enterobacter* spp. were the most frequent pathogens. Reactivation of toxoplasmosis, histoplasmosis, pneumocystosis, and staphylococcal infections are some of the other infections that are now frequent.

Diagnosis

Two elements must be considered: visiting or residence in an endemic area and a compatible clinical picture with demonstration of the bacteria in the blood film. Fluorescence antibody test, indirect haemagglutination, immunoblot, and enzyme-linked immunosorbent assay (ELISA) are the new serological tests, but they are not generally available.

Laboratory features

Bartonella can be isolated from the blood during the anaemic stage and sometimes during the eruptive stage. The enriched media may be positive in 4 to 28 days at 28 °C. As fever develops, intraerythocytic bacteria are visible in thick and thin films stained with Giemsa, Wright, or other variants of the Romanovsky stain. Organisms can also be seen and cultivated in the skin lesion of verrucous tissue. The haemolytic anaemia is Coombs' test negative. The blood picture is a macrocytic and hypochromic anaemia with polychromasia, anisocytosis, and poikilocytosis. The reticulocytosis is marked (average 11 per cent). The marrow is hyperactive and megaloblastic with erythrophagocytosis. The white cell count is not markedly elevated unless there is a secondary infection. Thrombocytopenia is quite common. After the crisis, the intracellular organisms become coccoid and later disappear, the white cell count rises, and there is lymphocytosis. Eosinophils, which are usually absent during the acute stage, reappear in differential counts of peripheral blood.

Prognosis and treatment

Death is usually during the anaemic phase, and in the preantibiotic era varied between 20 and 95 per cent. At present it varies between 1.1 and 2.4 per cent in endemic areas and around 9 per cent in patients admitted to hospital. During outbreaks, especially when the disease in not promptly recognized and treated, the mortality can reach 88 per cent. Alterations of consciousness (excitement, stupor, and coma) and progressive or focal neurological features, biochemical evidence of hepatic dysfunction (increased serum aspartate and alanine transaminases and alkaline phosphatase), pulmonary complications (non-cardiogenic pulmonary oedema), anasarca (severe hypoalbuminaemia), and pregnancy are associated with a higher mortality.

Chloramphenicol, penicillin, erythromycin, co-trimoxazole, tetracycline, and ciprofloxacin are dramatically effective, usually eliminating the fever in less than 48 h. Because of the common association with salmonellosis, chloramphenicol is the treatment of choice in a dose of 50 mg/kg per day for 10 days. An alternative is ciprofloxacin in a dose of 500 mg twice a day for 10 days. Supportive treatment includes transfusion of packed red cells and dexamethasone (if there is severe neurological involvement). Rifampicin (300 mg twice a day in adults or 10 mg/kg per day in children, orally for 14 to 21 days) is indicated for treatment of the verrucous form.

Prevention

When transmission is around dwellings, sandflies can be temporarily eliminated by spraying inside and outside with DDT or pyrethroids. Bites usually occur after dusk. They can be prevented by insect repellents, impregnation of clothes with pyrethroids, sleeping inside fine-meshed or impregnated nets, or by avoiding sleeping in highly endemic areas.

Further reading

Birtles RJ *et al.* (1999). Survey of *Bartonella* species infecting intradomicillary animals in the Huayllacallan valley, Ancash-Perú, a region endemic for human bartonellosis. *American Journal of Tropical Medicine and Hygiene* **60**, 799–805.

Gray GC *et al.* (1990). An epidemic of Oroya fever in the Peruvian Andes. *American Journal of Tropical Medicine and Hygiene* **42**, 215–21.

Maguiña C (1998). *Bartonellosis o enfermedad de Carrión.* AFA Editores Importadores SA Lima, Peru.

Maguiña C, Gotuzzo E (2000). Bartonellosis new and old. In: Emerging and re-emerging diseases in Latin America. *Infectious Diseases Clinics of North America* **14**, 1–22.

Walker DH, Guerra H, Maguiña C (1999). Bartonellosis. In: Guerrant RL, Walker DH, Weller PF, eds. *Tropical infectious diseases, principles, pathogens and practice,* pp 492–7. Churchill Livingstone, Philadelphia.

7.11.40 Chlamydial infections including lymphogranuloma venereum

D. Taylor-Robinson and D. C. W. Mabey

Trachoma is discernible as a cause of blindness in ancient Chinese and Egyptian writings. However, it was not until 1907 that L. Halberstaedter and S. von Prowazek first described intracytoplasmic inclusions in conjunctival scrapings from patients with trachoma and recognized the involvement of an infectious agent. In 1930, the first isolation of a chlamydial agent (*Chlamydia psittaci*) from psittacosis was made, that is about 27 years before the genomically and biologically different agent, *Chlamydia trachomatis*, was isolated in fertile hens' eggs from trachoma. The advent of the cell-culture technique in the late 1950s paved the way for the isolation of *C. trachomatis* in 1965 by this means and, together with immunological developments, made it possible to explore the nature, range, prevalence, and pathogenesis of clinical conditions associated with chlamydial infection. The complete sequencing of the chlamydial genome, accomplished recently, provides an even greater opportunity to define many unfathomed aspects of the biology and pathogenesis of chlamydial infections.

Classification

Chlamydial organisms, or chlamydiae, are ubiquitous pathogens infecting many species of mammals and birds. The genus *Chlamydia* comprises at least four species, of which three can infect humans. *C. trachomatis* is pathogenic for humans and causes ocular, genital, and systemic infections that affect millions of people worldwide. *C. pneumoniae* causes mainly human respiratory disease, has been associated with atherosclerosis, and equine and koala strains exist. *C. psittaci* infects birds and other animals, resulting in major economic losses and occasionally is transmitted to humans The fourth chlamydial species, *C. pecorum*, causes pneumonia, polyarthritis, encephalomyelitis, and diarrhoea in cattle and sheep.

Taxonomic reclassification based on 16S RNA analysis has been proposed recently. In this, the order Chlamydiales contains four families, the first of which, Chlamydiaceae, comprises two genera, namely *Chlamydia* (for example, *Chlamydia trachomatis*) and *Chlamydophila* (for example, *Chlamydophila pneumoniae*). This proposal has generated considerable debate.

Growth cycle, serovars, and protein profile

Chlamydiae probably evolved from host-independent, Gram-negative ancestors that contained peptidoglycan in their cell wall. The chlamydial

Fig. 1 Elementary bodies (E) and reticulate bodies (R) of *C. trachomatis* forming an inclusion in oviduct cell shown by transmission electron microscopy.

envelope, like that of Gram-negative bacteria, has inner and outer membranes. Indeed, chlamydiae are best considered as bacteria that are specialized for an intracellular existence. The infectious elementary body is electron dense, deoxyribonucleic acid rich, and approximately 300 nm in diameter. Elementary bodies of *C. pneumoniae* often, but not always, have a wide periplasmic space and appear pear shaped, whereas those of the other chlamydial species have a narrow periplasmic space and are spherical. The elementary body begins its eukaryotic intracellular lifecycle by binding to the host cell and entering by 'parasite-specified' endocytosis. Inside the host cell, fusion of the chlamydia-containing endocytic vesicle with lysosomes is inhibited and the elementary body begins its unique developmental cycle. After about 10 h it has differentiated into the larger (800 to 1000 nm), noninfectious, metabolically active, reticulate body. This divides by binary fission and by 20 h there is the beginning of reorganization into a new generation of elementary bodies (Fig. 1), which reach maturation 20 to 30 h after entry into the cell. Their rapid accumulation within the endocytic vacuole precedes release from the cell between 30 and 48 h after the start of the cycle.

All species within the genus *Chlamydia* contain a common, heat-stable, lipopolysaccharide antigen, which is exposed on the surface of the reticulate body, but not on that of the elementary body. The major outer membrane protein (**MOMP**) is immunodominant in the elementary body and it contains epitopes that exhibit genus, species, and serovar specificity.The serovar-specific epitope is the basis of the microimmunofluorescence test by which *C. trachomatis* has been separated into 15 serovars: A, B, Ba, and C are responsible mainly for endemic trachoma, and D to K for oculogenital infections. Serovars L1, L2, and L3 of *C. trachomatis* cause the genital disease, lymphogranuloma venereum. At present, only one *C. pneumoniae* serovar has been identified, although minor geographical serovar variations have been described. The loosely defined *C. psittaci* species is likely to contain a wide variety of host-related serovars. Amino acid sequences of the MOMPs of all *C. trachomatis* serovars are now known and epitope maps of different antigenic domains have been elucidated. It appears that the MOMP genes consist of five highly conserved regions punctuated by four short variable sequences. Serovar-specific epitopes have been demonstrated in variable sequence in I and II, while species-specific epitopes have been found in variable sequence IV. It is also probable that these variable sequences have some role in chlamydial pathogenesis. *C. trachomatis*, *C. psittaci*, and *C. pneumoniae* species have been compared and, although there is only 10 per cent DNA homology between each of them, MOMP gene analysis of the respective species reveals up to 65 per cent amino acid homology, indicating a probable common ancestor. A common chlamydial 57-kDa protein has been described and its possible role in disease pathogenesis is considered below.

Trachoma

Trachoma is a chronic keratoconjunctivitis believed to affect some 500 million people, of whom 7 million are blind and 10 million have some visual impairment. After cataract, it is the most common cause of blindness worldwide, but is now confined largely to developing countries. Trachoma is a disease of poverty rather than of hot climates, and in some respects the relation between genital and ocular chlamydial infections resembles that between syphilis and non-venereal treponematoses. In poor communities where hygienic standards are low, there is direct transfer of chlamydiae from eye to eye (compare with skin to skin for non-venereal treponematoses), and trachoma is endemic. As standards of hygiene improve, this mode of transmission is no longer possible and trachoma becomes less of a problem.

Clinical features

The active (inflammatory) stage of the disease, a follicular conjunctivitis, affects chiefly the subtarsal conjunctiva, but follicles occur elsewhere on the conjunctiva and at the limbus, where on resolution they leave characteristic shallow depressions known as Herbert's pits. New vessels (pannus) may be seen at this stage in the cornea, usually at the superior margin, and punctate keratitis may also be a feature. Since symptoms are mild or absent, the disease may not be suspected unless the upper eyelid is everted. Active trachoma affects mainly children in endemic areas. Among older children and adults in such areas, conjunctival fibrosis often develops as the follicles resolve and, if severe, it may distort the upper lid margin, turning it inward (entropion). Lashes rubbing against the globe (trichiasis) cause continuous discomfort and sometimes blindness due to corneal damage.

The World Health Organization (**WHO**) has proposed criteria for the clinical diagnosis of active trachoma and its potentially blinding sequelae and for grading their severity as follows:

(1) trachomatous inflammation—follicular (**TF**): five or more follicles, each at least 0.5 mm in diameter, in the upper tarsal conjunctiva;

(2) trachomatous inflammation—intense (**TI**): pronounced inflammatory thickening of the tarsal conjunctiva that obscures more than half the normal deep tarsal blood vessels;

(3) trachomatous conjunctival scarring (**TS**): easily visible scarring in the tarsal conjunctiva;

(4) trachomatous trichiasis (**TT**): at least one eyelash rubbing on the eyeball—evidence of recent removal of inturned eyelashes also graded as trichiasis; and

(5) corneal opacity (**CO**): easily visible corneal opacity over the pupil, so dense that at least part of the pupil margin is blurred when viewed through the opacity.

Epidemiology

The reservoir of infection in endemic areas is the eye and possibly the nasopharynx of children with active disease. Active cases tend to cluster by household where there is prolonged intimate contact within the family. The higher prevalence of active disease and scarring in women than in men is probably due to the closer contact between women and children. *C. trachomatis* may be transferred from the eye of one individual to that of another via fingers, fomites, coughing, and sneezing, and by eye-seeking flies. Severe conjunctival scarring probably occurs only among individuals repeatedly exposed to reinfection. The availability and use of water are important determinants of the development of trachoma. When living conditions improve trachoma tends to disappear.

Diagnosis

In trachoma-endemic areas the diagnosis is generally made on clinical grounds, as most cases of follicular conjunctivitis are due to trachoma and laboratory facilities are usually lacking. Trachomatous follicles may be confused with the giant papillas of vernal conjunctivitis, in which pannus may also be seen. A number of viruses, notably adenoviruses, can cause follicular conjunctivitis. Intense cases of trachoma (TI), in which follicles may not be visible, should be distinguished from bacterial conjunctivitis. The diagnosis of trachomatous scarring is usually obvious, as few other conditions cause conjunctival scarring of the upper lid.

Laboratory diagnosis depends on the detection of *C. trachomatis*, which may be found in about 50 per cent of cases of active disease (TF or TI), but in only a minority of cases of scarring disease (TS). The microbiological diagnostic procedures are discussed later in this chapter.

Treatment

Inflammatory trachoma (TF and TI) responds to treatment with antimicrobial agents active against *C. trachomatis* (see Table 2). Until recently, the WHO has recommended 1 per cent topical tetracycline ointment, to be applied to both eyes daily for 6 weeks. This has proved impractical on a wide scale in trachoma-endemic communities. More recently, a single oral dose of azithromycin (20 mg/kg, to a maximum of 1 g) has been shown to be equally effective. When only individual cases are treated, reinfection is usually rapid; treatment of whole communities may reduce the rate of reinfection. Trichiasis and entropion require surgical correction. Several lid operations have been described, but few have been evaluated prospectively. Tarsal rotation is probably the operation of choice.

Prevention

The WHO has launched an initiative for the global elimination of blinding trachoma by the year 2020. The recommended strategy is based on the acronym 'SAFE': Surgery for trichiasis; Antibiotics for the treatment of inflammatory disease and the elimination of the reservoir of infection; promotion of Face washing, and Environmental improvement, to reduce fly populations, both of which are likely to reduce the rate of transmission of ocular *C. trachomatis* infection. In Mexico, children who washed their faces seven or more times per week were less likely to have trachoma than those who washed less often, and this intervention was also effective among rural villagers in Tanzania.

Genital tract infections

Infections of the genital tract due to *C. trachomatis* (Table 1) occur worldwide and, at least in developed countries, are much more common than gonococcal infections. The economic burden on health services due to genital chlamydial infections is enormous; for example, more than 3 billion dollars per year for pelvic inflammatory disease in the United States, based on 1994 incidence data. In Sweden, widespread and effective diagnostic testing, coupled with aggressive contact tracing and treatment, has greatly reduced genital chlamydial infections. This has not been achieved in other developed countries, but screening programmes are being or have been developed and implemented in some.

Non-gonococcal urethritis

C. trachomatis is detectable in the urethra of not more than 50 per cent of men with non-gonococcal urethritis and in up to 25 per cent of those with asymptomatic urethral infections. It is also likely that chlamydiae are a cause of some cases of chronic non-gonococcal urethritis

In women, there is no doubt that chlamydial urethral infection may cause urethritis but, in contrast to men, infection and inflammation are almost always asymptomatic. Thus, the dysuria and frequency of the urethral syndrome are rarely of chlamydial origin.

Prostatitis and epididymo-orchitis

There is no evidence that *C.trachomatis* causes acute symptomatic prostatitis. In chronic abacterial prostatitis diagnosed by the Stamey procedure, biopsy tissues taken transperineally to avoid the urethra have shown chronic inflammation, but chlamydiae have not been detected in them by culture and direct immunofluorescence techniques, although about 10 per cent have proved positive using polymerase chain-reaction technology. These largely negative observations, and the failure to detect chlamydial antibody, suggest that chlamydiae are not often implicated directly in the chronic disease. However, the possibility cannot be excluded that a portion, at least, of chronic disease is chlamydial in origin, maintained perhaps by immunological means. A predominance of CD8 cells in the tissues is consistent with this notion.

C. trachomatis is responsible for epididymitis primarily in young men (35 years of age or less) in developed countries, being detected in at least one-third of epididymal aspirates. Furthermore, there is a strong correlation between IgM and IgG chlamydial antibodies, measured by micro-immunofluorescence, and chlamydia-positive disease. In developing

Table 1 Assessment of the extent to which *C. trachomatis* is involved in various oculogenital and associated diseases

Disease	Evidence that *C. trachomatis* is a cause*	Proportion of disease due to *C. trachomatis*
In men		
Acute NGU	++++	Up to 50%
Postgonococcal urethritis	++++	Up to 50%
Persistent and recurrent NGU	++	?
Acute and chronic prostatitis	+	?
Acute epididymo-orchitis	++++	Up to 50%
Infertility	−	
In women		
Urethritis	+++	?
Bartholinitis	+	?
Vaginitis	−	
Bacterial vaginosis	−	
Cervicitis	++++	About 50%
Cervical dysplasia	+	
Endometritis	+++	?
Salpingitis	++++	40–60%
Periappendicitis	++	?
Perihepatitis	+++	?
Infertility	+++	≥ 8% due to chlamydial salpingitis
Ectopic pregnancy	+++	?
Abortion	−	
In men or women		
Conjunctivitis	++++	?
Otitis media	++	?
Arthritis (Reiter's syndrome)	+++	About 40%
Endocarditis	++	?
Pharyngitis	−	
Proctitis	++	?
Lymphogranuloma venereum	++++	100% (by definition)
In infants		
Conjunctivitis	++++	Up to 50%
Pneumonia	++++	30%?
Chronic lung disease	++	?
Gastroenteritis	−	

* ++++, overwhelming; +++, good; ++, moderate; +, weak; −, none.
NGU, non-gonococcal urethritis.

countries, although chlamydiae are important, *Neisseria gonorrhoeae* is still the major cause of acute epididymitis. In patients older than 35 years, an age boundary that, of course, is not strict, epididymo-orchitis tends to be caused by urinary-tract pathogens.

Convincing evidence that chlamydiae have been detected in the testes or that a previous chlamydial urethral infection or asymptomatic chlamydial infection causes male infertility has not been forthcoming.

Bartholinitis, vaginitis, and cervicitis

C. trachomatis has been weakly associated with bartholinitis, but is not regarded as a major cause. Chlamydiae are often detected more frequently in women with bacterial vaginosis than in those without this condition, but there is no evidence that they are causally associated or in any way contribute to the disease. It is apparent that the squamous epithelium of the vagina is not susceptible to chlamydial infection and that the cervix is the primary target for *C. trachomatis*. Indeed, it is a well known cause of mucopurulent/follicular cervicitis, although infection often may be asymptomatic. Women younger than 25 years, unmarried, using oral contraceptives, and who have signs of cervicitis are the most likely to have a chlamydial infection.

An association between cervical chlamydial infection and cervical intraepithelial neoplasia has been seen, but a causal link has not been established.

Pelvic inflammatory disease

Canalicular spread of chlamydiae to the upper genital tract leads to endometritis, which is often plasma-cell associated and sometimes intensely lymphoid. Further spread causes salpingitis, perihepatitis (the Curtis Fitz-Hugh syndrome), sometimes confused with acute cholecystitis in young women, in addition to periappendicitis and other abdominal complaints. Surgical termination of pregnancy or insertion or removal of an intrauterine contraceptive device may predispose to dissemination of the organisms.

Chlamydiae are the major cause of pelvic inflammatory disease in developed countries. Infertility is the outcome in about 10 per cent of such disease and may be the first indication of asymptomatic tubal disease. Fertility is influenced adversely by an increasing number and severity of upper genital tract chlamydial infections and infertility could result from endometritis, blocked or damaged tubes, or perhaps abnormalities of ovum transportation. Other consequences of salpingitis are ectopic pregnancy and chronic pelvic pain.

Other diseases associated with *C. trachomatis*

Adult paratrachoma (inclusion conjunctivitis) and otitis media

Adult chlamydial ophthalmia is distinguished from trachoma because it is caused by serovars D to K of *C. trachomatis* and commonly results from the accidental transfer of infected genital discharge to the eye. Chlamydiae can be detected in conjunctival specimens and in this respect the condition is different from the 'reactive' conjunctivitis seen in Reiter's syndrome (see below), where isolation from the conjunctiva is extremely unusual. Adult chlamydial ophthalmia usually presents as a unilateral follicular conjunctivitis of acute or subacute onset, the incubation period ranging from 2 to 21 days. The features are swollen lids, mucopurulent discharge, papillary hyperplasia due to congestion and neovascularization and later, follicular hypertrophy, and occasionally punctate keratitis. About one-third of patients have otitis media, complaining of blocked ears and hearing loss. The disease is generally benign and self-limited, but pannus formation and corneal scarring may occur unless systemic treatment is given. Patients and

their sexual contacts should be investigated for the existence of genital chlamydial infections and managed accordingly.

Arthritis

Arthritis occurring with or soon after non-gonococcal urethritis is termed sexually acquired reactive arthritis (**SARA**); in about one-third of cases, conjunctivitis and other features characteristic of Reiter's syndrome are seen. At least one-third of cases of such disease are initiated by chlamydial infection and *C. trachomatis* elementary bodies and chlamydial DNA and antigen may be detected in the joints. *C. trachomatis* has also been associated in the same way with 'seronegative' arthritis in women. Viable chlamydiae have not been detected in the joints of patients with SARA and the pathogenesis of the disease is probably immunologically based (see below). Despite this, early tetracycline therapy is advocated by some investigators.

Immunocompromised states

C. trachomatis has been isolated from the lower respiratory tract of a few immunocompromised adults with pneumonia, some after renal transplantation, but its role has been obscured by the recovery of other agents from some. However, neither *C. trachomatis* nor *C. pneumoniae* is an important respiratory-tract pathogen in patients with AIDS. Nor does genital chlamydial disease seem to be more widely prevalent or severe in HIV-infected patients and hypogammaglobulinaemic patients do not appear to be especially prone to infection with any of the chlamydial species.

Neonatal infections

Although intrauterine chlamydial infection can occur, the major risk of infection to the infant is from passing through an infected cervix. The proportion of neonates exposed to infection depends, of course, on the prevalence of maternal cervical infection, which varies widely. However, between one-fifth and one-half of infants exposed to *C. trachomatis* serovars D to K infecting the cervix at the time of birth develop conjunctivitis, which occurs usually 1 to 3 weeks after birth. A mucopurulent discharge and occasionally pseudomembrane formation occur, but it is usually self-limited, resolution occurring without visual impairment. If complications do arise, however, they tend to be in untreated infants.

About half of the infants who develop conjunctivitis develop pneumonia, although the latter is not always preceded by conjunctivitis. A history of recent conjunctivitis and bulging eardrums is found in only about half of the cases. Chlamydial pneumonia occurs usually between the fourth and eleventh week of life, preceded by upper respiratory symptoms, and has an afebrile, protracted course in which there is tachypnoea and a prominent, stacatto cough. Hyperinflation of the lungs with bilateral, diffuse, and symmetrical interstitial infiltration and scattered areas of atelectasis are the radiographic findings. The occurrence of serum IgM antibody to *C. trachomatis* in infants with pneumonia is pathognomonic. Children so affected during infancy are more likely to develop obstructive lung disease and asthma than are those who have had pneumonia due to other causes.

The vagina and rectum also may be colonized by *C. trachomatis* at birth. However, vaginal colonization has not been associated with clinical disease, nor has there been evidence for chlamydial gastroenteritis in infants.

Lymphogranuloma venereum

This is a systemic, sexually transmitted disease caused by serovars L1, L2, L2a, and L3 of *C. trachomatis*. These chlamydiae are more invasive than the other serovars and cause disease primarily in lymphatic tissue. Although a small papule or necrotic genital lesion may be the first sign of infection, with the rectosigmoid colon also a primary site, the chlamydiae are soon carried to regional lymph nodes. These enlarge rapidly and inflammation of the capsule causes them to mat together. Multiple minute abscesses form in the parenchyma and in the absence of treatment they may coalesce and form sinus tracts, which rupture through the overlying skin. Scar tissue may obstruct lymphatic flow causing lymphoedema and elephantiasis of the genitalia and strictures, ulcers, and fistulas may develop.

Clinical features

Three stages of infection are usually recognized. After an incubation period of 3 to 21 days, a small, painless, papular, vesicular, or ulcerative lesion develops and disappears spontaneously within a few days without scarring. In men the lesion is on the penis, and in women most commonly on the fourchette, often going unnoticed, especially if it is in the rectum of homosexual men. Extragenital primary lesions on fingers or tongue are rare.

The secondary stage is conventionally separated into inguinal and genitoanorectal syndromes. The former is more common and is usually seen in men as an acute painful inguinal bubo. The lymphadenopathy is unilateral in two-thirds of cases, and rarely may be so extensive that the inguinal mass is cleaved by the inelastic Poupart's ligament—the almost pathognomonic 'groove sign' of the disease. Buboes are accompanied by fever, malaise, chills, arthralgia, and headache and about 75 per cent of them suppurate and form cutaneous draining sinus tracts. In women, the external and internal iliac lymph nodes and the sacral lymphatics are involved more often than are the inguinal lymph nodes. Signs include a hypertrophic suppurative cervicitis, backache, and adnexal tenderness. In both sexes, but more frequently in women, a genitoanorectal syndrome characterized by a haemorrhagic proctitis or proctocolitis may occur. Inflammation is limited to the rectosigmoid colon and is accompanied by fever, a mucopurulent or bloody anal discharge, tenesmus, and diarrhoea. Histopathological changes in such cases may mimic Crohn's disease. The process usually resolves spontaneously after several weeks but, rarely, anal, rectovaginal, rectovesical, and ischiorectal fistulas occur and, late in the disease, a rectal stricture. Rare manifestations of the secondary stage are acute meningoencephalitis, synovitis, pneumonia, cardiac involvement, and follicular conjunctivitis, which is self-limited.

Lesions of the tertiary stage appear after a latent period of several years. They include genital elephantiasis, occurring predominantly in women as a sequel to the genitoanorectal syndrome and often accompanied by fistula formation, and rectal stricture, which is found almost exclusively in women or homosexual men. Gross ulceration and granulomatous hypertrophy of the vulva ('esthiomene') is very rare. Indeed, all late complications are rare today because of broad-spectrum antibiotics.

Epidemiology

Lymphogranuloma venereum is found worldwide, but its major incidence is limited to endemic foci in sub-Saharan Africa, South-East Asia, South America, and the Caribbean. All races are equally susceptible to infection, but the reported sex ratio is usually greater than 5:1 in favour of men because early disease is recognized much more easily in them. In North America and Europe, the disease is usually diagnosed in travellers, seamen, and military personnel returning from endemic areas, and in male homosexuals. The reservoir of infection is presumed to be asymptomatically infected women and male homosexuals.

Diagnosis

The differential diagnosis of lymphogranuloma venereum includes genital herpes, syphilis, chancroid, donovanosis, extrapulmonary tuberculosis, cat-scratch disease, plague, filariasis, lymphoma, and other malignant diseases. Of these, primary genital herpes can be the most difficult to distinguish. Lymphadenitis of the deep iliac nodes may mimic appendicitis or pelvic inflammatory disease and tuberculosis and certain parasitic and fungal infections of the genital tract cause lymphoedema and elephantiasis of the genitalia that may cause confusion.

The classic Frei skin test is no longer used for diagnosis. Staining of infected tissues to detect elementary bodies or inclusions (see later section on diagnosis) is not often used because the frequent bacterial contamination makes detection difficult. The use of cell culture is preferable, but only 25 to 40 per cent of patients with lymphogranuloma venereum have positive cultures of bubo aspirate, endourethral or endocervical scrapings,

or of other infected material. The much more sensitive DNA amplification methods are being used with increasing frequency.

Of the serological tests (see later section on diagnosis), complement fixation is not specific for lymphogranuloma venereum. The microimmunofluorescence test is also not entirely specific, but is the method of choice and antibody titres of 1:1024 or more are not uncommon and can be regarded as diagnostic, particularly in a patient with typical signs and symptoms.

Treatment

Of the several antimicrobial drugs available, oral tetracycline is usually recommended (Table 2) although azithromycin is finding a place. Fever and bubo pain rapidly subside after antibiotic treatment is started, but buboes may take several weeks to resolve. Suppuration and rupture of buboes with sinus formation is usually prevented by antibiotic treatment. Surgical incision and drainage is neither necessary nor recommended. How long treatment needs to be continued to prevent relapse or progression of disease is debated but a minimum of 2 weeks is recommended. Fistulas, strictures, and elephantiasis may require plastic repair but surgery should not be attempted until the patient has had weeks or months of antimicrobial treatment to reduce inflammation and necrosis.

Chlamydia pneumoniae infections

It is interesting that the prototype strains of *C. pneumoniae* were isolated from conjunctival material collected in the mid-1960s from patients in trachoma-endemic areas. It was not until 1983, however, that a third *C. pneumoniae* strain was isolated, this time from the throat of a patient with acute pharyngitis. The two original isolates (TW-183 and IOL-207) were found to be identical serologically and distinct from *C. trachomatis* and *C. psittaci* and, in 1989, *C. pneumoniae* was defined as the third species of the genus *Chlamydia*. At present only one serovar of *C. pneumoniae* has been identified, although minor geographical serovar variations have been described.

Clinical features

Respiratory tract disease

At the outset of acute disease, pharyngitis is often present, more than 80 per cent of patients with lower respiratory-tract disease developing a sore throat. A cough may take some time to develop and fever is uncommon. Bronchitis is associated with some infections and in young adults about 5 per cent of primary sinusitis is associated with *C. pneumoniae*. Mild respiratory infections are probably frequent but, overall, pneumonia has been the most common feature; in mild cases, radiographs usually reveal a unilateral pneumonia, whereas in patients needing hospital care, bilateral pneumonia is quite common. This is often difficult to distinguish clinically from that caused by other micro-organisms, for example *Mycoplasma pneumoniae*.

Arthritis

An exaggerated synovial lymphocyte response to *C. pneumoniae* has been found in some adults with reactive arthritis and *C. pneumoniae* DNA and high titres of specific antibody have been detected in the joints of a few children with juvenile chronic arthritis, suggesting the possibility of a causal role.

Atherosclerosis

Patients with chronic coronary heart disease and acute myocardial infarction were noted first by Finnish investigators and later by others to have antibody to *C. pneumoniae* significantly more often than age-matched controls. The possibility that *C. pneumoniae* infection might be a risk factor for such disease was enhanced by detection of the organisms or their DNA in at least 40 per cent of atheromatous coronary and other major arteries of adults and subjects as young as 15 years. In addition, specific DNA has been found in at least 40 per cent of peripheral blood mononuclear cells, raising the possibility that they transmit the organisms to the arterial wall, atheromatous or otherwise, from the respiratory tract. Inoculation of mice and rabbits with *C. pneumoniae* has initiated or potentiated atherosclerotic-like changes, observations that are provocative but insufficient to determine the significance of the human findings.

Epidemiology

C. pneumoniae organisms are transmitted from person to person, apparently without any intermediate host. Serological evidence indicates that *C. pneumoniae* is widespread and endemic in many areas, although localized epidemics have been recorded in both military and civilian groups in Scandinavia, the United States, the United Kingdom, and elsewhere. *C. pneumoniae* probably causes many mild respiratory infections that were previously thought to be viral in origin and it is also likely that many infections labelled 'human psittacosis/ornithosis' in the past were in reality due to *C. pneumoniae*.

Chlamydia psittaci infections

The *C. psittaci* species comprises a diverse group of organisms that have been isolated from a variety of mammals and frogs and many avian species.

Nine serovars have been proposed from mammals and seven from birds, and two biovars from koala bears. The relatively low degree of homology between serovars exhibited in DNA–DNA hybridization analyses signals the possibility of further speciation among organisms currently assigned to the species. This, in fact, has happened with the separation of strains causing pneumonia, polyarthritis, encephalomyelitis, and diarrhoea in cattle and sheep and the constitution of the fourth chlamydial species, *C. pecorum*.

The spectrum of animal diseases caused by *C. psittaci* species includes enteritis, abortion, sterility, pneumonia, and encephalitis, all of which cause economic loss. Occasionally, the organisms are transmitted to humans through contact with infected animals or birds or from contact with faecal materials from an infected source. Psittacosis may be a hazard to those who keep pet birds or who work in poultry processing plants, or in animal husbandry. Many birds are known to harbour the organisms, but psittacine species (parrots), poultry, and pigeons are probably the major sources of human infection.

Clinical features

Human respiratory infection with *C. psittaci* (psittacosis) is equally common in either sex. It is uncommon and mild in childhood and usually affects adults, particularly those in the 30- to 60-year age group. After an incubation period of 1 to 2 weeks, the clinical presentation can vary from a mild influenza-like illness to a fulminating toxic state with multiple organ

Table 2 Recommended treatment schedules for chlamydial infections and associated diseases

Disease/infection	Antibiotic	Dose schedule[a]	Duration (days)
Trachoma	Topical tetracycline	1% ointment daily	6 weeks
	Azithromycin alone	20 mg/kg (up to 1 g)	Single dose
Adult inclusion conjunctivitis	Tetracycline HC1	500 mg 4 times daily	14
	or doxycycline	100 mg twice daily	14
	or erythromycin stearate	500 mg 4 times daily	14
	or azithromycin	1 g	Single dose
Non-gonococcal urethritis (NGU)	Antibiotics and regimens as for treatment of adult inclusion conjunctivitis		7
Epididymo-orchitis	Ampicillin	3.5 g	
	then antibiotics as for NGU		10
Cervicitis/urethritis	Antibiotics and regimens as for NGU		7
Pelvic inflammatory disease			
For ambulatory patient	Ceftriaxone	250 mg intramuscularly	Single dose
	then doxycycline	100 mg twice daily	14
For patient admitted to hospital	(a) Doxycycline	100 mg twice daily intravenously	≥ 4
	then doxycycline	100 mg twice daily	14
	or (b) clindamycin	600 mg 4 times daily intravenously	≥ 4
	and gentamicin	2 mg/kg intravenously	≥ 4
	and then	1.5 mg/kg 3 times daily	
	clindamycin	450 mg 4 times daily	10[b]
Neonatal infections	Erythromycin syrup	50 mg/kg daily in 4 divided doses	14
Lymphogranuloma venereum	Antibiotics and regimens as for NGU[c]		21
C. pneumoniae infections	Antibiotics and regimens as for NGU except doxycycline twice daily		7–21[d]
C. psittaci infections	Antibiotics and regimes as for NGU except doxycycline twice daily		≥ 14

[a] All antibiotics orally unless otherwise indicated.
[b] Total duration of therapy 14 days.
[c] Azithromycin likely to be effective but multiple doses probably required.
[d] Relapse more often with short course.

involvement. The disease may be insidious in onset over a few days or start abruptly with high fever, rigors, and anorexia. Headache occurs in most, a cough, often dry, in over two-thirds, and arthralgia and myalgia in over one-third. Inspiratory crepitations are more common than classic signs of consolidation. Chest radiographs usually show patchy shadowing, most often in the lower lobes. Homogeneous lobar shadowing is less common, and miliary and nodular patterns even less so. Hilar lymphadenopathy has been reported in up to two-thirds of patients and a pleural reaction in more than half, but significant pleural effusions are infrequent. Extrapulmonary complications, mostly rare, include endocarditis, myocarditis, pericarditis, a toxic confusional state, encephalitis, meningitis, tender hepatomegaly, splenomegaly, pancreatitis, haemolysis, and disseminated intravascular coagulation. The advent of superior laboratory tests should not allow disease caused by *C. psittaci* to be confused with that due to *C. pneumoniae*, as occurred in the past.

Ovine *C. psittaci* strains have caused abortion, albeit rarely, in pregnant women, often farmers' wives, after exposure to sheep suffering from enzootic abortion during the lambing season. The feline keratoconjunctivitis agent, isolated from the genital tract of female cats, has caused follicular conjunctivitis in humans similar to that caused by *C. trachomatis* serovars D to K.

Diagnosis of chlamydial infections

The laboratory diagnosis of chlamydial infection depends on detection of the organisms or their antigens or DNA and to a much lesser extent on serology. The procedures mentioned, with some of their advantages and disadvantages, are summarized in Table 3. Certain swabs, for example those that are cotton tipped, are superior to others, and swabs provided in commercial enzyme immunoassay kits may be toxic if used for collecting specimens for culture. Examination of two or more consecutive swabs from patients rather than one improves the chlamydial detection rate and this may be achieved in women by pooling cervical and urethral specimens. However, in recent times attention has turned to the use of 'first-catch' urine specimens, which were ignored for years because they were found not to be suitable for chlamydial culture. Nevertheless, they are unquestionably valuable samples from both men and women, provided that the centrifuged deposits are tested by molecular methods. The same comment applies to the use of meatal samples in men and of vulvar/vaginal samples.

Culture and staining of chlamydia

The growth of chlamydiae about 40 years ago in cultured cells, rather than in embryonated eggs, revolutionized both their detection and chlamydial research. *C. pneumoniae* is particularly difficult to isolate and this may be facilitated by using a line of human lung cells. The method of detection used widely for *C. trachomatis* involves the centrifugation of specimens on to cycloheximide-treated McCoy cell monolayers. Inoculation of cell cultures is followed by incubation and staining with a fluorescent monoclonal antibody or with a vital dye, usually Giemsa, to detect inclusions; one blind passage may increase sensitivity. However, the cell-culture technique is no more than 70 per cent sensitive and is slow and labour intensive, drawbacks that have hastened the development of non-cultural methods.

Staining of epithelial cells in ocular and genital specimens with vital dyes was used first to detect chlamydial inclusions, but the method is insensitive and often non-specific. Papanicolaou-stained cervical smears provide an excellent example of these drawbacks. In contrast, detection of elementary bodies by using species-specific fluorescent monoclonal antibodies is rapid and, for *C. trachomatis* oculogenital infections, sensitivities ranging from 70 to 100 per cent and specificities from 80 to 100 per cent have been achieved. Skilled observers, capable of detecting a few elementary bodies, even one, provide values at the top of these ranges. However, the test is most suited for dealing with a few specimens and for confirming positive results obtained with other tests.

Enzyme immunoassays and DNA amplification techniques

The popularity of enzyme immunoassays that detect chlamydial antigens is due to their ease of use and not to their sensitivity. Indeed, it is rarely possible to detect small numbers of chlamydial organisms (less than 10) of whatever species. Since at least 30 per cent of genital swab specimens and a larger proportion of urine samples from women contain such small numbers, some chlamydia-positive patients are misdiagnosed. Despite this, immunoassays still occupy a diagnostic niche largely because of cost saving.

By enabling enormous amplification of a DNA sequence specific to the chlamydial species, polymerase chain reaction (PCR), ligase chain reaction (LCR), transcription mediated, and some other molecular assays have overcome the problem of poor sensitivity and may provide evidence for the existence of chlamydiae in chronic or treated disease when viable or intact organisms no longer exist. These sensitive assays have replaced culture as the 'gold standard' and have a place not only in research, but also in routine diagnosis and in promoting and maintaining effective screening programmes.

Serological tests

The complement fixation test tends not to distinguish between the chlamydial species and, therefore, is used infrequently. Most of the pertinent diagnostic information has come through the use of the microimmunofluorescence test by which class-specific antibodies (IgM, IgG, IgA, or secretory) may be measured. However, a fourfold or greater increase in the titre

Table 3 Advantages and disadvantages of chlamydial detection procedures

Factor considered	Culture	Direct fluorescent antibody	Enzyme immunoassay	DNA amplification
Speed/temperature for transport of specimen	Rapid or at low temperature	Unimportant if fixed	Unimportant if in buffer	Speed not crucial if at low temperature; may use fixed specimens
Storage requirements	4°C if overnight; liquid nitrogen if long term	4°C if short term; −20°C and fixed if long term	4°C if 3 to 5 days; freezing if longer	4°C if short term; −70°C if long term
Evaluation of adequacy of specimen	Not practical	Evaluate during test	Not practical	Determine whether DNA present
Special equipment or procedure	Centrifuge	Fluorescence microscope	ELISA reader	Thermocycling machine and electrophoresis equipment
Processing of specimen	Tedious	Simple	Relatively simple	Requires precautions against DNA contamination
Reading of test	Subjective and moderately tedious	Subjective and tedious	Objective and simple	Objective and simple
Duration of test	48–72 h	30 min	3 h	12–24 h
Sensitivity of test	60–70%	70–100%	50–70%	Up to 100%

of antibody (IgM and/or IgG) is detected infrequently so that the value of serology in the diagnosis of chlamydial infections in individual patients is limited. A good correlation has been found between the presence of IgG and/or IgA antibody in tears and the isolation of *C. trachomatis* from the conjunctiva in endemic trachoma and adult ocular paratrachoma. In genital infections, serum antibodies are found frequently in the absence of a current chlamydial infection of the cervix, so that reliance cannot be put on a single serum or local IgA-specific antibody titre to denote a current infection. In pelvic inflammatory disease, especially in the Curtis Fitz-Hugh syndrome, antibody titres tend to be higher than in uncomplicated cervical infections. A very high IgG antibody titre, for example 512 or greater, suggests causation in pelvic disease, but high titres do not always correlate with detection of chlamydiae and are associated more with chronic or recurrent disease. However, specific *C. trachomatis* IgM antibody in babies with pneumonia is pathognomonic of chlamydia-induced disease.

In primary respiratory infections with *C. pneumoniae*, IgM antibody is considered to develop within a few weeks and IgG antibody by 2 months. In repeat infections, IgG but not IgM antibody develops more rapidly and to a greater titre than before. However, when only a single serum is available, it may be difficult to interpret information complicated by cross-reacting antibodies to the other species. Only in children is the finding of *C. pneumoniae* antibody in a single serum sample an assurance of infection with this species. Although the complement fixation test has been used in the past to diagnose lymphogranuloma venereum and psittacosis, as indicated above it is unwise to do so because of its lack of specificity.

Treatment of chlamydial infections

Chlamydiae are particularly sensitive to tetracyclines and macrolides, but also to a variety of other drugs. The rifampicins are probably more active than the tetracyclines *in vitro* but there is evidence for chlamydial resistance to the rifampicins which, in any case, are usually reserved for mycobacterial infections. Tetracycline resistance has been reported but is insufficiently widespread to cause a problem clinically. However, vigilance should be kept for resistant strains that might jeopardize clinical practice, particularly as the move away from cultural diagnostic procedures has made their detection less easy. Of the macrolides, erythromycin is used most often, particularly to treat chlamydial infections in infants, young children, and in pregnant and lactating women. Azithromycin in a single dose has gained popularity because it seems to be effective and enhances compliance. Other alternatives, such as some of the quinolones, particularly ofloxacin, are effective but have not found regular use.

More detailed recommendations for dose and duration of antibiotic treatment are presented in Table 2. The principle of giving systemic treatment as well as topical to eradicate nasopharyngeal carriage in trachoma applies also in neonatal chlamydial conjunctivitis, where topical treatment provides no additional benefit. Oral erythromycin should be given to treat the conjunctivitis and to prevent the development of pneumonia. Azithromycin in a single oral dose (20 mg/kg) has been shown to be as effective as 6 weeks of topical tetracycline for active trachoma and may well be the drug of choice. Azithromycin as a single 1-g oral dose has also been shown to be effective in treating non-gonococcal urethritis. In complicated genital tract infections such as epididymo-orchitis and pelvic inflammatory disease, treatment will almost certainly be needed before a microbiological diagnosis can be established, following which additional broad-spectrum antibiotic cover may be required. In the case of *C. pneumoniae* and *C. psittaci* infections, treatment follows the same principles as for *C. trachomatis* infections. Finally, it should be kept in mind that treatment is likely to be most effective when given over a long rather than short time, suboptimal doses are avoided, compliance is strict, and when, in the case of genital infections, partners of patients are also treated.

Immune response and pathogenesis

The immune response to chlamydial infections may be protective or damaging, much of the pathology being immunologically mediated. The hallmark of chlamydial infection, whatever the anatomical site, is the lymphoid follicle. Follicles contain typical germinal centres, consisting predominantly of B lymphocytes, with T cells, mostly CD8 cells, in the parafollicular region. Between follicles the inflammatory infiltrate contains plasma cells, dendritic cells, macrophages, and polymorphonuclear leucocytes in addition to T and B lymphocytes. The late stage of chlamydial infection is characterized by fibrosis, seen typically in trachoma and pelvic inflammatory disease. T lymphocytes are also present and outnumber B cells and macrophages. Biopsies taken from patients with cicatricial trachoma and persisting inflammatory changes show a predominance of CD4 cells, but those from patients in whom inflammation has subsided contain mainly CD8 cells.

Repeated ocular infection by chlamydiae induces progressively worse disease with a diminished ability to isolate the organisms, features noted both naturally and experimentally. There is also experimental evidence that such events occur in the genital tract. For example, primary inoculation of the oviducts of pig-tailed macaques with *C. trachomatis* produced a self-limiting salpingitis with minimal residual damage, whereas repeated tubal inoculation caused hydrosalpinx formation with adnexal adhesions. In the cynomolgus monkey model, a similar exaggerated inflammatory response was effected by the genus-specific 57-kDa protein that has sequence homology with the GroEL heat-shock protein of *Escherichia coli*. It is thought that the damaging sequelae of chlamydial infections, such as scarring in trachoma, tubal adhesions following pelvic inflammatory disease, and reactive arthritis consequent to urethritis, may result from soluble mediators of inflammation in response to the 57-kDa protein. Thus, it is possible that interferon-γ secreted by lymphocytes from immune subjects, together with other cytokines, particularly those that stimulate fibroblast activity, such as interleukin 1 and tumour necrosis factor-β, may play a part in the scarring process.

The epidemiology of trachoma suggests that protective immunity follows natural infection, as active disease is uncommon in adults in endemic areas, and *C. trachomatis* can rarely be isolated from them. Similarly, the chlamydial isolation rate for men with non-gonococcal urethritis is lower in those who have had previous episodes. Furthermore, women who have had cervical chlamydial infections accompanied by IgM and IgG antibodies to *C. trachomatis* are less likely to develop salpingitis than those without such antibodies. These observations and the results of animal experiments indicate that chlamydial infection of the eye, the genital tract, and also the respiratory tract provides moderate resistance to reinfection. Nevertheless, attempts to develop an effective vaccine against any of the chlamydial species have, so far, been unsuccessful, although DNA vaccines hold out some hope.

Further reading

Black CM (1997). Current methods of laboratory diagnosis of *Chlamydia trachomatis* infection. *Clinical Microbiology Reviews* **10**, 160–84.

Grayston JT *et al.* (1990). A new respiratory tract pathogen: *Chlamydia pneumoniae* strain TWAR. *Journal of Infectious Diseases* **161**, 618–25.

Mabey DCW, Bailey RL, Hutin YJF (1992). The epidemiology and pathogenesis of trachoma. *Review of Medical Microbiology* **3**, 1–8.

Perine PL, Stamm WE (1999). Lymphogranuloma venereum. In: Holmes KK *et al.*, eds. *Sexually transmitted diseases*, 3rd edn, pp 423–32. McGraw-Hill, New York.

Rasmussen SJ (1998). Chlamydial immunology. *Current Opinion in Infectious Diseases* **11**, 37–41.

Schachter J *et al.* (1999). Azithromycin in control of trachoma. *Lancet* **354**, 630–5.

Stephens RS *et al.* (1998). Genome sequence of an obligate intracellular pathogen of humans: *Chlamydia trachomatis*. *Science* **282**, 754–9.

Stephens RS, ed. (1999). *Chlamydia. Intracellular biology, pathogenesis and immunity.* American Society for Microbiology, Washington DC.

Taylor-Robinson D (1991). Genital chlamydial infections: clinical aspects, diagnosis, treatment and prevention. In: Harris JRW, Forster SM, eds. *Recent advances in sexually transmitted diseases and AIDS*, pp 219–62. Churchill Livingstone, Edinburgh.

Taylor-Robinson D (1997). Evaluation and comparison of tests to diagnose *Chlamydia trachomatis* genital infections. *Human Reproduction* **12**, 113–20.

Taylor-Robinson D, Thomas BJ (1998). *Chlamydia pneumoniae* in arteries: the facts, their interpretation, and future studies. *Journal of Clinical Pathology* **51**, 793–7.

Thylefors B *et al.* (1987). A simple system for the assessment of trachoma and its complications. *Bulletin of the World Health Organization* **65**, 477–83.

Zhang D-J *et al.* (1997). DNA vaccination with the major outer membrane protein gene induces acquired immunity to *Chlamydia trachomatis* (mouse pneumonitis) infection. *Journal of Infectious Diseases* **176**, 1035–40.

7.11.41 Mycoplasmas

D. Taylor-Robinson

Characteristics of mycoplasmas

Mycoplasmas, originally called pleuropneumonia-like organisms (**PPLO**), are the smallest free-living micro-organisms. They lack a rigid cell wall seen in other bacteria so that they are resistant to penicillins and other antimicrobials which act on this structure. Instead, they are bounded by a pliable unit membrane (Fig. 1), which encloses the cytoplasm, DNA, RNA, and other metabolic components necessary for propagation in cell-free media. Despite their general similarity, mycoplasmas comprise a heterogeneous group of micro-organisms that differ from one another in DNA composition, nutritional requirements, metabolic reactions, antigenic composition, and host specificity. Taxonomically, mycoplasmas are divided into four orders, namely the Mycoplasmatales, the Entomoplasmatales comprising those from insects and plants, the Acholeplasmatales, which do not require sterol for growth, and the oxygen-sensitive, strictly anaerobic Anaeroplasmatales, one genus of which also does not need sterol. The mycoplasmas isolated commonly from humans belong to the family Mycoplasmataceae within the order Mycoplasmatales. This family comprises the genus *Mycoplasma*, which contains organisms that metabolize glucose or arginine or both, but not urea, and the genus *Ureaplasma*, the organisms of which hydrolyse urea uniquely. The latter originally were termed T-strains or T-mycoplasmas because of the tiny (T) colonies they form on agar medium, in contrast to the larger characteristic 'fried-egg'-like colonies produced by most other mycoplasmas (Fig. 2).

The small size of the mycoplasma genome restricts their metabolic capabilities. Nevertheless, apart from their importance in humans, certain mycoplasma species are of economic importance because of the pneumonia, arthritis, keratoconjunctivitis, and mastitis they cause among livestock and poultry in Africa, Australia, and other parts of the world. Furthermore, a number of species are a laboratory nuisance as occult contaminants of cell cultures.

Occurrence of mycoplasmas in man

Sixteen mycoplasma species have been isolated from humans, but only 14 constitute the normal flora or behave as pathogens (Table 1). Most of them are found in the oropharynx. There is little information, as yet, about the

(a)

(b)

Fig. 2 (a) 'Fried-egg'-like mycoplasma colonies (one not well formed) and a larger bacterial colony. Transmission light microscopy, × 43. (b) Section through mycoplasma colonies illustrating growth in the depth of the agar. × 78.

Fig. 1 Electron micrograph of *M. pulmonis* (murine origin), illustrating that the organism does not have a bacterial cell wall but has a trilaminar unit membrane (arrow); also note what appears to be a terminal structure (T). × 66 000.

Table 1 The biological features, occurrence, and disease association of mycoplasmas of human origin[a]

Mycoplasma	Metabolism of:	Preferred atmosphere	Haemadsorption	Frequency of detection in the:					Cause of disease
				Respiratory tract	Genitourinary tract	Rectum	Eye	Blood	
M. buccale	Arginine	Anaerobic[b]	No	Rare	–[c]	–	–	–	No
M. faucium	Arginine	Anaerobic	Yes[d]	Rare	–	–	–	–	No
M. fermentans	Glucose, arginine	Anaerobic	No	Common	Rare	–	–	Rare	?Yes
M. genitalium	Glucose	Anaerobic	Yes	Rare	Common	Rare	?	?	Yes
M. hominis	Arginine	Aerobic	No	Rare	Common	Common	Rare	Very rare	Yes
M. lipophilum	Arginine	Anaerobic	No	Rare	–	–	–	–	No
M. orale	Arginine	Anaerobic	Yes[d]	Common	–	–	–	–	No
M. penetrans	Glucose, arginine	Anaerobic	Yes	–	Rare	Very rare	–	?	?
M. pirum	Glucose	Anaerobic	?	?	–	Rare	?	Very rare	?
M. pneumoniae	Glucose	Aerobic	Yes	Rare[e]	Very rare	–	–	–	Yes
M. primatum	Arginine	Anaerobic	No	–	Rare	–	–	–	No
M. salivarium	Arginine	Anaerobic	No	Common	Rare	–	–	–	No[f]
M. spermatophilum	Arginine	Anaerobic	No	–	?Rare	?	?	?	?
Ureaplasma urealyticum	Urea	Anaerobic	Serotype 3 only	Rare	Common	Common	Rare	Very rare	Yes

[a] Acholeplasma laidlawii and A. oculi have also been recovered very rarely, but are not of human origin.
[b] 5% carbon dioxide, 95% nitrogen.
[c] No reports of detection.
[d] With chick erythrocytes only.
[e] Except in disease outbreaks.
[f] Except in hypogammaglobulinaemia.

distribution or significance of *M. penetrans*, *M. pirum*, and *M. spermatophilum*.

Respiratory infections

The relation between mycoplasmas and respiratory disease

M. pneumoniae is the most important mycoplasma found in the respiratory tract (see below), most of them behaving as commensals (Table 1). *M. genitalium* was found originally in the male genitourinary tract but was subsequently isolated from a few respiratory specimens, which also contained *M. pneumoniae*. However, the significance of *M. genitalium* in the respiratory tract remains to be determined. *M. fermentans* has been detected in the throat more often than hitherto because of the use of the polymerase chain reaction (**PCR**) (see later) and has been recovered from adults with an acute influenza-like illness, which sometimes deteriorates rapidly with development of an often fatal respiratory distress syndrome. *M. hominis*, on the other hand, shows little virulence. Despite it causing a mild exudative pharyngitis in adult male volunteers given large numbers of organisms orally, it has not been shown to cause naturally occurring sore throats in children or adults.

In the late 1930s, non-bacterial pneumonias were first recognized and brought under the heading of primary atypical pneumonia to distinguish them from typical lobar pneumonia. Gradually, primary atypical pneumonia was recognized to be aetiologically heterogeneous and, in one variety, cold agglutinins often developed. It was from this form of disease that an infectious agent was isolated in embryonated eggs. This micro-organism, the 'Eaton agent', produced pneumonia in cotton rats and hamsters, and was thought first to be a virus. However, this was seriously doubted when it was found to be affected by chlortetracycline and gold salts, and its mycoplasmal nature was established finally by cultivation on a cell-free agar medium. The agent was subsequently called *M. pneumoniae* and its ability to cause respiratory disease was established fully by studies based on isolation, serology, volunteer inoculation, and vaccine protection.

M. pneumoniae disease manifestations

M. pneumoniae produces a spectrum of effects ranging from inapparent infection and mild, afebrile, upper respiratory-tract disease to severe pneumonia. Clinical manifestations are often not sufficiently distinctive to permit an early definitive diagnosis of mycoplasmal pneumonia. Indeed, this shares the features of other non-bacterial pneumonias in that general symptoms, such as malaise and headache, often precede chest symptoms by 1 to 5 days, and radiographic examination frequently reveals evidence of pneumonia before physical signs, such as rales, become apparent. Usually, only one of the lower lobes is involved and the radiograph most often shows patchy opacities. About 20 per cent of patients suffer bilateral pneumonia, but pleurisy and pleural effusions are unusual. The course of the disease is variable but often protracted. Thus, cough, abnormal chest signs, and changes in the radiograph may persist for several weeks and relapse is a feature. The organisms may also persist in respiratory secretions despite antibiotic therapy, particularly in patients with hypogammaglobulinaemia, where excretion may continue for months or years rather than weeks. Although a few very severe infections have been reported, occurring usually in patients with immunodeficiency or sickle-cell anaemia, death has been rare. In children, infection has been characterized occasionally by a prolonged illness with paroxysmal cough followed by vomiting, thus simulating the features of whooping cough.

Extrapulmonary manifestations

Disease caused by *M. pneumoniae* is limited usually to the respiratory tract, but various extrapulmonary conditions may occur during the course of the respiratory illness or as a sequel to it. These complications and an estimation of their frequency are shown in Table 2. Whether any of them might be due to *M. genitalium* is a moot point. Haemolytic anaemia with crisis is brought about by the development and action of cold agglutinins (anti-I antibodies), the organisms apparently altering the I antigen on erythrocytes sufficiently to stimulate an autoimmune response. It is possible that some of the other clinical conditions, such as the neurological complications, may arise in a similar way. However, invasion of the central nervous system

Table 2 Extrapulmonary manifestations of *M. pneumoniae* infections

System	Manifestations	Estimated frequency
Cardiovascular	Myocarditis, pericarditis	< 5%
Dermatological	Erythema multiforme; Stevens–Johnson syndrome; other rashes	Some skin involvement in about 25%
Gastrointestinal	Anorexia, nausea, vomiting, and transient diarrhoea; hepatitis; pancreatitis	14–44%
		?
		?
Genitourinary	Tubo-ovarian abscess; acute glomerulonephritis	Insignificant
		?
Haematological	Cold agglutinin production; haemolytic anaemia; thrombocytopenia; intravascular coagulation	About 50%
		?
		?
		> 50 reported cases
Musculoskeletal	Myalgia, arthralgia; arthritis	14–45%
		?
Neurological	Meningitis, meningoencephalitis, ascending paralysis, transient myelitis, cranial-nerve palsy, poliomyelitis-like illness	6–7%

cannot be discounted as *M. pneumoniae* has been isolated from cerebrospinal fluid.

Microbiological diagnosis of *M. pneumoniae* infection

This depends on detection by culture or molecular methods and/or serology. The usual medium employed for isolation of *M. pneumoniae* consists of PPLO broth, 20 per cent horse serum, and 10 per cent (v/v) fresh yeast extract (25 per cent w/v). However, a more sensitive medium (SP4) is that used first for the isolation of spiroplasmas, comprising a conventional mycoplasma broth medium with fetal calf serum and a tissue-culture supplement. Either medium is supplemented with a broad-spectrum penicillin, and glucose, with phenol red as a pH indicator. The fluid medium, inoculated with sputum, throat washing, pharyngeal swab, or other specimen, is incubated at 37 °C and a colour change (red to yellow), which occurs usually within 4 to 21 days, signals the fermentation of glucose (Table 1), with production of acid, owing to multiplication of the organisms. This preliminary identification may be confirmed after subculturing to agar medium, usually by demonstrating inhibition of colony development around discs impregnated with specific antiserum (Fig. 3) or by immunofluorescence of colonies with an *M. pneumoniae*-specific antibody.

Culture and identification are slow, but rapid PCR determination of *M. pneumoniae* positivity and then continued culture of only those specimens that are PCR-positive makes for a speedier diagnosis. However, this approach, or the use of the PCR to test specimens directly, is not routine,

reliance still being placed on serology for diagnosis. Testing by complement fixation is undertaken in many laboratories and a fourfold or greater rise in antibody titre with a peak at about 3 to 4 weeks after the onset of disease is said to occur in about 80 per cent of cases and be indicative of a recent infection. A titre of 1:128 or greater in a single serum is suggestive but not proof of infection in the previous few weeks or months; a fourfold or greater fall in antibody titre, perhaps over 6 months, may be helpful but, sometimes, may be difficult to relate to a particular prior illness. It must be remembered that the complement-fixation test does not distinguish between *M. pneumoniae* and *M. genitalium* and the occasional occurrence of the latter in the respiratory tract may jeopardize a specific diagnosis of *M. pneumoniae* infection. More specific, perhaps, is the microimmunofluorescence test in which IgM antibody is sought; its presence provides some confidence in making an accurate diagnosis of a current infection or one within the previous few weeks. The same comment applies to a commercially available enzyme immunoassay specific for IgM. Cold agglutinins, detected by agglutination of O Rh-negative erythrocytes at 4 °C, develop in about half the patients and a titre of 1:128 or greater is suggestive of a recent *M. pneumoniae* infection. However, such agglutinins are occasionally induced by a number of other conditions, but the ability of *M. genitalium* to do so is unknown.

Epidemiology of *M. pneumoniae* infections

The consequence of infection depends on age, about a quarter of infections in persons 5 to 15 years old resulting in pneumonia, with about 7 per cent of infections in young adults doing so. Thereafter, pneumonia is even less frequent, but generally is more severe the older the patient.

Although *M. pneumoniae* causes inapparent and mild upper respiratory-tract infections more commonly than severe disease, it is responsible for only a small proportion of all upper respiratory-tract disease, most of it being of viral or streptococcal aetiology. It plays a relatively greater part in producing lower respiratory-tract disease together with *Chlamydia pneumoniae* and various other bacteria. Thus, in the United States, it has been calculated that in a large general population, the proportion of all pneumonias due to *M. pneumoniae* is about 15 to 20 per cent, and in certain populations, for example military recruits, it has been responsible for as much as 40 per cent of acute pneumonic illness.

M. pneumoniae infections have been reported from every country where appropriate diagnostic tests have been undertaken. Infection is endemic in most areas and occurs during all months of the year, with a predilection for late summer and early autumn. However, epidemic peaks have been observed about every 4 to 7 years in some countries. The incubation period ranges from 2 to 3 weeks and spread from person to person occurs slowly, usually where there is continual or repeated close contact, for example in a family.

Fig. 3 Mycoplasma identification by agar growth inhibition. Colony development inhibited around a filter-paper disc impregnated with specific antiserum. Note also antibody–antigen precipitation at edge of inhibition zone.

Immunopathological factors in the development of *M. pneumoniae* pneumonia

Adherence of *M. pneumoniae* organisms to respiratory mucosal epithelial cells (Fig. 4) is a crucial factor in the pathogenesis of disease. After cytadsorption, mediated by P1, P30, and possibly up to seven other proteins on the surface of the organisms, immune mechanisms are important in the development of *M. pneumoniae* pneumonia in humans, which rarely causes death. Thus, the histopathological picture is derived mainly from infection in other animals. The pneumonic infiltrate is predominantly a peribronchiolar and perivascular accumulation of lymphocytes, most of which are thymus dependent (Fig. 5). The importance of cell-mediated immune mechanisms is indicated by the fact that immunosuppression in hamsters results in ablation of the pneumonia or a decrease in its severity. The development of a cell-mediated immune response to *M. pneumoniae* has been shown further by positive lymphocyte transformation, macrophage migration inhibition, and delayed-hypersensitivity skin tests. A polysaccharide–protein fraction of the organisms is involved in this response rather than the glycolipid that is the main antigenic determinant in complement-fixation and other serological reactions. The initial lymphocyte response is followed by a change in the character of the bronchiolar exudate, with polymorphonuclear leucocytes and macrophages predominating. The rather slow development of these events on primary infection contrasts with an accelerated and often more intense host response seen on reinfection. To at least some extent, therefore, the pneumonia caused by *M. pneumoniae* is an immunopathological process. Children of 2 to 5 years of age often possess mycoplasmacidal antibody, suggesting infection at an early age and the notion that the pneumonia that occurs in older persons is an immunological over-response to reinfection, the lung being infiltrated by previously sensitized lymphocytes.

Treatment

M. pneumoniae, like other mycoplasmas, is sensitive to the tetracyclines and apparently more sensitive to erythromycin than the other mycoplasmas of human origin. It is also inhibited by the newer macrolides, such as clarithromycin and azithromycin, and the newer quinolones, such as sparfloxacin. The value of tetracyclines was shown first in a controlled trial of dimethylchlortetracycline in United States marine recruits, a dose of 300 mg three times daily for 6 days significantly reducing the duration of fever, pulmonary infiltration, and other signs and symptoms. Planned trials are the most favourable for determining the value of antimicrobials but in civilian practice they prove less effective, probably because disease is often well established before treatment is instituted. Despite this, treatment with an antimicrobial is worthwhile. For pregnant women and children it is advisable to use erythromycin rather than a tetracycline, and the former has sometimes proved more effective than a tetracycline in adults. Successful treatment of clinical disease, however, is not always accompanied by early eradication of the organisms from the respiratory tract, probably because they can become intracellular and the drugs only inhibit their multiplication and do not kill them. These are possible reasons for relapse in some patients and plausible ones for recommending a 2- to 3-week course of treatment. It is a moot point whether early treatment prevents some of the complications but, nevertheless, it should commence as soon as possible. As laboratory confirmation of *M. pneumoniae* infection sometimes may be slow, it would seem wise to start antimicrobial treatment on the basis of the clinical evidence and a suggestive antibody titre in a single serum sample despite the drawbacks, mentioned previously, of making a diagnosis serologically.

The true value of corticosteroids is in doubt, although, in conjunction with antimicrobials, they appear to have been helpful in patients with severe pneumonia and erythema multiforme.

Prevention

M. pneumoniae infection or disease may occur despite high titres of serum mycoplasmacidal antibody. Furthermore, mycoplasmal infection of the respiratory tract of laboratory animals may stimulate only a weak antibody response and yet induce greater resistance to reinfection and disease than parenteral inoculation with organisms that stimulate much higher titres of serum antibodies. Such observations have led to the belief that local immune factors are crucial in resistance. The correlation between the resistance of adult volunteers to *M. pneumoniae* disease and the presence of IgA antibody in respiratory secretions is consistent with this contention. This antibody could provide the first line of defence by preventing attachment of the organisms to respiratory epithelial cells.

Fig. 4 Electron micrograph of ciliated epithelial cells in the tracheal mucosa of a hamster infected with *M. pneumoniae*. Note cilia (c) and individual organisms (m), some with specialized terminal structure oriented towards the membrane of the host cell (arrows). × 9880.

Fig. 5 Pneumonia 2 weeks after intranasal inoculation of a hamster with *M. pneumoniae*. Note peribronchiolar and perivascular infiltration of mononuclear cells, predominantly lymphocytes. Haematoxylin and eosin, × 98.

So far as vaccination is concerned, the efficacy of formalin-inactivated *M. pneumoniae* vaccines in preventing pneumonia caused by this mycoplasma has ranged from 28 to 67 per cent in field trials. The failure of some killed *M. pneumoniae* vaccines to protect fully may have been due to poor antigenicity, but others induced serum antibody levels similar to those that develop after natural infection. This suggests that the relatively poor protection afforded by the killed vaccines may have been due to their inability to stimulate cell-mediated immunity and/or local antibody. With local antibodies in mind, live attenuated vaccines, particularly those based on temperature-sensitive mutants of *M. pneumoniae*, were developed. The organisms could multiply at the temperature of the upper, but not the lower, respiratory tract and some vaccines produced pulmonary infection in hamsters without causing pathological changes, and induced significant resistance to subsequent challenge with virulent wild strains of *M. pneumoniae*. However, because the same mutants produced some disease in human volunteers they were considered unacceptable for general human use. Recombinant DNA vaccines involving P1 and other proteins, or a recombinant vaccine developed by cloning a component of the *M. pneumoniae* P1 gene into an adenovirus vector may offer greater success.

Chronic respiratory disease

As mycoplasmas of animals are frequently involved in chronic illnesses, the possible role of mycoplasmas in human chronic respiratory disease, particularly chronic bronchitis, is worthy of consideration.

M. pneumoniae frequently persists in the respiratory tract long after clinical recovery and occasionally the respiratory disease it causes has a protracted course. Furthermore, tracheobronchial clearance is very much reduced soon after infection and there is a tendency for slower clearance, in comparison with that in healthy subjects, even 1 year later. Despite this, there is no evidence that *M. pneumoniae* is a primary cause of chronic bronchitis, or that it is responsible for maintaining chronic disease other than by possibly causing some acute exacerbations. This is perhaps the case in some patients, experiencing an acute exacerbation of chronic bronchitis, from whom *M. pneumoniae* has been isolated and in whom a serological response has been seen.

There is no doubt that *M. salivarium*, *M. orale*, and perhaps other mycoplasmas present in the oropharynx of healthy persons spread to the lower respiratory tracts of some who suffer from chronic bronchitis. There is no substantial evidence that these mycoplasmas are a cause of acute exacerbations, but antibody responses to them occur in association with such exacerbations more frequently than at other times, which suggests that the organisms are more antigenic during exacerbations. It is tempting to think that this is probably due to increased mycoplasmal multiplication and participation in tissue damage brought about primarily by viruses and bacteria, and that in this way the mycoplasmas may play some part in perpetuating a chronic condition.

Mycoplasmas in the vagina are transmitted rarely to the infant *in utero*, but often during birth and *U. urealyticum* organisms (ureaplasmas), in particular, may be isolated from the throats and tracheal aspirates of some neonates. Ureaplasma-infected infants of very low birth-weight (under 1000 g), have died or have developed chronic lung disease twice as often as uninfected infants of similar birth weight or those of over 1000 g. *M. hominis* has also been implicated in pneumonia soon after birth, albeit even more rarely. However, whether these organisms are a cause of the disease in their own right or only together with the various bacteria that are associated with maternal bacterial vaginosis is unresolved. It remains to be seen whether *M. genitalium* might be involved, a possibility that exists because it has been detected in the vagina and cervix.

Genitourinary and related infections

Clinical conditions in which there is evidence strongly suggesting that mycoplasmas have an aetiological role, at least in part, will be considered in some detail. Other diseases in which the role of mycoplasmas is minimal, or the evidence for a mycoplasmal cause is weak and/or contentious, are mentioned briefly. All are summarized in Table 3.

Non-gonococcal urethritis and complications

There have been many studies concerned with the role of large-colony-forming mycoplasmas. It is clear that most of them cannot be considered as causes of non-gonococcal urethritis because they are isolated so rarely from the genitourinary tract either in health or disease (Table 1). However, *M. genitalium* (Fig. 6a) is associated strongly with acute non-gonococcal urethritis, having been detected by use of the PCR in about 25 per cent of such cases compared with a significantly smaller proportion (about 6 per cent) of healthy controls, and almost independently of *Chlamydia trachomatis*. Experimentally, it also causes urethritis in male chimpanzees and, like *M. pneumoniae*, adheres to and enters epithelial cells (Fig. 6b). Such a location could, at least, partially protect *M. genitalium* from antimicrobials and account for its occurrence in about one-quarter of men with persistent or recurrent non-gonococcal urethritis, in some of whom it may be a cause. Although *M. hominis* has been isolated from about 20 per cent of patients with acute non-gonococcal urethritis, it has not been implicated as a cause. Nevertheless, the fact that some cases are associated with bacterial vaginosis in sexual partners in whom *M. hominis* organisms are found in large numbers should not be overlooked. The role of ureaplasmas in non-gonococcal urethritis has been contentious for many years and is discussed below.

The results of most studies, based on qualitative estimations, have failed to demonstrate a significant difference between the prevalence of ureaplasmas in men with or without acute non-gonococcal urethritis. However, if ureaplasmas are involved in the pathogenic process, it would be reasonable to expect them to be present in larger numbers in men with disease than if they were behaving only as commensals; a few workers have provided quantitative data to support this idea. In addition, some patients with hypogammaglobulinaemia develop a prolonged urethrocystitis in which persistent ureaplasmal infection seems to be responsible. In support of ureaplasmal pathogenicity in non-gonococcal urethritis are the results of several antimicrobial trials. For example, in one of these a larger proportion of patients responded to minocycline (active against ureaplasmas and *C. trachomatis*) than to rifampicin (active against *C. trachomatis* only), and those infected with ureaplasmas failed to respond to rifampicin significantly more often than those who were not infected. Although these findings might be difficult to explain if ureaplasmas had no involvement in non-gonococcal urethritis, the failure to take *M. genitalium* into account tends to jeopardize this conclusion. About 10 per cent of ureaplasmas are resistant to tetracyclines and the urethritis of patients infected by them sometimes responds only to treatment with antimicrobials, such as erythromycin, to which the organisms are susceptible.

Finally, some ureaplasma strains, unpassaged in the laboratory, produced a mild urethritis and an antibody response in male chimpanzees inoculated intraurethrally, the disease responding to tetracycline therapy. Furthermore, four investigators inoculated themselves intraurethrally and each developed urethritis. In one detailed study, two of them received cloned *U. urealyticum*, serotype 5, which had been isolated from a patient with acute non-gonococcal urethritis in whom no other potentially pathogenic micro-organisms could be detected, although *M. genitalium* was not sought at that time. Both developed symptoms and signs of urethritis which responded to treatment with minocycline. The results of the most recent volunteer experiment suggest that ureaplasmas may cause disease the first few times they gain access to the urethra but later insults result in colonization without disease, accounting perhaps for their frequent occurrence in the urethra of healthy men.

Ureaplasmas have been recovered from the urethra and directly from epididymal aspirate fluid, accompanied by a specific antibody response, in a patient with acute non-chlamydial, non-gonococcal epididymitis, and they may be a rare cause. *M. genitalium* has not been sought. Information suggesting that the prostate becomes infected during the course of an acute ureaplasmal infection of the urethra is scanty, although ureaplasmas have been isolated more frequently and in greater numbers from patients with acute urethroprostatitis than from controls, and most of those with more than 10³ organisms in expressed prostatic fluid responded to tetracycline therapy. In contrast, ureaplasmas have not been found, and *M. genitalium* only rarely, in prostatic biopsy specimens from patients with chronic abacterial prostatitis, and, in most studies, *M. hominis* has not been associated with prostatitis of any kind.

Pyelonephritis

M. hominis has been isolated, sometimes in pure culture, from the upper urinary tract of almost 10 per cent of patients with acute pyelonephritis. In addition, antibody to *M. hominis*, measured by indirect haemagglutination, has been demonstrated in serum and urine of some of these patients. In contrast, the mycoplasma has not been found in the upper urinary tract of patients with non-infectious urinary-tract diseases, nor has antibody been detected in their urine. These data have not been confirmed recently, but they suggest that *M. hominis* causes a few cases of acute pyelonephritis or acute exacerbations of chronic pyelonephritis and that ureaplasmas are involved less often if at all.

Pelvic inflammatory disease

Micro-organisms in the vagina and lower cervix may ascend to and cause inflammation of the fallopian tubes and adjacent pelvic structures. Like non-gonococcal urethritis, non-gonococcal pelvic inflammatory disease does not have a single cause and the possibility that infection by genital mycoplasmas might be one cause has engaged the attention of numerous investigators.

M. hominis has figured prominently among reports of the isolation of large-colony-forming mycoplasmas from inflamed fallopian tubes, tubo-ovarian abscesses, and pelvic abscesses or fluid. Swedish workers collected specimens by laparoscopy and found *M. hominis* in the tubes of about 10 per cent of women with salpingitis but not in those of women without signs of the disease, an observation that has found some support with investigators in the United Kingdom.

It is likely, but not certain, that this happens mostly when large numbers of *M. hominis* organisms occur in the vagina as a consequence of bacterial vaginosis. The same comment applies to hysterosalpingography, which may occasionally stimulate inflammation of the fallopian tubes in women who carry *M. hominis* in the lower genital tract.

Table 3 The association of *M. genitalium*, *M. hominis*, and *U. urealyticum* with human genitourinary, reproductive, and perinatal disease

| Disease | Evidence suggesting a causal relation of: | | | Comments on the relation |
	M. genitalium	*M. hominis*	*U. urealyticum*	
Non-gonococcal urethritis (NGU)	Strong	None	Some	The proportion of NGU caused by ureaplasmas is unknown
Urethroprostatitis	None	None	Some	Ureaplasmas may cause some acute but not chronic disease; *M. hominis* appears not to cause either acute or chronic disease
Epididymitis	?	None	Some	Ureaplasmas involved in one case of acute disease
Urinary calculi	?	None	Weak	Experimentally, ureaplasmas cause bladder calculi in male rats but so far little evidence for a cause of natural human disease
Pyelonephritis	?	Strong	None	*M. hominis* causes some cases of acute pyelonephritis and exacerbations
Reiter's disease	Weak	None	Some	*M. genitalium* detected in joint of one case; ureaplasmas are related on the basis of lymphocytic response to specific antigen
Abscess of Bartholin's gland	?	Very weak	None	Doubtful whether *M. hominis* is involved
Vaginitis, vaginosis, and cervicitis	Some	None	None	*M. hominis* and to a lesser extent ureaplasmas are associated with bacterial vaginosis, but a causal relation is unproved; *M. genitalium* is associated with cervicitis
Pelvic inflammatory disease	Some	Some	Very weak	*M. genitalium* is related serologically; *M. hominis* probably causes a small proportion of cases, but very doubtful that ureaplasmas do
Postabortal fever	?	Strong	None	*M. hominis* is responsible for some cases, but the proportion is unknown
Postpartum fever	?	Strong	Some	*M. hominis* and to a much lesser extent ureaplasmas cause some cases
Infertility	Some	None	None	*M. genitalium* is related serologically to tubal factor infertility; ureaplasmas are associated with reduced sperm motility, but a causal relation is unproved
Premature labour	?	Some	None	*M. hominis* is involved, possibly as part of bacterial vaginosis
Spontaneous abortion and stillbirth	?	None	None	Maternal and fetal infections are associated with spontaneous abortion, but a causal relation is unproved
Chorioamnionitis	?	None	Some	An association exists with ureaplasmas, but a causal relation is unproved
Low birth weight	?	None	Some	An association exists with ureaplasmas in some studies, but a causal relation is unproved
Neonatal meningitis	?	Some	Some	A rare event
Neonatal lung disease	?	Weak	Some	*M. hominis* has been involved in pneumonia soon after birth; ureaplasmas possibly involved in premature infants of < 1000 g

Fig. 6 (a) Electron micrograph of *M. genitalium*, negatively stained, to show flask-shaped appearance and terminal specialized structure (arrow). × 90 000. (Reproduced from Tully *et al.*, 1983, *International Journal of Systematic Bacteriology* **33**, 387, with permission.) (b) Electron micrograph of *M. genitalium* adhering to Vero cell by the terminal structure. × 60 000. (Reproduced from Tully *et al.*, 1983, *International Journal of Systematic Bacteriology* **33**, 387, with permission.)

Ureaplasmas have been studied less intensively, but they have been isolated directly from the fallopian tubes of a very small proportion of patients with acute salpingitis, from pelvic fluid, and from a tubo-ovarian abscess. *M. pneumoniae* is reported to have been isolated also from such an abscess and from the cervix. The significance of these findings is unclear but it would seem that ureaplasmas, at least, are of little importance. Examination of specimens for *M. genitalium* by PCR technology is needed to establish whether it is involved in pelvic inflammatory disease, which is possible since it has been found in the cervix.

Antibody to *M. hominis*, measured by the indirect haemagglutination technique, was found by Swedish workers in about half the patients they studied with salpingitis, but in only 10 per cent of healthy women. Furthermore, a significant rise or fall in antibody titre occurred during the course of disease in more than half of the women who had *M. hominis* in the lower genital tract. Others found that patients with gonococcal pelvic inflammatory disease responded serologically to *M. hominis* more often than those without such disease; they suggested that damage incurred by the gonococci was a factor in the serological response and questioned the primary role of *M. hominis*. However, a response to *M. hominis* has been seen quite often in women in whom gonococci are not the cause of pelvic inflammation. In addition, a significant antibody response to *M. genitalium* has been detected in about one-third of women with pelvic inflammatory disease in whom antibody responses to *M. hominis* and *C. trachomatis* could not be detected. In contrast, antibody responses to *U. urealyticum* have been detected rarely, consistent with the impression that ureaplasmas are of little importance in acute pelvic inflammatory disease.

Fallopian-tube organ cultures, in which the tissues are maintained in a condition similar to that *in vivo*, are particularly useful in assessing the effect of micro-organisms. In such cultures, gonococci destroy the epithelium, and *M. genitalium* causes some damage, whereas *M. hominis* organisms, although multiplying, produce no more than swelling of some of the cilia. No damage has been caused by ureaplasmas of human origin. This differential effect may be a true reflection of the pathogenic potential of these micro-organisms *in vivo*. However, failure to demonstrate damage does not mean necessarily that the organisms are avirulent, because organ-culture studies do not account for the role of the immune system in pathogenesis. Studies in intact animals may be helpful in elucidating this aspect. It is of interest, therefore, that the introduction of *M. hominis* into the oviducts of grivet monkeys and *M. genitalium* into the oviducts of these monkeys, as well as those of marmosets, resulted in a self-limited acute salpingitis and parametritis with an antibody response, whereas ureaplasmas had no effect.

These various data indicate that *M. hominis* and perhaps *M. genitalium* are likely to have a role in some cases of acute pelvic inflammatory disease.

Postabortal fever

The results of various studies suggest a role for *M. hominis* in fever after abortion (see Section 13), the mycoplasma having been isolated from the blood of about 10 per cent of women who had such fever but not from aborting women without fever, nor from normal pregnant women. However, the key point of whether the mycoplasma was isolated in pure culture was not always clear. A rise in the titre of antibody to *M. hominis* has been detected in half the women who become febrile but in only a small proportion of those who have abortions and remain afebrile. Thus, despite the caveat mentioned, on balance the evidence seems in favour of *M. hominis* causing some cases of postabortal fever, whereas there is none to suggest that ureaplasmas do likewise, possibly because studies have not been focused on this micro-organism.

Postpartum fever

Genital mycoplasmas found transiently in maternal blood a few minutes after normal vaginal delivery are not associated with postpartum fever. However, *M. hominis* isolated from the blood a day or more after delivery has been associated in 5 to 10 per cent of women who develop fever, often with an antibody response. As the organisms are seldom isolated from the blood of afebrile postpartum women, the inference is that *M. hominis* induces postpartum fever, assuming they are recovered in pure culture. Whether fever occurs predominantly in women who have bacterial vaginosis in pregnancy, in which there is proliferation of *M. hominis* together with various bacteria in the vagina, has not been resolved. Patients with postpartum or postabortal fever recover usually without antibiotic treatment.

Microbiological diagnosis of genitourinary and related infections

Swabs from the urethra or vagina provide a slightly more sensitive means of collecting specimens for mycoplasmal isolation than urine specimens. The basic medium is similar to that described for the isolation of *M. pneumoniae*, SP4 medium, mentioned previously, being best for *M. genitalium*. Advantage is taken of the metabolic activity of the mycoplasmas (Table 1) in order to detect their growth. Clinical material is added to separate vials of liquid medium containing phenol red and 0.1 per cent glucose, arginine, or urea. *M. genitalium* metabolizes glucose and changes the colour of the medium from red to yellow. *M. fermentans* does this also but, in addition, converts arginine to ammonia, as do *M. hominis* and *M. primatum*. Ureaplasmas possess a urease that breaks down urea to ammonia too. In each case, the pH of the medium increases and there is a colour change from yellow to red. Ureaplasmas change the colour usually within 1 to 2 days, while *M. genitalium* may take 50 days or longer. Indeed, it soon became clear that attempts to culture this mycoplasma failed and detection was salvaged only by the implementation of PCR technology. Introduction of specimens into Vero cell cultures with subculture to mycoplasmal medium when the PCR signifies multiplication is laborious but has been a successful strategy. A PCR assay is also useful for the detection of *M. fermentans* and *U. urealyticum*. Conventionally, however, when colour changes have occurred in liquid medium, subculture to agar medium results in the formation of colonies of about 200 to 300 μm diameter by most genital mycoplasmas; those of *M. genitalium* are usually smaller. Ureaplasma colonies are very small (15 to 60 μm) (Fig. 7(a)) and on medium containing manganous sulphate are brown in colour and, therefore, are detected more easily (Fig. 7(b)). On ordinary blood agar, *M. hominis*, but not ureaplasmas, produces non-haemolytic pinpoint colonies, the nature of which can be established by the methods outlined above. The metabolism-inhibition technique may be used to detect antibodies to *M. hominis* and the ureaplasmas. Antibody inhibits multiplication and metabolism of homologous organisms, thus preventing a change in colour of the medium due to organism multiplication. The indirect haemagglutination technique has been used to detect antibody to *M. hominis* and the microimmunofluorescence test to detect antibody to *M. genitalium*, but these and other tests, such as the enzyme immunoassay, tend to be used as research tools only.

Joint infections

Rheumatoid arthritis

The fact that mycoplasmas cause several animal arthritides, and that gold salts inactivate mycoplasmas and have had a beneficial effect on rheumatoid arthritis, provided the impetus to search for mycoplasmas in the joints of persons suffering from this disease. However, numerous attempts over the second half of the twentieth century failed to detect mycoplasmas in rheumatoid joints or produced inconsistent or unrepeatable results, those mycoplasmas (*M. hyorhinis*, *M. hominis*) that were recovered by means of cell-culture techniques being nothing more than culture contaminants. The case made in the late 1960s and early 1970s, based on apparent isolation and immunological observations, that *M. fermentans* was important in

(a)

(b)

Fig. 7 (a) Colony of *Ureaplasma urealyticum* (15 μm diameter) (arrow) adjacent to colonies of *M. hominis* (90 μm diameter) grown from urethral exudate. Oblique light, × 68. (b) Dark colonies of *U. urealyticum* with colonies of *M. hominis* on agar containing manganous sulphate. × 136.

rheumatoid arthritis was not substantiated in the next 30 years. However, renewed interest has been generated because this mycoplasma, and ureaplasmas, have been found by PCR technology in the joints of more than 20 per cent of patients with rheumatoid arthritis and other chronic inflammatory disorders, that is significantly more than in those with non-inflammatory disorders. The significance of the findings needs to be determined.

M. pneumoniae and other mycoplasmal infections

A feature of the mycoplasmal arthritides of animals is that the mycoplasmas isolated from the joints are found often in the respiratory tract. The question arises, therefore, of whether the known human respiratory pathogenic mycoplasma, namely *M. pneumoniae*, causes arthritis. There is no doubt that respiratory infection is often accompanied by non-specific arthralgia or myalgia (Table 2) during the acute phase, and occasionally it leads to migratory polyarthritis affecting middle-sized joints in adults. A fourfold or greater rise in the titre of antibody to *M.pneumoniae* has been seen occasionally in juvenile chronic arthritis, but an aetiological association has not been demonstrated.

M. hominis has been isolated from septic joints, usually hip, that have developed in mothers after childbirth. The arthritis responds to tetracycline therapy and the diagnosis should be considered in a postpartum arthritis which is unaffected by penicillin.

Reiter's disease (see also Section 21)

Arthritis may occur soon after or concomitant with non-gonococcal urethritis (sexually acquired reactive arthritis; SARA) or the arthritis may be associated with conjunctivitis and urethritis (Reiter's disease). In defining the role of mycoplasmas, a difficulty is that the patients have often been treated with antimicrobials before microbiological investigation. However, the possible role of *M. genitalium* and ureaplasmas should not be ignored in view of the strong involvement of the former and the weaker involvement of the latter in uncomplicated non-gonococcal urethritis. *M. genitalium* has been detected in the synovial fluid of a patient with SARA, but further evidence is required to establish a causal link in the case of this mycoplasma, and ureaplasmas too. The latter have not been isolated from involved joints but synovial lymphocytes from some patients have been shown to proliferate *in vitro* in response to ureaplasmal antigens.

Arthritis in patients with hypogammaglobulinaemia

Arthritis of mycoplasmal aetiology (Fig. 8(a and b)) should be considered in patients with hypogammaglobulinaemia (see Section 5) who develop an abacterial septic arthritis. Thus, *M. pneumoniae* (together with *M. genitalium* in one instance), *M. hominis*, *M. salivarium*, and, in particular, ureaplasmas have been isolated from synovial fluids of at least two-fifths of these patients. Furthermore, in view of diminished immunity, vigilance should be kept for infection by mycoplasmas of non-human origin. The arthritis usually responds to tetracyclines or other antimicrobials to which the organisms are sensitive, an indication that they are a cause of the disease. Intravenous therapy may be required and administration of antiserum prepared specifically against the mycoplasma in question may be helpful in the few patients whose disease does not respond to antimicrobial therapy.

Conditions of rare or equivocal mycoplasmal aetiology

The occurrence of *M. hominis* or ureaplasmas in cerebrospinal fluid from cases of neonatal meningitis or brain abscess is due presumably to infection *in utero* or to colonization at birth with subsequent invasion. This is a rare

Fig. 8 (a) Damage to the knee joint of a hypogammaglobulinaemic patient caused by *U. urealyticum* infection. (b) Sinus connected with the shoulder joint of a patient with hypogammaglobulinaemia; ureaplasmas were isolated repeatedly from the sinus exudate. (By courtesy of A.D.B. Webster.)

event but should be considered in cases of neonatal disease of the central nervous system in which the results of bacteriological staining and culture are negative.

M. hominis organisms, apart from inducing fever after abortion or childbirth, have been associated with fever attributed to burns and trauma, and have been implicated in some wound infections. Whether they have any role in the pathogenesis of bacterial vaginosis in which they occur in large numbers is difficult to define because they do so together with a variety of bacteria, which are found also in profusion. *M. hominis* has been associated with premature labour, but in view of this pregnancy outcome being associated strongly with bacterial vaginosis, the involvement of the mycoplasma would seem to be as part of the latter condition.

Data on ureaplasmas in urinary calculi suggest that they could be involved aetiologically, and these organisms have been associated also with infertility, chorioamnionitis, spontaneous abortion, and low birth weight. It is noteworthy, however, that like *M. hominis* organisms, ureaplasmas are found in larger numbers in the vagina of women with bacterial vaginosis than in those without disease. Thus, it cannot be ignored that, in the reproductive problems referred to, ureaplasmas may be involved, at least in part, as a component of bacterial vaginosis and to attribute the problems to ureaplasmas alone may sometimes be misleading.

Association of mycoplasmas with AIDS

The idea that mycoplasmas might act as a cofactor, enhancing human immunodeficiency virus type 1 (**HIV-1**) replication and accelerating progression to AIDS, was fuelled initially by studies *in vitro*. In these, treatment of HIV-infected cell cultures with tetracyclines or fluoroquinolones, active against mycoplasmas, inhibited cell killing without affecting virus replication. In other studies, certain mycoplasmas (*M. fermentans, A. laidlawii*) enhanced cytopathic changes by HIV-1. Such *in vitro* observations, however, were preceded by attempts to identify a virus in Kaposi's sarcoma tissue which culminated in the recovery of a mycoplasma in cell culture, possibly a cell-culture contaminant. This was termed initially '*M. incognitus*', but identified later as *M. fermentans*, and was found to be distributed widely in tissues taken at autopsy from patients with AIDS. Subsequently, it was shown to be linked strongly with AIDS-associated nephropathy. In addition, some investigators, who used PCR technology, detected *M. fermentans* in peripheral blood monocytes, throat, and urine of 10, 23, and 8 per cent of HIV-seropositive patients, respectively, almost all of whom were homosexual men. They probably had the mycoplasma before acquiring the virus because the former was detected with similar frequency in samples taken from HIV-seronegative patients, a large proportion of whom were homosexual men, attending a sexually transmitted disease clinic. The interaction of mycoplasmas with the immune system could induce cytokines and so enhance HIV replication with increased loss of CD4+ cells, in this way the mycoplasma acting as a cofactor. Nevertheless, no association was found between infection by *M. fermentans* and the stage of the disease, the patients' CD4+ count, or the viral load. This does not eliminate the possibility that a mycoplasmal infection could influence the speed of disease progression. However, this seems unlikely as no significant difference has been found between the proportion of non-progressors, slow progressors, or rapid progressors of HIV-associated disease who have peripheral blood monocytes that are positive for *M. fermentans*.

A recently discovered mycoplasma of human origin, *M. penetrans*, was isolated from urine sediments of a small number of homosexual men infected with HIV-1, most of whom had AIDS. This mycoplasma avidly invades eukaryotic cells, and antibody to it, detected by an enzyme-linked immunosorbent assay, was found in the sera of 40 per cent of patients with AIDS, but in only a very small proportion of HIV-seronegative subjects, or subjects attending sexually transmitted disease clinics, and in none of a group of patients with other immune dysfunctions. However, the mycoplasma has not been found by PCR technology in the peripheral blood monocytes of a large number of HIV-positive homosexual men. Thus, despite its ability to penetrate cells and its apparent association with HIV infection and AIDS, there is no evidence that *M. penetrans* behaves as a cofactor in the development of AIDS.

Further reading

Maniloff J, ed. (1992). *Mycoplasmas. Molecular biology and pathogenesis.* American Society for Microbiology, Washington, DC.

Razin S, Tully JG, ed. (1996). *Molecular and diagnostic procedures in mycoplasmology*, Vol. 1, *Molecular characterization*. Academic Press, London.

Razin S, Yogev D, Naot Y (1998). Molecular biology and pathogenicity of mycoplasmas. *Microbiology and Molecular Biology Reviews* **62**, 1094–156.

Taylor-Robinson D (1989). Genital mycoplasma infections. In: Judson FN, ed. *Clinics in laboratory medicine. Sexually transmitted diseases*, Vol. 9, pp 501–23. Saunders, Philadelphia.

Taylor-Robinson D (1996). Infection due to species of *Mycoplasma* and *Ureaplasma*: an update. *Clinical Infectious Diseases* **23**, 671–84.

Taylor-Robinson D (1996). Mycoplasmas and their role in human respiratory tract disease. In: Myint S, Taylor-Robinson D, eds. *Viral and other infections of the human respiratory tract*, pp 319–39. Chapman & Hall, London.

Taylor-Robinson D, Bebear C (1997). Antibiotic susceptibilities of mycoplasmas and treatment of mycoplasmal infections. *Journal of Antimicrobial Chemotherapy* **40**, 622–30.

Taylor-Robinson D, Keat A (2001). How can a causal role for small bacteria in chronic inflammatory arthritis be established or refuted? *Annals of Rheumatic Diseases* **60**, 177–84.

Taylor-Robinson D, Gilroy CB, Jensen JS (2000). The biology of *Mycoplasma genitalium*. *Venereology* **13**, 119–27.

Tully JG, Razin S, ed. (1996). *Molecular and diagnostic procedures in mycoplasmology*, Vol. 2, *Diagnostic procedures*. Academic Press, London.

7.11.42 Newly identified and lesser known bacteria

J. Paul

Specialists in clinical microbiology and infectious diseases aim, among other things, to detect and characterize novel pathogens and their disease associations and to refine our knowledge regarding the natural history and treatment of known infections. At the time of writing, at least 890 species of bacteria, with names which have standing in nomenclature, in 193 genera, plus a number of other less well characterized taxa, have been reported to be associated in some way with human disease (Table 1). The list includes a core assemblage of bacteria long known to be associated with infection, some of which are widely known (e.g. *Staphylococcus aureus*), others of which are of restricted geographical distribution (e.g. *Bartonella bacilliformis*, the agent of Oroya fever) or seldom encountered (e.g. *Erysipelothrix rhusiopathiae*, the cause of erysipeloid). Advances in laboratory methods have made it possible to associate novel pathogens with well-known clinical conditions (e.g. *Tropheryma whippelii* and *Arthrobacter* spp. with Whipple's disease; and *Bartonella henselae* and *Afipia felis* with cat scratch disease). Members of the human commensal flora from various body sites have been associated with localized infections (e.g. *Acidaminococcus fermentans, Bilophila wadsworthia*, and *Buttiauxella agrestis* from the faecal flora with abdominal sepsis; *Catonella morbi, Centipeda periodontii*, and *Cryptobacterium curtum* with periodontal disease). In such cases it is difficult to distinguish between aetiological agents and colonists of pre-existing disease foci. In addition to well-known zoonotic agents (e.g. *Mycobacterium bovis*, the agent of bovine tuberculosis), increasing numbers of species have been associated with contact with animals or animal products (e.g. *Capnocytophaga canimorsus* from dog bites). Some rarely encountered conditions have been associated with exposure to environmental organisms (e.g. humidifier fever following inhalation of *Parachlamydia acanthamoebae*; actinomycetoma following inoculation injury with *Actinomadura* spp.). Invasive medical procedures and devices and immunosuppressive therapies have allowed relatively non-pathogenic organisms (e.g. *Acinetobacter* spp.

and *Staphylococcus epidermidis*) to cause infection, making it harder to distinguish between contaminants and isolates of clinical significance.

Clinicians cannot be expected universally to be familiar with more than a small proportion of the known potentially pathogenic bacteria. Hence, it is necessary to develop strategies that allow assessment of the likely significance of bacterial names encountered in the literature and laboratory reports. Table^1 lists genera in alphabetical order. Within genera, species are grouped according to associated clinical features, alongside which are given reported antimicrobial susceptibilities and treatments, concise notes, and selected references. The names used are those which have standing in nomenclature at the time of writing; that is to say, names that appear in the *Approved lists of bacterial names* (Skerman VBD, McGowan V, Sneath PHA (1989) American Society for Microbiology, Washington DC; amended edition), or the *Index of the bacterial and yeast nomenclature changes* (Moore WEC, Moore LVH (1992) American Society for Microbiology, Washington DC), or have been validated by publication in the *International Journal of Systematic Bacteriology*. Issues up to and including Part 4 of Volume 49 (October 1999) have been consulted. To check a taxon's standing in nomenclature, an extremely useful reference source is the *List of bacterial names with standing in nomenclature* (www.bacterio.cict.fr). The use of correct names allows accurate communication between specialists, but name changes resulting from reclassification (e.g. the splitting of *Pseudomonas* into several genera) or from the correction of Latin (e.g. *Streptococcus sanguinis* instead of *S. sanguis*) may cause confusion. Table 1 includes some recently used synonyms (stated in parentheses) and CDC alphanumeric groups (e.g. CDC group DF-3) which await designation of scientific names. A useful list of such terms may be found in the *Summary of current nomenclature, taxonomy and classification* in *Clinical Infectious Diseases* 1999, **29**, 713–27. Names not validly published are stated in inverted commas (e.g. '*Flexispira rappini*'). An updated version of this chapter is available at (http://homepages.pavilion.co.uk/tetrix/).

The antimicrobial susceptibility and treatment notes are based on a wide range of sources and are no more than a rough guide. In the absence of well-established regimens for particular situations, treatment should take into account susceptibility data from the strain causing the infection and the monitoring of treatment response. Caution should be exercised in interpreting the significance of unusual isolates, especially from normally non-sterile sites.

Table 1 Bacteria associated with infection in humans

Nomenclature Genus (synonyms, CDC alphanumeric groups)	Species and subspecies	Associated infections	Reported susceptibilities and treatments	Notes	Refs
Abiotrophia	*A. adiacens, A. defectiva, A. elegans*	Endophthalmitis, brain abscess, osteomyelitis	Vancomycin, ceftriaxone	Previously known as nutritionally variant streptococci	1–3
Achromobacter (*Alcaligenes*)	*A. xylosoxidans xylosoxidans, A. x. denitrificans, A. piechaudii, A. ruhlandii*	Septicaemia, CAPD peritonitis, pneumonia, ear infection	Ureidopenicillins, ceftazidime		4–9, 108
Acidaminococcus	*A. fermentans*	Abscesses, postsurgical infections	Metronidazole		10–11
Acidovorax (*Pseudomonas*)	*A. delafieldii, A. facilis, A. temperans*	Wound infection, UTI, bacteraemia, meningitis, septic arthritis			12
Acinetobacter	*A. baumannii, A. calcoaceticus, A. haemolyticus, A. johnsonii, A. junii, A. lwoffi, A. radioresistens*	Septicaemia, UTI, wound infections, abscesses, endocarditis, meningitis, osteomyelitis	Aminoglycosides, ureidopenicillins, ceftazidime, imipenem	May be multiresistant. Nosocomial outbreaks reported. Infections associated with debilitated patients	13–18

Table 1 Continued

Nomenclature Genus (synonyms, CDC alphanumeric groups)	Species and subspecies	Associated infections	Reported susceptibilities and treatments	Notes	Refs
Actinobacillus	A. actinomycetemcomitans (Haemophilus actinomycetemcomitans)	Periodontitis, endocarditis, abscesses, pericarditis, meningitis	Penicillin (plus gentamicin for endocarditis)	Human oral commensal. Validly published transfer to Haemophilus generally ignored	19–20
	A. equuli, A. lignieresii, A. suis	Wound infection, abscesses, endocarditis, meningitis	Ampicillin (plus gentamicin for endocarditis)	Associated with animal contact and bites	21–22
	A. hominis	Septicaemia, empyema	Amoxicillin–clavulanate		23
	A. ureae (Pasteurella ureae)	Meningitis, pneumonia, endocarditis, hepatitis, peritonitis	Ampicillin (plus gentamicin for endocarditis), chloramphenicol	Respiratory tract commensal in humans	24–25
Actinobaculum	A. schaali	Pyelonephritis			26
Actinomadura	A. latina, A. madurae, A. pelletieri	Actinomycetoma, Madura foot	Co-trimoxazole, dapsone		27
Actinomyces	A. europaeus, A. georgiae, A. gerencseriae, A. graevenitzii, A. israelii, A. meyeri, A. naeslundii, A. neuii neuii, A. neuii anitratus, A. odontolyticus, A. radingae, A. turicensis, A. viscosus	Actinomycosis	β-Lactams		28–29
Aerococcus	A. urinae, A. viridans	Endocarditis, UTI, wounds, meningitis, abscesses	Penicillin (plus gentamicin for endocarditis)		30–31
Aeromonas	A. allosaccharophila, A. bestiarum, A. caviae, A. enteropelogenes, A. hydrophila, A. jandaei, A. media, A. salmonicida, A. schubertii, A. trota, A. veronii	Wound infection, abscesses, septicaemia, meningitis, leech-bite infection, alligator-bite infection, acute diarrhoea	Aminoglycosides, chloramphenicol, ceftazidime, co-trimoxazole	Infections associated with aquatic exposure. A. veronii includes biovars veronii and sobria	32–43
Afipia	A. felis	Cat-scratch disease	Aminoglycosides, imipenem, ceftriaxone	Cat-scratch disease is associated also with Bartonella spp.	44
	A. broomeae	Bone marrow infection, septic arthritis	Imipenem, ceftriaxone	Role as pathogen uncertain	44
	A. clevelandensis	Bone infection	Imipenem, ceftriaxone	Role as pathogen uncertain	44
Agrobacterium	A. radiobacter (A. tumefaciens)	Endocarditis, CAPD peritonitis, UTI, line sepsis	Co-trimoxazole, gentamicin		45–48
[Alcaligenes dentrificans—see Achromobacter xylosoxidans dentrificans]					
Alcaligenes	A. faecalis, A. latus	Pneumonia, otitis, UTI, osteomyelitis, bacteraemia	Amoxicillin–clavulanate, cephalosporins, fluoroquinolones		49

[Alcaligenes xylosoxidans—see Achromobacter xylosoxidans xylosoxidans]
[Alcaligenes piechaudii—see Achromobacter piechaudii]
[Alcaligenes ruhlandii—see Achromobacter ruhlandii]

Table 1 Continued

Nomenclature Genus (synonyms, CDC alphanumeric groups)	Species and subspecies	Associated infections	Reported susceptibilities and treatments	Notes	Refs
Alloiococcus	*A. otitidis (A. otitis)*	Otitis media	Vancomycin		50–52
[*Alteromonas putrefaciens*— see *Shewanella putrefaciens*]					
[*Amycolata autotrophica*—see *Pseudonocardia autotrophica*]					
Amycolatopsis	*A. orientalis* (*Nocardia orientalis*)			Role as pathogen uncertain	53
Anaerobiospirillum	*A. succiniproducens, A. thomasii*	Diarrhoea, bacteraemia	Cefuroxime, tetracycline, chloramphenicol	Infection may be related to exposure to cat or dog faeces	54–59
Anaerorhabdus (*Bacteroides*)	*A. furcosus*	Lung abscess, appendix and abdominal abscesses			60
['*Anguillina coli*'—see *Brachyspira pilosicoli*]					
[*Arachnia propionica*—see *Propionibacterium propionicus*]					
Arcanobacterium	*A. haemolyticum* (*Corynebacterium hemolyticum*)	Tonsillitis, cellulitis, lymphadenopathy, brain abscess, septicaemia, osteomyelitis	Penicillin, erythromycin		61–64
	A. bernardiae (*Actinomyces bernardiae*)	UTI, septicaemia, septic arthritis	β-Lactams	Previously known as CDC coryneform group 2	64–68
	A. pyogenes (*Actinomyces pyogenes*)	Septic arthritis	β-Lactams		64, 69, 70
Arcobacter (*Campylobacter*)	*A. butzleri, A. cryaerophilus*	Abdominal cramps, diarrhoea		Self-limiting	71–73
Arthrobacter	*A. creatinolyticus, A. cumminsii, A. woluwensis, A. sp.*	UTI, bacteraemia, Whipple's disease	Vancomycin, penicillins	Whipple's disease is associated with *Tropheryma whippelii*	74–76
Atopobium	*A. minutum* (*Lactobacillus minutus*), *A. parvulum* (*Streptococcus parvulus*), *A. rimae* (*Lactobacillus rimae*), *A. vaginae*	UTI, dental abscesses, pelvic abscesses, wound infection		Isolates from periodontal sites suggest possible role in periodontal disease	77–80
[*Aureobacterium*—see *Microbacterium*]					
Bacillus	*B. anthracis*	Anthrax	Penicillin, erythromycin		81–82
	B. circulans, B. coagulans, B. megaterium, B. mycoides, B. sphaericus, B. thuringiensis	Pneumonia, septicaemia, corneal infections, meningitis, food poisoning, eye infection, lung infection	Vancomycin, clindamycin, aminoglycosides, imipenem, penicillin	Other than the well-known *B. anthracis* and *B. cereus*, *Bacillus* spp. ar rare causes of focal and systemi sepsis. Some isolates are resistant to vancomycin. Isolates may represent specimen or laboratory contamination. *B. thuringiensis* is a biological insecticide which has caused corneal infection	48, 81–86
	B. cereus, B. licheniformis, B. pumilus, B. subtilis	Food poisoning, wound infection, bacteraemia, endocarditis, eye infection	Clindamycin, vancomycin, gentamicin	Diarrhoea is self-limiting. *B. cereus* is resistant to β-lactams	48, 81–83, 87

Table 1 Continued

Nomenclature Genus (synonyms, CDC alphanumeric groups)	Species and subspecies	Associated infections	Reported susceptibilities and treatments	Notes	Refs
Bacteroides	B. caccae, B. capillosus, B. coagulans, B. distasonis, B. eggerthii, B. forsythus, B. fragilis, B. merdae, B. ovatus, B. putredinis, B. pyogenes, B. splanchinicus, B. stercoris, B. tectus, B. thetaiotaomicron, B. uniformis, B. ureolyticus, B. vulgatus	Abscesses, bacteraemia, bite infections, wound infections, chronic otitis media, pelvic inflammatory disease	Ureidopenicillins, carbapenems, metronidazole	Many of the species still currently included in Bacteroides are of uncertain taxonomic position. Resistance to metronidazole and β-lactams has been reported	88, 89
Balneatrix	B. alpica	Pneumonia, bacteraemia, meningitis	Ceftriaxone, ofloxacin, amoxicillin, netilmicin	Infection associated with exposure to hot spring water	90, 91
Bartonella	B. bacilliformis	Oroya fever, verruga peruana	Chloramphenicol, streptomycin		92
	B. elizabethae (Rochalimaea elizabethae)	Endocarditis	Gentamicin, imipenem, co-trimoxazole		93
	B. clarridgeiae B. henselae (Rochalimaea henselae),	Cat-scratch disease, bacillary angiomatosis	Aminoglycosides, doxycycline	Cat scratch disease is associated also with Afipia felis	94–96
	B. quintana (Rochalimaea quintana)	Trench fever, bacillary angiomatosis	Aminoglycosides, doxycycline		95, 96
	B. vinsonii	Bacteraemia	Ceftriaxone	Zoonosis from rodents	97
Bergeyella	B. zoohelcum (Weeksella zoohelcum)	Wound infection, septicaemia, meningitis	Cefotaxime, penicillins, ciprofloxacin, tetracycline	Associated with dog and cat bites	98
Bifidobacterium	B. adolescentis, B. angulatum, B. bifidum, B. dentium, B. infantis, B. inopinatum, B. longum, B. pseudocatenulatum	Bacteraemia, abscesses, peritonitis, otitis, paronychia	Clindamycin, penicillins, cefoxitin	Reported risk factors include surgery, malignancy, steroid therapy, intravenous drug use and acupuncture	99– 102
Bilophila	B. wadsworthia	Appendicitis, abscesses, bacteraemia, biliary tract sepsis	Metronidazole, amoxicillin/clavulanate, ureidopenicillins, cephalosporins	Reported from faecal flora	103, 104
[Branhamella catarrhalis—see Moraxella catarrhalis]					
Borrelia	B. afzelii, B. andersonii, B. bissettii, B. burgdorferi, B. garinii, B. japonica, B. lusitaniae, B. tanukii, B. turdi, B. valaisiana	Lyme disease	Amoxicillin, doxycycline, ceftriaxone		105
	B. caucasica, B. crocidurae, B. duttoni, B. graingeri, B. hermsii, B. hispanica, B. latyschewii, B. mazzottii, B. parkeri, B. persica, B. recurrentis, B. turicatae, B. venezuelensis	Relapsing fever	Tetracycline, erythromycin, chloramphenicol, penicillin	B. recurrentis is louse-borne; other agents are tick-borne	106
Bordetella	B. bronchiseptica	Respiratory tract infection	Tetracycline, fluoroquinolones	Zoonosis from dogs and other animals	107
	B. hinzii, B. holmseii, B. trematum	Bacteraemia, otitis, wound infection		B. hinzii is a pathogen of poultry	108– 110
	B. parapertussis, B. pertussis	Whooping cough, respiratory tract infection	Erythromycin	B. parapertussis causes less severe disease	111

Table 1 Continued

Nomenclature Genus (synonyms, CDC alphanumeric groups)	Species and subspecies	Associated infections	Reported susceptibilities and treatments	Notes	Refs
Brachyspira	*B. aalborgi, B. pilosicoli* (*Serpulina pilosicoli*, 'Anguillina coli')	Intestinal spirochaetosis		Of uncertain significance	112–114
[*Branhamella catarrhalis*—see *Moraxella catarrhalis*]					
Brevibacillus (*Bacillus*)	*B. agri, B. brevis, B. laterosporus*	Endophthalmitis, food poisoning, bacteraemia	Vancomycin		115–117
Brevibacterium	*B. casei, B. epidermidis, B. mcbrellneri, B. otitidis*	Bacteraemia, meningitis, chest infection	Glycopeptides		48, 118, 119
Brevundimonas (*Pseudomonas*)	*B. diminuta, B. vesicularis*	Septicaemia			120
Brucella	*B. abortus, B. canis, B. melitiensis, B. suis*	Brucellosis	Doxycycline (plus streptomycin or rifampicin)		121
Burkholderia (*Pseudomonas*)	*B. cepacia* (*Pseudomonas cepacia*), *B. gladioli* (*Pseudomonas gladioli*), *B. multivorans*, *B. vietnamiensis*	Lung infection, bacteraemia, endocarditis, septic arthritis, UTI	Ureidopenicillins, ceftazidime, aztreonam, carbapenems, fluoroquinolones, co-trimoxazole	Resistant to aminoglycosides. Infection in cystic fibrosis may follow chronic course or result in acute necrotizing pneumonia. Clinical significance of the various taxa is unclear	122, 123
	B. mallei (*Pseudomonas mallei*)	Glanders	Sulfadiazine	Other antibiotics should be considered and evaluated	124
	B. pseudomallei (*Pseudomonas pseudomallei*)	Melioidosis	Ceftazidime, co-trimoxazole, chloramphenicol, imipenem		125, 126
Buttiauxella	*B. agrestis, B. noackiae*	Appendicitis, wound infection	Aminoglycosides, doxycycline	Cephalosporin resistance reported	127, 128
Butyrivibrio	*B. fibrisolvens*	Endophthalmitis	Penicillin, chloramphenicol	From rumina of farm animals	129
[*Calymmatobacterium granulomatis*—see *Klebsiella granulomatis*] [*Campylobacter butzleri*—see *Arcobacter butzleri*] [*Campylobacter cinaedi*—see *Helicobacter cinaedi*]					
Campylobacter	*C. coli, C. jejuni jejuni, C. jejuni doylei, C. mucosalis C. concisus, C. curvus* (*Wolinella curva*), *C. gracilis* (*Bacteroides gracilis*), *C. rectus* (*Wolinella recta*), *C. showae, C. sputorum*	Gastroenteritis, bacteraemia Periodontitis, appendicitis, peritonitis, head and neck infections	Erythromycin, fluoroquinolones Ureidopenicillins, amoxicillin/clavulanate, carbapenems, fluoroquinolones, metronidazole	Infections are usually self-limiting	130, 131 129
[*Campylobacter fennelliae*—see *Helicobacter fennelliae*]					
Campylobacter	*C. fetus fetus*	Fever, diarrhoea, meningoencephalitis, endocarditis, abscesses	Erythromycin, ampicillin, chloramphenicol, gentamicin		132
	C. fetus venerealis	Bacterial vaginosis		Role as human pathogen poorly defined. Reported from faeces of homosexual men	130
	C. hyointestinalis, C. lari (*C. laridis*), *C. upsalensis*	Diarrhoea, bacteraemia, abscess	Erythromycin, ampicillin, gentamicin	Zoonoses from mammals and birds	133–137

Table 1 Continued

Nomenclature Genus (synonyms, CDC alphanumeric groups)	Species and subspecies	Associated infections	Reported susceptibilities and treatments	Notes	Refs
[*Campylobacter pyloridis*—see *Helicobacter pylori*]					
Capnocytophaga	*C. canimorsus* (CDC DF-1), *C. cynodegmi* (CDC DF-2)	Wound infection, septicaemia, abscesses, meningitis, endocarditis	Penicillin	From dog bites	138–140
	C. gingivalis, *C. granulosa*, *C. haemolytica*, *C. ochracea*, *C. sputigena*	Periodontitis, septicaemia	Penicillins, ciprofloxacin, tetracycline, chloramphenicol	From oral flora. Infections associated with malignancy and malignancy	141, 142
Cardiobacterium	*C. hominis*	Endocarditis, meningitis	Penicillin (plus gentamicin for endocarditis)		143, 144
Catonella	*C. morbi*	Periodontitis		Role as pathogen unclear	145
CDC group DF-3		Diarrhoea, bacteraemia	Tetracycline	Genus awaiting scientific name, related to *Capnocytophaga*	146–149
Cedecea	*C. davisae*, *C. lapagei*, *C. neterii*	Bacteraemia	Chloramphenicol, cefamandole, gentamicin	Two other spp. (sp. 3 and sp. 5) have been isolated from clinical specimens	150, 151
Cellulomonas	*C. hominis*	Bacteraemia, meningitis	Tetracycline, vancomycin	Clinical significance poorly defined	152
	C. turbata (*Oerskovia turbata*)	Bacteraemia, endocarditis	Amikacin, co-trimoxazole, chloramphenicol	Vancomycin resistance reported	153, 154
Centipeda	*C. periodontii*	Periodontitis		Role as pathogen unclear	155
Chlamydia	*C. trachomatis*	Trachoma, genital infection, neonatal infection, lymphogranuloma venereum	Erythromycin, tetracycline, azithromycin	Includes 18 serovars clustered into two biovars: trachoma and lymphogranuloma venereum	156
Chlamydophila	*C. abortus* (*Chlamydia psittaci*)	Abortion		Associated with contact with infected ruminants	156
	C. pneumoniae (*Chlamydia pneumoniae*)	Chest infection	Tetracycline	Infections in humans associated with biovar TWAR	156
	C. psittaci (*Chlamydia psittaci*)	Psittacosis	Tetracycline	Zoonosis from birds	156
Chromobacterium	*C. violaceum*	Septicaemia, osteomyelitis, abscesses, eye infection	Erythromycin, tetracycline, chloramphenicol, gentamicin	Associated with exposure to soil and water	157–159
Chryseobacterium (*Flavobacterium*)	*C. gleum*, *C. indologenes*, *C. meningosepticum*	Bacteraemia, meningitis, abdominal sepsis, wound infection, line infection	Minocycline, fluoroquinolones, rifampicin	Susceptibilities vary. Often multiresistant	160–162
[*Chryseomonas luteola*—see *Pseudomonas luteola*]					
Citrobacter	*C. amalonaticus*, *C. braakii*, *C. diversus*, *C. farmeri*, *C. freundii*, *C. gilenii*, *C. koseri*, *C. murliniae*, *C. rodentium*, *C. sedlakii*, *C. werkmanii*, *C. youngae*,	UTI, meningitis, haemolytic–uraemic syndrome	Aminoglycosides, β-lactams	Variable susceptibility. May be multiresistant. Nosocomial outbreaks of infection reported. *Citrobacter* spp. are part of the normal faecal flora	37, 163

Table 1 Continued

Nomenclature Genus (synonyms, CDC alphanumeric groups)	Species and subspecies	Associated infections	Reported susceptibilities and treatments	Notes	Refs
Clostridium	*C. absonum, C. argentinense, C. baratii, C. beijerinckii, C. bifermentans, C. butyricum, C. cadaveris, C. carnis, C. celatum, C. clostridioforme, C. cochlearium, C. cocleatum, C. fallax, C. ghonii, C. glycolicum, C. haemolyticum, C. hastiforme, C. histolyticum, C. indolis, C. innocuum, C. irregulare, C. leptum, C. limosum, C. malenominatum, C. novyi, C. oroticum, C. paraputrificum, C. piliforme, C. putrefasciens, C. ramosum, C. septicum, C. sordelii, C. sphenoides, C. sporogenes, C. subterminale, C. symbiosum, C. tertium,*	Wound infection, bacteraemia, abscesses	Penicillin, clindamycin, metronidazole	Many *Clostridium* spp. have been isolated form clinical specimens. For most, their clinical significance is poorly defined. *C. baratii* and *C. butyricum* are rare causes of botulism. *C. fallax, C. histolyticum, C. novyi, C. septicum,* and *C. sordellii* are gas-gangrene agents. Treatment of gas gangrene includes debridement and penicillin, clindamycin, or metronidazole	164
	C. botulinum	Botulism		Antitoxin and respiratory support as treatment	164
	C. difficile	Diarrhoea, pseudomembranous	Metronidazole, vancomycin	Infection associated with antibiotic exposure	164
	C. perfringens	Food poisoning, necrotizing enterocolitis, gas gangrene		Debridement and penicillin, clindamycin or metronidazole for treatment of gas gangrene	164
	C. tetani	Tetanus	Metronidazole, penicillin	Antitoxin and supportive treatment	164
Collinsella	*C. aerofaciens*			From faecal flora. Clinical significance is undefined	165
[*Comamonas acidovorans*—see *Delftia acidovorans*]					
Comamonas (*Pseudomonas*)	*C. avenae, C. terrigena, C. testosteroni*	Bacteraemia, conjunctivitis	Ureidopenicillins, ceftazidime, ciprofloxacin, aminoglycosides	Infections in neutropenic patients	48, 166, 167
Corynebacterium	*C. accolens, C. afermentans, C. amycolatum, C. argentoratense, C. auris, C. bovis, C. confusum, C. coyleae, C. durum, C. falsenii, C. glucuronolyticum, C. imitans, C. jeikeium, C. kroppenstedtii, C. kutscheri, C. lipophilum, C. macginleyi, C. matruchotii, C. mucifaciens, C. pilosum, C. propinquum, C. renale, C. riegelii, C. sanguinis, C. singulare, C. striatum, C. sundsvallense, C. thomssenii,*	Septicaemia, peritonitis, eye infection, wound infection, endocarditis, osteomyelitis, septic arthritis, meningitis, abscesses	Glycopeptides, β-lactam, erythromycin, rifampicin	More than 40 *Corynebacterium* species have been isolated from clinical specimens. For many of them, clinical significance and empirical therapy are poorly defined. Many isolates are susceptible to β-lactams. Multiresistant, vancomycin-susceptible isolates of CDC coryneform group G-2, *C. jeikeium* and *C. urealyticum* have been reported. Nosocomial outbreaks have been reported. *Corynebacterium* spp. may	64, 68, 168– 186

Table 1 Continued

Nomenclature Genus (synonyms, CDC alphanumeric groups)	Species and subspecies	Associated infections	Reported susceptibilities and treatments	Notes	Refs
	C. urealyticum, C. xerosis			be specimen or laboratory contaminants. CDC coryneform groups 1, E, F-1, and G-2 await designation of scientific names	
	'C. aquaticum'	UTI, endocarditis, meningitis, CAPD peritonitis	Ampicillin, chloramphenicol, gentamicin	Not in approved lists of bacterial names. Confused with Aureobacterium (which has been united with Microbacterium)	64, 187
	C. diphtheriae	Diphtheria, cutaneous infection	Penicillin, erythromycin	Toxigenic infection requires treatment with antitoxin	64
[Corynebacterium hemolyticum—see Arcanobacterium haemolyticum]					
	C. minutissimum	Erythrasma, bacteraemia, endocarditis		Role as an agent of erythrasma is poorly defined	64, 188
	C. mycetoides	Tropical ulcer, septicaemia			
	C. pseudodiphtheriticum	UTI, endocarditis, lymphadenopathy, necrotizing tracheitis	Penicillin		189
	C. pseudotuberculosis	Lymphadenitis, pulmonary infection	Penicillin, erythromycin	Associated with sheep contact. May require drainage or excision	190
	C. ulcerans	Diphtheria-like disease, pharyngitis	Penicillin, erythromycin	Toxigenic infection requires teatment with antitoxin	191
[Corynebacterium CDC groups A-4 and A-5—see Microbacterium]					
[Corynebacterium group 2—see Arcanobacterium bernardiae]					
Coxiella	C. burnettii	Q fever	Tetracycline, ciprofloxacin, co-trimoxazole, rifampicin		192
Cryptobacterium	C. curtum	Periodontitis			193
Delftia	D. acidovorans (Comamonas acidovorans) (Pseudomonas acidovorans)	Bacteraemia, endocarditis	Ureidopenicillins, fluoroquinolones		194
Dermabacter	D. hominis	Brain abscess, bacteraemia, wound infection	Cephalosporins, glycopeptides		64, 195
Dermatophilus	D. congolensis	Cutaneous infection	Penicillin	Zoonosis from cattle, sheep, goats, and horses	196
Desulfomonas	D. pigra	Pilonidal cyst abscess, peritonitis		From faecal flora	197
Desulfovibrio	D. desulfuricans, D. vulgaris	Bacteraemia, liver abscess	Penicillin, clindamycin		198– 200
Dialister	D. pneumosintes	Periodontitis			201
Dichelobacter	D. nodosus (Bacteroides nodosus)	Pilonidal cyst, rectal fistula, wound infection		Cause of ovine footrot. Isolates reported from humans may not be D. nodosus	202

Table 1 Continued

Nomenclature Genus (synonyms, CDC alphanumeric groups)	Species and subspecies	Associated infections	Reported susceptibilities and treatments	Notes	Refs
Dolosicoccus	*D. paucivorans*	Bacteraemia	Cephalosporins		203
Dolosigranulum	*D. pigrum*	Spinal cord infection, eye infection		Significance as a pathogen poorly defined.	204, 205
Edwardsiella	*E. hoshinae, E. ictaluri, E. tarda*	Wound infection, abscesses, gastroenteritis	β-Lactams, aminoglycosides, fluoroquinolones	Aquatic exposure, penetrating fish injury	206–210
Eggerthella	*E. lenta* (*Eubacterium lentum*)	Rectal abscess		From faecal flora	211
Ehrlichia	*E. chaffeensis, E. sennetsu, E. sp.*	Erhlichiosis	Tetracycline		212, 213
Eikenella	*E. corrodens*	Septicaemia, endocarditis, abscesses, septic arthritis	Penicillin (plus gentamicin for endocarditis)		214–217
Empedobacter	*E. brevis* (*Flavobacterium breve*)			Role as human pathogen poorly characterized	218
Enterobacter	*E. aerogenes, E. amnigenus, E. asburiae, E. cancerogenus, E. cloacae, E. gergoviae, E. hormaechei, E. kobei, E. sakazakii*	Bacteraemia, respiratory tract infections, UTI	Carbapenems, fluoroquinolones, aminoglycosides, ureidopenicillins	May be multiresistant. Common cause of nosocomial infection	219
Enterococcus	*E. avium, E. casseliflavus, E. cecorum, E. dispar, E. durans, E. faecalis, E. faecium, E. flavescens,* *E. gallinarum, E. hirae, E. malodoratus, E. mundtii, E. pseudoavium, E. raffinosus, E. solitarius*	Bacteraemia, abscesses, endocarditis, meningitis, UTI, peritonitis, osteomyelitis, wound infection	Penicillins, glycopeptides	May be resistant to penicillins and glycopeptides. Nosocomial outbreaks reported	220
Erwinia	*E. persicinus*	UTI	Cephalosporins, fluoroquinolones, aminoglycosides	The causative agent of necrosis of bean pods	221
Erysipelothrix	*E. rhusiopathiae*	Erysipeloid, septicaemia, endocarditis	Penicillin	Animal contact	222, 223
[*Escherichia adecarboxylata*—see *Leclercia adecarboxylata*]					
Escherichia	*E. coli*	UTI, bacteraemia, wound infection, meningitis, enteric infection, haemolytic fluoroquinolones, uraemic syndrome	β-Lactams, aminoglycosides, co-trimoxazole	Susceptibilities variable	224
	E. fergusonii	Bacteraemia, wounds, UTI	Chloramphenicol, gentamicin	Ampicillin-resistant	225
	E. hermanii	Wounds	Chloramphenicol, cephalosporins, gentamicin		226
	E. vulneris	Wounds	Ampicillin, cephalosporins, gentamicin		227
Eubacterium	*E. brachy, E. combesii, E. contortum, E. infirmum, E. limosum, E. minutum, E. moniliforme, E. nitrotogenes, E. nodatum,*	Wounds, abscesses, septicaemia, periodontitis	Penicillins, clindamycin, metronidazole		228, 229

Table 1 Continued

Nomenclature Genus (synonyms, CDC alphanumeric groups)	Species and subspecies	Associated infections	Reported susceptibilities and treatments	Notes	Refs
	E. saburreum, E. saphenum, E. sulci, E. tenue, E. timidum, E. yurii yurii, E. y. mararetiae, E. y. schtitka				
Ewingella	E. americana	Septicaemia, wounds, UTI	Ureidopenicillins, aminoglycosides		230
Exiguobacterium	E. acetylicum, E. aurantiacum	Wound infection		Role as pathogen unclear	64
Facklamia	F. hominis, F. ignava, F. languida, F. sourekii	UTI, bacteraemia, abscess			231
Filifactor	F. alocis, F. vilosus	Gingivitis, periodontitis			232, 233
[Flavimonas oryzihabitans—see Pseudomonas oryzihabitans]					
Flavobacterium spp. (CDC groups IIe, IIh, IIi)				Rare causes of infections in debilitated patients	218
[Flavobacterium gleum—see Chryseobacterium gleum] [Flavobacterium indologenes—see Chryseobacterium indologenes] [Flavobacterium meningosepticum—see Chryseobacterium meningosepticum]					
'Flexispira'	'F. rappini'	Bacteraemia, diarrhoea		Not in approved lists of bacterial names	234, 235
Francisella	F. philomiragia (Yersinia philomiragia)	Septicaemia, invasive systemic infection	Fluoroquinolones, aminoglycosides, chloramphenicol, cefoxitin		236
	F. tularensis	Tularaemia	Streptomycin, tetracycline		237
Fusobacterium	F. gonidiaformans, F. mortiferum, F. naviforme, F. necrogenes, F. necrophorum necrophorum, F. n. fundiliforme, F. nucleatum nucleatum, F. n. fusiforme , F. n. polymorphum, F. n. vincentii, F. periodonticum, F. russii, F. ulcerans, F. varium	Abscesses, bacteraemia, periodontitis, endocarditis, necrobacillosis	Metronidazole, penicillins, carbapenems, cephalosporins		238, 239
Gardnerella	G. vaginalis	Intrauterine and neonatal sepsis	β-Lactams, clindamycin	Associated with bacterial vaginosis	240
Gemella	G. bergeri, G. haemolysans, G. morbillorum, (Streptococcus morbillorum), G. sanguinis	Bacteraemia. endocarditis	Penicillin or vancomycin (plus gentamicin for endocarditis)		241, 242
Globicatella	G. sanguinis	Bacteraemia, UTI, meningitis	Vancomycin		243
Gordona (Rhodococcus)	G. aichensis, G. bronchialis, G. rubropertinctus, G. sputi, G. terrae	Pulmonary infection, sternal wound sepsis, brain abscess, bacteraemia	Co-trimoxazole, imipenem, fluoroquinolones		244–247

Table 1 Continued

Nomenclature Genus (synonyms, CDC alphanumeric groups)	Species and subspecies	Associated infections	Reported susceptibilities and treatments	Notes	Refs
Haemophilus	*H. aegyptius*	Brazilian purpuric fever	Ampicillin, cephalosporins, chloramphenicol	Treated by some authors as a biotype of *H. influenzae*	248, 249
	H. aphrophilus, *H. parainfluenzae*, *H. paraphrophilus*, *H. segnis*	Sinusitis, otitis media, pneumonia, abscesses, endocarditis	Cefotaxime, chloramphenicol ampicillin, aminoglycosides	Ampicillin (plus gentamicin to treat endocarditis)	250–254
	H. ducreyi	Chancroid	Macrolides, ceftriaxone, fluoroquinolones		255
	H. influenzae	Bacteraemia, meningitis, epiglottitis	Cephalosporins, penicillins, fluoroquinolones	Many strains produce penicillinases	256
Hafnia	*H. alvei*	Bacteraemia		Associated with diarrhoea Susceptibility variable	257
Helicobacter	*H. canis*	Gastroenteritis		Zoonosis from dogs	258
	H. cinaedi (*Campylobacter cinaedi*), *H. fennelliae* (*Campylobacter fennelliae*)	Proctitis in homosexual men, septicaemia	Ampicillin, gentamicin	Zoonosis from hamsters	259–261
	'*H. heilmannii*'	Gastritis		May be conspecific with *H. bizzozeronii* from dogs	262
	H. pullorum	Gastroenteritis		Zoonosis from poultry	263
	H. pylori (*Campylobacter pyloridis*)	Gastritis	Omeprazole plus clarithromycin and metronidazole	Numerous similar treatment combinations have been recommended	264
Helcococcus	*H. kunzii*	Sebaceous cyst infection, breast abscess	Penicillins, vancomycin	From skin flora	265, 266
Holdemania	*H. filiformis*			From faecal flora. Clinical significance is unclear	267
Ignavigranum	*I. ruoffiae*	Wound infection, ear abscess		Role as pathogen poorly defined	268
Johnsonella	*J. ignava*	Periodontitis			268a
Kingella	*K. denitrificans*, *K. kingae*, *K. oralis*	Septic arthritis, endocarditis	Penicillins (plus gentamicin for endocarditis)		269–272
[*Kingella indologenes*—see *Suttonella indologenes*]					
Klebsiella	*K. granulomatis* (*Calymmatobacterium granulomatis*)	Donovanosis	Tetracycline, co-trimoxazole		273
	K. ornithinolytica, *K. oxytoca*, *K. planticola*, *K. pneumoniae*, *K. ozaenae*, *K. terrigena*	UTI, bacteraemia, wound infection, respiratory tract infection	β-Lactams, aminoglycosides, fluoroquinolones	Susceptibilities vary. Nosocomial outbreaks reported	274
	K. rhinoscleromatis	Rhinoscleroma	Ciprofloxacin, rifampicin, co-trimoxazole		275
Kluyvera	*K. ascorbata*, *K. cryocrescens*, *K. georgiana*	Bacteraemia, UTI, mediastinitis, line sepsis	Aminoglycosides, ceftazidime, imipenem, ciprofloxacin		276, 277
Kocuria (*Micrococcus*)	*K. kristinae*, *K. varians*			From skin flora and of doubtful clinical significance	278
[*Koserella trabulsii*—see *Yokenella regensburgii*]					

Table 1 Continued

Nomenclature Genus (synonyms, CDC alphanumeric groups)	Species and subspecies	Associated infections	Reported susceptibilities and treatments	Notes	Refs
Kurthia	'K. bessonii' K. gibsonii, K. zopfii	Bacteraemia, endocarditis	Penicillin	Not in approved lists of bacterial names Isolated from faeces of patients with diarrhoea	280, 281 282
Kytococcus (*Micrococcus*)	K. sedentarius			From skin flora and of doubtful clinical significance	278
Lactobacillus	L. acidophilus, L. brevis, L. casei, L. catenaforme, L. crispatus, L. fermentum, L. gasseri, L. iners, L. jensenii, L. leichmannii, L. oris, L. paracasei, L. paraplantarum, L. plantarum, L. rhamosus, L. salicinius, L. salivarius, L. uli, L. vaginalis	Abscesses, bacteraemia, endometritis, endocarditis, lung infection, UTI	Cephalosporins, vancomycin, penicillins, aminoglycosides, clindamycin	Reported risk factors for infection include surgery, malignancy, diabetes, and immunodeficiency. May be vancomycin-resistant	283–286
Lactococcus (Streptococcus)	L. garviae, L. lactis	Bacteraemia, endocarditis, UTI	Penicillin (plus gentamicin for endocarditis)		287
Lautropia	L. mirabilis			Role as potential pathogen unclear. From oral flora of HIV patients and sputum of cystic fibrosis patient	288
Leclercia	L. adecarboxylata (*Escherichia adecarboxylata*)	Bacteraemia, wound infection		Variable susceptibility	289
Legionella	L. anisa, L. birminghamensis, L. bozemanii, L. cincinnatiensis, L. dumoffii, L. feeleii, L. gormanii, L. hackeliae, L. israelensis, L. jordanis, L. lansingensis, L. longbeachae, L. maceachernii, L. micdadei, L. oakridgemsis, L. pneumophila, L. sainthelensi, L. tucsonensis, L. wadsworthii	Legionnaires' disease, Pontiac fever	Macrolides, fluoroquinolones, rifampicin	Infections caused by species other than L. pneumophila and L. micdadei are seldom reported	290
Leminorella	L. grimontii, L. richardii	UTI	Chloramphenicol, tetracycline, gentamicin	Isolated from faeces but of uncertain significance	291
Leptospira	L. biflexa, L. borgpetersenii, L. inadai, L. interrogans, L. kirschneri, L. noguchii, L. santarosai, L. weilii	Leptospirosis	Penicillin, tetracycline	L. interrogans is composed of a number of named serogroups	292
Leptotrichia	L. buccalis, L. sanguinegens	Bacteraemia, endocarditis	β-Lactams, metronidazole		293
Leuconostoc	L. citreum, L. cremoris, L. dextranicum, L. lactis, L. mesenteroides, L. pseudomesenteroides	Meningitis, bacteraemia, pulmonary infection	Penicillin and gentamicin or clindamycin	Vancomycin-resistant	294–296

Table 1 Continued

Nomenclature Genus (synonyms, CDC alphanumeric groups)	Species and subspecies	Associated infections	Reported susceptibilities and treatments	Notes	Refs
Listeria	*L. ivanovii*, *L. monocytogenes*	Septicaemia, meningitis, intrauterine infection, enteric infection	Ampicillin and gentamicin		297
[*Listonella damsela*—see *Photobacterium damselae*]					
Megasphaera	*M. elsdenii*	Endocarditis	Metronidazole		298
Methylobacterium	*M. extorquens*, *M. mesophilicum* (*Pseudomonas mesophilica*)	Bacteraemia, CAPD peritonitis	Ureidopenicillins, imipenem, aminoglycosides, chloramphenicol		299–302
Microbacterium (*Aureobacterium*)	*M. arborescens*, *M. imperiale* (CDC coryneform groups A-4 and A-5), *M. liquefaciens* (*Aureobacterium liquefaciens*), ('*Corynebacterium aquaticum*')	Endophthalmitis, UTI, endocarditis, soft tissue infection, hypersensitivity pneumonitis, meningitis, CAPD peritonitis	Glycopeptides, β-lactams, chloramphenicol, gentamicin	The genus *Aureobacterium* was united with *Microbacterium* but *A. resistens* (which is vancomycin-resistant) was not listed in the reclassification. *Aureobacterium* isolates have been misidentified as '*Corynebacterium aquaticum*'	303–307
Micrococcus	*M. luteus*, *M. lytae*	Bacteraemia, endocarditis, septic arthritis	Vancomycin, penicillin, rifampicin	From skin flora. Common specimen contaminants	308
Mitsuokella	*M. multacida* (*Bacteroides multiacidus*)			Role as human pathogen poorly defined	309
Mobiluncus	*M. curtisii curtisii*, *M. curtisii holmesii*, *M. mulieris*	Endometritis, chorioamnionitis	Ampicillin, cephalosporins, clindamycin	Associated with bacterial vaginosis	310–312
Moellerella	*M. wisconsensis*	Diarrhoea		Of uncertain significance	313
Moraxella	*M. atlantae*, *M. lacunata*, *M. nonliquefaciens*, *M. osloensis*, *M. phenylpyruvica*	Conjunctivitis, wound infection, endocarditis, abscesses, osteomyelitis	Penicillin	Penicillin resistance has been reported	314–318
	M. catarrhalis (*Branhamella catarrhalis*)	Respiratory infections, endocarditis, bacteraemia	Cefuroxime	Some authors retain *Branhamella catarrhalis*	192
[*Moraxella urethralis*—see *Oligella urethralis*]					
Morganella	*M. morganii morganii*, *M. morganii sibonii*	Bacteraemia, UTI, wound infection	β-Lactams, aminoglycosides	Susceptibilities vary	319
Mycobacterium	*M. abscessus*, *M. africanum*, *M. alvei*, *M. asiaticum*, *M. aurum*, *M. avium*, *M. bohemicum*, *M. bovis*, *M. branderi*, *M. brumae*, *M. celatum*, *M. chelonae*, *M. chubuense*, *M. confluentis*, *M. conspicuum*, *M. cookii*, *M. flavescens*, *M. fortuitum*, *M. gadium*, *M. gastri*, *M. genavense*, *M. gordonae*, *M. goodii*, *M. haemophilum*, *M. hassicum*, *M. heidelbergense*,		Isoniazid, rifampicin, ethambutol, pyrazinamide, streptomycin, azithromycin, clarithromycin, ciprofloxacin, dapsone, clofazimine, imipenem, co-trimoxazole, amikacin	Many *Mycobacterium* spp. have been associated with infection. *M. tuberculosis*, *M. africanum*, and *M. bovis* are the agents of tuberculosis. *M. scrofulaceum* causes cervical adenitis. The agent of Buruli ulcer is *M. ulcerans*. *M. marinum* causes fish-tank granuloma. *M. leprae* causes leprosy. *M. malmoense*, *M. szulgai*,	320

Table 1 Continued

Nomenclature Genus (synonyms, CDC alphanumeric groups)	Species and subspecies	Associated infections	Reported susceptibilities and treatments	Notes	Refs
	M. interjectum, M. intracellulare, M. kansasii, M. lentiflavum, M. leprae, M. malmoense, M. marinum, M. microgenicum, M. microti, M. mucogenicum, M. neoaurum, M. nonchromogenicum, M. peregrinum, M. phlei, M. scrofulaceum, M. shimoidei, M. simiae, M. smegmatis, M. szulgai, M. terrae, M. thermoresistibile, M. triplex, M. triviale, M. tuberculosis, M. tusciae, M. ulcerans, M. vaccae, M. wolinskyi, M. xenopi			M. shimoidei, M. kansasii, and M. xenopi cause pulmonary infection. M. intracellulare and M. avium cause systemic infection mainly in immunocompromised patients. The rapid growers, M. chelonae, M. abscessus, and M. fortuitum cause local postinoculation injury and systemic infection	
Mycoplasma	M. buccale, M. faucium, M. fermentans, M. genitalium, M. hominis, M. lipophilum, M. orale, M. penetrans, M. pirum, M. pneumoniae, M. primatum, M. salivarium, M. spermatophilum	Respiratory infection, postpartum fever, pyelonephritis, pelvic inflammatory disease, myocarditis, pericarditis, meningitis	Tetracycline, macrolides, fluoroquinolones	May be resistant to macrolides. M. pneumoniae infection may be complicated by haemolytic anaemia, intravascular coagulation, Stevens–Johnson syndrome, or erythema multiforme	321
Myroides (Flavobacterium)	M. odoratimimus, M. odoratus	UTI, wound infection	Minocycline	May be multiresistant	322
Neisseria	N. canis, N. weaveri (CDC M-5)	Wound infections, abscesses	Amoxicillin	From dog and cat bites	323
	N. cinerea, N. elongata elongata, N. elongata glycolytica, N. elongata nitroreductens, N. flavescens, N. kochii, N. lactamica, N. mucosa, N. parelongata, N. polysaccharea, N. sicca, N. subflava	Meningitis, bacteraemia, endocarditis, osteomyelitis	Penicillin, cephalosporins	Bacteraemia in AIDS reported for several species. Penicillin resistance rarely reported in commensal Neisseria spp. N. subflava includes biovars, flava, perflava, and subflava	324– 328
	N. gonorrhoeae	Gonorrhoea, septicaemia, ophthalmia neonatorum	Penicillin, ciprofloxacin	Susceptibility varies geographically	329
	N. meningitidis	Septicaemia, meningitis, conjunctivitis, genital infection, epiglottitis	Penicillin, cefotaxime	Rifampicin, ciprofloxacin, or ceftriaxone to clear carriage	330
Nocardia	N. asteroides, N. brasiliensis, N. farcinica, N. nova, N. otitidiscaviarum, N. pseudobrasiliensis, N. transvalensis	Nocardiosis	Sulphonamides, co-trimoxazole, amikacin, imipenem,		331
Nocardiopsis	N. dassonvillei, N. synnemataformans	Mycetoma, cutaneous infection, pulmonary infection, conjunctivitis	Fluoroquinolones, piperacillin		332

Table 1 Continued

Nomenclature Genus (synonyms, CDC alphanumeric groups)	Species and subspecies	Associated infections	Reported susceptibilities and treatments	Notes	Refs
Ochrobactrum	*O. anthropi* (*Achromobacter* group Vd), *O. intermedium*	Bacteraemia, endophthalmitis, liver abscess	Imipenem, fluoroquinolones, aminoglycosides	Nosocomial infections in debilitated patients	333, 334
[*Oerskovia turbata*—see *Cellulomonas turbata*]					
Oerskovia	*O. xanthinolytica*	Meningitis, pyonephrosis, CAPD peritonitis, endophthalmitis	Vancomycin and gentamicin		335– 339
Oligella	*O. ureolytica* (CDC IVe) *O. urethralis* (*Moraxella urethralis*)	UTI, Septicaemia	Aminoglycosides, cephalosporins	Associated with urinary catheters	340, 341
Orientia	*O. tsutsugamushi* (*Rickettsia tsutsugamushi*)	Scrub typhus	Tetracycline, chloramphenicol		342
Paenibacillus	*P. alvei*, *P. macerans*, *P. polymyxa*	Septicaemia, meningitis, pneumonia	Vancomycin		343
Pantoea	*P. agglomerans* (*Enterobacter agglomerans*), *P. dispersa*	Bacteraemia, endocarditis, wound infection, cellulitis, alligator-bite infection, endophthalmitis	Carbapenems, fluoroquinolones, ureidopenicillins, aminoglycosides	Susceptibilities vary. May be multiresistant	37, 344
Parachlamydia	*P. acanthamoebae*	Humidifier fever			156
Pasteurella	*P. aerogenes*, *P. bettyae*, *P. canis*, *P. dagmatis*, *P. gallinarum*, *P. haemolytica*, *P. multocida multocida*, *P. m. gallicida*, *P. m. septica*, *P. pneumotropica*, *P. stomatis*	Wound infection, septicaemia, abscesses, pneumonia, endocarditis, meningitis	Penicillin, tetracycline, ciprofloxacin	*Pasteurella* infections in humans relate to species usually associated with animals. There may no history of an animal bite or contact	345– 350
(+ CDC EF-4)					
[*Pasteurella ureae*—see *Actinobacillus ureae*]					
Pediococcus	*P. acidilactici*, *P. damnosus*, *P. dextrinicus*, *P. parvulus*, *P. pentosaceus*	Bacteraemia, abscesses, pulmonary infection	Imipenem, gentamicin, chloramphenicol	Debilitated hospital patients. Resistant to vancomycin	351– 354
Peptococcus	*P. niger*	Abdominal sepsis	Penicillin, clindamycin		355
Peptostreptococcus	*P. anaerobius*, *P. asaccharolyticus*, *P. harei*, *P. hydrogenalis*, *P. indolicus*, *P. ivorii*, *P. lacrimalis*, *P. lactolyticus*, *P. magnus*, *P. micros*, *P. octavius*, *P. prevotii*, *P. tetradius*, '*P. trisimilis*', *P. vaginalis*	Mixed anaerobic infections, arthroplasty infection, dentoalveolar abscess, postsurgical sepsis	Penicillins, cephalosporins, carbapenems, metronidazole, chloramphenicol	Clinical significance of some *Peptostreptococcus* spp. is uncertain	355– 359
Photobacterium	*P. damselae* (*Listonella damsela*) and *Vibrio damsela*)	Necrotizing wound infection	Penicillins, tetracycline, chloramphenicol	Infection associated with penetrating fish injury. May require debridement	360
Photorhabdus (*Xenorhabdus*)	*P. luminescens*	Bacteraemia, wound infection	Cefoxitin, oxacillin, gentamicin		361
Plesiomonas	*P. shigelloides*	Gastroenteritis, septicaemia, meningitis, endophthalmitis	Ciprofloxacin, trimethoprim, cephalosporins	Infections associated with contaminated food and water	362, 363

Table 1 Continued

Nomenclature Genus (synonyms, CDC alphanumeric groups)	Species and subspecies	Associated infections	Reported susceptibilities and treatments	Notes	Refs
Porphyromonas (*Bacteroides*)	*P. asaccharolytica, P. cangingivalis, P. canoris, P. cansulci, P. catoniae, P. circumdentaria, P. crevioricanis, P. endodontalis, P. gingivalis, P. gingivicanis, P. levii, P. macacae*	Mixed anaerobic infections at various sites, periodontitis, human and animal bites	Metronidazole, ureidopenicillins, amoxicillin/clavulanate, carbapenems, cephalosporins, chloramphenicol	Members of the oral flora of humans and animals	364
Prevotella (*Bacteroides*)	*P. bivia, P. buccae, P. buccalis, P. corporis, P. dentalis, P. denticola, P. disiens, P. enoeca, P. heparinolytica, P. intermedia, P. loeschii, P. melaninogenica, P. nigrescens, P. oralis, P. oris, P. oulora, P. tannerae, P. veroralis, P. zoogleoformans*	Abscesses, bacteraemia, wound infection, bite infections, genital tract infections, periodontitis	Metronidazole, amoxicillin/clavulanate, ureidopenicillins, carbapenems, cephalosporins, clindamycin, chloramphenicol	A genus that includes the well-known former *Bacteroides melaninogenicus* and allied species of anaerobes	365, 366
Propionibacterium	*P. acnes, P. avidum, P. granulosum, P. lymphophilum, P. propionicus* (*Arachnia*)	Abscesses, endocarditis, bacteraemia, septic arthritis, endophthalmitis	Glycopeptides, penicillin, macrolides	Associated with acne vulgaris	64, 367, 368
Proteus	*P. mirabilis, P. penneri, P. vulgaris*	UTI, bacteraemia, wound infection, abscesses	β-Lactams, aminoglycosides, fluoroquinolones,	Susceptibilities vary	369
Providencia	*P. alcalifaciens, P. rettgeri, P. rustigianii, P. stuartii*	UTI, wound infection, bacteraemia	β-Lactams, aminoglycosides, fluoroquinolones	Susceptibilities vary. *P. alcalifaciens* has been associated with gastroenteritis	370
[*Pseudomonas acidivorans*—see *Delftia acidivorans*]					
Pseudomonas	*P. aeruginosa, P. alcaligenes, P. chlororaphis, P. fluorescens, P. mendocina, P. monteilii, P. pertocinogena, P. pseudalcaligenes, P. putida, P. stutzeri*	Bacteraemia, UTI, wound infection, abscesses, septic arthritis, conjunctivitis, endocarditis, meningitis	Ureidopenicillins, aminoglycosides, ceftazidime, fluoroquinolones, carbapenems	Nosocomial infections associated with invasive devices in debilitated patients. Nosocomial outbreaks reported. May be multiresistant	371, 372
[*Pseudomonas cepacia*—see *Burkholderia cepacia*] [*Pseudomonas diminuta*—see *Brevundimonas diminuta*] [*Pseudomonas mallei*—see *Burkholderia mallei*] [*Pseudomonas maltophilia*—see *Stenotrophomonas maltophilia*] [*Pseudomonas mesophilica*—see *Methylobacterium mesophilicum*]					
Pseudomonas	*P. luteola* (*Chryseomonas luteola*)	Bacteraemia, endocarditis, CAPD peritonitis	Ureidopenicillins, ceftazidime, ciprofloxacin, aminoglycosides		373
Pseudomonas	*P. oryzihabitans* (*Flavimonas oryzihabitans*)	Septicaemia, eye infection, CAPD peritonitis	Ampicillin, tetracycline, gentamicin, cefotaxime		373–376
[*Pseudomonas paucimobilis*—see *Sphingomonas paucimobilis*] [*Pseudomonas pickettii*- see *Ralstonia pickettii*] [*Pseudomonas pseudomallei*—see *Burkholderia pseudomallei*] [*Pseudomonas putrefaciens*—see *Shewanella putrefaciens*] [*Pseudomonas terrigena*—see *Comamonas terrigena*]					

Table 1 Continued

Nomenclature Genus (synonyms, CDC alphanumeric groups)	Species and subspecies	Associated infections	Reported susceptibilities and treatments	Notes	Refs
[*Pseudomonas testosteroni*—see *Comamonas testosteroni*]					
[*Pseudomonas vesicularis*—see *Brevundimonas vesicularis*]					
Pseudonocardia	*P. autotrophica* (*Amycolata autotrophica*)			Role as pathogen uncertain	53, 377
Pseudoramibacter	*P. alactolyticus*	Periodontal disease, wound infection, abscesses	Penicillin, clindamycin, chloramphenicol		378
Psychrobacter	*P. immobilis*, *P. phenylpyruvicus*	Meningitis, bacteraemia, eye infection	Penicillins, aminoglycosides, chloramphenicol		379, 380
Rahnella	*R. aquatilis*	UTI, septicaemia	Ciprofloxacin	Immunocompromised patients	381, 382
Ralstonia	*R. gilardii* (*Alcaligenes faecalis*), *R. paucula* (CDC group IV c-2), *R. pickettii* (*Pseudomonas pickettii*)	Bacteraemia, UTI, meningitis, wound infection, peritonitis	Cephalosporins, ureidopenicillins, chloramphenicol, imipenem	Aminoglycoside resistance reported	383–387
Rhodococcus	*R. equi* (*Corynebacterium equi*)	Bacteraemia, osteomyelitis lung abscesses	Vancomycin, erythromycin, aminoglycosides	In immunocompromised patients, including AIDS	388–390
Rickettsia	*R. africae*, *R. akari*, *R. australis*, *R. conorii*, *R. felis*, *R. honei*, *R. japonica*, '*R. mongolotimonae*,' *R. prowazekii*, *R. rickettsiae*, *R. sibirica*, *R. slovaca*, *R. typhi*	Rickettsial spotted fever, tick typhus, tick-bite fever, rickettsialpox	Tetracycline	Transmitted by arthropods. Agents of Astrakhan fever, Israeli tick typhus, and Thai tick typhus await designation of scientific names	391
[*Rochalimea*—see *Bartonella*]					
Roseomonas	*R. cervicalis*, *R. fauriae, R. gilardii*	Bacteraemia, wound infection, peritonitis	Aminoglycosides, imipenem	Genomospecies 4, 5, and 6 await scientific names	392
Rothia	*R. dentocariosa*	Endocarditis, abscesses	Penicillin and gentamicin		64, 393
Ruminococcus	*R. flavefaciens, R. hansenii* (*Streptococcus hansenii*), *R. productus* (*Peptostreptococcus productus*)	Abdominal sepsis, abscesses	Penicillins	Current nomenclature is controversial	394–396
Salmonella	*S. cholersuis choleraesuis*, *S. c. arizonae, S. c. bongori*, *S. c. diarizonae*, *S. c. houtenae, S. c. indica*, *S. c. salamae, S. enteritidis*, *S. typhi, S. typhimurium*	Gastroenteritis, enteric fever, osteomyelitis	β-Lactams, fluoroquinolones, chloramphenicol	The names listed are those with standing in nomenclature at the time of writing. It is likely that all salmonellas belong to one species for which the name '*S. enterica*' has been proposed. Meanwhile, a number of systems is widely used, including the representation of serotypes (e.g. *S. enteritidis*, '*S. virchow*') as Linnaean binomials	397

Table 1 Continued

Nomenclature Genus (synonyms, CDC alphanumeric groups)	Species and subspecies	Associated infections	Reported susceptibilities and treatments	Notes	Refs
Selenomonas	*S. artemidis, S. dianae, S. flueggei, S. infelix, S. noxia, S. sputigena*	Bacteraemia, lung abscess	Clindamycin, chloramphenicol, metronidazole	Malignancy and alcohol abuse reported as risk factors for infection	129, 398– 400
Serpulina	*S. intermedia, S. murdochii*	Intestinal spirochaetes		Intestinal spirochaetes of uncertain significance	114
[*Serpulina pilosicoli*—see *Brachyspira pilosicoli*]					
Serratia	*S. ficaria, S. fonticola, S. grimesii, S. liquefaciens, S. marcescens, S. odorifera, S. plymuthica, S. proteamaculans proteamaculans, S. p. quinovora, S. rubidea*	Septicaemia, abscesses, burn infections, osteomyelitis	Imipenem, aminoglycosides, fluoroquinolones, ureidopenicillins, ceftazidime	Nosocomial outbreaks reported. May be multiresistant	401– 405
Shewanella	*S. algae, S. putrefaciens (Alteromonas putrefaciens) (Pseudomonas putrefaciens)*	Abdominal sepsis, meningitis, bacteraemia	Ampicillin, cefotaxime, gentamicin, chloramphenicol	Debilitated patients	406– 407
Shigella	*S. boydii, S. dysenteriae, S. flexneri, S. sonnei*	Enteric infection	Co-trimoxazole, fluoroquinolones		408
Simkania	*S. negevensis*	Bronchiolitis, pneumonia			409
Slackia	*S. exigua (Eubacterium exiguum)*	Periodontitis			410
Sphingobacterium (Flavobacterium)	*S. mizutae, S. multivorum, S. spiritivorum, S. thalpophilum*	Bacteraemia, UTI, peritonitis	Ampicillin, perfloxacin, co-trimoxazole		411– 413
Sphingomonas	*S. parapaucimobilis, S. paucimobilis (Pseudomonas paucimobilis), S. sanguis, S. yanoikuyae*	Septicaemia, UTI, wound infections, CAPD peritonitis	Ceftazidime, aminoglycosides	Nosocomial infections	414
Spirillum	*S. minus*	Rat-bite fever	Penicillin	*Streptobacillus monilliformis* is also a rat-bite fever agent	415
Staphylococcus	*S. aureus, S. auricularis, S. capitis capitis, S. c. ureolyticus, S. caprae, S. cohnii cohnii, S. c. urealyticus, S. epidermidis, S. equorum, S. gallinarum, S. haemolyticus, S. hominis hominis, S. h. novobiosepticius, S. hyicus, S. intermedius, S. lugdunensis, S. pasteuri, S. saccharolyticus, S. saprophyticus, S. schleiferi schleiferi, S. s. coagulans, S. sciuri, S. simulans, S. warneri, S. xylosus,*	Bacteraemia, wound infection, endocarditis, catheter-related sepsis, UTI, toxic shock syndrome, food poisoning, eye infection, osteomyelitis	Glycopeptides, β-lactams, aminoglycosides, tetracycline, macrolides, rifampicin, fluoroquinolones, fucidin, mupirocin	Staphylococci are surface commensals of humans and animals. *S. aureus* is also a major pathogen, causing focal and systemic sepsis, toxic shock syndrome, and food poisoning. *S. epidermidis* infection is often associated with foreign bodies (e.g. catheters and implants). *S. saprophyticus* causes UTI. *S. lugdenensis* is a rare cause of endocarditis. *S. intermedius, S. hyicus,* and others are from animals. Susceptibilities are variable but glycopeptide resistance is as yet rare	416

Table 1 Continued

Nomenclature Genus (synonyms, CDC alphanumeric groups)	Species and subspecies	Associated infections	Reported susceptibilities and treatments	Notes	Refs
Stenotrophomonas	*S. maltophilia* (*Pseudomonas maltophila*) (*Xanthomonas maltophila*)	Bacteraemia, meningitis, wound infection, UTI, pneumonia	Fluoroquinolones, chloramphenicol, co-trimoxazole	Resistance to aminoglycosides, penicillins, and carbapenems reported AIDS-associated	417
	S. africana	Meningitis	Ciprofloxacin, netilmicin, co-trimoxazole		418
Stomatococcus	*S. mucilaginosus* (*Micrococcus mucilaginosus*)	Endocarditis, meningitis, neutropenic sepsis	Glycopeptides, imipenem, rifampicin, ceftriaxone		419–422
Streptobacillus	*S. moniliformis*	Rat-bite fever, Haverhill fever	Penicillin, erythromycin	*Spirillum minus* is also a causative agent of rat-bite fever	423
Streptococcus	*S. acidominimus*	Pneumonia, pericarditis, meningitis	β-Lactams	From cattle	424
	S. agalactiae, S. canis, S. dysgalactiae dysgalactiae, S. d. equisimilis, S. equi equi, S. e. zooepidemicus, S. iniae (S. shiloi), S. porcinus, S. pyogenes	Pharyngitis, bacteraemia, pyogenic infection, necrotizing infection, septic arthritis, glomerulonephritis, meningitis	β-Lactams, macrolides	*S. pyogenes* (Lancefield group A), *S. agalactiae* (group B), and *S. d. equisimilis* (groups C and G) are commensals and pathogens of humans. *S. iniae* is from fish. Others are from mammals	425, 426
	S. anginosus, S. constellatus constellatus, S. c. pharyngis, S. intermedius	Abscesses, bacteraemia, endocarditis, pharyngitis	β-Lactams, macrolides	Often termed 'S. milleri' or microaerophillic streptococci. From human oral flora	427
	S. bovis, S. equinus	Endocarditis, CAPD peritonitis	β-Lactams	Intestinal streptococci from animals and humans	428
	S. criceti, S. mutans, S. ratti, S. sobrinus	Dental caries, endocarditis	β-Lactams	From the tooth-surface flora of humans and mammals	429
	S. cristatus, S. gordonii, S. mitis, S. oralis, S. parasanguinis, S. pneumoniae, S. salivarius, S. sanguinis, S. vestibularis,	Bacteraemia, endocarditis, wound infection	β-Lactams, macrolides	Human oral streptococci including taxa sometimes termed 'S. viridans'	429
		Pneumonia, bacteraemia, sinusitis, peritonitis, otitis, conjunctivitis	β-Lactams, macrolides, chloramphenicol	Penicillin resistance locally common	430
	S. suis	Meningitis	β-Lactams	Associated with pig contact	431
Streptomyces	*S. anulatus, S. paraguayensis, S. somaliensis*	Actinomycetoma	Dapsone, co-trimoxazole		432
Succinivibrio	*S. dextrinosolvens*	Bacteraemia	Penicillin	From faecal and gingival flora	200
Sutterella	*S. wadsworthensis*	Appendicitis, peritonitis, abscesses, osteomyelitis	Amoxicillin/clavulanate, ticarcillin/clavulanate, meropenem, ceftriaxone	One-third of isolates reported to be metronidazole-resistant	433–435
Suttonella	*S. indologenes* (*Kingella indologenes*)	Endocarditis, eye infection	Penicillin (plus gentamicin for endocarditis)		436
Tatumella	*T. ptyseos*	Bacteraemia, UTI	Ampicillin, tetracycline, chloramphenicol, gentamicin	The significance of isolates from sputum is unclear	437

Table 1 Continued

Nomenclature Genus (synonyms, CDC alphanumeric groups)	Species and subspecies	Associated infections	Reported susceptibilities and treatments	Notes	Refs
Tissierella	T. praeacuta (Bacteroides praeacuta)	Bacteraemia	Metronidazole		438
Trabulsiella	T. guamensis	Diarrhoea	Co-trimoxazole, gentamicin, chloramphenicol	Role as possible pathogen uncertain	439
Treponema	T. amylovorum, T. denticola, T. lecithinolyticum, T. maltophilum, T. medium, T. pectinovorum, T. scoliodontum, T. socranskii, T. vincentii			Associated with periodontal disease. Role as potential pathogens unclear	440, 441
	T. carateum	Pinta	Penicillin		442
	T. minutum, T. phagedenis, T. refringens			From genital flora. Considered non-pathogenic but have been isolated from genital lesions	443
	T. pallidum pallidum, T. p. endemicum	Syphilis	Penicillin	T. p. endemicum is the agent of non-venereal endemic syphilis	442, 444
	T. pallidum pertenue	Yaws	Penicillin		442
Tropheryma	T. whippelii	Whipple's disease		Uncultured organism	445
Tsukamruella	T. inchonensis, T. paurometabola, T. pulmonis, T. tyrosinosolvens	Septicaemia, cutaneous infections, lung infections	β-Lactam (plus aminoglycoside)	Line-associated infections in debilitated patients. T. pulmonis isolated from the sputum of a tuberculosis patient	446–449
Turicella	T. otitidis	Otitis, cervical abscess	Glycopeptides, β-lactams		64, 176, 450
Ureaplasma	U. parvum, U. urealyticum	Urethritis	Tetracycline, erythromycin		451
Vagococcus	V. fluvialis		Ampicillin, vancomycin cefotaxime	Possible role as pathogen poorly defined	452
Veillonella	V. atypica, V. dipsar, V. parvula	Abscesses, bacteraemia	Metronidazole		80, 453
Vibrio	V. alginolyticus	Wound infection, ear infection	Chloramphenicol, tetracycline	Infection associated with aquatic exposure	454
	V. carchariae	Wound infection	Cephalosporins, chloramphenicol, gentamicin	Infection associated with shark bite. May require debridement	455
	V. cholerae	Cholera	Tetracycline		454
	V. cincinnatiensis	Bacteraemia	Moxalactam, chloramphenicol, cephalosporins	Risk factors for infection not defined	456
[Vibrio damsela—see Photobacterium damselae]					
	V. fluvialis, V. furnissii, V. hollisae, V. metschnikovii, V. mimicus, V. parahaemolyticus	Diarrhoea, septicaemia	Tetracycline, chloramphenicol	Infection associated with ingestion of contaminated water or shellfish	454, 456–458
	V. vulnificus	Wound infection, septicaemia, meningitis, endometritis	Tetracycline, penicillins, gentamicin, chloramphenicol	Risk factors include aquatic exposure and penetrating fish injury. May require debridement	459, 460

Table 1 Continued

Nomenclature Genus (synonyms, CDC alphanumeric groups)	Species and subspecies	Associated infections	Reported susceptibilities and treatments	Notes	Refs
Weeksella	*W. virosa*	Peritonitis	Imipenem, ampicillin	From vaginal flora	461, 462
[*Weeksella zoohelcum*—see *Bergeyella zoohelcum*]					
[*Wolinella curva*—see *Campylobacter curvus*]					
[*Wolinella recta*—see *Campylobacter rectus*]					
Xanthomonas	*X. campestris*	Bacteraemia			463
[*Xanthomonas maltophilia*—see *Stenotrophomonas maltophilia*]					
[*Xenorhabdus luminescens*—see *Photorhabdus luminescens*]					
Yersinia	*Y. aldovae, Y. bercovieri, Y. enterocolitica, Y. frederiksenii, Y. intermedia, Y. kristensenii, Y. mollaretii, Y. pseudotuberculosis, Y. rohdei*	Enterocolitis, soft tissue infections, mesenteric lymphadenitis	Tetracycline, chloramphenicol, aminoglycosides, fluoroquinolones, cephalosporins	Medical significance of many *Yersinia* spp. is unclear. Antibiotic treatment is not indicated for uncomplicated enteric infection	464
	Y. pestis	Plague	Streptomycin, tetracycline		464
Yokenella	*Y. regensburgei* (*Koserella trabulsii*)	Bacteraemia, wound infection	Aminoglycosides, chloramphenicol		279, 465

CAPD, continual ambulatory peritoneal dialysis; UTI, urinary tract infection; HIV, human immunodeficiency virus; AIDS, acquired immunodeficiency syndrome.

References

1. Heath CH, *et al.* (1998). Vertebral osteomyelitis and discitis associated with *Abiotrophia adiacens* (nutritionally variant streptococcus) infection. *Australian and New Zealand Journal of Medicine* **28**, 663.

2. Biermann C, *et al.* (1999). Isolation of *Abiotrophia adiacens* from a brain abscess which developed in a patient after neurosurgery. *Journal of Clinical Microbiology* **37**, 769–71.

3. Namdari H, *et al.* (1999). *Abiotrophia* species as a cause of endophthalmitis following cataract extraction. *Journal of Clinical Microbiology* **37**, 1564–6.

4. Yabuuchi E, *et al.* (1998). Emendation of genus *Achromobacter* and *Achromobacter xylosoxidans* (Yabuuchi and Yano) and proposal of *Achromobacter ruhlandii* (Packer and Vishniac) comb. nov., *Achromobacter piechaudii* (Kiredjian *et al.*) comb. nov., and *Achromobacter xylosoxidans* subsp. *denitrificans* (Ruger and Tan) comb. nov. *Microbiology and Immunology* **42**, 429–38.

5. Rolston KVI, Messer M (1990). The *in-vitro* susceptibility of *Alcaligenes denitrificans* subsp. *xylosoxidans* to 40 antimicrobial agents. *Journal of Antimicrobial Chemotherapy* **26**, 857–60.

6. Peel MM, *et al.* (1988). *Alcaligenes piechaudii* from chronic ear discharge. *Journal of Clinical Microbiology* **26**, 1580–1.

7. Igra-Siegman Y, Chmel H, Cobbs C (1980). Clinical and laboratory characteristics of *Achromobacter xylosoxidans* infection. *Journal of Clinical Microbiology* **11**, 141–5.

8. Holmes B, Snell JJS, Lapage SP (1977). Strains of *Achromobacter xylosoxidans* from clinical material. *Journal of Clinical Pathology* **30**, 595–601.

9. Reverdy ME, *et al.* (1984). Nosocomial colonisation and infection by *Achromobacter xylosoxidans*. *Journal of Clinical Microbiology* **19**, 140–3.

10. Sugihara PT, *et al.* (1974). Isolation of *Acidaminococcus fermentans* and *Megasphaera elsdenii* from normal human feces. *Applied Microbiology* **27**, 274–5.

11. Chatterjee BD, Chakraborti CK (1995). Non-sporing anaerobes in certain surgical group of patients. *Journal of the Indian Medical Association* **93**, 333–5, 339.

12. Willems A, *et al.* (1990). *Acidovorax*, a new genus for *Pseudomonas facilis*, *Pseudomonas delafieldii* E Falsen (EF) group 13, EF group 16, and several clinical isolates, with the species *Acidovorax facilis* comb. nov., *Acidovorax delafieldii* comb. nov., and *Acidovorax temperans* sp. nov. *International Journal of Systematic Bacteriology* **40**, 384–98.

13. Rosenthal SL, Freundlich LF (1977). The clinical significance of *Acinetobacter* species. *Health Laboratory Science* **14**, 194–8.

14. French GL, *et al.* (1980). A hospital outbreak of antibiotic-resistant *Acinetobacter anitratus*: epidemiology and control. *Journal of Hospital Infection* **1**, 125–31.

15. Bouvet PJM, Grimont PAD (1986). Taxonomy of the genus *Acinetobacter* with recognition of *Acinetobacter baumanni* sp. nov., *Acinetobacter haemolyticus* sp. nov., *Acinetobacter johnsonii* sp. nov., and *Acinetobacter junii* sp. nov. and emended descriptions of *Acinetobacter calcoaceticus* and *Acinetobacter lwoffii*. *International Journal of Systematic Bacteriology* **36**, 238–40.

16. Haley S, *et al.* (1990). *Acinetobacter* sp. L-form infection of a cemented Charnley total hip replacement. *Journal of Clinical Pathology* **43**, 781.

17. Bergogne-Bérézine E, Joly-Guillou ML (1991). Hospital infection with *Acinetobacter* spp.: an increasing problem. *Journal of Hospital Infection* **18A**, 250–5.

18. Urban C, *et al.* (1993). Effect of sublactam on infections caused by imipenem-resistant *Acinetobacter calcoaceticus* biotype *anitratus*. *Journal of Infectious Diseases* **167**, 448–51.

19. Ellner JJ, *et al.* (1979). Infective endocarditis caused by slow-growing, fastidious, Gram-negative bacteria. *Medicine* (Baltimore) **58**, 145–58.

20. Kristinsson KG, Thorgeirsson G, Holbrook WP (1988). *Actinobacillus actinomycetemcomitans* and endocarditis. *Journal of Infectious Diseases* **157**, 599.

21. Peel MM, *et al.* (1991). *Actinobacillus* spp. and related bacteria in infected wounds of humans bitten by horses and sheep. *Journal of Clinical Microbiology* **29**, 2535–8.

22. Dibb WL, Digranes A, Tønjum S (1981). *Actinobacillus lignieresii* infection after a horse bite. *British Medical Journal* **283**, 583.

23. Wust J, *et al.* (1991). *Actinobacillus hominis* as a causative agent of septicemia in hepatic failure. *European Journal of Clinical Microbiology and Infectious Diseases* **10**, 693–4.

24. Marriott DJ, Brady LM (1983). *Pasteurella ureae* meningitis. *Medical Journal of Australia* **2**, 455–6.

25. Noble RC, Marek BJ, Overman SB (1987). Spontaneous peritonitis caused by *Pasteurella ureae*. *Journal of Clinical Microbiology* **25**, 442–4.

26. Lawson PA, *et al.* (1997). Characterization of some Actinomyces-like isolates from human clinical specimens: reclassification of *Actinomyces suis* (Soltys and Spratling) as *Actinobaculum suis* comb. nov. and description of *Actinobaculum schaalii* sp. nov. *International Journal of Systematic Bacteriology* **47**, 899–903.

27. Venugopal PV, Venugopal TV (1990). *Actinomadura madurae* mycetomas. *Australasian Journal of Dermatology* **31**, 33–6.

28. Smego RA Jr, Foglia G (1998). Actinomycosis. *Clinical Infectious Diseases* **26**, 1255–63.

29. Funke G, *et al.* (1997). *Actinomyces europaeus* sp. nov., isolated from human clinical specimens. *International Journal of Systematic Bacteriology* **47**, 687–92.

30. Colman G (1967). *Aerococcus*-like organisms isolated from human infections. *Journal of Clinical Pathology* **20**, 294–7.

31. Nathavitharana KA, *et al.* (1983). Acute meningitis in early childhood caused by *Aerococcus viridans*. *British Medical Journal* **286**, 1248.

32. Mercer NSG, *et al.* (1987). Medicinal leeches as sources of wound infection. *British Medical Journal* **294**, 937.

33. Gluski I, *et al.* (1992). A 15-year study of the role of *Aeromonas* spp. in gastroenteritis in hospitalised children. *Journal of Medical Microbiology* **37**, 315–18.

34. Joseph SW, *et al.* (1991). *Aeromonas jandaei* and *Aeromonas veronii* dual infection of a human following aquatic exposure. *Journal of Clinical Microbiology* **29**, 565–9.

35. Ong KR, Sordillo E, Frankel E (1991). Unusual case of *Aeromonas hydrophila* endocarditis. *Journal of Clinical Microbiology* **29**, 1056–7.

36. Janda JM, Duffey PS (1988). Mesophilic aeromonads in human disease: current taxonomy, laboratory identification, and infectious disease spectrum. *Reviews of Infectious Diseases* **10**, 980–97.

37. Flandry F, *et al.* (1989). Initial antibiotic therapy for alligator bites: characterization of the oral flora of *Alligator mississippiensis*. *Southern Medical Journal* **82**, 262–6.

38. Hickman-Brenner FW, *et al.* (1988). *Aeromonas schubertii*, a new mannitol-negative species found in human clinical specimens. *Journal of Clinical Microbiology* **26**, 1561–4.

39. Hickman-Brenner FW, *et al.* (1987). *Aeromonas veronii*, a new ornithine decarboxylase-positive species that may cause diarrhea. *Journal of Clinical Microbiology* **25**, 900–6.

40. Wolff RL, Wiseman SL, Kitchens CS (1980). *Aeromonas hydrophila* bacteremia in ambulatory immunocompromised hosts. *American Journal of Medicine* **68**, 238–40.

41. Young DF, Barr RJ (1981). *Aeromonas hydrophila* infection of the skin. *Archives of Dermatology* **117**, 244.

42. Champsaur H, *et al.* (1982). Cholera-like illness due to *Aeromonas sobria*. *Journal of Infectious Diseases* **145**, 248–54.

43. Motyl MR, McKinley G, Janda JM (1985). *In vitro* susceptibilities of *Aeromonas hydrophila*, *Aeromonas sobria*, and *Aeromonas caviae* to 22 antimicrobial agents. *Antimicrobial Agents and Chemotherapy* **28**, 151–3.

44. Brenner DJ, *et al.* (1991). Proposal of *Afipia* gen. nov., with *Afipia felis* sp. nov. (formerly the Cat Scratch Disease Bacillus), *Afipia clevelandensis* sp. nov. (formerly the Cleveland Clinic Foundation Strain), *Afipia broomeae* sp. nov., and three unnamed genospecies. *Journal of Clinical Microbiology* **29**, 2450–60.

45. Plotkin GR (1980). *Agrobacterium radiobacter* prosthetic valve endocarditis. *Annals of Internal Medicine* **93**, 839–40.

46. Hammerberg O, Bialowska-Hobrzanska H, Gopaul D (1991). Isolation of *Agrobacterium radiobacter* from a central venous catheter. *European Journal of Clinical Microbiology and Infectious Diseases* **10**, 450.

47. Freney J, *et al.* (1985). Septicemia caused by *Agrobacterium* sp. *Journal of Clinical Microbiology* **22**, 683–5.

48. Castagnola E, *et al.* (1997). Broviac catheter-related bacteraemias due to unusual pathogens in children with cancer: case reports with literature review. *Journal of Infection* **34**, 215–18.

49. Bizet J, Bizet C (1997). Strains of *Alcaligenes faecalis* from clinical material. *Journal of Infection* **35**, 167–9.

50. Hendolin PH, *et al.* (1999). High incidence of *Alloiococcus otitis* in otitis media with effusion. *Pediatric Infectious Disease Journal* **18**, 860–5.

51. Faden H, Dryja D (1989). Recovery of a unique bacterial organism in human middle ear fluid and its possible role in chronic otitis media. *Journal of Clinical Microbiology* **27**, 2488–91.

52. Aguirre M, Collins MD (1992). Development of a polymerase chain reaction-probe test for identification of *Alloiococcus otitis*. *Journal of Clinical Microbiology* **30**, 2177–80.

53. Lechevalier MP, *et al.* (1986). Two new genera of nocardioform actinomycetes: *Amycolata* gen. nov. and *Amycolatopsis* gen. nov. *International Journal of Systematic Bacteriology* **36**, 29–37.

54. Malnick H, *et al.* (1983). *Anaerobiospirillum* species isolated from humans with diarrhoea. *Clinical Pathology* **36**, 1097–101.

55. Goddard WW, Bennett SA, Parkinson C (1998). *Anaerobiospirillum succiniciproducens* septicaemia: important aspects of diagnosis and management. *Journal of Infection* **37**, 68–70.

56. Lee JI, Hampson DJ (1994). Genetic characterisation of intestinal spirochaetes and their association with disease. *Journal of Medical Microbiology* **40**, 365–71.

57. Tee W, *et al.* (1998) Three cases of *Anaerobiospirillum succiniciproducens* bacteremia confirmed by 16S rRNA gene sequencing. *Journal of Clinical Microbiology* **36**, 1209–13.

58. Malnick H (1997). *Anaerobiospirillum thomasii* sp. nov., an anaerobic spiral bacterium isolated from the feces of cats and dogs and from diarrheal feces of humans, and emendation of the genus *Anaerobiospirillum*. *International Journal of Systematic Bacteriology* **47**, 381–4.

59. Malnick H, *et al.* (1990). Description of a medium for isolating *Anaerobiospirillum* spp, a possible cause of zoonotic disease, from diarrheal feces and blood of humans and use of the medium in a survey of human, canine, and feline feces. *Journal of Clinical Microbiology* **28**, 1380–4.

60. Shah HN, Collins MD (1986). Reclassification of *Bacteroides furcosus* Veillon and Zuber (Hauduroy, Ehringer, Urbain, Guillot and Magrou) in a new genus *Anaerorhabdus*, as *Anaerorhabdus furcosus* comb. nov. *Systematic Applied Microbiology* **8**, 86–8.

61. Fell HWK, *et al.* (1977). *Corynebacterium haemolyticum* infections in Cambridgeshire. *Journal of Hygiene, Cambridge* **79**, 269–74.

62. Jobantputra RS, Swain CP (1975). Septicaemia due to *Corynebacterium haemolyticum*. *Journal of Clinical Pathology* **28**, 798–800.

63. Greenman JL (1987). *Corynebacterium hemolyticum* and pharyngitis. *Annals of Internal Medicine* **106**, 633.

64. Funke G, *et al.* (1997). Clinical microbiology of coryneform bacteria. *Clinical Microbiology Reviews* **10**, 125–59.

65. Lepargneur JP, *et al.* (1998). Urinary tract infection due to *Arcanobacterium bernardiae* in a patient with a urinary tract diversion. *European Journal of Clinical Microbiology and Infectious Diseases* **17**, 399–401.

66. Adderson EE, *et al.* (1998). Septic arthritis due to *Arcanobacterium bernardiae* in an immunocompromised patient. *Clinical Infectious Diseases* **27**, 211–12.

67. Ieven, M (1996). Severe infection due to *Actinomyces bernardiae*: case report. *Clinical Infectious Diseases* **22**, 157–8.

68. Na'was TE, *et al.* (1987). Comparison of biochemical, morphologic, and chemical characteristics of Centers for Disease Control fermentative coryneform groups 1, 2, and A-4. *Journal of Clinical Microbiology* **25**, 1354–8.

69. Lynch M, *et al.* (1998). *Actinomyces pyogenes* septic arthritis in a diabetic farmer. *Journal of Infection* **37**, 71–3.

70. Drancourt M, *et al.* (1993). Two cases of *Actinomyces pyogenes* infection in humans. *European Journal of Clinical Microbiology and Infectious Diseases* **12**, 55–7.

71. Vandamme P, *et al.* (1992). Outbreak of recurrent abdominal cramps associated with *Arcobacter butzleri* in an Italian school. *Journal of Clinical Microbiology* **30**, 2335–7.

72. Tee W, *et al.* (1988). *Campylobacter cryaerophila* isolated from a human. *Journal of Clinical Microbiology* **26**, 2469–73.

73. Vandamme P, *et al.* (1991). Revision of *Campylobacter*, *Helicobacter* and *Wolinella* taxonomy: emendation of generic descriptions and proposal of *Arcobacter* gen. nov. *International Journal of Systematic Bacteriology* **41**, 88–103.

74. Bodaghi B, *et al.* (1998). Whipple's syndrome (uveitis, B27-negative spondylarthropathy, meningitis, and lymphadenopathy) associated with *Arthrobacter* sp. infection. *Ophthalmology* **105**, 1891–6.

75. Hou XG, *et al.* (1998). Description of *Arthrobacter creatinolyticus* sp. nov., isolated from human urine. *International Journal of Systematic Bacteriology* **48**, 423–9.

76. Hsu C-L, *et al.* (1998). Septicaemia due to *Arthrobacter* species in a neutropenic patient with acute lymphoblastic leukemia. *Clinical Infectious Diseases* **27**, 1334–5.

77. Collins MD, Wallbanks S (1992). Comparative sequence analyses of the 16S rRNA genes of *Lactobacillus minutus*, *Lactobacillus rimae* and *Streptococcus parvulus*: proposal for the creation of a new genus *Atopobium*. *FEMS Microbiology Letters* **95**, 235–40.

78. Olsen I, *et al.* (1991). *Lactobacillus uli* sp. nov. and *Lactobacillus rimae* sp. nov. from the human gingival crevice and emended descriptions of *Lactobacillus minutus* and *Streptococcus parvulus*. *International Journal of Systematic Bacteriology* **41**, 261–6.

79. Rodriguez Jovita M, *et al.* (1999). Characterization of a novel *Atopobium* isolate from the human vagina: description of *Atopobium vaginae* sp. nov. *International Journal of Systematic Bacteriology* **49**, 1573–6.

80. Meijer-Severs GJ, *et al.* (1979). The presence of antibody-coated anaerobic bacteria in asymptomatic bacteriuria during pregnancy. *Journal of Infectious Diseases* **140**, 653–8.

81. Ihde DC, Armstrong D (1973). Clinical spectrum of infection due to bacillus species. *American Journal of Medicine* **55**, 839–45.

82. Slimans R, Rehm S, Shlaes DM. (1987). Serious infections caused by *Bacillus* species. *Medicine* (Baltimore) **66**, 218–23.

83. Weber DJ, *et al.* (1988). *In vitro* susceptibility of *Bacillus* spp. to selected antimicrobial agents. *Antimicrobial Agents and Chemotherapy* **32**, 642–5.

84. Isaacson P, *et al.* (1976). Pseudotumour of the lung caused by infection with *Bacillus sphaericus*. *Journal of Clinical Pathology* **29**, 806–11.

85. Samples JR, Buettner H (1983). Corneal ulcer caused by a biological insecticide (*Bacillus thuringiensis*). *American Journal of Ophthalmology* **95**, 258–60.

86. Samples JR, Buettner H (1983). Ocular infection caused by a biological insecticide. *Journal of Infectious Diseases* **148**, 614.

87. Reller LB (1973). Endocarditis caused by *Bacillus subtilis*. *American Journal of Clinical Pathology* **60**, 714–18.

88. de Carvalho CB, Moreira JL, Ferreira MC (1996). Epidemiology and antimicrobial resistance of *B. fragilis* group organisms isolated from clinical specimen and human intestinal microbiota. *Revista do Instituto de Medicina Tropical de Sao Paulo* **38**, 329–35.

89. Rasmussen BA, Bush K, Tally FP (1993). Antimicrobial resistance in *Bacteroides*. *Clinical Infectious Diseases* **16**(Suppl 4), 390–400.

90. Dauga C, *et al.* (1993). *Balneatrix alpica* gen. nov., sp. nov. a bacterium associated with pneumonia and meningitis in a spa therapy centre. *Research in Microbiology* **144**, 35–46.

91. Casalta JP, *et al.* (1989). Pneumonia and meningitis caused by a new nonfermentative unknown gram-negative bacterium. *Journal of Clinical Microbiology* **27**, 1446–8.

92. Ellis BA, *et al.* (1999). An outbreak of acute bartonellosis (Oroya fever) in the Urubamba region of Peru, 1998. *American Journal of Tropical Medicine and Hygiene* **61**, 344–9.

93. Daly JS, *et al.* (1993). *Rochalimaea elizabethae* sp. nov. isolated from a patient with endocarditis. *Journal of Clinical Microbiology* **31**, 872–81.

94. Regnery RL, *et al.* (1992). Serological response to 'Rochalimaea henselae' antigen in suspected cat-scratch disease. *Lancet* **339**, 1443–5.

95. Relman DA, *et al.* (1990). The agent of bacillary angiomatosis: an approach to the identification of uncultured pathogens. *New England Journal of Medicine* **323**, 1573–80.

96. Koeler JE, *et al.* (1992). Isolation of *Rochalimaea* species from cutaneous and osseous lesions of bacillary angiomatosis. *New England Journal of Medicine* **327**, 1625–31.

97. Welch DF, *et al.* (1999). Isolation of a new subspecies, *Bartonella vinsonii* subsp. *arupensis*, from a cattle rancher: identity with isolates found in conjunction with *Borrelia burgdorferi* and *Babesia microti* among naturally infected mice. *Journal of Clinical Microbiology* **37**, 2598–601.

98. Reina J, Borrell N (1992). Leg abscess caused by *Weeksella zoohelcum* following a dog bite. *Clinical Infectious Diseases* **14**, 1162–3.

99. Ha GY, *et al.* (1999). Case of sepsis caused by *Bifidobacterium longum*. *Journal of Clinical Microbiology* **37**, 1227–8.

100. Brook I (1996). Isolation of non-sporing anaerobic rods from infections in children. *Journal of Medical Microbiology* **45**, 21–6.

101. Brook I, Frazier EH (1993). Significant recovery of nonsporulating anaerobic rods from clinical specimens. *Clinical Infectious Diseases* **16**, 476–80.

102. Bourne KA, *et al.* (1978). Bacteremia due to *Bifidobacterium*, *Eubacterium* or *Lactobacillus*; twenty-one cases and review of the literature. *Yale Journal of Biology and Medicine* **51**, 505–12.

103. Kasten MJ, Rosenblatt JE, Gustafson DR (1992). *Bilophila wadsworthia* bacteremia in two patients with hepatic abscesses. *Journal of Clinical Microbiology* **30**, 2502–3.

104. Summanen P, *et al.* (1989). *Bilophila wadsworthia*, gen. nov. and sp. nov., a unique gram-negative anaerobic rod recovered from appendicitis specimens and human faeces. *Journal of General Microbiology* **135**, 3405–11.

105. Wang G, *et al.* (1999). Molecular typing of *Borrelia burgdorferi sensu lato*: taxonomic, epidemiological, and clinical implications. *Clinical Microbiology Reviews* **12**, 633–53.

106. Fukunaga M, *et al.* (1996). Phylogenetic analysis of *Borrelia* species based on flagellin gene sequences and its application for molecular typing of Lyme disease borreliae. *International Journal of Systematic Bacteriology* **46**, 898–905.

107. Dworkin MS, *et al.* (1999). *Bordetella bronchiseptica* infection in human immunodeficiency virus-infected patients. *Clinical Infectious Diseases* **28**, 1095–9.

108. Vandamme P, *et al.* (1996). *Bordetella trematum* sp. nov., isolated from wounds and ear infections in humans, and reassessment of *Alcaligenes denitrificans* Rüger and Tan 1983. *International Journal of Systematic Bacteriology* **46**, 849–58.

109. Vandamme P, *et al.* (1995). *Bordetella hinzii* sp. nov., isolated from poultry and humans. *International Journal of Systematic Bacteriology* **45**, 37–45.

110. Weyant RS, *et al.* (1995). *Bordetella holmesii* sp. nov., a new gram-negative species associated with septicemia. *Journal of Clinical Microbiology* **33**, 1–7.

111. Bergfors E, *et al.* (1999). Parapertussis and pertussis: differences and similarities in incidence, clinical course, and antibody responses. *International Journal of Infectious Diseases* **3**, 140–6.

112. Mikosza AS, *et al.* (1999). PCR amplification from fixed tissue indicates frequent involvement of *Brachyspira aalborgi* in human intestinal spirochetosis. *Journal of Clinical Microbiology* **37**, 2093–8.

113. Lee JI, Hampson DJ (1994). Genetic characterisation of intestinal spirochaetes and their association with disease. *Journal of Medical Microbiology* **40**, 365–71.

114. Stanton TB, *et al.* (1997). Recognition of two new species of intestinal spirochetes: *Serpulina intermedia* sp. nov. and *Serpulina murdochii* sp. nov. *International Journal of Systematic Bacteriology* **47**, 1007–12.

115. Shida O, *et al.* (1996). Proposal for two new genera, *Brevibacillus* gen. nov. and *Aneurinibacillus* gen. nov. *International Journal of Systematic Bacteriology* **46**, 939–46.

116. Wen RR (1984). [A preliminary study of food poisoning by *Bacillus brevis* Migula]. *Chung Hua Yu Fang I Hsueh Tsa Chih* **18**, 168–9. [In Chinese]

117. Yabbara KF, Juffali F, Matossian RM (1977). *Bacillus laterosporus* endophthalmitis. *Archives of Ophthalmology* **95**, 2187–9.

118. Gruner E, *et al.* (1994). Human infections caused by *Brevibacterium casei*, formerly CDC groups B-1 and B-3. *Journal of Clinical Microbiology* **32**, 1511–18.

119. Funke G, Punter V, von Graevenit A (1996). Antimicrobial susceptibility patterns of some recently established coryneform bacteria. *Antimicrobial Agents and Chemotherapy* **40**, 2874–8.

120. Segers P, *et al.* (1994). Classification of *Pseudomonas diminuta* Leifson and Hugh 1954 and *Pseudomonas vesicularis* Büsing, Döll, and Freytag 1953 in *Brevundimonas* gen. nov. as *Brevundimonas diminuta* comb. nov. and *Brevundimonas vesicularis* comb. nov., respectively. *International Journal of Systematic Bacteriology* **44**, 499–510.

121. Lulu AR, *et al.* (1988). Human brucellosis in Kuwait: a prospective study of 400 cases. *Quarterly Journal of Medicine* **66**, 39–54.

122. Gessner AR, Mortensen JE (1990). Pathogenic factors of *Pseudomonas cepacia* isolates from patients with cystic fibrosis. *Journal of Medical Microbiology* **33**, 115–20.

123. Glass S, Govan JRW (1986). *Pseudomonas cepacia*—fatal pulmonary infection in a patient with cystic fibrosis. *Journal of Infection* **13**, 157–8.

124. Miller R, Pannell L, Ingalls MS (1948). Experimental chemotherapy in glanders and melioidosis. *American Journal of Hygiene* **47**, 205–13.

125. Dance DAB (1990). Melioidosis. *Reviews in Medical Microbiology* **1**, 143–50.

126. Dance DAB (1991). Melioidosis: the tip of the iceberg? *Clinical Microbiology Reviews* **4**, 52–60.

127. Dionisio D, *et al.* (1992). Appendicite: interazioni microbiche e nuovi patogeni. *Recenti Progressi in Medicina* **83**, 330–6.

128. Freney J, *et al.* (1988). Susceptibilities to antibiotics and antiseptics of new species of the family *Enterobacteriaceae*. *Antimicrobial Agents and Chemotherapy* **32**, 873–6.

129. Johnson CC, Finegold SM (1987). Uncommonly encountered, motile, anaerobic gram-negative bacilli associated with infection. *Reviews of Infectious Diseases* **9**, 1150–62.

130. Blazer MJ (1990). *Campylobacter* species. In: Mandell GL, Douglas RG, Bennett JE, eds. *Principles and practice of infectious diseases*, 3rd edn. Churchill Livingstone, New York.

131. Figura N, *et al.* (1993). Two cases of *Campylobacter mucosalis* enteritis in children. *Journal of Clinical Microbiology* **31**, 727–8.

132. Francioli P, *et al.* (1985). *Campylobacter fetus* subspecies *fetus* bacteremia. *Archives of Internal Medicine* **145**, 289–92.

133. Edmonds P, *et al.* (1987). *Campylobacter hyointestinalis* associated with human gastrointestinal disease in the United States. *Journal of Clinical Microbiology* **25**, 685–91.

134. Simon AE, Wilcox L (1987). Enteritis associated with *Campylobacter laridis*. *Journal of Clinical Microbiology* **25**, 10–12.

135. von Graevenitz A (1990). Revised nomenclature of *Campylobacter laridis*, *Enterobacter intermedium*, and '*Flavobacterium branchiophila*.' *International Journal of Systematic Bacteriology* **40**, 211.

136. Walmsley SL, Karmali MA (1989). Direct isolation of atypical thermophilic *Campylobacter* species from human feces on selective agar medium. *Journal of Clinical Microbiology* **27**, 668–70.

137. Gaudreau C, Lamothe F (1992). *Campylobacter upsalensis* isolated from a breast abscess. *Journal of Clinical Microbiology* **30**, 1354–6.

138. Decoster H, Snoeck J, Pattyn S (1992). *Capnocytophaga canimorsus* endocarditis. *European Heart Journal* **13**, 140–2.

139. Brenner DJ, *et al.* (1989). *Capnocytophaga canimorsus* sp. nov. (formerly CDC group DF-2), a cause of septicemia following dog bite, and *C. cynodegmi* sp. nov., a cause of localised wound infection following dog bite. *Journal of Clinical Microbiology* **5**, 231–5.

140. Anderson HK, Pedersen M (1992). Infective endocarditis with involvement of the tricuspid valve due to *Capnocytophaga canimorsus*. *European Journal of Clinical Microbiology and Infectious Diseases* **11**, 831–2.

141. Bilgrami S, *et al.* (1992). *Capnocytophaga* bacteremia in a patient with Hodgkin's disease following bone marrow transplantation: case report and review. *Clinical Infectious Diseases* **14**, 1045–9.

142. Sundqvist G (1992). Associations between microbial species in dental root canal infections. *Oral Microbiology and Immunology* **7**, 257–62.

143. Savage DD, *et al.* (1977). *Cardiobacterium hominis* endocarditis: description of two patients and characterisation of the organism. *Journal of Clinical Microbiology* **27**, 75–80.

144. Wormser GP, Bottone EJ (1983). *Cardiobacterium hominis*: review of microbiologic and clinical features. *Reviews of Infectious Diseases* **5**, 680–91.

145. Moore LVH, Moore WEC (1994). *Oribaculum catoniae* gen. nov., sp. nov.; *Catonella morbi* gen. nov., sp. nov.; *Hallella seregens* gen. nov., sp. nov.; *Johnsonella ignava* gen. nov., sp. nov.; and *Dialister pneumosintes* gen. nov., comb. nov., nom. rev, anaerobic gram-negative bacilli from the human gingival crevice. *International Journal of Systematic Bacteriology* **44**, 187–92.

146. Gill VJ, Travis LB, Williams DY (1991). Clinical and microbiological observations on CDC group DF-3, a Gram-negative coccobacillus. *Journal of Clinical Microbiology* **29**, 1589–92.

147. Blum RN, *et al.* (1992). Clinical illness associated with isolation of dysgonic fermenter 3 from stool samples. *Journal of Clinical Microbiology* **30**, 396–400.

148. Aronson N, Zbick CJ (1988). Dysgonic fermenter 3 bacteremia in a neutropenic patient with acute lymphocytic leukemia. *Journal of Clinical Microbiology* **26**, 2213–15.

149. Bangsborg JM, Frederiksen W, Bruun B (1990). Dysgonic fermenter 3-associated abscess in a diabetic patient. *Journal of Infection* **20**, 237–40.

150. Farmer JJ III, *et al.* (1982). Bacteremia due to *Cedecea neteri* sp. nov. *Journal of Clinical Microbiology* **16**, 775–8.

151. Grimont PAD, *et al.* (1981). *Cedecea davisae* gen. nov., sp. nov. and *Cedecea lapagei* sp. nov., new *Enterobacteriaceae* from clinical specimens. *International Journal of Systematic Bacteriology* **31**, 317–26.

152. Funke G, Ramos CP, Collins MD (1995). Identification of some clinical strains of CDC coryneform group A-3 and A-4 bacteria as *Cellulomonas* species and proposal of *Cellulomonas hominis* sp. nov. for some group A-3 strains. *Journal of Clinical Microbiology* **33**, 2091–7.

153. Le Prowse C, McNeil MM, McCarty JM (1989). Catheter-related bacteremia caused by *Oerskovia turbata*. *Journal of Clinical Microbiology* **27**, 571–2.

154. Reller LB, *et al.* (1975). Bacterial endocarditis caused by *Oeskovia turbata*. *Annals of Internal Medicine* **83**, 664–6.

155. Lai CH, *et al.* (1983). *Centipeda periodontii* gen. nov., sp. nov., from human periodontal lesions. *International Journal of Systematic Bacteriology* **33**, 628–35.

156. Everett KDE, Bush RM, Andersen AA (1999). Emended description of the order *Chlamydiales*, proposal of *Parachlamydiaceae* fam. nov. and *Simkaniaceae* fam. nov., each containing one monotypic genus, revised taxonomy of the family *Chlamydiaceae*, including a new genus and five new species, and standards for the identification of organisms. *International Journal of Systematic Bacteriology* **49**, 415–40.

157. Tucker RE, Winter WG, Wilson HD (1979). Osteomyelitis associated with *Chromobacterium violaceum* sepsis: a case report. *Journal of Bone and Joint Surgery* **61**, 949–51.

158. Feldman RB (1984). *Chromobacterium violaceum* infection of the eye: a report of two cases. *Archives of Ophthalmology* **102**, 711–13.

159. Sorensen RU, Jacobns MR, Shurin SB (1985). *Chromobacterium violaceum* adenitis acquired in the northern United States as a complication of chronic granulomatous disease. *Pediatric Infectious Disease* **4**, 701–2.

160. Thong ML, Puthucheary SD, Lee EL (1981). *Flavobacterium meningosepticum* infection: an epidemiological study in a newborn nursery. *Journal of Clinical Pathology* **34**, 429–33.

161. Hsueh PR, *et al.* (1997). Increasing incidence of nosocomial *Chryseobacterium indologenes* infections in Taiwan. *European Journal of Clinical Microbiology and Infectious Diseases* **16**, 568–74.

162. Fraser SL, Jorgensen JH (1997). Reappraisal of the antimicrobial susceptibilities of *Chryseobacterium* and *Flavobacterium* species and methods for reliable susceptibility testing. *Antimicrobial Agents and Chemotherapy* **41**, 2738–41.

163. Doran TI (1999). The role of *Citrobacter* in clinical disease of children: review. *Clinical Infectious Diseases* **28**, 384–94.

164. Bittner J (1980). The clinical significance, taxonomy and special methodological problems of the pathogenic clostridia. *Infection* **8**(**Suppl** 2), 117–22.

165. Kageyama A, Benno Y, Nakase T (1999). Phylogenetic and phenotypic evidence for the transfer of *Eubacterium aerofaciens* to the genus *Collinsella* as *Collinsella aerofaciens* gen. nov., comb. nov. *International Journal of Systematic Bacteriology* **49**, 557–65.

166. Atkinson BE, Smith DL, Lockwood WR (1975). *Pseudomonas testosteroni* septicemia. *Annals of Internal Medicine* **83**, 369–70.

167. Tamaoka J, Ha D-M, Komagata K (1987). Reclassification of *Pseudomonas acidovorans* den Dooren de Jong 1926 and *Pseudomonas testosteroni* Marcus and Talalay 1956 as *Comamonas acidovorans* comb. nov. and *Comamonas testosteroni* comb. nov., with an emended description of the genus *Comamonas*. *International Journal of Systematic Bacteriology* **37**, 52–9.

168. Lipsky BA, *et al.* (1982). Infections caused by non-diphtheria corynebacteria. *Reviews of Infectious Diseases* **4**, 1220–35.

169. Funke G, Lawson PA, Collins MD (1995). Heterogeneity within human-derived centers for disease control and prevention (CDC) coryneform group ANF-1-like bacteria and description of *Corynebacterium auris* sp. nov. *International Journal of Systematic Bacteriology* **45**, 735–9.

170. Vale JA, Scott GW (1977). *Corynebacterium bovis* as a cause of human disease. *Lancet* **2**, 682–4.

171. Philippon A, Bimet F (1990). *In vitro* susceptibility of *Corynebacterium* Group D2 and *Corynebacterium jeikeium* to twelve antibiotics. *European Journal of Clinical Microbiology and Infectious Diseases.* **9**, 892–5.

172. Gill VL, *et al.* (1981). Antibiotic-resistant group JK bacteria in hospitals. *Journal of Clinical Microbiology* **13**, 472–7.

173. Quinn JP, *et al.* (1984). Outbreak of JK diphtheroid infections associated with environmental contamination. *Journal of Clinical Microbiology* **19**, 668–71.

174. Messina OD, *et al.* (1989). *Corynebacterium kutscheri* septic arthritis. *Arthritis and Rheumatism* **32**, 1053.

175. Wilhelmus KR, Robinson NM, Jones DB (1979). *Bacterionema matruchotii* ocular infections. *American Journal of Ophthalmology* **87**, 143–7.

176. Funke G, Punter V, von Graevenitz A (1996). Antimicrobial susceptibility patterns of some recently established coryneform bacteria. *Antimicrobial Agents and Chemotherapy* **40**, 2874–8.

177. Barr JG, Murphy PG (1986). *Corynebacterium striatum*: an unusual organism isolated in pure culture from sputum. *Journal of Infection* **13**, 297–8.

178. Chomarat M, Breton P, Dubost J (1991). Osteomyelitis due to *Corynebacterium* group D2. *European Journal of Clinical Microbiology and Infectious Diseases* **10**, 43.

179. Soriano F, Ponte C (1992). A case of urinary tract infection caused by *Corynebacterium urealyticum* and coryneform group F1. *European Journal of Clinical Microbiology and Infectious Diseases* **11**, 626–8.

180. Soriano F, Fernandez-Roblas R (1988). Infections caused by antibiotic-resistant *Corynebacterium* group D2. *European Journal of Clinical Microbiology and Infectious Diseases* **7**, 337–41.

181. Porschen RK, Goodman Z, Rafai B (1977). Isolation of *Coryebacterium xerosis* from clinical specimens. *American Journal of Clinical Pathology* **68**, 290–3.

182. Liakim R, *et al.* (1983). *Corynebacterium xerosis* endocarditis. *Archives of Internal Medicine* **143**, 1995.

183. Krish G, *et al.* (1989). *Corynebacterium xerosis* as cause of vertebral osteomyelitis. *Journal of Clinical Microbiology* **27**, 2869–70.

184. Guillard F, Appelbaum PC, Sparrow FB (1980). Pyelonephritis and septicemia due to Gram-positive rods similar to *Corynebacterium* Group E (aerotolerant *Bifidobacterium adolescentis*). *Annals of Internal Medicine* **92**, 635–6.

185. Austin GE, Hill EO (1983). Endocarditis due to *Corynebacterium* CDC group G2. *Journal of Infectious Diseases* **147**, 1106.

186. Malanoski GJ, Parker R, Eliopoulos GM (1992). Antimicrobial susceptibilities of a *Corynebacterium* CDC group I1 strain isolated from a patient with endocarditis. *Southern Medical Journal* **80**, 923.

187. Tendler C, Bottone EJ (1989). *Corynebacterium aquaticum* urinary tract infection in a neonate and concepts regarding the role of the organism as a neonatal pathogen. *Journal of Clinical Microbiology* **27**, 343–5.

188. Golledge CL, Phillips G (1991). *Corynebacterium minutissimum* infection. *Journal of Infection* **23**, 73–6.

189. Colt HG, *et al.* (1991). Necrotizing tracheitis caused by *Corynebacterium pseudodiphtheriticum*: unique case and review. *Reviews of Infectious Diseases* **13**, 73–6.

190. Goldberger AC, Lipsky BA, Plorde JJ (1981). Suppurative granulomatous lymphadenitis caused by *Corynebacterium ovis (pseudotuberculosis)*. *American Journal of Clinical Pathology* **76**, 486–90.

191. Meers PD (1979). A case of classical diphtheria, and other infections due to *Corynebacterium ulcerans*. *Journal of Infection* **1**, 139–42.

192. Maurin M, Raoult D (1999). Q fever. *Clinical Microbiology Reviews* **12**, 518–53.

193. Nakazawa F, *et al.* (1999). *Cryptobacterium curtum* gen nov., sp. nov., a new genus of Gram-positive anaerobic rod isolatated from human oral cavities. *International Journal of Systematic Bacteriology* **49**, 1193–200.

194. Horowitz H, *et al.* (1990). Endocarditis associated with *Comamonas acidovorans*. *Journal of Clinical Microbiology* **28**, 143–5.

195. Bavbek M, *et al.* (1998). Cerebral *Dermabacter hominis* abscess. *Infection* **26**, 181–3.

196. Pal M (1995). Prevalence in India of *Dermatophilus congolensis* infection in clinical specimens from animals and humans. *Revue Scientifique et Technique* **14**, 857–63.

197. Gibson GR, Macfarlane GT, Cummings JH (1988). Occurrence of sulphate-reducing bacteria in human faeces and the relationship of dissimilatory sulphate reduction to methanogenesis in the large gut. *Journal of Applied Bacteriology* **65**, 103–11.

198. McDougall R, *et al.* (1997). Bacteremia caused by a recently described novel *Desulfovibrio* species. *Journal of Clinical Microbiology* **35**, 1805–8.

199. Tee W, *et al.* (1996). Probable new species of *Desulfovibrio* isolated from a pyogenic liver abscess. *Journal of Clinical Microbiology* **34**, 1760–4.

200. Porschen RK, Chan P (1977). Anaerobic vibrio-like organisms cultured from blood: *Desulfovibrio desulfuricans* and *Succinivibrio* species. *Journal of Clinical Microbiology* **5**, 444–7.

201. Willems A, Collins MD (1995). Phylogenetic placement of *Dialister pneumosintes* (formerly *Bacteroides pneumosintes*) within the *Sporomusa* subbranch of the *Clostridium* subphylum of the gram-positive bacteria. *International Journal of Systematic Bacteriology* **45**, 403–5.

202. Liu D, Yong WK (1997). Improved laboratory diagnosis of ovine footrot: an update. *The Veterinary Journal* **153**, 99–105.

203. Collins MD, *et al.* (1999). *Dolosicoccus paucivorans* gen. nov., sp. nov., isolated from human blood. *International Journal of Systematic Bacteriology* **49**, 1439–42.

204. Aguirre M, *et al.* (1993). Phenotypic and phylogenetic characterization of some *Gemella*-like organisms from human infections: description of *Dolosigranulum pigrum* gen. nov., sp. nov. *Journal of Applied Bacteriology* **75**, 608–12.

205. Miller PH, Facklam RR, Miller JM (1996). Atmospheric growth requirements for *Alloiococcus* species and related gram-positive cocci. *Journal of Clinical Microbiology* **34**, 1027–8.

206. Maskell R, Pead L (1990). A cluster of *Edwardsiella tarda* infection in a day-care center in Florida. *Journal of Infectious Diseases* **162**, 282.

207. Hargreaves JE, Lucey DR (1990). Life-threatening *Edwardsiella tarda* soft tissue infection associated with catfish puncture wound. *Journal of Infectious Diseases* **162**, 1416.

208. Janda JM, *et al.* (1991). Pathogenic properties of *Edwardsiella* species. *Journal of Clinical Microbiology* **29**, 1997–2001.

209. Murphey DK, Septimus EJ, Waagner DC (1990). Catfish-related injury and infection: report of two cases and review of the literature. *Clinical Infectious Diseases* **14**, 689–93.

210. Reger PJ, Mockler DF, Miller MA (1993). Comparison of antimicrobial susceptibility, beta-lactamase production, plasmid analysis and serum bactericidal activity in *Edwardsiella tarda* E *ictaluri* and *E. hoshinae*. *Journal of Medical Microbiology* **39**, 273–81.

211. Kageyama A, Benno Y, Nakase T (1999). Phylogenetic evidence for the transfer of *Eubacterium lentum* to the genus *Eggerthella* as *Eggerthella lenta* gen. nov., comb. nov. *International Journal of Systematic Bacteriology* **49**, 1725–32.

212. McDade JE (1990). Ehrlichiosis—disease of animals and humans. *Journal of Infectious Diseases* **161**, 609–17.

213. Anderson BE, *et al.* (1991). *Ehrlichia chaffeensis*, a new species associated with human ehrlichiosis. *Journal of Clinical Microbiology* **29**, 2838–42.

214. Dupon M, *et al.* (1991). Sacro-iliac joint infection caused by *Eikenella corrodens*. *European Journal of Clinical Microbiology and Infectious Diseases* **10**, 529–30.

215. Stoloff AL, Gillies ML (1986). Infections with *Eikenella corrodens* in a general hospital: a report of 33 cases. *Reviews of Infectious Diseases* **8**, 50–3.

216. Suwangol S, *et al.* (1983). Pathogenicity of *Eikenella corrodens* in humans. *Archives of Internal Medicine* **143**, 2265–8.

217. Pérez-Pomata MT, *et al.* (1992). Spleen abscess caused by *Eikenella corrodens*. *European Journal of Clinical Microbiology and Infectious Diseases* **11**, 162–3.

218. Dees SB, *et al.* (1986). Chemical characterization of *Flavobacterium odoratum*, *Flavobacterium breve*, and *Flavobacterium*-like groups IIe, IIh, and IIf. *Journal of Clinical Microbiology* **23**, 267–73.

219. Sanders WE Jr, Sanders CC (1997). *Enterobacter* spp.: pathogens poised to flourish at the turn of the century. *Clinical Microbiology Reviews* **10**, 220–41.

220. Morrison D, Woodford N, Cookson B (1997). Enterococci as emerging pathogens of humans. *Society for Applied Bacteriology Symposium Series* **26**, S89–99.

221. O'Hara CM, *et al.* (1998). First report of a human isolate of *Erwinia persicinus*. *Journal of Clinical Microbiology* **36**, 248–50.

222. MacGowan AP, Reeves DS (1991). Tricuspid valve infective endocarditis and pulmonary sepsis due to *Erysipelothrix rhusiopathiae* successfully treated with high doses of ciproflaxacin but complicated by gynaecomastia. *Journal of Infection* **22**, 100–1.

223. Venditti M, *et al.* (1990). Antimicrobial susceptibilities of *Erysipelothrix rhusiopathiae*. *Antimicrobial Agents and Chemotherapy* **34**, 2038–40.

224. Brook MG, Bannister BA (1993). Diarrhoea-causing *Escherichia coli*. *Digestive Diseases* **11**, 288–97.

225. Farmer JJ III, *et al.* (1985). *Escherichia fergusonii* and *Enterobacter taylorae*, two new species of *Enterobacteriaceae* isolated from clinical specimens. *Journal of Clinical Microbiology* **21**, 77–81.

226. Brenner DJ, *et al.* (1982). Atypical biogroups of *Escherichia coli* found in clinical specimens and description of *Escherichia hermanii* sp. nov. *Journal of Clinical Microbiology* **15**, 703–13.

227. Brenner DJ, *et al.* (1982). *Escherichia vulneris*: a new species of Enterobacteriaceae associated with human wounds. *Journal of Clinical Microbiology* **15**, 1133–40.

228. Sans MD, Crowder JG (1973). Subacute bacterial endocarditis caused by *Eubacterium aerofaciens*: report of a case. *American Journal of Clinical Pathology* **59**, 576–80.

229. Tew JG, *et al.* (1985). Serum antibody reactive with predominant organisms in the subgingival flora of young adults with generalized severe periodontitis. *Infection and Immunity* **49**, 487–93.

230. Devreese K, Claeys G, Verschraegen G (1992). Septicaemia with *Ewingella americana*. *Journal of Clinical Microbiology* **30**, 2746–7.

231. Collins MD, *et al.* (1997). Phenotypic and phylogenetic characterization of some *Globicatella*-like organisms from human sources: description of *Facklamia hominis* gen. nov., sp. nov. *International Journal of Systematic Bacteriology* **47**, 880–2.

232. Collins MD, *et al.* (1994). The phylogeny of the genus *Clostridium*: proposal of five new genera and eleven new species combinations. *International Journal of Systematic Bacteriology* **44**, 812–26.

233. Jalava J, Eerola E (1999). Phylogenetic analysis of *Fusobacterium alocis* and *Fusobacterium sulci* based on 16S rRNA gene sequences: proposal of *Filifactor alocis* (Cato, Moore and Morre) comb. nov. and *Eubacterium sulci* (Cato, Moore and Moore) comb. nov. *International Journal of Systematic Bacteriology* **49**, 1375–9.

234. Weir S, *et al.* (1999). Recurrent bacteremia caused by a '*Flexispira*'-like organism in a patient with X-linked (Bruton's) agammaglobulinemia. *Journal of Clinical Microbiology* **37**, 2439–45.

235. Sorlin P, *et al.* (1999). Recurrent '*Flexispira rappini*' bacteremia in an adult patient undergoing hemodialysis: case report. *Journal of Clinical Microbiology* **37**, 1319–23.

236. Hollis DG, *et al.* (1989). *Francisella philomiragia* comb. nov (formerly *Yersinia philomiragia*) and *Francisella tularensis* biogroup novicida (formerly *Francisella novicida*) associated with human disease. *Journal of Clinical Microbiology* **27**, 1601–8.

237. Evans ME, *et al.* (1985). Tularemia: a 30-year experience with 88 cases. *Medicine* (Baltimore) **64**, 251–69.

238. Moore-Gillon J, *et al.* (1984). Necrobacillosis: a forgotten disease. *British Medical Journal* **288**, 1526–7.

239. George WL, Kirby BD, Sutter VL (1981). Gram-negative anaerobic bacilli: their role in infection and patterns of susceptibility to antibiotic agents. II Little-known *Fusobacterium* species with miscellaneous genera. *Reviews of Infectious Diseases* **3**, 599–626.

240. Hillier SL (1993). Diagnostic microbiology of bacterial vaginosis. *American Journal of Obstetrics and Gynecology* **169**, 455–9.

241. Chatelain R, *et al.* (1982). Isolement de *Gemella haemolysans* dans trois cas d'endocardites bacteriennes. *Médecine et Maladies Infectieuses* **12**, 25–30.

242. Kilpper-Bälz R, Schleifer KH (1988). Transfer of *Streptococcus morbillorum* to the *Gemella* genus, *Gemella morbillorum* comb. nov. *International Journal of Systematic Bacteriology* **38**, 442–3.

243. Collins MD, *et al.* (1992). *Globicatella sanguis* gen. nov., sp. nov., a new gram-positive catalase-negative bacterium from human sources. *Journal of Applied Bacteriology* **73**, 433–7.

244. Drancourt M, *et al.* (1994). Brain abscess due to *Gordona terrae* in an immunocompromised child: case report and review of infections caused by *G. terrae*. *Clinical Infectious Diseases* **19**, 258–62.

245. Drancourt M, *et al.* (1997). *Gordona terrae* central nervous system infection in an immunocompetent patient. *Journal of Clinical Microbiology* **35**, 379–82.

246. Richet HM, *et al.* (1991). A cluster of *Rhodococcus (Gordona) Bronchialis* sternal-wound infections after coronary-artery bypass surgery. *New England Journal of Medicine* **10**, 104–9.

247. Riegel P, *et al.* (1996). Bacteremia due to *Gordona sputi* in an immunocompromised patient. *Journal of Clinical Microbiology* **34**, 2045–7.

248. Brenner DJ, *et al.* (1988). Biochemical, genetic, and epidemiologic characterization of *Haemophilus influenzae* biogroup aegyptius (*Haemophilus aegyptius*) strains associated with Brazilian purpuric fever. *Journal of Clinical Microbiology* **26**, 1524–34.

249. Brazilian Purpuric Fever Study Group (1987). *Haemophilus aegyptius* bacteremia in Brazilian purpuric fever. *Lancet* **2**, 761–3.

250. Bieger RC, Brewer NS, Washington JA II (1978). *Haemphilus aphrophilus*: a microbiologic and clinical review and report of 42 cases. *Medicine* (Baltimore) **57**, 345–55.

251. Goldberg R, Washington JA II (1978). The taxonomy and antimicrobial susceptibility of *Haemophilus* species in clinical specimens. *American Journal of Clinical Pathology* **70**, 899–904.

252. Julander I, Lindberg AA, Swanbom M (1980). *Haemophilus parainfluenzae*: an uncommon cause of septicemia and endocarditis. *Scandinavian Journal of Infectious Diseases* 12, 85–9.

253. Jones RN, Slepack J, Bigelow J (1976). Ampicillin-resistant *Haemophilis paraphrophilus* laryngo-epiglottitis. *Journal of Clinical Microbiology* 4, 405–7.

254. Visvanathan K, Jones PD (1991). Ciprofloxacin treatment of *Haemophilus paraphrophilus* brain abscess. *Journal of Infection* 22, 306–7.

255. Schmid GP (1999). Treatment of chancroid, 1997. *Clinical Infectious Diseases* 28(Suppl 1), 14–20.

256. Jordens JZ, Slack MP (1995). *Haemophilus influenzae*: then and now. *European Journal of Clinical Microbiology and Infectious Diseases* 14, 935–48.

257. Washington JA III, Birk RJ, Ritts RE (1971). Bacteriologic and epidemiologic characteristics of *Enterobacter hafniae* and *Enterobacter liquefaciens*. *Journal of Infectious Diseases* 124, 379.

258. Stanley J, et al. (1993). *Helicobacter canis* sp. nov., a new species from dogs: an integrated study of phenotype and genotype. *Journal of General Microbiology* 139, 2495–504.

259. Orlicek SL, Welch DF, Kuhls TL (1993). Septicemia caused by *Helicobacter cinaedi* in a neonate. *Journal of Clinical Microbiology* 31, 569–71.

260. Vandamme P, et al. (1990). Identification of *Campylobacter cinaedi* isolated from blood and faeces of children and adult females. *Journal of Clinical Microbiology* 28, 1016–20.

261. Totten PA, et al. (1985). *Campylobacter cinaedi* (sp. nov.) and *Campylobacter fennelliae* (sp. nov.): two new campylobacter species associated with enteric disease in homosexual men. *Journal of Infectious Diseases* 151, 131–9.

262. Meining A, Kroher G, Stolte M (1998). Animal reservoirs in the transmission of *Helicobacter heilmannii*. Results of a questionnaire-based study. *Scandinavian Journal of Gastroenterology* 33, 795–8.

263. Stanley J, et al. (1994). *Helicobacter pullorum* sp. nov.—genotype and phenotype of a new species isolated from poultry and from human patients with gastroenteritis. *Microbiology* 140, 3441–9.

264. Marshall BJ (1986). *Campylobacter pyloridis* and gastritis. *Journal of Infectious Diseases* 153, 650–7.

265. Chagla AH, et al. (1998). Breast abscess associated with *Helcococcus kunzii*. *Journal of Clinical Microbiology* 36, 2377–9.

266. Peel MM, et al. (1997). *Helcococcus kunzii* as sole isolate from an infected sebaceous cyst. *Journal of Clinical Microbiology* 35, 328–9.

267. Willems A, et al. (1997). Phenotypic and phylogenetic characterization of some *Eubacterium*-like isolates containing a novel type B wall murein from human feces: description of *Holdemania filiformis* gen. nov., sp. nov. *International Journal of Systematic Bacteriology* 47, 1201–4.

268. Collins MD, et al. (1999). *Ignavigranum ruoffiae* sp. nov., isolated from human clinical specimens. *International Journal of Systematic Bacteriology* 49, 97–101.

268a. Moore LV, Moore WE (1994). *Orbiculum catoniae* gen. nov., sp. nov.; *Catonella morbi* gen. nov., sp. nov.; *Hallella seregens* gen. nov., sp. nov.; *Johnsonella ignava* gen. nov., sp. nov.; and *Dialister pneumosintes* gen. nov., comb. nov., nom. rev.; anaerobic Gram-negative bacteria from the human gingival crevice. *International Journal of Systematic Bacteriology* 44, 187–92.

269. Yagupsky P, et al. (1992). High prevalence of *Kingella kingae* in joint fluid from children with septic arthritis revealed by the BACTEC blood culture system. *Journal of Clinical Microbiology* 30, 1278–81.

270. Goldman IS, et al. (1980). Infective endocarditis due to *Kingella denitrificans*. *Annals of Internal Medicine* 93, 152–3.

271. Jenny DB, Letendre PW, Iverson G (1988). Endocarditis due to *Kingella* species. *Reviews of Infectious Diseases* 10, 1065–6.

272. Namnyak SS, Quinn RJM, Ferguson JDM (1991). *Kingella kingae* meningitis in an infant. *Journal of Infection* 23, 104–6.

273. Carter JS, et al. (1999). Phylogenetic evidence for reclassification of *Calymmatobacterium granulomatis* as *Klebsiella granulomatis* comb. nov. *International Journal of Systematic Bacteriology* 49, 1695–700.

274. Chetoui H, et al. (1999). Epidemiological typing of extended-spectrum beta-lactamase-producing *Klebsiella pneumoniae* isolates by pulsed-field gel electrophoresis and antibiotic susceptibility patterns. *Research in Microbiology* 150, 265–72.

275. Miller RH, et al. (1979). *Klebsiella rhinoscleromatis*: a clinical and pathogenic enigma. *Otolaryngology—Head and Neck Surgery* 87, 212–21.

276. Farmer JJ III, et al. (1981). *Kluyvera*, a new (redefined) genus in the family Enterobacteriaceae: identification of *Kluyvera ascorbata* sp. nov. and *Kluyvera cryocrescens* sp. nov. in clinical specimens. *Journal of Clinical Microbiology* 13, 919–33.

277. Sierra-Madero J, et al. (1990). *Kluyvera* mediastinitis following open-heart surgery: a case report. *Journal of Clinical Microbiology* 28, 2848–9.

278. Stackenbrandt E, et al. (1995). Taxonomic dissection of the genus *Micrococcus*: *Kocuria* gen. nov., *Nesterenkonia* gen. nov., *Kytococcus* gen. nov., *Dermacoccus* gen. nov., and *Micrococcus* Cohn 1872 gen. emend. *International Journal of Systematic Bacteriology* 45, 682–92.

279. Hickman-Brenner FW, et al. (1985). *Koserella trabulsii*, a new genus and species of Enterobacteriaceae formerly known as enteric group 45. *Journal of Clinical Microbiology* 21, 39–42.

280. Elston HR (1961). *Kurthia bessonii* isolated from clinical material. *Journal of Pathology and Bacteriology* 81, 245–7.

281. Pancoast SJ, et al. (1979). Endocarditis due to *Kurthia bessonii*. *Annals of Internal Medicine* 90, 936–7.

282. Keddie RM, Shaw S (1986). Genus *Kurthia* Trevisan 1885, 92^AL Nom. cons. Opin. 13 Jud. Comm. 1954, 152. In: Sneath PHA, et al., eds. *Bergey's manual of systematic bacteriology*, Vol. 2. Williams and Willkins, Baltimore, MD.

283. Chomarat M, Espinouse D (1991). *Lactobacillus rhamosus* septicemia in patients with prolonged aplasia receiving ceftazidime–vancomycin. *European Journal of Clinical Microbiology and Infectious Diseases* 10, 44.

284. Rahman M (1982). Chest infection caused by *Lactobacillus casei* ss *rhamosus*. *British Medical Journal* 284, 471–2.

285. Sussman JI, et al. (1986). Clinical manifestation and therapy of *Lactobacillus* endocarditis: report of a case and review of the literature. *Reviews of Infectious Diseases* 8, 771–6.

286. Bantar CE, et al. (1991). Abscess caused by vancomycin-resistant *Lactobacillus confusus*. *Journal of Clinical Microbiology* 29, 2063–4.

287. Elliott JA, et al. (1991). Differentiation of *Lactococcus lactis* and *Lactococcus garviae* from humans by comparison of whole-cell protein patterns. *Journal of Clinical Microbiology* 29, 2731–4.

288. Rossmann SN, et al. (1998). Isolation of *Lautropia mirabilis* from oral cavities of human immunodeficiency virus-infected children. *Journal of Clinical Microbiology* 36, 1756–60.

289. Tamura K, et al. (1986). *Leclercia adecatrboxylata* gen nov., comb. nov., formerly known as *Escherichia adecarboxylata*. *Current Microbiology* 13, 179–82.

290. Benson RF, Fields BS (1998). Classification of the genus *Legionella*. *Seminars in Respiratory Infections* 13, 90–9.

291. Hickman-Brenner F, et al. (1985). *Leminorella*, a new genus of Enterobacteriaceae: identification of *Leminorella grimontii* sp. nov. and *Leminorella richardii* sp. nov. found in clinical specimens. *Journal of Clinical Microbiology* 21, 234–9.

292. Lecour H, et al. (1989). Human leptospirosis: a review of 50 cases. *Infection* 17, 8–11.

293. Vemelen K, et al. (1996). Bacteraemia with *Leptotrichia buccalis*: report of a case and review of the literature. *Acta Clinica Belgica* 51, 265–70.

294. Friedland IR, Snipelisky M, Khoosal M (1990). Meningitis in a neonate caused by *Leuconostoc* sp. *Journal of Clinical Microbiology* 28, 2125–6.

295. Bernaldo de Quirós JCL, et al. (1991). *Leuconostoc* species as a cause of bacteremia: two case reports and a literature review. *European Journal of Clinical Microbiology and Infectious Diseases* 10, 505–9.

296. Horowitz HW, Handwerger S, van Horn KG (1987). *Leuconostoc*, an emerging vancomycin-resistant pathogen. *Lancet* 1, 1329–30.

297. Hof H, Nichterlein T, Kretschmar M (1997). Management of listeriosis. *Clinical Microbiology Reviews* 10, 345–57.

298. Brancaccio M, Legendri GG (1979). *Megasphaera eldenii* endocarditis. *Journal of Clinical Microbiology* **10**, 72–4.

299. Kaye KM, Macone A, Kazanjian PH (1992). Catheter infection caused by *Methylobacterium* in immunocompromised hosts: report of three cases and review of the literature. *Clinical Infectious Diseases* **14**, 1010–14.

300. Gould FK, Venning MC, Ford M (1990). Successful treatment with chloramphenicol of *Pseudomonas mesophilica* peritonitis not resonding to aztreonam and gentamicin. *Journal of Antimicrobial Chemotherapy* **26**, 458–9.

301. Rutherford PC, *et al.* (1988). Peritonitis caused by *Pseudomonas mesophilica* in a patient undergoing continuous ambulatory peritoneal dialysis. *Journal of Clinical Microbiology* **26**, 2441–3.

302. Smith SM, Eng RHK, Forrester C (1985). *Pseudomonas mesophilica* infections in humans. *Journal of Clinical Microbiology* **21**, 314–17.

303. Funke G, *et al.* (1997). Endophthalmitis due to *Microbacterium* species: case report and review of microbacterium infections. *Clinical Infectious Diseases* **24**, 713–16.

304. Funke G, *et al.* (1998). *Aureobacterium resistens* sp. nov., exhibiting vancomycin resistance and teicoplanin susceptibility. *FEMS Microbiology Letters* **158**, 89–93.

305. Saweljew P, *et al.* (1996). Case of fatal systemic infection with an *Aureobacterium* sp.: identification of isolate by 16S rRNA gene analysis. *Journal of Clinical Microbiology* **34**, 1540–1.

306. Nolte FS, *et al.* (1996). Vancomycin-resistant *Aureobacterium* species cellulitis and bacteremia in a patient with acute myelogenous leukemia. *Journal of Clinical Microbiology* **34**, 1992–4.

307. Hagiwara S, *et al.* (1995). [Hypersensitivity pneumonitis caused by a home humidifier]. *Nihon Kyobu Shikkan Gakkai Zasshi* **33**, 1024–9. [In Japanese]

308. Peces R, *et al.* (1997). Relapsing bacteraemia due to *Micrococcus luteus* in a haemodialysis patient with a Perm-Cath catheter. *Nephrology, Dialysis, Transplantation* **12**, 2428–9.

309. Shah HN, Collins MD (1982). Reclassification of *Bacteroides multiacidus* (Mitsuoka, Terada, Watanabe and Uchida) in a new genus *Mitsuokella*, as *Mitsuokella multiacidus* comb. nov. *Zentralblatt fur Bakteriologie, Parasitenkunde, Infektionskrankhe und Hygiene. Abstract 1, Orig.* **C3**, 491–4.

310. Schwebke JR, *et al.* (1991). Identification of two new antigenic subgroups within the genus *Mobiluncus*. *Journal of Clinical Microbiology* **29**, 2204–8.

311. Glupczynski T, *et al* (1984). Isolation of *Mobiluncus* in four cases of extragenital infection in adult women. *European Journal of Clinical Microbiology* **3**, 433–5.

312. Spiegel CA (1987). Susceptibility of *Mobiluncus* species to 23 antimicrobial agents and 15 other compounds. *Antimicrobial Agents and Chemotherapy* **31**, 249–52.

313. Hickman-Brenner FW, *et al.* (1984). *Moellerella wisconsensis*, a new genus and species of *Enterobacteriaceae* found in human stool specimens. *Journal of Clinical Microbiology* **19**, 460–3.

314. Silverfarb PM, Lawe JE (1968). Endocarditis due to *Moraxella liquefaciens*. *Archives of Internal Medicine* **122**, 512–13.

315. Ebright JR, Lentino JR, Juni E (1982). Endophthalmitis caused by *Moraxella nonliquefaciens*. *American Journal of Clinical Pathology* **77**, 362–3.

316. Bøvre K, Henriksen SD (1967). A new *Moraxella* species, *Moraxella osloensis*, and a revised description of *Moraxella nonliquefaciens*. *International Journal of Systematic Bacteriology* **17**, 127–35.

317. Bøvre K, Fuglesang JE, Hagen N (1976). *Moraxella atlantae* sp. nov. and its distinction from *Moraxella phenylpyruvica*. *International Journal of Systematic Bacteriology* **26**, 511–21.

318. Percival A, *et al.* (1977). Pathogenicity of and beta-lactamase production by *Branhamella (Neisseria) catarrhalis*. *Lancet* **2**, 1175.

319. Salen PN, Eppes S (1997). *Morganella morganii*: a newly reported, rare cause of neonatal sepsis. *Academic Emergency Medicine* **4**, 711–14.

320. Falkinham JO 3rd (1996). Epidemiology of infection by nontuberculous mycobacteria. *Clinical Microbiology Reviews* **9**, 177–215.

321. Taylor-Robinson D, Bebear C (1997). Antibiotic susceptibilities of mycoplasmas and treatment of mycoplasmal infections. *Journal of Antimicrobial Chemotherapy* **40**, 622–30.

322. Vancanneyt M, *et al.* (1996). Reclassification of *Flavobacterium odoratum* (Stutzer 1929) strains to a new genus, *Myroides*, as *Myroides odoratus* comb. nov. and *Myroides odoratimimus* sp. nov. *International Journal of Systematic Bacteriology* **46**, 926–32.

323. Guidbourdenche M, Lambert T, Riou JY (1989). Isolation of *Neisseria canis* in mixed culture from a patient after a cat bite. *Journal of Clinical Microbiology* **27**, 1673–4.

324. Herbert DA, Ruskin J (1981). Are the 'non-pathogenic' neisseriae pathogenic? *American Journal of Clinical Pathology* **75**, 739–43.

325. Morla N, Guibourdenche M, Riou J-Y (1992). *Neiseria* spp. and AIDS. *Journal of Clinical Microbiology* **30**, 2290–4.

326. Wong JD, Janda JM (1992). *Neisseria* species, *Neisseria elongata* subsp. *nitroreductens*, with bacteremia, endocarditis, and osteomyelitis. *Journal of Clinical Microbiology* **30**, 719–20.

327. Berger SA, *et al.* (1988). Bartholin's gland abscess caused by *Neisseria sicca*. *Journal of Clinical Microbiology* **26**, 1589.

328. Gay RM, Sevier RE (1978). *Neisseria sicca* endocarditis: report of a case and review of the literature. *Journal of Clinical Microbiology* **8**, 729–32.

329. Lind I (1997). Antimicrobial resistance in *Neisseria gonorrhoeae*. *Clinical Infectious Diseases* **24**(Suppl 1), 93–7.

330. Oppenheim BA (1997). Antibiotic resistance in *Neisseria meningitidis*. *Clinical Infectious Diseases* **24**(Suppl 1), 98–101.

331. Boiron P, *et al.* (1998). *Nocardia*, nocardiosis and mycetoma. *Medical Mycology* **36**(Suppl 1), 26–37.

332. Yassin AF, *et al.* (1997). Description of *Nocardiopsis synnemataformans* sp. nov., elevation of *Nocardiopsis alba* subsp. *prasina* to *Nocardiopsis prasina* comb. nov., and designation of *Nocardiopsis antarctica* and *Nocardiopsis alborubida* as later subjective synonyms of *Nocardiopsis dassonvillei*. *International Journal of Systematic Bacteriology* **47**, 983–8.

333. Holmes B, *et al.* (1988). *Ochrobactrum anthropi* gen. nov., sp. nov. from human clinical specimens and previously known as group Vd. *International Journal of Systematic Bacteriology* **38**, 406–16.

334. Moller LVM, *et al.* (1999). *Ochrobactrum intermedium* infection after liver transplantation. *Journal of Clinical Microbiology* **37**, 241–4.

335. Rihs JD, *et al.* (1990). *Oerskovia xanthineolytica* implicated in peritonitis associated with peritoneal dialysis: case report and review of *Oerskovia* infections in humans. *Journal of Clinical Microbiology* **28**, 1934–7.

336. Cruikshank SJ, Gawler AH, Shaldon G (1979). *Oerskovia* species: rare opportunistic pathogens. *Journal of Medical Microbiology* **12**, 513–15.

337. Truant AL, *et al.* (1992). *Oerskovia xanthinolytica* and methicillin-resistant *Staphylococcus aureus* in a patient with cirrhosis and variceal hemorrhage. *European Journal of Clinical Microbiology and Infectious Diseases* **11**, 950–1.

338. Kailath EJ, Goldstein E, Wagner FH (1988). Case report: meningitis caused by *Oeskovia xanthinolytica*. *American Journal of Medical Sciences* **295**, 216–17.

339. Hussain Z, *et al.* (1987). Endophthalmitis due to *Oeskovia xanthinolytica*. *Canadian Journal of Ophthalmology* **22**, 234–6.

340. Mesnard R, *et al.* (1992). Septic arthritis due to *Oligella urethralis*. *European Journal of Clinical Microbiology and Infectious Diseases* **11**, 195–6.

341. Rossau R, *et al.* (1987). *Oligella*, a new genus including *Oligella urethralis* comb. nov (formerly *Moraxella urethralis*) and *Oligella ureolytica* sp. nov (formerly CDC group IVe): relationship to *Taylorella equigenitalis* and related taxa. *International Journal of Systematic Bacteriology* **37**, 198–210.

342. Silpapojakul K (1997). Scrub typhus in the Western Pacific region. *Annals of the Academy of Medicine Singapore* **26**, 794–800.

343. Coudron PE, Payne JM, Markowitz SM (1991). Pneumonia and empyema infection associated with a *Bacillus* species that resembles *B. alvei*. *Journal of Clinical Microbiology* **29**, 1777–9.

344. Olenginski TP, Bush DC, Harrington TM (1991). Plant thorn synovitis: an uncommon cause of monoarthritis. *Seminars in Arthritis and Rheumatism* **21**, 40–6.

345. Sneath PHA, Stevens M (1990). *Actinobacillus rossii* sp. nov., *Actinobacillus seminis* sp. nov., nom. rev, *Pasteurella bettii* sp. nov., *Pasteurella lymphangitidis* sp. nov., *Pasteurella mairi* sp. nov., and *Pasteuerella trehalosi* sp. nov. *International Journal of Systematic Bacteriology* **40**, 148–53.

346. Johnson RH, Rumans LW (1977). Unusual infections caused by *Pasteurella multocida*. *Journal of the American Medical Association* **237**, 146–47.

347. Rogers BT, *et al.* (1973). Septicaemia due to *Pasteurella pneumotropica*. *Journal of Clinical Pathology* **26**, 396–8.

348. Pouëdras P, *et al.* (1993). *Pasteurella stomatis* infection following dog bite. *European Journal of Clinical Microbiology and Infectious Diseases* **12**, 65.

349. Yaneza AL, *et al.* (1991). *Pasteurella haemolytica* endocarditis. *Journal of Infection* **23**, 65–7.

350. Holst E, *et al.* (1992). Characterization and distribution of *Pasteurella* species recovered from infected humans. *Journal of Clinical Microbiology* **30**, 2984–7.

351. Mastro TD, *et al.* (1990). Vancomycin-resistant *Pediococcus acidilactici*: nine cases of bacteremia. *Journal of Infectious Diseases* **161**, 956–60.

352. Sire JM, *et al.* (1992). Septicaemia and hepatic abscess caused by *Pediococcus acidilactici*. *European Journal of Clinical Microbiology and Infectious Diseases* **11**, 623–5.

353. Sarma PS, Mohanty S (1998). *Pediococcus acidilactici* pneumonitis and bacteremia in a pregnant woman. *Journal of Clinical Microbiology* **36**, 2392–3.

354. Colman G, Efstratiou A (1987). Vancomycin-resistant leuconostocs, lactobacilli and now pediococci. *Journal of Hospital Infection* **2**, 1–3.

355. Petrini B, Welin-Berger T, Nord CE (1979). Anaerobic bacteria in late infections following orthopedic surgery. *Medical Microbiology and Immunology* (Berlin) **167**, 155–9.

356. Sklavounos A, *et al.* (1986). Anaerobic bacteria in dentoalveolar abscesses. *International Journal of Oral and Maxillofacial Surgery* **15**, 288–91.

357. Murdoch DA, Mitchelmore IJ, Tabaqchali S (1994). The clinical importance of gram-positive anaerobic cocci isolated at St. Bartholomew's Hospital, London, in 1987. *Journal of Medical Microbiology* **41**, 36–44.

358. Murdoch DA, *et al.* (1997). Description of three new species of the genus *Peptostreptococcus* from human clinical specimens: *Peptostreptococcus harei* sp. nov., *Peptostreptococcus ivorii*, sp. nov., and *Peptostreptococcus octavius* sp. nov. *International Journal of Systematic Bacteriology* **47**, 781–7.

359. Pelz K, Mutters R (1997). Taxonomic update and clinical significance of species within the genus *Peptostreptococcus*. *Clinical Infectious Diseases* **25**(Suppl), 94–7.

360. Coffey JA, *et al.* (1986). *Vibrio damsela*: another potentially virulent marine vibrio. *Journal of Infectious Diseases* **153**, 800–2.

361. Farmer JJ III, *et al* (1989). *Xenorhabdus luminescens* (DNA hybridization group 5) from human clinical specimens. *Journal of Clinical Microbiology* **27**, 1594–600.

362. Clark RB, *et al.* (1990). *In vitro* susceptibilities of *Plesiomonas shigelloides* to 24 antibiotics and antibiotic-β-lactamase-inhibitor combinations. *Antimicrobial Agents Chemotherapy* **34**, 159–60.

363. Brenden RA, Miller MA, Janda JM (1988). Clinical disease spectrum and pathogenic factors associated with *Plesiomonas shigelloides* in humans. *Clinical Infectious Diseases* **10**, 303–16.

364. Shah HN, Collins MD (1988). Proposal for reclassification of *Bacteroides asaccharolyticus*, *Bacteroides gingivalis*, and *Bacteroides endodontalis* in a new genus, *Porphyromonas*. *International Journal of Systematic Bacteriology* **38**, 128–31.

365. Shah HN, Collins DM (1990). *Prevotella*, a new genus to include *Bacteroides melaninogenicus* and related species formerly classified in the genus *Bacterioides*. *International Journal of Systematic Bacteriology* **40**, 205–8.

366. Flynn MJ, Li G, Slots J (1994). *Mitsuokella dentalis* in human periodontitis. *Oral Microbiology and Immunology* **9**, 248–50.

367. Riley TV, Ott AK (1981). Brain abscess due to *Arachnia propionica*. *British Medical Journal* **i**, 1035.

368. Brock DW, *et al.* (1973). Actinomycosis caused by *Arachnia propionica*. *American Journal of Clinical Pathology* **59**, 66–77.

369. Mobley HL, Belas R (1995). Swarming and pathogenicity of *Proteus mirabilis* in the urinary tract. *Trends in Microbiology* **3**, 280–4.

370. Hawkey PM (1984). *Providencia stuartii*: a review of a multiply antibiotic-resistant bacterium. *Journal of Antimicrobial Chemotherapy* **13**, 209–26.

371. Pallerono NJ (1984). Family 1. *Pseudomonadaceae*. In: Krieg NR, Holt JG, eds. *Bergey's manual of systematic bacteriology*, Vol. 1. Williams and Willkins, Baltimore, MD.

372. Woese CR (1987). Bacterial evolution. *Microbiological Reviews* **51**, 221–71.

373. Holmes B, *et al.* (1987). *Chryseomonas luteola* comb. nov. and *Flavimonas oryzihabitans* gen. nov. comb. nov. *Pseudomonas*-like species from human clinical specimens and formerly known respectively as groups Ve-1 and Ve-2. *International Journal of Systematic Bacteriology* **37**, 245–50.

374. Podbielski A, *et al.* (1990). *Flavimonas oryzihabitans* septicaemia in a T-cell leukaemic child: a case report and review of the literature. *Journal of Infection* **20**, 135–41.

375. Bendig JWA, *et al.* (1989). *Flavimonas oryzihabitans* (*Pseudomonas oryzihabitans*; CDC group Ve-2): an emerging pathogen in peritonitis related to continuous ambulatory peritoneal dialysis? *Journal of Clinical Microbiology* **27**, 217–18.

376. Levett PN, Garrett DA, Wickramasuriya T (1991). *Flavimonas oryzihabitans* as a cause of ocular infection. *European Journal of Clinical Microbiology and Infectious Diseases* **10**, 594–5.

377. Warwick S, *et al.* (1994). A phylogenetic analysis of the family *Pseudonocardiaceae* and the genera *Actinokineospora* and *Saccharothrix* with 16S rRNA sequences and a proposal to combine the genera *Amycolata* and *Pseudonocardia* in an emended genus *Pseudonocardia*. *International Journal of Systematic Bacteriology* **44**, 293–9.

378. Willems A, Collins MD (1996). Phylogenetic relationships of the genera *Acetobacterium* and *Eubacterium* sensu stricto and reclassification of *Eubacterium alactolyticum* as *Pseudoramibacter alactolyticus* gen. nov., comb. nov. *International Journal of Systematic Bacteriology* **46**, 1083–7.

379. Lloyd-Puryear M, *et al.* (1991). Meningitis caused by *Psychrobacter immobilis* in an infant. *Journal of Clinical Microbiology* **29**, 2041–2.

380. Gini GA (1990). Ocular infection caused by *Psychrobacter immobilis* acquired in a hospital. *Journal of Clinical Microbiology* **28**, 400–1.

381. Alballaa SR, *et al.* (1992). Urinary tract infection due to *Rahnella aquatilis* in a renal transplant patient. *Journal of Clinical Microbiology* **30**, 2948–50.

382. Goubau P, *et al.* (1988). Septicaemia caused by *Rahnella aquatilis* in an immunocompromised patient. *European Journal of Clinical Microbiology and Infectious Diseases* **7**, 697–9.

383. Lacey S, Want SV (1991). *Pseudomonas pickettii* infections in a paediatric oncology unit. *Journal of Hospital Infection* **17**, 45–51.

384. Fujita S, Yoshida T, Matsubara F (1981). *Pseudomonas pickettii* bacteremia. *Journal of Clinical Microbiology* **13**, 781–2.

385. Zapardiel J, *et al.* (1991). Peritonitis with CDC group IVc-2 bacteria in a patient on continuous ambulatory peritoneal dialysis. *European Journal of Clinical Microbiology and Infectious Diseases* **10**, 509–11.

386. Dan M, *et al.* (1986). Septicaemia caused by the Gram-negative bacteria CDC IVc-2 in an immunocompromised human. *Journal of Clinical Microbiology* **23**, 803.

387. Crowe HM, Brecher SM (1987). Septicaemia with CDC group IVc-2, an unususal gram-negative bacillus. *Journal of Clinical Microbiology* **25**, 2225–6.

388. Sane DC, Durack DT (1986). Infection with *Rhodococcus equi* in AIDS. *New England Journal of Medicine* **314**, 56–7.

389. Berg XX, *et al.* (1977). *Corynebacterium equi* infection complicating neoplastic disease. *American Journal of Clinical Pathology* **68**, 73–7.

390. Van Etta LL (1983). *Corynebacterium equi*: a review of twelve cases of human infection. *Reviews of Infectious Diseases* **5**, 1012–18.

391. Xu W, Raoult D (1998). Taxonomic relationships among spotted fever group rickettsiae as revealed by antigenic analysis with monoclonal antibodies. *Journal of Clinical Microbiology* **36**, 887–96.

392. Struthers M, Wong J, Janda JM (1996). An initial appraisal of the clinical significance of *Roseomonas* species associated with human infections. *Clinical Infectious Diseases* **23**, 729–33.

393. **Broeren SA, Peel MM** (1984). Endocarditis caused by *Rothia dentocariosa*. *Journal of Clinical Pathology* **37**, 1298–300.

394. **Willems A, Collins MD** (1995). Phylogenetic analysis of *Ruminococcus flavefaciens*, the type species of the genus *Ruminococcus*, does not support the reclassification of *Streptococcus hansenii* and *Peptostreptococcus productus* as ruminococci. *International Journal of Systematic Bacteriology* **45**, 572–5.

395. **Nakatani S, et al.** (1998). [A case report of epidural abscess due to anaerobic bacteria, producing a mass of gas]. *Rinsho Shinkeigaku* **38**, 224–7. [In Japanese]

396. **Botha SJ, et al.** (1993). Anaerobic bacteria in orofacial abscesses. *Journal of the Dental Association of South Africa* **48**, 445–9.

397. **Threlfall J, Ward L, Old D** (1999). Changing the nomenclature of salmonella. *Communicable Disease and Public Health* **2**, 156–7.

398. **Bisiaux-Salauze B, et al.** (1990). Bacteremias caused by *Selenomonas artemidis* and *Selenomonas infelix*. *Journal of Clinical Microbiology* **28**, 140–2.

399. **Westh H, et al.** (1991). Fatal septicaemia with *Selenomonas sputigena* and *Acinetobacter calcoaceticus*. A case report. *Acta Pathologica, Microbiologica et Immunologica Scandinavica (APMIS)* **99**, 75–7.

400. **Pomeroy C, Shanholtzer CJ, Peterson LR** (1987). *Selenomonas* bacteraemia: case report and review of the literature. *Journal of Infection* **15**, 237–42.

401. **Yu VL** (1979). *Serratia marcescens*: historical perspective and clinical review. *New England Journal of Medicine* **300**, 887–92.

402. **Pfyffer GE** (1991). *Serratia fonticola* as an infectious agent. *European Journal of Clinical Microbiology and Infectious Diseases* **11**, 199–200.

403. **Zbinden R, Blass R** (1988). *Serratia plymuthica* osteomyelitis following a motorcycle accident. *Journal of Clinical Microbiology* **26**, 1409–10.

404. **Clark RB, Janda JM** (1985). Isolation of *Serratia plymuthica* from a human burn site. *Journal of Clinical Microbiology* **21**, 656–7.

405. **Horowitz HW, et al.** (1987). *Serratia plymuthica* sepsis associated with infection of central venous catheter. *Journal of Clinical Microbiology* **25**, 1562–3.

406. **Marne C, Pallarés R, Sitges-Sera A** (1983). Isolation of *Pseudomonas putrefaciens* in intraabdominal sepsis. *Journal of Clinical Microbiology* **17**, 1173–4.

407. **Laudat P, et al.** (1983). *Pseudomonas putrefaciens* meningitis. *Journal of Infection* **7**, 281–3.

408. **Kotloff KL, et al.** (1999). Global burden of *Shigella* infections: implications for vaccine development and implementation of control strategies. *Bulletin of the World Health Organization* **77**, 651–66.

409. **Kahane S, et al.** (1999). *Simkania negevensis* strain ZT: growth, antigenic and genome characteristics. *International Journal of Systematic Bacteriology* **49**, 815–20.

410. **Wade WG, et al.** (1999). The family *Coriobacteriaceae*: reclassification of *Eubacterium exiguum* (Poco et al. 1996) and *Peptostreptococcus heliotrinreducens* (Lanigan 1976) as *Slackia exigua* gen. nov., comb. nov. and *Slackia heliotrinireducens* gen. nov., comb. nov., and *Eubacterium lentum* (Prevot 1938) as *Eggerthella lenta* gen. nov., comb. nov. *International Journal of Systematic Bacteriology* **49**, 595–600.

411. **Reina J, Borrell N, Figuerola J** (1992). *Sphingobacterium multivorum* isolated from a patient with cystic fibrosis. *European Journal of Clinical Microbiology and Infectious Diseases* **11**, 81–2.

412. **Holmes B, et al.** (1983). *Flavobacterium thalpophilum*, a new species recovered from human clinical material. *International Journal of Systematic Bacteriology* **33**, 677–82.

413. **Freney J, et al.** (1987). Septicemia caused by *Sphingobacterium multivorum*. *Journal of Clinical Microbiology* **25**, 1126–8.

414. **Southern PM, Kutscher AE** (1981). *Pseudomonas paucimobilis* bacteremia. *Journal of Clinical Microbiology* **13**, 1070–3.

415. **Bhatt KM, Mirza NB** (1992). Rat bite fever: a case report of a Kenyan. *East African Medical Journal* **69**, 542–3.

416. **Kloos WE, Bannerman TL** (1994). Update on clinical significance of coagulase-negative staphylococci. *Clinical Microbiology Reviews* **7**, 117–40.

417. **Zuravleff JJ, Yu VL** (1982). Infections caused by *Pseudomonas maltophilia* with emphasis on bacteremia: case reports and a review of the literature. *Reviews of Infectious Diseases* **4**, 1236–46.

418. **Drancourt M, Bollet C, Raoult D** (1997). *Stenotrophomonas africana* sp. nov., an opportunistic human pathogen in Africa. *International Journal of Systematic Bacteriology* **47**, 160–3.

419. **von Eiff C, Peters G** (1998). *In vitro* activity of ciprofloxacin, ofloxacin, and levofloxacin against *Micrococcus* species and *Stomatococcus mucilaginosus* isolated from healthy subjects and neutropenic patients. *European Journal of Clinical Microbiology and Infectious Diseases* **17**, 890–2.

420. **Condron PE, et al.** (1987). Isolation of *Stomatococcus mucilaginosus* from drug user with endocarditis. *Journal of Clinical Microbiology* **25**, 1359–63.

421. **Gruson D, et al.** (1998). Severe infection caused by *Stomatococcus mucilaginosus* in a neutropenic patient: case report and review of the literature. *Hematology and Cell Therapy* **40**, 167–9.

422. **Park MK, et al.** (1997). Successful treatment of *Stomatococcus mucilaginosus* meningitis with intravenous vancomycin and intravenous ceftriaxone. *Clinical Infectious Diseases* **24**, 278.

423. **Hagelskjaer L, Sorensen I, Randers E** (1998). *Streptobacillus moniliformis* infection: 2 cases and a literature review. *Scandinavian Journal of Infectious Diseases* **30**, 309–11.

424. **Akaike T, et al.** (1988). *Streptococcus acidominimus* infections in a human. *Japanese Journal of Medicine* **27**, 317–20.

425. **Schugk J, et al.** (1997). A clinical study of beta-haemolytic groups A B, C and G streptococcal bacteremia in adults over an 8-year period. *Scandinavian Journal of Infectious Diseases* **29**, 233–8.

426. **Weinstein MR, et al., and S. iniae Study Group** (1997). Invasive infections due to a fish pathogen, *Streptococcus iniae*. *New England Journal of Medicine* **337**, 589–94.

427. **Bert F, et al.** (1998). Clinical significance of bacteremia involving the 'Streptococcus milleri' group: 51 cases and review. *Clinical Infectious Diseases* **27**, 385–7.

428. **Elliott PM, Williams H, Brooksby IA** (1993). A case of infective endocarditis in a farmer caused by *Streptococcus equinus*. *European Heart Journal* **14**, 1292–3.

429. **De Gheldre Y, et al.** (1999). Identification of clinically relevant viridans streptococci by analysis of transfer DNA intergenic spacer length polymorphism. *International Journal of Systematic Bacteriology* **49**, 1591–8.

430. **Crook DW, Spratt BG** (1998). Multiple antibiotic resistance in *Streptococcus pneumoniae*. *British Medical Bulletin* **54**, 595–610.

431. **Kohler W, et al.** (1989). *Streptococcus suis* Typ 2 (R-Streptokokken) als Erreger von Berufskrankheiten. Bericht über eine Erkrankung und Literaturübersicht. *Zeitschrift fur die Gesamte Innere Medizin* **44**, 144–8.

432. **Nasher MA, et al.** (1989). *In vitro* studies of antibiotic sensitivities of *Streptomyces somaliensis*: a cause of human actinomycetoma. *Transactions of the Royal Society of Tropical Medicine and Hygiene* **83**, 265–8.

433. **Molitoris E, Wexler HM, Finegold SM** (1997). Sources and antimicrobial susceptibilities of *Campylobacter gracilis* and *Sutterella wadsworthensis*. *Clinical Infectious Diseases* **25**(Suppl 2), 264–5.

434. **Finegold SM, Jousimies-Somer H** (1997). Recently described clinically important anaerobic bacteria: medical aspects. *Clinical Infectious Diseases* **25**(Suppl 2), 88–93.

435. **Wexler HM, et al.** (1996). *Sutterella wadsworthensis* gen. nov., sp. nov., bile-resistant microaerophilic *Campylobacter gracilis*-like clinical isolates. *International Journal of Systematic Bacteriology* **46**, 252–8.

436. **Jenny DB, Letendre PW, Iverson G** (1987). Endocarditis caused by *Kingella indologenes*. *Reviews of Infectious Diseases* **9**, 787.

437. **Hollis DG, et al.** (1981). *Tatumella ptyseos* gen. nov., sp. nov., a member of the family *Enterobacteriaceae* found in clinical specimens. *Journal of Clinical Microbiology* **14**, 79–88.

438. **Farrow JA, et al.** (1995). Phylogenetic evidence that the gram-negative nonsporulating bacterium *Tissierella (Bacteroides) praeacuta* is a member of the *Clostridium* subphylum of the gram-positive bacteria and description of *Tissierella creatinini* sp. nov. *International Journal of Systematic Bacteriology* **45**, 436–40.

439. McWhorter AC, *et al.* (1991). *Trabulsiella guamensis*, a new genus and species of the family *Enterobacteriaceae* that resembles *Salmonella* subgroups 4 and 5. *Journal of Clinical Microbiology* **29**, 1480–5.

440. Willis SG, *et al.* (1999). Identification of seven *Treponema* species in health- and disease-associated dental plaque by nested PCR. *Journal of Clinical Microbiology* **37**, 867–9.

441. Wyss C, *et al.* (1999). *Treponema lecithinolyticum* sp. nov., a small saccharolytic spirochaete with phospholipase A and C activities associated with periodontal diseases. *International Journal of Systematic Bacteriology* **49**, 1329–39.

442. Koff AB, Rosen T (1993). Nonvenereal treponematoses: yaws, endemic syphilis, and pinta. *Journal of the American Academy of Dermatology* **29**, 519–38.

443. Wallace AL, Harris A, Allen JP (1967). Reiter treponeme. A review of the literature. *Bulletin of the World Health Organization* **36**(Suppl), 1–103.

444. Singh AE, Romanowski B (1999). Syphilis: review with emphasis on clinical, epidemiologic, and some biologic features. *Clinical Microbiology Reviews* **12**, 187–209.

445. Relman DA, *et al.* (1992). Identification of the uncultured bacillus of Whipple's disease. *New England Journal of Medicine* **327**, 293–301.

446. Granel F, *et al.* (1996). Cutaneous infection caused by *Tsukamurella paurometabolum*. *Clinical Infectious Diseases* **23**, 839–40.

447. Yassin AF, *et al.* (1996). *Tsukamurella pulmonis* sp. nov. *International Journal of Systematic Bacteriology* **46**, 429–36.

448. Chong Y, *et al.* (1997). *Tsukamurella inchonensis* bacteremia in a patient who ingested hydrochloric acid. *Clinical Infectious Diseases* **24**, 1267–8.

449. Shapiro CL, *et al.* (1992). *Tsukamurella paurometabolum*: a novel pathogen causing catheter-related bacteremia in patients with cancer. *Clinical Infectious Diseases* **14**, 200–3.

450. Funke G, *et al.* (1994). *Turicella otitidis* gen. nov., sp. nov., a coryneform bacterium isolated from patients with otitis media. *International Journal of Systematic Bacteriology* **44**, 270–3.

451. Hudson MM, Talbot MD (1997). *Ureaplasma urealyticum*. *International Journal of STD and AIDS* **8**, 546–51.

452. Teixeira LM, *et al.* (1997). Phenotypic and genotypic characterization of *Vagococcus fluvialis*, including strains isolated from human sources. *Journal of Clinical Microbiology* **35**, 2778–81.

453. Rogosa M (1984). Family I. *Veillonellaceae* Rogosa 1971, 232. In: Krieg NR, Holt JG, eds. *Bergey's manual of systematic bacteriology*, Vol. 1. Williams and Willkins, Baltimore, MD.

454. West PA (1989). The human pathogenic vibrios—a public health update with environmental perspectives. *Epidemiology and Infection* **103**, 1–34.

455. Pavia AT, *et al.* (1989). *Vibrio carchariae* infection after a shark bite. *Annals of Internal Medicine* **111**, 85–6.

456. Bode RB, *et al.* (1986). *Vibrio cincinnatiensis* causing meningitis: successful treatment in an adult. *Annals of Internal Medicine* **104**, 55–6.

457. Hickman-Brenner FW, *et al.* (1982). Identification of *Vibrio hollisae* sp. nov. from patients with diarrhea. *Journal of Clinical Microbiology* **15**, 395–400.

458. Jean-Jacques W, *et al.* (1981). *Vibrio metschnikovii* bacteremia in a patient with cholecystitis. *Journal of Clinical Microbiology* **14**, 711–12.

459. Bonner JR, *et al.* (1983). Spectrum of *Vibrio* infections in a Gulf coast community. *Annals of Internal Medicine* **99**, 464–9.

460. Levine WC, Griffin PM, Gulf Coast *Vibrio* Working Group (1993). *Vibrio* infections on the Gulf Coast: results of first year of regional surveillance. *Journal of Infectious Diseases* **167**, 479–83.

461. Boixeda D, *et al.* (1998). A case of spontaneous peritonitis caused by *Weeksella virosa*. *European Journal of Gastroenterology and Hepatology* **10**, 897–8.

462. Faber MD, *et al.* (1991). Response of *Weeksella virosa* peritonitis to imipenem/cilastin. *Advances in Peritoneal Dialysis* **7**, 133–4.

463. Li ZX, *et al.* (1990). First isolation of *Xanthomonas campestris* from the blood of a Chinese woman. *Chinese Medical Journal* **103**, 435–9.

464. Bercovier H, Mollaret HH (1984). Genus XIV *Yersinia* Van Loghem 1944, 15. In: Krieg NR, Holt JG, eds. *Bergey's manual of systematic bacteriology*, Vol. 1. Williams and Willkins, Baltimore, MD.

465. Kosako Y, Sakazaki R, Yoshizaki E (1984). *Yokenella regensburgei* gen. nov., sp. nov.: a new genus and species in the family *Enterobacteriaceae*. *Japanese Journal of Medical Science and Biology* **37**, 117–24.

7.12 Fungal infections (mycoses)

7.12.1 Fungal infections

R. J. Hay*

Introduction

Fungi are saprophytic or parasitic organisms that are normally assigned to a distinct Kingdom. As eukaryotes, they have the complex subcellular organization and highly organized genetic material seen in both animal and plant cells. The cell wall is a distinctive feature of fungi and has a complex skeleton based on mannan and glucan subunits. The arrangement and reproduction of individual cells is also characteristic. Most fungi form new cells terminally, which remain connected to form long, branching filaments or hyphae (the mould fungi). Some reproduce in a similar manner but each new cell separates from the parent by a process of budding (the yeast fungi). It is a feature of certain fungi to be yeast-like during one phase of their life history but hyphal at another, a phenomenon known as dimorphism. In culture, mould fungi usually form a cottony growth on laboratory media while yeasts normally have a smooth, shiny appearance.

Fungi adversely affect humans in a number of ways. They cause disease indirectly by spoilage and destruction of food crops with subsequent malnutrition and starvation. Many of the common moulds produce and release spores, which may act as airborne allergens to produce asthma or hypersensitivity pneumonitis. Fungi elaborate complex metabolic by-products, some of which are useful to humans, such as the penicillins. However, others are toxic. Disease caused by the ingestion of fungal toxins includes both poisoning by eating certain mushrooms (mycetism) and damage caused by the ingestion of minute quantities of toxin (mycotoxicosis), for instance in contaminated grain. The contribution of the latter mechanism to human disease remains largely unexplored and, in addition, whether inhalation of toxic fungal spores may cause pathology. Finally, fungi may invade human tissue. Medical mycology is largely concerned with this last group. Invasive fungal diseases are normally divided into three groups: the superficial, subcutaneous, and deep mycoses. In superficial infections, such as ringworm or thrush, fungi are confined to the skin and mucous membranes. Extension deeper than the surface epithelium is rare. Subcutaneous infections are usually tropical: the main site of involvement is within subcutaneous tissue, although secondary invasion of adjacent structures such as bone or skin may occur. In deep or systemic infections, deep organs such as the lung, spleen, or brain are invaded. This classification of mycoses is based on the main 'sphere of involvement' by the causal organisms, but there are exceptions. For instance, brain involvement has been recorded in patients with chromoblastomycosis, which is normally a subcutaneous infection.

* Dr M.A.H. Bayles prepared the chapter on Chromoblastomycosis for the third edition of this textbook. Much of her text has been included in this chapter and we acknowledge her contribution with grateful thanks.

The fungi causing systemic mycoses are often classified in two groups: the opportunists and the endemic pathogens. The former cause disease in overtly compromised individuals. These contrast with the true pathogens, which cause infection in all subjects inhaling airborne spores.

Further reading—general

Ajello L, Hay RJ, eds (1997). *Mycology. Topley and Wilson's microbiology and microbial infections*, 9th edn, Vol 4. Arnold, London.

Kibbler CC, MacKenzie DWR, Odds FC (1996). *Principles and practice of clinical mycology.* John Wiley & Sons, Chichester.

Midgley G, Clayton YM, Hay RJ (1997). *Diagnosis in colour. Medical mycology.* Mosby-Wolfe, London.

Warnock DW, Richardson MD, ed. (1990). *Fungal infection in the compromised patient.* Wiley, Chichester.

Superficial fungal infections

The main superficial mycoses are the dermatophyte infections, superficial candidosis, and tinea versicolor (see Section 23). These are both common and widespread. Rare superficial infections include tinea nigra, and black or white piedra.

Dermatophyte infections (dermatophytoses)

Aetiology

The dermatophyte or ringworm infections are caused by a group of organisms capable of existing in keratinized tissue such as stratum corneum, nail, or hair. The mechanism of invasion is thought to be linked to production of extracellular enzymes, such as the three distinct keratinases produced by *Trichophyton mentagrophytes*, but other proteases may also be involved.

Epidemiology

Some dermatophyte fungi have a worldwide distribution; others are more restricted. The most common and most widely distributed is *Trichophyton rubrum*, which causes different types of infection in different parts of the world. It is commonly associated with athlete's foot (tinea pedis) in temperate areas as well as tinea corporis or tinea cruris in the tropics. This distinction is not based solely on climatic factors, as immigrants from tropical countries, particularly the Far East, may still have tinea corporis caused by *T. rubrum* when living in northern Europe. Certain dermatophytes are limited to defined areas. For instance, tinea imbricata caused by *Trichophyton concentricum*, is found in hot, humid areas of the Far East, Polynesia, and South America. Scalp ringworm tends to occur in well-defined endemic areas in Africa and elsewhere. In different regions, different species of dermatophytes may predominate. Thus, in North Africa, the most common cause of tinea capitis is *Trichophyton violaceum*; in southern parts of the continent, the major agents may be *Microsporum audouinii*, *Microsporum ferrugineum*, and *Trichophyton soudanense*. Not all dermatophyte infections are endemic and dominant species may disappear to be replaced by others. *M. audouinii*, once endemic and common in the United Kingdom, is now infrequent, probably because of improved treatment and detection of carriers. By contrast *Trichophyton tonsurans* is now established as a major cause of tinea capitis in urban areas in both the United Kingdom and the United States. Dermatophytes may be passed from person to person (anthropophilic infections), from animal to person (zoophilic), or soil to person (geophilic). Sources of zoophilic organisms in Europe include cats and dogs, cattle, hedgehogs, and small rodents. Rarer sources include horses, monkeys, and chickens. Lesions produced by zoophilic species may be highly inflammatory.

Factors governing the invasion of stratum corneum are largely unknown, but heat, humidity, and occlusion have all been implicated. Susceptibility to certain infection, such as tinea imbricata, may be genetically determined.

Clinical features

The clinical features of dermatophyte infections are best considered in relation to the site involved. Often the term tinea, followed by the Latin name of the appropriate part (such as *corporis*—body) is used to describe the clinical site of infection.

Tinea pedis

Scaling or maceration between the toes, particularly in the fourth interspace, is the most common form of dermatophytosis seen in temperate countries. Itching is variable, but may be severe. Sometimes blisters may form both between the toes and on the soles of the feet. The causative organisms are commonly *T. rubrum* and *Trichophyton interdigitale*, the latter being responsible for the vesicular forms. Similar appearances can be caused by *Candida albicans* and in the bacterial infection, erythrasma. Gram-negative bacterial infection causes erosive interdigital disease associated with discomfort.

'Dry type' infections of the soles and palms

These are normally caused by *T. rubrum*. Palms or soles have a dry, scaly appearance, which in the soles may encroach on to the lateral or dorsal surfaces of the foot. The palmar involvement is often unilateral, an important diagnostic feature (Plate 1). Nail invasion is often seen (see below). Itching is not prominent, and infections are usually chronic.

Tinea cruris

Infections of the groin, most often caused by *T. rubrum* or *Epidermophyton floccosum*, are relatively common. They occur in both tropical and temperate climates, although in the former the infection may spread to involve the whole waist area in both males and females. Tinea cruris in females is uncommon in Europe. An erythematous and scaly rash with a distinct margin extends from the groin to the upper thighs or scrotum. Itching may be severe. Coincident tinea pedis is common, and patients should be examined for this. The rash of crural erythrasma shows uniform scaling without a margin, whereas in candidosis, satellite pustules occur distal to the rim.

Onychomycosis (caused by dermatophytes)

Invasion of the nail plate is most often seen with *T. rubrum* infections. The plate is invaded distally and becomes thickened and friable with terminal loss of the nail plate. Onycholysis may be seen. More rarely, and most often with *T. interdigitale*, the dorsal surface of the plate is invaded, causing superficial white onychomycosis.

Tinea corporis (body ringworm)

Dermatophyte or ringworm infection on the trunk or limbs may produce the characteristic annular plaque with a raised edge and central clearing (Plate 2). Scaling and itching is variable. Lesions caused by zoophilic organisms may be highly inflammatory and in certain cases, particularly those caused by *Trichophyton verrucosum*, intense itching, oedema, and pustule formation (kerion) may develop. This reaction is seldom secondarily infected by bacteria but is a response to the fungus on hairy skin. Infections of the beard, tinea barbae, are often highly refractory to treatment. Facial dermatophyte infections may mimic a variety of non-fungal skin diseases, including acne, rosacea, and discoid lupus erythematosus. However, the underlying annular configuration can usually be distinguished. The term tinea incognito is used to describe such atypical lesions.

Tinea capitis (scalp ringworm)

In the United Kingdom as in the United States, the most common cause of scalp ringworm is *Trichophyton tonsurans*, an anthropophilic fungus which mainly occurs in inner cities, particularly in black Caribbean or African children. This has now replaced *Microsporum canis*, originating from an infected cat or dog, although this dermatophyte is dominant elsewhere. Scalp ringworm is mainly a disease of childhood, with rare infections occurring in adult women. Spontaneous clearance at puberty is the rule. *M. canis* causes an 'ectothrix' infection where spores form on the outside of the hair shaft and the scalp hair breaks above the skin surface. Scaling, itching, and loss of hair occur. Other causes of ectothrix infection include *M. audouinii*, which is becoming more common in Europe, and is still seen in the tropics. This infection can be spread from child to child and causes serious social handicap. The infection may occur in epidemic form, particularly in schools. By contrast, infections with *M. canis* are acquired from a primary animal source rather than by spread from human lesions. In endothrix infections where sporulation is within the hair shaft, scaling is less pronounced and hairs break at scalp level (black dot ringworm). Examples include *T. tonsurans* and *T. violaceum*, the latter being most prevalent in the Middle East, parts of Africa, and India, although it also is being recognized with increasing frequency in Europe.

Favus, now most often seen in isolated foci in the tropics, is a particularly chronic form of ringworm where hair shafts become surrounded by a necrotic crust or scutulum. Individual crusts coalesce to form a pale, unpleasant-smelling mat over parts of the scalp. Such infections may cause extensive and permanent hair loss.

Tinea imbricata (tokelau)

This infection is endemic in parts of the Far East, West Pacific, and Central and South America, and is caused by *Trichophyton concentricum*. In many cases the trunk is covered with scales laid down in concentric rings producing a 'ripple' effect. Alternatively, large, loose scales (tiled, Latin—*imbricata*) may form. The infection is often chronic, and may constitute a serious social handicap. There is some evidence that susceptibility of this disease in Papua New Guinea may be inherited as an autosomal recessive trait.

Infection in HIV and immunocompromised patients

While dermatophyte infections are no more common in the immunocompromised patient, they may differ clinically. In patients with HIV infections there may be (i) more tinea facei, (ii) more widespread and atypical skin lesions, and (iii) a distinct pattern of nail infection characterized by white discoloration spreading rapidly through the nail plate from the proximal nail fold.

Laboratory diagnosis

The mainstays of diagnosis are direct microscopy of skin scales mounted in potassium hydroxide (20 per cent) to demonstrate hyphae, and culture. Scalp hairs may also be examined in a similar way, and the site of arthrospore formation, inside or outside the shaft, determined. Fluorescent whitening agents (Calcofluor) or chlorazol black stain have been used to highlight fungi in scales. Further tests, such as the ability to penetrate hair, may be used to separate similar cultures. Identification of organisms is important, as it will indicate the source of infection in scalp ringworm, for example. When large numbers of children are involved, screening of scalp infections with a filtered ultraviolet (Wood's light) lamp is useful. Certain species, including *M. canis* and *M. audouinii*, cause infected hair to fluoresce with a vivid greenish light. Scalps can also be screened for infection by passing a sterile brush or scalp massager through the hair and plating this directly on to an agar plate.

Treatment

The treatment of dermatophyte infections depends to an extent on the nature and severity of infection. Topical therapy is reserved for circumscribed infections such as athlete's foot and tinea corporis, not involving hair or nail keratin. Scalp and nail infections, severe or widespread ringworm, and failures of topical therapy are usually treated orally with griseofulvin, itraconazole, or terbinafine.

Specific antifungal drugs in topical form are effective and well tolerated. The important compounds in this group are miconazole, clotrimazole, ketoconazole, and econazole, which are imidazole derivatives, undecenoic acid, and tolnaftate and the allylamine, terbinafine. Generally treatment is given for 7 to 30 days. They are all very similar in their clinical efficacy, but topical terbinafine is particularly rapid in foot infection (7 days or less). Adverse reactions are rare.

For oral therapy the main alternatives are terbinafine, itraconazole, or fluconazole. Terbinafine (250 mg daily) is rapidly effective in most forms of dermatophytosis that require oral therapy and also produces rapid responses in toe nail (12 weeks) and sole infections (2 to 4 weeks), without a high rate of relapse. Side-effects include headache and nausea, but loss of taste may also occur. Itraconazole is somewhat similar in its profile, but is given intermittently (200 mg twice daily for 7 days). This course is given once for sole infections but repeated three times at monthly intervals for toe nail infections, as pulsed therapy. Side-effects include nausea and abdominal discomfort. Fluconazole is also active and is given in a dose of 150 mg weekly; 300 mg may be necessary for toe nail infections. This side-effect profile is similar to itraconazole. All three drugs are extremely rare causes of hepatic toxicity. Griseofulvin is still used for tinea capitis in a dose of 10 to 20 mg/kg daily. Treatment should be continued for at least 6 weeks in tinea capitis. Side-effects are not common, but include headache, nausea, and urticaria. The drug can also precipitate acute intermittent porphyria and systemic lupus erythematosus in predisposed subjects.

Further reading—dermatophytosis

de Vroey C (1985). Epidemiology of ringworm (dermatophytosis). *Seminars in Dermatology* 4, 185–200.

Hay RJ (1982). Chronic dermatophyte infections I. Clinical and mycological features. *British Journal of Dermatology* 106, 1–6.

Hay RJ (1997). Fungal infections. In: Bos JD, ed. *Skin immune system (SIS)*, pp 593–604. CRC Press, Florida.

Hay RJ et al. (1996). Tinea capitis in south-east London—a new pattern of infection with public health implications. *British Journal of Dermatology* 135, 955–8.

Torssander J et al. (1988). Dermatophytosis and HIV infection—study in homosexual men. *Acta Dermatologica et Venereologica* 68, 53–9.

Scytalidium infections

The organisms, *Scytalidium dimidiatum* (*Hendersonula toruloidea*) and *Scytalidium hyalinum*, can cause a superficial scaly condition that resembles the 'dry type' of dermatophyte infection on the palms or soles. Nail plate destruction may also occur, the lateral border of the nail being the initial site of invasion. The disease has been seen in Europe, almost invariably in immigrants from the tropics, particularly the Caribbean, West Africa, and India or Pakistan. Its prevalence in the tropics is unknown, although in some surveys it has been shown to be relatively common. In skin scrapings the tortuous hyphae may resemble those of a dermatophyte, but the organisms do not grow on media containing cycloheximide, which is often incorporated into agar for routine dermatophyte isolation.

Treatment is difficult, but some improvement may follow the use of keratolytic compounds such as salicylic acid. Nail infections do not respond to terbinafine, griseofulvin, or azoles.

Further reading—*Scytalidium*

Hay RJ, Moore MK (1984). Clinical features of superficial fungal infections caused by *Hendersonula toruloidea* and *Scytalidium hyalinum*. *British Journal of Dermatology* 110, 677–83.

Miscellaneous nail infections

Occasionally, fungi other than dermatophytes or *Scytalidium* species are isolated from dystrophic nails. These include *Scopulariopsis brevicaulis*, *Onychocola canadensis*, *Acremonium*, and *Fusarium* species, and certain types of *Aspergillus*. These infections are usually seen in the elderly. It is often difficult, particularly with *Aspergillus* species, to establish that the organism is playing a pathogenic role.

Pityriasis versicolor (tinea versicolor)

Aetiology

Pityriasis versicolor is a superficial infection caused by *Malassezia* species. Although most common in tropical countries, it has a worldwide distribution. Dermal penetration does not occur.

There are six species of *Malassezia* that can be found on normal skin, the commonest of which are *M. sympodialis* and *M. globosa*. In pityriasis versicolor there is transformation of yeast cells to produce hyphae. It is likely that the state of host immunity plays some part in pathogenesis and depression; for instance, endogenous or exogenous corticosteroids potentiate the disease in some individuals. However, it is also commonly seen in normal individuals, and climatic factors or sun exposure are believed to trigger the infection in many cases. There is no effective animal model for studies of this disease.

Epidemiology

Pityriasis versicolor is very common in the tropics, where it may be widespread on the body. Its incidence in temperate climates has increased over the last 20 to 30 years. It is not more common in HIV infected subjects.

Clinical features

The rash of pityriasis versicolor is asymptomatic or mildly pruritic. Its presents with scaling, confluent macules on the trunk, upper arms, or neck. These may be hypopigmented or hyperpigmented. In some individuals and in the tropics, other areas including face, forearms, and thighs may be involved.

The diagnosis is rarely confused with other complaints, although eczema or ringworm infections are sometimes considered. Patients are often anxious to exclude leprosy, but the two are unlikely to be mistaken. In vitiligo, depigmentation is complete and there is no scaling.

Laboratory diagnosis

The diagnosis is made by demonstration of the yeasts and hyphae of *Malassezia* in skin scales removed by scraping. Culture is difficult and unnecessary.

Treatment

Topical ketoconazole, miconazole, clotrimazole, or econazole are effective. Oral itraconazole may be used in recalcitrant cases. Alternatives include 2 per cent selenium sulphide or 20 per cent sodium hyposulphate lotions. Whatever the treatment, relapse is common.

Other *Malassezia*-associated conditions

Malassezia yeasts have been implicated in the pathogenesis of a number of other skin diseases such as seborrhoeic dermatitis and a form of itchy folliculitis, *Malassezia* folliculitis. The evidence connecting seborrhoeic dermatitis, one of the most common of skin diseases, and *Malassezia* is largely concerned with the response of antifungal drugs and the observation that improvements in the rash mirror disappearance of organisms from the skin. Severity of the skin condition does not appear to reflect the numbers of yeasts on the skin surface.

Further reading—*Malassezia*

Mathes BM, Douglas MC (1985). Seborrheic dermatitis in patients with acquired immunodeficiency syndrome. *Journal of the American Academy of Dermatology* **13**, 947–51.

Superficial candidosis (candidiasis)

Aetiology

Superficial candidosis is a term used to describe a group of infections of skin or mucous membranes caused by species of the genus *Candida*. They range in severity from oral thrush to chronic mucocutaneous candidosis, a chronic infection refractory to conventional antifungal treatment.

Candida albicans is the species most frequently involved. It is a saprophytic yeast often found as a commensal in the mouth and gastrointestinal tract, and is commonly present in the vagina. Several factors may influence the incidence of carriage. For instance, oral colonization is more common in hospital staff than in equivalent non-hospital subjects. Vaginal carriage is more common in pregnancy. Other factors (Table 1) are known that predispose to conversion from a commensal to a parasitic role with the causation of disease—candidosis. The list includes factors that influence host immunological response, such as carcinoma, AIDS, or cytotoxic therapy; those that disturb the population of other micro-organisms, such as antibiotics; and those that affect the character of the epithelium, such as dentures.

Other species of *Candida* may also cause superficial infections, but are less common. They include *C. glabrata*, *C. dubliniensis*, and *C. parapsilosis*. There is evidence that the first two species are more common now in oral infection in patients with HIV and *C. glabrata* in vaginal candidosis.

Epidemiology

Superficial *Candida* infections are seen in all countries.

Clinical features

There are a number of clinically distinct types of superficial infection caused by *Candida* species, as follows.

Oral candidosis (thrush)

Oral infection by *Candida* is fairly common, particularly in infancy and old age, or in association with antibiotic or cytotoxic therapy, or in diseases where the neutrophil or T-lymphocyte responses may be impaired. In the older age group, the wearing of dentures is a predisposing factor. The lesions present with discomfort both in the mouth and at the corners of the lips. The mouth and buccal mucosa show patchy or confluent, white adherent plaques; less commonly the mucosa and tongue are sore and glazed—erythematous candidosis. Angular cheilitis usually accompanies the oral

Table 1 Predisposing factors in superficial candidosis

1. Local epithelial defects, occlusion, constant immersion in water, e.g. damaged nail folds, beneath dentures
2. Defects of immunity (primarily T cell or phagocytosis)
   (i) primary immunological disease, e.g. chronic granulomatous disease
   (ii) immunodefects secondary to intercurrent illness, e.g. leukaemia
   (iii) immunodefects secondary to therapy, e.g. cytotoxic therapy in organ transplantation
3. Drug therapy, e.g. antibiotics
4. Carcinoma or leukaemia
5. Endocrine disease
   (i) diabetes mellitus
   (ii) hypothyroidism, hypoparathyroidism, hypoadrenalism (all in chronic mucocutaneous candidosis)
6. Physiological changes, e.g. infancy, pregnancy, old age
7. Miscellaneous disorders, e.g.
   (i) iron deficiency
   (ii) zinc deficiency
   (iii) malabsorption

lesions. In long-standing cases, the plaque may become hypertrophic, with oedema of the mucosal surfaces, or the mucosa may appear glazed and raw.

There is a significant correlation between leucoplakia and oral candidosis, and it has been suggested that the infection may lead to epithelial dysplasia.

The diagnosis is made by the demonstration of yeasts and hyphae of *Candida* in smears, and by culture.

Vaginal candidosis (thrush)

See Chapter 21.3 for further details.

Paronychia

Infection around the nail fold is seen in people whose occupations involve frequent wetting of the hands (such as cooks) or in those with eczema or psoriasis. The aetiology is complicated and there may be a mixture of bacterial infection and irritant or allergic contact dermatitis as well as *Candida* infection. The condition presents with painful, red swelling of the nail fold. Pus may be discharged. Secondary invasion of the lateral border of the nail plate by *Candida* may occur from this site.

Candida intertrigo

Infection of the moist folds of the skin in the groin or under the breasts causes itching and discomfort. The area becomes macerated and erythematous. Candida may contribute to this condition, but is certainly not the only factor. It may also superinfect the napkin area in infants. The presence of satellite pustules (see above) is a useful indicator of involvement by *Candida* in the disease process.

Direct invasion of toe-web folds by *Candida* closely resembles 'athlete's foot' caused by dermatophytes. A similar erosive infection may occur in the finger webs—interdigital candidosis—and is seen most commonly in the tropics.

Chronic superficial candidosis

Chronic *Candida* infections of the mouth, vagina, and nail present problems in management. Chronic oral candidosis, for instance, is associated with leucoplakia. Predisposing causes should be searched for. The most serious of this group of infections is chronic mucocutaneous candidosis, a rare condition in which chronic skin, nail, and mucosal infection coexist (Plate 3). A series of underlying genetic, endocrine (hypoparathyroidism, hypoadrenalism, or hypothyroidism), and immunological abnormalities has been found. Extensive human papilloma virus (wart) or dermatophyte infections may also be present in these patients, whose condition is normally diagnosed in childhood.

Oral candidosis is one of the earliest signs of untreated AIDS, occurring in a high proportion of patients. The appearances are similar to those seen with other groups, although plaque formation may be very extensive. Oesophageal infection is common in this group.

Laboratory diagnosis

All these infections are diagnosed by microscopy and culture. When associated with the condition, *Candida* cells are always evident on microscopy. Culture establishes the specific identity and is important particularly where non-*albicans Candida* species may be involved.

Treatment

Two groups of drugs are effective in superficial candidosis. The polyenes such as nystatin and amphotericin B are topically active in many forms of candidosis. They are often less effective in oral candidosis in immunodeficient patients including those with AIDS. Likewise, topical azole drugs such as miconazole and clotrimazole are usually effective in superficial candidosis. For resistant cases, oral therapy with fluconazole, itraconazole, or ketoconazole may be necessary.

For vaginal infections, topical creams or vaginal preparations should be used—many requiring only a single treatment. Single-dose oral fluconazole is an alternative. In recalcitrant cases it may be necessary to use longer courses of fluconazole or itraconazole.

Further reading—candidosis

Bodey GP, ed. (1993). *Candidiasis. Pathogenesis, diagnosis and treatment.* Raven Press, New York.

Greenspan D, Greenspan JS (1987). Oral mucosal manifestations of AIDS. *Dermatologic Clinics* **5**, 733–7.

Torssander J *et al.* (1987). Oral *Candida albicans* in HIV infection. *Scandinavian Journal of Infection* **189**, 291–5.

Miscellaneous superficial mycoses

There are a number of relatively rare, superficial fungal infections such as tinea nigra, and black or white piedra. They never cause invasive disease, and are mainly confined to the tropics.

Tinea nigra

Tinea nigra is a superficial infection confined to the epidermis of the palms or soles, and more rarely elsewhere. The initial lesion is a dark macule without scaling, which resembles a brown stain on the skin and spreads slowly over the palmar or plantar surface. The disease is normally asymptomatic.

On scraping the skin, brown pigmented hyphae can be seen by direct microscopy, and the causative organism, *Phaeoannellomyces werneckii*, isolated.

The lesion responds to Whitfield's ointment.

Black piedra

Black piedra is a disease of the tropics in which small, dark nodules form on hair shafts in the scalp or, less commonly, elsewhere. There are no symptoms. Each nodule consists of a dense mat of hyphae containing the sexual spores (ascospores) of the fungus.

The diagnosis is made by direct microscopy of infected hair, and the isolation of *Piedraia hortae*. Treatment using formalin solution or amphotericin B lotion is usually effective.

White piedra

White piedra occurs in both temperate and tropical climates, and is rare. It produces pale nodules on the hair of the beard, groin, or scalp. The hair shaft may fracture. The nodule consists of hyphae, arthrospores (spores formed by fragmentation of hyphae), and blastospores (budding yeast cells). The organism *Trichosporon beigelii* can be readily cultured. The treatment is similar to that for black piedra.

The subcutaneous mycoses

Subcutaneous infections caused by fungi are rare, and are mainly seen in the tropics. The organisms gain entry via the skin; in mycetoma, organisms may be implanted subcutaneously via a thorn. The majority of the causative organisms in this group of infections can be isolated from vegetation or soil. Involvement of deep viscera is rare. Attempts to establish experimental infections that resemble the human diseases have been largely unsuccessful. A clearer understanding of the pathogenesis therefore awaits such a model system. These infections tend to be chronic, chemotherapy may be lengthy, and in the case of mycetoma, often unsuccessful.

Mycetoma (Madura foot)

Aetiology

Mycetoma is a chronic infection involving subcutaneous tissue, bone, and skin, in which colonies of infecting fungi or actinomycetes (grains) are found within a network of burrowing abscesses and sinuses (Plate 4).

A list of the more common organisms that cause mycetoma is shown in Table 2. The organisms are divided into two groups, the actinomycetomas

Table 2 Causes of mycetoma

Fungi, e.g.
Madurella mycetomatis
Madurella grisea
Scedosporium apiospermum
Exophiala jeanselmei
Leptosphaeria senegalensis
Species of *Acremonium*, *Aspergillus*, *Fusarium*
Actinomycetes, e.g.
Nocardia brasiliensis
Actinomadura madurae
Actinomadura pelletieri
Streptomyces somaliensis

and the eumycetomas, caused by actinomycetes and fungi, respectively. The size and colour of the grains (red, pale, or dark) are important clues to their identification. The organisms can be found in the natural environment, and some have even been identified in association with acacia thorns in an endemic area. The infection is initiated when an infected thorn is implanted in deep tissue. However, many years may elapse before the formation of a clinically apparent mycetoma.

Epidemiology

The disease is seen primarily in the tropics, although rare cases, apart from imported ones, may occur in temperate areas. Countries with the most reported cases include Sudan, India, Senegal, Mexico, and Venezuela. However, the disease is widely distributed in the tropics, particularly to the south and east of the Sahara Desert in Africa.

The pattern of prevalence of infections caused by certain organisms differs strikingly in different parts of the world. For instance, *Streptomyces somaliensis* is most common in the Sudan and Middle East. *Madurella grisea* is mainly found in the New World. Altogether about 60 per cent of reported infections are caused by actinomycetes, of which *Nocardia brasiliensis* is the most common (Chapter 7.11.27).

Clinical features

Early mycetomas may present with a circumscribed area of hard subcutaneous swelling (Plate 5). Later, sinus tracts open on to the skin surface and visible grains may be discharged, along with serosanguinous fluid (Plate 6). Bone erosion and destruction, leading to deformity, may occur. However, severe pain is rarely a problem. Local lymph node invasion may occur, but more widespread involvement is very rare.

Feet and lower legs are the areas most commonly involved, but the arms, buttocks, chest, and head may all be sites of infection. Mycetoma caused by *N. brasiliensis* may occur in any site, but one favoured area is the chest wall.

The radiological features of mycetoma are cortical erosion, followed by the development of lytic deposits in bone. Periosteal proliferation and destruction, leading to deformity, may follow. MRI provides a clearer picture of bone involvement and may be positive earlier than radiography.

Laboratory diagnosis

The diagnosis is made by the demonstration and identification of grains obtained from the sinus openings by gentle pressure or curettage. If these measures are not successful, tissue should be obtained by deep surgical biopsy. Grains can be mounted in potassium hydroxide and examined microscopically. Those containing filaments of 3 to 4 μm in diameter or more are caused by true fungi (eumycetomas), and those with filaments of less than 1 μm by actinomycetes (actinomycetomas). These features can usually be distinguished by direct microscopy.

The morphology of grains fixed, sectioned, and stained with haematoxylin and eosin is typical. Special stains are less helpful. Grains can be used for culture, although several attempts at isolation may have to be made.

Serology (such as immunodiffusion) can also be helpful, although the tests are not widely available.

Treatment

Actinomycetomas may respond to sulphones such as dapsone (50 to 100 mg daily) or sulphonamides such as sulphadiazine. The treatment of choice for many is long-term co-trimoxazole (two to three tablets twice daily) with an initial 2 to 3 months of streptomycin or rifampicin. Treatment may have to be continued for many months or years. Dapsone is an effective and cheaper alternative to co-trimoxazole. Extensive actinomycetomas may respond poorly and additional treatment with amikacin or fucidin may be necessary. The eumycetomas seldom respond to antifungal therapy. About 50 per cent of *Madurella mycetomatis* infections respond to ketoconazole. In other infections griseofulvin, amphotericin B, ketoconazole, and itraconazole have rarely produced remission or cure. A trial of therapy may be attempted, where the patient can be monitored closely in outpatient departments. Otherwise, radical surgery or amputation is usually necessary. Small, local excisions are rarely successful.

Mycetoma is slowly progressive and increasingly disabling. However, wider dissemination is very rare, and therefore cases are seldom fatal, except where the skull is involved. However, the deformity caused by the disease may be severely disabling.

Further reading—mycetoma

Hay RJ (1997). Granule forming pathogenic mould fungi. In: Ajello L, Hay RJ, eds. *Mycology. Topley and Wilson's Microbiology and Microbial Infections*, 9th edn, Vol 4, pp 487–98. Arnold, London.

Mahgoub ES (1976). Medical management of mycetoma. *WHO Bulletin* **54**, 303–10.

Chromoblastomycosis

Aetiology

Chromoblastomycosis, one of the intermediate subcutaneous mycoses, is a chronic granulomatous fungal infection characterized histologically by the presence of brown, spherical fungal cells known as sclerotic cells or fumagoid bodies. In most cases, the lesions are confined to the skin and subcutaneous tissues. In the past there has been great confusion over nomenclature of the aetiological agents of chromoblastomycosis. At present, five agents assigned to four genera are recognized as causing chromoblastomycosis. They are:

(1) *Fonsecaea pedrosoi*, which occurs in high rainfall areas and is found worldwide;

(2) *Cladophialophora carrionii*, the sole cause of chromoblastomycosis in arid areas;

(3) *Phialophora verrucosa*, the first agent to be described;

(4) *Fonsecaea compactum*, an uncommon cause and isolated only a few times;

(5) *Rhinocladiella aquaspersa*, the rarest cause.

Sporadic cases caused by other dematiaceous fungi such as *Cladosporium trichoides* and *Taeniolélla boppii* have been reported from Uganda and Brazil.

Epidemiology

The principal endemic areas for chromoblastomycosis are the tropical and subtropical countries including Central and South America, Costa Rica, Africa, Japan, Australia, Malagasy, and Indonesia. Curiously, sporadic cases have been reported from Finland and Russia.

Although soil itself does not seem to be a particularly good substrate, the various agents of chromoblastomycosis occur as saprobic fungi in the environment and have been isolated from soil, decaying vegetation and rotting wood. Strains of *F. pedrosoi* and *P. verrucosa* have been isolated from the atmosphere but proved less virulent than those isolated from human lesions or organic material.

Infection occurs as a result of trauma, however minor, the fungi gaining entrance through a cut, abrasion, or thorn prick. Farmers and labourers in agricultural areas are most likely to be exposed to contaminated material. Although lesions on exposed areas may be accounted for in this way it was suggested by Wilson in 1958 that lesions on non-exposed areas may result from a previously unrecognized pulmonary focus. Bacquero later demonstrated the presence of *F. pedrosoi* in bronchial washings and subsequently proved their pathogenicity by inoculating those strains into normal skin of human volunteers and recovering the fungus from the ensuing skin lesions. Other methods of transmission have included metal particles from automobiles, and acupuncture. Person-to-person and animal-to-man transmission have not so far been reported. Chromoblastomycosis has rarely been reported in children and it may be that factors other than trauma and exposure to contaminated material are necessary for its development.

Pathogenesis

Host resistance and virulence of the organism are the two main factors associated with the pathogenesis of this disease. Chromoblastomycosis occurs mainly in healthy individuals. However, it has been found in patients where immunosuppression has occurred either from underlying disabling disease or from chemotherapy. Although the mechanism of granuloma formation is not well understood, it appears that lipids extracted from these fungi and cell-wall constituents may be responsible for this reaction.

Clinical features

The initial lesion of chromoblastomycosis is a small papule at the site of trauma, which gradually enlarges. Nodules and tumours develop, producing a malodorous discharge; eventually, over a period of years, a wide variety of morphological patterns may emerge including dry, hyperkeratotic plaques, verrucose lesions, and large, cauliflower-like masses. Extensive cicatricial plaques, surrounded by peripherally spreading vegetative lesions, may also be present. Evolution is slow and lesions usually involve the lower limb. However, any part of the body may be involved and the sites may be multiple.

Dissemination occurs by (i) surface spread, (ii) the lymphatics, the most common method, (iii) autoinoculation from scratching, and (iv) haematogenously, resulting in subcutaneous lesions at sites distant from the primary. Visceral metastases are known to occur and involvement of the central nervous system, respiratory system, larynx, and vocal chords has been recorded. Therapeutically, therefore, early diagnosis is important.

Complications of long-standing chromoblastomycosis include lymphoedema, flexion deformity of joints, and development of squamous carcinoma.

Diagnosis

Although the history and clinical presentation may suggest the diagnosis, the varied clinical presentation of chromoblastomycosis necessitates consideration of other granulomatous diseases such as sporotrichosis, cutaneous tuberculosis, Hansen's disease, blastomycosis, candidosis, leishmaniasis, paracoccidioidomycosis, rhinosporidiosis, tertiary syphilis, squamous carcinoma, and even psoriasis, sarcoidosis, and discoid lupus erythematosus.

Therefore, to establish a definitive diagnosis, histological and mycological investigations are essential. Diagnosis is confirmed by the presence of the characteristic brown, sclerotic bodies in histological sections. From both epidemiological and therapeutic points of view, culture is necessary as *F. pedrosoi* is the most difficult of the causative fungi to eradicate whereas *C. carrionii* responds rapidly to treatment.

Treatment

Small, single, localized lesions are satisfactorily eradicated by cryosurgery, but long-term follow-up is needed to assess accurately the success of this treatment. Thermotherapy has been found effective by some, again principally in the management of small, single lesions, but here the possibility of a burn must be borne in mind. Rapid spread of the disease has been associated with inadequate surgery, curettage, and electrodesiccation.

Oral monotherapy has been unsuccessful in some cases and drug resistance remains a problem. However itraconazole and terbinafine have both been reported as effective agents. A combination of 5-flucytosine with either thiabendazole or itraconazole may also be efficacious., particularly in long-standing disease

Whatever method of treatment is used, chromomycosis although clinically healed, should be followed-up for at least 2 years before its total eradication can be assumed.

Further reading—chromoblastomycosis

Bayles MAH (1989). Chromomycosis. In: Tropical fungal infections, *Baillière's clinical tropical medicine and communicable diseases*, Vol. 4, pp. 45–70. Baillière Tindall, London.

Bacquero GF, Lopez BP, Lescay BR (1961). Cromoblastomicosis experimental: cromoblastomicosis producida experimentalmente con cepas de *Hormodendrum pedrosoi* obtenida por lavado bronquial de enfermos que padecen la affecion. *Boletin de la Sociedad Cubana de Dermatologia y Sifilografia* 18, 19–28.

Grigoriu D, Delacretaz J, Borelli D (1987). In *Medical mycology*, (English edn), pp. 333–42. Hans Huber, Toronto.

McGinnis MR, Ajello L, Schell WA (1985). Mycotic diseases: a proposed nomenclature. *International Journal of Dermatology* 24, 9–15.

Silva CL, Ekizlerian SM (1985). Granulomatous reaction induced by lipids extracted from *Fonsecaea pedrosoi, Fonsecaea compactum, Cladosporium carrionii* and *Phialophora verrucosum. Journal of General Microbiology* 131, 187–94.

Silva CL, Fazioli RA (1985). Role of the fungal cell wall in the granulomatous response of mice to the agents of chromomycosis. *Journal of Medical Microbiology* 20, 299–305.

Wilson JW (1958). Importancia de las enfermedades fungosas en imunologia. *Boletin de la Sociedad Cubana de Dermatologia y Sifilografia* 15, 115–24.

Sporotrichosis

Aetiology

The most common clinical form of sporotrichosis is a subcutaneous infection, which may spread proximally from its initial site in a series of nodules along the course of a lymphatic. More rarely, systemic involvement is seen, for example in the lung (see Systemic mycoses, below).

The causative organism *Sporothrix schenckii* can be found in soil, vegetation, or in association with plants or bark. People who develop the subcutaneous infection may have had contact with material that harbours the organism, such as moss or flowers (for example florists). It is assumed that the pathogen gains entry via an abrasion and in some endemic areas there is often a preceding history of a scratch or insect bite.

Epidemiology

Although sporotrichosis was once prevalent in Europe, particularly France, non-imported cases are now very rare in this area. However, the disease is seen in the United States, Mexico, Central and South America, and Africa. In the late 1930s, there was a remarkable epidemic of sporotrichosis in workers in the Witwatersrand gold mines. The source of infection was a large number of wooden pit props contaminated with the organism. Other, smaller 'epidemics' have been described in certain groups, such as Mexican pottery workers packing ceramics in straw. Normally, however, cases are sporadic in incidence. There are also 'hyperendemic' areas where there is an unexpectedly high incidence of this infection.

Systemic sporotrichosis is much rarer, and cases have mainly been described from the United States.

Clinical features

There are two main clinical types of subcutaneous sporotrichosis.

The first, the fixed type, presents with a solitary cutaneous ulcer or nodule. In this form of the disease, infection does not spread along lymphatics.

It has been suggested that it is most common in children, and it has been described most frequently in Central and South America.

In the lymphangitic form, an initial nodule forms on a limb or extremity, such as a finger. This may break down and ulcerate. Subsequently, one or more secondary nodules develop along the draining lymphatic channel, which may ulcerate through the skin. Other variants include the psoriasiform or verrucous types or a superficial granuloma that resembles lupus vulgaris. These usually represent chronic infection.

Rarer forms include secondary spread via scratching, which may present with multiple widespread ulcers or multiple cutaneous lesions secondary to systemic disease. In HIV-positive individuals, widespread cutaneous lesions may develop.

Fixed-type sporotrichosis may resemble many other forms of cutaneous ulceration. However, in endemic areas a major source of confusion is cutaneous leishmaniasis. The lymphangitic variety may also resemble other infections, notably atypical mycobacterial infections, particularly fish-tank granuloma, or 'sporotrichoid' leishmaniasis.

Treatment

Some cases of sporotrichosis may heal spontaneously. However, treatment is usually advised to prevent scar formation. The cheapest treatment is potassium iodide, which is administered in a saturated aqueous solution. The starting dose is 0.5 to 1 ml, given three times daily, and this is increased drop by drop per dose to 3 to 6 ml, three times daily. The mixture is more palatable if given with milk. Treatment should be given for a month after clinical resolution. However, both itraconazole and terbinafine are also effective; minimal durations of treatment for these agents have not been defined.

Further reading—sporotrichosis

Bibler MR *et al.* (1986). Disseminated sporotrichosis in a patient with HIV infection after treatment for acquired factor VIII inhibitor. *Journal of the American Medical Association* 256, 3125–6.

de Albornoz MCB (1989). Sporotrichosis. In: Hay RJ, ed. *Tropical fungal infections, Baillière's clinical tropical medicine and communicable diseases*, Vol. 4, pp. 71–96. Baillière Tindall, London.

Subcutaneous zygomycosis due to *Basidiobolus*

Subcutaneous zygomycosis is an infection primarily seen in children in Africa or the Far East (Indonesia). It is characterized by the development of localized woody swellings on the limbs or trunk. The swelling is rarely inflammatory, but has a well-defined leading edge, and is hard. Progression is slow. The causative organism *Basidiobolus haptosporus* can be cultured or demonstrated histologically in biopsy material. Although resolution has been recorded without treatment, therapy is normally given. Potassium iodide solution is the treatment of choice, and is given in as high a dose as possible (see Sporotrichosis, above). Itraconazole may also be effective.

Subcutaneous zygomycosis due to *Conidiobolus* (conidiobolomycosis or rhinoentomophthoromycosis)

Conidiobolomycosis is a similar infection confined to subcutaneous tissue and presenting with painless swelling. The infection is mainly seen in West Africa, but a case has been seen in the Caribbean. There are important differences from the subcutaneous zygomycosis caused by *Basidiobolus*. The disease is most common in young adults, and is confined to facial tissues around the nose, the forehead, and the upper lip. The initial site of infection is in the region of the inferior turbinate in the nose. The diagnosis is established by biopsy or culture. The causative organism is *Conidiobolus coronatus*. Treatment with itraconazole or ketoconazole is effective, but an alternative is high-dose potassium iodide. Relapse after treatment is common, and residual fibrosis may be severely disfiguring.

Lobo's disease (lobomycosis)

Lobo's disease is a subcutaneous infection. The organism, in tissue, appears to be a yeast. It has a tendency to form chains of four to six yeast cells with prominent nucleoli, joined by a narrow, intercellular bridge. However, the organism has never been cultured from human cases and can only be identified by biopsy and histology. The disease is seen in countries of South America around, and north of, the Amazon basin, and cases are also seen in Central America. Apart from humans the only other species affected are freshwater dolphins. Often, exposed sites (such as ear lobes) are invaded and small nodules containing the organisms develop. These may resemble keloids (Plate 7). More diffuse plaques may also be seen. Deep invasion has not been documented. The treatment is excision, and there is no effective chemotherapy.

Systemic mycoses

The systemic or deep visceral mycoses include some of the rare and more serious of the fungal infections. There are two main types of infection in this group, those caused by organisms which invade normal hosts, the endemic mycoses, and those which only cause disease in compromised patients, the opportunistic mycoses. The fungi associated with these two types of infection differ in their innate levels of pathogenicity, but an element of opportunism, depending on host susceptibility, is usually recognizable in all cases of systemic mycoses.

The endemic pathogens cause infections such as histoplasmosis or coccidioidomycosis. These diseases have well-defined endemic zones and the majority of those exposed remain symptomless but usually develop positive skin tests. However, in certain patients, chronic local or disseminated disease may occur. In the systemic infections caused by opportunistic fungi, there is usually a serious underlying abnormality in the patient affecting T lymphocytes (such as HIV) or neutrophils (such as cancer chemotherapy). Such infections are worldwide in occurrence: where tissue invasion occurs the mortality is high. Cryptococcosis, a systemic yeast infection, has features of both types of systemic disease and occurs in both normal and immunosuppressed subjects.

The systemic endemic infections are histoplasmosis, coccidioidomycosis, blastomycosis, paracoccidioidomycosis, and infections due to *Penicillium marneffei*. The significance of various laboratory tests in these infections is shown in Table 3.

Further reading—systemic mycoses

de Pauw BE, Meunier F (1999). The challenge of invasive fungal infection. *Chemotherapy* **45**(Suppl 1), 1–14.

Histoplasmosis (see also Section 17)

There are two forms of histoplasmosis. In both types, the organism is present in tissue in its yeast phase. In small-form or classic histoplasmosis, the diameter of the yeast cells is between 3 and 4 μm. Infections are most common in the United States, but sporadic cases are reported widely from the New World, Africa, and the Far East. By contrast, large-form or African histoplasmosis is most common in Central Africa, south of the Sahara and north of the Zambezi river. Yeast forms in infected tissue are much larger, 10 to 15 μm in diameter. Both infections are clinically distinct (see below), but cultural isolates are indistinguishable.

Histoplasmosis (classic or small-form histoplasmosis)

Aetiology

Histoplasmosis is a systemic infection caused by *Histoplasma capsulatum*. The main route of infection is pulmonary. The majority of those exposed are sensitized without overt signs of infection, but more rarely chronic pulmonary or disseminated forms of the disease are seen.

The organism, *H. capsulatum*, can be found in soil in endemic areas. Its growth is facilitated by the presence of bird excreta, for instance in old chicken houses, bird roosts, and barns. In tropical and some temperate areas, bat guano plays a similar role. Exposure to a suitable source, such as a cave containing bats, is often recorded in acute epidemic histoplasmosis (see below). It is rarely identified in more slowly evolving cases.

The condition of the host is important in determining the clinical course and manifestations of histoplasmosis. Slowly evolving (chronic), disseminated disease may occur in normal individuals. However, infants, elderly

Table 3 Laboratory tests in systemic mycoses

	Direct microscopy	Significance of positive cultures	Serology	Histopathology
Histoplasmosis				
1. Classic (small form)	Sometimes positive	Significant	ID, CIE, CFT	Yeasts (3–4 μm)
2. African histoplasmosis	Positive in pus (valuable)	Significant	ID, CFT	Yeasts (10–15 μm)
Coccidioidomycosis	Positive in pus, sputum etc. (valuable)	Significant NB Handle with caution	ID, CFT, TP, CIE	Spherules (50–150 μm)
Blastomycosis	Positive in pus, sputum etc. (valuable)	Significant	ID, CFT, CIE (unreliable)	Yeasts (4–10 μm) Broad-based buds
Paracoccidioidomycosis	Positive in pus, sputum etc. (valuable)	Significant	ID, CFT, TP Antigen detection	Yeasts (5–15 μm) Multiple buds
Cryptococcosis	Often positive in CSF (rare in urine, pus) NB Indian ink	Significant	ID, CFT, WCA, IF, Latex agglutination-antigen	Encapsulated yeasts (5–10 μm) Mucicarmine positive
Systemic candidosis	Positive in oral smears, sputum etc. (interpret with caution)	Significance depends on site and presence of positive microscopy	ID, CFT, WCA, CIE Antigen detection e.g. RAMCO	Yeasts (5–10 μm) and hyphae
Invasive aspergillosis	Rarely positive, depends on site	Positive sputum cultures not always significant	ID, CIE, rarely positive Antigen detection e.g. Pasteurex	Hyphae—dichotomous branching
Invasive zygomycosis	Rarely positive	Depends on site	ID, CIE, rarely positive	Hyphae—broad and aseptate

CFT, complement fixation test; CIE, counterimmunoelectrophoresis; CSF, cerebrospinal fluid; ID, immunodiffusion; IF, immunofluorescence; RIA, radioimmunoassay; TP, tube precipitation; WCA, whole-cell agglutination.

people, or those with untreated AIDS appear to be more likely to develop the more rapidly progressive forms of disseminated infection.

Epidemiology

The major endemic area, as shown by skin testing, is in the central region of the United States around the Ohio and Mississippi valley basins. Prevalence is highest in the states of Tennessee, Kentucky, and Ohio. Up to 95 per cent of those skin tested in certain parts of these areas have positive delayed reactions to intradermal histoplasmin (compare Mantoux test). Scattered cases of active disease, healed calcified foci in chest radiographs, and foci found at autopsy representing inactive histoplasmosis also provide evidence of spread within this area. However, the disease also occurs in other parts of the United States, Mexico, Central and South America, Africa, the Far East, and Australia. Outside the major endemic areas in the United States, human cases are less frequent, and much of the evidence of the endemicity comes from positive skin tests or the presence of the organism in selected sites, such as caves. Although there has been considerable discussion on the nature of soil factors responsible for the growth of *H. capsulatum*, the conditions limiting its occurrence to certain areas are largely unknown.

Clinical features

The clinical forms of histoplasmosis can be placed in several groups:

(1) asymptomatic;

(2) acute symptomatic pulmonary:

    (i) acute epidemic,

    (ii) acute reinfection;

(3) chronic pulmonary;

(4) disseminated (acute, subacute, and chronic); and

(5) primary cutaneous (by inoculation).

Asymptomatic infection

Over 99 per cent of patients becoming infected in endemic areas record no overt symptoms but develop a positive skin test. The incidence of positive skin tests declines in individuals above the age of 60 years.

Acute (symptomatic) pulmonary histoplasmosis

Acute epidemic histoplasmosis Groups of individuals exposed to a source of infection, for instance during cave exploration, or those who may have inhaled a large infecting dose, often develop a symptomatic illness 12 to 21 days after exposure. The main features are pyrexia, cough, chest pain, and malaise. Flitting arthralgia and, less commonly, erythema nodosum or multiforme may occur. The radiological appearances may be much more severe than would be supposed from the symptoms, and enlargement of hilar lymph nodes and diffuse or patchy consolidation suggesting pneumonitis may occur (Plate 6).

These patients develop precipitating or complement-fixing antibody, but this often follows the peak of illness. About 50 per cent of those with symptoms do not develop positive antibody responses. Likewise, skin test conversion is often too late to be of diagnostic value, and its use is normally contraindicated, as a single histoplasmin test may cause the development of false-positive serological results. Cultures are often negative. The symptoms and history of exposure to a suitable source, combined with a rising antibody titre, are often the best evidence of infection.

The majority of cases require no specific therapy apart from rest. Those with severe or prolonged symptoms or impaired gas exchange require intravenous amphotericin B or itraconazole. The lung lesions often heal to leave multiple scattered pulmonary calcifications.

Acute reinfection histoplasmosis Massive acute exposure to *H. capsulatum* in sensitized individuals is believed by some physicians to cause a less severe infection associated with bilateral pulmonary infiltrates. The incubation period is shorter than with acute epidemic histoplasmosis, namely 5 to 10 days.

Chronic pulmonary histoplasmosis

Chronic pulmonary disease caused by *H. capsulatum* is mainly seen in the United States. It is more common in males and smokers, and there is often underlying pulmonary disease such as emphysema. Early cases may present with pyrexia and cough, but malaise and weight loss occur later. Lesions may heal initially, but relapse is common, leading to established consolidation and cavitation. The most common radiological appearance of early lesions is of unilateral, wedge-shaped, segmental shadows in the apical zones. Subsequently, the disease may become bilateral, with fibrosis and cavitation. In some cases, extensive and progressive destruction of lung tissue may occur.

Culture and serology are both helpful methods of diagnosis in this form of histoplasmosis, but repeated attempts may be required before positive results are obtained.

In early cases, resolution may occur on rest alone. However, relapse occurs in at least 25 per cent of cases, and these patients may require amphotericin B therapy or itraconazole. Although chemotherapy may virtually sterilize lesions, fibrosis persists and relapse may occur. Surgical excision or lobectomy is sometimes effective.

Solid lung tumours may persist after the primary infection. These may be single (coin lesions) or multiple, and have to be distinguished from carcinomas. The diagnosis is normally made at surgery, although the presence of calcification may give a clue to the nature of the lesion (histoplasmoma). The organisms can be demonstrated by histopathology, but they are seldom viable.

Disseminated histoplasmosis

There is considerable variation in the rate of progression of histoplasmosis that has spread beyond the initial focus in the lung. In rapid or acutely disseminated cases, widespread infiltration of reticuloendothelial cells of bone marrow, spleen, and liver may occur. Gastrointestinal lesions, endocarditis, and meningitis are less common, and meningitis is more usually associated with a slower course of disseminated disease. Infants, elderly people, or immunosuppressed patients are more susceptible to acute dissemination. The most prominent symptoms are fever and weight loss, with accompanying hepatosplenomegaly. Extensive purpura and bruising secondary to thrombocytopenia may occur. The blood picture may reflect marrow infiltration with organisms, leading to pancytopenia. Disseminated histoplasmosis is also seen in patients with AIDS. The clinical manifestations are not significantly different, although skin papules and ulcers have been reported in many; isolation of *Histoplasma* from blood has also been reported more frequently in these patients. Cultures, including sputum or bone marrow, should be taken. Serology is often positive, with high titres of complement-fixing antibodies occurring in some patients. However, new antigen detection systems in serum or urine provide a better means of confirming the diagnosis and monitoring treatment.

A much more slowly progressive form of disseminated histoplasmosis may present with fewer localized lesions, such as persistent oral ulcers, chronic laryngitis, or adrenal insufficiency. Granulomas, few of which contain organisms, can be found in the liver in some patients. Such cases may present up to 30 years after the patient has left an endemic area. Outside endemic areas this form is the most widely recognized presentation of histoplasmosis, occurring in Europeans, for instance, who have worked in Africa or the Far East.

The diagnosis of disseminated histoplasmosis is made on culture or biopsy of affected areas. Antibodies may only be positive in low titres and in all cases adrenal involvement should be looked for.

Treatment is required in all forms of disseminated histoplasmosis. Itraconazole is preferred by most physicians, although amphotericin B may be necessary in some patients. Oral ketoconazole is an alternative. In patients with AIDS who are acutely ill, the disease is often controlled by a short (2 week) course of amphotericin B and thereafter patients receive continuous itraconazole indefinitely.

Primary cutaneous histoplasmosis

Primary infection sometimes follows accidental inoculation of viable organisms in a laboratory or autopsy room. This type of infection is normally associated with a chancre at the site of inoculation and regional lymphadenopathy. The condition is self-limiting.

African histoplasmosis

Overt pulmonary involvement is rare in this form of histoplasmosis, and the normal portal of entry of the pathogen is not known. The most common presenting features are skin lesions (papules, nodules, abscesses, or ulcers) (Plate 8) or lytic bone deposits. Solitary or multiple foci may be present, and in the latter instances rapid progression and death may occur. In such cases, gastrointestinal and lung lesions may develop.

The diagnosis is normally made by culture, smear, or biopsy. The organism *H. capsulatum* var. *duboisii* is identical to that causing classic histoplasmosis in culture, but in lesions the yeast forms are considerably larger (10 to 15 μm).

While local excision of skin nodules has been reported to be curative, treatment with itraconazole, ketoconazole, or amphotericin B is usual. Some patients will respond to co-trimoxazole. A skeletal scan should be made to detect occult foci of infection.

Further reading—histoplasmosis

Ashford DA *et al.* (1999). Outbreak of histoplasmosis among cavers attending the National Speleological Society Annual Convention, Texas, 1994. *American Journal of Tropical Medicine and Hygiene* **60**, 899–903.

Goodwin RA, Loyd JE, DesPrez RM (1981). Histoplasmosis in normal hosts. *Medicine* **60**, 231–66.

Khalil MA, Hassan AW, Gugnani HC (1998). African histoplasmosis: report of four cases from north-eastern Nigeria. *Mycoses* **41**, 293–5.

Mandell W, Goldberg DM, Neu HC (1986). Histoplasmosis in patients with the acquired immune deficiency syndrome (AIDS). *Annals of Internal Medicine* **111**, 655–9.

Blastomycosis (see also Section 23)

Blastomycosis (North American blastomycosis) caused by *Blastomyces dermatitidis* is a systemic fungal infection in which skin and lung involvement are common features.

The infective organism, *B. dermatitidis*, has only been isolated from the environment on rare occasions. Positive sites have included soil and rotten timbers. The organism infects humans and domestic animals, particularly the dog.

Epidemiology

Blastomycosis was originally thought to be confined to North America, where it occurs sporadically throughout the south and east-central area, and in areas of central Canada. 'Epidemics' of acute disease are rare, and where these occur a source of infection is rarely demonstrated. There is evidence that sources may include areas exposed to flooding.

More recently, cases have been found in Africa. Again, these are widely scattered from the north coast to the southern parts of the continent, and are rare in all areas. Patients with the disease have also been reported from the Middle East and Central Europe.

Clinical features

The clinical forms of blastomycosis differ from histoplasmosis in a number of important aspects. The existence of an asymptomatic form has not been proved conclusively, because there is no reliable skin test. Acute infections or infections in groups are rare, and the features are often similar to histoplasmosis (acute pulmonary). However, specific serological tests may be negative in 30 to 50 per cent of cases. The demonstration of the organisms in sputum and positive cultures are more reliable diagnostic criteria. Although some cases undoubtedly resolve without sequelae, some phys-

icians advise chemotherapy, with a short course of amphotericin B in acute cases of blastomycosis.

Chronic pulmonary blastomycosis

Chronic consolidation or cavitation of the upper or mid-zones occur with chronic pulmonary infections. Fever, malaise, and cough with sputum are seen. Weight loss may be prominent. Culture is again the most reliable method of diagnosis.

The mainstays of treatment are itraconazole or amphotericin B.

Disseminated blastomycosis

Although generalized infiltration in skin, lungs, and liver may occur over a short period, leading to rapid death, signs of chronic extrapulmonary dissemination are more usual.

The skin is an area that is frequently involved (chronic cutaneous blastomycosis). The face or forearms and hands are common sites for skin lesions. These are slow, spreading, verrucose plaques with central scarring. The initial lesion is often a dermal nodule. Many such cases have underlying pulmonary consolidation, or cavities. The diagnosis is established by biopsy and culture. Bone deposits in the form of lytic lesions, and involvement of the genitourinary tract, particularly the epididymis, are also seen in chronic disseminated blastomycosis. Unlike tuberculosis, the kidneys are often spared.

In slowly progressive forms of blastomycosis, itraconazole (200 to 400 mg daily) has proved to be very effective. Alternatively, amphotericin B can be given intravenously and is indicated where there is rapidly progressive disease.

Further reading—blastomycosis

Emerson PA, Higgins E, Branfoot A (1984). North American blastomycosis in Africans. *British Journal of Diseases of the Chest* **78**, 286–91.

Sarosi GA, Davies SF (1979). Blastomycosis. *American Reviews of Respiratory Diseases* **120**, 911–38.

Coccidioidomycosis

See Chapter 7.12.3.

Paracoccidioidomycosis

See Chapter 7.12.4.

Systemic sporotrichosis

In addition to causing cutaneous disease, *Sporothrix schenckii* may be responsible for a systemic mycosis. The infection is rare and has been mainly reported from the United States. Involvement may be confined to a single site such as a lung or a joint, or it may be multifocal. Cavitation in the lung associated with weight loss and pyrexia is probably the most common variety of systemic sporotrichosis. Unlike cutaneous forms of the disease, systemic sporotrichosis responds poorly to potassium iodide, and amphotericin B is the treatment of choice.

Rare systemic infections

These include pulmonary invasion by *Geotrichum candidum* (geotrichosis) and adiaspiromycosis, a respiratory infection caused by *Emmonsia crescens* or *Emmonsia parva*. Isolated examples of human disease caused by fungi are consistently reported and almost always occur in the immunosuppressed host. In these patients many fungi that are normally saprophytes in the environment may invade and cause disease.

Systemic mycoses caused by opportunistic fungi

The opportunistic mycoses are a worldwide problem, although fortunately rare in most countries. In recent years they have been recognized more frequently with the increase in transplantations of organs such as heart or bone marrow and in the more effective but immunocompromising regimes of cancer chemotherapy. Opportunistic invasion by organisms such as *Candida* or zygomycetes (*Mucor, Absidia*) may also occur in cases of malnutrition. One of the recent trends in the management of the patient with neutropenia has been the emergence of new pathogens such as non-*albicans* species of *Candida* or other organisms such as *Fusarium, Trichosporon,* or *Hansenula* species.

The opportunists present particular problems in diagnosis and management. Because many of the organisms are normally saprophytic, it has to be positively established that they have assumed an invasive role. Mere isolation may not provide sufficient evidence and in some instances low titres of antibody may be present even in normal hosts. The significance of various laboratory tests in these infections is shown in Table 3. Treatment is also difficult and it is important in most cases to attempt to reverse the process that led to the establishment of the infection.

Systemic candidosis

Aetiology

In addition to their role in superficial infections, yeasts of the genus *Candida* may also cause invasive systemic disease. The clinical forms described range from bloodstream isolation or candidaemia to disseminated invasive disease, sometimes with involvement of a single organ, site, or body cavity (deep focal candidosis) as may occur in peritonitis or meningitis. Urinary tract infections may also be caused by *Candida* species.

The factors underlying systemic *Candida* infections are shown in Table 4. All these factors are important in disrupting the balance by which *Candida* is maintained as a saprophyte. Intravenous or central venous pressure lines may serve as a portal of entry or as a nidus for circulating yeasts in a candidaemia. Antibiotic therapy may upset the balance by inhibiting a potentially competitive bacterial flora.

Candida albicans is the most common species involved but other species may be isolated, particularly in cases of endocarditis, for example *Candida parapsilosis. Candida tropicalis* has been implicated in infections of patients with neutropenia. These non-*albicans Candida* species are now more frequent causes of systemic infection and are important to recognize as their antifungal susceptibility may differ from *C. albicans.* Portals of entry include the gastrointestinal tract (common), skin, and urinary tract (rare). However, superficial candidosis or saprophytic colonization of mouth, skin, or airways may also occur in compromised patients and does not necessarily indicate systemic invasion.

Epidemiology

Systemic infections caused by *Candida* species are worldwide in distribution. However, they are particularly associated with a number of predisposing factors such as neutropenia, antibiotic usage, indwelling lines, and abdominal surgery.

Table 4 Predisposing factors in deep *Candida* infections

1. Local defects, foreign bodies, e.g. prosthetic heart valves, intravenous lines
2. Defects of immunity (primarily T cell or phagocytosis), e.g. cytotoxic therapy or systemic lupus erythematosis
3. Drug therapy, e.g. antibiotics
4. Carcinoma or leukaemia
5. Endocrine disease, e.g. diabetes mellitus in urinary tract candidosis
6. Physiological changes, e.g. infancy, old age, and pregnancy (urinary tract)
7. Miscellaneous disorders, e.g.
    (i) malnutrition
    (ii) surgery such as gastrointestinal resections
    (iii) drug addiction

Clinical features

Candidaemia

The isolation of *Candida* in blood culture may be linked to any of the factors listed in Table 4. Common predisposing features are the presence of intravenous lines, previous surgery (mainly gastrointestinal), antibiotic therapy, hepatic failure, or neutropenia. Patients develop a swinging fever and feel generally unwell. Clinical shock may occur.

Some such cases resolve following removal of predisposing factors, particularly the intravenous lines. Generally, however, all such patients receive treatment and a careful investigation should be made to identify the presence of established invasive disease. Other sites should be searched for evidence of infection; for example urine by culture or the presence of white cells. Signs of muscle invasion (tenderness) or metastatic skin nodules should be excluded (Plate 9). Other signs of invasion include the development of new cardiac murmurs or of soft, white, retinal plaques caused by *Candida.* Persistently positive blood cultures or serum *Candida* antigen levels or high antibody titres may also indicate possible deep invasion.

Disseminated candidosis

Although multiorgan invasive candidosis may follow candidaemia, at least 50 per cent of disseminated infections develop in patients without initially positive blood cultures. The features of some forms of invasive candidosis are listed above (under Candidaemia). Although *Candida* may be isolated from the sputum in these patients, there is rarely objective evidence of lung invasion. Moreover, there is no radiological appearance that is diagnostic of pulmonary candidosis and, indeed, chest radiographs may even appear normal. General localizing signs may be a late feature of disseminated candidosis.

Laboratory diagnosis of disseminated candidosis The diagnosis may be made by culture and repeated attempts to isolate should be made where cultures are initially negative. Numerous techniques have been used to detect antibody or antigen in disseminated candidosis. However, in many patients, particularly those with neutropenia, it may not be possible to confirm the diagnosis using laboratory tests and treatment is often initiated on the basis of clinical suspicion (empirical therapy) as the risk of delaying antifungal therapy is great.

By themselves, positive cultures, particularly from sputum, or the presence of antibodies do not necessarily prove the existence of deep-seated candidosis. A positive isolation may simply indicate the presence of colonization and normal individuals may have low titres of antibody to *Candida.* If there is a readily accessible lesion from which to take a biopsy, such as a skin nodule or even a pulmonary infiltrate, this may provide the best evidence of invasion, although such procedures may carry their own risk (Plate 8).

Treatment of disseminated candidosis Untreated disseminated candidosis is normally progressive and fatal. The signs must be separated from, for instance, bacterial septicaemia, which may coexist with the *Candida* infection.

The treatment of invasive candidosis is intravenous amphotericin B or intravenous or oral fluconazole given until there is a clinical and mycological response. This may take between 2 and 20 weeks depending on the site of infection and the underlying state of the patient. Fluconazole is usually used in infections where the patient is not neutropenic. Lipid-associated forms of amphotericin B are also useful and carry a lower risk of renal impairment. An alternative approach is to add flucytosine in doses of 150 to 200 mg/kg body weight daily to amphotericin B in serious infections or where cure may be hampered by poor penetration of amphotericin B, such as in the eye.

Deep focal candidosis

Candida infections in the peritoneum or meninges most often follow direct implantation after dialysis or surgery. Alternatively, secondary invasion from the middle ear or a perforated bowel is also possible. The signs and symptoms are similar to bacterial meningitis or peritonitis but *Candida* is isolated. Sometimes these infections clear spontaneously, but normally treatment is instituted with fluconazole, which penetrates areas such as peritoneum, or amphotericin B.

Candida endocarditis

Invasion of heart valves, mainly the mitral or aortic valves, most commonly follows homograft replacement, but it may occur also in patients with neutropenia or drug addicts. The symptoms are similar to bacterial endocarditis. However, *Candida* vegetations may reach considerable size. Embolic phenomena may involve obstruction of large vessels including the femoral artery or large cerebral vessels. The detection of large vegetations using an echo scanning device, particularly in cases with negative blood cultures, should raise the possibility of fungal endocarditis. Blood cultures are usually positive at some stage in the illness but repeated sampling may be necessary. High antibody titres are usually seen in such cases and serological tests are therefore of considerable value.

Untreated *Candida* endocarditis is uniformly fatal. There is also a high mortality associated with cases in which early surgical intervention is precipitated by impending heart failure. Normally, treatment consists of amphotericin B given intravenously and, where possible, valve replacement. There is no evidence to suggest that the addition of flucytosine to the regimen increases the effectiveness of treatment. However, the relapse rate is high and combination therapy may therefore be a reasonable approach on theoretical grounds.

Urinary tract candidosis

Candida species may be isolated from the urine, particularly in conditions associated with urinary stasis such as neurogenic bladder or where there is an indwelling catheter. Maturity-onset diabetes mellitus is another predisposing factor. There is no value in using the presence of pyuria or quantitative yeast-colony counts to assess the significance of infection. Treatment is normally given where there are symptoms such as dysuria or frequency or where there is a potential risk of invasion such as in immunosuppressed patients. Fluconazole is very useful in these patients as urinary levels are above inhibitory concentrations.

Further reading—opportunistic systemic mycoses

Krcmery V, Krupova I, Denning DW (1999). Invasive yeast infections other than *Candida* spp. in acute leukaemia. *Journal of Hospital Infection* **41**, 181–94.

Reiss E *et al.* (1998). Molecular diagnosis and epidemiology of fungal infections. *Journal of Medical Mycology* **36**(Suppl 1), 249–57.

Wingard JR (1999). Fungal infections after bone marrow transplant. *Biology of Blood and Marrow Transplantation* **5**, 55–68.

Aspergillosis (see Section 8.4)

Cryptococcosis

Aetiology

Cryptococcosis is a systemic infection caused by *Cryptococcus neoformans*. Its most common clinical feature is meningitis, but pulmonary, cutaneous, and widely disseminated forms of the infection are also recognized. There are two varieties of *C. neoformans* called *C. neoformans neoformans* and *C. neoformans gattii*. They differ in their geographical range and ecology. The *neoformans* variety is the most common in patients with AIDS.

C. neoformans neoformans is a yeast that can be isolated from the environment, although it is most often found in pigeon excreta. Its growth from soil appears to be enhanced by certain nitrogenous compounds, such as creatinine in the pigeon droppings. The birds are not infected, although their crops may be heavily colonized. Very large numbers of organisms (1×10^7 yeasts/g of droppings) may be found in densely populated urban areas. *C. neoformans gattii* has been detected in leaf and bark debris of certain eucalyptus species.

The portal of entry is usually the lung, from where the organism spreads to involve other organs or sites such as the meninges. Although many isolates from natural sources have small cells, one sequel to tissue invasion is the development of a large, mucoid capsule *in vivo*, a feature that may confer some protection to the organism. Infections with *C. neoformans* are seen in both normal and immunocompromised hosts. The main underlying processes are sarcoidosis, Hodgkin's disease, collagen disease, carcinoma, and the administration of systemic corticosteroid therapy, but AIDS is the commonest predisposition.

Epidemiology

Cryptococcosis has been recorded from most countries, although it is most prevalent in the United States and Australia. Before the AIDS epidemic in the United States approximately 50 per cent of cases were said to occur in normal persons. By contrast, in the United Kingdom, 85 per cent of cases were found in patients with underlying disorders. There is no skin-test reagent widely available, but some pilot studies in the United States suggest that workers exposed to the organism (for example in laboratories) are more likely than other groups to have a positive skin test without any overt sign of infection. It is probable, therefore, that there is an asymptomatic form of cryptococcosis (compare histoplasmosis). Additional evidence for the existence of subclinical infection is provided by the repeated isolation of *C. neoformans* in sputum from individuals without evidence of disease.

Clinical features

Pulmonary cryptococcosis

Acute or subacute respiratory disease caused by *C. neoformans* is seen in both HIV-positive and healthy individuals. The disease consists of a chest infection with fever and cough and scattered, often well-circumscribed, areas of pulmonary infiltration seen on radiographs. Pleural involvement can occur and sometimes massive pulmonary infiltrates may occur. Before the advent of the azoles, in some patients the whole process resolved without treatment, although it is probably advisable to give fluconazole to those with isolated pulmonary disease. More often, lung lesions accompany disseminated cryptococcosis or cryptococcal meningitis and the treatment is discussed below. The laboratory diagnosis is made by biopsy or culture. Isolated cryptococcal granulomas (cryptococcoma) may present as coin lesions and are removed surgically to exclude carcinoma. Once the correct diagnosis is made, many workers advise a short course of amphotericin B or fluconazole as there is a small risk of dissemination to other organs following surgery.

Disseminated cryptococcosis

The best-recognized form of extrapulmonary cryptococcosis is meningitis. This may present with signs of acute meningism. However, more usually the features are less specific. Pyrexia, headache, and mental changes such as confusion or drowsiness occur. The mental changes probably follow the development of hydrocephalus. Blurring of vision and papilloedema may also occur. Cranial nerve involvement is less common. Patients with AIDS often present with widely disseminated disease. The signs of meningeal involvement may be very subtle and the infection has often spread to other sites such as liver and spleen as well as skin.

The cerebrospinal fluid shows pleocytosis that is highly variable. Often there are excessive numbers of lymphocytes, but sometimes polymorphonuclear leucocytes abound. In some cases only small numbers of white cells (4 to 10/ml) are seen. Characteristically, but not invariably, the glucose concentration falls and protein rises. Cryptococci can be seen in some cases in an India ink or nigrosin preparation, which is used to highlight the capsule. A spun sediment is best for this purpose. The organism can also be cultured from the cerebrospinal fluid. The latex test for antigen is usually positive for cerebrospinal fluid, but on rare occasions this is negative. The antigen titre has both diagnostic and prognostic value. Initial high (> 100) titres are likely to correlate with relapse following therapy and with a poor prognosis. In patients with AIDS, antigen titres over 1:1000 convey poor prognosis and blood cultures are often positive. Extrameningeal disease should be looked for by sputum or urine culture and serology in patients presenting with meningitis.

Other sites

Cryptococci may disseminate to other sites including liver and spleen, kidney, skin, or bone. Infection in skin and bone are most often seen in patients with sarcoidisis. In every case, underlying deep disseminated lesions (such as meningitis) may be found. The methods of diagnosis and treatment are similar to those seen with meningitis. Only a small proportion of cases with solitary disseminated lesions of cryptococcosis, such as bone or skin, may have detectable antigen (15 to 30 per cent), and this may occur late in the course of therapy. In patients with AIDS the organism spreads widely involving bone marrow, liver, and spleen as well as other sites. Positive blood cultures are not uncommon. The serum antigen titres are often very high, for example over 500, and may not return to normal even during antifungal treatment.

It is important in all cases where cryptococcosis presents with lesions in an extrameningeal site to exclude occult meningitis by lumbar puncture.

Treatment

In the patient without AIDS the combination of flucytosine (150 to 180 mg/kg daily) and intravenous amphotericin B (0.3 to 0.6 mg/kg daily) is the most widely used treatment. It is possible to induce recovery with this approach and treatment is generally continued for at least 6 weeks or longer if necessary. The clinical response and antigen levels are useful for monitoring progress.

The situation is different in patients with AIDS because in patients not receiving combination antiretrovirals it is impossible to achieve complete recovery. The object of therapy is to induce the most rapid remission possible, followed by long-term suppressive therapy. There are various regimens used for induction of remission. The use of amphotericin B with or without flucytosine is favoured by many. This is given for 2 weeks and is then followed by indefinite treatment with fluconazole to prevent relapse. Itraconazole is an alternative. In patients on highly active antiretroviral therapy (MAART) it may be possible to discontinue treatment but guidelines are awaited.

Further reading—cryptococcosis

Clark RA *et al.* (1990). Spectrum of *Cryptococcus neoformans* infection in 68 patients infected with acquired immunodeficiency virus. *Reviews of Infectious Diseases* **12**, 768–77.

Seaton A *et al.* (1996). Exposure to *Cryptococcus neoformans* var *gattii*—a seroepidemiological study. *Transactions of the Royal Society of Tropical Medicine and Hygiene* **90**, 508–12.

Stevens DA (1990). Fungal infections in AIDS patients. *British Journal of Clinical Practice* **44**(Suppl 71), 11–22.

Invasive zygomycosis (mucormycosis, phycomycosis)

Aetiology

Invasive disease caused by mucor-like (zygomycete) fungi is rare. In the compromised host it may lead to paranasal destruction, necrotic lung or skin lesions, and disseminated disease.

The causative organisms commonly belong to three genera, *Absidia*, *Rhizopus*, and *Rhizomucor*. More rarely other organisms such as *Cunninghamella* or *Saksenaea* have been implicated. Most of the agents are associated with decaying vegetable matter and are common airborne moulds. The route of infection is highly variable: they may invade via the lungs, paranasal sinuses, gastrointestinal tract, or damaged skin. The predisposing illness may in some way determine the site of clinical invasion. Underlying factors include diabetic ketoacidosis (rhinocerebral involvement), leukaemia and immunosuppressive therapy (lung and disseminated infection), malnutrition (gastrointestinal infection), and burns or wounds (cutaneous invasion). These patterns are not always strictly followed.

Epidemiology

Invasive zygomycosis is rare but has a worldwide distribution. Its invasive nature, particularly the tendency to involve blood vessels and its selection of compromised hosts, distinguishes this form of infection from subcutaneous zygomycosis, which is also caused by zygomycete species.

Clinical features

The most characteristic features of this type of infection are the extensive necrosis and infarction that may follow blood vessel invasion leading to thrombosis. A similar type of invasion may occur with invasive aspergillosis, but is usually less prominent. Invasive zygomycosis follows a number of different patterns.

The infection may initially localize in one of several sites. The most common is in the paranasal sinuses and this is most often seen in diabetic patients with ketoacidosis. The patient presents with fever and unilateral facial pain. Subsequently, there may be facial swelling with nasal obstruction and proptosis. There may be invasion into the orbit leading to blindness, into the brain, and the palate. Palatal ulceration should be searched for. Widespread dissemination with infarction of major organs or limbs may occur subsequently. A similar pattern of invasion of surgical wounds or burns may occur and has on occasions been associated with contamination of dressing packs. Infections are initially localized causing extensive necrosis around the original wound. Gastrointestinal invasion may be heralded by perforation of viscera, and diarrhoea or haemorrhage.

Alternatively, a patient may present with established pulmonary or widespread dissemination. Such patients are usually leukaemic or are severely immunosuppressed. Neutropenia is often seen.

Once infection has spread beyond the original site, invasive zygomycosis is almost invariably fatal with or without treatment.

Laboratory diagnosis

The diagnosis is suggested by the combination of infection and extensive infarction, particularly if it occurs in any of the sites mentioned. The organisms may be difficult to culture even from biopsy and histology is often the quickest way of establishing the diagnosis. Serology is frequently negative.

Treatment

Treatment should be initiated as soon as possible and extensive surgical debridement combined with intravenous amphotericin B in maximum daily dosage offers the best chance of success. Local instillations of amphotericin B may also be used where appropriate (such as nasal sinuses). Some physicians also recommend anticoagulation with heparin to forestall thrombosis. Despite therapy, the mortality remains high. Liposomal amphotericin B also has been used with some success is cases of mucormycosis.

Further reading—zygomycosis

Nenoff P *et al.* (1998). Rhinocerebral zygomycosis following bone marrow transplantation in chronic myelogenous leukaemia. Report of a case and review of the literature. *Mycoses* **41**, 365–72.

Rhinosporidiosis

Rhinosporidiosis is an infection found in India, Sri Lanka, parts of East Africa, and South America. It is characterized by polypoid growth from the nose or conjunctiva. The causative organism can be demonstrated in tissue and consists of aggregates of large sporangia containing spores in various phases of development. However, they have never been successfully cultured and their fungal nature has only been assumed from their morphological appearance in histology.

The treatment is surgical excision.

Otomycosis and oculomycosis

External otitis is often multifactorial, but in some cases dense fungal colonization can contribute to the picture. In severe cases, the external ear may be plugged by a dense mat of mycelium. *Aspergillus* species are the most common organisms cultured, particularly *A. niger*, but *Candida*, *Penicillium*, and *Mucor* may all contribute. Intensive ear toilet may eradicate the infection without recourse to antifungal agents.

Infections of the eye, particularly the cornea, caused by fungi (oculomycosis) are rare. They often follow penetrating injuries to the globe or contamination of lacerations. An opacity develops within the cornea with associated pain and chemosis. An exudate is usually present in the aqueous humour. Prompt treatment with intensive topical instillation of drugs containing an antifungal drug such as miconazole or econazole is necessary every 2 to 4 h. Perforation of the eye may occur in advanced cases.

Approaches to management of fungal infections

Antifungal agents can be considered in four main groups: the polyenes, azoles, morpholines, and allylamines, and an assortment of drugs of specific activity that are not related.

The polyene antifungals are macrolide substances derived originally from species of *Streptomyces*. They include amphotericin B, natamycin, and nystatin. More recent additions to this group are partricin and mepartricin. Amphotericin B is the only one widely used as a parenterally administered drug. Nystatin and natamycin are purely topical. Amphotericin B is metabolized in the liver with low penetration of body cavities, cerebrospinal fluid, and urine. The polyenes have broad activity against a wide range of fungi. The mode of action of the polyenes appears to involve inhibition of sterol synthesis in the fungal cell membrane.

The combination of an amphotericin B with a lipid, for instance a liposome, has been proposed as a means of reducing the nephrotoxicity of this drug. Three commercial lipid amphotericins are available: AmBisome (a true liposome), amphotericin B lipid complex—ABLC or Abelcet (a ribbon-like lipid binding amphotericin B), and amphotericin B colloidal dispersion (ABCD) (a dispersion of lipid discs).

The imidazoles are synthetic antifungal agents. They include miconazole, clotrimazole, econazole, isoconazole, ketoconazole, tioconazole, and bifonazole. The triazole series contains two potent oral agents, fluconazole and itraconazole. A third, voriconazole, is in clinical trial. Most are used topically except for ketoconazole (oral), itraconazole (oral), and miconazole (intravenous). These are metabolized in the liver and, like amphotericin B, affect fungal cell-membrane synthesis and penetrate cerebrospinal fluid and urine in low concentrations. The imidazoles have a broad spectrum of activity against many fungi, although neither miconazole nor ketoconazole are useful for aspergillus infections. By contrast, itraconazole is active *in vitro* against aspergilli. Fluconazole is less active against moulds and there are instances of both primary (*Candida krusei*, *C. glabrata*) and secondary resistance to this compound. The allylamines such as terbinafine are primarily active against superficial fungi, but *in vitro* appear to have fungicidal activity at low concentrations.

Other antifungal drugs include flucytosine, which is a synthetic pyrimidine analogue. Given either intravenously or orally it is mainly useful for chromomycosis and certain yeast infections. Drug resistance is a major problem with flucytosine, particularly with cryptococcus. The drug shows a number of modes of action including disruption of RNA transcription following uptake by the cell. Griseofulvin is derived from a species of *Penicillium*. It can be given orally and is only useful against dermatophytes. It is best absorbed when given with a meal and selectively accumulates in stratum corneum in concentrations approximately 10 times greater than serum levels. Griseofulvin acts by inhibiting intracellular microtubule formation. There are a large number of unrelated antifungal drugs, such as tolnaftate, haloprogin, and chlorphenesin, that are only used topically.

Management of superficial infections

Specific details of therapy are included under the separate diseases. Benzoic acid compound (Whitfield's ointment), which contains 2 per cent salicylic acid and 2 per cent benzoic acid, acts as a keratolytic agent by causing exfoliation of the superficial layers of the stratum corneum. Other topical agents with only weak antifungal activity include gentian violet (candidosis or dermatophytosis), Castellani's paint, which contains magenta and resorcinol (candidosis or dermatophytosis), and brilliant green (dermatophytosis). Two per cent selenium sulphide remains a highly effective method of treating pityriasis versicolor by application once daily for 2 weeks.

The more specific antifungals such as the polyenes, amphotericin B, nystatin, and natamycin (candidosis) or the imidazoles (candidosis, dermatophytosis, and pityriasis versicolor) are highly effective and probably quicker, although more expensive, than the keratolytics or dyes. Local irritancy can be a problem particularly with Whitfield's ointment, which is usually given as a half-strength preparation. Allergic contact dermatitis is rare but has been recorded from some imidazoles (miconazole, clotrimazole, tioconazole) and tolnaftate. Topical terbinafine is highly active in tinea pedis with cures being effected with less than 1 week of therapy.

Terbinafine or itraconazole are more effective in many forms of dermatophytosis requiring oral therapy than griseofulvin. In onychomycosis they are preferred. Terbinafine has occasional side-effects, mainly related to gastrointestinal intolerance, although it may also cause transient loss of taste. It is given in daily doses of 250 mg. Itraconazole is usually given in 'pulses', for example 200 mg twice daily for one week monthly. Itraconazole likewise can cause gastrointestinal discomfort and nausea. Both drugs rarely cause hepatic injury, with a frequency of less than 1 in 70 000–120 000. This is in contrast with ketoconazole, which also causes hepatitis but in around 1 in 8000 cases. Liver function tests should be monitored if ketoconazole is used extensively over any length of time. In high doses, ketoconazole may block human androgen biosynthesis causing side-effects such as gynaecomastia. Fluconazole is also effective in dermatophytosis and is given in weekly doses of 150 to 300 mg. Griseofulvin is still the principal treatment for tinea capitis (10 to 20 mg/kg per day).

In onychomycosis caused by dermatophytes both terbinafine and itraconazole lead to remission of toe-nail infections in only 3 months. Terbinafine is used on a daily basis, whereas itraconazole is given in a pulsed regimen, 200 mg twice daily for 1 week every month for 3 to 4 months. There is one study which shows better responses with terbinafine for toe-nail disease. Amorolfine, a morpholine drug, is used in the topical treatment of nail disease where there is less than complete involvement of the nails. It can be given together with other drugs, such as terbinafine.

Management of deep mycoses

There are very few drugs that are effective in systemic fungal infections and those that are used should always be accompanied by supportive measures and, if possible, an attempt to eliminate any predisposing conditions. For instance, if their condition permits, patients who have developed a candidaemia while a central venous line is in place should be managed by removal of the line. However, fluconazole is also usually given as well. In the patient with neutropenia, a positive blood culture would be regarded as evidence of dissemination and antifungal therapy would be required.

Amphotericin B is given intravenously in a 5 per cent dextrose infusion not containing additional drugs, if possible. A test dose of 1 to 5 mg is given over 2 h and this is followed by gradually increasing doses over the next 3 to 9 days to the normal maximum of 0.6 to 1.0 mg/kg body weight daily depending on the infection. In some cases this slow approach may help the patient to tolerate the drug better or may define the dose at which side-effects such as pyrexia start. In severely ill patients, half of the full dose may be given 4 h after a test dose of 5 mg, usually under hydrocortisone cover. The full dose is given 24 h later. Side-effects include thrombophlebitis, nausea, hypotension, and pyrexia. Renal clearance may fall in the initial period but this usually returns to normal after a temporary halt in therapy. More permanent renal tubular damage may follow a total dose of 4 g or more. Amphotericin B does not penetrate urine, cerebrospinal fluid, or peritoneal fluid in significant concentrations. Local instillations (such as the peritoneum) can be used, but can be highly irritant. Amphotericin B is normally given until clinical or mycological cure is induced. This is often difficult to judge accurately and in many of the mycoses caused by the systemic pathogens a course of at least 2 g is often used on an empirical basis. In the opportunistic infections, lower total doses are probably effective and the length of treatment should depend on the clinician's judgement.

This approach is not necessary with the lipid-associated amphotericin B formulations, which can be given without the slow build-up. The initial dose is usually 1 mg/kg but standard daily doses of 3 mg/kg are common. Patients are less likely to develop renal impairment although it can occur. There have been a few clinical trials comparing these formulations with amphotericin B and these show equal efficacy with less toxicity; however, these formulations are expensive. The main lipid-associated formulations are given above.

The azole drugs are also used in systemic mycoses. Fluconazole is given in systemic candidosis, urinary tract infections, and as a long-term suppressive, in addition to primary therapy, in cryptococcosis in patients with AIDS. Side-effects are uncommon, although it can cause nausea and vomiting. Fluconazole can be given orally or intravenously. It penetrates urine in effective concentrations. Its daily dosage varies from 100 to 200 mg for oropharyngeal infections to 600 to 800 mg for disseminated candidosis. It is highly active in *Candida* infections. It can also be used in some endemic mycoses such as histoplasmosis. Resistance to fluconazole has mainly been recorded with oropharyngeal candidosis, principally in HIV-positive patients, although it can occur with other *Candida* infections; *C. krusei* and *C. glabrata*, for instance, are often primarily resistant to this drug.

Itraconazole has been evaluated in a variety of systemic mycoses from aspergillosis to cryptococcosis. Its active range includes histoplasmosis, sporotrichosis, chromoblastomycosis, blastomycosis, coccidioidomycosis, and paracoccidioidomycosis. Itraconazole is used as an oral preparation, but a new intravenous formulation is now available. Oral absorption is often defective in individuals with AIDS and patients after bone marrow transplantion and in these groups the mean daily dosage is doubled (200 mg). An itraconazole suspension is also available for treatment of oral infections.

Flucytosine (5-fluorocytosine) is an effective oral and intravenous antifungal agent that is primarily active against yeasts such as *Candida* and *Cryptococcus*. It enters urine, cerebrospinal fluid, and peritoneal fluid. Its excretion is reduced in renal failure and the daily dose should be reduced accordingly and blood levels monitored. The main disadvantage of flucytosine is the development of either primary or secondary drug resistance in a significant number of isolates, and when given in toxic doses it may cause bone marrow depression. The serum level should not be allowed to rise above 100 to 120 µg/ml.

Combination amphotericin B and flucytosine therapy may offer an alternative but effective method of treatment. Theoretically, as the drugs synergize, the dose of amphotericin B may be reduced. In cryptococcal meningitis, combination therapy using a dose of 0.3 to 0.6 mg/kg body weight of amphotericin B with the normal dose of flucytosine is more effective at sterilizing the cerebrospinal fluid and preventing relapse. In other forms of systemic infection such as candidosis there is little evidence that it is more effective than amphotericin B alone, although this may be the case. Combinations of other drugs have not been evaluated *in vivo*.

The use of leucocyte growth factors has been reported to improve the recovery from fungal infections. The most effective combination has been a mixture of granulocyte and granulocyte–monocyte colony-stimulating factors. Further studies of these compounds in patients with neutropenia are warranted.

Further reading—therapy

Bohme A, Karthaus M, Hoelzer D (1999). Antifungal prophylaxis in neutropenic patients with hematologic malignancies: is there a real benefit? *Chemotherapy* **45**, 224–32.

Elweski B, ed. (1996). *Cutaneous fungal infections*. Marcel Dekker, New York.

Medoff G, Kobayashi GA (1980). The polyenes. In: Speller DCE, ed. *Antifungal chemotherapy*, pp 3–34. Wiley, Chichester.

Root RK, Dale DC (1999). Granulocyte colony-stimulating factor and granulocyte–macrophage colony-stimulating factor: comparisons and potential for use in the treatment of infections in non-neutropenic patients. *Journal of Infectious Diseases* **179**(Suppl 2), S342–52.

Vanden Bossche H *et al.* (1998). Antifungal drug resistance in pathogenic fungi. *Medical Mycology* **36**(Suppl 1), 119–28.

7.12.2 Cryptococcosis
William G. Powderly

Aetiology and epidemiology

Infection with the fungus *Cryptococcus neoformans* occurs mainly in patients with impaired cell-mediated immunity. It is the most common, systemic, fungal infection in patients infected with human immunodeficiency virus (HIV), and is also seen as a complication of solid organ transplantation, lymphoma, and corticosteroid therapy. *C. neoformans* is found world-wide as a soil organism; it is an encapsulated yeast measuring 4 to 6 µm with a surrounding polysaccharide capsule ranging in size from 1 to over 30 µm. Two varieties exist, distinguishable by serology—*C. neoformans* var. *neoformans* (serotypes A and D) and *C. neoformans* var. *gattii* (serotypes B and C). Virtually all HIV-associated infection is caused by *C. neoformans* var. *neoformans*. About 5 per cent of HIV-infected patients in the Western World develop disseminated cryptococcosis; the disease is more prevalent in sub-Saharan Africa and southeast Asia. *C. neoformans* var. *gattii* infection is more common in tropical and subtropical areas (Australia, New Guinea, the Philippines) in apparently immunocompetent people. It has rarely been reported in HIV-immunosuppressed patients.

The exact mechanism of infection is unknown. It is assumed that transmission occurs via inhalation of the organism leading to colonization of the airways and subsequent respiratory infection. Throughout the world, the excreta of birds such as pigeons is the richest environmental source of *C. neoformans* var. *neoformans*. The ecological association of *C. neoformans* var. *gattii* is with red river and forest river gum trees (*Eucalyptus camaldulensis* and *E. tereticonrnis*) and it has been suggested that infective basidiospores are released at flowering.

In the case of *C. neoformans* var. *neoformans*, the absence of an intact cell-mediated response results in ineffective clearance with subsequent dissemination. The polysaccharide capsule, composed mainly of glucuronoxylomannan, is thought to be its primary virulence factor. It is unclear whether cryptococcal infection in immunocompromised patients represents acute primary infection or reactivation of previously dormant disease.

Clinical features

The most common presentation of cryptococcosis is a subacute meningitis or meningoencephalitis with fever, malaise, headache, and altered behaviour and level of consciousness. Symptoms are usually present for 2 to 4 weeks before diagnosis. Classic meningeal symptoms and signs (such as neck stiffness or photophobia) occur in only about a quarter to a third of patients. Papilloedema and cranial nerve palsies (especially VI and VII) are common. Patients may present with encephalopathic symptoms such as lethargy, altered mentation, personality changes, and memory loss. Analysis of the cerebrospinal fluid (CSF) usually shows a mildly elevated serum protein, normal or slightly low glucose, and a lymphocytic pleocytosis. India ink staining of the CSF will usually reveal the yeast. Cryptococcal antigen is almost invariably detectable in the CSF. The opening pressure in the CSF is elevated in a majority of patients.

Infection with *C. neoformans* can involve sites other than the meninges. Isolated pulmonary disease has been well described and usually presents as a solitary nodule in the absence of other symptoms. Cryptococcal pneumonia also occurs. In immunocompromised patients, especially those with AIDS, subsequent dissemination is common but presentations such as cough or dyspnoea and abnormal chest radiographs may be the initial finding. Many patients have positive blood cultures. Skin involvement is common; several types of skin lesion have been described but the most common form is that resembling molluscum contagiosum. Osteolytic bone lesions and prostatic involvement have also been described.

In New Guinea, *C. neoformans* var. *gattii* is the commonest cause of chronic meningitis. Immunocompetent people are affected. Compared to *C. neoformans* var. *neoformans* meningitis in AIDS patients, victims of var. *gattii* have more aggressive retinal involvement with papilloedema and haemorrhagic papillitis in more than a half, leading to blindness in one-third of survivors.

Diagnosis

The latex agglutination test for cryptococcal polysaccharide antigen in the serum is highly sensitive and specific in the diagnosis of infection with *C. neoformans* and a positive serum cryptococcal antigen titre of greater than 1:8 is presumptive evidence of cryptococcal infection. Such patients should be evaluated for possible meningeal involvement. Culture of *C. neoformans* from any body site should also be regarded as significant and is an indication for further evaluation and initiation of therapy.

Treatment

Management of patients with cryptococcal infection depends on the extent of the disease and the immune status of the patient. The finding of a solitary pulmonary nodule in a normal host may not need treatment, provided patients have careful follow-up. Fluconazole, 200 to 400 mg/day can be given for 3 to 6 months in most patients with localized pulmonary disease. Extrapulmonary disease is generally managed in the same way as meningitis. In patients who are not known to be immunosuppressed, a search for underlying problems should be initiated. An HIV antibody test should be performed as cryptococcal meningitis may be the initial AIDS-defining event. Additionally, a CD4 lymphocyte count should be considered, as cryptococcal infection has been described as one of the manifestations of so-called 'isolated CD4 T-lymphocytopenia'.

Untreated, cryptococcal meningitis is fatal. In patients with AIDS, amphotericin B (0.7 mg/kg intravenously) given for 2 weeks followed by fluconazole 400 mg orally for a further 8 weeks is associated with the best outcome to date in prospective trials, with a mortality of less than 10 per cent and a mycological response of approximately 70 per cent. This regimen is also reasonable for treatment of meningitis in other circumstances. Concomitant use of flucytosine (100 mg/kg per day in four divided doses) with amphotericin B may be considered. In patients with AIDS, it does not improve immediate outcome but may decrease the risk of relapse. In other hosts, more prolonged use (4 to 6 weeks) of amphotericin B and flucytosine may be curative but is also toxic. The combination of fluconazole (400 to 800 mg/day) with flucytosine and liposomal formulations of amphotericin B are options for patients unable to tolerate the usual formulation of amphotericin B.

Clinical deterioration in patients with meningitis may be due to cerebral oedema, which may be diagnosed by a raised opening pressure of the CSF.

All patients with cryptococcal meningitis should have the opening pressure measured when a lumbar puncture is performed, and if the opening pressure is high (>25 cm of water) pressure should be reduced by repeated lumbar punctures, a lumbar drain, or a shunt. In var. *gattii* meningitis, corticosteroid treatment is helpful in reducing intracranial pressure and reducing retinal damage.

Cryptococcal meningitis in AIDS requires life-long suppressive therapy unless the immunosuppression is reversed. In other immunocompromised patients, suppressive treatment for 6 to 12 months may be given. Fluconazole, 200 mg daily, is the suppressive treatment of choice. Fluconazole, in dosages ranging from 400 mg weekly to 200 mg daily, and itraconazole, 100 mg twice daily, are very effective in preventing invasive cryptococcal infections, especially in HIV-positive patients with CD4 counts less than 50 to 100 cells/mm³. However, because of the relative infrequency of invasive fungal infections, antifungal prophylaxis does not prolong life and is not routinely recommended.

Further reading

Ellis DH, Pfeiffer TJ (1990). Ecology, lifecycle, and infections propagule of *Cryptococcus neoformans*. *Lancet* **36**, 923–5.

Graybill JR, *et al.* (2000). Diagnosis and management of increased intracranial pressure in patients with AIDS and cryptococcal meningitis. *Clinical Infectious Diseases* **30**, 47–54.

Lalloo D, Fisher D, Naraqi S, *et al.* (1994). Crytococcal meningitis (*C. neoformans* var *gattii*) leading to blindness in previously healthy Melanesian adults in Papua new Guinesa. *Quarterly Journal of Medicine* **87**, 343–9.

Mundy LM, Powderly WG (1997). Invasive fungal infections: Cryptococcosis. *Seminars in Respiratory and Critical Care Medicine* **18**, 249–57.

Van Der Horst CM, *et al.* (1997). Treatment of cryptococcal meningitis associated with the acquired immunodeficiency syndrome. *New England Journal of Medicine* **337**, 15–21.

7.12.3 Coccidioidomycosis

John R. Graybill

Aetiology and epidemiology

Coccidioides immitis was initially named by Gilchrest in 1986, because its round spherule form appears similar to coccidia, which are protozoans. Although traditionally associated with the southwest United States, the pathogen was initially discovered by Alejandro Posadas in Buenos Aires. Although the Argentine Pampas remains an important focus for *Coccidioides*, the desert southwest of the United States and northern Mexico is better known as the endemic zone. Fifty years ago, German prisoners of war who were held in Arizona developed coccidioidomycosis, and were mistakenly thought to be the victims of 'medical research'. This illness still plagues German airmen who train in Arizona.

Coccidioides immitis is dimorphic, and grows as a mycelium in desert soil where winters are mild. After spring rains, mycelia form myriads of small barrel-shaped arthroconidia. The mycelium disrupts readily, and the conidia are wafted for many kilometres. Earthquakes and desert sand-storms in California have caused large epidemics. Infection follows inhalation of just a few conidia. Over the course of several days the fungus converts to the pathognomonic spherule. This enlarges to as much as 60 μm in diameter, and is commonly filled with maturing endospores. Endospores are released after several days of growth; they are chemoattractive to neutrophils, which ingest but cannot kill them. Endospores enlarge into spherules and the growth cycle repeats itself. Although the spherule does not directly transmit disease, it is important to destroy all contaminated materials to prevent this most infectious of the endemic mycoses from converting back to the mycelium and causing secondary infections.

Clinical features

In no mycosis is the interplay of pathogen and host defences more important than coccidioidomycosis. The uncomplicated infection progresses through 3 to 6 weeks in the lungs, during which time protective cell-mediated immune responses develop. A strong immune response may cause arthralgias, fever, eosinophilia, and various rashes, including erythema multiforme or erythema nodosum ('desert fever'). A rise in IgM precipitin antibodies is diagnostic. Initial pulmonary infiltrates are later replaced by granulomas, which may condense to cicatrices or nodules. Cavitation of nodules may occur within weeks, or be a much later consequence of smouldering disease. The skin test to either spherulin or coccidioidin antigens commonly converts to positive. Illness resolves over weeks or months, to leave lifelong immunity. Low titres of IgG 'complement-fixation' antibody are generated 1 to 2 months after infection, and may persist for months.

Immunity and dissemination

Although immune suppression (by steroids or AIDS) is associated with dissemination, there are subtle factors of race (Blacks, American Indians, Filipinos) and gender (pregnancy) which also favour dissemination. The course of the disease may be strung out over years, with responses to treatment being followed by relapses. If the host is severely immune depressed, the course may evolve rapidly over weeks to persistent worsening pulmonary infiltrates and haematogenous dissemination to almost any tissue. Favourite locations are the bones (especially vertebral osteomyelitis), the skin (papular verrucous or proliferative), the lymph nodes, and the central nervous system. Coccidiodal meningitis presents insidiously (or rarely acutely after exposure) with headache, nausea, vomiting, seizures, and focal signs. Hydrocephalus and brain infarcts may develop. In general the association of skin or deep tissue abscesses draining pus with neutrophils and coccidioides indicates a poor host immune response, while granulomas showing spherules in Langerhans giant cells suggest better control of the organism.

Diagnosis

The IgG antibodies tend to rise to levels associated with the severity of disease (titres of ≥ 1:16 suggest worsening disease), and may remain elevated for many months. The erythrocyte sedimentation rate also rises. Coccidioidal meningitis is associated with lymphocytic and eosinophilic pleocytosis, hypoglychoracchia, and positive cerebrospinal fluid culture and/or serology for IgG.

The diagnosis of coccidioidomycosis may be made by culture or histopathology of tissues showing the characteristic spherule, or may be inferred from positive IgM or IgG serum (or IgG cerebrospinal fluid) antibody titres. The oganism is biphasic and converts readily to the mycelium in most culture media. Coccidioides is susceptible *in vitro* to most polyene and azole antifungals. Nevertheless, coccidioidomycosis is the most difficult of the endemic mycoses to treat.

Treatment

Clinical response is assessed using a scoring system developed by the Mycoses Study Group. This includes clinical symptoms and signs, cultures, radiographic changes, and serology. For non-meningeal disease, amphotericin B is reserved for those patients with the most fulminant courses, and even then there may be only a 70 per cent response rate. One troubling site of disease is vertebral osteomyelitis. This site is commonly refractory to medical therapy alone, and usually requires surgical stabilization of the spine for cure. For most patients the treatment of choice may be itraconazole, with a loading dose of 800 mg followed by 400 mg per day (capsules) until the illness resolves and then 9 to 12 months more for consolidation. A solution of itraconazole improves absorption but is less well tolerated than capsules. Resolution may require months or years, and occurs in fewer than 70 per cent of patients. Post-treatment relapses occur in 30 to 40 per cent of patients and may require repeated courses or higher doses. Fluconazole at 400 to 800 mg per day is an alternative for non-meningeal coccidioidomycosis, and is the drug of choice for meningeal coccidioidomycosis. Fluconazole allows highly toxic intrathecal amphotericin B to be avoided, but for coccidioidal meningitis it must be administered for the rest of the patient's life. More than two-thirds of patients relapse if fluconazole is stopped, even after many years of therapy. Cerebrospinal fluid abnormalities normalize very slowly on fluconazole; chemistries may improve more rapidly with intrathecal amphotericin B. However, amphotericin B causes arachnoiditis, and patients may even have cerebrovascular accidents complicating this therapy.

Two recently developed thiazoles, voniconazole and posaconazole, may be superior to itraconazole. Posaconazole has shown very rapid improvement in most patients but there are still relapses when treatment is dropped.

Further reading

Galgiani JN *et al.* (1993). Fluconazole therapy for coccidioidal meningitis. *Annals of Internal Medicine* **119**, 28–35.

Graybill JR *et al.* (1990). Itraconazole treatment of coccidioidomycosis. *American Journal of Medicine* **89**, 292.

Stevens DA (1995). Current concepts: coccidioidomycosis. *New England Journal of Medicine* **332**, 1077–82.

7.12.4 Paracoccidioidomycosis
M. A. S. Yasuda

Definition

Paracoccidioidomycosis is a systemic granulomatous disease caused by a dimorphic fungus, *Paracoccidioides brasiliensis*, that involves mainly the lungs, phagocytic mononuclear system, mucous membranes, skin, and adrenals.

History

The disease was first described in 1908 by Lutz, a Brazilian scientist. In 1912, Splendore classified the organism as a yeast of the genus *Zymonema* and in 1928, Almeida and Lacaz suggested the name Paracoccidioides. In 1930, Almeida named the fungus *Paracoccidioides brasiliensis*. Formerly the disease was known as South American blastomycosis, or Lutz–Splendore–Almeida' s disease. In 1977 it was renamed paracoccidioidomycosis.

Epidemiology

Paracoccidioidomycosis is the most common endemic human mycosis in Latin America and is geographically restricted to Central and South America, ranging from Mexico to Argentina. The disease is prevalent in Brazil,

Colombia, Venezuela, Argentina, Uruguay, Paraguay, Guatemala, Equador, Peru, and Mexico. No cases have been reported in Chile, Belize, Nicaragua, Guyana, Surinam, or French Guyana. Imported cases have been recorded in the United States, Europe, and Asia.

Prevalence, inferred from the result of intradermal paracoccidioidin testing, ranges from 6 to 60.6 per cent among rural and urban populations of endemic and non-endemic areas. It is equally prevalent in both sexes.

The disease occurs mainly among 20- to 50-year-olds, who are agricultural workers or who have lived in rural endemic areas. The sex ratio of clinical cases is 10 or more males to each female among adults, while it is equally distributed among prepubescent boys and girls. This may be explained by the ability of oestrogens to inhibit the transformation of mycelium or conidia to yeast. Spouses of patients are rarely affected by the disease, which suggests that hormonal and genetic factors play a part in the distribution of this mycosis. Transmission from one person to another has not been shown.

Ecology

The geographical regions in which paracoccidioidomycosis is most commonly found are humid areas where the soil is more frequently acidic and the temperature ranges from 15 to 30 °C.

P. brasiliensis has been isolated from soil, animals such as armadillos and bats, dog food, and penguin faeces. It has also been isolated from the intestinal contents of bats. Efforts to maintain the fungus in bat intestines have been unsuccessful. The saprophytic habitat of *P. brasiliensis* has yet to be discovered.

Aetiology

Mycology

P. brasiliensis is a dimorphic fungus, which can be cultivated either as a mould or a yeast. When cultured at 25 °C it appears after 15 to 30 days as white colonies. When Sabouraud's dextrose agar is used the mycelium shows hyaline septate hyphae with branches.

P. brasiliensis also grows as a yeast in human and animal tissues (Fig. 1) and in cultures maintained at 37 °C. Colonies can be observed after 7 to 20 days. Under direct microscopy, yeast forms can be observed as oval or spherical cells with doubly refractile walls; the cells vary in size from buds of 2 to 10 μm in diameter to mature cells of 20 to 30 μm. Mother cells may produce 10 to 12 uniform or variably sized buds (Fig. 2), forming the characteristic 'pilot wheel' shape observed in biological samples or in infected tissues.

Fig. 1 Small and large yeast forms of *Paracoccidioides brasiliensis* in the lung of a transplant recipient. Methenamine silver stain.

Fig. 2 Scanning electron micrograph of a multiple budding yeast cell of *Paracoccidioides brasiliensis*. (By courtesy of C. S. Lacaz.)

Genomic clones that encode a 70 kDa heat shock protein from this dimorphic fungus have been studied. A differential expression of this gene was observed between mycelial and yeast forms, with a higher level of expression in the yeast form.

Virulence

Virulence is defined as the ability to produce disseminated infection in experimental animals. Variation in the virulence of different fungal isolates has been documented but little is understood of the biochemical basis for these differences.

The presence of higher levels of α-1,3 glucan in virulent strains of *P. brasiliensis* compared with avirulent strains was initially related to virulence, but no correlation has been shown between glucans and virulence in experimentally induced infections.

Pathogenesis

Several experimental and clinicopathological observations provide evidence that the respiratory route is the main portal of entry and the lung is the primary site of infection.

The first fungus–host contact occurs through inhalation of airborne conidia. When mice are experimentally infected through the respiratory route, conidia have been observed in the alveoli soon after inoculation. Some 12 to 18 h after the exposure, yeast forms can be observed in the alveoli. There is an initial inflammatory response, which is mediated by polymorphonuclear cells, followed by granuloma formation.

The primary infective complex develops at the inoculation site and involves the surrounding lymphatic vessels and regional lymph nodes. The fungus spreads to other parts of the lung through peribronchial lymphatic vessels and drains into regional lymph nodes. Haematogenous dissemination to a variety of organs and tissues may occur at this time. The lesions usually undergo involution and the fungi remain dormant if the host's immune response can control their proliferation. A balanced host–fungus relationship is associated with the absence of symptoms, although in some children or young adults, acute disease may arise, primarily affecting the phagocytic mononuclear system. In adult life, previously quiescent lesions may become reactivated, especially in the lungs, leading to the adult or chronic form of the disease.

Pathology

The characteristic lesion is a granuloma containing *P. brasiliensis* cells. The infected tissue may exhibit a predominantly proliferative, granulomatous inflammatory response, and/or an exudative reaction, sometimes resulting in necrosis, with variable numbers of neutrophils and large numbers of extracellular yeast cells, leading to a chronic epithelioid granuloma.

Autopsy studies, mainly of adult patients, indicate that the organs most frequently involved are the lungs (42 to 96 per cent), adrenals (44 to 80 per cent), lymph nodes (28 to 72 per cent), pharynx/larynx (18 to 60 per cent), and skin/other mucosal surfaces (2.7 to 64 per cent).

Host–fungus interaction

Non-specific immune response

The influence of genetic factors on the individual susceptibility to this mycosis is suggested by the observation of higher rates of HLA phenotypes A9, B13, B40, and Cw3 among patients than in controls. In isogenic mice, resistance to *P. brasiliensis* is controlled by a single autosomal gene.

The ability of circulating human neutrophils obtained by bronchoalveolar washing to digest the yeast forms of fungi was impaired in severe cases, while this defect was absent in uninfected family members of patients.

Specific immune response

The relation of the severity of the human disease to deficient late hypersensitivity was established through intradermal testing for ubiquitous antigens and paracoccidioidin, or through lymphoblastic transformation tests to mitogens and to *P. brasiliensis* antigens, including the 43 kDa glycoprotein.

The different distribution of T-lymphocyte subpopulations according to the clinical form of the disease (decreased CD4 in chronic form and increased CD8 in acute form) suggests that different mechanisms might be involved in each form.

The deficient T-cell response is followed by a decreased ability of macrophages to control fungal multiplication and to kill the fungus. This capacity of murine pulmonary macrophages in intratracheal infection is increased *in vivo* and *in vitro* by treatment with interferon-γ. Neutralization of endogenous interferon-γ by monoclonal antibodies induced exacerbation of the pulmonary infection, earlier fungal dissemination to the liver and spleen, and impairment of the specific cellular immune response and increased levels of IgG1 and IgG2b specific antibodies.

In severe human disease there are decreased levels of T helper 1 type cytokines (interferon-γ and interleukin 2 (**IL-2**)) and preserved T helper 2 type cytokines (IL-10 and IL-13 or IL-4). This pattern is associated with poor granuloma formation, spreading of the fungus and high levels of antibody production (immunoglobulins IgG1, IgG4, and IgE). The importance of late hypersensitivity in protection has been observed recently in patients receiving cytotoxic therapy for associated neoplasms and in those with AIDS.

Antibodies may enhance phagocytosis through opsonization of the fungus, but their role in resistance is not established.

Clinical features

The clinical picture ranges from an asymptomatic course to severe disseminated disease, which can lead to death. The incubation period is unknown except in a laboratory worker, who developed a skin lesion some days after an accidental inoculation. The disease has been reported in children 3 years of age or older who had lived for some years in the endemic area.

The following classification of clinical forms of paracoccidioidomycosis has been proposed:

(1) paracoccidiodomycosis infection;

(2) regressive (self-healing) paracoccidioidomycosis;

(3) paracoccidioidomycosis disease;

    (a) acute form (juvenile type): moderate or severe;

    (b) chronic form (adult type): mild, moderate, or severe;

Fig. 3 Lymph node and skin involvement in a patient with the acute form of paracoccidioidomycosis. (Courtesy of C. S. Lacaz.)

(4) sequelae.

Localization in a particular tissue or organ and the degree of severity of the disease according to established criteria make this classification easily and uniformly applicable. General and nutritional debility and organ dysfunction (lung, brain, adrenals, bone marrow) indicate the severity of the disease.

Acute form (juvenile type)

Children, adolescents, and young adults (under 30 years old) are affected; males and females being affected in equal numbers. Only 1 to 20 per cent of the patients fall into this group. There is progression for 2 to 3 months or more, characterized by involvement of the phagocytic mononuclear system. Cervical, axillary, and inguinal nodes are the most commonly enlarged (Fig. 3). Nodes are initially hard but are sometimes fluctuant and drain pus rich in fungi. Less frequently, deep-seated lymph nodes may also be affected. When the hepatic perihilar lymph nodes are enlarged, they may produce symptoms of obstructive jaundice.

The liver and spleen are usually moderately enlarged. Bones (clavicle, scapulae, ribs, skull, long, and flat bones) and, rarely, the bone marrow may be involved. Radiographs show lytic lesions without periosteal reaction. Involvement of the small bowel may be asymptomatic or produce abdominal pain, diarrhoea, constipation, and even intestinal obstruction. Radiological studies of the digestive tract reveal intestinal tract involvement in about 50 per cent of clinical cases.

Fever and weight loss are common. Multiple mucocutaneous lesions are more frequent in some geographical areas. High transient blood eosinophilia (up to 30 000/mm³) has sometimes been described.

Clinical lung involvement is rarely described in this form of paracoccidioidomycosis. In some case reports either bronchopneumonia or primary complex-like disease was observed.

Chronic form

This form of the disease usually occurs in 30- to 50-year-old men who have worked in agricultural areas. The male:female ratio varies from 10:1 to 25:1. The evolution is insidious and in many cases clinically mild.

The organ most frequently involved is the lung, followed by skin and mucous membranes, mainly pharynx, larynx, and trachea. Lymph nodes and adrenals may be compromised. More than one organ or tissue is usually involved. Less frequently, intestine, spleen, bones, central nervous system (brain, cerebellum, meninges), eyes, genitourinary system, myocardium, pericardium, and arteries are involved.

The patients may be asymptomatic or complain of dyspnoea, cough, sometimes purulent sputum, and rarely haemoptysis. Fever is unusual. Physical examination is frequently normal or there may be scattered rales. In contrast, chest radiography commonly reveals bilateral, asymmetrical, reticulonodular infiltrates in the middle and lower parts of the lungs (Fig. 4). Apical cavities and pleural effusions are less frequently observed.

Fig. 4 Alveolar and interstitial infiltrates in both lungs in a patient with chronic paracoccidioidomycosis.

Cutaneous lesions include papules, pustules, ulcers, crusted ulcers, vegetations, tuberculoids, verrucoids, or acneiform lesions mainly on the face (Fig. 5) or limbs. Multiple, scattered lesions result from haematogenous dissemination. Subcutaneous cold abscesses, more commonly associated with bone lesions, can occur.

Mucosal lesions are usually in the mouth and/or oropharynx, including the palate, uvula, and tonsils, or in the respiratory tract, involving mainly the larynx (vocal cords, glottis, and epiglottis) and trachea. Pain is usually intense, and may hamper mastication and swallowing. Hoarseness and dysphonia result from laryngeal lesions, and may lead to obstruction of the upper respiratory tract. Examination shows ulcerative, verrucous, vegetant, and infiltrative 'moriform' stomatitis, resembling a raspberry, with papules, vesicles, and haemorrhagic spots. The last is characteristic of this mycosis and appears as shallow ulcers, with a granular surface showing multiple, fine, haemorrhagic points.

Few lymph nodes may be involved, in contrast to the acute form of the disease.

Uni- or bilateral lesions in the adrenal glands have been found in about half of patients coming to autopsy. Partial adrenal insufficiency has been documented in about 40 per cent of the cases but only 7.4 per cent were symptomatic.

Concomitant tuberculosis is observed in about 10 to 15 per cent of cases of pulmonary paracoccidioidomycosis and has also been described in cases of lymph node involvement by *P. brasiliensis*. Carcinomas may arise in pulmonary or mucosal mycotic lesions.

Fig. 5 Mucocutaneous lesions in a patient with chronic paracoccidioidomycosis. (By courtesy of C. S. Lacaz.)

Fig. 6 Ascites, cachexia, and immunodeficiency due to malabsorption and protein-losing enteropathy as sequelae of acute paracoccidioidomycosis. (By courtesy of M. Shiroma.)

Sequelae

Nowadays these constitute one of the most important problems in the management of paracoccidioidomycosis. Although fungal multiplication can been controlled by chemotherapy, impairment of vital functions might prove fatal.

Acute form

Lesions in the small intestine and mesenteric lymph nodes may fibrose causing lymphatic obstruction, intestinal malabsorption, or protein-losing enteropathy. A clinical picture of severe malnutrition and immunodeficiency has been reported (Fig. 6).

Chronic form

As the lesions usually tend to heal by fibrosis, sequelae such as microstomy and laryngeal, tracheal, or even bronchial stenosis may be observed. Corrective surgery is indicated.

Pulmonary emphysema, fibrosis, respiratory insufficiency, and, finally, cor pulmonale are frequent sequelae. Obstructive and restrictive patterns of ventilatory defect have been found in about 36 and 16 per cent of patients respectively. As many as 30 per cent of these patients may die as a result of respiratory or cardiorespiratory failure.

Diagnosis

Microbiological identification

Isolated or budding (single or multiple) mother cells are observed under direct microscopy in sputum, pus from lymph nodes, and material from the skin or mucous membrane lesions.

Specimens are cultured at 37 °C on blood, chocolate, or yeast extract agar. The colonies are produced after 7 days, usually in 10 to 20 days. Cultures can be maintained, at 25 °C, on Sabouraud's dextrose agar, where the colonies may be noticed after 15 to 30 days.

Histopathology

Silver or periodic acid-Schiff staining is required to detect the fungus on sputum. Diagnostic features are the variable size (1 to 30 μm) of the yeast cells, and their multiple budding. Proliferative or exudative reactions, as described in the section on pathology, may be observed.

Immunological test

Serological reactions

Immunodiffusion (Ouchterlony) and counterimmunoelectrophoresis are the best techniques initially. Sensitivities and specificities are as high as 95 per cent. Cross reactions are mainly with other deep mycoses such as histoplasmosis, aspergillosis, cryptococcosis, and candidiasis.

Complement fixation and indirect immunofluorescence are less reliable tests for diagnosis, but they can be employed in patients under treatment.

Recently, enzyme immunoassays employing *P. brasiliensis* antigens, including a 43 kDa glycoprotein have shown high sensitivity and specificity. Antibody titres tend to decrease about 3 to 6 months after starting specific therapy and to disappear after 9 months to 5 years or more.

Antigenaemia and antigenuria have been considered useful indications in patients presenting low levels of antibodies in the sera, both for diagnosis and follow-up after treatment, particularly in an immunocompromised host.

The correlation between immunological and histopathological findings and clinical forms is outlined in Table 1.

Therapy

Clinically active disease is treated for 3 to 6 months, followed by maintenance therapy with sulfamethoxipiridazine after the resolution of clinical signs and symptoms, continued for many months or until 1 to 2 years after antibody levels have fallen to normal.

Severe cases of acute or chronic disease should be treated with intravenous infusion of amphotericin B. The daily dose begins at 0.1 to 0.2 mg/kg, increasing up to 1.0 mg/kg. The total dose ranges from 1 to 3 g or more. Toxic reactions to amphotericin B include fever, chills, headache, anaemia, and nephrotoxicity characterized by tubular acidosis and potassium urinary excretion and resultant hypokalaemia and azotaemia. In most cases, these reactions can be controlled until the end of the course of therapy. Liposomal amphotericin has been used in severe cases of paracoccidioidomycosis, but this treatment was followed by relapses.

In milder cases, sulphonamides or imidazoles (ketoconazole 200 to 400 mg/day or itraconazole 100 to 200 mg/day) have been shown to be effective. In a randomized trial, sulphadiazine (150 mg/kg per day), itraconazole (50 to 100 mg/day), and ketoconazole (200 to 400 mg/day) were equally effective in patients with moderately severe disease. The combination of 160 mg of trimethoprim and 800 mg of sulfamethoxazole is also effective. Fluconazole has been used in a few cases and although it achieves high levels in cerebrospinal fluid, there is no conclusive experience in neuroparacoccidioidomycosis.

Prognosis

Even though the disease is easily controlled in the majority of cases, the course of treatment is long and in Brazil, for example, abandonment of treatment is the most important cause of therapeutic failure. Normalization of cellular specific responses, particularly of the skin test (paracoccidioidin) indicates a good prognosis.

Death may occur in severe acute or chronic cases and severe cases with sequelae.

Further reading

Bueno JP *et al.* (1997). IgG, IgM and IgA antibody response for the diagnosis and follow-up of paracoccidioidomycosis:comparison of counterimmunoelectrophoresis and complement fixation. *Journal of Medical and Veterinay Mycology* **35**, 213–17.

Calich VLG *et al.* (1985).Susceptibility and resistance of inbred mice to *P. brasiliensis*. *British Journal of Experimental Pathology* **66**, 585–94.

Restrepo A (1985). The ecology of *Paracoccidioides brasiliensis*: a puzzle still unsolved. *Journal of Medical Mycology* **23**, 323–34.

Table 1 Correlation between the immunological histopathological findings and the clinical forms of paracoccidioidomycosis

	Clinical form Severe, acute/ chronic	Moderate, chronic/acute	Mild, chronic
Intradermal tests:			
Paracoccidioidin	–	+/–	+
Ubiquitous antigen/PHA*	–	+/–	+
'In vitro' tests[†]			
PHA*	–	+/–	+
Suppressive factor (patient's serum/plasma)	+	–/+	–
Increased T-cell subpopulation	CD8 (acute)	CD8 (acute)	
Decreased T-cell subpopulation	CD4 (chronic)	CD4 (chronic)	CD4 (chronic)
Cytokines IL-10 + IFNγ[‡]			
Histopathology			
Epithelioid granuloma	–	+/–	+
Loose granuloma	+	+	+
Fungi	+++	++	++/–
Antibodies			
Immunoglobulins (IgG4)	+++	++	+
Specific antibodies	+++	++	+
Immune complexes	++	+/–	–

* Antigen: PHA, phytohaemagglutinin.

[†] Lymphoblastic transformation test.

[‡] IL-10 = interleukin 10; IFNγ = interferon-γ.

7.12.5 *Pneumocystis carinii*

Robert F. Miller and Ann E. Wakefield

Who gets *Pneumocystis carinii* pneumonia?

Most patients have abnormalities of T-lymphocyte function or numbers, but rarely *Pneumocystis carinii* pneumonia develops in patients with isolated B-cell defects and in individuals without evidence of immunosuppression. In non-HIV immunosuppressed individuals, glucocorticoid administration is an independent risk factor for development of *P. carinii* pneumonia irrespective of the type or intensity of immunosuppression or the nature of the underlying disease process. In HIV-infected individuals, those at greatest risk have CD4+ T lymphocyte counts less than 200 cells/μl. *P. carinii* pneumonia in HIV-infected patients in Europe, United States, and Australasia is now largely confined to patients who are unaware of their HIV serostatus at presentation or to those who are non-compliant with, or intolerant of, prophylaxis and antiretroviral therapy. The incidence of *P. carinii* pneumonia in HIV-infected individuals in Africa is lower than in the West.

Aetiology

Until recently, *P. carinii* was regarded taxonomically as a protozoan, based on its morphology and lack of response to antifungal agents such as amphotericin B. *P. carinii* pneumonia cannot be cultured *in vitro*, but molecular biological techniques demonstrate clearly that it is a fungus. *P. carinii* from different mammalian host species show antigenic, karyotypic, and genetic heterogeneity. Cross infection between host species has not been successful, suggesting host specificity and that *P. carinii* infection in man is not a zoonosis. In the human host, *P. carinii* shows lower levels of genetic diversity than occurs between *P. carinii* from different mammalian hosts. Over 30 genotypes of human type *P. carinii* have been described; some types are associated with a mild pneumonia, others with severe hypoxic pneumonia.

The demonstration of antibodies against *P. carinii* in the majority of healthy children and adults has been regarded previously as supportive of the hypothesis that *P. carinii* arises in an immunocompromised individual by reactivation of a childhood-acquired, symptomless, latent infection. However, this hypothesis is challenged by the failure to demonstrate *P. carinii* in bronchoalveolar lavage (BAL) fluid or necropsy lung tissue of immune competent individuals, and the observation that *P. carinii*-specific DNA is detectable only at low levels in less than 25 per cent of HIV-infected individuals with low CD4+ T lymphocyte counts presenting with respiratory episodes and diagnoses other than *P. carinii* pneumonia. Human *P. carinii* infection is now thought to arise from *de novo* infection from an exogenous source. The finding of different *P. carinii* genotypes in each episode in patients with recurrent *P. carinii* pneumonia supports the reinfection model.

Pathogenesis

After inhalation of *P. carinii*, the organism reaches the alveoli where the trophozoite form attaches to type 1 pneumocytes. In an immune-competent individual the organism is eliminated, in the immune-deficient host *P. carinii* pneumonia will develop.

The major surface glycoprotein of *P. carinii* binds macrophages and induces T-lymphocyte proliferation and increases secretion of IL-1 and -2 and TNF-α. Monocytes respond to major surface glycoprotein by releasing IL-8 and TNF-α. *P. carinii* induces changes in the quantity and quality of

pulmonary surfactant: total cholesterol, glycerol, and phospholipase A-2 are increased while phospholipid is reduced.

Clinical presentation

This is non-specific. Patients typically present with progressive exertional dyspnoea, a non-productive cough, and fever of several days or weeks duration. Patients often report an inability to take in a deep breath, not due to pleural pain. Purulent sputum, haemoptysis, and pleural pain are atypical for *P. carinii* and suggest a bacterial or mycobacterial pathogen. In HIV-infected patients, the presentation is usually more insidious than in patients immunosuppressed by other causes, however in a small proportion of HIV-infected patients the disease course of *P. carinii* is fulminant with an interval of 7 days or less between onset of symptoms and progression to respiratory failure. Occasionally *P. carinii* may have an indolent presentation with respiratory symptoms worsening almost imperceptibly over many months. Rarely, *P. carinii* may present as pyrexia of undetermined origin.

Examination of the chest is usually normal; occasionally fine bibasal end-inspiratory crackles are heard. Signs of focal consolidation or pleural effusion suggest an alternative diagnosis.

Pathology

Within the lung, *P. carinii* infection is characterized by an eosinophilic, foamy intra-alveolar exudate, associated with a mild plasma cell interstitial pneumonitis. Morphologically, two forms of *P. carinii* may be identified: thick-walled cysts (6–7 μm diameter) which lie freely within the alveolar exudate are demonstrated by Grocott's methenamine silver, toluidine blue O, or cresyl violet stains. The exudate consists largely of thin-walled, irregularly shaped, single-nucleated trophozoites (2–5 μm diameter) which are shown by Geimsa stain but lack distinctive features. Rarely, interstitial fibrosis, diffuse alveolar damage, granulomatous inflammation, nodular and cavitary lesions, and pneumatocoele formation may occur.

Rarely *P. carinii* infection extends beyond the air spaces; extrapulmonary pneumocystosis involving liver, spleen, gut, or eye may occur and is strongly associated with use of nebulized pentamidine for prophylaxis or treatment.

Investigations

The chest radiograph may be normal in early or mild pneumonia. With more severe disease or later presentation, diffuse perihilar interstitial infiltrates are seen. These may progress to diffuse bilateral alveolar (air space) consolidation that mimics pulmonary oedema. In the late stages the lungs may be massively consolidated and almost airless. Radiographic deterioration from near normal at presentation to being markedly abnormal may occur over 48 h or less. Up to 20 per cent of chest radiographs are atypical, showing intrapulmonary nodules, cavitary lesions, lobar consolidation, pneumatocoeles, or hilar/mediastinal lymphadenopathy. Predominantly apical change may be seen in patients who develop *P. carinii* pneumonia having received *P. carinii* prophylaxis with nebulized pentamidine. All these typical and atypical radiographic appearances may also be seen in bacterial, mycobacterial, and fungal infection, and in non-specific pneumonitis and Kaposi's sarcoma.

With treatment and clinical recovery the chest radiograph in some individuals may remain abnormal for many months in the absence of symptoms. In others postinfectious bronchiectasis or fibrosis occurs.

Arterial blood gases/oximetry

Less than 10 per cent of patients with *P. carinii* pneumonia have a normal Pao_2 and a normal $PAo_2–Pao_2$. These measures are sensitive though not specific for *P. carinii* pneumonia and may also occur in bacterial pneumonia, Kaposi's sarcoma, and tuberculosis.

Computed tomography

High resolution computed tomography scanning of the chest may be useful in the symptomatic patient with a normal or equivocal chest radiograph. Areas of ground glass shadowing indicate active pulmonary disease. These appearances may be caused by *P. carinii*, cytomegalovirus, or fungal pneumonia.

Induced sputum

Spontaneously expectorated sputum is inadequate for diagnosis of *P. carinii* pneumonia. Sputum induction by inhalation of ultrasonically nebulized hypertonic (3N) saline may provide a suitable sample. *P. carinii* is usually found in clear 'saliva-like' samples. Purulent samples suggest an alternative diagnosis. The sensitivity varies between 55 and 90 per cent and a negative result for *P. carinii* should prompt further diagnostic tests.

Bronchoscopy

Fibreoptic bronchoscopy with BAL has a sensitivity of more than 90 per cent for detection of *P. carinii*. Immunoflourescence staining increases the diagnostic yield compared to conventional histochemical staining. Transbronchial biopsies add very little to the diagnostic yield and are associated with a relatively high complication rate (pneumothorax in ≈ 8 per cent). As *P. carinii* persists in the lung for many days after the start of antimicrobial therapy, bronchoscopy may be performed up to 1 week after commencing anti-*P. carinii* therapy without a reduction in diagnostic yield.

Molecular diagnostic tests

Detection of *P. carinii*-specific DNA by the polymerase chain reaction (PCR) on BAL fluid and induced sputum is superior to conventional histochemical methods. Detection of *P. carinii* DNA by PCR may also be achieved on oropharangeal samples obtained by gargling with normal saline; this technique compared to conventional staining of BAL fluid has a sensitivity of 89 per cent and a specificity of 94 per cent for *P. carinii*. These molecular techniques are not widely available.

Empirical therapy

Many centres in the United Kingdom and North America seek to confirm a diagnosis in every suspected case of *P. carinii* pneumonia. Other centres treat HIV-infected patients empirically who present with symptoms, chest radiographic abnormalities, and hypoxaemia, features typical of *P. carinii* pneumonia. Bronchoscopy is reserved for those who fail to respond to empirical therapy by day five or those who have atypical presentations. Both strategies are equally effective in clinical practice.

Treatment

It is important to stratify *P. carinii* pneumonia as mild (Pao_2 (on air) > 11.0 KPa, Sao_2 > 96 per cent) moderate (Pao_2 = 8.0–11.0 KPa, Sao_2 = 91–96 per cent), or severe (Pao_2< 8.0 KPa, Sao_2 < 91 per cent) as some drugs are unproven or ineffective in severe disease.

First choice treatment is high-dose co-trimoxazole (sulfamethoxazole 100 mg/kg per day and trimethoprim 20 mg/kg per day) in two to four divided doses, orally or intravenously. In HIV-infected patients with *P. carinii* pneumonia 21 days are given, in those with other causes of immunosuppression 14 to 17 days are frequently given. In mild disease oral medication may be given throughout, in moderate/severe disease intravenous therapy is usually given for the first 7 to 10 days, then orally.

Other treatments in patients with severe disease include clindamycin 450 to 600 mg orally or intravenously, four times daily, with primaquine 15 mg once daily orally, or trimetrexate 45 mg/m² intravenously, daily, with foli-

nic acid 20 mg/m² four times daily. Despite its toxicity, pentamidine 4 mg/kg daily, intravenously, may be used if other treatments have failed. In patients with mild or moderate disease, alternatives to co-trimoxazole include clindamycin with primaquine (doses as above), dapsone 100 mg orally once daily, with trimethoprim 20 mg/kg per day, or atovaquone 750 mg orally twice daily.

Adjuvant steroids

HIV infected patients with moderate/severe *P. carinii* pneumonia benefit from adjuvant glucocorticoids which reduce the risk of respiratory failure, need for mechanical ventilation, and risk of death. Many non-HIV infected patients with *P. carinii* pneumonia are already receiving glucocorticoids as part of their immunosuppression/chemotherapy and the benefits of adjunctive dose increases have not clearly been demonstrated. Adjunctive glucocorticoid regimens include prednisolone 40 mg twice daily orally for 5 days, then 40 mg once daily on day 6 to 10, 20 mg once daily on days 11 to 21 (or methylprednisolone intravenously at 75 per cent of these doses). An alternative regimen is methylprednisolone 1 g intravenously for 3 days, then 0.5 g intravenously on days 4 and 5, followed by prednisolone reducing from 40 mg orally once daily to zero over 10 days.

Adverse reactions

Adverse reactions to co-trimoxazole, which usually occur between day 6 and day 14 of treatment, are commoner in HIV-infected patients than in patients with other causes of immunosuppression. Anaemia and neutropenia (up to 40 per cent of patients), rash and fever (up to 30 per cent), and biochemical hepatitis (up to 15 per cent) are the most frequent adverse reactions. Coadministration of folic or folinic acid does not prevent or attenuate haematological toxicity and may be associated with increased therapeutic failure.

Glucose-6-phosphate dehydrogenase deficiency

Patients with glucose-6-phosphate dehydrogenase deficiency should not receive co-trimoxazole, dapsone, or primaquine.

Prophylaxis

HIV-infected patients are at increased risk of *P. carinii* pneumonia as the CD4+ lymphocyte count decreases. Primary prophylaxis (to prevent a first episode of *P. carinii* pneumonia) is given when the CD4 count falls below 200/µl or the CD4:total lymphocyte ratio is less than 1:5, to patients with HIV- associated constitutional features such as unexplained fever of 3 weeks' or more duration, or oral candida, irrespective of CD4 count, and to patients with other AIDS-defining diagnoses, for example Kaposi's sarcoma. Secondary prophylaxis is given after an episode of *P. carinii* pneumonia.

The first choice agent for primary and secondary prophylaxis is co-trimoxazole 960 mg daily. Lower doses, that is 960 mg three times weekly or 480 mg daily, may be equally effective and have fewer side effects. Co-trimoxazole may also protect against bacterial infections and reactivation of cerebral toxoplasmosis.

Adverse reactions, including rash with or without fever, occur in up to 20 per cent of patients receiving co-trimoxazole as prophylaxis. Desensitization may be attempted in those unable to tolerate co-trimoxazole; alternative less effective options include nebulized pentamidine 300 mg once per month via jet nebulizer (once per fortnight if the CD4 count is 50/µl or less), dapsone 100 mg daily with pyrimethamine 25 mg once weekly (pyrimethamine may also protect against cerebral toxoplasmosis), or atovaquone 750 mg twice daily.

Non-HIV infected patients with high attack rates of *P. carinii* pneumonia should receive prophylaxis (drug choice and doses as above). At risk groups include those with acute lymphoblastic leukaemia, severe combined immunodeficiency syndrome, Hodgkin's disease, rhabdomyosarcoma, primary and secondary central nervous system tumours, Wegener's granulomatosis, and organ transplantation including allogenic bone marrow, renal, heart, heart/lung, and liver.

Areas of uncertainty/future research

The mode of transmission of *P. carinii* infection is unclear, but recent molecular data suggest that transmission from infected patients to susceptible immunocompromised individuals may occur. The drug target for sulfamethoxazole and dapsone is dihydropteroate synthase. The possibility that *P. carinii* may develop resistance to sulpha drugs is suggested by the finding of non-synonymous single nucleotide polymorphisms (which are associated with resistance in other organisms) in the dihydropteroate synthase gene of human *P. carinii* which occur more frequently in those who have received prophylaxis with co-trimoxazole or dapsone. The limited availability of other equally effective drugs for prophylaxis restricts the use of 'drug switching' as a strategy for preventing emergence of resistance of *P. carinii* to sulpha drugs.

Of new anti *P. carinii* drugs under development, and most promising are sordarin derivatives which target translation elongation factor-2 and inhibit fungal protein synthesis.

Further reading

Dei-Cas E, Cailliez JC, eds (1998). *Pneumocystis* and pneumocystosis: advances in *Pneumocystis* research. *FEMS Immunology and Medical Microbiology* **22**, 1–189. A summary of current knowledge about the molecular biology of the organism.

Miller RF (1999). Pneumocystis carinii infection in non-AIDS patients. *Current Opinion in Infectious Diseases* **12**, 371–7. Comprehensive review of non-AIDS-associated *Pneumocystis carinii* pneumonia.

Miller RF, Lipman MCI (1999). Pulmonary infections (AIDS). In: Albert R, Spiro S, Jett J, eds. *Comprehensive respiratory medicine*. Mosby, London, pp. 32.1–22. Comprehensive review of *Pneumocystis carinii* pneumonia and other infections in AIDS.

Miller RF, Lenoury J, Corbett EL, Felton JM, DeCock KM (1997). Pneumocystis carinii infection: current treatment and prevention. *Journal of Antimicrobial Chemotherapy* **77** (Suppl. B), 33–53. A comprehensive review of treatment and prophylaxis regimens for *Pneumocystis carinii* pneumonia.

7.12.6 Infection due to *Penicillium marneffei*

Thira Sirisanthana

Introduction

Penicillium marneffei was first isolated from bamboo rats (*Rhizomys sinensis*) in Vietnam in 1956. The fungus is endemic in southeast Asia, northeast India, south China, Hong Kong, and Taiwan. Fewer than 40 cases of infection with *P. marneffei* were reported prior to the HIV epidemic. The incidence of disseminated *P. marneffei* infection has increased markedly over the past few years. This increase is mainly due to infection in patients already infected with HIV. The majority of patients have been reported from Thailand, Hong Kong, and Taiwan. Cases have also been reported in HIV-infected individuals from the United States, the United Kingdom, The Netherlands, Italy, France, Germany, Switzerland, Sweden, and Australia following visits to the endemic region.

Aetiology

P. marneffei is the only dimorphic fungus of the genus *Penicillium*. The fungus grows in a mycelial phase at 25 °C on Sabouraud dextrose agar. Mould-to-yeast conversion is achieved by subculturing the fungus on to brain–heart-infusion agar and incubating at 37 °C. In its mycelial form, the colony is greyish white and downy. The colour of the colony may vary during differentiation. The reverse side becomes cerise to brownish red, as a soluble red pigment diffuses into the agar medium. Microscopic examination of the mycelial form shows structures typical of the genus *Penicillium*. Colonies of the yeast form of *P. marneffei* have a wrinkled or cerebriform surface. They are light tan to brown in colour. Microscopic examination of the yeast form reveals unicellular, pleomorphic, ellipsoidal-to-rectangular cells, about 2 μm by 6 μm in size, that divide by fission and not by budding.

Natural history

Many features of the natural reservoir, mode of transmission, and natural history of *P. marneffei* infection remain unknown. The fungus has been isolated from several species of bamboo rats in the endemic area. Since bamboo rats usually live near the forest and have limited contact with people, it is believed that both humans and bamboo rats become infected with *P. marneffei* from a common source, rather than the patients being infected by the rats. By analogy with other endemic systemic mycoses, such as histoplasmosis, it is likely that *P. marneffei* conidia are inhaled from a contaminated reservoir in the environment and subsequently disseminate from the lungs when the host experiences immunosuppression. The disease is more likely to occur in the rainy season, suggesting that there may be an expansion of the environmental reservoirs with favourable conditions for growth at this time.

In endemic areas it is likely that a certain proportion of the population is infected, but remains asymptomatic. Patients have been reported with long periods of asymptomatic infection before presentation with clinical *P. marneffei* infection. In other cases, clinical manifestation of *P. marneffei* infection occurred within weeks of exposure to the fungus.

Clinical features

Patients with *P. marneffei* infection commonly present with symptoms and signs of infection of the reticuloendothelial system. These include fever, chills, lymphadenopathy, hepatomegaly, and splenomegaly. Cough, dyspnoea, and lung crepitations may be present. Other manifestations are secondary to dissemination of the fungus via the bloodstream. Cutaneous and subcutaneous lesions are observed in up to two-thirds of patients. Arthritis and osteomyelitis are not uncommon. Cases with mesenteric lymphangitis, colitis, genital or oropharyngeal ulceration, retropharyngeal abscess, or pericarditis have been reported.

In HIV-infected patients, *P. marneffei* infection occurs late in the course of the disease. The patient's CD4+ cell count at presentation is usually below 50 cells per microlitre. HIV-infected patients with *P. marneffei* infection have a more acute onset and higher fever. They are more likely to have fungaemia and shock and their skin lesions are more numerous and tend to be papules with central necrotic umbilication. Patients who are not infected with HIV are more likely to have one or several subcutaneous nodules which may develop into abscesses and cause skin ulceration.

Biochemical and haematological laboratory findings are non-specific and include elevation of liver enzymes, anaemia, and leucocytosis. Chest radiographs may show diffuse interstitial, localized alveolar, or diffuse alveolar infiltrates. Cases with cavitary lesions or lung masses have been reported.

Diagnosis

Presumptive diagnosis can be made by microscopic examination of Wright's-stained samples of bone marrow aspirate, and/or touch smears of skin biopsy specimens, and/or lymph node biopsy specimens. Many intracellular and extracellular basophilic, spherical, oval, and elliptical yeast cells can be seen using this staining technique. Some of these cells had clear central septation, which is a characteristic feature of *P. marneffei*. The diagnosis is confirmed by histopathological section and/or by culturing the fungus from the blood, skin biopsy specimens, bone marrow, or lymph nodes. Cases of *P. marneffei* infection can clinically resemble tuberculosis, histoplasmosis, and cryptococcosis. Tests to detect antibodies or *P. marneffei* antigens have been developed. Clinical trials are needed to show their usefulness in the diagnosis of active *P. marneffei* infection and in predicting relapses. They may also be used to identify HIV-infected individuals who are infected with *P. marneffei* but who are still asymptomic. These persons may then benefit from pre-emptive treatment with an antifungal agent.

Treatment

P. marneffei infection is potentially fatal. The fungus is sensitive to ketoconazole, fluconazole, itraconazole, and amphotericin B. The recommended treatment is to give amphotericin B intravenously in a dose of 0.6 mg/kg/day for 2 weeks, followed by itraconazole 400 mg/day orally in two divided doses for the next 10 weeks. The majority of patients respond well, with resolution of fever and other signs of infection within the first 2 weeks. After initial treatment, HIV-infected patients should be given 200 mg/day of itraconazole orally as secondary prophylaxis for life.

Further reading

bibliography
Deng Z *et al.* (1988). Infection caused by *Penicillium marneffei* in China and Southeast Asia: review of eighteen published cases and report of four more Chinese cases. *Review of Infectious Diseases* **10**, 640–52. A review of *Penicillium marneffei* infection in patients not infected with the human immunodeficiency virus.

Sirisanthana T, Supparatpinyo K (1998). Epidemiology and management of penicilliosis in human immunodeficiency virus-infected patients. *International Journal of Infectious Diseases* **3**, 48–53. A review of the epidemiology and management of penicilliosis.

Supparatpinyo K *et al.* (1994). Disseminated *Penicillium marneffei* infection in southeast Asia. *The Lancet* **344**, 110–13. A report of the clinical findings in patients with disseminated *Penicillium marneffei* infection.

Supparatpinyo K *et al.* (1998). A controlled trial of itraconazole to prevent relapse of *Penicillium marneffei* infection in patients infected with the human immunodeficiency virus. *New England Journal of Medicine* **339**, 1739–43. A report on the means to prevent relapse of *Penicillium marneffei* infection.

7.13 Protozoa

7.13.1 Amoebic infections

R. Knight

The amoebic species infecting humans belong to two very different groups. First, the obligate parasitic species of the gut that include the major pathogen *Entamoeba histolytica*, several non-pathogenic species including *E. dispar*, and a minor pathogen *Dientamoeba fragilis*. The second group are free-living, water and soil amoebae, which can become facultative tissue parasites. All motile feeding amoebae are called trophozoites; they move with pseudopodia and divide by binary fission. The hyaline external cytoplasm, the ectoplasm, is a contractile gel that surrounds the sol endoplasm containing numerous phagocytic and pinocytic vacuoles. Most species can form environmentally resistant cysts by rounding up and secreting a chitinous cyst wall.

Entamoeba histolytica infection

Biology and pathogenicity

Following ingestion of infective cysts a population of trophozoites becomes established in the caecum and proximal colon. Some degree of tissue invasion occurs in all subjects with at least low-titre seroconversion. Tissue invasion is frequently mild, self-limiting, and with minimal symptoms, but at the other end of the clinical spectrum it can lead to extensive destruction of the colonic mucosa. Invasive trophozoites have a characteristic morphology; they may reach 30 to 40 µm in diameter and are very active with apparently purposeful, unidirectional movements during which they become considerably elongated. Their most important diagnostic characteristic is the presence of host erythrocytes within the endoplasm, which otherwise appears clear and contains no bacteria. Trophozoites containing red blood cells are described as erythrocytophagous. Progression through tissues is by active movement, facilitated by secreted collagenase; leucocytes are drawn chemotactically towards the amoebae but most are rapidly destroyed on contact.

The transmissive cystic form of the parasite is derived entirely from a commensal population within the colonic lumen. Live commensal amoebae measure 10 to 20 µm in diameter, the endoplasm is granular and contains bacteria; the pseudopodia are blunt and movement is sluggish. Intestinal hurry from any cause, including the use of laxatives, can lead to the appearance of commensal trophozoites in the faeces. Cysts are spherical and measure 11 to 14 µm in diameter; when mature they contain four nuclei, several chromatoid bodies that are a ribosome store, and a glycogen vacuole.

Host factors may increase susceptibility to overt disease. Steroid therapy given systemically or locally into the rectum carries great risk, as may cytotoxic therapy. Severe bowel disease is particularly common in late pregnancy and the puerperium. Before puberty both sexes are equally susceptible to hepatic amoebiasis, but in adults this condition is at least seven times more common in males. Local disease can also favour tissue invasion; thus amoebic ulceration may be superimposed upon colonic and rectal cancers, or those of the uterine cervix. Colonic disease is favoured by concurrent *Trichuris* infection and intestinal schistosomiasis. Infection with human immunodeficiency virus appears to have little effect on outcome.

The taxonomic separation of *E. dispar* as a discrete non-pathogenic species from *E. histolytica* was formally made in 1993. Characterization of cultures by zymodeme, using isoenzyme electrophoresis of a small set of glycolytic enzymes, was the first convincing biochemical distinction between these two species, but many genomic differences have now been identified. All strains of *E. histolytica* are now regarded as pathogenic.

Epidemiology

The incidence of disease is particularly high in Mexico, South America, Natal, the west coast of Africa, and South-East Asia. In most temperate countries *E. histolytica* is now rare and nearly all amoebic disease seen in such countries will have been acquired elsewhere. Symptomless or convalescent carriers are the main source of infection; patients with dysentery normally pass only trophozoites in their stool, and are therefore non-infectious. Cysts remain viable in the environment for up to 2 months. The infection is eventually self-limiting and rarely exceeds 4 years. Tissue invasion can occur at any time during an infection, but is much more common during the first 4 months; the incubation period may be as short as 7 days.

The incidence of amoebiasis in a population is best estimated from seropositivity surveys. Surveys for cysts are of no value as differentiation from *E. dispar* is impossible. All the modes of faeco-oral transmission occur in amoebiasis; of special importance are the food handler and contaminated vegetables; transmission by flies and drinking water is less common. Drinking water can be contaminated in the home or at surface-water sources. Direct spread can produce outbreaks; it occurs within institutions for children and the mentally handicapped, and with contaminated colonic irrigation equipment. Household clustering is common; hand-fed infants are frequently infected from the fingers of their mother. Contamination of piped water supplies can lead to serious disease outbreaks as happened in the Chicago hotels epidemic in 1933. Nearly all *Entamoeba* infections among male homosexuals are due to *E. dispar*, *E. coli*, or *E. hartmanni*.

Pathology

The basic lesion is the result of cell lysis and tissue necrosis, which, by creating locally anoxic and acidic conditions, favours further penetration of the parasite; most amoebae are seen at the advancing edge of the lesion with little inflammatory cell response. In tissue sections amoebae stain indistinctly with haematoxylin and eosin but appear bright red with periodic acid–Schiff stain; iron haematoxylin is necessary to show nuclear detail. Cysts of *E. histolytica* are never seen in tissue.

Amoebic lesions of the gut are most common in the rectosigmoid and caecum but can occur anywhere in the large bowel; involvement may be patchy or continuous, less commonly the appendix or terminal ileum are affected. The initial lesions are either small, discrete erosions of the mucosa, or minute crypt lesions. Unrestrained, the lesions extend through the mucosa, across the muscularis mucosa, and into the submucosa, where they expand laterally to produce lesions that are typically flask shaped in cross-section. Further lateral spread of the submucosal lesions leads to their coalescence, and later, to denudation of overlying mucosa. The bowel wall may become appreciably thickened. Blood vessels involved in the disease may thrombose, bleed into the gut lumen or, in the case of portal-vein radicles, provide a vehicle for the dissemination of amoebae to the liver. In very severe lesions, and usually in association with toxic megacolon, there is an irreversible coagulative necrosis of the bowel wall.

Amoebomas are tumour-like lesions of the colonic wall measuring up to several centimetres in length; they are most common in the caecum and may be multiple. Histologically there is tissue oedema, with a mixed picture of healing and new areas of epithelial loss and tissue destruction; round-cell infiltration is patchy. Lesions may be annular and rarely an amoeboma initiates an intussusception; narrow, stricture-like amoebomas may occur in the anorectal region.

Amoebae reach the liver in the portal vein. Once initiated the amoebic lesion extends progressively in all directions to produce the liver-cell necrosis and liquefaction that constitute an 'amoebic liver abscess'. The lesions are well demarcated from surrounding liver tissue; untreated, nearly all will eventually extend into adjacent structures. Secondary bacterial infection is rare and usually follows rupture or aspiration.

Clinical manifestations

Invasive intestinal amoebiasis (Plates 1, 2)

The clinical features show a wide spectrum from minimal changes in bowel habit to severe dysentery. Lesions may be limited to a small part of the large bowel or extend throughout its length. A relapsing course is common.

Amoebic colitis with dysentery

Dysentery, the passage of loose or diarrhoeal stools containing fresh blood, occurs when there is generalized colonic ulceration, or when more localized lesions occur in the rectum or rectosigmoid. Onset may be gradual, intermittent, or much less commonly, acute. Typically, constitutional upset is initially mild and the patient remains ambulant; mild or moderate abdominal pain is common, often colicky and maximal over affected parts of the gut. Tenesmus can occur but is rarely severe. Stools vary in consistency from semiformed to watery. They are foul-smelling and always contain visible blood; even when watery, faecal matter is nearly always present. Symptoms frequently wax and wane over a period of weeks or even months and such patients can become debilitated and wasted. In a few patients the disease runs a fulminating course. The most frequent physical sign is abdominal tenderness in one or both iliac fossas; but tenderness may be generalized. Affected gut may be palpably thickened. A low fever is common, but dehydration is uncommon. Abdominal distension occurs in the more severely ill patients, who sometimes pass relatively small amounts of stool.

When stool microscopy reveals no erythrocytophagous trophozoites, a careful proctoscopy or sigmoidoscopy should be done. The endoscopic appearances may be non-specific in early, acute, or very severe colitis; the findings are hyperaemia, contact bleeding, or confluent ulceration. In more chronic cases the presence of normal-looking intervening mucosa is highly suggestive of amoebiasis; early lesions are often elevated, with a pouting opening only 1 to 2 mm in diameter; later, ulcers may reach 1 cm or more in diameter, with an irregular outline and often a loosely adherent, yellowish or grey exudate. Mucosal scrapings or superficial biopsies taken at endoscopy should be examined immediately by wet-preparation microscopy.

Special forms of amoebic colitis

Fulminant colitis This may arise *de novo*, for example in pregnant women or during steroid therapy, or it may evolve during a dysenteric illness.

Patients show progressive abdominal distension, vomiting, and watery diarrhoea. Bowel sounds are absent and there may be little or no abdominal tenderness, guarding, or rigidity. Plain radiographs may reveal free peritoneal gas, together with acute gaseous dilatation of the colon; affected segments of bowel may appear relatively narrow and show visible musosal pathology. Barium enema and full sigmoidoscopy are contraindicated. Stools contain erythrocytophagous trophozoites.

Amoebic colitis without dysentery When ulceration is limited to the caecum or ascending colon, or when early, mild, or localized lesions occur elsewhere in the colon there may be no dysenteric symptoms. Patients complain of change in bowel habit, blood-staining of the stool, flatulence, and colicky pain. Often the only physical sign is tenderness in the right iliac fossa, or elsewhere along the course of the colon. Some patients eventually go into complete remission; others progress to a dysenteric illness.

The most important diagnostic measure is repeated stool examination for erythrocytophagous amoebae; the finding of cysts or commensal trophozoites is of little diagnostic value, especially in endemic areas. Sigmoidoscopy is often normal when the distal bowel is not involved but colonoscopy may reveal typical lesions.

Amoeboma These present as an abdominal mass, most frequently in the right iliac fossa. The lesion may be painful, tender, and associated with fever. Bowel habit is altered and some patients have intermittent dysentery, especially if lesions are multiple or distal. Evidence of partial or intermittent bowel obstruction may be present, particularly when lesions are distal and annular.

Localized perforation and amoebic appendicitis Sudden perforation with peritonitis can occur from any deep amoebic ulcer; alternatively, leakage may lead to a pericolic abscess or retroperitoneal cellulitis. Amoebic appendicitis is an uncommon but important condition that occurs when amoebic lesions are confined to the appendix and caecum. The clinical presentation can resemble that of simple appendicitis, often with some clinical evidence of dysentery. If unrecognized at appendicectomy, the outcome can be disastrous with gut perforation; fresh smears should be made from the resected appendix, and examined immediately.

Rectal bleeding Some patients with amoebiasis present with rectal bleeding, with or without tenesmus; this occurs particularly in children. Massive bleeding into the gut lumen can occur in any form of amoebic colitis but is rare.

Differential diagnosis

Amoebic colitis must be differentiated from other causes of infective colitis. High-volume diarrhoea, copious mucus, and severe tenesmus are all uncommon in amoebiasis. In temperate countries, non-specific ulcerative colitis and colorectal carcinoma create the greatest diagnostic problems. Parasitic conditions to be considered are intestinal schistosomiasis, heavy *Trichuris* infection, and balantidiasis. More chronic amoebic pathology may clinically resemble Crohn's disease, ileocaecal tuberculosis, diverticulitis, or anorectal lymphogranuloma venereum.

Hepatic amoebiasis

Less than half of all patients give any convincing history of dysentery and few have concurrent dysentery. In those with no dysenteric history the interval between presumed infection and presentation may be as short as 3 weeks, or as long as 15 years; for most it is between 8 weeks and a year.

The dominant symptoms are fever and sweating, liver or diaphragmatic pain, and weight loss. Onset of constitutional symptoms is often insidious; but pain may begin abruptly. Most patients seek medical help within 1 to 4 weeks. Fever is typically remittent, with a prominent evening rise, brief rigors, and very profuse sweating. Liver pain may be poorly localized initially and later become pleuritic, referred to the right shoulder tip, or localized to the abdominal wall. Within a few weeks, patients lose much weight and often become anaemic; a painful dry cough is common.

The most important clinical finding is liver enlargement (Fig. 1) with localized tenderness, which should be searched for in the right hypochondrium, the epigastrium, and along all the intercostal spaces overlying the liver. Liver pain, on compression or heavy digital percussion, is a less useful sign. Left-lobe lesions can present as an epigastric mass. Hepatomegaly may be difficult to detect by abdominal palpation when enlargement is mainly upwards, but bulging of the right chest wall may be noted, together with a raised upper level of liver dullness on percussion. Reduced breath sounds or crepitations may be heard at the right lung base.

Important radiological findings are a raised, or locally upward-bulging, right diaphragm (Fig. 2) with immobility on screening, areas of lung collapse or consolidation, and sometimes a pleural effusion. A neutrophil leucocytosis is almost invariable, the erythrocyte sedimentation rate is raised, and normochromic normocytic anaemia is common. 'Liver function tests' are frequently completely normal, or there may be a raised alkaline phosphatase; less commonly the serum transaminase or bilirubin is elevated. Liver scanning to demonstrate a filling defect is of great value; about 70 per cent of lesions are solitary, but multiple lesions are common in children and those with concurrent dysentery. Ultrasonographic scans and computed tomography are the most useful. Lesions appear round or oval, and are usually 4 to 10 cm in diameter at the time of presentation. On ultrasonography most are hypoechoic with well-defined walls without enhanced echoes. Even when concurrent dysentery is absent the stools are frequently, but not always, positive for *E. histolytica*. Colonoscopy may reveal unsuspected lesions.

Complications

Most complications involve extension of hepatic lesions into adjacent structures: usually the right chest, the peritoneum, and the pericardium. Upward extension usually produces adhesions between the liver, the diaphragm, and the lung; in consequence, subphrenic rupture and amoebic empyema are rare, although a right serous pleural effusion is not uncommon. Untreated, the disease process advances upwards through lung tissue leading to hepatobronchial fistula and expectoration of brownish, necrotic liver tissue, the so-called 'anchovy sauce' sputum. Rupture into the peritoneum can occur at any time; it is sometimes the mode of presentation of an amoebic liver abscess, the cause of peritonitis being discovered only at laparotomy. Amoebic pericarditis usually results from upward extension of a left-lobe liver lesion. Initially patients have retrosternal pain, a pericardial friction rub, or a serous effusion; later rupture produces cardiac tamponade. The diagnosis is most difficult when an underlying liver abscess was not suspected.

Less commonly the lesion extends through the skin producing a sinus and cutaneous lesion. The gut, stomach, vena cava, spleen, and kidney are occasionally involved by direct spread. Bloodborne spread to the lung produces a lesion resembling an isolated pyogenic lung abscess. Amoebic brain abscesses due to *E. histolytica* are rare; most are discovered after death (Fig. 3). Jaundice occurs when a large lesion compresses the common bile duct or when multiple lesions compress several intrahepatic bile ducts. Rupture into a major bile duct can cause haemobilia. Portal-vein compression occasionally produces portal hypertension and congestive splenomegaly.

Differential diagnosis

Amoebic serology and scanning have now greatly simplified diagnosis. However, a few patients, generally less than 5 per cent, are initially seronegative; scanning patterns may be atypical before lesions have liquefied. Pyogenic abscess, especially when cryptogenic, may be clinically indistinguishable and this condition is quite common in some Asian countries. Other conditions to be distinguished are primary and secondary carcinoma of the liver, lesions of the right lung base and right pleura, subphrenic

Fig. 1 Amoebic liver abscess. Hepatic enlargement with focal tenderness in a Thai woman. (By courtesy of Professor S. Looareesuwan.)

(a)   (b)   (c)

Fig. 2 Amoebic liver abscess, radiographic changes: (a) elevated right diaphragm; (b) enormous abscess in the right lobe of the liver outlined with air (fluid level) after the aspiration of more than 1 litre of pus; (c) lateral view, same patient as (b). (By courtesy of Professor S. Looareesuwan.)

Fig. 3 Metastatic brain abscess in a patient with an amoebic liver abscess. (By courtesy of Professor S. Looareesuwan.)

Fig. 5 Aspirate from amoebic liver abscess showing margin of hepatocytes and erythrocytophagous trophozoites of *E. histolytica*. (By courtesy of Professor S. Looareesuwan.)

Laboratory diagnosis

Microscopy and culture

The identification of live erythrocytophagous trophozoites in temporary wet mounts is of prime importance because it confirms the diagnosis of invasive amoebic disease. Amoebae should be sought in dysenteric bowel-wall scrapings, the last portion of aspirate from a liver abscess (Fig. 5), sputum, and tissue smears from skin lesions. In non-dysenteric stools, flecks of pus, blood, or mucus should be looked for and examined. The amoebae remain active for about 30 min at room temperature and so recently voided stool samples should be examined without delay ('hot stool'). Other microscopical features of faeces in amoebic colitis are scanty or absent leucocytes (methylene blue staining), clumped or degenerating red cells, and sometimes Charcot–Leyden crystals. If wet preparations are not made, or are negative, a portion of the specimen should be preserved in polyvinyl alcohol or SAF (sodium acetate–acetic acid–formalin) fixative for later smear preparation; alternatively, drying faecal smears should be fixed in Schaudinn's solution. In either case fixed smears should be stained with Gomori trichrome or Heidenhain's iron haematoxylin.

Cysts and commensal trophozoites of *E. histolytica* found in wet faecal mounts are indistinguishable from those of *E .dispar*. The cysts of both species can be differentiated from the smaller *E. hartmanni* using an eyepiece micrometer. Direct mounts are made by emulsifying a small portions of stool in 1 per cent eosin, and in Lugol's iodine; however, the diagnostic sensitivity, per specimen, is only about 30 per cent. Concentration methods for cysts such as formol-ether sedimentation give a 70 per cent sensitivity per specimen. Cultivation of intestinal amoebae with bacterial associates in Robinson's medium is relatively easy; species identification requires immunofluorescent staining. Culture lysates provide material for zymodeme assay. Positive cultures from extraintestinal sites confirm invasive *E. histolytica*; amoebae are often difficult to find microscopically in liver aspirates.

Unless invasive trophozoites are found, differentiation of *E. histolytica* from *E. dispar* is only possible using zymodeme assay, or immunofluorescent staining of trophozoites in fixed faecal or amoebic culture smears.

Immunological tests

E. histolytica antigen can now be detected in faecal specimens and where this test is available it greatly simplifies diagnosis in both amoebic disease and in carriers; sensitivity and specificity of these tests is good. Assays for antigen in serum have also been used.

Many serodiagnostic methods have been applied to amoebiasis, most detectable antibody is IgG, with some IgM in active disease. However, seropositivity does not distinguish current and past tissue invasion. The more sensitive methods are indirect haemagglutination, enzyme immunoassay,

abscess, cholecystitis, septic cholangitis including that resulting from aberrant *Ascaris* worms, and liver hydatid cysts.

Needle aspiration of the liver (Fig. 4) may be necessary for diagnostic or therapeutic purposes (see below). Suspected pyogenic abscess is the main indication for the former; blood cultures should also be taken. Typically the aspirate in hepatic amoebiasis is pinkish-brown ('anchory sauce') (Plate 3), odourless, and bacteriologically sterile; a thinner, malodorous, or frothy aspirate suggests bacterial infection. A therapeutic amoebicide trial is generally preferable to diagnostic needling of the liver.

Cutaneous and genital amoebiasis

Skin ulceration due to *E. histolytica* produces deep, painful, and foul-smelling lesions that spread rapidly. Secondary bacterial infection is common and may mask the amoebic pathology. Lesions are most frequent in the perianal area, but also occur at colostomy stomas, laparotomy scars, and at the site of skin rupture by a hepatic lesion.

Female genital involvement results from faecal contamination, the extension of perianal lesions, or by the formation of internal fistulas from the gut, which can involve the bladder. Lesions of the vulva and uterine cervix may resemble carcinoma. Male genital lesions follow rectal coitus, the lesion beginning as a balanoposthitis and progressing rapidly.

Fig. 4 Diagnostic/therapeutic aspiration of 'anchovy sauce pus' from a patient with amoebic liver abscess. (Copyright Professor D.A. Warrell.)

and indirect immunofluorescence. Latex agglutination and gel-diffusion precipitation are also used, the former being commercially available as a slide test, taking only minutes to perform. Using sensitive tests, over 95 per cent of patients with liver abscess are seropositive, as are about 60 per cent of those with invasive bowel disease; patients with amoeboma are nearly all seropositive. All patients with tissue invasion eventually become seropositive. Titres decline after therapy but may remain positive for 2 years or more with the most sensitive tests.

Patient management

Chemotherapy

Nitroimidazoles are tissue amoebicides, and metronidazole for 5 days will be the first choice in most patients. The usual adult dose of metronidazole is 800 mg three times daily for 5 or 8 days; the paediatric dose is 35 to 50 mg/kg in three divided doses. An alternative is tinidazole, which has the advantage of a single daily dose of 2 g in adults and 50 to 60 mg/kg in children. A 5- or even a 3-day course may be sufficient for tissue amoebae but rates of parasitological cure may be low. When nitroimidazoles are contraindicated, or not available, erythromycin is useful in non-severe colitis.

The alkaloid emetine hydrochloride is a potent tissue amoebicide but has cumulative cardiotoxicity. Where appropriate nitroimidazoles are unavailable, as continues to be the case in many tropical contexts, this drug will continue to be life-saving, especially when a parenteral drug is needed. Emetine at 1 mg/kg daily (maximum 60 mg) by intramuscular injection for 5 days is usually sufficient; the synthetic derivative dehydoemetine hydrochloride is less toxic and more rapidly excreted in the urine, the daily intramuscular dose is 1.25 mg/kg (maximum 90 mg). Chloroquine is an effective alternative amoebicide in hepatic amoebiasis but is now little used; for adults a course of 150 mg of base twice daily is necessary.

Cutaneous and genital amoebiasis respond well to metronidazole, partly perhaps because these lesions often contain anaerobic bacteria. Amoebiasis at other sites is nearly always secondary to hepatic lesions and the chemotherapy will be the same. Metronidazole crosses the blood–brain barrier and should be used in the desperate situation of amoebic brain abscess due to *E. histolytica*.

Elimination of carrier state ('cyst'-passers)

All patients with *E. histolytica* infection treated with a tissue amoebicide should also be given diloxanide to eliminate all infection from the bowel and so prevent recurrence of tissue invasion or transmission to others. The dosage of diloxanide for adults is 500 mg three times daily for 10 days; the daily dose in children is 20 mg/kg in three divided doses.

Convalescent carriers should always be treated and also infected family contacts. Persons entering temperate countries from the tropics or new residents from such countries should be screened if there is a significant risk of infection; those with *E. histolytica* faecal antigen, or who are seropositive and have four-nucleated *Entamoeba* cysts in their stools, should be treated. In such cases, diloxanide is the drug of choice. Metronidazole is less effective, even using an 8-day course, and side-effects are troublesome. Unfortunately, cure rates with tinidazole are very low when followed up at 1 month.

Supportive and surgical management

Intestinal amoebiasis

Supportive management plays a major role in patients with complicated amoebic colitis, with emphasis on fluid and electrolyte replacement, gastric suction, and blood transfusion as necessary. Gut perforation in the context of extensive colitis carries a very poor prognosis; management may have to be medical. Parenteral metronidazole is invaluable in these contexts because of its activity against anaerobic bacteria in the peritoneum and bloodstream. Gentamicin plus a cephalosporin will normally be given as well.

Amoebomas respond well to metronidazole; a slow response should arouse suspicion that the amoebic lesion is superimposed upon other pathology, particularly a carcinoma. Surgical management is important in several situations. Acute colonic perforation in the absence of diffuse colitis, or ruptured amoebic appendicitis may be amenable to local repair. In the case of diffuse colitis, local repair, or end-to-end anastomosis, may not be possible because of the poor condition of the gut wall: temporary exteriorization with an ileostomy may be necessary. In fulminant colitis with multiple perforation the viability of the gut wall is uncertain and the only definitive option is total colectomy.

Hepatic amoebiasis

Parenteral metronidazole can be used in patients who undergo laparotomy. A favourable response to medical treatment alone can be expected in about 85 per cent of patients. Liver abscesses may rupture before, during, or after chemotherapy. Intra-abdominal rupture will always require laparotomy. Extension into the pleural or pericardial cavities necessitates drainage of these structures, together with aspiration of the liver lesion; pericardial drainage is most urgent when tamponade is present. Hepatopulmonary lesions generally require drainage of the liver lesion but medical treatment alone has been successful in some cases. Antimicrobials will always be needed when the abscess ruptures into the peritoneum or lung.

The most common management problem is slow response to the amoebicide. Patients whose pain and fever do not subside within 72 h are at significantly greater risk of rupture or therapeutic failure, and aspiration is generally to be recommended. A likely explanation of poor initial response is a tense lesion that restricts drug entry. Regular ultrasonographic monitoring is of great value as it will indicate the risk of rupture and guide the aspiration procedure. No change in lesion size on ultrasound can be expected during the first 2 weeks, although its outline may become clearer. Percutaneous aspiration with a wide-bore needle will be possible in most patients; if unsuccessful or anatomically contraindicated, then surgical help should be sought. Resolution time for small or moderate lesions is unaffected by aspiration. All patients with hepatic amoebiasis should be given a 10-day course of diloxanide to elimanate bowel infection.

Prognosis

Uncomplicated invasive intestinal disease and uncomplicated hepatic amoebiasis should normally have a mortality rate of less than 1 per cent. In complicated disease the mortality is much greater and may reach 40 per cent for amoebic peritonitis with multiple gut perforation. Prognosis is usually better in centres where the disease is common and more likely to be recognized early. Late diagnosis increases the probability of complicated disease and mortality rises accordingly.

Unless parasitological cure is achieved, and the gut completely freed of *E. histolytica*, clinical relapse is quite common, although probably limited by immunological responses. There is so far no evidence of naturally occurring strains of *E. histolytica* being resistant to normally used drugs. Hepatic scans show that nearly all liver abscesses completely disappear within 2 years; the median resolution time is 8 months. In secondarily infected lesions, bizarre hepatic calcification may be seen years afterwards. Healing of the bowel is remarkably rapid and complete; occasionally fibrous strictures persist after severe dysentery.

Prevention

Chlorination of water supplies does not destroy amoebic cysts, but adequate filtration will remove them. Regular stool screening of food handlers and domestic staff is of no value, but health education is important with encouragement to have a medical check if diarrhoea occurs.

Visitors to the tropics should not attempt chemoprophylaxis; in particular, long-term unsupervised use of hydroxyquinoline drugs must be strongly deprecated. Simple hygienic measures provide considerable protection. Boiling water for 5 min kills cysts. Routine examinations in temperate countries for returning visitors from the tropics or for new residents coming from such countries is of no value unless *E. histolytica* can be differentiated from *E. dispar*. Amoebic serology is particularly useful in those with gut symptoms or a history of dysentery.

Other parasitic gut amoebae including *Dientamoeba fragilis*

In addition to *E. histolytica* five species of *Entamoeba* infect humans, all have a nucleus with a small central endosome and abundant peripheral chromatin. *E. gingivalis* has no cystic stage and lives in the mouth within gingival pockets and tonsillar crypts. It is spread by kissing or more indirect oral contact. Its possible role in periodontal disease was formerly dismissed but there is now renewed interest following recognition of its high prevalence in individual lesions in people with this condition; it may act as a bacterial vector within the lesions. It has been found on intrauterine devices removed because of symptoms. Both in the uterus and in the mouth this amoeba occurs in association with the bacterium *Actinomyces israeli*.

The other *Entamoeba* species are non-pathogenic colonic commensals. *E. coli* has eight nuclei and is the commonest species in most surveys. *E. dispar* and *E. hartmanni* both have cysts with four nuclei; the former was previously known as 'non-pathogenic *E. histolytica*', and the latter as 'small race *E. histolytica*'; size is the only simple diagnostic criterion for *E. hartmanni*, its cysts are less than 10 μm in diameter. The global prevalence of *E. dispar* is about 10 per cent; even in the tropics the prevalence ratio of *E. dispar* to *E. histolytica* is often between 4:1 and 10:1. Lastly there is *E. polecki*, which is primarily a pig parasite; the cyst has one nucleus and an 'inclusion body'. Human infections are common in highland Papua New Guinea where humans and pigs may share a peridomestic environment; elsewhere it is rare.

Endolimax nana and *Iodamoeba buetchlii* both have nuclei with large endosomes and no visible peripheral chromatin. Cysts of the former are oval in shape with four nuclei; those of the latter are somewhat irregular in shape with a single nucleus and a large glycogen vacuole that stains prominently with iodine. Neither species is pathogenic.

Dientamoeba fragilis is overlooked in most parasitological laboratories and most reports are from developed countries. There is good evidence that it can cause colonic inflammation; however, this is not severe and there is no ulceration or systemic spread. It has no cystic stage and unless this organism is specifically looked for it will be missed. In fixed stained smears, about 60 per cent of trophozoites have two nuclei; the endosome is large and lobulated without peripheral chromatin. Alternatively it may be identified in faeces or cultures using immunofluorescence with specific antibody. Transmission is believed to be nearly always within the eggs of the threadworm *Enterobius*. It causes a relatively mild diarrhoeal illness that may persist for several weeks, sometimes there is a superficial eosinophilic colitis. Blood eosinophilia is quite common and seropositivity is reported. This infection is common in some institutional contexts, but sudden outbreaks are not reported, presumably because of its mode of transmission. It is found within some resected appendices but a causal role is unlikely. Electron micrographs indicate that *D. fragilis* is an amoeboflagellate or a trichomonad rather than a true amoeba. The infection responds to metronidazole.

Free-living amoebae

Several species produce cytopathic changes in cultured cell monolayers and cerebral invasion after intranasal inoculation into mice and other animals. These amoebae are aerobic and their cytoplasm contains mitochondria, Golgi complexes, and a contractile vacuole; their natural food is bacteria. A shared feature is the very large central nuclear endosome, quite different from that of *E. histolytica*, from which differentiation may be necessary in tissue sections. Under dry conditions, trophozoites form resistant cysts that permit survival and also airborne dispersal; cysts can resist chlorination. Many species are thermophilic and they are one of the causes of 'humidifier fever', a form of extrinsic allergic alveolitis presenting with fever, cough, and sometimes progressive pulmonary fibrosis and dyspnoea. Some bacteria including *Legionella* and *Listeria* may live symbiotically within amoebae persisting within the phagosome, being resistant to lyzosomal enzymes. Surprisingly, *Legionella* can survive encystment: the amoebae provide a refuge for these bacteria when chlorination or other antibacterial measures are applied. The following three genera of free-living amoebae cause human infections.

Naegleria is an amoeboflagellate with two trophozoite forms. The amoeba moves rapidly with a single pseudopodium, it can transform into a non-feeding flagellate in hypotonic media and these free-swimming forms facilitate dispersal. Cysts are thin walled and spherical. It may be cultured aerobically on a confluent growth of *Escherichia coli*.

Acanthamoeba has no flagellate form. The small pseudopodia are multiple, thin, and spike-like (Fig. 6); they are called acanthopodia. Cysts are thick walled, angulated, and buoyant (Fig. 7); their dispersal may be windborne. It can be cultured on a confluent growth of *Escherichia coli*.

Balamuthia is a leptomyxid amoeba; it shows little directional movement and has an irregular or branched shape. Cysts are thick walled and wrinkled. Human infections formerly attributed to *Hartmanella* are now all thought to be due to *B. mandrillaris*, a species described in 1993 from a

Fig. 6 Trophozoite of *Acanthamoeba* showing spike-like acanthopodia. (Copyright V. Zaman.)

Fig. 7 Cysts of *Acanthamoeba*. (Copyright V. Zaman.)

mandrill baboon that died of meningoencephalitis in San Diego zoo. *Balamuthia* can only be cultured on tissue culture monolayers.

Primary amoebic meningoencephalitis due to *Naegleria fowleri*

Epidemiology and pathology

Nearly all patients give a history of swimming or diving in warm fresh water, or spa water, between 2 and 14 days before the illness began. Common-source outbreaks occur during warm summer months in temperate countries. Amoebic trophozoites cross the cribriform plate from the nasal mucosa to the olfactory bulbs and subarachnoid space. At autopsy the brain shows cerebral softening and damage to the olfactory bulbs; cysts are never formed in the tissues. So far only about 200 cases have been documented since the first human case was reported in 1965. However, some are missed clinically and discovered at autopsy, or in preserved pathologcal material. Specific antisera enable amoebae to be recognized by immunofluorescence staining.

Clinical features and diagnosis

Most patients are young adults and children. Initial nasal symptoms and headache are soon followed by fever, neck rigidity, coma, and later, convulsions; most die within a few days. Cerebrospinal fluid is often turbid, and bloodstained with high protein and low glucose levels and neutrophils. Amoebae must be urgently looked for in wet specimens using phase-contrast microscopy. Unless amoebae are seen, bacterial meningitis will be suspected; on Gram staining, amoebae appear as indistinct smudges. Fixed preparations stained with iron haematoxylin will show full details of nuclear structure. Confirmation is by culture at 37°C. Amphotericin B is the only effective drug. It should be given by daily intravenous infusion, and intrathecally, with the dosage regimens used for cryptococcal meningitis. So far, very few patients have survived, but this may partly be due to diagnostic delays.

Amoebic keratitis due to *Acanthamoeba*

Corneal lesions are painful and present as indolent and progressive ulcers leading eventually to perforation. Recognition may be in the context of lesions unresponsive to antibiotics or corticosteroids; differention must be made from herpes simplex. Inflammatory cells are mainly neutrophils. Infection may be by wind-borne cysts upon a damaged epithelium or from contact lenses. Solutions used to store, or wash, lenses can be contaminated by these amoebae, many of which are resistant to some antiseptics, especially as cysts.

Five species of *Acanthamoeba* are recognized to cause keratitis, the most common are *A. castellani* and *A. polyphaga*. Amoebae are found in corneal scrapings or histologically in corneal tissue but can be missed unless stained with iron haematoxylin or immunofluorescence using specific antisera. Cysts may be seen in tissue. Cultures from fresh material should be at 30°C.

Lesions usually respond to local propamidine and neomycin, but the latter is not cysticidal; combinations of topical propamidine with chlorhexidine, or with polyhexamethylene, have recently been successful. Alternatives are topical miconazole and oral ketoconazole. Corneal grafting may be necessary. Wearers of contact lenses must take especial care to avoid contamination, especially when storage cases are used; raw tap water may contain *Acanthamoeba*. The most appropriate disinfectants are chlorhexidine and hydrogen peroxide.

Granulomatous amoebic encephalitis due to *Acanthamoeba*

Humans become infected by swallowing or inhaling cysts or amoebae; or these may contaminate wounds, or skin or mucosal ulcers. *Acanthamoeba* species are sometimes isolated from throat or nasal swabs, or from stool specimens.

Many patients have predisposing factors such as craniofacial trauma, vascular brain infarct, or a systemic disorder such as lymphoma, other malignancy, collagen disorder, alcoholism, or diabetes mellitus. Relatively acute cerebral lesions are described in a few patients with AIDS. Cerebral lesions arise haematogenously, by direct spread, or rarely from the nasal mucosa as with *Naegleria*. Pathologically, lesions resemble chronic bacterial brain abscesses or localized subacute haemorrhagic necrosis; involvement of the meninges is common. Some patients present with headache and meningism, others with evidence of a focal brain lesion. Primary lesions have been described from the lung, orbit and other cranial structures, and the gastric wall.

Unless these amoebae are found in wet-tissue preparations or cerebrospinal fluid, the diagnosis will be based upon histology. Cysts may be seen in tissue, but trophozoites may be missed unless stained with iron haematoxylin or immunofluorescence using specific antisera. Cultural diagnosis from fresh biopsies or cerebrospinal fluid is sometimes possible.

Survival of patients with this condition is very rarely reported. Total excision of cerebral lesions is occasionally possible. The drug sensitivities are poorly defined; a wide spectrum of resistance is common. Systemic amphotericin B or flucytosine will be the initial choice, but ketoconazole is an alternative.

Amoebic meningoencephalitis due to *Balamuthia mandrillaris* infection

Since 1990, when this condition was recognized in a non-human primate, more than 60 human cases have been reported, in the Americas, Europe, and Australia. Immunocompetent as well as immunocompromised patients may be infected. Exposure may be associated with contact with fresh water in pools. Cerebral lesions may be subacute and necrotizing, with prominent vasculitis, or chronic and granulomatous. Some patients have associated granulomatous facial lesions (Plate 4). Prolonged treatment with albendazole and itroconazole has proved effective in Peru. Diagnosis is made by finding amoebic trophozoites and cysts in infected tissue and by indirect immunofluorescence.

Further reading

Gut amoebae

Clark CG (1998). Amoebic disease: *Entamoeba dispar*, an organism reborn. *Transactions of the Royal Society of Tropical Medicine and Hygiene* **92**, 361–4.

Cuffari C, Oligny L, Seidman EG (1998). *Dientamoeba fragilis* masquarading as allergic colitis. *Journal of Paediatric Gastroenterology and Nutrition* **26**, 16–20.

Diamond LS, Clark CG (1993). A redescription of *Entamoeba histolytica* Schaudinn, 1903 (emended Walker 1911) separating it from *Entamoeba dispar* Brumpt, 1925. *Journal of Eukaryote Microbiology* **40**, 340–4.

Irusen EM *et al.* (1992). Asymptomatic intestinal colonization by pathogenic *Entamoeba histolytica* in amebic liver abscess: prevalence, response to therapy, and pathogenic potential. *Clinical Infectious Diseases* **14**, 889–93.

Jackson TF (1998). *Entamoeba histolytica* and *Entamoeba dispar* are distinct species; clinical, epidemiological and serological evidence. *International Journal of Parasitology* **28**, 181–6.

Martinez-Palomo A, ed. (1986). *Amoebiasis*. Elsevier, New York.

Ockert G (1990). Symptomatology, pathology, epidemiology, and diagnosis of *Dientamoeba fragilis*. In: Honigberg BM, ed. *Trichomonads parasitic in humans*, pp 395–410. Springer, New York.

Ravdin JI, ed. (1988). *Amebiasis. Human infection by* Entamoeba histolytica. Wiley, New York.

Ravdin JI (1995). Amebiasis. [Review.] *Journal of Infectious Diseases* **20**, 1453–64.

Ravdin JI, ed. (2000). *Amebiasis*. Imperial College Press, London.

Sachdev GK, Dhol P (1997). Colonic involvement in patients with amoebic liver abscess: endoscopic findings. *Gastrointestinal Endoscopy* **46**, 37–9.

Free-living amoebae

Carter RF (1972). Primary amoebic meningo-encephalitis. *Transactions of the Royal Society of Tropical Medicine and Hygiene* **66**, 193–208.

Denney CF *et al.* (1997). Amebic meningoencephalitis caused by *Balamuthia mandrillaris*: case report and review. *Clinical Infectious Diseases* **25**, 1354–8.

Harf C (1996). Amoebae in relationship with bacteria in their environment. In: Özcel MA, Alkan MZ, eds. *Parasitology for the 21st century*, pp 253–60. CAB International, Wallingford, UK.

Illingworth CD *et al.* (1995). *Acanthamoeba* keratitis: risk factors and outcome. *British Journal of Ophthalmology* **79**, 1078–82.

Visvesvara GS, *et al.* (1990). Leptomyxidameba, a new agent of amebic meningoencephalitis in humans and animals. *Journal of Clinical Microbiology* **28**, 2570–6.

Visvesvara GS, Schuster FL, Martinez AJ (1993). *Balamuthia mandrillaris*, N.G., N. Sp., agent of amebic meningoencephalitis in humans and other animals. *Journal of Eukaryote Microbiology* **40**, 504–14.

7.13.2 Malaria

D. J. Bradley and D. A. Warrell*

Introduction

Malaria is the most important human parasitic disease globally, causing over 170 million clinical cases annually, of which over a million die, mostly in Africa. It has had large effects on the course of history and settlement in tropical regions. In recent years malaria has been subject to massive control efforts, with varying degrees of success but the disease has been resurgent for the last two decades. Resistance of falciparum malaria parasites to the main antimalarial drugs is now a serious problem in SE Asia. Malaria epidemics are an increasing problem. Malaria remains the dominant tropical vector-borne disease but, after decades of neglect, international interest in its control has recently revived.

Parasitology

There are over a hundred species of malarial parasite (*Plasmodium* spp.), but only four species have humans as their natural vertebrate host: *P. falciparum*, *P. malariae*, *P. vivax*, and *P. ovale* (Plate 1). Rare zoonotic infections

* Contains same material by C. Newbold from previous editions.

have been recorded from non-human primate malarias such as *P. knowlesi*, *P. simium*, and *P. cynomolgi*.

Although each of the human malarias has distinguishing biological, morphological, and clinical characteristics (Table 1), their overall biology and lifecycles are similar (Fig. 1).

In both the mosquito and mammalian hosts the lifecycle of *Plasmodium* spp. has alternating stages of invasion and intracellular asexual division. The sexual stage, by facilitating the exchange of genetic information between different parasite strains or genotypes, assists in the generation of genetic diversity within the parasite population.

Infection is initiated when sporozoites from the salivary glands of a female *Anopheles* mosquito are inoculated during a blood meal into the human bloodstream. These organisms invade hepatic parenchymal cells within a few minutes, the process being largely complete within 30 min. Once inside the liver cell, two pathways of differentiation are possible.

In all species there is intracellular asexual multiplication. In addition, in *P. vivax* and *P. ovale* infections some parasites enter a cryptobiotic phase termed 'hypnozoites', which may lie dormant for months or even years before starting to divide and giving rise to late relapses. In *P. falciparum* and *P. malariae* infections there is no cryptobiotic phase and so relapses from the liver do not occur, although blood infections may persist for a few years in the case of *P. falciparum* or decades in the case of *P. malariae*.

The time required to complete the intrahepatic multiplication depends on the parasite species (Table 1). The products of the liver stage (extra-erythrocytic merozoites) are liberated in their thousands into the bloodstream. Here they attach to and invade circulating erythrocytes. Inside the erythrocyte, asexual division begins and, over a period of 48 h (*P. falciparum*, *P. vivax*, *P. ovale*) or 72 (*P. malariae*), the parasites develop through a series of morphological changes from 'ring' forms to trophozoites and finally to schizonts containing daughter erythrocytic merozoites. These are liberated by red-cell lysis and immediately invade uninfected erythrocytes, producing a repetitive cycle of invasion and multiplication. Because the intraerythrocytic division cycle is usually fairly synchronous (particularly in *P. vivax* and *P. ovale* infections) and also tied to the diurnal cycle of the host, red-cell lysis and merozoite release occur at approximately the same time of day for a given individual. 'Malarial pyrogens' released at this time induce cytokine production (for example, tumour necrosis factor-α (**TNF-**α) and interleukin-1 (**IL-1**)) giving rise to the periodic 'agues' or paroxysms of fever that have long been a diagnostic feature of malaria infection. The asexual blood forms are the only forms of the parasite that give rise to clinical symptoms.

A small proportion of the merozoites within red cells develop into male and female gametocytes. Once mature, these gametocytes may return to the mosquito if ingested during a blood meal.

Inside the mosquito's midgut, male and female gametes are liberated from their host red cells and fuse to form a zygote which develops into an ookinete, able to penetrate the gut wall and form an oocyst. At this point a further series of asexual divisions takes place, giving rise to sporozoites that migrate to the insect's salivary glands to complete the lifecycle.

Table 1 Developmental characteristics of human malaria parasites

Species	P. falciparum	P. vivax	P. ovale	P. malariae
Prepatent period[a]	8–25 days	8–27 days	9–17 days	15–30 days
Length of asexual erythrocytic cycle	48 h	48 h	48 h	72 h
Red cells parasitized	All	Retics	Retics	Mature erythrocytes
Merozoites per schizont	8–32	12–24	4–16	6–12
Relapse from persistent liver infection	No	Yes	Yes	No, but persistent red-cell infection up to 30 years
Drug resistance	Yes	Yes	No	No

[a] Time from infective mosquito bite to appearance of parasites in the blood.

Retics, reticulocytes.

Fig. 1 Development cycle of *Plasmodium* spp. (redrawn by permission of F. Hoffman-la-Roche Ltd, Basel).

Genetics of the parasite

Variation has been found in isoenzyme types, antigenic markers, drug-resistance markers, and in the virulence of different isolates. Such genetic diversity has an important bearing on the disease, for an individual infection may consist of different parasite genotypes of varying drug resistance and exposure to a variety of antigenic types that may be needed before clinical immunity develops. During the intraerythrocytic cycle in the blood, the parasites are haploid. The diploid phase of the lifecycle occurs after gamete fusion in the mosquito where meiosis takes place.

Resistance to chloroquine and pyrimethamine results from mutations at unlinked loci. However, in the case of resistance to chloroquine alone, multiple mutations at independent loci may give rise to resistance. In some cases, resistance is stable in the absence of drug pressure. A locus on chromosome 7 segregates with the resistant phenotype.

Molecular biology

DNA from *P. falciparum* has proved to have an unusual base composition with an average A+T content of approximately 80 per cent. A very high proportion of genes, including 'housekeeping genes', contain large blocks of tandemly repeated amino acid sequences. It has been proposed that these sequences may act as immunological decoys by acting as T-independent antigens. The presence of multiple, low-affinity cross-reactivities between different repeats may serve to prevent the affinity maturation of specific B cells.

Comparison of rRNA sequences of different species of *Plasmodium* shows that *P. falciparum* is more closely related to avian malarias than to other mammalian species.

Proteins/antigens

The surface proteins of the sporozoite and sexual stages are dealt with in the section on vaccination below. Some of the molecules expressed on the surface of the merozoite, the invasive free-living form, are involved in the process of invasion of new erythrocytes. Other proteins bind specifically to the surface of normal red cells, but not to cells rendered refractory to invasion. Because red-cell invasion is an essential step in asexual parasite multiplication, understanding its molecular basis could lead to new forms of therapy.

Molecules on the surface of the infected red cell determine the adherence of infected cells to vascular endothelium and are a target of the protective immune response. Biochemical, immunochemical, and cell biological data reveal that a family of high molecular-weight molecules undergo a process of rapid, clonal, antigenic variation. The genes for this group of proteins (**PfEMP-1**, *Plasmodium falciparum* erythrocyte membrane protein-1), have recently been cloned.

Many other parasite-derived proteins are secreted into the host red cell, but do not find their way to the cell surface. Some interact specifically with the red-cell cytoskeleton modifying the host-cell environment in favour of the parasite.

In vitro culture

Since 1975 it has been possible to grow asexual forms of *P. falciparum* in long-term culture, using a suitable growth medium with uninfected red cells in an atmosphere of low oxygen and high carbon dioxide tension. The availability of large numbers of *P. falciparum* parasites, without recourse to patients or experimental non-human primates, has speeded up much of the basic research on malaria and has permitted the development of *in vitro*

Fig. 2 Feeding posture of different types of adult mosquito. (a) Culicine, (b) anopheline.

tests for sensitivity to certain antimalarial drugs. The complete development of the hepatic stage of *P. falciparum* has also been achieved *in vitro*. Gametocytes can also be produced from *in vitro* culture of asexual blood forms.

Biology of the mosquito vector

Human malarial parasites are transmitted only by Anopheles mosquitoes. There are many species with varying habits, breeding places, and effectiveness as malaria vectors. Anopheles can be distinguished from other adult mosquitoes by the way that the female, when taking a blood feed, inclines her whole body at an angle to her victim, while in the other, culicine mosquitoes, the body is parallel to the skin surface (Fig. 2). The culicine and anopheline larval stages are also distinguishable (Fig. 3).

Since the female Anopheles needs a blood meal before egg laying, her adult life consists of finding a suitable blood meal, resting while it is digested, flying off to lay eggs at a suitable body of water, and then repeating this cycle every few days. The eggs, larvae, and pupae develop in water and the winged adults emerge. For ecological reasons, only a few species of Anopheles in a given locality are likely to be important malaria vectors, because to transmit malaria the mosquitoes need to be sufficiently abundant, to bite people rather than only some other vertebrate host, and to live long enough for ingested gametocytes to develop through to sporozoites. Identification of the main vector species in an area determines the design of specific control measures. Since most species are selective in their breeding sites, knowledge of the larval ecology permits engineering and other measures to be directed at the selective removal of the vector habitat, a process called 'species sanitation'.

The behaviour of the adult mosquito will dictate which insecticidal strategies are most likely to succeed. Anophelines vary in their preferred feeding and resting locations, though the majority bite in the evening and night. They may bite indoors (endophagic) or outside (exophagic). This determines whether the use of bednets and screened doors and windows will protect, or whether long sleeves and protective footwear when outside the house are more relevant. Of greater importance is where the female rests

Fig. 3 Resting posture of different types of mosquito larva. (a) Culicine, (b) anopheline.

overnight to digest the blood meal. Endophilic mosquitoes, which rest on the inside walls of houses and in the roof, are thereby exposed to residual insecticides previously sprayed on the walls, whereas exophilic mosquitoes, resting outside houses, may escape the effects of insecticidal attack. The success of many antimalarial efforts has depended on the major vectors in several continents being endophilic, and failures of attempted eradication have sometimes resulted from exophilic vector species being present, as in many forested areas of SE Asia. Anopheline mosquitoes extend into temperate countries, and in the United Kingdom several indigenous species, notably *A. atroparvus*, were responsible for transmitting the historical English 'agues' (*P. vivax* and *P. malariae*).

Epidemiology

Malaria is widely distributed throughout the tropics (Fig. 4) except for the south-central Pacific islands from which anopheline mosquitoes are absent. *P. falciparum* is the predominant species in the highly endemic areas of Africa, New Guinea, and Haiti, while *P. vivax* is more common in Central America, North Africa, and southern and western Asia. Both species are prevalent in South America, the rest of Asia, and Oceania. *P. malariae* is widespread but often overlooked, and in West Africa *P. ovale* largely replaces *P. vivax*, to which the indigenous inhabitants are resistant.

The epidemiological features of human malaria differ markedly even between endemic areas. At one extreme, as in tropical Africa, everyone is infected shortly after birth, parasitaemia is almost universal throughout childhood, and the brunt of mortality falls in early childhood; epidemics do not occur except at high altitude. By contrast, as in parts of India, malaria is an epidemic disease affecting all ages and causing temporary dislocation of community life due to the concurrent illness of the people. These differences result from differing levels of malaria transmission affecting the pattern of immunity in the human population, so that to understand even the clinical spectrum of malaria seen in patients from a given locality it is essential to understand the local epidemiological situation. The epidemiology of malaria is complex but relatively well understood. Attempts at control in recent years have changed the epidemiological pattern in many areas.

Climate and mosquito ecology are the primary determinants of malarial epidemiology. Once the biology of the relevant anopheline mosquito is understood, much of the complex epidemiology of malaria falls into place. There is some variation in susceptibility to malaria within the anophelines, so that *P. falciparum* from Africa may fail to develop in some European anophelines even under optimal conditions, but usually in a given locality the indigenous anopheline mosquitoes will be capable of transmitting the local malaria strains, so that the importance of a vector species depends particularly on their behaviour and ecology.

The epidemiological pattern is determined by the density, human-biting habit, and longevity of the mosquito. Density is the number of vectors present in a locality relative to the human population. Malaria transmission will tend to be proportional to mosquito density, as might be expected. The human-biting habit combines two features: the frequency with which the female mosquito feeds and the choice of host. The human-biting frequency rises to as high as 0.5/day in *A. gambiae*, an African mosquito that feeds on alternate days and preferentially on people; while *A. culicifacies*, a vector in South Asia, may feed only every third day and as few as 10 per cent of its meals may be from people, giving a human-biting habit of 15-fold less. Because malaria transmission is proportional to the square of the human-biting habit, and as transmission involves both parasite uptake by bite and subsequent inoculation to human by a second bite, this factor has a large effect on malaria transmission.

Mosquito longevity has an even greater effect. The duration of the 'extrinsic cycle', the interval between when a mosquito ingests infective gametocytes and the first day on which sporozoites are present in the salivary glands ready for transmission, depends on the ambient temperature (Fig. 5), but it will rarely be less than 10 days. Only mosquitoes that become infected and then survive for longer than the duration of the extrinsic cycle (say 10 days) can pass on the infection. As mosquitoes of a given species have a relatively constant probability of dying during a day, regardless of their age, the longevity may be described by the probability of surviving through one day, and it varies greatly between mosquito species and environments. It will affect transmission very greatly indeed: if the chance of survival through one day is p and the duration of the extrinsic cycle n days, then transmission is proportional to pn, that is, something like the tenth power of p. Thus the most effective transmission of malaria will be by a long-lived mosquito that occurs at high density and frequently bites people. *A. gambiae* and *A. funestus* best fit this description well and are the predominant African malaria vectors.

Malaria transmission is most conveniently measured in terms of the basic case reproduction rate (**BCRR**). This is the average number of new cases of malaria that will result from one human case of malaria in a locality, assuming all the other people are non-immune and uninfected. The BCRR may vary from over 1000 in some areas of Africa to below 1. Where the BCRR is less than 1, the infection will not replace itself and the disease will die out. In the 'real world', the BCRR will vary considerably about a mean value. In areas with a very high BCRR everyone will become infected,

the variation will be immaterial, and the amount of malaria seen will be determined by acquired human immunity. This is the situation called 'stable malaria' (Table 2) and is seen in sub-Saharan Africa and New Guinea particularly. Because the BCRR is so high, control methods aimed at breaking transmission have to reduce it by a factor of perhaps 1000 to bring the BCRR below 1. By contrast, in places where the BCRR is, say, 3, natural variations will cause the BCRR to be below 1 for much of the time. There will be intermittent periods of transmission, and epidemics will occur from time to time. This is called 'unstable malaria'. Because human immunity will be much less, people of all ages will become ill during the epidemics, but the transmission will be much easier to control. Unstable malaria is dramatically evident but kills fewer people than stable malaria, in which the brunt of the mortality falls on young children.

Even in stable malaria, seasonal variation may occur. In the African savannah, no mosquitoes may bite during the hot dry season and in more temperate zones it may be too cold for transmission for part of the year, but the annual peaks will be comparable, with all children infected each year. While the division between stable and unstable malaria is the most useful (Table 2), an earlier classification of areas by the parasite prevalence in children or by the proportion of children aged 2 to 9 years with enlarged

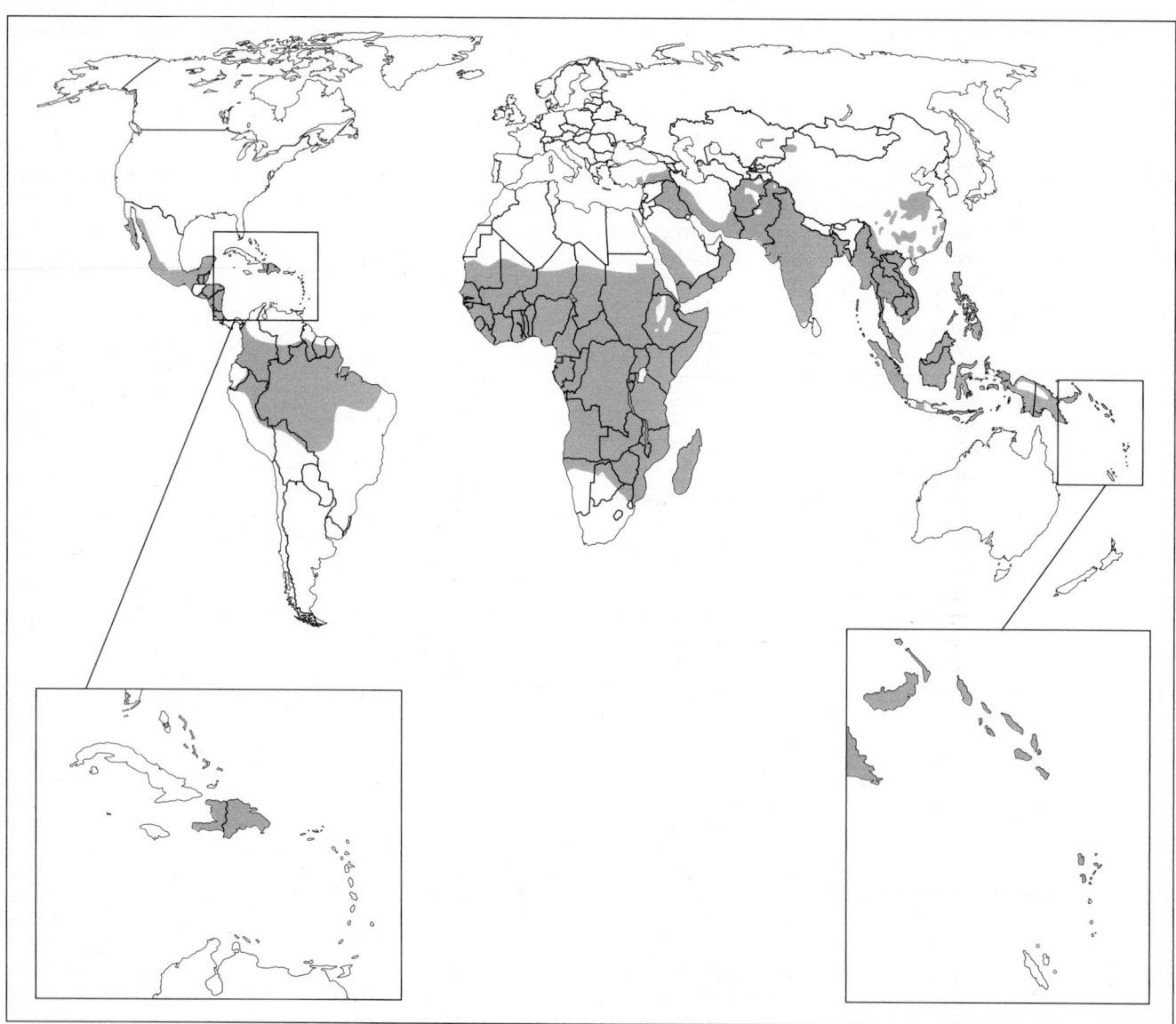

Fig. 4 Malarious areas of the world.

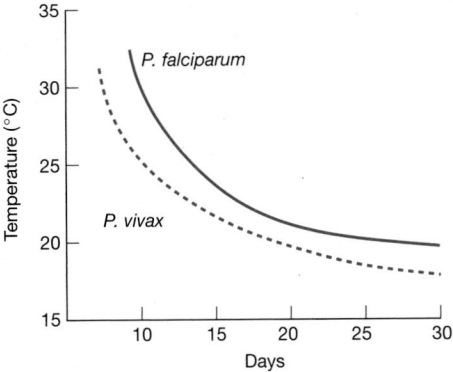

Fig. 5 The period of extrinsic development of *P. falciparum* and *P. vivax*.

spleens is often still used (Table 3). The prevalence of splenic enlargement gives a better cumulative picture of the amount of malaria than does the parasite prevalence, which is influenced by casual chemotherapy.

Under endemic conditions there is still a great deal of variation in risk to a non-immune visitor. At one extreme, in some parts of rural Africa an unprotected person is likely to be bitten on average by more than one infective mosquito nightly, whilst in a highly malarious part of India the corresponding rate is perhaps five times yearly or less. Yet both will be rightly perceived as highly malarious places by the local inhabitants.

The epidemiological background to clinical malaria is likely to change over time in most places due to environmental changes (often man-made, whether local or global), changing resistance of parasites to drugs, and the consequences of attempts at malaria control.

The widespread availability of chloroquine and other effective chemotherapeutic agents in endemic areas has resulted in the early treatment of a proportion of infections. This often leads to disparities between a high spleen rate in children and an artificially low parasite rate. With the increasing use of chemotherapy and of bed nets for personal protection, the acqui-

Table 2 The major differences between stable and unstable malaria

	Unstable	Stable
Basic case reproduction rate (BCRR)	Lowish, variable	High
Endemicity	Usually low	Usually high
Epidemics	Likely	Not seen except in migrants
Seasonal changes	Marked	Fall only in cold or dry season
Predominant parasite	*P. vivax*	*P. falciparum*
Incidence changes	Uneven and large	Small and only seasonal
Immunity population	Variable	High
Clinical effects most in	All ages	Young children
Determinants:		
Mosquito life	Short	Long
Human-biting habit	Low	High
Climate suitable	Short periods	Long periods
Anopheline density for transmission	High	Low is sufficient
Control	Feasible	Extremely difficult

Table 3 The traditional terminology for levels of malaria endemicity

Term	Spleen rate in children (%)
Hypoendemic	<10
Mesoendemic	11–50
Hyperendemic	51–75, >25 in adults
Holoendemic	>75, low in adults

sition of immunity is somewhat deferred. Under the most intense transmission, severe and often fatal anaemia in infants predominates. With rather less transmission, cerebral malaria in early childhood may be more apparent. Cerebral malaria will also be the main hazard in falciparum malaria epidemics and in non-immune individuals who contract it. Human migration is commonly associated with malaria epidemics, because population pressure in hilly areas drives the inhabitants down into malarious regions, or the aggregation of workers at new sites mixes infected people with those who are susceptible, or refugees may have impaired resistance to infection and public health measures may have collapsed. Migrants are commonly blamed for introducing malaria, but more usually they are non-immune individuals suffering from the disease acquired from the indigenous inhabitants.

Susceptibility to infection and innate resistance

People of West African origin are strikingly resistant to *P. vivax* infection. This correlates with the extreme rarity of the Duffy blood-group antigen alleles *Fya* and *Fyb*, which are receptors for penetration of the red cell by the merozoites.

Other genetic determinants affect the course and outcome of infection. Although *P. falciparum* is responsible for around 1 million deaths of African children annually, the mortality would be much greater but for a number of inherited resistance factors, and for the processes of acquired resistance discussed in the next section.

The high mortality associated with malaria is perhaps best illustrated by the way in which a number of otherwise disadvantageous genes have been selected in chronically exposed populations because of the resistance to malaria that they confer. In 1948, J.B.S. Haldane first suggested that heterozygotes of thalassaemia might be 'fitter than the normal [and] more resistant to attacks by the sporozoa that cause malaria'.

It has since become clear for several mutations affecting haemoglobin production or structure that these have reached their present frequencies by this selective mechanism. The best-known example is sickle-cell disease, due to a point mutation in position six of the β-globin chain. Here the mutant-gene frequency is stabilized because the enhanced survival of heterozygotes is counterbalanced by the lethal consequences of homozygosity in developing countries. Protection afforded to heterozygotes is seen most dramatically in case-control studies, which show that the relative risk of contracting severe malaria by heterozygotes and controls is about 1 to 10, respectively. Perhaps surprisingly, parasite rates and densities at the population level are very similar in normal and AS individuals, except in very young children, indicating that heterozygotes are resistant to disease rather than to infection.

Table 4 lists the genotypes for which there is either epidemiological or clinical evidence of selection by malaria. Despite this often clear evidence of protection, the mechanisms involved are still controversial.

Acquired resistance

Those exposed to repeated malarial infection in endemic areas gradually acquire immunity in several stages, but it is rarely complete. Immunity is species-specific and largely strain-specific. The first change observed is a reduction in clinical symptoms and signs for a given level of parasitaemia. This is sometimes known as 'tolerance' but the mechanism is not understood.

Acquired resistance to the parasites takes months to develop and first affects the density of gametocytes in the peripheral blood. Subsequently, the density of asexual erythrocytic parasites, trophozoites, and schizonts falls and gradually reaches very low levels, so that under conditions of holoendemic transmission the prevalence of infection falls by half in those aged 15 years compared with children. Infected older children and adults from

Table 4 Human genetic polymorphisms associated with resistance to malaria

α-Thalassaemia	SE Asian ovalocytosis	Duffy blood gp	Glycophorin B deficiency
β-Thalassaemia	G6PD deficiency	S–s U blood gp	TNF-α promoter
Haemoglobin S	ABO blood groups	HLABw53	IFN-γ receptor
Haemoglobin E	Class 1 MHC	HLADRB1* 1302	
Haemoglobin F	Class 2 MHC		

MHC, major histocompatibility complex; G6PD, glucose 6-phosphate dehydrogenase; TNF-α, tumour necrosis factor-α, IFN-γ, interferon-γ

highly endemic areas often have very low-level, persistent, asymptomatic parasitaemias combined with relative resistance to superinfection.

It is clear that in a highly endemic area for *P. falciparum* there are several parasite strains circulating, and concepts of why resistance is so slowly acquired may either emphasize a balance in immune responses or the successive infection with various strains combined with a largely strain-specific response. The latter is favoured at present. Severe malaria in very young children is ascribed to multiple infections over a short time, and the cerebral malaria that predominates in slightly older children is possibly due to some more virulent strains.

Infants born to immune mothers are partially protected against severe malaria attacks by transplacental antibodies and those acquired from breast milk, for a few months, after which the infant suffers from severe malaria attacks with only gradual acquisition of resistance. Adult non-immune people, including visitors to the tropics from non-malarious areas, are equally susceptible to high mortality in their first few attacks, while women from an endemic area become more susceptible during pregnancy (second trimester), especially the first pregnancy. Splenectomy, for any reason, also increases susceptibility to malaria, which may have a fatal outcome.

Immunity is stage-specific, in that immunity to either sporozoite challenge or to gametocyte transmission does not protect against asexual parasites. It also has components that are specific for the parasite species, strain (genome), and antigenic variant within a strain. Thus protection against infection by sporozoites appears to be mediated largely by cytotoxic T cells, which can kill infected hepatocytes, although antibody to the repeat regions of the circumsporozoite protein may also have a role. Specific T and B cells, in addition to non-antigen-specific mechanisms, are involved in the control of asexual parasitaemia. The central role of antibody has been demonstrated by a variety of passive transfer experiments in people and experimental animals. Pooled immunoglobulin from highly immune donors is extremely effective in rapidly reducing parasitaemia, but not in the long-term control of infection. Maintaining parasite numbers below subclinical levels requires the involvement of T cells, as shown by adoptive transfer experiments in animals. Work in rodents suggests that early in infection, TH1 cells are critical but that later during the course of infection cells of a TH2 phenotype are more important. High levels of cytokines, such as TNF-α, during acute infection are a feature of severe malaria and are associated with a poor outcome. The acute response in non- or semi-immune individuals, while vital to the control of parasitaemia, may also contribute to the pathogenesis of disease by triggering a variety of non-specific effector mechanisms.

Clinical immunity takes many years and several infections to be effectively induced. It is also a non-sterilizing response, as immune adults are constantly and demonstrably reinfected. Several explanations have been put forward for these observations. Generalized, parasite-induced immunosuppression certainly does occur and may be clinically relevant in the response to certain non-malarial antigens such as meningococcal vaccine. It is not clear, however, whether overall it is any more severe than in other acute viral or bacterial infections. One area where it does seem to play a definite part is in the development of Burkitt's lymphoma, in which case it has been shown that individuals with acute *P. falciparum* infection have impaired T-cell control of endogenous, Epstein–Barr virus-infected, B-cell proliferation. Other explanations for the difficulty in inducing effective immunity have involved interference by the parasite in the development of specific responses. This could either be by the presence of important T-independent antigens, which induce a relatively poor response with no memory, or by the effect of crossreactive, tandem-repeat elements in inhibiting affinity maturation of specific B cells. Perhaps the most likely explanation is the extreme polymorphism or clonal variation of immunologically relevant antigens, such that the host requires exposure to a variety of 'strains' before a broadly effective response can develop. If the latter is true, then it presents formidable problems to vaccine development.

Malaria and HIV-immunosuppression

For at least 20 years, falciparum malaria and HIV-immunosuppression have coexisted in Africa, but the effects of their interaction on the clinical course of both diseases is still uncertain. Early studies that suggested an association between HIV and falciparum malaria in African children were vitiated by the greater risk of HIV-contaminated blood transfusions in children with severe malaria-related anaemia in this region. However, *P. falciparum* parasitaemia has been found to be more frequent among HIV-1-infected multigravidae than controls in malaria holoendemic areas of Central/Southern Africa, associated with increased perinatal mortality. Both HIV and malaria contribute to maternal anaemia and low birthweight babies and, in Lusaka, Zambia, a dramatic increase in maternal morbidity over the last 20 years has been attributed to malaria, HIV-immunosuppression, AIDS-associated tuberculosis, and chronic respiratory illnesses. Recently, in a study of 613 adults with microscopically confirmed falciparum malaria in an area of unstable transmission in Kwa-Zulu Natal, South Africa, the results suggested that underlying HIV infection might double the risk of severe malaria and increase the risk of fatal malaria by five- to sevenfold.

Molecular pathology

All the pathology associated with malaria infection is attributable to asexual parasite multiplication in the bloodstream. No adverse effects are caused by the quantitatively small degree of parasite invasion and multiplication within hepatocytes, nor by the presence of relatively small numbers of circulating gametocytes. The consequences to the host of the intraerythrocytic multiplication of parasites range from a variety of severe, but not life-threatening, symptoms common to all the species that infect humans, to the potentially lethal complications associated with acute *P. falciparum* infection and the chronic renal damage caused by some infections with *P. malariae*. The relative severity of *P. falciparum* infections, as well as the ability to culture this parasite *in vitro*, has meant that it has been the focus of most experimental effort.

It had been noted for centuries that malaria was characterized by periodic fevers. Once the causative organism was identified, it was clear that the bouts of fever generally followed the synchronous release of new merozoites into the bloodstream as each cycle of erythrocytic multiplication was completed. While it was assumed that the release of infected cell contents that occurs at this time was responsible for fever induction, it was not until very recently that it was proven that components of the infected cell such as the lipid, glycosyl phosphatidyl inositol anchor of a parasite membrane protein (perhaps **MSP-1**, merozoite surface protein-1) could directly induce the release of cytokines such as TNF-α and IL-1 from macrophages. Moreover, it was demonstrated that the older stages of parasites within erythrocytes were differentially sensitive to physiological increases in temperature, so that the effect of fever was both to limit parasite multiplication and to maintain synchronous development. Measurements of TNF-α in children suffering from severe malaria also demonstrated that very high levels of this cytokine were associated with a lethal outcome, although the correlation was not sufficient to be a useful prognostic indicator.

The principal life-threatening complications of *P. falciparum* in African children are cerebral malaria and severe anaemia often associated with metabolic acidosis and respiratory distress. The clinical picture in non-immune adults is more complex and can include single or multiple organ failure. Mechanisms responsible for severe malarial anaemia are poorly understood, but include parasite-induced dyserythropoiesis and accelerated red-cell clearance of both normal and infected cells by both immune and non-immune mechanisms (see below). However, the central event underlying the pathology of most other manifestations of severe falciparum malaria is the cytoadherence and resulting sequestration of infected cells, which is unique to this organism (Figs 6 and 7 and Plate 2). Only the younger developmental stages of the parasite circulate, as the more mature forms adhere to specific receptors on venular endothelium. The distribu-

Fig. 6 Brain section of a patient who died of cerebral malaria, showing a blood vessel packed with red blood corpuscles, the majority of which were identifed as being infected by the presence of parasites (P), or at a higher magnification, the presence of knobs (by courtesy of Dr D. Ferguson, Oxford).

Fig. 7 Human cerebral malaria. Electron micrograph showing endothelial cell microvilli making contact with a parasitized erythrocyte via electron-dense strands (upper right). (Copyright N. Francis.)

tion of infected cells found in tissue sections suggests that the chief sites of infected cell sequestration correlate with specific organ dysfunction. It is assumed, but not formally proven, that the reduction in, or obstruction of, local blood flow associated with the partial occlusion of small vessels with infected cells results in reduced perfusion and tissue damage. Some have suggested that the sequestered cells may induce the local release of a number of potentially toxic or pharmacologically active compounds (such as reactive oxygen species or nitric oxide) from macrophages, neutrophils, or endothelium, and that these may affect tissues locally.

While the detailed mechanisms by which sequestered cells result in the specific symptoms seen in cases of severe falciparum malaria remain largely unresolved, much more progress has been made in understanding the molecular interactions that lead to sequestration. Several endothelial receptors have been identified, including CD36 (formerly platelet glycoprotein IV), thrombospondin, intercellular adhesion molecule-1 (**ICAM-1**), and more recently, vascular cell-adhesion molecule (**VCAM**) and E-selectin (Table 5). Most field isolates bind to CD36 and thrombospondin and the majority bind to ICAM-1; to date there are insufficient data on VCAM and E-selectin. *In vitro* assays of purified proteins reveal great variability in the absolute levels of adhesion between isolates. No good correlation has yet emerged between the ability of parasites to bind to individual receptors and disease pattern. These studies are, however, fraught with difficulty and many more data are needed to resolve this point. The parasite molecules involved in adhesion are well characterized biochemically but have not yet been cloned, so that primary-sequence data are not available. They form a family of red-cell surface proteins that undergo clonal antigenic variation during a single infection and that also appear to be targets of a host-protective antibody response.

Some parasite isolates show two other properties: the rosetting of uninfected erythrocytes around red cells containing mature developmental forms of the parasite (Fig. 8) and autoagglutination of infected erythrocytes in the absence of immune serum. Rosetting has been linked to cerebral malaria in some, but not all, studies. It is presumed that the multicellular aggregates, if they occur *in vivo*, may exacerbate vascular obstruction caused by sequestration.

Despite the life-threatening nature of severe falciparum malaria, and the enormous number of childhood deaths that it causes in sub-Saharan Africa, the mortality rate of all malaria infections is extremely low. In holo-endemic areas, infections in children are universal and constant, yet only a small proportion of those infected show clinical symptoms at any one time and only a fraction of these go on to develop severe illness. This is probably only partially explained by the known innate resistance factors and acquired immunity, and so it is likely that unidentified factors are also important in determining how far individual infections progress from parasitaemia to clinical illness and finally to severe disease.

Table 5 Cerebral malaria: cytoadherence and rosetting candidate receptors

Infected erythrocyte surface	Vascular endothelium		
Cytoadherence			
PfEMP-1	Thrombospondin	)	
Sequestratin	CD36	)	all parasites
Modified red blood cell band 3	ICAM-1 (cerebral malaria)	)	
Rosetting	VCAM		
Pf332	E-selectin (ELAM-1)		
CR1	Chondroitin sulphate	)	placenta
ABO	Hyaluronic acid	)	
PfEMP-1	CD31 (PECAM-1)		
	$\alpha_v \beta_3$ integrin		

PfEMP, *Plasmodium falciparum* erythrocyte membrane protein; ICAM, intercellular adhesion molecule; VCAM, vascular cell adhesion molecule; ELAM, endothelial leucocyte adhesion molecule; CR1, complement receptor 1; PECAM, platelet–endothelial cell adhesion molecule.

Fig. 8 Rosetting *in vitro*. The central parasitized erythrocyte shows many electron-dense protruberances (knobs) beneath its membrane (bar = 1 μm). (Copyright D. Ferguson.)

Pathology

Brain

Only falciparum malaria causes cerebral pathology. At autopsy, the brain is sometimes oedematous but evidence of cerebral, cerebellar, or medullary herniation is rarely seen. The small blood vessels, including those of the leptomeninges, are congested with parasitized red blood cells containing malaria pigment (Figs 6 and 7). This gives the surface of the brain its characteristic leaden or plum-coloured appearance and the cut surface a slatey-grey hue. Many of the parasites are schizonts and other mature forms. In larger vessels, parasitized red cells form a layer along the endothelium ('margination'). Up to 70 per cent of erythrocytes in the cerebral vessels are parasitized and these are more tightly packed than in other organs. The cerebrovascular endothelium shows pseudopodial projections, which may be in close apposition to electron-dense, knob-like protruberances on the surface of parasitized red cells (Fig. 7). Numerous petechial haemorrhages are seen in the white matter, resulting from haemorrhages from end arterioles, proximal to occlusive plugs of parasitized red cells and fibrin. Focal ring haemorrhages can be found centred on small subcortical vessels. Dürck's granulomas, small collections of microglial cells surrounding an area of demyelination, may develop at the site of these haemorrhages, but an inflammatory cell response is generally lacking.

Bone marrow

There is evidence of iron sequestration, erythrophagocytosis, dyserythropoiesis, and cytoadherence with plugging of sinusoids in the acute phase of falciparum malaria. Maturation defects are present in the marrow for at least 3 weeks after clearance of parasitaemia. Increased numbers of large, abnormal-looking megakaryocytes have been found in the marrow and the circulating platelets may also be enlarged, suggesting dyspoietic thrombopoiesis. Malaria pigment and parasites can be found in monocytes and phagocytes in the marrow, even when they are not detectable in peripheral blood.

Liver

The liver is affected by all four species of human malaria parasites, but changes are most severe in falciparum malaria. The liver is enlarged and oedematous, and coloured brown, grey, or even black as a result of malaria pigment deposition. Hepatic sinusoids are dilatated, containing hypertrophied Kupffer cells and parasitized red cells that appear to obstruct the circulation. Parasitized and uninfected red cells are phagocytosed by Kupffer cells, endothelial cells, and sinusoidal macrophages. Small areas of centrilobular necrosis, which are occasionally seen in severe cases, may be attributable to shock or disseminated intravascular coagulation. Hepatocytes usually show only mild abnormalities but may be depleted of glycogen in some patients who are hypoglycaemic. Lymphocytic infiltration of portal tracts has been described (see also Tropical splenomegaly syndrome, below).

Gastrointestinal tract

Cytoadherent, sequestered, parasitized red cells may be found in the small and large bowel, especially in capillaries of the lamina propria and larger submucosal vessels. The bowel may appear congested, with mucosal ulceration and haemorrhage.

Kidney

Glomerular lesions range from the acute transient glomerular nephritis of falciparum malaria to the chronic lesions of quartan malarial nephrosis. In severe falciparum malaria, with or without 'blackwater fever', acute renal failure is associated with the histopathological changes of acute tubular necrosis. Parasitized red cells may be found in glomerular and peritubular capillaries, with fibrin thrombi and pigment-laden macrophages. Tubular pigment casts are prominent in cases of blackwater fever.

Lung

The lungs are oedematous in almost all patients dying of malaria. Pulmonary capillaries and venules are packed with inflammatory cells including neutrophils, plasma cells, and pigment-laden macrophages, and with parasitized red cells. The vascular endothelium is oedematous, causing narrowing of the capillary lumen, and there is interstitial oedema and hyaline-membrane formation. Secondary bronchopneumonia is a common finding.

Spleen

The spleen is large, engorged, and dark-red or greyish-black in colour. The red and white pulp is congested and hyperplastic, and the splenic cords and sinuses are filled with phagocytic cells containing pigment, parasitized red cells, and non-infected red cells. Tropical splenomegaly syndrome is described below.

Heart

There is no evidence of myocarditis. Subendocardial and epicardial petechial haemorrhages are unusual. The myocardial capillaries are congested with parasitized red cells, pigment-laden macrophages, lymphocytes, and plasma cells. However, the parasitized cells are not tightly packed and there is no evidence of cytoadherence.

Pathophysiology

Anaemia

This is attributable mainly to the destruction or phagocytosis of parasitized red cells, but other mechanisms contribute. The bone marrow shows dyserythropoietic changes. Initial iron sequestration and hypoferraemia may be explained by the very marked hyperferritinaemia, an acute-phase reaction. There is evidence of immune-mediated haemolysis in some populations. Erythrocyte survival is reduced even after the disappearance of parasitaemia. Increased splenic clearance of non-parasitized as well as parasitized red cells has been demonstrated.

Intravascular haemolysis occurs in patients whose erythrocytes are congenitally deficient in enzymes such as glucose 6-phosphate dehydrogenase

(**G6PD**) in response to oxidant drugs such as primaquine. However, in classical blackwater fever, G6PD levels are, by definition, normal and the mechanism of haemolysis is unknown, although quinine-mediated haemolysis has been suspected.

Thrombocytopenia

This is attributable to sequestration in the spleen, failure of production by the marrow, and immune-mediated lysis.

Cerebral malaria

Mechanical obstruction to the microcirculation of the brain by cytoadherent, parasitized red cells, and perhaps 'rosettes' of uninfected red cells stuck around a parasitized red cells, is thought to be the principal mechanism leading to coma. Red blood cells infected with some strains of *P. falciparum* develop adhesive properties as they mature. Parasite-derived protein such as PfEMP-1 expressed on the surface of the parasitized red cell may act as a ligand that binds to receptors such as ICAM-1 on cerebral venular endothelium (Table 5). The expression of ICAM-1, and some other receptors involved in the cytoadherence of parasitized red cells, may be increased by TNF-α and other cytokines. Obstruction to cerebral blood flow could result in 'stagnant anoxaemia', leading to coma. In Thai adults with cerebral malaria, it was found that global cerebral blood flow was inappropriately low and there was evidence of cerebral anaerobic glycolysis with increased lactate concentrations in the cerebrospinal fluid. In African children with cerebral malaria, plasma concentrations of TNF-α, IL-1α, and other cytokines correlate closely with disease severity, as judged by parasitaemia, hypoglycaemia, case fatality, and the incidence of neurological sequelae. As well as enhancing cytoadherence, cytokines may have other effects on cerebral function, perhaps by releasing nitric oxide, which interferes with neurotransmission, or by leading to the generation of free oxygen radicals. Cytokines may also be responsible for fever, hypoglycaemia, coagulopathy, dyserythropoiesis, and leucocytosis in falciparum malaria.

In SE Asian adults, the opening pressure of cerebrospinal fluid at lumbar puncture was usually normal and cerebral oedema was demonstrable (by computed tomography (**CT**) scanning) during life in only a small minority, and usually as an agonal phenomenon. In these patients there was little evidence that brain swelling contributed to coma. However, in African children with cerebral malaria, intracranial pressure is usually elevated and there is evidence of brain swelling in the majority of those examined by CT scan. Ischaemic damage resulting from a critical reduction in cerebral perfusion pressure and other factors such as hypoglycaemia and status epilepticus are thought to be important in the mechanism of brain damage in these children.

Pulmonary oedema

This may develop in patients who have been overloaded with fluid in hospital and have elevated central venous and pulmonary-artery wedge pressures. More commonly, the clinical picture is of adult respiratory distress syndrome, with normal or low hydrostatic pressures in the pulmonary vascular bed. In these cases, the mechanism is likely to be increased pulmonary capillary permeability resulting from leucocyte products and cytokines. The histological appearances of neutrophil sequestration in the pulmonary capillaries, increased permeability, and hyaline membrane formation are consistent with this hypothesis.

Hypoglycaemia

This can be caused by cinchona alkaloids (quinine or quinidine), which are potent stimulators of insulin secretion by the pancreatic β-cells. The resulting reduction in hepatic gluconeogenesis and increased peripheral glucose uptake by tissues results in hypoglycaemia. In malaria, glucose consumption is increased by fever, infection, anaerobic glycolysis, and the metabolic demands of the malaria parasites. Glycogen reserves may be depleted, especially in children and pregnant women, as a result of fasting and 'acceler-

ated starvation'. In African children with severe malaria, adult patients with severe disease, and pregnant women, hypoglycaemia develops spontaneously (without treatment with cinchona alkaloids) and is associated with appropriately low plasma insulin concentrations. Plasma lactate and alanine concentrations are elevated and ketone bodies are moderately increased. Counter-regulatory hormone levels are usually very high. The mechanism of hypoglycaemia in these cases may be inhibition of hepatic gluconeogenesis by TNF-α and other cytokines.

Acute renal failure

Hypovolaemia, from dehydration, is responsible for acute renal failure in the majority of patients whose acute oliguria and renal dysfunction is reversible by fluid replacement. Hyperparasitaemia, jaundice, and haemoglobinuria are associated with a high risk of acute tubular necrosis. Renal cortical perfusion is reduced during the acute stage of the disease. Renal cortical necrosis must be rare, as survivors rarely show evidence of chronic renal impairment. Cytoadherence of parasitized red blood cells in the renal microvasculature, deposition of fibrin microthrombi, and prolonged hypotension ('algid malaria') may contribute to acute renal failure. Quartan malarial nephrosis is discussed below.

Hyponatraemia

In patients with relatively normal plasma osmolalities, hyponatraemia has been attributed to the inappropriate secretion of ADH triggered by fever or reduced effective plasma volume. However, the levels of ADH were appropriately high in Thai patients who were proved to be grossly hypovolaemic by carefully monitored fluid-repletion studies. Mild hyponatraemia is often attributable to intravenous therapy with 5 per cent dextrose alone in patients who are salt-depleted and dehydrated.

Hypovolaemia and 'shock' ('algid malaria')

This may result from hypovolaemia (dehydration and, rarely, haemorrhagic shock following splenic rupture or gastrointestinal haemorrhage) but is most often associated with a secondary Gram-negative bacteraemia. The source may be an intravenous cannula, urethral catheter, or aspiration pneumonia. Transient immunosuppression, impaired macrophage function, or 'blockade' of the reticuloendothelial system may increase the susceptibility of patients to severe secondary bacterial infections.

Clinical features

The pathogenic species of *Plasmodium* cause acute febrile illnesses characterized by periodic febrile paroxysms occurring every 48 or 72 h, with afebrile asymptomatic intervals and a tendency to recrudesce or relapse over periods of months or even years. The severity of the attack is determined by the species and strain, and hence the geographical origin, of the infecting parasite; on the age, genetic constitution, state of immunity, general health, and nutritional state of the patients, and on their use of antimalarial drugs.

Falciparum malaria ('malignant' tertian or subtertian malaria)

The shortest interval between an infecting mosquito bite and parasitaemia is 5 days, but this prepatent period is usually 9 to 10 days. The incubation period (the interval between infection and the first symptom) usually ranges from 7 to 14 days (mean 12 days) but may be prolonged further by immunity, chemoprophylaxis, or partial chemotherapy. In Europe and North America, 98 per cent of patients with imported falciparum malaria present within 3 months of arriving back from the malarious area. A few present up to 1 year later, but none after more than 4 years.

Several days of prodromal symptoms such as malaise, headache, myalgia, anorexia, and mild fever are interrupted by the first paroxysm. Suddenly the patient feels inexplicably cold (in a hot climate) and apprehensive. Mild shivering quickly turns into violent shaking with teeth-chattering. There is intense peripheral vasoconstriction and gooseflesh. Some patients vomit. The rapid increase in core temperature may trigger febrile convulsions in young children. The rigor lasts up to 1 h and is followed by a hot flush with throbbing headache, palpitations, tachypnoea, prostration, postural syncope, and further vomiting while the temperature reaches its peak. Finally, a drenching sweat breaks out and the fever defervesces over the next few hours. The exhausted patient sleeps. The whole paroxysm is over in 8 to 12 h, after which the patient may feel remarkably well. These symptoms are typical of a classical 'endotoxin reaction' produced by typhoid vaccine, infection with Gram-negative bacteria, or the release of TNF-α and other cytokines by other agents. Classical tertian or subtertian periodicity (48 and 36 h between fever spikes) is rarely seen with falciparum malaria. A high irregularly spiking, continuous or remittent fever, or daily (quotidian) paroxysm, is more usual. Other common symptoms are headache, backache, myalgias, dizziness, postural hypotension, nausea, dry cough, abdominal discomfort, diarrhoea, and vomiting. The non-immune patient with falciparum malaria usually looks severely ill, with 'typhoid' facies and, in dark-skinned races, a curious greenish complexion. Commonly, there is anaemia and a tinge of jaundice, with moderate tender enlargement of the spleen and liver. Useful negative findings are the lack of lymphadenopathy and rash (apart from herpes simplex 'cold sores') and focal signs.

Cerebral malaria and other severe manifestations and complications

The global case fatality of falciparum malaria is probably around 1 per cent or 1 to 3 million deaths per year. Cerebral malaria is the most important of the severe manifestations of *P. falciparum* infection, accounting for 80 per cent of these deaths. Patients who have been feverish and ill for a few days may have a generalized convulsion from which they do not recover consciousness, or their level of consciousness may decline gradually over several hours. High fever alone can impair cerebral function causing drowsiness, delirium, obtundation, confusion, irritability, psychosis, and, in children, febrile convulsions. The term 'cerebral malaria', implying encephalopathy specifically related to *P. falciparum* infection, should be restricted to patients in an unrousable coma (no appropriate verbal response and no purposive motor response to noxious stimuli—Glasgow Coma Scale ≤9/14) and evidence of acute *P. falciparum* infection, in whom other encephalopathies, including hypoglycaemia and transient postictal coma, have been excluded. Patients with cerebral malaria may have mild meningism but neck rigidity and photophobia are rare. Retinal haemorrhages (Plate 3) are present in about 15 per cent of African and SE Asian cases, but exudates are rare. (In Papua New Guinea these changes are not confined to patients with severe falciparum malaria.) Papilloedema is very rare (0.5 per cent of cases). Dysconjugate gaze is common. In adult patients the pupillary, corneal, oculocephalic, and oculovestibular reflexes are normal. Muscle tone and tendon reflexes are usually increased and there is ankle clonus. The plantar responses are extensor and abdominal reflexes are absent. In African children, brainstem reflexes may be abnormal and there may be neurological evidence of severe intracranial hypertension with rostrocaudal progression suggesting cerebral, cerebellar, and medullary herniation. Hypotonia is more common than in adults. In patients of all ages, abnormal flexor or extensor posturing (decerebrate or decorticate rigidity), associated with sustained upward deviation of the eyes (not the transient upward gaze of oculogyric crisis), pouting and stertorous breathing, is sometimes, but not always, associated with hypoglycaemia (Figs 9(a) and (b)). About half of adult patients and more children have generalized convulsions. In children, seizures may be subtle and detectable only as twitching of the facial muscles, deviation with nystagmus of the eyes, irregularities of breathing, and sometimes posturing of one arm. Less than 5 per cent of adult survivors have persisting neurological sequelae; these include cranial-nerve lesions, extrapyramidal tremor, and transient paranoid psychosis. However, more than 10 per cent of African children who

survive an attack of cerebral malaria suffer from sequelae such as hemiplegia, cortical blindness, epilepsy, ataxia, and mental retardation.

Anaemia (see above) is an inevitable consequence of all but the mildest infections. It is most common and severe in pregnant women, children (Plate 4), and in patients with high parasitaemia, schizontaemia, secondary bacterial infections, and renal failure.

Spontaneous bleeding, from the gums (Plate 5) and gastrointestinal tract, is seen in less than 5 per cent of adult patients with severe malaria. It is rare in children.

Jaundice (Plate 6) is common in adults but rare in children. Biochemical evidence of severe hepatic dysfunction is unusual. Hepatic failure suggests concomitant viral hepatitis or another diagnosis.

Hypoglycaemia is being increasingly recognized in patients with malaria. Pregnant women with severe or uncomplicated falciparum malaria and other patients with severe disease may become hypoglycaemic a few hours to 6 days after starting treatment with quinine or quinidine, even after the parasitaemia has cleared. Pregnant women and children with malaria, and other patients with hyperparasitaemia and complicating bacteraemias, may all become hypoglycaemic early in their illness and without quinine therapy. The symptoms and signs of hypoglycaemia—anxiety, tachycardia, breathlessness, feeling cold, confusion, sweating, light-headedness, restlessness, fetal bradycardia, other signs of fetal distress, coma, convulsions, and extensor posturing—may be misinterpreted as merely manifestations of malaria.

Hypotension and shock ('algid malaria') is seen in patients who develop pulmonary oedema, metabolic acidosis, complicating bacteraemias, and massive gastrointestinal haemorrhage. Mild supine hypotension with a marked postural drop in blood pressure is usually attributable to vasodilatation and relative hypovolaemia. Cardiac arrhythmias are rare but may be

(a)

(b)

Fig. 9 (a) and (b) Extensor posturing (decerebrate rigidity) in a Thai woman with cerebral malaria and profound hypoglycaemia (Copyright D. A. Warrell).

precipitated by rapid infusion or excessive doses of antimalarial drugs such as chloroquine, quinine, or quinidine. Patients with coronary insufficiency may develop angina during febrile crises of malaria. Patients with severe malaria sometimes develop complicating bacterial infections such as aspiration pneumonia, urinary-tract infections, infected bedsores, and phlebitis at intravenous drip sites.

Oliguria, with increased blood urea and serum creatinine concentrations, is seen in about one-third of patients with severe malaria. Although most of these patients respond to cautious rehydration, 10 per cent develop renal failure requiring dialysis.

In patients whose red blood cells are deficient in G6PD (and other enzymes), intravascular haemolysis and haemoglobinuria (Plate 7) may be precipitated by oxidant antimalarial drugs, especially primaquine, whether or not they have malaria. Classical blackwater fever is the association of haemoglobinuria with severe manifestations of falciparum malaria—including renal failure, hypotension and coma—in a non-immune patient who is not G6PD deficient.

Metabolic acidosis is seen in association with hyperparasitaemia, hypoglycaemia, and renal failure. Usually it results from lactic acidosis, even in patients with renal failure. In African children, respiratory distress manifested as deep (Kussmaul) breathing, associated with severe anaemia and metabolic acidosis, is emerging as a syndrome, and which carries a higher mortality than cerebral malaria.

Pulmonary oedema (Fig. 10) appears to be the terminal event in most fatal cases of falciparum malaria in adults. It may develop late in the clinical course as a result of fluid overload or in patients with severe disease in the absence of fluid overload. It may also appear suddenly after delivery in pregnant women who are in positive fluid balance. The earliest sign is an increase in respiratory rate. Pulmonary oedema may be difficult to differentiate from aspiration pneumonia, a common complication in comatose patients, and metabolic acidosis. Radiography may be needed to make this distinction with confidence. The patients who are not fluid-overloaded resemble those with adult respiratory distress syndrome with a normal jugular venous, central venous, or pulmonary-artery wedge pressure.

Cerebellar dysfunction

A rare presentation of falciparum malaria is cerebellar ataxia with unimpaired consciousness. Similar signs may be seen in patients recovering from cerebral malaria and, in Sri Lanka, delayed cerebellar ataxia has been described 3 to 4 weeks after an attack of fever attributable to falciparum malaria. Complete recovery is the rule.

Malarial psychosis

Acute psychiatric symptoms in patients with malaria may be attributable to their drug treatment, including antimalarial drugs such as chloroquine,

mefloquine, and the obsolete mepacrine, and to exacerbation of pre-existing functional psychoses. However, in some patients, organic mental disturbances associated with malaria infection have been the presenting feature or, more often, have developed during convalescence after attacks of otherwise uncomplicated malaria or cerebral malaria. Depression, paranoia, delusions, and personality changes should probably be classified as brief reactive psychoses. These symptoms rarely last for more than a few days.

Vivax, ovale, and malariae malarias

The prepatent and incubation periods are given in Table 1. Some strains of *P. vivax*, especially those from temperate regions (*P. v. hibernans* from Russia, *P. v. multinucleatum* from China) may have very long incubation periods (250–637 days). Only about one-third of imported cases of vivax malaria present within a month of returning from the malarious area; 5 to 10 per cent will present more than a year later.

The 'benign' malarias cause paroxysmal, feverish symptoms no less hectic and distressing than those of falciparum malaria. Prodromal symptoms are said to be more severe with *P. malariae* infection. In untreated cases, the characteristic tertian (48–50 h) interval between fever spikes may be seen with *P. vivax* and *P. ovale* and the quartan (72 h) pattern in *P. malariae* infections.

This periodicity is established after several days of irregular fever. Vivax and ovale malarias have a persistent hepatic cycle, which may give rise to relapses every 2 to 3 months for 5 to 8 years in untreated cases. *P. malariae* does not relapse but a persisting, undetectable parasitaemia may cause recrudescences for more than 50 years.

Although symptoms may be severe and temporarily incapacitating, especially in non-immune individuals, the acute mortality is very low. For example, during the 1967 to 1969 Sri Lankan epidemic of predominantly vivax malaria, there were more than half a million cases with a case fatality of only 0.1 per cent. Only in immunocompromised, splenectomized or debilitated patients are the 'benign' malarias likely to prove life-threatening. However, acute pulmonary oedema has been documented in several cases of vivax malaria in non-immune travellers (Fig. 11).

An important practical point is that indigenous West Africans are very rarely infected with *P. vivax*. Patients suffering from vivax malaria may become anaemic, thrombocytopenic, and mildly jaundiced with tender hepatosplenomegaly. Splenomegaly may be particularly gross in areas of *P. malariae* infection (see also Tropical splenomegaly syndrome, below). In debilitated patients with vivax malaria, anaemia rarely may be severe enough to be life-threatening. Splenic rupture, which carries a mortality of 80 per cent, is said to be more common with vivax than falciparum malaria. It results from acute, rapid enlargement of the spleen, with or without trauma; chronically enlarged spleens are less vulnerable. A ruptured spleen

Fig. 10 Pulmonary oedema in a Vietnamese woman with cerebral malaria (copyright D. A. Warrell).

Fig. 11 Pulmonary oedema in a 20-year-old woman with vivax malaria and bilateral pleural effusions (copyright D. A. Warrell).

presents with abdominal pain and guarding, haemorrhagic shock (tachy-cardia, postural hypotension, and prostration), fever, and a rapidly falling haematocrit. These features may be misattributed to malaria itself.

Cerebral vivax malaria has occasionally been reported especially with the long incubation period strain in China. Mixed falciparum infection or another encephalopathy must be adequately excluded in such cases. The same strictures apply to cerebral *P. malariae* malaria, especially as this parasite coexists with *P. falciparum* throughout most of its range. The acute symptoms of ovale and malariae malarias may be as severe as those of vivax infection, but anaemia is less severe and the risk of splenic rupture is lower. *P. ovale* causes negligible mortality, but *P. malariae* causes many deaths from nephrotic syndrome (see below).

Malaria in pregnancy and the puerperium

Malaria is a major cause of maternal anaemia, death, abortion, stillbirth, premature delivery, low birth weight, and neonatal death in those areas of the tropics where malaria transmission is unstable and women of child-bearing age have little acquired immunity. Even in some hyperendemic areas, clinical symptoms and parasitaemia are worse in primiparous than in multiparous women and other patients. In non-immune individuals, cerebral and other forms of severe falciparum malaria are more common in pregnancy. In the great epidemic of falciparum malaria in Sri Lanka during 1934 to 1935 the mortality among pregnant women was 13 per cent, twice that in non-pregnant women, and in Thailand, where malaria has been the most important cause of maternal mortality, cerebral malaria in late pregnancy had a mortality of 50 per cent. In some parts of Africa, one-quarter to one-half of all placentas are parasitized. The incidence is highest in primiparae. Changes in humoral and cell-mediated immunity in pregnancy do not explain this vulnerability, but it is clear that the placenta is a privileged site for parasite multiplication. An adhesion receptor for some strains (genotypes) of *P. falciparum*, chondroitin sulphate A, is expressed on the surface of the syncytiotrophoblast. This may explain sequestration in the placenta.

In most endemic regions, birth weights of neonates born to women with malaria are significantly less than those of controls. Fetal distress was observed in 6 out of 12 Thai women with malaria who were beyond the twenty-ninth week of pregnancy. Painless uterine contractions were detected in seven out of eight who were not in labour. This uterine activity subsided as the patients' temperatures were reduced by simple cooling.

Special risks to the mother of malaria during pregnancy are hyperpyrexia, hypoglycaemia, anaemia, cerebral malaria, and pulmonary oedema.

Severe anaemia, exacerbated by malaria, is an important complication of pregnancy in many tropical countries. Especially in communities where chronic hookworm anaemia is prevalent, high output anaemic cardiac failure may develop in late pregnancy.

Asymptomatic hypoglycaemia may occur in pregnant women with malaria before antimalarial treatment, and pregnant women with severe uncomplicated malaria are particularly vulnerable to quinine-induced hypoglycaemia (see above).

There is an increased risk of pulmonary oedema precipitated by fluid overload or by the sudden increase in peripheral resistance, or autotransfusion of hyperparasitaemic blood from the placenta, which occurs just after delivery (Fig. 10).

Prevention

Malaria is so dangerous in pregnancy that pregnant women who cannot leave the area of transmission must be given intermittent preventive treatment with sulfadoxine–pyrimethamine or antimalarial prophylaxis extending into the early puerperium. This is a most important part of antenatal care.

Congenital and neonatal malaria

Vertical transmission of malaria can be diagnosed by detecting parasitaemia in the neonate within 7 days of birth, or later if there is no possibility of postpartum, mosquito-borne infection. Save for a few discordant reports, most evidence from malarious parts of the world indicates that congenital malaria is rarely symptomatic, despite the high prevalence of placental infection. This confirms the adequacy of protection provided by IgG from the immune mother, which crosses the placenta to active immunization from exposure to soluble malarial antigens *in utero* and to the high proportion of fetal haemoglobin in the neonate, which retards parasite development. Congenital malaria is, however, much more common in infants born to non-immune mothers, and there is an increased incidence during malaria epidemics. It can cause stillbirth or perinatal death. All four species can produce congenital infection, but because of its very long persistence *P. malariae* causes a disproportionate number of cases in non-endemic countries. Fetal plasma quinine and chloroquine concentrations are about one-third of the simultaneous maternal levels. Thus, antimalarial concentrations that are adequate to cure the mother might result in subtherapeutic concentrations in the fetus. Quinine and chloroquine are excreted in breast milk, but the suckling neonate would receive only a few mg/day. Maternal hypoglycaemia, a common complication of malaria or its treatment with quinine, may produce marked fetal bradycardia and other signs of fetal distress.

Differential diagnosis

The clinical features of congenital malaria include fever, irritability, feeding problems, hepatosplenomegaly, anaemia, and jaundice. Unless parasites are found in a smear from a heel prick or cord blood, the patient may be misdiagnosed as having rhesus incompatibility or another congenital infection such as cytomegalovirus, herpes simplex, rubella, toxoplasmosis, or syphilis.

Transfusion malaria, 'needlestick', and nosocomial malaria

Malaria—like trypanosomiasis, Colorado tick fever, HIV, hepatitis viruses, and some other pathogens—can be transmitted in blood from apparently healthy donors. Exceptionally, donors may remain infective for up to 5 years with *P. falciparum* and *P. vivax*, 7 years with *P. ovale*, and 46 years with *P. malariae*. Because the infecting forms are erythrocytic (not sporozoites), no exoerythrocytic (hepatic) cycle will be established and so vivax and ovale malarias will not relapse. Theoretically, parasitaemia might be detectable immediately and hence the incubation period should be shorter than with mosquito-transmitted malaria. However, the incubation period tends to be longer because of the time needed to build up parasitaemias sufficient to cause symptoms. Mean incubation periods are 12 (range 7–29) days for *P. falciparum*, 12 (range 8–30) days for *P. vivax*, and 35 (range 6–106) days for *P. malariae*. Whole blood, packed cells (blood products), leucocyte or platelet concentrates, fresh plasma, marrow transplants, and haemodialysis have been responsible for transfusion malaria. As patients requiring transfusion are likely to be debilitated and may be immunosuppressed, and there may be a long delay before making the diagnosis because malaria is not suspected, unusually high parasitaemias may develop with *P. falciparum* and *P. malariae*. With *P. ovale* and *P. vivax* infections, the parasitaemia is usually limited to 2 per cent because only reticulocytes are invaded. Severe manifestations are common, mortality may be high, for example 8 out of 11 in a group of heroin addicts, and even acute *P. malariae* infections may prove fatal.

Nosocomial malaria has resulted from contamination of saline used for flushing intravenous catheters, contrast medium, and intravenous drugs. Malaria has complicated parenteral drug abuse.

Prevention

Outside the malaria endemic area, donors who have been in the tropics during the previous 5 years should be screened for malarial antibodies (indirect fluorescent antibody) (see below). In the endemic area, recipients of blood transfusions can be given antimalarial chemotherapy, or at least should be watched carefully for evidence of infection.

Monkey malarias

Human erythrocytes can be infected with at least six species of simian plasmodia. There have been rare cases of natural infections or accidental laboratory infections by *P. brazilianum*, *P. cynomolgi*, *P. inui*, *P. knowlesi*, *P. schwetzi*, and *P. simium*. Severe feverish and systemic symptoms have been described, but no cerebral or other severe complications. No patient has died. Parasitaemia may remain undetectable for 2 to 6 days after the start of symptoms. Periodicity is quotidian (*P. knowlesi*) or tertian (*P. simium* and *P. cynomolgi*). Infectivity and virulence may be enhanced by repeated passage in humans. Chloroquine is the treatment of choice.

Diagnosis

Malaria can present with a wide range of symptoms and signs, none of them diagnostic. **It must be excluded by repeated thick and thin blood smears in any patient with acute fever and an appropriate history of exposure.** Until malaria is confirmed or an alternative diagnosis emerges, smears should be repeated every 8 to 12 h. **However, if the patient is severely ill, or the symptoms persist or deteriorate, a therapeutic trial of antimalarial chemotherapy must not be delayed.** Antimalarial chemoprophylaxis should be stopped while the patient is under investigation for malaria, as this may make microscopical diagnosis more difficult. Patients should be asked about travel to malaria endemic countries during the previous year. The possibility of malaria must not be dismissed because the patient took prophylactic drugs, for none is completely protective. Short airport stopovers, even on the runway, or working in or living near an international airport, may allow exposure to an imported, infected mosquito. Transmission by blood transfusion, 'needlestick', or nosocomial infection should be borne in mind. Those who grew up in an endemic area will probably lose their immunity to disease after living for a few years in the temperate zone and become vulnerable when they return to their homeland on holiday. In malaria endemic regions, a large proportion of the immune population may have asymptomatic parasitaemia and it cannot be assumed that malaria is the cause of the patient's symptoms even if parasitaemia is detected. The diagnosis of malaria may be missed, even in the endemic zone, during an epidemic of some other infection (for example, meningitis, pneumonia, cholera).

Differential diagnosis (Table 6)

Malaria should be considered in the differential diagnosis of any acute febrile illness until it can be excluded by a definite lack of exposure, by repeated examination of blood smears, or by a therapeutic trial of antimalarial chemotherapy. In Europe and North America, imported malaria has been misdiagnosed as influenza, viral hepatitis, viral encephalitis, or travellers' diarrhoea, sometimes with fatal consequences. Cerebral malaria must be distinguished from other infective meningoencephalitides. Cerebrospinal fluid (**CSF**) examination will identify most of these infective causes (see Chapter 24.14.1). Abdominal reflexes are brisk in patients with psychotic stupor and hysteria but absent in cerebral malaria. Recognition of poisoning will depend largely on the history or the clinical circumstances. Overdose of antimalarial drugs (chloroquine and quinine) can be confused with cerebral malaria. Intravenous drug abusers are at risk both from severe malaria and drug overdose. Alcoholism may be confused with cerebral malaria, whether the patient presents simply as 'drunk', with delirium tremens, or encephalopathy.

Misdiagnosis of a viral haemorrhagic fever in a case of imported malaria is potentially dangerous, for patients may be placed in a high-containment unit where they may be denied basic investigations such as examination of a blood smear because of a fear of infection. Jaundice is a common feature of yellow fever, but not other viral haemorrhagic fevers.

Malaria in pregnancy may be confused with viral hepatitis, acute fatty liver with liver failure or eclampsia, and in the puerperium with puerperal sepsis or psychosis.

Laboratory diagnosis

Microscopy

It is most important to confirm the diagnosis by examining thick and thin blood films on several occasions (Plate 1). Parasites may be found in blood taken by venepuncture, finger-pulp or ear-lobe stabs, and from the umbilical cord and impression smears of the placenta. In fatal cases, cerebral malaria can be confirmed rapidly as the cause of death by making a smear from cerebral grey matter obtained by needle necropsy through the foramen magnum, superior orbital fissure, ethmoid sinus via the nose, or through a fontanelle in young children. Sometimes no parasites can be found in peripheral blood smears from patients with malaria, even in severe infections. This may be explained by partial antimalarial treatment or by sequestration of parasitized cells in deep vascular beds. In these cases, parasites or malarial pigment may be found in a bone marrow aspirate.

Table 6 Differential diagnosis of malaria

Symptom	Diagnosis
Acute fever	Heat stroke, hyperpyrexia of other causes, other infections, other causes of fever
Fever and impaired consciousness (cerebral malaria)	Viral, bacterial, fungal, protozoal (e.g. African trypanosomiasis) or helminthic meningoencephalitis, cerebral abscess. Head injury, cerebrovascular accident, intoxications (e.g. insecticides), poisonings (e.g. antimalarial drugs), metabolic (diabetes, hypoglycaemia, uraemia, hepatic failure, hyponatraemia). Septicaemias
Fever and convulsions	Encephalitides, metabolic encephalopathies, hyperpyrexia, cerebrovascular accidents, epilepsy, drug and alcohol intoxications, poisoning, eclampsia, febrile convulsions, and Reye's syndrome (children)
Fever and haemostatic disturbances	Septicaemias (e.g. meningococcaemia), viral haemorrhagic fever, rickettsial infection, relapsing fevers, leptospirosis
Fever and jaundice	Viral hepatitis, yellow fever, leptospirosis, relapsing fevers, septicaemias, haemolysis, biliary obstruction, hepatic necrosis (drugs, poisons)
Fever with gastrointestinal symptoms	Travellers' diarrhoea, dysentery, enteric fever, other bacterial infections, inflammatory bowel disease
Fever with haemoglobinuria ('blackwater fever')	Drug-induced haemolysis (e.g. oxidant antimalarials in glucose 6-phosphate-dehydrogenase-deficient patient), favism, transfusion reaction, dark urine of other causes (e.g. myoglobinuria, urobilinogen, porphobilinogen)
Fever with acute renal failure	Septicaemias, yellow fever, leptospirosis, drug intoxications, poisonings, prolonged hypotension
Fever with shock ('algid malaria')	Septicaemic shock, haemorrhagic shock (e.g. massive gastrointestinal bleed, ruptured spleen), perforated bowel, dehydration, hypovolaemia, myocarditis

Pigment may be seen in circulating neutrophils. A number of Romanowski stains, including Field's, Giemsa, Wright's, and Leishman's, are suitable for malaria diagnosis. The rapid Field's technique, which can yield a result in minutes, and Giemsa are recommended. Smears may be unsatisfactory because the slides are not clean; stains are unfiltered, old, or infected; the buffer pH is incorrect (it should be 7.0–7.4); drying is too slow, especially in a humid climate (producing heavily crenated erythrocytes); or the blood has been stored in anticoagulant causing lysis of parasitized erythrocytes. It is difficult to make a good smear if the patient is very anaemic. Common artefacts resembling malaria parasites are superimposed platelets, particles of stain and other debris, and pits in the slide. Other erythrocyte infections such as bartonellosis and babesiosis may be misdiagnosed as malaria. Parasites should be counted in relation to the total white-cell count (on thick films when the parasitaemia is relatively low) or erythrocytes (on thin films). An experienced microscopist can detect as few as 5 parasites/μl (0.0001 per cent parasitaemia) in a thick film and 200/μl (0.004 per cent parasitaemia) in a thin film.

Fluorescent microscopy

Becton-Dickinson's QBC (quantitative buffy coat) method involves spinning blood in special capillary tubes in which parasite DNA is stained with Acridine Orange and a small float presses the parasitized red blood cells against the wall of the tube where they can be viewed by ultraviolet microscopy. In expert hands, the sensitivity of this method can be as good as with conventional microscopy of thick blood films but species diagnosis is difficult, and the method is much more expensive.

Malarial antigen detection

Becton-Dickinson's 'Para Sight F' and ICT Diagnostics' 'ICT Malaria Pf' dipstick antigen-capture assays employ monoclonal antibody detecting *P. falciparum* histidine-rich protein-2 (**PfHRP-2**) antigen. These tests are rapid (taking about 20 min), sensitive, and specific for *P. falciparum*. A number of other, species-specific, antigen-detection methods are now marketed, such as OptiMAL (Flow Laboratories) which detects parasite lactate dehydrogenase.

Other methods

Enzyme and radioimmunoassays, DNA probes (using chemoluminescence for detection), and polymerase chain reaction (**PCR**) methods now approach the sensitivity of classical microscopy. They take much longer (up to 72 h), are much more expensive, and are unlikely to replace microscopy for routine diagnosis. However, some of these newer methods could be automated for screening blood donors or for use in epidemiological surveys and, in the case of PCR, identification of parasite strains as well as species is possible.

Serological techniques

Malarial antibodies can be detected by immunofluorescence, enzyme immunoassay, or haemagglutination for epidemiological surveys, for screening potential blood donors, and occasionally for providing evidence of recent infection in non-immune individuals. These tests are not useful in making an acute diagnosis of malaria. In future, detection of protective antibodies will be important in assessing the response to malaria vaccines (see below).

Other laboratory investigations

Anaemia is usual, with evidence of haemolysis. Serum haptoglobins may be undetectable. The direct antiglobulin (Coombs') test is usually negative. Neutrophil leucocytosis is common in severe infections whether or not there is a complicating bacterial infection, but the white-cell count can also be normal or low. The presence of visible malarial pigment in more than

5 per cent of circulating neutrophils is associated with a bad prognosis. Thrombocytopenia is common in patients with *P. falciparum* and *P. vivax* infections; it does not correlate with severity. Prothrombin and partial thromboplastin times are prolonged in up to one-fifth of patients with cerebral malaria. Concentrations of plasma fibrinogen and other clotting factors are normal or increased, and serum levels of fibrin(ogen) degradation products are normal in most cases. Fewer than 10 per cent of patients with cerebral malaria have evidence of disseminated intravascular coagulation. However, antithrombin III concentrations are often moderately reduced and have prognostic significance. Total and direct (unconjugated) plasma bilirubin concentrations are usually increased, consistent with haemolysis, but in some patients with very high total bilirubin concentrations there is a predominance of conjugated bilirubin, indicating hepatocyte dysfunction. Some patients have cholestasis. Serum albumin concentrations are usually reduced, often grossly. Serum aminotransferases, 5'-nucleotidase, and especially lactic dehydrogenase are moderately elevated, but not into the range seen in viral hepatitis. Hyponatraemia is the most common electrolyte disturbance. Mild hypocalcaemia (after correction for hypoalbuminaemia) and hypophosphataemia have been described, especially when the patient has been given blood or a glucose infusion. Biochemical evidence of generalized rhabdomyolysis (elevated serum creatine kinase concentration, myoglobinaemia, and myoglobinuria) has been found in some patients. In about one-third of patients with cerebral malaria, the blood urea concentration is increased above 80 mg/dl (13 mmol/l) and serum creatinine above 2 mg/dl (176 μmol/l). Lactic acidosis occurs in severely ill patients, especially those with hypoglycaemia and renal failure. It may be suspected if there is a wide 'anion gap'. Blood glucose must be checked frequently, especially in children, pregnant women, and severely ill patients, even if the patient is not receiving quinine treatment and is fully conscious. A 'stix' method, with or without photometric quantification, is rapid and convenient. Microscopy and culture of cerebrospinal fluid is important in patients with cerebral malaria to exclude other treatable encephalopathies. In cerebral malaria the cerebrospinal fluid may contain up to 15 lymphocytes/μl and an increased protein concentration. Pleocytosis of up to 80 cells/μl, mainly leucocytes, may be found in patients who have had repeated generalized convulsions. The CSF glucose level will be low in hypoglycaemic patients and this result may be the first hint of hypoglycaemia. In view of the finding of cerebral compression and high opening pressures in many African children with cerebral malaria, some paediatricians prefer to delay lumbar puncture, while covering the possibility of bacterial meningoencephalitis with empirical antimicrobial treatment. Blood cultures should be performed in patients with a high white-cell count, shock, persistent fever, or an obvious focus of secondary bacterial infection. Gram-negative rod bacteria (*E. coli*, *Pseudomonas aeruginosa*, etc.) have been cultured from the blood of adult patients with 'algid' malaria. In Gambian children an association was found between malaria and nontyphoid salmonella septicaemia.

Urine should be examined by microscope and dipstix. Common abnormalities are proteinuria, microscopic haematuria, haemoglobinuria, and red-cell casts. The urine is literally black in patients with severe intravascular haemolysis. Urine specific gravity should be measured: the optical method is most convenient when urine output is small. Rapid measurement of plasma quinine or quinidine concentrations is possible in some hospitals. This is a valuable way of monitoring chemotherapy.

Treatment

Antimalarial drugs

Antimalarial drugs can be grouped as follows:

(1) arylaminoalcohols, comprising quinoline methanols such as the cinchona alkaloids, quinine and quinidine (extracted from the bark of the cinchona tree), mefloquine, halofantrine, and lumefantrine;

(2) 4-aminoquinolines, such as chloroquine and amodiaquine;

(3) folate-synthesis inhibitors, including type 1 antifolate drugs, which compete for dihydropteroate synthase (e.g. sulphones and sulphonamides), and type 2 antifolate drugs, which inhibit malarial dihydrofolate reductase (e.g. the biguanides, proguanil and chlorproguanil, and the diaminopyrimidine, pyrimethamine);

(4) 8-aminoquinolines, such as primaquine and tafenoquine (Etaquine, WR238,605);

(5) antibiotics, such as tetracycline, doxycycline, clindamycin, azithromycin, and fluoroquinolones;

(6) peroxides (sesquiterpene lactones)—artemisinin (qinghaosu) derivatives from the Chinese medicinal plant, *Artemisia annua*, and its semisynthetic analogues (artemether, arteether, artesunate, and artelinic acid); and

(7) naphthoquinones, such as atovaquone (BW566C80).

The stages of the lifecycle sensitive to some of the principal antimalarial drugs are shown in Fig. 12. Among blood schizonticides, artemisinin derivatives can prevent the development of rings or trophozoites, but quinine and mefloquine cannot stop development before the stage of mature trophozoites, and pyrimethamine–sulphadoxine combinations do not prevent the development of schizonts.

Mechanism of action of antimalarial drugs

The mode of action of the antifolate drugs is well understood and described above. Chloroquine is concentrated in the parasite's lysosomes, where haemoglobin is digested, and may act by inhibiting the haempolymerase that converts toxic haemin into insoluble haemozoin (malarial pigment). Alternatively, the drug may interfere with parasite feeding by disrupting its food vacuole. Antimalarial antibiotics are all inhibitors of ribosomal protein synthesis and probably act on the parasite's mitochondria. In the case of artemisinin derivatives, iron within the parasite probably catalyses the cleavage of the endoperoxide bridge leading to the generation of free radicals, which then form covalent bonds with parasite proteins (alkylation). Naphthoquinones, such as atovaquone, act on the electron-transport chain in malarial mitochondria through their structural similarity to coenzyme Q. No satisfactory explanation of the mode of action of the other antimalarial drugs is yet available.

The alarming spread of drug resistance has prompted great experimental effort to reveal the mechanism of resistance. The observation that chloroquine resistance could be reversed *in vitro* by high concentrations of drugs such as the calcium-channel blocker verapamil, which in other situations could reverse the multidrug resistance (**mdr**) phenotype acquired by some tumour cells, focused attention on a malarial homologue of the human *mdr* gene. Recent work suggests involvement of the *P. falciparum mdr1* gene early in the development of resistance, but segregation of resistance in the cloned progeny of a cross showed that the product of a second, uncharacterized gene product from chromosome 7 was also required.

Chloroquine

Despite the widespread resistance of *P. falciparum* to this drug, and the recent emergence of chloroquine-resistant *P. vivax* in New Guinea and adjacent areas of Indonesia, chloroquine is still the most widely used antimalarial drug. It remains the treatment of choice for vivax, ovale, and malariae infections, and for uncomplicated falciparum malaria acquired in the few areas where the parasite remains sensitive to this drug (Central America north-west of the Panama Canal, Haiti and the Dominican Republic, and parts of the Middle East). In the rest of the malaria-endemic region, the emergence of chloroquine resistance is having a devastating effect on malarial morbidity and mortality. For example, in Senegal, mortality form malaria in children under 5 years old, increased up to 11-fold between 1984 and 1995. After oral administration, chloroquine is rapidly and almost completely absorbed, peak plasma concentrations being reached in about 2 h. Absorption after intramuscular or subcutaneous injection is very rapid, which can produce dangerously high plasma concentrations unless small doses are given frequently. This probably explains the deaths of some children soon after they had received intramuscular injections of chloroquine. About half the absorbed dose is excreted unchanged by the kidney, the remainder being converted to active metabolites in the liver. Therapeutic blood concentrations persist for 6 to 10 days after a single dose and the terminal elimination half-time is 1 to 2 months. Plasma concentrations above about 250 ng/ml produce unpleasant symptoms such as dizziness, headache, diplopia, disturbed visual accommodation, dysphagia, nausea, and malaise. Chloroquine, even in small doses, may cause pruritus in dark-skinned races. Chloroquine may exacerbate epilepsy and photosensitive psoriasis. Cumulative, irreversible retinal toxicity from chloroquine has been reported after lifetime prophylactic doses of 50 to 100 g base (i.e. after 3–6 years of taking 300 mg of base per week), although this is most unusual. Chloroquine overdose is described in Chapter 8.1. Chloroquine is safe during pregnancy and lactation.

Amodiaquine, a 4-aminoquinoline that is structurally similar to chloroquine, retains activity against chloroquine-resistant strains of *P. falciparum* in some geographical areas. Unlike chloroquine, it is metabolized to a toxic quinoneimine that can produce a toxic hepatitis and potentially lethal agranulocytosis (which occurred in up to 1 in 2000 people taking amodiaquine prophylactically). Amodiaquine is still quite widely used, but, because of its risks and the limited therapeutic advantage over chloroquine, its use for prophylaxis and repeated treatment is now discouraged by the World Health Organization.

Quinine

The advent of chloroquine-resistant *P. falciparum* restored quinine to being the treatment of choice for falciparum malaria. Its antimalarial properties were discovered in Peru around 1600. Given by mouth it is rapidly and almost completely absorbed, producing peak plasma concentrations within 1 to 3 h. Some 20 per cent is excreted in the urine and the rest is metabolized in the liver. The elimination half-time in healthy people is approximately 11 h, and in patients with malaria approximately 16 h. Intravenous injection of quinine is dangerous as high plasma concentrations may result during the distribution phase, causing fatal hypotension or arrhythmias. However, quinine can be given safely if it is diluted and infused intravenously over 2 to 4 h. When intravenous infusion is not possible, but parenteral treatment is needed, quinine may be given by intramuscular

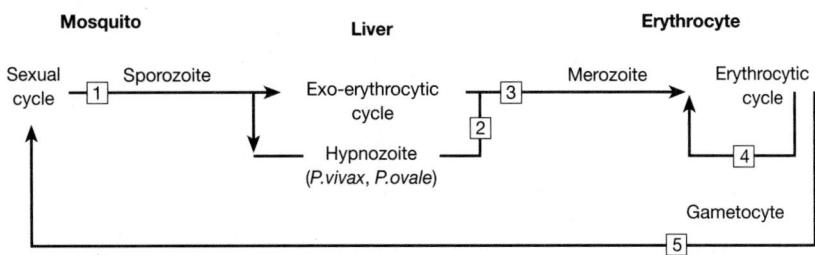

Fig. 12 Stage specificity of antimalarial drugs. 1. Sporontocidal (e.g. proguanil, pyrimethamine, atovaquone); 2. hypnozoitocidal (e.g. primaquine WR238,605); 3. tissue schizontocidal (e.g. proguanil, pyrimethamine); 4. blood schizontocidal (e.g. chloroquine, quinine, artemisinin); 5. gametocytocidal (e.g. primaquine, tafenoquine; chloroquine for *P. vivax, P. malariae*, and *P. ovale*).

injection divided between the anterior part of the thighs. For intramuscular injection, the stock solution of quinine dihydrochloride (300 mg/ml) should be diluted to 60 mg/ml. It is well absorbed from this site and complications are rare provided that strict sterile precautions are observed. Because most deaths from severe falciparum malaria occur within the first 96 h of starting treatment, it is important to achieve parasiticidal plasma concentrations of quinine as quickly as possible. This can be accomplished safely by giving a loading dose of twice the maintenance dose. A loading dose of 20 mg of the salt per kg of body weight and an 8- to 12-hourly maintenance dose of 10 mg/kg have proved safe and effective in children and adults in many tropical countries. The initial dose of quinine should not be reduced in patients who are severely ill with renal or hepatic impairment, but in these cases the maintenance dose should be reduced to between 3 and 5 mg/kg if parenteral treatment is required for longer than 48 h. Little is known about the optimal and safe quinine dosage in elderly and obese patients outside malaria endemic areas.

The minimum inhibitory concentration of quinine for *P. falciparum* in SE Asia and other areas of the tropics has risen steadily. Longer courses of quinine and in combination with other drugs, such as Fansidar, tetracycline, or clindamycin, have been required for complete cure. Recently, cases of RII and RIII resistance (failure to clear or failure to reduce parasitaemia in the first 7 days of treatment) to quinine have been documented in Thailand and Vietnam. Quinine should not be withheld or stopped in patients who are pregnant or haemolysing. In the doses used to treat malaria it does not stimulate uterine contraction or cause fetal distress. Hypoglycaemia is the most important complication of quinine treatment (see above). Plasma quinine concentrations above 5 mg/l produce a characteristic group of symptoms—'cinchonism'—transient high-tone deafness, giddiness, tinnitus, nausea, vomiting, tremors, blurred vision, and malaise. Rarely, quinine may give rise to haemolysis, thrombocytopenia, disseminated intravascular coagulation, hypersensitivity reactions, vasculitis, and granulomatous hepatitis. Blindness, deafness, and central nervous depression are commonly observed in patients who have attempted suicide by taking overdoses of quinine. These features are rarely seen in patients being treated for malaria, even though their plasma quinine concentrations may exceed 20 mg/l. This discrepancy may be explained by the increased binding of quinine to α-1 acid glycoprotein (orosomucoid) and to other acute-phase reactive serum proteins in patients with malaria.

Quinidine, the dextrorotatory stereoisomer of quinine, is more effective against resistant strains of *P. falciparum* but is more cardiotoxic than quinine. Because of its use for treating cardiac arrhythmias, it is more generally available (as quinidine gluconate injection) than parenteral quinine in continental Europe and North America, and in the United States has replaced quinine for the parenteral treatment of malaria. It must be infused slowly while the electrocardiogram and blood pressure are monitored. Infusion should be slowed if the blood pressure falls, the plasma concentration exceeds 22 μmol/l (7 mg/ml), or if the Q–Tc interval increases by more than 25 per cent.

Mefloquine ('Lariam')

This synthetic drug is effective against some *P. falciparum* strains resistant to chloroquine, pyrimethamine–sulphonamide combinations, and quinine. It is too irritant to be given parenterally, but is well absorbed when given by mouth, reaching peak plasma concentrations in 6 to 24 h. The elimination half-time is 14 to 28 days. The drug can be given as a single dose but, to reduce the risk of vomiting and other gastrointestinal side-effects, the dose is best divided into two halves given 6 to 8 h apart. Gastrointestinal symptoms occur in 10 to 15 per cent of patients but are usually mild. Less frequent side-effects include nightmares and sleeping disturbances, dizziness, ataxia, sinus bradycardia, sinus arrhythmia, postural hypotension, and an 'acute brain syndrome' consisting of fatigue, asthenia, seizures, and psychosis. Mefloquine treatment should be avoided in pregnant women, especially during the first trimester, and pregnancy should be avoided within 3 months of stopping mefloquine. People taking β-blockers and those with a past history of epilepsy or psychiatric disease should also avoid the drug. Unfortunately, *in vitro* resistance to mefloquine and treatment failures have now been reported in SE Asia, Africa, and South America.

Halofantrine

This synthetic antimalarial compound is active against multiresistant, including mefloquine-resistant, *P. falciparum*, but is no longer recommended because of its cardiotoxicity.

Artemisinin

Artemisinin or qinghaosu (pronounced 'ching-how-soo') is the active principle of the Chinese medicinal herb *Artemisia annua*—family Compositae (sweet wormwood), which has been used as a treatment for fevers in China for more than 1000 years. The active principle was isolated in China during 1971 to 1972. It is a sesquiterpene lactone with an endoperoxide (trioxane) active group. It destroys young trophozoites as well as other blood stages of *P. falciparum,* including chloroquine-resistant strains, and clears parasitaemia more rapidly than any other antimalarial drug. Dihydroartemisinin, the active metabolite, is cleared rapidly. In severe falciparum malaria, most experience has been gained with intramuscular artemether, given in a loading dose of 3.2 mg/kg on the first day (as a single dose or divided, 12 h apart) followed by 1.6 mg/kg per day until the patient is able to take an oral drug such as mefloquine. The efficacy and safety of artemether was compared with quinine in a series of large randomized trials in children and adults with severe falciparum malaria in Africa, Asia, and Papua New Guinea. A meta-analysis of trials involving nearly 2000 patients confirmed it to be as effective as quinine, judged by case fatality and incidence of neurological sequelae, but it cleared parasitaemia more rapidly and was significantly superior in preventing 'adverse outcome' (either death or neurological sequelae). Artesunate, although inherently unstable in aqueous solution, can be made up with 5 per cent bicarbonate just before injection and given by intravenous or intramuscular injection (2 mg/kg on the first day followed by 1 mg/kg until the patient can take oral treatment). An extra dose of 1 mg/kg can be given 4 to 6 h after the initial loading dose in hyperparasitaemic patients. Suppository formulations of artemisinin have proved effective in severe falciparum malaria and should prove particularly valuable in treating children at peripheral levels of the health service. A combination of artemether and lumefantrine (Riamet, Co-artemether) is being marketed for the oral treatment of multiresistant falciparum malaria.

The severe neurotoxicity reported in animals given large doses of artemisinin has not been detected in any of the tens of thousands of human patients treated with these compounds.

Primaquine

This is the only readily available drug effective against exoerythrocytic (hepatic) forms of *P. vivax* and *P. ovale*, and is essential for the radical cure of these infections. It is also gametocytocidal for all species of malaria. Mass treatment of patients with *P. falciparum* infection could eliminate the sexual cycle in mosquitoes by sterilizing gametocytes. Its elimination half-time is 7 h. The principal drawback of primaquine is that it causes haemolysis in patients with congenital deficiencies of erythrocyte enzymes, notably G6PD. However, severe intravascular haemolysis is unusual even in G6PD-deficient patients, except in certain areas of the world such as the Mediterranean (for example, Sardinia) and Sri Lanka. Primaquine can cross the placenta and cause severe haemolysis in a G6PD-deficient fetus, most commonly a boy. It is also excreted in breast milk. It should not be used during pregnancy or lactation in areas where G6PD deficiency is prevalent. Primaquine, like sulphonamides and sulphones (for instance, dapsone) can produce severe haemolysis and methaemoglobinaemia in patients with congenital deficiency of **NADH** (the reduced form of nicotinamide adenine dinucleotide) methaemoglobin reductase. The patient quickly develops dusky cyanosis, noticed first in the nail beds. In patients with G6PD deficiency, weekly dosage with 45 mg of primaquine is better tolerated than the usual daily dose of 15 mg. In the Solomon Islands, Indonesia, Thailand, and Papua New Guinea a total dose of 6.0 mg/kg (twice the usual dose) or even more may be needed to eliminate the primaquine-resistant Chesson-type strain of *P. vivax*. This is usually given as 15 mg base/day for 28 days. Tafenoquine (Etaquine), a new 8-aminoquinoline, is now in clinical trials. As a hypnozoiticide, it is over 10 times more active than primaquine, and is also a potent schizontocide.

Pyrimethamine–sulphonamide combinations (Fansidar, Metakelfin, etc.)

These synergistic combinations were once valuable in the treatment of chloroquine-resistant falciparum infections worldwide. A single adult dose of three Fansidar tablets (75 mg pyrimethamine, 1500 mg sulfadoxine) proved safe and effective, and is useful as an emergency standby for travellers out of the reach of medical facilities and as an adjunct to quinine in the treatment of *P. falciparum* infections in areas of increasing quinine resistance. However, in most of SE Asia, China, Oceanea, Latin America, and Africa already troubled by chloroquine resistance, resistance to pyrimethamine–sulphonamide combinations is also spreading. It results from mutations at residues 108, 51, 59, 16, and 164 of the parasite's dihydrofolate reductase gene. An intramuscular formulation has proved effective against *P. falciparum* in southern Africa. Pyrimethamine is a folate inhibitor and so may cause folic acid deficiency in pregnant women and others unless folinic acid supplements are given. The sulphonamide components of these combinations are potentially dangerous. In patients who are hypersensitive to sulphonamide they may cause systemic vasculitis, the Stevens–Johnson syndrome, or toxic epidermal necrolysis. In the United States the risk of fatal reactions has been calculated as 1 in 18 000–26 000 prophylactic courses. Aplastic anaemia and agranulocytosis can also occur. Both pyrimethamine and sulphonamide cross the placenta and are excreted in milk. In the fetus and neonate, sulphonamides can displace bilirubin from plasma protein-binding sites, thus causing kernicterus. For these reasons, pyrimethamine–sulphonamide combinations are not recommended for treatment during pregnancy or lactation unless no alternative drug is available, nor for prophylaxis at all.

P. vivax and *P. malariae* parasitaemias are generally cleared by all the drugs effective against *P. falciparum*. However, in some scattered areas, pyrimethamine–sulphonamide combinations may not be effective because of pyrimethamine resistance.

Chlorproguanil–dapsone ('lapdap')

This combination has been developed as an alternative to pyrimethamine–sulphonamide combinations (**PSD**) to replace chloroquine for the treatment of uncomplicated falciparum malaria in Africa. It has proved more effective than PSD in treating parasites with 108, 51, and 59 mutations, but should probably be further combined with an artemisinin to extend its useful therapeutic life.

Hydroxynaphthoquinones

Atovaquone (BW566C80) is marketed in combination with proguanil as 'Malarone' for the treatment and prevention of multiresistant *P. falciparum*. It inhibits the parasite's mitochondrial respiration by binding to the cytochrome bc, complex. The drug is poorly and variably absorbed, but bioavailability is greatly enhanced by a fatty meal. Its elimination half-life is between 50 and 70 h.

Antibiotics

Tetracycline, clindamycin, azithromycin, quinolones, and sulphonamides such as co-trimoxazole, have some antimalarial activity. Generally, they kill parasites too slowly to be used alone. In an emergency, in the absence of quinoline antimalarials, they could be used to treat malaria.

Practical antimalarial chemotherapy

Prescribing quinoline antimalarial drugs

The various salts of quinoline compounds contain greatly differing amounts of base. If the prescription fails to specify salt or base, or which particular salt is intended, serious problems can arise. Where possible, the dose of base should be prescribed. This is generally accepted for chloro-

Table 7 Salt and base equivalents of common quinoline antimalarial drugs

Antimalarial drug	Salt (mg)	Base (mg)
Amodiaquine sulphate	130	100
Chloroquine hydrochloride	123	100
Chloroquine phosphate	161	100
Chloroquine sulphate	136	100
Halofantrine hydrochloride	107	100
Mefloquine hydrochloride	110	100
Primaquine phosphate	18	10
Quinidine gluconate	145	100
Quinidine sulphate	108	100
Quinine bisulphate	137	100
Quinine dihydrochloride	105	100
Quinine hydrochloride	105	100
Quinine sulphate	103	100

quine, amodiaquine, mefloquine, and primaquine, but, in the case of quinine and quinidine, weights of salts are usually quoted. Conversions are given in Table 7.

Treatment of uncomplicated malaria (Table 8)

Chloroquine is the treatment of choice for *P. vivax*, *P. ovale*, *P. malariae*, and uncomplicated *P. falciparum* malarias in those geographical areas where this drug can still achieve a satisfactory clinical response. Chloroquine-resistant *P. vivax* has so far been reported only from New Guinea and adjacent islands of Indonesia. It should be treated by increasing the dose of oral chloroquine. Chloroquine resistant *P. falciparum* is very widespread.

Chloroquine is cheap, safe, and in the usual 3-day course well tolerated. However, despite the clinical improvement following chloroquine treatment, attributable to its anti-inflammatory action, its failure to eliminate parasitaemia and the subsequent recrudescences may eventually lead to the development of profound anaemia. Patients with *P. vivax* or *P. ovale* malarias who will not subsequently reside in malarious areas should be given a course of primaquine (or the new 8-aminoquinoline drug, tafenoquine) to destroy persistent exoerythrocytic stages (see Table 8) unless they are G6PD-deficient.

For the treatment of *P. falciparum* malaria in most parts of the malaria endemic area, chloroquine has been replaced by pyrimethamine–sulphonamide combinations such as 'Fansidar' and 'Metakelfin'. These have the great advantage of being single-dose treatments that are usually well tolerated. In Africa, chlorproguanil–lapudrine ('lapdap') is more effective than PSD against parasites with dihydrofolate reductase gene mutations. Quinine is an effective replacement for chloroquine in most areas where multidrug-resistant strains of *P. falciparum* are prevalent. However, it has the disadvantage of producing unpleasant symptoms. In some countries a short course (3–5 days) of quinine followed by a single dose of pyrimethamine–sulphonamide is still effective. Quinine has also been combined with antibiotics such as tetracycline and clindamycin to improve its efficacy. Mefloquine, given as a single dose, or in divided doses 6 to 8 h apart to reduce the risk of vomiting, was initially highly effective against multiresistant strains of falciparum malaria throughout the world. However, in some areas, notably in the border regions of Thailand, mefloquine resistance has developed rapidly and this drug is now used in combination with artemisinin derivatives such as artesunate. The newer combination drugs 'Malarone' and 'Co-artemether' are effective against multiresistant *P. falciparum*

Patients with uncomplicated malaria can usually be given antimalarial drugs by mouth. However, feverish patients may vomit the tablets. The risk of vomiting can be reduced if the patient lies down quietly for a while after taking an antipyretic such as paracetamol. The initial dose of antimalarial drug may have to be given by injection for those who vomit persistently.

Treatment of severe falciparum malaria (Table 9)

Appropriate chemotherapy should be started as soon as possible as there is a highly significant relationship between delay in chemotherapy and mor-

tality. **In sick and deteriorating patients, a therapeutic trial is indicated even if initial smears have proved negative.** Whenever possible, the dosage should be calculated according to the patient's body weight. The parenteral administration of drugs is the rule for patients with severe and complicated falciparum malaria and in any patient who vomits and is unable to retain swallowed tablets. In the case of cinchona alkaloids, this is most safely and

Table 8 Antimalarial chemotherapy in adults or children with uncomplicated malaria who can swallow tablets

Chloroquine-resistant *P. falciparum* or where origin of species unknown		Chloroquine-sensitive *P. falciparum*[†] or *P. vivax*, *P. ovale*, *P. malariae*, or monkey malarias	
1 *Mefloquine*		1 *Chloroquine*[×]	
Adults:	15–25 mg **base**/kg[+] given as 2 doses 6–8 h apart	Adults:	600 mg **base** on the 1st and 2nd days; 300 mg on the 3rd day
Children:	25 mg **base**/kg given as 2 doses 6–8 h apart	Children:	~10 mg base/kg on the 1st and 2nd days; 5 mg base/kg on the 3rd day
OR			
2 *Proguanil with atovaquone* ('Malarone')		For radical cure of vivax/ovale add:	
Adults:	4 tablets (each containing 100 mg proguanil and 250 mg atovaquone) once daily for 3 days	2 *Primaquine*	
		Adults:	(except pregnant and lactating women as well as G6PD-deficient patients): 15 mg **base**/day on days 4–17; *or* 45 mg/week for 8 weeks[*]
Children:	11–20 kg, one tablet; 21–30 kg, 2 tablets; 31–40 kg, 3 tablets; **all** once daily for 3 days		
OR			
3 *Artemether with lumefantrine* ('Riamet', 'Coartemether')		Children:	0.25 mg/kg per day on days 4–17; *or* 0.75 mg/kg per week for 8 weeks[*]
Adults:	4 tablets (each containing 20 mg artemether and 120 mg lumefantrine) twice daily for 3 days		
Children:	<15 kg body weight, 1 tablet; 15–<25 kg, 2 tablets; 25–<35 kg, 3 tablets; **all** twice daily for 3 days		
OR			
4 *Quinine*			
Adults:	600 mg **salt**, 3 times daily for 7 days[++]		
Children:	Approx. 10 mg **salt**/kg, 3 times daily for 7 days		
OR			
5 *Chlorproguanil with dapsone* ('LAPDAP')			
Adults and children	Chlorproguanil 2.0 mg/kg + dapsone 2.5 mg/kg once daily for 3 days		
OR			
6 *Sulphonamide–pyrimethamine*[**] Pyrimethamine (25 mg) plus sulfadoxine (500 mg per tablet) or sulfalene(500 mg)			
Adults:	3 tablets as a single dose		
Children:	<5 years, ½ tablet; <9 years, 1 tablet; <15 years, 2 tablets; **all** as single doses		

For **salt/base** equivalents see Table 7.

[×] For chloroquine-resistant *P. vivax*, repeat the course.

[+] Depending on geographical area and presumed immunity.

[++] In areas where 7 days of quinine is not curative (e.g. Thailand), **add** tetracycline 250 mg four times each day or doxycycline 100 mg daily for 7 days, except for children under 8 years and pregnant women, **or add** clindamycin 5 mg/kg three times daily for 7 days

[*] For Chesson-type strains (SE Asia, W Pacific) use double the dose or double the duration up to a total dose of 6 mg **base**/kg in daily doses of 15–22.5 mg for adults.

[**] Pyrimethamine+sulfadoxine ('Fansidar'); pyrimethamine+sulfalene ('Metakelfin'). Contraindicated if patient has known sulphonamide hypersensitivity

[†] Currently restricted to Haiti, Dominican Republic, Central America, and parts of the Middle East.

Table 9 Antimalarial chemotherapy for adults or children with severe malaria or for those who cannot swallow tablets

Chloroquine-resistant *P. falciparum* or original unknown		Chloroquine-sensitive *P. falciparum*[*] or *P. vivax*, *P. ovale, P. malariae*, or monkey malarias	
1	*Quinine* Adults: 20 mg **salt**/kg (loading dose)++ diluted in 10 ml/kg isotonic fluid by IV infusion over 4 h, followed 8 h after the start of the loading dose with 10 mg **salt**/kg over 4 h, every 8 h until patients can swallow+++	1	*Chloroquine*[×] 25 mg **base**/kg diluted in isotonic fluid by continuous IV infusion over 30 h (*or* 5 mg **base**/kg over 6 h every 6 h)
	Children: 20 mg **salt**/kg (loading dose)++ diluted in 10 ml/kg isotonic fluid by IV infusion over 2 h, followed 12 h after the start of the loading dose with 10 mg **salt**/kg over 2 h, every 12 h until patients can swallow+++	OR 2	*Quinine* (see left-hand column above)
	The 7-day course should be completed with quinine tablets, approximately 10 mg **salt**/kg (maximum 600 mg) every 8–12 h[××]		
OR 2	*Quinine* (in intensive care unit) 7 mg **salt**/kg (loading dose)++ IV by infusion pump over 30 min, followed immediately with 10 mg **salt**/kg (maintenance dose) diluted in 10 ml/kg isotonic fluid by IV infusion over 4 h, repeated every 8 h until patient can swallow, etc.[××+++]		
OR 3	*Artesunate*[×××] 2.4 mg/kg (loading dose) intravenously on the first day, followed by 1.2 mg/kg daily for a minimum of 3 days until the patient can take oral therapy or another effective antimalarial		
OR 4	*Artemether* 3.2 mg/kg (loading dose) IM on the first day, followed by 1.6 mg/kg daily for a minimum of 3 days until the patient can take oral treatment or another effective antimalarial. In children, the use of a 1 ml tuberculin syringe is advisable since the injection volumes will be small		
OR 5	*Quinidine* (in intensive care unit) 15 mg **base**/kg (loading dose)++ IV by infusion over 4 h, followed 8 h after the start of the loading dose with 7.5 mg **base**/kg over 4 h every 8 h, until the patient can swallow,+++ then quinine tablets to complete 7 days of treatment[××] *or* Give a single dose of 25 mg/kg sulfadoxine and 1.25 mg/kg pyrimethamine		
If it is not possible to give drugs by intravenous infusion 1 *Quinine* 20 mg **salt**/kg diluted to 60–100 mg/ml (loading dose)++ IM into anterolateral thigh (half given into each leg), followed by 10 mg **salt**/kg, every 8 h until patient can swallow etc.[××+++]		1	*Chloroquine*[×] Total dose 25 mg **base**/kg given as either: (a) IM or SC 2.5 mg **base**/kg, every 4 h; (b) IM or SC 3.5 mg **base**/kg, every 6 h

Table 9 continued

		OR	
		2	*Quinine* IM (see above left-hand column)

If it is not possible to give drugs by injection (IM/IV) or infusion			
1	*Suppositories of artemisinin*‡ 40 mg/kg loading dose as suppositories intrarectally, followed by 20 mg/kg at 4, 24, 48, and 72 h followed by an oral antimalarial drug°	1	*Chloroquine* 10 mg **base**/kg of body weight as tablets/syrup by mouth or nasogastric tube, *then* refer the patient to a higher level of healthcare for parenteral treatment *or* Continue 5 mg **base**/kg 5, 24, and 48 h later°
	Suppositories of artesunate‡ One 200 mg suppository intrarectally at 0, 4, 8, 12, 24, 36, 48, and 60 h followed by an oral antimalarial drug‡‡°		

OR		OR	
2	*Tablets of artemisinin* (artesunate, artemether, artemether with lumefantrine), quinine, mefloquine or other appropriate antimalarials˙	2	*Suppositories of artemisinin or artesunate, oral quinine, mefloquine or sulfadoxine/pyrimethamine* (see left-hand column)˙

For **salt/base** equivalents see Table 7.

˙ Currently restricted to Haiti, Dominican Republic, Central America, and parts of the Middle East.

ˣ Parenteral chloroquine should be used with great caution in young children.

⁺⁺ Loading dose must not be used if the patient has received quinine, quinidine, or halofantrine within preceding 24 h.

⁺⁺⁺ In patients requiring more than 48 h of parenteral therapy reduce the dose to 5.7 mg **salt**/kg every 8 h or 3.75 mg quinidine **base**/kg every 8 h.

ˣˣ In areas where 7 days of quinine is not curative (e.g. Thailand) **add** tetracycline 250 mg four times each day or doxycycline 100 mg daily for 7 days except for children under 8 years and pregnant women, **or add** clindamycin 5 mg/kg three times daily for 7 days.

ˣˣˣ Artesunic acid 60 mg is dissolved in 0.6 ml of 5 per cent sodium bicarbonate diluted to 3–5 ml with 5 per cent (w/v) dextrose and given immediately by intravenous ('push') bolus injection.

˙ Transfer the patient to hospital as soon as possible after initiating chemotherapy.

‡ Artemisinin and artesunate suppositories are registered for use in a few countries. If suppository formulations are not available, tablets of artemisinins should be given orally if possible, or crushed and given by nasogastric tube.

‡‡ In Vietnam; 4 mg/kg of artesunate in suppository form (China) intrarectally as a loading dose, followed by 2 mg/kg at 4, 12, 48, and 72 h followed by an oral antimalarial drug, proved as effective as artemisinin suppositories.

IV, intravenous; IM, intramuscular; SC, subcutaneous.

effectively achieved by infusing the drug, diluted in isotonic fluid, intravenously over a period of 2 to 4 h.

The therapeutic response must be carefully monitored by frequent clinical assessments, measurement of temperature, pulse, and blood pressure, and examination of blood films. Patients should be switched to oral treatment as soon as they are able to swallow and retain tablets. They must be watched carefully for signs of drug toxicity. In the case of cinchona alkaloids, the most common toxicity during antimalarial treatment is the development of hypoglycaemia. The blood sugar should, therefore, be checked frequently.

General management

Patients with severe malaria should be transferred to the highest level of care available, preferably the intensive care unit. They must be nursed in bed because of their postural hypotension and because of the risk of splenic rupture were they to fall. Body temperatures above 38.5 °C are associated with febrile convulsions, especially in children, and between 39.5 and 42 °C with coma and permanent neurological sequelae. In pregnant women, hyperpyrexia contributes to fetal distress. Temperature should therefore be controlled by fanning, tepid sponging, a cooling blanket, or antipyretic drugs such as paracetamol (15 mg/kg in tablets by mouth, or powder washed down a nasogastric tube, or as suppositories). As the slight prolongation of parasitaemia associated with the use of paracetamol (and possibly other methods for controlling fever) is clinically insignificant, this possible disadvantage and theoretical arguments against lowering the temperature are outweighed by the symptomatic benefits. Pyrazolones such as metamizole sodium (Dipyrone) are widely used in tropical countries but carry an unacceptable risk of inducing agranulocytosis.

Cerebral malaria

Convulsions, vomiting, and aspiration pneumonia are common, so patients should be nursed in the lateral position with a rigid oral airway or endotracheal tube in place. They should be turned at least once every 2 h to avoid bed sores. Vital signs, Glasgow coma score, and occurrence of convulsions should be recorded frequently. Convulsions can be controlled with diazepam given by slow intravenous injection (adults 10 mg, children 0.15 mg/kg) or intrarectally (0.5–1.0 mg/kg), or with paraldehyde drawn in a glass syringe and given by intramuscular injection (0.1 ml/kg). Anaphylactic use of phenobarbital was associated with increased case fatality in a placebo-controlled study in African children and is not recommended. Stomach contents should be aspirated through a nasogastric tube to reduce the risk of aspiration pneumonia. Elective endotracheal intubation is indicated if coma deepens and the airway is jeopardized. Deepening coma with signs of cerebral herniation is an indication for CT or magnetic resonance imaging, or a trial of treatment to lower intracranial pressure, such as an intravenous infusion of mannitol (1.0–1.5 g/kg of a 10–20 per cent solution over 30 min) or mechanical hyperventilation to reduce the arterial $P\text{CO}_2$ to below 4.0 kPa (30 mmHg).

A number of potentially harmful remedies of unproven value have been recommended for the treatment of cerebral malaria. Two double-blind trials of dexamethasone (2 mg/kg and 11 mg/kg intravenously over 48 h) in adults and children in Thailand and Indonesia showed no reduction in mortality but prolongation of coma and an increased incidence of infection and gastrointestinal bleeding. Low molecular-weight dextrans, osmotic agents, heparin, adrenaline (epinephrine), ciclosporin A, prostacyclin, and pentoxifylline (oxpentifylline), malarial hyperimmune globulin, and anti-TNF-α monoclonal antibodies have proved ineffective in the treatment of cerebral malaria. Most of these interventions were associated with serious side-effects.

Anaemia

Indications for transfusion—preferably with fresh, compatible whole blood or packed cells—include a low (less than 20 per cent or rapidly falling) haematocrit, severe bleeding or predicted blood loss (for example, imminent parturition or surgery), hyperparasitaemia, and failure to respond to conservative treatment with oxygen and plasma expanders. When the screening of transfused blood is inadequate and infections such as human immunodeficiency virus (**HIV**), human T-cell leukaemia virus-1 (**HTLV-1**), and hepatitis viruses are prevalent in the community, the criteria for blood transfusion must be even more rigorous. Exchange transfusion is a safe way of correcting the anaemia without precipitating pulmonary oedema in those who are fluid-overloaded or chronically and severely anaemic. The volume of transfused blood must be included in the fluid-balance chart. Diuretics such as furosemide (frusemide) can be given intravenously in a dose of 1 to 2 mg/kg body weight to promote diuresis during the transfusion, and in all cases transfusion must be cautious with frequent observations of the jugular or central venous pressure and auscultation for pulmonary crepitations. Survival of compatible donor red cells is greatly reduced during the acute and convalescent phases of falciparum malaria.

Disturbances of fluid and electrolyte balance

Fluid and electrolyte requirements must be assessed individually in patients with malaria. Circulatory overload with intravenous fluids or blood transfusion may precipitate fatal pulmonary oedema, but untreated hypovolaemia may lead to fatal shock, lactic acidosis, and renal failure. Hypovolaemia may result from salt and water depletion through fever, diarrhoea, vomiting, insensible losses, and poor intake. The state of hydration is assessed clinically from the skin turgor, peripheral circulation, postural change in blood pressure, peripheral venous filling, and jugular or central venous pressure. The history of recent urine output and measurement of urine volume and specific gravity may be useful. Adult patients with severe falciparum malaria usually require between 1000 and 3000 ml of intravenous fluid during the first 24 h of hospital admission. Fluid replacement should be controlled by observations of jugular, central venous, or pulmonary artery wedge pressures. Hyponatraemia (plasma sodium concentration 120–130 mmol/l) usually requires no treatment, but these patients should be cautiously rehydrated with isotonic saline if they are clinically dehydrated, have low central venous pressures, a high urinary specific gravity, and a low urine sodium concentration (below 25 mmol/l).

Renal failure

Patients with falling urine output and elevated blood urea nitrogen and serum creatinine concentrations can be treated conservatively at first, but established acute renal failure must be treated with haemofiltration or dialysis. Hypovolaemia is corrected by the cautious infusion of isotonic saline until the central venous pressure is in the range +5 to +15 cmH$_2$O. If urine output remains low after rehydration, increasing doses of slowly infused intravenous furosemide (frusemide) (up to a total dose of 1 g) and finally an intravenous infusion of dopamine (2.5–5 µg/kg per min) can be tried. If these measures fail to achieve a sustained increase in urine output, a strict fluid balance should be enforced with particular emphasis on fluid restriction. Indications for haemoperfusion/dialysis include a rapid increase in serum creatinine level, hyperkalaemia, fluid overload, metabolic acidosis, and clinical manifestations of uraemia (diarrhoea and vomiting, encephalopathy, gastrointestinal bleeding, and pericarditis). Haemofiltration is the most effective technique in malaria but haemodialysis or peritoneal dialysis are also effective. The initial doses of antimalarial drug should not be reduced in patients with renal failure but, after 48 h of parenteral treatment, the maintenance dose should be reduced by one-third to one-half.

Metabolic acidosis

This is usually attributable to lactic acidosis and is an important life-threatening complication, especially in anaemic children. It should be treated by improving perfusion and oxygenation by blood transfusion and correcting hypovolaemia, clearing the airway, increasing the inspired oxygen concentration, and by treating septicaemia, a frequently associated complication.

Pulmonary oedema

This must be prevented by propping the patient up at an angle of 45 degrees and controlling fluid intake so that the jugular or central venous pressure is kept below +5 cmH$_2$O. Those who develop pulmonary oedema should be propped upright and given oxygen to breathe. In a well-equipped intensive care unit, the judicious use of vasodilator drugs can be controlled by monitoring haemodynamic variables, fluid overload can be corrected by haemoperfusion, and oxygenation can be improved by mechanical ventilation with positive end-expiratory pressure.

Hypotension and 'shock' ('algid malaria')

This should be treated as for bacteraemic shock. The circulatory problems should be corrected with blood transfusion (for example, in anaemic children with respiratory distress and acidosis), plasma expanders, dopamine, and broad-spectrum antimicrobial treatment (such as gentamicin with ceftazidime or cefuroxime plus metronidazole) should be started immediately, bearing in mind that likely routes of infection include the urinary tract, lungs, and the gut. Other causes of shock in patients with malaria include dehydration, blood loss (for instance, following splenic rupture), and pulmonary oedema.

Hypoglycaemia

This may be asymptomatic, especially in pregnancy, and its clinical manifestations may be confused with those of malaria. Blood sugar must be checked every few hours, especially in patients being treated with cinchona alkaloids. Hypoglycaemia may arise despite continuous intravenous infusions of 5 or even 10 per cent dextrose. A therapeutic trial of dextrose (1 ml/kg by intravenous bolus injection) should be given if hypoglycaemia is proved or suspected. This should be followed by a continuous infusion of 10 per cent dextrose. Glucose may be given by nasogastric tube to unconscious patients or by peritoneal dialysis in those undergoing this treatment for renal failure. Among agents that block insulin release, diazoxide was ineffective, but octreotide (Sandostatin), a synthetic somatostatin analogue, proved effective in some severe cases of quinine-induced hypoglycaemia.

Hyperparasitaemia and exchange blood transfusion

In non-immune patients, mortality increases with parasitaemia, exceeding 50 per cent with parasitaemias above 500 000/µl. Exchange transfusion reduces parasitaemia more rapidly than optimal chemotherapy alone, although this advantage will be less when artemisinins are used, and could have the additional benefit of removing harmful metabolites, toxins, cytokines and other mediators, and restoring normal red-cell mass, platelets, clotting, factors, albumin, etc. Potential dangers of the procedure include electrolyte disturbances (for example, hypocalcaemia), cardiovascular complications, and the introduction of infectious agents into the blood and through infection of intravascular lines. The use of exchange transfusion, haemopheresis, and plasmapheresis has been reported in more than 100 patients, the vast majority of whom survived. There was undoubtedly some reporting bias. Some patients showed clinical improvement, such as recovery of consciousness, and restoration of urine flow, soon after the procedure. A meta-analysis discovered no higher survival rate compared to chemotherapy alone and there have been a few recent reports of adult respiratory distress syndrome developing during the procedure. The efficacy of exchange transfusion is never likely to be put to the test of a randomized comparative study, but, where facilities allow and screening of donor blood is adequate, the procedure should be considered in non-immune patients who are severely ill, who have deteriorated on conventional treatment, and who have parasitaemias in excess of 10 per cent. The introduction of antimalarial agents, such as artemisinins, which clear parasitaemia very rapidly, may obviate the need for exchange transfusion.

Splenic rupture

Acute abdominal pain and tenderness with left shoulder-tip pain and shock in patients with vivax and falciparum malaria should suggest the possibility of splenic rupture, especially if there is a history of abdominal trauma. Free blood in the peritoneal cavity and a torn splenic capsule can be detected by ultrasound or CT and confirmed by needle aspiration of the peritoneal cavity, laparoscopy, or laparotomy. Conservative management with blood transfusion and close observation in an intensive care unit is sometimes successful but access to surgical help is essential in case there is a sudden deterioration.

Disseminated intravascular coagulation

Patients with evidence of a coagulopathy should be given vitamin K (adult dose 10 mg by slow intravenous injection). Prothrombin complex concentrates, cryoprecipitates, platelet transfusions, and fresh-frozen plasma should be considered.

Management of the pregnant woman with malaria

Malaria must be diagnosed and treated rapidly in pregnant women. Unwarranted fears of abortifacient and fetus-damaging effects of antimalarial drugs have led to the delay or even withdrawal of treatment, but experience since the nineteenth century has confirmed the safety of quinine in pregnancy. Chloroquine has been used extensively without ill effect to mother or fetus. However, pyrimethamine–sulphonamides, tetracycline, primaquine, and aspirin (but not paracetamol) are contraindicated in late pregnancy and mefloquine should be avoided if possible. In pregnant women, the total apparent volume of distribution of quinine is reduced and the drug is eliminated more rapidly. Initial dosage is the same as in non-pregnant patients, but in severe cases requiring prolonged parenteral treatment, the dose, but not the frequency of administration, should be reduced. The main danger of quinine in pregnancy is its stimulation of insulin secretion with resulting hypoglycaemia (see above). Blood glucose must be checked at least once a day in pregnant women with malaria, whether or not they are receiving quinine. Maternal fever should be reduced as soon as possible. Induction of labour, caesarean section, or speeding up of the second stage of labour with forceps or vacuum extractor should be considered in patients with severe falciparum malaria. Fluid balance is particularly critical in these patients. If possible, the central venous pressure should be monitored. Exchange transfusion of 1000 to 1500 ml of blood in late pregnancy proved an effective way of managing severe anaemia with high-output cardiac failure in Nigeria. Circulating volume could be reduced and the risk of postpartum pulmonary oedema lessened by replacing exfused blood with a smaller volume of packed cells.

Prognosis

The mortality of acute vivax, ovale, and malariae malarias is negligible. Strictly defined cerebral malaria has a mortality of about 10 to 15 per cent when medical facilities are good, and may be less than 5 per cent in Western intensive care units. Antecedent factors that predispose to severe falciparum malaria include the lack of acquired immunity or lapsed immunity, splenectomy, pregnancy, and immunosuppression. There is a strong correlation between the density of parasitaemia and disease severity. Severe clinical manifestations, such as impaired consciousness, retinal haemorrhages,

renal failure, hypoglycaemia, haemoglobinuria, metabolic acidosis, and pulmonary oedema, carry a bad prognosis. The case fatality of pregnant women with cerebral malaria, especially primiparae in the third trimester, is approximately 10 times greater than in non-pregnant patients. The following laboratory findings carry a poor prognosis: peripheral schizontaemia, peripheral leucocytosis exceeding 12 000/μl, malarial pigment in >5 per cent of circulating neutrophils, high CSF lactate or low glucose, low plasma antithrombin III, serum creatinine exceeding 265 μmol/l, or a blood urea nitrogen of more than 21.4 mmol/l, haematocrit less than 20 per cent, blood glucose less than 2.2 mmol/l, and elevated serum enzyme concentrations (for example, aspartate and alanine aminotransferases, lactate dehydrogenase).

Chronic immunological complications of malaria

Quartan malarial nephrosis

In parts of East and West Africa, South America, India, South-East Asia, and Papua New Guinea, there is epidemiological evidence linking *P. malariae* infection to immune-complex glomerulonephritis, leading to nephrotic syndrome. Few of those exposed to repeated *P. malariae* infections develop nephrosis, suggesting that additional factors are involved. The histological changes, which are not entirely specific, are of a progressive focal and segmental glomerulosclerosis with fibrillary splitting or flaking of the capillary basement membrane, producing characteristic lacunae. Electron-dense deposits beneath the endothelium can be seen by electron microscopy. Immunofluorescence reveals glomerular deposits of immunoglobulins and C3, and *P. malariae* antigen, in about 25 per cent of cases. More than half the patients present by the age of 15 years with typical features of nephrotic syndrome. *P. malariae* is frequently found in blood smears and *P. malariae* antigen in renal biopsies in children but not in adults. The renal lesions may be perpetuated by autoimmune mechanisms. The pattern of immunofluorescent staining has some prognostic significance. Few patients respond to corticosteroids, but some are helped by azathioprine and cyclophosphamide, especially those whose renal biopsies show the coarse or mixed patterns of immunofluorescence. Antimalarial treatment is not effective. This condition could be prevented by antimalarial prophylaxis and has disappeared in countries such as Guyana during a period of malaria eradication.

Tropical splenomegaly syndrome (hyper-reactive malarial splenomegaly)

Transient splenomegaly is a feature of acute attacks of malaria in non-immune or partially immune patients, while progressive splenomegaly is seen in children resident in malarious areas during the process of their acquiring immunity to the infection. However, a separate entity has been described in Africa (especially Nigeria, Uganda, and Zambia), the Indian subcontinent (Bengal, Sri Lanka), South-East Asia (Vietnam, Thailand, and Indonesia), South America (Amazon region), Papua New Guinea, and the Middle East (Aden). The defining features are residence in a malarious area, chronic splenomegaly, elevated serum IgM and malarial antibody levels, hepatic sinusoidal lymphocytosis, and a clinical and immunological response to antimalarial prophylaxis. This condition is thought to result from an aberrant immunological response to repeated infection by any of the species of malaria parasite.

Pathophysiology

In Flores, Indonesia, *P. vivax* infection leads to the production of IgM lymphocytotoxic antibodies specific for the suppressor T lymphocytes, which normally regulate IgM production. The resulting disinhibition of B lymphocytes leads to their overproduction of IgM, forming macromolecular aggregates of IgM (cryoglobulins). The need to clear these aggregates stimulates the reticuloendothelial system and causes the progressive and eventually massive splenomegaly and hepatomegaly. The decrease in suppressor/cytotoxic (CD8) lymphocytes increases the helper:suppressor (CD4:CD8) ratio. Antimalarial chemoprophylaxis, by removing the antigenic stimulus provided by repeated malarial infections, allows the patient's immune system to return to normal. There are some differences between tropical splenomegaly syndrome in Africa, Flores, and Papua New Guinea. In Africa, but not in Flores or Papua New Guinea, there is a peripheral lymphocytosis resulting from an increase in B lymphocytes, and distinction from chronic lymphatic leukaemia may be difficult. In Ghana, clonal rearrangements of the JH region of the immunoglobulin gene were found in patients with tropical splenomegaly who failed to respond to proguanil chemoprophylaxis, suggesting that the syndrome may evolve into a malignant lymphoproliferative disorder. Some of these patients had features of splenic lymphoma with villous (hairy) lymphocytes. In Africa and Papua New Guinea, IgG levels were significantly increased, but not in Flores. In Flores only the titres of *P. vivax* IgM antibodies were higher in patients with the splenomegaly syndrome, but in Papua New Guinea titres of *P. falciparum*, *P. vivax*, and *P. malariae* were increased, and in Africa *P. falciparum* and *P. malariae* are the species involved. The familial tendency of the tropical splenomegaly syndrome in Africa and Papua New Guinea suggests a genetic factor.

Clinical features

In malaria endemic areas, patients with tropical splenomegaly syndrome are distinguishable by their progressive splenic enlargement persisting beyond childhood. The spleen may be enormous, filling the left iliac fossa, extending across the midline and anteriorly, producing a visible mass with an obvious notch. The liver is usually enlarged, especially its left lobe. Symptoms attributable to the spleen include a vague dragging sensation and occasional episodes of severe pain with peritonism, suggesting perisplenitis or splenic infarction. Anaemia may become severe enough to cause the features of high-output cardiac failure. Acute haemolytic episodes are described. These patients are vulnerable to infections, especially of the skin and respiratory system, and most deaths are attributable to overwhelming infection. Chronic hypersplenic neutropenia or failure to mobilize neutrophils in response to acute bacterial infections may be the cause. In Papua New Guinea, 57 per cent of those with massive splenomegaly were dead within 7 years.

Patients with splenic lymphoma with villous lymphocytes (Ghana) had splenic discomfort, anorexia, and hepatosplenomegaly, with infiltration of the bone marrow with villous lymphocytes.

Laboratory findings

Severe chronic anaemia is the result of destruction and pooling in the spleen and dilution in an increased plasma volume. Thrombocytopenia may also be caused by splenic sequestration; it rarely causes bleeding. There is neutropenia and, in African patients, peripheral lymphocytosis and lymphocytic infiltration of the bone marrow. Serum IgM is greatly elevated.

The essential histopathological feature is lymphocytosis of the hepatic sinusoids with Kupffer-cell hyperplasia. In some cases, round-cell infiltration of the portal tracts is associated with fibrosis, leading to portal hypertension. In the spleen there is dilatation of the sinusoids, hyperplasia of the phagocytic cells with evident erythrophagocytosis, and infiltration with lymphocytes and plasma cells. No histopathological explanation has been found for the episodes of acute splenic pain.

In patients with splenic lymphoma and villous lymphocytes, more than 30 per cent of circulating lymphocytes are villous. These cells can be distinguished from hairy-cell leukaemia by their lack of CD25, CD11c, and tartrate-resistant acid phosphatase markers.

Differential diagnosis

Tropical splenomegaly syndrome must be distinguished from other causes of chronic, painless, massive splenomegaly, including leukaemias, lymph-omas, myelofibrosis, thalassaemias, haemoglobinopathies, visceral leishmaniasis (by examination of bone marrow or splenic aspirates), and schistosomiasis (by liver biopsy, rectal snip, and stool examination). Lymphomas (especially chronic lymphatic leukaemia and follicular lymphoma—see above) and even leukaemias may develop in patients with tropical splenomegaly syndrome. Non-tropical idiopathic splenomegaly (normal serum IgM) and Felty's syndrome produce a similar histological picture in the liver. Many cases of splenomegaly in the tropics remain undiagnosed.

Treatment

Prolonged antimalarial chemoprophylaxis is the most important element of treatment. In Papua New Guinea, 70 per cent of the patients showed marked improvement after 12 months of chemotherapy. The choice of drug will depend on the local sensitivity of whichever species or group of species of malaria parasite are thought to be responsible for this syndrome (see Chemoprophylaxis below). The short- and long-term dangers of splenectomy rule out this procedure in the rural tropics. Similarly, splenic irradiation and antimitotic agents are dangerous and unnecessary. Folic acid may be needed. Diagnosis of patients with splenic lymphoma with villous lymphocytes (Ghana) is important as, in this condition, the risks of splenectomy are outweighed by the benefits.

Endemic Burkitt's lymphoma (see Chapter 7.10.3)

Endemic Burkitt's lymphoma, a tumour of the jaw, abdomen, and other areas that spreads to the bone marrow or meninges, is the most common type of childhood malignant disease in many parts of East and West Africa and Papua New Guinea. It has also been reported from Brazil, Malaysia, and the Middle East. Burkitt noticed that its distribution (by altitude, temperature, and rainfall) and even its seasonal incidence followed that of holoendemic falciparum malaria. Outside the malaria endemic area, Burkitt's lymphoma occurs sporadically. There is a suggestion that the B-cell line in Caucasian cases comes from lymphoid tissue, whereas in African cases it comes from the bone marrow. Epstein–Barr virus (**EBV**) produces a lifelong infection of B lymphocytes. In normal individuals this is controlled by specific, HLA-restricted, cytotoxic T cells, which recognize a virus-induced, lymphocyte-detected membrane antigen (**LYDMA**) on B cells. Immunosuppression, as in recipients of renal allografts, allows uncontrolled proliferation of the EBV-infected B-cell line, which may give rise to one of the three chromosomal translocations [t(8;14), t(2;8), t(8;22)] that activate the c-*myc* oncogene on chromosome 8 responsible for malignant transformation. Acute *P. falciparum* infection leads to a reduction in the numbers of suppressor T (CD8) lymphocytes and a decrease in the helper:suppressor (CD4:CD8) ratio, allowing proliferation and increased immunoglobulin secretion by EBV-infected B cells. No lymphocytotoxic antibody is found in acute plasma samples to explain the decrease in suppressor T cells. These tumours may grow so rapidly that massive local tissue destruction results in urate nephropathy and acute renal failure. Cyclophosphamide, vincristine, methotrexate, and prednisolone are used in chemotherapy, producing remissions in 80 to 90 per cent of patients and a long-term survival of 20 to 70 per cent. Breakdown of large tumours during the first week of chemotherapy may be so dramatic that the acute tumour lysis syndrome may be precipitated. This consists of metabolic acidosis, hyperuricaemia, hyperphosphaturia, hyperphosphataemia, hyperproteinaemia, and hyperkalaemia, which may result in fatal cardiac arrhythmia and acute uric-acid nephropathy with renal failure.

Malaria control

Malaria control relies on breaking the chain of transmission, often by attacks on the vector. As the insecticide resistance of mosquitoes and drug resistance of parasites increase, the environmental methods previously used to control anopheline breeding are being revived. The use at night of insecticide-treated bed nets (**ITNs**) has been a major innovation, combining personal protection with population protection (the mass effect) in some situations. No vaccine is yet available for operational use. There is currently a more balanced approach to malaria control than in the past, with emphasis on the early diagnosis and prompt treatment of infected people, selective and sustainable use of antivector measures, and epidemic control. The importance of malaria control has been acknowledged at the political level and available methods are being more energetically applied than for some decades, for example, in the WHO's 'Roll back malaria' programme.

Transmission control

Mosquitoes may be controlled in two ways: by removing, poisoning, or otherwise changing their larval habitats and so reducing their numbers; or by killing the adult mosquitoes by means of insecticides. These may be sprayed into the air for a transient effect or put on to the surfaces where mosquitoes rest to obtain a persistent or residual effect. Other methods may simply deter mosquitoes from biting people. Combination methods whereby insecticide is put on a mechanical barrier such as a bednet are currently much favoured and are discussed separately. For the future, there is also much interest in finding ways to transfect mosquitoes with genes to render them unable to transmit malaria, incorporating them into an infective agent that will spread through mosquito populations. Although killing the adult mosquitoes or their larvae will reduce mosquito numbers, and malaria transmission proportionately, residual insecticides have a greater effect on the survival of infected mosquitoes to the age at which they can pass on the infection, thereby reducing malaria transmission much more than might otherwise be expected.

Mosquito species are highly selective in their choice of larval habitat, and there are usually few major vector species in a given locality. The selective destruction of vector breeding sites (species sanitation), is a long-term method of mosquito control. Sites can be made unsuitable for vector breeding by drainage, changing the rate of water flow, and adding or removing shade, cutting emergent vegetation, and altering the margins of bodies of water. Near the sea, salinity changes may be relevant. For small reservoirs and irrigation canals, cyclical changes in water level by means of a large siphon may control larvae by alternately stranding and flushing. Intermittent drying out of irrigation channels may be of value. No generalizations are possible as, for example, water fluctuations that control vectors in the southern United States would increase breeding in sub-Saharan Africa. Enough local information is available to guide public-health engineering interventions in most endemic areas. As these and other measures against breeding reduce mosquito density, to which transmission is proportional, environmental control is most effective in areas of unstable malaria. Because costs of environmental measures are related to the area involved, and the resources and benefits are related to the human population, environmental control is most likely to be feasible in areas of high population density. In cities it needs to extend beyond the periurban fringe where the poor are concentrated. Control of mosquitoes such as *A. gambiae,* which utilize temporary pools as small as hoof prints, is very difficult by environmental means without ruthless discipline.

Where habitats cannot be drained or rendered structurally unsuitable, chemical larvicides may be used. Diesel oil, at 40 1/hectare of water surface with or without the addition of insecticides, will prevent the larvae breathing when it is spread on the water surface with the addition of a spreading agent. In the correct formulation, 1 kg/hectare of Paris Green is effective, but 2 to 20 kg/hectare of temephos (Abate) granules is a safer alternative, usually needing to be repeated weekly or fortnightly.

The use of residual insecticides applied to walls and other indoor surfaces gives a far more persistent effect, so that **DDT** (dichlorodiphenyltrichloethane) at 2 g/m² will remain toxic to endophilic anophelines for 6 months or more on a non-absorbent wall material, as may λ-cyhalothrin at a much lower dosage, while organophosphorus insecticides such as malathion, propoxur, and fenitrothion at the same dosage last about 3 months.

This approach is a community one, requiring coverage of all houses and shelters, as it relies on killing the mosquito after it has fed. Where the aim is individual or family protection, a knock-down insecticide used before evening in a screened house is more relevant.

Prudent behaviour can greatly reduce the risk of an infective mosquito bite, especially for the visitor to an endemic area. As anophelines bite mostly in the evening, remaining in a screened area from dusk, wearing long sleeves and leg coverings, and sleeping beneath a mosquito net are of real, if underestimated, benefit. Recently, the use of bednets impregnated with synthetic pyrethroids such as permethrin or λ-cyhalothrin has been found to give substantial malaria protection in endemic areas, reducing the number of clinical attacks even in areas of high transmission by 50 per cent, and where high coverage is achieved reducing the all-cause infant mortality rate by up to 27 per cent. The effect is due to a combination of reduced access of mosquitoes to people because of the net, a repellent and lethal effect of the insecticide on the mosquitoes trying to bite, and sometimes an effect on mosquito density so that even those outside the nets may get some protection. Nets are most effective when mosquito biting is concentrated late at night, and they can give good protection to babies in cots. The large-scale operational use of impregnated bednets in endemic areas is currently expanding, but as the net is a commodity rather than a health service, the best economic basis for sustainable high coverage by ITNs, and for their regular retreatments, are still being explored. ITNs appear to be one of the most hopeful means of control pending development of an operational vaccine.

As engineering methods are costly, though long lasting, and insecticides can be viewed as polluting the environment, other methods of mosquito control have been sought, with variable success. Genetic control of anophelines is not feasible at present; biological control is often a useful accessory method and usually relies on small fish, especially of such genera as *Gambusia* and *Lebistes* that preferentially feed on mosquito larvae. Species of fish that survive drying out of the habitat as eggs are now of interest. The micro-organism *Bacillus thuringiensis* is used in control, but it effectively functions as a biological insecticide because it produces a toxin.

Prevention of malaria in travellers

Advice to travellers

The prevention of malaria in travellers, particularly those usually resident in non-malarious areas but visiting endemic regions, is becoming increasingly difficult, owing to the spread of resistance to the commonly available antimalarial agents, which means that prevention cannot be completely successful. The four components of advice to travellers must therefore be: (1) to be aware of the risk; (2) to reduce exposure to being bitten by anopheline mosquitoes; (3) to take chemoprophylaxis where appropriate; (4) to seek immediate medical advice in the event of any fever or 'flu-like illness developing while in the area, or within 3 or more months of leaving it, and to consider malaria as a possibility regardless of the precautions taken. The first two of these are at least as important as the third in preventing mortality from malaria.

Preventive advice is subject to uncertainty. This is because unequivocal data on efficacy are often unavailable, published studies are conflicting, and the distribution of resistance to many prophylactics is not well mapped. The balance between the risk of malaria and the risk of side-effects involves value judgements on which experts differ. Moreover, prospective travellers consult several sources of advice, obtain different opinions, and compliance with any regimen thus falls. Published advice is usually by country (the World Health Organization annually produces the most useful list of risk areas) and is inevitably directed towards prophylaxis for the areas of greatest transmission. Consultation with someone who knows the country and the traveller's itinerary may well lead to good advice that differs and is more specific. Intelligent travellers need to be made aware of these issues but they also require clear advice that must include the general points discussed in the following paragraph.

For any traveller to an endemic area there is a risk of malaria. No prophylactic regimen will give total protection, but many will reduce the risk of a malaria attack substantially. In the event of a fever while travelling, or afterwards, malaria must be considered as a diagnosis. Strict compliance, even with a suboptimal prophylactic regimen, is more important than vacillation over finding the optimal one.

Prevention of mosquito bites

There are many additional ways to reduce the risk of malaria. Bednets impregnated with a pyrethroid insecticide (permethrin, deltamethrin, or λ-cyhalothrin) should be used, properly tucked in, and without tears or other holes through which mosquitoes might enter. A well-screened bedroom and other accommodation, combined with use of a knock-down insecticide when the doors are closed, will give substantial protection. Clothes that deter mosquito bites, repellent sprays and soaps (containing N, N-diethyl-m-toluamide (**DEET**) or permethrin), and avoiding exposure to bites in the evenings will also help.

Chemoprophylaxis

Chloroquine and/or proguanil

In malarious areas from which chloroquine-resistant P. falciparum is absent, mainly in Western Asia, North Africa, and Central America, chloroquine 300 mg (base), usually two tablets taken once a week, will give good protection. However, since it acts as a suppressive of the blood forms of Plasmodium it will not prevent late attacks of P. vivax or P. ovale. Proguanil, 100 mg daily, or 200 mg daily in areas of intense transmission, will act as a true causal prophylactic but is poorly protective against P. vivax in these doses. The extremely low incidence of adverse side-effects from proguanil makes it acceptable to long-term residents in endemic areas. Chloroquine is suitable for up to 6 years of use, but beyond this proguanil may be substituted. Recommendations are summarized in Tables 9 and 10.

By 1993, chloroquine-resistant P. falciparum had been reported from most malarious countries, and it constitutes a massive and increasing problem in sub-Saharan Africa and in SE Asia (where multiple drug resistance is common). Newer drugs and the more effective drug combinations for prophylaxis against chloroquine-resistant P. falciparum carry a significant risk of severe toxic side-effects that has to be balanced against the malaria risk, which varies greatly within countries, especially in Asia. Where the proportion of malaria resistant to chloroquine is low or the degree of resistance limited, the combination of chloroquine and proguanil ((b)1, Table 10) has the advantage of low toxicity and appears to be effective in many areas, including India and the rest of South Asia. These two drugs also have a good safety record in pregnant women and in young children. Long-term use of prophylactic chloroquine only carries a risk of retinopathy (probably very small) once the total cumulative dose exceeds 100 g of base (over 6 years at the standard prophylactic dose). Pruritis can be a problem in those with dark skins.

However, the combination of chloroquine and proguanil no longer provides adequate protection in sub-Saharan Africa where the malaria challenge in rural areas may exceed one infective bite per night and resistance is common, nor in SE Asia where there is a much lower transmission rate but a greater range of drugs to which P. falciparum is resistant.

Other prophylactic drugs

Other prophylactic regimens involve the use of mefloquine, doxycycline, and the combination of atovaquone and proguanil. Mefloquine was the most widely used of these three regimens and there are far more data on its use in malaria prevention than for the other two. Doxycycline was only recently licensed in the United Kingdom for the chemoprophylaxis of malaria, although it has been in use for the prevention of acne for many years; it has also been used as an antimalarial agent outside the license. There is much less experience with the combination of atovaquone and proguanil, though each of its component medicines has been used without high resistance and without high levels of side-effects. Trials of the efficacy of all three regimens demonstrate good protection against chloroquine-resistant falciparum malaria and the choice between them depends on the traveller, destination, and duration of travel. In the absence of specific resistance, mefloquine has a prophylactic efficacy of around 90 per cent against falciparum malaria, and doxycycline is almost as effective in trials in Asia. However, the data on the combination of atovaquone and proguanil come mainly from studies of semi-immune people and are less extensive. Although the atovaquone/proguanil regimen gives a similar level of efficacy to the other two prophylactics, more information is needed: its particular advantage lies in the low level of serious adverse effects observed in studies to date.

Mefloquine ('Lariam')

Mefloquine has a long half-life and on a weekly dosage schedule the blood level rises to a plateau from about 7 weeks. The majority of the side-effects, which are the main problem with its use, are associated with the initial three doses of mefloquine. The drug should therefore be started 2½ weeks prior to departure for a malarious place, so that if side-effects are troublesome an alternative may be used. Although it is usual to avoid taking mefloquine for longer than a year, American experience suggests that no additional problems arise after 2 to 3 years. The main serious early side-effects of mefloquine are neuropsychiatric, and include anxiety, depression, delusions, fits, and psychotic attacks. The frequency of these is disputed. Airline passenger surveys have shown a frequency of 1:10 000, but experienced doctors in the United Kingdom assert a much higher frequency and further data are needed. As its safety during early pregnancy is uncertain, it is not recommended for those in the first trimester of pregnancy or those at risk of pregnancy during the 3 months after the end of chemoprophylaxis There is some evidence from SE Asia of an increased stillbirth rate in those taking it in later pregnancy, but the risk from malaria is also great in pregnancy. It is contraindicated in people with a history of epilepsy or psychiatric disease. Sporadic cases of mefloquine resistance are already reported from Africa, and on the border between Thailand and Cambodia up to 40 per cent of cases of falciparum malaria are mefloquine-resistant.

Doxycycline

Doxycycline has been shown to give good protection against drug-resistant falciparum malaria in trials in Oceania, and it is being increasingly used, especially for those with adverse reactions to, or who are unwilling to take, mefloquine. It should not be used in children or pregnant women. The main side-effects are photosensitization, which occurs in up to 3 per cent of users making it less than ideal for beach holidays in the tropics, a tendency

Table 10 Recommended malaria prophylaxis (adult dose) in addition to general measures specified in text

(a)	Where chloroquine-resistant P. falciparum is absent:	
	1.	Chloroquine 300 mg **base** weekly (best for short-term visitors)
	2.	Proguanil 200 mg daily (best for long-term residents)
(b)	Where chloroquine-resistant P. falciparum is not widespread and is predominantly of low degree:	
	1.	Chloroquine 300 mg **base** weekly plus proguanil 200 mg daily
(c)	Where highly chloroquine-resistant P. falciparum occurs:[a]	
	1.	Mefloquine 250 mg weekly
	or	
	2.	Doxycycline 100 mg daily
	or	
	3.	Atovoquone/proguanil (Malarone) 1 tablet daily
	or	
	[4.	Chloroquine 300 mg **base** weekly plus proguanil 200 mg daily will give some, albeit limited, protection.]

[a] (c)1, (c)2 and (c)3 are more effective in some areas of SE Asia, Africa, and South America, but there is a low but significant risk of severe side-effects with (c)1 and (c)2; (c)4 is the safest of the four (c) regimens, so far as toxic side-effects are concerned, and is preferred for pregnant women and, with reduced dose, for young children (Table 11).

to precipitate attacks of candidiasis in women (hence it is helpful for women to take doxycycline with a one-dose therapy for candidal infections), and the rare risk of *Corynebacterium difficile* diarrhoea. However, doxycycline is likely to reduce the risk of the commoner travellers' diarrhoeas; but gastrointestinal discomfort from the doxycycline itself is not uncommon. The drug is taken daily with food, taking care not to miss any days, but avoiding lying down too soon after taking it to avert a real risk of acute pain from ulceration of the lower oesophagus. It is best to start a few days before travel: this is to get accustomed to taking the daily medication rather than for pharmacological reasons.

Atovaquone–proguanil ('Malarone')

This combination, which has been successfully used for malaria treatment for several years, has now been licensed in the United Kingdom (and previously in the United States) and Europe for malaria prophylaxis. It appears to have two great advantages: the level and severity of adverse effects has so far been lower than for the mefloquine and doxycycline; and, in part, it acts as a causal prophylactic, attacking the pre-erythrocytic stages of the malarial parasites. As a consequence, it is continued for 7 days after leaving the malarious area, so that the chance of compliance with this shorter period is improved. There are two concerns over it at present: although it appears to afford comparable protection as the alternative drugs against falciparum malaria, the evidence in non-immune individuals is scanty, and it is uncertain how soon resistance to this drug combination will emerge. Although resistance to atovaquone alone readily occurs, resistance to the combination is a much rarer event. Malarone is extremely expensive. However, since it is taken daily the different overall regimen means that the cost for short visits is more comparable to the alternatives, but the cost rises greatly for longer visits (and it is currently licensed for up to 4 weeks abroad). There is no experience of its use in pregnancy and the licence for its use in Europe currently excludes pregnancy and childhood, though it is used for children in the United States where paediatric tablets are available.

Continuation of chemoprophylaxis after leaving the malarious area

All antimalarial agents except Malarone must be continued for 4 weeks after leaving the malarious area.

Choice of chemoprophylaxis (Table 10)

Where there is a substantial risk of chloroquine-resistant falciparum malaria, either mefloquine, doxycycline, or Malarone are appropriate, so providing a better range of protective options than a few years ago for healthy adults. However, of these only mefloquine is licensed for children, and none is ideal for pregnant women who are best advised to avoid such areas. Doses of prophylactic antimalarial drugs for children are given in Table 11.

Chemoprophylaxis in people with epilepsy

In patients with epilepsy, proguanil or atovaquone/proguanil or doxycycline do not increase the risk of fits and can be used for prophylaxis, depending on the particular geographical area and level of risk.

The fixed drug combination Maloprim (12.5 mg pyrimethamine and 100 mg dapsone per tablet), marketed as Deltaprim in parts of Africa, has been of value in patients with epilepsy and for others unable to take the first-line drugs. It is now hard to obtain, and it is important not to confuse Malarone and Maloprim. Maloprim alone gives poor protection against *P. vivax* and chloroquine may be given concurrently. The dose of Maloprim must not exceed one tablet a week or the incidence of the otherwise uncommon side-effect, agranulocytosis, rises. Methaemoglobinaemia occasionally occurs with Maloprim chemoprophylaxis.

Rejected chemoprophylactic drugs

The following drugs are unsuitable for chemoprophylaxis (but Fansidar has a role in treatment): amodiaquine because of the high risk of agranulocytosis; Fansidar (25 mg pyrimethamine and 100 mg sulfadoxine per tablet) because of the frequency of severe skin reactions; and pyrimethamine on its own, because it is ineffective in most malarial areas.

Risk of malaria and need to take chemoprophylaxis

The risk of malaria is much higher in sub-Saharan Africa than elsewhere and it would be folly not to take prophylactics, except where the altitude is too great for transmission to occur or in the non-endemic southern parts of the continent (see Fig. 4). In Asia, the risk is usually much lower. Visitors to the air-conditioned hotels of the larger cities of SE Asia do not need prophylaxis but elsewhere in Asia there may be urban malaria. Mefloquine does not protect adequately against malaria in SE Asia, and travellers to the areas of higher transmission will need regimens (c)2 or (c)3 (Table 10). Those residing for long periods in such areas may prefer to adopt vigilance and the early treatment of fevers, but awareness of the risk is essential. Freedom from malaria in Asia by travellers does not mean that they will escape infection in Africa!

Because no prophylactic is completely effective in chloroquine-resistant *P. falciparum* areas, travellers who may be in remote areas and away from prompt medical assistance should carry a therapeutic dose of Fansidar, Malarone, mefloquine, or Riamet/Co-artem ether. Resistance to Fansidar has been reported from many countries with highly chloroquine-resistant malaria. The prophylactic regimen used should be continued for the appropriate time, usually 4 weeks, after returning to a non-endemic area. Compliance is hard to achieve, but this will prevent most cases of imported malaria. However, no regimen is 100 per cent protective and whatever precautions are taken, the possibility of malaria must, however, be borne in mind by the traveller and pointed out to any medical adviser, whom he or she must seek in case of a fever.

Malarial vaccines

Difficulties facing the development of a malaria vaccine

No satisfactory vaccine has emerged from the many attempts, over the last 70 years, to immunize animals and humans against malaria. A major problem is the impracticability of producing large quantities of attenuated micro-organisms, the basis for most effective viral and bacterial vaccines. The alternative, a subunit vaccine, has proved much more difficult to produce. Other problems are attributable to biological features of the malaria parasite, selected by evolutionary pressure to enable it to persist long enough in the human host to be taken up by a mosquito and propagated. During the different stages of its lifecycle—in the bloodstream, hepatocytes, and erythrocytes of the human host and in mosquitoes—*P. falciparum* expresses a variety of antigens. Antibodies elicited against sporozoites, the infective stage inoculated by the mosquito, will not recognize blood-stage antigens. A different set of immunizing antigens is therefore needed to target each stage of the lifecycle. The large and complex genome of *P. falciparum* (25–30 megabases with 5–6000 genes, many of them polymorphic, on 14 chromosomes) shows great diversity, and an attack of malaria may involve simultaneous infection with as many as eight different *P. falciparum* genomes. Antigenic variation of some parasite proteins, such as the high molecular weight PfEMP-1 on the surface of infected erythrocytes, enables *P. falciparum* to evade the host's immune response. Another problem facing the widespread use of a malaria vaccine is the variation in the innate genetic resistance of humans to the pathological effects of malaria infection, related, for example, to their MHC class I polymorphism (Table 4). The immune response to vaccines may also be determined genetically.

Pre-erythrocytic stage vaccines

Irradiation-attenuated sporozoites

The first successful attempt to immunize a human against malaria was reported by DF Clyde and his colleagues in 1973. Their technique was based on studies in mice infected with *P. berghei*, in which protective immunity had been achieved by repeated intravenous injections of live, irradiation-attenuated sporozoites or by exposure to bites by irradiated infected mosquitoes. In mice, protection was associated with the development of precipitating antibodies to circumsporozoite antigens. Over a period of 84 days, three healthy adult volunteers were exposed, on six occasions, to bites by *Anopheles stephensi* mosquitoes which had been irradiated after becoming heavily infected with sporozoites of the Burma (Thau.) strain of *P. falciparum*. After being challenged through bites by non-irradiated mosquitoes bearing the same strain of *P. falciparum*, 98 days after the start of immunization, two of them developed malaria but one remained uninfected. This uninfected man was exposed to bites by irradiated mosquitoes on five further occasions, after which he was challenged again on day 327. Again, he failed to develop parasitaemia but was not protected against an intravenous injection of blood-stage parasites of the same strain, illustrating the stage-specific nature of malarial immunity. Work over the next 20 years confirmed the principle that protective immunity could be induced in humans by bites of irradiated infected mosquitoes. Between 1989 and 1999 further studies were carried out of immunization by the bites of irradiated *P. falciparum*-infected mosquitoes. A group of 11 volunteers, immunized by receiving more than a thousand bites from irradiated mosquitoes harbouring infectious sporozoites of *P. falciparum* strain NF54 and the 3D7 clone of NF54, were protected against 33 out of 35 challenges through bites by non-irradiated infected mosquitoes. Protection lasted for at least 36–42 weeks and extended to parasitic strains from geographical areas different from the immunizing strains.

These studies of artificial infections by mosquito-borne attenuated sporozoites provided the first evidence that vaccination against malaria was possible. However, such a prolonged, intensive, and laborious process could never become a practicable way of immunizing even small groups of non-immune travellers, let alone endemic populations. The immunological mechanism of protection conferred by irradiated sporozoite immunization has been studied in the mouse model and in human volunteers. In mice, CD8+ T-cell recognition of infected hepatocytes, by targeting sporozoite proteins expressed within the cell, is the most important mechanism. Humoral antibodies to proteins on the sporozoite's surface and CD4+ T-cells may also play a role.

Effector T-cell vaccines

An encouraging recent development, based on these findings, has been the preparation and testing of effector T-cell vaccines targeting pre-erythrocytic stages of the lifecycle, in infected hepatocytes. Theoretically, these vaccines could prevent both blood-stage infection and transmission in malaria endemic areas. The two most productive strategies have been the use of protein-adjuvants (for example, in RTS,S/(SB)AS02 vaccine) and heterologous prime–boost immunization.

RTS,S/(SB)AS02 malaria vaccine

RTS,S is a fusion protein combining most of the circumsporozoite protein of *P. falciparum* with Hb$_s$Ag with a complex adjuvant (AS02) capable of inducing strong antibody and CD4+ T-cell responses. This vaccine protected 50 per cent of volunteers challenged within 2 to 3 weeks of their last immunization, but after 6 months, only one in five was protected. Field trials in The Gambia showed an overall efficacy against infection during the whole surveillance period of 34 per cent (95 per cent confidence interval (CI), 8.0–53 per cent; $p = 0.014$). Efficacy was 71 per cent (46–85 per cent) during the first 9 weeks but there was no protection after that. A single booster vaccination led to similar protection during the next malaria season (efficacy, 47 per cent (3.8–71 per cent); $p = 0.037$). Protection correlated with a short-lived vaccine peptide-specific CD4+ T-cell response. It is hoped to improve this vaccine by modifying the adjuvant, by boosting with a vaccinia recombinant circumsporozoite protein, and by the addition of a blood-stage (MSP-1) antigen. Trials in Gambian children are underway.

Heterologous prime–boost immunization

AVS Hill and his colleagues have pioneered the strategy of priming with a DNA-based vaccine and boosting with a recombinant poxvirus. This is particularly effective in inducing CD8+ cytotoxic T lymphocytes and in enhancing TH1-type CD4+ T-cell responses, both of which are associated with protection. The DNA vaccine encodes a number of sporozoite epitopes together with the entire thrombospondin-related adhesion protein (**TRAP**), while the poxvirus recombinant consists of a highly attenuated vaccinia virus strain (Modified Vaccinia [Virus] Ankara, **MVA**)—which does not replicate in mammalian cells—containing the same malaria insert. Phase I and II studies in Oxford and The Gambia have confirmed the safety and immunogenicity of the regime and challenge studies are in progress. An even more promising regimen, based on mouse studies, consists of priming with a Fowlpox (Avipox FP9) recombinant, and boosting with the MVA recombinant. (Table 11)

Table 11 Doses of prophylactic antimalarial drugs for children[a]

Age	Weight (kg)	Fraction of adult dose Chloroquine with proguanil	Maloprim (pyrimeth-amine and dapsone	Mefloquine
Term to 12 weeks		1/8	NR	NR
6 weeks to 11 months		1/4	1/8[b]	NR
1–5 years	10–19 15–19	1/2	1/4	NR under age 2 years 1/4 (2–5 years)
6–11 years	20–39	3/4	1/2	1/2 (6–8 years) 3/4 (9–11 years)
≥ 12 years	>40	Adult dose	Adult dose	Adult dose

NR, not recommended.

[a] For children aged under 2 years in areas of chloroquine resistance the appropriate medication is chloroquine plus proguanil. Chloroquine is available as a syrup but the proguanil has to be powdered on to jam or food. Measures against mosquito bites are specially important.

[b] Not feasible to prepare unless a paediatric formulation is available.

Further reading

Bates I, *et al.* (1991). Use of immunoglobulin gene rearrangements to show clonal lymphoproliferation in hyper-reactive malarial splenomegaly. *Lancet* **337**, 505–7.

Beadle C, *et al.* (1994). Diagnosis of malaria by detection of *Plasmodium falciparum* HRP-2 antigen with a rapid dipstick antigen-capture assay. *Lancet* **343**, 564–8.

Berendt AR, *et al.* (1994). Molecular mechanisms of sequestration in malaria. *Parasitology* **108**, S19–28.

Bradley DJ, Bannister B (2001). Guidelines for malaria prevention in travellers from the United Kingdom for 2001. *Communicable Disease and Public Health* **4**, 84–101.

Hill AVS, Weatherall DJ (1998). Host genetic factors in resistance to malaria. In: Sherman IW, ed. *Malaria: parasite biology pathogenesis protection*, pp 445–55. ASM Press, Washington DC.

Hoffman SL, *et al.* (2002). Protection of humans against malaria by immunization with radiation-attenuated *Plasmodium falciparum* sporozoites. *Journal of Infectious Diseases* **185**, 1150–64.

Koch O, *et al* (2002). IFNGRI gene promotor polymorphisms and susceptibility to cerebral malaria. *Journal of Infectious Disease* **185**, 1684–7.

Kwiatkowski D, *et al* (1990). TNF concentration in fatal cerebral, non-fatal cerebral, and uncomplicated *Plasmodium falciparum* malaria. *Lancet* **336**, 1201–4.

MacPherson GG, *et al.* (1985). Human cerebral malaria: a quantitative ultrastructural analysis of parasitized erythrocyte sequestration. *American Journal of Pathology* **119**, 385–401.

Marsh K, *et al* (1995). Indicators of life-threatening malaria in African children: clinical spectrum and simplified prognostic criteria. *New England Journal of Medicine* **332**, 1399–404.

Miller LH (1994). Impact of malaria on genetic polymorphism and genetic diseases in Africans and African Americans. *Proceedings of the National Academy of Sciences (USA)* **91**, 2415–19.

Nardin EH, Nussenzweig RS (1993). T cell responses to pre-erythrocytic stages of malaria: role in protection and vaccine development against pre-erythrocytic stages. *Annual Reviews of Immunology* **11**, 687–727.

Ockenhouse CF (1993). The molecular basis for the cytoadherence of *Plasmodium falciparum*-infected erythrocytes to endothelium. *Seminars in Cell Biology* **4**, 297–303.

Riddle MS, *et al* (2002). Exchange transfusion as an adjunct therapy in severe *Plasmodium falciparum* malaria: a meta-analysis. *Clinical Infectious Diseases* **34**, 1192–8.

The Artemether–Quinine Meta-analysis Study Group (2001). A meta-analysis using individual patient data of trials comparing artemether with quinine in the treatment of severe falciparum malaria. *Transactions of the Royal Society of Tropical Medicine and Hygiene* **95**, 1–14.

Turner GDH, *et al* (1994). An immunohistochemical study of the pathology of fatal malaria. *American Journal of Pathology* **145**, 1057–69.

Warrell DA, Gilles HM (2002). *Essential malariology*, 4th edn. Arnold, London.

Warrell DA, *et al* (1982). Dexamethasone proves deleterious in cerebral malaria. A double-blind trial in 100 comatose patients. *New England Journal of Medicine* **306**, 313–19.

Wernsdorfer WH, McGregor IA (1988). *Malaria. Principles and practice of malariology*. Churchill Livingston, Edinburgh.

White NJ and Ho M (1992). The pathophysiology of malaria. *Advances in Parasitology* **31**, 83–173.

White NJ, *et al* (1983). Severe hypoglycemia and hyperinsulinaemia in falciparum malaria. *New England Journal of Medicine* **309**, 61–6.

World Health Organization (2000). Severe falciparum malaria. *Transactions of the Royal Society of Tropical Medicine and Hygiene* **94**(Suppl. 1), 51–90.

World Health Organization (2002). *International travel and health*. WHO, Geneva.

7.13.3 Babesia

P. Brasseur

Babesia are intraerythrocytic, tick-transmitted, protozoan parasites that infect a broad variety of wild and domestic animals including cattle, horses, dogs, and rodents. Human babesial infection may occur occasionally.

Epidemiology

Two species of *Babesia*, *B. microti* and *B. divergens*, are responsible for most human cases. More than 200 cases of *B. microti* infections have been reported since 1966 along the north-east coast of the United States, especially in Massachusetts including Nantucket Island, Martha's Vineyard, and Cape Cod. *B. microti* is transmitted by *Ixodes dammini* and the reservoir host of parasites is the common white-footed mouse, *Peromyscus leucopus*. The zoonotic *Borrelia burgdorferi* causing Lyme disease is also transmitted by *I. dammini*; coinfections are documented among residents of coastal New England, where the risk of both babesiosis and Lyme disease is highest in June when nymphal *I. dammini* are most abundant. *B. microti* babesiosis may occur in people with intact spleens as well as in asplenic subjects.

After the first description of a case in 1957, 28 additional cases have been documented in Europe. Seventy six per cent of cases were due to *B. divergens*, a common cattle pathogen transmitted by *Ixodes ricinus* and responsible for economic losses, by reducing weight gains and milk production. France, the British Isles, and Ireland account for more than 50 per cent of European cases. They usually occur between May and October, the season of activity of tick vectors such as *I. ricinus*, which often seems to be responsible for human transmission. Most patients were residents of rural areas such as farmers and foresters, or visitors such as campers and hikers. Splenectomized people are at highest risk, comprising 24 out of 29 patients with babesiosis including all 22 *B. divergens* cases. Although no transfusion-associated case has been reported in Europe, this route of transmission is possible because *B. divergens* survives in packed red blood cells for several weeks at 4°C. No case has been recorded among HIV-infected patients.

Pathogenesis

Ticks infected with *Babesia* inoculate parasites while feeding on a vertebrate, the parasites enter red blood cells directly and multiply by budding to form two or four parasites, rarely more, in about 8 to 10 h. These are released and will invade other erythrocytes. The spleen plays a major role in resistance to babesial infections, especially for *B. divergens* babesiosis.

Clinical features

Human *B. microti* babesiosis is characterized by a gradual onset of malaise, anorexia, and fatigue with subsequent development of fever, drenching sweats, and generalized myalgia appearing 1 to 4 weeks after a tick bite. Other clinical manifestations such as headache, shaking chills, nausea, depression, and hyperaesthesia have been observed less frequently. The only finding on clinical examination is occasional mild hepatosplenomegaly. Anaemia, thrombocytopenia, and generally a low or normal white blood cell count is observed. A mild to severe haemolytic anaemia is frequent. Lactate dehydrogenase, liver enzymes, and bilirubin levels may be increased. Parasites are found in the peripheral blood of 1 to 20 per cent of patients with intact spleens, but in up to 80 per cent of asplenic patients. Most patients infected with *B. microti* have no history of splenectomy, but splenectomized patients generally have a more severe illness. Babesiosis is more severe in people over 40 years old and in HIV-infected patients. The acute illness lasts from 1 to 4 weeks, but weakness and malaise often persist for several months. A low and asymptomatic parasitaemia may persist several weeks after recovery.

In Europe, babesial infections are usually more severe (in 76 per cent of cases, with 38 per cent mortality) than in North America. After an incubation period of 1 to 3 weeks, severe intravascular haemolysis begins suddenly, causing haemoglobinuria, severe anaemia, and jaundice, associated with non-periodic high fever (40 to 41°C), hypotension, shaking chills, intense sweats, headache, myalgia, lumbar pain, abdominal pain, vomiting, and diarrhoea (Plate 1). Peripheral blood *B. divergens* parasitaemia may vary from 5 to 80 per cent. Patients rapidly develop renal failure which may be associated with pulmonary oedema, coma, and death. In severe cases, haemoglobin falls to 7 to 8 g/dl, sometimes to 4 g/dl, in spite of blood transfusions. Plasma haemoglobin levels may exceed 4 g/dl, haptoglobin decreases dramatically, and bilirubin and liver enzymes are markedly elevated.

Diagnosis

Babesiosis should be suspected in any patient with fever and a history of tick bite from any area. Initially, *Plasmodium falciparum* infection may be suspected, but splenectomy, lack of recent travel to a malaria-endemic area, or blood transfusion should lead to suspicion of babesiosis. Diagnosis is based on discovery of parasites in Giemsa-stained thin blood smears. Although the variable morphology of the parasites may be confusing, *Babesia* species can be distinguished from malaria parasites by the absence of gametocytes and pigment in erythrocytes containing mature stages.

B. microti is characterized by multiple basket-shaped parasites. In some cases, parasitaemia is sparse and inoculation of patient's blood into hamsters may facilitate diagnosis. This method may detect parasitaemias as low as 300 parasites/ml. Amplification by polymerase chain reaction using species-specific primers may establish the diagnosis in 24 h with high specificity and sensitivity.

B. divergens infection is suspected if there are symptoms of intravascular haemolysis and renal failure. The presence of double piriform intraerythrocytic parasites or tetrads is typical of *B. divergens*, but annular, punctiform, and filamentous forms may also be encountered. Inoculation of infected blood in gerbils (*Meriones unguiculatus*) may confirm the diagnosis. Serological tests may be useful especially in *B. microti* infections, but correlation between antibody titres and severity is poor. Using an indirect immunofluorescent test, antibody titres rise during the first weeks and fall after 6 months. Serology is not used for rapid diagnosis of *B. divergens* infection.

Treatment and prevention

Chloroquine, sulphadiazine, pyrimethamine, co-trimoxazole, pentamidine, and berenil (diminazene aceturate) appear ineffective in completely eliminating *B. microti*. A combination of quinine and clindamycin is effective except in immunocompromised individuals, especially those with HIV. Quinine should be given orally in doses of 650 mg every 6 to 8 h daily and clindamycin intravenously at 1200 to 2400 mg in three or four divided doses daily for at least 7 to 10 days. In fulminating infection, exchange transfusion is recommended.

In Europe, babesiosis should be treated as a medical emergency. Immediate chemotherapy should reduce parasitaemia and prevent extensive haemolysis. Exchange transfusion should be considered at the first sign of *B. divergens* infection. Massive exchange transfusion (2 to 3 total blood volumes) followed by administration of intravenous clindamycin at a dose of 600 mg four times daily for at least 10 days has proved successful. Imidocarb, which is used to treat babesiosis in cattle, has been used successfully in two patients in Ireland, although this drug has not been approved for human use. Atovaquone is active *in vitro* and in gerbils, but has not yet been used in human *B. divergens* infections.

Further reading

Telford III SR *et al.* (1993). Babesial infections in human and wildlife. In: Kreier JP, ed. *Parasitic protozoa*, Vol. 5. Academic Press, New York.
Pruthi RK *et al.* (1995). Human babesiosis. *Mayo Clinic Proceedings* **70**, 853.

7.13.4 Toxoplasmosis

J. Couvreur and Ph. Thulliez

Parasitology, epidemiology, transmission

Toxoplasma gondii is a ubiquitous coccidian parasite. Its definitive host is the cat. It exists in three forms: (i) the oocyst, which is excreted with the cat faeces, can remain viable for months in the soil under certain conditions of temperature and humidity; (ii) the tachyzoite, which multiplies intracellularly (Fig. 1); and (iii) cysts, the result of this intracellular multiplication, which can persist as viable parasites in the brain and striated muscles throughout the life of the host.

The prevalence of toxoplasma antibodies is high in most populations. It depends mostly upon eating habits. Prevalence is well defined in fertile women—for instance 72 per cent seropositivity in Paris, 36 per cent in Stuttgart, 54 per cent in Padua, and 21 per cent in London.

Toxoplasmosis is usually acquired by ingestion of cysts. There are four stages: acute, subacute, chronic, and relapses. Organisms spread from the gut by lymphatics and the bloodstream, reaching every organ, where they multiply intracellularly (acute stage). Termination of this stage depends upon the development of both cellular and humoral immunity. In immunocompetent hosts, the parasite encysts and will persist without any inflammatory process as long as the cysts are not disrupted (chronic stage). If the host is or becomes immunocompromised, there is a tendency for the cysts to release bradyzoites and toxoplasma becomes an opportunistic agent. Congenital infection occurs through transplacental transmission of tachyzoites when a previously uninfected woman is infected during pregnancy.

Acute acquired toxoplasmosis

Acquired toxoplasmosis is usually subclinical. The typical presentation is lymphadenopathy affecting posterior cervical, suboccipital, retroauricular, or submental nodes. Supraclavicular, axillary, pectoral, epitrochlear, and inguinal localizations are less frequent. Lymphadenopathy is usually localized but it can be generalized. Nodes can be painful and tender for 1 or 2 weeks. They are rarely larger than walnuts, smooth, well defined, and mobile. They never suppurate; they can persist for months and even a year. Mesenteric lymphadenopathy has been observed. Other clinical signs and symptoms are fatigue for several weeks, headache, myalgias, low-grade fever for one or several weeks, and rarely, a transient rash. Ocular involvement can be observed. Hepatomegaly and splenomegaly are rare. Neurological signs and myocarditis are exceptional in immunocompetent patients.

The blood count shows a relative neutropenia with lymphocytosis. Atypical lymphocytes indistinguishable from those of infectious mononucleosis may be seen. Inversion of the CD4/CD8 ratio has been noted more often in clinical than in subclinical toxoplasmosis. Features suggesting toxoplasmosis rather than infectious mononucleosis are absence of pharyngitis, oral petechias, and splenomegaly and a less marked but more persistent lymphadenopathy. The histological pattern is characteristic when there are groups of epithelioid cells scattered throughout the node, or immature sinus histiocytosis and follicular hyperplasia with phagocytosis and nuclear debris. Inflammatory infiltrates sometimes extend into perinodal tissues and may be misinterpreted as lymphangioma, lymphoma, or sarcoidosis.

Toxoplasmosis of the central nervous system

In acquired toxoplasmosis, central nervous system involvement is observed most commonly in the immunodeficient patient. The selectivity of toxoplasma for brain tissue has been ascribed to low local immunity. In animal experiments, tachyzoites are demonstrable in brain 5 days after intraperitoneal inoculation, with ensuing perivascular inflammation with mononuclear cells. Tachyzoite-infected cells provoke multiple foci of micronecrosis. Mononuclear cells gather into microglial nodules associated with toxoplasma antigen. Cysts appear away from the inflammatory process. Intermediate appearances are observed between disseminated foci of microglial nodules, more or less numerous large necrotic areas, and large space-occupying masses.

Clinical features of central nervous damage are protean and may develop insidiously: generalized encephalitis with meningeal involvement and localizing signs with fever, headache, drowsiness progressing into coma, and death within a few days or weeks; encephalitis with low-grade meningeal involvement; 'pseudotumour cerebri' syndrome with transient intracranial hypertension; space-occupying mass mimicking a tumour or a brain abscess; multiple mass lesions; miscellaneous patterns—confusion, psychiatric features, seizures, and signs of brainstem or spinal cord injury. The above patterns can progress to death fulminantly within 2 weeks or persist for months or even years with or without therapy (chronic relapsing encephalitis).

The diagnosis of toxoplasmosis of the nervous system is often difficult. Clinical signs and results of imaging are not specific and can be misleading. Serological data are often perplexing. Biopsy is advocated whenever the diagnosis is uncertain. It is mandatory to look for an underlying disease or an immunodeficiency.

Ocular toxoplasmosis

Toxoplasma infection is the most common cause of retinochoroiditis and posterior uveitis. The focal necrotizing retinitis in its acute or subacute stage appears as cottonwool-like patchy areas of the fundus with vitreous exudate. The lesion heals within 3 to 6 weeks leaving a punched-out scar with central atrophy and a peripheral black pigmentation. The lesion can be peripheral or central, single or multiple. It may reach the size of the optic disc. Atypical presentations include retinal detachment, haemorrhage, and optic nerve injury.

The natural history of ocular toxoplasmosis suggests that the first retinal lesion occurs more commonly during the subacute stage, weeks or months after the begining of the infection, than later during the chronic stage of the infection. It results from a previous colonization of the retina. The immediate cause is the rupture of a cyst. Its mechanism involves delayed sensitivity to toxoplasma antigens, and secondary proliferation of parasites.

Congenital toxoplasmosis is currently considered the major cause of ocular toxoplasmosis. Ninety per cent of retinochoroiditis discovered in infants and young children, and at least 20 per cent in adults, is attributable to congenital toxoplasmosis. It can be seen at birth or may occur much later, even in a previously normal retina, as is the case for 35 to 85 per cent of children with untreated congenital toxoplasmosis. There is a peak frequency of new lesions during puberty and adolescence. The common presenting signs are amblyopia or strabismus. There is some evidence that early treatment of even subclinical congenital toxoplasmosis decreases this risk. Ocular disease can complicate acquired toxoplasmosis more often

Fig. 1 Algorithm for neonates at risk of toxoplasmic fetopathy (mother infected during pregnancy).

than was previously considered. It can occur early following the acute stage of the infection, or after 2 years or more in one-third of cases. It is unilateral, with relapses in one-third of cases. It is generally isolated, being associated with neurological signs in no more than 10 per cent of cases, and most often without underlying immunodeficiency.

The diagnosis of ocular toxoplasmosis cannot be based on fundoscopic examination alone. The fact that it occurs mainly during the chronic stage of the infection while the antibody titre is low is a major problem. This can be solved by the demonstration of a local synthesis of antibodies in the aqueous humour.

Toxoplasmosis and immunodeficiency

Any patient with severe toxoplasmosis should be investigated for an immune defect, even subtle, and for an underlying disease, particularly AIDS. Conversely an immunodeficiency, either spontaneous or iatrogenic, can be complicated by severe toxoplasmosis. The last is generally related to chronic infection. The long persistence of cysts, particularly in brain, striated muscles, and myocardium is a well documented fact. In animals with chronic infection, corticoids, irradiation, or immunodeficiency can induce cyst rupture and proliferation of toxoplasma in the nervous tissue.

Among malignancies, the most common condition associated with cerebral toxoplasmosis is Hodgkin's disease and less often lymphoproliferative disorders such as lymphosarcoma, non-Hodgkin's lymphoma, and angioimmunoblastic lymphadenopathy. All types of leukaemia are involved.

Severe toxoplasmosis can occur in organ transplant recipients. It is rare in renal, liver, and bone marrow transplantations but is more frequent in heart and heart–lung transplantations in which the risk can reach 57 per cent in mismatched transplantations of a serologically positive donor and negative recipient. This risk is mainly related to the infected heart-tissue transplant. It is increased by the use of steroids for graft rejection. Conversely, cyclosporin has an antiparasitic activity. The risk is reduced by antiparasitic treatment in all recipients.

Severe toxoplasmosis of the central nervous system, lungs, and heart appeared as a major problem in patients with AIDS. Toxoplasma encephalitis was observed in 25 to 80 per cent of patients with signs of cerebral injury. The risk of such an encephalitis was 6 to 12 per cent in toxoplasma seropositive patients and it was definitely increased by several factors: late stage of the disease; the presence of antibodies, particularly if the IgG titre was more than 150 IU; and a CD4 lymphocyte count of less than 200 per m. The risk of cerebral toxoplasmosis has been markedly reduced by the administration of co-trimoxazole for prevention of pneumocystis in these patients.

It is often difficult to prove that clinical manifestations encountered in immunocompromised patients are attributable to toxoplasmosis. Antibody titres may not be significantly elevated. Attempts to isolate toxoplasma from cerebrospinal fluid, from myocardial or cerebral biopsies, or from bronchoalveolar lavage may be necessary.

Congenital toxoplasmosis

Maternofetal transmission

Following seroconversion during pregnancy, 31 per cent of infants are infected, 2 per cent suffer intrauterine death, but 67 per cent are uninfected. These overall data vary according to the date of maternal infection: before pregnancy, 0 per cent; during the first month, 1 per cent; during the second and third month, 17 per cent; from the fourth to the sixth month, 45 per cent as an average; and later an increased risk up to 80 per cent during the ninth month. The date of the maternal infection is also important for the clinical pattern of the fetopathy: 83 per cent of the fetuses infected during the first trimester have clinical involvement, often severe, while clinical signs, mostly mild and ocular, are seen in only 12 per cent of

the infants whose mothers were infected during the ninth month. The risk of fetopathy is reduced by more than 50 per cent if spiramycin is given to the mother. Very rare cases of transmission following chronic infection even years before pregnancy have been observed in immunocompromised mothers.

The placenta is the transmitting organ and placental infection is synonymous with fetopathy. If maternofetal transmission occurs early after maternal infection, fetopathy will be severe. If it is delayed, the fetus will be protected by passively transmitted maternal antibodies and toxoplasma will have a tendency to encyst in fetal tissues without causing serious early injury. Serological and clinical progression may thus be delayed for months after birth.

Clinical patterns

Five patterns can be identified in the protean presentation of congenital toxoplasmosis.

1. Systemic disease of the newborn baby with rash, jaundice, thrombocytopenic purpura, hepatosplenomegaly, pneumonia, progressive uveitis, high protein content of cerebrospinal fluid, cerebral ventricular dilation, and encephalomyelitis.

2. Neurological disease: hydrocephalus or microcephaly, microphthalmia, retinochoroiditis, and cerebral calcification. Hydrocephaly, always related to a stenosis of the duct of Sylvius, can be discovered *in utero* or several months after birth as well as in an infant initially considered as normal. Shunting is required.

3. Mild disease with isolated retinochoroiditis or mild cerebral calcification without any clinical signs of cerebral injury.

4. Subclinical infection. Prospective studies of women with acquired infection during pregnancy revealed that this is the most common pattern encountered in more than 70 per cent of the infected babies. The differentiation between subclinical toxoplasmosis and absence of infection is a common challenge for the paediatrician.

5. Relapses: flare-ups of retinochoroiditis can occur in infants, children, adolescents, or adults even in a previously intact retina in up to 85 per cent of cases (see Ocular toxoplasmosis). The possibility of late relapses in cerebral tissue is confirmed by the frequency of increased local synthesis of antibodies in the cerebrospinal fluid (see Laboratory diagnosis). Complete work-up, particularly examination of the cerebrospinal fluid is mandatory in any form of congenital toxoplasmosis even when subclinical.

Laboratory diagnosis

Serological methods are the main tools for diagnosis, but in the fetus and the immunocompromised patient the demonstration of parasites in body fluids and tissues is the preferred method of diagnosis.

Serology

In a non-immune pregnant woman who is tested repeatedly throughout pregnancy, seroconversion definitely proves the acquisition of infection. In the absence of seroconversion, the diagnosis of recent infection requires the demonstration of a significant rise of IgG antibody titre and the presence of IgM in serial samples obtained at 3-week intervals and tested in parallel. A stable IgG titre is consistent with an infection acquired at least 2 months before the first specimen was obtained. Since IgM antibodies may be detected for over a year after the infection, the use of complementary methods, based on acute-phase IgG antibodies, is necessary to rule out a recent infection, particularly in women who are evaluated late in pregnancy. The differential AC/HS agglutination test and the measurement of IgG avidity in enzyme immunoassay are suitable for this purpose.

In the newborn baby, the detection of specific IgM after 2 days of life or of specific IgA after 10 days is diagnostic of congenital infection. Synthesis of anti-toxoplasma IgG antibodies can be demonstrated by comparing the ratio: specific IgG titre/total IgG on monthly serial samples. In the absence of infection, this ratio decreases as the infant produces IgG that does not contain toxoplasma-specific antibodies. If the ratio remains the same or increases, the diagnosis is proved. Synthesis of specific IgG, IgM, or IgA can also be demonstrated by immunoblotting or by using enzymze-linked immunofiltration assay. In some cases, the only marker of congenital infection is production of specific IgG which may be delayed for several months. Consequently, in infants born to women infected during pregnancy, serological tests must be repeated until specific IgG disappears within the first 12 months of life, before ruling out a congenital infection.

In HIV-infected patients, tests for determination of specific antibodies must be sensitive enough to avoid underdiagnosing a latent infection which should be considered for specific prophylaxis.

Intrathecal or intraocular production of specific antibodies can be determined by comparing the ratio of specific to total IgG in cerebrospinal fluid or aqueous humour with that of serum. A coefficient higher than 3 is considered positive.

Detection of *Toxoplasma gondii*

Parasites can be isolated from tissues or biological fluids by inoculation into mice or into cell cultures. Isolation from blood or cerebrospinal fluid indicates the presence of an acute infection. Conversely, positive isolation from muscle after enzymatic digestion, from brain, or from heart tissues is possible in old, chronic infections and does not prove a recent or progressing infection. Positive isolation from the placenta is indicative of congenital infection.

Polymerase chain reaction can be used to detect toxoplasma DNA in various clinical samples. It has proved reliable for diagnosis in immunocompromised patients. It is the method of choice for prenatal diagnosis of congenital infection on a single sample of amniotic fluid. The method is rapid and specific provided that carry-over contamination of the samples and contamination risks associated with handling steps are avoided. This is the most sensitive diagnostic method although all congenital infections cannot be identified prenatally because a delayed transmission of toxoplasma from the placenta to the fetus may occur after the date of the amniocentesis.

Treatment

Drugs

The combination of pyrimethamine and sulpha drugs is the mainstay of treatment. Pyrimethamine is given orally in a daily dose of 1 mg/kg or 50 mg in adults. The dosage of sulphadiazine, the sulpha drug currently used, is 50 to 100 mg/kg per day in infants, up to 2 to 6 g in adults in two to four divided doses. It is necessary to monitor weekly the antiparasitic treatment with blood counts because of the risk of bone marrow depression resulting in leucopenia with pyrimethamine or leucopenia and granulopenia with sulphadiazine. Folinic acid at a dose of 50 mg by oral or intramuscular route every 3 to 6 days can prevent the pyrimethamine side-effects.

The combination of 25 mg of pyrimethamine and 500 mg of sulphadoxine (Fansidar) may be given orally in a dose of one tablet per 20 kg every 7 to 10 days for months. Other drugs of interest are atovaquone, co-trimoxazole, or macrolides—spiramycin given in a daily oral dose of 3 g to infected pregnant women to prevent maternofetal transmission of the parasite or clarithromycin, clindamycin, and azithromycin in various combinations.

Indications

Acquired toxoplasmosis

Indications for treatment are marked systemic symptoms, and evidence of organ involvement. The pyrimethamine–sulphadiazine combination can be given for one or several weeks according to the clinical pattern.

Immunocompetent pregnant women

Seroconverters are given spiramycin throughout pregnancy. A positive *in utero* diagnosis of fetopathy warrants pyrimethamine–sulphadiazine treatment with written consent. Serial ultrasound examination of the fetus is mandatory to detect cerebral involvement as a guide to elective termination.

Congenital toxoplasmosis

Any case, even if subclinical, must be treated to control active disease and/or to prevent the risk of secondary retinochoroiditis. The combination pyrimethamine–sulphadiazine is given daily for 3 to 6 months according to the clinical data, followed by treatment three times a week until 1 year of age.

Cerebral toxoplasmosis in AIDS

In the acute stage of infection, the regimen of choice is 50 mg of pyrimethamine, 6 to 8 g sulphadiazine, and 20 mg folinic acid per day for 3 to 6 weeks. Maintenance therapy is necessary throughout life. The risk of toxoplasma encephalitis is markedly reduced by routine administration of co-trimoxazole.

Ocular toxoplasmosis

A flare-up requires emergency treatment with pyrimethamine–sulphadiazine together with steroids. The pyrimethamine–sulphadoxine combination can then be given for 6, 12, or more months if there is a tendency for repeated relapses.

Prevention

Any patient at risk should avoid contact with cats, as their faeces is potentially infectious (litter, soil, garden sand pits, vegetables), and eat meat that is well cooked or preserved by deep freeze.

Further reading

Couvreur J (1991). Foetopathie toxoplasmique: Traitement in utero par l'association pyrimethamine– sulfamides. *Archives Françaises de Pediatrie* **48**, 397–403.

Couvreur J, Desmonts G (1962). Congenital and maternal toxoplasmosis; a review of 300 congenital cases. *Developmental Medicine and Child Neurology* **4**, 519–30.

Couvreur J, Leport C (1998). *Toxoplasma gondii*. In: Yu VL, Meignan TC, Barriere NJS, eds. *Antimicrobial chemotherapy and vaccines*, pp 600–12. William & Wilkins, Baltimore.

Couvreur J *et al.* (1984). La production locale accrue d'anticorps dans le liquide cephalo-rachidien au cours de la toxoplasmose congénitale. *Annales de Pédiatrie (Paris)* **3**, 839–45.

Desmonts G, Couvreur J (1985). Congenital toxoplasmosis: a prospective study of 378 pregnancies. *New England Journal of Medicine* **318**, 271–5.

Hohlfeld P *et al.* (1994). Prenatal diagnosis of congenital toxoplasmosis with a polymerase-chain-reaction test on amniotic fluid. *New England Journal of Medicine* **331**, 695–9.

Leport C, Raffi F, Matheron S (1998). Treatment of central nervous system toxoplasmosis with pyrimethamine–sulfadiazine combination in 35 AIDS patients. Efficacy of long term continuous therapy. *American Journal of Medicine* **84**, 94–100.

McAuley J *et al.* (1994). Early and longitudinal evaluations of treated children and untreated historical patients with congenital toxoplasmosis; the

Chicago Collaborative Treatment Trial. *Clinical Infectious Diseases* **18**, 38–72.

Remington JS, McLeod R, Thulliez P, Desmonts G (2001). Toxoplasmosis. In: Remington JS, Klein JO, eds. *Infectious diseases of the fetus and newborn infant*, 5th edn, pp. 205–346. Saunders, Philadelphia.

7.13.5 Cryptosporidium and cryptosporidiosis

D. P. Casemore and D. A. Warrell

Introduction

The cryptosporidia are obligate intracellular parasites of which primarily one species, *Cryptosporidium parvum*, is associated with infection in man, young livestock, and other mammalian species. First described in laboratory mice, by Tyzzer in 1912, *C. parvum* was first recognized as a cause of human infection in 1976. In the 1980s it emerged worldwide as a common cause of severe or life-threatening infection in severely immunocompromised patients, especially those with AIDS, and of acute, self-limiting gastroenteritis in otherwise healthy subjects, especially children.

Biology

Cryptosporidium spp. are members of the coccidia (phylum Apicomplexa) with oocysts that contain four sporozoites. The oocysts, an environmentally robust transmissible stage, are fully sporulated and infective when excreted. Cryptosporidia are monoxenous, that is, they complete their lifecycle in a single individual (Fig. 1). *C. parvum* is not tissue specific but shows a predilection for the lower ileum during the primary stages of infection.

Following ingestion of oocysts, the motile sporozoites are released, through a suture in the oocyst wall, in the lumen of the small bowel. They quickly attach superficially to cells, rounding up to form fixed trophozoites

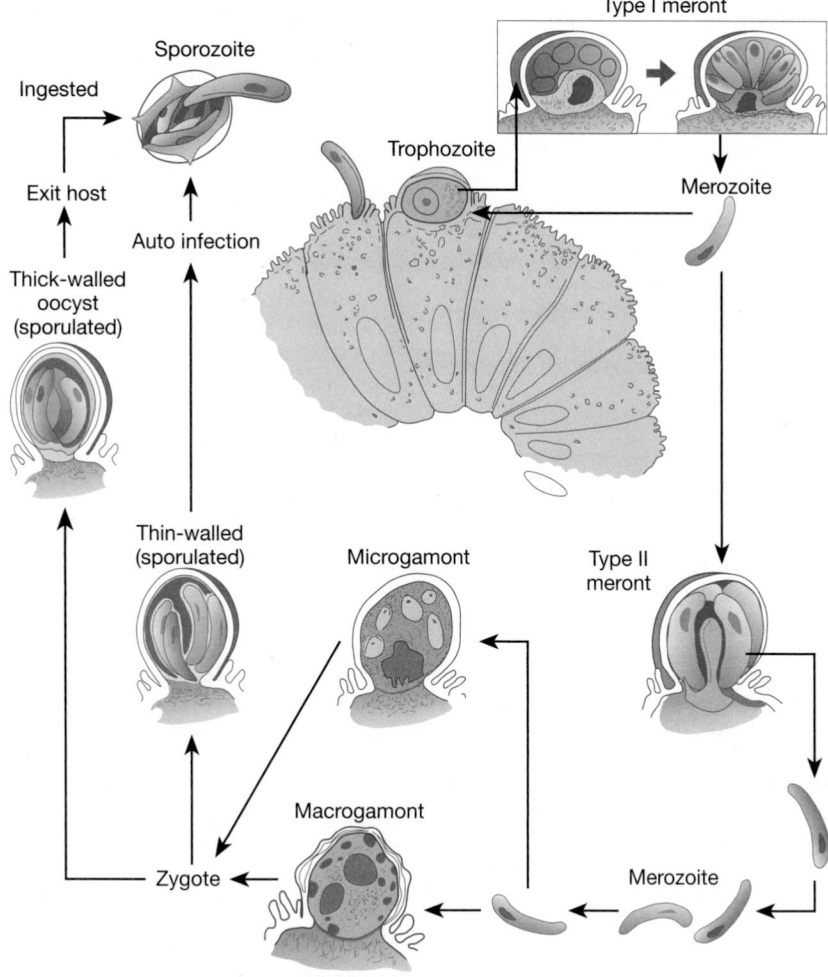

Fig. 1 Diagrammatic representation of the lifecycle of *C. parvum*. Following ingestion, the motile sporozoites are released, attach to cells, and develop into fixed trophozoites (uninucleate meronts) in an intracellular but extracytoplasmic location. These undergo schizogony (asexual multiple budding), the first-stage meronts producing eight merozoites, some of which recycle to form further type I meronts. Type II meronts produce four merozoites, which form gamonts (sexual stages) that mature as either macrogametes, or as microgamonts containing 16 motile microgametes. Most of the zygotes formed after fertilization develop into thick-walled, environmentally resistant, transmissible oocysts, which then sporulate, usually by the time they are excreted. Some have only a thin unit membrane, which ruptures to release the sporozoites *in situ* to produce an autoinfective cycle. (Adapted from a drawing by Kip Carter, University of Georgia, and shown by courtesy of Dr W.I. Current and CRC Press, Inc., Boca Raton.)

Fig. 2 Electron micrograph of a transverse section of small bowel of a mouse infected with *C. parvum*. The section shows numerous developmental stages: uninucleate meronts (trophozoites); type I meronts (schizonts) containing merozoites in which may be seen the darker granules of the apical complex organelles; the degenerate remains of a schizont and a free-swimming merozoite within the lumen; macrogamonts showing dark wall-forming granules and electron-lucent amylopectin (polysaccharide) food-storage granules. The parasitophorous vacuole can be clearly seen surrounding the parasite stages. Some of the intracellular stages appear to be free within the lumen because of the plane of sectioning.

(meronts). The initial site of infection is the brush border of enterocytes in the small bowel, but the parasite is able to infect other epithelial and parenchymal cells. The complex lifecycle includes both asexual and sexual stages of replication (Figs 1 and 2). The endogenous (tissue) stages develop within a parasitophorous vacuole, the outer layer of which is derived from the host cell's outer membranes, in a unique intracellular but extracytoplasmic location.

Molecular biology

Various genes and sequences have been studied and some have been cloned; chromosomes have been identified. Sequences coding for structural proteins such as actin and tubulin involved in parasite motility and attachment have been identified and may prove useful targets for the development of anticryptosporidial compounds. Nucleic acid sequences have differentiated recognized species and isolates within species, while some of the genotypes found may represent cryptic species. Differences between isolates of *C. parvum* from various sources show that those derived from animal hosts (genotype 2 or C) may, as expected, also be found in humans, but some isolates from humans appear to be relatively specific for humans (genotype 1 or H). Several other less common genotypes have been described, including from cats and dogs, the latter also having been found in a few immunocompromised humans. These findings have considerable public health significance and may also account for some of the variable responses seen in trials of specific anticryptosporidial therapy. Sensitive, genetically based probes are being applied to the detection of the parasite in clinical and environmental samples.

Epidemiology

C. parvum occurs worldwide and is common in humans and in livestock animals, especially lambs and calves, and has been reported from goats, horses, pigs, and farmed deer, as well as in mammalian wildlife. Prevalence in humans varies both geographically and temporally. Because of the diversity of host species, the epidemiology of the human infection is complex and involves both direct and indirect routes of transmission from animals

to man (zoonotic transmission) and from person to person ('urban' cycle).

Direct zoonotic infection

Transmission from livestock is common, particularly in children, including those from urban homes and schools visiting educational farms and rural activity centres. Household pets are an infrequent source of infection in otherwise healthy subjects. Cryptosporidiosis is rarely seen in adults in rural areas, presumably as a result of frequent exposure and the development of immunity.

Urban transmission

Infection is common in children attending playgroups and day-care centres and outbreaks have been reported in the United Kingdom and the United States. This results mainly from direct (person-to-person) faecal–oral transmission, although the infection may be introduced in the first instance through zoonotic contact. Affected adults may acquire infection from young children in the home or occupationally. Infection may be transmitted sexually where this involves faecal exposure. Cryptosporidium is a cause of travellers' diarrhoea although apparently not as frequently as is the case with giardia.

Waterborne infection

In the United Kingdom, the United States, and elsewhere, there have been numerous well-documented outbreaks resulting from contamination of public drinking-water supplies. Some have been associated with human-specific isolates and thus are likely to have been the result of contamination of the supply by human sewage. Other outbreaks have been associated with the zoonotic type, while isolates from endemic (sporadic) cases, some of which will be waterborne, fall into both categories. Oocysts have been demonstrated widely in both raw and treated water and legislation has been introduced in the United Kingdom in an attempt to limit the latter.

Cryptosporidiosis associated with swimming pools has been reported from several countries, including the United Kingdom, America, and Australia, resulting from accidental faecal contamination from bathers, and may also be acquired from recreational use of natural waters.

Foodborne infection

Foods associated with infection include unpasteurized milk, sausage meat, and salad. Isolation of oocysts from such foods is generally extremely difficult. In the United States infection has resulted from the consumption of fresh-pressed apple juice.

Nosocomial infection

Transmission has been reported between health-care staff and patients and between patients, particularly the immunocompromised. Large numbers of oocysts may be present in patients' stools and in vomit; transmission via fomites occurs although this route of transmission is limited by the susceptibility of oocysts to desiccation. Poor hand-washing practice has been identified as an important factor. In an outbreak with high mortality in a ward of immunocompromised patients in Denmark, transmission was probably by patients' hands via a ward ice-making machine.

Demography

Age and sex distribution

In the United Kingdom approximately two-thirds of *Cryptosporidium*-positive samples are from children 1 to 10 years of age, with a secondary peak in adults under 45 years; the infection is uncommon in infants less than 1 year old and in the elderly. Distribution appears to be the same in both sexes. A relative increase in adult cases is often seen in waterborne outbreaks. In developing countries, infection is common in infants less than 1 year old and asymptomatic infection is common in older subjects.

Temporal distribution

In the United Kingdom there are peaks in the spring and in the autumn, which do not necessarily both occur in any one locality, nor recur year by year, which coincide generally with lambing and calving. The zoonotic genotype is more prevalent in humans in the spring, some of which may result from secondary spread. Similar seasonal peaks are seen in patients with AIDS. The human-specific type shows some increase in frequency later in the year and this may be associated with foreign travel.

Frequency of occurrence

Laboratory rates of detection in non-immunocompromised subjects average about 2 per cent (range: less than 1 to 5 per cent) in developed countries and about 8 per cent in developing countries (range: 2 to 30 per cent), about fourth in the list of pathogens detected in stools submitted to the laboratory. In the United Kingdom about 5000 to 6000 confirmed cases are reported annually, somewhat less frequent generally than giardiasis. Among young children in the United Kingdom, cryptosporidiosis is more common than salmonella infection and during peak periods detection rates may exceed 20 per cent.

Cryptosporidiosis is one of the most common causes of diarrhoea in patients with AIDS and in some studies prevalence has exceeded 50 per cent. The infection rate in patients with AIDS in the United Kingdom has been falling in recent years, which has been attributed to infection control advice and the use of multiple antiretroviral therapy. Infection rates are not generally increased for most other immunocompromised groups.

Clinical aspects

Pathology

Histopathology

There is mucosal involvement of the small bowel, other parts of the gastrointestinal tract, and sometimes beyond. Moderate to severe abnormalities of villous architecture occur, with stunting and fusion of villi and lengthening of crypts. There may be evidence of mild inflammation, with some cellular infiltration into the lamina propria.

The endogenous stages of the parasite in the luminal surface are generally inconspicuous and appear as small (2 to 8 μm) bodies, apparently superficially attached to the brush border, unevenly distributed over the apical cells and within the crypts of the villi (Figs 1 and 2). Peaking and apoptosis of infected cells have been reported. There is usually little intracellular change at the ultrastructural level beyond the attachment zone of the parasite. Rectal biopsy may reveal mild, non-specific proctitis. Extensive and chronic involvement of the bile duct and gallbladder is seen in some patients with AIDS.

Immunological response

The particular immunodeficient conditions in which cryptosporidiosis has been reported to show increased severity or persistence suggest that both humoral and cellular factors have a role in limiting infection. An immune response has been demonstrated in the main immunoglobulin classes, although the initial IgG response may be poor. Serological diagnostic tests are, however, of little clinical value. Seroprevalence studies indicate that the infection is common, even in developed countries, and this may reflect water supply quality or other exposures.

Reports differ on the effect of breast feeding on incidence in infancy; some studies suggest a protective effect although protection from the environment by breast feeding may also be important.

Although functioning humoral and cellular immunity seem to be important in limiting or controlling infection, it currently appears that, in animal models, CD4+ and CD8+ T lymphocytes and interferon-γ are especially important in this respect. In humans, CD4 cell counts of fewer than 200 cells/mm³ probably indicate the need to take special care to avoid exposure to Cryptosporidium, and fewer than 100 cells/mm³ indicates a poor prognosis if infection occurs.

Possible pathogenic mechanisms

The watery diarrhoea is characteristic of non-inflammatory infection of the small bowel, especially that associated with toxin-producing organisms and enteric viruses. Several mechanisms have been suggested to explain the symptoms: reduction in absorptive capacity, particularly for water and electrolytes; increase in secretory capacity from crypt hypertrophy; osmotic effects from loss of brush-border enzymes (e.g. disaccharidases) resulting in malabsorption of sugars, increased osmolality of chyme, and subsequent microbial fermentation of sugars in the colon (which may account for the characteristic offensive smell); toxic activity has been described.

Clinical presentation in otherwise healthy (immunocompetent) people

Cryptosporidiosis in the immunocompetent person is a self-limiting, acute gastroenteritis with a variety of presenting symptoms. In cases where the time of exposure has been known the incubation period was about 5 to 7 days (range probably 2 to 14 days; wider limits have been suggested but are unlikely). There may be a prodrome of one to a few days, with malaise, abdominal pain, nausea, and loss of appetite. Gastrointestinal symptoms start suddenly, the stools being described as watery, greenish with mucus in some cases, without blood or pus, and very offensive. Patients may open their bowels more than 20 times a day but more usually 3 to 6 times. Other symptoms include colicky, abdominal pain, especially after meals, anorexia, nausea and vomiting, abdominal distension, and marked weight loss. 'Flu-like' systemic effects, including malaise, headache, myalgias, and fever, commonly occur. Gastrointestinal symptoms usually last about 7 to 14 days, but weakness, lethargy, mild abdominal pain, and intermittent loose bowels sometimes persist for up to a further month.

There is no evidence of transplacental transmission but infection during late pregnancy may cause metabolic disturbances in the mother, leading to the infant's failure to thrive. Failure to thrive has also been observed in older infants and children, and may be associated with persistent infection and enteropathy, especially in underdeveloped countries.

Reported sequelae include pancreatitis (associated with severe abdominal pain), toxic megacolon, and reactive arthritis. In immunocompetent patients, deaths are rarely attributable to cryptosporidiosis.

Clinical presentation in immunocompromised patients

Susceptibility to cryptosporidiosis and the severity of the disease is increased in patients who are immunocompromised as a result of AIDS, hypo- or agammaglobulinaemia, severe combined immunodeficiency, leukaemia, malignant disease, and bullous pemphigoid. Disease susceptibility and severity are also increased during immunosuppressive treatment with cyclophosphamide and corticosteroids as in patients undergoing bone marrow transplantation, and in children immunosuppressed by measles and chickenpox, especially where there is associated malnutrition. Infection in patients with leukaemia may be unusually severe and has sometimes proved fatal, particularly when associated with aplastic crisis, and may then require modification of chemotherapy to control the infection.

Symptoms of cryptosporidiosis are generally similar but often develop insidiously in immunocompromised patients. In those with late-stage AIDS with very low CD4 cell counts, or in some other profound deficiency states, diarrhoea may be frequent, profuse, and watery, like cholera. Patients may open their bowels frequently, passing up to 20 litres of infected fluid stool per day; persistent nausea and vomiting is usually associated with severe diarrhoea and suggests a poor prognosis. Associated symptoms include colicky, abdominal pain often associated with meals, severe weight loss, weakness, malaise, anorexia, and low-grade fever. Cryptosporidial infection in immunocompromised patients may involve the pharynx, oesophagus, stomach, duodenum, jejunum, ileum, appendix, colon, rectum, gallbladder, bile duct, pancreatic duct, and the bronchial tree. Cryptosporidial cholecystitis (presenting with severe right upper-quadrant abdominal pain), sclerosing cholangitis, pancreatitis, hepatitis, and respiratory-tract symptoms may occur, with or without diarrhoea. The clinical picture may include other features of HIV infection and there is often coinfection with other pathogens such as cytomegalovirus, *Pneumocystis carinii*, and *Toxoplasma*.

Patients with less severe impairment of immunity may experience resolution or a more chronic course, with less profuse diarrhoea, sometimes with remission and then recurrence, possibly associated with biliary tract involvement. Except in those patients whose immune suppression can be relieved by stopping immunosuppressant drugs, or, in the case of HIV, intensifying antiretroviral therapy, severe symptoms may persist until the patient dies. This is either as a result of dehydration, acid–base or electrolyte disturbances, and cachexia, from some other opportunistic infection or malignant disease, or a combination of these.

Laboratory investigations

In early acute cases the stools are usually watery, greenish with mucus in some cases, without blood or pus.

Peripheral leucocytosis and eosinophilia are found rarely. Serum electrolyte abnormalities will develop in patients who become severely dehydrated. In immunocompromised patients with cryptosporidial cholecystitis, serum alkaline phosphatase and γ-glutamyl transpeptidase levels are raised, while aminotransferases and bilirubin levels may remain normal.

In patients with AIDS, common associated infections are with cytomegalovirus and *Isospora belli*. Mixed infection with *Campylobacter* and *Giardia* species may be found in immunocompetent patients.

In the bowel mucosa there is histological evidence of enterocyte damage, villous blunting, and inflammatory-cell infiltration of the lamina propria; cell peaking and apoptosis have been reported. Histopathological appearances of the affected biliary tract resembles primary sclerosing cholangitis. Radiographic abnormalities include dilatation of the small bowel, mucosal thickening, prominent mucosal folds, and abnormal motility, and in the biliary system, dilated distal biliary ducts, stenosis with an irregular lumen, and other changes reminiscent of primary sclerosing cholangitis.

Differential diagnosis

The absence of blood, pus, cells, or Charcot–Leyden crystals may distinguish cryptosporidiosis from some acute bacterial diarrhoeas and that associated with amoebiasis and isosporiasis. In immunocompetent patients, the symptoms of cryptosporidiosis resemble those of giardiasis or cyclosporiasis. Intense abdominal pain and cramps are generally more common in cryptosporidiosis, but bloating and weakness less common. In immunocompromised patients, especially in those with AIDS, isosporiasis is clinically indistinguishable, but can be diagnosed by finding the organisms in the stool, when Charcot–Leyden crystals may also be found. This infection responds to treatment with trimethoprim and sulphamethoxazole, as does cyclosporiasis.

Treatment of cryptosporidiosis

In immunocompetent patients, the illness is self-limiting, but they may become dehydrated and require intravenous fluids, electrolytes, and symptomatic treatment for their vomiting and diarrhoea.

Immunocompromised patients with persistent severe diarrhoea, malabsorption, and other complications may require prolonged palliative treatment. They should avoid excess milk, as lactose intolerance may develop. Parenteral feeding and fluid, electrolyte, and nutrient replacement may be needed. Antiperistaltic agents such as loperamide, diphenoxylate, or opiates may increase abdominal pain and bloating. Antiemetics may be needed for symptomatic relief. Temporary relief of biliary obstruction has been achieved by endoscopic papillotomy and of cholecystitis by cholecystectomy. Diarrhoea and vomiting may, however, prove intractable.

Some reports suggest possible activity with letrazuril/diclazuril, somatostatin, azidothymidine, diloxanide furoate, furazolidone, amprolium, the macrolides, roxithromycin, and nitazoxanide. Paromomomycin has also been suggested as an active agent although a very recent report indicates that it is no more effective than placebo for cryptosporidiosis in patients with advanced HIV infection. Zydovudine (Retrovir™) therapy may result in remission or amelioration of symptoms, as may treatment of coinfecting agents. Separating the effect of the drugs on copathogens or of fluctuations in immune competence, both spontaneous and drug-induced, may be difficult. Immunotherapy (e.g. with bovine colostrum, hyperimmune immunoglobulin, transfer factor, and interleukin 2) has been attempted, with variable results.

Laboratory detection and diagnosis

The characteristic endogenous stages (Figs 1 and 2) may be found in histological sections, using light and electron microscopy, but diagnosis is usually by detection of oocysts in stools. (Plates 1–10) Oocysts have also been found in vomit and sputum in some cases, especially those associated with AIDS. The oocysts of *C. parvum* are spherical or slightly ovoid, about 4 to 6 µm, and appear refractile in wet faecal preparations with a highly refractile inner body, the cytoplasmic residuum; the four sporozoites within may be distinguished with difficulty using special optical systems. Several conventional stains have been adapted for diagnostic purposes, such as the modified Ziehl–Neelsen method and phenol–auramine fluorescent stain. Immunofluorescent antibody and enzyme immunoassay methods, using monoclonal antibodies, are commercially available but are expensive. Standardization of approach to screening and of reporting is essential for epidemiological purposes. Ideally, all stool samples from cases of diarrhoea should be screened; restriction, where unavoidable, should be based on age group (see demography) and not on factors such as stool consistency. Concentration of stool specimens is not usually required for diagnosis in acute cases.

Fungal spores, yeasts, cysts of *Balantidium*, sporocysts of *Isospora*, and oocysts of *Clyclspora* may readily be mistaken for cryptosporidial oocysts.

Infectivity, resistance, and control

Infectivity

In studies using monkeys and lambs, the infective dose for *C. parvum* was fewer than 10 oocysts. Human volunteer studies in the United States, initially with the zoonotic genotype, suggest the minimum infective dose varies from fewer than 10 oocysts to more than 1000, varying with the isolate. Symptomatic reinfection was achieved in some subjects despite the presence of antibody. Studies with the human-specific genotype are now in progress.

Resistance and disinfection

Oocysts can survive for many months in a cool, moist environment but are highly susceptible to desiccation, prolonged freezing, and moderate heat (pasteurization temperatures). They are remarkably resistant to most disinfectants and antiseptics, including chlorine at concentrations far greater than those used in water treatment and even to glutaraldehyde under normal use conditions. Some disinfectants may be more effective if used at elevated temperature (37°C or higher). Oocysts are sensitive to 10 volume (3 per cent) hydrogen peroxide, and to appropriate levels of ozone and medium or high-pressure ultraviolet. The adequate disinfection of instruments such as endoscopes is difficult and prolonged immersion in

7.13.9 *Blastocystis hominis* infection

R. Knight

This is an anaerobic protist of the caecum and colon, its taxonomic affinity has long been uncertain. Sequencing of ribosomal RNA genes indicates that it is a stramenopile, a group that includes certain unicellular, mostly flagellated, algae. The form commonly described in faeces, and also in cultures, is spherical, 5 to 8 μm in diameter, with a prominent central body surrounded by peripheral cytoplasm containing granules; electron microscopy reveals a nucleus, with a crescentic cap of heterochromatin, and mitochondria with tubular cristae (Figs 1, 2, and 3). The organism grows readily in cultures with mixed bacteria but axenic cultures can be established; division is by binary fission and also probably by schizogony within the central body. Electron microscopy of faeces reveals a multivacuolar form with multiple small vesicles that can either form cysts or transform into the familiar form. Colonoscopy specimens have shown an amoeboid form that ingests bacteria with pseudopodia. Bizarre environmentally induced forms with huge vacuoles may develop in cultures. The common 'univacuolar form' was named *Blastocystis* by Brumpt in 1912, who considered it to be a yeast, although it was first described by Alexieff in 1911 as a protozoan cyst.

Fig. 1 *B. hominis* from culture showing binary fission; the cytoplasm is lying at the periphery. v, vacuole. Phase contrast, × 400.

Fig. 2 *B. hominis* from culture showing the great variation in size. v, vacuole. Dark field, × 400.

Fig. 3 *B. hominis*. Electron micrograph showing the peripheral cytoplasm (c) and the central vacuole (v); the inclusions in the cytoplasm are mitochondria. × 5000.

Epidemiology

Prevalence is high in many human populations in contexts of high faeco-oral transmission. This infection is associated with travel and institutions and may occur in outbreaks. Similar *Blastocystis* organisms of uncertain pathogenicity occur in birds, pigs, and monkeys. The recently recognized cysts are the transmissive stage.

Diagnosis

It is usually recognized in direct wet faecal smears or formol ether concentrates; wet mounts can be stained with iodine giving a brownish central body; or with toluidine blue. The organism is often numerous in symptomatic subjects. Permanent mounts stain well with trichrome. *Blastocystis* can resemble amoebic cysts but lacks their characteristic nuclei. In fixed smears stained specifically for *Cryptosporidium* there is no oocyst wall.

Clinical features and treatment

A diarrhoeal illness lasting 3 to 10 days is attributed to this organism. Sometimes symptoms continue for weeks or months. Associated features are abdominal bloating, flatulence, and anorexia. Symptoms are more prolonged in immunocompromised subjects. There is no association with irritable bowel syndrome. Illnesses are self-limiting in most people but infection can be eliminated with metronidazole or tinidazole; the organism is also sensitive to furazolidine and co-trimoxazole.

Evidence for pathogenicity

Serum antibody is detectable in symptomatic subjects; preliminary studies suggest *in vitro* cytotoxicity to tumour cell monolayers, and local lesions have been produced in mice after intramuscular injection.

The situation with *Blastocystis* in humans may be similar to that of several anaerobic lumen-dwelling protozoa infecting vertebrates in which a self-limited non-invasive pathogenicity is followed by a longer carrier state. Such a relationship remains very difficult to prove or disprove, especially as there is genetic heterogeneity between *Blastocystis* isolates. Clinical response to metronidazole is hardly compelling evidence for pathogenicity since concurrent infection with other enteropathogens is common and this drug has a wide spectrum of activity, including an effect upon small bowel bacterial overgrowth. More well-documented outbreaks and cytopathic evidence are needed.

Further reading

Boreham PF, Stenzel DJ (1993). *Blastocystis* in humans and animals: morphology, biology, and epizootiology. *Advances in Parasitology* **32**, 1–70.

Moe KT *et al.* (1998). Cytopathic effect of *Blastocystis hominis* after intramuscular inoculation into laboratory mice. *Parasitology Research* **84**, 450–4.

Stenzel DJ, Boreham PF (1996). *Blastocystis hominis* revisited. *Clinical Microbiology Reviews* **9**, 563–84.

7.13.10 Human African trypanosomiasis

August Stich

Introduction

Sleeping sickness or human African trypanosomiasis (HAT) is caused by subspecies of the protozoan haemoflagellate *Trypanosoma brucei* transmitted to man and animals by tsetse flies (*Glossina* spp.). The distribution of the vector restricts sleeping sickness to the African continent between 14° north and 29° south (Fig. 1). Human disease occurs in two clinically and epidemiologically distinct forms, *gambiense* or West African and *rhodesiense* or East African sleeping sickness (Table 1). A third subspecies of the parasite, *T.b. brucei*, causes disease in cattle but is non-pathogenic in humans.

First reports of the disease go back to the fourteenth century. In the past, the impact on health in Africa has been enormous. Many areas had long been rendered uninhabitable for people and livestock. During the first decades of the twentieth century, millions may have died in Central Africa around Lake Victoria and in the Congo basin (Fig. 2). The success of control programmes in the 1960s promised the disappearance of sleeping sickness as a public health problem. However, recent epidemics in the Democratic Republic of Congo, Northern Angola, Sudan, Uganda, and other countries confirm a major resurgence of HAT. According to current estimates by WHO, the achievements in sleeping sickness control during colonial times will be completely reversed in the near future.

Today, 60 million people in some 40 African countries are exposed to the risk of HAT. Half a million are believed to be infected (almost all with *T.b. gambiense*). They are doomed if left untreated. For tourists and expatriates, sleeping sickness has always been a rare disease, but a recent cluster of cases in tourists to Tanzania re-emphasizes that it is also important in travel medicine.

Aetiology

In 1895, Sir David Bruce (1855–1931) suggested an association between trypanosomes and 'cattle fly fever', a major problem for livestock in southern Africa. In 1902, Robert M. Forde and Everett Dutton identified trypanosomes in the blood of a patient during a research expedition in The Gambia, and in 1903, Aldo Castellani isolated trypanosomes from the cerebrospinal fluid. In the same year, tsetse flies were identified as the vector.

Trypanosoma brucei (phylum Sacromastigophora, order Kinetoplastida) is an extracellular protozoal parasite. Like *Leishmania*, it possesses a centrally placed nucleus and a kinetoplast, a distinct organelle with extranuclear DNA. The kinetoplast is the insertion site of an undulating membrane, which extends over nearly the whole cell length and ends as a free flagellum.

The three subspecies of *Trypanosoma brucei* are indistinguishable morphologically. However, they differ considerably in their interaction with their mammalian host and the epidemiological pattern of the diseases they cause. Formerly, *T.b. gambiense* and *T.b. rhodesiense* isolates were characterized either by isoenzyme analysis or by animal inoculation. The advent of molecular techniques created expectations of more reliable tools for their differentiation. However, genomic characterization has revealed several more subdivisions rather than the three expected. Whereas West African isolates proved relatively homogeneous, East African isolates from humans and animals did not simply conform to what is still called *T.b. rhodesiense* and *T.b. brucei* but showed a complex relationship with evidence of sexual genetic exchange in the vector. Further molecular research may soon lead to a comprehensive phylogenetic tree and a deeper insight into trypanosomal evolution and biology.

Transmission

Although congenital, blood-borne, and mechanical transmission have been reported and may play an occasional role, the main mode of transmission is through the bite of infected tsetse flies (*Glossina* spp., order Diptera; Fig. 3 and Plate 1). These are biologically unique insects, which occur only in Africa in 31 distinct species and subspecies. Less than half are potential vectors of HAT. Their distinctive behaviour, ecology, and chosen habitat explain many epidemiological features of sleeping sickness. Tsetse flies can live for many months in the wild, but give birth to only about eight to 10 larvae per lifetime. Both sexes feed on blood. They are fastidious in requiring warm temperatures, shade, and humidity for resting and larviposition and so their distribution is highly localized. Recently, the mapping and monitoring of possible HAT transmission foci has become possible with the use of satellite imaging techniques.

During the blood meal on an infected mammalian host, the tsetse fly takes up trypanosomes ('short-stumpy form') into its mid-gut, where they develop into procyclic forms and multiply. After about 2 weeks, they migrate to the salivary glands as epimastigotes where they finally develop into infective metacyclic forms. With the next blood meal, they are then injected into the new vertebrate host where they appear and multiply as 'long-slender' trypomastigotes.

Fig. 1 The geographical distribution of human African trypanosomiasis.

Table 1 The principal features of West and East African sleeping sickness

Disease	West African sleeping sickness	East African sleeping sickness
Parasite	*Trypanosoma brucei gambiense*	*Trypanosoma brucei rhodesiense*
Vector	Transmitted by riverine tsetse flies (*Palpalis* group)	Transmitted by savannah tsetse flies (*Morsitans* group)
Clinical course	Insidious onset, slow progression, death in stage II after many months or years	Acute onset, chancre frequent, rapid course, death frequently in stage I (cardiac failure)
Diagnosis	Parasitaemia scanty, Winterbottom's sign, serology	Parasitaemia usually higher, serological tests unreliable
Treatment	See Table 3	
Epidemiology	Tendency for endemicity, man as main reservoir, growing public health problem in many West and Central African countries	Wild animals (bushbuck) as reservoir and source of epidemics

Molecular and immunological aspects

The cyclic changes of the trypanosome into different developmental stages are accompanied by variations in morphology, metabolism, and antigenicity. Several unique metabolic pathways have been described in trypanosomes, distinct from their host and thus qualifying as potential drug targets.

The blood stream forms of *T. brucei* are covered with a dense coat of identical glycoproteins, numbering up to about 500 aminoacids per molecule. Being highly immunogenic, they stimulate the production of specific antibodies, mainly of the IgM subclass. Once the surface glycoproteins have been recognized by host antibodies, the parasitic cell will be attacked and destroyed through complement activation and cytokine release.

However, about 2 per cent of *T. brucei* in each new generation change the expression of their specific surface glycoprotein. The 'coat' will then be dif-

ferent in the new clone ('variant' surface glycoprotein: VSG). This phenotypic switch is done mainly by programmed DNA-rearrangements, moving a transcriptionally silent VSG gene into an active, telomerically located expression site. Within a trypanosome population, the potential repertoire of such different VSG copies seems to be virtually infinite.

Every new VSG copy is antigenically different, thus stimulating the production of a new IgM population. This antigenic variation is the major immune evasion strategy of the parasite, enabling the trypanosome to persist in its vertebrate host. It also reduces parasite load and prolongs the infection. But the inevitable outcome is immune exhaustion of the host, penetration of trypanosomes into immune-privileged sites such as the central nervous system, and finally death.

Clinical features

Sleeping sickness is a dreadful disease, causing great suffering to patients, their families, and the affected community. The infection often has an insidious onset, but *T. brucei*, whether the East or West African subspecies, will invariably kill if the patient is not treated in time. The natural course of HAT can be divided into different and distinct stages. Their recognition and differentiation is important for the management of the patient.

The trypanosomal chancre

Tsetse bites can be quite painful, usually leaving a small and self-healing mark. In the case of a trypanosomal infection, the local reaction can be quite pronounced and longer lasting. A small raised papule will develop after about 5 days. It increases rapidly in size, surrounded by an intense erythematous tissue reaction (Fig. 4 and Plate 2) with local oedema and regional lymphadenopathy. Although some chancres have a very angry appearance, they are not usually very painful unless they become ulcerated and superinfected. They heal without treatment after 2 to 4 weeks, leaving a permanent, hyperpigmented spot.

Trypanosomal chancres occur in about half the cases of *T.b. rhodesiense*. In *T.b. gambiense*, they are much less common. They often go undetected in endemic populations.

Haemolymphatic stage (HAT stage I)

After local multiplication at the site of inoculation, the trypanosomes invade the haemolymphatic system, where they can be detected after 7 to 10 days. During this period of spread, they are exposed to vigorous defence mechanisms of the host, which they evade by antigenic variation. This continuous battle between antigenic switches and humoral defence results in a fluctuating parasitaemia with parasites frequently becoming undetectable, especially in *gambiense* HAT. The cyclic release of cytokines during periods of increased cell lysis results in intermittent, non-specific symptoms: fever, chills, rigors, headache, and joint pains. These can easily be misdiagnosed as malaria, viral infection, typhoid fever, or many other conditions. Hepatosplenomegaly and generalized lymphadenopathy are common, indicating activation and hyperplasia of the reticuloendothelial system.

A reliable sign, particularly in *T.b. gambiense* infection, is the enlargement of lymph nodes in the posterior triangle of the neck (Winterbottom's

Fig. 2 Sleeping sickness patients on an island in Lake Victoria; historical photograph taken during Robert Koch's research expedition to East Africa.

Fig. 3 Adult tsetse fly (*Glossina morsitans*). (See also Plate 1.)

Fig. 4 Trypanosomal chancre on the shank of a missionary returning from the Congo. (See also Plate 2.)

Fig. 5 Patient with late-stage trypanosomiasis. (See also Plate 3.)

Diagnosis

HAT can never be diagnosed with certainty on clinical grounds alone. Definitive diagnosis requires the detection of the parasite in chancre aspirate, blood, lymph juice, or cerebrospinal fluid using various parasitological techniques. The methods for diagnosis are essentially the same for *gambiense* and *rhodesiense* HAT (Table 2).

Lymph node aspirate

Lymph node aspiration is widely used, especially for the diagnosis of *gambiense* HAT. Fluid of enlarged lymph nodes, preferably of the posterior triangle of the neck (Winterbottom's sign), is aspirated and examined immediately at 400 × magnification. Mobile trypanosomes can be detected for a few minutes between the numerous lymphocytes.

Wet preparation, thin, and thick blood film

During all stages of the disease, trypanosomes may appear in the blood where they can be detected in unstained wet or in stained preparations. The yield of detection is highest in the thick blood film, a technique widely used

sign). Other typical signs are a fugitive patchy rash, a myxoedematous infiltration of connective tissue ('puffy face syndrome'), and an inconspicuous periostitis of the tibia with delayed hyperaesthesia (Kérandel's sign).

In *T.b. rhodesiense* infection, this haemolymphatic stage is very pronounced with severe symptoms, sometimes even resulting in early death through cardiac involvement (myocarditis). In the early stage of *T.b. gambiense* infection, symptoms are usually infrequent and mild. Febrile episodes become less severe as the disease progresses.

Meningoencephalitic stage (HAT stage II)

Within weeks in *T.b. rhodesiense* and months in *T.b. gambiense* infection, cerebral involvement will invariably follow; trypanosomes cross the blood–brain barrier. In children, HAT progresses even more rapidly towards this meningoencephalitic stage.

The onset of stage II is insidious. The exact time of central nervous system involvement cannot be determined clinically. Histologically, perivascular infiltration of inflammatory cells ('cuffing') and glial proliferation can be detected, resembling endarteritis. As the disease progresses, patients complain of increasing headache, and their families may detect a marked change in behaviour and personality. Neurological symptoms, which follow gradually, can be focal or generalized, depending on the site of cellular damage in the central nervous system. Convulsions are common, usually indicating a poor prognosis. Periods of confusion and agitation slowly evolve towards a stage of distinct perplexity when patients lose interest in their surroundings and their own situation. Sleep abnormalities result finally in a somnolent and comatose state. Progressive wasting and dehydration follows the inability to eat and drink.

There is no unique, clinical sign of late HAT, opening up a wide range of possible neurological and psychiatric differential diagnoses. However, the appearance of the patient, with apathy and the typical expressionless face, is a very characteristic sight in endemic areas (Fig. 5 and Plate 3).

Table 2 Detection limits of various techniques in the diagnosis of HAT

Technique	Detection limit (no. of parasites/ ml sample)
In vitro isolation	100
Lymph node aspirates	50–100
Thin blood film	33
Wet blood film	25
Thick blood film	17
Capillary tube centrifugation	16
Quantitative buffy coat	16
Inoculation in mice	3–5
Inoculation in immunosuppressed mice	< 1
Mini anion exchange centrifugation technique	3–4
Cerebrospinal fluid with double centrifugation	1

Fig. 6 Trypanosomes in thin human blood film (Giemsa stain, ×1000 magnification). (See also Plate 4.)

for the diagnosis of blood parasites such as *Plasmodia* or microfilaria. Giemsa or Field staining techniques are appropriate (Fig. 6 and Plate 4).

Especially in *gambiense* HAT, parasitaemia is usually scanty and fluctuating, often being undetectable. Repeated examinations on successive days are sometimes necessary until trypanosomes can be documented.

Concentration methods

To increase the sensitivity of blood examinations, various concentration assays have been developed. Trypanosomes tend to accumulate in the buffy coat layer after centrifugation of a blood sample. The best results in the field have been obtained with the m-AECT (mini anion exchange column technique), where trypanosomes are concentrated after passage through a cellulose column, and the QBC method (quantitative buffy coat), which was originally developed for the diagnosis of malaria.

Serological assays

Serology is a useful tool to detect antibodies against trypanosomiasis. Various test methods have been described and are now commercially available. They are mainly based on ELISA technique or immunofluorescence, but provide reliable results only in *gambiense* HAT.

For rapid screening under field conditions, the CATT (card agglutination test for trypanosomiasis) is an excellent tool in areas of *T.b. gambiense* infestation. It is easy to perform and delivers results within 5 min. A visible agglutination in the CATT suggests the existence of antibodies, but does not necessarily imply overt disease.

Non-specific laboratory findings

Anaemia and thrombocytopenia are caused by systemic effects of cytokine release, especially of TNF-α. Hypergammaglobinaemia can reach extreme levels as a result of polyclonal activation of immunoglobulins. IgM levels detected in HAT are among the highest observed in any infectious disease.

Diagnosis of stage II

Stage determination is crucial for the correct management of a patient. This cannot be done on clinical grounds alone. Therefore, a lumbar puncture for the examination of the cerebrospinal fluid has to be performed in every patient found positive for trypanosomes in blood or lymph aspirate. In addition, a lumbar puncture should be performed in all patients with the clinical suspicion of HAT even if peripheral examinations had proved negative. A minimum of 5 ml of cerebrospinal fluid is required to examine for:

- Leucocytes—cerebral involvement in HAT stage II is accompanied by pleocytosis, mostly lymphocytes, in the cerebrospinal fluid. By convention a number of more than five cells per mm³ cerebrospinal fluid defines central nervous system involvement even if the patient does not (yet) have neurological symptoms. Pathognomonic for HAT is the appearance of activated plasma cells with eosinophilic inclusions in the cerebrospinal fluid, the morular cells of Mott (Fig. 7 and Plate 5).

- Trypanosomes—the chances of detecting trypanosomes in the cerebrospinal fluid increase with the level of pleocytosis and the technique used. The highest yield is obtained by cerebrospinal fluid double centrifugation.

- Protein—in patients with HAT, a level of 37 mg of protein per 100 ml cerebrospinal fluid (dye-binding protein assay) is highly suggestive of the advanced stage. Stage II HAT is characterized by an autochthonous production of IgM antibodies in the cerebrospinal fluid, which can be selectively detected if suitable laboratory facilities exist (e.g. latex IgM test).

Treatment

General considerations

HAT is curable, especially if the diagnosis is made in an early stage of the disease and treatment is administered correctly. In the stark reality of the African situation, however, there are many major obstacles to successful patient management:

1. Sleeping sickness is a disease of rural, remote places. The active foci of sleeping sickness are usually in far-away and insecure places, which are difficult to reach. Numerous treatment centres work under emergency

Fig. 7 Morular cell of Mott in a histological brain section of a stage II HAT patient (haematoxylin and eosin stain, ×1000 magnification). (See also Plate 5.)

conditions with extremely restricted resources. Many affected patients, without proper access to health care, are left unattended.

2. The diagnosis is difficult. Initial diagnosis and exact staging of trypanosomiasis requires sophisticated and dangerous methods, justified only in the hands of experienced personnel. Repetitive training programmes, constant supervision, and continuous quality control are necessary but in reality are rarely available.

3. The treatment of trypanosomiasis is extremely costly. Invariably it exceeds the locally available resources. However, external funding and a sustainable donor commitment for Africa is generally diminishing.

4. The treatment is complicated. Treatment of HAT is dangerous, prolonged, and usually requires hospitalization. Most patients with late-stage trypanosomiasis are severely ill and malnourished. Adverse drug reactions during treatment are difficult to assess due to concomitant pathologies. Their management requires considerable medical skill and good nursing care. Hospitals in rural Africa are often not sufficiently equipped to accomplish good patient care.

5. Many drugs are unavailable. Treatment of HAT is hampered by the limited availability of essential drugs on the international market. Many trypanosomicidal agents are on the verge of disappearance despite increasing demand. Many are no longer produced, as the affected patient populations cannot pay. The range of drugs is diminishing, and hardly any new treatments are in sight. This is especially worrying in view of the reported spread of drug resistance.

6. HAT treatment is not standardized. Trypanosomiasis treatment regimens vary considerably between countries and treatment centres. Results from different centres are comparable to only a very limited extent. Few properly conducted and sufficiently powerful clinical trials are available to evaluate duration, dosage, and possible combinations of drugs. There are few suitable research sites at major trypanosomiasis foci.

Stage I drugs

The treatment of HAT varies according to the trypanosome subspecies and the stage of the disease (Table 3).

Pentamidine

Since its introduction in 1937, pentamidine has become the drug of first choice for *gambiense* HAT stage I, achieving cure rates as high as 98 per cent. However, there are frequent failures in *rhodesiense* HAT. Lower rates of cellular pentamidine uptake in *T.b. rhodesiense* may explain these differences. Some cures of stage II infections have also been reported, but cerebrospinal fluid drug levels are usually not sufficiently high to guarantee a reliable trypanosomicidal effect in the central nervous system.

Pentamidine is usually given by deep intramuscular injection, manageable even in outpatients. If hospital care and reasonable monitoring conditions are available, an intravenous infusion, given in normal saline over 2 h, might be used instead. The main advantage of pentamidine over other drugs is the short treatment course and ease of administration. Adverse effects are related to the route of administration or its dose and are usually reversible (Table 4).

Pentamidine is also used as second-line therapy for visceral leishmaniasis and especially in the prophylaxis and treatment of opportunistic

Pneumocystis carinii pneumonia in AIDS. Since the advent of the HIV pandemic, the cost of pentamidine was increased more than tenfold by producers, making it unaffordable by health institutions in low-income countries. After an intervention by WHO, a limited amount of pentamidine is now made available for use in HAT at a subsidised rate.

Suramin

In the early twentieth century, the development of suramin, resulting from German research on the trypanosomicidal activity of various dyes ('Bayer 205'), was a major break-through in the field of tropical medicine. For the first time, African trypanosomiasis, at least in its early stages, became treatable.

Suramin is still used to treat stage I HAT, especially *rhodesiense*. Like pentamidine it does not reach therapeutic levels in cerebrospinal fluid. Suramin is injected intravenously after dilution in distilled water.

Adverse effects depend on nutritional status, concomitant illnesses (especially onchocerciasis) and the patient's clinical condition. Although life-threatening reactions have been described, serious adverse effects are rare and the drug remains one of the safest in trypanosomiasis treatment (Table 4).

Stage II drugs

Melarsoprol

Until the introduction of the arsenical compound melarsoprol in 1949, late stage trypanosomiasis was untreatable. Since then, it has remained the most widely used stage II antitrypanosomal drug both for *T.b. gambiense* and *rhodesiense* infections. It has saved many lives, but has a high rate of dangerous adverse effects. Increasing frequency of relapses and resistance has been reported in some parts of Uganda, Congo, and Angola.

Melarsoprol clears trypanosomes rapidly from the blood, lymph, and cerebrospinal fluid. Its toxicity usually restricts its use to late-stage disease. It is given by slow intravenous injection; extravascular leakage must be avoided.

A new, simpler regimen is based on recently acquired knowledge of the drug's pharmacokinetics (Table 4). The most important adverse effect is an acute encephalopathy, provoked around day 8 of the treatment course in 5 to 14 per cent of all patients. There is severe headache, convulsions, rapid neurological deterioration, or deepening of coma. Characteristically, the comatose patient's eyes remain open. Most probably, this is an immune-mediated reaction precipitated by release of parasite antigens in the first days of treatment. The overall case fatality ranges between 2 and 12 per cent, depending on the stage of disease and the quality of medical and nursing care. Simultaneous administration of glucocorticosteroids (prednisolone 1 mg/kg body weight; maximum 40 mg daily) reduces mortality, especially in cases with high cerebrospinal fluid pleocytosis. However, in areas where tuberculosis, amoebiasis, or strongyloidiasis are highly prevalent, corticosteroids have dangers of their own!

Eflornithine (DFMO)

Initially developed as antitumour agent, eflornithine was introduced in 1980 as an antitrypanosomal drug, in the hope that it might replace melarsoprol for treatment of stage II trypanosomiasis. However, exorbitant

Table 3 The choice of drugs in the treatment of sleeping sickness

		Gambiense sleeping sickness		*Rhodesiense* sleeping sickness
HAT	1st line:	Pentamidine	1st line:	Suramin
Stage I	2nd line:	Suramin Melarsoprol	2nd line:	Melarsoprol
HAT	1st line:	Melarsoprol	1st line:	Melarsoprol
Stage II	2nd line:	Eflornithine Nifurtimox	2nd line:	+ Nifurtimox

Table 4 Dosage and principal adverse reactions of antitrypanosomal agents

	Dosage regimen	Adverse drug reactions
Pentamidine	4 mg/kg body weight intramuscular daily or on alternate days for 7 to 10 injections	Hypotensive reaction with tachycardia, dizziness, even collapse and shock, especially after intravenous administration, close monitoring of pulse rate and blood pressure after injection is mandatory; inflammatory reactions at the site of injection (sterile abscesses, necrosis); renal, hepatic, and pancreatic dysfunction; neurotoxicity: peripheral polyneuropathy; bone marrow depression
Suramin	Day 1: Test dose of 4–5 mg/kg body weight Day 3, 10, 17, 24, and 31: 20 mg/kg body weight, maximum dose per injection 1 g	Pyrexia (very common); early hypersensitivity reactions such as nausea, circulatory collapse, urticaria; late hypersensitivity reactions: skin reactions (exfoliative dermatitis), haemolytic anaemia; renal impairment: albuminuria, cylinduria, haematuria (high renal tissue concentrations); regular urine checks during treatment are mandatory; neurotoxicity: peripheral neuropathy; bone marrow toxicity: agranulocytosis, thrombocytopenia
Melarsoprol	New regimen: Day 1–10: 2.2 mg/kg body weight	Treatment-induced encephalopathy; pyrexia; neurotoxicity: peripheral motor or sensory polyneuropathy; dermatological reactions: pruritus, exfoliative dermatitis; cardiotoxicity; renal and hepatic dysfunction
Eflornithine	Most commonly used dosage regimen: 100 mg/kg body weight at 6-hourly intervals for 14 days	Gastrointestinal symptoms such as nausea, vomiting and diarrhoea; bone marrow toxicity: anaemia, leucopenia, thrombocytopenia; alopecia, usually towards the end of the treatment cycle; neurological symptoms such as convulsions
Nifurtimox	5 mg/kg body weight 3 times daily for 30 days	Abdominal discomfort such as nausea, pains, and vomiting in half of the treated patients, often leading to a disruption of the treatment course; neurological complications: convulsions, impairment of cerebellar function, polyneuropathy; skin reactions

costs and limited availability have restricted its use to melarsoprol-refractory cases of *gambiense* sleeping sickness. *T.b. rhodesiense* isolates are normally much less sensitive.

It can be taken orally, but intravenous administration is preferred as it achieves a much higher bioavailability and success rate. Eflornithine should be administered slowly over a period of at least 30 min. Continuous 24-h administration is preferable if facilities allow.

The range of adverse reactions to eflornithine is wide, as with other cytotoxic drugs in cancer treatment. Their occurrence and intensity increase with the duration of treatment and the severity of the patient's general condition. Generally, all adverse effects of eflornithine are reversible (Table 4).

No pharmaceutical company has produced eflornithine for use against HAT since 1999, despite pressure by WHO. The discovery of its therapeutic effect in cosmetic creams against facial hair might help to restimulate production and thus have a beneficial 'spin-off effect' for HAT. In 2001 agreements were signed between WHO and two major drug producing companies which might help to assure a sufficient supply of eflornithine and other drugs essential for the treatment of HAT for the next few years.

Nifurtimox

Ten years after its introduction for the treatment of American trypanosomiasis in 1967, nifurtimox was found to be effective in the treatment of *gambiense* sleeping sickness. It has a place as second line treatment in melarsoprol-refractory cases or in a combination chemotherapy. Experience is limited to few cases treated on compassionate grounds. Prospective clinical trials in HAT are currently in progress.

Nifurtimox is generally not well tolerated, but adverse effects are usually not severe. They are dose-related and rapidly reversible after discontinuation of the drug (Table 4).

Combination treatments in HAT

Melarsoprol, eflornithine, and nifurtimox interfere with trypanothione synthesis and activity at different stages. There is also experimental evidence that combinations of suramin and stage II drugs might be beneficial. Therefore, by reducing the overall dosage of each individual component, drug combinations could perhaps reduce the frequency of serious side-effects, and the development of resistance, which are such common problems in the treatment of sleeping sickness.

Drug combination treatment of HAT is virtually confined to single-case reports. Properly conducted clinical trials are overdue.

Individual protection

HAT among tourists and occasional visitors of endemic areas is a rare event. Pentamidine or suramin chemoprophylaxis is historical, and can no longer be recommended. Long-sleeved, bright clothing and insecticide repellents are the best defence against attacking tsetse flies.

Prevention and control

In the past, tremendous efforts have been undertaken to control sleeping sickness as a threat to human lives and rural development. Control programmes are based on the five complementary pillars given in Table 5.

Table 5 Control of HAT

1. Diagnosis and treatment of patients
2. Active case finding
3. Vector control
4. Implementation and continuation of a surveillance system
5. Health education and community participation

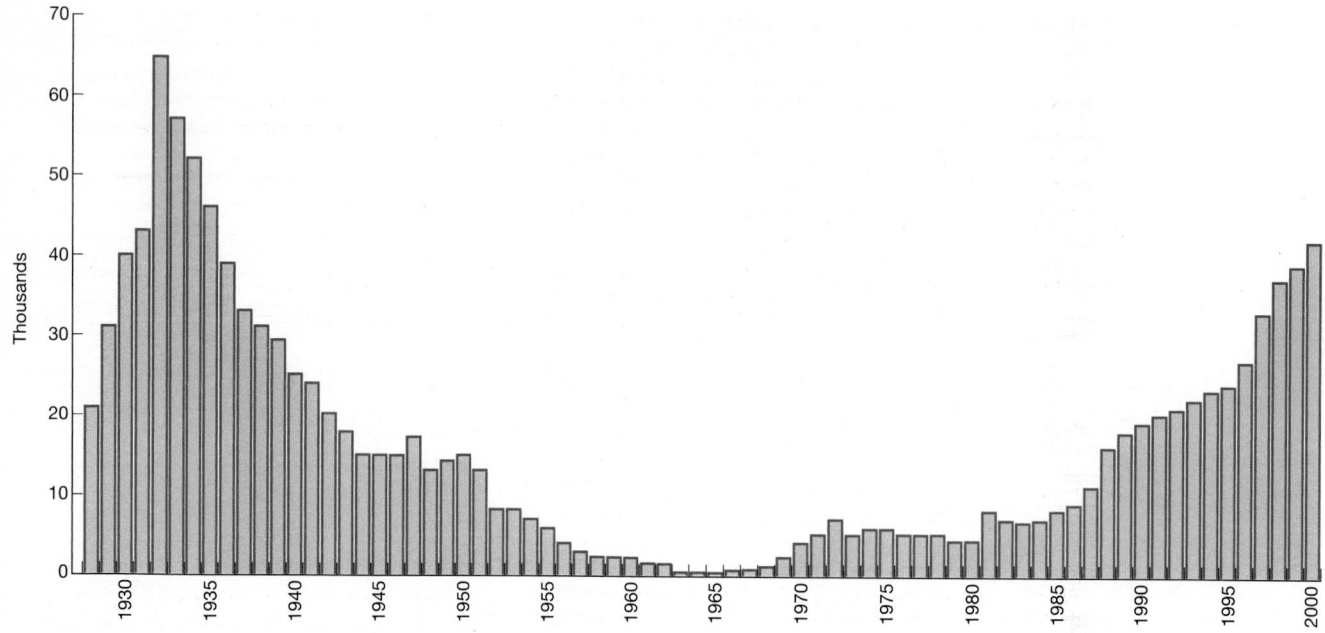

Fig. 8 Number of annually reported cases of HAT (source: WHO Report on Global Surveillance and Epidemic-prone Infectious Diseases); according to WHO, the actual patient numbers are about 10-fold higher.

The most important strategy is active case finding. This requires mobile teams, which regularly visit villages in endemic areas. Mostly based on the results of CATT screening, patients, preferably in the early stage of the disease, are identified and treated. Gradually, the parasite reservoir is depleted. As *Glossina* is a relatively incompetent vector and susceptible to control measures such as insecticide application or trapping, the combination of various approaches can lead to a complete break of the transmission cycle. This was achieved in the past in many places. However, the recent resurgence of sleeping sickness in areas ridden by war and civil unrest, in combination with the decreasing availability of drugs on the international market and the general loss of interest in health in Africa, gives rise to the fear that HAT will soon be again uncontrollable and untreatable (Fig. 8).

Trypanosomiasis in the twenty-first century

There is hardly any other tropical disease which demonstrates more clearly the dichotomy characterizing our modern age. On one side, trypanosomes are kept in culture and studied extensively in numerous research laboratories. Their genome is sequenced, and many molecular, biochemical, and immunological phenomena have been discovered as a result of basic science research. General interest in this disease is usually restricted to research aspects only. On the other hand, diagnostic and especially therapeutic tools are increasingly unavailable, because the hundreds of thousands of infected people in Africa are not commercially viable consumers. The prospects for fighting trypanosomiasis look grim. African countries are less and less able to implement effective control programmes, because of political instability or financial incapacity. Global concern about the crisis of human trypanosomiasis in Africa is a question of scientific ethics and international solidarity.

Further reading

Bailey JW, Smith DH (1992). The use of the acridine orange QBC technique in the diagnosis of African trypanosomiasis. *Transactions of the Royal Society of Tropical Medicine Hygiene* **86**, 630.

Burri C, Nkunku S, Merolle A, Smith T, Blum J, Brun R (2000). Efficacy of new, concise schedule for melarsoprol in treatment of sleeping sickness caused by *Trypanosoma brucei gambiense*: a randomised trial. *Lancet* **355**, 1419–25.

Dumas M, Bouteille B, Buguet A, eds. (1999). *Progress in human african trypanosomiasis, sleeping sickness.* Springer-Verlag, France.

Keiser J, Stich A, Burri C (2001). New drugs for the treatment of human African trypanosomiasis: research and development. *Parasitology Today* **17**, 42–9.

Pepin J, Milord F, Guern C, Mpia B, Ethier L, Mansinsa D (1989). Trial of prednisolone for prevention of melarsoprol-induced encephalopathy in gambiense sleeping sickness. *Lancet* **i**, 1246–50.

Smith DH, Pepin J, Stich A (1998). Human African trypanosomiasis: an emerging public health crisis. *British Medical Bulletin* **54**, 341–55.

World Health Organization (1998). *Control and surveillance of african trypanosomiasis.* WHO Technical Report Series 881. WHO, Geneva.

7.13.11 Chagas' disease

M. A. Miles

A poeira de Curvelo	The dust of Curvelo does not harm anybody
Não faz mal para ninguém não	
Do pulmão lá ninguém morre	No-one dies there of lung disease
O que mata é o coração	What kills is the heart

[From the poem 'O galo cantou na serra' by Luiz Claudio and Guimarães Rosa]

Introduction and aetiology

The Brazilian scientist, Carlos Chagas, discovered the disease that bears his name, and the entire lifecycle of the causative organism during a few months in 1907. Chagas first found the protozoan agent, *Trypanosoma*

Fig. 1 Adult female triatomine bug (*Panstrongylus megistus*), with a single egg shown adjacent to the tip of the abdomen. (By courtesy of Dr T.V. Barrett.) (See also Plate 1.)

(a)

(b)

Fig. 2 (a) Pseudocyst of *Trypanosoma cruzi* in heart muscle. (By courtesy of J.E. Williams.) (b) Pseudocyst of *Trypanosoma cruzi* in umbilical cord, from a congenital case of Chagas' disease. (By courtesy of Dr Hipolito de Almeida.) (See also Plate 2.)

cruzi, in the gut of the large blood-sucking insect vector—the triatomine bug (Hemiptera: Reduviidae, subfamily Triatominae) (Fig. 1 and Plate 1). Later he returned to bug-infested houses and detected *T. cruzi* in the blood of sick children.

T. cruzi is a kinetoplastid protozoan. In addition to the nucleus, it has a second, microscopically visible, DNA-containing organelle—the kinetoplast. The main lifecycle stages (trypomastigote, amastigote, epimastigote) are distinguished by the position of the kinetoplast relative to the nucleus, and by the presence or absence of a free flagellum.

Vector-borne transmission of *T. cruzi* is by contamination of the mammal host with infected faeces of triatomine bugs, not by their bite. During or shortly after feeding, bugs release liquid faeces and urine on to the skin of the host. Infective forms (metacyclic trypomastigotes) penetrate mucous membranes or abraded skin. Inside the mammal, *T. cruzi* is primarily an intracellular parasite. Trypomastigotes enter non-phagocytic or phagocytic cells, in which they transform to ovoid or round amastigotes (no flagellum). Amastigotes multiply inside the cell by binary fission to produce a pseudocyst (Fig. 2 and Plate 2). After 5 days or more, the pseudocyst ruptures to release numerous new trypomastigotes, which reinvade cells or circulate in the blood. Multiplication may occur at the site of infection, but pseudocysts subsequently predominate in muscle, especially heart and smooth muscle. In the blood, trypomastigotes are small, often C-shaped, with a large terminal kinetoplast (Fig. 3 and Plate 3). Trypomastigotes do not multiply in the blood. Triatomine bugs become infected by taking a blood meal from an infected mammal; birds and reptiles are not susceptible to infection. Infection in the bug is confined to the alimentary tract, where *T. cruzi* multiplies by binary fission as epimastigotes (kinetoplast adjacent to the nucleus). Metacyclic trypomastigotes are produced in the hindgut and rectum of the bug. All stages of the *T. cruzi* lifecycle can be cultured *in vitro*. *T. cruzi* can also be transmitted by blood transfusion, organ transplantation, transplacentally, to the infant via breast milk (rarely), and orally through food contaminated by triatomine faeces and the raw meat of infected mammals. Sexual transmission has not been documented.

Fig. 3 *Trypanosoma cruzi* C-shaped trypomastigote in blood, note large posterior kinetoplast. (See also Plate 3.)

Epidemiology

T. cruzi is confined to the Americas, although closely related organisms of the same subgenus (*Schizotrypanum*) are cosmopolitan in bats. The vast majority of the 133 triatomine bug species are also restricted to the Americas. Their natural habitats are the refuges of mammals, birds, and reptiles, in trees, in burrows, and among rocks. All mammals are thought to be susceptible to *T. cruzi*, which has been reported from at least 150 mammal species. The opossum (*Didelphis* spp.) is the most common sylvatic host. A few triatomine species thrive as domestic colonies. More than 10 000 bugs have been found in a single house. *Triatoma infestans* is widespread in Southern Cone countries of South America (Argentina, Bolivia, Brazil, Chile, Paraguay, Uruguay, and in southern Peru). *Rhodnius prolixus* is the common vector in northern South America and Central America, with *Triatoma dimidiata* as secondary vector in that region. *Panstrongylus megistus* infests central and eastern Brazil, and *Triatoma brasiliensis* north-eastern Brazil. Animals that share human dwellings, such as guinea-pigs, dogs, cats, rats, and mice are domestic reservoirs of *T. cruzi* infection. Chickens, although not susceptible to *T. cruzi*, encourage bug infestation and can sustain large colonies.

Serological surveys suggest that up to 20 million people are infected with *T. cruzi* in South and Central America. In some communities seropositivity rates exceed 70 per cent. As expected from the precarious contaminative route of transmission, prevalence rises with age. Based on prevalence, it is estimated that up to 300 000 new infections might occur in Latin America each year. Less than 200 cases are known from the Amazon Basin, but that is because the local forest vectors do not colonize houses. For the same reason, autochthonous infection is very rare in the United States.

Initial acute infections are frequently asymptomatic or overlooked. It is thought that less than 10 per cent of acute infections in children are fatal. Morbidity due to Chagas' disease arises primarily from the chronic infection. Once acquired, infection is usually carried for life. Around 30 per cent of those infected will subsequently display electrocardiograph (**ECG**) abnormalities and chagasic cardiomyopathy, and a proportion of those have associated megaoesophagus or megacolon.

There are marked regional differences in the epidemiology of Chagas' disease. Mega syndromes are common in central and eastern Brazil but virtually unknown in northern South America and Central America. Molecular genetics' research has shown that *T. cruzi* is not a single entity, but a species with a vast subspecific heterogeneity. There are at least two radically distinct strain groups, TC1 and TC2. TC1 predominates in sylvatic and domestic transmission cycles, north of the Amazon. TC2 predominates in domestic transmission cycles in Southern Cone countries.

Pathogenesis and pathology

At the portal of entry, local multiplication of *T. cruzi* may lead to unilateral conjunctivitis or to a skin lesion (Fig. 4 and Plate 4). Unruptured pseudocysts in muscle apparently generate no inflammatory response. Pseudocyst rupture is followed by infiltration of lymphocytes, monocytes, and/or polymorphonuclear cells. Antigens released from pseudocysts may spread and be adsorbed on to adjacent uninfected cells. Such uninfected cells may be attacked by the immune response of the host, and destroyed. In this way expanded focal lesions may be produced. Postmortem histology on human hearts and experimental studies in dogs have demonstrated a clear association between ECG abnormalities and focal lesions in the conducting system of the heart. Much damage may occur in the acute phase of infection, particularly if pseudocysts are numerous. Postmortem histology has demonstrated that neurone loss is a feature of chagasic cardiopathy and of mega syndromes. Neurone loss may be exacerbated by further disease or age-related loss. Thus a threshold may be reached, often many years after the acute infection, at which organ function is perturbed. Further ECG abnormalities, aperistalsis, and organ enlargement may ensue. This 'neurogenic' pathogenesis has been linked to sudden death.

Fig. 4 Romaña's sign in acute Chagas' disease. (See also Plate 4.)

Pathological exposure of normal host sequestered antigens, or sharing of antigens between *T. cruzi* and its host, may precipitate autoimmune pathogenesis. Some chronic chagasic cardiomyopathy is said to display a renewed intense inflammatory response and a progressive diffuse myocarditis, and a slow decline in cardiac function.

The contribution of the lifelong infection to the pathogenesis of chronic Chagas' disease is controversial. After the initial acute phase, trypomastigotes are only detectable in the blood by sensitive indirect methods. Similarly, pseudocysts in the tissues are infrequent, but are detectable immunologically and by amplification of *T. cruzi* DNA.

T. cruzi infection is controlled primarily by a cell-mediated immune response, especially the TH1 arm of the immune response. Patients immunocompromised by **AIDS** (acquired immunodeficiency syndrome) have impaired TH1 responses. Thus **HIV** (human immunodeficiency virus)-positive patients chronically infected with *T. cruzi* may suffer reactivated acute Chagas' disease, with microscopically patent parasitaemia, and poor prognosis.

At the level of gross pathology, substantial megacardia may be seen. Thinning of the myocardium may be present, with focal aneurysms visible upon transillumination, especially at the apex of the left ventricle (Fig. 5) and thrombus in the right atrial appendage (Fig. 6). Apical aneurysm is considered to be a pathognomonic sign of chronic chagasic cardiomyopathy. Megaoesophagus (Fig. 7) and megacolon (see Fig. 9) may show enormous dilatation and thinning of the wall. Chagasic megaoesophagus is more frequent than chagasic megacolon, but both are known from single individuals and each is often accompanied by chagasic heart disease. Chagasic megaoesophagus may be a prelude to carcinoma.

Clinical features

There are classically three clinical phases of Chagas' disease. Clinical signs in the acute phase may be fever, myalgia, headache, hepatosplenomegaly, generalized lymphadenopathy, facial or generalized oedema, rash, vomiting, diarrhoea, and anorexia. If *T. cruzi* has infected the eye, Romaña's sign may be present, with unilateral conjunctivitis and periophthalmic oedema (Fig. 4). If the portal of entry is the skin, an indurated oedematous cutaneous lesion (chagoma) may be seen. Regional lymphadenopathy may be

Fig. 5 Apical aneurysm of the left ventricle in chronic Chagas' disease. (By courtesy of Dr J.S. de Oliveira.) (See also Plate 5.)

Fig. 7 Megaoesophagus seen by radiography in chronic Chagas' disease. (By courtesy of Dr J.S. de Oliveira.) (See also Plate 7.)

present. Multiple chagomas may occasionally occur in acute-phase infections in infants. ECG abnormalities may include sinus tachycardia, increased P–R interval, T-wave changes, and low QRS voltage. The incubation period may be as short as 2 weeks, or as long as several months if infection is due to transfusion of contaminated blood. General lymphadenopathy and splenomegaly are frequent in blood transfusion-acquired infections.

Congenital acute infection may display fever, oedema, metastatic chagomas, neurological signs such as convulsions, tremors, and weak reflexes, and apnoea. Hepatosplenomegaly is frequent. The ECG is usually normal but low-voltage complexes, reduced T-wave height, and longer atrioventricular (AV) conduction time may be present.

Meningoencephalitis is rare in adults, more frequent in infants, common in immunocompromised patients, and carries a poor prognosis.

The clinical picture of AIDS-associated chagasic meningoencephalitis may be similar to toxoplasmosis. Haemorrhagic necrotic encephalitis is described in the nests of trypanosomes in microglia. Congenital infection may resemble toxoplasmosis, cytomegalic inclusion disease, or syphilis, with an increased likelihood of abortion and premature birth.

Symptomatic or asymptomatic acute infection may be followed by a symptom-free indeterminate phase of unpredictable length, which may be lifelong.

Chronic-phase symptoms may emerge in up to 30 per cent of patients recovering from the acute phase. Cardiac symptoms include arrhythmias, palpitations, chest pain, oedema, dizziness, syncope, and dyspnoea. The cardiac enlargement may be massive with chronic congestive cardiac failure, apical aneurysm (Fig. 5 and Plate 5), and thrombus in the right atrial appendage (Fig. 6 and Plate 6). The cardiac conducting system is involved, especially the sinus node, bundle of His and AV node, in which there is mononuclear and mast-cell infiltration, inflammation, and fibrosis. Characteristic ECG abnormalities are right bundle-branch block (**RBBB**) and left anterior hemiblock (**LAH**). AV conduction abnormalities, including AV block, may be present. Arrhythmias may include sinus bradycardia, sinoatrial block, ventricular tachycardia, primary T-wave changes, and abnormal Q-waves. The severity of heart disease is graded by the degree of disturbance. Sudden death is attributable, not to ruptured aneurysm but to arrhythmias often precipitated by exercise (e.g. on the football field). Radiography may reveal megacardia (Fig. 8). Signs of oesophageal involvement include loss of peristalsis, regurgitation, and dysphagia (Fig. 7 and Plate 7). Parotid enlargement may be associated. In megacolon there may be failure of defaecation, constipation, and faecaloma (Fig. 9 and Plate 8). Progressive dilatation of either organ can be graded clinically according to severity and may be detectable by radiography. Megaduodenum and megaureter are also described. The lymph nodes between the pulmonary trunk and the aorta are frequently enlarged.

A differential diagnosis requires distinction from other types of heart disease and ECG abnormality. RBBB and LAH are indicative, but a history of exposure to *T. cruzi* infection and laboratory diagnostic evidence must be considered (see below).

Laboratory diagnosis

A history of exposure to triatomine bugs, to potentially contaminated transfused blood, or a prolonged stay in endemic regions must be considered.

Fig. 6 Mural thrombus filling the right atrial appendage. (Copyright D.A. Warrell.) (See also Plate 6.)

Fig. 8 Chest radiograph showing gross cardiac enlargement in a Brazilian woman with chronic Chagas' disease. (Copyright D.A. Warrell.)

Motile trypomastigotes might be seen in unstained, wet blood preparations examined by microscopy. Nevertheless, parasitaemia is often scanty or undetectable by this method. The sensitivity of parasitological diagnosis may be enhanced by concentration methods, such as: microscopy of the centrifugation pellet from separated serum (Strout's method), microscopy of the haematocrit buffy coat layer, microscopy of Giemsa-stained thick films, or microscopy of the centrifugation sediment after lysis of red blood cells with 0.87 per cent ammonium chloride. All these tests may be negative if parasitaemia is low. Potentially infected blood must be handled with care, especially during haematocrit centrifugation, as a single trypomastigote can give rise to infection. Multiple blood cultures may also be performed, with a sensitive blood agar-based medium and physiological saline overlay. Even more sensitive than blood culture is xenodiagnosis, in which hungry fourth or fifth instar bugs from a triatomine colony, raised from bug eggs and fed only on birds, are allowed to feed on the patient. Bugs are applied in a plastic pot contained in a discrete black bag, which is tied beneath the patient's forearm. The bugs are dissected 20 to 25 days later. The hindgut and rectum are drawn out into a drop of sterile physiological saline, mixed with a blunt instrument (microspatula), and observed microscopically for motile epimastigotes and trypomastigotes. Dissection should be performed behind a small, Perspex safety screen or in a microbiological safety cabinet. *R. prolixus* is the most avid feeder for xenodiagnosis but may cause delayed

Fig. 9 Megacolon postmortem in chronic Chagas' disease. (By courtesy of Dr J.S. de Oliveira.) (See also Plate 8.)

hypersensitivity reactions in sensitized patients. The local vector should be used as the susceptibility of triatomine species varies with the strain of *T. cruzi*.

After the acute-phase infection, all the above methods of parasitological diagnosis will fail except xenodiagnosis, and possibly multiple blood cultures. Up to 50 per cent of patients in chronic phase may yield a positive xenodiagnosis, providing at least 10 triatomine bugs are used. Although polymerase chain reaction (**PCR**) amplification of *T. cruzi* DNA is sensitive and specific, it not available as a routine diagnostic test. Serum antibody is produced within a few days of *T. cruzi* infection and persists for life in untreated patients. There is an early IgM response, but it is not sustained at the high levels seen in African trypanosomiasis. Persistent IgG may be detected by the enzyme-linked immunosorbent assay (**ELISA**), by the indirect fluorescent-antibody test (**IFAT**), or by the indirect haemagglutination test (**IHAT**). Complement fixation, developed in 1913, is effective but now seldom used. Recombinant antigens are under trial but have not yet been adopted. Cross-reactions may occur, with visceral and mucocutaneous leishmaniasis, treponematoses, and possibly with other hyperimmune responses or autoimmune diseases. Serological assays must be standardized with negative and positive control sera, and by reference to experienced external reference centres to check reproducibility. Transplacentally acquired IgG may persist for up to 9 months in infants born of seropositive mothers. However, IgM specific seropositivity in such infants is an indicator of congenital infection.

Treatment

Proven acute cases must be treated promptly in an effort to minimize tissue damage and neurone loss. The synthetic oral nitrofuran, nifurtimox (LAMPIT®) from Bayer was the first successful drug for the treatment of Chagas' disease but it is no longer readily available. Benznidazole (Rochagan®) from Roche is now the sole first-line chemotherapy. An oral nitroimidazole, the adult dosage is 5 to 7 mg/kg for adults, in two divided doses, for 60 days; for children, 10 mg/kg also in two divided doses for 60 days. Adverse effects may demand interruption of treatment. These include rashes, fever, nausea, peripheral polyneuritis, leucopenia, and (rarely) agranulocytosis. Children tolerate treatment better than adults. Double or even higher doses have been used for immunocompromised patients, especially if meningoencephalitis is present. There is no guarantee that a full course of treatment will eliminate the infection. Although the value of drug treatment for chronic infections is still debated, it is favoured for children.

Chemotherapy is an important part of supportive treatment. In acute-phase heart failure, sodium intake is restricted and diuretics and digitalis may be indicated. Meningoencephalitis may require anticonvulsants, sedatives, and intravenous mannitol. Heart failure due to Chagas' disease may require vasodilatation (angiotensin-converting enzyme inhibitors) and maintenance of normal serum potassium levels; digitalis is a last resort because it may aggravate arrhythmias. A pacemaker may be fitted to improve bradycardia not responding to atropine, or for atrial fibrillation with a slow ventricular response that is not responsive to vagolytic drugs, or for complete AV block. Amiodarone has been suggested as the most useful drug to treat arrhythmias but it may still be aggravating. For ventricular extrasystoles lidocaine (lignocaine), mexiletine, propafenone, flecainide, and β-adrenoreceptor antagonists may be effective. Lidocaine may be used intravenously in emergencies. It is essential to consult detailed WHO expert reports and physicians with substantial experience in the management of chagasic heart disease.

Surgery is a vital part of case management for Chagas' disease. Resection of ventricular aneurysms has been suggested. Specialized surgery has been developed in Brazil for the treatment of megaoesophagus and megacolon. Early megaoesophagus may respond to balloon dilatation. The Heller–Vasconcelos operation, in which a portion of muscle at the junction of the oesophagus and stomach is removed, may alleviate megaoesophagus. Severe megaoesophagus requires replacement of the distal oesophagus, for example with a portion of jejenum. The modified Duhamel–Haddad operation has been considered the most successful surgery for correction of a megacolon: after resection, the colon is lowered through the retrorectal stump as a perineal colostomy. Subsequent suturing, under peridural anaesthesia, gives a wide junction between the colon and the rectal stump.

Prognosis, even in treated patients who show serological reversion, is unpredictable as the sequelae of damage due to the acute phase of Chagas' disease cannot be foreseen.

Prevention and control

There is no vaccine against Chagas' disease and no immunotherapy.

Chagas' disease flourishes on the back of poverty and in poor housing conditions. There are proven methods of controlling domestic triatomine bugs. These depend on insecticide spraying, health education, community support, and house improvement. Synthetic pyrethroids are the insecticides of choice, and several commercial sources are available. Vector control programmes consist of preparatory, attack, and vigilance phases. In the preparatory phase, the distribution of all dwellings must be mapped, the presence of infested houses assessed, and the attack and vigilance phases costed and planned. The attack phase involves spraying all houses and peridomestic buildings, irrespective of whether bugs have been found. During the vigilance phase, the community plays an essential role in reporting residual bug infestations, which elicit a rapid respraying response for the affected sites. Serology is vital for monitoring the success of control programmes. Children born after control programmes begin should be serologically negative beyond 9 months of age (to exclude transplacental transfer of IgG) except for infrequent cases of congenital transmission.

Blood donors in, or from, endemic areas should be screened serologically. If conditions demand the use of seropositive blood it can be decontaminated with crystal violet (250 mg per litre) and storage at 4 °C for at least 24 h. Potentially infected organ donors or recipients should be screened serologically. Seropositive immunosuppressed recipients are likely to suffer reactivated acute-phase infection. Prophylactic chemotherapy with benznidazole may be effective.

The Southern Cone Programme launched a massive effort to eliminate *T. infestans* from Argentina, Bolivia, Brazil, Chile, Paraguay, Uruguay, and from southern Peru. Domestic infestation in Brazil has been reduced by 85 per cent. Uruguay and Chile are essentially free of vector-borne and blood-transfusion transmission. Substantial progress has also been made in the other participating countries. Similar international collaborations are planned for the Andean Pact countries and for Central America. Reinvasion of sylvatic bugs into domestic habitats may complicate vector control in some regions. A surveillance programme and rapid responses to new domestic triatomine populations are planned to protect the Amazon against domiciliation of vectors.

T. cruzi is of immense research interest. It is not entirely clear how the organism evades the host immune response. Furthermore, the pathogenesis of Chagas' disease is not fully understood. Molecular methods have radically changed our understanding of the epidemiology of *T. cruzi* infection. Molecular features unique to trypanosomatids (trypanosomes and leishmanias) make *T. cruzi* an attractive model for molecular biologists. Further research is required to produce a non-toxic, low-cost oral drug, which would eliminate the reservoir of infection in humans, and to clarify further the population genetics and epidemiological significance of diverse strains. The origins and evolution of the organism and its vectors are also of considerable academic interest.

Trypanosoma rangeli

The second human trypanosomiasis in the New World is due to *T. rangeli* infection. *T. rangeli* is also transmitted by triatomine bugs, in particular the genus *Rhodnius*. In *Rhodnius* spp., however, *T. rangeli* traverses the wall of

the alimentary tract, infects the haemocoel, and reaches the salivary glands, in which the metacyclic infective trypomastigotes are produced. *T. rangeli* is thus transmitted by the bite of the triatomine bug and not by contamination with bug faeces. Although enzootic *T. rangeli* infection is widespread in Latin America, transmission to humans is virtually confined to areas in which *R. prolixus* is the domestic vector of *T. cruzi*. Co-infections of *T. cruzi* and *T. rangeli* may occur. The organism appears to be non-pathogenic in humans. *T. rangeli* can be pathogenic to *Rhodnius* spp. The importance of *T. rangeli* lies in the fact that it may confuse xenodiagnosis to detect *T. cruzi*. With care and experience, *T. rangeli* can be distinguished from *T. cruzi* either by its long slender epimastigotes (up to 80 μm in length), or by its smaller kinetoplast, or by its presence in the haemolymph or salivary glands of some xenodiagnosis bugs. The lifecycle in the mammalian host is uncertain, but *T. rangeli* is thought to divide in the peripheral blood. Trypomastigotes are rarely seen in human blood: they are much larger than *T. cruzi*, with a small subterminal kinetoplast. Antibodies to *T. cruzi* certainly crossreact strongly with *T. rangeli*. Based on experimental work in mice, *T. rangeli* infections are thought to induce very low crossreactive antibody titres to *T. cruzi*.

Further reading

Lent H, Wygodzinsky P (1979). Revision of the Triatominae (Hemiptera, Reduviidae) and their significance as vectors of Chagas disease. *Bulletin of the American Museum of Natural History.* **163**, 123–520. [An essential taxonomic monograph for all those interested in triatomine bugs, with keys for identification, but note that more species have since been described.]

Miles MA (1997). New World trypanosomiasis. In: Cox FEG, Kreier JP, Wakelin D, eds. *Topley and Wilson's microbiology and microbial infections*, pp. 283–302. London, Arnold. [A detailed account of the causative agent, the disease, and control efforts.]

Pan American Health Organization (1994). *Chagas disease and the nervous system*, Scientific publication No. 547. PAHO, Washington, DC. [An entire volume devoted to the interaction between *T. cruzi* and the nervous system.]

Raia AA (1983). *Manifestações Digestivas da Moléstia de Chagas*. Sarvier, São Paulo, Brasil. [For the surgeon, fascinating accounts of the development of lifesaving procedures, especially correction of megaoesophagus and megacolon (in Portuguese).]

World Health Organization (1991). *Control of Chagas disease*, Technical Report Series 811. WHO, Geneva. [Not strictly on control, but one of the best clinical reviews of Chagas' disease in the English language.]

7.13.12 Leishmaniasis

A. D. M. Bryceson

Leishmaniasis is caused by parasites of the genus *Leishmania*, which are transmitted by phlebotomine sandflies. The infection may be anthroponotic or zoonotic. In humans, the disease is usually either cutaneous or visceral. The most important variant is mucosal leishmaniasis of South and Central America. In certain places the disease is common and important, but there are few accurate statistics. The World Health Organization estimates 500 000 cases of visceral leishmaniasis and 1.5 to 2 million cases of cutaneous leishmaniasis annually, with 200 million people at risk of each disease.

Aetiological agent and lifecycle

In its vertebrate host the oval amastigote form of the parasite, which is 2 to 3 μm in diameter, is found in cells of the reticuloendothelial system

Fig. 1 Amastigotes of *Leishmania donovani* in a reticuloendothelial cell from the splenic aspirate of a patient with visceral leishmaniasis.

(Fig. 1). In the sandfly or in culture medium it is in the elongated, motile, promastigote form with an anterior flagellum.

The most important species of *Leishmania* that cause disease in humans and their own reservoir hosts are shown in Table 1; isoenzyme patterns and DNA hybridization are used to distinguish species.

Sandflies require a precise microclimate that is provided in certain places in each endemic focus at particular seasons of the year. Transmission is often seasonal. Amastigotes are ingested from blood or tissues of the mammalian host by the female fly, and transform into promastigotes in the gut, rendering the fly infective after about 10 days.

Cutaneous leishmaniasis

Epidemiology (see Table 1)

The vectors of *Leishmania major* live in rodent burrows. Hunters, travellers, tourists, and dwellers at oases or in new settlements are affected. The disease may be sporadic or epidemic. The vectors of *L. tropica* live in crevices in buildings and walls. The disease may be endemic or epidemic. The vector of *L. aethiopica* bites people sleeping in their huts. The disease is endemic and most people are affected by early adulthood. *L. infantum* causes simple,

self-healing skin lesions in some parts of southern Europe and North Africa. *L. donovani* causes post-kala-azar dermal leishmaniasis in India.

In the New World, transmission is usually in the forest. *L. brasiliensis*, the major cause of American cutaneous and mucosal leishmaniasis, is the most widely distributed of the New World species. Its vectors are highly anthropophilic and human infection is common. Periurban and urban foci of infection are increasing. Infection with *L. peruviana* occurs in high Andean valleys, where it may be locally common.

Pathogenesis and pathology

Leishmania inoculated by the sandfly invade and multiply in macrophages in the skin. The parasitized macrophage granuloma is infiltrated by lymphocytes and plasma cells. Piecemeal or focal necrosis destroys parasitized cells. The overlying epidermis shows hyperkeratosis, and ulcerates. In chronic lesions epithelioid cells and Langhans giant cells produce a picture similar to that of non-caseous tuberculosis. Rarely, the cellular immune response is suppressed and histology shows heavily parasitized macrophages with little or no lymphocytic infiltrate, characteristic of diffuse cutaneous leishmaniasis.

L. aethiopica, *L. mexicana*, and *L. brasiliensis* may invade cartilage. Cartilaginous lesions are extremely chronic. *L. brasiliensis*, and occasionally *L. panamensis* or *L. guyanensis*, may metastasize through the bloodstream to sites deep in the mucosa of the upper respiratory tract, where they may lie dormant. After months or years a lesion develops characterized by necrosis, vasculitis, and tissue destruction.

Immunity to a given species of *Leishmania* is usually lifelong. Second infections occur occasionally, especially in the elderly or immunosuppressed.

Clinical features

After an incubation period of a few days to several months an erythematous nodule develops at the site of the infected sandfly bite. A golden crust forms. The sore reaches its final size, usually 1 to 5 cm in diameter, over weeks or months. The crust may fall away leaving an ulcer with a raised edge (Fig. 2 and Plate 1). Satellite papules are common. After months or years the lesion starts to heal leaving a depressed, mottled scar. Secondary infection is unimportant. The lesion is not normally painful, but may disfigure or disable if scarring is severe or over a joint. Draining lymphatic vessels may be thickened or nodular.

Table 1 Epidemiology of leishmaniasis

Organism	Geographical location	Reservoir	Vector
Old World			
L. donovani	Northeast India, Bangladesh, Nepal	Humans	*Phlebotomus argentipes*
L. infantum	Mediterranean basin, Middle East, China, central Asia	Dogs, foxes, jackals	*P. perniciosus, P. major, P. chinensis* etc.
L. donovani (Africa)	Sudan, Kenya, Horn of Africa, ?Senegambia	?Rodents in Sudan, ?canines ?humans	*P. orientalis, P. martini*
L. major	Semideserts in Middle East, north India, Pakistan, North Africa, central Asia	Gerbils (especially *Rhombomys, Meriones* etc.)	*P. papatasi*
L. major	Sub-Saharan savannah, Sudan	Rodents (especially *Arvicanthus, Tatera*)	*P. duboscqi*
L. tropica	Towns in Middle East, Mediterranean basin, central Asia	Humans, ?dogs	*P. sergenti*
L. aethiopica	Highlands of Kenya, Ethiopia	Hyraxes (*Procavia, Heterohyrax*)	*P. longipes, P. pedifer*
New World			
L. chagasi, (=*L. infantum*)	Most of Central and South America, especially Brazil	Dogs, foxes opossums (*Didelphis*)	*Lutzomyia longipalpis, Lu. evansi*
L. mexicana	Central and northern South America	Forest rodents (especially *Ototylomys*)	*Lu. olmeca*
L. amazonensis	Tropical forests of South America	Forest rodents (especially *Proechimys, Oryzomys*)	*Lu. flaviscutellata*
L. brasiliensis	Tropical forests and cultivated land throughout South and Central America	?Forest rodents, dogs and equines	*Lu. wellcomei, Lu. whitmani,* etc., *Lutzomyia* spp.
L. guyanensis	Northern South America	Sloths (*Choleopus*), arboreal anteaters (*Tamandua*)	*Lu. umbratilis*
L. panamensis	Central America, Ecuador, Colombia	Sloths (*Choleopus*)	*Lu. trapidoi* etc.
L. peruviana	West Andes of Peru	Dogs, ?rodents, ?opossums	*Lu. verrucarum, Lu. peruensis*

Fig. 2 Shallow ulcer with raised edge due to *L. brasiliensis* (copyright A.D.M. Bryceson). (See also Plate 1.)

There are many variations on this classical pattern. Sores due to *L. major* form and heal rapidly (mean 3–5 months) and may be inflamed and exudative: the so-called wet or rural sore. Sores due to *L. tropica* tend to be less inflamed and to heal more slowly (mean 10–14 months): the so-called dry or urban sore. Lesions due to *L. infantum* have an incubation period of many months, and may persist over several years. In *L. aethiopica* infections lesions are usually central on the face. Satellite papules accumulate to produce a slowly growing, shiny tumour or plaque that may not crust or ulcerate, taking 2 to 5 years to heal (Fig. 3); mucocutaneous leishmaniasis may develop, producing swelling of the lips and expansion and elongation of the nose.

L. brasiliensis often causes deep, spreading ulcers, which heal over 6 to 24 months. Up to 15 per cent of patients will relapse after spontaneous or therapeutic cure. *L. mexicana* lesions are commonly on the limbs or side of the face, and heal in 6 to 8 months. Sores on the pinna of the ear may invade the cartilage, persist for many years, and destroy the pinna.

Fig. 3 Spreading nodular lesion, typical of *L. aethiopica*, Kenya.

Fig. 4 Diffuse cutaneous leishmaniasis, caused by *L. aethiopica*, Ethiopia.

Three forms of cutaneous leishmaniasis do not heal spontaneously: diffuse cutaneous leishmaniasis, leishmaniasis recidivans, and American mucosal leishmaniasis.

Diffuse cutaneous leishmaniasis

This occurs with *L. aethiopica* and *L. amazonensis* infections, but is rare. The primary nodule spreads locally without ulceration, and secondary blood-borne lesions appear on other sites in the skin, affecting especially the face and the cooler extensor surfaces of the limbs (Fig. 4). The eye, mucosae, viscera, and peripheral nerves are spared, in contrast with lepromatous leprosy with which it may be confused. The infection proceeds gradually over many years.

Leishmaniasis recidivans or lupoid leishmaniasis

This is a rare complication of *L. tropica* infection. The initial sore heals, but papules recrudesce in the edge of the scar and the lesion spreads slowly over many years (Fig. 5 and Plate 2).

Fig. 5 Lupoid or recidivans leishmaniasis in a citizen of Baghdad. (By courtesy of Dr Ahmed.) (See also Plate 2.)

Fig. 6 Swollen upper lip and nose due to mucosal leishmaniasis in Peru (copyright A.D.M. Bryceson). (See also Plate 3.)

American mucosal leishmaniasis, espundia

Up to 40 per cent of patients with untreated cutaneous ulcers due to *L. brasiliensis* may develop mucosal lesions, half of them within 2 years of the appearance of the original lesion, and 90 per cent within 10 years. About one in six patients gives no history of a previous skin lesion. In most cases the nasal mucosa is affected, and in one-third another site is also involved: the pharynx, palate, larynx, and upper lip, in order of frequency. The initial lesion is a nodule and the initial symptom is of nasal obstruction. It commonly presents as protuberant new growth of the nose or lips (Figs. 6 and 7 and Plates 3, 4), or cicatrization which causes an elongated 'tapir' nose. Mucosal leishmaniasis is slowly destructive, the septum perforates, and eventually the whole nose and mouth may be destroyed. Death may result from secondary sepsis, starvation, or laryngeal obstruction.

Fig. 7 Infiltration of lip and palate due to mucosal leishmaniasis in Peru (copyright A.D.M. Bryceson). (See also Plate 4.)

Laboratory findings

Parasitological diagnosis

Leishmania may normally be isolated from 80 per cent of sores during the first half of their natural course. The nodular part of the lesion is grasped firmly between the finger and thumb until it blanches. An incision a few millimetres long is made into the dermis with the point of a scalpel, which is used to scrape dermal tissue and juice. Material obtained may be used to inoculate special diphasic culture medium and to prepare smears for staining with Giemsa, Wright's, or Leishman's stain (Fig. 1). Biopsy material may be used to make impression smears, for culture and for histology. Diagnosis of mucosal leishmaniasis requires deep punch biopsy. Species diagnosis is desirable for American parasites, to assess the risk of mucosal leishmaniasis.

Immunological diagnosis

The leishmanin test is an intradermal test of delayed hypersensitivity which becomes positive in over 90 per cent of cases of self-healing forms of cutaneous leishmaniasis and mucosal leishmaniasis and is 95 per cent specific. Evaluation of a positive test must take into account naturally acquired positivity in the population at risk. Serology is unhelpful.

Treatment

Old World sores or those due to *L. mexicana*, *L. amazonensis*, and *L. peruviana* that are not troublesome may be left to heal naturally. But those that are disfiguring, potentially disabling, inconvenient, or around the ankle, where they heal slowly, should be treated either locally or systemically. Systemic treatment is required when there is risk that the sore may be due to *L. brasiliensis*, *L. panamensis*, or *L. guyanensis*, when the sore is too large or badly sited for local treatment, and for mucosal leishmaniasis, diffuse cutaneous leishmaniasis, and recidivans leishmaniasis.

Local treatment

Surgery, curettage, and cryotherapy are methods of removing small sores. Infiltration into the lesion with a pentavalent antimonial, twice weekly for 2 or 3 weeks, may be successful. Leishmanicidal ointments are under evaluation.

Systemic treatment (see Tables 2 and 3 for dosage regimens)

All cutaneous species of *Leishmania* are sensitive to pentavalent antimonials in conventional dosage except *L. aethiopica*, when pentamidine or paromomycin may be used. Ketoconazole may be useful for *L. major* and *L. mexicana* infections. Patients with diffuse cutaneous leishmaniasis should be treated for at least 2 months longer than it takes to clear parasites from

Table 2 Dosage regimens for the treatment of leishmaniasis (see text for choice of drug regimen)

Drug	Dose
Sodium stibogluconate or meglumine antimoniate	10–20 mg Sb/kg body weight once daily for 21 days (visceral or cutaneous disease) or 28 days (visceral or mucosal disease)—see Table 3 for dosage
Amimosidine	16 mg/kg body weight daily for 21 days
Pentamidine	4 mg salt/kg body weight once weekly to once monthly
Ketoconazole	60 mg/day (adult) for 4–6 weeks
Amphotericin B desoxycholate	1 mg/kg body weight on alternate days for 2 weeks (visceral disease) or 4–6 weeks (mucosal disease)
Liposomal amphotericin B (AmBisome®, NeXtar)	Ampoules of 50 mg, 2–3 mg/kg body weight daily for 7–10 doses, using whole ampoules to avoid waste, to total at least 21 mg/kg. In India a total dose of 6–9 mg/kg is sufficient

Table 3 Simplified dosage regimens for pentavalent antimonials based on body surface area according to the formula body surface area in m² = 0.1³/kg², whereby a 20 kg child receives 20 mg Sb/kg at 542 mg Sb/m². (Adapted from Anabwani GM and Bryceson ADM (1982). *Indian Paediatrics* **19**, 819–22)

Nearest weight of patient (kg)	Calculated dose (mg Sb)	Recommended dose as ml of	
		Pentostam (mg Sb)	Glucantime (mg Sb)
90	1088	11.0 (1100)	13.0 (1105)
80	1006	10.0 (1000)	12.0 (1220)
70	925	9.5 (950)	11.0 (935)
60	832	8.5 (850)	10.0 (850)
50	737	7.5 (750)	9.0 (765)
40	635	6.5 (650)	7.5 (637)
30	524	5.0 (500)	6.0 (510)
20	400	4.0 (400)	5.0 (425)
10	252	2.5 (250)	3.0 (255)
5	159	2.0 (200)	2.5 (212)

Pentostam (Wellcome Foundation) = sodium stibogluconate solution, containing 100 mg Sb/ml. Glucantime (Specia) = meglumine antimoniate solution containing 85 mg Sb/ml.

the skin, and relapses should be treated again promptly. Relapsed cases of mucosal leishmaniasis have usually become unresponsive to antimonials and should be treated with amphotericin B desoxycholate for at least 4 to 6 weeks or liposomal amphotericin B for 3 weeks. In addition they may require antibiotics for secondary sepsis, attention to nutrition, and later plastic surgery.

Visceral leishmaniasis

Epidemiology

Visceral leishmaniasis is found in four main zoogeographical zones (Table 1). Around the Mediterranean littoral, across the Middle East and central Asia, and in northern and eastern China human disease is endemic in many places. Children under 5 years of age are especially affected. In other places the disease is sporadic. Non-immune adults such as tourists, hunters, and soldiers are susceptible. The Ganges and Brahmaputra river valleys of India and Bangladesh are the home of epidemic visceral leishmaniasis, or kala-azar, which returns approximately every 15 to 20 years. The majority of cases are in young people under 15 years of age. In the interepidemic period the parasite survives in patients with post-kala-azar dermal leishmaniasis. Visceral leishmaniasis is endemic in parts of Sudan and Kenya. Older children and teenagers are most commonly affected. Sporadic cases also occur in nomads and visitors. An epidemic that began in southern Sudan in the late 1980s is still raging, and has caused over 100 000 deaths. It has been especially severe among refugees from the civil war.

In South America the disease is most common in northeastern Brazil, where older children are affected. Previously a rural disease, it is becoming increasingly important in towns.

Visceral leishmaniasis may be transmitted by blood transfusion from subclinical cases and appears unexpectedly in immunosuppressed patients, for example after renal transplantation, or as an opportunistic infection with HIV.

Pathogenesis and pathology

For every case of classical visceral leishmaniasis, there are about 30 subclinical infections that cause leishmanin positivity and lifelong immunity to *L. donovani*. Malnutrition predisposes to clinical disease. Established visceral infections are characterized by the failure of specific cell-mediated immunity. The leishmanin test is negative. The parasite multiplies freely in macrophages in the spleen, bone marrow, lymphoid tissues, and jejunal submucosa and Kupffer cells of the liver. Histology shows a variable degree

of granuloma formation, and of interstitial inflammation in the liver that may lead to fibrosis. In the spleen especially there is massive reticuloendothelial hyperplasia and infiltration with plasma cells. Small splenic infarcts may develop.

Antibodies, polyclonal IgG, and immune complexes circulate at high concentration but rarely cause complications. About half of patients have mild malabsorption but seldom diarrhoea. Jaundice when present is usually due to intercurrent viral hepatitis. Spontaneous bleeding is unusual and is associated with hypoprothrombinaemia. Visceral leishmaniasis is characterized by anaemia, leucopenia, thrombocytopenia, and hypoalbuminaemia. The anaemia results mainly from shortened red-cell survival with destruction of cells in the spleen, together with splenic pooling and sequestration (hypersplenism). In young children, profound anaemia may develop rapidly as a result of severe haemolysis. Death is usually due to secondary infection.

Clinical features

The male/female ratio is between 3:1 and 4:1. The incubation period is usually 2 to 8 months. In endemic areas the onset is usually ill defined. The patient develops fever, discomfort from an enlarged spleen, abdominal swelling, weight loss, cough, or diarrhoea. Classically the fever spikes twice daily, usually without rigors, but daily, irregular, or undulant fevers are common. During an epidemic or in visitors to an epidemic area, the onset may be abrupt with high fever and rapid progression of illness with toxaemia, weakness, dyspnoea, and acute anaemia.

Physical examination of early cases may show only symptomless splenomegaly. Late cases are wasted with hair changes and pedal oedema typical of hypoalbuminaemia. Hyperpigmentation is characteristic of visceral leishmaniasis in India (kala-azar means black sickness). The spleen is huge, smooth, and non-tender unless there has been a recent infarct. The liver is moderately enlarged in one-third of cases. In Africa generalized lymphadenopathy is common.

Over months or years the patient becomes emaciated, with a distended abdomen (Fig. 8). Intercurrent infections are common, especially pneumococcal otitis, pneumonia, septicaemia, tuberculosis, measles, dysentery, other locally important infections, and rarely, cancrum oris. Untreated, 80 to 90 per cent of patients die.

Post-kala-azar dermal leishmaniasis

Twenty per cent of Indian patients and 5 per cent of African patients develop a rash on the face and extensor surfaces of the arms and legs after recovery from visceral leishmaniasis. In India the rash begins after an interval of 1 or 2 years and progresses over many years: pale macules become erythematous plaques or nodules resembling lepromatous leprosy, and almost all the body surface may be involved (Fig. 9). In Africa the rash

Fig. 8 Visceral leishmaniasis in a Kenyan child. Note the wasting and massive enlargement of spleen and liver.

Fig. 9 Post-kala-azar dermal leishmaniasis in an Indian child, showing the typical hypopigmented macular rash. Note also the nodules on the lower lip.

appears while the patient is still recovering, as discrete nodules which show a tuberculoid histology. It heals spontaneously within 6 months.

Visceral leishmaniasis and AIDS

Visceral leishmaniasis may be associated with HIV infection and is an AIDS-defining illness in adults in southern Europe, where it is commonest among intravenous drug users. It may be due to reactivation of latent infection with *Leishmania* or to a recent infection. In Spain, over 50 per cent of adults with visceral leishmaniasis are HIV positive, and it is estimated that 9 per cent of HIV-infected individuals will acquire visceral leishmaniasis. The presentation may not be typical. Often the parasite is found by chance, for example in a rectal or skin biopsy taken for other purposes, or in bronchoscopic lavage. The bone marrow is teeming with parasites, but two-thirds of cases have no detectable antileishmanial antibodies. In 90 per cent of cases the CD4 count is less than 0.2×10^6/litre.

Laboratory diagnosis

Parasitological diagnosis

Leishmania may be isolated from reticuloendothelial tissue. Yields are of the order: spleen over 95 per cent, bone marrow or liver 85 per cent, African lymph node 65 per cent, and buffy coat 70 per cent. Bone marrow aspiration is most commonly used, but splenic aspiration is simple, painless, and safe if the prothrombin time is normal and the platelet count above 40 $\times 10^9$/litre. Occasionally, the diagnosis is made accidentally on biopsy of bone marrow, liver, lymph node, or bowel mucosa. Antibodies are present in high titre. Indirect immunofluorescence is suitable for individual cases. Enzyme-linked immunosorbent assay or direct agglutination are the techniques of choice for field diagnosis. The leishmanin test is negative.

Other findings

There is normochromic, normocytic anaemia without reticulocytosis, and neutropenia, eosinopenia, and thrombocytopenia. Serum albumin is low (~20 g/litre) and globulin high (~70 g/litre), IgG and IgM being approximately thrice and twice the normal population values. Hepatic enzymes and prothrombin and partial thromboplastin times are usually normal.

Treatment

Chemotherapy (see Tables 2 and 3 for dosage regimens)

Liposomal amphotericin B (AmBisome) by intravenous infusion is the best drug for visceral leishmaniasis. It is concentrated and retained in reticuloendothelial cells and is not toxic. All patients respond promptly, but HIV-coinfected patients relapse. At the moment it is far too costly for most countries where visceral leishmaniasis is endemic. Therefore, a pentavalent antimonial remains the drug of choice in most situations.

Sodium stibogluconate containing 100 mg antimony (Sb) per millilitre and meglumine antimoniate containing 85 mg Sb/ml, are of equal efficacy and toxicity. The drug is administered by intramuscular injection, which may be painful, or by intravenous injection through a fine-gauge needle, slowly or by infusion in 50 to 100 ml of 5 per cent dextrose over 20 min to reduce the risk of venous thrombosis. Treatment is given daily for 21 days. Usually the drug is well tolerated, but towards the end of treatment there may be malaise, anorexia, nausea, vomiting, and muscle pains. Should toxic effects develop, rest for 1 day and reduce each dose by 2 mg Sb/kg. Hepatic and pancreatic enzyme levels may rise and haemoglobin levels fall, but they return to normal when treatment is stopped. The electrocardiogram develops unimportant T-wave changes. At higher doses the corrected QT interval may be prolonged, heralding the development of a serious arrhythmia. If it is essential, for example during an epidemic, to give a shorter course of treatment, 10 mg Sb/kg may safely be given every 8 h for 10 days.

The aminoglycoside antibiotic paromomycin or aminosidine (IDA Pharmamed) is equally effective and well tolerated. It is given by intramuscular injection or intravenous infusion over 90 min.

In India, conventional amphotericin B desoxycholate is particularly effective. A new oral drug miltefosine is undergoing trials

Patients who are immunosuppressed as a result of HIV coinfection or immunosuppressive drugs respond slowly, require longer treatment, and are more liable to relapse than immunocompetent patients. Ideally, treatment of such patients should be monitored by splenic aspirate counts of parasites, and continued for 2 to 3 weeks beyond parasitological cure. Aminosidine is the drug of choice, as it is well tolerated and not prohibitively expensive. Renal function and hearing should be monitored. Clinical pancreatitis has been reported with the antimonials. Liposomal amphotericin B, although well tolerated, does not prevent relapse.

Supportive treatment

Intercurrent infection must be sought and treated, and nutritional deficiencies corrected. Blood transfusion is rarely needed.

Response to treatment

Fever, splenic size, haemoglobin, serum albumin, and body weight are useful monitors of progress. Proof of parasitological cure is not usually necessary. Reassessment at 6 weeks and 6 months will detect over 90 per cent of relapses. Relapse rates should be almost zero in Mediterranean and Indian disease and about 2 per cent in African disease. Relapsed patients are slower to respond, and run a 40 per cent chance of further relapse(s) and of becoming unresponsive to antimony. Primary resistance to antimonials is increasing in India where the first choice lies between aminosidine and amphotericin B desoxycholate.

Prevention and control of cutaneous and visceral leishmaniasis

Prevention is a matter of controlling reservoir hosts and sandfly vectors, or of avoiding bites by vectors. Successful control requires an accurate knowledge of transmission in each ecological focus.

In the Old World, urban cutaneous leishmaniasis is controlled by case-finding and treatment, better housing, and domestic spraying with residual insecticides, while rural leishmaniasis is controlled in the Middle East and

North Africa by the destruction of gerbil colonies. Mediterranean and urban visceral leishmaniasis in South America may be controlled by the destruction or treatment of dogs. In India, mass campaigns to spray houses and cattle sheds are needed. In the interepidemic period, cases of post-kala-azar dermal leishmaniasis should be sought and treated.

Individuals may take precautions to prevent infection during the season of transmission by the use of insect repellent creams and fine mesh bed nets or chadors impregnated with permethrin.

Further reading

Alvar J *et al.* (1997). Leishmania and human immunodeficiency virus coinfection: the first 10 years. *Clinical Microbiology Review* **10**, 298–319.

Berman JD *et al.* (1998). Efficacy and safety of liposomal amphotericin B (AmBisome) for visceral leishmaniasis in endemic developing countries. *Bulletin of the World Health Organization* **76**, 25–32.

Grimaldi G Jr, Tesh RB, McMahon-Pratt D (1989). A review of the geographic distribution and epidemiology of leishmaniasis in the New World. *American Journal of Tropical Medicine and Hygiene* **41**, 687–725.

Jha TK *et al.* (1998). Randomised controlled trial of aminosidine (paromomycin) v sodium stibogluconate for treating visceral leishmaniasis in North Bihar, India [see comments]. *British Medical Journal* **316**, 1200–5.

Jha TK *et al.* (1999). Miltefosine, an oral agent, for the treatment of Indian visceral leishmaniasis [see comments]. *New England Journas of Medicine* **341**, 1795–800.

Seaman J, Mercer AJ, Sondorp E (1996). The epidemic of visceral leishmaniasis in western Upper Nile, southern Sudan: course and impact from 1984 to 1994. *International Journal of Epidemiology* **25**, 862–71.

WHO Expert Committee (1990). Control of the leishmaniases. *World Health Organization Technical Reports Series* **793**, 1–158.

7.13.13 Trichomoniasis

J. P. Ackers

Urogenital trichomoniasis is caused by infection with the protozoan *Trichomonas vaginalis*. About 170 million new cases each year may well make it the world's commonest non-viral sexually transmitted infection.

In clinical specimens or culture *T. vaginalis* is a motile, round or oval flagellate 10 to 13 μm long and 8 to 10 μm wide; fixed and stained it is about 25 per cent smaller (Fig. 1 and Plate 1). Diagnostic features include the jerky motility, undulating membrane, and microtubular rod (axostyle), which runs through the body and projects as a thin spine from the pos-

Fig. 1 Trichomonads, Giemsa stain, in vaginal secretions. (Copyright J.P. Ackers.) (See also Plate 1.)

terior end. In contact with vaginal epithelial cells *in vitro* the organism becomes extremely flattened and adherent. The lifecycle is simple; no resistant cysts are formed and there are no intermediate or reservoir hosts.

Two other trichomonads—*T. tenax* and *Pentatrichomonas hominis*—are uncommon and probably harmless human parasites of the mouth and large bowel, respectively. All three species are site specific. Urogenital trichomoniasis is not due to contamination from other sites.

Epidemiology

Although it is often difficult to isolate the organism from male contacts of infected women, all epidemiological evidence suggests that the vast majority of infections are sexually acquired. *T. vaginalis* has been shown to survive for many hours at room temperature if kept damp so the theoretical possibility of non-venereal transmission exists. It is also known that a very small proportion of female babies of infected mothers will become infected during birth, but the infection is transient and trichomoniasis discovered in a child should immediately raise the suspicion of sexual abuse.

Very few studies have been made of genuinely unselected populations; the majority have examined either pregnant women or those attending sexually transmitted disease clinics. There are wide variations but most report that 10 to 25 per cent of patients are infected, although the full range is 0 to 63 per cent. Usually female cases outnumber males by 5 or 10 to 1. In several developed countries there has been a steady decline in the incidence of trichomoniasis in the past two decades, but this has not occurred in less-developed countries nor in deprived inner-city areas in industrialized nations. Human trichomoniasis is becoming a disease of the underprivileged.

Pathogenesis

In vitro, *T. vaginalis* has a well defined, contact-mediated, cytotoxic effect, but the relationship of this to pathogenesis *in vivo* is not known. The organism activates complement and attracts neutrophils; several together can kill the parasite, but their presence in large numbers may be responsible for much of the pathology observed. It seems likely that differences in clinical severity are due to both host and parasite factors.

Symptoms

In women trichomoniasis may present as anything from an asymptomatic infection (10 to 50 per cent of cases) to an acute inflammatory diseases with a copious and malodorous discharge; vulvovaginal soreness and irritation, dysuria, and dyspareunia are also frequently mentioned. The discharge may vary over time and, untreated, the infection may be spontaneously lost or persist for months or years. A recent study showed trichomoniasis significantly associated with symptoms of yellow vaginal discharge and vulvar itching and signs of colpitis macularis (strawberry cervix), purulent vaginal discharge, and vulval and vaginal erythema. Colpitis was seen frequently if colposcopy was undertaken, but hardly ever by naked-eye examination. Vaginal pH is usually elevated.

The majority of men with trichomoniasis are asymptomatic, but the parasite is responsible for a small but increasing proportion of cases of non-gonococcal urethritis.

Pathology

In women, *T. vaginalis* may be found in the vagina and the exterior cervix in over 95 per cent of infections, but is recovered from the endocervix in only 13 per cent. The urethra and Skene's glands are also commonly infected. In men the urethra is the most common site of infection, but the organism has also been recovered from epididymal aspirates. Dissemination beyond the lower urogenital tract is extremely rare even in severely immunocompromised patients.

Previously regarded as unpleasant but harmless, epidemiological studies have recently linked trichomoniasis in women with a modest increase in the risk of heterosexual HIV transmission and with adverse pregnancy outcome and have suggested that it might cause a few per cent of cervical neoplasias.

Laboratory diagnosis

The symptoms and signs are not sufficient to establish the diagnosis, which must be made by detecting the parasite. This is most frequently achieved by wet-film microscopic examination of vaginal (not endocervical) secretions, urethral scrapings, centrifuged urine sediment, or prostatic fluid. The specimen should be examined as soon as possible—a motile trichomonad is unmistakable. Sensitivity is moderate, 50 to 70 per cent in women but only 10 to 20 per cent in men.

Culture provides significantly greater sensitivity; media vary in efficiency but Diamond's TYM and the very convenient if rather expensive InPouch® system are amongst the best.

Antigen detection, DNA probe, and polymerase chain reaction (**PCR**)-based tests have been developed; none has yet found widespread acceptance but the sensitivity of the PCR-based methods offers new possibilities for making an accurate diagnosis on specimens obtained in less invasive ways including self-administered tampons.

Treatment

The 5-nitroimidazole drugs provided the first and so far only group of effective chemotherapeutic agents. Doses given here are for metronidazole and should be adjusted to give the equivalent amount of other compounds. Two regimens are used—the original one of 250 mg three times a day for 7 days, or a single 1.6 or 2 g dose. Cure rates in women are similar (about 95 per cent) with both regimens if male sexual partners are also treated, but appear to be lower with the single-dose regimen if they are not. Only the 7-day regimen has been extensively evaluated in males, where it is equally effective. Treatment failures with any of the 5-nitroimidazole drugs are rare, but a proportion is due to resistant parasites.

Further reading

Honigberg BM, ed. (1989). *Trichomonads parasitic in humans*. Springer-Verlag, New York.

Krieger JN (1995). Trichomoniasis in men: old issues and new data. *Sexually Transmitted Diseases* **22**, 83–96.

Petrin D *et al.* (1998). Clinical and microbiological aspects of *Trichomonas vaginalis*. *Clinical Microbiology Review* **11**, 300–17.

7.14 Nematodes (roundworms)

7.14.1 Cutaneous filariasis

G. M. Burnham

Filarial infections of the skin and soft tissues

Filarial infections of man and animal are worldwide. Of the filarias which primarily affect the skin or subcutaneous tissues of man—*Onchocerca volvulus*, *Loa loa*, and *Mansonella streptocerca*—the burden imposed by *O. volvulus* is by far the greatest. *Loa loa* produces self-limited swellings of the extremities and the migrating adult worm may be seen subcutaneously. *Mansonella perstans* and *Mansonella ozzardi* cause minimal if any symptoms.

Onchocerciasis

Onchocerciasis, or river blindness, occurs in 34 countries in Africa, Latin America, and the Arabian Peninsula. An estimated 17.7 million people are infected, the vast majority in Africa. Infection has caused blindness in 270 000 and left another 500 000 with severe visual impairment. Besides eye changes, onchocerciasis has chronic systemic effects, causing extensive and disfiguring skin changes, musculoskeletal complaints, weight loss, changes to the immune system, and perhaps epilepsy and growth arrest as well. Of all the manifestations of onchocerciasis, skin lesions are the most common. These include acute and chronic itchy papular disease, and intensely pruritic lichenification. Lesions may be localized or widespread. In later stages, degenerative skin disease develops with a loss of elastic tissue, and extensive pigmentary changes.

The disease, endemic to some of the world's poorest areas, has great impact on the economic and social fabric of communities. A complex human–parasite tolerance allows people who host millions of parasites to continue daily existence. The discovery of ivermectin treatment has brought untold benefits to victims of the disease and to their communities.

Epidemiology

The microfilariae of *O. volvulus* were first observed by O'Neill in Ghana in 1875 in an intensely pruritic chronic skin condition called 'Craw-craw,' Leuckart described the adult worm 20 years later, and in 1923 Blacklock in Sierra Leone showed the blackfly, *Simulium damnosum*, to be the vector. Hissette in the Congo, and Robles in Guatemala linked blindness with onchocerciasis. Long before, Ghanians along the Red Volta river had associated the biting flies with skin lesions and blindness.

Vector control has now interrupted onchocerciasis transmission in the Volta river basin of West Africa, leaving the largest numbers of infected people in Nigeria, Cameroon, Chad, Ethiopia, Uganda, and the Congo.

Most African foci are fairly stable, but in South America, foci continue to enlarge and new ones are found. Within foci, the disease may occur unevenly due to differences in both distribution of flies and exposure to bites. In the Americas, onchocerciasis is most common in the highland areas of Guatemala. Other countries with disease foci are Mexico, Venezuela, Colombia, Brazil, and Ecuador

In Africa, blindness was noted to be more common in savannah and woodland than rain forest areas, but people in forest areas had more depigmented skin disease. Parasite DNA probes have shown the existence of different strains or forms of the parasite, particularly in West Africa, although migration may now be blurring this geographical distribution. Other factors such as population density, genetic factors, transmission patterns, and perhaps nutrition may contribute to the risk of blindness. Onchocercal skin disease may reduce marital prospects (and dowry size), disrupt social relationships, and decrease the productivity of agricultural workers.

Experimental studies suggested considerable variation in the efficiency with which sibling species of *Simulium* flies transmitted forest and savannah strains of the parasite. This has given rise to the concept of vector–parasite complexes in which forest strains of parasites are preferentially transmitted by forest sibling species of flies and savannah strains by savannah sibling species. However, recent studies using polymerase chain reaction (**PCR**)-amplified *O. volvulus* larval DNA have questioned the importance of transmission complexes.

Parasitology

Larvae of *O. volvulus* enter the human during the blood meal taken by an infected female *Simulium* fly. Within 1 to 3 months larvae develop into male or female adult worms within palpable nodules commonly located over bony prominences of the thorax, pelvic girdle, or the knees (Fig. 1 and

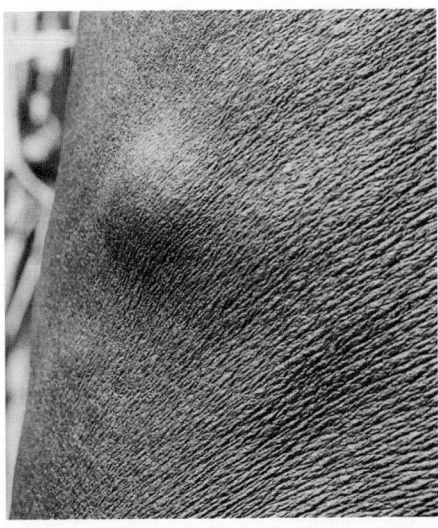

Fig. 1 A 3-cm subcutaneous nodule. (See also Plate 1.)

Plate 1). Nodules may be found on the head, particularly among children. These average 3 cm in diameter and are easily palpable, but some are deep, particularly around the pelvis.

A female worm may release 1300 to 1900 microfilariae per day for 9 to 11 years. From the nodules, these microfilariae find their way mainly to the skin and eye. In the skin they are found predominantly in the lymphatics of the subepidermis. In the eye, most are in the anterior chamber, but they are also found in the retina and optic nerve. When an infected human is bitten, anticoagulants from the *Simulium* fly create a pool of blood from which blood and microfilariae are ingested. Within the fly, those microfilariae that survive moult twice over the following 6 to 12 days to become infective larvae.

Microfilariae are about 250 to 300 µm in length and may live up to 2 years. They move easily through the skin and connective tissue ordinarily remaining within lymphatic vessels and provoking little reaction while alive. They have been seen in blood, urine, cerebrospinal fluid, and internal organs. One hundred million or more microfilariae may be present in heavily infected people. While live microfilariae are tolerated by their human hosts, dead and dying microfilariae may evoke intense inflammatory reactions which are responsible for the eye and skin damage. Tolerance of microfilariae may be regulated by MHC-encoded molecules.

Important species of *Simulium* are really complexes made up of sibling species, identifiable through banding patterns of their larval chromosomes. In Africa the main vectors are members of the *S. damnosum* complex or *sensu lato* (*s.l.*), which can fly long distances. The vector in areas of Uganda, Tanzania, Ethiopia, and the Congo are members of the *S. neavei* complex. In the Americas complexes of *S. ochraceum*, *S. metallicum*, and *S. exiguum* are the principal vectors, and these cover shorter distances. Some *Simulium* will bite humans almost exclusively while others are to varying degrees zoophilic.

Simulium develop in water courses varying from broad rivers to small streams, depending on the individual sibling species. Rapid flowing water provides the oxygenation needed for development of the immature stages. Most larvae and pupae develop on rocks or vegetation just below the water surface, but those of *S. neavei* develop on amphibious *Potamonautes* crabs. During this development period, the larvae are susceptible to insecticides.

Clinical features

Manifestations of onchocerciasis are almost entirely due to localized host inflammatory responses to dead or dying microfilariae. In a heavily infected person, 100 000 or more microfilariae die every day. The predominant immune response in onchocerciasis is antibody mediated, but with an important cellular component. Inflammatory responses may vary considerably between groups of people depending on length of exposure to antigens and the down-regulating activities by the host's immune system.

Eosinophils play an important role in the inflammatory responses. Cellular proteins derived from eosinophils are deposited on connective tissues throughout the dermis and are attached to elastic fibres causing skin changes.

In the eye, eosinophils are present in the anterior segment but lymphocytes and macrophages are more numerous. There is an activation of vascular endothelium, pericytes, and fibroblasts in people with chronic eye changes. Autoantibodies have been found to cells in the inner retina and to the retinal photoreceptors. The roll of these antibodies in causing retinal damage is uncertain. There is extensive evidence for a down-regulating of the immune response in chronically infected eye tissue by suppressor T cells and lymphocytes secreting interleukin 4.

Adult worms elaborate substances that inhibit the host's normal immune response. Exposure to filarial antigens *in utero* and through breast milk may induce an immune tolerance in residents of endemic areas. This could explain the difference in the disease patterns seen in people from non-endemic areas who become infected.

Fig. 2 (a) Sclerosing keratitis in a distorted eccentric pupil from anterior uveitis in a person blind from onchocerciasis. (b)Onchocerciasis producing a Hissette–Ridley fundus and optic atrophy in a person with central keyhole vision remaining.

Among those coinfected with HIV, there is a lessened reactivity to *O. volvulus* antigens, but no difference in adverse reactions following ivermectin treatment.

Eye damage

The risks of visual impairment increase as prevalence and intensity of infection rises in a community. Microfilariae enter the cornea from the skin and conjunctiva, and a punctate keratitis develops around dead microfilariae which clears when inflammation settles. In those exposed to years of heavy infection, sclerosing keratitis and iridocyclitis are likely to develop, causing permanent visual impairment or blindness (Fig. 2).

The first sign of sclerosing keratitis appears as a haziness at the medial and lateral margins of the cornea. This is followed by a migration of pigment on to the cornea accompanied by a progressive ingrowth of vessels. Gradually the cornea becomes opacified. The central and superior areas are the last involved. Although eye lesions can be found wherever onchocerciasis occurs, in West Africa blindness is most common in savannah areas. Before control efforts began in Burkina Faso, 46 per cent of men and 35 per cent of women would eventually become blind.

Posterior segment lesions, which can coexist with anterior eye lesions, may be caused by inflammation around microfilariae entering the retina along the posterior ciliary vessels. Choroidoretinal lesions are commonly seen at the outer side of the macula or encircling the optic disc. Active optic neuritis is reported as an important cause of blindness in Nigeria. Optic atrophy has been reported to be present in 1 to 4 per cent of people with onchocerciasis in Cameroon and 6 to 9 per cent in northern Nigeria. Loss of peripheral vision is well recognized in onchocerciasis.

Skin disease

Of all the consequences of onchocerciasis, skin lesions are the most pervasive. Surveys of seven endemic sites in five African countries reported that between 40 and 50 per cent of adults had troublesome itching, which in some cases was so intense that people slept on their elbows and knees to minimize this symptom.

In its mildest form, onchocerciasis presents as itching with a localized maculopapular rash. These reactive lesions and itching may be evanescent, clearing completely without treatment in a few months. In other instances the papular lesions may become chronic and generalized, and accompanied by severe itching (Fig. 3 and Plate 2). Oedema and excoriations can be associated, and lesions may heal with hyperpigmentation. Particularly distressing are lichenified, hyperkeratotic lesions which may be widespread, and intensely itchy (Fig. 4 and Plate 3). A localized form of chronic papular dermatitis, often confined to one extremity, is known as *Sowdah*, Arabic for dark. In this condition, first described from Yemen, there is an exceptionally strong IgG antibody response.

Fig. 3 Excoriated papular lesions of onchocerciasis with hyperpigmentation. (See also Plate 2.)

Light-skinned expatriates infected while visiting an endemic area may present a year or later with intensely itchy and red macular or maculopapular lesions. These may be confined to one area of the body or be more generalized, and may be associated with fever, muscle, joint pain, and sometimes oedema. Rash may sometimes persist for several months following ivermectin treatment.

In endemic areas, degenerative skin changes may develop in some people with long-standing infection. Elastic fibres are destroyed leaving the skin thinned with a wrinkled cigarette-paper appearance. The atrophied skin begins to sag, the most extreme state being 'hanging groin' with its apron-like skin folds. Depigmentation of the pretibial areas, or 'leopard skin', is a characteristic finding in older people living in endemic areas (Fig. 5 and Plate 4).

Fig. 4 Lichenified skin lesions with atrophy. (See also Plate 3.)

Fig. 5 Depigmented 'leopard skin'. (See also Plate 4.)

Other conditions associated with onchocerciasis

Both men and women with onchocerciasis weigh less than an uninfected cohort, and report more musculoskeletal pains. Evidence from Uganda and Burundi have suggested a possible association between epilepsy and onchocerciasis.

A peculiar pattern of growth arrest beginning between the age of 6 to 10 years was reported from a Ugandan onchocerciasis focus near Jinja in 1951. This Naklanaga syndrome, as it was called, now seems to have disappeared from there following elimination of onchocerciasis, but has been noted in western Uganda, and perhaps in Burundi.

Diagnosis

Finding microfilariae in skin snips is the time-honoured, though not very sensitive, method of diagnosis. Microfilariae lie close to the surface and are most plentiful in the iliac crest area, except in Latin America where they are more common in the shoulder and scapular areas. Using either a scalpel blade or a sclerocorneal punch, four to six snips (about 5 mg each) are taken under sterile conditions and immersed in normal saline. Microfilariae swimming free of the skin fragments can be counted easily with a dissecting microscope at 24 h or sooner. Examination of excised onchocercal nodules shows sections of adult worms. Enzyme immunoassay and PCR diagnostic methods have a high degree of sensitivity and specificity. Eosinophilia is common in onchocerciasis.

The Mazzotti test, in which people with onchocerciasis react with itching and a skin rash to 50 mg of diethylcarbamazine (DEC or Banocide), is seldom needed for diagnosis and is dangerous in heavy infections.

For community assessment, the prevalence of nodules in 30 to 50 males over the age of 20 years multiplied by 1.5 gives the approximate community prevalence of onchocerciasis. Where the prevalence of nodules is over 40 per cent the risk of blinding disease is high.

Treatment

The introduction of ivermectin for onchocerciasis in 1987 was one of the milestones of tropical disease treatment. Symptoms of onchocerciasis can be controlled effectively in individuals in a clinic or through mass treatment of endemic communities.

Ivermectin is derived from *Streptomyces avermitilis*. A single dose of 150 µg/kg clears microfilariae from the skin for several months. Annual treatment controls microfilarial counts and prevents progression of clinical findings, though in some locations it is given twice yearly. Treatment can be repeated if itching returns before the next dose is due. In the absence of reinfection, treatment should probably be continued for 10 or more years, or until adult worms stop producing microfilariae. In Ghana, after 5 years of annual ivermectin, the number of microfilariae was reduced to 7 per cent of the pretreatment baseline count.

Limiting the numbers of microfilariae through annual treatment improves early and advanced anterior-segment eye lesions, halts development of optic nerve disease, and improves severe onchocercal skin lesions. Adverse reactions to ivermectin commonly consist of increased itching, swelling of the face or extremities, and headache and body pains. Hypotension has been reported rarely after treatment in heavily infected people. Bullas have been seen occasionally. The most pronounced adverse reactions occur after the first ivermectin treatment, decreasing after subsequent treatment cycles. Ivermectin has no adverse effects in uninfected people. Although ivermectin temporarily reduces the release of microfilariae by adult worms, it does not destroy the adults. Care should be exercised in treating people coinfected with *Loa loa*, particularly those with counts above 10 000 microfilariae/ml blood, as potentially fatal central nervous system events can occur.

Ivermectin acts primarily on parasite neurotransmitters producing paralysis. This action appears to be mediated by potentiation or direct opening of glutamate-gated chloride channels. Although some ivermectin resistance has developed in animal parasites, no drug resistance has been reported in humans.

Prevention and control

Methods have included insecticides added to rivers to interrupt *Simulium* breeding, mass distribution of ivermectin, and nodulectomy in an attempt to prevent blindness.

Vector control

Killing *Simulium* larvae by adding DDT to rivers eliminated onchocerciasis in Kenya and the Mabari forest of Uganda. In 1974 the Onchocerciasis Control Programme (OCP) was formed to control *Simulium* through the larviciding of rivers in the Volta basin of West Africa with ecologically suitable compounds. This highly successful vector control programme, later supplemented with ivermectin distribution, has now permitted tens of millions of people to live free of disease. Mass distribution of ivermectin is now the principal method for onchocerciasis control, though vector control may still be appropriate in some locations.

Ivermectin mass distribution

After the effectiveness of ivermectin had been shown, its manufacturers, Merck and Co., established the Mectizan® Donation Program to provide the drug free 'for as long as necessary to as many as necessary'. By mid-1998 over 100 million ivermectin treatments had been given in 33 of 34 endemic countries.

The goal of a control programme may be either complete eradication of the parasite reservoir or elimination of the public health and socio-economic consequences of continuing infection. In Guatemala, where high population coverage with 6-monthly treatment has reduced parasite transmission by 80 to 100 per cent after 3 years, eradication may ultimately be possible, and this could be true elsewhere in Latin America where sustained treatment is implemented.

The Onchocerciasis Elimination Program in the Americas (OEPA) and the African Programme for Onchocerciasis Control (APOC) have been formed with support by the World Bank and other United Nations agencies to eliminate the public consequences of infection. These programmes focus on regular mass administration of ivermectin through community-based distributors and mobile teams.

Because of the lifespan of adult worms, ivermectin distribution programmes must be sustained for a period of 15 years or more. In some places, the duration may have to be longer because of the difficulty in achieving good coverage, often because of insecurity.

Nodulectomy

A third form of onchocerciasis control has been the nodulectomy programmes of Mexico and Guatemala. For many years health workers have moved from village to village removing nodules, especially around the head. The evidence for this preventing blindness is not strong.

Areas needing further research

Although ivermectin brings great relief to the individual, and has a clear impact on the disease in mass distribution programmes, its does not kill adult worms. While symptoms and risks are controlled through annual treatment, the disease itself is not eradicated. A number of macrofilaricidal drugs, capable of killing adult worms, have been tested, but none has so far proved suitable for either individual or mass treatment. Diagnostic methods, although dramatically improved in recent years, are still not in a form suitable for practitioners in developing countries. Our basic knowledge of *O. volvulus* and the disease it causes still contains many gaps. These include a fuller understanding of the parasite and its relationship with the host, the nature of the systemic effects of *O. volvulus* infection, and better knowledge of the natural history of a disease which continues to affect millions worldwide.

Loa loa

Introduction

Loa loa is a filaria transmitted by the *Chrysops* fly in West Africa. The adult worm migrates beneath the skin, and sometimes across the eye, moving at about 1 cm/min. Periodically the infection causes sudden but transient localized inflammatory oedema known as Calabar swellings.

Parasitology

Larvae of *L. loa* burrow into the human skin during feeding of the *Chrysops* or 'mangrove fly' (*C. silacea* or *C. dimidiata*). In humans the parasites mature and live in the fascial layers. After a year or more, microfilariae are produced. Microfilariae are present in the blood during the day, when the *Chrysops* fly bites. Once taken up by the fly, microfilariae go through developmental stages in the fly's thoracic muscles. After 10 days the fly is able to infect a human, and can do so for another 5 days.

Epidemiology

Infection is most common around the Gulf of Guinea, particularly in Nigeria and Cameroon, but extends through Central Africa into Sudan, and Uganda, and south to Angola and the Congo (Fig. 6). Man is the only host, although a similar parasite is found in monkeys in the same areas. The fly lives in the rain forest canopy, and descends to bite humans, attracted perhaps by movement. Transmission may be most intense during the rainy season when flies are breeding on the muddy banks of forest streams.

Clinical features

The first clinical symptoms of loiasis may be delayed for several years after infection. Calabar swellings appear suddenly, most commonly in the forearms or wrists, and sometimes following heavy exercise. These oedematous lesions are red and itchy, and may be associated with fever and irritability. After a few hours, or 1 to 2 days at most, the affected part returns to normal. Swellings are not confined to the arms, but may be present in the face, breasts, or legs. They appear more commonly in hot seasons.

Fig. 6 Map of the approximate distribution of *Loa loa*.

Calabar swellings are a hypersensitivity reaction to worm antigens which may be released in the process of migration or perhaps during the maturation of the worm. A high proportion of eosinophils are seen in peripheral blood smears, often exceeding 70 per cent.

A second common feature is the appearance of a migrating worm (Fig. 7 and Plate 5). This may be under the skin in any location, but is most dramatic when it crosses the eye ('eye worm', Fig. 8). Other than local irritation of the conjunctiva while the worm is passing, and the obvious concern of the host, there are no serious consequences.

Rare but potentially serious consequences of *L. loa* are meningioencephalitis, renal disease, and endomyocardial fibrosis. The meningioencephalitis may occur spontaneously, though usually after treatment with diethycarbamazine or ivermectin. Recovery is common following support-

Fig. 8 *Loa loa* crossing the bulbar conjunctiva.

ive treatment, although fatalities have been reported. Those at most risk have microfilarial counts above 10 000/ml of blood. The renal and endocardial complications of loiasis may have an immune origin.

Laboratory diagnosis

Diagnosis has traditionally been by the finding of microfilariae in a daytime blood sample, or by a history or typical clinical findings. Use of more sensitive PCR methods has shown that many, even perhaps the majority of those infected, do not have microfilariae in their peripheral blood.

Treatment

The standard treatment has been diethycarbamazine (DEC), which kills microfilariae and many adult worms. The treatment is given as 50 mg on the first day, and the dose doubled each subsequent day until 2 to 3 mg/kg is reached (maximum 600 mg). This is then continued for up to 21 days. During treatment, fever, arthralgias, and itching can occur. Ivermectin at 200 µg/kg dramatically decreases the number of microfilariae and decreases some of the loiasis symptoms. As with diethycarbamazine, there is a risk of potentially fatal meningioencephalitis in those with high microfilarial counts. It might be prudent to initiate any ivermectin treatment at half dose, particularly in those with higher (more than 10 000 microfilariae/ml) parasite counts. Since many people with loiasis also have onchocerciasis, careful monitoring for severe eye and skin inflammation is important when giving diethycarbamazine. Treatment is unlikely to eradicate all adult worms, and in endemic areas reinfection is probable. Blood films for microfilariae or PCR examinations should be followed to indicate the need for retreatment.

Prevention

The best prevention is avoiding *Chrysops* fly bites. Having window screens on dwellings, wearing clothing to protect legs and forearms, and avoiding high biting areas can reduce risks.

The Mansonellas

Introduction

The mansonellas are a group of filarial infections common to many countries, and are of negligible clinical importance under most circumstances. Infection is transmitted by *Culicoides* midges.

Epidemiology

Mansonella (formerly *Dipetalonema*) *perstans* is found in much of tropical Africa as well as Trinidad and several parts of South America. Adult worms live free in the abdominal cavity, and microfilariae are found in the blood.

Fig. 7 Migrating *Loa loa*. (See also Plate 5.)

Mansonella ozzardi is found in the West Indies and Central and South America. Microfilariae are found in the blood and skin. Adult worms have been found in the peritoneal cavity. In addition to *Culicoides*, *Simulium* flies have been reported to transmit *M. ozzardi* in the Amazon basis. *Mansonella* (formerly *Dipetalonema*) *streptocerca* is a common infection in West and Central Africa extending into western Uganda. Both microfilariae and adult worms are found in the skin, but without the nodules seen in onchocerciasis. Unless *M. streptocerca* microfilariae are differentiated parasitologically from those of *O. volvulus*, inappropriate mass treatment programmes for onchocerciasis could be implemented.

Clinical manifestions

Of the mansonellas, only *M. streptocerca* produces clear-cut symptoms, although even these can be confused with those of *O. volvulus* which may be a coinfection. Chronic papular lesions are commonly present, often associated with postinflammatory hyperpigmentation. Lichenification may occur less commonly. Hypopigmentation has been noted in areas of skin overlying the location of adult worms in the skin. In general these findings are not easily distinguishable from those of onchocerciasis.

M. perstans has been reported to produce Calabar-like swellings, and in Zimbabwe, central nervous system symptoms. *M. ozzardi* infections are generally without symptoms, though fever, arthralgias, headache, and itching have been associated in the Amazon area.

Diagnosis

A diagnosis is made by the finding of characteristic microfilariae in the blood or the skin. The microfilaria has a distinctive 'walking stick' shape to its tail, and four prominent nuclei in the tail, both of which distinguish it from the microfilaria of *O. volvulus*. Recently a PCR assay has been described for *M. streptocerca* and both QBC-fluorescence and ELISA methods for *M. perstans*. Eosinophilia is a characteristic finding.

Treatment

In asymptomatic persons no treatment is required. *M. streptocerca* responds well to ivermectin, often with mild reactions similar to those seen in onchocerciasis. Treatments of *M. perstans* with diethycarbamazine, and albendazole, have all been disappointing, though mebendazole given as 100 mg once or twice daily for 28 to 45 days has been reported to clear microfilariae. Ivermectin was able to lower microfilarial counts to 60 per cent of pretreatment values.

Further research

Little attention has been given to the mansonellas, ubiquitous in many places. A reliable, inexpensive field test kit for mass screening could help determine the extent of infection and any association with the ill-defined clinical symptoms often reported.

Further reading

Mectizan and onchocerciasis: a decade of accomplishment (1998). *Annals of Tropical Medicine and Parasitology* 92(Suppl.), S1–174.

Alley ES *et al.*(1994). The impact of five years of annual ivermectin treatment on skin microfilarial loads in the onchocerciasis focus of Asubende, Ghana. *Transactions of the Royal Society of Tropical Medicine and Hygiene* 88, 581–84.

Brieger WR *et al.* (1998). The effects of ivermectin on onchocercal skin disease and severe itching: results of a multicentre trial. *Tropical Medicine and International Health* 3, 951–61.

Chan CC *et al.*(1989). Immunopathology of ocular onchocerciasis. I. Inflammatory cells infiltrating the anterior segment. *Clinical Experimental Immunology* 77, 367–73.

Cooper PJ *et al.* (1999). Eosinophil sequestration and activation are associated with the onset and severity of systemic adverse reactions following the treatment of onchocerciasis with ivermectin. *Journal of Infectious Diseases* 179, 738–42.

Fischer P, Bamuhiiga J, Büttner DW (1997). Occurrence and diagnosis of *Mansonella streptocerca* in Uganda. *Acta Tropica* 63, 43–55.

Garcia A *et al.* (1995). Longitudinal survey of *Loa loa* filariasis in southern Cameroon. *American Journal of Tropical Medicine and Hygiene* 52, 370–5.

Mudroch ME *et al.* (1997). HKA-DQ alleles associate with cutaneous features of onchocerciasis. *Human immunology* 55, 46–52.

Ottesen EA (1995). Immune responsiveness and the pathogenesis of human onchocerciasis. *Journal of Infectious Diseases* 171, 659–71.

World Health Organization (1995). *Onchocerciasis and its control*. Geneva

Yameogo L *et al.* (1999). Pool screen polymerases chain reaction for estimating the prevalence of *Onchocerca volvulus* infection in *Simulium damnosum sensu lato*: results of a field trial in an area subject to successful vector control. *American Journal of Tropical Medicine and Hygiene* 60, 124–8.

7.14.2 Lymphatic filariasis

R. Knight

Wuchereria bancrofti, *Brugia malayi*, and *Brugia timori* are mosquito-borne nematodes. They are important causes of morbidity in the tropics and subtropics between latitudes 41°N and 28°S in the Old World and 30°N and 30°S in the Americas (Fig. 1). Bancroftian filariasis due to *W. bancrofti* infects 110 million people; it was introduced into the Americas from Africa by the Atlantic slave trade. The two *Brugia* species infect about 13 million people in South and South-East Asia. Approximately 700 million people live in countries where these infections are endemic. *Brugia timori*, which was first described in 1964, has a very localized distribution but causes severe disease.

Aetiology—the biology of the parasite

Adult worms live in the larger lymphatic vessels and lymph nodes. They are smooth, creamy-white, and threadlike; females measure 80 to 100 mm in length, and males 40 mm; their lifespan is normally 2 to 5 years, but exceptionally much more. Mated females produce numerous microfilariae throughout their lives; these actively motile embryonic worms are sheathed by the remnants of the egg shell. They are 180 to 290 μm in length and 7 to 10 μm in diameter. Different species can be distinguished morphologically in stained films. Microfilariae migrate via the lymphatic system to the blood where they have a lifespan of up to 12 months (Plate 1). Their numbers in the peripheral blood vary during the day and night—a phenomenon known as periodicity; when not circulating they are sequestered in lung and reticuloendothelial capillaries. Maximal counts in the blood coincide with the biting cycle of the vector. The species and strain of parasite determine the periodicity; most common is nocturnally periodic with maximal counts between 22.00 and 02.00 h and virtual absence during the day. Alternatively, microfilariae may be present throughout the 24 h cycle with prominent peaks during the day or the night: diurnally and nocturnally subperiodic, respectively.

After uptake by the vector, microfilariae penetrate the gut and migrate to thoracic muscles where they mature over 9 to 15 days to infective third-stage larvae, which then migrate to the mosquito head and escape from the proboscis during a blood meal. Larval worms enter the puncture wound made by the vector, reach the peripheral lymphatic system, and move to larger lymph vessels below a lymph node. Sexual maturity and appearance of microfilariae in the blood usually takes 8 to 18 months, but sometimes only 3 months.

Epidemiology and transmission

In endemic areas microfilarial prevalence rates increase steadily from early childhood to reach a maximum in early adult life, when in highly endemic areas 10 to 30 per cent prevalences are not unusual; rates in males are generally higher, perhaps due to greater vector exposure. The cord blood of some infants shows microfilariae.

In some locations *Brugia malayi* is a zoonosis with an animal reservoir; elsewhere it is an anthroponosis with only a human source of infection.

Geographical distribution and mosquito vectors

W. bancrofti infection

Culex transmission

This vector breeds mostly in organically polluted water, usually in urban and suburban areas but also villages when there are suitable latrine and cesspit habitats. This is the commonest type of transmission and is increasing with urbanization; it occurs in India, Sri Lanka, Central and South America, some Caribbean Islands, urban and coastal villages in East Africa, Egypt, and parts of China. *Culex* bites at night, mostly on the legs, the

(a)

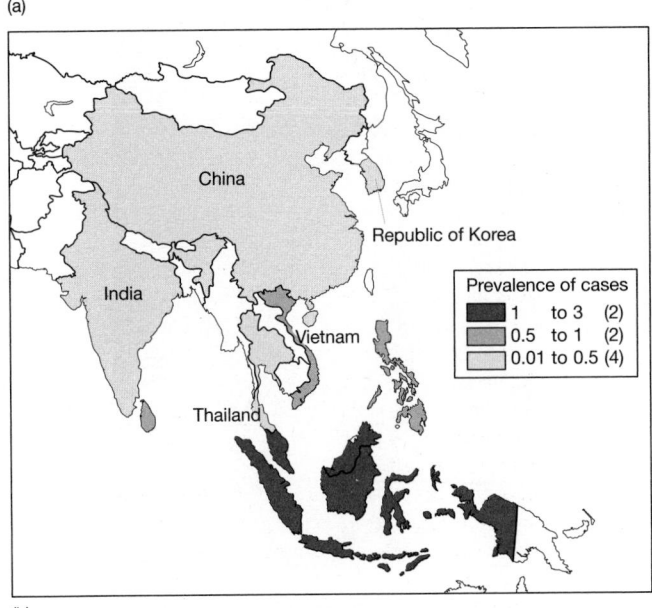

(b)

Fig. 1 Distribution of lymphatic filariasis; case prevalences (percentages) due to (a) *Wuchereria bancrofti* and (b) *Brugia* spp. The figures in parentheses indicate the number of countries. Circles denote Pacific Island prevalences. (By courtesy of E.Michael and D.A.P. Bundy.)

microfilariae are nocturnally periodic. *Culex* is the most efficient vector and can maintain transmission at low microfilarial densities, making control difficult.

Anopheles transmission

The same vector species commonly transmit both filariasis and malaria. This occurs in East and West Africa, Papua New Guinea and Vanuatu, limited areas in South America, and parts of China. *Anopheles* bites nocturnally, mainly on the legs; microfilariae are nocturnally periodic.

Aedes transmission

This is limited to Southern Oceania, especially Fiji, Samoa, Tonga, the Cook Islands, and New Caledonia, but also patchily in Thailand, the Philippines, Vietnam, and the Nicobar Islands. *Aedes* feeds throughout the 24 h cycle with a daytime peak, and bites all over the body; the microfilariae are diurnally subperiodic.

B. malayi infection

Zoonotic Mansonia transmission in swamp forests

This occurs in Malaysia, Indonesia, and southern Thailand; monkeys and carnivores are reservoir hosts. *Mansonia* bites mainly by night but also by day, usually on legs below the knee; the microfilariae are nocturnally subperiodic.

Transmission in agricultural areas

In parts of Malaysia, Buru in Indonesia, and southern Thailand a mixed anthroponosis and zoonosis occurs in transitional zones with monkeys and cats as reservoirs, and both *Anopheles* and *Mansonia* as vectors. Microfilariae have periodicities intermediate between nocturnally periodic and nocturnally subperiodic.

In India (mainly Kerala), Malaysia, Sulawesi, southern Thailand, Vietnam, China, and Korea infection involves humans only with *Anopheles* as the main vector and *Mansonia* as the accessory vector; the microfilariae are nocturnally periodic.

B. timori infection

This is confined to Timor and other islands in the Lesser Sundas group in eastern Indonesia. *Anopheles barbirostris* is the vector. The microfilariae are nocturnally periodic.

Pathogenesis

Local immunological reactions to worm antigens provoke acute and subacute responses with oedema of lymphatic tissue and infiltration with eosinophils and monocytes. Antigens derive from moulting fluids of developing worms, excretory products, microfilariae trapped within the lymphatic system, and also dying worms including those killed by chemotherapy. Dead and disintegrating worms become surrounded by granulation tissue with giant cells and epithelioid cells. Stenosis or blockage of lymph vessels leads to distal dilatation with varicosities and valve incompetence. Prolonged or recurrent lymph stasis leads to accumulation of protein-rich interstitial fluid and fibroblast proliferation, dilated dermal lymphatics, and epithelial acanthosis and hyperkeratosis.

Determinants of pathology include duration of exposure, intensity of transmission, anatomical sites of infective mosquito bites, and the species and strain of parasite. Prenatal exposure to filarial antigen is of great importance and induces immunological tolerance. Residents in high-transmission areas often show patent microfilariaemia but little immunopathology. However, in many adults a later decline in microfilarial prevalence parallels increased host immunological reactivity and pathology. New residents and visitors show marked local reactivity to worms and often no blood microfilariae; the latter situation was well documented among

American troops in the Pacific in 1942 to 1944 and French troops in former Indochina.

Clinical manifestations

Acute lymphatic filariasis

In endemic areas acute episodes are recurrent from the age of 10 years and most frequent 4 to 8 months after the peak of seasonal transmission. Episodes last several days or weeks; fever and malaise are common but blood eosinophilia is not marked. People leaving endemic areas cease to have acute episodes after 1 year although they may experience recurrent pain in previously affected tissues, especially after unusual exercise.

Filarial lymphadenitis and lymphangitis

Tender lymphadenopathy is most common in the inguinal and femoral nodes, but axillary and epitrochlear nodes are also affected. Tender retrograde lymphangitis typically spreads peripherally below the node.

Acute genital filariasis

This is uncommon in boys before puberty but common thereafter. The typical lesion is funiculitis with a tender fusiform or cylindrical swelling of the spermatic cord; epididymitis and orchitis are less common.

Filarial abscess and filarial fever

Affected nodes in the groin or elsewhere may break down producing an open ulcer that heals slowly leaving characteristic scars. Pelvic and retroperitoneal lymphadenitis can produce a febrile illness that is difficult to diagnose.

Chronic lymphatic filariasis

Lymphoedema and elephantiasis

Initially, transient pitting oedema occurs during inflammatory episodes in proximal nodes. Later, oedema persists between episodes becoming non-pitting distally. Eventually, brawny non-pitting oedema becomes permanent (Fig. 2). In patients with leg involvement epidermal thickening,

Fig. 2 Chronic elephantiasis in a man in Belém, northern Brazil. Note the scars of unsuccessful surgery. (Copyright Pedro Pardal.)

Fig. 3 Chronic elephantiasis with epidermal thickening, fissuring, and papillomatosis in a man in north-east Nigeria. (Copyright D.A. Warrell.)

Fig. 4 Gross hydrocele in a patient with chronic filariasis. (By courtesy of the late P.E.C. Manson-Bahr.)

papillomatosis, and fissuring are common (Fig. 3), and bacterial infection becomes an important complication.

Chronic genital filariasis

Hydrocele is the commonest lesion and prevalence rates may reach 30 per cent in men over 35 years in highly endemic areas; many patients give a history of preceding episodes of funiculitis or epididymitis. The tunica vaginalis is often thickened. Nodular lesions of the spermatic cord and epididymis are common and the testis itself becomes enlarged and indurated. Lymphoceles occur on the cord. Dilated dermal lymphatics in the scrotal wall associated with atrophic epidermis produce lymph scrotum, the skin having a velvety appearance. Rupture of these lymphatics leads to weeping skin lesions and often secondary infection, occasionally complicated by Fournier's gangrene.

Lymphoedema of the scrotum is a late sequel (Fig. 4), often the testes are unaffected; penile lesions are rare. Vulval lymphoedema is under-recognized; it is associaeted with dilated retroperitoneal lymphatics and must be distinguished from lymphogranuloma venereum.

Chronic lymphadenitis and lymphangitis

Recurrent episodes of acute inflammation lead to persisting and sometimes massive lymph node enlargement. Thickened lymphatic cords may be palpable connecting the axillary and epitrochlear, or the femoral and popliteal nodes. Varicose lymph vessels may be visible in these areas. Lymph varices are fluctuant sacs of lymphatic tissue derived usually from the capsule of a node, hence the alternative term lymphadenocele. They partially empty when the part is raised; aspiration reveals lymph or occasionally chyle. They occur in the medial thigh, groin, axilla, and sometimes even the neck.

Chyluria and lymphuria

Dilated pelvic and retroperitoneal lymphatics may rupture into the urinary tract in the renal pelvis, ureter, or bladder. When there is lymph stasis above the cisterna chyli then small bowel chyle may reflux into the urine postprandially. Chyluria is often intermittent and blood stained (Fig. 5). Con-

tinued loss of protein and lipids in the urine may lead to weight loss and cachexia. Chyluria may eventually be self-limited.

Non-lymphatic pathology

Tropical pulmonary eosinophilia

This presents as a subacute or chronic illness with cough, wheezing, and reticular or miliary pulmonary shadowing. Microfilariae are absent from the blood, but eosinophilia is marked and titres of filarial antibody are very high. Some patients have features of lymphadenopathic or genital filariasis, but many do not. Lung functional loss is restrictive. Response to antifilarial treatment is good but untreated the condition leads to pulmonary fibrosis and pulmonary hypertension. The syndrome is due to a heightened immunological response to dead microfilariae which may be found, in biopsies of lung and other tissue, surrounded by eosinophilic microabscesses. It occurs in most endemic areas, but is rare in Africa; it is commoner in men and rare in children; many patients are not long-term residents.

Fig. 5 Chyluria and haematuria in a patient with chronic filariasis. (By courtesy of the late P.E.C. Manson-Bahr).

Filarial arthritis

Joint involvement is subacute and often recurrent with effusion; it usually affects the knee.

Filarial glomerulonephritis

The incidence of clinically significant disease is uncertain; it results from immune complex deposition on the glomerular basement membrane. Recurrent streptococcal infection associated with filarial lymphoedema is also implicated.

Diagnosis

Clinical

Many patients will have several clinical features that, together with history of preceding acute episodes, will be strongly suggestive diagnostically: manifestations such as varicose lymphatics, lymphadenocele, retrograde lymphangitis, and lymph scrotum are highly specific to filariasis. Genital lesions are rare in *Brugia* infections, which usually present with lymphoedema below the knee. In *B. timori* infections lymph node pathology in the legs is often severe, sometimes with skin ulceration. Upper limb and breast lesions are common in diurnally subperiodic *W. bancrofti* infections in the Pacific; but they do occur elsewhere with other strains of this parasite.

Parasitological

Microfilariae are typically found in blood films but also in aspirates from a lymph varix, hydrocele, lymphocele of the cord, or in urine. Blood should be taken to coincide with the expected microfilarial periodicity. Measured 10 or 20 µl volumes are used to prepare thick blood films stained by Giemsa. Counting chambers taking 100 µl of lysed blood can be used or larger volumes may be lysed and the spun deposit examined. Alternatively, 1 ml of lysed or unlysed blood is passed through a Millepore filter; the filter is then stained. Nocturnally periodic *W. bancrofti* microfilariae appear transiently in the blood 30 to 60 min after a 100 mg dose of diethylcarbamazine and this forms the basis of the 'provocation test'. Stained microfilariae can be identified by their sheaths, but these may be lost by *Brugia* parasites during staining; *B. timori* has distinctive sheath staining. The arrangement of nuclei at the caudal end allows species diagnosis; *B. malayi* has two subterminal nuclei separated by a space. The microfilariae of *Loa loa* also have sheaths and must be distinguished from those of species causing lymphatic filariasis.

Immunodiagnosis

Positive skin tests and filarial antibody are common in those exposed to infection and may be of value in visitors to an endemic area. Several tests for filarial antigen in serum are now available and a positive test indicates persisting adult worms. Antigen may be present in the absence of microfilariaemia.

Imaging of lymphatic vessels

Lymphangiography will delineate anatomical details of abnormal lymphatic tissues such as lymph varices and lymphatic connections to the urinary tract in chyluria. They are not usually diagnostic for filariasis. Scrotal ultrasound can show live worms—the 'filarial dance' sign.

Lymphoscintigraphy using technetium-labelled dextran or albumin is a less invasive and useful technique that can demonstrate lymphatic pathology. Abnormal dermal lymphatics occur in many asymptomatic infected persons in endemic areas but, so far, few local control subjects have been examined and comparisons with normal lymphatic studies in Western countries may not be justified.

Treatment

Individual chemotherapy

Diethylcarbamazine remains the treatment of choice. Adequate dosage will kill adult worms. Even a small single dose will clear blood microfilariae temporarily. Sensitivity reactions to filarial antigen, both local and systemic, are common in infected people and simulate some of the acute manifestations of the infection; they necessitate care and supervision in the initial stages, especially in *Brugia* infections. Treatment should be started at 1 mg/kg on the first day, increasing over 3 or more days to 6 mg/kg in divided doses; this dose then being continued for 21 days. Coinfection with *Loa loa* and *Onchocerca volvulus* must be excluded before diethylcarbamazine is given to avoid dangerous reactions.

Indications for curative treatment are acute manifestations with or without microfilariaemia, and chronic disease in patients who are either microfilaria positive or positive for filarial antigen identified serologically. Treatment often reduces the size of hydroceles but has little effect on chronic lymphoedema.

Surgical and supportive treatment

Acute manifestations of filariasis can mimic strangulated hernia and testicular torsion. Surgical treatment of filarial hydrocele is the same as that for non-filarial disease. Scrotal lymphoedema can be treated surgically, usually with preservation of the testes. Lymphosaphenous anastomosis is being used for leg elephantiasis; many other procedures have been used in the past, often with disappointing results (Fig. 2).

Bacterial infection is common in those with lymphoedema, especially when the skin is fissured, breached in an interdigital cleft, or when there is minor injury, ulcer, or insect bite. Early use of antibiotics and resting of the affected limb lessens the risk of increasing lymphoedema; supportive bandaging applied each morning or wearing elastic stockings reduces chronic oedema.

Filariasis at the community level

Surveys for lymphatic filariasis

These are carried out to assess the importance to public health and plan intervention programmes. Current clinical features together with history of acute features in the preceding 6 months are documented, and blood is taken to measure microfilarial density. Serum collected on such surveys has been the source of many immunopathological studies. The following disease groups are recognized, but the availabilty of tests for filarial antigen will add a new dimension to such surveys.

(1) Asymptomatic without microfilariaemia—in highly endemic areas most of these people will have been exposed to infection; they are sometimes called 'endemic normals';

(2) asymptomatic with microfilariaemia;

(3) acute filariasis—many will show microfilariaemia, but this is absent in prepatent infections and in people with strong immunological responses, including visitors; and

(4) chronic filariasis—in some geographical areas many subjects will be microfilaria negative, especially those with chronic lymphoedema; in other areas they are positive; negativity may be due to a decline in transmission over several years or to host immune responses.

Social and economic consequences of lymphatic filariasis

Surgical care of patients with hydrocele and other manifestations places a great burden on health care in highly endemic areas. In agricultural communities acute manifestations and episodes of secondary bacterial infection impair productivity. Social stigma is a major problem and may lead to divorce or make a woman unable to marry.

Vector control

These campaigns are targeted at the local vector. Larval *Aedes* breeding sites such a discarded tins, tyres, or coconut shells can be removed. *Culex* numbers can be reduced by improved sanitation, larvicides, and polystyrene beads applied to the water surface of latrines and cesspits. Bednets and repellants are universally applicable. Where *Anopheles* is the vector, malaria control can interrupt filariasis transmission as in Samoa, Vanuatu, and parts of southern China.

Population-based chemotherapy

Different dosage regimens of diethylcarbamazine have been used in many endemic areas; with annual or 6-monthly administration either to the whole population or to those found to be infected; medicated salt is an alternative. The main aim is to eliminate microfilariaemia and hence transmission; however, with repeated and higher doses many adult worms are eventually killed. Ivermectin offers an alternative method of reducing microfilaraemia. A single dose of 6 mg/kg of diethylcarbamazine is as effective as one 200 or 400 μg/kg dose of ivermectin. Both will reduce microfilariaemia to almost nil for 6 or 12 months. Sensitivity reactions are much commoner with diethylcarbamazine. Annual dosage with both of these drugs continued for 4 or 6 years—the lifespan of adult worms—should interrupt transmission. Albendazole is also effective as a microfilaricide and has some activity against adult worms; a 600 mg dose can replace either diethylcarbamazine or ivermectin in a two-drug annual regimen; diethylcarbamazine must not be used where onchocerciasis is co-endemic.

Further reading

Dreyer G *et al.* (1999). Acute attacks in the extremities of persons living in an area endemic for bancroftian filariasis: differentiation of two syndromes. *Transactions of the Royal Society of Tropical Medicine and Hygiene* **93**, 413–7.

Freedman DO (1998). Immune dynamics in the pathogenesis of human lymphatic filariasis. *Parasitology Today* **14**, 229–34.

Freedman DO *et al.* (1994). Lymphoscintographic analysis of lymphatic abnormalities in symptomatic and asymptomatic human filariasis. *Journal of Infectious Diseases* **170**, 927–33.

Ismail MM *et al.* (1998). Efficacy of single dose combinations of albendazole, ivermectin and diethylcarbamazine for the treatment of bancroftian filariasis. *Transactions of the Royal Society of Tropical Medicine and Hygiene* **92**, 94–7.

Michael E, Bundy DAP, Grenfell BT (1996). Re-assessing the global prevalence and distribution of lymphatic filariasis. *Parasitology* **112**, 409–28.

Michael E, Bundy DAP (1997). Global mapping of lymphatic filariasis. *Parasitology Today* **13**, 472–6.

Norões J *et al.* (1996). Occurrence of living adult *Wuchereria bancrofti* in the scrotal area of men with microfilariaemia. *Transactions of the Royal Society of Tropical Medicine* **90**, 55–6.

Nutman TB, ed. (2000). *Lymphatic filariasis*. Imperial College Press, London.

Southgate BA (1992). Intensity and efficiency of transmission and the development of microfilaraemia and disease: their relationship in lymphatic filariasis. *Journal of Tropical Medicine and Hygiene* **95**, 1–12.

Weil GT, Lammie PJ, Weiss N (1997). The ICT filariasis test: a rapid format antigen test for the diagnosis of bancroftian filariasis. *Parasitology Today* **13**, 401–4.

7.14.3 Guinea worm disease: dracunculiasis

R. Knight

The clinical manifestations of Guinea worm and its surgical removal were known in antiquity. Attention was drawn to the seasonal occurrence of painful limb blisters that broke down to reveal a 'worm' in the floor of an ulcer. *Dracunculus medinensis* is the longest nematode infecting humans; in the Bible it is described as the 'fiery serpent'. It was the first human parasite to be shown to have an arthropod intermediate host: in 1869 the Russian naturalist Fedtschenko described the worm's early development in *Cyclops*—the 'water flea'. Recent attention is directed at eradication, for despite its complex lifecycle this can be achieved by public health measures alone.

Aetiology—the biology of the parasite (Fig. 1)

Mature female worms, 70 to 120 cm in length, migrate along fascial planes and subcutaneous tissue to reach the skin, usually below the knee. Tissue damage caused by worm products produces a blister that soon ulcerates. Immersion of the affected part in water causes the worm to contract and expel numerous rhabditiform first-stage larvae from the uterus at the ruptured anterior end of the worm. Larvae swim vigorously in water for up to 7 days and some are ingested by predatory copepod crustaceans of the

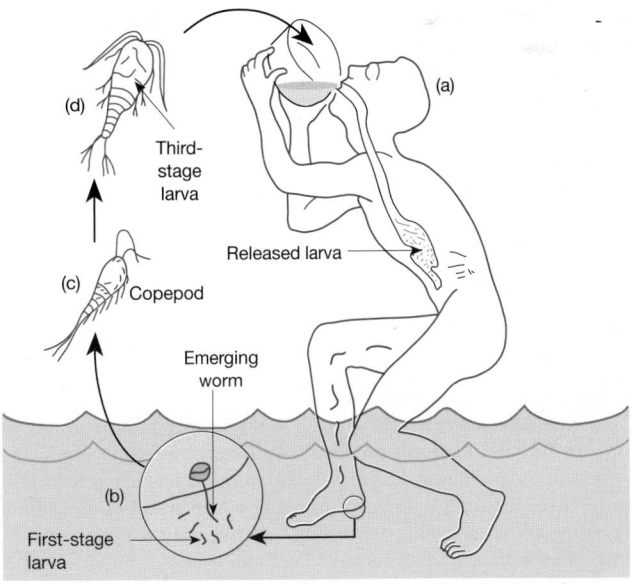

Fig. 1 Lifecycle of Guinea worm in man. (a) Copepods infected with third-stage larvae are ingested in drinking water; larvae are released in the intestine, migrate to the body cavity, mature, and mate. (b) Gravid female worms migrate to the limbs, cause a blister to form and release first-stage larvae into water. (c) First-stage larvae are ingested by copepods. (d) Larvae undergo two moults in the copepod and are infective after 2 weeks.

genus *Cyclops*. They penetrate the gut of the intermediate host and develop with two moults in the haemocele over a period of 14 days to become infective third-stage larvae. When water containing infected *Cyclops* is swallowed, the released infective larvae burrow though the wall of the duodenum to reach retroperitoneal tissue. After about 100 days the worms mate and the females begin their migration towards the limbs; the male worms die and may later calcify. Ten months after infection most female worms, containing fully formed larvae, have reached their destination; within the next month they will rupture through the skin to begin the cycle anew (Plate 1).

Epidemiology

Guinea worm transmission is predominantly rural with an annual cycle that often coincides with the planting or harvesting season. The seasonal morbidity causes great economic hardship. Water sources containing *Cyclops* are easily contaminated by infected people, including those seeking relief by immersion of their painful lesion. In semi-arid areas, transmission occurs in temporary ponds during the rainy season; in wetter areas, flooding and water turbidity limits transmission during the rains and infection occurs in shallow wells during the dry season. For practical purposes there is no zoonotic reservoir although infected dogs have been found in endemic areas and primates can be experimentally infected. Related species of *Dracunculus* are found in mink, raccoons, and otters in North America.

Geographic distribution

This infection was previously endemic over wide areas of the Middle East and the Indian subcontinent. Largely as a result of improved and protected water sources the infection disappeared from the Central Asian Republics between 1926 and 1933, from Iran in the 1970s, and Yemen and Saudi Arabia in the 1980s; India and Pakistan have recently become free of infection. It is now limited to the Sahel and Guinea savannah, between 2° and 18° north, in sub-Saharan Africa with most cases in southern Sudan, Niger, Nigeria, Mali, Burkina Faso, Chad, Ghana, and Uganda (Fig. 2). Formerly it was also present in the Americas having been introduced with the slave trade. By the 1880s it disappeared.

Clinical features

The blister is the first sign of infection in most patients (Plate 1). In others pre-emergent worms may be seen or felt under the dermis, some are actively motile. Allergic prodromal symptoms with urticaria, facial oedema, dyspnoea, and gastrointestinal manifestations may precede the blister by a few days; they disappear when the blister ruptures. Most patients have one or two worms each season, but up to 50 have been recorded. While most gravid worms emerge from a limb, other sites include the trunk, scrotum, and vulva (Plate 3).

Uncomplicated cases resolve within 4 weeks; local complications derive from sensitization to worm products and bacterial infection producing severe pain and prolonged disability. Gravid worms failing to reach the skin release larvae inducing vigorous tissue reactions and abscesses, sometimes presenting as bubos, epididymo-orchitis, or acute arthritis. Joint involvement, often with secondary bacterial infection, is also common near the site of emergence: this leads to ankylosis and tendon contractures with deformities and permanent disability. Immature female worms may die before reaching the skin and become encapsulated by host tissue, where some calcify; they may also enter ectopic sites including the orbit, pericardium, and central nervous system. Mortality is usually less than 1 per cent. It results from systemic or local bacterial infection; tetanus is a significant risk when spores contaminate open lesions.

Fig. 2 Distribution of dracunculiasis – endemic villages in Africa. (Reproduced from Peries H, Cairncross S (1997). *Parasitology Today* **13**, 434, with permission: data from Joint WHO-UNICEF Programme on Mapping and Geographic Information Systems for Dracunculiasis Eradication (Health Map), WHO/CTD, Geneva.)

Diagnosis

Most patients in endemic areas recognize their condition. Worms release larvae on contact with water and these can be seen as a milky cloud. When the worm is not visible, ulcers may be irrigated with saline and the centrifuged deposit examined for larvae.

Patient management

Local treatment can be very painful and often must be repeated. Warm moist packs should be applied for several hours, followed by gentle massage along the tract of the worm towards the ulcer. Light traction is then applied to the worm; breakage must be avoided as this greatly aggravates the situation. Analgesics and antibacterial soaks are useful; oral antibiotics are often necessary. Between local treatments the lesion must be bandaged to reduce the risk of bacterial infection and contamination of water sources.

Pre-emergent worms can be surgically removed, a practice originating in India. A small incision is made adjacent to the worm near its mid-point, and a loop of worm is lifted out with a blunt curved probe (Plate 2). Massage is applied along the length of the worm towards the incision and by gentle traction the whole worm can usually be removed; in the event of breakage the worm ends should be ligated to minimize contact between host tissue and worm antigens. Deep abscesses require surgical treatment. Anthelmintics have no role in the treatment of Guinea worm.

Control and eradication

Several factors facilitate control: Guinea worm is recognized by local communities as a major health problem, there are no carriers beyond the annual cycle, and there is no animal reservoir. Provision of save water for drinking is the key to control; piped water supplies are unrealistic in most endemic areas, but covered tube wells or hand dug wells provided with parapets are appropriate. Additional measures are filtration of household water with finely woven cloth and the application of temephos (Abate) to ponds to kill copepods.

National programmes have played a major role in many endemic areas. Case detection surveys and health education can be integrated into existing primary health care systems. Unhygienic local treatments such as mud or leaf poultices and crude methods of worm extraction must be discouraged.

Several international health agencies took up the challenge of Guinea worm eradication in the mid-1980s with the target eradication date of 1995. Much has been achieved but the target was missed. Initial expensive hydrological programmes were later replaced by training of local cadres who could conduct health education, case detection, and management, partly independent of local health care services. In some areas private sector initiatives have been able to gain commercially from the publicity achieved by adopting control in a defined area.

There has been a decline of about 95 per cent in the incidence of Guinea worm in the last 15 years. The last stages of eradication will be the most difficult as vertical programmes then become inefficient. Unfortunately many of the major residual foci are in situations of civil disorder and mobile refugees; in others, lack of resources or an absence of democratic institutions will slow progress.

Further reading

Cairncross S *et al.* (1996). Community participation in the eradication of Guinea worm disease. *Acta Tropica* **61**, 121–36.

Hopkins DR *et al.* (1995). Eradication of dracunculiasis from Pakistan. *Lancet* **346**, 621–4.

Issakah-Tinorgah A *et al.* (1994). Lack of effect of ivermectin on prepatent Guinea-worm: a single-blind, placebo-controlled trial. *Transactions of the Royal Society of Tropical Medicine* **88**, 346–8.

Muller R (1971) *Dracunculus* and dracunculiasis. *Advances in Parasitology* **9**, 73–151.

Periès H, Cairncross S (1997). Global eradication of Guinea worm. *Parasitology Today* **13**, 431–7.

7.14.4 Strongyloidiasis, hookworm, and other gut strongyloid nematodes

R. Knight

Strongyloidiasis

The parasitic female *Strongyloides* worms are parthenogenetic. They measure 2 to 2.5 mm in length and normally live in tunnels between the enterocytes of the crypts of Lieberkühn in the duodenum and jejunum. In the external environment larvae may develop directly, through two moults, into infective larvae, in a manner similar to that of the hookworm (Fig. 1). Alternatively, they may follow the indirect cycle, develping into free-living male and female adult worms, about 1 mm in length, that produce a second generation of infective larvae. In either case the cycle is completed when infective filariform larvae penetrate the skin and are carried in the venous circulation to the lungs, from where they ascend the bronchi to be swallowed and so reach the upper small bowel, where they mature.

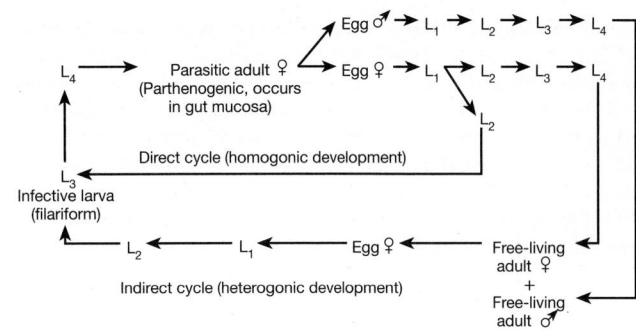

Fig. 1 Basic lifecycle in the genus *Strongyloides*; L₁, L₂, L₃, and L₄ are the larval stages. The indirect cycle occurs in the soil or faecal mass. Eggs of the parasitic female *S. stercoralis* hatch in the gut lumen and direct development may occur not only in the external environment but also on the perianal skin to produce external autoinfection, or in the gut lumen to produce internal autoinfection. The eggs of the parasitic female *S. fuelleborni* appear in the faeces and internal autoinfection is not possible.

Strongyloides stercoralis

Biology and epidemiology

Eggs hatch immediately on reaching the gut lumen, and the first-stage larvae (Fig. 2) then normally pass down the gut without moulting. Direct development in faecally contaminated soil takes 24 to 48 h; free-living adults mature in 72 to 96 h, and live for up to 10 days. Infective larvae can persist in the soil for 3 weeks. There is no second generation of free-living adults. Two types of autoinfection enable infection to persist in the host for long periods. In external autoinfection, infective larvae penetrate the perianal skin after rapid direct development on soiled skin. In internal autoinfection, larvae mature to the infective stage within the lumen of the gut and invade the mucosa of the small intestine or colon, they then pass via the gut lymphatics and portal vein to the lungs and back to the gut. In some patients, uncontrolled internal autoinfection leads to hyperinfection with massive worm loads and severe pathology.

S. stercoralis is widely distributed in the tropics, where prevalence may be 5 to 10 per cent or higher in humid lowlands. It remains endemic in the southern United States, Japan, and in parts of southern Europe, for example, among Swiss and Italian horticulturalists. It also occurs in institutions when soil temperatures are high enough. Transmission among male homosexuals is very rare. Host risk factors are of great importance for

Fig. 2 First-stage larvae of *S. stercoralis* in stool.

internal autoinfection. Patients on steroid and cytotoxic therapy are at most risk, but also those with lymphomas and some other malignancies, hypochlorhydria, diabetic ketosis, hypogammaglobulinaemia, and malnutrition. Despite coprevalence with human immunodeficiency virus type 1 over much of its range, this viral infection does not predispose significantly to *S. stercoralis* hyperinfection, except in patients with advanced AIDS. Servicemen in the Second World War became infected in Thailand and other parts of South-East Asia, mostly as prisoners of war. Many of these infections still persist and such people are at risk of hyperinfection if given steroids.

Pathology

In most persistent infections the parasite load is very low, evokes little pathological response, and the patient is free of symptoms. In some primary infections and when worm loads are higher there is villous blunting with oedema and cellular infiltration of the mucosa, leading to malabsorption and protein-losing enteropathy. In more severe infections and in hyperinfection the small-gut wall becomes oedematous and thickened with impaired motility, and the mesenteric lymph nodes are enlarged. In massive autoinfection there is patchy mucosal loss and some adult worms are found deep in the mucosa from where larvae may invade directly without entering the gut lumen (Plate 1). Invading infective larvae can produce a diffuse or haemorrhagic colitis; migrating or ectopic larvae may be found in any organ of the body. Rarely, adult female worms develop ectopically in the lungs, and these account for the occasional presence of eggs and rhabditiform larvae in sputum.

Clinical manifestations

Light persistent infections

Symptoms, if any, are usually intermittent, with episodes of upper abdominal pain, wheezy cough, and pruritus ani. Blood eosinophilia is common, and may be the only clinical finding. A pathognomonic sign is a rapidly migrating urticaria known as 'larva currens' that occurs on the buttocks, thighs, and lower trunk; it is a form of cutaneous larva migrans, arising from external autoinfection (Plate 2).

Moderate infections

Gut symptoms predominate, with diarrhoea and malabsorption. Weight loss and anorexia are prominent and not infrequently there is leg oedema. Pulmonary and skin lesions are not common. In primary infections a Loeffler's pneumonitis can occur, with high eosinophilia.

Hyperinfection

Diarrhoea is often severe, and sometimes bloody if there is colitis. Vomiting and abdominal distension may progress to pseudo-obstruction. Other manifestations are upper gastrointestinal bleeding, perforation, peritoneal and pleural effusions, pneumonitis (Fig. 3), and terminally, alveolar haemorrhages. Patients are often afebrile and without blood eosinophilia; they can deteriorate rapidly and develop Gram-negative septicaemia with shock, or meningitis, especially if they are immunosuppressed. Hypoglycaemia is a feature of autoinfection in malnourished children.

Diagnosis

Rhabditiform larvae should be sought in the stool (Fig. 2). They may be scanty and numbers do not necessarily correlate with symptoms. Live larvae are seen in fresh, wet, preparations or Baermann concentrates. Agar-plate coprocultures give a result in 48 h, earlier than with conventional charcoal cultures. Formol-ether concentrates are useful, but sensitivity can be low. When stool specimens are not fresh, filariform *Strongyloides* larvae may be found. Duodenal aspiration is another useful technique. In hyperinfection, larvae may be found in sputum (Fig. 4) and in pleural, peritoneal, or cerebrospinal fluids.

Fig. 3 Chest radiograph of a Thai patient who developed pneumonia as part of hyperinfection precipitated by corticosteroid treatment. (Copyright A.J.H. Simpson.)

Serodiagnosis is useful, especially as a screening test in non-endemic areas. In heavy infections, small-bowel barium studies show segmental dilatation, narrowing, and abnormal motility; in hyperinfection, plain abdominal films may show fluid levels.

Treatment

Thiabendazole remains the drug of choice; 25 mg/kg is given twice daily (maximum 3 g/day), usually for 3 days. Intolerance is common and drug-induced hepatitis is reported. Treatment may fail in hyperinfection, which continues to have a high mortality. Such patients need supportive care and parenteral antimicrobials. Invermectin kills adult worms but not migrating tissue larvae; a single oral dose of 200 μg/kg, repeated after 1 week, or 200 μg/kg daily for 3 days are used, but experience in patients with hyperinfection remains limited. Albendazole is an alternative in non-urgent cases but cure rates are rather low.

Strongyloides fuelleborni

In this species eggs do not hatch in the gut lumen so there can be no internal autoinfection. The eggs are thin-walled and contain a larva. In

Fig. 4 Gram stain of sputum from the patient whose chest radiograph is shown in Fig. 3, showing larvae of *S. stercoralis*. (Copyright A.J.H. Simpson.)

Africa this parasite is common in non-human primates. In the forests of West and Central Africa, particularly Zaire, people are commonly infected, mainly from zoonotic sources. Elsewhere, for instance in Zambia and adjacent countries, there is person-to-person transmission. Infected volunteers have developed wheezing, upper abdominal pain, and loose stools, but symptomatology in natural human infections is poorly defined.

In Papua New Guinea a subspecies of this parasite, *S. f. kellyi*, is focally common in both children and adults. In a few communities a distinctive 'swollen belly syndrome' is associated with enormously high faecal egg counts and protein-losing enteropathy. Infants aged 2 weeks to 6 months are affected and show abdominal distension, diarrhoea, breathing difficulties, weight loss, hypoproteinaemia, and peripheral oedema; untreated, the mortality is high. There are no non-human primates in Papua New Guinea and no animal reservoir for this parasite is known. In infants, external autoinfection occurs when they are nursed in soiled string-bag cradles; transmammary transmission is suspected.

S. fuelleborni infection should be treated with thiabendazole. Supportive care including plasma infusion or blood transfusion, plus antibiotic cover, is needed for 'swollen belly syndrome' in Papua New Guinea.

Hookworm and other gut strongyloid nematodes

Adult strongyloid worms live attached to, or buried within, the bowel mucosa (Fig. 5). The ovoid eggs of all genera are similar in appearance, with thin, transparent shells containing a segmented embryo, commonly a 4-, 8- or 16-cell morula. Eggs hatch in the soil and development proceeds through three stages with two moults. The first and second larval stages feed upon bacteria. They are described as rhabditiform, because of resemblance to the soil nematode *Rhabditis*; the pharynx is short, muscular, and constricted in the posterior third, just anterior to a posterior bulb. The third stage, the infective filariform larva, does not feed and may retain the cuticle of the second stage; the pharynx is long and slender, without any constriction. In adults the buccal capsule and its oral armature, and the male copulatory bursa and spicules are used for species identification. Filariform larvae from cultures are generically distinct.

Fig. 5 Adult worm of *Necator americanus* showing relationship of its pharynx to a jejunal villus.

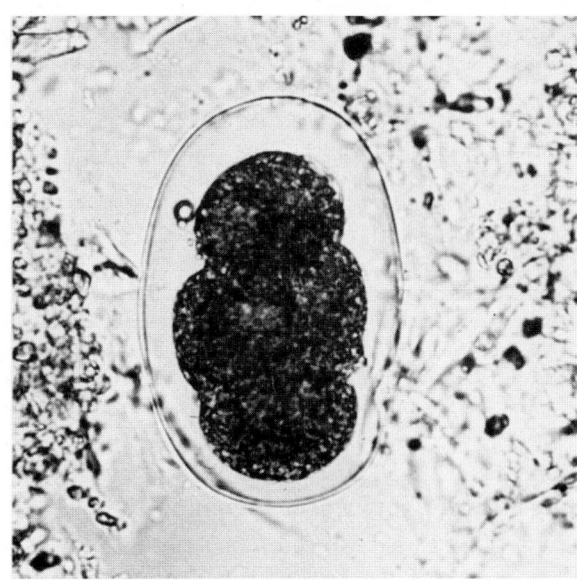

Fig. 6 Egg of *N. americanus*.

The hookworms

Aetiology—the biology of the parasites

Adult worm infections are due to *Ancylostoma duodenale* and *Necator americanus*. Several species that normally infect carnivores may accidentally infect humans and produce zoonotic cutaneous larva migrans or an eosinophilic enteritis in the case of *A. caninum*.

Adult worms measure 8 to 13 mm in length and taper at both ends (Plate 3). Anteriorly the worms are flexed dorsally, giving them their hooked appearance. They attach themselves to the jejunum by drawing mucosa into the buccal cavity (Fig. 5). A vigorous pharyngeal pump enables blood and tissue fluids to be ingested. Worms move frequently in response to host immunological responses. Females produce 5000 to 20 000 eggs per day, but output per worm declines as worm load rises. In the soil, development is temperature dependent. Under optimum conditions eggs hatch within 2 days and larvae develop to the infective stage in 5 days; they can persist in sandy soil for up to a month. Larvae penetrate host skin after soil contact, most commonly between the toes. After entry into dermal venules and lymphatics they are carried to the lung, ascend the bronchi and trachea, and after being swallowed, re-enter the gut where the final moult occurs. Eggs (Fig. 6) can appear in the faeces 50 to 60 days after cutaneous exposure.

Epidemiology

N. americanus is found in the warm, moist tropics where transmission is sometimes perennial. Its introduction to the Americas dates from the transatlantic slave trade. It is a smaller worm than *A. duodenale* and the mouth is guarded by two cutting plates. The mean egg output per female is 8000 per day and the lifespan may exceed 5 years; transmission is exclusively by the percutaneous route.

A. duodenale is primarily a subtropical and temperate species with development in the soil at lower temperatures. It is widely distributed in North Africa, the Middle East, the Indian subcontinent, central and northern China, and in parts of Latin America. Formerly, it was endemic in southern Europe and Japan; it was responsible for 'miner's anaemia' in Cornish tin mines and the Gotthard tunnel. The mouth is guarded by two pairs of sharp teeth. Females produce 15 000 eggs per day. The lifespan is usually less than 2 years. In addition to the percutaneous route, larvae on vegetables can penetrate the buccal mucosa and undergo transpulmonary migration, or they can be swallowed and develop directly within the gut mucosa. Infection may also be transplacental; in China severe hookworm disease is reported in very young infants. Another lifecycle feature is arrested development when larval maturation is delayed at the third or fourth stage within skeletal muscle, or more commonly, in the gut mucosa. This postpones the onset of patent infection and is an adaptive mechanism to irregular or seasonal transmission.

In most populations where these parasites are endemic the prevalence and worm load both rise with age to reach a plateau in adults. Prevalence is highest in rural agricultural communities. Aridity and coolness at higher altitudes limit transmission, but irrigation schemes favour it by raising the water table. Children commonly acquire clinically significant infections between the ages of 5 and 10 years. Within communities, individuals differ greatly in worm load; behavioural factors are important but immune responses, including IgE antibody and eosinophils, limit the proportion of larval worms that mature to adults, the adult lifespan, and also female fecundity.

Pathogenesis of hookworm anaemia

Hookworms damage the mucosa mechanically and by the inflammatory response they evoke; bleeding continues at former attachment sites. Gut motility is affected, especially in primary infections and in children, and this may affect digestive and absorptive function. The major pathogenic mechanism is ingestion of plasma, interstitial fluid, and red cells by the adult worms. A. duodenale ingests about 0.15 ml of blood daily, and N. americanus 0.05 ml. Most red cells pass through the worm's gut and a proportion of the iron content, variously estimated at 10 to 50 per cent, is reabsorbed by the host. Because worm loads are commonly above 50, and may reach 500 or more, the cumulative effect can be serious. The main nutritional effects are iron deficiency and hypoproteinaemia. The rate at which blood loss leads to anaemia is determined by worm load, the duration of infection, iron stores, other blood loss, and dietary iron. Children, and pregnant or lactating women, with little reserve iron, can become anaemic in a few months; in a previously healthy adult male it can take 2 years or more. Loss of albumin into the gut may exceed the capacity of the liver to replace it; synthesis is depressed by low dietary protein, and by the anaemia. Hypoproteinaemia limits the normal, compensatory expansion of plasma volume that occurs in chronic anaemia. While the risk of pulmonary oedema is less, transition to a state of low cardiac output is made more likely.

Clinical features attributable to adult worms

In acute primary infections and in children, epigastric pain is common and may be associated with poor appetite and sometimes diarrhoea. Anorexia is an important mechanism leading to nutritional deficit in children. A few patients develop overt gut bleeding, and melaena is reported in transplacentally infected infants in China.

Most patients present with slowly progressive iron-deficiency anaemia, many have no gut symptoms. Exertional dyspnoea may begin at a haemoglobin level of 8 g/dl, but may not be noted until it falls to 5 g/dl. Palpitations, weakness, and faintness on exertion are common; and sometimes precordial pain or leg claudication. A puffy oedema of the face, arms, and hands is typical, and often unaccompanied by dependent oedema. Other features in heavy infections are mental apathy and depression, and in adults, amenorrhoea or impotence. Pica is common, especially in pregnancy.

Milder degrees of anaemia reduce physical work performance in adults. In children, growth and development may be slowed and cognitive impairment leads to reduced scholastic achievement.

Assessment of cardiovascular status is essential in anaemic patients, to differentiate a well-compensated, high-output state from a dangerous low-output one.

Clinical features attributable to larval worms: cutaneous larva migrans

Cutaneous lesions take the form of migrating, itchy, red, serpiginous papules, known as creeping eruption or cutaneous larva migrans (Plate 4). They commonly become vesiculated and excoriated, with bacterial pyoderma. A. duodenale or N. americanus cause 'ground itch' among estate workers and prominent lesions occur in experimental human infections; however, in many endemic areas they are unnoticed.

Zoonotic hookworms produce more vigorous lesions that may continue to move for several months. Most infections are due to A. braziliense, which is common in dogs throughout the tropics, subtropics, and warmer temperate regions. Less common are infections by two other dog parasites, A. caninum and Uncinaria stenocephala, and the cattle hookworm Bunostomum phlebotomum. Infections occur on sandy bathing beaches, in children's play areas, and by contact with pet sandboxes. Lesions are most common on the lower legs and buttocks, but also occur on the arms, hands, and face.

Wheezy cough due to pneumonitis is more common with A. duodenale; symptoms can continue for many months after one exposure, owing to remobilization of larvae arrested in muscle. Lung symptoms are most prominent in heavy primary infections.

In Queensland it is now recognized that larvae of the dog hookworm A. caninum can reach the gut to produce an eosinophilic enteritis with abdominal pain and vomiting; immature adult worms are found at laparotomy or colonoscopy.

Diagnosis

Stool microscopy will reveal eggs (Fig. 6), except in prepatent infections; examination of stool concentrates is rarely necessary. Faecal egg counts per gram of stool enable the intensity of infection to be estimated. The simplest method is a semiquantitative wet smear, using 2 mg of stool. For more precise results the use of the McMaster counting chamber is recommended. An alternative is the modified Kato technique, but this requires special care as hookworm eggs can overclear and become invisible. Isotope studies indicate that, with either species, 1000 eggs per gram is equivalent to 2.2 ml of blood loss per day. Culture to the infective larval stage, using the Harada Mori technique, will differentiate the two major species and the other genera of gut strongyloid nematodes.

Treatment

A single 400-mg dose of albendazole, or mebendazole at 100 mg twice daily for 3 days, are both very effective. Alternatives are pyrantel at 10 mg/kg daily for three or four doses, or bephenium at 5 g daily for three doses, the latter being less effective for N. americanus.

To replace iron reserves, oral ferrous sulphate will suffice in most patients, but several weeks of medication may be necessary. When compliance is doubted, consideration should be given to intramuscular iron or total-dose intravenous infusion of iron dextran.

Transfusion of packed or sedimented red cells may be necessary in pregnancy and when cardiac output is compromised. Frusemide may be necessary to cover the transfusion, but in other circumstances diuretics should be used with caution. Depletion of plasma volume in patients with hookworm anaemia together with hypoproteinaemia can compromise cardiac output. Even bed rest in formerly ambulant patients can lead to significant diuresis. Chemotherapy should generally be avoided in pregnancy.

Cutaneous lesions can be treated with thiabendazole at 25 mg/kg in two divided doses, for 2 days, and, if necessary, after 2 days' rest a further 5 days at the same dose. Alternatively, a single dose of ivermectin at 200 μg/kg may be given; this is more effective than a single dose of 400 mg albendazole.

Topical treatment avoids systemic effects (usually nausea). One 0.5-g tablet of thiabendazole can be ground up in 5 g of petroleum jelly or dimethylsulphoxide base and applied daily over the worm track for 5 days.

Control

Population-based measures are necessary when endemicity and morbidity are high. Latrines are generally beneficial, but can create foci for transmission when the water table is high. Provision of piped water reduces contact with soil polluted by promiscuous defaecation. Where human excreta is used as fertilizer, composting and chemical ovicides are needed. Cash-crop estates, plantations, and irrigation schemes should provide safe latrines and subsidized footwear.

Anthelmintic drugs can be deployed in several ways. Certain target groups such as agricultural and sewage workers, clinic outpatients with pallor, and anaemic blood donors can be treated empirically because of their likelihood of infection. Population chemotherapy, repeated twice yearly, aims to reduce both prevalence and mean worm load. It may include those with positive stool tests—selective chemotherapy; or whole communities—mass chemotherapy. The relative costs of drugs and diagnosis will change during the course of a programme. Single-dose medication is best and possible with mebendazole at a dose of 600 mg or albendazole at 400 mg.

Other gut strongyloids

Trichostrongylus spp.

These are common and economically important gut parasites of domestic ungulates. Infection is by ingestion of filariform larvae on vegetation. Development in the gut is direct, without lung migration. Adults are reddish-brown, 5 to 10 mm in length, and live with their anterior ends embedded in the jejunal mucosa where they feed on tissue fluid, not blood.

Human infection has been recorded with eight species; *T. colubriformis* and *T. orientalis* being the most important. Prevalence rates are highest in Iran, Iraq, Egypt, and Japan. Most infection is derived from sheep, goats, cattle, and camels, but in Iran *T. orientalis* is non-zoonotic. Worms cause mucosal damage, and loss of protein and some blood. Clinical features include abdominal pain, eosinophilia, and sometimes anaemia. The eggs are longer and narrower than those of hookworm, but larval culture is required for reliable differentiation. Infections respond to drugs used for hookworm.

Ternidens deminutus

Human infection is locally common in parts of Central and southern Africa. Infection is direct following oral ingestion of larvae; adult worms are 8 to 16 mm long. They live partly embedded in the colonic mucosa, where they produce superficial ulceration and cystic nodules. The worm is sometimes referred to as 'false hookworm', because of the similarity of its eggs; differentiation is important both clinically and epidemiologically. Non-human primates are infected in much of Africa, but most human infections are non-zoonotic. Infections respond to drugs used for hookworm.

Oesophagostomum spp.

These are important parasites of primates and ungulates: in veterinary practice they are known as the 'nodular worms'. Fourth-stage larvae and immature adults live in the colonic wall, often deeply situated or in the subserosa; lesions may become bacterially infected or perforate. Normally, adult worms return to the gut lumen. Most human infections are reported from forested parts of West and Central Africa. In some remote villages of north Togo and Ghana faecal surveys, using larval culture, have shown prevalences reaching 30 per cent. Most cases have presented surgically with masses, or abscesses, located in the caecum or other parts of the colon; or with bowel obstruction, or ectopic lesions in the peritoneum or abdominal wall. Clinically the lesions simulate carcinoma, tuberculosis, appendicitis, and amoeboma. Diagnosis in such cases has been histological.

The eggs resemble those of hookworm and are absent in prepatent surgical cases. Chemotherapy has been little studied in man, but albendazole

has been successfully used. In Africa most human infections are with the monkey parasite *O. bifurcatum*, or *O. stephanostomum*, a parasite of anthropoid apes; in Asia, *O. aculeatum* is the likely cause. The ungulate species do not appear to infect humans.

Further reading

Adeneusi AA (1997). Cure by ivermectin of a chronic, persistent, intestinal strongyloidosis. *Acta Tropica* 66, 163–7.

Ashford RW, Barnish G, Viney ME (1992). *Strongyloides fuelleborni kellyi*: infection and disease in Papua New Guinea. *Parasitology Today* 8, 314–18.

Croese J *et al.* (1994). Human enteric infection with canine hookworms. *Annals of Internal Medicine* 120, 369–74.

Grove DI, ed. (1989). *Strongyloidiasis: a major roundworm infection in man*. Taylor & Francis, London.

Grove DI (1996). Human strongyloidiasis. *Advances in Parasitology* 38, 251–309.

Gulletta M *et al.* (1998). AIDS and strongyloidiasis. *International Journal of Sexually Transmitted Diseases and AIDS* 9, 427–9.

Jongwutiwes J *et al.* (1999). Increased sensitivity of routine laboratory detection of *Strongyloides stercoralis* and hookworm by agar-plate culture. *Transactions of the Royal Society of Tropical Medicine and Hygiene* 93, 398–400.

Krepel HP *et al.* (1995). Reinfection patterns of *Oesophagostomum bifurcum* after anthelmintic treatment. *Tropical and Geographic Medicine* 47, 160–3.

Mahmoud AAF (1996). Strongyloidiasis. *Clinical Infectious Diseases* 23, 949–53.

Roche M, Layrisse M (1966). The nature and causes of hookworm anaemia. *American Journal of Tropical Medicine and Hygiene* 15, 1029–102.

Schad GA, Warren KS, eds (1990). *Hookworm disease: current status and new directions*. Taylor & Francis, London.

7.14.5 Nematode infections of lesser importance

David I. Grove

From time to time, a patient may be encountered who harbours an unusual nematode. Some of these organisms are free-living parasites and the patient has a spurious infection, usually as the result of ingestion of the worm or following the *in vitro* contamination of a clinical specimen such as faeces or urine. Other individuals may have true infections with worms being found either in the gastrointestinal tract or in the tissues. Many of these infections are with parasites of animals that are adapted poorly to the human host and are unable to complete their development in man. Thus, worms in varying stages of development including larvae, adults, and eggs may be found in specimens. Some parasites may be recovered from fluids and are viewed intact whereas others are seen only in histological sections. If there is uncertainty in identifying the worm in the former circumstance, help may often be obtained from a veterinary parasitologist who may be more used to dealing with the species concerned. In the latter instance, definitive diagnosis may be very difficult but excellent resources are available.[13,39] A summary of rarely reported nematodes is shown in Table 1. *Dirofilaria* species and unusual microfilariae in blood and tissues have been reviewed elsewhere.[40]

Nematodes found in the gastrointestinal tract may respond to a benzimidazole agent such as mebendazole (100 mg orally, twice daily, for up to 3 days) or albendazole (10 mg/kg orally, daily, for up to 1 week). Thiabendazole (25 mg/kg twice daily for several days) has been used traditionally orally for the treatment of systemic larval infections but its effectiveness is very variable; albendazole may be more active than thiabendazole and is absorbed better from the gut than mebendazole. If these drugs fail, iver-mectin (0.15 mg/kg orally, daily, for several days) may be tried. Other drugs that have been used in these unusual nematode infections include levami-sole and diethylcarbamazine. Unfortunately, some infections are refractory

Table 1 A summary of rarely reported nematodes found infecting humans

Nematode	Geographical distribution	Usual host	Mode of transmission	Stage of development	Clinical features	Suggested treatment	Refs
Agamomermis species	?	Free-living, grasshoppers	? Ingestion	Larvae, adults	Spurious; worms in mouth, faeces, urethra	Manual removal if necessary	2
Anatrichosoma cutanea	Asia, Africa	Monkeys	?	Larvae	Cutaneous larva migrans	Thiabendazole/ albendazole	33
Ancylostoma caninum	Widespread	Dogs	Cutaneous penetration	Larvae, ? Adults	Cutaneous larva migrans, myositis, pulmonary infiltrates, eosinophilic enteritis	Mebendazole (enteritis), thiabendazole (other)	34, 44
Ancylostoma malayanum	Asia	Bear	?	?	?	Mebendazole	51
Ascaris suum	Widespread	Pigs	Ingestion of eggs	Larvae, ? Adults	Pneumonitis, abdominal discomfort	Albendazole	36, 41
Baylisascaris procyonis	North America	Raccoons	Ingestion of eggs in soil	Larvae	Visceral and ocular larva migrans, eosinophilic meningo-encephalitis	Albendazole	6, 19
Bunostomum trigonocephalum	Widespread	Sheep	Cutaneous penetration	Larvae	Cutaneous larva migrans	Albendazole	35
Brugia species (not *malayi, timori*)	Widespread	Monkeys, raccoons, rabbits	Mosquito-borne	Larvae, Adults	Lymph node swelling	Excision	40
Cheilospirura species	Widespread	Birds	? Ingestion of arthropods	Larvae	Conjunctival nodule	Excision	1
Contracaecum species	Widespread	Fish, birds	Ingestion of undercooked fish	Larvae	See anisakiasis	See anisakiasis	47
Cyclodontostomum purvisi	Asia	Rats	?	Adults	Worms in faeces	Mebendazole	4
Dioctophyma renale	Widespread	Mammals	Ingestion of aquatic annelids, amphibia, crustacea, fish	Larvae, adults	Haematuria, retroperitoneal mass, subcutaneous nodule	Excision	23
Diploscapter coronata	Widespread	Free-living	Ingestion in vegetation	Adults	Spurious; worms in stomach contents, urine	Unnecessary	11
Eustrongylides species	Widespread	Fish, birds	Ingestion of undercooked fish	Larvae	Peritonitis	Laparotomy and surgical removal	17, 50
Gongylonema pulchrum	Worldwide	Ruminants, swine	Ingestion of beetles, cockroaches etc.	Adults	Migrating worm, especially in the oral cavity	Surgical removal	24
Haemonchus contortus	Widespread	Sheep, cattle	? Ingestion of larvae on vegetation	Adults	?	Mebendazole	48
Lagochilascaris minor	Central and South America	?	?	Adults, eggs, larvae	Subcutaneous abscess in head and neck; nasopharyn-geal or sinus lesions, encephalitis	Surgical removal; levamisole, diethylcarb-amazine, thiabendazole	10, 46
Mammomonogamus (= Syngamus) laryngeus	Central and South America	Cattle, felines	?	Adults	Cough, pharyngeal lesion	Endoscopic removal	38

Table 1 *Continued*

Nematode	Geographical distribution	Usual host	Mode of transmission	Stage of development	Clinical features	Suggested treatment	Refs
Meloidogyne (= *Heterodera*) species	Widespread	Plant parasite	Ingestion of vegetation; contamination of faecal specimen	Eggs, larvae	Spurious; eggs and larvae in faeces	Unnecessary	29
Meningonema peruzzii	Africa	Monkeys	?	Larvae	Meningo-encephalitis	Albendazole	7
Mermis nigrescens	North America	Grasshoppers	? Ingestion of adult worm	Adults	Worm in mouth	Manual removal	43
Metastrongylus elongatus	Widespread	Pigs	Ingestion of earthworms	Adults	Worm in gut or respiratory tract	Albendazole	2, 35
Metastrongylid nematode	Italy	?	?	Larvae, adults	Pulmonary arteritis	? Anthelmintics	42
Micronema deletrix	Widespread	Free-living; horses	Trauma or skin lesions	Adults, larvae, eggs	Meningo-encephalitis; generalized spread	Albendazole	21
Muscipeoid nematode	Australia	?	?	Larvae, adults	Polymyositis	Albendazole	15
Necator suillis	Central America	Pigs	Percutaneous	Adults	?	Mebendazole	8
Onchocerca species (not *volvulus*)	Widespread	Cattle, horses	Insect-borne	Adults,	Subcutaneous nodule; eye lesions	Surgical excision	9, 40
Ostertagia species	Widespread	Cattle, sheep	? Ingestion of adult worms in undercooked abomasum	Adults	? Spurious; worms in gut	Mebendazole	27
Pelodera (= *Rhabditis*) *strongyloides*	Widespread	Free-living	Cutaneous	Larvae	Papular dermatitis	Albendazole, topical corticosteroid	25
Philometra species	Widespread	Fish	Cutaneous injury	Adults	Worms in laceration	Manual removal	14
Phocanema species	Widespread	Fish	Ingestion of undercooked fish	Larvae	See anisakiasis	See anisakiasis	28
Physaloptera caucasica	Europe, Africa	Primates	? Ingestion of beetles, cockroaches	Adults, eggs	Sometimes spurious; abdominal pain; small bowel gangrene	Mebendazole; surgical removal	18, 37
Rhabditis species	Widespread	Free-living	Ingestion	Adults	Spurious; worms in faeces, urine, skin	Unnecessary	2
Rictularia species	Widespread	Mammals, birds	? Ingestion	Adults	Found in an appendix		30
Spirocerca lupi	Widespread	Dogs, wolves	? Ingestion of beetle	Adults	Intestinal obstruction and peritonitis in a baby	Surgery	5
Spiruroid nematode	Japan	Fish, squid	Ingestion of undercooked food	Larvae	Creeping eruption, ileal granuloma	Excision; ? anthelmintics	22, 26
Syphacia species	Widespread	Mice	Ingestion	Eggs, adults	? Spurious; worms in faeces	Mebendazole if necessary	45
Terranova species	Widespread	Fish	Ingestion of undercooked fish	Larvae	See anisakiasis	See anisakiasis	32
Tetrameres fissispina	Widespread	Birds	? Ingestion of grasshoppers, cockroaches	Adults	? Spurious; worms in gut	Mebendazole	35
Thelazia californiensis	North America	Mammals	Deposition on eye by fly	Adults	Conjunctivitis	Manual removal	16
Thelazia callipaeda	Asia	Dogs, rabbits	Deposition on eye by fly	Adults	Conjunctivitis	Manual removal	12
Trichuris suis	Widespread	Pigs	Ingestion of eggs	Eggs, larvae, adults	Usually asymptomatic	Mebendazole	3
Trichuris vulpis	Widespread	Dogs	Ingestion of eggs	Eggs, larvae, adults	Usually asymptomatic	Mebendazole	31

Table 1 *Continued*

Nematode	Geographical distribution	Usual host	Mode of transmission	Stage of development	Clinical features	Suggested treatment	Refs
Turbatrix (= *Anguillula*) *aceti*	Widespread	Free-living (including vinegar, acetic acid)	Accidental inoculation	Larvae, adults	Spurious; urine, vaginal discharge, blood smears (in stains)	Unnecessary	49
Uncinaria Stenocephala	Widespread	Dogs, cats	Cutaneous penetration	Larvae	Cutaneous larva migrans	Thiabendazole, albendazole	20

to all anthelmintics. Nevertheless, these worms generally cannot multiply in humans and the parasites will die spontaneously after months or years.

Further reading

1. **Africa CM, Garcia EY** (1936). A new nematode parasite (*Cheilospirura* sp.) of the eye of man in the Philippines. *Journal of the Philippine Islands Medical Association* **16**, 603–7.

2. **Beaver PC, Jung RC, Cupp WE** (1984). *Clinical parasitology*, 9th edn. Lea & Febiger, Philadelphia.

3. **Beer RJ** (1971). Experimental infection of man with pig whipworm. *British Medical Journal* i, 44.

4. **Bhaibulaya M, Indrangarm S** (1975). Man, as an accidental host of *Cyclodontostomum purvisi* (Adams, 1933), and the occurrence in rats in Thailand. *Southeast Asian Journal of Tropical Medicine and Public Health* **6**, 391–4.

5. **Biocca E** (1959). Infestazione umana prenatale da *Spirocerca lupi* (Rud. 1809). *Parassitologia* **1**, 137–42.

6. **Boschetti A, Kasznica J** (1995). Visceral larva migrans induced cardiac pseudotumor: a cause of sudden death in a child. *Journal of Forensic Science* **40**, 1097–9.

7. **Boussinesq M** *et al.* (1995). A new zoonosis of the cerebrospinal fluid of man probably caused by *Meningonema peruzzii*, a filaria of the central nervous system of Cercopithecidae. *Parasite* **2**, 173–6.

8. **Buckley JJ** (1933). *Necator suillis* as a human infection. *British Medical Journal* i, 699–700.

9. **Burr WE, Brown,MF, Eberhard ML** (1998). Zoonotic *Onchocerca* (Nematoda: Filarioidea) in the cornea of a Colorado resident. *Ophthalmology* **105**, 1494–7.

10. **Calvopina M** *et al.* (1998). Treatment of human lagochilascariasis with ivermectin: first case report from Ecuador. *Transactions of the Royal Society of Tropical Medicine and Hygiene* **92**, 223–4.

11. **Chandler AC** (1938). *Diploscapter coronata* as a facultative parasite of man, with a general review of vertebrate parasitism by rhabditoid worms. *Parasitology* **30**, 40–5.

12. **Cheung WK** *et al.* (1998). Conjunctivitis caused by *Thelazia callipaeda* infestation in a woman. *Journal of the Formosa Medical Association* **97**, 425–7.

13. **Connor DH** *et al.*, eds (1997). *Pathology of infectious diseases*, Vol 2, pp 1305–588. Appleton & Lange, Stamford.

14. **Deardorff TL** *et al.* (1986). Piscine adult nematode invading an open lesion in a human hand. *American Journal of Tropical Medicine and Hygiene* **35**, 827–30.

15. **Dennett X** *et al.* (1998). Polymyositis caused by a new genus of nematode. *Medical Journal of Australia* **168**, 226–7.

16. **Doezie AM** *et al.* (1996). *Thelazia californiensis* conjunctival infestation. *Ophthalmic Surgery Lasers* **27**, 716–19.

17. **Eberhard ML** *et al.* (1989). Intestinal perforation caused by larval *Eustrongylides* (Nematoda: Dioctophymatoidae) in New Jersey. *American Journal of Tropical Medicine and Hygiene* **40**, 648–50.

18. **Evans AC, Markus MB, Steyne E** (1990). A survey of the intestinal nematodes of bushmen in Namibia. *American Journal of Tropical Medicine and Hygiene* **42**, 243–7.

19. **Fox AS** *et al.* (1985). Fatal eosinophilic meningoencephalitis and visceral larva migrans caused by the raccoon ascarid *Baylascaris procyonis*. *New England Journal of Medicine* **312**, 1619–23.

20. **Fülleborn F** (1927). Durch Hakenwurmlarven des Hundes (*Uncinaria stenocephala*) beim Menschen erzeugte 'Creeping Eruption'. *Abhandlungen aus dem Gebiet der Auslandskunde, Hamburg Universität (Fetschrift Nocht)* **26**, 121–33.

21. **Gardiner CH, Koh DS, Cardella TA** (1981). *Micronema* in man: third fatal infection. *American Journal of Tropical Medicine and Hygiene* **30**, 586–9.

22. **Goto Y** *et al.* (1998). Creeping eruption caused by a larva of the suborder Spiruna type X. *British Journal of Dermatology* **139**, 315–18

23. **Gutierrez Y, Cohen M, Machiaco CN** (1989). *Dioctophyme* [*sic*] larva in the subcutaneous tissues of a woman in Ohio. *American Journal of Surgical Pathology* **13**, 800–2.

24. **Jelinek T, Loscher T** (1994). Human infection with *Gongylonema pulchrum*: a case report. *Tropical Medicine and Parasitology* **45**, 329–30.

25. **Jones CC, Rosen T, Greenberg C** (1991). Cutaneous larva migrans due to *Pelodera strongyloides*. *Cutis* **48**, 123–6.

26. **Kagei N** *et al.* (1992). A case of ileus caused by a spiruroid nematode. *International Journal for Parasitology* **22**, 839–41.

27. **Kasimov GB** (1941). (The first case of ostertagiasis in man). *Meditsinskaya Parazitologiya i Parazitarnye e Bolezni* **10**, 121–3. In Russian. Abstracted in (1943). *Tropical Diseases Bulletin* **40**, 326.

28. **Kates S, Wright KA, Wright, R** (1973). A case of human infection with the cod nematode *Phocanema* sp. *American Journal of Tropical Medicine and Hygiene* **32**, 606–8.

29. **Keller AE** (1935). The occurrence of eggs of *Heterodera radicicola* in human feces. *Journal of Laboratory and Clinical Medicine*, **20**, 390–2.

30. **Kenney M** *et al.* (1975). A case of *Rictularia* infection of man in New York. *American Journal of Tropical Medicine and Hygiene* **24**, 596–9.

31. **Kenney Y, Yermakov V** (1980). Infection of man with *Trichuris vulpis*, the whipworm of dogs. *American Journal of Tropical Medicine and Hygiene* **29**, 1206–8.

32. **Koyama, T** *et al.* (1973). *Terranova* (Nematoda: Anisakidae) infection in man. II. Morphological features of *Terranova* sp. larva found in human stomach wall. *Japanese Journal of Parasitology* **21**, 257–61.

33. **Le VH, Duong HM, Nguyen, LV** (1963). Premier cas de capillariose cutanée humaine. *Bulletin de la Société de Pathologie Exotique* **56**, 121–6.

34. **Little MD** *et al.* (1983). *Ancylostoma* larva in a muscle fiber of man following cutaneous larva migrans. *American Journal of Tropical Medicine and Hygiene* **32**, 1285–8.

35. **Mao SP** (1991). Protozoan and helminth parasites of humans in mainland China. *International Journal for Parasitology* **21**, 347–51.

36. **Maruyama H** *et al.* (1996). An outbreak of visceral larva migrans due to *Ascaris suum* in Kyushu, Japan. *Lancet* **348**, 1766–7.

37. **Nicolaides NJ** *et al.* (1977). Nematode larvae (Spirurida: Physalopteridae) causing infarction of the bowel in an infant. *Pathology* **9**, 129–35.

38. **Nosanchuk JS, Wade SE, Landolf M** (1995). Case report of and description of parasite in *Mammomonogamus laryngeus* (human syngamosis) infection. *Journal of Clinical Microbiology* **33**, 998–1000.

39. **Orihel TC, Ash LR** (1995). *Parasites in human tissues*. American Society of Clinical Pathologists, Chicago.

40. **Orihel TC, Eberhard ML** (1998). Zoonotic filariasis. *Clinical Microbiology Reviews* **11**, 366–81.

41. Phills JA *et al.* (1972). Pulmonary infiltrates, asthma and eosinophilia due to *Ascaris suum* infestation in man. *New England Journal of Medicine* **286**, 965–70.

42. Pirisi M *et al.* (1995). Fatal human pulmonary infection caused by an *Angiostrongylus*-like nematode. *Clinical Infectious Diseases* **20**, 59–65.

43. Poinar GO Jr, Hoberg EP (1988). *Mermis nigrescens* (Mermithidae: Nematoda) recovered from the mouth of a child. *American Journal of Tropical Medicine and Hygiene* **39**, 478–9.

44. Prociv P, Croese J (1996). Human enteric infection with *Ancylostoma caninum*: hookworm reappraised in the light of a 'new' zoonosis. *Acta Tropica* **62**, 23–44.

45. Riley WA (1920). A mouse oxyurid, *Syphacia obvelata*, as a parasite of man. *Journal of Parasitology* **6**, 89–92.

46. Rosemberg S *et al.* (1986). Fatal encephalopathy due to *Lagochilascaris minor* infection. *American Journal of Tropical Medicine and Hygiene* **35**, 575–8.

47. Schaum E, Müller W (1967). Die Heterocheilidiasis. Eine Infektion des Menschen mit Larven von Fisch-Ascariden. *Deutsche medizinische Wochenschrift* **92**, 2230–3.

48. Sweet WC (1924). The intestinal parasites of man in Australia and its dependencies as found by the Australian Hookworm Campaign. *Medical Journal of Australia* **i**, 405–7.

49. Todd JC, Sanford AH (1943). *Clinical diagnosis by laboratory methods.* W.B. Saunders, Philadelphia.

50. Wittner M *et al.* (1989). Eustrongylidiasis—a parasitic infection acquired by eating sushi. *New England Journal of Medicine* **320**, 1124–6.

51. Yorke W, Maplestone RA (1926). *The nematode parasites of vertebrates.* J&A Churchill, London.

7.14.6 Other gut nematodes

V. Zaman

Ascariasis (roundworm)

Ascariasis is an infection caused by *Ascaris lumbricoides*. Normally, the adult worms are located in the small intestine. In unusual circumstances, such as fever, irritation due to drugs, anaesthesia, and bowel manipulation during surgery, the worms may migrate to ectopic sites where they may give rise to severe disease.

Geographical distribution

The distribution is cosmopolitan but the parasite occurs more frequently in moist and warm climates. In some rural tropical areas, the entire population may be infected. It is relatively more common in children, who also carry higher worm loads.

Morphology

The mature worm is cylindrical with tapering ends (Plate 1). It is creamy white to light brown in colour. The female measures 20 to 35 cm in length and 3 to 6 mm in breadth. The male measures 12 to 31 cm in length and 2 to 4 mm in breadth and has a curved tail. The head has three lips at the anterior end, which carry minute teeth or denticles along their margins. The lips can be closed or extended, allowing the worm to ingest food. In cross section, the worm reveals a thick cuticle, adjacent to which is the hypodermis which projects into the body cavity in the form of lateral cords (Fig. 1(a)). The somatic muscle cells are large and elongated and lie adjacent to the hypodermis. The worm is able to maintain its position in the small intestine by the activity of these muscles. If the somatic muscles are paralysed by anthelminthics, it is expelled by peristalsis.

Fig. 1 (a) *Ascaris lumbricoides* in the bile duct (× 125). (b) Anisakis larva in cross section in the human stomach showing large bulbous lateral cords.

The fertilized eggs are ovoidal and measure 60 to 70 by 30 to 50 μm. When freshly passed they are not infective and contain a single cell. The larva becomes infective in the soil. The cell is surrounded by a thin vitelline membrane. Around the membrane is a thick, translucent shell, which in turn is surrounded by an irregular, albuminous coat (Fig. 2). The albuminous coat is sometimes lost or can be removed by chemical treatment, resulting in a decorticated egg. It was once assumed that the brown coloration of the egg was due to bile pigment, but tannins in the egg shell are probably responsible. The unfertilized eggs are 88 to 94 by 40 to 44 μm and have disorganized contents. The larvae of *A. lumbricoides* may be seen in infected lungs and measure up to 2 mm in length, and 75 μm in diameter (Fig. 3). The larvae have a central intestine, paired excretory columns, and prominent lateral alae.

Lifecycle (see Fig. 4)

The gravid female produces 200 000 to 250 000 eggs daily. These take 3 or 4 weeks to develop into the infective stage, which is probably the third-stage rather than the second-stage larva as was previously thought. The eggs are resistant to chemicals and low temperatures and may remain viable for years in moist soil. On ingestion, the infective larva hatches out in the small intestine and penetrates the intestinal wall to enter the portal circulation. From the liver it is carried to the heart and via the pulmonary artery to the lungs. In the lungs, it breaks out of the capillaries into the alveoli and undergoes another moult to become a fourth-stage larva. From the lungs

Fig. 2 Ascaris ovum seen by scanning electron micrography. (Copyright Viqar Zaman.)

Fig. 3 Decorticated ova of Ascaris showing emergence of larvae. (Copyright Viqar Zaman.)

the larva moves up to the bronchi and then crawls over the epiglottis to enter the digestive tract. In the intestine, it moults again to become a sexually mature worm. The lifespan of an adult worm is approximately 1 year, after which it is spontaneously expelled. In hyperendemic areas, children are being continuously infected so that as some worms are being expelled, others are maturing to take their place.

Clinical aspects

In most cases, the infected person remains asymptomatic. However, there is much evidence to indicate that the presence of *Ascaris* causes nutritional problems and hinders the normal development of children. Occasionally, patients may develop fever, malaise, urticaria, intestinal colic, nausea, vomiting, diarrhoea, and central nervous system disorders.

The migration of larval *Ascaris* through the lungs may produce varying degrees of pneumonitis and bronchospasm known as Loeffler's syndrome

(Plate 2). Chest radiographs may show diffuse mottling and increased prominence of peribronchial markings. There is generally high eosinophilia and the condition subsides after 7 to 10 days unless reinfection occurs. In areas where pig farming is common the larvae of *A. suum* (pig *Ascaris*) may also produce severe pneumonitis and bronchospasm.

Occasionally, ascariasis can cause severe, life-threatening disease. This could happen in the following situations.

1. When large numbers of worms get entangled to form a bolus and block the intestinal lumen producing signs and symptoms of acute intestinal obstruction.

2. When ectopic migration results in the entry of the worm into the appendix, common bile duct, or pancreatic duct. When the biliary tract is invaded, there is severe abdominal pain, often followed by suppurative cholangitis and multiple liver abscesses resulting from the disintegration of the trapped worm and secondary bacterial infection. Disintegration of the female worm releases a large number of eggs in the liver that can be recognized on histological examination.

3. When a worm blocks in the ampulla of Vater causing acute pancreatitis and pancreatic necrosis.

Diagnosis

This is usually made by detecting *Ascaris* eggs in the faeces. Sometimes, the patient brings developing or adult worms that have been passed in the faeces or have emerged from the anus or the nose in a sick child. They are roughly the same size as and have the appearance of earthworms. Occasionally, adult worms are outlined in the intestines during barium-meal examination.

Treatment

Whenever possible, all positive cases, irrespective of the worm load, should be treated, as even a few worms can undergo ectopic migration with dangerous consequences.

Pyrantel pamoate

A single dose of 11 mg/kg body weight (maximum 1 g) is effective in curing over 90 per cent of cases of ascariasis. Side-effects are mild, if any, and the drug is well tolerated. It is also active against *Enterobius vermicularis* and hookworms (*Ancylostoma duodenale* and *Necator americanus*) but not against *Trichuris trichiura*. Its use in pregnant women and children of under 2 years is not recommended.

Mebendazole

This drug is a broad-spectrum anthelminthic with good host tolerance. It is active against *Ascaris*, *Trichuris*, *Enterobius*, and hookworms. This broad-spectrum activity is useful in endemic areas where multiple nematode infections are common. It is given as 100 mg twice daily for 3 days, for both adults and children of more than 2 years of age. Mebendazole should not be given to pregnant women, especially in the first trimester.

Albendazole

Like mebendazole this drug is also safe and effective against infections with *Ascaris*, *Trichuris*, *Enterobius*, and hookworms. The drug is given as a single oral dose of 400 mg for adults and children of more than 2 years of age. It should not be given to pregnant women.

Piperazine salts

These are old anthelminthics but still widely used because of their low cost and high degree of efficacy against *Ascaris* and *Enterobius*. The dose is 75 mg/kg (maximum of 3.5 g) given as a single dose daily for two consecutive days. It is not necessary to fast beforehand. Occasionally, symptoms involving the central nervous system, such as unsteadiness and vertigo, have been reported.

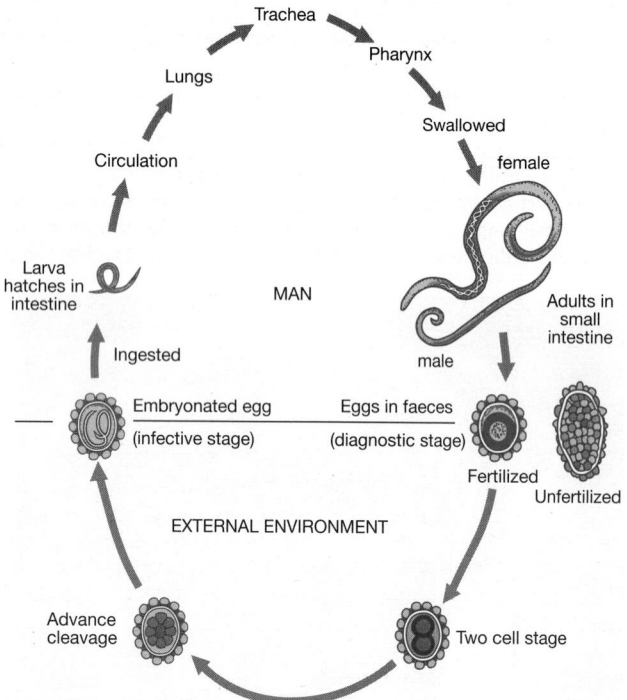

Fig. 4 Lifecycle of *Ascaris lumbricoides*. (Adapted from Centers for Disease Control, Atlanta, Georgia, United States.)

If signs of intestinal obstruction develop in a child living in an endemic area, ascariasis is a distinct possibility. The child should be admitted to hospital and prepared for surgical intervention. To start with the measures should be:

1. Decompression of the bowel through an intestinal tube with constant suction.
2. Rehydration and restoration of electrolyte balance by intravenous drip.
3. Antipyretics if fever is present.
4. Introduction of an appropriate dose of piperazine citrate through an intestinal tube. This induces flaccid paralysis of the worm.

In most cases this conservative therapy will relieve the obstruction and the child will rapidly recover. If, however, the signs of obstruction persist and the child's general condition worsens, laparotomy is required. Acute obstructive jaundice or pancreatitis due to obstruction of the common bile duct by *Ascaris* also requires urgent surgical intervention.

Prevention and control

As *Ascaris* eggs can survive in the soil for many years, prevention and control in endemic areas is difficult. Mass chemotherapy given at intervals of 6 months along with environmental sanitation can break the cycle. The prevalence of ascariasis and other soil-transmitted helminths is greatly reduced by improving housing. Infection is prevented by eating only cooked food and by avoiding green vegetables and salads in countries where human faeces are used as a fertilizer and where this parasite is endemic.

Anisakiasis

Anisakiasis is an infection caused by the larvae of nematodes belonging to the family Anisakidae.

Geographical distribution

The adult worms are commonly found in cetaceans (whales, dolphins, and porpoises) in many parts of the world. Human beings are infected when they eat raw or improperly cooked fish or squid. The incidence is highest in Japan, followed by Holland, Scandinavia, and countries along the Pacific coast of South America. A few cases have also been reported from California and the western United States.

Morphology

Complete speciation of the adults and larvae of this large group of parasites has not been done. In larval stages found in man the presence of large lateral cords which are bulbous in cross section is diagnostic of the family Anisakidae (Fig. 1(b)). Scanning electron microscopy shows the ventral side of the mouth to have a triangular boring tooth (Fig. 5).

Fig. 5 Anisakis larva: third-stage larva of *A. simplex* showing the tip of the boring tooth (arrow) (× 400).

Lifecycle

Adults live in the lumen of the intestine of cetaceans. Eggs are passed in water and second-stage larvae are ingested by crustaceans, which are then ingested by fish or squid where they enter the muscles; cetaceans and man become infected by eating the fish or squid. In man, larvae do not develop to maturity but attach themselves to the mucosa of the stomach or intestine.

Clinical aspects

Most patients present with gastric symptoms that develop 4 to 24 h after eating infected fish. The symptoms are due to ulceration produced by the larvae as they burrow into the mucous membrane. There is epigastric pain, nausea, and vomiting, and sometimes haematemesis during the acute stage of the disease. If symptoms are mild and the patient is left untreated, the infection can become chronic with tumour formation. The small intestine may be involved, resulting in severe pain in the lower abdomen, which may be misdiagnosed as appendicitis.

Diagnosis

Gastroscopy often reveals the lesion and the presence of larvae attached to the mucous membrane. Radiographs with a barium meal may show the presence of single or multiple ulcers and outline the worm. Serological tests are now available in some specialized centres.

Treatment

In acute infection an attempt should be made to remove all the larvae through a gastroscope. In chronic cases, surgical removal of the ulcerated areas or the tumour may be required. No effective chemotherapy is available. Prevention is by not eating raw fish and squid.

Capillariasis

Capillariasis is an infection by parasites belonging to the genus *Capillaria*. Two species infect man, *C. philippinensis*, which produces intestinal capillariasis, and *C. hepatica*, which produces hepatic capillariasis.

Geographical distribution

C. philippinensis has been described from the Philippines and Thailand. In the Philippines, the distribution of the disease includes the western and northern coastal areas of Luzon and the northeast of Mindanao. In Thailand, the infection is mostly sporadic and widely scattered. Infection has also been reported from Japan and recently from Dubai in the Middle East. *C. hepatica* is a rare human parasite but is commonly found in rodents in many parts of the world.

Morphology

Adult *C. philippinensis* are thin, small worms measuring 2.5 to 4.3 mm in length. They have a row of stichocytes at the anterior end, as in *Trichuris*. The eggs measure 36 to 45 μm in length and 19 to 21 μm in breadth, and have bipolar plugs, also like *Trichuris* (Fig. 6). However, unlike *Trichuris*, the eggs are not barrel shaped and the plugs do not protrude from the lateral ends. The adults of *C. hepatica* measure 52 to 104 mm in length and the anterior region contains the stichocytes. The eggs measure 48 to 66 by 28 to 36 μm and have bipolar plugs. The eggshell is thick and distinctly striated.

Lifecycle

The lifecycle of *C. philippinensis* has not been completely worked out. Humans are infected by eating freshwater fish and especially their succus entericus containing the infective larvae. Fish-eating birds act as a natural

Fig. 6 *Capillaria philippinensis* egg (× 1400).

or reservoir host. Humans become involved accidentally in this natural fish–bird cycle. The main danger is of autoinfection, leading to very heavy worm loads.

    C. hepatica is found in the liver of rodents and other mammals. The eggs are discharged in the liver tissue and remain there until the animal dies (Fig. 7). They eventually reach the soil by the decay of the carcass. Human beings are infected by accidentally swallowing embryonated eggs from the soil.

Clinical aspects

C. philippinensis can produce severe and even fatal disease. Patients often present with abdominal pain, diarrhoea, and borborygmi. As the worm load increases through autoinfection, diarrhoea becomes more severe, with anorexia, nausea, and vomiting. Prolonged diarrhoea leads to cachexia and muscular wasting. There may also be signs of hypotension and cardiac failure. In untreated cases, the mortality rate approaches 20 per cent.

    In *C. hepatica* infection, symptoms of visceral larva migrans may be present. The patient may have an enlarged tender liver with low-grade fever and eosinophilia.

Diagnosis

With *C. philippinensis*, diagnosis is made by finding the typical eggs in the faeces. Larvae or adult worms may also be present and repeated stool examination may be required in some cases. The parasite may also be found in jejunal aspirate or biopsy. With *C. hepatica*, diagnosis is made by identifying the parasite or eggs in a liver biopsy.

Fig. 7 *Capillaria hepatica* eggs in the liver (× 250).

Treatment

All cases of *C. philippinensis* should be treated with mebendazole 200 mg, twice daily, until the symptoms subside and the eggs completely disappear from the faeces after repeated stool examination. This may take up to 20 days or more. Alternatively, albendazole 400 mg can be given daily for 10 days. Supportive measures to overcome malnutrition and diarrhoea will be required in severely ill patients. There is no specific treatment for *C. hepatica* infection. Infection with *C. philippinensis* is prevented by not eating raw fish in the endemic regions of Southeast Asia.

Trichinosis

Trichinosis is an infection caused by *Trichinella spiralis*.

Geographical distribution

The infection is endemic in many parts of the world where pork is consumed, including Central and Eastern Europe, Central, South, and North America, and parts of Africa and Asia. Infection is also endemic in the Arctic regions resulting from eating polar bear meat.

Morphology

The adult males are small nematodes measuring 1.4 to 1.6 mm. The female is viviparous and about twice as long as the male. The anterior part contains a row of glandular cells (stichocytes) as in *Trichuris trichiura*. The male worm lacks a spicule but has two copulatory papillae on the sides of the cloacal opening.

Lifecycle (see Fig. 8)

Human beings become infected by eating improperly cooked pork or pork products such as sausages. In some parts of the world, wild boars are heavily infected. After ingestion, the larvae are liberated in the small intestine and mature into adults. The female deposits larvae in the intestinal tissues from where they find their way into the bloodstream and then into the striated muscles of the body (Fig. 9). The most heavily parasitized muscles are the diaphragm, tongue, laryngeal, and abdominal muscles. After penetration, the larva undergoes three moults and coils into a spiral, which eventually becomes enclosed in a thick-walled cyst. In this form, the larva may remain viable for many years.

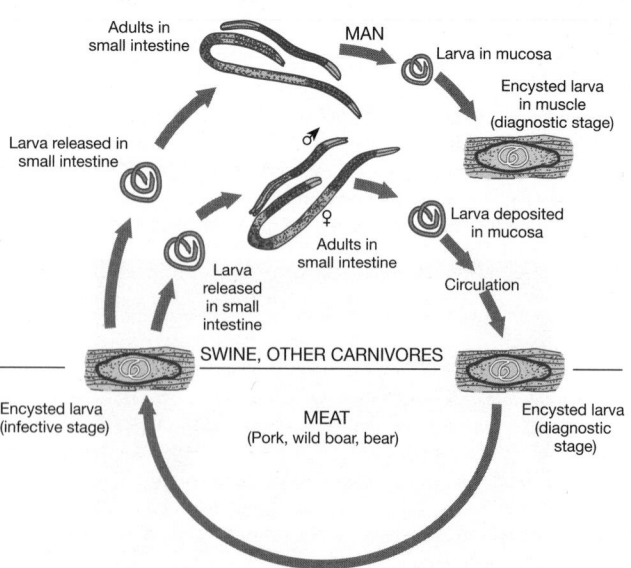

Fig. 8 Lifecycle of *Trichinella spiralis*. (Adapted from Centers for Disease Control, Atlanta, Georgia, United States.)

Fig. 9 *Trichinella spiralis* in human muscle (× 100).

Pigs become infected by eating infected scrap and garbage from slaughterhouses or farms. Occasionally, they may become infected by eating carcasses of infected rats.

Clinical aspects

Most people with light infections remain asymptomatic. In cases of heavy infection, there are three clinical stages.

The invasion stage

This is seen during the first week of infection and is due to juveniles and adults burrowing into the intestinal tissues. The patient complains of abdominal pain, nausea and vomiting, and diarrhoea of varying intensity. There may be fever, profuse sweating, and tachycardia.

The migration stage

This usually begins after the first week of infection. During this period, the larvae are liberated into the circulation by the gravid female and find their way to the muscles. Symptoms are attributable to toxic effects of the larvae and hypersensitivity reactions triggered by the liberation of parasite antigens. There is oedema of the face and periorbital tissues, fever, muscular tenderness, and hypereosinophilia. Complications involving the myocardium, lungs, and the central nervous system may occur due to the migrating larvae. However, the larvae do not encyst in the myocardium. A fine, macular skin rash, particularly on the trunk, may appear and last for a few days.

The encystment stage

This usually begins after the third week of infection. There is usually a gradual recovery from the symptoms. In a few cases with heavy infection, the symptoms may get worse and death may occur due to myocardiac failure, and respiratory and central nervous involvement. All serological tests become positive during this stage.

Diagnosis

This is based on a combination of clinical and epidemiological evidence. In a characteristic case, the patient will give a history of gastrointestinal disturbances (invasion stage) within 48 h of eating pork products, wild boar, or bear meat. If the patient presents in the later stage (migration stage), there is periorbital oedema, myositis, irregular fever, and hyperosinophilia.

Among the various tests that become positive during the encystment stage, the two most commonly used are the skin test and the slide flocculation test. Recently, enzyme immunoassay has also been used. The skin test antigen is made from larvae and gives an immediate type reaction in positive cases. The test is very good for surveys but unsuitable for the detection of acute disease as it remains positive for many years after infection. The slide flocculation test is also prepared from larval antigen, which is attached to cholesterol particles. In a positive reaction, flocculation is seen under the microscope. The test remains positive for about 10 months after infection. Serum enzymes such as aminotransferases are elevated. Muscle biopsy is positive in approximately 90 per cent of clinically positive cases.

Treatment

The prognosis is good and most patients recover after the larvae have encysted. The mainstays of treatment are bedrest and salicylates. For myocarditis and severe myalgia, oral prednisone for 3 to 5 days (0.5–1.0 mg/kg per day) is useful and provides symptomatic relief. In experimental animals, thiabendazole is able to kill encysted larvae. In man, its efficacy against larvae is doubtful but a dose of 25 to 50 mg/kg per day for 2 to 5 days usually brings down the fever and eosinophilia. Mebendazole appears to be a good alternative to thiabendazole as it has fewer side-effects, and is given at a dosage of 300 mg daily for 7 days. A higher dose of 1000 mg daily for 10 to 14 days is recommended by some authorities to ensure complete killing of the larvae. Even with this high dosage, side-effects appear not to be serious, consisting of mild Jarisch–Herxheimer type reactions at the start of therapy. The manufacturer does not recommend giving mebendazole to children under 2 years of age or pregnant women.

Control and prevention

Trichinosis in the pig population can be greatly reduced or eliminated by hygienic rearing methods. Larvae in pork can be killed by freezing at −18 °C for 24 h. Thorough cooking of pork is the best safeguard against infection in all endemic areas.

Enterobiasis (pinworm, threadworm)

Enterobiasis is an infection caused by *Enterobius vermicularis*.

Geographical distribution

This is one of the few parasites that is more prevalent in the temperate regions of the world than in the tropics. Children are more often involved than adults. It occurs in groups such as families living together, inmates of hostels, and in army camps.

Morphology

The male is approximately 5 mm long and 0.1 to 0.2 mm in diameter (Plate 3). The female is approximately 13 mm long and 0.3 to 0.5 mm in diameter. The gravid female has two distended uteri that practically fill the whole body. The male has a single spicule and a curved tail. The cervical alae of the cuticle allows easy recognition. The eggs are generally flattened on one side and measure approximately 50 to 60 µm in length and 20 to 30 µm in breadth. They have a thick, transparent shell. The eggs are unembryonated when passed but become infective within a few hours.

Lifecycle

The adults are mainly located in the caecal region (Fig. 10). The female deposits its eggs on the anus and perianal skin. Direct person-to-person infection occurs by inhalation and swallowing of the eggs. In addition, autoinfection occurs by contamination of fingers. It may occur as a sexually transmitted disease among male homosexuals. There is no visceral migration and the larva matures into an adult in the lumen of the intestinal tract. The lifecycle of the parasite is completed in about 6 weeks. Unlike *Ascaris* and *Trichuris* eggs, which need many days of development in soil before becoming embryonated, *Enterobius* eggs are embryonated when passed, hence there is rapid transmission from person to person.

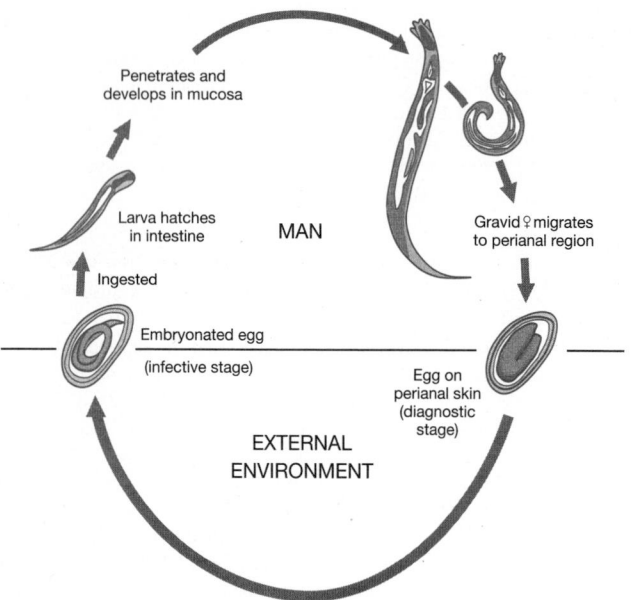

Fig. 10 Lifecycle of *Enterobius vermicularis*. (Adapted from Centers for Disease Control, Atlanta, Georgia, United States.)

Clinical aspects

The most common presenting symptom is pruritus ani. This can be very troublesome and occurs more often during the night. Persistent itching may lead to inflammation and secondary bacterial infection of the perianal region. Infected children may suffer from insomnia, emotional disturbance, anorexia, weight loss, and enuresis. Occasionally, adult worms may migrate, entering the female genital tract. Inside the uterus or the Fallopian tube they may get encapsulated and produce symptoms of salpingitis. In adolescents and children it is an important cause of vulvovaginitis. The parasite may also get lodged in the lumen of the appendix, leading to appendicitis (Fig. 11). The lifespan of the parasite is 3 to 6 weeks.

Diagnosis

The eggs are not usually found in the faeces. They are most easily found around the anus, by swabbing or using cellulose adhesive tape. The anal examination for eggs should be done before defaecation or bathing. Sometimes intact worms are passed in the faeces and can be easily recognized by their size and shape.

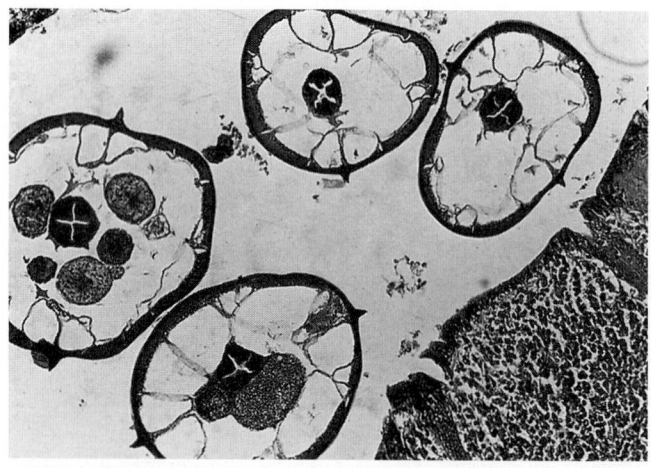

Fig. 11 *Enterobius vermicularis* in the lumen of the appendix (× 250).

Treatment

Attention to personal hygiene is an important part of treatment and prevention. The patient should be instructed to keep nails short and wash hands with soap and water after defaecating. The bed cover and sleeping garments should be changed every day and the floor in the bedroom kept clean. With these simple hygienic measures, infection will disappear on its own, due to the short lifespan of the parasite.

All the children and adults in a household should be treated at the same time. Many drugs are available to treat the infection. Piperazine citrate is given in a dose of 65 mg/kg for 7 days. The course is repeated after 2 weeks. Piperazine is contraindicated in renal and liver disease and epilepsy. Pyrantel pamoate is equally effective in a single dose of 11 mg/kg (maximum 1 g) and its side-effect profile is better than piperazine. The drug is repeated after 2 weeks. Mebendazole is effective in a single dose of 100 mg, repeated after 2 weeks. Alternately, albendazole in a single does of 400 mg can be given, repeated after 2 weeks. Both mebendazole and albandazole should not be given to pregnant women.

Trichuriasis (whip worm)

Trichuriasis is an infection caused by *Trichuris trichiura*.

Geographical distribution

It has a worldwide distribution and is the most common intestinal nematode in some tropical regions such as Southeast Asia.

Morphology

The adult male measures 30 to 45 mm and the female 35 to 50 mm in length. The parasite is commonly known as the whip worm because the anterior three-fifths is thin and elongated and the posterior two-fifths is bulbous and fleshy. One important feature of this group of worms is the possession of a thin, elongated oesophagus that is surrounded by gland cells known as stichocytes. The adults are mainly located in the caecum and produce barrel-shaped eggs, 22 to 50 μm long. At the lateral ends, they have transparent, blister-like plugs, which are single celled when freshly passed. In the soil the eggs become infective in about 3 weeks.

Lifecycle (see Fig. 12)

Infection occurs by the ingestion of the embryonated egg. The larva does not undergo visceral migration but penetrates the gut for a short period before returning to the lumen to mature into the adult stage. The worms attach themselves to the large intestine by threading their anterior end into the epithelium (Fig. 13). The posterior end hangs free in the lumen of the bowel. The whole period of development in the host takes about 3 months to complete.

Clinical aspects

Light infections are generally asymptomatic. In heavy infections, there is colitis with the passage of blood and mucus in faeces. The clinical picture is often similar to that of amoebic dysentery. Heavy infection in children leads to anaemia that may cause oedema, and cardiac failure. There may be marked clubbing of the fingers. The anaemia is probably due to bleeding from the damaged and inflamed mucous membrane rather than sucking of blood by the parasite itself. In some cases, prolapse of the rectum occurs, probably due to constant irritation produced by the worms and the weakness of the levator ani muscle. Occasionally, the worm may lodge itself in the lumen of the appendix and cause acute appendicitis. The subtler form of trichuriasis is associated with long-term failure of children to grown in height, although they may not appear emaciated.

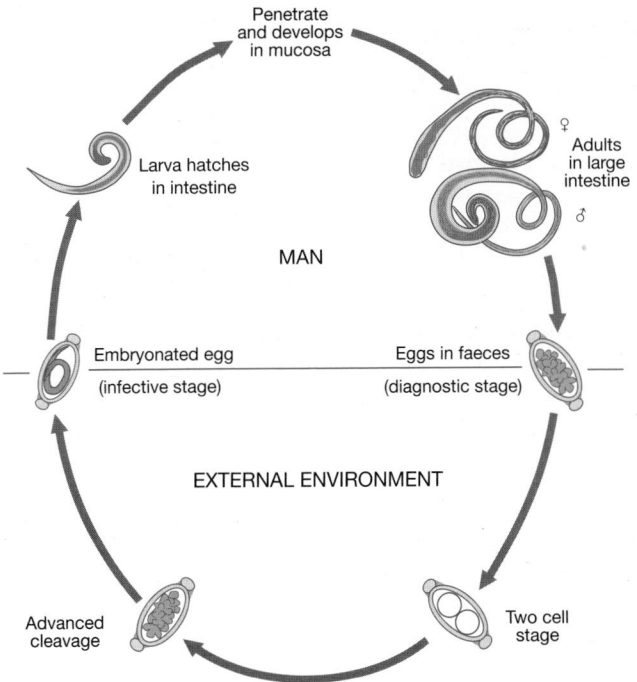

Fig. 12 Lifecycle of *Trichuris trichiura*. (Adapted from Centers for Disease Control, Atlanta, Georgia, United States.)

Diagnosis

This is based on finding characteristic barrel-shaped eggs in the faeces. Eosinophils and Charcot–Leyden crystals are often present. Sigmoidoscopy or proctoscopy may show worms attached to the mucous membrane and sometimes intact worms may be passed out in the faeces.

Treatment

Mebendazole

Mebendazole is the drug of choice and is given in a dose of 100 mg, twice daily for 3 days for both adults and children of not less than 2 years of age. Side-effects are few and it is well tolerated. During therapy, abnormal *Trichuris* eggs are produced as the drug interferes with embryogenesis of the worm. The drug should not be given to pregnant women, especially in the first trimester.

Fig. 13 *Trichuris trichiura*: anterior end embedded in the superficial layer of intestinal epithelium (× 250).

Albendazole

Albendazole is effective in a single dose of 400 mg for both adult and children of not less than 2 years of age. It should not be given the pregnant women. As with mebendazole, abnormal parasite eggs are produced during therapy.

Oxantel plus pyrantel pamoate

Oxantel is an analogue of pyrantel and a combination is effective against *Ascaris*, *Enterobius*, hookworms, and *Trichuris*. Dosage is 10 to 20 mg/kg body weight of each component as a single dose. In heavy infections, the drug may be repeated two or three times.

Preventive measures are the same as in ascariasis.

Further reading

Ascariasis

Crompton DWT, Nesheim MC, Pawlowski ZS, eds. (1989). *Ascariasis and its prevention.* Taylor and Francis, London.

Anisakiasis

Kliks MH (1986). Human anisakiasis: an update. *Journal of the American Medical Association* **255**, 2605.

Capillariasis

Cross JH, Basaca-Sevilla V (1983). Experimental transmission of *Capillaria philippinensis* to birds. *Transactions of the Royal Society of Tropical Medicine and Hygiene* **77**, 511–14.

Trichinosis

Campbell WC (1983). Trichenella *and trichinosis.* Plenum, New York.

Trichuriasis

Cooper ES, Bundy DAP (1987). Trichuriasis. *Baillière's Clinical Tropical Medicine and Communicable Disease* **2**, 629–43.

7.14.7 Toxocariasis and visceral larva migrans

V. Zaman

Visceral larva migrans is the name given to a syndrome characterized by hepatomegaly, fever, respiratory symptoms, and high eosinophilia. It is caused mainly by the migrating larvae of *Toxocara canis* and *T. cati*. Other parasites that may cause this syndrome are *Ancylostoma* spp., *Spirometra*, *Gnathostoma*, and *Alaria*.

Geographical distribution

Toxocarial infection occurs wherever there are large domestic dog and cat populations. Many cases have been reported from the United States and other Western countries. They result from close association between these animals and man. Surveys in Great Britain have shown that approximately 2 to 3 per cent of the population possess antibodies to these parasites.

Lifecycle

Infection with *T. canis* is maintained in the dog population by direct transmission from the soil containing embryonated eggs, from transplacental

Fig. 1 Granuloma formation in an experimentally infected monkey showing a large number of giant cells and some fibroblastic reaction. The arrow marks the larva. Haematoxylin and eosin, × 400.

transmission from bitch to puppies, through the maternal milk to puppies, and by dogs eating infected meat containing larvae. These multiple routes of infection ensure that almost all puppies are born infected. Human beings become infected by ingesting embryonated eggs from the soil. Toddlers and young children are usually involved because of their habit of eating soil and dirt. The larvae hatch out in the small intestine and migrate to various organs of the body including the liver, lungs, eye, and brain. They do not mature into adult worms in man. After some time a granuloma forms around the larvae.

Morphology

The larva of *T. canis* is approximately 18 to 20 μm in diameter and that of *T. cati* is about 15 to 17 μm in diameter; they are otherwise indistinguishable. Both species have pointed lateral alae and two lateral excretory columns. The posterior region of the larva contains the intestinal tract. Larvae of *Toxocara* spp. are much smaller than these *Ascaris* spp. This may be the reason why *Ascaris* larvae are not widely dispersed in the tissues as they are unable to enter the small blood vessels. Eggs of *Toxocara* spp. are similar in size to those of *Ascaris* but their surface is pitted, making identification easy. Eggs are never seen in human faeces as adults mature only in dogs and cats.

In animals and man the migrating toxocarae larvae eventually became surrounded by a granuloma. Various cell types are involved in granuloma formation, including macrophages, lymphocytes, eosinophils, and fibroblasts. In a fully formed granuloma the larvae are surrounded by layers of fibrous tissue and inflammation subsides. It is now accepted that granuloma formation is caused by the immune system, especially T cells. It is an attempt by the host to limit disease, but it also favours the larva by ensuring its survival for a long time in a circumscribed area (Figs. 1 and 2).

Fig. 2 Granuloma formation in the same animal as in Fig. 1 at a later stage, when the larva is completely surrounded by fibroblasts. Haematoxylin and eosin, × 400.

Clinical aspects

Toxocariasis may cause two different clinical pictures: classical visceral larva migrans syndrome and ocular toxocariasis.

Classical visceral larva migrans

This is seen most often in young children because of pica (dirt or soil eating). Most people remain asymptomatic. In a minority, symptoms consist of muscular pain, lassitude, anorexia, cough, and urticarial rashes. Physical signs include rhonchi, hepatomegaly, splenomegaly, and enlargement of the lymph glands. The acute phase generally lasts for 2 to 3 weeks followed by recovery. Sometimes the resolution of all the signs may take up to 18 months. Convulsions, paralysis, and other neurological disorders result when larvae enter the central nervous system. Rarely the infection may end fatally if a massive dose of parasites has been ingested.

Ocular larva migrans

This is caused by granuloma formation in the eye. If this is near to the macula, impairment of vision or even blindness may result. Patients may present visual difficulty in one eye, with or without strabismus. As the generalized manifestation of visceral larva migrans may not be present, diagnosis is often difficult. Unlike in visceral larva migrans, eosinophilia may be absent. On fundoscopy a rounded swelling, often near the optic disc, may be detected.

Diagnosis

In classical visceral larva migrans there is leucocytosis with marked eosinophilia (20 to 80 per cent). In ocular larva migrans there may be no peripheral eosinophilia.

Serological tests are useful. An enzyme immunoassay using extracts of excretory–secretory products of *T. canis* larvae is positive in the majority of patients with visceral larva migrans. In ocular larva migrans the vitreous fluid is shown to have antibodies to the parasite.

Biopsy of the liver may show larvae with granulomas and eosinophilic infiltration. However, biopsy is rarely done because the chances of obtaining the appropriate specimen are remote, unless it is a massive infection. If facilities are available, laparoscopy may permit direct biopsy of a granuloma, which appears as a white dot on the surface of the liver.

Treatment

No antihelminthic drug is completely effective in killing the larvae and most patients recover without specific therapy. Diethylcarbamazine in a dosage of 6 mg/kg a day in three divided doses for 2 to 3 weeks has given equivocal results. Albendazole 400 mg twice a day for 3 to 5 days for both adults and children of more than 2 years of age, and mebendazole 100 to 200 mg twice a day for 5 days for both adults and children of more than 2 years of age may be of some value. The use of antihelminthics may sometimes provoke a greater inflammatory response, with worsening of the clinical picture, due to injury of the parasite. In severe cases, corticosteroids have been used with reports of improvement.

In ocular larva migrans, visible larvae can be photocoagulated by laser. Vitrectomy has been used in some cases, and local and intraocular steroids also appear to be of some value.

Prevention and control

Most cases of human toxocariasis are preventable by careful personal hygiene, not allowing children to play in environment likely to contain parasite eggs, and eliminating roundworms from pets, especially puppies and kittens. Unfortunately, people are often not aware that the infection can be transmitted from pets to humans. Efforts must be directed towards increasing this awareness.

Further reading

Schantz PM (1989). Toxocara larva migrans then and now. *American Journal of Tropical Medicine and Hygiene* **41** (Suppl.), 21–34.

Small KW *et al.* (1989). Surgical management of retinal retraction caused by toxocariasis. *American Journal of Ophthamology* **108**, 10–14.

7.14.8 Angiostrongyliasis

R. Knight

Human disease caused by two nematode species of the genus *Angiostrongylus* has been recognized comparatively recently. Both parasites normally infect rodents; molluscs are the primary intermediate hosts. They were initially thought to be rare and of limited distribution in humans, but these assumptions have proved incorrect. The epidemiology is complex because of multiple potential routes of transmission.

Angiostrongylus cantonensis

This is the rat lungworm; it causes cerebrospinal angiostrongyliasis. The first known case, reported in 1944, was a 15-year-old Taiwanese boy with meningoencephalitis in whose cerebrospinal fluid an immature adult worm was found. Detailed clinicopathological studies were made in 1962 during epidemics of eosinophilic meningitis in Tahiti.

Aetiology—the biology of the parasite

Adult worms live in the pulmonary arteries of rats; larvae from hatched eggs ascend the airways and so reach the faeces. Molluscs ingest these larvae and after two moults they are infective when eaten by a rodent. In the rat, infective larval worms migrate to the cerebral grey matter where they start to mature, move to the meninges, and then enter the venous sinuses and so reach the pulmonary arteries where maturation is completed. Infective larvae from a mollusc can also enter a second or third intermediate host in which they undergo no further development until they enter a mammalian host; such supernumerary hosts are termed paratenic or transport hosts, they are important sources of infection to humans.

Development in humans reaches the immature adult stage, measuring 11 to 15 mm in length. Nearly all will die in the superficial cortex, brainstem, and meninges causing vigorous tissue reactions; very few reach the lungs.

Epidemiology

Human infections occur throughout Oceania, especially Hawaii, Samoa, the Solomons, Papua New Guinea, Indonesia, the Philippines, and Northern Australia; and in south-east Asia, especially Thailand, Taiwan, and south Japan, but also India; a few infections are reported from Ivory Coast, Egypt, Madagascar, Cuba, the Caribbean, and South America. All ages can be affected and outbreaks have occurred after weddings and feasts; infections are often seasonal.

The principal rodent hosts are *Rattus rattus*, *R.norvegicus*, *R.alexandrinus*, and *R.exulans*. The prevalence in rats in endemic areas may be 40 per cent or more. The geographic spread and population increase of these peridomestic rodents has increased the zoonotic reservoir. Another factor leading to the increase in human infection has been the dispersal by human agency of the edible giant African snail *Achatina fulica* eastwards across the Indian Ocean and the Pacific, from Madagascar in 1800 to reach Hawai in 1936.

Many species of snail and slug act as intermediate hosts, and paratenic hosts include freshwater prawns, land and coconut crabs, frogs, and land planarians; in Thailand the yellow tree monitor is an important paratenic host. Common modes of transmission to humans include eating raw *Achatina* snails as a delicacy and for medicinal purposes; eating salads containing small undetected molluscs, their slime trails, or planarians; eating raw freshwater prawns and crabs; or drinking water containing tiny immature prawns, especially after heavy rains.

The modes of transmission differ geographically, by age and social group, and with time. In Thailand, *Pila* snails are a seasonal delicacy eaten by all the family, but young men take them raw with alcohol; another edible snail *Ampullaria canaliculatus* is infected in Taiwan and Japan. In the Ryuku islands of Japan, patients are usually infected by eating raw snails or toad liver for medicinal purposes.

Pathology

Inflammatory, granulomatous, and sometimes track-like lesions occur predominantly in the cortical grey matter and the meninges, but also in the brainstem and cerebellum; nerve roots and spinal cord may also be affected. Live worms are occasionally found at autopsy and dead worms are found in many of the lesions. The number of worms found varies greatly and may reach several hundred; worm tracks in the tissue and meninges are surrounded by a cuff of eosinophils; Charcot–Leyden crystal derived from eosinophils are numerous. Rarely adult worms have been found in human lung at autopsy. Ocular infection derives from worms that have migrated across the cribriform plate.

Clinical features

After an incubation period of 2 to 4 weeks the onset is acute with headache, intermittent at first, together with nausea and vomiting. There is constitutional upset and frequently meningism; fever is unusual. The illness is often self-limiting over a period of 4 weeks. Cranial nerve lesions include optic, abducens, and facial nerve damage. Less common are seizures, confusion, or radiculopathy with parasthesias, root pains, or weakness. Long tract signs and impaired consciousness are uncommon except in severe cases, but spinal cord damage can cause sphincter disturbance.

Ocular complications include retinal haemorrhages and larval worms in the vitreous or anterior chamber (Plate 1). Rarely migration to the lungs produces clinical evidence of pneumonitis. Numerous eosinophils occur in the cerebrospinal fluid and there is a blood eosinophilia.

Diagnosis

Lumbar puncture reveals high opening pressure with a clear or lightly turbid cerebrospinal fluid containing 500 to 2000 cells/mm of which 10 to over 90 per cent are eosinophils. Protein levels are high with normal glucose. Detailed examination at low power reveals larval or immature adult worms in up to 25 per cent of cases; they measure 5 to 15 mm in length. Cerebrospinal fluid changes may persist for up to 3 months. Computed tomography or magnetic resonance imaging may reveal focal cortical abnormalities. Serology using antigens from fourth-stage larvae is useful, but cross-reactions with other nematodes can cause difficulty. Techniques to detect worm antigen in cerebrospinal fluid and serum have also been developed.

Differential diagnosis is from other helminthic infections affecting the nervous system as eosinophils are otherwise rare in cerebrospinal fluid. A detailed geographic and dietary history is essential; conditions to be considered include gnathostomiasis, paragonimiasis, schistosomiasis, and neurocysticercosis. Confusion with *Gnathostoma spinigerum* is a particular problem in Thailand, the latter more commonly causes long tract signs, bloody or xanthochromic cerebrospinal fluid, neck stiffness, and clouding of consciousness.

Treatment, prognosis, and control

Specific anthelmintic treatment is not useful and worm death aggravates the clinical condition. Headache can be relieved by repeated lumbar tap, analgesics, and sedatives. Steroids have been used in patients with focal neurological signs, but benefit is poorly substantiated. Larvae in the eye chambers should be removed surgically. Reported mortality rates vary from 0.5 to 30 per cent and depend mainly on the number of infective larvae ingested; some patients pass into coma after about 2 weeks and their prognosis is then very poor. Most patients improve in 2 to 4 weeks, but focal neurological deficits can persist longer; partial relapse after 2 months of illness may represent a reaction to dying worms. Some patients have relatively mild illnesses and can be discharged within a few days; during epidemics these patients may need only outpatient care.

Control measures include health education to limit ingestion of raw high-risk dietary items and unwashed salads. Warnings may be necessary regarding raw molluscs, amphibians, and reptiles used for medicinal purposes. Rodents in vegetable gardens and the peridomestic environment should be controlled.

Angiostrongylus costaricensis

This causes abdominal angiostrongyliasis. It was first recognized in Costa Rica in 1950 in surgical specimens simulating bowel malignancy. The parasite was described from such specimens in 1967 and the complete lifecycle in rodents was elucidated during the next 3 years.

Aetiology—the biology of the parasite

In both the rodent and human hosts the worms are located in the ileocaecal mesenteric arteries. The cotton rat *Sigmodon hispidus* is the principal reservoir host, but other species of rodents including the coatimundi are also involved, and even dogs and marmosets. In the rodent hosts, worm eggs embolize to gut wall capillaries and the hatched larvae pass into the gut lumen. Veronicellid slugs, especially *Vaginalus plebeius*, eat rodent faeces containing larvae and these develop with two moults in fibromuscular tissue of the mollusc into infective larvae over a period of 18 days. Infective larvae can persist in the slug for several months or be shed in slime trails. The prepatent period in rats eating infected slugs is 24 days.

In human infections the worms reach maturity but the embryonated eggs do not hatch.

Epidemiology

Infections occur especially in Costa Rica, Nicaragua, Guatemala, and Honduras, but also sporadically in the Americas from the United States to Argentina, and some Caribbean Islands. Recently, infections are being increasingly recognized from Brazil. Small veronicellid slugs are the main source of infection to humans; infection rates in these hosts can reach 85 per cent. Slugs may be unnoticed on fallen fruits or in salads, especially when small or chopped; their mucus also contains infective larvae. Many cases are in school children, but infants and older persons are also affected; an outbreak after eating mint is reported. Seropositivity in endemic areas suggests that there are unrecognized infections.

Pathology and clinical features

Lesions primarily affect small arteries; they produce subacute or chronic granulomatous inflammatory masses in the wall of the caecum (Fig. 1) and right colon; sometimes the predominant feature is ischaemic infarction. The finding of an adult nematode measuring 18 to 42 mm in length within a gut arterial vessel is diagnostic of this infection; eggs may be seen in vessels or in tissue where they are surrounded by eosinophil granulomas. Lesions also occur elsewhere in the colon or terminal ileum, in regional abdominal lymph nodes, or the omentum. Some larvae enter the hepatic

Fig. 1 Section of a human caecum showing three eggs of *A. costaricensis* with cellular infiltration mostly of eosinophils (by courtesy of Dr Pedro Morera, University of Costa Rica).

artery and cause granulomatous or necrotic lesions in the liver; others enter testicular arteries causing similar lesions of the testis.

Clinically, most patients present with right-sided or right iliac fossa pain, with tenderness and sometimes a palpable mass in this region. Other features are eosinophilia, fever, diarrhoea, or rectal bleeding. Tender hepatomegaly with high blood eosinophilia occurs in some patients and sometimes focal necrotic lesions in the liver. Serious complications are bowel obstruction and perforation, and testicular infarction.

Diagnosis and treatment

Confirmation of diagnosis is usually made histologically on resected material. The condition can mimic appendicitis, bowel neoplasm, Meckel's diverticulitis, testicular torsion, or other surgical problems. Parasite eggs are not found in faeces, but serology using enzyme immunoassay or latex agglutination is useful. Contrast radiology reveals filling defects and altered motility of terminal ileum, caecum, or ascending colon. Laparoscopy can reveal the bowel and hepatic lesions; biopsy may be diagnostic.

The value of anthelmintic treatment remains unproven; thiabendazole or high doses of mebendazole have been used. Surgery is often necessary but can sometimes be deferred in uncomplicated cases when the diagnosis is strongly suspected, as spontaneous remission is common.

Preventive measures include washing and careful inspection of vegetables, and hand washing before meals by children and those preparing salads.

Further reading

Alicata JE (1991). The discovery of *Angiostrongylus cantonensis* as a cause of human eosinophilic meningitis. *Parasitology Today* **7**, 151–3.

Graeff-Teixeira C *et al.* (1997). Seroepidemiology of abdominal angiostrongyliasis: the standardization of an immunoenzymatic assay and prevalence of antibodies in two localities in southern Brazil. *Tropical Medicine and International Health* **2**, 254–60.

Kramer MH *et al.* (1998). First reported outbreak of abdominal angiostrongyliasis. *Clinical Infectious Diseases* **26**, 365–72.

Mackerras MJ, Sandars DF (1995). The life history of the rat lungworm, *Angiostrongylus cantonensis* (Chen). *Australian Journal of Zoology* **3**, 1–25.

Morera P (1996). Importance of abdominal angiostrongylosis in the Americas. In: Özcel MA, Alkan MZ, eds. *Parasitology for the 21st century*, pp 253–60. CAB International, Wallingford, UK.

Punyagupta S, Juttijudata P, Bunnag T (1975). Eosinophilic meningitis in Thailand. Clinical studies of 484 typical cases probably caused by *Angiostrongylus cantonensis*. *American Journal of Tropical Medicine and Hygiene* **24**, 921–31.

7.14.9 Gnathostomiasis

Pravan Suntharasamai

Gnathostomiasis is an extraintestinal infection with larval or immature nematodes of the genus *Gnathostoma* (order Spirurida). It is characterized by intermittent and migratory space-occupying lesions in the skin or the internal organs, resulting in inflammation and/or haemorrhage.

Aetiology

Four species of gnathostomes are known to infect man. Adult parasites live in the upper gastrointestinal tract of the definitive hosts: *Gnathostoma spinigerum*, the most common infection, in dogs, cats, and other mammals; *G. hispidum* and *G. doleresi* in pigs; and *G. nipponicum* in weasels. Larvae, hatched in water from ova shed with the host's faeces and ingested by cyclops, are eaten by freshwater fish, amphibians, reptiles, crustaceans, birds, or mammals. Third-stage larvae are found in the walls of the viscera and in the muscles of these second intermediate hosts. Unless they are eaten by definitive hosts, the parasites cannot developed into reproductive adults but they remain infectious to man and other paratenic hosts.

Consumption of the raw or undercooked flesh of second intermediate and paratenic hosts is the most common mode of transmission. Skin penetration after contact with infected material is less important. Prenatal transmission can occur, as larvae have been recovered in neonates as young as 3 days old.

Epidemiology

Isolated cases of *G. spinigerum* infections have been reported frequently in Thailand and Japan and sporadically in Australia, Bangladesh, Cameroon, China, Ecuador, India, Mexico, Southeast Asian countries, and Sri Lanka. Infections with the other three species have been reported from Japan.

Gnathostomiasis can present in places far away from these endemic areas due to migration of the latently infected human host or importation of the infective flesh of paratenic hosts. Consumption of a raw fish dish at a party can result in an outbreak.

Pathogenesis

The ingested larva penetrates the gut wall and migrates to the liver before wandering through almost any tissue except bone. Symptoms and signs vary according to the sites and sizes of the inflammatory or haemorrhagic lesions induced intermittently along the migratory route.

Clinical features

Nausea, vomiting, and epigastric pain may develop within 1 or 2 days after consumption of the infective food. Fever, pain in the right upper quadrant of the abdomen, chest pain, dry cough, and hypereosinophilia may develop within 1 to 2 weeks.

The primary invasive illness usually passes unnoticed and so the incubation period is not known in most cases. General health is scarcely impared and fever is uncommon. The illnesses can be categorized according to the affected organs as follows.

Cutaneous forms

Gnathostomal creeping eruption (Fig. 1)

This is rare in *G. spinigerum* infection but frequent with the other three species. The serpiginous track (Fig. 1) is similar to but bigger and more

Fig. 1 Creeping eruption around the left thigh. (Reproduced from Bhaibulya and Charoenlarp (1983), with permission.)

variable in depth than that caused by dog or cat hookworm larvae (see Chapter 7.14.9). A trail of subcutaneous haemorrhage is sometimes observed.

Cutaneous migratory swelling

This most common manifestation of human gnathostomiasis is usually intermittent. The first swelling may develop 3 to 4 weeks after infection. Swelling can occur anywhere and may recur close to or distant from the original site (Fig. 2). It develops rapidly and usually lasts for about 1 to 2 weeks. Frequently it is extensive, involving the whole wrist or hand for example. Swelling of digits or plantar surfaces can be very painful and incapacitating. Itching is the main associated symptom. Regional lymphadenitis is usually absent. When swelling involves the eyelid, chemosis and conjunctival haemorrhage may be observed.

The worms can escape spontaneously through the skin or the conjunctiva. The interval between episodes of swelling varies from a few days to a

(a)   (b)

Fig. 2 Migratory swelling in a 23-year-old male. (a) At the eyelids for 5 days when seen on 5 June 1986. (b) At the right side of the upper lip on 9 June 1986 when the larva was picked out by needle puncture and squeezing.

few months and rarely 1 to 2 years. Intermittent cutaneous migratory swelling can go on for more than 5 years.

Visceral forms

Visceral invasion as described below for *G. spinigerum* infection has not been reported in infections with other *Gnathostoma* species.

Spinocerebral gnathostomiasis

Involvement of the spinal cord commonly starts with intermittent, agonizing, shooting pains in a limb or a segment of trunk, followed by paraplegia with urinary retention and, rarely, quadriplegia. Sensation is correspondingly impaired and the Brown–Séquard syndrome is sometimes seen. A few patients with haematoma and inflammation due to brain invasion (Fig. 3) present with severe headache and vomiting, followed very quickly by coma, cranial nerve palsies, and/or hemiplegia. A rapidly advancing or changing pattern of neurological deficits is characteristic of the infection. Eosinophilic meningitis without focal neurological deficit or subarachnoid haemorrhage occasionally occurs.

The cerebrospinal fluid can be bloody, xanthochromic, or slightly turbid with a minor increase in protein content. The proportion of eosinophils is higher than expected from haemorrhage *per se.*

Ocular gnathostomiasis

The gnathostome can be found in the anterior chamber (Fig. 4) and the vitreous. The parasite usually migrates through the sclera or the cornea. It can induce uveitis, iritis, intraocular haemorrhage, retinal detachment and scarring, and blindness.

Intra-abdominal and oral gnathostomiasis

These uncommon forms can present with intestinal obstruction or a painful intra-abdominal mass. Worms may emerge from the tongue, soft palate, gum, and cheek mucosa.

Pulmonary gnathostomiasis

Worms may be found in the sputum of patients with bronchitis, eosinophilis pneumonitis, pleurisy, pleural effusion, or pneumohaemothorax.

Genitourinary gnathostomiasis

The parasites have been recovered from blood-stained urethral discharge and urine, the glans penis, adnexal masses, and the cervix.

Auditory gnathostomiasis

The worms have been found in the external auditory canal in a patient with hearing loss and tinnitus, and penetrating the tympanic membrane in another patient.

(a)

(b)

(c)

Fig. 3 Magnetic resonance image of a case of cerebral gnathostomiasis. (a), (b) Coronal T₂-weighted sections at the level of the brainstem and basal ganglion demonstrate a serpiginous mixed hyposignal with a hypersignal track (* *) along the right lateral upper pons and midbrain penetrating into the lentiform nucleus (arrow head). (c) Axial T₁-weighted section of the brain at the basal ganglion level demonstrates a small hypersignal T₁ subacute haemorrhage (short arrow) along the track of the parasite at the posterior limb of the internal capsule and adjacent serpiginous hyposignal T₁ track (long arrows). (By courtesy of Dr Jiraporn Laothamatas, Ramathibodi Hospital, Bangkok, Thailand.)

Fig. 4 Gnathostome larva in the anterior chamber. (By courtesy of Dr Nesit Leelawong.)

Laboratory diagnosis

The diagnosis is definitive if the worm can be identified in sections of surgical specimens. The whole worm may be available if it emerges through the skin, in excretions and discharges, or from eye operations. Their sizes ranged from 0.34×2.2 mm to 1.0×16.25 mm. Their stage of development does not correlate with the duration of clinical illness. Infections with more than one worm are uncommon.

Enzyme immunoassay and Western blot tests are sometimes available in Thailand and Japan. Western blot is specific.

Blood eosinophilia (7 to 76 per cent) occurs irregularly in about 60 per cent of cases and therefore is not necessary for presumptive diagnosis.

Magnetic resonance imaging can show tortuous tracks and haemorrhage in cerebral gnathostomiasis (Fig. 3).

Differential diagnosis

Diagnosis of cutaneous forms is based on clinical characteristics, geographical and dietary history, and by excluding other causes. Differential diagnoses include contact dermatitis, angioedema and urticaria, Calabar swellings (caused by *Loa loa*), fascioliasis, paragonimiasis, sparganosis, dirofilariasis, and from non-infectious causes.

Gnathostomal aetiology is highly likely if rapidly advancing myelitis follows root pain, or if features of cerebral or subarachnoid haemorrhage occur in a person who is healthy apart from a history of cutaneous migratory swelling. Eosinophil pleocytosis is essential for the diagnosis, as is exclusion of eosinophilic meningoencephalitis caused by *Angiostronglus cantonensis*, *Baylisascaris procyonis*, and non-helminthic encephalomyelitis.

In intraocular infections, the larvae of *A. cantonensis* can be distinguished as they are thinner, longer, and folding. They usually appear in the eyeball 2 to 3 weeks after the manifestation of eosinophilic meningoencephalitis.

Visceral gnathostamiasis usually depends on identifying the worm in surgical specimens (at autopsy the worms may have migrated away from the site of the main pathological lesion), or in secretions such as sputum, urine, or vaginal discharge.

Treatment

Surgical removal is curative but advisable only in accessible areas such as the eye or skin. Blind exploration of subcutaneous tissues in areas of diffuse swelling is not productive.

Oral therapy with albendazole at an adult dosage of 400 mg twice daily for 2 to 3 weeks induces migration of the gnathostome to the skin. The worms are frequently recovered between days 2 and 14 of treatment by picking with a needle, excisional biopsy, or even by pinching with the patient's nails. However, the success rate is only 6 to 7 per cent. Recurrence of swelling in patients whose worms do not migrate to the skin is less frequent after albendazole treatment. Aminotransferases should be measured before this treatment even though hepatotoxicity at this dosage is usually mild and reversible.

Prognosis

Cerebral gnathostomiasis can be fatal and blindness is frequent after intraocular gnathostomiasis. Patients can be reassured that central nervous or intraocular involvement occur in less than 1 per cent of patients with cutaneous migratory swelling.

Prevention

All dishes that contain raw or poorly cooked flesh of animals in or imported from endemic areas must be avoided. Those who prepare potentially infected flesh should use gloves if prolonged exposure is likely.

Further reading

Bhaibulya M, Charoenlarp P (1983). Creeping eruption caused by *Gnathostoma spinigerum*. *Southeast Asian Journal of Tropical Medicine and Public Health* **14**, 226–8.

Inkatanuvat S *et al.* (1998). Changes of liver functions after albendazole treatment in human gnathostomiasis. *Journal of the Medical Association of Thailand*, **81**, 735–40.

Mijyazaki I (1991). *An illustrated book of helminthic zoonoses.* SEAMIC Publication No. 62, pp. 368–409. Southeast Asian Medical Information Centre, International Medical Foundation of Japan, Tokyo.

Rusnak JM and Lucey DR (1993). Clinical gnathostomiasis: case report and review of the English language literature. *Clinics in Infectious Diseases*, **16**, 33–50.

Suntharasamai P *et al.* (1992). Albendazole stimulates outward migration of *Gnathostoma spinigerum* to the dermis in man. *Southeast Asian Journal of Tropical Medicine and Public Health*, **23**, 716–22.

Swanson VL (1971). Gnathostomiasis. In: Marcial-Rojas RA, ed. *Pathology of protozoal and helminthic diseases with clinical correlation*, pp. 871–9. Williams and Wilkins, Baltimore.

7.15 Cestodes (tapeworms)

7.15.1 Cystic hydatid disease (*Echinococcus granulosus*)

Armando E. Gonzalez, Pedro L. Moro, and Hector H. Garcia

Introduction

Cystic hydatid disease is a zoonotic disease caused by infection with the larval stage (hydatid cyst) of the tapeworm *Echinococcus granulosus*. Hydatid cysts in liver and lung are frequent causes of human morbidity in endemic zones.

Aetiology

The lifecycle of *E. granulosus* requires two hosts. The adult tapeworm is found in the small intestine of the definitive host, usually dogs or other canids. It consists of only three to five proglottids, and measures between 3 and 7 mm long when fully mature. *E. granulosus* has remarkable biological potential; there may be as many as 40 000 worms in a heavily infected dog, each one of which sheds about 1000 eggs every 2 weeks. Dogs infected with *Echinococcus* tapeworms pass eggs in their faeces that contaminate the soil and vegetation and remain viable for long periods in cold humid places. Intermediate hosts (sheep, cattle, horses, pigs, and other mammals, including man) acquire hydatid disease by ingesting viable eggs of *E. granulosus*. Eggs hatch in the intestine freeing oncospheres which penetrate the intestinal mucosa and are transported by the blood and lymphatic systems to the liver, lungs, and other organs, where they develop into unilocular cysts.

Taxonomic studies have identified different strains of *Echinococcus*. Tapeworms developed from horse and sheep cysts are distinguishable, and *E. granulosus* from horse cysts is unlikely to infect humans. Wild cycles involving wolves with moose, caribou, and reindeer have been described in North America. In Africa, adult tapeworms have been identified in lions, hyenas, and jackals and cysts in antelopes and wild pigs.

Epidemiology

Hydatid disease is an important cause of human morbidity requiring costly surgical treatment. The infection is widely distributed in most parts of the world where sheep are raised and dogs are used to herd livestock. In the Americas most cases have been reported from Argentina, Chile, Uruguay, Peru, and southern Brazil. Recent studies in Peru have revealed prevalences of hydatid disease ranging from 5.7 to 8.9 per cent in highland villagers, and as high as 32 and 89 per cent in dogs and sheep, respectively. High prevalence of liver hydatid disease, with rates of up to 5.6 per cent, have also been reported in north-western Turkana in Kenya. *Echinococcus* is widespread in the Old World, particularly in Greece, Cyprus, Bulgaria, Lebanon, and Turkey. In the United States, most infections are seen in immigrants from endemic countries. However, sporadic autochthonous transmission is currently recognized in Alaska, California, Utah, Arizona, and New Mexico.

Communities at higher risk of infection include those where sheep are raised extensively and where dogs are used to care for large flocks of livestock. Known risk factors for infection include feeding dogs with raw offal and access of dogs to sheep that die in the field (Fig. 1). The risk of infection is also linked to poor hygiene and intimate contact with dogs. In north-western Turkana, dogs are allowed to stay within the house, and are used to clean up women's menses and lick vomit from faces and diarrhoea from the anal regions of their children.

Pathogenesis

The incubation period of human hydatid infections is highly variable and often prolonged for several years. Cysts have been reported to grow continuously between 1 and 5 cm per year. However, recent studies suggest that cyst growth is highly variable. Some cysts grow as much as 1 cm per year while other viable cysts showed no growth during 3 to 12 years of follow-up.

Fig. 1 Epidemiological conditions for completion of the lifecycle of *Echinococcus*: free dog waiting for sheep offal at a slaughterhouse.

Most human infections remain asymptomatic; hydatid cysts are found incidentally at autopsy much more frequently than the reported local morbidity rates. The locality of the cysts, their size, and their condition determine the particular manifestations.

Clinical features

Hydatid cysts are most frequently seen in the liver (60 to 70 per cent) followed by the lungs (30 to 40 per cent). Signs of hepatic hydatid disease include hepatomegaly with or without the presence of a mass in the upper right quadrant. Obstructive jaundice, mild epigastric pain, indigestion, and nausea may occur occasionally. Hydatid cysts may become secondarily infected with bacteria presenting as a hepatic abscess. Features of lung involvement (Fig. 2) are cough, haemoptysis, dyspnoea, and fever. The ratio of liver to lung cysts may vary from one geographical region to another: a liver to lung ratio of 1.4:1 has been observed in Peru, in contrast to the 3:1 to 13:1 ratio reported in Argentina and Uruguay. Differences in *Echinococcus* strains may account for this variation. Brain cysts produce intracranial hypertension and epilepsy. Vertebral cysts compress the spinal cord causing paraplegia; bone cysts produce spontaneous fractures (Fig. 3 and Plate 1) and deformity. Sudden rupture of cysts in the peritoneal cavity may result in peritonitis, and rupture in the lungs may cause pneumothorax and empyema. Rupture may also cause allergic manifestations such as pruritus, oedema, dyspnoea, anaphylactic shock, and even death.

Diagnosis

Clinical findings such as a space-occupying lesion and residence in an endemic region are suggestive of hydatid disease. Abdominal ultrasonography is an important aid to the diagnosis of abdominal cysts. Portable ultrasonography machines are used with good results in field surveys. Chest radiography is useful for diagnosis of lung cysts. CT scanning is very helpful, especially for diagnosis of non-typical lesions.

Serology

Efforts to develop sensitive and specific immunodiagnostic tests in humans have been relatively successful. A number of serological tests have been developed for diagnosis of hydatid disease, including an enzyme immunoassay, which identify antibodies against antigen B or components of this antigen. A Western blot assay based on the identification of three specific antigens of 8, 16, and 21 kDa is currently used. Major drawbacks in serological diagnosis are low sensitivity for detection of lung hydatid cysts and

Fig. 3 Pathological fracture of the femur caused by hydatid infection (copyright D.A. Warrell).

cross-reactivity with sera of patients with *Taenia solium* infection. In field surveys, serological tests should be used in combination with imaging techniques in order to detect most cases of hydatid disease.

Parasitological diagnosis

Although uncommon, this can be done from sputum samples of patients whose lung cysts have recently ruptured. Scolices have four spherical suckers and a rostellum with two rows of hooks.

Treatment

Surgery

Surgical removal of hydatid cysts remains the treatment of choice in many countries. The usual surgical approach involves injection of a protoscolicidal agent into the cyst, usually 20 per cent hypertonic saline solution or 90 per cent alcohol, followed by evacuation of the fluid, prior to surgical excision. Major risks of surgical treatment include accidental spillage of fluid and scolices into the peritoneal cavity, which may lead to anaphylaxis or secondary peritoneal hydatidosis. Recurrence rates following surgery may be as high as 30 per cent. Antihistamines are given as prophylxis and suction cones have been used to prevent spillage. The efficacy of these methods is uncertain.

Chemotherapy

Benzimidazole compounds have been shown to be effective against hydatid disease. Courses of albendazole in a dose of 10 to 15 mg/kg body weight per day for 28 days are interspersed with drug-free periods of 2 weeks. This regime cures approximately one-third of cases of liver hydatid disease and causes partial regression of cysts in another third of patients. However, many courses may be needed to achieve complete or partial cyst regression. Small liver or lung hydatid cysts should be treated with albendazole. Because of its high scolicidal activity, albendazole is recommended as a prophylactic agent 1 to 3 months prior to surgical intervention. Albendazole is indicated when surgery is contraindicated. Mebendazole may also be used, although it is less effective than albendazole. Albendazole, mebendazole, and other benzimidazole compounds should not be used in pregnant

Fig. 2 Plain chest radiographs showing a lung hydatid cyst.

women because of their potentially teratogenic effects. Since benzimida-zoles are potentially hepatotoxic, liver enzymes should be monitored before and during treatment.

Recent experimental studies in animals have shown that another benzi-midazole compound, oxfendazole, has strong parasiticidal activity. Inter-mittent weekly therapy with oxfendazole was effective in sheep hydatid disease, suggesting the possibility that daily therapy as currently used with albendazole may not be needed. Future studies will explore the effect of oxfendazole in the treatment of human hydatid disease.

PAIR (percutaneous aspiration, injection, reaspiration)

PAIR consists of percutaneous puncture using sonographic guidance, aspiration of substantial amounts of the cyst fluid, and injection of a proto-scolicidal agent, usually hypertonic saline for at least 15 min, followed by reaspiration of cyst contents. Albendazole should be administered before PAIR treatment, and antihistamines should be given to reduce the risk of allergic reactions if there is spillage of fluid. Good results have been reported with this procedure with no major complications. A recent study comparing the use of PAIR and surgical treatment for liver hydatid cysts found less complications and a shorter hospital stay in the PAIR-treated group.

Prevention and control

The earliest successful programme against echinococcosis was carried out in Iceland. It was based on a health educational campaign that eradicated the parasite. Control programmes have been aimed at educating dog owners to prevent their animals from having access to infected offal. This approach includes periodic treatment of sheepdogs with praziquantel (every 45 days), reduction in the dog population, close veterinary inspec-tion of slaughterhouse facilities for the presence of dogs, and cremation of infected offal. Control programmes are in force in Argentina, Chile, and Uruguay. Partial success has been achieved in the first two countries. How-ever, hydatid disease remains a serious problem in Uruguay. Control pro-grammes in New Zealand and Tasmania have reduced the number of infected animals and the incidence of human infection.

Serological tests such as the Western blot for diagnosis of sheep hydati-dosis and the coproantigen ELISA for canine echinococcosis are potentially useful for measuring the burden of disease and monitoring control pro-grammes in endemic regions. A recent major advance has been the devel-opment of a recombinant vaccine (EG95) which seems to confer 96 to 98 per cent protection against challenge infection. Recent trials in Australia and Argentina using this vaccine have reported that 86 per cent of immun-ized sheep were completely free of viable hydatid cysts when examined 1 year later. The number of viable cysts was reduced by 99.3 per cent. Although the results of these initial trials seem promising, further research is needed to assess the cost-benefit of using this vaccine.

Further reading

Allan JC et al. (1992). Coproantigen detection for immunodiagnosis of echinococcosis and taeniasis in dogs and humans. Parasitology 104, 347–55.

Frider B, Larrieu E, Odriozola M (1999). Long-term outcome of asymptomatic liver hydatidosis. Journal of Hepatology 30, 228–31.

Khuroo MS, Wani NA, Javid G (1997). Percutaneous drainage compared with surgery for hepatic hydatid cysts. New England Journal of Medicine 337, 881–3.

Macpherson CNL et al. (1987). Portable ultrasound scanner versus serology in screening for hydatid cysts in a nomadic population. Lancet ii, 259–91.

Moro PL et al. (1997). Epidemiology of Echinococcus granulosus infection in the Central Andes of Peru. Bulletin of the World Health Organization 75, 553–61.

Schantz PM, Williams JF, Posse CR (1973). Epidemiology of hydatid disease in southern Argentina. Comparison of morbidity indices, evaluation of immunodiagnostic tests, and factors affecting transmission in southern Rio Negro Province. American Journal of Tropical Medicine and Hygiene 22, 629–41.

Thompson RCA, ed. (1986). The biology of Echinococcus and hydatid disease. George Allen and Unwin, London.

Verastegui M et al. (1992). Enzyme-linked immunoelectrotransfer blot test for the diagnosis of human hydatid disease. Journal of Clinical Microbiology 30, 1557–61.

7.15.2 Gut cestodes

R. Knight

Two groups of tapeworms infect man: the cyclophyllidean species which are covered in this chapter, and the pseudophyllidea (see Chapter 7.15.4).

The cyclophyllidean tapeworms maintain anchorage to the host small-gut mucosa by means of the scolex, a holdfast structure bearing a circlet of four suckers and usually a central evertible rostellum with one or more circlets of minute hooks (Fig. 1(a and b)). The rest of the body forms the strobila and consists of a chain of flattened proglottids, which bud behind the scolex. The worms change their site of attachment regularly, and are surprisingly motile. Gravid proglottids are lost from the end of the worm and are replaced by others that have matured as they pass down the stro-bila. Each proglottid possesses a complete set of hermaphroditic sex organs and marginal genital openings. Eggs accumulate in the uterus of gravid proglottids and only enter the faecal stream when the proglottids are dis-rupted. In many species the eggs enter the environment within intact pro-glottids. In either case the eggs are embryonated and contain a hexacanth embryo (onchosphere) that bears three pairs of hooks. The egg shells have two membranes; but in Taenia the outer is lost early and the inner forms the thick embryophore.

After ingestion by the intermediate host, eggs hatch and the released hexacanth embryos bore their way into the mucosa. The larval stages of the parasite are generally cystic with an invaginated embryonic scolex—the protoscolex. The cycle is completed when the larval stage, within the inter-mediate host or its tissues, is eaten by the definitive host; the protoscolex evaginates and attaches to the gut mucosa.

In three species, humans are an obligatory part of the lifecycle (Table 1; Figs 2, 3, and 4), in the rest they are an accidental host (see Table 2). The two Taenia species cause anthropozoonoses because the cycle is maintained by an obligatory alternation between human and non-human hosts. Symp-toms result from local hypersensitivity reactions to the worm and its scolex, and altered gut motility due to the physical mass of the worm. Patients often become aware of proglottids in their faeces. Some patients report poorly defined systemic symptoms, which may have an immunological basis. A blood eosinophilia up to 10 per cent can occur with any gut cest-ode.

Taenia saginata (beef tapeworm)
Geographic distribution

The beef tapeworm is prevalent where cattle have access to human faeces and where humans eat undercooked beef. The highest prevalence is in Africa, particularly in eastern and north-eastern parts; it is also common in many countries in the Middle East, South America, and South-East Asia. Prevalence is now very low in the United States, Canada, and Australia. It still persists endemically in Western Europe; but eastwards prevalence increases progressively across Europe and into the former USSR.

Epidemiology

Gravid proglottids are passed at defaecation, often in short chains; free eggs also occur in faeces. The whitish proglottids, approximately 2 to 3 cm long, are actively motile, elongating and contracting (Fig. 5). Viable eggs persist on pasture for many months and can survive most forms of sewage treatment. Cattle have access to human faeces on farms, at camp sites and recreation areas, and on railway lines. Infected herdsmen can initiate epizootics. Eggs may be dispersed by flies and dung beetles, and seabirds can ingest proglottids in estuarine waters and deposit them in their faeces on inland pastures.

In cattle, cysticerci occur in striated muscle; they are whitish, ovoid, and measure 8 by 5 mm; they contain an invaginated protoscolex with no hooks. They become infective within 12 weeks and remain viable in the living host for 2 years; they are viable in stored, chilled meat for several weeks but are killed at −20°C within 1 week. The prepatent period in humans is 3 months and worms may live 30 years. Cattle develop protective immunity to new infection.

(a)

(b)

Fig. 1 (a) *Taenia solium* showing scolex with four suckers and a double row of hooks (× 250). (b) *Taenia saginata* showing scolex with four suckers and no hooks (× 250). (By courtesy of Professor V. Zaman.)

A subspecies *T. saginata asiatica* occurs in Taiwan, Korea, Indonesia, Thailand, and Burma. Infection follows ingestion of raw pig or wild boar liver; the protoscolex of the cysticercus bears hooks.

Clinical features

Most worms are solitary. Multiple worms are smaller, more common in high-transmission areas, and probably arise by simultaneous infection. Most patients are first aware of the worm by seeing proglottids on faeces (Fig. 5). Many will experience active worm migration through the anus, and this may induce an anxiety response. Many have no other symptoms, but others complain of nausea and upper abdominal pains, often relieved by food. A few patients eat to relieve symptoms. In children, impaired appetite can have nutritional consequences. Some patients have symptoms suggestive of hypoglycaemia, namely dizziness and sweating. Pruritus ani is common. The worm may be visible on small-bowel barium studies.

Proglottids have been found in a variety of surgical specimens including resected appendices, but a pathogenic role is usually difficult to establish. They occasionally obstruct the small intestine, pancreatic duct, or bile duct. After gut perforation they can occur in the peritoneum. Proglottids are recorded in the gallbladder, and eggs have been found in gallstones.

Diagnosis

The typical eggs may be found in faeces, but this is an insensitive method; perianal swabs are also useful. Eggs are indistinguishable from those of *T. solium*; patients should be asked to bring worm specimens. Unless the proglottid is fully gravid the number of uterine branches is an unreliable diagnostic character. A better morphological distinction is the presence of a vaginal sphincter; this is absent in *T. solium*. In human surveys in endemic areas a 24-h faecal collection after an anthelmintic will give the most reliable prevalence.

Treatment

A single morning dose of 2 g niclosamide is given to adults and older children on an empty stomach; the tablets should be chewed. Children of 2 to 6 years should receive 1 g, and those below 2 years, 500 mg. The alternative is praziquantel given in a single dose of 10 to 20 mg/kg after a light breakfast. After either drug the proximal part of the worm disintegrates in the gut and the scolex cannot be found. Failure of proglottids to reappear within 3 to 4 months indicates cure.

Control

This includes health education about raw beef, meat inspection, sanitation and hygiene on cattle farms, and proper sewage treatment and disposal. Mass treatments of herd contacts, or whole adult populations, are the most effective short-term measures when endemicity is high. *T. saginata* causes great economic loss to the beef industry in some developing countries.

Taenia solium (pork tapeworm)

The clinical importance of the pork tapeworm relates mainly to cysticercosis, the occurrence of larval forms in human tissue (see Chapter 7.15.3). This arises when eggs hatch in the upper gut and humans become an accidental intermediate host. The source of such eggs is the faeces of persons infected with adult worms.

T. solium is generally less common than the beef tapeworm; it is now very rare in North America and Western Europe, but it remains common in much of sub-Saharan Africa, Mexico, South America, and in China, India, and other parts of Asia.

Epidemiology

In the pig muscle cysticerci produce 'measly pork' (Fig. 6). The cysts are most numerous in the tongue, masseter, heart, and diaphragm, but also

Table 1 Major gut cestodes infecting man

Species	*Taenia saginata* **Beef tapeworm (excluding T. s. asiatica)**	*Taenia solium* **Pork tapeworm**	*Hymenolepis nana* **Dwarf tapeworm**
Intermediate hosts	Cattle, water buffalo, other bovids, reindeer	Pig, wild boar, accidentally in man	None; but see Table 2 for murine subspecies
Length	4–12 m	3–5 m	25–40 mm
Number of proglottids	2000 (mean)	700–1000	200 (mean)
Gravid proglottid	Longer than wide, 20–30 × 5–7 mm	Longer than wide, 18–25 × 5–7 mm	Transverse 0.8 × 0.2 mm
Scolex	No rostellum No hooks	Rostellum with double circlet of 22–32 large and small hooks	Rostellum with single circlet of 20–30 minute hooks
Gravid uterus	15–20 lateral branches	7–13 lateral branches	Bilobed
Testes	800–1200	394–534	3
Ovary	Two-lobed	Three-lobed	Two-lobed
Egg (contains hexacanth embryo)	Embryophore shell is radially striated and 31–40 mm in diameter	Embryophore shell is radially striated and 31–40 mm in diameter	Oval, 30–47 mm long; two shell membranes; 4–8 filaments arise from each pole of inner membrane

occur in the brain. When eaten by humans in undercooked pork the worms mature in 5 to 12 weeks. The eggs have the same resistant qualities as *T.saginata*.

Human cysticercosis is much more limited geographically than *T. solium* implying that internal autoinfection from disrupted proglottids is rare. Conditions favouring cysticercosis include poor personal hygiene, which facilitates external autoinfection and contaminated fingers among food handlers. Faecal pollution of the peridomestic environment, irrigation water, or cultivated vegetables is also important. In parts of Africa, tapeworm proglottids are used in traditional medicine. In the absence of these factors, cases of cysticercosis may be very sporadic even when *T. solium* is common. Cysticercosis is a major health problem in Mexico, some South American countries, and to a lesser extent in Africa and Asia. In 1969, *T. solium* was introduced from Bali into the highlands of Irian Jaya, New Guinea, where the disease is now of great importance.

Pathology of cysticercosis

Cysts occur especially in striated muscle, subcutaneous tissue, the nervous system, and the eye. Many remain clinically silent until the parasite dies after 3 to 5 years, when vigorous inflammatory and hypersensitivity reactions can occur; later lesions may calcify. In the brain, particularly in the subarachnoid and the ventricular system, atypical racemose cysts may occur. They appear as irregular or grape-like clusters of cysts that have no protoscolex; they can be mistaken pathologically for non-parasitic cysts.

Clinical features

Symptoms due to the adult worms are similar to those of *T. saginata* but are often milder and not associated with pruritus ani. The proglottids do not migrate actively *per anum*.

Diagnosis

Adult worm infection is detected as for *T. saginata*. Methods for detecting faecal antigen are available and have great potential use in epidemiological studies. Proglottid fragments can be identified using DNA probes.

Treatment and control

Adult worms are treated as for *T. saginata*. Vomiting must be avoided and an antiemetic is recommended, together with a purgative 2 h after the medication, which should be given after a light breakfast. It should be remembered that the faeces will be potentially highly infective for several days, both for the patient and attendants. Control measures are similar to

Fig. 2 Lifecycle of *Taenia saginata*. (Adapted by Professor V. Zaman from Centers for Disease Control, Atlanta, Georgia, USA.)

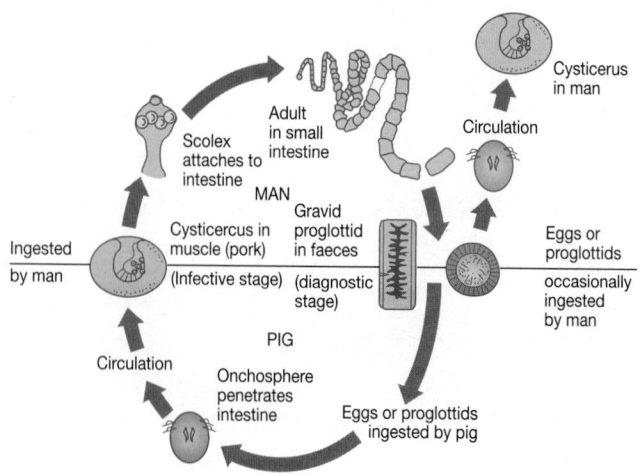

Fig. 3 Lifecycle of *Taenia solium*. (Adapted by Professor V. Zaman from Centers for Disease Control, Atlanta, Georgia, USA.)

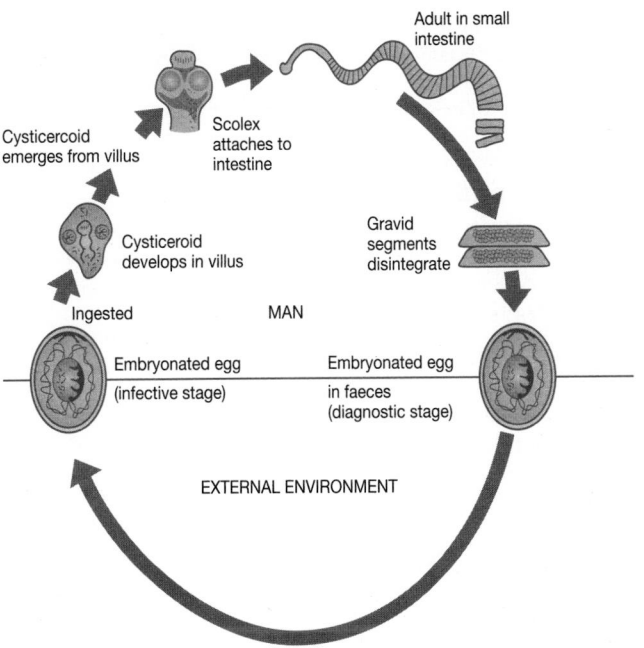

Adult in small intestine

Cysticercoid emerges from villus

Scolex attaches to intestine

Cysticeroid develops in villus

Gravid segments disintegrate

Ingested

MAN

Embryonated egg (infective stage)

Embryonated egg in faeces (diagnostic stage)

EXTERNAL ENVIRONMENT

Fig. 4 Lifecycle of *Hymenolepsis nana*. (Adapted by Professor V. Zaman from Centers for Disease Control, Atlanta, Georgia, USA.)

those of *T. saginata* but local risk factors for human cysticercosis must receive special attention.

Hymenolepis nana (dwarf tapeworm)

The dwarf tapeworm is the most common cestode in man; it is also the smallest. When worm loads are high it causes more gut pathology than any other species. It is common in most developing and tropical countries. The lifecycle normally involves only humans (Fig. 4). Fully embryonated infective eggs are passed in the faeces; gravid proglottids normally disintegrate completely in the gut. Infection is commonly direct, but also by the other faecal–oral routes. Eggs hatch in the jejunum and the hexacanth embryo bores into a villus where it transforms into a cysticercoid larva. After 4 to 6 days it re-enters the gut, everts the scolex, and attaches to the mucosa; eggs appear in the faeces within 12 days. The lifespan is 3 months. The eggs are delicate and survive less than 10 days in the environment. Prevalence is usually much higher in children than adults; outbreaks can occur in families and institutions. External autoinfection is common in high-risk groups and enables high worm loads to build up. In addition, internal autoinfection occurs when there is gut stasis or retroperistalsis. Because of the importance of direct transmission, this infection may be common even in arid environments such as Western Australia.

Clinical features

In heavily infected people, especially children, up to 1000 or more worms may be present. Mucosal damage caused by both larval and adult worms leads to protein loss and sometimes malabsorption. Abdominal pains and anorexia are common.

Immunosuppressant or steroid therapy, particularly in patients with lymphoma, can lead to the development of bizarre cystic larval forms in the gut wall, mesenteric nodes, liver, and lungs. A similar condition can be produced in immunosuppressed mice.

Diagnosis and treatment

Eggs can be detected in faeces using concentration methods. Proglottids are rarely found in faeces, except after treatment.

Praziquantel in a single dose of 25 mg/kg is the most effective drug. If niclosamide is used, a 7-day course is needed to ensure that larval stages are killed when they re-enter the gut lumen. The dose on the first day is as for *T. saginata*; on the remaining days one-half of this dose is given. Relapses often result from persistence of eggs in the patient's environment.

Table 2 Accidental gut cestodes that infect man

Species	Geographic distribution	Definitive hosts	Intermediate hosts	Length, and width	Shape of gravid proglottid	Other features
Hymenolepis nana fraterna	Worldwide	Mouse, rat	Fleas, beetles	2.5–9 cm, 0.5–1 mm	Very transverse	Murine form of *H. nana*; the egg is identical
H. diminuta (rat tapeworm)	Worldwide	Rat	Fleas, beetles, cockroaches	20–60 cm, 3–4 mm	Very transverse	Egg like *H. nana* but yellow outer membrane and no filaments; 60–85 mm
Dipylidium caninum	Worldwide	Dog, cat	Fleas and dog louse	10–70 cm, 2.5–3 mm	Elongate, wider in middle	Double set of sex organs; egg capsules with 8–15 eggs
Bertiella studeri	S. and S.E. Asia, Africa, Cuba	Primates	Oribatid mites	27–30 cm, 6–10 mm	Much wider than long	Inner egg shell bears bicornuate knob
B. mucronata	S. and C. America	Primates	Oribatid mites	15–45 cm, 5–10 mm	Transverse	As above
Mathevotaenia symmetrica	Thailand	Rats	Beetles	13 cm, 1–2 mm	Elongate	Capsule surrounds individual egg
Inermicapsifer madagascariensis	Malagasy, Africa, C. America, Cuba	Rats	'Arthropod'	26–42 cm, 2.6 mm	Slightly elongate, white and opaque	Egg capsules with 6–11 eggs
Raillietina celebensis	East Asia, Australia	Rats	Ant	16–60 cm, 3 mm	As above	Egg capsules with 1–4 eggs
R. demerariensis	Guyana, Cuba, Ecuador	Rats	'Insect'	16–60 cm, 2–3 mm	As above	Egg capsule with 8–10 eggs
R. siriraji	Thailand	Rats	Cockroach	As above	As above	As above
Mesocestoides variabilis	Rwanda, Japan, Greenland, United States, Korea	Carnivores (fox, skunk, etc.); birds of prey	Mites (1st host) Amphibia, reptiles, birds, and mammals (2nd hosts)	40 cm, 2 mm	Longer than broad	Larval worms can occur in humans, in muscle and subcutaneous tissue

Fig. 5 Actively motile, contracting proglottid of *Taenia saginata* found by a patient in the stool. (Copyright D.A. Warrell.)

Accidental gut cestodes

Many species have been recorded in humans (see Table 2). All have arthropods as intermediate hosts, the larval cysticercoid stage being in the haemocele; the full lifecycles of some species are still uncertain. The normal definitive host becomes infected by eating the arthropod intentionally or accidentally. The means by which humans become infected is sometimes not clear, but fleas, small beetles, and mites are easily overlooked in food. *Dipylidium caninum* infection occurs in children who have groomed their pet. Infections with *Bertiella* are mostly in owners of pet monkeys, but oribatid mites are common in fallen fruit, especially mangoes. Children may eat insects deliberately, and this appears to be the mode of infection by *Raillietina siriraji* in Bangkok. Beetles are used for medicinal purposes in parts of Thailand and Malaysia, and this is the most likely route by which *Mathevotaenia* is acquired.

Hymenolepis nana fraterna is the murine strain of the human parasite and *H. diminuta* also infects rodents; both are rare in human beings. Both human and murine subspecies of *H. nana* will infect *Tribolium* beetles. In many of these species the eggs are in capsules that are released when the proglottid disintegrates in the gut, or more commonly, in the faecal mass. *Mesocestoides* is unique among these parasites in three respects: two intermediate hosts are required; the genital opening is medioventral rather than at the margin of the proglottid as in all other cyclophyllidean tapeworms; and larval worms can occur in man when mites are ingested.

Many patients will present because they have passed proglottids. *Dipylidium caninum* actively migrates out of the anus, like *T. saginata*. Faecal examinations of persons with abdominal complaints may reveal unusual eggs or egg capsules. Poorly defined systemic and allergic complaints are common. Treatment is as for *T. saginata*.

Fig. 6 'Measly pork' showing numerous cysts in the pig's muscle. (Copyright Sornchai Looareesuwan.)

Recognition of these parasites is of epidemiological interest and may indicate potential transmission of other zoonotic pathogens. It is certain that all these parasites are underreported. Unusual proglottids or eggs should be preserved in formol saline and sent to a parasitologist.

Further reading

Chitchang S *et al.* (1985). Relationship between the severity of the symptom and the number of *Hymenolepis nana* after treatment. *Journal of the Medical Association of Thailand* **68**, 424–6.

Fan PC (1988). Taiwan *Taenia* and taeniasis. *Parasitology Today* **4**, 86–8.

Fan PC (1997). Annual economic loss caused by *Taenia saginata asiatica* taeniasis in three endemic areas of east Asia. *Southeast Asian Journal of Tropical Medicine and Public Health* **28**(Suppl 1), 217–21.

Fan PC *et al.* (1995). Morphological description of *Taenia saginata asiatica* (Cyclophyllidea: Taeniidae) from man in Asia. *Journal of Helminthology* **69**, 299–303.

Flisser A (1988). Neurocysticercosis in Mexico. *Parasitology Today* **4**, 131–7.

Flisser A *et al.* (1990). New approaches in the diagnosis of *Taenia solium* cysticercosis and taeniasis. *Annales de Parasitologie Humaine et Comparée* **65**(Suppl 1), 95–8.

Harrison LJ (1990). Differential diagnosis of *Taenia saginata* and *Taenia solium* with DNA probes. *Parasitology* **100**, 459–61.

Lucas SB *et al.* (1979). Aberrant forms of *Hymenolepis nana*: possible opportunistic infections in immunosuppressed patients. *Lancet* **ii**, 1372–3.

Mason PR, Patterson BA (1994). Epidemiology of *Hymenolepis nana* in primary school children in urban and rural communities in Zimbabwe. *Journal of Parasitology* **80**, 245–50.

Pawlowski Z, Schultz MG (1972). Taeniasis and cysticercosis (*Taenia saginata*). *Advances in Parasitology* **10**, 269–343.

Subianto DB, Tumada LR, Morgono SS (1978). Burns and epileptic fits associated with cysticercosis in mountain people of Irian Jaya. *Tropical and Geographic Medicine* **30**, 275–8.

7.15.3 Cysticercosis
Hector H. Garcia and Robert H. Gilman

Introduction

Known since the Hippocratic era, cysticercosis is the commonest helminthic infection of the human central nervous system. It is probable that the suspicion of its origins led some religions expressly to forbid the consumption of pork. Socio-economic improvements eradicated the infection in Europe and North America. However, endemic *Taenia solium* taeniasis/cysticercosis persists in most developing countries, where human cysticercosis is an important cause of epilepsy and other neurological morbidity, and porcine infections cause important economical losses to peasants.

Aetiology

Cysticercosis is infection with the larval stage (cysticercus) of *T. solium*, the pork tapeworm. In the lifecycle (Fig. 1) of this two-host zoonotic cestode, humans are the only definitive host and harbour the adult tapeworm, whereas pigs are intermediate hosts. The hermaphroditic adult *T. solium* inhabits the small intestine. Its head or scolex bears four suckers and a double crown of hooks, connected by a narrow neck to a large body (strobila) between 2 and 4 m long, composed of several hundred proglottids. Gravid proglottids, each containing 50 000 to 60 000 fertile eggs, detach from the distal end of the worm and are excreted in the faeces. The cycle is

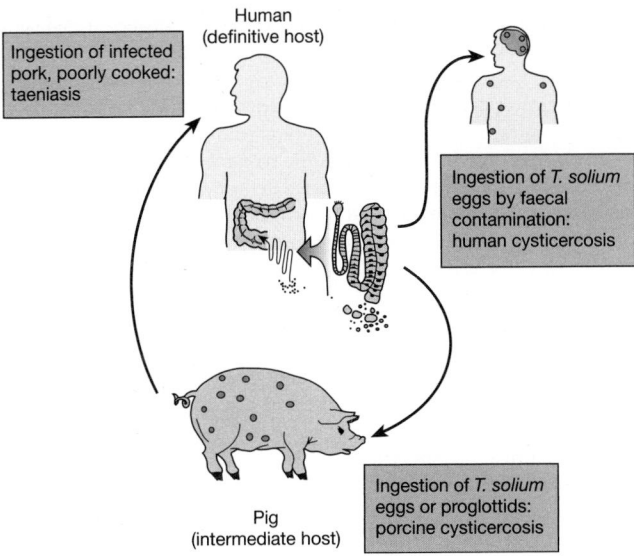

Fig. 1 Lifecycle of *T. solium*.

completed when pigs ingest stools contaminated with *T. solium* eggs. Once ingested by the pig, the invasive oncospheres in the eggs are liberated by the action of gastric acid and intestinal fluids and actively penetrate the bowel wall, enter the bloodstream, and are carried to the muscles and other tissues where they develop into larval cysts. When humans ingest undercooked pork containing cysticerci, the larvae evaginate in the small intestine, their scolices attach to the intestinal mucosa, and they begin forming proglottids. By accidentally ingesting *Taenia* eggs, humans may also act as intermediate hosts for *T. solium* and develop cysticercosis.

Epidemiology

The availability of neuroimaging studies and the subsequent development of specific serodiagnostic tests resulted in identification of neurocysticercosis as a frequent neurological disorder in Latin America, Africa, and Asia, where the prevalence of active epilepsy is almost twice that in Western countries. Neurocysticercosis is an emerging problem in industrialized countries, seen mainly in immigrants from endemic areas, some of whom may spread the infection as tapeworm carriers.

The main sources of human cysticercosis are ingestion of food contaminated with *T. solium* eggs and faecal–oral contamination in those carrying the tapeworm. Epidemiological studies suggest that almost every newly diagnosed patient with cysticercosis has been infected by someone in their close environment who is harbouring a *T. solium* and tends to dismiss the role of environment or water in transmission. Airborne transmission of *T. solium* eggs or internal autoinfection by regurgitation of proglottids into the stomach have been suggested but not proved.

Pathogenesis

Any organ may be infected but parasites survive more frequently in the nervous system, possibly because the immune response there is limited. Signs and symptoms are caused by perilesional inflammation and oedema, mass effect, or obstruction of cerebrospinal fluid circulation. Although complete development of cysts takes about 2 months, symptoms usually develop years after the initial infection. This clinically silent period and finding inflammation around cysts in symptomatic cases suggest that symptoms are due to inflammatory processes associated with death of the parasite rather than to the presence of the parasite itself.

Meningeal cysticerci elicit an intense inflammatory reaction causing thickening of basal leptomeninges. The optic chiasma and other cranial nerves are usually entrapped within this dense exudate, resulting in visual field defects and other cranial nerve dysfunctions. The foramens of Luschka and Magendie may be occluded by the thickened leptomeninges leading to hydrocephalus. Blood vessels may be affected by the inflammatory reaction. The walls of small penetrating arteries are invaded by inflammatory cells, leading to a proliferative endarteritis with occlusion of the lumen, and which may result in cerebral infarction.

Clinical features

Neurocysticercosis is a pleomorphic disease, whose manifestations vary with the number, size, and topography of the lesions and the intensity of the host's immune response to the parasites. Patients can be classified by the number and location of the cysticerci, and the presence or absence of associated inflammation or calcifications.

Epilepsy, the most common presentation of neurocysticercosis, is usually the primary or sole manifestation of the disease. Seizures occur in 50 to 80 per cent of patients with parenchymal brain cysts or calcifications but are less common in other forms of the disease. Other common focal signs include pyramidal tract signs, sensory deficits, signs of brainstem dysfunction, and involuntary movements. These manifestations usually follow a subacute or chronic course, making neurocysticercosis difficult to differentiate clinically from neoplasms or other infections of the central nervous system. Focal signs may occur abruptly in patients who develop a cerebral infarct as a complication of subarachnoid neurocysticercosis. Subarachnoid cysticerci may reach 10 cm or more in diameter ('giant' cysticercosis, Fig. 2), and exert a mass effect.

Neurocysticercosis may present with increased intracranial pressure, usually from hydrocephalus secondary to cysticercotic arachnoiditis, granular ependymitis, or ventricular cysts. In these cases, intracranial hypertension develops subacutely and progresses slowly. An encephalitic picture may result from overwhelming inflammation around many parasitic cysts, a syndrome that occurs more frequently in younger people, especially women. In contrast, some patients may tolerate hundreds of intraparenchymal cysticerci with only minor symptoms.

Muscular pseudohypertrophy, a rare presentation, is caused by heavy cysticercal infection of skeletal muscles (Fig. 3) giving a 'Herculean' appearance. The few cases reported are all from India. Other apparent differences

Fig. 2 Giant cysticercotic cyst (brain CT).

Fig. 3 Heavy cysticercal infection of skeletal muscles (copyright Sornchai Looareesuwan).

in clinical manifestations between Asia and Latin America include a high frequency of subcutaneous cysts and single degenerating brain lesions in Asia.

Pathology

The cysticerci are liquid-filled vesicles consisting of vesicular wall and scolex (Fig. 4). The vesicular wall is composed of an outer or cuticular layer, a middle or cellular layer with pseudoepithelial structure, and an inner or reticular layer. The invaginated scolex has a head or rostellum armed with suckers and hooks, and a rudimentary body or strobila that includes the spiral canal.

The macroscopic appearance of cysticerci varies in different locations within the central nervous system. Cysticerci within the brain parenchyma are usually small and tend to lodge in the cerebral cortex or basal ganglia. Subarachnoid cysts may be small if located in the depths of cortical sulci, or grow to 5 cm or more in the basal cisterns or sylvian fissures. Ventricular cysticerci are usually single, may or may not have a visible scolex, and may be attached to the choroid plexus or float freely in the ventricle. Spinal cysticerci are usually located in the subarachnoid space (rarely intramedullary). Their morphology is similar to cysts located within the brain.

Basal cysticerci may undergo a disproportionate growth of their membrane, with extension processes, resembling a brunch of grapes (racemose cysticercosis, Fig. 5). In these cases, the scolex is frequently unidentifiable even by microscopy.

Viable, vesicular cysticerci elicit little inflammatory change in surrounding tissues because of active immune evasion mechanisms. The appearance of symptoms is interpreted as the result of immunological attack from the host, in a process of degeneration that ends with the death of the parasite. Inflammatory changes in the parasite membrane and increased density of cyst fluid mark the transition between four defined stages: viable, colloidal, granular nodular, and calcified cyst. Viable cysts may coexist with degenerating cysts or calcifications.

Laboratory/imaging diagnosis

The pleomorphism of neurocysticercosis makes it impossible to diagnose on clinical grounds alone. In endemic regions, late-onset seizures in otherwise healthy individuals are highly suggestive of neurocysticercosis. Most of these patients are normal on neurological examinations. Routine neuroimaging and serological studies are, therefore, mandatory. Finding cysticerci outside the central nervous system (eye, subcutaneous tissue, muscle) assists the diagnosis of neurocysticercosis. Muscular and subcutaneous cysticerci are far less common in American than in African or Asian patients with neurocysticercosis.

Neuroimaging

CT and MRI have drastically improved diagnostic accuracy by providing objective evidence about the topography of the lesions and the degree of the host inflammatory response to the parasite. Imaging findings in parenchymal neurocysticercosis depend on the stage of involution of cysticerci.

Fig. 4 Uncontrasted T_1 MR image showing two intraparenchymal cysticerci with visible scolices.

Fig. 5 Basal 'racemose' cysticercosis.

Fig. 6 Calcified neurocysticercosis.

Viable cysticerci appear as rounded cystic lesions on CT (Fig. 2), hypointense on MRI (Fig. 4), without associated enhancement, whereas degenerating parasites are seen as focal enhancing lesions surrounded by oedema, and calcifications as hyperdense dots or nodules (Fig. 6). Disappearance of cyst fluid signals the degenerative phase and calcified nodules the residual phase. Single or multiple ring-like or nodular enhancing lesions are non-specific and present a diagnostic challenge. Pyogenic brain abscesses, fungal abscesses, tuberculomas, toxoplasma abscesses, and primary or metastatic brain tumours may produce similar findings on CT or MRI.

CT and MRI findings in subarachnoid neurocysticercosis are less specific. They include hydrocephalus, abnormal meningeal enhancement, and subarachnoid cysts. Cerebral angiography may show segmental narrowing or occlusion of major intracranial arteries in patients with cerebral infarcts secondary to parasitic vasculitis. In neurocysticercosis there is rarely fever or signs of meningeal irritation; glucose levels of cerebrospinal fluid are usually normal. MRI is generally better than CT for the diagnosis of neurocysticercosis, particularly in patients with basal lesions, brainstem or intraventricular cysts, and spinal lesions. MRI is, however, less sensitive than CT for the detection of small calcifications.

Immunological tests

Immunoblot (Western blot) is the best available serological test for *T. solium* antibodies. It is 98 per cent sensitive in cases with more than one active lesion, and 100 per cent specific. Its sensitivity may drop in patients with a single cyst. Other assays using unfractionated antigens (e.g. enzyme immunoassay) suffer from poor specificity but are more reliable when performed with cerebrospinal fluid than serum. Antigen-detection tests may provide a tool for serological monitoring of antiparasitic therapy. Although results of serology and imaging studies may be similar, they evaluate different aspects of the disease and may be discordant in some patients. Intestinal tapeworm carriers, naturally cured patients, or non-neurological infections may have normal brain images but be positive serologically. Those with only inactive lesions or a single cerebral lesion may be seronegative.

A proportion (about 10 to 15 per cent) of patients with neurocysticercosis are tapeworm carriers at the time of diagnosis, and in another 10 per cent or so a carrier can be detected in the household. Parasitological diagnosis is difficult: eggs and proglottids are shed only intermittently in stool and are usually missed by routine stool examination. Stool assays to detect parasite antigens are more sensitive than microscopy, but are not widely available. A recently described serological test for tapeworm carriers may improve detection.

A set of diagnostic criteria based on neuroimaging studies, serological tests, clinical presentation, and exposure history has been proposed by Del Brutto and colleagues. Besides absolute demonstration of the presence of the parasite, 'major' criteria (including typical findings on neuroimaging, demonstration of specific anticysticercal antibodies, or the presence of typical cigar-shaped calcifications in muscle) are combined with 'minor' criteria and epidemiological data to suggest a probable or possible diagnosis. Application of these criteria should improve the consistency of diagnosis.

Treatment

Because of the clinical and pathological pleomorphism of neurocysticercosis, precise assessment of the viability and size of cysts, the location of parasites, and the severity of the host's immune response is important before planning treatment.

Symptomatic treatment is very important. Seizures secondary to parenchymal neurocysticercosis can usually be controlled with anticonvulsants. However, the optimal length of anticonvulsant therapy in patients with neurocysticercosis has not been determined, and it is difficult to withdraw this treatment. Prognostic factors associated with recurrence of seizures include the development of parenchymal brain calcifications, and occurrence of recurrent seizures or multiple brain cysts before starting antiparasitic therapy.

Antiparasitic agents destroy viable cysts, although their long-term clinical benefit in seizures due to parenchymal neurocysticercosis has not been proved. Currently, albendazole is the drug of choice for antiparasitic treatment of cerebral cysticercosis (15 mg/kg.day for 7 days, with steroids), although a recently described single-day praziquantel regimen (75 to 100 mg/kg, in three doses at 2-h intervals, followed by steroids 6 h later) demonstrated similar cestocidal activity with few cysts. Longer courses may be required in patients with many lesions or subarachnoid cysticercosis. Transient worsening of neurological symptoms can be expected during antiparasitc therapy, secondary to the perilesional inflammatory reaction. There is no role for antiparasitic drugs in inactive neurocysticercosis (i.e. calcifications with or without enhancement on CT scan) since the parasites are dead.

Between the second and fifth day of antiparasitic therapy there is usually an exacerbation of neurological symptoms, attributed to local inflammation caused by the death of the larvae. For this reason, albendazole or praziquantel are generally given simultaneously with steroids in order to control the oedema and intracranial hypertension. Serum levels of praziquantel decrease when steroids are administered simultaneously, an effect that does not occur with albendazole. However, there is no evidence that cysticidal efficacy is decreased. Serum levels of phenytoin and carbamazepine may be lowered by simultaneous praziquantel administration. There are no data in patients receiving albendazole.

Some forms of neurocysticercosis should not be treated with antiparasitic agents. In patients with severe cysticercotic encephalitis these drugs may result in worsening cerebral oedema and fatal herniation. In this case, the mainstay of therapy is high doses of corticosteroids to decrease the inflammatory response. In patients with both hydrocephalus and parenchymal brain cysts, antiparasitic drugs should be started only after placement of a ventricular shunt in case the intracranial pressure increases as a result of drug therapy. Antiparasitic drugs must be used with caution in patients with giant subarachnoid cysticerci. In such patients, concomitant steroid administration is mandatory to avoid cerebral infarction. Albendazole can successfully destroy ventricular cysts, but the surrounding inflammatory reaction may cause acute hydrocephalus if the cysts are located within the fourth ventricle or near the foramens of Monro and Luschka.

Surgery is limited to ventriculoperitoneal shunts to relieve obstructive hydrocephalus, and excision of single cysticerci (in the fourth ventricle or giant intraparenchymal cysts). However, shunts frequently dysfunction. The protracted course in these patients and their high mortality rates (up to 50 per cent in 2 years) is directly related to the number of surgical interventions required to change the shunts. Recently, neuroventriculoscopy has been employed as a less invasive option for resection of ventricular cysticerci.

Prognosis

Parenchymal cysticercosis has a good prognosis. Seizures usually subside in time without sequelae. In contrast, extraparenchymal cysticercosis and especially racemose cysticercosis have a poor prognosis, responding poorly to antiparasitic therapy, and leading to progressively deteriorating disease and death.

Prevention and control

Cysticercosis would not exist if pigs had no access to human faeces. However, this approach is hampered in endemic zones by the lack of sanitary facilities, veterinary inspection, and more importantly, because farmers tend to raise pigs under free-range conditions in order to reduce the cost of feeding them. Intervention programmes have concentrated on mass chemotherapy to eliminate human taeniasis, but their results have not been sustained. New tools for controls are oxfendazole, an effective and cheap single-dose therapy for porcine cysticercosis, and the candidate porcine vaccines under trial by several groups.

Monitoring the effect of an intervention requires suitable indicators. Human seroprevalence does not reflect changes in infection patterns because antibodies persist for years, even after successful treatment. Studies in Peru have shown that serological monitoring of porcine infection is a useful marker for both prevalence and changes in infection intensity over time. Similarly, the rate of infection in uninfected (sentinel) pigs over time can be used to estimate intensity of *T. solium* infection in the community. The prevalences of human and porcine infection are strongly correlated.

Areas of uncertainty/controversy

Although most cysts disappear after antiparasitic treatment, it remains uncertain whether this is associated with better control of seizures. Retrospective trials suggested that seizures were better controlled in treated patients. An open-label controlled trial failed to find a beneficial effect for albendazole or praziquantel in either clinical control or radiological evolution. However, the methodology of this study has been questioned, and data from double-blind randomized studies are not yet available.

Areas needing further research

A recent report suggests an association between brain calcifications secondary to cysticercosis and glial neoplasms. This has not yet been confirmed or rejected. Systematic long-term evaluation is needed to determine whether hydrocephalus is a late complication of antiparasitic therapy. The efficacy and costs of comprehensive human–porcine eradication programmes must be assessed.

Further reading

Corona T *et al.* (1996). Single-day praziquantel therapy for neurocysticercosis. *New England Journal of Medicine* **334**, 125.

Del Brutto OH (1997). Albendazole therapy for subarachnoid cysticerci: clinical and neuroimaging analysis of 17 patients. *Journal of Neurology, Neurosurgery and Psychiatry* **62**, 659–61.

Del Brutto OH *et al.* (2001). Proposed diagnostic criteria for neurocysticercosis. *Neurology* **57**, 177–83. [A guide to systematic diagnosis.]

Evans C *et al.* (1997). Controversies in the management of cysticercosis. *Emerging Infectious Diseases* **3**, 403–5.

Garcia HH, Martinez SM, eds (1999). Taenia solium *taeniasis/cysticercosis*, 2nd edn. Ed. Universo, Lima.

Garcia HH *et al.* (1993). Cysticercosis as a major cause of epilepsy in Perú. *Lancet* **341**, 197–200.

Garcia HH *et al.* (1997). Albendazole therapy for neurocysticercosis: a prospective double-blind trial comparing 7 versus 14 days of treatment. Cysticercosis Working Group in Peru. *Neurology* **48**, 1421–7.

Gonzalez AE *et al.* (1997). Treatment of porcine cysticercosis with oxfendazole: a dose–response trial. *Veterinary Record* **141**, 420–2.

White AC, Jr (1997). Neurocysticercosis: a common cause of neurologic disease worldwide. *Clinical Infectious Diseases* **24**, 101–13. [Comprehensive review.]

Wilkins PP *et al.* (1999). Development of a serologic assay to detect *Taenia solium* taeniasis. *American Journal of Tropical Medicine and Hygiene* **60**, 199–204.

7.15.4 Pseudophyllidean tapeworms: diphyllobothriasis and sparganosis

Seung-Yull Cho

Diphyllobothriasis

Diphyllobothriasis is a fish-borne infection of the intestine with tapeworms that belong to the genus *Diphyllobothrium*. The type species is *D. latum*.

Plerocercoid larvae of *D. latum* in fish can infect humans. In the intestine, the 1 cm long plerocercoid develops into a 5–6 m long adult, which produces a million eggs each day. In fresh water, a cycle is maintained—the egg embryonates to a coracidium, which becomes a procercoid larva in the copepod *Cyclops strenuus*, and then a plerocercoid in fish.

Human infections occur worldwide. The incidence is high in Siberia and in Baltic countries such as Finland. In Switzerland, the Lake Regions of North America, and in East Asia, cases of diphyllobothriasis are not uncommon. Humans may also be infected by zoonotic species of *Diphyllobothrium*. For instance, *D. yonagoense* and *D. nihonkaiense* in Japan and *D. pacificum* in Chile and Peru are intestinal parasites of seals while *D. ursi* and *D. dendriticum* in Alaska are parasites of bears and birds respectively. The habit of eating sliced raw fish, such as pike, burbot, perch, salmon, and other freshwater fish, creates the opportunity for infection. Prevention is achieved by freezing fish for 1 day at − 18 °C or lower.

Infection usually causes few symptoms. Abdominal discomfort, fatigue, diarrhoea, and urticaria may be the vague presenting symptoms. Vomiting up a tapeworm and intestinal obstruction due to a mass of worms occurs very rarely. A strip of gravid segments may pass out through the anus. Tapeworm pernicious anaemia may be associated with *D. latum* infection. In these patients, elimination of the tapeworm results in improvement of the anaemia. Clinically, haematological and neurological manifestations are the same as in pernicious anaemia.

Clinical symptoms are rarely responsible for raising the suspicion of diphyllobothriasis. The diagnosis can be confirmed by identifying eggs in the stool by microscopy. Discharged chains of gravid segments are also

Fig. 1 A sparganum surgically removed from a subcutaneous mass.

diagnostic. In endemic areas, all patients with pernicious anaemia should have their stools examined. Treatment is simple and effective. Niclosamide in a single adult dose of 2 g or praziquantel in a single dose of 10 mg/kg body weight are the drugs of choice.

Sparganosis

Sparganosis is a zoonotic infection caused by the larval tapeworm of *Spirometra mansoni* or *S. mansonoides*. The larvae invade a variety of human tissues (Fig. 1).

The sparganum (plerocercoid) is a 1–30 cm long, white, slender tapeworm larva without round suckers. It is found in terrestrial vertebrates. Carnivorous mammals are infected with the adult stage in their small intestine. In fresh water, the egg embryonates, becoming a coracidium. The swimming coracidium is taken up by zooplankton, such as *Cyclops leuckarti*, and develops into a procercoid larva. When terrestrial vertebrates including man ingest the procercoid, it transforms into a tissue-invading sparganum.

Human sparganosis occurs sporadically worldwide. The procercoid larva in *Cyclops* can be inadvertently drunk in unfiltered water. Sparganum-infected frog, snake, poultry, or pork meat are important sources of human infection in endemic areas such as Japan, Korea, China, Vietnam, and Southeast Asian countries due to traditional habits. Some people believe that eating raw meat is a tonic or is beneficial for patients with tuberculosis. Rural people in Vietnam practise applying poultices of frog or snake skin to an inflamed eye. In this case a sparganum in the frog or snake skin can directly penetrate the conjunctiva.

Ingested larvae penetrate the intestinal wall and migrate systemically. The worm usually lodges in subcutaneous tissue or muscle of the chest or abdominal walls, breast, limbs, or scrotum. A lump may appear and then spontaneously disappear, only to reappear some weeks or months later at a site remote from the first. The sparganum secretes at least six different serine and cysteine proteases, which facilitate worm migration and evasion of the host's immune response. Orbital, chest, and abdominal cavities are involved. Sparganosis of the central nervous system is increasingly recognized.

A granuloma is formed along the tortuous migration track. Zones of necrosis and intense lymphohistiocytic reaction with eosinophilic infiltration surround the larva and its track. The disintegrated worm may be found in a granuloma, leaving behind calcareous corpuscles. Local bleeding and suppuration may complicate sparganosis. The sparganum can survive for more than 5 years. In general, one or only a few infect each patient.

Sparganum proliferum is an acephalic, branched, proliferating larva that is histologically similar to a non-proliferating sparganum. In very rare human infections the larvae are found in thousands in subcutaneous tissue and internal organs. The human infection has been found in Japan, the United States, and Venezuela. The biology of this larva is still unknown. The patient's serum reacts with sparganum antigen.

Diagnosis of sparganosis is rarely made preoperatively. Incidental recovery of the worm at surgery makes a definitive diagnosis. Preoperative diagnosis of cerebral sparganosis is made with high confidence when computed tomography or magnetic resonance imaging of the brain shows an enhancing nodule with changing shape or position in the sequential images, degeneration of white matter, and ventricular dilatation together with positive antibody tests in serum and cerebrospinal fluid (Fig. 2).

Excision of the mass or removal of the worm from the lesion is curative. Repeated surgery is necessary when the patient has multiple lesions. There are no drugs which are are known to be effective against sparganosis. The prognosis is excellent in almost all cases when treated surgically. However, all cases of *S. proliferum* infection have proved fatal.

Further reading

Kim DG *et al.* (1996). Cerebral sparganosis: clinical manifestations, treatment, and outcome. *Journal of Neurosurgery* **85**, 1066–71.

Moulinier R *et al.* (1982) Human proliferative sparganosis in Venezuela: report of a case. *American Journal of Tropical Medicine and Hygiene* **31**, 358–63.

Von Bonsdorff B (1977). *Diphyllobothriasis in man*. Academic Press, London.

Fig. 2 A MRI finding of cerebral sparganosis. Coronal contrast-enhanced T_1-weighted image shows a tortuous curvilinear enhancing lesion (arrow) with surrounding low density of oedema and degeneration in right frontal lobe.

7.16 Trematodes (flukes)

7.16.1 Schistosomiasis

D. W. Dunne and B. J. Vennervald

Introduction

Schistosomiasis, also known as bilharzia, is caused by infection with parasitic trematode worms (flukes) of the genus *Schistosoma*. Disease is usually associated with chronic infections contracted by exposure to fresh water containing infective cercarial larvae that penetrate intact skin and develop into blood-dwelling worms. Most human infections are caused by one of three species, *S. mansoni*, *S. haematobium*, or *S. japonicum*. Two species, *S. intercalatum* and *S. mekongi*, are less important. Schistosomiasis is patchily distributed in parts of South America, Africa, the Middle East, China, and Southeast Asia. An estimated 600 million people in 74 countries are at risk of infection and some 200 million are infected. Of these, the World Health Organization estimates that 120 million may be symptomatic, while 20 million are suffering severe consequences of infection. Although simple diagnosis and effective drug treatment is available for individual uncomplicated cases, the world disease burden caused by these parasites has increased from the estimated 114 million human infections in 1947. Diagnosis and treatment are often not available to exposed rural populations, and drug-based control programmes are hampered by the continued susceptibility of treated individuals, particularly children, to reinfection. Human schistosomiasis is most often an insidious and chronic disease with a range of pathological manifestations involving the intestine and liver, or the urogenital tract. Mortality estimates are difficult, but 20 000 to 200 000 deaths may be directly associated with schistosomiasis each year.

Parasite lifecycle

The schistosome lifecycle requires two host species: a 'definitive' vertebrate host, in which adult male and female worms develop and sexual reproduction occurs, and an 'intermediate' freshwater snail host, in which the parasite multiplies asexually. Transmission between these hosts is achieved by two different free-swimming larval stages. For species that infect man, miracidia hatch from eggs excreted in the faeces or urine of the vertebrate host, and then seek out and infect snails. Cercariae are released from the snail and are able actively to penetrate intact human skin. Different schistosome species have their own, often very restricted, range of snail hosts. Schistosomiasis is thus closely associated with particular freshwater habitats, and its geographical distribution is restricted by the availability of particular snail species. *S. mansoni* and *S. haematobium* are confined to aquatic snails (genera *Biomphalaria* and *Bulinus* respectively) that inhabit ponds, lakes, irrigation canals, slow-flowing streams, and rivers. *S. japonicum* is transmitted by amphibious snails of the genus *Oncomelania* that, in addition to a variety of freshwater habitats, are also present in damp soil and

Fig. 1 The infective larva (cerceria) of *Schistosoma mansoni*, length approximately 200 μm. The head region has characteristic suckers; the muscular forked tail propels the free-swimming larva, but is discarded during skin penetration. This larva will develop into an adult worm in a human host.

vegetation, such as paddy fields. Schistosomes that infect man can also infect other mammals. This is important in the transmission of *S. japonicum*, a zoonotic infection in which cattle, water buffalo, pigs, dogs, and rodents can act as reservoir hosts of the human parasite. *S. mansoni* infects a narrower range of mammals and only a few rodent species and baboons have any potential to act as occasional reservoirs. In nature *S. haematobium* is essentially specific to man. The sites of maturation of the adult worms vary between schistosome species, affecting both the transmission of the infection and its clinical sequelae.

Once shed from freshwater snails, cercariae (Fig. 1) live for about 24 h, but their effective period of infectivity is probably shorter under field conditions. Cercarial behaviour and the timing of their release enhance their chance of contacting their vertebrate host of choice. Light and increasing temperature trigger the release of *S. mansoni* and *S. haematobium* cercariae during the day and their tails are used actively to maintain their position near the water surface. *S. japonicum* cercariae are shed late in the day and are closely associated with the meniscus, perhaps reflecting their wider host range, as species specific for rodents are shed at night. Contact with skin triggers adherence mechanisms and proteolytic enzymes and muscular

Fig. 2 Adult worms of *S. mansoni*. The shorter male encloses the female in its gynaecophoric canal, the characteristic haematin-like pigment can be seen in the female worm's gut.

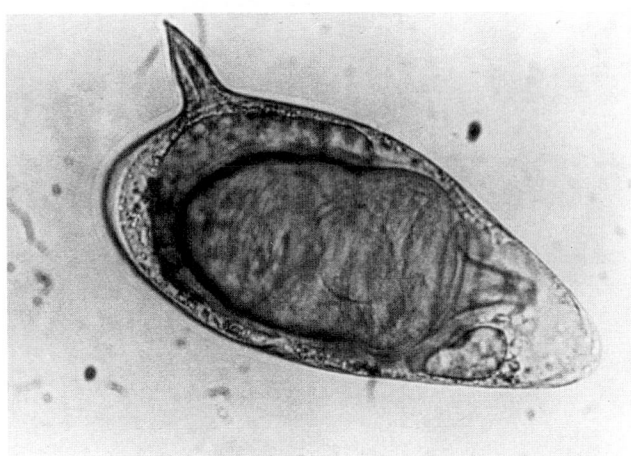

Fig. 3 Egg of *S. mansoni* containing a fully developed miracidium and showing the characteristic lateral spine of this species.

movements allow penetration of the skin in minutes. Penetration initiates transformation into a schistosomular larva, with loss of the tail and of the protective outer glycocalyx layer, and the addition of an extra lipid bilayer to the surface membrane of the parasite's syncytial outer tegument. This tegument now forms the main parasite–host interface and so has physiological and immunological functions vital to long-term survival in the hostile environment of the bloodstream. These include uptake of nutrients, response to injury, and surface adsorption of host antigens to provide an immunological disguise.

Newly transformed schistosomula remain in the epidermis for several days before migrating, via the bloodstream, lungs, and systemic circulation, to the hepatic portal system. Here the schistosomula mature and differentiate into adult worms, pair, and migrate against the portal blood flow to the small venules draining the genitourinary tract (*S. haematobium*) or the large and, to a lesser extent, small intestine (*S. mansoni*, *S. japonicum*, *S. intercalatum*, *S. mekongi*). Male and female worms are 1 to 2 cm long and morphologically distinct. Paired worms remain permanently coupled, with the shorter, flatter, more muscular male gripping the female in its gynaecophoric canal (Fig. 2). Worms ingest blood cells into their blind-ending bifurcated gut, producing a haematin-like pigment that is regurgitated into the blood. Adult worms have average lifespans in man of 3 (*S. haematobium*) to 7 (*S. mansoni*) years, although active infections are reported in individuals who have left endemic areas more than 20 years previously. Female worms start to produce eggs between 5 and 12 weeks after infection, at rates of 300 (*S. mansoni*) to 3000 (*S. japonicum*) per day. A few days after an egg is laid, a single miracidium develops within the rigid eggshell, the shape and size of which is characteristic for each species. *S. mansoni* (Fig. 3) and *S. haematobium* eggs are ellipsoid, 65 by 150 μm, the former having a lateral spine and the latter a terminal spine. *S. japonicum* eggs are more spherical, 70 by 90 μm, with a small lateral knob that is not always apparent microscopically. Embryonated eggs pass from the venules into the gut or bladder lumen. This is facilitated by host immune responses to secreted egg antigens, as egg excretion is inhibited in immunosuppressed experimental hosts. The passage of the eggs causes tissue damage, as does the granulomatous reactions to eggs that fail to escape from the bloodstream and get swept into the liver by the portal blood flow.

Eggs deposited in fresh water rapidly hatch in response to osmotic changes, releasing the miracidium. This ciliated and actively swimming larva lives for about 6 h, and is able to detect chemically the proximity of snails, modifying its swimming behaviour as it approaches a potential host. The parasite actively penetrates the snail's tissues and transforms into a primary sporocyst. Asexual replication gives rise to daughter sporocysts that migrate to the snail's hepatopancreas where cercariae are asexually generated within each sporocyst. Thus, snails infected with a single mira-

cidium release cercariae that are all of the same sex. Cercariae are first released from snails 3 to 6 weeks after infection, depending on parasite species and ambient temperature. Infected snails can shed hundreds of cercariae daily over several months.

Distribution (Fig. 4)

Schistosomiasis is associated with poor living conditions and inadequate sanitation and water supply. Its distribution has changed over the last 50 years. In some areas sustained control strategies have been successful. However, environmental changes, development of water resources, population increases, and migration, have led to its spread into previously non-endemic areas or areas with a low rate of infection. *S. japonicum* and *S. haematobium* have decreased, whereas *S. mansoni* has increased to become the most prevalent and widespread species. *S. japonicum* has been controlled effectively in many areas and is now endemic only in China, where it is much reduced, Indonesia, the Philippines, and Thailand. *S. mekongi* is found in Kampuchea and Laos, while *S. intercalatum* is found in 10 countries within the rainforest belt of central Africa. *S. mansoni* is present in most countries of sub-Saharan Africa, and in Madagascar, the Nile delta and valley, as well as Saudi Arabia, Yemen, Oman, Libya, northern and eastern Brazil, Surinam, Venezuela, and some Caribbean islands. *S. haematobium* is widespread in sub-Saharan Africa and Madagascar, and is more prevalent than *S. mansoni* in North Africa and the Middle East. Information on the geographical distribution of schistosomiasis is available from the World Health Organization website: http://www.who.int/ctd/html/schistoepidat.html.

Clinical features

Stage of invasion: cercarial dermatitis or 'swimmer's itch'

When cercariae penetrate the skin they can cause a skin reaction, called cercarial dermatitis or 'swimmer's itch'. This is frequently seen after exposure to avian schistosomes, and is associated with the death of cercariae in the skin. It is seen both in areas endemic for human schistosomiasis and in non-endemic areas. In previously unexposed people, the invasion causes a transient immediate hypersensitivity reaction with intense itching. Within 12 to 24 h it is followed by a delayed reaction characterized by a small, red, pruritic, macular rash progressing to papules after 24 h. The rash may persist for up to 15 days and residual pigmentation may persist for months. Following repeated exposure, the signs and symptoms increase dramatically and start earlier. A similar reaction can be seen after re-exposure to

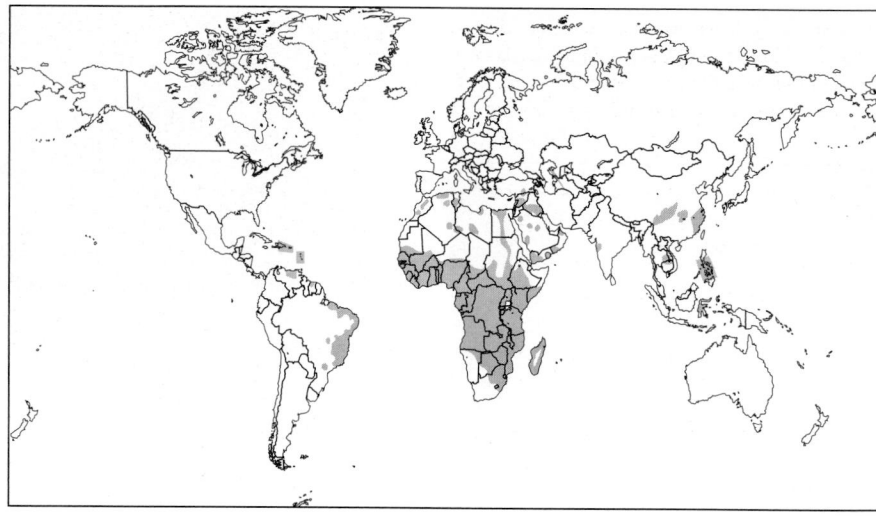

Fig. 4 Global distribution of the schistosomes that affect humans.

human cercariae, predominantly *S. mansoni* and *S. japonicum*. Treatment, if needed, is symptomatic.

Stage of maturation: acute schistosomiasis or Katayama fever

The early stages of a primary infection can be associated with a severe systemic reaction that resembles serum sickness. This acute illness, called acute toxaemic schistosomiasis or Katayama fever, can occur following initial infection with any schistosome infecting humans, although it is more common in *S. japonicum* and *S. mansoni* infections. Acute schistosomiasis is most marked in primary infections in non-immune adults, but acute *S. japonicum* infection can occur in re-exposed individuals. Symptoms appear 2 to 6 weeks after exposure. The clinical picture resembles an acute pyrexial illness with fever as a prime characteristic. The patient feels ill, and may have rigors, sweating, headache, malaise, muscular aches, profound weakness, weight loss, and a non-productive irritating cough. Anorexia, nausea, abdominal pain, and diarrhoea can occur. Physical examination may reveal a generalized lymphadenopathy, an enlarged tender liver, and, sometimes, a slightly enlarged spleen and an urticarial rash (Plate 1). Eosinophilia is almost always present. Patients may become confused or stuporose or present with visual impairment or papilloedema. Severe cerebral or spinal cord manifestations may occur, and this is an indication for urgent investigative measures. Even light infections may cause severe illness and the syndrome can, in rare cases, be fatal.

Differential diagnosis includes infections such as typhoid (leucopenia, no eosinophilia), brucellosis, malaria, infectious mononucleosis, miliary tuberculosis, leptospirosis, and other conditions with fever of unknown origin. Fever and eosinophilia occur in trichinosis, tropical eosinophilia, invasive ankylostomiasis, strongyloidiasis, visceral larva migrans, and infections with *Opisthorchis* and *Clonorchis* species.

Established infections

Urinary schistosomiasis (*Schistosoma haematobium*)

The signs and symptoms due to *S. haematobium* infection relate to the worms' predilection for the veins of the genitourinary tract, and result from deposition of eggs in the bladder, ureters, and to some extent the genital organs. In the phase of established infection two stages can be recognized:

(a) An active stage mainly in children, adolescents, and younger adults with egg deposition in the urinary tract, egg excretion in the urine with proteinuria and macroscopic or microscopic haematuria.

(b) A chronic stage in older patients with sparse or absent urinary egg excretion but the presence of urinary tract pathology.

In the active stage many patients will have minimal symptoms. The most frequently encountered complaint is a painless, characteristically terminal, haematuria, the prevalence and severity of which is related to the intensity of infection. In communities where *S. haematobium* is highly endemic, macroscopic haematuria among boys is considered a natural sign of puberty. Dysuria, frequency, and suprapubic discomfort or pain is associated with schistosomal cystitis and may continue throughout the course of active infection. Initially the eggs may give rise to an intense inflammatory response in the mucosa. This may cause ureteric obstruction leading to hydroureter and hydronephrosis. Cytoscopy reveals friable masses or polyps extending into the bladder, petechiae, and granulomas. These early inflammatory lesions, including the obstructive uropathy, are usually reversible after treatment with antischistosomal drugs. The bladder lesions and obstructive uropathy can be visualized by ultrasonography (Fig. 5).

As the infection progresses, the inflammatory component decreases, possibly due to modulation by the host immune response, and fibrosis increases. Various changes occur in the bladder including calcification, ulceration, and the development of papillomas. Cytoscopy reveals 'sandy

Fig. 5 Bladder pseudopolyps as seen by ultrasound in *S. haematobium* infection. (Photograph by courtesy of Dr J. Richter, Heinrich-Heine-Universität Düsseldorf, Germany.)

patches' composed of large numbers of calcified eggs surrounded by fibrous tissue and an atrophic mucosal surface. The bladder lesions may lead to nocturia, precipitancy, retention of urine, dribbling, and incontinence. Calculus formation is common, as is secondary bacterial infection, usually due to *Escherichia coli*, *Pseudomonas*, *Klebsiella*, *Enterobacter*, or *Salmonella* species. The ureters are less commonly involved, but ureteric fibrosis can cause irreversible obstructive uropathy which can progress to uraemia. Bilateral ureteric involvement is common, although lesions may predominate on one side. Despite damage to the ureters, symptoms may be absent or minimal.

Egg deposition may also cause granulomas and lesions to develop in the genital organs, most commonly in the cervix and vagina in females and the seminal vessels in males. Dyspareunia, contact bleeding, and lower back pain may result in women, and perineal pain and painful ejaculation in males. Symptoms such as haematospermia and perineal discomfort have been described in travellers returning from Mali. In some of these patients, eggs have been demonstrated in seminal fluid but not in urine. The impact of genital lesions caused by *S. haematobium* infection on the spread of HIV needs to be elucidated. Although small numbers of *S. haematobium* eggs are frequently detected in faeces and rectal biopsies, intestinal symptoms are uncommon.

In some areas in Africa an association between *S. haematobium* infection and squamous cell carcinoma of the urinary bladder has been described. The aetiological significance of the parasite in the causation of this cancer is not proven, but is suggested by the finding that the prevalence of carcinoma of the bladder is correlated with intensity of *S. haematobium* infection. In the established stage *S. haematobium* should be distinguished from renal tuberculosis with haematuria, haemoglobinuria, and cancer of the urogenital tract.

Intestinal schistosomiasis

In most early *S. mansoni* and *S. japonicum* infections few, if any, minimal symptoms are apparent. Clinical features are generally encountered in those with high-intensity infections, and are diarrhoea, sometimes with blood or mucus in the stool, abdominal discomfort, and hypogastric pain or colicky cramps. Severe dysentery is rare, but can occur. The liver, especially the left lobe, may be enlarged and tender; the spleen may also be enlarged, but is usually soft. At this stage, the condition is entirely reversible by antischistosomal treatment, but the relative lack of symptoms may cause it to pass unnoticed until irreversible complications set in. Later stages present as intestinal or hepatosplenic disease. Intestinal schistosomiasis is associated with granuloma formation (Plate 2), inflammation, and fibrosis, primarily in the large intestine. Focal dense deposits of eggs of *S. mansoni* or *S. japonicum* in the large intestine can induce the formation of inflammatory polyps. The major clinical manifestation is intermittent diarrhoea with or without passage of blood or mucus, occasionally associated with protein-losing enteropathy and anaemia. Intestinal schistosomiasis in *S. japonicum* infection may also involve the stomach, with gastric bleeding and pyloric obstruction.

The differential diagnosis includes irritable bowel syndrome, amoebiasis, giardiasis, intestinal helminth infection, ulcerative colitis, Crohn's disease, and tuberculosis.

Hepatosplenic disease is the most severe chronic manifestation of *S. mansoni* and *S. japonicum* infection. The development of presinusoidal periportal fibrosis (clay pipe stem or Symmers' fibrosis) (Fig. 6) leads to portal hypertension, but hepatic function usually remains normal (Plate 3). Patients with periportal fibrosis may not excrete eggs in faeces. During the early stages the liver is enlarged, especially the left lobe; it is smooth, firm, and sometimes tender. Later, in many cases, it becomes small firm and nodular. The spleen is enlarged, often massively, due to passive congestion and reticuloendothelial hyperplasia (Fig. 7). The patient may be asymptomatic or may complain of a left hypochondrial mass with discomfort and anorexia. Anaemia may be present. Ascites, attributable both to the portal hypertension and to hypoalbuminaemia, may be seen, especially in *S. japonicum* infection. There may be reduced growth, infantilism, and amenor-

Fig. 6 Periportal fibrosis as seen by ultrasound in *S. mansoni* infection.

rhoea. Most importantly, 80 per cent of patients with hepatosplenic disease have oesophageal varices detectable by endoscopy. These patients may experience repeated bouts of haematemesis, melaena, or both. This is the most severe, potentially fatal, complication of hepatosplenic schistosomiasis, and death may result from massive loss of blood.

The differential diagnosis of hepatosplenic schistosomiasis includes kalaazar (visceral leishmaniasis), tropical splenomegaly syndrome associated with malaria, leukaemia, lymphoma, alcoholic, or viral cirrhosis, and some of the haemoglobinopathies. Some regression of periportal fibrosis may occur after specific antischistosomal therapy, as judged by ultrasonography examination of the liver, but in most individuals with periportal fibrosis and clinical manifestations of hepatosplenic disease, regression does not occur.

In comparison with *S. japonicum* and *S. mansoni* infections, clinical symptoms of disease in *S. intercalatum* infection are commonly mild or absent, and it is not regarded as a serious public health problem. Active

Fig. 7 Kenyan child with severe hepatosplenic schistosomiasis mansoni.

infection is seen in children and adolescents and pathology is detected only in those with egg excretion exceeding 400 eggs per gram of faeces. The usual clinical presentation is one of diarrhoea, often with blood in the stool and lower abdominal pain or discomfort. *S. mekongi* infections are usually asymptomatic but may produce a clinical picture similar to that of *S. japonicum*, although the infections are usually milder. Hepatosplenomegaly can occur.

Other manifestations

Central nervous system manifestations

Central nervous system involvement in *S. mansoni* and *S. haematobium* infections most frequently affect the spinal cord following acute infection. This manifestation is not related to the intensity of infection. A myelopathy results from the inflammatory reaction, caused by the deposition of eggs around the spinal cord, and presents with ascending motor and sensory symptoms. The lesion is usually in the region of the canda equina. Although paraparesis is seen most commonly during acute schistosomiasis, it may also be a late stage complication of *S. mansoni* infection in endemic areas with high rates of transmission. Myelography, computed tomography, and magnetic resonance imaging are of diagnostic value. In acute cases lesions are seen on magnetic resonance imaging scans as a diffuse swelling of the lumbar cord with central softening or cyst formation.

The brain is the major site of central nervous system involvement in *S. japonicum* infections, with about 2 per cent of acutely infected patients experiencing symptoms that mimic acute encephalitis or a focal neurological process. Computed tomography shows multiple enhancing lesions. In chronic infections, patients may present with focal brain lesions that can resemble tumours and present as focal epilepsy. These lesions contain masses of eggs and granulomas. Uncontrolled studies suggest that treatment with a combination of antischistosomal drugs and glucocorticoids is effective.

Pulmonary manifestations

Deposition of eggs can also occur in the lungs. Granulomatous reactions and fibrosis develop in the pulmonary vasculature leading to pulmonary hypertension and/or cor pulmonale (Plate 4). This is normally seen secondary to hepatosplenic schistosomiasis in patients with portal fibrosis and portal hypertension, but pulmonary hypertension may also result from accumulation of *S. haematobium* eggs in the lungs. A syndrome of cough with multiple small radiographic lesions and eosinophilia has been described. Symptoms include fatigue, palpitations, dyspnoea, cough, and sometimes haemoptysis. Patients may progress to decompensation with congestive cardiac failure. In endemic areas schistosomiasis must always be considered as a possible cause of cor pulmonale.

Renal manifestations

Glomerulonephritis is a common occurrence in chronic *S. mansoni* infection in Brazil, especially in patients with hepatosplenic disease. Immunoglobulins, complement components, and schistosome antigens are deposited in the mesangial area. The condition is manifested clinically as proteinuria and/or nephrotic syndrome, sometimes with hypertension.

Miscellaneous manifestations

Patients infected with any of the three major schistosome species and subsequently infected with *Salmonella* may develop a prolonged intermittent febrile illness. Prolonged excretion of *Salmonella* in the urine and intermittent bacteraemia has been demonstrated in *S. haematobium* infection. Treatment for the *Salmonella* infection alone is often not effective without treatment of the underlying schistosome infection.

Diagnosis and investigations

Information about geographical area and history of exposure to potentially contaminated fresh water is important for diagnosis of schistosomiasis, especially in travellers. This can indicate the likelihood of infection and point to the schistosome species involved. A definitive diagnosis is made by the direct demonstration of schistosome eggs by microscopy of urine or stool samples, biopsies or, on rare occasions, secretions such as seminal fluid. In epidemiological studies it is usually important to obtain quantitative estimates of egg output to provide information about intensity of infection within a population.

Direct parasitological methods

In *S. haematobium* infection eggs can be detected in urine after filtration, sedimentation, or centrifugation followed by microscopy. Ideally, urine should be passed around midday and the terminal part of the stream examined. The most commonly used method in epidemiological studies in endemic areas is filtration of 10 to 20 ml of urine using a syringe and a polycarbonate (Nucleopore®), polyamide (Nytrel®), or paper filter. Infection intensity is expressed as eggs per 10 ml of urine. This may not be sufficiently sensitive for detection of low-intensity infections in travellers. In such cases, diagnosis is often based on filtration of 24-h urine samples.

For *S. mansoni*, *S. japonicum*, *S. mekongi*, and *S. intercalatum* eggs in the faeces, sedimentation of the eggs followed by microscopy is a useful and simple technique. However, the Kato thick smear technique is the most widely used method in epidemiological studies. This is based on microscopic examination of a smear of a small but fixed amount of faecal sample (usually 20 to 50 mg). Coarse particles and fibrous material are first removed from the sample by passing it through a sieve. A fixed sample volume is obtained by the use of a template. This is placed on a microscope slide and squashed with either a piece of cellophane soaked in glycerol or a glass coverslip. After leaving the slide for 6 to 24 h to allow the preparation to clear, the eggs are counted and the level of infection expressed as eggs per gram of faeces. Unfortunately, watery or diarrhoeal stools cannot be processed this way, and low-intensity infections may not be detected, since only small faecal samples are examined and eggs may be clumped unevenly in the stool. Increased sensitivity is obtained by increasing the number of samples examined. For diagnosis of light infections in previously unexposed travellers, microscopic examination of a rectal tissue snip crushed between glass slides is often the most sensitive direct diagnostic method. This method can also be used for biopsies. The crushed tissue sample is far better than a sectioned biopsy for the detection and identification of eggs.

Other direct methods

Recently, sensitive enzyme immune assays have been developed to detect circulating schistosome antigens in serum or urine. These antigens, circulating anodic antigen and circulating cathodic antigen, are derived from the gut of the adult schistosomes. The assays have almost 100 per cent specificity and very high sensitivity, and are excellent epidemiological tools as they provide a direct estimate of worm burden and can be used to monitor the efficacy of chemotherapy. They are less well suited for diagnosis of light infections in travellers.

Indirect diagnostic techniques

In *S. haematobium* infections, chemical reagent strips for detection of microhaematuria are widely used in endemic areas as a diagnostic measure. The method can be used in areas of both high and low transmission and there is a consistent significant correlation between microhaematuria and intensity of infection. In intestinal schistosomiasis, blood may be found in the stools, but it is not as useful an indicator of infection. In urinary schistosomiasis, eosinophiluria, with high numbers of eosinophil granulocytes in the urine, is a characteristic finding. Recently, detection of the eosinophil granule protein **ECP** (eosinophil cationic protein) in urine has been used for the qualitative assessment of eosinophil infiltration of the bladder mucosa, and hence local inflammation. Measurement of ECP in urine has proved useful in following post-treatment resolution of urinary tract morbidity in endemic areas. Eosinophilia is often found in acutely infected travellers. In cases where eggs are difficult to find, eosinophilia plus a history of exposure may suggest the need for further examination for schistosomiasis including serodiagnosis.

Immunodiagnosis

In cases of suspected schistosomiasis in which eggs have not been detected, serology can be used to demonstrate specific antibodies. An indirect immunofluorescence test using sections of adult worms for detection of specific immunoglobulins (IgM and IgG) is widely used. For travellers, a positive antibody result combined with a history of exposure should lead to treatment. Serodiagnosis is not useful in endemic areas because of the high levels of specific antibodies found in naturally exposed populations.

Ultrasonography

Ultrasonography is non-invasive, portable, has no biological hazards for the patient, and can be used to either complement or replace many invasive diagnostic techniques. It is the technique of choice for grading schistosomal periportal fibrosis, portal hypertension, hydronephrosis, and urinary bladder lesions. A protocol for standardized investigations and methods of reporting has been produced by the World Health Organization. Ultrasonography is especially useful for monitoring decreases in morbidity after chemotherapy programmes.

Pathophysiology/pathogenesis

Schistosome eggs can be trapped in the tissues, often the walls of the intestines or, depending on species, the urinary bladder or ureters. The eggs of *S. mansoni* and *S. japonicum* are swept into the liver via the portal system, where they embolize into the portal radicles and give rise to vascular and granulomatous changes. Granulomatous pyelophlebitis and peripyelophlebitis is responsible for development of portal hypertension, while granulomata with subsequent fibrosis may be responsible for the periportal fibrosis. The characteristic lesion in the liver is a presinusoidal periportal fibrosis (Symmers' fibrosis). There is typically no bridging between the fibrous tracts, no nodule formation, and no hepatic cell damage. Increased portal pressure can result in the development of portosystemic collaterals and eggs may pass directly from the portal vein to the pulmonary circulation. Here the combination of vascular and granulomatous changes is responsible for pulmonary hypertension.

Treatment

Today the drug of choice is praziquantel, available as 600 mg tablets (e.g. Biltricide®, Distocide®). It is administered orally, normally in a single dose, and is effective against all schistosome species infecting man. It is also effective for most other trematode infections and against adult cestodes. The drug is safe and well tolerated. Drug dosages are shown in Table 1. Complete cure is achieved in up to 85 per cent of those treated, and egg counts are reduced by 95 per cent or more in others. In endemic areas, this level of efficacy is acceptable since very light residual infections do not lead to severe morbidity. In patients who are not cured by the initial treatment, the same dose can be repeated at weekly intervals for 2 weeks or on two successive days.

Although praziquantel has not been shown to be teratogenic, it is not recommended for use during pregnancy. Apart from this there are no contraindications. Any side-effects are generally mild, resolving spontaneously over a few hours and rarely requiring medication. Gastrointestinal side-effects include abdominal pain or discomfort and sometimes vomiting. They occur more frequently in individuals with high infection intensities. Urticarial skin reactions and periorbital oedema may occur in about 2 per cent of treated individuals. General side-effects including headache, dizziness, fever, and fatigue can also occur, but less frequently. As a general principle, all patients with acute schistosomiasis should be treated with praziquantel. It is disputed whether steroids should be added to specific drug treatments. A beneficial effect has been demonstrated in some studies where corticosteroids have been added to praziquantel treatment. Use of praziquantel for cerebral *S. japonicum* infections is safe and effective, resulting in rapid dissipation of cerebral oedema and resolution of cerebral masses. Chemotherapy is only part of the management of schistosomiasis-associated portal hypertension, since the main complications are due to obstructive pathology. Management of portal hypertension and prevention of bleeding from oesophageal varices is beyond the scope of this chapter. Praziquantel has largely replaced other drugs for treatment of schistosomiasis. However, metrifonate (Biarcil®) and oxamniquine (Mansil® (South America), Vansil® (Africa)) are still used sometimes.

Prognosis

Most infected people have few, if any, overt symptoms. Acute schistosomiasis can be fatal or can lead to severe residual damage to the nervous system if not treated, but responds well to antischistosomal therapy if started early. Early infections respond extremely well to treatment and the pathological lesions regress leaving little residual damage. However, in endemic areas individuals, particularly young children, are rapidly re-exposed and reinfected unless control measures are taken at the community level. Chronic infections with fibrosis respond less well to specific antischistosomal treatment, although some regression of hepatosplenic disease has been seen after treatment. The lifetime prognosis is worst in patients with severe hepatosplenic schistosomiasis and oesophageal varices. Previous episodes of haematemesis indicates a 70 per cent risk of rebleeding.

Transmission and epidemiology

Each successful cercarial penetration of human skin has the potential to give rise to a single male or female adult worm, but it is probable that many cercariae die naturally in the epidermis. People tend to accumulate worms with continued exposure to infection. However, human populations in

Table 1 Dosage of drugs for treating schistosomiasis

Species	Drug	Total dose (mg/kg body weight)	Administration
Schistosoma haematobium	Praziquantel	40	Single oral dose or two doses of 20 mg/kg
	Metrifonate	22.5—30	Three oral doses of 7.5 to 10 mg/kg given at an interval of 14 days
Schistosoma intercalatum	Praziquantel	40	Single oral dose
Schistosoma mansoni			
Americas and Caribbean	Praziquantel	40	Single oral dose with food
	Oxamniquine	15	Single oral dose with food
Africa and Middle East	Praziquantel	40	Single oral dose with food
	Oxamniquine	60	Oral dose of 15 mg/kg twice a day for 2 days with food
Schistosoma japonicum and *Schistosoma mekongi*	Praziquantel	60	Oral dose of 20 mg/kg every 4 h with food

endemic areas do not just continue to accumulate worms with age. Intensities of infection increase in children during their younger years (as estimated by numbers of excreted eggs), peaking around the age of 12 years, before falling to lower levels in adulthood (Fig. 8(a)). This is probably due to the death of older worms, which are not replaced at a similar rate in older people. This age–infection intensity profile is more pronounced if study populations are given chemotherapy to remove existing infections and then monitored for levels of reinfection over several subsequent years. In these circumstances, it is clear that young children are much more susceptible to reinfection than older children or adults, and that a striking change in susceptibility to reinfection occurs after 12 years of age. The slower acquisition of worms in adulthood could be due to reduced exposure to infection or to age-dependent changes in innate resistance or acquired immunity. In many endemic areas children have more contact with water than adults, but careful observation of water-associated behaviour has shown that age profiles of water contact are variable between communities, whereas profiles of reinfection intensities are remarkably consistent (Fig. 8(b)). This suggests that host-related factors other than

exposure influence susceptibility to reinfection. This has been most convincingly shown in fishing communities in areas with high *S. mansoni* transmission on Lake Albert, Uganda. Here occupational water contact results in adults having greater exposure to infection than their children, yet, within 12 months of treatment, it is the children under 12 years of age that suffer much higher reinfection intensities. Current research is focused on assessing the relative roles of innate resistance and acquired immunity in this age-dependent resistance and whether the onset of puberty or the length of time spent living in endemic areas might be important. For example, it is not known if this age-dependent resistance to infection holds true for travellers exposed to infection for the first time. Immune responses to schistosomes also differ between children and adults. Specific IgE and other characteristically T helper 2 type responses against the parasite are associated with resistance to reinfection. Whatever mechanisms underlie the contrasting susceptibilities of children and adults, continued exposure can be expected to result in reinfection, especially amongst younger children.

Prevention and control

Despite the high risk of reinfection, chemotherapy is usually highly beneficial at both the individual and population levels, as those suffering high intensities of infection are at greatest risk of the more severe forms of schistosomiasis. Various chemotherapy-based control strategies can be employed depending on intensity of transmission and the available resources. In areas of high transmission, population-based chemotherapy can avoid the time and expense required for diagnosis and reduce the prevalence and severity of morbidity. Alternatively, schoolchildren can be targeted for treatment, as they invariably have the heaviest worm burdens and contribute most to on-going transmission. In areas of less intense transmission, treatment can be restricted to diagnosed cases. The provision of safe water supplies and sanitation, where it can be achieved, will make an important additional contribution. Mortality can be prevented and morbidity best controlled by a combination of health education, chemotherapy, provision of safe water supplies and sanitation, and, where appropriate, snail control. Health education should be aimed at improving practices of water use and preventing indiscriminate urination and defaecation. The role of molluscicides in control programmes depends on the local epidemiological and ecological circumstances and the resources available. Within the context of a larger concerted intervention, focal mollusciciding of major transmission sites can be useful. Eradication of host snail species is not usually feasible, although modification of the environment to eliminate snails has been successful in parts of China. In general, it has only been through sustained effort with integrated control strategies that disease control has been achieved. Schistosomiasis control strategies are guided by the Second Report of the WHO Expert Committee on the Control of Schistosomiasis (1993). Recognition that the available control methods, including effective chemotherapy, have failed to reduce the world burden of schistosomiasis has led to renewed efforts to develop an effective vaccine. Recombinant schistosome antigens have been partially successful in protecting experimental animals and several are progressing towards phase I and II human trials.

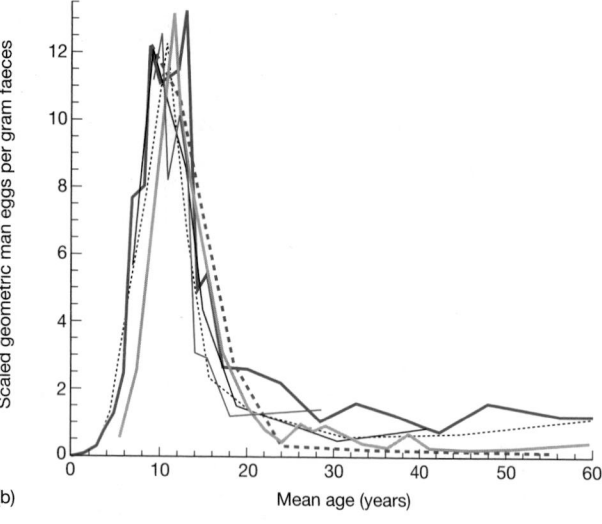

Fig. 8 (a) Age–intensity profiles of *S. mansoni* infection from six communities in Kenya. (Reproduced from Fulford *et al.* (1992) with permission.) (b) Age–reinfection intensity profiles of *S. mansoni* after chemotherapy in the same six communities in Kenya, assessed between 12 and 36 months after treatment. (By courtesy of AJC Fulford.)

Further reading

Day JH *et al.* (1996). Schistosomiasis in travellers returning from sub-Saharan Africa. *British Medical Journal* **313**, 268–9. [A review on schistosomiasis in travellers with emphasis on most common symptoms and clinical findings.]

Fairley J (1991). *Bilharzia. A history of imperial tropical medicine*. Cambridge University Press, Cambridge. [An excellent and detailed history of schistosomiasis, including developments in research and control up until the 1970s.]

Feldmeier H, Poggensee G (1993). Diagnostic techniques in schistosomiasis control. A review. *Acta Tropica* **52**, 205–20. [A review of diagnostic techniques, also considering the constraints and drawbacks relating to the various diagnostic methods.]

Ferrari TC (1999). Spinal cord schistosomiasis. A report of 2 cases and review emphasising clinical aspects. *Medicine (Baltimore)* **78**, 176–90. [Review of 231 cases including clinical and treatment aspects.]

Jordan P, Webbe G, Sturrock RF, eds (1993). *Human schistosomiasis.* CAB International, Wallingford. [The definitive text on human schistosomiasis. Including: A comprehensive review of pathology and clinical aspects of *Schistosoma mansoni* infection by Lambertucci; of *S. haematobium* and *S. intercalatum* by Farid; and of *S. japonicum* and *S. japonicum*-like infections by Gang.]

Kabatereine NB *et al.* (1999). Adult resistance to schistosomiasis: age-dependence of reinfection remains constant in communities with diverse exposure patterns. *Parasitology* **118**, 101–6. [The demonstration that children are more susceptible to reinfection than adults.]

Mahmoud A, ed. (2001). *Tropical Medicine: Science and Practice*, Vol. 3 Schistosomiasis, Imperial College Press, London. [A recent book with reviews on various aspects of clinical and experimental schistosomiasis.]

Saconato H, Atallah A (1999). Interventions for treating schistosomiasis mansoni (Cochrane Review). In: *The Cochrane Library*, Issue 3. Update Software, Oxford.

Squires N (1999). Interventions for treating schistosomiasis haematobium (Cochrane Review) In: *The Cochrane Library*, Issue 3. Update Software, Oxford.

7.16.2 Liver fluke infections

David I. Grove

Liver flukes, otherwise known as trematodes, are leaf-like hermaphroditic flatworms. The hepatobiliary system of humans is commonly infected by flukes of the genera *Clonorchis* and *Opisthorchis* and occasionally by other species (Table 1). In addition, *Eurytrema pancreaticum* has been found rarely in the pancreatic duct. These infections are usually diagnosed by finding eggs in the faeces. Unfortunately, eggs of many of these species cannot be differentiated from each other nor can they be distinguished reliably from the eggs of certain intestinal trematodes. In such cases, definitive diagnosis can only be made if adult worms are recovered from the stools after anthelmintic treatment, at surgery, or at autopsy; parasitological textbooks should be consulted for diagnostic details.

Clonorchiasis

Lifecycle

Clonorchis sinensis adult worms, 10 to 25 mm long by 3 to 5 mm wide, live in the bile ducts or occasionally the gallbladder attached to the mucosa. They produce eggs which are passed in the faeces (Fig. 1). The miracidium within the egg hatches after ingestion by a suitable species of aquatic snail; nine species belonging to the families Hydrobidae, Melanidae, Assimineidae, and Thiaridae are known to be susceptible but *Parafossarulus manchouricus* is perhaps the most common. The miracidia develop into sporocysts then in turn become rediae which produce larvae known as cercariae. After 6 to 8 weeks, the cercariae emerge from the snail and swim about in the water until they encounter certain freshwater fishes (over 100 species, mostly of the family Cyprinidae, i.e. carp, are susceptible). They attach to the surface of the fish, lose their tails, penetrate under the scales, encyst in the skin or flesh, and develop into infective metacercariae over several weeks. When raw or undercooked infected fish is eaten by humans, the metacercariae excyst in the stomach, enter the common bile duct through the ampulla of Vater, and ascend into the biliary passages where they mature in 1 month. Adult worms may live for up to 40 years.

Epidemiology and control

Fish-eating mammals including humans, dogs, cats, and rats may be infected with *C. sinensis*. Human clonorchiasis is endemic in Japan, Korea, China, and Vietnam where the first and second intermediate hosts are found and where the population habitually consumes raw fish. In endemic areas, fish are kept in ponds and fertilized with human and animal faeces. Over 20 million people are thought to be infected in China. Control programmes include proper waste disposal, measures to control snail numbers, and mass treatment with praziquantel, but the most important is health education to discourage the habit of eating raw or undercooked fish.

Pathology

Pathological changes are related to the intensity and duration of infection. They are produced by mechanical irritation, toxin production, immunological responses, and secondary bacterial infection. Inspection of the cut surface of the liver often reveals dilated, thick-walled bile ducts with adult worms visible within their lumens. Adult flukes may be found in the gallbladder but they are usually killed by bile. Histologically, there is desquamation and hyperplasia of epithelial cells, formation of adenomatous tissue and proliferation of periductal connective tissue, and infiltration with eosinophils and mononuclear cells. This may be complicated by epithelial metaplasia then mucinous cholangiocarcinoma. Recurrent pyogenic cholangitis is a common complication and the worms and eggs act as a nidus for gallstone formation. Some patients have flukes in the pancreatic duct which may cause pancreatitis.

Table 1 Liver flukes infecting humans

Species	Geographical distribution	Source of infection	Size of eggs (µm)
Clonorchis sinensis	Eastern Asia	Freshwater fish	28–35 × 12–19[a]
Dicrocoelium dendriticum	Widespread	Ants accidentally ingested with food	38–45 × 22–30[b]
Eurytrema pancreaticum	Eastern Asia	Grasshoppers	38–45 × 22–30 [b]
Fasciola gigantica	Asia, Africa	Vegetation, e.g. watercress	130–150 × 60–90[c]
Fasciola hepatica	Widespread	Vegetation, e.g. watercress	130–150 × 60–90 [c]
Metorchis conjunctus	Canada	Freshwater fish	28–35 × 12–19 [a]
Opisthorchis felineus	Europe, Asia	Freshwater fish	28–35 × 12–19 [a]
Opisthorchis guayaquilaris	Ecuador	Freshwater fish	28–35 × 12–19 [a]
Opisthorchis viverrini	Indochina	Freshwater fish	28–35 × 12–19 [a]

[a, b, c] Superscripts indicate that eggs within each group are indistinguishable.

Fig. 1 Egg of *Clonorchis sinensis*: this is identical with that of *Opisthorchis viverrini*. (By courtesy of Prayong Radomyos, Faculty of Tropical Medicine, Mahidol University, Bangkok.)

Clinical features

Most patients are asymptomatic and are diagnosed incidentally on stool examination. Symptoms are more common in older patients with heavy worm burdens. It is difficult to differentiate these symptoms from other conditions but they include right hypochondrial or epigastric pain or discomfort, lassitude, anorexia, and flatulence. Some patients complain of a peculiar, hot sensation on the skin of the abdomen or back. Cholangitis causes fever, right upper quadrant pain, and jaundice. Cholangiocarcinoma is associated with pain, jaundice, and weight loss.

Diagnosis

The diagnosis is suggested by finding eggs in faeces or in duodenal aspirates. They are yellow-brown, 25 to 35 µm long by 12 to 19 µm wide, and have a seated operculum with a small knob at the other end (Fig. 2). They cannot be differentiated from ova of *Opisthorchis* species. Furthermore, they are extremely difficult to differentiate from eggs of flukes in the family Heterophyidae (see Chapter 7.16.4), although the latter tend to have a smoother egg shell, a less prominent shoulder at the operculum, and the knob may be absent. The diagnosis can only be confirmed by examination of adult flukes. Serological tests have been described but are not routinely used for individual patient diagnosis. Imaging techniques such as ultrasound or computed tomography may disclose adult worms in the gallbladder or bile ducts, which are often dilated and may contain sludge. Liver function tests may be abnormal, often with an obstructive picture.

Treatment

Praziquantel is the treatment of choice and in a dose of 25 mg/kg three times daily after meals for 2 days has a cure rate of close to 100 per cent; eggs should disappear from the stool within 1 week. Biliary tract abnormalities may reverse after treatment as this has been shown in opisthorchiasis. Triclabendazole may prove to be useful but there is insufficient documentation at present. Bacterial cholangitis is treated with antibiotic therapy such as a combination of amoxicillin, gentamicin, and metronidazole. Surgery may be required in some patients with obstructive jaundice.

Opisthorchiasis viverrini

This infection is very similar to clonorchiasis. The adult *Opisthorchis viverrini* is smaller than *C. sinensis*, measuring 7 to 12 mm by 2 to 3 mm, although there is some discrepancy in the literature over its size, perhaps reflecting different methods of preparation and fixation. It may live for over 10 years. The lifecycle is similar to that of *Clonorchis* with various species of the genus *Bithynia*, particularly *B. goniomphalus*, *B. funiculata*, and *B. siamensis* (= *laevis*), being the snail first intermediate host. Many species of carp serve as the second intermediate host. Humans, dogs, cats, and other fish-eating mammals are definitive hosts. This parasite is endemic in northern Thailand and adjacent Laos and Cambodia where 10 million people are estimated to be infected because of the popularity of chopped raw cyprinoid fish as a foodstuff.

The pathology and clinical features are similar to those induced by *C. sinensis*. The association with cholangiocarcinoma may be even more striking with this infection. The diagnosis is made as discussed under clonorchiasis. Praziquantel is the drug of choice; 25 mg/kg three times after meals for 1 day gives close to 100 per cent cure rate. Mebendazole (30 mg/kg daily) or albendazole (400 mg twice daily) may be effective if given for several weeks. Triclabendazole may prove to be useful but there is insufficient documentation at present. A control programme is underway in Thailand which includes detection and treatment of infected people together with intensive health education.

Opisthorchiasis felineus

This infection is very similar to clonorchiasis. The adult *Opisthorchis felineus* is morphologically very similar if not identical to *O. viverrini* (the two species have been distinguished by the pattern of flame cells in the cercariae). The lifecycle is similar with *Bithynia leachi* being the only known molluscan intermediate host. Many species of carp serve as the second intermediate host. Humans, dogs, cats, rats, foxes, seals, and other fish-eating mammals are definitive hosts. Infection is acquired by eating raw or undercooked fish; in Siberia, raw, slightly salted, and frozen fish is often consumed. This parasite is endemic particularly in Russia and adjacent countries but also in parts of southern Europe and eastern Asia with several million people probably being infected overall. Eggs are indistinguishable from those of *O. viverrini* and *C. sinensis*. The pathology, clinical features, diagnosis, and treatment are similar to *O. viverrini* and *C. sinensis* infections.

Fascioliasis

Lifecycle

Fascioliasis is due to infection with the sheep liver fluke, *Fasciola hepatica* or with *F. gigantica*. Adult *F. hepatica* flukes, 20 to 30 mm by 8 to 13 mm in

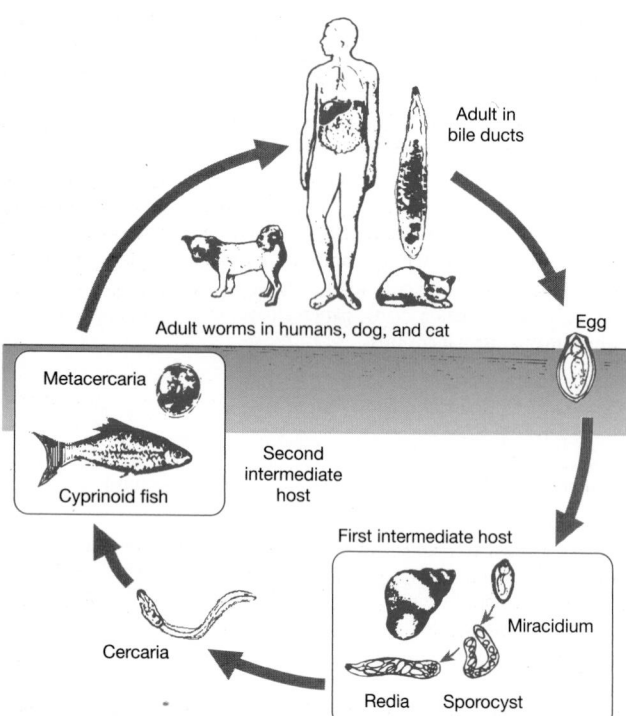

Fig. 2 Lifecycle of *Clonorchis sinensis* and *Opisthorchis* species.

size, live in the large bile ducts and produce eggs which are passed in the stools. The eggs require a period of 9 to 15 days for the miracidia to develop and hatch in water at 22 to 25°C, but remain viable for up to 9 months if kept moist and cool. The miracidia penetrate the tissues of various species of amphibious snails of the family Lymnaeidae and develop over the next 4 to 5 weeks through the stages of sporocyst, rediae, daughter rediae, and cercariae. The cercariae emerge from the snails and encyst on various kinds of aquatic vegetation to become metacercariae. A wide range of mammals is susceptible to infection, but sheep and cattle are the most important. Human infections are usually acquired by eating watercress or by drinking water contaminated with metacercariae. Metacercariae excyst in the duodenum, penetrate the intestinal wall, and pass into the peritoneal cavity. They then invade the liver capsule and migrate through the hepatic parenchyma to the bile ducts where they mature in about 3 to 4 months. The lifespan of these flukes is several years.

F. gigantica is large attaining a size of up to 7.5 cm. The eggs are difficult to distinguish from those of *F. hepatica* and the lifecycle of the two parasites is similar.

Epidemiology and control

Because of the wide range of susceptible definitive and intermediate hosts, the infection is geographically widespread. Human infections with *F. hepatica* have been reported from all continents. Fascioliasis gigantica is less frequent and has been seen in Africa and Asia. Infection is prevented by not eating fresh aquatic plants, particularly watercress (*Nasturtium officinale*) and by boiling drinking water. Veterinary control measures include elimination of the snail intermediate hosts by drainage of pastures and treatment with molluscicides and by eradication of infection from infected herds.

Pathology

In the early stages of infection, larvae migrating through the liver parenchyma may cause considerable destruction with necrosis, abscess formation, and haemorrhage. The number of tunnels lined by ragged walls of necrotic, bleeding, and inflamed liver tissue is proportional to the number of worms. In the chronic stages, the walls of the bile ducts become thickened by fibrous tissue and inflammatory infiltration, the epithelium becomes hyperplastic, and the bile ducts dilate. Occasionally the lumina of the bile ducts may become obliterated causing obstructive jaundice. These structural changes predispose to secondary bacterial infection which exacerbates the problem. Sclerosing cholangitis and biliary cirrhosis may follow prolonged heavy infection. There is no apparent association with cholangiocarcinoma.

Clinical features

Human fascioliasis is usually mild and related to the phase of infection. There are three phases.

1. In the migratory phase, symptoms usually begin about 1 month after infection. Patients may develop abdominal discomfort or pain (especially in the epigastrium and right upper quadrant), anorexia, nausea, vomiting, fever, headache, tender hepatomegaly, and urticaria. These initial symptoms may persist for several months.

2. The latent phase is asymptomatic and may last for months to years.

3. The obstructive phase is characterized by the recurrence or appearance for the first time of epigastric and right upper quadrant abdominal pain, biliary colic, anorexia, nausea, vomiting, tender hepatomegaly, fever, and jaundice. These features are frequently due to complicating bacterial cholangitis or cholecystitis and may be associated with bacteraemia.

Flukes occasionally migrate to other sites, especially the anterior abdominal wall. Acute oedematous nasopharyngitis ('halziun') may be an allergic response to larval flukes which attach to the pharyngeal wall after ingestion of infected, raw sheep or goat liver.

Diagnosis

In enzootic areas, early fascioliasis is suspected in patients with fever, tender hepatomegaly, and eosinophilia who give a history of consuming freshwater plants. If available, serological tests may be useful early in the illness before egg production begins. Liver biopsy may be helpful in some cases.

Chronic fascioliasis is diagnosed by finding the characteristic eggs in stools or fluid obtained by duodenal or biliary drainage. The eggs of *F. hepatica* and *F. gigantica* cannot be distinguished reliably from each other or from those of the intestinal fluke, *Fasciolopsis buski*; differentiation of these two infections requires identification of adult flukes. Liver function tests are often abnormal and may show an obstructive picture. Radiolucent shadows of flukes may be seen by cholangiography. Ultrasonography and computed tomography are useful in the demonstration of lesions in the liver and biliary tracts. If the patient has recently consumed liver, spurious infection (ingestion of eggs) should be ruled out by placing the patient on a liver-free diet for a few days and repeating the stool examination.

Treatment

The treatment of fascioliasis has been problematic. Success has been claimed for bithiniol and emetine but these drugs are not generally available. Chloroquine at 5 mg/kg per day orally for 3 weeks has limited effectiveness. Praziquantel, which is active against many trematodes, is often ineffective in fascioliasis but may be tried if other agents are not available. Recent studies have shown that triclabendazole in a single oral dose of 10 mg/kg is very effective although some patients require a second dose after a few weeks. This drug appears to have few side-effects. It is available in some countries but not others; further information can be sought from the manufacturer (Novartis, Basle, Switzerland). Flukes are evacuated through the intestinal tract. Another drug under investigation which shows promise is nitazoxanide administered in a dose of 500 mg orally twice daily for 6 days.

Dicrocoeliasis

Dicrocoelium dendriticum adult worms measuring 5 to 15 mm by 1.5 to 2.5 mm live in the biliary passages. Eggs passed in the stools are ingested by certain land snails (e.g. species of *Zebrina* and *Helicella*) in which they develop through two stages of sporocysts with the eventual production of cercariae. The snail leaves slime balls of cercariae on the ground and these are ingested by ants (*Formica* species) in which they develop into metacercariae.

This organism is primarily an infection of sheep, goats, deer, and other herbivores which ingest ants. Humans are rarely infected, usually by accident. Cases have been reported from Europe, Asia, and Africa. Spurious infections result from the consumption of raw, infected liver. Patients may be asymptomatic but may complain of dyspepsia, flatulence, and abdominal colic. The diagnosis is made by finding the eggs in faeces, bile, or duodenal fluid; they cannot be differentiated from those of *Eurytrema pancreaticum*. Definitive diagnosis is made by identification of adult worms. Treatment is with praziquantel at 25 mg/kg three times after meals for 1 day.

Metorchiasis

Many fish-eating mammals of North America serve as definitive hosts for *Metorchis conjunctus*. The aquatic snail *Amnicola limosa* is the first intermediate host; eggs are ingested, hatch into miracidia, and ultimately release cercariae. Metacercariae develop in the flesh of several species of freshwater fish. Ingested metacercariae hatch in the duodenum and migrate up the biliary tree.

A point source outbreak of this disease has been reported in 19 people who ate raw fish prepared from the white sucker (*Catostomus commersoni*) caught in a river north of Montreal. The illness was characterized by upper abdominal pain, low-grade fever, eosinophilia, and abnormal liver function tests. Ten days after ingestion of infected fish, eggs indistinguishable from those of *O. viverrini* were seen in the stools. The patients responded to treatment with praziquantel.

Further reading

Arjona R *et al.* (1995). Fascioliasis in developed countries: a review of classic and aberrant forms of the disease. *Medicine (Baltimore)* **74**, 13–23.

Bronstein AM, Zavoikin VD. Brief update on *Opisthorchis felineus* in Russia. http://www.cfound.to.it/html/bronste.htm.

Connor DH *et al.*, eds (1997). *Pathology of infectious diseases*, Vol 2, pp 1305–588. Appleton & Lange, Stamford.

el-Karaksy H *et al.* (1999). Human fascioliasis in Egyptian children: successful treatment with triclabendazole. *Journal of Tropical Paediatrics* **45**, 135–8.

Jongsuksuntigul P, Imsomboon T (1998). Epidemiology of opisthorchiasis and national control program inThailand. *Southeast Asian Journal of Tropical Medicine and Public Health* **29**, 327–32.

Kino H *et al.* (1998). Epidemiology of clonorchiasis in Ninh Binh Province, Vietnam. *Southeast Asian Journal of Tropical Medicine and Public Health* **29**, 250–4.

MacLean JD *et al.* (1996) Common-source outbreak of acute infection due to the North American liver fluke *Metorchis conjunctus*. *Lancet* **347**, 154–8.

Pungpak S *et al.* (1997). *Opisthorchis viverrini* infection in Thailand: studies on the morbidity of the infection and resolution following praziquantel treatment. *American Journal of Tropical Medicine and Hygiene* **56**, 311–4.

Rossignol JF, Abaza H, Friedman H (1998). Successful treatment of human fascioliasis with nitazoxanide. *Transactions of the Royal Society of Tropical Medicine and Hygiene* **92**, 103–6.

Watanapa P (1996). Cholangiocarcinoma in patients with opisthorchiasis. *British Journal of Surgery* **83**, 1062–4.

7.16.3 Lung flukes (paragonimiasis)

Sirivan Vanijanonta

Lung fluke infection is caused by *Paragonimus* spp. At least 15 species cause disease in humans (Table 1). *Paragonimus westermani* is the most common and widespread, but *P. africanus*, *P. uterobilateralis* (West Africa), *P. ilokstuenensis* (China), and *P. peruvianus* (South America) are also causative. *P. heterotremus* (Thailand, Laos, Vietnam), *P. szechuanensis*, and *P. hueitungensis* also cause cutaneous paragonimiasis.

The adult flukes are reddish-brown and pea-shaped (Plate 1). They are 0. 8 to 1. 6 cm in length, 0. 4 to 0. 8 cm in width, and 0. 3 to 0. 5 cm thick with cuticular spines on the integument. Typically they are encapsulated in cysts adjacent to the bronchi. The eggs are golden brown and ovoid in shape (80–120 × 50–60 μm) (Plate 2).

Lifecycle

Adult flukes encyst in the lung. Ova are expelled through the bronchi and expectorated with sputum or swallowed and passed with faeces. They hatch in fresh water after a few weeks. The resulting miracidia then infect various species of freshwater snail in which they form sporocysts, rediae, and daughter rediae. Metacercariae develop in susceptible freshwater crabs and crayfish (Plates 3, 4). Infection results from ingestion of viable metacercariae in raw or insufficiently cooked crabs and crayfish. Metacercariae excyst in the peritoneal cavity, where they grow and become young flukes. Most of these will then reach the lung by passing through the peritoneal cavity, diaphragm, and pleural cavity, before finally encysting in the lung parenchyma. Tunnels may be formed during their migration. Encysted flukes mature over a period of 6 to 8 weeks and eggs are produced in 10 to 12 weeks. The circuitous routes of migration allow young flukes to lodge and mature in ectopic locations. The reservoir hosts are wild and domestic felines that feed on crabs and crayfish. Freshwater snails that serve as the first intermediate hosts belong to the Thiaridae, Hydrobilidae, and Pleuroceridae families. The second intermediate hosts are the freshwater and brackish-water crabs *Eriocheir japonicus*, *Larnaudia beusekomae* (*Tiwaripotamon beusekomae*), and *Potamon smithiasis*, or crayfish of the genus *Cambaroides*, such as *C. japonicus* in Japan, and *C. similis*, *C. dauricus*, and *C. sckrenki* in China and Korea.

Epidemiology

Paragonimiasis is an important zoonosis. Human beings enter the lifecycle accidentally. However, in some areas human paragonimiasis may be common enough for person-to-person transmission to occur. Human infection is limited in its distribution to places where there are contributory factors that facilitate the lifecycle: reservoir hosts, suitable environment, first and second intermediate hosts, and permissive dietary habits. The three major foci of this disease are in Asia, Africa, and Central and South America. In Asia, endemic areas are to be found in China, Japan, Taiwan, Korea, The Philippines, Thailand, Laos, Vietnam, and Burma, in which the principal parasites are *P. westermani*, *P. skjabini*, and *P. heterotremus*. In Africa, the disease is endemic in eastern Nigeria, the Cameroons, the Congo valley, and the Republic of Congo. In Nigeria the dominant parasite is *P. uterobilateralis*, while in the Cameroons and the Republic of Congo, *P. africanus* predominates. *P. mexicanus*, *P. peruvianus*, and *P. caliensis* are causative agents in Mexico, Guatemala, Honduras, Costa Rica, Ecuador, Colombia, Peru, and Paraguay.

Transmission of *Paragonimus* spp. to man occurs mostly through ingestion of metacercariae in the second intermediate host. Paratenic hosts infected with immature worms also contribute to animal and human disease.

Pathology and pathogenesis

The pathogenesis of human paragonimiasis is unknown. In experimental animals the larval flukes penetrate the intestinal wall and reach the peritoneal cavity, then pass through the diaphragm and pleura to the lung. They cause irritation, acute inflammatory reactions, traumatic tracts, pressure effects, haemorrhage, and necrosis in affected tissues. Pathological findings in the pleural cavity include turbid and haemorrhagic fluid containing numerous pus cells and eosinophils. Acute, diffuse, fibrinoexudative peritonitis may also occur. Abscess cavities containing young flukes are then formed and become enclosed in a fibrous capsule. Mature cysts adjacent to the bronchial system may rupture into it and the cystic contents are then expectorated with sputum or swallowed and passed with faeces. Single or multiple cysts may occur, usually in the lower lobes of the lungs.

Extrapulmonary pathological changes may be caused by aberrant migratory flukes. Cysts, abscesses, and granulomas may be found in the abdominal viscera, subcutaneous tissue, muscles, genital organs, and the brain. *P. heterotremus* and *P. skjabini* also create migratory subcutaneous swellings.

Clinical manifestation

The clinical manifestations are divided into acute and chronic phases. The acute phase occurs after the consumption of an improperly cooked, infected crab or crayfish. The incubation period varies from a few days to weeks. The severity of symptoms usually correlates with the worm load.

Table 1 Human lung flukes (and other tissue trematodes)

Species	Geographical distribution	Definite hosts other than humans	Source of infection	Size of adults (mm)	Size of ova (µm)
Paragonimus africanus	Cameroons	Mongoose, civet cat, dog	Freshwater crabs (Sudanautes africanus, S. pelii)	16–17 × 10	65.1–113 × 36.8–62.3
P. caliensis	Peru, Ecuador, Colombia, Mexico, Honduras, El Salvador	Didelphys marsupialis Philander opossum	Freshwater crabs	7.6–13.3 × 4.2–6.4	70–92 × 38–54
P. compactus	India	Herpestes myula Mungos mungo	–	4.7–9 × 3.5–5.6	
P. heterotremus (P. tuanshanensis)	Thailand, Laos, Vietnam, China	Cat, dog, leopard, rat	Freshwater crabs	11–14.2 × 5.5–7.1	77–80.1 × 40.4–55.5
P. hueitungensis	China –	Cat, dog –	Freshwater crabs crayfish, shrimps	–	–
P. kellicotti	Peru, Ecuador, other Latin American countries	Mink, crayfish-eating mammals, cat, dog, pig	Freshwater crabs Cambarus spp.	3–20 × 2.0–7.7	77.5–87.5 × 52.5–65
P. mexicanus	Mexico, Guatemala, Panama, Ecuador, Peru, Costa Rica	Opossum	Freshwater crabs	13.5–14.8 × 6.6–7.9	59.5–78.5 × 38.5– 49
P. miyazakii	Japan	Cat, dog, rat, boar	Freshwater crabs	9.2–12.5 × 5.0–6.0	62–81 × 39–52
P. ohirai	Japan	Pig, dog, rat	Freshwater crabs	7.2–10.11 × 4.1–5.0	64–87 × 42–54
P. peruvianus	Peru	Cat	Freshwater crabs	11.6–13.3 × 5.8–7.6	75–86 × 44–53
P. philippinensis (P. filipinus)	Philippines	Cat, dog	Freshwater crabs	–	–
P. pulmonalis	Japan, Korea, Taiwan	Cat, dog	Freshwater crabs, crayfish, shrimps		
P. rudis	Brazil Guatemala	Lutra braziliensis Mustela vison Mephitis macroura	Freshwater crabs	12.72 × 6.94	67–71 × 46
P. skjabini (P. szechuanensis)	China	Paguma larvata, cat, dog	Freshwater crabs, crayfish, shrimps	13.13 × 5.43	71 × 48
P. uterobilateralis	Cameroons, Liberia, Nigeria	Cat, dog	Freshwater crabs	5–7 × 4–5	62.3–73.6 × 34–50.9
P. westermani	Worldwide	Tiger, cattle, crayfish-eating mammals	Freshwater crabs, crayfish, shrimps	7.5–16 × 4–6	80–100 × 48–60
P. westermani ichunensis	China	Cat, dog, tiger, leopard, wolf, carnivorous animals of Felidae and Canidae families	Freshwater crabs, crayfish, shrimps	–	–
Other tissue trematodes: Achillurbania nouveli	China,	Felis pardus	–	9.5–11 × 4.5–6.0	55–64 × 32–36
Poikilorchis congolensis	Republic of the Congo, Sarawak	Leopard, giant rat	Freshwater crabs?	7.6 × 3.9	56–68 × 33–41

Invasion and migration by young flukes cause inflammatory and allergic responses such as fever, rashes, urticaria, abdominal pain and discomfort, and a feeling of tightness in the chest. Acute symptoms are rarely serious and patients progress to the chronic stage.

Chronic manifestations are classified as pulmonary and extrapulmonary.

Pulmonary paragonimiasis

The most remarkable clinical feature is a chronic, productive cough with jam-like, brownish-red sputum. Other symptoms include breathlessness, chest pain, unilateral or bilateral pleural effusions, and empyema. Occasionally patients may experience haemoptysis following heavy work or exertion, while pneumothorax occurs rarely.

Pulmonary paragonimiasis is an insidious and persistent lung disease. Patients have surprisingly good general health and usually show few abnormalities on physical examination. A minority of symptomatic patients have normal chest radiographs. Abnormal findings include linear infiltrations, exudative pneumonia, localized pleural effusion, and nodular or cystic lesions. These lesions are predominantly found in the basilar and peripheral regions of both lower lung fields. Cysts may be single or multiple; the most characteristic radiographic feature is a ring shadow with a crescent-shaped opacity along one side of the border resembling the corona phase of a solar eclipse. Other findings are pleural effusion, pleural thickening, and calcification. Long-standing, extensive lesions with fibroatelectasis resemble the lesions of chronic pulmonary tuberculosis.

Extrapulmonary paragonimiasis

Extrapulmonary paragonimiasis is caused by the aberrant migration of larval and young adult flukes to any organ. Migratory swelling of cutaneous or subcutaneous tissues may also occur.

Cerebral paragonimiasis

The clinical symptoms are similar to those of a cerebral space-occupying lesion and are related to the site of the lesion. However, one or more syndromes may be present. Epileptic seizures are common, and patients may develop mental disturbances of the schizoid and paranoid type. Increased intracranial pressure induces persistent intense headache, nausea, vomiting, papilloedema, diplopia, and loss of visual acuity. Patients with paragonimus cysts in the basal meninges will present with meningeal symptoms that include increased intracranial pressure, obstructive hydrocephalus, arterial thrombosis, and stroke. On rare occasions, patients may suffer from cerebellopontine-angle syndrome with tinnitus, progressive deafness, nystagmus, dysphagia, and hiccups.

Spinal-cord paragonimiasis

Spinal involvement produces progressive weakness, sensory impairment of the lower extremities, paralysis, and back pain.

Intra-abdominal paragonimiasis

Paragonimus spp. may create migratory tracts or pressure effects leading to necrosis of the spleen, liver, small and large intestinal wall, and cause non-specific abdominal signs and symptoms.

Subcutaneous paragonimiasis

P. skjabini, *P. westermani*, and *P. heterotremus* cause migratory subcutaneous nodules or asymptomatic subcutaneous nodule(s) at any part of the body.

Fig. 1 Pulmonary paragonimiasis posteroanterior radiograph showing thick-walled cystic lesion in the right lower lobe and left lower lobe with pericystic fibrosis. (Copyright Professor Sirivan Vanijanonta.)

Diagnosis

Pulmonary paragonimiasis should be excluded in any patient from an endemic area who presents with a chronic productive cough and jam-like, brownish-red or 'rusty' sputum. The definitive diagnosis is made by observing the characteristic ova in sputum, pleural effusion, or stool, or flukes in biopsy specimens. Expectoration of intact flukes has been reported. Other supportive evidence is obtained by chest radiographs, which show the characteristic shadows of single or multiple cysts in the lungs (Fig. 1) Computed tomography of the chest is also helpful (Fig. 2).

Serology is essential for the diagnosis of extrapulmonary paragonimiasis. Enzyme immunoassay, and dot enzyme immunoassay, and monoclonal antibody tests are highly sensitive and specific, as is counterimmunoelectrophoresis using adult or free metacercariae as a source of antigen. Other

Fig. 2 Pulmonary paragonimiasis' CT scan, showing thick-walled lesion with pericystic fibrosis in the left upper lobe and a fibrocalcific lesion in the right upper lobe. (Copyright Professor Sirivan Vanijanonta.)

less sensitive but more specific tests include complement fixation and indirect haemagglutination. Intradermal skin tests have been used for epidemiological surveys.

Differential diagnosis

Pulmonary paragonimiasis should be differentiated from pulmonary tuberculosis, melioidosis, lung abscesses, and lung tumours.

Extrapulmonary paragonimiasis should be differentiated from other diseases that produce similar clinical manifestations in affected organs. For example, cerebral paragonimiasis should be differentiated from cerebral cysticercosis, hydatidosis, meningoencephalitis, brain abscesses, and tumours. Subcutaneous paragonimiasis may resemble gnathostomiasis, sparganosis, loiasis, or onchocerciasis.

Treatment
Specific

The drug of choice is praziquantel at a dosage of 75 mg/kg per day in three divided doses for 2 to 3 days. A cure rate of nearly 100 per cent has been reported in multicentre studies. Albendazole and tricarbendazole are also effective. The symptoms rapidly improve in a few days. Eggs disappear from the sputum in a few weeks. Radiological improvement takes months, depending on the extent and chronicity of the disease. Convulsions, seizures, coma, and behavioural changes may develop during treatment of cerebral paragonimiasis. As a result of parasite death, brain oedema and host–parasite interaction may cause increased intracranial pressure. Therefore, treatment should proceed with caution and the dose adjusted if necessary. Dexamethasone cover has been suggested in some cases.

Symptomatic and supportive treatment

These treatments, including blood transfusion, bronchodilators, anticonvulsants, and analgesics, are also important.

Prognosis

Pulmonary paragonimiasis is rarely fatal and the lesions may calcify or completely resolve in a few years. Cerebral paragonimiasis may cause chronic morbidity such as epilepsy, mental changes, and neurological sequelae.

Prevention and control

Effective control measures are directed towards interruption of the life-cycle. However, control and eradication of intermediate hosts is impracticable; therefore, health education, changes in social and dietary customs, and the mass treatment of infected people in an endemic area are more effective for prevention and control.

Further reading
Calvopina M, et al. (1998). Treatment of human paragonimisis with tricarbendazole: clinical tolerance and drug efficacy. *Transactions of the Royal Society of Tropical Medicine and Hygiene* 92, 566–9.

Chen GU, et al. (1986). Counterimmunoelectrophoresis in detecting antibodies in experimental paragonimiasis. *Chinese Journal of Zoonoses* 2, 58.

Chung HL, et al. (1981). Recent progresses in studies of paragonimus and paragonimiasis control in China. *Chinese Medical Journal* 94, 483–94.

Jun-ichi I (1987). Evaluation of ELISA for the diagnosis of paragonimiasis westermani. *Transactions of the Royal Society of Tropical Medicine and Hygiene* 81, 3–6.

Maleewong W (1997). Recent advance in the diagnosis of paragonimiasis. *Southeast Asian Journal of Tropical Medicine and Hygiene* 28, 134–8.

Miyazaki I (1982). Paragonimiasis. In *CRC handbook series in zoonoses, Section C: Parasitic zoonoses*, Vol. III, pp. 143–64. Lea and Febiger, Philadelphia.

Miyazaki I, Harinasuta T (1966). The first case of human paragonimiasis caused by *Paragonimus heterotremus* (Chen and Hsia 1964). *Annals of Tropical Medicine and Parasitology* 60, 509.

Pariyananda S, et al. (1990). Serodiagnosis of human paragonimiasis caused by *Paragonimus heterotremus*. *Southeast Asia Journal of Tropical Medicine and Public Health* 21, 103–7.

Queuche F, et al. (1997). Endemic area of paragonimiasis in Vietnam. *Sante* 7, 155–9.

Vanijanonta S, Bunnag D, Harinasuta T (1984). *Paragonimus heterotremus* and other paragonimus spp. in Thailand: pathogenesis, clinical and treatment. *Drug Research* 34, 1186–8.

Vanijanonta S, Bunnag D, Harinasuta T (1984). Radiological findings in pulmonary paragonimiasis heterotremus. *Southeast Asia Journal of Tropical Medicine and Public Health* 15, 122–8.

Zhang YQ, et al. (1986). The significance of dot-ELISA in diagnosis of paragonimiasis. *Chinese Journal of Internal Medicine*, 25, 679–81.

7.16.4 Intestinal trematode infections
David I. Grove

Intestinal trematode infections of humans other than intestinal schistosomiasis are widespread but are most common in Asia. This is a reflection of cultural factors, particularly the consumption of raw or undercooked vectors, most frequently freshwater fish and molluscs, but also water plants. More than 50 million people are estimated to harbour one or more species of these hermaphroditic flukes. In many instances, the extent of morbidity due to these infections is uncertain.

Diagnosis

The diagnosis of intestinal fluke infections is usually based upon recovery of eggs from stools. Unfortunately, ova from species within a given family often look very similar and it may be possible when using routine laboratory methods to identify an infection only to family level, such as a heterophyid or echinostomatid egg. Definitive identification relies upon recovery of adult worms after anthelmintic treatment. Identifying characteristics are provided in parasitology texts.

Treatment

Praziquantel has been shown to be effective with a number of these infections and is the drug of first choice. It is given in a dose of 20 mg/kg orally after a meal, perhaps repeated once or twice. Flukes are usually expelled the following day. The role of triclabendazole, for instance in a dose of 10 mg/kg orally, in the treatment of intestinal trematodiases is not yet clear. Other possibilities which are less likely to be effective include niclosamide at 150 mg/kg orally for 1 or 2 days and albendazole at a dose of 200 mg orally for 2 days.

Prevention

These fluke infections can be prevented by thoroughly cooking potentially infected foodstuffs.

Echinostomiasis

This term may be conveniently used to include all infections with flukes of the family Echinostomatidae. There are more than 30 genera in this family and so far 18 species have been reported to infect humans (Table 1). These species vary in size from 1 to 20 mm in length. Echinostomes live in the intestines of various birds and mammals. When eggs are passed in the stools and reach water, the miracidium develops, hatches, and enters a snail, the first intermediate host. It then develops through the stages of sporocyst, mother redia, and daughter redia to release cercariae. The cercariae in turn infect second intermediate hosts which include various species of snails, tadpoles, and fish or they encyst on vegetation. Humans are infected after ingestion of inadequately cooked food containing these metacercariae.

In humans, they live in the small bowel, particularly the jejunum, and attach to the mucosa where they may cause a variable amount of damage. Heavy worm loads may cause abdominal discomfort, flatulence, and diarrhoea. Eggs 80 to 150 by 50 to 75 μm in size are passed in the stools (Fig. 1). They are yellow-brown, ellipsoidal, thin-shelled, and operculate and contain an immature embryo; eggs of the various species cannot be reliably differentiated from each other or from those of the intestinal fluke *Fasciolopsis buski* or the liver flukes *Fasciola hepatica* and *F. gigantica*.

Fasciolopsiasis

This infection is caused by *Fasciolopsis buski* (see Table 3). The adult fluke (Fig. 2) is found in the small intestine of humans and pigs. When eggs are passed in the stools and reach water, the miracidium develops, hatches, and enters a snail, the first intermediate host; snail hosts include species of *Segmentina*, *Hippeutis*, and *Gyraulus*. The miracidium then develops through the stages of sporocyst and redia to release cercariae after 8 weeks or so. The cercariae swim out and encyst on water plants and develop into metacercariae over 4 weeks. Infection is acquired by ingestion of infected uncooked edible plants such as water caltrop (*Trapa bicornis*), water chestnut (*Eliocharis tuberosa*), water bamboo (*Zizania aquatica*), and watercress (*Neptunia oleracea*).

Fifty years ago it was estimated that 10 million people were infected with this parasite. The current prevalence is unknown. Fasciolopsiasis occurs most commonly in areas where people keep pigs and raise and eat freshwater plants.

The adult worms attach themselves to the mucosa of the upper small bowel where they may cause inflammation and erosion and provoke a mucous intestinal discharge. Light infections are generally asymptomatic but heavy worm burdens may be associated with anorexia, nausea, abdominal discomfort, and diarrhoea or even intestinal obstruction. Stools may be foul-smelling and contain undigested food. In severe cases, a protein-losing enteropathy is associated with ascites, generalized oedema, and prostration.

Eggs 130 to 140 by 80 to 85 μm in size are passed in the stools (Fig. 3). They are yellow-brown, ellipsoid, thin-shelled, and operculate and contain an immature embryo; they cannot be reliably differentiated from those of the intestinal echinostomes or of the liver flukes *Fasciola hepatica* and *F. gigantica*.

Table 1 Intestinal trematodes infecting humans that belong to the family Echinostomatidae

Species	Geographical distribution	Definitive hosts other than man	Source of infection	Size of adults (mm)	Size of eggs (μm)
Acanthoparyphium tyosenense (=kuragamo)	Korea	Ducks	Clams	2–4 × 0.5–0.7	84–110 × 60–69
Artyfechinostomum mehrai	India	Rats, pigs	Freshwater snails	4.8–8.4 × –?	96 × 64
Echinochasmus japonicus	China, Korea	Cats, dogs, rodents, chickens	Fish	0.6–0.9 × 0.16–0.18	77–90 × 51–57
Echinochasmus perfoliatus	Europe, northern and eastern Asia, Egypt	Cats, dogs, foxes, rats, pigs	Freshwater fish (carp)	4.0–5.5 × 0.85–1.1	99–125 × 58–74
Echinoparyphium paraulum	Russia and surrounds	Ducks, geese, swans, doves			
Echinochasmus recurvatum	Egypt, Taiwan, Indonesia	Birds, mammals	Tadpoles, frogs, snails	1.9–7.3 × 0.4–0.9	88–111×54–75
Echinostoma cinetorchis	Japan, Taiwan	Rats	Tadpoles, frogs	5.6–21.2 × 1.3–3.7	96–100 × 61–70
Echinostoma hortense	Japan	Dogs, rats	Loaches, frogs	8.2–14 × 0.9–1.6	110–126 × 61–70
Echinostoma ilocanum	South-east Asia, China	Dogs, rats, mice	Freshwater snails	4–8 × 0.55–1.0	86–116 × 52–72
Echinostoma jassyense (= melis)	Romania, China		Tadpoles	5.5–7.5 × 1.2	132–154 × 75–85
Echinostoma lindoense	Indonesia, Brazil	Rats, birds	Freshwater snails	13–22 × 2.5–3.0	92–124 × 65–76
Echinostoma macrorchis	Japan	Rats	Freshwater snails	3.3–4.2 × 0.68–0.86	81–89 × 54–58
Echinostoma malayanum	South-east Asia, China	Rats	Freshwater snails, tadpoles, fish	5–10 × 2.5	137 × 75.5
Echinostoma revolutum	South-east Asia, China	Ducks, geese, chickens, rats	Clams, tadpoles, freshwater snails	21–26 × 2.0–3.5	104–112 × 64–72
Episthmium caninum	Thailand	Dogs	Fish	1.0–1.5 × 0.40–0.75	84 × 50–60
Himasthla muehlensi	Germany	Birds	Clams, molluscs	11–18 × 0.41–0.67	114–149 × 62–85
Hypoderaeum conoideum	Thailand	Ducks, fowl	Freshwater snails, tadpoles	6–12 × 1.3–2.0	95–108 × 61–68
Paryphostomum sufrartyfex	India	Pigs, dogs, rats	Snails	9.0 × 2.5	90–125 × 60–75

Fig. 1 Egg of *Echinostoma ilocanum* (by courtesy of P. Radomyos). All echinostome eggs look similar, as do those of *Fasciolopsis* and *Fasciola* species.

Fig. 2 Adult *Fasciolopsis buski*, 6.5 cm in length (by courtesy of P. Radomyos).

Heterophyiasis

This term may be conveniently used to include all infections with flukes of the family Heterophyidae although some infections are more precisely known by the generic name of the infecting organism, for instance metagonimiasis. These are small flukes, generally less than 1 to 2 mm in length. So far 37 species in this family have been reported to infect humans (Table 2). These infections are found in many places but are most common in Asia. *Metagonimus yokogawai* is believed to be the most common heterophyid infection.

Heterophyids live in the intestines of various mammals and birds. When eggs are passed in the stools, they contain a ciliated miracidium which hatches when ingested by a freshwater or brackish-water snail, the first intermediate host. Snails susceptible to *Heterophyes* include *Pirenella conica*, *Cerithidea cingulata*, and *Tympanotonus micropterus* while *Semisulcospira libertina* and *Thiara granifera* are host to *Metagonimus*. The miracidium then develops through the stages of sporocyst and one or two generations of rediae to release cercariae. The cercariae in turn infect various species of salmonoid and cyprinoid fish as the second intermediate hosts. These include mullet (e.g. *Mugil cephalus*) and minnow (*Gambusia* spp.) for *Heterophyes* species and carp (e.g. *Carassius carrasius*) and sweet fish (*Plecoglossus altivelis*) in the case of *Metagonimus* species. Humans are infected after ingestion of inadequately cooked fish containing metacercariae which mature in the flesh or scales of the fish.

The adult worms attach to or invade the mucosa of the upper small bowel where they may cause granulomatous inflammation and erosion. Light infections are generally asymptomatic but heavy worm burdens may be associated with anorexia, nausea, abdominal discomfort, and mucous diarrhoea. Occasionally ova deposited in the bowel wall enter blood vessels and embolize to other tissues. Eggs have been found in the heart and central nervous system. In cases of heterophyiasis described in the Philippines, cardiac failure was associated with subepicardial haemorrhages, myocardial damage caused by occlusion of vessels by ova, and eggs were stuck to a thickened, calcified mitral valve. Neurological features include focal cerebral disturbances and transverse myelitis.

Eggs 20 to 40 by 10 to 20 µm in size are passed in the stools (Fig. 4). They are yellow-brown, elongated, operculate, and contain a miracidium. Eggs of members of the family Heterophyidae cannot be reliably differentiated from each other. Furthermore, they are extremely difficult to differentiate from eggs of *Clonorchis sinensis* and *Opisthorchis* species although heterophyids tend to have a smoother egg shell, a less prominent shoulder at the operculum, and the abopercular knob may be absent.

Fig. 3 Egg of *Fasciolopsis buski* (by courtesy of P. Radomyos). Note its similarity to ova of *Fasciola* species and echinostomes.

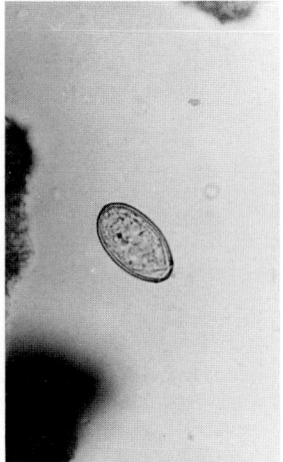

Fig. 4 Egg of *Metagonimus yokogawai* (by courtesy of P. Radomyos). All heterophyid eggs look similar, as do those of *Clonorchis sinensis* and *Opisthorchis viverrini*.

Other intestinal fluke infections

There are another dozen or so species of intestinal fluke belonging to various families that have been reported to infect humans (Table 3). As with other fluke infections, definitive diagnosis depends upon recovery of the adult worms; this is most commonly achieved by treatment with praziquantel. *Gastrodiscoides hominis* is unusual in that it attaches to the mucosa of the large bowel.

Alariasis

In North America, various species of the fluke *Alaria* are found in the intestines of wild carnivores such as wolves, foxes, bobcats, and skunks. The first intermediate hosts are snails and the second intermediate hosts are frogs and tadpoles. Cases of visceral larva migrans (sometimes fatal), ocular disease, and subcutaneous nodules due to *Alaria* mesocercariae have been described, usually following ingestion of undercooked frogs' legs. Other than surgical excision, no treatment has been described.

Further reading

Africa CM, De Leon W, Garcia EY (1940). Visceral complications in intestinal heterophydiasis of man. *Monographic series, Acta Medica Philippina*, No. 1 June.

Butcher AR *et al.* (1998). First report of the isolation of an adult worm of the genus *Brachylaima* (Digenea: Brachylaimidae) from the gastrointestinal tract of a human. *International Journal of Parasitology* 28, 607–10.

Chai JY *et al.* (1991). Intestinal trematodes infecting humans in Korea. *Southeast Asian Journal of Tropical Medicine and Public Health* 22(Suppl), 163–70.

Chai JY *et al.* (1997). Two endemic foci of heterophyids and other intestinal fluke infections in southern and western coastal areas in Korea. *Korean Journal of Parasitology* 36, 155–61.

Table 2 Intestinal trematodes infecting humans that belong to the family Heterophyidae

Species	Geographical distribution	Definitive hosts other than man	Source of infection	Size of adults (mm)	Size of eggs (µm)
Apophallus donicus	United States	Dogs, cats, rats, foxes, rabbits	Fish	1.1–1.3 × 0.58–0.72	35 × 25
Centrocestus armatus	Japan	Cats, dogs, rodents, herons	fish	0.35–0.63 × 0.18–0.29	28–32 × 16–17
Centrocestus caninus	Taiwan	Dogs, cats, rats	Fish	0.4–0.45 × 0.21–0.25	32–35 × 17–20
Centrocestus cuspidatus	Egypt, Taiwan	Chickens, rats	Fish	0.5–0.8 × 0.25–0.35	30–35 × 15–20
Centrocestus formosanus	China, Philippines	Rats, cats, dogs, chickens, ducks	Fish, frogs	0.42–0.47 × 0.21–0.25	0.24–0.42 × 0.21–0.25
Centrocestus kurokawai	Japan	Dogs, rodents (experimental)	Fish	0.35–0.51 × 0.18–0.23	33–40 × 17–21
Centrocestus longus	Taiwan	Dogs, cats (experimental)	Mullet and brackish-water fish	0.6 × 0.15	41 × 22
Cryptocotyle lingua	Greenland	Cats, dogs, rats	Fish	1.2–2.0 × 0.4–0.9	42–48 × 20–22
Diorchitrema formosanus	Taiwan	Cats, rats	Fish	0.32–0.56 × 0.13–0.21	18–24 × 12–15
Diorchitrema pseudocirratum	Hawaii, Philippines	Dogs, cats	Fish	0.3–0.6 × 0.2–0.3	18–21 × 9–12
Haplorchis microrchia	Japan	Dogs, cats,	Fish	0.40–0.76 × 0.17–0.29	27–30 × 14–16
Haplorchis pleurolophocerca	Egypt	Cats	Fish	0.32–0.42 × 0.14–0.17	29–32 × 15–18
Haplorchis pumilio	South-east Asia, Egypt	Dogs, cats, birds	Fish	0.45–0.89 × 0.2–0.4	24–28 × 12–15
Haplorchis taichui	Eastern Asia, Pakistan	Dogs, cats	Fish	0.47–0.64 × 0.18–0.22	20–33 × 11–17
Haplorchis vanissimus	Philippines		Fish	0.38–0.51 × 0.25–0.31	25–30 × 18–21
Haplorchis yokogawai	South-east Asia, China	Dogs, cats	Fish	0.47–0.64 × 0.18–0.22	20–33 × 10–17
Heterophyes heterophyes	Egypt, China, south-east Asia	Cats, dogs, rats, foxes, weasels, birds	Fish	1.0–1.7 × 0.3–0.4	28–30 × 15–17
Heterophyes katsuradai	Japan	Dogs	Fish	0.61–0.89 × 0.40–0.47	25–26 × 14–15
Heterophyes nocens	Japan	Dogs, cats, rats	Fish	0.9–1.1 × 0.4–0.5	28 × 15.5
Heterophyopsis continua	Japan	Dogs	Fish	2.0–2.1 × 0.24–0.28	25–26 × 14–16
Metagonimus minutus	Taiwan	Cats, mice	Fish	0.43–0.50 × 0.25–0.40	21–24 × 12–15
Metagonimus miyatai	Korea		Fish		
Metagonimus takahashii	Korea	Dogs, cats, rats, birds	Fish	0.84–1.48 × 0.42–0.72	28–34 × 17–21
Metagonimus yokogawai	Eastern Asia, south-east Asia, Europe	Dogs, cats, pigs, pelicans	Fish	1.0–2.5 × 0.40–0.75	26–28 × 15–17
Procerovum calderoni	Philippines	Cats, dogs	Fish	0.47–0.55 × 0.25–0.26	21–25 × 11–15
Procerovum varium	Japan	Cats, birds	Fish	0.26–0.38 × 0.13–0.16	25–29 × 12–18
Pygidiopsis summa	Korea	Birds, cats, dogs, rats	Fish	0.49–0.76 × 0.25–0.44	21–23 × 11–14
Stellantchasmus amplicaecus (=Diorchitrema amplicacaecale)	Taiwan	Dogs, cats, rats (experimental)	Fish (mullet)	0.45–0.65 × 0.20–0.34	22–24 × 8–14
Stellantchasmus falcatus	Japan, south-east Asia, Hawaii	Dogs, cats	Fish	0.59 × 0.23	21–23 × 12–13
Srictodora fuscata	Japan	Cats, birds	Fish	0.59 × 0.23	36–38 × 22–23

Table 3 Families of intestinal trematodes containing lesser numbers of species that are human pathogens.

Species	Geographical distribution	Definitive hosts other than man	Source of infection	Size of adults (mm)	Size of eggs (µm)
Brachylaimidae					
Brachylaima cribbi	South Australia	Mice, birds	Land snails	6–12 × 0.3–0.5	28–30 × 16–17
Fasciolidae					
Fasciolopsis buski	Asia	Dogs, pigs	Water plants	20–75 × 8–20	130–140 × 80–85
Gymnophallidae					
Gymnophalloides seoi	Korea	Birds	Oysters	0.4–0.5 × 0.2–0.3	20–25 × 11–15
Lecithodendriidae					
Phaneropsulus bonnei	Thailand, Indonesia	Bats, monkeys	Dragonflies	0.48–0.78 × 0.22–0.35	27–29 × 10–12
Phaneropsulus spinicirrus	Thailand			0.55–0.76 × 0.43–0.63	27–33 × 13–16
Prosthodendrium molenkampi	Thailand, Indonesia	Bats, monkeys, rats	Dragonflies, damsel flies		30 × 15
Microphallidae					
Spelotrema (=Carneophallus) brevicaeca	Philippines	Birds	Crabs	0.5–0.7 × 0.3–0.4	15–16 × 9 –10
Neodiplostomidae					
Neodiplostomum (=Fibricola) seoulensis	Korea	Freshwater snails	Frogs, snakes		
Paramphistomatidae					
Gastrodiscoides hominis	Asia, Guyana	Pigs, rats, monkeys, deer	Water plants	4–8 × 3–4	150 × 72
Watsonius watsoni	Southern Africa	Monkeys	Water plants?	8–10 × 4–5	120–130 × 75–80
Plagiorchidae					
Plagiorchis harinasutai	Thailand		Insect larvae	1.75–1.87 × 0.60–0.65	32–34 × 16–18
Plagiorchis javensis	Indonesia	Birds, bats	Insect larvae	1.8 × 0.7	36 × 22–24
Plagiorchis muris	Japan	Birds, dogs, rats	Snails, aquatic insects	0.8–2.0 × 0.24–0.84	36 × 21
Plagiorchis philippinensis	Philippines	Birds, rats	Insect larvae	1.5–2.0 × 0.39–0.44	28–30 × 19–21

Connor DH *et al.*, eds (1997). *Pathology of infectious diseases*, Vol 2, pp 1305–588. Appleton & Lange, Stamford.

Cross JH, ed. (1991). *Emerging problems in food-borne parasitic zoonosis: impact on agriculture and public health.* Thai Watana Panich Press Co. Ltd.

Department of Parasitology, Chiang Mai University, Thailand. http://www.medicine.cmu.ac.th/ dept/parasite/official.p_image.htm/trematodes

Hong SJ *et al.* (1996). One case of natural infection by *Heterophyopsis continua* and three other species of intestinal trematodes. *Korean Journal of Parasitology* **34**, 87–9.

Huffman JE, Fried B (1990). *Echinostoma* and echinostomiasis. *Advances in Parasitology* **29**, 215–69.

Kaewkes S *et al.* (1991). *Phaneropsulus spinicirrus* n. sp. (Digenea: Lecithodedriidae), a human parasite in Thailand. *Journal of Parasitology* **77**, 514–6.

McDonald HR *et al.* (1994). Two cases of intraocular infection with *Alaria* mesocercaria (Trematoda). *American Journal of Ophthalmology* **117**, 447–55.

Pungpak S *et al.* (1998). Treatment of *Opisthorchis viverrini* and intestinal fluke infections with praziquantel. *Southeast Asian Journal of Tropical Medicine and Public Health* **29**, 246–9.

Radomyos P, Bunnag D, Harinasuta T (1985) Report of *Episthmium caninum* (Verma, 1935) Yamaguti 1958 (Digenea: Echinostomatidae) in man. *Southeast Asian Journal of Tropical Medicine and Public Health* **16**, 508–11.

7.17 Non-venomous arthropods

J. Paul

Almost one million arthropod species have been described and it is likely that millions more await description. Most arthropods are of no medical importance. Medical problems they pose include envenoming, biting, transmission of infectious agents, allergy, infestation, and phobias. Arthropods may act as intermediate hosts of parasites and may cause nuisance by crawling over the skin, by making loud monotonous noises, or by invading dwellings. Most medically important arthropods are in the classes Insecta or Arachnida. Arthropod-related problems commonly present either as a particular clinical manifestation, such as bites or infestation, without an obviously visible causative agent, or as a problem visibly related to a specific kind of arthropod. Schemes of classification based on clinical manifestations and their likely causes and on the taxonomic arrangement of arthropods and their medical significance provide two useful approaches towards understanding arthropod-related problems.

Bites

Arthropod bites are common. They may be important because of the immediate physical discomfort of the bite, sensitization leading to pruritus, excoriation and secondary infection, other immunological phenomena including anaphylaxis, the transmission of infectious agents, and in exceptional circumstances blood loss. Reaction to bites varies with age, past exposure, and other factors which influence immune response. When the patient is able to associate bites with a particular kind of arthropod, management may be directed towards treatment of the bite if necessary (topical corticosteroids, systemic antihistamines), consideration of the risk of transmitted infection, and prevention of further bites (eradication of ectoparasites, change in behaviour to avoid exposure, repellents, special clothing, insecticide-impregnated bednets). It is often possible to associate bites with infesting ectoparasites, to arthropods which remain attached (ticks), and to predatory bloodsuckers which are highly visible (mosquitoes, midges, and black flies, when swarming) and which cause immediately painful bites (tsetse flies, some mosquitoes, tabanid flies). In is harder to ascribe a cause to bites from arthropods which bite at night or when the patient is asleep (some mosquitoes, sand flies, bedbugs, triatomine bugs) or from arthropods which are inconspicuous and which do not cause immediately painful bites (harvest mites, some fleas, some biting flies). Bites of larger arthropods typically have a central punctum and a surrounding area of inflammation and are pruritic. In cases of uncertainty it may be necessary to obtain a dermatological opinion to exclude other diagnoses, including organic disorders, artefact, and delusion.

Blood-sucking flies (Diptera)

Many flies are haematophagous (Table 1). Most blood-sucking flies are in the suborder Nematocera (mosquitoes, sand flies, black flies, biting midges) and the family Tabanidae of the suborder Brachycera (horse flies, clegs). The tsetse flies, *Glossina* spp., are in the suborder Cyclorrhapha. All blood-sucking flies are at least a nuisance: the bites are often painful and associated with sensitization. More importantly, biting flies may transmit infection. Mosquitoes (Culicidae) are vectors of filariasis and numerous viral diseases, including yellow fever and dengue. Mosquitoes of the genus *Anopheles* transmit malaria. Depending on species and location, mosquitoes bite at different times of the day. Mosquitoes need stagnant water for the development of their larval stages. Mosquitoes may be controlled by reducing their access to stagnant water and by application of insecticides to dwellings. Use of permethrin-impregnated bednets has been shown to reduce malaria transmission. Sand flies (Phlebotominae) are mainly tropical and subtropical in distribution and transmit leishmaniasis. In South America, sand flies of the genus *Lutzomyia* transmit *Bartonella bacilliformis*. Black flies (Simuliidae) occur worldwide but in Britain are rarely troublesome to humans except in certain localities, notably by the River Stour, Dorset. In Africa, simuliids transmit onchocerciasis, and in South America they are associated with the haemorrhagic syndrome of Altimira, but in Britain they are merely a nuisance (Blandford fly, *Simulium posticatum*). Black flies pierce the skin and suck blood from the edge of the puncture. The bites, oozing blood, have a characteristic appearance and may be associated with severe reaction by the host. Black fly larvae require fast-flowing water. Biting midges (Ceratopogonidae) are vectors of the filarial worms *Dipetalonema perstans* and *Mansonella ozzardi*. In Africa, tabanid flies transmit *Loa loa*. Tsetse flies, are vectors of African trypanosomiasis. When visiting locations where biting flies are troublesome, bites may be avoided to some extent by wearing clothing which covers the skin and by use of repellents.

True bugs (Hemiptera)

The two main groups of medically important Hemiptera are the bedbugs, *Cimex* spp., and the triatomine reduviid bugs, including *Rhodnius prolixus* and *Triatoma infestans*. The common bedbug *Cimex lectularius* (Plate 1) is cosmopolitan. The tropical bedbug *Cimex hemipterus* occurs in tropical and subtropical countries. There is no clear evidence to implicate bedbugs as vectors of disease. Bedbugs are nocturnal, hiding during the day and feeding at night. Although in some cases, bites may go unnoticed and there may be no allergic reaction, bedbugs may cause sleeplessness and the bites may cause pain and swelling (Fig 1). Where a room is heavily infested, patients may complain of an unpleasant odour produced by the bugs. Bugs may be found by making special searches at night or by searching their hiding places during the day. Bedbugs superficially resemble lentils, being round and flat. Adults reach a length of about 5 mm. Nymphs pass through five instars to reach adulthood after about 4 months. Bedbugs can live for 6 months without feeding, becoming paper-thin. Bedbugs may be translocated in furniture and personal effects. Control relies on removal or steam cleaning of infested mattresses and treatment of infested rooms with insecticides. Related bugs which occasionally bite humans are the pigeon bug *Cimex columbarius*, the bat bug *Cimex pipistrelli*, and the martin bug, *Oeciacus hirundinis*. Infestation may be managed by restricting the access of host species to dwellings. In Britain, bats are protected under the Wildlife and Countryside Act.

Table 1 Blood-sucking flies and the infectious diseases transmitted by them

Family	Genus (and species)	Associated agent or condition
Suborder Nematocera		
Culicidae (mosquitoes)		
subfamily Anophelinae	*Anopheles*	Malaria, Brugian, and Bancroftian filariasis
subfamily Culicinae	*Culiseta*	Western equine encephalitis
	Culex	Bancroftian filariasis
	Mansonia	Brugian filariasis
	Aedes	Eastern equine encephalitis, dengue fever, yellow fever, Bancroftian filariasis
	Haemagogus	Yellow fever
	Sabethes	Yellow fever
Phlebotomidae (sand flies)	*Phlebotomus*	*Leishmania* spp.
	Lutzomyia	*Leishmania* spp., *Bartonella bacilliformis*
Simuliidae (black flies)	*Simulium*	*Onchocerca volvulus*, *Mansonella ozzardi*, haemorrhagic syndrome of Altimira
Ceratopogonidae (biting midges)	*Culicoides*	*Dipetalonema perstans*, *Mansonella ozzardi*
Suborder Brachycera		
Tabanidae (horse flies, clegs)	*Haematopota*	
	Tabanus	
	Pangonia	
	Chrysops	*Loa loa*
Rhagionidae (snipe flies)	*Symphoromyia*	
	Atherix	
	Spaniopsis	
	Austroleptis	
Suborder Cyclorrhaphia		
Glossinidae (tsetse flies)	*Glossina*	African trypanosomiasis
Calliphoridae (Congo floor maggot)	*Auchmeromyia luteola*	
Muscidae (stable fly)	*Stomoxys calcitrans*	
Hippoboscidae (sheep ked)	*Melophagus ovinus*	

Most of the 129 species of cone-nose bugs (family Reduviidae, subfamily Triatominae) occur in the Americas. Seven species occur in Asia and one species, *Triatoma rubrofasciata*, is cosmotropical. Many triatomines are obligate feeders on the blood of vertebrates. Triatomines transmit South American trypanosomiasis. Important vector species are *Rhodnius prolixus*, *Triatoma infestans*, *Triatoma brasiliensis*, *Triatoma dimidiata*, and *Panstrongylus megistus*. The bugs infest dwellings, hiding in crevices during the day and biting at night. Dwellings may be heavily infested: in Colombia, 11 403 specimens of *Rhodnius prolixus* were reported from one house, occupied by nine people, all seropositive for trypanosomiasis. As well as transmitting trypanosomiasis, triatomines may cause significant blood loss to occupants

Fig. 1 Erythematous macules of bedbugs. (Reproduced by courtesy of D. Hill, Adelaide.)

of infested buildings. Control depends on deinfestation of dwellings with insecticides and on the construction of buildings which offer few hiding places for the bugs.

Ticks (Ixodoidea)

Ticks bites are often recognized as such because ticks may remain attached to the skin for days. Hard ticks (Ixodidae) and soft ticks (Argasidae) occur worldwide. Stages of the lifecycle are egg, larva (six-legged), and nymph and adult (both eight-legged). Ticks attach and feed with a barbed hypostome and detach when engorged. Smaller stages and ticks in inconspicuous sites, such as on the perineum, may feed unobserved. Bites are usually painless but may result in local sensitization, secondary infection, and transmission of infectious agents, including numerous viruses, rickettsias, and Lyme disease (Table 2). Local reaction to bites may be confused with erythema migrans of Lyme disease, (which expands and typically develops a cyanosed centre). Ticks may be removed by gripping with forceps (or in the field, with finger and thumbnail), between the skin and the tick's head and pulling gently. One should avoid squeezing the tick. Careless removal may detach the hypostome, a potential source of secondary infection or inflammation. In Britain, ticks most often found on humans are the sheep tick *Ixodes ricinus* (a vector of Lyme disease), and the hedgehog tick *Ixodes hexagonus* (Plate 3). When visiting tick-infested places, bites may be avoided by tucking trousers into boots and by wearing light-coloured clothing which makes ticks highly visible. After visiting tick-infested habitats, searches of the body allow prompt removal of ticks which reduces the chance of disease transmission.

Harvest mites (Tromboculidae)

In Britain, larvae of the harvest mite *Neotrombicula autumnalis* are a common cause of bites in late summer. The mites are tiny and seldom noticed. They crawl rapidly on to the body, attach (often under tight-fitting

Table 2 Ticks and tick-borne diseases

Genus and species	Geographical distribution	Associated infections
Argasidae (soft ticks)		
Ornithodoros spp.	Widely distributed	Endemic relapsing fever
Ixodidae (hard ticks)		
Amblyomma hebraeum	Africa	Tick typhus
Amblyomma cajennense	Americas	Rocky mountain spotted fever
Dermacentor andersoni	North America	Colorado tick fever, rocky mountain spotted fever
Dermacentor marginatus	Palaearctic	Tick typhus, Omsk haemorrhagic fever
Dermacentor silvarum	Eastern Palaearctic	Tick typhus, tick-borne encephalitis
Dermacentor variabilis	North America	Rocky mountain spotted fever
Haemaphysalis concinna	Palaearctic	Tick typhus
Haemaphysalis spinigera	India	Kyasanur Forest disease
Haemaphysalis turturis	India	Kyasanur Forest disease
Hyalomma spp.	Old World	Crimean–Congo haemorrhagic fever
Ixodes scapularis	Eastern North America	Lyme disease
Ixodes holocyclus	Australia	Queensland tick typhus
Ixodes pacificus	Western North America	Lyme disease
Ixodes ricinus	Western Palaearctic	Lyme disease, tick-borne encephalitis, louping ill
Ixodes persulcatus	Eastern Palaearctic	Tick-borne encephalitis, Omsk haemorrhagic fever
Rhipicephalus sanguineus	Cosmopolitan	Tick typhus

clothes), inject proteolytic enzymes, feed on tissue fluid and detach, causing pruritic, sometimes bullous lesions hours later. Red bugs or chiggers (a term also applied to *Tunga penetrans*) are names given to tromboculids in the Americas. In Asia, trombolucids are vectors of scrub typhus. Where tromboculids are troublesome, tucking trousers into boots and application of diethyltoluamide and other repellents may be partially effective.

Accidental bites

Some arthropods which do not normally bite man can inflict painful but usually trivial bites when provoked by handling, as by children and entomologists: these include predatory true bugs such as the water boatman *Notonecta glauca* and the assasin bug *Reduvius personatus* in Britain and wheel bugs, *Arilus* spp., in the Americas; larger beetles (Coleoptera); dragonflies (Odonata); and bush-crickets (Orthoptera) such as the wart-biter *Decticus verrucivorus*. Spines used in defence by the great silver diving beetle *Hydrous piceus* and larger tropical grasshoppers of the subfamily Cyrtacanthridinae can cause penetrating injury when handled. Pincers of larger crabs and lobsters (Crustacea) can cause crushing injuries of digits and their spines may cause penetrating injury.

Infestation

Sites of infestation include the hair, body surface and immediate environment (ectoparasites: lice, fleas), the skin and subdermis (scabies, tungosis, dermal myiasis), wounds, tissues, and orifices (myiasis), and the gastrointestinal tract (myiasis, canthariasis). With ectoparasites, the main problems are related to their bites: diagnosis and management may be based on the identification of the ectoparasite. Delusory parasitosis is a condition in which the patient becomes convinced of infestation by parasites despite reassurance by the doctor and absence of clinical or laboratory evidence.

Scabies

The agent of human scabies, a chronic infestation, is the human scabies mite *Sarcoptes scabiei* var. *hominis*. Scabies mites adapted to other hosts, such as *Sarcoptes scabiei* var. *canis* cause a self-limiting pruritus in man. Clinical manifestations of scabies are caused by the adult female mite which burrows through the epidermis. The adult female is oval and about a third of a millimetre long (Fig. 2). The female lives for about a month, burrowing and ovipositing daily. The burrow may extend to a centimetre in length. Six-legged larvae hatch after a few days and moult to become eight-legged nymphs and later eight-legged adults. Adult males are smaller than females,

do not burrow, and die after mating on the epidermis. Scabies is cosmopolitan in distribution. Prevalence rates vary but may be higher in conditions of overcrowing and following social disruption in wartime. Outbreaks may occur in nursing homes and in hospitals. Most cases must be acquired by close contact as the mites do not survive long away from the body. The main presenting symptom is pruritus which occurs with sensitization about a month after the onset of infestation. Symptoms may be worse at night and after a hot bath or shower. Burrows commonly occur in web spaces between the fingers and on the wrists but may be very widespread. There is often evidence of excoriation but the appearance of the

Fig. 2 Adult specimen of *Sarcoptes scabiei*. (Reproduced by courtesy of R.V. Southcott, Adelaide, South Australia.)

Fig. 3 Secondarily infected scabies in mother and child.

skin is variable and may show secondary infection, eczematization, lichenification, and papulovesicles (Fig. 3). Careful examination may reveal burrows and mites. Diagnosis may be confirmed by microscopy of scrapings from affected areas, especially interdigital spaces, but many cases are atypical and a dermatological opinion may be required to exclude other causes (Fig. 4). Immunosuppressed patients, including transplant recipients and patients with AIDS, are prone to crusting or so-called Norwegian scabies in which crusting lesions of scales and mites accumulate over the hands, feet, and other sites such as the eyebrows, but the patient suffers relatively little discomfort. Such cases and presumably their fomites are highly contagious. Treatment of scabies is by topical application of acaricides. Malathion and permethrin are currently recommended, applied twice, one week apart, in the United Kingdom. Gamma benzene hexachloride is also effective. To prevent reinfection, close contacts should be treated simultaneously. During outbreaks, it may be necessary to treat whole cohorts of patients or healthcare teams. Ivermectin, by mouth, has been used to treat cases of crusting scabies in immunosuppressed patients. Occasionally, the mites *Dermanyssus gallinae* and *Ornithonyssus* spp. whose normal hosts are birds, bite humans, causing lesions which resemble scabies.

Fig. 4 Papulovesicular lesions of scabies.

Louse infestation

Lice are obligate parasites of animals. They bite using piercing mouthparts to feed on blood or tissue fluids. Three species, of cosmopolitan distribution, are associated with man: *Pthirus pubis*, the pubic louse, the body louse (or clothing louse) *Pediculus humanus*, and the head louse *Pediculus capitis*. Body and head lice are morphologically similar and are treated by some authors as subspecies or forms of *P. humanus*. Lice complete their lifecycle on their host. Adult females deposit eggs (nits) on hairshafts (pubic and head lice) or on clothing (body louse). Larvae hatch after about 1 week, begin to feed, and over the course of about 2 weeks undergo several moults before reaching adulthood. Adult females live for about a month and may lay about a hundred eggs. Egg cases remain where attached and may persist after successful treatment of infestation. Most infestations are probably acquired through close contact with an infested case but some cases may result from contact with clothing, bedclothes, or hairbrushes containing living lice or their eggs which may be attached to shed hairs. In addition to the aesthetic and social drawbacks of louse infestation, medical problems common to all three taxa, relate to sensitization of the host to louse antigens from bites and the resulting pruritus which may lead to excoriation and secondary infection. Louse bites have a central punctum and surrounding small red macule. Body lice may transmit a number of agents, including those of endemic typhus (*Rickettsia prowazekii*), trench fever (*Bartonella quintana*), and relapsing fever (*Borrelia recurrentis*). Louse infestation may be treated by topical application of pediculocides. Pediculocides should be used with caution in children and asthmatics.

Pubic lice (crab lice)

The lice attach themselves to pubic hairs. Rarely they may be found on eyebrows, eyelashes (phthirus palpebrarum), axillary, head, or chest hair. Eggs are deposited on hair shafts. Most infestations are probably acquired through sexual contact with an infested case. Children may acquire phthirosis at atypical sites through close contact with adults. Lice seldom stray from the body. Transmission is possible but unlikely without close contact with an infested case. The main symptom is pruritus, sometimes with excoriation and secondary infection. Bluish-grey patches (maculae caeruleae) may occur on the skin. Diagnosis is by observation of the lice, which may be difficult to find, or of eggs or egg cases attached to hairshafts. Adults are 1 to 2 mm long. The anterior legs are smaller than the other two pairs. The body is squat and crablike (body length, excluding head, about 1.2 times body width) (Fig. 5). Infestation may be treated by topical application of carbaryl or malathion to the whole body, repeated a week later to kill newly hatched larvae. (The original description contained a printing error (*Pthirus*) for phthirus (Greek for 'louse').)

Head lice

Head lice infest the scalp and rarely other body sites. They lay their eggs at the base of hair shafts. Infestation is more common in children than in adults and more common in females than in males. Prevalence rates vary but may be very high in certain communities or institutions, such as schools. Prevalence rates may be high despite good standards of hygiene. Most cases occur probably as a result of close contact. The main symptom is pruritus which may be associated with excoriation, secondary infection, and lymphadenopathy. Diagnosis is by observation of lice, which generally remain close to the scalp, or of eggs or egg cases attached to hairs (Fig. 6). A fine comb (nit comb) may be used to collect material to make the diagnosis. Adults are 3 to 4 mm long. Infestation may be treated by application of pediculicide lotion to the scalp overnight and repeated a week later to destroy newly hatched larvae. Currently available pediculocides in the United Kingdom include malathion, permethrin, phenothrin, and carbaryl. Treatment failure with permethrin has been reported from many parts of the world. Compared with laboratory reference strains, lice collected from infestations failing to respond to permethrin have shown relative resistance to the agent. There is evidence that in Israel permethrin resistance may be

Fig. 5 Adult specimen of *Pthirus publis*. (Reproduced by courtesy of R.V. Southcott, Adelaide, South Australia.)

due to mono-oxygenase plus nerve insensitivity resistance mechanisms. Malathion resistance has been reported and may be due to a malathion-specific esterase. Regular and fastidious use of a nit comb may be used (on its own or in combination with a pediculocide) to treat infestation. There is much anecdotal evidence that combing can be effective. Combing avoids concerns of pediculocide toxicity and resistance, but a study in Wales showed combing to be less effective that chemical treatment. In institutions, co-ordinated treatment campaigns may be required to prevent reinfestation.

Fig. 6 Nits attached to hair. (Reproduced by courtesy of D. Hill, Adelaide.) Photograph from a patient with pediculosis showing several hair fibres with numerous egg cases attached.

Body lice

Body lice infest clothing and body hair. They lay their eggs on clothing, often along seams. Body lice are morphologically like head lice but they are slightly larger (Plate 4). Body louse infestation is associated with poor hygiene and social deprivation, as may occur in wartime. Transmission occurs as a result of close contact or through contact with infested clothing. Bites occur on the body, resulting in pruritus which may be associated with excoriation, eczematization, and secondary infection. Diagnosis is confirmed by finding lice, usually on the clothing. Infestation may be treated by topical application of carbaryl or malathion to the whole body, repeated a week later to kill newly hatched larvae. Hot washing of clothing will destroy adults and early stages.

Fleas (Siphonaptera)

Fleas are bloodsucking ectoparasites. There are thousands of species, adapted to various host animals. Adults are a few millimetres long, brown, laterally compressed, and typically very active. Adults move through the fur or under clothing but can survive in the environment for long periods without feeding. Eggs are dropped to the ground, where the larvae develop, feeding on organic matter. The pupa may remain in the environment for long periods before the adult emerges. Increasing standards of hygiene in developed countries have made the human flea, *Pulex irritans*, a rarity. Most flea bites in Britain are due to cat and dog fleas, *Ctenocephalides felis* (Plate 2) and *C. canis*, either through direct exposure to an infested animal or to an environment exposed to an infested animal, possibly months previously. Flea bites result in intense pruritus at the bite site. There is a central punctum and there may be bulla formation (Fig. 7). Flea bites often occur in groups. Although patients may not witness fleas, clues that bites have been caused by fleas include intense pruritus, the appearance of bites in small groups and a history of exposure to a flea-ridden animal or its domain. Troublesome bites may be treated with topical corticosteroids and systemic antihistamines. Prevention of bites is by good domestic hygiene

Fig. 7 Fleabites. Erythematous macropapule with central bite point visible. (Reproduced by courtesy of D Hill, Adelaide.)

and treatment of infested animals and environments with insecticides. Certain species of flea are vectors of a number of infectious diseases including plague and murine typhus.

Tungosis

Tungosis is infestation by a flea, *Tunga penetrans*, the jigger, chigger, or chigoe (but popular names are shared with trombiculid mites). The gravid female, about 1 mm long, burrows into exposed skin (usually the foot) or under a toenail and swells to about 1 cm in diameter, causing local discomfort. Lesions may be enucleated surgically, the diagnosis being confirmed by histology. Local remedies in endemic areas (tropical Africa and the Americas) of shelling out fleas may leave cavities prone to secondary infection and tetanus. The wearing of footwear prevents infestation.

Myiasis

Myiasis is the infestation of living animals by the larvae of flies (Diptera). Useful schemes of classification of myiasis include those based on the anatomical site (dermal, subdermal, wound, nasopharyngeal, orbital, ophthalmic, aural, urogenital, pulmonary, intestinal) and on the species of fly involved. Myiasis caused by flies whose larvae are obligate parasites of living tissues may be termed specific or primary myiasis. Myiasis associated with larvae which feed on decaying organic matter may be termed opportunistic or secondary myiasis. Myiasis due to larvae which find there way into the body (especially the gastrointestinal tract) by chance may be called accidental myiasis. Of the many species listed as possible agents (Table 3), most are opportunists whose saprophagous larvae feed on decaying organic matter, which might include necrotic wound tissue. Opportunists usually confine themselves to dead tissue and may even benefit the healing process.

There is no dipterous obligate intestinal parasite of man. Intestinal myiasis may be caused by coprophagous larvae which invade the rectum or by resilient maggots, such as those of the false stable fly *Muscina stabulans* and the cheese skipper *Piophila casei* which survive when swallowed in food and may cause intestinal disturbance and scarring. Intestinal myiasis may be spurious following diagnosis based on observation of rapidly hatching larvae on freshly passed faeces. Flies from several genera, notably *Fannia*, may cause urogenital myiasis. Scuttle flies (Phoridae) have been reported to cause pulmonary myiasis, possibly following inhalation of the gravid female fly. A small number of flies are obligate parasites of living tissues and a few species are closely associated with, but not specific to, humans. Many cases of myiasis are benign, self-limiting, and relatively harmless, but aural, nasopharyngeal, and malign wound myiasis are potentially lethal entities that may require removal of the larvae and possibly reconstructive surgery. Myiasis is diagnosed by observing dipterous larvae in a lesion. Identification of larvae may require entomological expertise but management of the patient, which depends on the type of lesion, may involve the removal of larvae, surgical exploration, debridement, or treatment of secondary infection and should be based on clinical assessment.

Dermal myiasis

Dermatobia hominis, the human bot fly, is a common cause of dermal myiasis in the American tropics. The female fly lays her eggs on biting arthropods such as mosquitoes. The eggs hatch when in contact with skin into which the larva burrows. The larval stage lasts about 10 weeks (Fig. 8), a boil with a small aperture forming as the larva grows. Such boils are not infrequently seen in Europeans returning from the neotropics. The larva may grow to more than a centimetre in length. An early symptom is sporadic pain caused by the spiny larva. Unless in an unusual anatomical site,

Table 3 Flies associated with myiasis in humans

Genus and species	Common name	Distribution	Type of myiasis
Phoridae			
Megaselia spp.	Scuttle flies	Cosmopolitan	Wound, intestinal, urogenital, pulmonary
Syrphidae			
Eristalis tenax	Common drone fly	Widely distributed	Rectal
Piophilidae			
Piophila casei	Cheese skipper	Widely distributed	Intestinal
Muscidae			
Fannia canicularis	Lesser house fly	Cosmopolitan	Urogenital
Musca domestica	House fly	Cosmopolitan	Wound, intestinal
Muscina stabulans	False stable fly	Cosmopolitan	Intestinal
Stomoxys calcitrans	Stable fly	Cosmopolitan	Intestinal
Calliphoridae			
Auchmeromyia luteola	Congo floor maggot	Africa	Sanguinivorous
Calliphora spp.	Bluebottles	Widely distributed	Wound, intestinal
Cochliomyia hominivora	New World screw worm	Americas	Primary
Cochliomyia macelleria	Secondary screw worm	Americas	Wound
Cordylobia anthropophaga	Tumbu fly	Africa	Subdermal
Cordylobia rodhaini	Lund's fly	Africa	Subdermal
Chrysomya bezziana	Old World screw worm	Africa, Asia	Wound
Lucilia spp.	Green bottles	Widely distributed	Wound
Sarcophagidae			
Wohlfahrtia magnifica	Wohlfahrt's myiasis fly	Southern Palaearctic	Primary
Wohlfahrtia vigil		North America	Dermal
Wohlfahrtia nuba		Southern Palaearctic	Wound
Sarcophaga spp.	Flesh flies	Widely distributed	Intestinal, wound
Gasterophilidae			
Gasterophilus spp.	Horse bot flies	Widely distributed	Dermal (creeping)
Cuterebridae			
Cuterebra sp.	Rabbit bot fly	Americas	Nasal
Dermatobia hominis	South American bot fly	Neotropics	Subdermal
Oestridae			
Oestrus ovis	Sheep nasal bot fly	Widely distributed	Ocular myiasis
Hypoderma spp.	Warble flies	Holarctic	Dermal (creeping), ophthalmic

854

7 INFECTION

such as close to the eye, infestation is generally harmless. Secondary infection of the wound is the most common complication. Larvae may be removed through a simple incision. Remedies which include application of raw meat or glue to the lesion may not be successful. Squeezing may rupture the larva to evoke a local granulomatous reaction.

The tumbu fly, *Cordylobia anthropophaga*, is widespread in the Afrotropical region. The female oviposits on sand and also on drying clothes. Ironing destroys eggs. Contact with viable ova on clothing leads to infestation. The larvae (Plate 6) pierce the skin and grow rapidly. An uncomfortable boil forms which oozes serosanguinous fluid. Fever and lymphadenopathy may occur. Larvae reach maturity in about 10 days. Larvae may be removed through a simple incision, but with care it may be possible to express larvae following application of petroleum jelly.

The larvae of warble flies, *Hypoderma* spp., occasionally cause dermal myiasis in man. Larvae of horse bot flies, *Gasterophilus* spp., cannot complete their lifecycle in man but they can pierce human skin, where they wander for a week or so, causing intense itching (creeping eruption).

(a)

(b)

Fig. 8 Two third larval instars of the human bot fly (*Dermatobia hominis*) (approximately 13 mm long) extracted from a facial 'boil' in a European who had been visiting Guyana. (b) Larva of *Dermatobia hominis* initially infesting the scalp of a young child in Panama. The larva made a 4-mm hole in the anterior fontanelle and entered the frontal lobe of the brain. The child died of malaria. (Armed Forces Institute of Pathology photograph, neg. no. 50807.)

Wound myiasis

Many dipterous species are known to cause wound myiasis, but most of them are facultative feeders on necrotic tissue and are rarely destructive to the host, although the presence of maggots in a wound may cause distress. Debridement of nectrotic tissue will control such infestation. In contrast, under controlled conditions, clinicians may introduce maggots to promote healing.

Causes of malign myiasis include the New World screw-worm *Cochliomyia hominivorax*, in the Americas and the Old World screw-worm *Chrysomya bezziana* and Wohlfahrt's wound myiasis fly *Wohlfahrtia magnifica* in the Old World. Their larvae are obligate parasites of living tissue. Eggs are laid on wounds, in ears, and on mucous membranes. The larvae (Fig. 9) burrow in groups into healthy tissue, causing widespread destruction which may be mutilating or fatal (Fig. 10). Secondary bacterial infection or secondary wound myiasis may ensue. All species may cause nasopharyngeal, aural, orbital, genital, and malign wound myiasis. Infestation is best avoided by cleaning and dressing wounds as they occur. Treatment involves surgical removal of the larvae, debridement of affected tissue, and treatment of secondary infection. Reconstructive surgery may be required.

Ophthalmic myiasis

Nasal bot flies, *Oestrus* spp., naturally parasitize various herbivorous mammals. They are larviparous and drop their larvae into the nostrils of the host. Dropped into human eyes they cause a self-limiting conjunctivitis. Larvae of warble flies, *Hypoderma* spp., are more dangerous: they may burrow into the eye, resulting in pain, nausea, and much damage and must be surgically removed.

Canthariasis

Infestation of the body by beetles (Coleoptera) or their larvae is called canthariasis. Clinically, it may resemble myiasis but is much rarer. Larvae swallowed with food may dwell temporarilly in the intestines, causing discomfort and may be detected in excreta. Beetles occasionally invade orifices. In Sri Lanka, scarabid dung beetles have been reported to invade the rectum. A specimen of the ground beetle *Sciates sulcatus* was recovered from the vagina of a women complaining of vaginal discharge who had visited Pakistan (Plate 5). In Israel, the dung beetle *Maladera matrida* has been reported to invade the external auditory canal. In Oman, two cases of invasion of the external auditory canal by the ground beetle *Crasydactylus*

Fig. 9 Larvae of the New World screw-worm (*Cochliomyia hominivorax*) (approximately 8 mm long) extracted from the wound illustrated in Fig. 10. These were sent to the Natural History Museum, London, where they were identified. Larvae of the second myiasis species (*C. macellaria*) were also found in the sample and were probably collected from the edges of the wound. (By courtesy of Dr Martin JR. Hall, Medical and Veterinary Division, The Natural History Museum, London .)

Fig. 10 Fatal myiasis (New World screw-worm): historical illustration of a 50-year-old Honduran woman who complained of a small chronic ulcer on the right cheek; on admission to hospital she was found to have a huge ulcer exposing the bones of the face and forehead and destroying the tissues of the cheek and face, right eye, and orbit; more than 300 larvae were removed (see Fig. 9). (Harrison JHH (1908). A case of myiasis. *Journal of Tropical Medicine and Hygiene*, **XI**, 20.)

punctatus have been reported. In one case, the beetle reached the middle ear causing sensorineural hearing loss.

Allergy

A wide range of immunological responses to arthropod bites has been described, from local pruritus to anaphylaxis. The dead remains, cast skins (exuviae), and faeces of many arthropods include sensitizing agents. They may act as contact or inhalant allergens following domestic or occupational exposure, resulting in dermatitis, conjunctivitis, rhinitis, and asthma. Allergic patients may show specific IgE antibodies to a wide range of domestic pests including house flies, clothes moths, cockroaches, carpet beetles, *Anthrenus* spp., silverfish, *Ctenolepisma longicaudata*, and house dust mites *Dermatophagoides* spp. *Dermatophagoides* spp. are a common cause of allergy in Britain and exposure to cockroach allergens in household dust has been associated with asthma in the United States. Following mass emergence, the exuviae of mayflies (Ephemeroptera) and caddis flies (Trichoptera) may act as inhalant allergens. Entomologists who collect insects by sucking them into pooters may develop inhalant allergy to their subject of study. Larvae of the beetles *Tenebrio molitor* (mealworm) and *Alphitobius diaperinus* (lesser mealworm), which are reared for fish bait and animal food, have been associated with rhinoconjunctivitis, contact urticaria, and asthma. Beetles which infest stored grain, including *Tenebrio molitor*, *Tribolium confusum* (confused flour beetle), *Sitophilus* sp. (grain weevil), and *Alphitobius diaperinus* have been associated with occupational allergy in grain workers or bakers. Allergy has been associated with other beetles, including *Dermestes peruvianus* (hide beetle), *Gibbium psylloides* (mite beetle), and *Harmonia axyridis* (Asian ladybird). Insect allergy can be investigated by skin prick tests, measurement of allergen-specific serum IgE, and by monitoring respiratory function following allergen exposure.

Insects and hygiene

Synanthropic insects which feed or wander over faeces, wounds, and food may serve as passive vectors of bacterial and viral diseases. Such insects include pharaoh's ants, *Monomorium pharaonis*, flies, and cockroaches (Dictyoptera). Despite many reports of the isolation of pathogenic bacteria and viruses from these insects, there have been few epidemiological studies to define their importance as passive vectors but is generally accepted that the presence of these insects in hospitals should be monitored and controlled.

Flies

Many species of fly (especially of the suborder Cyclorrhapha), frequent human and animal food, wounds, eyes, and faeces. Such flies vomit and defaecate where they feed. Numerous pathogenic bacteria and viruses have been isolated from flies, suggesting that they may act as passive vectors of bacterial and viral diseases. A controlled study in The Gambia where fly control was associated with fewer new cases of trachoma, suggested that flies may act as vectors of the trachoma agent, *Chlamydia trachomatis*. In The Gambia *Musca sorbens* is the most common eye-visiting fly. In Pakistan, a controlled study showed fly control to be significantly associated with a reduction in incidence of childhood diarrhoeal illness. In Israel, fly control was associated with a reduction in cases of shigellosis. Flies may be controlled by using insecticides or fly traps in dwellings and latrines.

Pharaoh's ants

Pharaoh's ants, *Monomorium pharaonis* L., commonly infest hospitals, where they invade sterile packs and wound dressings. They are potential passive vectors: bacteria, including *Salmonella* spp. and *Staphylococcus* spp. have been isolated from these ants, which should, therefore, be controlled with insecticides.

Cockroaches

Cockroaches are omnivorous scavengers. A few of the 3500 described species have become cosmopolitan synanthropes. The main pest species are the common cockroach, *Blatta orientalis*, the American cockroach, *Periplaneta americana*, the German cockroach, *Blattella germanica*, and the banded cockroach, *Supella longipalpa*. Other species may be locally important, for example *Ectobius lapponicus*, described by Linnaeus as infesting dried fish in Lapland. The common pest species are mostly of tropical origin and require temperatures of 25 to 33 °C but *B. orientalis* will tolerate 20 °C. In cooler climates they are restricted to permanently heated areas and can occur in large numbers in hospitals and in sewers. Many pathogenic viruses, including poliomyelitis virus and Coxsackie A virus, and bacteria, including *Shigella* spp., have been isolated from cockroaches. There is evidence that cockroaches acted as vectors of hepatitis A during an outbreak in California and of *Salmonella typhimurium* on a paediatric ward in Belgium. Cockroaches are potential allergens, 7.5 per cent of healthy persons having a positive skin test in one study. Cockroaches wander over sleepers and are attracted to nasal and oral secretions. Herpes blattae is a dermatitis described from Réunion and attributed to cockroach allergy. Cockroaches sometimes wander into the ears and nostrils, where they become trapped or reluctant to leave. Lidocaine spray is reported to hasten the exit of such visitors.

Eye-frequenting moths and beetles

Some nocturnal moths of the families Pyralidae, Noctuidae, and Geometridae in Africa and Southeast Asia habitually feed on the lachrymal secretions of animals. They may visit human eyes, causing a certain amount of discomfort, and may transmit eye infections, including trachoma and viral conjunctivitis. They may also cause mechanical damage to the cornea. The moths stimulate the flow of secretions by vibrating and probing with their probosces. Implicated species include *Lobocraspis griseifulva, Arcyophora* spp., and *Filodes fulvidorsalis. Calyptra eustrigata* is a skin-piercing, blood-sucking noctuid moth from Malaya. Such Lepidoptera may be avoided by sleeping under a net. In Australia a beetle, *Orthoperus* sp., has been associated with corneal erosion.

Further reading

Alexander JO'D (1984). *Arthropods and the human skin.* Springer, Berlin.

Auerbach PS, ed. (1995). *Wilderness medicine: management of wilderness and environmental emergencies.* Mosby, St Louis, MO.

Baker AS (1999). *Mites and ticks of domestic animals: an identification guide and information source.* The Stationery Office, London.

Hope FW (1840). On insects and their larvae occasionally found in the human body. *Transactions of the Royal Entomological Society* 2, 256–71.

James MT (1947). *The flies that cause myiasis in man.* United States Department of Agriculture, Washington.

Roberts DT, ed. (2000). *Lice and scabies: a health professional's guide to epidemiology and treatment.* Public Health Laboratory Service, London.

Rosenstreich DL *et al.* (1997). The role of cockroach allergy and exposure to cockroach allergen in causing morbidity among inner-city children with asthma. *New England Journal of Medicine* 336, 1356–63.

Roth LM, Willis ER (1957). The medical and veterinary importance of cockroaches. *Smithsonian Miscellaneous Collection* 134, 1–147.

Smith KGV, ed. (1973). *Insects and arthropods of medical importance.* British Museum (Natural History), London.

Zumpt F (1965). *Myiasis in man and animals in the Old World.* Butterworth, London.

7.18 Pentastomiasis (porocephalosis)

D. A. Warrell

The Pentastomida, pentastomes or 'tongue worms', inhabit the respiratory tracts of vertebrates where they feed on blood and other tissues. There are more than one hundred species, classified into two orders, Cephalobaenida (e.g. genus *Raillietiella*) and Porocephalida (e.g. genera *Linguatula*, *Armillifer*, *Leiperia*, and *Sebekia*). About ten species are known to be capable of causing zoonotic infections in humans. Pentastomida are probably arthropods, but they have also been classified as Branchiuran crustacea, annelids, and in a separate phylum. The name pentastome derives from their having two pairs of anterior hooks and a mouth, giving the impression of five stomata (Fig. 1). In humans, visceral pentastomiasis is most often caused by *Linguatula serrata* or *Armillifer armillatus* and nasopharyngeal pentastomiasis (halzoun or Marrara syndrome) by *L. serrata*.

Aetiology

Linguatula species

Linguatula serrata occurs in Europe, the Middle East, Africa, and North, Central, and South America, but not Asia. The names 'Linguatula' and 'tongue worm' describe the flattened shape, particularly of the adult female. Their surface bears numerous annular grooves. Dogs, foxes, and wolves, the definitive hosts, harbour adults and nymphs in their upper respiratory tract and shed them in their nasal secretions, saliva, and faeces. Herbivorous animals ingest the ova which hatch in the lumen of the gut releasing larvae that burrow into the tissues and encyst. When these intermediate hosts are eaten by the definitive host, nymphs hatch from the cysts and migrate to the lungs and nasopharynx where they mature.

Clinical features

If humans ingest ova of *Linguatula* spp., cysts usually develop in the liver but do not cause symptoms unless they obstruct or compress, for example, the filtration angle of the anterior chamber of the eye (2nd- or 3rd-instar larvae), biliary, gastrointestinal or respiratory tracts, meninges, or brain.

Fig. 1 Adult pentastomid showing mouth (arrowed) and lateral hooks giving the appearance of five stomata. Scanning electron micrograph, 400 ×. (By courtesy of Professor Viqar Zaman.)

Fig. 2 *Armillifer armillatus*. Left: two adults found in the lungs of a Gaboon viper (*Bitis gabonica*). Right: calcified nymph from the mesentery of a Ghanaian patient. (By courtesy of Dr G. M. Ardran.)

Ingestion of cysts containing third-stage larvae in raw liver and lymphnodes of sheep, goats, cattle, and lagomorphs can result in acute nasopharyngitis, known as halzoun, Marrara syndrome, or nasopharyngeal pentostomiasis. This has been reported from the Middle East, especially Lebanon, Greece, and the Sudan. In the human stomach, larvae escape from the cysts and migrate up the oesophagus to the nasopharynx mucosa. Within a few hours of eating the infected viscera there is intense irritation of the upper respiratory and gastrointestinal tracts associated with coughing, sneezing, rhinorrhoea, retching, vomiting, lacrimation, haemoptysis, epistaxis, cervical lymphadenopathy, transient deafness, difficulty in speaking, dysphagia, wheezing, and dyspnoea. Larvae can be found in sputum and vomitus. Patients usually recover in 1 or 2 weeks, but deaths have resulted from acute upper airway obstruction. These features suggest a hypersensitivity reaction. Halzoun has also been attributed to flukes (*Fasciola hepatica*) and nematodes (*Mammomonogamus laryngeus*) ingested in raw sheep and goat liver and to leeches (*Limnatis nilotica* and *Dinobdella ferox*). Very rarely, larvae may develop into adults in the human nasal cavity.

Armillifer (*Porocephalus*) species

These are also annulated, non-segmented parasites (Fig. 2). The adults, up to 20 cm long, inhabit the respiratory and digestive tracts of snakes, especially those of the genera *Python*, *Boaedon*, *Naja*, and *Bitis*, and other vertebrates. Ova are shed in the snake's nasal secretions and are picked up by herbivorous mammals. Larvae encyst in the tissues of these intermediate hosts and will develop to the nymph stage if ingested by another animal, but develop to adults only in snakes. Humans may ingest ova by drinking water contaminated by snakes, or they may ingest living encysted larvae in raw snake meat eaten as part of *ju ju* rituals (West Africa), or from inadequately cooked snake (Temuan tribe of Malaysian aborigines and in Benin and other West African countries). Ingested eggs hatch in the gut releasing larvae which burrow into the tissues where they develop into nymphs. Hundreds of wriggling nymphs have been discovered beneath the visceral peritoneum at laparotomy.

Human infections with the larvae or nymphs of the following species of *Armillifer* have been reported:

- *A. agkistrodontis*—China (in the snake *Deinagkistrodon acutus*);
- *A. armillatus* (18–22 annular rings)—Africa: Egypt, Senegal, The Gambia, Ghana, Benin, Nigeria, Cameroon, Congo, and Zimbabwe;
- *A. grandis*—Congo;
- *A. moniliformis* (30 annular rings)—Malaysia, Philippines, Indonesia, Tibet, and Australia;
- *A. najae*—India.

Clinical features

The commonest evidence of infection by *Armillifer* spp. is the discovery of calcified nymphs (Fig. 2) on radiographs of the abdomen and chest (Fig. 3). These appear as discrete, crescent-shaped, soft tissue calcifications, 4 × 4 mm in size. In West Africa they are seen particularly in the right upper quadrant and are situated beneath the peritoneum covering the liver. In Ibadan, Nigeria, these shadows were seen in 2 per cent of adult males and 4 per cent of adult females. Hundreds of calcified encysted nymphs have been found in the peritoneum at laparotomy or at autopsy in the liver (Fig. 4), spleen, gut wall and lumen, lungs, cirrhosal cavities, central nervous system, eye, and elsewhere in 27 per cent of cases in The Congo (*A. armillatus* and *A. grandis*), in 6 to 13 per cent in Cameroon (*A. armillatus*), and in 45 per cent in Malaysian Orang Asli (*A. moniliformis*).

Armillifer spp. infection is usually symptomless or causes vague abdominal pain. Serious inflammatory and obstructive effects have been described in the gut, lungs, biliary tract, pericardium, central nervous system, and anterior chamber of the eye. Severe acute reactions may be related to hypersensitivity or perhaps to massive infection such as might follow ingestion of a gravid female. Migration of large numbers of larvae from the gut into the tissue might produce abdominal pain and obstructive jaundice. A few fatal

Fig. 4 Encysted nymph/larva of *Armillifer armillatus* in human liver. The outer layer of the parasite (arrowed) lines the cyst wall. Acidophilic glands (ag), intestine (in), 21 ×. (Armed Forces Institute of Pathology photograph, negative number 75–2703.)

cases have been reported, including one patient who died from intestinal obstruction caused by nymphs of *A. armillatus*. It has been suggested (Nigeria and The Congo) that infection by *Armillifer* spp. might be associated with malignancy of the colon and elsewhere.

Other pentastomid infections

Human infections with *Leiperia cincinnalis* have been described in Africa, and subcutaneous infections by *Railliettiella gehyrae* and *R. hemidactyli* in Vietnam and by *Sebekia* species in Costa Rica. In Vietnam, infection with *Railliettiella* spp. follows the swallowing of small live lizards for medicinal purposes.

Diagnosis

The radiographical appearances of calcified pentastomid nymphs are distinctive (Fig. 3). Pentastomes may be discovered at surgery or autopsy. In the liver (Fig. 4), intestinal wall, mesentery, mesenteric lymph nodes, peritoneum, or lung, viable encysted larvae or granulomas containing necrotic pentastomes or their moulted cuticles may be identified. Initially, encysted larvae excite little or no tissue reaction, but the granulomas are surrounded by hyalinized or calcified fibrous tissue. In tissue sections, pentastomes can be distinguished from helminths. Antibodies to *Armillifer* spp. have been detected by fluorescence in infected patients.

Treatment

There is no specific treatment, although mebendazole has been suggested. Obstruction and compression should be relieved surgically. Hypersensitivity phenomena should be treated with adrenaline (epinephrine), antihistamines, and corticosteroids. Infections can be prevented if all meat is thoroughly cooked.

Fig. 3 Typical radiographic appearance of calcified nymphs of *Armillifer armillatus* in the abdominal cavity of a Ghanaian patient. (By courtesy of Dr G. M. Ardran.)

Other zoonoses transmitted from reptiles to humans

The most important of these is salmonellosis transmitted to humans by the faecal–oral route or by scratches and bites, from chelonians (tortoises, turtles, terrapins) and from snakes and lizards, especially iguanas. In Britain, 38 per cent of imported tortoises (*Testudo* species) contain *Salmonella* spp.; in the United States, where 8 million reptiles are kept as pets, 14 per cent of reported salmonellosis cases (280 000 per year) were attributable to pet terrapins, as were up to 17 per cent of cases of infant salmonellosis in Puerto Rico. The species include *S. typhimurium, S. muenchen, S. ealing, S. volta, S. alachua, S. stanley, S. marina, S. poona, S. pomona,* and *S. java.*

Other infections transmissible from reptiles to humans include *Arizona hinshawii* (in snake powder, Pulvo de Vibora, made from rattlesnakes), *Plesiomonas shigelloides, Edwardsiella tarda,* leptospirosis, Q fever, sparganosis, capillariasis, strongyloidiasis, mesocestoidiasis, and infestation with the mite *Ophionyssus natricis.* Potential zoonoses include *Mycobacteria, Pseudomonas,* other *Aeromonas* species, *Proteus* spp., and some togaviruses (such as western equine encephalitis in garter snakes in western North America) and herpesviruses.

Further reading

Drabick JJ (1987). Pentastomiasis. *Reviews of Infectious Diseases* **9**, 1087–94.

Fain A (1975). The Pentastomida parasitic in man. *Annales de la Societé Belge de Medecine Tropicale* **55**, 59–64.

Faisy C, *et al.* (1995). La porocéphalose, parasitose méconnue revue de la litérature à propos d'un cas congolais. *Médecine Tropicale (Marseille)* **55**, 258–62.

Haugerud RE (1989). Evolution in the pentastomids. *Parasitology Today* **5**, 126–32.

Lavarde V, Fornes P (1999). Lethal infection due to *Armillifer armillatus* (Porocephalida): a snake-related parasite. *Clinical Infectious Diseases* **29**, 1346–7.

Riley J (1986). The biology of pentastomids. *Advances in Parasitology* **25**, 45–128.

Self JT, Hopps HC, Williams AO (1975). Review. Pentastomiasis in Africans. *Tropical and Geographical Medicine* **27**, 1–13.

Warwick C, *et al.* (2001). Reptile-related salmonellosis. *Journal of the Royal Society of Medicine* **94**, 124–6.

Yagi H, *et al.* (1996). The Marrara syndrome: a hypersensitivity reaction of the upper respiratory tract and buccopharyngeal mucosa to nymphs of *Linguatula serrata. Acta Tropica* **16**, 127–34.

7.19 Chronic fatigue syndrome (postviral fatigue syndrome, neurasthenia, and myalgic encephalomyelitis)

Michael Sharpe

Historical introduction

Illness characterized by chronic fatigue but without a clear pathological basis has a long history. In the nineteenth century it attracted a diagnosis of 'neurasthenia' but by the early twentieth century this diagnosis fell into disuse. It is probable that since that time patients have continued to present to doctors with similar symptoms but have received other diagnoses such as depression, brucellosis, and Epstein–Barr virus infection. Apparent epidemics of fatiguing illness have been occasionally reported over the last 50 years and attributed to infection by various agents. One occurred among staff at the Royal Free Hospital, London in 1955 giving rise to the term myalgic encephalomyelitis. More recently, it has become accepted that the cause of many cases of chronic disabling fatigue is not an infection. The purely descriptive term chronic fatigue syndrome was consequently introduced in 1988. The cause and treatment of chronic fatigue syndrome remain controversial.

Introduction

The terms chronic fatigue syndrome, postviral fatigue syndrome, neurasthenia, and myalgic encephalomyelitis have all been used to describe an idiopathic syndrome characterized by disabling fatigue occurring chronically after minimal exertion. The current international consensus definition is shown in Table 1. It is now clear that there is considerable overlap between chronic fatigue syndrome and other 'functional' syndromes such as irritable bowel syndrome and fibromyalgia.

- What is fatigue? Fatigue is an imprecise term with many meanings. In clinical medicine, the symptom of fatigue implies a subjective feeling of lack of both energy and endurance.
- When is fatigue abnormal? Fatigue after exertion is a normal phenomenon. It is abnormal when it is disproportionate to the exertion, persistent, and associated with impaired function.
- Why 6 months? Six months is used to define chronicity for purposes of research. It excludes the short-lived fatigue that can follow any illness.

Table 1 International consensus definition of chronic fatigue syndrome

1. Principal complaint of fatigue
2. At least four of the following additional symptoms:
    Subjective memory impairment
    Sore throat
    Tender lymph nodes
    Muscle pain-Joint pain
    Headache
    Unrefreshing sleep
    Post-exertional malaise lasting more than 24 h
3. Impairment of functioning
4. Duration at least 6 months
5. Other conditions excluded

- Which other symptoms? Patients with chronic fatigue syndrome commonly complain of additional symptoms, which are described below under clinical features.
- What conditions must be excluded? Chronic fatigue may be a symptom of many, if not most, medical and psychiatric illnesses. The term chronic fatigue syndrome has been reserved for patients in whom the fatigue remains medically unexplained or 'idiopathic' after clinical assessment.

Aetiology

No specific aetiology has been identified. However, a number of psychological and biological factors have been identified that may play a role in the onset and/or perpetuation of illness. It is likely that different and perhaps multiple factors operate in different cases.

Infection

Patients frequently give a history suggestive of acute infection at the outset. Fatigue states lasting several months can follow infections such as Epstein–Barr virus and Q fever. Infection may therefore trigger chronic fatigue syndrome, but the available evidence does not support the hypothesis that chronic infection is the cause of chronic fatigue syndrome.

Immune dysfunction

Minor immune abnormalities have been detected in a proportion of patients. Cytokines can cause fatigue. However, no consistent immune abnormality or casual link of these with symptoms has been established in patients with chronic fatigue syndrome. The role of immune factors remains of interest but is unclear.

Stress and emotional disorder

More than half of the patients seen in hospital clinics who meet criteria for chronic fatigue syndrome also meet criteria for depressive and anxiety disorders. Many patients describe major life stresses. It has therefore been suggested that at least some cases of chronic fatigue syndrome are due to emotional disorder that is expressed somatically (somatization). This is undoubtedly true in some cases, but in many others these syndromes are either absent or are an inadequate explanation of the illness.

Psychological and behavioural factors

There is evidence that psychological and behavioural factors play a role in perpetuating chronic fatigue syndrome. They include misconceptions about the nature of the illness, excessive avoidance of physical activities so that the person becomes inactive, repeated seeking of (ineffective) medical care, and failure to resolve continuing psychological and social problems.

Inactivity

Some patients with chronic fatigue syndrome are profoundly inactive. This may lead to muscle wasting, changes in the cardiovascular response to exertion, and postural hypotension. The consequent intolerance of activity may perpetuate the illness.

Dysfunction of the central nervous system

Abnormalities have been found in tests of cognitive function. There is also evidence for abnormalities in neuroendocrine tests and in functional neuroimaging. However, abnormalities in similar domains have been found in patients with depression and anxiety disorders. Consequently the specificity and clinical utility of such tests remains to be established.

Endocrine dysfunction

A slightly reduced 24-h cortisol excretion has been reported. Replacement therapy with low-dose hydrocortisone has been reported to produce short-term symptomatic relief. However, the balance of risks and benefits of this treatment is not yet established.

Idiopathic postural hypotension (neurally mediated hypotension)

A tendency to postural hypotension has been reported in a proportion of patients with chronic fatigue syndrome. At present the aetiological and treatment implications of this observation remain unclear.

Sleep disorder

Various sleep abnormalities have been found in patients with chronic fatigue syndrome. They include both specific sleep disorders such as sleep apnoea syndrome and non-specific abnormalities such as fragmentation of sleep. These may contribute to daytime fatigue in at least some cases.

Social and iatrogenic factors

Information about chronic fatigue syndrome or myalgic encephalomyelitis, whether from doctors, patient groups, or the media, that leads patients to see their illness as mysterious with a hopeless prognosis and best treated by rest is likely to be unhelpful.

Epidemiology

Prevalence

One-quarter of the general population complain of persistent fatigue. In contrast, recent population studies in the United Kingdom and United States suggest that only approximately 0.5 per cent could be regarded as having chronic fatigue syndrome. Most of these persons are aged between 20 and 40 with a predominance of females. The syndrome is also seen in children and adolescents.

Epidemics

Epidemics of a chronic fatigue-like syndrome have been described from various parts of the globe. This observation is compatible with, but does not establish, an infective cause. It remains unclear whether these were true epidemics and also whether the clinical picture reported is similar to that of cases of sporadic chronic fatigue syndrome.

Pathogenesis

A number of explanations have been proposed (see section on aetiology above). These are best considered in the categories of predisposing, precipitating and perpetuating factors:

- Predisposing factors: Certain individuals may be predisposed to develop chronic fatigue syndrome by virtue of genetics, personality, or other vulnerability.
- Precipitating factors: The condition may be precipitated by factors such as infection or psychological stress (life events).
- Perpetuating factors: For practical management the most important factors are those that perpetuate the illness and consequently act as barriers to recovery. Perpetuating factors include the modifiable psychological and behavioural factors described above as well as biological factors.

Clinical features

Main symptoms

The principal symptom of chronic fatigue syndrome is chronic mental and physical fatigue, tiredness, or exhaustion that is exacerbated by activity. Patients often report being able to perform activities for brief periods, but subsequently experiencing severe fatigue for hours or days thereafter.

Other symptoms

Other common symptoms include muscular pain, unrefreshing sleep, dizziness and breathlessness, headache, tender lymph glands, and symptoms of irritable bowel syndrome. Patients often describe day-to-day fluctuations in their symptoms, irrespective of activity. Periods of almost complete recovery may be followed by relapse, often sufficiently severe to make normal daily activity impossible. Depression and anxiety are common, and a proportion of patients suffer panic attacks. Patients and their relatives may hold strong beliefs about the nature and aetiology of their illness (see section on aetiology), and these may be of importance when planning management.

Physical signs

Physical examination is typically unremarkable. Complaints of fever and lymphadenopathy are generally not confirmed on examination. The presence of definite physical signs (such as objectively measured fever) should not be ascribed to the syndrome and alternative diagnoses should be sought.

Differential diagnosis

Almost any disease may present with unexplained fatigue. The differential diagnosis of idiopathic chronic fatigue syndrome is correspondingly large (see Table 2). The nature of the fatigue may offer useful clues. Muscular disease should be considered if the patient has objective weakness, no psychological symptoms, and a family history. If the patient's complaint of fatigue includes prominent sleepiness, a sleep disorder should be considered. In particular, prominent snoring and morning headaches in the obese patient raise the possibility of obstructive sleep apnoea.

It is important to also assess the mental state. Depression is suggested by fatigue that is worse in the morning and accompanied by loss of motivation, interest, and pleasure. Other symptoms of depression should be sought including sadness, loss of appetite and weight, and feelings of pessimism and failure. If there is evidence of depression it is essential to ask about suicide plans. Chronic anxiety is also associated with fatigue and may

Table 2 Conditions to be considered in the differential diagnosis of chronic fatigue syndrome

Nature of symptoms	Possible condition
General	Occult malignancy
	Autoimmune disease
	Endocrine disease
	Cardiac, respiratory or renal failure
Gastroenterological	Malabsorption including coeliac disease
Neurological	Disseminated sclerosis
	Myasthenia gravis
	Parkinson's disease
	Early dementia
	Cerebrovascular disease
Infectious disease	Chronic active hepatitis (B or C)
	Lyme borreliosis
	HIV
	Tuberculosis
Respiratory disease	Nocturnal asthma
	Obstructive sleep apnoea
Chronic toxicity	Alcohol
	Solvents
	Heavy metals
	Irradiation
Psychiatric	Major depressive disorder
	Dysthymia
	Anxiety and panic disorder
	Somatization disorder

also give rise to many of the somatic symptoms of chronic fatigue syndrome such as muscle pain, impaired concentration, and poor sleep.

Pathology

There is no established pathology other than muscular and other changes associated with inactivity. Reports of abnormal structural brain scans have not been confirmed.

Laboratory diagnosis

There are no diagnostic tests and no characteristic abnormalities on laboratory investigation. These are conducted purely to exclude other diseases. All patients should have a full blood count, erythrocyte sedimentation rate or C-reactive protein, basic biochemistry screen, urine analysis, and possibly thyroid function and antinuclear antibody tests. Further investigation depends on the clinical findings and differential diagnoses under consideration.

Treatment

General management

The doctor should listen to the patient's story and ask about his or her own understanding of the illness in all cases. It is usually also worth seeing the partner or relevant family members. This provides opportunities to correct misconceptions. It is especially important to explain that the illness is not progressive or life threatening (see below). A more positive and less sinister explanation of chronic fatigue syndrome as a 'reversible dysfunction of the central nervous system' with a cautiously optimistic prognosis may be offered. The adverse physiological and psychological effects of prolonged bed rest should be explained if necessary. The patient should be encouraged

to adopt a consistent but gradually increasing level of activity, avoiding extremes of both inactivity and exertion. An evidence-based self-help book may be useful (such as *CSF/ME: the facts*; see Further reading). An initial hospital appointment that achieves all the above usually requires at least 45 min.

Drug therapy

A trial of an antidepressant drug may be considered, especially if there is evidence of depression. It is advisable to choose a non-sedating type and to start with a low dose. Low doses of antidepressant drugs may reduce anxiety, improve the quality of sleep, and reduce pain. If there is evidence that the patient has a depressive disorder it is important to give an adequate dose for an adequate period.

Psychological aspects of care

Many patients have ongoing difficulties in their work or personal relationships. Whether contributors to or consequences of the illness, they may need help to improve their ability to cope with these. For some patients long-term follow-up provides an opportunity to encourage them to persevere with rehabilitation and to minimize the risk of multiple referrals and resulting iatrogenic harm from conflicting advice, repeated medical investigation, and failed attempts at treatment.

Rehabilitation and cognitive behavioural treatment

A systematic review has found that rehabilitative psychological therapy (cognitive behavioural therapy) is more effective than conventional management, with significant improvement rates of 60 per cent and 25 per cent respectively at 12 months. Two trials have suggested that supervised and gradually increased physical activity alone may be effective for willing patients. If available, a general hospital liaison psychiatry or psychology service may be best placed to offer treatment in a setting acceptable to the patient. General rehabilitation services are of value for chronic severe disability.

Other treatments

Many other treatments have been proposed but none has been adequately evaluated. Patients should be discouraged from pursuing unproven treatments unless they are part of a clinical trial.

Prognosis

The prognosis for functional recovery is relatively good for patients seen in general practice. It is poor for those severe enough to be referred to hospital clinics. A long history, multiple symptoms, and entrenched belief that the illness is irreversible predict a particularly poor prognosis. Effective treatment can improve the patient's ability to function. There is no mortality associated with chronic fatigue syndrome other than suicide, which may reflect unrecognized depressive illness.

Prevention

As the cause is unknown there is no specific primary prevention. Secondary prevention is important as it is likely that good early management and avoidance of iatrogenesis will reduce the risk of chronicity.

Other aspects

Occupational, quality of life, and psychological aspects

Chronic fatigue syndrome can be associated with a markedly reduced quality of life. Occupational issues are often prominent. Occupational stress may be an aetiological factor and having chronic fatigue syndrome makes it difficult to sustain employment. The ambiguous status of chronic fatigue syndrome as an accepted disease makes it especially difficult for patients with this diagnosis to negotiate with employers, insurers, and other agencies.

Areas of controversy

Almost all aspects of chronic fatigue syndrome are controversial. Most controversy has centred on whether it is most appropriately regarded as a medical or a psychiatric syndrome. This debate should be seen in the context of the stigma associated with psychiatric illness.

Areas needing further research

Further work is needed into both aetiology and treatment. In particular a refinement of the definition of the syndrome to enable the identification of more homogeneous groups will be important in developing effective treatment.

Further reading

Campling F, Sharpe M (2000). *CFS/ME: the facts.* Oxford University Press, Oxford.

Fukuda K *et al.* (1994). Chronic fatigue syndrome: a comprehensive approach to its definition and management. *Annals of Internal Medicine* **121**, 953–9.

Komaroff AL, Buchwald DS (1998) Chronic fatigue syndrome: an update. *Annual Review of Medicine* **49**, 1–13.

Wessely S, Sharpe M, Hotopf M (1998). *Chronic fatigue and its syndromes.* Oxford University Press, Oxford.

Whiting P, Bagnall A, Sowden A, Cornell JE, Mulrow C, Ramirez G (2001). Interventions for the treatment and management of chronic fatigue syndrome: a systematic review. *Journal of the American Medical Association,* **286**, 1360–8.

7.20 Infection in the immunocompromised host

J. Cohen

One of the most distressing experiences in medicine is to see a patient cured of a serious underlying disease only to die as a result of a complication of the treatment. While the benefits of immunosuppression have been enormous, there is no doubt that unwanted effects, and in particular serious infection, have proved to be a major drawback.

Classification

The term 'immunocompromised host' has no formal definition, but embraces a group of overlapping conditions in which the ability to respond normally to an infective challenge is in some way impaired. Nevertheless, it is helpful to think of such patients falling into one of four broad groups (Fig. 1).

Primary immunodeficiency syndromes

These are patients with congenital defects in immunity that render them more susceptible to infection. At the most extreme, children with severe combined immunodeficiency have virtually no functioning cellular or humoral immunity, and if unprotected will die from infection within a few months of birth. In contrast, some patients with chronic granulomatous disease, an inherited defect of neutrophil function, remain undiagnosed until early adult life. A complete description of the diagnosis and management of this group of disorders is given elsewhere.

Secondary immunodeficiency syndromes

AIDS

AIDS is a model for an acquired defect of immunity leading to an increased risk of infection. Although there are inevitably parallels with other groups of immunocompromised patients, there are particular issues both in the diagnosis and management of infection in AIDS that warrant separate discussion (see Chapter 7.10.21).

Infection related to the underlying condition

The notion of opportunistic infection in the immunocompromised host is most familiar with haematological malignancies or organ transplantation, discussed in detail below. Less obvious, but probably more numerous, are the many physiological conditions and other diseases associated with an increased incidence of infection (Table 1). These immune defects are usually mixed, and frequently poorly characterized, but the clinical problem is real enough. In malnutrition, for example, infection due to mycobacteria and *Salmonella* is more common, and *Pneumocystis carinii* pneumonia was first described in children with protein-calorie malnutrition. There is an extensive literature documenting multiple defects of host defence in association with alcohol abuse; clinically, this is reflected in an excess of lower respiratory tract infections with *Streptococcus pneumoniae*, *M. tuberculosis*, and *Klebsiella pneumoniae*. In Cushing's disease, the excess endogenous steroid production can result in a pattern of opportunistic infections that mirrors that seen in patients receiving steroid therapy (see below). Diabetes mellitus is good example of a disease that is frequently complicated by infection, typically with staphylococcal skin abscesses.

Patients who have had their spleen removed, or who have functional (or more rarely congenital) asplenia, are at increased risk of certain infections. The degree of risk is related to the underlying cause; overall, 4 to 12 per cent will suffer a serious infection, but this varies from 1.5 per cent following traumatic splenectomy to as high as 25 per cent in patients with thalassaemia. Serious infections are most common during the first 5 years following splenectomy, and particularly during the first year; recurrent infections occur in about 20 per cent of those affected. Approximately 50 per cent of infections are meningitis or bacteraemias, and most of the remainder are pneumonias (see Chapter 22.4.4).

Table 1 Examples of conditions associated with impaired immune responses and an increased risk/severity of infection

Extremes of life
Pregnancy
Malnutrition
Trauma/surgery
Haemodialysis
Cushing's disease
Intravenous drug abuse
Down's syndrome
Splenectomy
Alcohol abuse
Spinal cord injury
Burns
Uraemia
Diabetes mellitus
Haemochromatosis
Severe liver disease

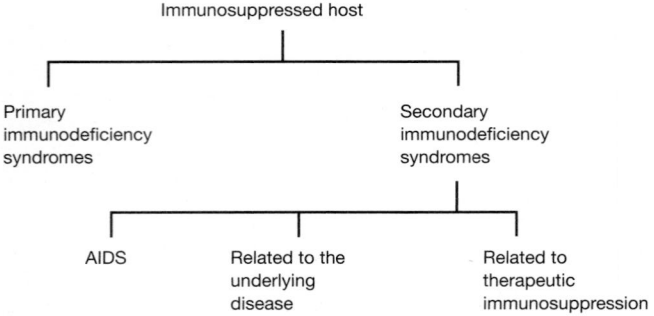

Fig. 1 A classification of the immunocompromised host.

In myeloma and chronic lymphocytic leukaemia the primary defect is hypogammaglobulinaemia, manifested clinically by an excess of bacterial infections, typically those caused by encapsulated organisms such as *Streptococcus pneumoniae* and *Haemophilus influenzae*. These patients (and others, such as those with rheumatoid arthritis, systemic lupus erythematosus, or polyarteritis nodosa) all have impaired immunity as a consequence of their underlying disease, but because they also commonly receive treatment with immunosuppressive drugs it can be very difficult to attribute cause and effect.

Infection complicating therapeutic immunosuppression

In addition to the well-recognized risk groups such as those with haematological malignancy or allograft recipients, infective complications of immunosuppression are now being recognized in a much broader range of patients. Conditions as diverse as severe skin disease, asthma, inflammatory bowel disease, and rheumatoid arthritis are routinely treated with drugs such as prednisolone (typically at doses of 5 to 25 mg/day), azathioprine, cyclosporin, and cyclophosphamide. These patients are not so profoundly immunosuppressed as the recipient of a bone marrow transplant, but they are certainly at risk of opportunistic infections. Any failure to recognize the risk may mean that diagnosis is delayed.

Immunosuppressed patients have multiple risk factors; a recipient of a bone marrow transplant may have been neutropenic, receiving corticosteroids and cyclosporin A for management of graft-versus-host disease, and have an indwelling right atrial catheter for feeding purposes. Clearly each of these factors represents a substantial and very different type of risk factor for infection, and it is important to remember that, in such patients, multiple pathogens can cause disease simultaneously. The following sections describe the management of some of the common clinical syndromes that present as infection in immunosuppressed patients.

Common clinical syndromes

A general approach to management

Infections in immunosuppressed patients can progress with frightening rapidity; the early physical signs are often muted and the microbiology can be confusing. Patients need to be reviewed frequently and will often need empirical therapy, but this need not be totally 'blind'; a structured and informed assessment will generally allow a logical response to what are the most likely pathogens.

The history

This may reveal exposure to community-acquired infections such as varicella zoster or tuberculosis, which can be particularly severe in the immunocompromised patient. Note should be made of any past history of infection; bronchiectasis, for instance, can be very troublesome in transplant recipients. A detailed travel history is important; patients who have visited certain parts of the United States may have been exposed to the systemic mycoses such as histoplasmosis or coccidioidomycosis, which are unfamiliar to many clinicians. Visitors to Central America or the Far East, even many years ago, may have acquired an asymptomatic infection with the helminth *Strongyloides stercoralis*; immunosuppression can lead to overt disease (the hyperinfection syndrome) with a high mortality (see below).

Physical examination

This may be unhelpful; immunosuppressed patients often do not mount a good inflammatory response. Thus there may only be a low-grade fever, a thin serous exudate may suffice for pus, and mild abdominal tenderness be the only sign of peritonitis. Nevertheless, careful, and if necessary repeated, clinical examination is worthwhile, as signs of inflammation may become apparent only when immune function returns. Particular attention should be paid to the presence of new skin lesions. In neutropenic patients bacteraemias may be accompanied by striking embolic lesions; *Pseudomonas*

Fig. 2 A scheme representing a timetable for the development of infective complications in renal transplant and bone marrow transplant recipients.

infections (and less commonly *Klebsiella* and *Aeromonas*) can cause a focal necrotic cellulitis called ecthyma gangrenosum. Fungal infections present as indolent, locally invasive lesions; *Aspergillus* infections often have a black eschar. The perianal area and the insertion sites of indwelling right atrial catheters repay careful examination. Aspiration and/or biopsy of any new skin lesion in immunosuppressed patients is well worthwhile, since it may quickly point to an otherwise inapparent diagnosis. Lymphadenopathy is always important and provides the opportunity for aspiration or biopsy. It is more usually seen as a feature of subacute or chronic complication of immunosuppression. It may be due to direct infection (for example tuberculosis), or as a manifestation of a lymphoproliferative condition secondary to Epstein–Barr virus. Post-transplant lymphoproliferative disease is emerging as one of the major causes of late death following renal transplantation.

Underlying disease

This can provide valuable clues. Neutropenia is a major risk factor for infection, conferring susceptibility to bacteraemias, particularly with Gram-negative organisms such as *Escherichia* and *Pseudomonas*. A patient with an obstructing bronchial neoplasm may develop a lung abscess due to inadequate drainage. Corticosteroids are used widely; when given in doses exceeding 15 to 20 mg daily for long periods they increase susceptibility to infections with viruses, fungi, parasites, and bacteria such as *M. tuberculosis*—all organisms normally associated with cellular immune defences.

Duration of immunosuppression

This often has a profound effect on the type of infection that occurs. This effect is well illustrated by comparing the 'timetables' of infections in renal transplant recipients with these receiving bone marrow transplants (Fig. 2). In the first 6 weeks after a renal transplant bacterial infections predominate, typically complicating the surgery or urinary infections. Between 6 weeks and 6 months post-transplant the patient is most at risk from the 'classical' opportunistic infections; as time continues and the intensity of immunosuppression declines, typical community-acquired infections become more common. In bone marrow transplantation, the initial period of neutropenia is characterized by bacterial infections; later, when many patients receive high-dose steroids for graft-versus-host disease, cytomegalovirus and fungal infections (*Candida* and *Aspergillus*) develop.

Speed of progression

An assessment of this is helpful in both differential diagnosis and in deciding on empirical therapy. In neutropenic patients, the onset of fever is usually an indication for immediate empirical antibiotic therapy (see below). In contrast, the response to a fever and new pulmonary infiltrates in a patient 8 months after renal transplant will depend on the pace of the illness. Rapid deterioration over the space of a few hours will suggest a bacterial infection or a non-infectious cause, and will need urgent therapy; a more indolent presentation would point to a fungal or mycobacterial aetiology, and treatment can be delayed for a short period to try and establish the diagnosis.

Investigations

It is important that the diagnostic laboratories be made aware of the clinical problem, since handling of specimens from immunosuppressed patients—and interpretation of the results—will often differ substantially from routine procedures. In addition, routine screening of transplant recipients and donors should include serological tests for cytomegalovirus, hepatitis B, and HIV.

Pyrexia of unknown origin

In neutropenic patients, fever is often the first and only sign of bacteraemia, and prompt action is necessary. In this situation, a pyrexia of unknown origin is defined as a fever of over 38 °C sustained for 2 h, and not obviously due to an identifiable cause such as concomitant blood transfusion.

The risk of bacteraemia is directly related to the severity of neutropenia; the incidence is greatest at below 1×10^9/litre, and particularly when the count falls to less than 0.1×10^9/litre (Fig. 3). Some years ago, the commonest isolates were Gram-negative bacteria such as *E. coli* and *Klebsiella*, generally derived from the patient's gut flora, and *Ps. aeruginosa*, a common environmental pathogen, especially in hospitals. Gram-negative bacteraemia in neutropenic patients carried a very high mortality, and led to the introduction of a number of preventive strategies such as the use of prophylactic antibiotics and colony stimulating factors. Although these approaches have not been entirely successful, the incidence of Gram-negative bacteraemias has declined substantially, and in most units Gram-positive organisms, notably coagulase negative staphylococci (*Staphylococcus epidermidis*) and viridans streptococci, are now the commonest isolates.

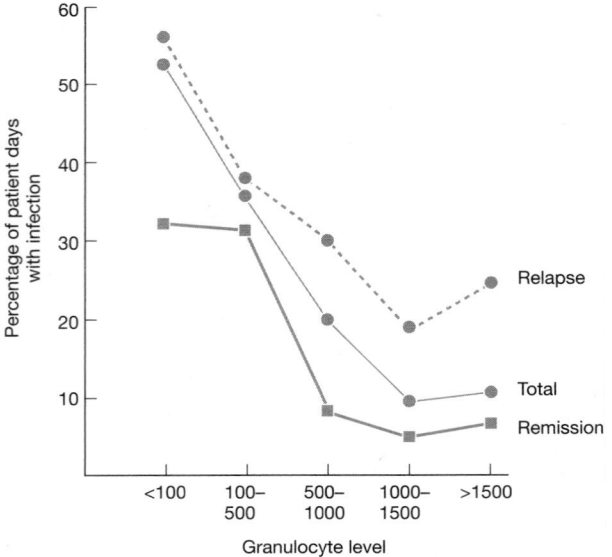

Fig. 3 The relationship between neutrophil count and the risk of invasive Gram-negative infection. (From Bodey G et al. (1966). *Annals of Internal Medicine* **64**, 328–40, with permission.)

The clinical features are entirely non-specific. Occasionally a focus will be suggested by erythema around the point of entry of an indwelling catheter, a finding often associated with staphylococcal infection. Septic shock is infrequent, although it can be associated with viridans streptococci; endocarditis is rare.

Blood cultures should be drawn before treatment is begun. Ideally two sets should be obtained, at least one of which should be from a peripheral vein (rather than an indwelling catheter), although this is not always possible. Culturing larger volumes of blood (for example 30 ml rather than the more conventional 10 ml) increases the yield. Appropriate samples must also be taken from other potential foci of infection. Nevertheless, it has been one of the enduring frustrations of this subject that even the most rigorous of microbiological investigations in the febrile neutropenic patient will yield only some 40 to 50 per cent of positive cultures. The explanation for this is unknown; some studies have suggested that it is due to endotoxaemia in the absence of bacteraemia, but the data are inconclusive. What is clear, however, is that treatment must begin before the results of the cultures are available; delay can kill.

The choice of the initial empirical antibiotic regimen for the febrile neutropenic patient has been the subject of intense investigation. The ideal regimen will be safe and have good bactericidal activity against all the common pathogens. No single regimen is perfect; much will depend on the availability (and cost) of antibiotics in a given institution, and on local patterns of antibiotic susceptibility. Well-validated regimens include the combination of an antipseudomonal penicillin plus an aminoglycoside (for example piperacillin plus gentamicin), or the use of single agents such as a third-generation cephalosporin (for example ceftazidime) or a penem such as meropenem. All these regimens are very active against the common Gram-negative organisms, but are relatively ineffective at treating Gram-positive bacteria such as coagulase negative staphylococci, nowadays a common problem. Unfortunately, the only drugs which are reliably active for these organisms are glycopeptides such as vancomycin, and some clinicians have advocated adding vancomycin to the initial empirical regimen. The disadvantage of this approach is the toxicity (and cost) of vancomycin, which may not be justified since unlike the Gram-negative infections, coagulase negative staphylococci rarely cause death. Several prospective clinical trials have concluded that vancomycin can usually be withheld until the results of blood cultures are known. An alternative strategy under investigation is to use a fourth-generation cephalosporin, such as cefepime, that has an improved spectrum of activity against Gram-positive bacteria while preserving good cover against Enterobacteriaceae and *Pseudomonas aeruginosa*.

In patients who respond to the initial regimen the treatment should be continued for at least 7 days, and ideally until the neutrophil count has returned to more than 0.5×10^9/litre. Sometimes this is not possible; the patient may have a persistent or unresponsive neutropenia (for example in aplastic anaemia or following bone marrow transplant). In these cases treatment is usually stopped cautiously after an arbitrary period such as 14 days; rebound bacteraemias will need further treatment.

A common problem is the patient who continues to have high swinging fevers in the absence of any obvious focus or positive microbiology. In this situation, deep fungal infection becomes more likely. The few clinical trials which have addressed this problem have concluded that persistent fever for 72 h should be treated by the addition of amphotericin B. For patients who are intolerant of amphotericin B or who develop nephrotoxicity, one of the liposomal formulations of the drug can be used; toxicity is greatly diminished and they are of at least equal efficacy, although they are extremely expensive.

Fever of unknown origin in the non-neutropenic immunosuppressed patient is a completely different problem. Fever in this situation is rarely immediately life-threatening, and since there is a wide differential diagnosis it is better to pursue the cause rather than embark on empirical therapy.

Table 2 The aetiology of the 'febrile pneumonitis' syndrome in different patient groups. (Modified from Wilson *et al*. 1985.)

Time since surgery	Renal transplant patients	Bone marrow transplant patients
Less than 1 month	Aspiration Nosocomial LRTI	Aspiration Nosocomial LRTI *Aspergillus*
1–3* months	Cytomegalovirus *Pneumocystis* *Aspergillus* *Nocardia* Mycobacteria *Mucor*	Cytomegalovirus *Pneumocystis* Aspergillus Respiratory syncytial virus Mycobacteria Mucor
More than 3* months	Influenza *Legionella* Common respiratory bacteria	Non-infective causes† Varicella zoster GVHD Common respiratory bacteria and viruses

Abbreviations: LRTI = lower respiratory tract infection; GVHD = graft-versus-host disease.
*6 months in renal transplants.
†Includes idiopathic interstitial pneumonitis in bone marrow transplant recipients.

Fever and new pulmonary infiltrates

The development of fever and new pulmonary infiltrates is one of the most challenging clinical problems in this group of patients. Pneumonia is the commonest infective cause of death in immunocompromised patients. In the presence of diffuse airspace disease the mortality approaches 50 per cent irrespective of the underlying defect in host defence, although the epidemiology varies between different patient groups and with the intensity of the immunosuppression (Table 2).

The condition can progress extremely quickly, and conventional diagnostic procedures may be unhelpful. The list of possible causes is so daunting (Table 3) that clinicians can be tempted to use multiple empirical antimicrobial agents, sometimes to the patient's detriment. It is often not possible to 'guess' with any certainty the precise cause of the problem and multiple causes may be present . But considering the available information it may be possible to construct a 'short-list' to guide further investigation and treatment.

The initial evaluation should follow the approach outlined above, in particular making an assessment of the intensity of the immunosuppression and the speed of progression of the pulmonary disease. The main purpose is to determine the need for empirical therapy, either because the clinical picture is suggestive of a 'simple' bacterial pneumonia, or because of a potentially more serious, progressive cause of uncertain aetiology. Factors favouring bacterial aetiology include neutropenia, a rapidly developing

Table 3 Causes of fever and new pulmonary infiltrates in the immunocompromised host

Causative agent	Organism/disease
Bacterial infection	
Conventional respiratory pathogens	*S. pneumoniae*, *H. influenzae*, *Klebsiella*
Nosocomial pathogens	*E. coli*; *Pseudomonas* spp. *Legionella* spp.
'Atypical' organisms	*Chlamydia psittaci*, *C. pneumoniae*, *Mycoplasma*
Mycobacteria and related organisms	*M. tuberculosis*, atypical mycobacteria, *Nocardia*
Other unusual organisms	*Listeria*, *Bacillus* spp.
Viral infection	
Herpes viruses	Cytomegalovirus, herpes simplex, varicella zoster
Respiratory viruses	Respiratory syncytial virus; (para)influenza; adenovirus; measles
Fungal infection	
Systemic mycoses	Blastomycosis, histoplasmosis, coccidioidomycosis
Opportunist mycoses	*Candida, Aspergillus, Mucor, Cryptococcus*
Other rare fungi	*Trichosporon, Pseudallescheria*
Parasitic infection	*Pneumocystis, Strongyloides, Toxoplasma*
Pulmonary pathology	Pulmonary oedema; pulmonary infarction/emboli
	Pulmonary haemorrhage
	Primary or secondary malignancy
Other causes	Drugs (e.g. busulfan)
	Activity of the underlying disease (e.g. SLE)
	Radiation pneumonitis

SLE = systemic lupus erythematosus.

Table 4 Organisms causing neurological infections in different patient groups

	Bacteria	Fungi	Parasites	Viruses
Neutropenia	Enterics	*Candida* *Aspergillus* *Mucor*		
T-cell/ monocyte defect	*Listeria* *Legionella* *Nocardia* Mycobacteria	*Cryptococcus* *Aspergillus* *Mucor* Coccidioides	*Toxoplasma* *Strongyloides*	Varicella zoster Herpes simplex Papovavirus
Splenectomy	*S. pneumoniae* *H. influenzae* *Neisseria*			

clinical evolution (for example deterioration over a period of 12 h), progressive hypoxia, a sputum Gram stain showing a marked predominance of a single bacterial morphology (even in the absence of neutrophils), or a chest radiographic appearance that has worsened over a short period. High fever is not necessarily a part of this syndrome; it is important to emphasize that this rapidly evolving clinical picture is not inevitably due to infection. Non-infective causes such as acute lung haemorrhage or pulmonary oedema can present in an identical fashion, and the most appropriate therapy may be diuretics rather than antimicrobials. However, antimicrobials will often need to be given as well because of what has been termed 'infection-provoked relapse'. In immunologically mediated diseases such as systemic lupus erythematosus or antiglomerular basement membrane disease (Goodpasture's syndrome) infection can precipitate a relapse of the underlying disease. Thus, the development of fever and new pulmonary shadows in a patient with antiglomerular basement membrane disease may be primarily due to lung haemorrhage associated with a rise in antiglomerular basement membrane antibodies, but this in turn can be precipitated by an infection that need not necessarily be in the lung. Treatment must be directed both towards improving oxygenation and the underlying infection.

Blood cultures should always be obtained, and attempts made to obtain sputum. A chest radiograph and arterial blood gas analysis are essential. The initial treatment will be dictated by the clinical circumstances, but it is best to avoid a complex regimen to provide very broad spectrum cover. Rapid clinical deterioration is usually attributable to bacterial infections; if community acquired, a combination of an extended-spectrum cephalosporin plus erythromycin is appropriate. For hospital-acquired infections, a cephalosporin (combined with an aminoglycoside if there is strong evidence of *Pseudomonas* infection) is reasonable. Where staphylococcal infection is suspected, flucloxacillin plus an aminoglycoside should be used. Unusual ('opportunist') organisms such as mycobacteria, *Nocardia*, or cytomegalovirus rarely cause such a rapid clinical deterioration and are difficult to distinguish on clinical grounds alone. For these reasons, the addition of further empirical agents is usually not warranted.

In patients in whom immediate empirical therapy is not necessary, additional diagnostic procedures can be performed. These should include serological tests for atypical organisms, and examination of blood and urine for cytomegalovirus (tests for cytomegalovirus early antigen are very helpful). The chest radiograph should be repeated, but it is not as sensitive as arterial blood gas measurements, which should be done twice daily. The radiographic appearances are rarely sufficiently specific to suggest a precise diagnosis, although they can be suggestive. Thus a bilateral interstitial midzone infiltrate associated with marked hypoxia is typical of *Pneumocystis* pneumonia, and a pleural based infarct is suggestive of *Aspergillus*. However, there are pitfalls in relying on the radiographic appearance alone in guiding the choice of therapy. First, no radiographic appearance is pathognomonic of any single pathological process; cytomegalovirus or pulmonary oedema can mimic *Pneumocystis* pneumonia, for example, and *Legionella* pneumonia cannot be distinguished from *Aspergillus*. Secondly, multiple agents can coexist, each requiring separate treatment. Other imaging techniques, such

as computed tomography (**CT**), can often provide useful additional information on the extent of the process, and will sometimes point to the cause (for example the 'halo sign' associated with invasive aspergillosis).

It is often appropriate to try and make a specific diagnosis by obtaining material directly from the bronchial tree. In most cases the method of choice is bronchoscopy with bronchoalveolar lavage. This will provide adequate material without incurring a serious risk of bleeding (many such patients are thrombocytopenic) or pneumothorax. In most series, bronchial brush or transbronchial biopsy specimens produce only a marginal increase in the diagnostic yield, and are usually not done unless the clinical picture is suggestive of a non-infective process such as an infiltrating tumour. The highest yield is from open lung biopsy, but this should not usually be done as a first-line procedure.

Acute neurological syndromes

A large number of conventional and opportunist pathogens can lead to neurological infection in immunocompromised patients. Although there is some degree of overlap, the underlying defect in host defence is a often a good indicator of the likely cause (Table 4).

The clinical features may help suggest the diagnosis. Meningitic syndromes are more likely to be associated with conventional bacterial infections, listeriosis, and tuberculosis, as well as fungi such as *Cryptococcus* and *Candida*. In contrast, infections with *Toxoplasma*, *Aspergillus*, or *Nocardia* more commonly present as space-occupying lesions. Pure encephalitic syndromes are less common, but can occur with herpes simplex. Rhinocerebral mucormycosis is a progressive, destructive infection caused by *Mucor* and related moulds, that usually begins in the paranasal sinuses and spreads caudally to involve the orbits or the frontal lobes of the brain. It is seen particularly in patients with uncontrolled diabetes mellitus or as a complication of neutropenia.

Bacterial infections generally proceed rapidly, while fungi and parasites pursue a more indolent course. However, exceptions to this are common, and there is no substitute for obtaining a precise diagnosis. Examination of the skin (see below) and fundoscopy may be valuable. Retinitis is not usually a feature of systemic infection with toxoplasma or cytomegalovirus; in contrast, *Candida* endophthalmitis may be the only manifestation of deep-seated infection.

Examination of the cerebrospinal fluid is mandatory. A high index of suspicion is necessary, since the clinical features of meningitis are often muted in these patients. An unexplained low-grade fever and mild headache may be the only clues; frank meningism, photophobia, or focal neurological signs occur late. Examination of the cerebrospinal fluid should include direct microscopy (neutrophil, lymphocyte, or eosinophil pleocytosis) and culture for (myco)bacteria and fungi, a cryptococcal latex agglutination test, antigen tests for pneumococcus, and a search for specific antibody production (for example for coccidioidomycosis) or DNA sequences by the polymerase chain reaction (for example for herpes simplex and papovaviruses).

Some organisms are rarely seen by direct microscopy: Mycobacteria are seen in fewer than 10 per cent of cases, *Nocardia* and *Aspergillus* only very rarely. A predominance of lymphocytes suggests partially treated bacterial infection, tuberculosis, or a viral aetiology but not infection with *Listeria*, despite its name. A low cerebrospinal fluid glucose points to tuberculosis but is not specific. Sometimes the only abnormality is a modest elevation of the cerebrospinal fluid protein; this should never be ignored, even in the seeming absence of other features of neurological infection. Where appropriate, cytological examination of the cerebrospinal fluid should be done to exclude carcinomatous or leukaemic meningitis, which can mimic an acute infective presentation.

Certain neurological infections are often associated with pulmonary disease; these include *Legionella*, tuberculosis, *Aspergillus*, *Mucor*, and *Nocardia*. A brain CT scan, which should be contrast-enhanced, is valuable. Focal, usually enhancing, lesions are particularly associated with pyogenic abscesses and toxoplasmosis. Tuberculomas can appear as single lesions. Magnetic resonance imaging is better then CT scanning for detecting abnormalities of the brainstem (for example the basal meningitis associated with cryptococcal infection), and frequently reveals lesions in toxoplasmosis which are not seen on CT scans. It may pre-empt the need for brain biopsy when a diagnosis of progressive multifocal leucoencephalitis is considered.

Any new skin lesions should be biopsied. Nasal biopsy may reveal *Mucor*. An electroencephalogram is not helpful, unless herpes encephalitis is suspected. Brain biopsy is done rarely; it should not be considered unless empirical therapy has failed, or there is a real prospect of therapeutic benefit to the patient.

If the cerebrospinal fluid is non-diagnostic but bacterial infection cannot be excluded, empirical antibiotics should be given immediately. An extended spectrum cephalosporin such as cefotaxime is suitable. Serological tests for toxoplasmosis are not specific in this setting, and if the infection is suspected it is better to start empirical therapy with pyrimethamine and sulphadiazine. Cerebral aspergillosis and mucormycosis have a very poor prognosis; treatment should be begun with high-dose amphotericin B, and surgical debridement considered if possible. There is no effective treatment for progressive multifocal leucoencephalitis.

Acute gastrointestinal syndromes

The organisms associated with specific gastrointestinal syndromes in these patients are shown in Table 5.

Severe stomatitis is a common complaint in immunosuppressed patients. The three commonest causes: *Candida*, herpes simplex, and chemotherapy-induced mucositis are clinically indistinguishable and indeed can coexist and cause disease together. For these reasons, the diagnosis should always be confirmed by microscopy and culture. Herpetic stomatitis in particular can be atypical in these patients; the classical appearance of groups of small vesicles is unusual, and a more common presentation is ulceration, which can be extensive. In profoundly immunosuppressed patients such as bone marrow transplant recipients, oral candidiasis is very common, and in patients who are seropositive before

transplant, reactivation of herpes simplex is almost universal. For these reasons, prophylaxis is usually given. Both herpes simplex and *Candida* can cause oesophagitis, generally (but not exclusively) as an extension of oral disease. Oesophagoscopy with brush cytology and/or biopsy is the investigation of choice. Proven oesophageal candidiasis should be regarded as 'invasive' disease and treated with systemic antifungals (amphotericin B or fluconazole).

A large number of organisms can cause acute diarrhoeal syndromes; in addition, non-infective conditions such as radiation enteritis, drugs, and graft-versus-host disease must be included in the differential diagnosis. There are no distinguishing clinical features of note, and diagnosis depends on microbiological examination of the faeces.

The diarrhoea caused by *Clostridium difficile* is usually due to a pseudomembranous colitis. However, patients with leukaemia or aplastic anaemia may develop neutropenic enterocolitis (previously called typhlitis), a fulminating invasive colitis characterized by diffuse dilation and oedema of the bowel walls, haemorrhage, ulceration, and a high mortality. Classically this has been associated with clostridial bacteraemia, in particular *C. septicum*, but other clostridia, including *C. difficile*, and even Gram-negative bacteria, can also be found.

Strongyloides stercoralis is a nematode that can be carried asymptomatically for many years after exposure (see Chapter 7.14.4). Strongyloidiasis has been recognized as a complication of HTLV-I infection, and also occurs secondary to immunosuppression (typically with high-dose steroids and in recipients of solid organ transplants). A rise in the worm burden results in the hyperinfection syndrome, which may present as pneumonitis or intermittent intestinal obstruction. Worms moving through the gut wall can carry with them enteric bacteria, resulting in polymicrobial bacteraemias and Gram-negative meningitis when the worms invade the cerebrospinal fluid.

Giardiasis is particularly associated with hypogammaglobulinaemia, and curiously is rarely seen in other groups. *Cryptosporidium*, *Microsporidia*, and *Isospora* are now well recognized causes of severe and sometimes chronic diarrhoea in AIDS patients, but may also occur in other less severely immunocompromised patients. Among the viruses, the most difficult problem is cytomegalovirus. Cytomegalovirus can cause a severe colitis, and in these cases ganciclovir is beneficial. The diagnosis should be confirmed by biopsy, but ultimately may depend on the result of a therapeutic trial since demonstration of the organism does not necessarily indicate that it is causing disease.

Mild abnormalities of liver function tests are a common accompaniment of many systemic infections, but hepatitis is a particular feature of both toxoplasmosis and cytomegalovirus infection. An increased prevalence of hepatitis B has been found in patients on chronic haemodialysis (10 per cent), and those with Hodgkin's disease (8 per cent) and lepromatous leprosy (20 per cent). The acute hepatitic episode is mild, often anicteric, and may pass unnoticed. However, persistent viral replication (hepatitis e antigenaemia) and the development of complications associated with chronic infection are more likely. Although it is likely that infection with the other

Table 5 Gastrointestinal syndromes in the immunocompromised host

	Bacteria	Fungi	Parasites	Viruses
Oral infection		Candida		Herpes simplex
Diarrhoeal syndromes	Neutropenic enterocolitis C.difficile Salmonella/Shigella Atypical mycobacteria	Candida	Giardia Isospora Cryptosporidia Microsporidia	Enterovirus Adenovirus Cytomegalovirus Rotavirus
Hepatic syndromes		Candida	Toxoplasma	Cytomegalovirus Hepatitis B and C Herpes simplex Varicella zoster

hepatitis viruses occurs in immunosuppressed patients there are as yet no detailed clinical or epidemiological data that define the problem.

A particular form of systemic candidiasis has been called chronic hepatosplenic candidiasis (although other organs can be involved, and the syndrome is better referred to as chronic systemic candidiasis). The patient presents with unremitting fever and occasionally abdominal pain; palpable hepatomegaly is unusual. Typically the neutrophil count has returned to normal after a recent course of chemotherapy for acute leukaemia; the liver function tests show a markedly raised alkaline phosphatase and there may be hyperbilirubinaemia, but microbiological investigations (including blood cultures) are negative. The diagnosis is made by ultrasonography or CT scan of the abdomen, which reveals multiple intrahepatic (or less commonly splenic) abscesses. Unfortunately biopsy of these lesions reveals histological or culture evidence of *Candida* in only about a third of cases. Treatment has been difficult; conventional therapy with amphotericin B (even with the addition of flucytosine) has often failed, but the use of a liposomal formulation of amphotericin B and fluconazole has produced encouraging results.

Further reading

Fishman JA, Rubin RH (1998). Infection in organ-transplant recipients. *New England Journal of Medicine* **338**, 1741–51.

Klastersky J (1995). *Infectious complications of cancer*. Kluwer Academic, Boston.

Meunier F (1995). *Invasive fungal infections in cancer patients. Baillière's clinical infectious diseases*. Baillière Tindall, London.

Pizzo PA (1999). Fever in immunocompromised patients. *New England Journal of Medicine* **341**, 893–900.

Rosenow EC, Wilson WR, Cockerill FR (1985). Pulmonary disease in the immunocompromised host I. *Mayo Clinic Proceedings* **60**, 473–87.

Rubin RH, Young LS (1994). *Clinical approach to infection in the compromised host*, 3rd edn. Plenum, New York.

Warnock DW, Richardson MD (1991). *Fungal infection in the compromised patient*, 2nd edn. Wiley, Chichester.

Wilson WR, Cockerill FR, Rosenow EC (1985). Pulmonary disease in the immunocompromised host II. *Mayo Clinic Proceedings* **60**, 610–31.

8

Chemical and physical injuries and environmental factors and disease

8.1 Poisoning by drugs and chemicals

A. T. Proudfoot and J. A. Vale

Introduction

In the minds of most people, not least those of doctors, the term poisoning suggests an acute event demanding immediate care and attention. This is often so, but poisoning may take other forms. The consequence is not always immediate even after a single dose—so-called acute poisoning. Prolonged uptake may result in accumulation, as with many heavy metals, and the damage may arise only after prolonged exposure—that is, chronic poisoning.

Exposure by oral, inhalational, cutaneous, or other routes, should not itself be equated with poisoning. Uptake is necessary for there to be a toxic effect, and even if this occurs, poisoning does not necessarily result, as the amount absorbed may be too small.

If true poisoning does occur, the ensuing clinical syndrome may be distinctive. For example, fixed dilated pupils, exaggerated tendon reflexes, extensor plantar responses, depressed respiration, and cardiac tachyarrhythmias suggest tricyclic antidepressant poisoning. Anaemia, constipation, colic, and motor nerve palsies are indicative of lead poisoning. However, with a whole range of psychotropic medications there may be only non-specific central nervous depression, respiratory impairment, and hypotension. In some instances, distinctive sequelae may not appear until many years have elapsed as, for example, with carcinoma of the oesophagus following ingestion of corrosives or hepatic haemangiosarcoma from vinyl chloride exposure.

Poisoning may be accidental or deliberate. It is usually accidental in small children, but in adults it is invariably deliberate with parasuicidal, suicidal, or rarely, homicidal intent.

Thus, the medical approach to poisoning should never be confined to the poison and its effects. All the circumstances surrounding the episode must be taken into account, especially in cases where litigation may follow, for example in the event of an occupational mishap with a chemical. It is therefore important that the doctor concerned, having instituted any necessary life-saving measures, should take a careful history, retain all pertinent evidence such as suicide notes and biological specimens, and make a meticulous record of symptoms, signs, progress, and outcome.

Epidemiology

Few health-care professionals would deny that poisoning, accidental or deliberate, is a common problem in most countries throughout the world. Yet it is remarkably difficult to obtain reliable statistics on the morbidity or mortality it causes, even in countries with comparatively advanced systems for collection of population health data. In the developing world, about 600 000 deaths/year are attributed to deliberate self-harm, the majority from poisoning with pesticides such as organophosphorus insecticides. The following observations are based primarily on statistics from the United Kingdom and the United States but, wherever appropriate, observed variations in patterns of poisoning in other countries are noted.

Hospital admissions due to poisoning

Poisoning from accidental or deliberate ingestion or inhalation of drugs or chemicals is a common acute medical emergency requiring hospital admission. In the period 1957 to 1976, the annual number of hospital admissions due to acute poisoning in England and Wales rose steadily from less than 20 000 to more than 125 000. Since then, there has been a decline in the incidence of self-poisoning in England to approximately 100 000 admissions each year. Despite this decline, self-poisoning still accounts for more than 10 per cent of acute adult medical admissions in the United Kingdom. However, the true incidence of self poisoning may be as much as three times that of the hospital admission rate.

In the United Kingdom, with the exception of young children, females predominate in all age groups in those admitted to hospital because of acute poisoning and there is a marked preponderance in those aged 15 to 44 years. Many paediatric episodes are poisoning scares, rather than true poisonings, though this often only becomes clear in retrospect. The majority of adults who poison themselves are not suicidal.

In Western Europe and North America, drugs have always been the most common agents taken by adults and rank second only to household products as the substances most often ingested by children. In the United Kingdom, alcohol is taken in addition to the drug overdose in 60 per cent of males and 40 per cent of females, and at least one-third of self-poisoning episodes involve one or more drugs. Approximately two-thirds of adults ingest drugs that have been bought in retail outlets or prescribed for themselves or a close relative. Therefore, the pattern of pharmaceutical agents used for self-poisoning reflects prescribing habits (particularly for illnesses occurring in those aged 15 to 44 years) and common symptoms that are self-treated. Barbiturate and non-barbiturate hypnotics are now seldom encountered causes of poisoning, while use of other psychotropic agents such as the benzodiazepines, tricyclic antidepressants, and selective serotonin-specific reuptake inhibitors in overdose is now more frequent; analgesic poisoning also occurs much more commonly than previously.

Within Europe there are variations from country to country. In Finland, for example, alcohol, cardiovascular drugs, and psychotropics are the most common causes of poisoning. Outside Europe, and in developing countries in particular, the situation is often very different. In Sri Lanka, for example, agrochemicals account for nearly 60 per cent of all poisonings; such agents account for less than 1 per cent of hospital admissions for poisoning in England and Wales. In South Africa, the pattern of poisoning in the white population mirrors that in North America and Western Europe, whereas that observed in black South Africans is very different, with kerosene (paraffin) and traditional medicines accounting for the majority of hospital admissions (and deaths) attributable to poisoning. In countries where malaria is prevalent, poisoning by antimalarials is an additional cause of morbidity and mortality.

Deaths from poisoning

The number of deaths from poisoning is to some extent determined by the lethality of the agents involved. This, in turn, results in regional differences with rates that are often much higher in developing countries.

In contrast to the rise in the number of hospital admissions for poisoning in England and Wales, deaths from acute poisoning have decreased over the last 40 years and, since 1972, they have remained virtually constant at 4000 per annum. The lack of change over the last 30 years is particularly striking because this period follows the substitution of 'natural gas' for 'town gas', which led directly to a fall in carbon monoxide deaths from nearly 4000 in 1963 to just over 1000 per annum 10 years later.

Despite relatively little change in the overall mortality statistics for acute poisoning in England and Wales, there have been very substantial changes in the agents responsible. Deaths from barbiturate and non-barbiturate hypnotics have fallen, while those due to analgesics and psychotropic agents have risen. Deaths from carbon monoxide have shown a slow but steady increase since 1975, reaching just over 1500 in 1991. Increasing numbers of young men (14 to 24 years) in the United Kingdom are killing themselves. Self-poisoning with car exhaust fumes (containing carbon monoxide) is currently the most common means of doing so.

In England and Wales, about 80 per cent of individuals who die as a result of poisoning do so at home, the inpatient mortality being less than 1 per cent of all cases admitted to hospital. The age and sex distribution of deaths attributed to acute poisoning is significantly different from that for admissions—there are fewer patients in the age range 15 to 44 years and more in the older age categories where males predominate. A similar pattern of causes of death has been observed elsewhere in Western Europe and in North America, but in many developing agricultural countries, agrochemicals (cholinesterase inhibitors, paraquat, aluminium phosphide, and other pesticides) more commonly predominate. On a global scale, it has been estimated that pesticides account annually for 1 million serious unintentional poisonings and 2 million people admitted to hospital for suicide attempts, predominantly in developing countries.

Childhood poisoning

It is estimated that in the United Kingdom as many as 41 000 poison exposures occur in children aged 4 years or less each year. In the United States, the Toxic Exposure Surveillance System (TESS) of the American Association of Poison Control Centers for 2000 records 1 142 796 poison exposures in children less than 6 years of age.

Children aged less than 5 years are particularly active and exploratory and have a strong impulse to put things into their mouths. These characteristics predispose to accidental poisoning, which in Western Europe is particularly likely to occur when parents are inattentive or neglectful, as at times of family crises. The vast majority (80 to 85 per cent) of cases occur in the child's own home, and in many instances the substances involved are out of their usual storage place or have been put into some other container; grandparents, for example, may find it convenient to remove drugs from child-resistant closures or leave the caps off containers because they themselves have difficulty opening this type of packaging.

A child may also be poisoned by an adult who administers a toxic substance by mistake, and rarely a parent or carer may poison a child as a form of abuse, sometimes with fatal consequences. In addition, older (typically 10 to 16 years) emotionally disturbed children may deliberately poison themselves. Abuse of volatile substances is a continuing problem in adolescents.

Further reading

Casey P, Vale JA (1994). Deaths from pesticide poisoning in England and Wales: 1945–1989. *Human and Experimental Toxicology* **13**, 95–101.

Eddleston M (2000). Patterns and problems of deliberate self-poisoning in the developing world. *Quarterly Journal of Medicine* **93**, 715–31.

Fingerhut LA, Cox CS (1998). Poisoning mortality 1985–1995. *Public Health Report* **113**, 218–33.

Hawton K, Fagg J, Simkin S (1996). Deliberate self-poisoning and self-injury in children and adolescents under 16 years of age in Oxford, 1976–1993. *British Journal of Psychiatry* **169**, 202–8.

Hoppe-Roberts JM, Lloyd LM, Chyka PA (2000). Poisoning mortality in the United States: comparison of national mortality statistics and poison control center reports. *Annals of Emergency Medicine* **35**, 440–8.

Kasilo OMJ, Nhachi CFB (1992). A pattern of acute poisoning in children in urban Zimbabwe: ten years experience. *Human and Experimental Toxicology* **11**, 335–40.

Litovitz TL *et al.* (2001). 2000 Annual Report of the American Association of Poison Control Centers Toxic Exposure Surveillance System. *American Journal of Emergency Medicine* **19**, 337–95.

Owens D *et al.* (1994). Outcome of deliberate self-poisoning. An examination of risk factors for repetition. *British Journal of Psychiatry* **165**, 797–801.

Pickett W *et al.* (1998). Suicide mortality and pesticide use among Canadian farmers. *American Journal of Industrial Medicine* **34**, 364–72.

Shepherd G, Klein-Schwartz W (1998). Accidental and suicidal adolescent poisoning deaths in the United States, 1979–1994. *Archives of Pediatric and Adolescent Medicine* **152**, 1181–5.

Tay SY *et al.* (1998). Patients admitted to an intensive care unit for poisoning. *Annals of the Academy of Medicine of Singapore* **27**, 347–52.

Woolf AD, Lovejoy FH Jr (1993). Epidemiology of drug overdose in children. *Drug Safety* **9**, 291–308.

Diagnosis

Ideally, the diagnosis of acute poisoning requires that the doctor establish the chemical composition of the poison, the magnitude of the exposure, and the route of exposure (whether by ingestion, injection, inhalation, or skin contamination), so that the features likely to develop can be anticipated and the risk assessed. As in any other branch of medicine, diagnosis of acute poisoning is based on the patient's history and on a combination of circumstantial evidence, the findings on physical examination, and appropriate investigations when a history is not available. However, in acute poisoning, there are many obstacles to establishing the information required. Young children may not be able to give a history and adults are often unreliable while physical signs are rarely diagnostic. Similarly, circumstantial evidence may not be available, be only tentative or misleading, and laboratory diagnosis can never be fully comprehensive.

History

Since accidental poison exposure in childhood is most common between the ages of 9 months and 5 years, an unequivocal history is unlikely to be forthcoming from the victim but may be obtainable from older witnesses. Clearly, however, statements about amounts must be interpreted with caution since knowledge of the quantities in original containers is frequently inaccurate or unknown.

In contrast, 90 per cent or more of adults presenting with acute poisoning are conscious or only slightly drowsy and there would seem little reason why diagnosis of self-poisoning on the basis of the history should be difficult. Indeed, while a small number of patients adamantly deny having taken a poison, the majority usually admit to it without hesitation, although problems often arise in trying to establish precisely the nature and quantity of what has been taken. Comparison of patients' statements with the agents detected by laboratory analysis of blood or urine consistently reveals major differences in about half the cases. In consequence, patients are often thought to be deliberately untruthful. However, surprise at these findings may merely reveal a lack of medical insight into the circumstances under which self-poisoning occurs. It is commonly an impulsive act; the patient ingests the contents of the first bottle that comes to hand, often when under the influence of alcohol. Moreover, although about 60 per cent of episodes involve drugs prescribed for the victims or their relatives, like many other patients, they are often ignorant of their names.

If these considerations make it difficult to establish the nature of the poison, it is hardly surprising that they should make the amounts involved even more suspect. Few patients count the number of tablets they consume and it is impossible for patient or doctor to know what constitutes a 'handful', 'bottleful', or similar arbitrary quantity.

Circumstantial evidence

Circumstantial evidence becomes important in the diagnosis of acute poisoning when patients are either unable to give a history (for example young children, adults who have severe learning difficulties or who are demented, and unconscious patients) or are unwilling to do so. However, although circumstantial evidence may strongly suggest poisoning, it is seldom incontrovertible. It takes several forms.

Circumstances under which found

The mother may return to the kitchen or bathroom to find her child with some substance all over his hands, face, and clothing, or surrounded by pills, one of which he is eating. The assumption that more has been ingested may or may not be correct and the amount swallowed is a matter of speculation. Similarly, adults may be found unconscious with tablet particles around the mouth or on clothing as the only clue to diagnosis. More often, the presence of empty drug containers with occasional tablets or capsules nearby suggests the diagnosis. Less commonly, they are found unconscious or dead in some remote location. The lack of personal effects to indicate who they are or where they live may suggest a desire not to be identified and should arouse suspicion of drug overdosage. Self-poisoning is a common cause of coma in previously healthy young adults. Protestations by relatives that patients would never take overdoses are usually wrong.

Suicide notes

Suicide notes are reliable indicators of drug overdose in the absence of physical violence as a cause of coma. The note may specify what has been taken in addition to expressing despair, futility, worthlessness, and remorse.

Features

There are few symptoms or physical signs that cannot be attributed to one poison or another. However, a clinical feature rarely arises in isolation and clusters of features are of much greater diagnostic value. Those most commonly encountered in present-day practice are given in Table 1.

Conscious patients with abnormal behaviour, who may be experiencing auditory and visual hallucinations, may have ingested amphetamines, phencyclidine, LSD (lysergic acid diethylamide), 'magic' (psilocybin-containing) mushrooms, and drugs such as the older antihistamines and tri-

cyclic antidepressants that have marked anticholinergic actions. Occasionally a patient with severe salicylate intoxication, who cannot give a history despite being conscious, is hyperventilating, sweating, flushed, and tachycardic, suggesting a diagnosis which can then be confirmed analytically.

Drowsiness, ataxia, dysarthria, and nystagmus are common after ingestion of benzodiazepines. Coma with hypotonia and hyporeflexia may follow, particularly if alcohol has also been taken. Hypotension, hypothermia, and respiratory depression are rare. All of these features, however, may occur after overdosage with outmoded drugs such as barbiturates, methaqualone, meprobamate, and ethchlorvynol that are still occasionally prescribed. In present-day clinical practice, tricyclic antidepressants remain among the most common central nervous system (CNS) depressants encountered in overdose. They cause hypertonia, hyperreflexia, extensor plantar responses, and dilated pupils. Sinus tachycardia and prolongation of the QRS interval on the electrocardiogram support a diagnosis of intoxication with these drugs. Hypotension and hypothermia are less common features. Tricyclic antidepressants and non-steroidal anti-inflammatory agents, particularly mefenamic acid, are the most common causes of seizures after drug overdosage. Coma with pinpoint pupils and a reduced respiratory rate is virtually diagnostic of overdosage with opioid analgesics and is an indication for a therapeutic trial of naloxone. Many patients with opioid poisoning will be habitual drug abusers and have venepuncture marks and evidence of venous tracking in the antecubital fossae. Alcohol may be smelt on the breath, as may solvents such as toluene, acetone, or xylene as the result of 'sniffing' glues, cleaning agents, or other preparations. Skin blisters occur in poisoning by many drugs (see below) but rarely in coma due to other causes. Burns around the lips or in the buccal cavity or pharynx indicate ingestion of corrosives, including paraquat.

Lateralizing neurological signs

Since most serious poisonings are associated with impairment of consciousness, neurological signs are particularly important. Lateralizing signs (unless they are attributable to a known neurological disease) virtually exclude a diagnosis of acute poisoning. Such findings have been recorded with barbiturate and phenytoin overdose but so rarely that the general rule is not significantly compromised. A possible exception is transient inequality of pupil size. This has been reported only rarely in acute poisoning but is not an uncommon finding in normal individuals (for instance due to Holmes–Adie pupils); clinical experience suggests that it occurs more frequently in poisoning than seems apparent from the literature.

Decerebrate and decorticate movements

Unconscious poisoned patients may respond to painful stimuli with flexor and extensor limb movements of the type seen in decorticate and decerebrate states. However, in poisoning, these signs do not indicate irreversible brain damage and patients showing them can be expected to recover fully. Hypoglycaemia must be excluded in these cases.

Strabismus, and internuclear and external ophthalmoplegia

A variety of ocular signs including strabismus, internuclear ophthalmoplegia, and total external opthalmoplegia, may be found in acutely poisoned patients. They are also features of Wernicke's encephalopathy in chronic alcohol abusers.

Strabismus has been described in poisoning with phenytoin, carbamazepine, and tricyclic antidepressants. Usually the optic axes diverge in the horizontal plane but in some patients there is additional vertical deviation. It is present transiently and only in patients who are unconscious. Dysconjugate, roving eye movements may also be seen if both eyes are observed for a period of time. It is important to know that such abnormalities occur so that they are not misattributed to intracranial vascular lesions or some other pathology requiring surgical intervention.

Table 1 Common feature clusters

Feature cluster	Likely poisons
Coma, hypertonia, hyperreflexia, extensor plantar responses, myoclonus, strabismus, mydriasis, sinus tachycardia	Tricyclic antidepressants—less commonly orphenadrine, thioridazine
Coma, hypotonia, hyporeflexia, plantar responses which are flexor or non-elicitable, hypotension	Barbiturates, benzodiazepine and alcohol combinations, severe tricyclic antidepressant poisoning
Coma, miosis, reduced respiratory rate	Opioid analgesics
Nausea, vomiting, tinnitus, deafness, sweating, hyperventilation, vasodilation, tachycardia	Salicylates
Restlessness, agitation, mydriasis, anxiety, tremor, tachycardia, convulsions, arrhythmias	Sympathomimetics

Dysconjugate eye movements may become apparent only when vestibulo-ocular reflexes are examined by caloric stimuli. Installation of ice-cold water into the external auditory meatus should make both eyes turn to the side irrigated and failure of one eye to deviate is evidence of internuclear ophthalmoplegia and a lesion of the medial longitudinal fasciculus. This has been reported in poisoning with a variety of drugs including tricyclic antidepressants, phenothiazines, benzodiazepines, barbiturates, and ethanol and can be detected in 10 per cent of cases if caloric tests are carried out. Both sides are usually affected but internuclear ophthalmoplegia also occurs on one side only in acute poisoning.

In some cases, cold-induced lateral eye movements are followed after an interval of 5 to 15 s by forced downward gaze lasting several minutes, but the suggestion that the latter may be diagnostic of drug-induced coma requires further study before acceptance.

It is widely accepted that absence of oculocervical (abnormal 'doll's eye' responses) and vestibulo-ocular responses indicates severe brainstem damage and the likelihood that the patient will not survive. However, this is not the case in acute poisoning where these reflexes may be abolished in patients who subsequently make a full recovery.

Management

Antidotes and methods to enhance elimination are available for very few poisons. Management of most poisoned patients is based on what has been called 'an orderly if unspectacular regimen of supportive therapy'.

Immediate treatment

A small but important number of poisoned patients arrive at hospital with respiratory obstruction, ventilatory failure, or in cardiorespiratory arrest. In these cases, conventional resuscitation takes precedence over detailed assessment of the patient and attempts to obtain a history. The opioid antagonist, naloxone, can be of inestimable value in emergency treatment. It is safe and should be used whenever there is the slightest suspicion that an opioid may be involved. Its use may transform a desperate situation for the better within seconds and even if it is given inappropriately, it is unlikely to have adverse effects.

Unconscious patients need scrupulous attention to respiration, hypotension, hypothermia, and other complications if they are to survive. Expert nursing is as important as medical measures.

Airway

Establishing and maintaining an adequate airway is of paramount importance in the management of the unconscious poisoned patient. The tongue falling back, dental plates being dislodged, other foreign bodies, buccal secretions, vomitus, and flexion of the neck may obstruct the airway. In the first instance, the neck should be extended and the tongue and jaw held forward. Secretions in the oropharynx must be removed and an oropharyngeal airway should be inserted before turning the patient into a semiprone position. If the cough reflex is absent, an endotracheal tube should be inserted to prevent aspiration into the lungs and allow regular aspiration of bronchial secretions. It is then important to ensure that the inspired air is adequately warmed and humidified.

Ventilation

Once a clear airway has been established the adequacy of spontaneous ventilation should be assessed from the results of arterial blood gas and pH measurements. These should be carried out in all patients who are unconscious irrespective of the presence or absence of features suggesting inadequate gas exchange. Unconscious poisoned patients often have a mild, mixed respiratory and metabolic acidosis with carbon dioxide tensions at the upper limit of normal and oxygen tensions that fall with increasing depth of coma. Increasing the oxygen content of the inspired air is often sufficient to correct hypoxia. Patients with acute respiratory failure should have an endotracheal tube inserted to reduce the respiratory dead space

and thereby increase alveolar ventilation. If this does not reduce carbon dioxide tensions, assisted ventilation is indicated. High-inspired oxygen concentrations are imperative in patients with carbon monoxide and cyanide poisoning and in pulmonary oedema resulting from inhalation of irritant gases.

Hypotension

Hypotension in acute poisoning can be due to a variety of factors including a relative reduction in the intravascular volume secondary to expansion of the venous capacitance bed, metabolic acidosis, arrhythmias, the cardiodepressant effects of some drugs, and blood or fluid loss into the gut. Correct management of individual cases obviously depends on accurate identification of the causes. Young patients are generally not at risk of cerebral or renal damage unless the systolic blood pressure falls below 80 mmHg, but in those over the age of 40 years it is preferable to keep the systolic blood pressure above 90 mmHg. Hypotension often responds to elevation of the foot of the bed by 15 cm and, if this is unsuccessful, a central venous line should be inserted and the intravascular volume expanded as necessary. Dobutamine 2.5 to 10 µg/kg.min or adrenaline (epinephrine) at 1 to 10 µg/kg.min are indicated if hypotension is resistant to these measures.

Arrhythmias

Although many poisons are potentially cardiotoxic, the incidence of serious cardiac arrhythmias in acute poisoning is very low. Tricyclic antidepressants, β-adrenoceptor blocking drugs, chloral hydrate, cardiac glycosides, amphetamines, cocaine, bronchodilators (particularly theophylline and its derivatives), and antimalarial drugs are the most likely causes. Cardiotoxicity usually occurs together with other features of severe poisoning including metabolic acidosis, hypoxia, convulsions, respiratory depression, and abnormalities of electrolyte balance that should be corrected before considering the use of antiarrhythmic drugs. The latter have narrow therapeutic ratios and their use may further impair myocardial function. In general, drug therapy should only be given for persistent, life-threatening arrhythmias associated with peripheral circulatory failure. The drug used must be selected from a knowledge of the pharmacology and toxicology of the poison involved and in such a way that it will not further compromise cardiac function. Lignocaine is probably the drug of choice for clinically important ventricular tachydysrhythmias since its half-life is short and the dose can be adjusted readily.

Convulsions

Convulsions are potentially life-threatening because they cause hypoxia and metabolic acidosis and may precipitate cardiac arrhythmias and arrest. Short isolated convulsions do not require treatment but those that are recurrent or protracted should be suppressed with diazepam intravenously 10 mg in an adult, repeated as necessary. This drug is highly effective in adequate doses and alternatives are seldom needed. However, it is important to remember that giving benzodiazepines in this way may potentiate the respiratory depressant effects of other poisons and further complicate management. The combination of convulsions, coma, and vomiting, which may occur with overdosage of theophylline derivatives, is particularly dangerous and in these circumstances it may be preferable to paralyse the patient, insert an endotracheal tube, and start assisted ventilation. However, although this ensures control of the airway and oxygenation, thus avoiding the risk of inhalation of gastric contents, it does not suppress seizure activity; cerebral function must therefore be monitored and parenteral anticonvulsants given as required.

Hypothermia

Any poison that depresses the central nervous system may impair temperature regulation and cause hypothermia, especially when discovery of the patient is delayed and environmental temperatures are low. This important complication may be missed unless temperature is recorded rectally using a low-reading thermometer. In severe cases, peripheral and core temperatures should be monitored. Treatment includes nursing the patient in a warm room (27 to 29°C) and a heat conserving 'space blanket'. Cold intravenous fluids should be avoided and bottles for use should be stored in the room or the lines should pass through a heating device.

Hyperthermia

Rarely, body temperature may increase to potentially fatal levels after overdosage with central nervous system stimulants such as cocaine, amphetamines, phencyclidine, monoamine oxidase inhibitors, butyrophenomes, and theophylline and its derivatives. In such cases, muscle tone is often grossly increased and convulsions and rhabdomyolysis are common. Cooling measures, including administration of chlorpromazine, may be indicated and dantrolene should be given to reduce muscle tone.

Acid–base abnormalities

Acid–base disturbances commonly accompany coma due to drugs. Acute respiratory acidosis is less common than might be expected but some elevation of arterial carbon dioxide tensions towards the upper limit of normal is usual. This, in combination with mild hypoxia in the deeper grades of coma, produces overall acidaemia. In general, acidosis should be prevented and managed by ensuring adequate ventilation, oxygenation, and tissue perfusion, and control of convulsions rather than by giving bicarbonate. However, a number of poisons, particularly methanol and ethylene glycol, cause life-threatening metabolic acidosis, which should be corrected by infusion of sodium bicarbonate.

Acute respiratory alkalosis, often in combination with a minor metabolic acidosis, is commonly found in acute salicylate poisoning. The metabolic component may require treatment if it is the dominant feature and is causing overall acidaemia. Respiratory alkalosis should not be treated.

Electrolyte abnormalities

Electrolyte abnormalities may result from acid–base disturbances or the direct effects of poisons. Massive tissue damage, usually rhabdomyolysis, may allow potassium to leak from cells leading to potentially lethal hyperkalaemia. Cardiac glycosides cause hyperkalaemia secondary to loss from cells due to inhibition of the membrane sodium–potassium pump while the reverse occurs with sympathomimetic drugs. Ingestion of potassium salts, even in sustained release formulations, may lead to hyperkalaemia and fatal arrhythmias. Oxalic acid and ethylene glycol (which is metabolized to oxalic acid) may cause hypocalcaemia by leading to the formation of insoluble calcium oxalate that is deposited in tissues. Similarly, ingestion of fluorides is also a possible cause of hypocalcaemia, but the amounts children tend to ingest in the form of tablets to prevent dental caries seldom cause serious problems.

Bladder care

Urinary retention is a common complication of acute poisoning, particularly with tricyclic antidepressants and other drugs that have marked anticholinergic actions. However, bladder catheterization is all too often an unthinking measure in unconscious poisoned patients. Coma per se is not an indication for catheterization in poisoned patients, the great majority of whom regain consciousness within 12 h. The bladder can usually be induced to empty reflexly (provided it is not allowed to become grossly overdistended) by applying gentle suprapubic pressure. Catheterization should be reserved for those patients in whom suprapubic pressure is insufficient to empty the bladder, and in those thought to be developing renal failure.

Skin, muscle, and nerve lesions

Skin blisters may be found after poisoning with a wide variety of drugs including barbiturates, tricyclic antidepressants, and benzodiazepines, and non-drug toxins. They often occur over bony prominences that have been subjected to pressure and less frequently at sites where two skin areas have been in contact, such as the the inner aspects of the knees. They should be managed as partial thickness burns. Rhabdomyolysis is a further possible result of immobility and may occur in combination with skin lesions or

independently. Drug overdose is the most common non-traumatic cause of this condition and it may lead to acute renal failure and, rarely, to ischaemic muscle contractures and long-term disability. Similarly, peripheral nerves such as the radial, ulnar, and common peroneal may be damaged by direct pressure while the patient is unconscious or by being entrapped in fibrosing muscle after rhabdomyolysis.

Antidotes

Naloxone for opioid analgesics, oxygen for carbon monoxide, and possibly, flumazenil for benzodiazepines are the only antidotes commonly needed in the management of unconscious poisoned patients. N-Acetylcysteine is used frequently for paracetamol poisoning. Other antidotes of proven value are listed in Table 2. They are seldom required and although their use in correct circumstances may be lifesaving, some are toxic in their own right and the reader is recommended to seek further advice from a poisons information service. Antivenoms for bites and stings by venomous animals are discussed in Chapter 8.2.

Reduction of poison absorption

Prevention of absorption of poisons through the lungs obviously requires removal from the toxic atmosphere and occasionally removal of soiled clothing as well. The latter is also necessary when absorption is thought to have been percutaneous. In addition, the contaminated skin should be thoroughly washed with soap and water.

Table 2 Antidotes of proven value in poisoning due to drugs and chemicals

Poison	Antidote
Aluminium (aluminum)	Desferrioxamine (deferoxamine)
Anticoagulants (oral)	Vitamin K
Arsenic	DMPS
	DMSA
	Dimercaprol
Benzodiazepines	Flumazenil
β-Adrenoceptor blockers	Atropine
	Glucagon
Carbon monoxide	Oxygen
Copper	D-Penicillamine
	DMPS
Cyanide	Oxygen
	Dicobalt edetate
	Hydroxocobalamin
	Sodium thiosulphate
	Sodium nitrite
Diethylene glycol	Ethanol
	Fomepizole
Digoxin	Digoxin-specific Fab antibodies
Ethylene glycol	Ethanol
	Fomepizole
Iron salts	Desferrioxamine (deferoxamine)
Lead (inorganic)	DMSA
	Sodium calcium edetate
Methaemoglobinaemia	Methylthioninium chloride (methylene blue)
Methanol	Ethanol
	Fomepizole
Mercury	DMPS
	DMSA
Opioids	Naloxone
Organophosphorus insecticides	Atropine
	Pralidoxime
Paracetamol (acetaminophen)	N-acetylcysteine
	Methionine

DMPS, dimercapto-1-propane sulphonate; DMSA, dimercaptosuccinic acid.

While it appears logical to assume that removal of unabsorbed drug from the gastrointestinal tract ('gut decontamination') will be beneficial, the efficacy of current methods remains unproven and efforts to remove small amounts of 'safe' drugs are clearly not worthwhile or appropriate. The two major international societies of clinical toxicology (American Academy of Clinical Toxicology and the European Association of Poisons Centres and Clinical Toxicologists) have produced Position Statements on each method. The Position Statements are summarized below.

Gastric lavage

Gastric lavage should not be employed routinely in the management of poisoned patients. In experimental studies, the amount of marker removed by gastric lavage was highly variable and diminished with time. There is no certain evidence that its use improves clinical outcome and it may cause significant morbidity. Gastric lavage should not be considered, therefore, unless a patient has ingested a potentially life-threatening amount of a poison and the procedure can be undertaken within 1 h of ingestion. Even then, clinical benefit has not been confirmed in controlled studies. Unless a patient is intubated, gastric lavage is contraindicated if airway protective reflexes are lost. It is also contraindicated if a hydrocarbon with high aspiration potential or a corrosive substance has been ingested.

Syrup of ipecacuanha

Syrup of ipecacuanha should not be administered routinely in the management of poisoned patients. In experimental studies the amount of marker removed by syrup of ipecacuanha was highly variable and diminished with time. There is no evidence from clinical studies that syrup of ipecacuanha improves the outcome of poisoned patients and its administration, even in children, should be abandoned. In particular, syrup of ipecacuanha should not be administered to a patient who has a decreased level or impending loss of consciousness as aspiration pneumonia might ensue. In addition, it should not be administered to a patient who has ingested a corrosive substance or hydrocarbon with high aspiration potential.

Single-dose activated charcoal

Single-dose activated charcoal should not be administered routinely in the management of poisoned patients. Based on volunteer studies, the effectiveness of activated charcoal decreases with time; the greatest benefit is within 1 h of ingestion. The administration of activated charcoal may be considered if a patient has ingested a potentially toxic amount of a poison (which is known to be adsorbed to charcoal) up to 1 h previously; there are insufficient data to support or exclude its use after 1 h of ingestion. However, there is no evidence that the administration of activated charcoal improves clinical outcome. Unless a patient has an intact or protected airway, the administration of charcoal is contraindicated.

Cathartics

The administration of a cathartic alone has no role in the management of the poisoned patient and is not recommended as a method of gut decontamination. Experimental data are conflicting regarding the use of cathartics in combination with activated charcoal. No clinical studies have been published to investigate the ability of a cathartic, with or without activated charcoal, to reduce the bioavailability of drugs or to improve the outcome of poisoned patients. Based on available data, the routine use of a cathartic in combination with activated charcoal is not endorsed. If a cathartic is used, it should be limited to a single dose in order to minimize adverse effects.

Whole bowel irrigation

Whole bowel irrigation should not be used routinely in the management of the poisoned patient. Although some volunteer studies have shown substantial decreases in the bioavailability of ingested drugs, no controlled clinical trials have been performed and there is no conclusive evidence that whole bowel irrigation improves the outcome of the poisoned patient. Based on volunteer studies, whole bowel irrigation may be considered for potentially toxic ingestions of sustained-release or enteric-coated drugs. There are insufficient data to support or exclude its use for potentially toxic ingestions of iron, lead, zinc, or packets of illicit drugs, but it remains a theoretical option for these ingestions. Whole bowel irrigation is contraindicated in patients with bowel obstruction, perforation, ileus, and in patients with haemodynamic instability or a compromised airway. Whole bowel irrigation should be used cautiously in debilitated patients, or in patients with medical conditions that may be further compromised by its use.

Methods to increase poison elimination

Once a poison has been absorbed and providing there is no antidote, it is reasonable to consider the use of treatments that might speed its elimination from the body. Formerly, forced diuresis, peritoneal and haemodialysis, charcoal haemoperfusion and, less commonly, plasmapheresis were the techniques employed most commonly. In recent years, however, it has been shown that multiple doses of oral activated charcoal given over many hours significantly shortened the plasma half-life of many drugs, at least in volunteers.

Forced diuresis

In the past, forced diuresis enjoyed extensive use in the treatment of acute poisoning if only because it did not require special equipment and could be instituted rapidly and in any hospital. However, there was considerable ignorance of its rationale and its use for many poisons was not justified. The efficacy of forced diuresis depends on the poison being excreted unchanged by the kidney or as an active metabolite. However, most drugs are either degraded by the liver to non-toxic metabolites or have such large volumes of distribution that there is insufficient active drug elimination in urine for forced diuresis to be of any clinical value as the amount removed is insignificant compared with that removed by hepatic metabolism. Urine pH is more important than urine flow and in recent years there has been a trend away from forcing a diuresis (i.e. infusing large volumes of fluid) to attempting to alter urine pH alone.

Urine alkalinization

Most drugs are partly reabsorbed from the urine as it flows through the renal tubules. Reabsorption is confined to unionized, lipid-soluble molecules. Increasing the concentration of ionized drug in the urine should reduce reabsorption and further enhance elimination. This is achieved by manipulating urine pH. Thus, rendering the urine alkaline enhances elimination of weakly acidic compounds such as salicylates, phenobarbital, chlorpromamide, fluoride, and phenoxyacetate herbicides such as 2,4-D and mecoprop.

In practice, inducing an alkaline urine is only used in cases of poisoning due to salicylates and phenoxyacetate herbicides as phenobarbital poisoning may be treated effectively with multiple-dose activated charcoal.

Before alkalinizing the urine, it is important to correct plasma volume depletion and electrolyte and metabolic abnormalities. Sodium bicarbonate, most conveniently administered as an 8.4 per cent solution (1 mmol bicarbonate/ml), is infused intravenously to ensure that the pH of the urine, which is measured by narrow-range indicator paper or a pH meter, is more than 7.5 and preferably close to 8.5.

As urine alkalinization is a metabolically invasive procedure requiring frequent biochemical monitoring, and medical and nursing expertise, it should be performed in a critical care area.

Acid diuresis

Although, theoretically, induction of an acid diuresis should increase the elimination of basic drugs such as amphetamines, there is seldom any need to use it and no evidence that it is of value in cases of poisoning.

Multiple doses of oral activated charcoal

Multiple doses of activated charcoal aid the elimination of some drugs from the circulation by interrupting their enterohepatic circulation and adsorbing that which diffuses into the intestinal juices. The rate of transfer of the latter is dependent upon the blood supply to the gut, the area of mucosa available for transfer, and the concentration gradient of the drug across the mucosa. The adsorptive capacity of charcoal is such that zero drug concentrations are present in luminal fluid and that the diffusion gradient remains as high as possible. The process has been termed 'gut dialysis' since, in effect, the intestinal mucosa is being used as a semipermeable membrane.

The American Academy of Clinical Toxicology and the European Association of Poisons Centres and Clinical Toxicologists have published a Position Statement on multiple-dose activated charcoal. This confirms that although many studies in animals and volunteers have demonstrated that multiple-dose activated charcoal increases drug elimination significantly, this therapy has not yet been shown in a controlled study in poisoned patients to reduce morbidity and mortality. Further studies are required to establish its role and the optimal dosage regimen of charcoal to be administered.

Based on experimental and clinical studies, multiple-dose activated charcoal should be considered only if a patient has ingested a life-threatening amount of carbamazepine, dapsone, phenobarbital, quinine, or theophylline. In all of these cases there are data to confirm enhanced elimination, though no controlled studies have demonstrated clinical benefit.

Although volunteer studies have demonstrated that multiple-dose activated charcoal increases the elimination of amitriptyline, dextropropoxyphene, digitoxin, digoxin, disopyramide, nadolol, phenylbutazone, phenytoin, piroxicam, and sotalol, there are insufficient clinical data to support or exclude the use of this therapy in patients poisoned with these drugs.

The use of multiple-dose charcoal in salicylate poisoning is controversial. One animal study and two of four volunteer studies did not demonstrate increased salicylate clearance with multiple-dose charcoal therapy. Data in poisoned patients are insufficient at present to recommend the use of multiple-dose charcoal therapy for salicylate poisoning.

Multiple-dose activated charcoal did not increase the elimination of astemizole, chlorpropamide, doxepin, imipramine, meprobamate, methotrexate, phenytoin, sodium valproate, tobramycin, and vancomycin in experimental and/or clinical studies.

Unless a patient has an intact or protected airway, the administration of multiple-dose activated charcoal is contraindicated. It should not be used in the presence of intestinal obstruction. The need for concurrent administration of cathartics remains unproven and is not recommended. In particular, cathartics should not be administered to young children because of their propensity to cause fluid and electrolyte imbalance.

In conclusion, based on experimental and clinical studies, multiple-dose activated charcoal should be considered only if a patient has ingested a life-threatening amount of carbamazepine, dapsone, phenobarbital, quinine, or theophylline.

Recommended adult doses of charcoal for this purpose are 50 to 100 g initially, followed by 50 g 4-hourly or 25 g 2-houly until charcoal appears in the faeces or recovery occurs.

Further reading

American Academy of Clinical Toxicology/European Association of Poisons Centres and Clinical Toxicologists (1997/1999). Position Statements. *Journal of Toxicology—Clinical Toxicology* **35**, 699–762; **37**, 731–51.

Dialysis

Haemodialysis in acute poisoning is indicated most commonly for the treatment of acute renal failure and only infrequently to increase the elimination of poisons. The rate of elimination across the dialysis membrane depends upon a number of variables including the molecular weight of the poison, the extent to which it is protein bound, the concentration gradient, and pH of blood and dialysate. Haemodialysis is of little value in patients who ingest poisons with large volumes of distribution (such as tricyclic antidepressants) because the plasma contains only a small proportion of the total amount of drug in the body. Haemodialysis is indicated in patients with severe clinical features and high plasma concentrations of salicylate, lithium, methanol, isopropanol, ethylene glycol, and ethanol. Peritoneal dialysis increases the elimination of poisons such as ethylene glycol and methanol but is much less efficient than haemodialysis.

Haemoperfusion

Haemoperfusion involves the passage of blood through an adsorbent material that retains the poison. Activated charcoal is the most popular adsorbent. Within 4 to 6 h haemoperfusion can reduce significantly the body burden of compounds with a low volume of distribution (less than 1 litre/kg). The technique effectively removes barbiturates, carbamazepine, disopyramide, ethchlorvynol, glutethamide, meprobamate, methaqualone, theophylline, and trichloroethanol derivatives. However, there is now evidence that multiple-dose activated charcoal is as effective as haemoperfusion in phenobarbital, carbamazepine, and theophylline poisoning, and is simpler to use. Furthermore, barbiturate and non-barbiturate hypnotics are now prescribed only rarely.

Acetone

Acetone is a clear liquid with a characteristic pungent odour and sweet taste, used widely in industrial and household products. Once absorbed either through the lungs, skin, or gut, acetone is exhaled unchanged or metabolized to carbon dioxide.

Clinical features

Acetone has an irritating effect on the mucous membranes of the eyes, nose, and throat. Intoxication results in headache, excitement, restlessness, chest tightness, incoherent speech, nausea, and vomiting. Occasionally, gastrointestinal bleeding, coma, and convulsions have been reported.

Treatment

If toxicity has followed inhalation, remove from exposure and give supportive treatment. After ingestion, gut decontamination is not useful.

Further reading

International Programme on Chemical Safety (1998). *Environmental Health Criteria 207. Acetone.* World Health Organization, Geneva.

Acids

Acids commonly involved in cases of poisoning include the inorganic acids such as hydrochloric, hydrofluoric, nitric, phosphoric, and sulphuric acids; and organic acids such as acetic, formic, lactic, and trichloroacetic acids. Car battery acid typically contains 28 per cent sulphuric acid. Proprietary cleaning agents and antirust compounds often contain a mixture of hydrochloric and phosphoric acids.

Clinical features

On the skin acids behave characteristically as corrosives leading to erythema and burns. In the eyes, intense pain and blepharospasm are common, and corneal burns may occur. When ingested, acids flow rapidly along the lesser curvature of the stomach to the prepyloric region where they pool because of spasm of the pylorus and antrum to cause almost instantaneous coagulative necrosis of one or more layers of the stomach. In many cases, acids spare the oesophagus because of rapid transit and resistant squamous epithelium.

There is immediate pain in the mouth, pharynx, and abdomen, intense thirst, vomiting, haematemesis, and diarrhoea. The pain and mucosal oedema cause dysphagia and drooling saliva. Gastric and oesophageal perforation may occur resulting in chemical peritonitis. Other effects include hoarseness, stridor, and respiratory distress secondary to laryngeal and epiglottic oedema, shock, metabolic acidosis, leucocytosis, acute tubular necrosis, renal failure, hypoxaemia, respiratory failure, intravascular coagulation, and haemolysis.

Hydrofluoric acid ingestion causes chelation of calcium, with resultant weakness, paraesthesiae, tetany, convulsions, cardiac arrhythmias, and disturbed coagulation.

Treatment

Acid burns to the skin should be irrigated liberally with water or saline. Dressings are applied as for a thermal burn. Skin grafting may be necessary.

After ocular exposure, the eye should be irrigated preferably with saline for 15 to 30 min. Topical local anaesthetic is usually required to relieve pain and to overcome blepharospasm. Ophthalmic advice should be sought.

After ingestion a clear airway should be established. Opioids are often necessary for analgesia. Dilution and/or neutralization is contraindicated. Urgent panendoscopy is needed and resection of necrotic tissue and surgical repair should be undertaken to ensure survival, particularly if inorganic acids have been ingested. Total parenteral nutrition is often required. Corticosteroids confer no benefit and may mask abdominal signs of perforation; antibiotics should be given for established infection only.

Acid ingestion may result in antral, pyloric, or jejunal strictures, achlorhydria, protein-losing enteropathy, and gastric carcinoma.

Further reading

Advisory Committee on Pesticides (1998). *Evaluation of fully approved or provisionally approved products. Evaluation number 174: sulphuric acid.* Advisory Committee on Pesticides, Pesticides Safety Directorate, York.

Boyce SH, Simpson KA (1996). Hydrochloric acid inhalation: who needs admission? *Journal of Accident and Emergency Medicine* **13**, 422–4.

Ochi K *et al.* (1996). Surgical treatment for caustic ingestion injury of the pharynx, larynx, and esophagus. *Acta Otolaryngologica* **116**, 116–19.

Stiff G *et al.* (1996). Corrosive injuries of the oesophagus and stomach: experience in management at a regional paediatric centre. *Annals of the Royal College of Surgeons of England* **78**, 119–23.

Alkalis

Those commonly encountered in cases of poisoning include drain, lavatory, and pipe cleaners (sodium hydroxide), dishwashing detergents (sodium carbonate, sodium silicate, sodium tripolyphosphate), denture cleaning tablets (sodium perborate, sodium phosphate, sodium carbonate), urinary glucose testing tablets (sodium hydroxide), water sterilizing tablets (sodium dichloroisocyanurate), alkaline batteries, and sodium hypochlorite (a bleaching agent).

Clinical features

The features of eye, skin, and laryngeal contamination with alkalis are similar to those produced by acids (above). When ingested, alkalis typically damage the oesophagus but usually spare the stomach. There is little immediate oral discomfort but subsequently a burning sensation develops in the mouth and pharynx, together with epigastric pain, vomiting, and diarrhoea. Oesophageal ulceration with or without perforation may occur with mediastinitis, pneumonitis, cardiac injury, and aorto-enteric fistula formation as secondary complications of perforation.

Treatment

The treatment of corrosive injuries caused by alkalis is largely the same as for those produced by acids.

Corticosteroids do not alter the incidence of stricture formation but may decrease the need for surgical repair of strictures if they are used in conjunction with either anterograde or retrograde oesophageal dilation. Methylprednisolone at a dose of 40 mg intravenously 8-hourly in adults or prednisolone at 2 mg/kg per day intravenously can be given, until oral intake is resumed, when an equivalent dosage of prednisolone is given orally and tapered off over a period of 3 to 6 weeks. A broad-spectrum antibiotic, such as amoxicillin, should be prescribed at the same time as the corticosteroid.

Alkali ingestion may result in stricture formation and there is a risk of malignancy. The mean latent period for development of carcinoma of the oesophagus following alkali ingestion is more than 40 years.

Further reading

Anderson KD, Rouse TM, Randolph JG (1990). A controlled trial of corticosteroids in children with corrosive injury of the esophagus. *New England Journal of Medicine* **323**, 637–40.

Davis AR *et al.* (1997). Topical steroid use in the treatment of ocular alkali burns. *British Journal of Ophthalmology* **81**, 732–4.

Gaudreault P *et al.* (1983). Predictability of esophageal injury from signs and symptoms: a study of caustic ingestion in 378 children. *Pediatrics* **71**, 767–70.

Keskin E *et al.* (1991). The effect of steroid treatment on corrosive oesophageal burns in children. *European Journal of Pediatric Surgery* **1**, 335–8.

Lee KAP, Opeskin K (1995). Fatal alkali burns. *Forensic Science International* **72**, 219–27.

Ochi K *et al.* (1996). Surgical treatment for caustic ingestion injury of the pharynx, larynx and oesophagus. *Acta Otolaryngologica* **116**, 116–19.

α-Chloralose

α-Chloralose is marketed as cereal baits containing 4 per cent rodenticide, while technical α-chloralose (about 90 per cent pure) is used against moles and is occasionally encountered in self-poisoning episodes. The toxic amount for an adult is approximately 1 g and for an infant, 20 mg/kg body weight.

Clinical features

Toxic amounts of α-chloralose cause severe CNS excitation with hypersalivation, increased muscle tone, hyperreflexia, opisthotonus, and convulsions. Rhabdomyolysis is a potential complication. Coma, generalized flaccidity, and respiratory depression may follow.

Treatment

No treatment is required for ingestion of α-chloralose baits. Supportive measures are necessary when large amounts of bait or the technical compound is involved. Gastric emptying should not be carried out since the stimulation may provoke seizures.

Further reading

Thomas HM, Simpson D, Prescott LF (1988). The toxic effects of α-chloralose. *Human Toxicology* **7**, 285–7.

Aluminium (aluminum)

Aluminium hydroxide is used as an antacid and as a phosphate binder in the management of chronic renal failure. Aluminium sulphate is employed in water purification and paper manufacture. Aluminium may be absorbed orally and by inhalation. More than 90 per cent of absorbed aluminium is bound to transferrin. Though some accumulates in brain tissue, most body aluminium is stored in bone and the liver. It is excreted mainly via the kidneys.

Clinical features

Acute poisoning

Ingestion of a significant quantity of soluble aluminium salts such as aluminium sulphate gives rise to burning in the mouth and throat, nausea, vomiting, diarrhoea, abdominal pain, hypotension, seizures, haemolysis, haematuria, and rarely, hepatorenal failure. Topical aluminium sulphate may be irritant to the skin and eyes. By contrast, insoluble aluminium salts, such as aluminium oxide, do not produce an acute toxic response.

Chronic poisoning

Inhalation of 'stamped aluminium powder' can cause a persistent cough and breathlessness due to lung fibrosis or occupational asthma. Workers involved in aluminium production may be at increased risk of developing lung cancer.

'Dialysis dementia' involves the accumulation of aluminium, mainly in the brain (see Section 20).

Aluminium has also been implicated in Alzheimer's disease and may contribute to osteomalacia in renal osteodystrophy. It may cause contact allergy.

Treatment

Desferrioxamine (deferoxamine) forms a stable complex with aluminium and mobilizes aluminium primarily from bone with subsequent urinary elimination of the chelate. Theoretically 100 mg of desferrioxamine can bind 4.1 mg of aluminium. As desferrioxamine is absorbed poorly from the gastrointestinal tract, parenteral therapy is preferred.

The desferrioxamine chelate is dialysable and all published clinical studies of aluminium chelation using desferrioxamine have involved patients in renal failure undergoing either dialysis or haemofiltration. Haemofiltration is probably superior to haemodialysis in enhancing aluminium elimination using desferrioxamine. As the aluminium–desferrioxamine chelate concentration reaches a maximum 12 to 24 h postinfusion, desferrioxamine should be administered shortly before dialysis for maximum benefit.

There is clinical evidence that desferrioxamine can improve aluminium-induced encephalopathy, bone disease, and anaemia in patients on dialysis. Desferrioxamine should therefore be prescribed when features of dialysis encephalopathy are present, when there is an increased body aluminium load, and there is clinical evidence of aluminium-related bone disease. In addition, desferrioxamine should be considered in the presence of severe, transfusion-dependent anaemia even in the absence of characteristic clinical or analytical features of aluminium overload. It has also been proposed that desferrioxamine should be employed in the presence of an increased (greater than 60 µg/l) serum aluminium concentration.

Conventionally, desferrioxamine at 40 to 80 mg/kg has been administered once weekly as a subcutaneous or intravenous infusion, reduced to 20 to 60 mg/kg when treatment is required for several months. However, recent studies suggest that desferrioxamine 5 mg/kg once weekly is an adequate alternative regime.

Further reading

International Programme on Chemical Safety (1997). *Environmental Health Criteria 194. Aluminium.* World Health Organization, Geneva.

McCarthy JT, Milliner DS, Johnson WJ (1990). Clinical experience with desferrioxamine in dialysis patients with aluminium toxicity. *Quarterly Journal of Medicine* **74**, 257–76.

Aluminium and zinc phosphides

Aluminium and zinc phosphides react with moisture in the air and the gastrointestinal tract to produce phosphine (see below), a gas with a garlic-like odour.

Clinical features

Exposure to phosphine causes lacrimation, rhinorrhoea, cough, breathlessness, chest tightness, dizziness, nausea, and drowsiness. Pulmonary oedema may develop later. Ingestion of aluminium phosphide causes vomiting, epigastric pain, peripheral circulatory failure, severe metabolic acidosis, and renal failure in addition to many of the features induced by inhalation of phosphine.

Treatment

Treatment is symptomatic and supportive. Gastric lavage should be considered if the poison has been ingested within 1 h.

Further reading

Gupta S, Ahlawat SK (1995). Aluminium phosphide poisoning: a review. *Journal of Toxicology—Clinical Toxicology* **33**, 19–24.

Ammonia

Ammonia, a colourless gas with a strong irritating odour, is used in aqueous solution in industry and in the home.

Clinical features

Ammonia may be absorbed by inhalation, ingestion, or percutaneously. It irritates the eyes, upper respiratory tract, and pharynx. Exposed surfaces may develop chemical burns, blisters, thrombosis of surface vessels, and severe local oedema that may lead to respiratory obstruction and death, if the larynx and glottis are involved. Inhaled high concentrations may cause dyspnoea, pulmonary oedema, and persistent lung damage.

Treatment

The casualty should be removed from the contaminated area. The eyes should be irrigated with water or 0.9 per cent saline for 15 to 30 min and an ophthalmic opinion sought as permanent blindness may result. Pulmonary complications should be treated with humidified supplemental oxygen, bronchodilators, and if necessary, assisted ventilation with positive end-expiratory pressure. Although widely employed, there is no conclusive evidence that diuretics and corticosteroids alter the prognosis. Patients who survive for 24 h are likely to recover fully.

Further reading

De La Hoz RE, Schlueter DP, Rom WN (1996). Chronic lung disease secondary to ammonia inhalation injury. *American Journal of Industrial Medicine* **29**, 209–14.

Wibbenmeyer LA *et al.* (1999). Our chemical burn experience: exposing the dangers of anhydrous ammonia. *Journal of Burn Care and Rehabilitation* **20**, 226–31.

Amfetamines and ecstasy (MDMA)

Amfetamine, dexamfetamine, methamfetamine, and 'ecstasy' (3,4-methylenedioxymethamfetamine, MDMA) stimulate the central nervous system.

Poisoning with them is usually the result of their use for pleasurable purposes rather than single massive doses.

Clinical features

These drugs cause increased alertness and self-confidence, euphoria, extrovert behaviour, increased talkativeness with rapid speech, lack of desire to eat or sleep, tremor, dilated pupils, tachycardia, and hypertension. More severe intoxication is associated with excitability, agitation, paranoid delusions, hallucinations with violent behaviour, hypertonia, and hyperreflexia. Convulsions, rhabdomyolysis, hyperthermia, and cardiac arrhythmias may also develop. In severe cases of MDMA poisoning, hyperthermia, disseminated intravascular coagulation, rhabdomyolysis, acute renal failure, and hyponatraemia are observed. Hepatic damage has also been reported. Rarely, poisoning due to amphetamines may result in intracerebral and subarachnoid haemorrhage and acute cardiomyopathy; these complications may be fatal. Hyperthyroxinaemia may be found in chronic amphetamine users.

Treatment

Gastric lavage should be considered if a substantial overdose has been ingested in the preceding 1 h. Sedation with diazepam, chlorpromazine, or droperidol may be required. β-Adrenoceptor blocking drugs will antagonize the peripheral sympathomimetic actions of amphetamines.

Further reading

Boot BP, McGregor LS, Hall W (2000). MDMA (ecstasy) neurotoxicity: assessing and communicating the risks. *Lancet* **355**, 1818–21.
Ernst T *et al.* (2000). Evidence for long-term neurotoxicity associated with methamphetamine abuse. A¹ H MRS study. *Neurology* **54**, 1344–9.
Maurer HH *et al.* (2000). Toxicokinetics and analytical toxicology of amphetamine-derived designer drugs ('Ecstasy'). *Toxicology Letters* **112–13**, 133–42.
McGuire P (2000). Long term psychiatric and cognitive effects of MDMA use. *Toxicology Letters* **112–13**, 153–6.
Ricaurte GA *et al.* (2000). Toxicodynamics and long-term toxicity of the recreational drug, 3,4-methylenedioxymethamphetamine (MDMA, 'ecstasy'). *Toxicology Letters* **112–13**, 143–6.

Angiotensin-converting enzyme (ACE) inhibitors

Clinical features

Anorexia, nausea, abdominal discomfort, headache, and paraesthesiae have been reported. In addition, hypotension (which may be mediated by the endogenous opioid system), sinus tachycardia, bronchospasm, and hyperkalaemia may develop. Fatalities have been reported.

Treatment

Gastric lavage or activated charcoal administration should be considered if the patient presents within 1 h of a substantial overdose. Supportive therapy should then be employed, including volume expansion with plasma expanders for hypotension. Naloxone in a dose of 0.8 to 1.2 mg may reverse ACE inhibitor-induced hypotension. Marked hyperkalaemia may require an intravenous infusion of glucose (50 g) and soluble insulin (15 units).

Further reading

Lip GYH, Ferner RE (1995). Poisoning with anti-hypertensive drugs: angiotensin converting enzyme inhibitors. *Journal of Human Hypertension* **9**, 711–15.

Antibacterial agents

Most patients develop no symptoms and require no treatment. Transient nausea, vomiting, and diarrhoea may occur. There have been rare reports of renal failure after overdosage with co-trimoxazole, pancreatitis with erythromycin, and haemorrhagic cystitis with amoxicillin.

Further reading

Berger TM *et al.* (1992). Acute pancreatitis in a 12 year old girl after an erythromycin overdose. *Pediatrics* **90**, 624–6.
Cohen H, Francisco DH (1994). Twelve-gram overdose of ciprofloxacin with mild symptomatology. *Annals of Pharmacotherapy* **28**, 805–6.
Jones DP *et al.* (1993). Acute renal failure following amoxycillin overdose. *Clinical Pediatrics* **32**, 735–9.

Anticholinergic substances

Anticholinergic substances are occasionally abused. Plants have been used for this purpose for many years.

A large number of drugs currently used in medicine also have anticholinergic properties and have been misused. They include antihistamines, particularly cyclizine, antiparkinsonian drugs such as benzhexol (trihexyphenidyl), benzatropine, orphenadrine, biperiden, and tricyclic antidepressants (see below).

Further reading

Burns MJ *et al.* (2000). A comparison of physostigmine and benzodiazepines for the treatment of anticholinergic poisoning. *Annals of Emergency Medicine* **35**, 374–81.
Ramirez M, Rivera E, Ereu C (1999). Fifteen cases of atropine poisoning after honey ingestion. *Veterinary and Human Toxicology* **41**, 19–20.
Thabet H *et al.* (1999). *Datura stramonium* poisoning in humans. *Veterinary and Human Toxicology* **41**, 320–21.

Anticoagulant rodenticides

Warfarin was widely used as a rodenticide until target species developed resistance to it. The newer anticoagulant rodenticides such as brodifacoum, bromodialone, chlorophacinone, coumatetralyl, difenacoum, diphacinone, and flocoumafen are more potent antagonists of vitamin K₁ than warfarin and reduce the synthesis of clotting factors II, VII, IX, and X. In the case of short-acting formulations, such as those containing warfarin, prolongation of the International Normalized Ratio (**INR**) will be evident within 24 h and patients can remain anticoagulated for several days. In contrast, the ingestion of the more potent anticoagulant rodenticides may result in prolongation of the INR for weeks or months.

Clinical features

Gastrointestinal bleeding, haematuria, and bruising are the commonest features, though the most common site of fatal haemorrhage is intracranial.

Treatment

If the patient is not receiving an anticoagulant therapeutically, is not bleeding, and if the INR is more than 8, give vitamin K₁ (phytomenadione) in a dose of 5 mg slowly intravenously. If there is active bleeding give prothrombin complex concentrate at 50 units/kg (or fresh frozen plasma 15 ml/kg if the concentrate is not available) and vitamin K₁ 5 to 10 mg intravenously. Treatment may be required for several weeks in the case of the more potent anticoagulant rodenticides. The INR should be monitored for at least 2 weeks after stopping vitamin K₁ therapy. If the patient is receiving warfarin therapeutically see below under Warfarin for further discussion.

Further reading

Casner PR (1998). Superwarfarin toxicity. *American Journal of Therapeutics* **5**, 117–20.

McCarthy PT *et al.* (1997). Covert poisoning with difenacoum: clinical and toxicological observations. *Human and Experimental Toxicology* **16**, 166–70.

Antihistamines

First-generation antihistamines include brompheniramine, chlorphenira-mine (chlorphenamine), cyclizine, diphenhydramine, mepyramine, methapyrilene, promethazine, and trimeprazine. Second-generation drugs include astemizole and terfenadine. The toxicity of the two groups varies.

Clinical features

The older antihistamines have anticholinergic actions and their effects are therefore similar to the tricyclic antidepressants (see below) although con-vulsions, coma, respiratory depression, arrhythmias (other than sinus tachycardia), and death are rare.

Astemizole and terfenadine lack anticholinergic actions but are cardio-toxic causing Q–T$_c$ interval prolongation and ventricular tachycardia, including the *torsade de pointes* type. Associated giant U waves have been described. Terfenadine in overdose can cause convulsions.

Treatment

Gastric lavage may be undertaken or oral activated charcoal may be given if the patient presents less than 1 h after the ingestion of a substantial over-dose of a first-generation antihistamine. The patient should be observed for about 12 h with cardiac monitoring if the Q–T interval is prolonged. Intra-venous magnesium sulphate may abolish serious ventricular arrhythmias.

Further reading

June RA, Nasr I (1997). Torsades de pointes and terfenadine ingestion. *American Journal of Emergency Medicine* **15**, 542–3.

Zareba W *et al.* (1997). Electrocardiographic findings in patients with diphenhydramine overdose. *American Journal of Cardiology* **80**, 1168–73.

Antiparkinsonian drugs

Amantadine, benzhexol, and orphenadrine have anticholinergic effects in overdosage. Orphenadrine is probably the most toxic and has caused deaths.

Clinical features and treatment

The features of poisoning are similar to those of the tricyclic antidepres-sants and should be managed in the same way.

Further reading

Jones AL, Proudfoot AT (1997). The features and management of poisoning with drugs used to treat Parkinson's disease. *Quarterly Journal of Medicine* **91**, 613–16.

Antiseptics and disinfectants

Once these solutions commonly contained phenol but phenol has been replaced largely by small quantities of either chlorophenol or chloroxylenol which, although less toxic than phenol, can be hazardous if ingested in large quantities. More dangerous are isopropanol and ethanol (see below).

Clinical features

Ingestion of a substantial quantity results in a sensation of burning in the mouth and throat, followed by drowsiness, stupor, depression of respir-ation, and coma.

Treatment

Management is supportive. (See also ethanol and isopropanol.)

Further reading

Chan TYK (1994). Poisoning due to Savlon (cetrimide) liquid. *Human and Experimental Toxicology* **13**, 681–2.

Chan TYK, Critchley JAJH (1996). Pulmonary aspiration following Dettol poisoning: the scope for prevention. *Human and Experimental Toxicology* **15**, 843–6.

Arsenic

Arsenic forms both trivalent and pentavalent derivatives. Inorganic arsen-ical compounds may generate arsine gas (see below) when in contact with acids, reducing metals, sodium hydroxide, and aluminium. Some 90 per cent of an ingested dose of most inorganic arsenicals is absorbed. The half-life is in the range of 1 to 3 days. Excretion is predominantly in the urine. Soluble arsenical compounds can also be absorbed by inhalation, but skin absorption is generally poor. In exposed individuals high concentrations of arsenic are present in bone, hair, and nails.

Clinical features

Acute poisoning

This can follow accidental, suicidal, or deliberate ingestion, the toxicity being largely dependent on the water solubility of the ingested compound. Within 2 h of substantial ingestion of a soluble arsenical compound, severe haemorrhagic gastritis or gastroenteritis may ensue with collapse and death usually within 4 days. A metallic taste, salivation, muscular cramps, facial oedema, difficulty in swallowing, hepatorenal dysfunction, convulsions, and encephalopathy are reported. A peripheral neuropathy (predominantly sensory), striate leuconychia (Mee's lines), and hyperkeratotic, hyperpig-mented skin lesions are common in those surviving a near-fatal ingestion. In moderate or severe arsenic poisoning investigations may show anaemia, leucopenia, thrombocytopenia, and disseminated intravascular coagula-tion. ECG abnormalities have been reported and include Q–T prolongation and ventricular arrhythmias.

Chronic poisoning

The ingestion of arsenic in contaminated drinking water (recently in Ban-gladesh) or 'tonics' has led to progressive weakness, anorexia, nausea, vomiting, stomatitis, colitis, increased salivation, epistaxis, bleeding gums, conjunctivitis, weight loss, and low-grade fever. Characteristically there is hyperkeratosis of the palms and soles of the feet, 'raindrop' pigmentation of the skin, and 'Mee's lines' on the nails. There is an increased risk of skin cancer (usually squamous cell epithelioma) in affected individuals. A sym-metrical peripheral neuropathy is typical. Hearing loss, psychological impairment, and electroencephalogram changes have been reported. Other chronic effects include disturbances of liver function and ulceration and perforation of the nasal septum. Chronic exposure to arsenic has been linked to lung cancer.

Treatment

Traditionally, dimercaprol (British Anti-Lewisite, BAL) has been the recommended chelator. However, DMPS (unithiol) and DMSA (succimer) are preferable, if available, as they are more effective in reducing the arsenic content of tissues and, unlike dimercaprol, they do not cause accumulation of arsenic in the brain. DMSA and DMPS may be given orally in a dose of 30 mg/kg body weight daily for 5 days, whereas dimercaprol must be given by a deep intramuscular injection in a dose of 2.5 to 5 mg/kg 4-hourly for 2 days followed by 2.5 mg/kg intramuscularly twice daily for 1 to 2 weeks.

Further reading

Cullen NM, Wolf LR, St Clair D (1995). Pediatric arsenic ingestion. *American Journal of Emergency Medicine* 13, 432–5.

Kingston RL, Hall S, Sioris L (1993). Clinical observations and medical outcome in 149 cases of arsenate ant killer ingestion. *Journal of Toxicology—Clinical Toxicology* 31, 581–91.

Wong SS, Tan KC, Goh CL (1998). Cutaneous manifestations of chronic arsenicism: review of seventeen cases. *Journal of the American Academy of Dermatology* 38, 179–85.

Arsine

Arsine is a colourless, non-irritating gas which binds with oxidized haemoglobin causing marked intravascular haemolysis. Haemoglobinuria and acute renal tubular necrosis then develop.

Clinical features

There is usually a delay of some 2 to 24 h after exposure before the onset of headache, malaise, weakness, dizziness, breathlessness, migratory abdominal pain, fever, tachycardia, tachypnoea, nausea, and vomiting. A bronze skin colour is noted in some patients but most have the typical appearance of a jaundiced patient. Acute renal failure is observed by the third day after substantial exposure and the urine is dark red then brown before anuria ensues. Investigations will show leucocytosis, reticulocytosis, elevated plasma haemoglobin, and haemoglobinuria.

Treatment

If haemolysis is severe, plasmapheresis or exchange transfusion should be undertaken and, if renal failure ensues, haemodialysis/filtration. Dimercaprol and other chelating agents are of no value.

Further reading

Romeo L *et al.* (1997). Acute arsine intoxication as a consequence of metal burnishing operations. *American Journal of Industrial Medicine* 32, 211–16.

Barbiturates

Amylobarbital, butobarbital, cyclobarbital, heptabarbital, hexabarbital, pentobarbital, and secobarbital are regarded as being short- or medium-acting. The more lipid soluble, shorter-acting preparations are associated commonly with more serious poisoning than phenobarbital and barbital, which are much more water-soluble.

Clinical features

Impairment of consciousness, respiratory depression, hypotension, and hypothermia are typical and potentiated by alcohol and benzodiazepines. There are no specific neurological signs. Hypotonia and hyporeflexia are the rule and the plantar responses are either flexor or absent. Hypotension, skin blisters, and rhabdomyolysis may develop. During recovery from coma, with or without hypothermia, it is common to observe a peak of temperature that cannot be explained by infection. Most deaths result from respiratory complications.

Treatment

Gastric lavage may be considered if it can be undertaken within 1 h of overdose; supportive measures should be used as appropriate. Although char-

coal haemoperfusion is very effective for severely poisoned patients, phenobarbital can be removed efficiently by multiple-dose oral activated charcoal.

Further reading

Hantson P *et al.* (1996). Severe hypoxia and hypothermia following barbiturate poisoning. *Intensive Care Medicine* 22, 998–9.

Benzene

Benzene is a colourless, volatile liquid with a pleasant odour. It is an ingredient in many paints and varnish removers and some petrols (gasolines). About 10 per cent of inhaled benzene is excreted unchanged in the breath. The remainder is metabolized by mixed function oxidase enzymes predominantly in the liver, but also in the bone marrow, the target organ of benzene toxicity.

Clinical features

Acute exposure

Following inhalation or ingestion, euphoria, dizziness, weakness, headache, blurred vision, mucous membrane irritation, tremor, ataxia, chest tightness, respiratory depression, cardiac arrhythmias, coma, and convulsions have been reported. Direct skin contact with liquid benzene may produce marked irritation.

Chronic exposure

The toxic effects of chronic poisoning may not become apparent for months or years after initial contact and may develop after all exposure has ceased.

Anorexia, headache, drowsiness, nervousness, and irritability are well described. Anaemia (including aplastic anaemia), leucopenia, thrombocytopenia, pancytopenia, leukaemia, lymphomas, chromosomal abnormalities, and cerebral atrophy have been reported. Patients have recovered after as long as a year of almost complete absence of formation of new blood cells. A dry, scaly dermatitis may develop on prolonged or repeated skin exposure to liquid benzene.

Treatment

Following removal from the contaminated atmosphere, treatment should be directed towards symptomatic and supportive measures. Gastric lavage is hazardous as aspiration is likely to occur.

Further reading

Barbera N, Bulla G, Romano G (1998). A fatal case of benzene poisoning. *Journal of Forensic Sciences* 43, 1250–1.

Ireland B *et al.* (1997). Cancer mortality among workers with benzene exposure. *Epidemiology* 8, 318–20.

Benzodiazepines

These are widely used as tranquillizers, hypnotics, and sedatives.

Clinical features

Although many benzodiazepines have active metabolites that account for their sometimes prolonged sedative effects, they all share a remarkable safety when taken alone in overdose. However, there is individual variation in response; some otherwise healthy elderly people respond to an overdose with prolonged toxicity. Benzodiazepines potentiate the effects of other CNS depressants, particularly alcohol, tricyclic antidepressants, and barbiturates. Dizziness, drowsiness, ataxia, and slurred speech are the usual features while coma, respiratory depression, and hypotension are uncommon and usually mild. Flurazepam is most likely to cause significant CNS depression.

Treatment

Gastric lavage is unnecessary unless the overdose exceeds 30 therapeutic doses in an adult and the patient presents within 1 h. In severe poisoning, the specific benzodiazepine antagonist, flumazenil, may be indicated; 0.5 mg is given intravenously over 30 s and, if necessary, a further 0.5 mg over 30 s. Most patients will respond to a total dose of between 1 and 3 mg.

Further reading

Hojer J, Baehrendtz S, Gustafsson L (1989). Benzodiazepine poisoning: Experience of 702 admissions to an intensive care unit during a 14-year period. *Journal of Internal Medicine* **226**, 117–22.

Weinbroum A *et al.* (1996). Use of flumazenil in the treatment of drug overdose: a double-blind and open clinical study in 110 patients. *Critical Care Medicine* **24**, 199–206.

Benzyl alcohol

Benzyl alcohol has been used as a preservative in intravascular flush solutions and in drug formulations. Benzyl alcohol is metabolized to benzoic acid that is then conjugated with glycine in the liver and excreted as hippuric acid. The immature liver's capacity to metabolize benzoic acid is limited and when exceeded leads to accumulation of this metabolite and metabolic acidosis.

Clinical features

In 1982, a syndrome consisting of metabolic acidosis, convulsions, neurological deterioration (due to intraventricular haemorrhage), gasping respirations, hepatic and renal abnormalities, cardiovascular collapse, and death was described in small premature infants between 2 and 14 days of age. The removal of benzyl alcohol solutions from neonatal units led to a considerable reduction both in morbidity and mortality and in particular there was a reduction in cases of kernicterus and intraventricular haemorrhage.

Further reading

Anderson CW *et al.* (1984). Benzyl alcohol poisoning in a premature newborn infant. *American Journal of Obstetrics and Gynecology* **130**, 344–6.

β-Adrenoceptor blocking drugs

β-Adrenoceptor blocking drugs antagonize the effects of endogenous catecholamines on the heart and other tissues by competitive inhibition at β-adrenoceptors. In overdose these drugs exhibit a marked negative inotropic action.

Clinical features

Sinus bradycardia may be the only feature following a small overdose, but if a substantial amount has been ingested, coma, convulsions (particularly with propranolol), profound bradycardia, and hypotension may occur. Other effects include drowsiness, delirium, hallucinations, low-output cardiac failure, and cardiorespiratory arrest (asystole or ventricular fibrillation). Bronchospasm and hypoglycaemia occur rarely.

First-degree heart block, intraventricular conduction defects, right and left bundle branch block, ST segment elevation, ventricular extrasystoles, and disappearance of the P wave may be noted on the electrocardiogram. Sotalol has been reported to cause Q–T interval prolongation and ventricular arrhythmias and asystole may follow severe overdose from any β-adrenoceptor blocking drug.

Treatment

A delay in treatment may be fatal in patients who are severely poisoned. The blood pressure and cardiac rhythm of the patient should be monitored immediately in an intensive care area and supportive measures implemented. Gastric lavage should be considered in adults who have ingested a substantial overdose less than 1 h previously; 0.6 to 1.2 mg of atropine intravenously may prevent vagal-induced cardiovascular collapse during this procedure.

Glucagon is the drug of choice for severe hypotension and should be given in a bolus dose of 50 to 150 µg/kg (typically 10 mg in an adult) over 1 min, followed by an infusion of 1 to 5 mg/h according to response.

Insertion of a temporary transvenous pacemaker wire, atropine, and isoprenaline 0.5 to 10 µg/min intravenously or other inotropic agents have been recommended but are probably less effective than glucagon. Occasionally, 5 to 10 mg of diazepam intravenously may be needed for convulsions. If bronchospasm supervenes, salbutamol (albuterol) by nebulizer, or aminophylline by intravenous infusion, should be employed. Hypoglycaemia should be corrected.

Further reading

Lip GYH, Ferner RE (1995). Poisoning with anti-hypertensive drugs: β-adrenoreceptor blocker drugs. *Journal of Human Hypertension* **9**, 213–21.

Taboulet P *et al.* (1993). Pathophysiology and management of self-poisoning with β-blockers. *Journal of Toxicology—Clinical Toxicology* **31**, 531–51.

β₂-Adrenoceptor stimulants

Poisoning with β$_2$-adrenoceptor stimulants, including fenoterol, pirbuterol, reproburerol, rimiterol, salbutamol, and terbutaline, has followed deliberate and accidental ingestion of these drugs and may also result from confusion over the difference between oral and parenteral doses.

Clinical features

These include a feeling of excitement, hallucinations, and agitation, accompanied by palpitations, tachycardia, tremor, and peripheral vasodilation. More serious complications such as hypokalaemia, ventricular tachyarrhythmias, ECG changes of myocardial ischaemia, pulmonary oedema, convulsions, hyperglycaemia, and lactic acidosis are uncommon.

Treatment

Gastric lavage may be considered or activated charcoal administered if the patient presents within 1 h of a substantial overdose. Hypokalaemia should be corrected as soon as possible by the administration of an infusion of potassium at a rate of 40 to 60 mmol/h diluted in 1 litre 5 per cent dextrose. A non-selective β-blocker, such as propanolol 1 to 5 mg by slow intravenous injection will also reverse hypokalaemia induced by β$_2$-adrenoceptor stimulants. However, its use may exacerbate pre-existing chronic air flow obstruction. Methods to increase elimination have no role.

Further reading

Leikin JB *et al.* (1994). Hypokalemia after pediatric albuterol overdose: a case series. *American Journal of Emergency Medicine* **12**, 64–6.

Bismuth chelate (tripotassium dicitratobismuthate)

Although bismuth absorption from bismuth chelate is low after a therapeutic dose, a significant quantity may be absorbed after overdose. Renal toxicity is dose-dependent in animals and is directed primarily towards the tubular epithelial cells.

Clinical features

Self-poisoning with large doses of bismuth chelate has caused reversible renal failure up to 10 days after overdose and at least one death. During prolonged (and sometimes high-dose) therapy, bismuth-induced encephalopathy has been reported.

Treatment

If a patient presents within 1 h of a substantial overdose, gastric lavage should be considered. Dimercaprol can lower brain bismuth concentrations though there is no evidence that it can prevent nephrotoxicity. DMSA and DMPS may be effective oral alternatives.

Further reading

Akpolat I *et al.* (1996). Acute renal failure due to overdose of colloidal bismuth. *Nephrology, Dialysis, Transplantion* **11**, 1890–1.

Bleaches and lavatory cleaners

Household bleach is normally a 3 to 6 per cent solution of sodium hypochlorite, whereas industrial bleaches contain more than 10 per cent. Some bleaches also contain sodium hydroxide. Household bleach may give rise to toxic gases such as chlorine if mixed with other cleaning agents in a lavatory bowl.

Clinical features

Ingestion may cause a burning sensation in the mouth, throat, and oesophagus, accompanied by a sensation of thirst, vomiting, and abdominal discomfort. Pharyngeal and laryngeal oedema and hypernatraemia may develop.

Treatment

When small quantities of household bleach have been ingested, liberal fluids by mouth are all that is required. Gastric lavage should only be considered if concentrated bleach has been swallowed less than 1 h previously. Endoscopy should be performed if industrial bleach has been ingested.

Inhalation of gases liberated by mixing bleach with other products may result in severe respiratory irritation and pulmonary oedema. Treat as for inhalation of chlorine.

Further reading

Hilbert G *et al.* (1997). Euro bleach: fatal hypernatremia due to 13.3 per cent sodium hypochlorite. *Journal of Toxicology—Clinical Toxicology* **35**, 635–6.

Kiristioglu I *et al.* (1999). Is it necessary to perform an endoscopy after the ingestion of liquid household bleach in children? *Acta Paediatrica* **88**, 233–4.

Butyrophenones

Benperidol, droperidol, haloperidol, and triperidol are used as antipsychotic and neuroleptic agents.

Clinical features

Overdosage may result in drowsiness and hypotension, but acute dystonic reactions are the most dramatic consequences. Neuroleptic malignant syndrome has also been reported.

Treatment

Treatment is supportive. Acute dystonic reactions should be treated with benztropine (benzatropine) 1 to 2 mg or procyclidine 5 to 10 mg intravenously for an adult.

Further reading

Yoshida I *et al.* (1993). Acute accidental overdosage of haloperidol in children. *Acta Paediatrica Scandinavica* **82**, 877–80.

Cadmium

Cadmium compounds are poorly absorbed orally but are well absorbed through the lungs. Cadmium is deposited in the liver and kidneys and very slowly excreted in the urine (half-life 10 to 30 years).

Clinical features

Acute poisoning

Inhalation of cadmium oxide fumes produced in welding or cutting has led to the development of severe lung damage and death. Often there are no initial symptoms but after some 4 to 10 h there is increasing respiratory distress. Chills and tremor accompany dyspnoea, cough, and chest pain. Severe pulmonary oedema may develop, or chemical pneumonitis in less severe cases. Recovery may be complicated by progressive pulmonary fibrosis.

The ingestion of cadmium salts (more than 3 mg/kg body weight) may lead to gastrointestinal disturbance which, in severe cases, may progress to circulatory collapse, acute renal failure, pulmonary oedema, and death.

Chronic poisoning

Repeated exposure to cadmium leads to renal tubular dysfunction with glycosuria, aminoaciduria, and hypercalciuria, an increased incidence of renal stones and osteomalacia. Less common features include anosmia, anaemia, teeth discoloration, and neuropsychological impairment. Later, emphysema may develop.

Workers repeatedly exposed to high concentrations of cadmium have developed carcinoma of the prostate or lung.

Treatment

There is no clinical evidence that any currently available antidote chelates a substantial body burden of cadmium.

Further reading

Järup L *et al.* (1998). Health effects of cadmium exposure—a review of the literature and a risk estimate. *Scandinavian Journal of Work, Environment and Health* **24**, 1–51.

Calcium-channel blockers

Calcium-channel blockers (amlodipine, diltiazem, felodipine, isradipine, nicardipine, nifedipine, nimodipine, verapamil) interfere with the inward transmembrane passage of calcium ions in myocardial cells, the cardiac conducting system, and vascular smooth muscle.

Clinical features

In overdose, calcium-channel blockers cause nausea, vomiting, dizziness, slurred speech, confusion, sinus bradycardia and tachycardia, prolonged atrioventricular conduction, atrioventricular dissociation, hypotension, pulmonary oedema, respiratory arrest, convulsions, coma, hyperglycaemia, and metabolic acidosis. Large overdoses carry a poor prognosis, particularly in patients with ischaemic heart disease and in those taking β-adrenoceptor blocking agents.

Treatment

Gastric lavage should be considered in all patients who present within 1 h of substantial overdose or, alternatively, 50 to 100 g of activated charcoal may be administered. Calcium gluconate in a dose of 10–20 ml of 10 per cent solution intravenously may reverse prolonged intracardiac conduction times but inotropic support with dobutamine at 2.5 to 10 µg/kg.min or isoprenaline at 0.5 to 10 µg/kg.min by intravenous infusion, will also be needed to maintain cardiac output in severe cases.

Further reading
Lip GYH, Ferner RE (1995). Poisoning with anti-hypertensive drugs: calcium antagonists. *Journal of Human Hypertension* 9, 155–61.

Yuan TH *et al.* (1999). Insulin-glucose as adjunctive therapy for severe calcium channel antagonist poisoning. *Journal of Toxicology—Clinical Toxicology* 37, 463–74.

Cannabis

Cannabis is obtained from the plant *Cannabis sativa* that contains many active substances of which the most important are the tetrahydrocannabinols.

Smoking is the common route of use of cannabis. It is occasionally ingested and, rarely, made into a 'tea' and injected intravenously.

Clinical features

Euphoria with drowsiness and distorted and heightened images, colours, and sounds are the usual effects of this compound. Tactile sensations may also be altered. A tachycardia is often present and heavy use may lead to conjunctival suffusion, hypotension, and ataxia. Higher doses induce auditory hallucinations, confusion, depersonalization, and panic. Some people find the distortion of perception pleasurable but novice users may panic and seek medical help. Long-term use may predispose to psychosis.

Intravenous injection of cannabis infusions causes serious illness. Within a few minutes, there is nausea, vomiting, and chills followed after an interval of 1 h or so by profuse watery diarrhoea, tachycardia, hypotension, and arthralgia. A marked neutrophil leucocytosis is often present and hypoglycaemia has been reported in some cases. There may also be transient renal failure.

Treatment

Most patients respond to reassurance. Sedation with intravenous diazepam may be required for those whose behaviour is disruptive or who are clearly very distressed. Those who have injected cannabis infusions should be treated supportively.

Further reading
Ashton CH (1999). Adverse effects of cannabis and cannabinoids. *British Journal of Anaesthesia* 83, 637–49.

Fant RV *et al.* (1998). Acute and residual effects of marijuana in humans. *Pharmacology, Biochemistry and Behavior* 60, 777–84.

Carbamate insecticides

Like many organophosphorus compounds, carbamate insecticides inhibit acetylcholinesterase. However, in comparison the duration of this effect is relatively short-lived since the carbamate–enzyme complex tends to dissociate spontaneously.

Clinical features

See organophosphorus insecticide poisoning (below).

Treatment

Symptomatic cases require atropine, but the use of oximes is usually unnecessary; rapid recovery within 24 h is the rule.

Further reading
Wagner SL (1997). Diagnosis and treatment of organophosphate and carbamate intoxication. *Occupational Medicine (Philadelphia)* 12, 239–49.

Carbamazepine

Carbamazepine is structurally related to the tricyclic antidepressants and has similar anticholinergic actions. Overdosage may therefore result in a dry mouth, drowsiness, coma, and convulsions. Cardiotoxicity similar to that seen in tricyclic antidepressant poisoning also occurs but is uncommon. Relapse into coma has been described during the course of recovery, probably due to continuing drug absorption. Treatment should include administration of activated charcoal or gastric lavage, if appropriate, and supportive therapy. Diazepam may be required to treat convulsions. Carbamazepine elimination is hastened by giving multiple doses of activated charcoal.

Further reading
Apfelbaum JD *et al.* (1995). Cardiovascular effects of carbamazepine toxicity. *Annals of Emergency Medicine* 25, 631–5.

Boldy DAR *et al.* (1987). Activated charcoal for carbamazepine poisoning. *Lancet* i, 1027.

Durelli L, Massazza U, Cavallo R (1989). Carbamazepine toxicity and poisoning. *Medical Toxicology and Adverse Drug Experience* 4, 95–107.

Montoya-Cabrera MA *et al.* (1996). Carbamazepine poisoning in adolescent suicide attempters. Effectiveness of multiple-dose activated charcoal in enhancing carbamazepine elimination. *Archives of Medical Research* 27, 485–9.

Carbon dioxide

Carbon dioxide is a colourless gas that is also available commercially as a solid for refrigeration purposes ('dry ice'). High concentrations may accumulate in wells, silos, manholes, and mines.

Clinical features

Dyspnoea, cough, headache, dizziness, sweating, restlessness, paraesthesiae, and sinus tachycardia are features after modest carbon dioxide exposure. Higher concentrations produce psychomotor agitation, myoclonic twitches, eye flickering, coma, and convulsions. Death occurs from acute cardiorespiratory depression.

Skin contact with 'dry ice' may result in frostbite and local blistering.

Treatment

The casualty should be removed from the contaminated environment. Thereafter, supportive care should be employed.

Further reading
Guillemin MP, Horisberger B (1994). Fatal intoxication due to an unexpected presence of carbon dioxide. *Annals of Occupational Hygiene* 38, 951–7.

Carbon disulphide

Carbon disulphide is used as a fumigant for grain and as a solvent, particularly in the rayon industry. It is a clear, colourless, volatile liquid with an odour like that of decaying cabbage.

Clinical features

Acute exposure

Acute poisoning is rare. Absorption occurs through the skin as well as by inhalation. Carbon disulphide, due to its potent defatting activity, causes reddening, cracking, and peeling of the skin and a burn may occur if contact continues for several minutes. Splashes in the eye cause immediate and severe irritation. Acute inhalation may result in irritation of the mucous membranes, blurred vision, nausea and vomiting, headache, delirium, hallucinations, coma, tremor, convulsions, and cardiac and respiratory arrest.

Chronic exposure

There is an increased incidence of cardiovascular disease among workers exposed to carbon disulphide. In addition, sleep disturbances, fatigue, anorexia, and weight loss are common complaints. Intellectual decline, depression, stereotyped behaviour, ocular changes, cerebellar and extrapyramidal signs, hepatic damage, and permanent impairment of reproductive performance have been described.

Treatment

Treatment involves removal from exposure, washing contaminated skin, irrigation of the eyes with water, and supportive measures. In the majority of cases, however, preventive measures to keep carbon disulphide concentrations in the workplace as low as possible are more important.

Further reading

Spyker DA, Gallanosa AG, Suratt PM (1982). Health effects of acute carbon disulfide exposure. *Journal of Toxicology—Clinical Toxicology* 19, 87–93.

Carbon monoxide

Carbon monoxide is a tasteless, odourless, colourless, non-irritating gas produced by incomplete combustion of organic materials. Normal endogenous carbon monoxide production is sufficient to maintain a resting carboxyhaemoglobin level of 1 to 3 per cent in urban non-smokers and 5 to 6 per cent in smokers.

Common sources of carbon monoxide are car exhaust fumes (in the absence of a catalytic converter), improperly maintained and vented heating systems, and smoke from all types of fire. Carbon monoxide derived from domestic heating systems is a major cause of accidental death in the developing world. Inhalation of methylene chloride (found in paint strippers) may also lead to carbon monoxide poisoning.

Mechanisms of toxicity

Symptoms and signs that follow inhalation of carbon monoxide are the result of tissue hypoxia. The affinity of haemoglobin for carbon monoxide is approximately 240 times greater than that for oxygen. Carbon monoxide combines with haemoglobin to form carboxyhaemoglobin, reducing the total oxygen-carrying capacity of the blood. In addition, the oxygen dissociation curve shifts to the left and modifies oxygen-binding sites. As a result, the affinity of the remaining haem groups for oxygen is increased, the oxygen dissociation curve is distorted as well as being shifted and the resulting tissue hypoxia is thus far greater than that which would result from simple loss of oxygen-carrying capacity.

Carbon monoxide may also inhibit cellular respiration as a result of reversible binding to cytochrome oxidase a_3. Brain lipid peroxidation mediated by carbon monoxide may play a role in the development of delayed neuropsychiatric sequelae.

Clinical features

The clinical features of carbon monoxide poisoning are summarized in Table 3.

Acute exposure

The symptoms of mild to moderate exposure to carbon monoxide are non-specific and may even be mistaken for a viral illness and for this reason it is

Table 3 Features of carbon monoxide poisoning

Agitation, confusion, headache (usually frontal and band-like, sometimes occipital)

Nausea and vomiting, incontinence (occasionally), haematemesis, melaena

Hyperventilation, pulmonary oedema, respiratory failure

Cheyne–Stokes respiration

Metabolic acidosis

Bullous lesions

Hyperpyrexia

Loss of consciousness, hypertonia, hyperreflexia

Extensor plantar responses, papilloedema, convulsions

Monoplegia or hemiplegia, peripheral neuropathies

Cerebral, cerebellar, and midbrain damage (parkinsonism, akinetic mutism)

Myocardial ischaemia and infarction

Arrhythmias and ECG changes: atrial fibrillation, prolonged P–R interval, atrioventricular block, bundle-branch block, ventricular extrasystoles, prolonged Q–T interval, ST depression

Decrease in light sensitivity and dark adaptation, retinal haemorrhages

Hearing loss (central type due to ischaemia of cochlea and brainstem nuclei)

Acute renal failure

Muscle necrosis

Thrombotic thrombocytopenic purpura

---

important that the diagnosis is always borne in mind. Elderly patients and those with pre-existing cardiorespiratory disease are at greater risk. A carboxyhaemoglobin concentration of less than 10 per cent is not normally associated with symptoms and 10 to 30 per cent carboxyhaemoglobin may result only in headache and mild exertional dyspnoea. Even low concentrations of carbon monoxide produce significant effects on cardiac function during exercise in subjects with coronary artery disease. Coma, convulsions, and cardiorespiratory arrest may be expected with carboxyhaemoglobin concentrations in excess of 60 per cent.

Delayed effects

Neuropsychiatric problems after recovery from carbon monoxide intoxication may develop insidiously over a number of weeks. They include intellectual deterioration, memory impairment, features of cerebral, cerebellar, and midbrain damage, parkinsonism, akinetic mutism, irritability, verbal aggressiveness, violence, impulsiveness, and moodiness.

Treatment

The patient should be removed from exposure and 100 per cent oxygen administered using a tightly fitting facemask. Endotracheal intubation and mechanical ventilation may be required in those who are unconscious. The administration of oxygen should be continued until the carboxyhaemoglobin concentration is less than 10 per cent.

Controlled studies of hyperbaric oxygen have not shown greater benefit than 100 per cent normobaric oxygen with elective ventilation.

General symptomatic and supportive measures will be required. Diazepam (5 to 10 mg intravenously) repeated as necessary is the agent of choice for the management of convulsions. The benefit of corticosteroids for the treatment of cerebral oedema has not been proved but mannitol may be useful.

Further reading

International Programme on Chemical Safety (1999). *Environmental Health Criteria 213. Carbon monoxide*, 2nd edn. World Health Organization, Geneva.

Thom SR *et al.* (1995). Delayed neuropsychologic sequelae after carbon monoxide poisoning; prevention by treatment with hyperbaric oxygen. *Annals of Emergency Medicine* 25, 474–80.

Carbon tetrachloride (tetrachloromethane)

Carbon tetrachloride was once widely used as a dry-cleaning chemical, degreasing agent, and fire extinguisher but international regulations have now restricted it to laboratory and industrial usage and it is no longer manufactured in most developed countries.

Clinical features

Acute exposure

The immediate effects include nausea, vomiting, abdominal pain, and diarrhoea. High concentrations cause dizziness, confusion, coma, respiratory depression, hypotension, and occasionally convulsions. Death may follow from respiratory failure or ventricular fibrillation due to cardiac sensitization to circulating catecholamines. Hepatorenal damage supervenes after a delay of up to 2 weeks. Hepatic enzyme activities increase before jaundice and a tender swollen liver develop. Maximal liver damage probably occurs within 48 h of an acute exposure and may progress to fulminant hepatic failure. Acute renal tubular necrosis is common and may develop in the absence of hepatic dysfunction 1 to 7 days after exposure. Rarely, cerebellar dysfunction, cerebral haemorrhage, optic atrophy, and parkinsonism may occur. Alcohol and previous liver damage render the individual more susceptible.

A plain film of the abdomen may confirm ingestion has occurred (Fig. 1).

Chronic exposure

Repeated exposure to low concentrations of carbon tetrachloride may also cause hepatic and renal damage. Hepatic cirrhosis and hepatoma may develop. Prolonged carbon tetrachloride exposure is associated with polyneuropathy, various visual disturbances, and anaemia, including fatal aplastic anaemia.

Fig. 1 Plain abdominal radiograph in a patient who ingested carbon tetrachloride.

Treatment

After ingestion, gastric emptying is probably best avoided because of the risk of aspiration. If the patient presents within 12 h of exposure, N-acetylcysteine should be given as for paracetamol overdose (see below). Renal and liver failure should be managed conventionally.

Further reading

International Programme on Chemical Safety (1999). *Environmental Health Criteria 208. Carbon tetrachloride*. World Health Organization, Geneva.

Chlorates

Clinical features

Sodium chlorate and potassium chlorate are powerful oxidizing agents and are highly toxic if ingested. The early features include nausea, vomiting, diarrhoea, abdominal pain, and cyanosis secondary to methaemoglobinaemia. Intravascular haemolysis occurs causing hyperkalaemia, jaundice, and oliguric renal failure.

Treatment

Gastric lavage should be considered if the patient presents within 1 h of ingestion. Methaemoglobinaemia can be corrected by slow intravenous injection of methylthioninium chloride (methylene blue) 2 mg/kg body weight, although antidotal efficacy is reduced in the presence of haemolysis. Blood transfusion may be required. Plasma potassium concentrations should be monitored and reduced if necessary. Haemodialysis will remove chlorate and may also be required for the management of renal failure and hyperkalaemia. Plasmapheresis has also been employed since it will remove chlorate, circulating free haemoglobin, and red cell stroma and thus help to prevent the development of renal failure.

Chlorine

Chlorine is a greenish-yellow gas normally transported as a pressurized liquid. Exposure after spillage may be prolonged because gaseous chlorine is heavier than air, causing it to remain near ground level. Chlorine has a pungent odour that can usually be detected by smell at concentrations of less than 0.5 ppm.

Molecular chlorine, a strong oxidizing agent, is known to react with many functional groups in cell components, forms chloramines, oxidizes thiol radicals, reacts with tissue water to form hypochlorite and hydrochloric acid, and it may generate oxygen free radicals.

Clinical features

Symptoms begin within minutes and include irritation of the mucous membranes of the eyes, nose, and throat, followed by cough, breathlessness, expectoration of white sputum (which may be bloodstained), chest pain and tightness, abdominal pain, nausea, headache, dizziness, and palpitation due to ventricular ectopic beats. Laryngeal oedema may cause hoarseness of the voice and stridor, and cardiac arrest may occur secondary to hypoxia.

Restrictive as well as obstructive ventilatory defects arise in those who have inhaled sublethal amounts. Diffusion is impaired, leading to arterial hypoxaemia. In very severe cases, non-cardiogenic pulmonary oedema and respiratory failure may develop. Survival is usually followed by complete resolution of the pulmonary defects.

Some workers chronically exposed to the gas become anosmic.

Treatment

The first priority is to remove the casualty from exposure. Conjunctival skin burns should be treated as for acids (see above).

Patients with respiratory symptoms persisting beyond the period of exposure should be admitted to hospital in case they require bronchodilators and humidified oxygen. Some will require mechanical ventilation, particularly if non-cardiogenic pulmonary oedema develops. Frusemide has been reported to be of value. Corticosteroids and prophylactic antibiotics have not been shown to be of value. Correction of serious metabolic acidosis with intravenous sodium bicarbonate may be necessary.

Further reading

Mvros R, Dean BS, Krenzelok EP (1993). Home exposures to chlorine/chloramine gas: review of 216 cases. *Southern Medical Journal* **86**, 654–7.

Schonhofer B, Voshaar T, Kohler D (1996). Long-term sequelae following accidental chlorine gas exposure. *Respiration* **63**, 155–9.

Chlorofluorocarbons (CFCs)

CFCs are derived by the partial or complete substitution of the hydrogen atoms in methane and ethane with chlorine and fluorine atoms. CFCs were developed as refrigerants some 60 years ago but have been used as propellants in aerosols, as blowing agents in foam insulation products, and as intermediates for plastics. The aerosol propellant market, which previously consumed half of the total production, is currently a minor application due to international restrictions imposed as a result of concerns that CFCs damage the ozone layer of the earth's atmosphere.

Clinical features

Acute exposure

Inhalation of CFCs may result in a tingling sensation, humming in the ears, apprehension, slurred speech, and decreased performance in psychological tests. Exposure to high concentrations may result in clinically significant arrhythmias, coma, and respiratory depression; fatalities have occurred particularly after CFC abuse (see volatile substance abuse).

Chronic exposure

A sensorimotor neuropathy developed in a laundry worker exposed for several years both to CFC 113 and tetrachloroethylene and in a refrigerator repair worker. However, epidemiological studies in exposed workers have not found evidence of a causal relationship.

Further reading

International Programme on Chemical Safety (1990). *Environmental Health Criteria 113. Fully halogenated chlorofluorocarbons.* World Health Organization, Geneva.

International Programme on Chemical Safety (1991). *Environmental Health Criteria 126. Partially halogenated chlorofluorocarbons (Methane derivatives).* World Health Organization, Geneva.

International Programme on Chemical Safety (1992). *Environmental Health Criteria 139. Partially halogenated chlorofluorocarbons (Ethane derivatives).* World Health Organization, Geneva.

Chlorophenoxy herbicides

The chlorophenoxy herbicides (Table 4) include the substances popularly referred to as 'hormone' weedkillers and are used widely in agriculture and by the public. Most instances of serious poisoning have been due to deliberate ingestion but few cases have been reported. These herbicides are often coformulated with the chemically related herbicide, dicamba, which is of low toxicity, and ioxynil and bromoxynil, which uncouple oxidative phosphorylation.

Table 4 Chlorophenoxyacetate herbicides

Chemical name	Other names
2,4-Dichlorophenoxy acetic acid	2,4-D
4-(2,4-Dichlorophenoxy) butyric acid	2,4-DB
2-(2,4-Dichlorophenoxy) propionic acid	2,4-DP, DCPP, dichlorprop
2,4,5-Trichlorophenoxy acetic acid	2,4,5-T
2-(2,4,5-Trichlorophenoxy) propionic acid	2,4,5-TP, fenoprop
4-Chloro-2-methylphenoxyacetic acid	MCPA
4-(4-Chloro-2-methylphenoxy) butyric acid	MCPB
2-(4-Chloro-2-methylphenoxy) propionic acid	MCPA, mecoprop

Clinical features

Ingestion causes burning in the mouth and throat, nausea, vomiting, and abdominal pain. The face may be flushed and there is often profuse sweating and fever. CNS depression leading to deep, prolonged coma, hyperventilation, metabolic acidosis, and pulmonary oedema may develop. ECG abnormalities and skeletal muscle damage leading to proximal myopathy have been reported.

Treatment

Gastric lavage should be considered if the patient presents within 1 h of overdose. Supportive measures should be employed as necessary. Alkalinization of the urine (see above) is indicated for severe poisoning since it considerably enhances elimination of 2,4-dichlorophenoxy acetic acid (2,4-D) and, to a lesser extent, mecoprop, particularly if combined with a high urine flow (>600 ml/h). Alkalinization of the urine probably does not have a beneficial effect on the elimination of other phenoxyacetates and does not affect that of ioxynil.

Further reading

Bradberry SM *et al.* (2000). Mechanisms of toxicity, clinical features and management of acute chlorophenoxy herbicide poisoning: A review. *Journal of Toxicology—Clinical Toxicology* **38**, 111–22.

Chloroquine

Chloroquine overdose is probably the most common form of self-poisoning with drugs in Africa, the Far East, and West Pacific and is a growing problem in Europe.

Clinical features

Toxicity can result from doses greater than 1 g (about six tablets) in adults. Cardiac arrest is commonly the first clinical manifestation of poisoning, but hypotension usually precedes it and may progress to cardiogenic shock and pulmonary oedema. Electrocardiographic abnormalities, bradyarrhythmias, and tachyarrhythmias are common and are similar to those of quinine (see below). Visual disturbance, agitation, drowsiness, acute psychosis, dystonic reactions, seizures, and coma may ensue. Hypokalaemia is common and is due to potassium channel blockade.

Treatment

Gastric lavage or activated charcoal (50 to 100 g) should be considered if the patient presents within 1 h. Supportive measures should be employed and hypokalaemia corrected. There is no specific antidote. There is evidence that mechanical ventilation, the administration of adrenaline (epinephrine) (0.25 µg/kg. min) and high-doses of diazepam (1 mg/kg as a loading dose and 0.25 to 0.4 mg/kg.h maintenance) may reduce the mortality to 10 per cent in severe poisoning. Multiple-dose activated charcoal may enhance chloroquine elimination.

Further reading

Clemessy JL *et al.* (1996). Treatment of acute chloroquine poisoning: a 5-year experience. *Critical Care Medicine* **24**, 1189–95.

McKenzie AG (1996). Intensive therapy for chloroquine poisoning—a review of 29 cases. *South African Medical Journal* **86**, 597–9.

Chromium

There is no good evidence that chromium(II), chromium(III) and chromium(IV) compounds are dangerous but chromium(III) compounds have produced skin sensitization. Chromium(VI) is the most important toxicologically because it can cross cell membranes readily. In contrast, chromium(III) compounds are confined to the extracellular space.

Chromium is absorbed mainly by inhalation and, to a lesser extent, via the skin or gastrointestinal tract. Hexavalent chromium compounds are generally better absorbed than trivalent chromium compounds and, understandably, soluble chromium compounds such as sodium (VI) chromate are absorbed more readily than insoluble compounds such as chromium(III) oxide. Chromium is excreted via the kidney.

Clinical features

Acute poisoning

Inhaled soluble chromium(VI) compounds, such as sodium and potassium chromate and dichromate, are highly irritant to mucous membranes and may lead to inflammation of the nasal mucosa. Inhalation of chromium(VI) trioxide (chromic acid) causes cough, headache, chest pain, dyspnoea, and cyanosis.

Ingestion of highly water-soluble chromium(VI) compounds leads within minutes to nausea, vomiting, abdominal pain, diarrhoea, and a burning sensation in the mouth, throat, and stomach; gastrointestinal haemorrhage is a frequent complication.

Methaemoglobinaemia, haemolysis, and disseminated intravascular coagulation, and renal and hepatic failure have been reported.

Chromic acid splashes produce severe burns. Percutaneous absorption may lead to kidney and liver failure; fatalities have occurred.

Chronic poisoning

'Chrome ulcers' may develop after repeated topical exposure to chromium(VI) compounds. They have a well-defined circular margin with raised edges and a central cavity that may penetrate to bone and is filled with exudate or a tenacious crust. Chromium(VI) compounds are also skin sensitizers and contribute to the development of cement dermatitis and contact dermatitis from paint primer, tanned leather, tattoo pigments, and matches.

Inhalation of chromium(VI) compounds has led to atrophy, ulceration, and perforation of the nasal septum. Pharyngeal and laryngeal ulcers may also occur. Asthma may be precipitated by exposure to fumes. Lung fibrosis, bronchitis, emphysema, and proximal tubular damage result from occupational exposure. There is an increased risk of lung cancer.

Treatment

Ascorbic acid reduces chromium(VI) to the less toxic chromium(III). Topical 10 per cent ascorbic acid, as an ointment or in solution, has led to dramatic resolution of occupational chromium dermatitis but there is no clinical evidence that the systemic administration of ascorbic acid, or any other reducing agent, lessens morbidity or mortality in severe chromium poisoning. Topical preparations containing sodium calcium edetate may also afford some protection to the skin but there is no evidence that systemic chelation treatment is beneficial in chromium poisoning. Haemodialysis effectively removes chromium from the blood but the high tissue uptake limits the value of this treatment when used alone.

Further reading

Barceloux DG (1999). Chromium. *Journal of Toxicology—Clinical Toxicology* **37**, 173–94.

Bradberry SM, Vale JA (1999). Therapeutic review: is ascorbic acid of value in chromium poisoning and chromium dermatitis. *Journal of Toxicology—Clinical Toxicology* **37**, 195–200.

Clomethiazole (chlormethiazole)

Clinical features

This hypnotic drug taken in overdose may cause coma, respiratory depression, reduced muscle tone, hypotension, and excessive salivation. The characteristic odour of clomethiazole is often detected on the breath.

Treatment

Treatment is supportive.

Clonidine

Clonidine exerts its hypotensive action by reduction of sympathetic tone mediated by a central effect on postsynaptic α_2-adrenoceptors in the medulla. Clonidine decreases heart rate, cardiac output, and total peripheral resistance. In the presence of high plasma clonidine concentrations, peripheral α_2-agonist activity predominates and accounts for those instances of vasoconstriction and hypertension reported following clonidine overdose.

Clinical features

Poisoning may be severe and life-threatening, particularly in children. Hypertension and severe vasoconstriction are unusual while bradycardia, hypotension, coma, and respiratory depression are common. Toxic effects last about 16 h, but may extend to several days in severe overdose.

Treatment

Gastric lavage should be considered or 50 to 100 g of activated charcoal administered if a patient presents within 1 h of a substantial overdose. Bradycardia is usually reversed by atropine in a dose of 0.6 to 2.4 mg intravenously. The use of α-adrenergic blocking drugs (tolazoline or phentolamine) has been advocated in severely poisoned patients but their action may be unpredictable. Severe hypotension should be treated with a plasma expander and then, if necessary, an inotropic agent such as, dobutamine 2.5 to 10 µg/kg.min may be given by intravenous infusion. The use of naloxone has been advocated but its benefit is inconsistent and it may produce hypertension. Sodium nitroprusside 0.5 to 8.0 µg/kg.min by intravenous infusion is the most effective agent for management of severe hypertension and peripheral vasoconstriction. Although forced diuresis has been employed in the treatment of clonidine poisoning, renal elimination is not increased.

Further reading

Erickson SJ, Duncan A (1998). Clonidine poisoning—an emerging problem: epidemiology, clinical features, management and preventative strategies. *Journal of Paediatrics and Child Health* **34**, 280–2.

Nichols MH, King WD, James LP (1997). Clonidine poisoning in Jefferson County, Alabama. *Annals of Emergency Medicine* **29**, 511–17.

Cobalt

Cobalt is a relatively rare element and usually exists in association with nickel, silver, lead, copper, and iron ores. It is used in steel alloys, in the manufacture of magnets, and in the hard metal industry as a binder for tungsten carbide. It is also an essential dietary trace element available as a component of vitamin B_{12} (cyanocobalamin).

Cobalt can be absorbed orally and by inhalation. Most absorbed cobalt is excreted within days but a small proportion is retained with a biological half-life of approximately 2 years. The normal body burden of cobalt is about 1.1 mg.

Clinical features

Acute poisoning
Cobalt salts are relatively non-toxic but their ingestion may lead to gastro-intestinal disturbance.

Chronic poisoning
Occupational exposure to cobalt dust occurs mainly in the tungsten carbide industry and causes 'hard metal' pneumoconiosis with interstitial fibrosis. This usually develops after several years of exposure to high concentrations of cobalt and may prove fatal. There is also a higher incidence of bronchitis and emphysema amongst cobalt workers and occupational asthma has been reported.

Chronic occupational exposure also leads to anosmia, auditory nerve damage, visual disturbance, irritability, headache, memory deficit, weakness, peripheral neuropathy, gastrointestinal disturbance, and weight loss. There is no firm evidence that cobalt is carcinogenic and assessment of its cancer risk is often confounded by a simultaneous exposure to nickel and arsenic.

Chronic ingestion of cobalt causes polycythaemia, inhibits the iodination of tyrosine (and therefore can cause goitre), and leads to cardiomegaly, congestive cardiomyopathy, pericardial effusion, and hypertrichosis, most of which are reversible when exposure is discontinued.

Simultaneous allergies to nickel and to cobalt are frequent and there is some evidence for a mutual enhancing effect of contact sensitization to one metal in the presence of the other.

Treatment
If the patient presents early after ingestion of a cobalt salt, gastric lavage should be considered. In two studies, DMSA (succimer) significantly reduced mortality in mice poisoned with cobalt chloride but in another study, DTPA (calcium trisodium pentetate) was more effective than DMSA. No satisfactory human studies have yet been performed.

Further reading
Mucklow ES *et al.* (1990). Cobalt poisoning in a 6-year-old. *Lancet* **335**, 981.

Cocaine

In recent years there has been a considerable increase in the recreational use of cocaine. Cocaine is a powerful local anaesthetic and vasoconstrictor and may be abused by smoking, ingestion, injection, or by 'snorting' it intranasally. Users, body packers, and those who swallow the drug to avoid being found in possession of it ('stuffers') are at risk of overdose. 'Street' cocaine (cocaine hydrochloride) is sometimes dissolved in an alkaline solution from which the cocaine is extracted into ether or other solvent that is then evaporated to leave crystals of relatively pure ('freebase') cocaine. 'Crack' is another type of freebase cocaine made by heating cocaine hydrochloride with baking soda. The hard paste which crackles when smoked is also used widely. Other drugs such as ethanol, cannabis, and conventional hypnotics and sedatives are frequently taken with cocaine to reduce the intensity of its less pleasant effects.

Clinical features

The features of cocaine overdosage are similar to those of amfetamine. In addition to euphoria, it also has sympathomimetic effects including agi-

tation, tachycardia, hypertension, sweating, and hallucinations. Prolonged convulsions with metabolic acidosis, hyperthermia, rhabdomyolysis, ventricular arrhythmias, and cardiorespiratory arrest may follow in the most severe cases. Less common features include dissection of the aorta, myocarditis, myocardial infarction, dilated cardiomyopathy, subarachnoid haemorrhage, cerebral haemorrhage, and cerebral vasculitis.

A number of rare complications of the method of use of cocaine have been reported. These include pulmonary oedema after intravenous injection of freebase cocaine and pneumomediastinum and pneumothorax after sniffing it. In addition, chronic 'snorting' has caused perforation of the nasal septum, cerebrospinal fluid rhinorrhoea due to thinning of the cribriform plate, and pulmonary granulomatosis.

Treatment
Users who are intoxicated may require sedation with diazepam to control agitation or convulsions. Measures to prevent further absorption are usually irrelevant. Active external cooling is required when body temperature exceeds 41°C. Myocardial ischaemia is best treated with intravenous glyceryl nitrite or a calcium channel blocker. Hypertension and tachycardia usually respond to sedation and cooling. β-Adrenoceptor blocking drugs are absolutely contraindicated because of the risk of precipitating paradoxical hypertension. Phentolamine in a dose of 2 to 5 mg intravenously or other vasodilator can be employed, if necessary. Accelerated idioventricular rhythm should not normally require treatment but ventricular fibrillation and asystole should be managed conventionally.

Further reading
Hatsukami DK, Fischman MW (1996). Crack cocaine and cocaine hydrochloride—are the differences myth or reality? *Journal of the American Medical Association* **276**, 1580–8.

Hollander JE (1996). Cocaine-associated myocardial infarction. *Journal of the Royal Society of Medicine* **89**, 443–7.

Kloner RA *et al.* (1992). The effects of acute and chronic cocaine use on the heart. *Circulation* **85**, 407–19.

Marzuk PM *et al.* (1995). Fatal injuries after cocaine use as a leading cause of death among young adults in New York city. *New England Journal of Medicine* **332**, 1753–7.

Rubin RB, Neugarten J (1992). Medical complications of cocaine: changes in pattern of use and spectrum of complications. *Journal of Toxicology—Clinical Toxicology* **30**, 1–12.

Co-phenotrope (Lomotil)

Co-phenotrope is a mixture of an opioid, diphenoxylate hydrochloride, and atropine.

Mechanism of toxicity

Gastric emptying is delayed and intestinal motility reduced. The onset of toxicity following an overdose may be delayed for up to 12 h.

Clinical features

Respiratory depression is the major complication of diphenoxylate poisoning. Vomiting, abdominal pain, drowsiness, and coma also occur. Even though co-phenotrope tablets incorporate only a small amount of atropine this is often toxic to children under 5 years and several deaths have been reported. Anticholinergic features are to be expected (see tricyclic antidepressants below).

Treatment

Repeated doses of naloxone may be necessary to reverse respiratory depression because of the long duration of action of diphenoxylate (see opiates and opioids below). Lavage may be appropriate in an adult presenting within 1 h of a substantial overdose before toxicity develops; activated charcoal (50 to 100 g) may also reduce absorption significantly if administered within that period.

Further reading

McCarron MM, Challoner KR, Thompson GA (1991). Diphenoxylate-atropine (Lomotil) overdose in children: An update (report of eight cases and review of the literature). *Pediatrics* **87**, 694–700.

Copper

Copper is used for pipes and roofing material, in alloys, and as a pigment. It is a component of several enzymes, including tyrosinase and cytochrome oxidase, and is essential for the utilization of iron. Copper sulphate is used as a fungicide, an algicide, and in some fertilizers.

Approximately one-third of an ingested copper salt is absorbed and in the blood 80 per cent is bound to caeruloplasmin. Most absorbed copper is deposited in the liver and eliminated mainly in bile.

Clinical features

Acute poisoning

Acute copper poisoning usually results from the ingestion of contaminated foods or from accidental or deliberate ingestion of copper salts. Following a substantial ingestion of a copper salt there is profuse vomiting with abdominal pain, diarrhoea, headache, dizziness, and a metallic taste. Gastrointestinal haemorrhage, haemolysis, and hepatorenal failure may ensue and fatalities have occurred. Body secretions may have a green or blue discoloration.

Occupational exposure to copper fumes (during refining or welding) or to copper-containing dust causes 'metal-fume fever' with upper respiratory tract symptoms, headache, fever, and myalgia.

Chronic poisoning

Chronic occupational copper poisoning causes general malaise, anorexia, nausea, vomiting, and hepatomegaly. Contact dermatitis, pulmonary granulomas, and pulmonary fibrosis have also been described. There is no convincing evidence that copper is carcinogenic in humans.

Treatment

Although vomiting occurs invariably following the ingestion of many copper salts, gastric lavage may be of value in reducing copper absorption if presentation is early. Blood copper levels correlate well with severity of intoxication, a concentration of less than 3 mg/l indicating mild to moderate poisoning and a concentration in excess of 8 mg/l severe intoxication. D-Penicillamine 25 mg/kg body weight daily until recovery enhances copper chelation in both acute and chronic copper poisoning. There is now animal evidence to suggest that *N*-acetylcysteine and DMPS (unithiol) are of similar efficacy.

Further reading

Barceloux DG (1999). Copper. *Journal of Toxicology—Clinical Toxicology* **37**, 217–30.

International Programme on Chemical Safety (1998). *Environmental Health Criteria 200. Copper.* World Health Organization, Geneva.

Cyanide

Hydrogen cyanide and its derivatives are used widely in industry and are released during the thermal decomposition of polyurethane foams. Cyanide poisoning may also result from the ingestion of the cyanogenic glycoside, amygdalin (vitamin B$_{17}$), which is found in the kernels of almonds, apples, apricots, cherries, peaches, plums, and other fruits.

Mechanisms of toxicity

Cyanide reversibly inhibits cellular enzymes which contain ferric iron, notably cytochrome oxidase a$_3$, so that electron transfer is blocked, the tricarboxylic acid cycle is paralysed, and cellular respiration ceases.

Clinical features

Acute exposure

The ingestion by an adult of 50 ml of (liquid) hydrogen cyanide or 200 to 300 mg of one of its salts is likely to prove fatal. Inhalation of hydrogen cyanide gas may produce symptoms within seconds and death within minutes.

Acute poisoning is characterized by dizziness, headache, palpitation, anxiety, a feeling of constriction in the chest, dyspnoea, pulmonary oedema, confusion, vertigo, ataxia, coma, and paralysis. Cardiovascular collapse, respiratory arrest, convulsions, and metabolic acidosis are seen in severe cases. Cyanosis may occur, and the classic 'brick-red' colour of the skin is noted occasionally. There is sometimes an odour of bitter almonds on the breath, but the ability to detect it is genetically determined and some 40 per cent of the population are unable to do so.

Chronic exposure

Chronic exposure results predominantly in neurological damage that can include ataxia, peripheral neuropathies, amblyopia, optic atrophy, and nerve deafness.

Treatment

Cyanide poisoning is a medical emergency, although specific antidotal treatment may not always be necessary. Where appropriate, the patient should be removed from the source of exposure, contaminated clothing discarded, and the skin washed with soap and water. Gastric lavage should be considered if a cyanide salt has been ingested less than 1 h previously, but this procedure must not delay treatment if symptoms or signs of toxicity are present. It may be difficult to differentiate between the genuine fear and anxiety of a patient and the early symptoms of cyanide poisoning. However, a patient who has been exposed to hydrogen cyanide gas and who is conscious 30 min later is unlikely to require antidotal therapy.

Oxygen

The administration of oxygen is of paramount importance in the treatment of cyanide poisoning. It is believed to prevent inhibition of cytochrome oxidase a$_3$ and to accelerate its reactivation.

Dicobalt edetate

Cobalt compounds form stable inert complexes with cyanide. Dicobalt edetate (Kelocyanor), if available, is the treatment of choice for confirmed cyanide poisoning and should be given intravenously in a dose of 300 to 600 mg over 1 min, with a further 300 mg if recovery does not occur within 1 min. It should be administered only if the diagnosis is certain because, in the absence of cyanide, Kelocyanor may cause serious side-effects including vomiting, tachycardia, hypertension, chest pain, and facial and palpebral oedema as it contains free cobalt, which is responsible in part for its efficacy.

Sodium thiosulphate

Cyanide is detoxified by conversion to thiocyanate. Thiosulphate is required for this reaction. Sodium thiosulphate 12.5 g (25 ml of a 50 per cent solution) should be given by intravenous injection over 10 min. Experimental studies have shown that the coadministration of sodium nitrite enhances the antidotal benefit of sodium thiosulphate.

Sodium nitrite, 4-dimethylaminophenol (4-DMAP)

Another means of inactivating cyanide is to convert a portion of the body's haemoglobin to methaemoglobin, which binds cyanide. Although the affinity of cyanide for methaemoglobin is less than that of cytochrome oxidase, the presence of a large circulating methaemoglobin pool diminishes cyanide toxicity by binding cyanide ion before tissue penetration occurs. Methaemoglobinaemia may be induced by the administration of either sodium nitrite or 4-dimethylaminophenol (**4-DMAP**). 4-DMAP may produce unexpectedly high methaemoglobin concentrations and cause acute tubular necrosis and Heinz-body haemolytic anaemia. Nitrites may also mitigate cyanide toxicity by virtue of their vasodilator actions and improvement of tissue perfusion. Sodium nitrite 300 mg (10 ml of a 3 per cent solution) should be administered by intravenous injection over 3 min.

Inhalation of amyl nitrite was recommended in the past but it produces only low circulating concentrations of methaemoglobin.

Hydroxocobalamin

One mole of hydroxocobalamin inactives one mole of cyanide but, on a weight-for-weight basis, 50 times more hydroxocobalamin is needed than cyanide because hydroxocobalamin is a far larger molecule. Concentrated formulations of hydoxocobalamin are not yet available in all countries. If available, give hydroxocobalamin in a dose of 5 g intravenously over 30 min. A second dose (5 g) may be required in severe cases of cyanide poisoning.

Conclusion

If dicobalt edetate or hydroxocobalamin are not available, a combination of sodium nitrite and sodium thiosulphate should be administered..

Further reading

Mueller M, Borland C (1997). Delayed cyanide poisoning following acetonitrile poisoning. *Postgraduate Medical Journal* **73**, 299–300.
Rosenow F *et al.* (1995). Neurological sequelae of cyanide intoxication—the patterns of clinical, magnetic resonance imaging and positron emission tomography findings. *Annals of Neurology* **38**, 825–8.
Yen D *et al.* (1995). The clinical experience of acute cyanide poisoning. *American Journal of Emergency Medicine* **13**, 524–8.

Dapsone

Dapsone is available formulated alone or in combination with pyrimethamine (as Maloprim).

Clinical features

Dapsone poisoning can be severe and result not only in methaemoglobinaemia but also in haemolysis, jaundice, drowsiness, coma, seizures, and metabolic acidosis.

Treatment

If presentation after overdose is within 1 h, gastric lavage should be considered or, alternatively, 50 to 100 g of activated charcoal may be administered. Administration of repeated doses of activated charcoal seems to have comparable efficacy to haemodialysis in increasing dapsone elimination. Methylthioninium chloride (methylene blue) at 1 to 2 mg/kg should be given intravenously over 5 min for severe methaemoglobinaemia.

Further reading

Ferguson AJ, Lavery GG (1997). Deliberate self-poisoning with dapsone—a case report and summary of relevant pharmacology and treatment. *Anaesthesia* **52**, 359–63.

Diethylene glycol

Diethylene glycol is used mainly in polyester resins and polyols, as a humectant in the tobacco industry, and as a solvent. It achieved notoriety in 1985 when it was discovered that for some years it had been added to some wines. Several pharmaceutical errors have also led to fatalities.

Mechanism of toxicity

Animal studies suggest that diethylene glycol is first oxidized by alcohol dehydrogenase to 2-hydroxyethoxyacetaldehyde and then to 2-hydroxyethoxyacetic acid.

Clinical features

Nausea, vomiting, and abdominal pain occur frequently and are followed by the development of jaundice and hepatomegaly, pulmonary oedema, metabolic acidosis, coma, and renal failure in most cases.

Treatment

Supportive measures to treat dehydration and to correct metabolic acidosis should be instituted promptly. Ethanol or fomepizole (4-methylpyrazole) should be administered to block diethylene glycol metabolism and dialysis should be employed if renal failure supervenes. A loading dose of 50 g of ethanol orally (conveniently given as 125 ml of gin, whisky, or vodka) should be administered followed by an intravenous infusion of 10 to 12 g ethanol/h to produce a blood ethanol concentration of 500 mg to 1 g/l. The infusion should be continued until diethylene glycol is no longer detectable in the blood. If dialysis is employed, the rate of ethanol administration will need to be increased to 17 to 22 g/h. The regimen for fomepizole is given in the section on ethylene glycol below.

Further reading

O'Brien KL *et al.* (1998). Epidemic of pediatric deaths from acute renal failure caused by diethylene glycol poisoning. *Journal of the American Medical Association* **279**, 1175–80.
Woolf AD (1998). The Haitian diethylene glycol poisoning tragedy—A dark wood revisited. *Journal of the American Medical Association* **279**, 1215–16.

Digoxin and digitoxin

Toxicity occurring during chronic administration of these cardiac glycosides is common. In contrast, acute poisoning from digoxin and digitoxin is infrequent, though the mortality may be as high as 20 per cent after a substantial overdose, particularly if digoxin-specific antibody fragments are not employed.

Clinical features

Nausea, vomiting, dizziness, anorexia, and drowsiness are common. Confusion, diarrhoea, visual disturbances, and hallucinations may also occur. Sinus bradycardia, often marked, is the earliest cardiotoxic effect and may be followed by supraventicular arrhythmias with or without heart block, ventricular premature beats, and ventricular tachycardia. Hyperkalaemia occurs due to inhibition of the Na^+-K^+ ATPase pump. The diagnosis may be confirmed by measurement of the serum digoxin concentration.

Treatment

Gastric lavage should be considered in patients with a history of a substantial overdose less than 1 h previously. Alternatively, 50 to 100 g of activated charcoal may be administered to reduce absorption and repeated doses will also enhance elimination. Potassium supplements should not be given until the serum potassium concentration is known, as severe poisoning is commonly associated with hyperkalaemia that should be treated conventionally.

Sinus bradycardia, ventricular ectopics, atrioventricular block, and sinoatrial standstill or block are often reduced or abolished by atropine in a dose of 1.2 to 2.4 mg. Ventricular ectopics alone should not be treated unless cardiac output is impaired. Ventricular tachydysrhythmias may be treated with intravenous lignocaine, atenolol, phenytoin, or amiodarone; if clinically significant and persistent, digoxin-specific antibody fragments should be considered. Failure to achieve a satisfactory cardiac output by drug therapy in patients with bradycardia, atrioventricular block, or sinus arrest is an indication for insertion of a right ventricular pacing wire or, if available, the administration of digoxin-specific antibody fragments (6 to 8 mg/kg body weight is sufficient in most cases of poisoning. In very severe cases consult the product literature to calculate the optimal dose). An improvement in the patient's condition should occur within 20 to 40 min.

Forced diuresis, peritoneal dialysis, haemodialysis, and haemoperfusion do not significantly increase the elimination of the drug.

Further reading

Kinlay S, Buckley NA (1995). Magnesium sulfate in the treatment of ventricular arrhythmias due to digoxin toxicity. *Journal of Toxicology—Clinical Toxicology* **33**, 55–9.

Williamson KM *et al.* (1998). Digoxin toxicity: an evaluation in current clinical practice. *Archives of Internal Medicine* **158**, 2444–9.

Dishwashing liquids, fabric conditioners, and household detergents

Most of these products including carpet shampoo, dishwashing rinse aid for dishwashing machines, fabric washing powder and flakes, scouring liquids, creams, and powders contain surfactants that have both hydrophilic and lipophilic groups to allow fat-soluble substances to be dispersed in aqueous media.

There are three types of surfactants of differing toxicity: anionic surfactants, which have a negative electrical charge on the lipophilic groups; cationic surfactants, which have a positive charge; and non-ionic surfactants that have no charge.

Clinical features

Anionic detergents irritate the skin by removing natural oils and cause redness, soreness, and even a papular dermatitis. Ingestion may cause mild gastrointestinal irritation, nausea, vomiting, and diarrhoea. Non-ionic surfactants irritate the skin only slightly and appear to be completely harmless when ingested. Cationic surfactants (e.g. quarternary ammonium compounds) are much more toxic than the others but are rarely found in household cleaning materials.

Treatment

After ingestion of products containing either a non-ionic or anionic surfactant, liberal amounts of water or milk should be administered.

Further reading

Cornish LS, Parsons BJ, Dobbin MD (1996). Automatic dishwasher detergent poisoning: opportunities for prevention. *Australian and New Zealand Journal of Public Health* **20**, 278–83.

Disulfiram (Antabuse)

Mechanism of toxicity

Disulfiram and its main metabolite diethyldithiocarbamate inhibit the activity of a wide range of enzymes, particularly aldehyde dehydrogenase. Carbon disulphide, another metabolite, may account for some of the side-effects observed during disulfiram therapy.

Clinical features

Adult cases are likely to be alcoholics who have been taking disulfiram before the overdose and to be malnourished, factors that may explain the frequency of neuropsychiatric features. Sensorimotor neuropathy, flaccid tetraparesis, and encephalopathy have been described after overdose though these features may have been exacerbated by pre-existing malnourishment. Vomiting for several days, abdominal pain, and diarrhoea were reported in a patient who ingested 18 g of disulfiram.

Several cases of paediatric poisoning have been reported. Drowsiness, pyrexia, hypotonia, ataxia, uncontrollable and inappropriate arm movements, irritability, speech difficulties, hallucinations, coma, and hyperreflexia were the major features.

Disulfiram–ethanol reaction

Nausea, vertigo, anxiety, blurred vision, hypotension, chest pain, palpitation, tachycardia, facial flushing, and throbbing headache are the usual features. Symptoms usually last for 3 to 4 days but may persist for 1 week. Occasionally the reaction is very severe with respiratory depression, cardiovascular collapse, cardiac arrhythmias, coma, cerebral oedema, hemiplegia, and convulsions; fatalities have been reported.

Further reading

Zorzon M *et al.* (1995). Acute encephalopathy and polyneuropathy after disulfiram intoxication. *Alcohol and Alcoholism* **30**, 629–31.

Diuretics

Most overdoses involving diuretics are minor, although inevitably some disturbance of fluid and electrolyte balance will result. When combined diuretic and potassium formulations are ingested, the potassium content is likely to pose the greater risk. More serious consequences are likely if a potassium-sparing diuretic has been ingested.

Clinical features

Symptoms and signs of toxicity include anorexia, nausea, vomiting, diarrhoea, profound diuresis, dehydration, and hypotension. In addition, dizziness, weakness, muscle cramps, tetany, and occasionally gastrointestinal bleeding may be seen. The electrolytic and metabolic disturbances that may be observed include hyponatraemia, hypoglycaemia or hyperglycaemia, hyperuricaemia, hypokalaemia, and metabolic alkalosis. Hyperkalaemia may develop following the ingestion of combined diuretic and potassium preparations and potassium-sparing diuretics, such as amiloride, spironolactone, or triamterene and small-bowel ulceration and stricture formation has followed poisoning due to diuretics with an enteric-coated core of potassium chloride.

Treatment

Symptomatic and supportive therapy should be employed with correction of fluid and electrolyte imbalance. Patients with hyperkalaemia may need a glucose and insulin infusion followed by oral or rectal administration of an ion-exchange resin.

Further reading

Lip GYH, Ferner RE (1995). Poisoning with anti-hypertensive drugs: diuretics and potassium supplements. *Journal of Human Hypertension* **9**, 295–301.

Ethanol

Ethanol is commonly ingested in beverages before, or concomitant with, the deliberate ingestion of other substances in overdose. It is also used as a

Table 5 Clinical features of ethanol poisoning

Mild intoxication (500–1500 mg/l)
Emotional lability, and mild impairment of visual acuity, muscular co-ordination, and reaction time

Moderate intoxication (1500–3000 mg/l)
Visual impairment, sensory loss, muscular incoordination, slowed reaction time, slurred speech

Severe intoxication (3000–5000 mg/l)
Marked muscular incoordination, blurred or double vision, sometimes stupor and hypothermia, and occasionally, hypoglycaemia and convulsions

Coma (> 5000 mg/l)
Depressed reflexes, respiratory depression, hypotension, and hypothermia. Death may occur from respiratory or circulatory failure or as the result of aspiration of stomach contents in the absence of a gag reflex

Table 6 Clinical features of ethylene glycol poisoning

Stage 1 (30 min to 12 h): Gastrointestinal and nervous system involvement
Apparent intoxication with alcohol (but no ethanol on breath)
Nausea, vomiting, haematemesis
Coma and convulsions (often focal)
Nystagmus, ophthalmoplegias, papilloedema, depressed reflexes, myoclonic jerks, V, VII, VIII nerve palsies
Tetanic contractions

Stage 2 (12–24 h): Cardiorespiratory involvement
Tachypnoea
Tachycardia
Mild hypertension
Pulmonary oedema
Congestive cardiac failure

Stage 3 (24–72 h): Renal involvement
Flank pain
Renal angle tenderness
Acute tubular necrosis

solvent and is found in many cosmetic and antiseptic preparations. It is rapidly absorbed through the gastric and intestinal mucosas and approximately 95 per cent is oxidized to acetaldehyde and then to acetate; the remainder is excreted unchanged in the urine and to a lesser extent in the breath and through the skin.

Ethanol is a central nervous depressant that exacerbates the effects of other central nervous system depressants, in particular, hypnotic agents. The fatal dose of ethanol alone is between 300 and 500 ml of absolute alcohol, if this is ingested in less than 1 h.

Clinical features

The clinical features of ethanol intoxication are well known and are generally related to blood concentrations (Table 5).

Severe hypoglycaemia may accompany alcohol intoxication due to inhibition of gluconeogenesis. This occurs more commonly in children than in adults and typically occurs within 6 to 36 h of ingestion of a moderate to large amount of alcohol by either a previously malnourished individual or one who has fasted for the previous 24 h. The patient is often in coma and hypothermic but flushing, sweating, and tachycardia are frequently absent. Rarely lactic acidosis, ketoacidosis, and acute renal failure have been described.

Treatment

Hypoglycaemia is usually unresponsive to glucagon and therefore intravenous glucose in a dose of 50 ml of 50 per cent solution should be given. Treatment is supportive. Gastric lavage has not been shown to be of benefit in ethanol poisoning. The use of haemodialysis should be considered if the blood ethanol concentration exceeds 5000 mg/l and/or if metabolic acidosis is present.

Further reading

Ernst AA *et al.* (1996). Ethanol ingestion and related hypoglycemia in a pediatric and adolescent emergency department population. *Academic Emergency Medicine* **3**, 46–9.

Ethylene glycol (1,2-ethanediol)

Ethylene glycol has a variety of commercial applications and is commonly used as an antifreeze fluid in car radiators. Its sweet taste and ready availability have contributed to its popularity as a suicide agent and as a poor man's substitute for alcohol.

It is thought that the minimum lethal dose of ethylene glycol is about 100 ml for an adult, although recovery after treatment has been reported following the ingestion of up to 1 litre.

Mechanism of toxicity

Ethylene glycol itself appears to be non-toxic. Metabolism takes place in the liver and kidneys. Accumulation of metabolites including aldehydes, glycolate, oxalate, and lactic acid may explain toxicity.

Clinical features

The clinical features of ethylene glycol poisoning may be divided into three stages depending on the time after ingestion (Table 6). In addition, hypocalcaemia, severe metabolic acidosis, and calcium oxalate crystalluria are observed in severe cases. The severity of each stage and the progression from one stage to the next depends on the amount of ethylene glycol ingested.

Death may occur during any of the three stages. A serum ethylene glycol concentration in excess of 500 mg/l indicates severe poisoning.

Treatment

Early diagnosis and appropriate therapy significantly reduce the mortality from ethylene glycol poisoning. Gastric lavage should be considered if presentation occurs less than 1 h after ingestion. Supportive measures to combat shock, respiratory distress, hypocalcaemia, and metabolic acidosis should be instituted. Thereafter, treatment has two main aims. First, the competitive inhibition of ethylene glycol metabolism, using ethanol or fomepizole (4-methylpyrozole), and, second, the increased elimination of the glycol from the body using dialysis. A loading dose of 50 g of ethanol (conveniently given as approximately 125 ml of gin, whisky, or vodka) should be administered followed by an intravenous infusion of 10 to 12 g of ethanol to provide blood ethanol concentrations of 500 mg to 1 g/l. The infusion should be continued until ethylene glycol is no longer detectable in the blood. If dialysis is also employed, the rate of ethanol administration will need to be increased (17 to 22 g/h). Alternatively, fomepizole at 15 mg/kg body weight can be administered over 30 min, followed by four 12-hourly bolus doses of 10 mg/kg until ethylene glycol concentrations are less than 200 mg/l. If treatment is needed for more than 48 h, the bolus dose should be increased to 15 mg/kg to compensate for the induction of fomepizole metabolism. If dialysis is employed, the frequency of dosing should be increased to 4-hourly during dialysis because fomepizole is dialysable.

Ethylene glycol, its aldehyde metabolites, and glycolate may be removed by either peritoneal or haemodialysis, though the latter is two to three times more efficient. Oxalate, however, is poorly dialysable. In addition, it may be necessary to treat the uraemic complications of ethylene glycol poisoning with dialysis and to use haemodialysis/ultrafiltration to correct the sodium overload that can result from the necessary, but sometimes overjudicious, correction of the metabolic acidosis with sodium bicarbonate. Dialysis should be continued until ethylene glycol is no longer detectable in the blood.

Further reading

Barceloux DG *et al.* (1999). American Academy of Clinical Toxicology practice guidelines on the treatment of ethylene glycol poisoning. *Journal of Toxicology—Clinical Toxicology* **37**, 537–60.

Glaser DS (1996). Utility of the serum osmol gap in the diagnosis of methanol or ethylene glycol ingestion. *Annals of Emergency Medicine* **27**, 343–6.

Jacobsen D, McMartin KE (1997). Antidotes for methanol and ethylene glycol poisoning. *Journal of Toxicology—Clinical Toxicology* **35**, 127–43.

Lewis LD, Smith BW, Mamourian AC (1997). Delayed sequelae after acute overdoses or poisonings: cranial neuropathy related to ethylene glycol ingestion. *Clinical Pharmacology and Therapeutics* **61**, 692–9.

Flecainide

Flecainide is a local anaesthetic-type antiarrhythmic drug that inhibits fast sodium channels of cardiac myocytes and markedly shortens action potential duration in the Purkinje system.

Clinical features

The features of overdose are predictable on the basis of the drug's known effects and include hypotension, bradycardia, intraventricular conduction abnormalities, atrioventricular block, and ventricular tachycardia. In severe cases convulsions and cardiorespiratory failure occur and fatalities have been reported.

Treatment

If the patient presents within 1 h of a substantial overdose, gastric lavage should be considered or, alternatively, activated charcoal (50 to 100 g) may be administered. Supportive measures should then be employed, as no specific antidote is available. Lignocaine has been found to be of value in controlling ventricular tachycardia after overdose. There is evidence from volunteer studies that acidification of the urine will increase flecainide elimination; haemodialysis and haemofiltration are of no benefit.

Folic acid

Overdosage with this vitamin does not cause toxic features. No treatment is necessary.

Formaldehyde

Formaldehyde is a flammable, colourless gas with a pungent odour. It is most commonly available commercially as a 30 to 50 per cent w/w aqueous solution and is an important raw material in the synthesis of organic compounds such as plastics and resins.

Metabolism

Formaldehyde is oxidized rapidly to formic acid then converted more slowly to carbon dioxide and water.

Clinical features

Acute exposure

Severe irritation of the mucous membranes of the eyes, nose, and upper airways occurs after minimal exposure to low (less than 5 ppm) formaldehyde concentrations, and tends to prevent higher exposure in even the most tolerant subjects. Substantial exposure may result in severe bronchospasm, pulmonary oedema, and death.

Formaldehyde solutions splashed into the eye have caused corneal damage and skin contamination has resulted in dermatitis. Spillage of phenol-formaldehyde resin on to the skin has produced extensive necrotic skin lesions, fever, hypertension, adult respiratory distress syndrome, proteinuria, and renal impairment. Ingestion of formaldehyde solution has resulted in severe corrosive damage to the buccal cavity and tonsils, oesophagus, and stomach with ulceration, necrosis, and subsequent fibrosis and contracture. Shock, metabolic acidosis (due in part to high formate concentrations), respiratory insufficiency, and renal impairment usually then ensue. Death may follow ingestion of less than 100 ml in an adult.

Treatment

Supportive measures, including the correction of acid–base disturbances, should be employed. Haemodialysis is only moderately effective in increasing formate elimination.

Further reading

Cohen N *et al.* (1989). Acute resin phenol-formaldehyde intoxication. A life threatening occupational hazard. *Human Toxicology* **8**, 247–50.

Glyphosate

Glyphosate-containing herbicides usually incorporate the isopropylamine salt together with a surfactant. The original surfactant was probably the main cause of toxicity but this is no longer present in currently marketed formulations.

Clinical features

The most prominent effects are on the alimentary tract with burning in the mouth and throat, nausea, vomiting, dysphagia, and diarrhoea being the main features. Upper gastrointestinal haemorrhage is a much less common complication. A polymorphic leucocytosis is usual. Hypotension, tachycardia, bradycardia, acute chemical pneumonitis, oliguria, haematuria, and metabolic acidosis may be seen in severe poisoning.

Treatment

Management is largely symptomatic and supportive. Intravenous fluids or blood transfusion may be required. Respiratory and renal failure should be managed conventionally. The toxicokinetics of glyphosate in man are not known and rational use of elimination procedures is therefore not possible.

Further reading

Chang C-Y *et al.* (1999). Clinical impact of upper gastrointestinal tract injuries in glyphosate-surfactant oral intoxication. *Human and Experimental Toxicology* **18**, 475–8.

n-Hexane

n-Hexane is an extremely volatile liquid that is used as a solvent.

Clinical features

When ingested it causes nausea, dizziness, CNS excitation and then depression and, as a result, presents an acute aspiration hazard resulting in chemical pneumonitis and non-cardiogenic pulmonary oedema. Following inhalation, either inadvertently or deliberately, similar symptoms occur. The development of a progressive sensorimotor neuropathy is the principal hazard of chronic exposure.

Treatment

Treatment is supportive and symptomatic.

Further reading

International Programme on Chemical Safety (1991). *Environmental Health Criteria 122. n-Hexane.* World Health Organization, Geneva.

Household products

There is a commonly held belief that household products contain a wide range of highly toxic chemicals, and so the ingestion of these substances by children is a frequent cause for alarm in parents and doctors alike. So-called poisoning from household products is more often the result of accidental than deliberate ingestion, mostly involves young children, and is not usually serious. Even when the toxicity of a household product is high, the risk it poses is usually low, certainly when ingested accidentally. However, adults intent on suicide may, by deliberately swallowing massive quantities, succeed in killing themselves. Antiseptics and disinfectants, dishwashing liquids, fabric conditioners, detergents, bleaches and lavatory cleaners, lavatory sanitizers, and deodorants are dealt with elsewhere.

Further reading

Gad-Johannsen H, Mikkelsen JB, Larsen CF (1995). Poisoning with household chemicals in children. *Acta Paediatrica* **83**, 62–5.

H₂-receptor antagonists

H_2-receptor antagonists such as cimetidine, famotidine, nizatidine, and ranitidine are very widely prescribed but few cases of overdose have been reported.

Clinical features

Most patients remain asymptomatic. In a few, drowsiness, dryness of the mouth, slurred speech, dizziness, confusion, vomiting, and abdominal discomfort have been reported. Rarely, bradycardia, respiratory depression, and coma may result.

Treatment

Gut decontamination is unnecessary and supportive and symptomatic measures should be employed if features develop. Although forced diuresis has been employed in one case, no supporting evidence of efficacy was given.

Further reading

Krenzelok EP *et al.* (1987). Cimetidine toxicity: an assessment of 881 cases. *Annals of Emergency Medicine* **16**, 1217–22.

Hydrogen fluoride

Hydrogen fluoride is a corrosive, fuming, nearly colourless liquid (hydrofluoric acid) at atmospheric pressures and temperatures below 19°C; above 19°C it is gaseous. Hydrogen fluoride is very soluble in cold water and for this reason it fumes strongly in moist air. Aqueous solutions dissolve glass.

Mechanisms of toxicity

Fluoride directly inhibits many enzyme systems, including glycolytic enzymes, cholinesterases, and those in which magnesium and manganese are present. In addition, fluoride appears to have a direct toxic effect on nerve tissue and muscle; depression of vasomotor and smooth muscle tone may also occur.

Clinical features

Inhalation or ingestion of hydrogen fluoride causes severe corrosive damage similar to other acids (see above). Following absorption by whatever route, fluoride chelates calcium and lowers the serum ionized calcium concentration and causes weakness, paraesthesiae, tetany, and convulsions. Hypotension and cardiac arrhythmias, including ventricular fibrillation, may be observed. Central effects of fluoride include confusion and coma. Hepatic and renal failure may develop.

Skin contact with anhydrous hydrogen fluoride produces liquefactive necrosis and severe burns that are felt immediately. Concentrated aqueous solutions also cause an early sensation of pain, but more dilute solutions may give no warning of injury. If the solution is not removed promptly, penetration of the skin by fluoride ion may occur, leading to painful ulcers that heal only slowly.

Treatment

Following inhalation of hydrogen fluoride, the casualty should be removed immediately from the contaminated atmosphere. Further treatment is symptomatic and supportive. Mechanical ventilation with positive end-expiratory pressure may be needed to treat pulmonary oedema.

If hydrofluoric acid has been ingested, 10 to 20 g of soluble calcium tablets should be given by mouth, followed by an intravenous injection of 10 ml of 10 per cent calcium gluconate solution. Symptomatic and supportive measures should be employed thereafter.

Skin contact requires thorough washing of the affected area with copious quantities of water for 20 min, even if there is no apparent burn or pain. Skin burns should be coated repeatedly with 2.5 per cent calcium gluconate gel, but if the gel is unavailable, immersion of the skin in iced water until the pain subsides is often helpful. If the pain does not subside, 10 per cent calcium gluconate solution (up to 0.5 ml/cm²) should be injected under the burn area, though calcium gluconate intra-arterially is more effective.

Further reading

Bentur Y *et al.* (1993). The role of calcium gluconate in the treatment of hydrofluoric acid eye burn. *Annals of Emergency Medicine* **22**, 1488–90.

Dunn BJ *et al.* (1996). Topical treatments for hydrofluoric acid dermal burns. *Journal of Occupational and Environmental Medicine* **38**, 507–14.

Henry JA, Hla KK (1992). Intravenous regional calcium gluconate perfusion for hydrofluoric acid burns. *Journal of Toxicology—Clinical Toxicology* **30**, 203–7.

Hydrogen sulphide

Hydrogen sulphide is a colourless gas that smells of rotten eggs, although high concentrations cause olfactory nerve paralysis. The gas is also found in mines and sewers and is liberated from decomposing fish (a hazard in fishing boats if the hold is filled with 'trash' fish used for making fish meal) and liquid manure systems.

Mechanisms of toxicity

It is now thought that the serious sequelae following exposure to high concentrations of hydrogen sulphide are due principally to inhibition of cytochrome oxidase a₃, in which respect it may be more potent than cyanide.

Clinical features

Exposure to low concentrations leads to blepharospasm, pain and redness of the eyes, blurred vision, and coloured haloes round lights. Headache, nausea, dizziness, drowsiness, sore throat, and cough may also occur. With exposure to higher concentrations, cyanosis, confusion, pulmonary oedema, coma, and convulsions are common. Six per cent of casualties die.

Treatment

The casualty should be moved to fresh air from the contaminated atmosphere by a rescuer who has donned breathing apparatus beforehand.

It has been shown in mice that the administration of sodium nitrite is superior to oxygen alone in the treatment of acute hydrogen sulphide poisoning. However, the mechanism of this benefit is disputed and the value of this treatment in humans has not been established.

Further reading

Guidotti TL (1996). Hydrogen sulphide. *Occupational Medicine* (Oxford) **46**, 367–71.

Milby TH, Baselt RC (1999). Hydrogen sulfide poisoning: clarification of some controversial issues. *American Journal of Industrial Medicine* **35**, 192–5.

Hypoglycaemic agents

Intentional overdose with insulin and oral hypoglycaemic agents is uncommon. However, deaths from insulin and sulphonylurea overdosage have been reported. Chlorpropamide and glyburide (available only in the United States) are the oral agents most commonly ingested. Chlorpropamide, because of its long half-life, may, in overdose, induce hypoglycaemia for a considerable period of time. In all cases of poisoning with hypoglycaemic agents prompt diagnosis and treatment are essential if death or cerebral damage from neuroglycopenia are to be prevented.

Clinical features

Features of overdosage include drowsiness, coma, twitching, convulsions, depressed limb reflexes, extensor plantar responses, hyperpnoea, pulmonary oedema, tachycardia, and circulatory failure. Hypoglycaemia is to be expected and hypokalaemia, cerebral oedema, and metabolic acidosis might occur. Neurogenic diabetes insipidus and persistent vegetative states are possible long-term complications. Cholestatic jaundice has been described as a late complication of chlorpropamide poisoning.

Treatment

The blood or plasma glucose concentration should be measured urgently and intravenous glucose given. Glucagon may be ineffective. If the blood sugar is normal, gastric lavage should be considered if the patient has presented within 1 h of the ingestion of an oral preparation.

Recurring hypoglycaemia is highly likely. A continuous infusion of glucose together with carbohydrate-rich meals is required in cases of severe insulin overdosage, though there may be difficulty in maintaining normoglycaemia. In the case of sulphonylurea overdosage, however, further glucose (although its administration may be unavoidable) only serves to increase already high circulating insulin concentrations. Diazoxide has therefore been recommended since it increases blood glucose concentrations and raises circulating catecholamine concentrations while blocking insulin release. The dose is 1.25 mg/kg body weight intravenously over 1 h, repeated at 6-hourly intervals if necessary.

Further reading

Palatnick W, Meatherall RC, Tenenbein M (1991). Clinical spectrum of sulfonylurea overdose and experience with diazoxide therapy. *Archives of Internal Medicine* **151**, 1859–62.

Roberge RJ, Martin TG, Delbridge TR (1993). Intentional massive insulin overdose: recognition and management. *Annals of Emergency Medicine* **22**, 228–34.

Iron

Most medicinal iron preparations are ferrous salts that must be oxidized to the ferric state before being absorbed and stored in the liver and reticuloendothelial system. Iron overdosage is much more common in preschool children than in adults. Toxic features are unlikely unless more than 60 mg of elemental iron/kg body weight has been ingested, probably because absorption is poor. Poisoning is therefore seldom severe and deaths are rare.

Mechanism of toxicity

Iron salts have complex actions, including direct corrosive effects on the upper gastrointestinal tract and potentially serious effects on the circulation; at a cellular level they tend to concentrate around mitochondrial cristae where they may act as an electron 'sink', thereby interfering with intermediary metabolism.

Clinical features

The course of iron poisoning is conventionally divided into four phases.

Phase 1

The first phase starts immediately after ingestion and lasts about 6 h. Nausea, vomiting, abdominal pain, and diarrhoea, all of which result from direct irritation of the gut, characterize it. The gastric and upper small bowel mucosas may be stained and impregnated with iron and become ulcerated, the severity of these changes decreasing with distance from the stomach. The disintegrating tablets may make the vomitus and stools grey or black in colour. Polymorphic leucocytosis and hyperglycaemia are common. Iron tablets in the upper gut may be visible in an abdominal radiograph, particularly if it is taken within 2 h of alleged ingestion.

A few patients develop haematemesis, hypotension, coma, and shock, which may be fatal.

Phase 2

This phase lasts from about 6 to 24 h after ingestion and is a period during which patients improve symptomatically. Indeed, most do not progress further.

Phase 3

During this phase, 12 to 48 h after ingestion, a small minority of patients deteriorate, often with profound shock, metabolic acidosis, and features which are due to acute renal tubular and hepatocellular necrosis. Liver failure and its complications develop and may be fatal. The extent of liver damage varies from almost complete necrosis in some areas to only periportal damage in others.

Phase 4

This is the period 2 to 6 weeks after ingestion. The features at this stage are those of high intestinal obstruction by a stricture formed at the site of corrosive damage to the mucosa, usually the pyloric antrum. Children are most likely to be affected.

Assessment of the severity of poisoning

The amount ingested is not reliable because of vomiting. Shock, coma, and acidosis indicate severe poisoning. Other clinical features are less useful. Emergency estimation of the serum iron concentration is essential. If the 4 to 6 h concentration exceeds the predicted normal iron-binding capacity (usually more than 90 μmol/l), free iron is circulating and treatment is needed. Measurement of the total iron-binding capacity in acute iron poisoning may give misleading results and is not recommended.

Treatment

Reducing absorption

Gastric lavage should be considered if more than 20 mg of elemental iron/kg body weight has been ingested in the previous 1 h. Addition of bicarbonate, phosphates, and desferrioxamine (deferoxamine) to lavage fluids does not reduce absorption further and may be dangerous. Whole bowel irrigation may have a role if a large amount (particularly of a slow release formulation) has been ingested and has already passed through the pylorus.

Severe poisoning with coma or shock

When coma or shock are present the specific iron-chelating agent desferrioxamine (deferoxamine) should be given without delay and without waiting for the result of the serum iron concentration. The dose is 15 mg/kg body weight/h intravenously and the total amount infused should not exceed 80 mg/kg in 24 h. Clinical improvement can be expected within 1 to 2 h, after which the rate of infusion may be reduced. There is no simple or readily available method of deciding when to stop desferrioxamine administration; the clinical state of the patient is probably the most appropriate guide. Desferrioxamine may also be given intramuscularly in a dose of 2 g for an adult and 1 g for a child.

Hypotension due to desferrioxamine-induced histamine release may develop if the recommended rate of administration is exceeded. Other adverse effects include hypersensitivity reactions and, rarely, anaphylaxis. Pulmonary oedema and adult respiratory distress syndrome attributed to desferrioxamine have been reported in patients given 15 mg/kg for 65 h and longer.

Poisoning without coma or shock

Routine administration of desferrioxamine cannot be recommended. Patients who are not in coma or shock but who have a serum iron concentration greater than 90 μmol/l should be given desferrioxamine.

Overdose without features

Patients who have not developed features of poisoning within 6 h have probably not ingested toxic amounts and therefore they do not require treatment. Those who present earlier than 6 h should be assessed as described above and treated accordingly.

Supportive measures

Only a small minority of patients will require supportive measures in addition to those described above. Attention to the airway and ventilation is obviously important if consciousness is impaired and fluid and electrolytes should be replaced as necessary. Blood transfusion may be required if there has been significant haemorrhage. Liver and renal function should be monitored and failure managed conventionally.

Overdosage in pregnancy

Overdosage with iron salts during pregnancy should be treated as under other circumstances. Limited evidence indicates that desferrioxamine is not fetotoxic or teratogenic and to withhold it when it is indicated may be fatal.

Further reading

Bosse GM (1995). Conservative management of patients with moderately elevated serum iron levels. *Journal of Toxicology—Clinical Toxicology* 33, 135–40.

Chyka PA, Butler AY, Holley JE (1996). Serum iron concentrations and symptoms of acute iron poisoning in children. *Pharmacotherapy* 16, 1053–8.

Tenenbein M (1996). Benefits of parenteral deferoxamine for acute iron poisoning. *Journal of Toxicology—Clinical Toxicology* 34, 485–9.

Isoniazid

Poisoning with isoniazid is potentially very serious, but uncommon.

Mechanisms of toxicity

Isoniazid depresses brain concentrations of γ-aminobutyric acid (GABA), thus leading to seizures.

Clinical features

The ingestion of 80 to 150 mg of isoniazid/kg body weight is likely to cause severe poisoning. Nausea, vomiting, slurred speech, dizziness, and visual hallucinations may develop. Stupor, coma, and convulsions follow rapidly and may be associated with hyperthermia, hyperreflexia, extensor plantar responses, and later, rhabdomyolysis. In addition, dilated pupils, sinus tachycardia, and urinary retention may be observed. In severe cases, hypotension, acute renal failure, and respiratory failure may ensure. Marked metabolic (lactic) acidosis is common. Less commonly, hyperglycaemia, ketoacidosis, glycosuria, and ketonuria are found.

Treatment

Supportive measures including the correction of metabolic acidosis should be instituted immediately if the patient is unconscious. If the airway can be protected, gastric lavage or the administration of 50 g of activated charcoal should be considered if presentation is less than 1 h after overdose. Pyridoxine (1 g for 1 g of isoniazid ingested) should be given intravenously to control convulsions. When the ingested dose of isoniazid is unknown, an initial intravenous dose of 5 g of pyridoxine should be given. Diazepam alone may be ineffective but the use of diazepam and pyridoxine is synergistic and both should be used in those with convulsions. Pyridoxine in a dose of 5 g may be repeated if convulsions persist (in one case 52 g of pyridoxine was given intravenously without ill effects).

Charcoal haemoperfusion is the most effective technique for elimination of isoniazid from the circulation but its use should rarely be necessary provided appropriate supportive measures and adequate and repeated doses of pyridoxine and diazepam are given.

Further reading

Blowey DL, Johnson D, Verjee Z (1995). Isoniazid-associated rhabdomyolysis. *American Journal of Emergency Medicine* 13, 543–4.

Gurnani A *et al.* (1992). Acute izoniazid poisoning. *Anaesthesia* 47, 781–3.

Wilcox WD, Hacker YE, Geller RJ (1996). Acute isoniazid overdose in a compliant adolescent patient. *Clinical Pediatrics* 35, 213–14.

Isopropanol (isopropyl alcohol; 2-propanol)

Isopropanol is used as a sterilizing agent and as rubbing alcohol. It is also found in aftershave lotions, disinfectants, and window-cleaning solutions. Intoxication can result both from ingestion and skin absorption. Isopropanol is oxidized in the liver to acetone.

Clinical features

Features of toxicity include coma and respiratory depression, the odour of acetone on the breath, gastritis, haematemesis, hypotension, hypothermia, renal tubular necrosis, acute myopathy, and haemolytic anaemia; cardiac arrest has occurred. The development of hypotension is a poor prognostic feature.

Treatment

Gastric lavage should be considered if the patient presents less than 1 h after ingestion. In addition to supportive measures, haemodialysis should be employed in severely poisoned patients as it not only removes isopropanol but also shortens the duration of coma.

Further reading

Pappas AA *et al.* (1991). Isopropanol ingestion: report of six episodes with isopropanol and acetone serum concentration time data. *Journal of Toxicology—Clinical Toxicology* **29**, 11–21.

Lavatory sanitizers and deodorants

Solid lavatory sanitizer or deodorant blocks normally contain paradichlorobenzene. Ingestion may cause nausea, vomiting, diarrhoea, and abdominal pain. Symptomatic and supportive treatment is all that is required unless many grams have been ingested in which case gastric lavage should be considered if the patient presents within 1 h of ingestion.

Lead

Exposure to lead occurs in the reclamation of lead from scrap metal, in the demolition and flame-cutting of old railway bridges previously painted with lead paint, and in the manufacture of storage batteries and ceramics. Children with pica who chew on lead-painted railings in homes, or who eat contaminated soil, have developed lead poisoning. As a consequence of lead leaching out of the glazing material, poisoning has also been described in individuals who have consumed drinks from lead-glazed mugs. Ingestion of lead-based powders in paints and imported baby tonics and application of lead-containing cosmetics such as 'surma' to the face in Asian communities has resulted in lead intoxication. Rarely, lead acetate has been injected intravenously with suicidal intent. Tetraethyl lead, which is used as an antiknock agent in leaded petrol, can be absorbed systemically by inhalation, ingestion, and through the skin. Transplacental transfer of lead from mother to fetus results in reduced viability of the fetus, reduced birth weight, and premature birth.

The Centers for Disease Control and Prevention in Atlanta have reduced the concentration of lead at which intervention is indicated from 150 µg/l as some adverse health effects have been observed in young children at a blood lead concentration of 100 µg/l.

Lead absorbed into the body is mainly (95 per cent) deposited in the bones and teeth. Of the lead in the blood, 99 per cent is associated with erythrocytes. As the body accumulates lead over many years and releases it into the urine only slowly, even small doses can in time lead to intoxication.

Clinical features

Mild intoxication may result in no more than lethargy and occasional abdominal discomfort, whereas abdominal pain (which is usually diffuse but may be colicky), vomiting, constipation, and encephalopathy develop in more severe cases. Lead colic was first described by Hippocrates and, on occasions, has been incorrectly managed surgically as a case of an acute abdomen. Encephalopathy (seizures, mania, delirium, coma) is more common in children than in adults. Classically, lead poisoning results in foot drop attributable to primary motor peripheral neuropathy; wrist drop occurs only as a late sign.

Renal effects include reversible renal tubular dysfunction causing glycosuria, aminoaciduria, and phosphaturia and irreversible interstitial fibrosis with progressive renal insufficiency leading to hypertension.

A bluish discoloration of the gum margins due to deposition of lead sulphide is observed occasionally.

Lead depresses the enzymes responsible for haem synthesis and shortens erythrocyte lifespan leading to microcytic or normocytic hypochromic anaemia. In severe intoxication haemolytic anaemia may occur. Basophilic stippling of erythrocytes is due to nuclear remnants. Lead blocks the conversion of δ-aminolaevulinic acid to porphobilinogen leading to an increase in δ-aminolaevulinic acid in blood and urine. Lead also inhibits ferrochelatase that results in elevated free erythrocyte protoporphyrin (**FEP**) concentrations. There is a concomitant increase in urinary coproporphyrins and FEP, commonly assayed as zinc protoporphyrin.

An elevated zinc protoporphyrin concentration (more than 350 µg/l) reaches a steady state in the blood only after the entire population of circulating erythrocytes has turned over (approximately 120 days). Consequently, it lags behind blood lead concentrations and is an indirect measure of long-term lead exposure. Moreover, zinc protoporphyrin is not a good screening test, as it is not sensitive at the lower levels of lead poisoning.

Medical surveillance

The current practice in the United Kingdom and some other European countries is to recommend stopping work with lead where a worker's blood lead concentration is shown to be above 700 µg/l although workers may be symptomatic below this concentration. In workers exposed to organic lead compounds, the urinary lead concentration (more than 150 µg/l) is a good indicator of exposure.

Treatment

Primary prevention aimed at eliminating lead hazards for children and workers must receive due public-health attention. The social dimension of the problem must also be recognized: simply giving children chelation therapy and then returning them to a contaminated home environment is of no value. Similarly, if an occupational source of lead exposure is implicated, a thorough evaluation of the workplace, other exposed workers, and the systems for handling lead at work is appropriate.

The decision to use chelation therapy is based not only on the blood lead concentration but also on the symptoms present and, if available, an estimate of the total body burden of lead using X-ray fluorescence. Sodium calcium edetate and DMSA (succimer) both increase lead excretion, though the former must be given intravenously and may result in increased uptake of lead into the brain. In severe acute lead poisoning, particularly of occupational origin, sodium calcium edetate 75 mg/kg body weight daily for 5 days provides rapid relief of symptoms with minimal risk of adverse effect; a second course may be given a week after the first. If hydration is maintained during chelation, proximal tubular damage is not usually observed. DMSA 30 mg/kg body weight orally for 5 days is an alternative though less efficient chelator than sodium calcium edetate.

Further reading

Centers for Disease Control and Prevention (1991). *Preventing lead poisoning in young children*, 4th edn. US Department of Health and Human Services, Washington DC.

Liftshitz M, Hashkanazi R, Phillip M (1997). The effect of 2,3 dimercaptosuccinic acid in the treatment of lead poisoning in adults. *Annals of Medicine* **29**, 83–5.

Lignocaine and related drugs

Lignocaine, mexiletine, and tocainide are sodium channel blockers. Intoxication with these agents, particularly lignocaine, occurs most often as a result of therapeutic overdose in intensive care areas or inadvertent intravenous administration during local anaesthesia. Topical absorption of lignocaine may result in systemic toxicity, particularly in children.

Clinical features

Poisoning induces nausea, vomiting, paraesthesias, tremor, drowsiness, dizziness, dysarthria, diplopia, nystagmus, ataxia, confusion, convulsions, and coma. Sinus bradycardia, heart block, and hypotension may develop in severe poisoning and cardiac arrest may ensue; mexiletine may also cause atrial fibrillation.

Treatment

Gastric lavage should be considered or 50 to 100 g of activated charcoal administered if an overdose has been ingested less than 1 h previously. Diazepam in a dose of 5 to 10 mg intravenously should be given for convulsions, if they are not short-lived, and atropine in a dose of 1 to 2 mg intravenously should be administered for sinus bradycardia. Inotropic support may become necessary if heart block or severe hypotension supervene. Pacing may be attempted but the ventricular response is usually poor. Tocainide elimination is increased significantly with haemodialysis.

Further reading

Denaro CP, Benowitz NL (1989). Poisoning due to class 1B antiarrhythmic drugs: Lignocaine, mexilitine and tocainide. *Medical Toxicology* 4, 412–28.

Lindane

Lindane is an organchlorine pesticide.

Clinical features

The main toxic effects following ingestion are on the central nervous system with rapid loss of consciousness and the development of myoclonus, hypertonia, hyperreflexia, convulsions, and rhabdomyolysis. Metabolic acidosis, disseminated intravascular coagulation, renal tubular and hepatocellular necrosis, pancreatitis, and proximal myopathy have been reported.

Treatment

Treatment is symptomatic and supportive. Gastric lavage should be considered if lindane has been ingested less than 1 h previously. Metabolic acidosis and convulsions should be treated conventionally.

Further reading

Aks SE *et al.* (1995). Acute accidental lindane ingestion in toddlers. *Annals of Emergency Medicine* 26, 647–51.

Fischer TF (1994). Lindane toxicity in a 24-year-old woman. *Annals of Emergency Medicine* 24, 972–4.

Liquefied petroleum gas (LPG 'bottled gas')

Liquefied petroleum gas (LPG 'bottled gas') contains propane and butane (and sometimes propylene and butylene). Propane and butane may cause vertigo and drowsiness and, at high concentrations, may act as asphyxiants.

Further reading

Gray MY, Lazarus JH (1993). Butane inhalation and hemiparesis. *Journal of Toxicology—Clinical Toxicology* 31, 483–5.

Lithium carbonate

The therapeutic index of lithium is low and toxicity is usually the result of therapeutic overdose rather than deliberate self-poisoning. However, individuals on or not on long-term treatment with the drug occasionally ingest single large doses.

Clinical features

Features of intoxication include thirst, polyuria, diarrhoea, and vomiting, and in more serious cases, impairment of consciousness, hypertonia,

tremor, and convulsions; irreversible neurological damage may occur. Measurement of the serum lithium concentration confirms the diagnosis, therapeutic toxicity usually being associated with concentrations above 1.5 mmol/l. However, acute massive overdosage may produce much higher concentrations without causing toxic features, at least initially.

Treatment

Gastric lavage may be considered if the patient presents less than 1 h after a substantial overdose. Thereafter, treatment is supportive together with measures to enhance the rate of lithium elimination. The decision to enhance elimination is based on the severity of features and a serum lithium concentration greater than 3 mmol/l, particularly in patients receiving lithium chronically. Forced diuresis with 0.9 per cent sodium chloride is effective but its use is commonly complicated by hypernatraemia and increased plasma osmolality; the infusion of low-dose dopamine at 2.5 µg/kg.min may be an effective alternative. Peritoneal dialysis or haemodialysis may be needed if renal function is impaired and in severe poisoning; peritoneal dialysis is much less effective. However, the relatively slow movement of lithium ions across cell membranes limits the efficacy of all these techniques. It is easy to reduce serum lithium concentrations but they frequently rebound when treatment is stopped and clinical improvement is much slower.

Further reading

Scharman EJ (1997). Methods used to decrease lithium absorption or enhance elimination. *Journal of Toxicology—Clinical Toxicology* 35, 601–8.

Lysergic acid diethylamide (LSD)

As with cannabis, individuals intoxicated with LSD rarely present to medical services.

Clinical features

The ability of LSD to distort reality is well known. Visual hallucinations, distortion of images, agitation, excitement, dilated pupils, tachycardia, hypertension, hyperreflexia, tremor, and hyperthermia are common; auditory hallucinations are rare. Time seems to pass very slowly and behaviour may become disturbed with paranoid delusions. Flashbacks in which the effects of LSD may be re-experienced without further exposure to the drug occur in about 15 per cent of users for several years and are not explained.

Treatment

Most individuals will require little more than reassurance and sedation. Supportive measures are all that can be offered to those who are seriously ill.

Mefenamic acid

Clinical features

Overdose of mefenamic acid produces nausea, vomiting, and occasionally, bloody diarrhoea. Drowsiness, dizziness, and headaches are common and hyperreflexia, muscle twitching, convulsions, cardiorespiratory arrest, hypoprothombinaemia, and acute renal failure have been reported. In a study of 29 cases of mefenamic acid poisoning, convulsions were noted in 38 per cent of patients, although only rarely were they persistent.

Treatment

Gastric lavage or activated charcoal may be considered if the patient presents less than 1 h after overdose. Symptomatic and supportive measures should be employed and haemodialysis/filtration undertaken for renal failure.

Further reading

Turnbull AJ, Campbell P, Hughes JA (1988). Mefenamic acid nephropathy—acute renal failure in overdose. *British Medical Journal* **296**, 46.

Mercury

Mercury is the only metal which is liquid at room temperature. It exists in three forms, metallic ($Hg°$), mercurous (Hg_2^{2+}), and mercuric (Hg^{2+}). Metallic mercury is very volatile and when spilt has a large surface area so that high atmospheric concentrations may be produced in enclosed spaces, particularly when environmental temperatures are high. In addition to simple salts, such as chloride, nitrate, and sulphate, mercuric mercury forms organometallic compounds where mercury is covalently bound to carbon, such as methyl-, ethyl-, phenyl-, and methoxyethyl mercury.

Non-occupational mercury exposure occurs principally from dietary intake and to a minor extent from dental amalgam. Many foodstuffs contain small amounts of mercury.

The absorption of mercury depends on its chemical form. Inhaled mercury vapour is absorbed rapidly and oxidized to Hg^{2+} in erythrocytes and other tissues. Prior to oxidation, absorbed mercury vapour can cross the blood–brain barrier, but the divalent ion oxidation product serves to trap mercury in the brain. Mercury vapour is also absorbed via the skin, at an average rate of 0.24 ng/cm². min. Less than 1 per cent of an ingested dose of metallic mercury reaches the systemic circulation. Organic mercuric salts are better absorbed following ingestion than are inorganic mercuric salts. Organic mercury compounds cross the blood–brain barrier readily to accumulate in the brain. In contrast the kidney is the main storage organ for inorganic mercury compounds. *In vivo* mercury is bound to metallothionein, which serves a protective role since renal damage is caused only by the unbound metal. Mercury is excreted mainly in urine and faeces although a small amount of absorbed inorganic mercury is exhaled as mercury vapour. The half-life of most body mercury is 1 to 2 months but a small fraction has a half-life of several years.

Clinical features

Acute poisoning

Acute mercury vapour inhalation causes headache, nausea, cough, chest pain, bronchitis, and pneumonia. In a few individuals renal damage from such acute exposure may produce gross proteinuria or nephrotic syndrome. In addition, a fine tremor and neurobehavioural impairment occurs and peripheral nerve involvement has also been observed.

Ingestion of metallic mercury is usually without systemic effects as metallic mercury is poorly absorbed from the gastrointestinal tract. However, mercuric chloride or other inorganic mercuric salts cause an irritant gastroenteritis with corrosive ulceration, bloody diarrhoea, and abdominal cramps and may lead to circulatory collapse and shock. The ingestion of disc batteries containing mercuric oxide usually results in uneventful spontaneous passage through the gastrointestinal tract, but potentially toxic mercury levels may result if the battery opens in transit. Mercury-containing batteries have been withdrawn from the European Union. Mercurous compounds are less soluble, less corrosive, and less toxic than mercuric salts. Ingestion of mercurous chloride in teething powder has led to 'pink disease' or acrodynia in infants.

There are reports of deliberate intravenous or subcutaneous metallic mercury injection. Accidental injection also has occurred after injury from broken thermometers and, in the past, following gas analysis procedures using mercury as a syringe sealant. Intravascular mercury may result in pulmonary venous or peripheral arterial embolism. Subcutaneous mercury initiates a soft-tissue inflammatory reaction with granuloma formation.

Signs of systemic mercury toxicity are rare following metallic mercury injection.

Chronic poisoning

Chronic poisoning from inorganic mercury compounds or mercury vapour is characterized by non-specific early symptoms such as anorexia, insomnia, abnormal sweating, headache, lassitude, increased excitability, tremor, gingivitis, hypersalivation, personality changes, and memory and intellectual deterioration. Glomerular and tubular damage may follow chronic exposure to mercury and renal tubular acidosis has been described in children.

Exposure to organic mercury compounds usually involves aromatic derivatives such as phenyl mercuric acetate and phenyl mercuric benzoate, or aliphatic compounds such as methylmercury and ethylmercury chloride. The main features of poisoning are paraesthesias of the lips, hands, and feet, ataxia, tremor, dysarthria, constriction of visual fields, deafness, and emotional and intellectual changes. There is often a latent period of several weeks between the last exposure and the development of symptoms.

Treatment

Even prompt removal from exposure to mercury vapour may not prevent the development of serious sequelae. Early intensive supportive measures are of paramount importance in the management of the severe gastrointestinal complications caused by the ingestion of mercuric salts, such as mercuric chloride. In these circumstances gastric lavage is best avoided as significant oesophageal erosions may be present.

Traditionally, dimercaprol (British Anti-Lewisite, BAL) has been used in the treatment of inorganic mercury poisoning, but it has to be administered intramuscularly and has adverse effects. Oral DMPS (unithiol) and DMSA (Succimer) in a dose of 30 mg/kg body weight daily have been shown to enhance mercury elimination significantly, protect against renal damage, and increase survival, at least in animal studies. In some of these experimental studies DMPS appears to be significantly better than DMSA in reducing the total body mercury burden, renal deposition of mercury, and mortality.

DMPS also appears to be of value in the treatment of acute methylmercury poisoning. Limited data suggest DMPS may improve the neurological features of chronic mercury poisoning.

Further reading

O'Carroll RE *et al.* (1995). The neuropsychiatric sequelae of mercury poisoning. The Mad Hatter's disease revisited. *British Journal of Psychiatry* **167**, 95–8.

Toet AE *et al.* (1994). Mercury kinetics in a case of severe mercuric chloride poisoning treated with dimercapto-1-propane sulphonate (DMPS). *Human and Experimental Toxicology* **13**, 11–16.

Torres-Alanis O, Garza-Ocanas L, Pineyro-Lopez A (1997). Intravenous self-administration of metallic mercury: report of a case with a 5 year follow-up. *Journal of Toxicology—Clinical Toxicology* **35**, 83–7.

Metaldehyde

Metaldehyde in the form of pellets is used widely for killing slugs and in some countries as a solid fuel.

Clinical features

Nausea, vomiting, abdominal pain, and diarrhoea often occur 1 to 3 h after ingestion of any amount, while more than 100 mg/kg body weight may cause hypertonia, convulsions, impairment of consciousness, and metabolic acidosis. Hepatic and renal tubular necrosis may become apparent after 2 to 3 days.

Treatment

Gastric lavage should be considered if more than 50 mg/kg has been ingested within 1 h. Treatment thereafter is supportive.

Further reading

Moody JP, Inglis FG (1992). Persistence of metaldehyde during acute molluscicide poisoning. *Human and Experimental Toxicology* **11**, 361–2.

Methanol (methyl alcohol)

Methanol is used widely as a solvent. It is also found in antifreeze solutions, paints, duplicating fluids, paint removers and varnishes, and shoe polishes. The ingestion of as little as 10 ml of pure methanol has caused permanent blindness and 30 ml is potentially fatal although individual susceptibility varies widely. Toxicity may also occur as a result of inhalation or percutaneous absorption.

Mechanisms of toxicity

In humans, methanol is metabolized by alcohol dehydrogenase and catalase enzyme systems to formaldehyde and formic acid (formate). The concentration of formate increases greatly and is accompanied by accumulation of hydrogen ions causing metabolic acidosis.

Clinical features

Ingested alone, methanol causes mild and transient inebriation and drowsiness. After a latent period of 8 to 36 h, nausea, vomiting, abdominal pain, headache, dizziness, and coma supervene. Blurred vision and diminished visual acuity may occur and the presence of dilated pupils, unreactive to light, suggests that permanent blindness is likely to ensue. A severe metabolic acidosis may develop and this may be accompanied by hyperglycaemia and raised serum amylase activity. A blood methanol concentration greater than 500 mg/l confirms serious poisoning. Mortality increases with the severity and duration of the metabolic acidosis. Survivors may show permanent neurological sequelae including blindness, rigidity, hypokinesis, and other parkinsonian-like signs; these features follow the development of optic neuropathy and necrosis of the putamen.

Treatment

Gastric lavage may be considered in patients who present less than 1 h after ingestion. Thereafter, the treatment of methanol poisoning is directed towards: first, the correction of metabolic acidosis; second, the inhibition of methanol oxidation; and third, the removal of circulating methanol and its toxic metabolites. Substantial quantities of bicarbonate (often as much as 2 mol) may be required and since this must be accompanied by sodium, hypernatraemia and hypervolaemia may result.

Ethanol and fomepizole (4-methylpyrazole) inhibit methanol oxidation. These antidotes should be given and monitored as for ethylene glycol. If admission plasma concentrations show that most of the methanol ingested has already been metabolized, ethanol or fomepizole administration will not be of benefit and ethanol might exacerbate the acidosis.

Dialysis is indicated when a patient has ingested more than 30 g of methanol, or develops metabolic acidosis, mental, visual, or fundoscopic abnormalities attributable to methanol, or a blood methanol concentration in excess of 500 mg/l. Folinic acid (30 mg intravenously 6-hourly) may protect against ocular toxicity by accelerating formate metabolism.

Further reading

Brent J *et al.* (2001). Fomepizole for the treatment of methanol poisoning. *New England Journal of Medicine* **344**, 44–90.

Jacobsen D, McMartin KE (1997). Antidotes for methanol and ethylene glycol poisoning. *Journal of Toxicology—Clinical Toxicology* **35**, 126–43.

Methyl bromide (bromomethane)

Methyl bromide is a colourless, odourless gas at ordinary temperatures and, therefore, dangerous concentrations may accumulate without warning. Methyl bromide has high penetrating power and is non-flammable and explosive; these features explain its increasing use as a disinfectant to fumigate soil, a wide range of commodities, grain, warehouses, and mills. Its high density causes it to settle at floor level.

Mechanism of toxicity

Methyl bromide is absorbed readily through the lungs and is excreted largely unchanged by the same route. The remainder is metabolized and inorganic bromide is excreted in the urine. The mechanism of toxicity is uncertain but methyl bromide appears to have an affinity for intracellular proteins, particularly those with sulphydryl groups.

Clinical features

There is a latent period of up to 12 h before toxic symptoms occur. Symptoms include dizziness, headache, nausea, vomiting, abdominal pain, malaise, transient blurring of vision, diplopia, and breathlessness. In severe cases, coma, status epilepticus, tremor, ataxia, hyporeflexia, paraesthesiae, hallucinations, acute psychosis, and polyneuropathy may be found. Proteinuria, oliguria (due to renal tubular and cortical necrosis), and jaundice have been described.

Long-term exposure to methyl bromide may lead to a chronic polyneuropathy, lethargy, personality changes, intolerance of alcohol, dysarthria, and epilepsy.

Treatment

The casualty should be removed promptly from the contaminated atmosphere and undressed, as methyl bromide can penetrate clothing and rubber gloves. Contaminated skin should be washed with water. Treatment is supportive.

Further reading

Hustinx WNM *et al.* (1993). Systemic effects of inhalational methyl bromide poisoning: a study of nine cases occupationally exposed due to inadvertent spread during fumigation. *British Journal of Industrial Medicine* **50**, 155–9.

Zwaveling JH *et al.* (1987). Exposure of the skin to methyl bromide: A study of six cases occupationally exposed to high concentrations during fumigation. *Human Toxicology* **6**, 491–5.

Methylene chloride (dichloromethane)

Methylene chloride is a common ingredient in paint removers and is used as a solvent for plastic films and cements and also as a degreaser and aerosol propellant.

Mechanism of toxicity

Methylene chloride is metabolized to carbon dioxide and carbon monoxide. Carboxyhaemoglobin concentrations of 3 to 10 per cent (exceptionally 40 per cent) are attained.

Clinical features

Skin contact with liquid methylene chloride can be painful. Following inhalation, dizziness, tingling and numbness of the extremities, throbbing headache, nausea, irritability, fatigue, and stupor have been reported. Severe and prolonged exposure may lead to irritative conjunctivitis, lacrimation, respiratory depression, and death. Hepatorenal dysfunction and pulmonary oedema have also been described. In addition, if high concentrations of carboxyhaemoglobin are present, the features of acute carbon monoxide poisoning may occur, although these tend to be mild even in the presence of very high carboxyhaemoglobin concentrations.

Treatment

Prompt removal from exposure prior to death usually results in complete recovery. Thereafter, treatment is supportive and should include the use of supplemental oxygen.

Further reading

McDonald W, Olmedo M (1996). Accidental deaths following inhalation of methylene chloride. *Applied Occupational and Environmental Hygiene* **11**, 17–19.

Metoclopramide

Overdose causes acute dystonic reactions affecting the eyes, tongue, and neck.

Treatment

Gastric lavage and activated charcoal may be considered if the patient presents less than 1 h after a substantial overdose. Benztropine in a dose of 1 to 2 mg for an adult should be given intravenously if extrapyramidal features are present. Alternatively, 5 to 10 mg of diazepam intravenously is effective and has the additional advantage of alleviating anxiety and agitation.

Further reading

Miller LG, Jankovic J (1989). Metoclopramide-induced movement disorders. *Archives of Internal Medicine* **149**, 2486–92.

Monoamine-oxidase inhibitors (MAOIs)

Phenelzine and tranylcypromine are now used less frequently in the treatment of depression, and poisoning with them is correspondingly uncommon. A new type A MAOI, moclobemide, is now marketed.

Clinical features

The onset of features may be delayed for 12 to 24 h after acute overdose and are due principally to increased sympathetic activity. They include excitement, restlessness (which may be extreme), hyperpyrexia, hyperreflexia, convulsions, opisthotonos, rhabdomyolysis, and coma. Cardiovascular effects include sinus tachycardia and either hypotension or hypertension.

Treatment

Gastric lavage and activated charcoal may be considered if the patient presents less than 1 h after a substantial overdose. Treatment of overdose is essentially supportive and includes control of convulsions and marked excitement with drugs such as diazepam. Dantrolene may be used to treat hyperpyrexia and extreme restlessness. Hypotension should, in the first instance, be treated by fluid replacement to restore a normal circulating blood volume. The use of sympathomimetic drugs should clearly be avoided. Hypertension, which persists despite diazepam administration, should be treated by the administration of an α-adrenoceptor blocker, such as chlorpromazine.

Further reading

Iwersen S, Schmoldt A (1996). Three suicide attempts with moclobemide. *Journal of Toxicology—Clinical Toxicology* **34**, 223–5.

Lichtenwalner MR *et al.* (1995). Two fatalities involving phenelzine. *Journal of Analytical Toxicology* **19**, 265–6.

Natural gas (methane, ethane)

Natural gas contains methane and ethane. Methane and ethane are pharmacologically inert and can be tolerated in high concentrations without producing any toxic effects. Both gases, however, if present in very high concentration (greater than 80 per cent), may produce asphyxia in poorly ventilated areas, as a result of oxygen deprivation. After removal from the asphyxia-inducing atmosphere, supplemental oxygen should be administered.

Nickel

Nickel is a ubiquitous trace metal and is mined in the form of sulphide ore. It is used primarily for producing stainless steel and other alloys. Nickel carbonyl, an intermediate compound in nickel purification, is used as a catalyst in the petroleum, plastic, and rubber industries. Nickel compounds have been divided into nickel carbonyl, soluble nickel salts (e.g. acetate, bromide, chloride, chloride hexahydrate, nitrate, sub-sulphide, sulphate), insoluble nickel compounds (e.g. arsenate, carbonate, hydroxide, oxide, phosphate) and metallic nickel. Nickel sulphate is used for electroplating and nickel hydroxide is a component of nickel–cadmium batteries.

Nickel can be absorbed both orally and by inhalation, and in the blood is transported bound principally to albumin. Nickel is concentrated in the kidneys, liver, and lungs and is excreted primarily in the urine.

Clinical features

Acute poisoning

Nickel carbonyl is a colourless, volatile liquid which when inhaled leads, within a few minutes, to dizziness, headache, vertigo, nausea, vomiting, cough, and dyspnoea. In many cases these symptoms disappear and there follows a symptom-free period lasting several days before the start of tachypnoea, dyspnoea, haemoptysis, cyanosis, chest pain, vomiting, tachycardia, weakness, and muscle fatigue. Paraesthesiae, diarrhoea, abdominal distension, delirium, and convulsions have also been reported. Death may occur 4 to 11 days after exposure from cardiorespiratory failure.

Urine nickel concentrations immediately following exposure to nickel carbonyl provide a guide as to the severity of exposure.

At high concentrations soluble nickel salts are primarily skin, gut, and eye irritants. Workers at an electroplating plant who drank water accidentally contaminated with nickel sulphate experienced nausea, vomiting, diarrhoea, abdominal pain, headache, cough, and breathlessness which persisted for up to 2 days. A 2-year-old child died 4 h after ingesting 15 g of nickel sulphate crystals.

Chronic poisoning

Chronic exposure to aerosols of nickel salts may lead to chronic rhinitis and sinusitis and, in rare cases, anosmia and perforation of the nasal septum. Inhaled nickel can produce a type I hypersensitivity respiratory reaction manifest as bronchial asthma with circulating IgE antibodies to nickel. Pulmonary eosinophilia (Loeffler's syndrome) due to a type III hypersensitivity reaction to nickel has also been described.

A significant increase in deaths from non-malignant respiratory disease or pneumoconiosis has also been observed in nickel refinery workers. There is evidence that occupational exposure to nickel may cause cancer of the lung and nasal sinuses.

Metallic nickel and nickel salts cause allergic contact dermatitis in up to 10 per cent of females and 1 per cent of males that is due to type IV delayed hypersensitivity.

Treatment

Severe acute nickel carbonyl poisoning requires intensive supportive care. Although chelation therapy with oral or parenteral diethyldithiocarbamate has been employed, its benefit remains uncertain. Ingestion of a substantial quantity of a nickel salt is likely to produce vomiting but if this does not occur, gastric lavage or activated charcoal may be considered if presentation is within 1 h.

Avoidance of exposure and symptomatic treatment of exacerbations with topical or systemic steroids, remain the mainstay of treatment of nickel allergy.

Further reading

Barceloux DG (1999). Nickel. *Journal of Toxicology–Clinical Toxicology* **37**, 239–58.

Bradberry SM, Vale JA (1999). Therapeutic review: do diethyldithiocarbamate and disulfiram have a role in acute nickel carbonyl poisoning? *Journal of Toxicology–Clinical Toxicology* **37**, 259–64.

Nitrates

Organic nitrates such as isosorbide mononitrate and isosorbide dinitrate relax smooth muscle cells and undergo extensive first-pass metabolism in the liver.

Clinical features

The symptoms and signs caused by nitrates in overdose are due primarily to *in vivo* conversion to nitrites causing excessive arteriolar and venous dilation. Headache and vomiting are common, accompanied by flushing of the skin and dizziness. Sinus tachycardia, severe orthostatic hypotension, and syncope may develop. Convulsions and coma may be seen in severely poisoned patients. Methaemoglobinaemia is seen very rarely with organic nitrates.

Treatment

Mild hypotension may be treated by placing the patient in a head-down position, but more severe hypotension will require plasma expanders or a vasopressor agent.

Further reading

Sanders P, Faunt J (1997). An unusual cause of cyanosis (isosorbide dinitrate induced methaemoglobinaemia). *Australian and New Zealand Journal of Medicine* **27**, 596.

Nitrogen dioxide

Combustion of fossil fuels yields nitric oxide and nitrogen dioxide (a largely insoluble, brown, mildly irritating gas). Fermentation of silage produces high concentrations of this gas within 2 days of filling the silo. It is also a by-product of many industrial processes.

Clinical features

The clinical features following acute exposure to high concentrations of nitrogen dioxide depend on the concentration and duration of exposure to the gas. Since nitrogen dioxide is only a mild upper respiratory tract irritant, modest acute exposure (less than 50 ppm) for a short time often produces no immediate symptoms, although throat irritation, cough, transient choking, tightness in the chest, and sweating have been observed. By contrast, exposure to a massive concentration of nitrogen dioxide such as that found in a silo can produce severe and immediate hypoxaemia, which may be fatal. In less severe cases, the onset of symptoms may be delayed for a few hours (typically 3 to 36 h) and the patient then develops dyspnoea, chest pain (which may be pleuritic), haemoptysis, tachycardia, headache, conjunctivitis, generalized weakness, and dizziness (which may be due to hypotension). Bronchiolitis obliterans may develop within 2 to 6 weeks.

Treatment

Bronchodilator and corticosteroid therapy is sufficient in most cases. Pulmonary oedema responds poorly to diuretics; corticosteroids and mechanical ventilation with positive end-expiratory pressure offer the best hope of reducing the mortality.

Further reading

Karlson-Stiber C *et al.* (1996). Nitrogen dioxide pneumonitis in ice hockey players. *Journal of Internal Medicine* **239**, 451–6.

Opiates and opioids

Acute opioid overdose occurs commonly in 'addicts' in whom the presence of venepuncture marks and thrombosed veins in the arms and legs should prompt the diagnosis.

Clinical features

The cardinal signs of opioid overdose are pinpoint pupils, reduced respiratory rate (often accompanied by cyanosis), and coma. These depressant effects are increased by alcohol. Hypotension, due to peripheral vasodilation, occurs in less than 10 per cent of cases. Hypothermia and hypoglycaemia may also complicate the clinical picture of opioid poisoning. As many as 50 per cent of heroin overdose victims develop non-cardiogenic pulmonary oedema, the majority of whom, in turn, develop bacterial pneumonia.

Methadone poses particular problems because of its long half-life (up to 50 h).

Codeine, dextropropoxyphene, and pethidine cause increased muscle tone, twitching, and convulsions. Rhabdomyolysis and its complications have been reported in association with poisoning due to diamorphine, dihydrocodeine, dipipanone, methadone, and morphine poisoning.

Diphenoxylate is used as an antidiarrhoeal agent in conjunction with atropine, and paediatric poisoning due to the ingestion of this antidiarrhoeal preparation is not uncommon (see Co-phenotrope).

Management

Naloxone is used to reverse severe respiratory depression and coma due to opioid poisoning. The adult dose is 0.8 to 1.2 mg given intravenously or, less satisfactorily, intramuscularly; the dose in children is 5 to 10 μg/kg body weight. If the diagnosis of opioid poisoning is correct, the patient should improve within 1 min with an increase in respiratory rate, an improvement in the level of consciousness, and dilation of the pupils. In severe opioid poisoning, larger initial doses of naloxone (e.g. 2.4 mg) may be required to obtain the desired response. The duration of action of naloxone (1 to 4 h) is often less than that of the drug taken in overdose and, for this reason, careful observation of the patient is necessary. Repeated doses of naloxone should be given as required.

The respiratory depressant effects of pentazocine and buprenorphine are only partially reversed by naloxone. Assisted ventilation may be necessary.

Gastric lavage and the administration of activated charcoal may be of value if an opioid had been ingested in overdose less than 1 h previously.

The development of non-cardiogenic pulmonary oedema may necessitate the use of assisted ventilation. Antibiotics will be required to treat secondary bacterial infection. Hyperkalaemia and renal failure, as a result of rhabdomyolysis, should be treated conventionally.

Organophosphorus insecticides

Organophosphorus insecticides are among the most extensively used pesticides throughout the world. They vary widely in their toxicity and while some (the phosphates) are directly toxic, others (the phosphorothioates) need biotransformation to become active.

Mechanisms of toxicity

Organophosphorus insecticides inhibit acetylcholinesterase causing accumulation of acetylcholine at central and peripheral cholinergic nerve endings, including neuromuscular junctions.

Clinical features

The features of organophosphorus insecticide poisoning are dose related. Minor exposure may produce subclinical poisoning in which there is reduction of cholinesterase activity but no symptoms or signs. Poisoning is characterized by anxiety, restlessness, insomnia, nightmares, tiredness, dizziness, headache, and muscarinic features such as nausea, vomiting, abdominal colic, diarrhoea, tenesmus, sweating, hypersalivation, and chest tightness. Miosis may be present. Nicotinic effects follow with muscle fasciculation and flaccid paresis of limb muscles, respiratory muscles, and occasionally, various combinations of extraocular muscles. Respiratory failure ensues and is exacerbated by the development of pulmonary oedema and by the retention in the bronchi of large amounts of respiratory secretions. Consciousness is impaired in severe poisoning and convulsions may occur. Hyperglycaemia and glycosuria have been reported though ketonuria is absent. Though bradycardia would be expected from the mode of action of organophosphates, it is present in only about 20 per cent of cases. Rarely, complete heart block and arrhythmias occur.

Diagnosis

Diagnosis of organophosphorus insecticide poisoning is difficult in the absence of a history of exposure and requires a high index of suspicion. Gastroenteritis is a common erroneous diagnosis and the findings of glycosuria and hyperglycaemia may prompt consideration of diabetes mellitus and its complications. Miosis is an important diagnostic sign but is not invariable. Once raised, the diagnosis can be confirmed by demonstrating reduced plasma, but preferably erythrocyte, cholinesterase activity. However, the extent of reduction correlates only crudely with the severity of poisoning. In subclinical poisoning cholinesterase activity may be reduced by up to 50 per cent while mild, moderate, and severe poisoning are associated with reduction of cholinesterase activity to approximately 20 to 50 per cent, 10 to 20 per cent, and less than 10 per cent of normal, respectively.

Treatment

Subclinical poisoning does not require treatment other than appropriate measures to prevent further absorption of the poison. The patient should be kept under observation for about 24 h to ensure that delayed toxicity does not develop. The management of symptomatic organophosphorus insecticide poisoning involves supportive measures and judicious administration of antidotes. Soiled clothing should be removed and contaminated skin washed with soap and water to prevent further absorption. Gastric lavage should be considered if the insecticide has been ingested less than 1 h previously. A clear airway, effective removal of respiratory secretions, and correction of hypoxia are essential using endotracheal intubation and assisted ventilation if necessary. The early use of diazepam may reduce morbidity and mortality; 5 to 10 mg intravenously for an adult reduces anxiety and restlessness but larger doses may be required to control convulsions.

Atropine in a dose of 2 mg intravenously every 10 to 30 min for an adult, depending on the severity of poisoning, should be given to reduce bronchorrhoea and bronchospasm or until signs of atropinization (flushed dry skin, tachycardia, and dry mouth) develop. As much as 30 mg and occasionally much more may be required in the first 24 h in severe cases. Children should be given atropine at 0.02 mg/kg body weight but may require up to 0.05 mg/kg.

Pralidoxime reactivates phosphorylated acetylcholinesterase and should be given together with atropine to every symptomatic patient. The dose (of the mesylate and chloride salts) is 30 mg/kg body weight by slow intravenous injection. Improvement will usually be apparent within 30 min.

Further bolus doses of pralidoxime may be required every 4 to 6 h. Alternatively, an infusion of pralidoxime at 8 to 10 mg/kg body weight per h may be administered. Monitoring of erythrocyte (not plasma) cholinesterase activity may be used together with clinical signs to guide the duration of therapy.

Complications

A small number of patients develop what has been called the intermediate syndrome that comprises cranial nerve and brainstem lesions and a proximal neuropathy starting 1 to 4 days after acute intoxication and persisting for 2 to 3 weeks. Respiratory failure secondary to muscle weakness is observed. The aetiology of this syndrome is uncertain but is probably due to inadequate oxime therapy.

A variety of longer-term complications may develop including tiredness, insomnia, inability to concentrate, depression, and irritability. A peripheral neuropathy starting 2 weeks after exposure and mainly affecting the lower limbs is also well recognized. Axonal degeneration of large myelinated motor and sensory fibres has been demonstrated and is thought to be caused by inhibition of neuropathy target esterase.

Further reading

Benson B, Tolo D, McIntyre M (1992). Is the intermediate syndrome in organophosphate poisoning the result of insufficient oxime therapy? *Journal of Toxicology—Clinical Toxicology* **30**, 347–9.

Committee on Toxicity of Chemicals in Food, Consumer Products and the Environment (1999). *Organophosphates*. Department of Health, London.

Okumura T *et al.* (1996). Report on 640 victims of the Tokyo subway sarin attack. *Annals of Emergency Medicine* **28**, 129–35.

Thiermann H *et al.* (1997). Cholinesterase status, pharmacokinetics and laboratory findings during obidoxime therapy in organophosphate poisoned patients. *Human and Experimental Toxicology* **16**, 473–80.

Oxicams

These include meloxicam, piroxicam, and tenoxicam.

Clinical features

The clinical features of oxicam overdose are summarized in Table 7.

Treatment

Treatment is symptomatic and supportive. Gastric lavage or activated charcoal may be considered if the patient presents within 1 h of a substantial overdose.

Paracetamol (acetaminophen)

Mechanism of toxicity

The toxicity of paracetamol is related to its metabolism. In therapeutic doses, 60 to 90 per cent is metabolized by conjugation to form paracetamol glucuronide and sulphate (Fig. 2). A much smaller amount (5 to 10 per cent) is oxidized by mixed function oxidase enzymes to form a highly reactive compound (*N*-acetyl-*p*-benzoquinoneimine, **NAPQI**) that is then

Table 7 Clinical features of oxicam poisoning

Nausea, vomiting, diarrhoea, abdominal (often epigastric) pain
Gastrointestinal bleeding (due to peptic erosions)
Dizziness, blurred vision, excitability, hyperventilation
Hyperreflexia, coma, convulsions
Haematuria, proteinuria, acute renal failure
Hepatic dysfunction, hypoprothrombinaemia

Fig. 2 Paracetamol metabolism in therapeutic dose and overdose.

immediately conjugated with glutathione and subsequently excreted as cysteine and mercapturate conjugates. Only 1 to 4 per cent of a therapeutic dose of the drug is excreted unchanged in urine.

In overdose, larger amounts of paracetamol are metabolized by oxidation because of saturation of the sulphate conjugation pathway. As a result, liver glutathione stores become depleted so that the liver is unable to 'deactivate' the toxic metabolite. The reactive metabolite has a high affinity for cell protein and binds to liver cell macromolecules. However, covalent binding of NAPQI to cell structure nucleophiles is not thought to be directly responsible for paracetamol-induced hepatic necrosis. NAPQI is believed to have two separate but complementary effects. First, it reacts with glutathione, thereby depleting the cell of its normal defence against oxidizing damage. Second, it is a potent oxidizing as well as arylating agent; it inactivates key sulphydryl groups in certain enzymes, particularly those controlling calcium homeostasis. Inhibition of membrane calcium translocase activity and impairment of microsomal calcium uptake leads to a marked increase in cytosolic calcium concentration, which causes depolymerization of microtubules and contraction of microfilaments, with consequent disruption of cellular architecture and function. The activity of the mixed function oxidase enzyme system and the size of liver glutathione stores may be modified by pharmacological means.

Paracetamol-induced renal damage probably results from a mechanism similar to that which is responsible for hepatotoxicity, that is by formation of NAPQI, although in the kidney this is generated by prostaglandin endoperoxide synthetase rather than by cytochrome P450-dependent mixed function oxidases.

Prediction of liver damage

In the early stages following ingestion of a paracetamol overdose, most patients have few symptoms and no physical signs. There is thus a need for some form of assessment that estimates the risk of liver damage at a time when the liver function tests are still normal. Details of the dose ingested may be used but, in many cases, the history is unreliable and, even when the dose is known for certain, it does not take account of early vomiting and individual variation in response to the drug. However, a single measurement of the plasma paracetamol concentration is an accurate predictor of liver damage provided that it is taken not earlier than 4 h after the overdose. Information gained from several studies has enabled the production of a graph which may be used for prediction of liver damage and which serves as a guide to the need for specific treatment (Fig. 3). Sixty per cent of patients whose plasma paracetamol concentration falls above a line drawn between 200 mg/l (1.32 mmol/l) at 4 h and 50 mg/l (0.33 mmol/l) at 12 h

after the ingestion of the overdose are likely to sustain liver damage (serum alanine or aspartate aminotransferase, **ALT** or **AST**, greater than 1000 iu/l) unless specific protective treatment is given. When more than 12 h have lapsed after ingestion, the plasma paracetamol concentration is still of value and should be considered in conjunction with changes in the prothrombin time (see below) when assessing the prognosis of an individual patient.

There is, however, some variation in individual susceptibility to paracetamol-induced hepatotoxicity and patients with pre-existing liver disease, those with a high alcohol intake particularly if malnourished, and those receiving enzyme-inducing drugs should be considered to be at greater risk ('High risk group'; Fig. 3). Individuals with HIV-related disease also appear to be more susceptible to paracetamol-induced hepatic damage. It is uncommon for young children to develop paracetamol-induced liver or renal damage, probably because they ingest relatively small amounts in overdose.

Clinical features

As would be expected from the mechanism of toxicity, the severity of paracetamol poisoning is dose-related. An absorbed dose of 15 g (approximately 200 mg/kg) or more is potentially serious in most patients.

Following the ingestion of an overdose of paracetamol, patients usually remain asymptomatic for the first 24 h or, at most, develop anorexia, nausea, and vomiting. Liver damage is not usually detectable by routine liver function tests until at least 18 h after ingestion of the drug, and hepatic tenderness and abdominal pain are seldom exhibited before the second day. Maximum liver damage, as assessed by plasma ALT or AST activity or prothrombin time, occurs 72 to 96 h after ingestion. Hepatic failure, manifest by jaundice and encephalopathy, may then develop between the third and fifth day (Table 8) with the rate of clinical deterioration reflecting the severity of the overdose. More usually there is prolongation of the prothrombin time and a marked rise in aminotransferase activity without the development of fulminant hepatic failure. Renal failure due to acute tubular necrosis develops in about 25 per cent of patients with severe hepatic damage and in a few without evidence of serious disturbance of liver function.

Other features, including hypoglycaemia and hyperglycaemia, cardiac arrhythmias, pancreatitis, gastrointestinal haemorrhage, and cerebral oedema, may all occur with hepatic failure due to any cause and are not direct consequences of paracetamol toxicity.

There are two additional metabolic complications of paracetamol overdosage: metabolic acidosis and hypophosphataemia. Paracetamol can cause metabolic acidosis at two distinct periods after overdosage. Transient hyperlactataemia is frequently found within the first 15 h of ingestion of

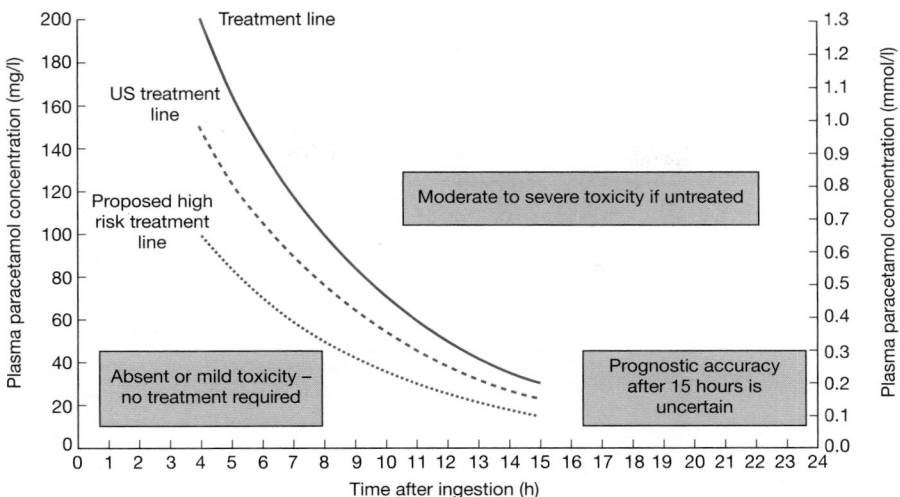

Fig. 3 Prediction of liver damage after paracetamol overdose.

paracetamol in all but minor overdoses. This appears to be due to inhibition of mitochondrial respiration at the level of ubiquinone and increased lactate production, and may be associated with a metabolic acidosis. It is rarely of clinical consequence, although in very severe paracetamol poisoning (plasma paracetamol concentration more than 500 mg/l at 4 h after ingestion) the acidosis may be associated with coma. The second phase of hyperlactataemia and acidosis occurs in those patients who present late and go on to develop hepatic damage. In this instance decreased hepatic lactate clearance appears to be the major cause, compounded by poor peripheral perfusion and increased lactate production. The development of lactic acidosis consequent upon paracetamol-induced liver damage is associated with a poor prognosis.

Hypophosphataemia is a recognized complication of acute liver failure, including that due to paracetamol, and may contribute to morbidity and mortality by inducing mental confusion, irritability, coma, and abnormalities of platelet, white cell, and erythrocyte function. Phosphaturia appears to be the principal cause of hypophosphataemia in paracetamol poisoning;

Table 8 Clinical, biochemical, and haematological features of paracetamol poisoning (> 200 mg/kg)

Day 1	Asymptomatic
	Nausea, vomiting, abdominal pain, anorexia
Day 2	May become asymptomatic
	Vomiting
	Hepatic tenderness ± generalized abdominal tenderness
	Occasionally, mild jaundice
Day 3	(In severe untreated poisoning)
	Jaundice → liver failure → hepatic encephalopathy
	Back pain + renal angle tenderness → renal failure
	Disseminated intravascular coagulation
	Cardiac arrhythmias → cardiac arrest
	Pancreatitis
Biochemical abnormalities	AST/ALT ↑ ↑
	Bilirubin ↑
	Blood sugar ↓
	Creatinine ↑
	Lactate ↑
	Phosphate ↓
	Amylase ↑
Haematological abnormalities	Prothrombin time ↑
	Platelets ↓
	Clotting factors II ↓ V ↓ VII ↓

it may occur in the absence of fulminant hepatic failure and indicates paracetamol-induced renal tubular damage.

Prognostic factors

The overall mortality of paracetamol poisoning in untreated patients is only of the order of 5 per cent. The prothrombin time is usually the first liver function test to become abnormal and, for this reason, it is of particular value in assessing the prognosis of an individual patient. The more rapid the increase in prothrombin time, the worse the prognosis of the patient. A prothrombin time of more than 20 s at 24 h after ingestion indicates that significant hepatic damage has been sustained, and a peak prothrombin time of more than 180 s is associated with a chance of survival of less than 8 per cent.

Acid–base disturbances are also a good guide to prognosis. Systemic acidosis developing more than 24 h after overdose indicates a poor prognosis; patients with a blood pH below 7.30 at this time have only a 15 per cent chance of survival. In addition, a rise in the serum creatinine concentration is associated with poor survival; patients with a serum creatinine concentration above 300 μmol/l have only a 23 per cent chance of survival.

A study of prognostic indicators in paracetamol-induced fulminant hepatic failure treated conventionally compared the sensitivity (percentage of patients who died with a positive test), predictive accuracy (percentage of patients whose outcome was predicted accurately), positive predictive value (percentage of patients with a positive test who died), and specificity (percentage of survivors with a negative test) of measurement of factors V and VIII with conventional tests. (Factor V is vitamin K dependent and concentrations fall in liver failure; levels of factor VIII rise in patients with liver failure.) An admission pH below 7.30 with a serum creatinine concentration above 300 μmol/l and a prothrombin time above 100 s in grade III to IV encephalopathy has a sensitivity, predictive accuracy, positive prediction value, and specificity of 91, 86, 83, and 91, respectively. However, a factor VIII/V ratio above 30 had comparable values of 91, 95, 100, and 100.

Treatment

Gastric lavage and activated charcoal may be of value within 1 h of overdose. Parenteral fluid replacement should be given if nausea persists or vomiting occurs.

From knowledge of the mechanism of toxicity, it may be predicted that replenishment of glutathione stores would be of value. Two substances, methionine and *N*-acetylcysteine have emerged as effective protection agents, provided that they are administered within 8 to 10 h of ingestion of

Table 9 Antidote regimens for paracetamol poisoning

Methionine (orally): 2.5 g initially, then 2.5 g 4-hourly for a further three doses. Total dose 10 g methionine over 12 h.

N-acetylcysteine (intravenously): 150 mg/kg over 15 min, then 50 mg/kg in 500 ml of 5 per cent dextrose in the next 4 h and 100 mg/kg in 1000 ml of 5 per cent dextrose over the ensuing 16 h. Total dose 300 mg/kg over 20–25 h

N-acetylcysteine (orally): 140 mg/kg initially, then 60 mg/kg every 4 h for 17 additional doses. Total dose 1330 mg/kg over 72 h.

the overdose; thereafter, the protective effects decline rapidly (Table 9). Both substances act by replenishing cellular glutathione stores, though N-acetylcysteine may also repair oxidation damage caused by NAPQI either directly or, more probably, through the generation of cysteine and/or glutathione. It may also act as a source of sulphate and so 'unsaturate' sulphate conjugation. Methionine appears more effective when given orally than when administered intravenously. As oral N-acetylcysteine induces vomiting in most patients, the intravenous route is preferred. Some 6 per cent of patients treated with intravenous N-acetylcysteine develop rash, angio-oedema, and bronchospasm. These reactions are seldom serious and no fatalities have so far been reported in those receiving the regimen outlined in Table 9. An antihistamine such as chlorpheniramine or terfenadine should be given if such anaphylactoid reactions do not settle after discontinuing the infusion of N-acetylcysteine for 30 to 45 min.

Forced diuresis, dialysis, or haemoperfusion have no role to play in the management of paracetamol poisoning, though dialysis or haemofiltration will be required if acute renal failure supervenes.

Fortunately, only a minority of patients present more than 12 to 24 h after an overdose of paracetamol but, in these cases, the morbidity and mortality is greater and the correct treatment is that intended to prevent or support hepatic failure, though the use of N-acetylcysteine has been advocated. Ten per cent glucose solution should be administered to prevent the onset of hypoglycaemia. Although there is no evidence that correction of severe coagulation abnormalities (prothrombin time greater than 100 s) with fresh frozen plasma improves the prognosis, bleeding can be catastrophic if it does occur. Fresh frozen plasma will be required to cover the insertion of intracranial pressure monitoring apparatus, if employed. An H$_2$-receptor antagonist or proton pump inhibitor may reduce the risk of gastrointestinal bleeding from 'stress' ulceration/erosion. If acute renal failure supervenes, this should be managed conventionally.

Current evidence suggests that if fulminant hepatic failure does supervene, the use of intravenous N-acetylcysteine (see Table 9 for 20.25 h regimen; the 16 h infusion is continued until recovery or death) will reduce morbidity and mortality. This beneficial effect is observed even after the onset of encephalopathy. In one study the survival rate in 25 patients with paracetamol-induced fulminant hepatic failure was 20 per cent, with an incidence of cerebral oedema and hypotension requiring inotropic support of 68 and 80 per cent, respectively. With N-acetylcysteine, the comparable figures in 25 matched patients were 48 per cent (survival rate), 40 per cent (cerebral oedema), and 48 per cent (hypotension), respectively.

Liver transplantation has been performed successfully in patients with paracetamol-induced fulminant hepatic failure, using criteria outlined above (see Prognostic factors) to identify those individuals who would otherwise be likely to die. However, there has been no formal study to compare the value of transplantation with N-acetylcysteine in fulminant hepatic failure.

Further reading

Keays P *et al.* (1991). Intravenous acetylcysteine in paracetamol induced fulminant hepatic failure: A prospective controlled trial. *British Medical Journal* **303**, 1026–9.

Makin AJ, Wendon J, Williams R (1995). A 7-year experience of severe acetaminophen-induced hepatotoxicity (1987–1993). *Gastroenterology* **109**, 1907–16.

Vale JA, Proudfoot AT (1995). Paracetamol (acetaminophen) poisoning. *Lancet* **346**, 547–52.

Paraffin oil (kerosene)

Paraffin oil has three physical properties accounting for its toxicity. Its low viscosity and surface tension allow it to spread rapidly throughout the lungs when aspirated after ingestion. Its low vapour pressure makes it unlikely to cause poisoning by inhalation.

Clinical features

Repeated local application to the skin results in dryness, dermatitis, and rarely, epidermal necrolysis. Pulmonary toxicity may occur within 1 h of ingestion and is characterized by pyrexia, cough, tachypnoea, tachycardia, basal crackles, and cyanosis. Non-segmental consolidation or collapse is seen radiologically. Pneumatocele formation, pneumothorax, pleural effusion, or pulmonary oedema may occur.

Paraffin ingestion causes respiratory symptoms, a burning sensation in the mouth and throat, vomiting, diarrhoea, abdominal pain, mild hepatomegaly with hepatic dysfunction, and in severe cases, atrial fibrillation and ventricular fibrillation.

Treatment

Gastric lavage and emesis should be avoided because of the increased risk of chemical pneumonitis, but lavage may be considered in those adults who ingest very large quantities of paraffin oil, if the airway can be protected and the procedure can be carried out within 1 h. There is no evidence that corticosteroids and antibiotics reduce morbidity or mortality; mechanical ventilation with positive end-expiratory pressure may be necessary in severe cases of aspiration.

Further reading

Baldachin BJ, Melmed RN (1964). Clinical and therapeutic aspects of kerosene poisoning: A series of 200 cases. *British Medical Journal* **2**, 28–30.

Nagi NA, Abdullah ZA (1995). Kerosene poisoning in children in Iraq. *Postgraduate Medical Journal* **71**, 419–22.

Paraquat and other bipyridyl herbicides

The bipyridilium herbicides include diquat, morfamquat, and paraquat, the last being the one most commonly encountered in clinical toxicology.

Clinical features

Occupational carelessness in handling paraquat has led to reversible changes in the fingernails and inhalation of spray may cause pain in the throat and epistaxis. Skin splashes that are promptly and thoroughly washed should not cause problems, but prolonged dermal exposure may cause burns and, very rarely, may enable enough paraquat to be absorbed to cause serious and fatal systemic poisoning. Splashes in the eye cause blepharospasm, lacrimation, and corneal ulceration.

Potentially lethal poisoning is most common after paraquat ingestion. Probably no more than 5 per cent of the ingested amount is absorbed but absorption is rapid, the volume of distribution is high, and there is energy-dependent accumulation in some organs (particularly the lungs). Elimination is mainly through the kidneys.

The features of toxicity are largely dependent on the amount of paraquat swallowed. Ingestion of 6 g or more of paraquat ion is likely to be fatal within 24 to 48 h, while 3 to 6 g is likely to lead to a more protracted, but still fatal, outcome. Nausea, vomiting, abdominal pain, and diarrhoea, rapidly followed by peripheral circulatory failure, metabolic acidosis, impaired consciousness, convulsions, and increasing breathlessness and cyanosis secondary to acute pneumonitis are the features of ingestion of large amounts of paraquat. With smaller amounts, the cardiovascular and CNS complications are not seen and alimentary features dominate the course of poisoning, particularly painful ulceration of the mouth, tongue, and throat, which makes it difficult to swallow, speak, and cough. Perforation of the oesophagus with subsequent mediastinitis has been reported. Mild jaundice may be seen and renal failure is usually severe. Breathlessness, tachypnoea, widespread crepitations, and central cyanosis may be present by 5 to 7 days after ingestion and progress relentlessly until the patient dies from hypoxia a few days later.

Ingestion of 1.5 to 2.0 g of paraquat causes nausea, vomiting and diarrhoea, mild renal tubular necrosis , and pain in the throat. Respiratory involvement may not be apparent until 10 to 21 days after ingestion, but may progress till the patient dies of respiratory failure as late as 5 or 6 weeks after taking the paraquat.

Diagnosis

The diagnosis of poisoning is usually made on the basis of the history and can be readily confirmed by a simple qualitative test on urine. This test is of particular value in accidental inhalation or ingestion of very small quantities and if performed on urine passed within 4 h of alleged ingestion; a negative test indicates that not enough has been taken to cause problems.

Treatment

There is no evidence that any form of intervention can alter the outcome of paraquat poisoning. It is traditional to empty the stomach despite the corrosive effects of the toxin, but administration of activated charcoal is probably more effective in reducing absorption.

Symptomatic measures including antiemetics, mouth washes, and analgesics are indicated and intravenous fluids may be necessary to replace gastrointestinal losses. Skin ulcers should be treated as burns. Unfortunately, currently available techniques for enhancing the elimination of poisons appear incapable of rapidly removing toxicologically significant quantities of paraquat. Equally there is no evidence that corticosteroids, drugs to prevent free radical formation, free radical scavengers, immunosuppressive agents, radiotherapy to the lungs, or lung transplantation reduce mortality. The prognosis in individual cases can be predicted from the plasma paraquat concentration related to the time from ingestion.

Further reading

Jones GM, Vale JA. Mechanisms of toxicity, clinical features and management of diquat poisoning: A review. *Journal of Toxicology—Clinical Toxicology* **38**, 123–8.
Pond SM (1990). Manifestations and management of paraquat poisoning. *Medical Journal of Australia* **152**, 256–9.

Petrol (gasoline)

Petrol is a complex mixture of hydrocarbons containing a small proportion of non-hydrocarbon additives.

Clinical features

Acute exposure

Following the inhalation of petrol, dizziness and irritation of the eyes, nose, and throat may occur within 5 min followed by euphoria, headache, and blurred vision. If inhalation continues, or if significant quantities of petrol are ingested, then excitement and depression of the nervous system occurs; incoordination, restlessness, excitement, confusion, disorientation, hallucinations, ataxia, nystagmus, tremor, delirium, coma, and convulsions may be seen. The inhalation of high concentrations of petrol may cause immediate death, probably from ventricular fibrillation or respiratory failure. Chemical pneumonitis may occur as in paraffin oil ingestion (see above) and the clinical features and management are then identical. In addition,

intravascular haemolysis, hypofibrinogenaemia, and cardiorespiratory arrest have been reported together with, in one patient, epiglottitis so severe that near total airway obstruction resulted.

Chronic exposure

Men engaged in cleaning storage tanks and those who habitually sniff may develop both hydrocarbon and lead poisoning.

Treatment

Following removal from exposure, supportive measures provide the basis of treatment. Gastric lavage and emesis will increase the risk of aspiration and chemical pneumonitis. Lavage could be considered, with protection of the airway, if an adult ingested a large amount of petrol and the procedure could be performed within 1 h of ingestion.

Further reading

Caprino L, Togna GI (1998). Potential health effects of gasoline and its constituents: a review of current literature (1990–1997) on toxicological data. *Environmental Health Perspectives* **106**, 115–25.

Phenol

Phenol (carbolic acid) is recognizable by its odour and, distinctively, the pain to which it gives rise is much less than might be expected. This is due to its ability to damage afferent nerve endings.

Clinical features

If phenol is spilt on the skin, pain is followed promptly by numbness. The skin becomes blanched, and a dry opaque eschar forms over the burn. When the eschar sloughs off, a brown stain remains. Phenol penetrates intact skin rapidly and is well absorbed through the lungs. After ingestion, vomiting and abdominal pain occur. Systemic toxicity may follow exposure by any route. Features include coma, loss of vasoconstrictor tone, and hypothermia together with cardiac and respiratory depression. An initial phase of CNS stimulation, and rarely convulsions, has sometimes been observed in children. Phenol poisoning is associated with grey or black urine and although this is due in part to metabolites of phenol, Heinz body haemolytic anaemia as well as methaemoglobinaemia and hyperbilirubinaemia are recognized features. Renal complications are seen frequently.

Treatment

Gastric lavage may be considered if the patient presents less than 1 h after ingestion and severe oropharyngeal burns are not suspected. Skin and eye contamination, renal failure, and methaemoglobinaemia are managed appropriately.

Further reading

Christiansen RG, Klaman JS (1996). Successful treatment of phenol poisoning with charcoal hemoperfusion. *Veterinary and Human Toxicology* **38**, 27–8.

Phenothiazines

The phenothiazines block peripheral cholinergic and α-adrenergic receptors, reuptake of amines, and the effects of histamine and serotonin.

Clinical features

The features of overdose include impairment of consciousness, hypotension, and respiratory depression. Chlorpromazine, perphenazine, and promazine seem more prone to cause hypothermia and hypotension, while anticholinergic effects with tachycardia, ECG abnormalities, and arrhythmias are most common with overdosage of thioridazine and mesoridazine,

Table 10 Clinical features of poisoning from phenylpropionic acid derivatives

Nausea, vomiting, abdominal pain and tenderness, haematemesis
Headache, tinnitus, hyperventilation, sinus tachycardia
Haematuria, proteinuria, renal angle tenderness, acute renal failure
Hypotension, hypothermia, hypoprothrombinaemia
Drowsiness, coma, respiratory depression
Nystagmus, diplopia

and acute spasmodic torticollis, oculogyric crises, and orolingual dyskinesias with trifluperazine and prochlorperazine.

Treatment

Treatment is supportive and symptomatic. Benztropine in a dose of 2 mg intravenously in an adult is required occasionally to reverse spasmodic torticollis and oculogyric crises.

Phenylpropionic (arylpropionic) acid derivatives

These include fenbufen, fenoprofen, flurbiprofen, ibuprofen, cetoprofen, naproxen, and tiaprofenic acid.

Clinical features

Propionic acid derivative poisoning causes nausea, vomiting, abdominal pain, drowsiness, headache, tinnitus, ataxia, stupor, and rarely, coma and convulsions. Hyperventilation, bronchospasm, and hypotension occur but gastrointestinal haemorrhage and renal failure are rare. These and additional clinical features are summarized in Table 10.

Treatment

Management is supportive.

Phenytoin

Clinical features

Acute overdose of phenytoin results in nausea, vomiting, headache, tremor, cerebellar ataxia, nystagmus, and rarely, loss of consciousness.

Treatment

Gastric lavage may be considered if the patient presents within 1 h after a substantial overdose. Multiple-dose activated charcoal may increase elimination although this has not been confirmed.

Further reading

Evers ML, Izhar A, Aqil A (1997). Cardiac monitoring after phenytoin overdose. *Heart and Lung* **26**, 325–8.

Manto M, Preiser JC, Vincent JC (1996). Hypoglycemia associated with phenytoin intoxication. *Journal of Toxicology—Clinical Toxicology* **34**, 205–8.

Phosgene

Phosgene is a colourless gas, which is now used in the synthesis of isocyanates, polyurethane and polycarbonate resins, dyes, and is produced in fires.

Mechanism of toxicity

Phosgene reacts with glutathione. When glutathione stores become depleted beyond a critical level covalent binding occurs between phosgene and cell macromolecules with resultant hepatic and renal necrosis.

Clinical features

Exposure to phosgene causes irritation of the eyes, dryness or burning sensation in the throat, cough, chest pain, and nausea and vomiting. There is usually a latent period lasting between 30 min and 24 h (rarely, 72 h) during which the casualty suffers little discomfort and has no abnormal chest signs. Subsequently, pulmonary oedema develops due to increased capillary permeability; circulatory collapse may follow.

Treatment

Administration of *N*-acetylcysteine may confer some protection. Oxygen should be administered. Mechanical ventilation may be life-saving in severe cases.

Further reading

Wyatt JP, Allister CA (1995). Occupational phosgene poisoning: a case report and review. *Journal of Accident and Emergency Medicine* **12**, 212–13.

Phosphine

Phosphine is a colourless gas with a fish-like odour and is used as a fumigant against insects and rodents in stored grain, particularly in grain elevators and, increasingly, aboard ships. It is also used to treat silicon crystals in the semiconductor industry.

Clinical features

Fatigue, nausea, vomiting, diarrhoea, chest tightness, breathlessness, productive cough, dizziness, and headache are common features of acute phosphine exposure. Acute pulmonary oedema, hypertension, cardiac arrhythmias, and convulsions have been described in severe cases. Ataxia, intention tremor, and diplopia may be found on examination. Focal myocardial infiltration with necrosis, pulmonary oedema, and widespread small-vessel injury were found at autopsy in a child who died.

Treatment

The casualty should be removed from exposure as soon as possible. Thereafter, treatment is supportive and symptomatic. The value of steroids in preventing pulmonary damage (which may be delayed) has not been established.

Further reading

Schoonbroodt D *et al.* (1992). Acute phosphine poisoning? A case report and review. *Acta Clinica Belgica* **47**, 280–4.

Primaquine

Clinical features

Primaquine poisoning is rare, though toxicity is frequent if more than 60 mg is ingested in 1 day. Headache, nausea, abdominal pain, and methaemoglobinaemia may occur and haemolytic anaemia and leucopenia have been observed, especially in patients with glucose-6-phosphate dehydrogenase deficiency.

Treatment

Gut decontamination should be considered if presentation is within 1 h of exposure. If methaemoglobinaemia exceeds 40 per cent, methylthioninium (methylene blue) at 1 to 2 mg/kg body weight should be administered intravenously over 5 min. Antidotal efficacy is NADPH dependent and therefore reduced in the presence of G6PD deficiency

Further reading

Jaeger A *et al.* (1987). Clinical features and management of poisoning due to antimalaria drugs. *Medical Toxicology* **2**, 242–73.

Propylene glycol (1,2-propanediol)

Propylene glycol is used widely as a preservative as a vehicle for both oral and intravenous medications and in preparations used for treating burns.

Mechanism of toxicity

Propylene glycol is oxidized to lactic acid and pyruvate.

Clinical features

The ingestion of substantial quantities of propylene glycol or its administration to neonates or those in renal failure may cause convulsions, coma, cardiac arrhythmias, hepatorenal damage, intravascular haemolysis, metabolic acidosis, and increased serum osmolality.

Treatment

Gastric lavage should be considered if the patient presents within 1 h after ingestion. Metabolic acidosis, renal failure, and respiratory depression should be treated conventionally. Haemodialysis removes propylene glycol efficiently.

Further reading

Levy ML *et al.* (1995). Propylene glycol toxicity following continuous etomidate infusion for the control of refractory cerebral edema. *Neurosurgery* **37**, 363–71.

Pyrethroids

Clinical features

Pyrethroids are best known for their ability to cause facial paraesthesiae following occupational exposure; these symptoms last only a few hours at most. Coma, convulsions, and pulmonary oedema may occur after substantial ingestion, percutaneous absorption, or inhalational exposure.

Treatment

Symptomatic and supportive measures should be employed and reassurance given that facial paraesthesiae will not be a long-term problem.

Further reading

Kühn K-H *et al.* (1999). Toxicokinetics of pyrethroids in humans: consequences for biological monitoring. *Bulletin of Environmental Contamination and Toxicology* **62**, 101–8.

Müller-Mohnssen H (1999). Chronic sequelae and irreversible injuries following acute pyrethroid intoxication. *Toxicology Letters* **107**, 161–76.

Wilkes MF (2000). Pyrethroid-induced paresthesia—a central or local toxic effect? *Journal of Toxicology—Clinical Toxicology* **38**, 103–5.

Pyridoxine

High doses (more than 2 to 3 g/day) have been used for the treatment of a variety of conditions including the premenstrual syndrome, carpal tunnel syndrome, schizophrenia, and hyperactivity in childhood.

Clinical features

Prolonged daily intake of 50 to 300 mg in women has been reported to cause headaches, irritability, tiredness, shooting pains, circumoral and limb paraesthesiae, numb extremities, clumsiness, and ataxia, indicating a sensory neuropathy.

Treatment

Improvement occurs within 2 months of stopping the drug. There is no specific treatment.

Quinidine and quinine

Though quinidine and quinine are optical isomers, quinine is more oculotoxic and quinidine more cardiotoxic in overdose. Poisoning with quinine is much more common than with quinidine and may be iatrogenic, suicidal, or from attempted abortion or adulterated heroin.

Clinical features

Doses as low as 2 g can be toxic in adults. Cinchonism (tinnitus, deafness, vertigo, nausea, headache, and diarrhoea) is common at plasma concentrations greater than 10 mg/l. In more serious poisoning, collapse with impairment of consciousness (due to ventricular arrhythmias), convulsions, rapid shallow breathing, hypotension, pulmonary oedema, and cardiorespiratory arrest may be observed. Ventricular tachycardia and fibrillation and depression of automaticity and intracardiac conduction are potentially lethal. Pulmonary oedema and acute renal failure have been described. About 40 per cent of patients develop ocular features, which may be unilateral, including blindness, contracted visual fields, scotomas, dilated pupils, blurred disc margins, macular oedema, arteriolar spasm, and late optic atrophy. Oculotoxicity is likely when plasma concentrations exceed 10 mg/l. Visual loss is permanent in about 50 per cent of cases. Hypoglycaemia resulting from insulin release is a common side-effect of quinine and quinidine, even when used in therapeutic doses.

Treatment

Gastric lavage may be indicated if the patient presents within 1 h of ingestion or, alternatively, 50 to 100 g of activated charcoal may be administered. Multiple doses of activated charcoal increase quinine clearance. Forced diuresis, charcoal haemoperfusion, haemodialysis, and stellate ganglion block are of no value. Electrolyte and acid–base disturbances and hypoglycaemia should be corrected. Bradyarrhythmias may respond to isoprenaline; overdrive pacing may be required if *torsade de pointes* occurs. Plasma expanders should be given for hypotension, but if the response is poor, an inotrope should be administered.

Further reading

Mackie MA, Davidson J, Clarke J (1997). Quinine—acute self-poisoning and ocular toxicity. *Scottish Medical Journal* **42**, 8–9.

Nordt SP, Clark RF (1998). Acute blindness after severe quinine poisoning. *American Journal of Emergency Medicine* **16**, 214–15.

Rifampicin

Clinical features

Poisoning with rifampicin results in the so-called 'red man syndrome' that can be fatal. The skin, and subsequently the sclerae, become yellow-orange in colour (the colour of a boiled lobster) and the skin discoloration may be removed by washing. These appearances are due to the intense colour of rifampicin and its metabolites that are distributed throughout the body. In addition, nausea, vomiting, abdominal pain, pruritis, a sensation of the skin burning, and convulsions have been observed. Less commonly, marked oedema of the forehead, cheeks, chin, and lips with associated eosinophilia has occurred. Elevations in serum activities of hepatic enzymes and bilirubin concentration have been noted. Sudden death has also been recorded in two patients, due probably to cardiorespiratory arrest.

Treatment

Treatment is supportive and symptomatic. Gastric lavage may be considered if the patient presents within 1 h of a substantial overdose.

Further reading

Holdiness MR (1989). A review of the red man syndrome and rifampicin overdose. *Medical Toxicology and Adverse Drug Experience* **4**, 444–51.

Salicylates

Despite the introduction of child-resistant packaging, the ingestion of aspirin by children still occurs, iatrogenic overdose is not uncommon, and moreover, aspirin remains the drug of choice for many adults who choose deliberately to poison themselves. Salicylate poisoning may also result from percutaneous absorption of salicylic acid (used in keratolytic agents), and ingestion of methyl salicylate (oil of wintergreen).

Mechanisms of toxicity

In therapeutic doses, aspirin is absorbed rapidly from the stomach and small intestine, but in overdose, absorption may occur more slowly and the plasma salicylate concentration may continue to rise for up to 6 to 12 h.

The pharmacokinetics of elimination of aspirin are an important determinant in the development of salicylate toxicity. The biotransformation pathways concerned with the formation of salicyluric acid and salicylphenolic glucuronide (Fig. 4) are saturable, a fact which has the following clinical consequences: (i) the time needed to eliminate a given fraction of a dose increases with increasing dose; (ii) the steady-state plasma concentration of salicylate, particularly that of the pharmacologically active non-

protein-bound fraction, increases more than proportionately with increasing dose; and (iii) as the metabolic pathways of elimination become saturated, renal excretion of salicylic acid becomes increasingly important, a pathway which is extremely sensitive to changes in urinary pH.

When ingested in overdose, salicylates directly stimulate the respiratory centre to produce both increased depth and rate of respiration, thereby causing a respiratory alkalosis (Fig. 5). At least part of this effect on the respiratory centre has been shown to be due to local uncoupling of oxidative phosphorylation within the brainstem. In an attempt to compensate, bicarbonate, accompanied by sodium, potassium, and water, is excreted in the urine. Dehydration and hypokalaemia result, but more importantly, the loss of bicarbonate diminishes the buffering capacity of the body and allows an acidosis to develop more easily. A very high salicylate concentration in the brain depresses the respiratory centre and may further contribute to the development of acidaemia.

Simultaneously, a variable degree of metabolic acidosis develops, not only because of the presence of salicylic acid itself, but also because of interference with carbohydrate, lipid, protein, and amino acid metabolism by salicylate ions (Fig. 5). Inhibition of citric acid cycle enzymes causes an

Fig. 4 The principal biotransformation pathways of aspirin.

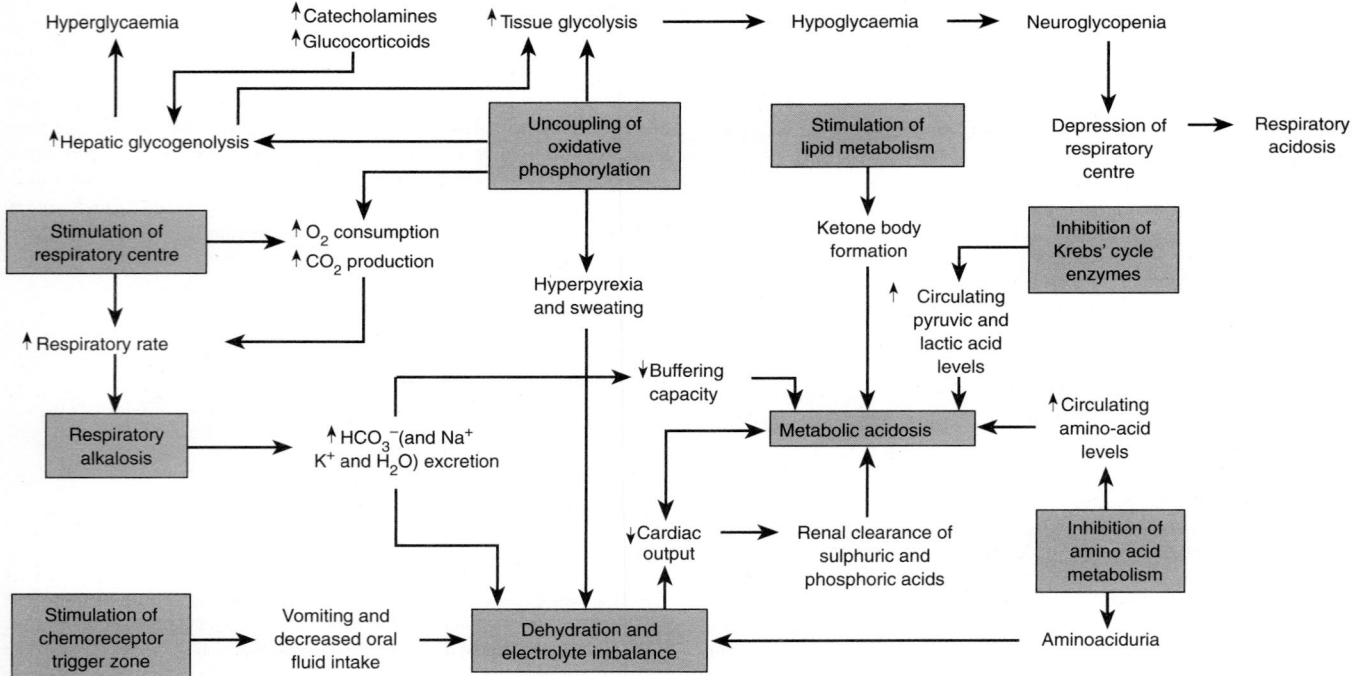

Fig. 5 The pathophysiology of salicylate poisoning.

increase in circulating lactic and pyruvic acids. Salicylates stimulate fat metabolism and cause increased production of the ketone bodies, β-hydroxybutyric acid, acetoacetic acid, and acetone. Dehydration and lack of food intake because of vomiting further contribute to the development of ketosis. Protein catabolism is accelerated, protein synthesis diminished, and aminotransferases (responsible for the interconversion of amino acids) inhibited. Increased circulating blood concentrations of amino acids result, together with aminoaciduria; this latter feature is further enhanced by inhibition of active tubular reabsorption of amino acids. The aminoaciduria increases the solute load on the kidneys and, thereby, increases water loss from the body.

A primary toxic effect of salicylates in overdose is uncoupling of oxidative phosphorylation (Fig. 5). ATP-dependent reactions are inhibited and oxygen utilization and carbon dioxide production increased. Energy normally used for the conversion of inorganic phosphate to ATP is dissipated as heat. Hyperpyrexia and sweating result causing further dehydration. Fluid loss is enhanced because salicylates stimulate the chemoreceptor trigger zone and induce nausea and vomiting and, thereby, diminish oral fluid intake. If dehydration is sufficiently marked, low cardiac output and oliguria will aggravate the metabolic acidosis already present which, if severe, can itself diminish cardiac output.

Glucose metabolism also suffers as a result of uncoupled oxidative phosphorylation because of increased tissue glycolysis and peripheral demand for glucose (Fig. 5). This is seen principally in skeletal muscle and may cause hypoglycaemia. The brain appears to be particularly sensitive to this effect and neuroglycopenia can occur in the presence of a normal blood sugar level when the rate of utilization exceeds the rate at which glucose can be supplied from the blood. Increased metabolism and peripheral demand for glucose activates hypothalmic centres resulting in increased adrenocortical stimulation and release of adrenaline. Increased glucose-6-phosphatase activity and hepatic glycogenolysis contribute to the hyperglycaemia that is sometimes seen following ingestion of large amounts of salicylate. Increased circulating adrenocorticosteroids exacerbate fluid and electrolyte imbalance.

Although rarely a practical problem, salicylate intoxication may be accompanied by hypoprothrombinaemia due to a warfarin-like action of salicylates on the physiologically important vitamin K_1 epoxide cycle. Vitamin K is converted to vitamin K 2,3-epoxide and then reconverted to vitamin K by a liver membrane reductase enzyme which is competitively inhibited by salicylates (and warfarin).

Clinical features and assessment of severity of salicylate intoxication

The dose of salicylate ingested and the age of the patient (see below) are the principal determinants of the severity of an overdose. The plasma salicylate concentration should be determined on admission, but it is important to repeat it 2 h later to ensure that the concentration is not rising. If the concentration has risen, the level should be repeated after a further 2 h. Generally speaking, plasma salicylate concentrations that lie between 300 and 500 mg/l some 6 h after ingestion of an overdose are associated with only mild toxicity, concentrations between 500 and 700 mg/l are associated with moderate toxicity, and concentrations in excess of 700 mg/l confirm severe poisoning.

Salicylate poisoning of any severity is associated with sweating, vomiting, epigastric pain, tinnitus, and deafness (Table 11).

Young children quickly develop metabolic acidosis following the ingestion of aspirin in overdose, but by the age of 12 years, the usual adult picture of a combined dominant respiratory alkalosis and mild metabolic acidosis is seen. Dehydration and electrolyte imbalance occur early. To some extent, the presence of an alkalaemia protects against serious salicylate toxicity because salicylate remains ionized and unable to penetrate cell membranes easily. Development of acidaemia allows salicylates to penetrate tissues more readily and leads, in particular, to CNS toxicity characterized by excitement, tremor, delirium, convulsions, stupor, and coma. Very

Table 11 Clinical features of salicylate poisoning

Nausea, vomiting, and epigastric discomfort
Irritability, tremor, tinnitus, deafness, blurring of vision
Hyperpyrexia, sweating, dehydration
Tachypnoea and hyperpnoea
Non-cardiogenic pulmonary oedema
Acute renal failure
Mixed respiratory alkalosis and metabolic acidosis (except in children who usually develop metabolic acidosis alone)
Hypokalaemia, hypernatraemia, or hyponatraemia
Hyperglycaemia or hypoglycaemia
Hypoprothrombinaemia (rare)
Confusion, delirium, stupor, and coma (in severe cases)

high plasma salicylate concentrations cause paralysis of the respiratory centre and cardiovascular collapse due to vasomotor depression.

Pulmonary oedema is seen occasionally in salicylate poisoning, and although this is often due to fluid overload as a result of treatment, it may be non-cardiac and occur in the presence of hypovolaemia. In these circumstances, the pulmonary oedema fluid has the same protein and electrolyte composition as plasma, suggesting increased pulmonary vascular permeability.

Although aspirin overdose may be complicated by inhibition of platelet aggregation and hypoprothrombinaemia, gastric erosions and gastrointestinal bleeding are rare following acute salicylate overdose.

Oliguria is sometimes seen in patients following the ingestion of salicylates in overdose. The most common cause is dehydration, but rarely, acute renal failure or inappropriate secretion of antidiuretic hormone may occur.

Whilst the urinary pH may be alkaline in the early stages of salicylate overdose, it soon becomes acid. Measurement of arterial blood gases, pH, and standard bicarbonate may show a respiratory alkalosis in the early stages of salicylate intoxication accompanied by the development of a metabolic acidosis. The plasma potassium concentration is often low; rarely, the blood sugar may be high.

Treatment

Gastric lavage and activated charcoal may be considered if the patient presents within 1 h of ingestion. Fluid and electrolyte replacement is particularly important and special attention should be paid to potassium supplementation. Severe metabolic acidosis requires at least partial correction with bicarbonate. Sedatives and respiratory depressant drugs should be avoided because they may hasten the development of acidaemia and CNS toxicity. Mild cases of salicylate poisoning may be managed with either oral or parenteral fluid and electrolyte replacement only.

Patients who exhibit marked symptoms or signs of salicylism and whose plasma salicylate concentration is in excess of 700 mg/l (or lower if acidaemia is present) should receive specific elimination therapy. Urine alkalinization is most often used for this purpose. The pH of the urine during this procedure is of far greater importance than the volume of urine excreted. The urinary pH should be in excess of 7.5 and should ideally lie between 8.0 and 8.5. Rarely, patients prove refractory to urine alkalinization, or this therapy may be contraindicated. Haemodialysis may then prove necessary to remove salicylate from the body. Haemodialysis is the treatment of choice for severely poisoned patients, particularly those with features of CNS toxicity and metabolic acidosis, and has the advantage that it enables simultaneous correction of the acid–base and fluid and electrolyte imbalances.

Pulmonary oedema occasionally complicates salicylate toxicity. Fluid overload should be excluded as far as possible, but if increased pulmonary vascular permeability is suspected, measurement of the pulmonary artery wedge pressure may be needed both for confirmation of the diagnosis and to monitor subsequent fluid administration. Positive and expiratory pressure ventilation appears to be beneficial in this form of pulmonary oedema.

Further reading

Chapman BJ, Proudfoot AT (1989). Adult salicylate poisoning: deaths and outcome in patients with high plasma salicylate concentrations. *Quarterly Journal of Medicine* **72**, 699–707.

Varela N *et al.* (1998). Salicylate toxicity in the older patient. *Journal of Clinical Rheumatology* **4**, 1–5.

Selective serotonin reuptake inhibitors (SSRIs)

Citalopram, fluoxetine, fluvoxamine, paroxetine, and sertraline are new antidepressants that inhibit serotonin reuptake (SSRIs). They lack the anticholinergic actions of tricyclic antidepressants.

Clinical features

Doses of up to 3.6 mg/kg body weight of fluoxetine and fluvoxamine do not appear to cause toxicity and even larger amounts are relatively safe unless potentiated by ethanol. Most patients will show no signs of toxicity but drowsiness, nausea, diarrhoea, and sinus tachycardia have been reported. Rarely, junctional bradycardia, seizures, and hypertension have been encountered and influenza-like symptoms may develop after a day or two.

Treatment

Supportive measures are all that are required. Activated charcoal may reduce absorption if administered within 1 h of overdose, but should only be considered if a substantial overdose has been ingested.

Further reading

Gross R *et al.* (1998). Generalized seizures caused by fluoxetine overdose. *American Journal of Emergency Medicine* **16**, 328–9.

Phillips S *et al.* (1997). Fluoxetine versus tricyclic antidepressants: a prospective multicenter study of antidepressant drug overdoses. *Journal of Emergency Medicine* **15**, 439–45.

Smoke

Smoke consists of a suspension of small particles in hot air and gases that are generated by thermal decomposition and combustion. The particles consist of carbon and are coated with combustion products such as organic acids and aldehydes. The gaseous phase of smoke has an extremely variable composition, depending on the materials involved in the fire. Carbon dioxide and carbon monoxide are always present and usually constitute major components.

Other toxic gases commonly contained in the gaseous phase, though not necessarily in high concentration, include acrolein, ammonia, chlorine, hydrogen bromide, hydrogen chloride, hydrogen cyanide, oxides of nitrogen, phosgene, phosphorus pentoxide, and sulphur dioxide.

Clinical features

The main effects are asphyxia and severe pulmonary irritation and oedema. Smaller particles, acids, and aldehydes cause lacrimation, burning of the throat, and nausea and vomiting when swallowed. Highly water-soluble gases (e.g. hydrogen chloride, sulphur dioxide) cause immediate irritation to the upper respiratory tract, whereas gases with low solubility (e.g. chlorine, nitrogen dioxide, phosgene) penetrate further into the lung and cause injury to the distal airways and alveoli.

Thus, features range from mild irritation of the eyes and upper airways to severe tracheobronchitis, bronchospasm, pulmonary oedema, and bronchopneumonia, which may result in pulmonary insufficiency and death. Laryngitis and laryngeal oedema can also occur and may progress to complete laryngeal obstruction over a period of several hours. Acute hypoxaemia may be associated with the occurrence of frequent ventricular premature beats; tissue hypoxia due to an elevated carboxyhaemoglobin concentration may lead to chest pain and cardiac arrhythmias in subjects with pre-existing ischaemic heart disease.

Treatment

Casualties should be removed from the smoke and resuscitated. Humidified oxygen should be administered, together with a nebulized bronchodilator such as salbutamol if bronchospasm is present. A carboxyhaemoglobin concentration should be obtained and arterial blood gases should be measured.

In the case of burning plastics, the possibility of cyanide poisoning should be considered. Early fibreoptic laryngoscopy or bronchoscopy may assist the diagnosis and enable the severity of any subglottal injury to be determined. Evidence that corticosteroids protect against pulmonary injury is lacking.

Further reading

Barillo DJ, Goode R, Esch V (1994). Cyanide poisoning in victims of fire: analysis of 364 cases and review of the literature. *Journal of Burn Care and Rehabilitation* **15**, 46–57.

Baud FJ *et al.* (1991). Elevated blood cyanide concentrations in victims of smoke inhalation. *New England Journal of Medicine* **325**, 1761–6.

Hantson P *et al.* (1997). Early complications and value of initial clinical and paraclinical observations in victims of smoke inhalation without burns. *Chest* **111**, 671–5.

Orzel RA (1993). Toxicological aspects of fire smoke: polymer pyrolysis and combustion. *Occupational Medicine* **8**, 415–29.

Shusterman D *et al.* (1996). Predictors of carbon monoxide and hydrogen cyanide exposure in smoke inhalation patients. *Journal of Toxicology—Clinical Toxicology* **34**, 61–71.

Sodium chloride

Poisoning with sodium chloride is uncommon but has occurred accidentally (e.g. addition of salt instead of sugar to infant feeds), as a result of deliberate intent (e.g. as a form of child abuse), or iatrogenically (e.g. use of hypertonic saline in gastric lavage or too rapid administration of saline during treatment of hyponatraemia).

Mechanism of toxicity

An increase in plasma sodium will increase plasma osmolality causing a shift of water from the intracellular to the extracellular space. CNS cell dehydration results in distended cerebral vessels. Subarachnoid, subdural, and intravascular haemorrhages may follow; these changes may be aggravated by overzealous rehydration.

Clinical features

Poisoning with sodium chloride can induce vomiting, increased thirst, anorexia, fever, hypotonia, lethargy, dehydration, peripheral vasoconstriction, irritability, muscular rigidity, convulsions, and coma. Hypernatraemia, increased plasma and urine osmolality, hyperglycaemia, metabolic acidosis, and hypocalcaemia may ensue. In severe cases pulmonary oedema and congestive heart failure may develop.

Treatment

The aim is to lower the serum sodium concentration slowly so that cerebral oedema, pulmonary oedema, convulsions, and coma are not provoked. Five per cent dextrose followed by hypotonic saline solutions should be given intravenously, but in severe cases complicated by renal insufficiency, haemodialysis (peritoneal dialysis is less efficient) should be considered. Hyperglycaemia should not be corrected by insulin as this may induce cerebral oedema.

Further reading

Addleman M, Pollard A, Grossman RF (1985). Survival after severe hypernatremia due to salt ingestion by an adult. *American Journal of Medicine* **78**, 176–8.

Sodium nitroprusside

This vasodilator is converted *in vivo* to nitric oxide and cyanide. Accumulation of cyanide occurs if too high an infusion rate of nitroprusside is used.

Clinical features

Hypotension is the major side-effect of treatment and may be corrected by a change in infusion rate. Metabolic (lactic) acidosis is usually the first indication of cyanide toxicity. Thiocyanate accumulation may lead to anorexia, nausea, lethargy, fatigue, and psychosis.

Treatment

During prolonged infusions the blood cyanide and thiocyanate concentrations should be measured and should not exceed 1 mg/l and 100 mg/l, respectively. The risk of toxicity can be avoided by not exceeding the recommended infusion rates and/or by giving sodium thiosulphate or hydroxocobalamin intravenously. Cyanide toxicity should be treated conventionally (see above).

Further reading

Johanning RJ *et al.* (1995). A retrospective study of sodium nitroprusside use and assessment of the potential risk of cyanide poisoning. *Pharmacotherapy* **15**, 773–7.

Sodium valproate

Clinical features

Sodium valproate in overdose causes impairment of consciousness and respiration. In severe cases, abnormal liver function tests, hyperammonaemia, increased anion gap acidosis, hypocalcaemia, and hypernatraemia have been reported. In addition, optic nerve atrophy, cerebral oedema, non-cardiogenic pulmonary oedema, renal failure, and pancreatitis have been observed.

Treatment

Gastric lavage may be considered if the patient presents less than 1 h after the ingestion of a substantial overdose. Treatment is symptomatic and supportive.

Further reading

Andersen GA, Ritland S (1995). Life threatening intoxication with sodium valproate. *Journal of Toxicology—Clinical Toxicology* **33**, 279–84.

Strychnine

Poisoning with strychnine, an alkaloid from *Strychnos* species (*Loganiaceae*), is now rare. It is no longer used as a medicine but has a continuing role for killing rodents, moles, and other vermin, and and has been used to 'cut' illicit drugs, especially cocaine and heroin. Strychnine is readily absorbed from the gastrointestinal tract and nasal mucosa and is highly toxic.

Clinical features

Systemic effects occur within 30 min of ingestion or inhalation. The threshold for CNS stimulation is lowered with the result that any sensory stimulus may produce violent muscular spasms reminiscent of tetanus. Features include stiffness of the neck and facial muscles, producing trismus and risus sardonicus. Increased muscle tone, hyperreflexia, agitation, restlessness, and convulsions lead to profound lactic acidosis, rhabdomyolysis, and hyperthermia. Painful muscle spasms and convulsions may be provoked by touch, pain, and noise. Opisthotonos may develop. Death usually results from contracture of respiratory muscles. Strychnine blocks glycine-mediated activation of chloride channels, especially in Renshaw cells of the spinal cord, disinhibiting reflex activity and leading to tetanus-like spasms and muscular rigidity.

Treatment

The patient should be kept at rest. Any type of stimulation must be reduced to a minimum and gastric lavage avoided. Oral activated charcoal, in a dose of 50 to 100 g for an adult, adsorbs strychnine and may reduce its absorption if given within 1 h of ingestion.

In severe poisoning, supportive measures to establish and maintain a clear airway and adequate ventilation are of prime importance. Convulsions should be controlled with intravenous diazepam and muscular spasms with neuromuscular blockade (e.g. with pancuronium) and mechanical ventilation. This, together with supplemental oxygen, will help correct metabolic acidosis. Hyperthermia, rhabdomyolysis, and renal failure should be managed conventionally. Patients may recover without apparent sequelae.

Further reading

Boyd RE *et al.* (1983). Strychnine poisoning. Recovery from profound acidosis, hyperthermia and rhabdomyoysis. *American Journal of Medicine* **74**, 507–12

Oberpaur B *et al.* (1999). Strychnine poisoning: an uncommon intoxication in children. *Pediatric Emergency Care* **15**, 264–5.

Styrene (vinyl benzene)

Styrene is a colourless to yellow liquid with a pleasant, sweet odour at low concentrations. Styrene monomer is an important agent in the production of plastic and a stabilizing agent in a variety of products.

Mechanism of toxicity

Styrene is oxidized to styrene oxide that binds covalently to cellular macromolecules, probably due to depletion of glutathione.

Clinical features

Although inhalation is the most common route of exposure, absorption of styrene may also occur through the skin and gut. It is irritant to the eyes, skin, mucous membranes, and respiratory system accompanied by mucous secretion, a metallic taste, drowsiness, and vertigo. Higher concentrations may cause CNS depression.

Treatment

If acute exposure has occurred, the subject should be removed from further exposure, the skin washed, and the eyes irrigated. CNS effects should be treated symptomatically and supportively. Potentially, *N*-acetylcysteine could be of value in preventing hepatic damage.

Further reading

Pahwa R, Kalra J (1993). A critical review of the neurotoxicity of styrene in humans. *Veterinary and Human Toxicology* **35**, 516–20.

Sulphur dioxide

Sulphur dioxide is a colourless gas which has a pungent irritating odour. The combustion of fuels for heating and power generation results in environmental pollution from this cause. Sulphur dioxide is also employed in the manufacture of sulphuric acid and is a potential occupational problem in paper mills, steel works, and oil refineries.

Mechanism of toxicity

The irritant effects of sulphur dioxide are thought to be caused by the rapidity with which it forms sulphurous acid on contact with moist membranes.

Clinical features

Following exposure to sulphur dioxide, lacrimation, rhinorrhoea, cough, increased bronchial secretions, bronchoconstriction, and in severe cases, pulmonary oedema and respiratory arrest occur. Corneal burns can follow eye exposure and liquified sulphur dioxide can cause skin burns. Survivors of massive sulphur dioxide exposure have shown a chronic obstructive defect in serial pulmonary studies along with bronchial hyperactivity.

Treatment

After removal from exposure, admission to hospital for observation is mandatory in severe cases to ensure that delayed pulmonary oedema is treated effectively. Symptomatic and supportive measures should be given and, if necessary, mechanical ventilation with positive end-expiratory pressure should be undertaken if diuretics alone do not control pulmonary oedema; the role of corticosteroids is uncertain. The eyes and skin should be irrigated with water if exposure has occurred.

Further reading

International Programme on Chemical Safety (1979). *Environmental Health Criteria 8. Sulfur oxides and suspended particulate matter.* World Health Organization, Geneva.

Tetrachloroethylene (perchloroethylene)

Tetrachloroethylene is a colourless, non-flammable liquid with a chloroform-like odour. It is used widely as an industrial solvent, particularly for dry cleaning and degreasing. Poisoning may occur by inhalation or ingestion.

Mechanisms of toxicity

A considerable proportion of an inspired dose is exhaled unchanged and that retained is excreted only slowly (half-life approximately 144 h), mainly by metabolism to trichloroacetic acid, the major urinary metabolite.

Clinical features

Following inhalation or ingestion, there is depression of the central nervous system; nausea and vomiting may occur and persist for several hours. Irritation of the eyes, nose, and throat may occur. Hepatic and renal dysfunction may also develop and ventricular arrhythmias and non-cardiogenic pulmonary oedema have been reported.

Treatment

After removal from exposure, treatment is supportive and symptomatic.

Further reading

Garnier R *et al.* (1996). Coin-operated dry cleaning machines may be responsible for acute tetrachloroethylene poisoning: report of 26 cases including one death. *Journal of Toxicology—Clinical Toxicology* **34**, 191–7.

Theophylline

Poisoning may complicate therapeutic use as well as being the result of deliberate self-poisoning. It is important to establish at an early stage the precise theophylline product involved in a poisoning incident since many of them are sustained-released formulations. As a consequence, peak plasma concentrations of the drug are frequently not attained until 6 to 12 h after overdosage and the onset of toxic features is correspondingly delayed.

Clinical features

Most symptomatic patients have concentrations in excess of 25 mg/l. Convulsions are seen more commonly when concentrations are greater than 50 mg/l.

Symptoms include nausea, vomiting, hyperventilation, haematemesis, abdominal pain, diarrhoea, sinus tachycardia, supraventricular and ventricular arrhythmias, hypotension, restlessness, irritability, headache, hyperreflexia, tremor, and convulsions. Hypokalaemia results predominantly from Na^+/K^+ ATPase activation. A mixed respiratory alkalosis and metabolic acidosis is common.

Assessment of the severity of poisoning

The severity of theophylline intoxication is important in deciding management. Plasma potassium concentrations of less than 2.6 mmol/l, acidaemia, hypotension, seizures, and arrhythmias are indications for urgent measurement of plasma theophylline concentrations. Patients require close observation to detect the onset of delayed toxicity and it may be necessary to repeat measurement of the plasma theophylline concentration a few hours after admission.

Treatment

Gastric lavage may be considered in patients who have ingested a significant overdose of theophylline and who present within 1 h; administration of 50 to 100 g of activated charcoal (by nasogastric tube if necessary) is an alternative. Multiple doses of charcoal (e.g. 50 g 4-hourly) will enhance the systemic elimination of theophylline. Intractable vomiting may be alleviated by ondansetron in a dose of 8 mg intravenously in an adult. Gastrointestinal haemorrhage may require blood transfusion and a proton pump inhibitor should be given intravenously. Tachyarrhythmias may be induced by the rapid flux of potassium across cell membranes and early correction of hypokalaemia may prevent their development. The plasma potassium concentration should therefore be measured on admission and at houry intervals thereafter while the patient is symptomatic. Potassium supplements will be needed in almost all cases and doses of up to 60 mmol/h may be required at the outset. Non-selective β-adrenoceptor blocking drugs, such as propranolol, may also be useful to treat tachyarrhythmias and reverse hypokalaemia. Convulsions should be managed conventionally.

Although charcoal haemoperfusion increases theophylline clearance, it should be reserved for those in whom intractable vomiting or recurrent seizures make oral charcoal impracticable or hazardous.

Further reading

Minton NA, Henry JA (1996). Acute and chronic human toxicity of theophylline. *Human and Experimental Toxicology* **15**, 471–81.

Thyroxine

Acute overdosage with thyroid hormones is uncommon. Not surprisingly, thyroxine is the agent most commonly involved.

Clinical features

Probably only a small percentage of patients who ingest large amounts of thyroid hormones develop features of toxicity. Symptoms develop within a few hours with tri-iodothyronine (T_3) and after 3 to 6 days with thyroxine (T_4). They tend to resolve in about the same time as they take to develop. Mental confusion, agitation, irritability, and hyperactivity with sinus tachycardia, tachypnoea, pyrexia, and dilated pupils are common while atrial fibrillation, sweating, loose stools, and the ocular features of hyperthyroidism are rare. Convulsions developed in one child.

Treatment

Gastric lavage may be considered if more than 2 mg of thyroxine has been ingested within the preceding 1 h; activated charcoal is an alternative. Serum T_4 and T_3 concentrations should be measured in blood taken 6 to 12 h after ingestion since a normal result precludes the possibility of delayed toxicity and allows the patient to be discharged. Those with high T_4 concentrations should be reviewed for evidence of toxicity on the fourth or fifth day after ingestion. Patients who develop toxicity should be given propranolol for 5 days.

Further reading

Hack JB *et al.* (1999). Severe symptoms following massive intentional L-thyroxine ingestion. *Veterinary and Human Toxicology* **41**, 323–6.

Toluene

Toluene has much lower volatility and toxicity than benzene. It is used extensively as a solvent in the chemical, rubber, paint, glue, and pharmaceutical industries and as a thinner for inks, perfumes, and dyes.

Metabolism

Following inhalation or ingestion, toluene is oxidized to benzoic acid then to hippuric acid benzoylglucuronates that are excreted in the urine.

Clinical features

Acute poisoning results in euphoria, excitement, dizziness, confusion, increased lacrimation, headache, nervousness, nausea, tinnitus, ataxia, tremor, and coma.

Chronic exposure

Chronic poisoning may give rise to muscle weakness, abdominal pain and haematemesis, cerebellar abnormalities, optic neuropathy, peripheral neuropathy, altered mental state, dementia, hearing loss, hypokalaemia, and hepatorenal disease, including distal renal tubular acidosis and urinary calculi.

Treatment

If poisoning results from inhalation, whether accidental or intentional as in volatile substance abuse (see below), the patient should be removed from the contaminated environment. Thereafter, treatment consists of symptomatic and supportive measures.

Further reading

Einav S *et al.* (1997). Bradycardia in toluene poisoning. *Journal of Toxicology—Clinical Toxicology* **35**, 295–8.

Hussain TF, Heidrenreich PA, Benowitz N (1996). Recurrent non-Q-wave myocardial infarction associated with toluene abuse. *American Heart Journal* **131**, 615–16.

1,1,1-Trichloroethane (methyl chloroform)

1,1,1-Trichloroethane is a colourless, non-flammable liquid of high volatility widely used as a solvent in industry, in the office (e.g. typewriter correction fluid), and at home (e.g. waterproofing aerosol products).

Mechanism of toxicity

1,1,1-Trichloroethane has low systemic toxicity because only small amounts of trichloroacetic acid and trichloroethanol are formed. Most of an inhaled dose is expired unchanged. Concomitant ingestion of ethanol is known to enhance toxicity.

Clinical features

Following inhalation of a sufficiently large dose, CNS depression occurs in proportion to the amount inhaled; hepatic and renal dysfunction may also result. Deaths have followed exposure to very high concentrations in unventilated tanks. In such cases death may either be due to CNS depression, culminating in respiratory arrest, or to fatal arrhythmias as a result of myocardial sensitization to circulating catecholamines in the presence of hypoxia. Inhalation of a weather-proofing aerosol containing 96.6 per cent 1,1,1-trichloroethane has been reported to give rise to transient shortness of breath, constricting chest pain, cough, and myalgia.

Treatment

The casualty should be removed from the contaminated environment. Thereafter treatment is symptomatic and supportive.

Further reading

House RA *et al.* (1996). Paresthesias and sensory neuropathy due to 1,1,1-trichloroethane. *Journal of Occupational and Environmental Medicine* **38**, 123–4.

Liss GM, House RA (1995). Toxic encephalopathy due to 1,1,1-trichloroethane. *American Journal of Industrial Medicine* **27**, 445–6.

Trichloroethylene

Trichloroethylene is a colourless, volatile liquid used widely as an industrial solvent, particularly in metal degreasing and extraction processes.

Mechanisms of toxicity

Trichloroethylene is absorbed readily from the gut and through the skin and lungs. Following inhalation, it is excreted unchanged in the breath and metabolized via chloral hydrate to trichloroethanol (by alcohol dehydrogenase) and trichloroacetic acid, which are excreted in the urine.

Clinical features

Following inhalation, ingestion, or dermal absorption, CNS depression occurs with nausea and vomiting, hepatic and renal dysfunction, and death. 'Degreaser's flush' (in which the skin on the face and arms becomes markedly reddened) may occur if ethanol is consumed shortly before or after exposure to trichloroethylene, as the metabolism of trichloroethylene is inhibited. Cranial nerve damage, cerebellar dysfunction, and convulsions have been described.

Treatment

Removal from exposure will reduce CNS depression, and thereafter, whether trichloroethylene has been inhaled, ingested, or absorbed through the skin, treatment is supportive and symptomatic.

Further reading

Szlatenyi CS, Wang RY (1996). Encephalopathy and cranial nerve palsies caused by intentional trichloroethylene inhalation. *American Journal of Emergency Medicine* **14**, 464–7.

Yoshida M *et al.* (1996). Concentrations of trichloroethylene and its metabolites in blood and urine after acute poisoning by ingestion. *Human and Experimental Toxicology* **15**, 254–8.

Tricyclic antidepressants

Tricyclic antidepressants have complex actions that account for the diverse nature of the features seen after overdosage. They block the reuptake of noradrenaline into peripheral and intracerebral neurones, thereby increasing the concentration of monoamines in these areas. They also have anticholinergic actions and class 1 antiarrhythmic (quinidine-like) activity.

Clinical features

Features of poisoning typically appear within 30 to 60 min after ingestion of an overdose and usually reach maximum intensity in 4 to 12 h. Drowsiness, sinus tachycardia, dry mouth, dilated pupils, urinary retention, increased reflexes, and extensor plantar responses are the most common features of mild poisoning. Severe intoxication leads to coma, often with divergent strabismus and convulsions. Plantar, oculocephalic ('doll's head'), and vestibulo-ocular reflexes may be temporarily abolished. Skin blisters and rhabdomyolysis may be present.

Sinus tachycardia is very common and the dose-related quinidine-like action decreases myocardial contractility and delays conduction producing a bizarre ECG; P–R and QRS intervals increase and the P waves diminish in amplitude and may be completely obscured by the preceding T wave. These changes, in conjunction with the increased heart rate, not infrequently make differentiation between ventricular tachycardia and supraventricular tachycardia with aberrant conduction difficult, if not impossible. Serious arrhythmias, particularly ventricular tachycardia, occur in only 4 per cent of cases. In severe cases the blood pressure and cardiac output fall; metabolic acidosis and cardiorespiratory depression are the major contributing factors to death.

Treatment

The great majority of patients poisoned with tricyclic antidepressants recover with supportive therapy alone. Potentially lethal complications such as convulsions and arrhythmias are most common within 6 h of overdosage. It is uncommon for coma to last for more than 24 h and most severely poisoned patients recover consciousness within 48 h.

Gastric lavage may be considered in adults when more than 250 mg of the drug has been ingested less than 1 h previously. Alternatively, 50 to 100 g of activated charcoal can be administered orally.

Management of tricyclic antidepressant-induced cardiotoxicity poses serious difficulties. In general, the natural inclination to use antiarrhythmic drugs to treat tachycardia and arrhythmias should be resisted. Attention to supportive measures, particularly adequate oxygenation, control of convulsions, and correction of acidosis will generally be rewarding; 50 mmol of sodium bicarbonate intravenously over 20 min should be given even if there is no acidosis. Lignocaine in a dose of 50 to 100 mg intravenously may be tried cautiously if ventricular tachycardia is compromising cardiac output.

Physostigmine salicylate, a cholinesterase inhibitor, has no role. When benzodiazepines have been taken in overdose together with tricyclic antidepressants, flumazenil may unmask the tricyclic antidepressant-induced seizure potential and should therefore be used with caution.

Forced diuresis and haemodialysis are of no value. Nor is there convincing evidence that charcoal haemoperfusion is effective.

Delirium with auditory and visual hallucinations is a frequent and troublesome complication during the recovery phase. Sedation with oral or intravenous diazepam may be required.

Further reading

Buckley NA *et al.* (1996). Interrater agreement in the measurement of QRS interval in tricyclic antidepressant overdose: implications for monitoring and research. *Annals of Emergency Medicine* **28**, 515–19.

Liebelt EL, Francis PD, Woolf AD (1995). ECG lead aVR versus QRS interval in predicting seizures and arrhythmias in acute tricyclic antidepressant toxicity. *Annals of Emergency Medicine* **26**, 195–201.

Taboulet P *et al.* (1995). Cardiovascular repercussions of seizures during cyclic antidepressant poisoning. *Journal of Toxicology—Clinical Toxicology* **33**, 205–11.

Vinyl chloride (monochloroethylene, chloroethene)

Vinyl chloride is a colourless, highly flammable, and explosive gas. It is usually handled as a liquid under pressure and in this form it polymerizes readily, at temperatures in the range of 40 to 70°C, to form polyvinyl chloride (PVC).

Mechanisms of toxicity

The main route of absorption of vinyl chloride is through the lungs, although some skin penetration does occur. Metabolism to a reactive metabolite appears to be necessary before toxic effects are seen. It has also been postulated that the various features of vinyl chloride disease may have an immunological basis.

Clinical features

Acute exposure

Acute exposure to vinyl chloride results in CNS depression, but concentrations need to be in excess of 10 000 ppm before this effect becomes noticeable. Exposure of volunteers to 20 000 ppm for 5 min caused dizziness, light-headedness, nausea, and dulling of vision.

Chronic exposure

Acro-osteolysis has been described in workers engaged in cleaning autoclaves by hand. The syndrome has three main components: (i) Raynaud's phenomenon, (ii) skin changes resembling scleroderma, and (iii) bony changes of the terminal phalanges of the fingers and sometimes the toes, radial and ulnar styloid processes, sacroiliac joints, and lower poles of patellas.

Angiosarcoma of the liver and hepatic fibrosis, often associated with splenomegaly and portal hypertension, have been reported in vinyl chloride workers.

Exposure to vinyl chloride may also be associated with the development of cancer of the liver and biliary tract and cancer of the brain, though the latter association has not been confirmed in some studies.

Treatment

Preventive measures, adopted worldwide, and designed to protect against angiosarcoma of the liver, should also prevent other adverse effects. Symptoms due to osteo-acrolysis do not improve significantly after removal from exposure, but radiographic improvement of the phalangeal lesions, with recalcification, has been demonstrated.

Further reading
Lewis R (1999). Vinyl chloride and polyvinyl chloride. *Occupational Medicine (Philadelphia)* **14**, 719–42.

Volatile substance abuse

Solvent abuse may be defined as the intentional inhalation of volatile organic chemicals other than conventional anaesthetic gases. These include organic solvents and vapours, hydrocarbon mixtures such as petrol (gasoline), and aerosol propellants.

Volatile substances are either 'bagged' (sprayed into a plastic bag and then inhaled until the subject passes out) or 'huffed' (sprayed on to a cloth held to the mouth). Glue is most often sniffed from a potato crisp bag and repeated abuse in this manner leads to the development of erythematous spots around the mouth and nose ('glue-sniffer's rash').

Clinical features

The clinical features of intoxication with volatile substances are similar to those of alcohol intoxication with initial CNS stimulation followed by depression. Other symptoms may include euphoria, blurring of vision, tinnitus, slurring of speech, ataxia, feelings of omnipotence, headache, abdominal pain, anorexia, nausea, vomiting, jaundice, chest pain, bronchospasm, impaired judgement, irritability, and excitement. Less often a delirious state is seen, with clouding of consciousness and hallucinations. Many chronic users report transient psychotic symptoms that often have an affective component. Convulsions, status epilepticus, and coma may occur. Those under the influence of volatile substances may carry out self-destructive and antisocial acts. Psychological dependence and tolerance may develop, but physical dependence is rare.

Unexplained listlessness, anorexia, and marked moodiness are suggestive of chronic abuse. Poor school adjustment and scholastic performance have been noted in chronic glue sniffers apparently due to lack of motivation.

'Glue sniffing'

Glues are volatile, semiliquid preparations that usually contain an aromatic hydrocarbon as the vehicle. The physical sequelae of prolonged glue sniffing include aplastic anaemia and acute hepatic and renal damage. Features of renal toxicity include proteinuria, haematuria, distal renal tubular acidosis, and recurrent urinary calculi. Irreversible neurological sequelae such as optic atrophy, encephalopathy, cerebellar degeneration, and equilibrium disorders have been reported in adults who are chronic abusers. Toluene inhalation may cause encephalopathy in children. Neurological damage may occur after 'sniffing' of less than 1 year's duration and symptoms may progress for up to 3 months after the habit has been abandoned. Glues containing *n*-hexane and toluene have been associated with the development of muscle weakness and atrophy and sensory impairment of either the 'glove and stocking' or sensorimotor type, with or without muscle atrophy.

A review of adults who had sniffed toluene indicated three major patterns of presentation: (i) muscle weakness, (ii) gastrointestinal complaints (abdominal pain, haematemesis), and (iii) neuropsychiatric disorders (altered mental status, cerebellar abnormalities, and peripheral neuropathy). In addition, hypokalaemia, hypophosphataemia, and hyperchloraemia were common. Rhabdomyolysis occurred in 40 per cent of cases. Cardiac and haematological toxicity due to toluene appears to be uncommon.

Petrol (gasoline) sniffing

Abusers of petrol have reported that 15 to 20 breaths of the vapour are sufficient to produce intoxication for 3 to 6 h.

The euphoria of mild intoxication may be accompanied by nausea and vomiting. After prolonged inhalation, or rapid inhalation of highly concentrated vapour, the 'sniffer' may experience a phase of violent excitement followed by loss of consciousness and coma. While unconscious, the subject may suffer convulsions and the pupils may become fixed and dilated or unequal. Nystagmus and conjugate deviation of the eyes may be observed. Cerebral and pulmonary oedema and renal and hepatic damage have been noted at autopsy. The greater danger from petrol 'sniffing' is related to the long-term effects of chronic exposure that include loss of appetite and loss of weight, neurasthenia, muscle weakness and cramps, and neuropsychological damage. Encephalopathy in petrol sniffers may also be due to tetraethyl lead.

Chlorinated hydrocarbon abuse

Inhalation of chlorinated hydrocarbons causes a sense of euphoria, and sometimes excitement, associated with headache, dizziness, nausea, vomiting, stupor, coma, and convulsions.

Aerosol inhalation

The most commonly abused aerosol propellants are the chlorofluorocarbons (CFCs). Several hundred teenagers have died from this cause. It is likely that the fatalities were due to cardiac arrhythmias.

Diagnosis and treatment

The clinical features described above and the circumstances in which patients are found usually point to the diagnosis, but confirmation may be obtained by detection of solvents in blood or metabolites in the urine.

Acute intoxication from volatile substance abuse is usually brief and self-limiting. If respiratory depression and cardiac arrhythmias supervene, they should be treated conventionally and renal and hepatic failure may require further supportive measures and dialysis.

Further reading
Brady WJ *et al.* (1994). Freon inhalation abuse presenting with ventricular fibrillation. *American Journal of Emergency Medicine* **12**, 533–6.
Cox MJ *et al.* (1996). Severe burn injury from recreational gasoline use. *American Journal of Emergency Medicine* **14**, 39–43.
Martinez JS *et al.* (1989). Renal tubular acidosis with an elevated anion gap in a 'glue sniffer'. *Human Toxicology* **8**, 139–40.
Steffee CH, Davis GJ, Nicol KK (1996). A whiff of death: fatal volatile solvent inhalation abuse. *Southern Medical Journal* **89**, 879–84.
Tenenbein M (1997). Leaded gasoline abuse: the role of tetraethyl lead. *Human and Experimental Toxicology* **16**, 217–22.

Warfarin

Warfarin toxicity is more likely to occur in the setting of therapeutic anticoagulation (as a result of a drug interaction) than as a consequence of acute overdose.

Clinical features

Epistaxis, gingival bleeding, spontaneous bruising, haematomas, haematuria, bilateral flank pain, rectal bleeding, and haemorrhage into any organ may occur. Spontaneous haemoperitoneum has been reported. Severe blood loss may result in hypovolaemic shock, coma, and death.

Treatment

If the intention is to continue anticoagulation

If the INR is less than 6.0 but more than 0.5 units above the target value, reduce the dose or stop warfarin; restart when the INR is less than 5.0. If the INR is 6.0 to 8.0 and the patient is not bleeding (or only minor bleeding is present), stop warfarin and restart when the INR is less than 5.0. If the INR is greater than 8.0 and the patient is not bleeding (or the bleeding is minor), stop warfarin and restart when the INR is less than 5.0. If there are other risk factors for bleeding, give 0.5 mg of vitamin K_1 intravenously slowly. If major bleeding occurs, give 5 mg of vitamin K_1 by slow intravenous injection together with prothrombin complex concentrate at 50 units/kg or, if the complex is not available, give fresh frozen plasma at 15 ml/kg.

If continued anticoagulation is unnecessary

If the INR is greater than 6.0, give 5 mg of vitamin K_1 and repeat if necessary. If active bleeding occurs, give prothrombin complex concentrate at 50 units/kg in addition or, if the complex is not available, give fresh frozen plasma at 15 ml/kg.

Further reading

Baglin T (1998). Management of warfarin (coumarin) overdose. *Blood Reviews* **12**, 91–8.

Xylenes

The three isomers of xylene, which possess similar properties, are used widely as solvents in paints, lacquers, pesticides, gums, resins, adhesives, and the paper-coating industry.

Metabolism

Xylene is oxidized and excreted in the urine either free or conjugated with glycine as methylhippuric acid. Ethanol inhibits xylene metabolism.

Clinical features

Following inhalation, dizziness, excitement, flushing of the face, eye irritation, drowsiness, incoordination, ataxia, tremor, confusion, coma, respiratory depression, and catecholamine-induced ventricular arrhythmias may occur. Hepatorenal damage also has been described. Immersion in liquid xylene may result in a burning feeling, erythema, and some scaling of the skin.

Treatment

Treatment is supportive.

Further reading

Ansari EA (1997). Ocular injury with xylene—a report of two cases. *Human and Experimental Toxicology* **16**, 273–5.

Hageman G *et al.* (1999). Parkinsonism, pyramidal signs, polyneuropathy, and cognitive decline after long-term occupational solvent exposure. *Journal of Neurology* **246**, 198–206.

Zinc

Zinc oxide fumes are emitted in any process involving molten zinc and are the most common cause of metal fume fever. Exposure to zinc chloride occurs in soldering, in the manufacture of dyes, paper, and deodorants, and on military exercises when it is used as a smoke screen.

Poisoning has followed the accidental or deliberate ingestion of elemental zinc and zinc chloride and fatal intoxication has followed inadvertent intravenous administration. Inhalation of zinc chloride and oxide may lead to nasopharyngeal and respiratory toxicity.

Zinc may be absorbed through broken skin when zinc oxide paste is used to treat wounds and burns.

Clinical features

Acute poisoning

Zinc sulphate ingestion causes gastrointestinal irritation, sometimes in association with headache and dizziness. Zinc chloride is highly corrosive and ingestion has led to erosive pharyngitis, oesophagitis, and haematemesis. Acute renal failure and pancreatitis have also been recorded after ingestion of zinc salts. Topical exposure to zinc chloride causes ulceration and dermatitis of the exposed skin. Zinc chloride is highly irritant to the eye.

Metal fume fever starts up to 24 h after exposure to zinc oxide fumes. It presents as an influenza-like illness with headache, fever, sweating, chest tightness and discomfort, and joint pains. Typically symptoms appear after the weekend. The illness usually has an excellent prognosis and the symptoms often improve towards the end of the working week as some short-term immunity from further symptoms develops.

In contrast to the relatively mild clinical course after zinc oxide inhalation, exposure to zinc chloride ammunition bombs (hexite) produces a chemical pneumonitis with marked dyspnoea, a productive cough, fever, chest pain, and cyanosis. The adult respiratory distress syndrome may ensue in the most severe cases; fatalities have been reported.

Chronic poisoning

Repeated topical exposure to zinc oxide may cause a papular folliculitis. Chronic excessive ingestion of zinc supplements (zinc sulphate) may induce reversible anaemia and leucopenia secondary to a relative copper deficiency.

Treatment

Symptomatic and supportive measures should be employed with treatment as for acids as appropriate (see above).

Further reading

Barceloux DG (1999). Zinc. *Journal of Toxicology—Clinical Toxicology* **37**, 279–92

Hantson P, Lievens M, Mahieu P (1996). Accidental ingestion of a zinc and copper sulfate preparation. *Journal of Toxicology—Clinical Toxicology* **34**, 725–30.

Hjortso E *et al.* (1988). ARDS after accidental inhalation of zinc chloride smoke. *Intensive Care Medicine* **14**, 17–24.

8.2 Injuries, envenoming, poisoning, and allergic reactions caused by animals

D. A. Warrell

Mechanical injuries caused by animals

Lions, tigers, leopards, jaguars, hyenas, wolves, dingoes, bears, elephants, hippopotamuses, buffaloes, rhinoceroses, musk oxen, wild pigs, and ostriches have mauled and killed humans. About 100 shark attacks are reported each year between latitudes 46 °N and 47 °S, half of which are fatal (Plate 1). Other fish capable of causing life-threatening mechanical trauma are barracuda, moray and conger eels, garfish, groupers, stingrays, and pirañas. Tiny Amazonian catfish (genus *Vandelia*; Spanish—'canero'; Portuguese—'candirú') are the only vertebrate parasites of humans. Attracted by urine, these 5-cm long fish may enter the urethra, vulva, or anus of swimmers causing pain, bleeding, and obstruction. Their spines make them difficult to remove. The 'electric eel' (*Electrophorus electricus*) of South American rivers can discharge up to 650 volts, 1 amp, 400 times per second, a shock capable of killing an adult. Marine torpedo rays can produce a dangerous 80-volt, high-amperage shock. Crocodiles (*Crocodilus niloticus*) kill about 1000 people each year in Africa, while in northern Australia 27 deaths from 60 attacks by the salt-water crocodile (*C. porosus*) have been reported since 1876. Giant pythons have attacked, killed, and even swallowed people in Indonesia (*Python reticulatus*) (Plate 2), Africa (*P. sebae*), and South America (*Eunectes murinus*). Collisions between vehicles and deer cause more than a 100 injuries each year in Kentucky and are also common in other areas. In the United States, injuries to horseback riders result in more than 46 000 visits to casualty departments each year and at least 20 deaths.

Bites by domestic dogs are common. An estimated 6 million dogs live in England and Wales. More than 200 000 patients bitten by dogs attend hospital each year. About 600 000 people are bitten by dogs each year in the United States. Other domestic animals which have caused severe injuries or deaths include camels, cattle, water buffalo, sheep, pigs, cats, and ferrets.

Treatment

First aid of severe injuries involves controlling bleeding, closing perforating injuries with pressure dressings, and rapid evacuation to hospital. All injuries inflicted by animals must be assumed to be infected by a range of organisms. Wounds may contain teeth and other foreign bodies and necrotic tissue, especially if treatment is delayed.

Wounds should be thoroughly cleaned with soap and water as soon as possible; suitable antiseptics include iodine and alcohol solutions. Prophylactic antimicrobials such as amoxicillin/clavulanic acid, doxycycline, or erythromycin have proved effective in dog- and cat-bite wounds and are indicated for multiple or severe wounds and bites on the face and hands.

Specific infections, such as tetanus, rabies, and herpes simiae virus must be considered and treated/prevented appropriately. Emergency surgery may be required, with: replacement of blood loss; attention to local mechanical complications such as fractures, tension pneumothorax, damage to large blood vessels, perforation of the bowel, and lacerations of other abdominal viscera; and thorough débridement or amputation of dead tissue with removal of foreign material, teeth, etc.; irrigation and drainage. Except for wounds on the head and neck, which can be sutured immediately, primary suturing should be delayed for 48 to 72 h, after which further débridement, suturing, or covering with split skin grafts should be considered. In these cases infection must be prevented by using a combination of penicillin, an aminoglycoside (such as gentamicin for 48 h), and metronidazole.

Venomous animals

For predation or defence, some animals inject venoms through fangs, chelicerae (venom jaws), stings, spines, hairs, nematocysts, and other specialized venom organs. 'Spitting' snakes, scorpions, and millipedes squirt venom on to absorbent mucous membranes. The flesh or skin of some animals contain poisons acquired through the food chain. Allergic reactions to injected venoms (for example, of *Hymenoptera* and cnidarians) and ingested poisons (for example, ciguatera) may create medical problems more commonly than their direct toxic effects.

Venomous mammals

Male duck-billed platypuses (*Ornithorhynchus anatinus*) have erectile venomous spurs on their hind limbs. These aquatic, egg-laying mammals of eastern Australia sting at least one person each year in Victoria, but only 17 cases have been reported since 1817. There is immediate, agonizing, persistent local pain, as well as prolonged local swelling, chronic pain on movement, hyperaesthesia, wasting, inflammation, and regional lymphadenopathy. These effects are not life-threatening in humans, but dogs have died of envenoming. In the absence of specific treatment, non-steroidal anti-inflammatory agents or corticosteroids have proved effective. The venom contains a C-type natriuretic peptide (which causes mast-cell degranulation), nerve growth factor, four defensin-like peptides, enzymes, and other peptides and proteins. Males of the echidna, the other egg-laying mammal, possess a similar but smaller venom apparatus. Several species of Insectivora produce venomous saliva conducted into bite wounds by curved and sometimes grooved lower incisors. Venomous species include the Hispaniolan and Cuban solenodons (*Solenodon paradoxus, S. (Apotogale) cubanus*), northern water shrew (*Neomys fodiens*), southern water shrew (*N. anomalus*), and the North American short-tailed shrew (*Blarina brevicauda*). Their bites can kill rodents and lagomorphs, but in humans the effect is local pain, swelling, and inflammation. The saliva of vampire bats (Desmodontinae) contains permeability increasing factors, a platelet inhibitor, draculin—an inhibitor of activated factors X and IX, and a plasminogen activator which is being developed as a thrombolytic drug.

Venomous snakes

Fewer than 200 species of venomous snake (families Colubridae, Atractaspididae, Elapidae, and Viperidae) have been responsible for severely envenoming humans resulting in death or permanent disability. Since it may be difficult to distinguish venomous from non-venomous species, unnecessary contact with snakes should be avoided and patients bitten by any species should be assessed carefully.

Distribution of venomous snakes

Free from venomous snakes are the Antarctic, most islands of the western Mediterranean, Atlantic, Caribbean, and Eastern Pacific (including Hawaii), Madagascar, New Caledonia, New Zealand, Ireland, Iceland, and the Atlantic Ocean, and Chile. Elsewhere, venomous snakes are widely distributed up to altitudes of more than 4000 m in the Himalayas (*Gloydius himalayanus*), within the Arctic Circle (*Vipera berus*), in the Indian and Pacific Oceans as far north as Siberia (*Pelamis platurus*), and in some freshwater lakes (*Hydrophis semperi*).

Classification

Medically important species have in their upper jaws one or more pairs of enlarged teeth (fangs) that inject venom into their victims through a groove or closed channel.

Colubridae

The short, immobile fangs are at the back of the maxilla (Fig. 1). Most familiar non-venomous snakes, such as the British grass snake and smooth snake, belong to this large family. However, some species have caused severe envenoming or death, including: three African species—the boomslang (*Dispholidus typus*) and the vine, twig, bird, or tree snake or Voëlslang (*Thelotornis kirtlandii* and *T. capensis*); the Japanese yamakagashi (*Rhabdophis tigrinus*); the Southeast Asian red-necked keelback (*R. subminiatus*); the Australasian brown tree snake (*Boiga irregularis*) introduced to Guam; and the South American green racer (*Philodryas olfersii*) (Fig. 1).

Atractaspididae

The African and Middle Eastern burrowing asps, stiletto snakes, burrowing or mole vipers or adders, strike sideways, impaling their victims on a long front fang protruding through the partially closed mouth (Fig. 2). Several species, including *Atractaspis microlepidota*, *A. engaddensis*, and *A. irregularis* have killed humans.

Elapidae

This family includes cobras (Fig. 3), kraits, mambas, shield-nose snakes, coral snakes, garter snakes, venomous Australasian snakes (Fig. 4), and sea snakes (Fig. 5). The short, front fangs are immobile (Figs 3(a) and 5). Several African and Asian species (rinkhals and spitting cobras) can eject their

Fig. 2 Burrowing asp (*Atractaspis engaddensis*) showing side-stabbing action with one of the long fangs (arrow) (in this case through a membrane). (Photograph by courtesy of Dr I. Golani and Professor E. Kochva, Tel Aviv.)

(a)

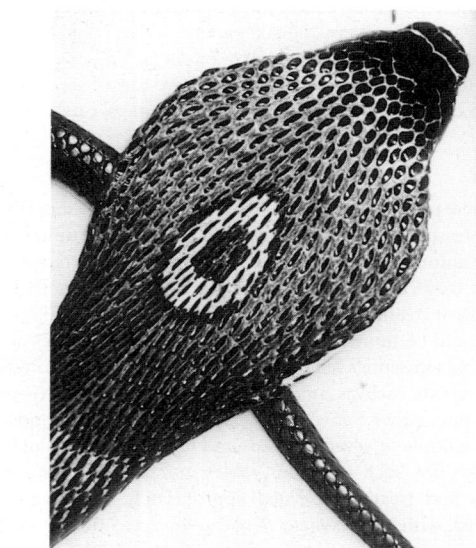

(b)

Fig. 3 Cobras. (a) Short front fang of the Sri Lankan cobra (*Naja naja*) a typical elapid snake. (b) Hood of monocellate Thai cobra (*Naja kaouthia*). (Copyright D.A. Warrell.)

Fig. 1 Back fangs of the green racer (*Philodryas olfersii*), a South American colubrid snake. A case of fatal envenoming has been reported from Brazil. (Copyright D.A. Warrell.)

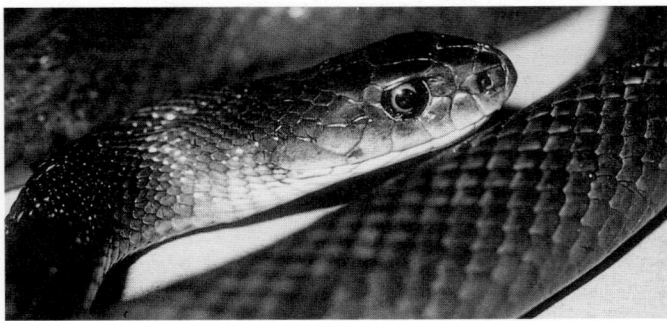

Fig. 4 Papua New Guinean taipan (*Oxyuranus scutellatus canni*), an Australasian elapid snake. (Copyright D.A. Warrell.)

venom from the tips of the fangs as a fine spray for a distance of a few metres into the eyes of an enemy.

Viperidae

The front fangs are long, curved, and capable of a wide range of movement (Fig. 6). The subfamily Crotalinae comprises the American rattlesnakes (Fig. 7), moccasins, lance-headed vipers, and Asian pit vipers which possess

Fig. 5 Short front fangs of the laticaudine sea snake (sea krait) *Laticauda colubrina*. (Copyright DA Warrell.)

a heat-sensitive pit organ behind the nostril (Plate 3). The Old World vipers and adders (subfamily *Viperinae*) have no pit organ.

Incidence and importance of snake bites

Snake bite is an important medical emergency in some parts of the rural tropics; its incidence is usually underestimated because most victims seek the help of traditional healers rather than practitioners of western-style medicine. In a rural population in Kenya, snake bites cause 6.7 deaths per 100 000 per year, 0.7 per cent of all deaths; it was found that 68 per cent of bitten people had sought treatment from traditional healers. In Africa, the saw-scaled or carpet viper (*Echis* spp.), puff adder (*Bitis arietans*), and spitting cobra (*Naja nigricollis, N. mossambica,* etc.) are the species of greatest medical importance. In the Benue Valley of NE Nigeria, *E. ocellatus* (Fig. 8) causes some 500 bites per 100 000 population per year, with a 12 per cent mortality. Vipers of the genus *Echis*, whose geographical range extends through the northern third of Africa, the Middle East, and Eastern Asia to India, are responsible for many bites and deaths. In India, the most important species are cobras (*Naja naja, N. oxiana, N. kaouthia*) (Fig. 3), common krait (*Bungarus caeruleus*), Russell's viper (*Daboia russelii*) (Fig. 6), and *E. carinatus*. An annual snake-bite mortality of 30 000 has been suggested. In Burdwan District, West Bengal, 8000 people are bitten and 800 die each year. In Southeast Asia, the Malayan pit viper (*Calloselasma rhodostoma*), *D. russelii*, green pit vipers (e.g. *Trimeresurus albolabris*) (Plate 3), and cobras (*N. kaouthia* and *N. siamensis*) cause most bites and deaths. In Burma, Russell's viper bite is the leading cause of acute renal failure and is responsible for most of the estimated 1000 snake-bite deaths each year. In Central and South America, medically important species include rattlesnakes (e.g. *C. durissus terrificus*) (Fig. 7) and the lance-headed vipers, *Bothrops atrox* ('barba amarilla' or 'fer de lance'), *B. asper* ('terciopelo'), and *B. jararaca* ('jararaca'). In the United States, 1370 bites were reported to Poisons Centers during 1995, but with only one death. Deaths are caused by rattlesnakes, especially eastern and western diamond-backs (*C. adamanteus* and *C. atrox*). In the Amami and Ryukyu islands of Japan, the habu (*T. flavoviridis*) inflicted an average of 610 bites with 5.6 deaths per year during the 1960s. In Britain, the adder or viper (*Vipera berus*) is the only venomous species (Fig. 9). More than 200 people are bitten each year but only 14 deaths have been reported since 1876, the last in 1975. In Sweden, this species causes between 150 and 200 hospital admissions each year: 44 deaths occurred between 1911 and 1978; and in Finland, 21 deaths in 25 years with an annual incidence of almost 200 bites. *V. aspis* causes most bites in France, while *V. ammodytes* is important in eastern Europe.

Australia harbours the deadliest snakes in the world, judging by the lethal potency of their venoms. However, only 3 or 4 people die each year from a snake bite. The most important species are the eastern brown snake

Fig. 6 Russell's vipers. (a) Thai Russell's viper (*Daboia russelii siamensis*), a typical viperine snake (scale in cm). (b) Long, hinged front fangs (reserve fang on the left side) in dental sheath. (Copyright D.A. Warrell.)

Fig. 7 South American tropical rattlesnake or cascabel (*Crotalus durissus cascavella*). (Copyright D.A. Warrell.)

Fig. 8 Saw-scaled or carpet viper from West Africa (*Echis ocellatus*). (Copyright D.A. Warrell.)

Fig. 9 European adder or viper (*Vipera berus*), Britain's only venomous snake. This specimen is 50 cm long. (Copyright D.A. Warrell.)

(*Pseudonaja textilis*), tiger snake (*Notechis scutatus*), taipan (*Oxyuranus scutellatus*) (Fig. 4), and death adder (*Acanthophis* spp.). The highest snake-bite mortalities, up to 24 per cent of all adult deaths, are recorded among the hunter–gatherer tribes of Brazil (Kashinawa), Venezuela (Yanomamo), Ecuador (Waorani), Tanzania (Hadza), and Papua New Guinea.

Epidemiology

Most snake bites are inflicted on the lower limbs of farmers, plantation workers, herdsmen, and hunters in rural areas. The snake is usually trodden on at night or in undergrowth. Some species such as the Asiatic kraits (*Bungarus* spp.) and African spitting cobras (*N. nigricollis*) enter human dwellings at night and may bite people who roll over on to them while sleeping on the floor. Snakes do not bite without provocation, but may strike if inadvertently trodden upon or touched. In Europe, North America, and Australia, snakes are increasingly popular 'macho' pets: in these countries many bites are inflicted on the hands of males who are picking up the snake. In the United States, 25 per cent of bites result from snakes being attacked or handled. Serious bites by back-fanged (colubrid) snakes usually occur only under these conditions. Seasonal peaks in the incidence of snake bite are associated with agricultural activities, such as ploughing before the annual rains in the West African Sahel and the rice harvest in Southeast Asia, or to fluctuations in the activity or population of venomous snakes. Severe flooding, by concentrating the human and snake populations, has given rise to epidemics of snake bite in Colombia, Pakistan, India, Bangladesh, Nepal, Burma, and Vietnam. Invasion of virgin jungle during construction of new highways and irrigation and hydroelectric schemes has led to an increased incidence of snake bite in Brazil and Sri Lanka. Snake bite or injection of snake venom has long been used for murder and suicide. Snake venoms or purified toxins have been used therapeutically.

Venom apparatus

The venom glands of Elapidae and Viperidae are situated behind the eye, surrounded by compressor muscles (Fig. 10). A venom duct opens within the sheath at the base of the fang and venom is conducted to its tip through a canal. In Colubridae, venom secreted by Duvernoy's gland tracks down grooves in the anterior surfaces of fangs at the posterior end of the maxilla (Fig. 1). The average dry weight of venom injected at a strike is approximately 60 mg in *N. naja*, 13 mg in *E. carinatus*, 63 mg in *D. russelii*, and 32 mg in *V. palaestinae*. The amount injected when a snake bites humans is very variable. A proportion of bites are 'dry bites', associated with negligible envenoming: more than 50 per cent of those bitten by Malayan pit vipers (*C. rhodostoma*) or Russell's vipers; less than 10 per cent bitten by *Echis* spp.; but more than 75 per cent bitten by common brown snakes in Australia (*Pseudonaja textilis*). The Palestine viper (*V. palaestinae*) expends only about one-tenth of the capacity of its venom gland at each consecutive strike, whereas *D. russelii* exhausts more than three-quarters of its supply at the first strike. There is no support for the popular belief that snakes are less dangerous after they have eaten.

Venom properties

Snake venoms may contain 20 or more components. More than 90 per cent of the dry weight of venom is protein, in the form of enzymes, non-enzymatic polypeptide toxins, and non-toxic proteins such as nerve growth factor. Between 80 and 90 per cent of viperid and 25 to 70 per cent of elapid venom consists of enzymes, including digestive hydrolases, hyaluronidase, and activators or inactivators of physiological processes. Most venoms contain L-amino acid oxidase, phosphomono- and diesterases, 5′-nucleotidase, DNAase, NAD-nucleosidase, phospholipase A_2, and peptidases. Elapid venoms, in addition, contain acetylcholine esterase, phospholipase B, and glycerophosphatase, while viperid venoms have endopeptidase, arginine ester hydrolase, kininogenase, as well as thrombin-like, factor X, and pro-thrombin-activating enzymes. Phospholipase A_2 (lecithinase) is the most widespread and extensively studied of all venom enzymes. It damages mitochondria, red blood cells, leucocytes, platelets, peripheral nerve endings, skeletal muscle, vascular endothelium, and other membranes, produces presynaptic neurotoxic activity, opiate-like sedative effects, and the autopharmacological release of histamine. The acetylcholinesterase found in most elapid venoms does not contribute to their neurotoxicity. Hyaluronidase promotes the spread of venom through tissues. Proteolytic enzymes (endopeptidases or hydrolases) are responsible for local changes in vascular permeability leading to oedema, blistering, and bruising, and to necrosis. L-amino acid oxidase, which gives yellow snake venoms their colour, is a digestive enzyme.

Polypeptide toxins (neurotoxins)

Postsynaptic (α) neurotoxins such as α-bungarotoxin and cobrotoxin, contain about 60 to 62 or 66 to 74 amino acids. They bind to acetylcholine receptors at the motor endplate. Presynaptic (β) neurotoxins such as β-bungarotoxin, crotoxin, and taipoxin, contain about 120 to 140 amino-acid residues and a phospholipase A subunit. These release acetylcholine at

the nerve endings at neuromuscular junctions and then damage the endings, preventing further release of transmitter.

Pharmacology

The neurotoxins of the Elapidae are rapidly absorbed into the bloodstream, whereas the much larger molecules of Viperidae venoms are taken up more slowly through the lymphatics. Venoms of the spitting cobras and rinkhals can be absorbed through the intact cornea, causing systemic envenoming and even death in animals. Envenoming after ingestion of snake venom has not been reported in humans. Most venoms are concentrated and bound in the kidney and some components are eliminated in the urine. Crotaline venoms are selectively bound in the lungs, concentrated in the liver, and excreted in bile, while polypeptide neurotoxins, such as α-bungarotoxin, are tightly bound at neuromuscular junctions. Most venom components do not cross the blood–brain barrier.

Pathophysiology

Swelling and bruising of the bitten limb result from increased vascular permeability induced by proteases, phospholipases, membrane-damaging polypeptide toxins, and endogenous autacoids released by the venom, such as histamine, 5-hydroxytryptamine, and kinins. Venoms of some of the North American rattlesnakes and viperine species cause a generalized increase in vascular permeability resulting in hypovolaemia, haemoconcentration, hypoalbuminaemia, albuminuria, serous effusions, pulmonary oedema, and, in the case of Burmese *D. russelii*, conjunctival and facial oedema (Fig. 11). Tissue necrosis near the site of the bite is caused by myotoxic and cytolytic factors: in some cases, ischaemia resulting from thrombosis, intracompartmental syndrome, or a tight tourniquet may contribute. Causes of hypotension and shock include hypovolaemia, vasodilatation, and myocardial dysfunction. Some venoms release vasodilating autacoids such as histamine and kinins. Venom of the Brazilian jararaca (*B. jararaca*) was found to activate bradykinin and, through a bradykinin-potentiating peptide, to prolong its hypotensive effect by inactivating the peptidyl dipeptidase responsible both for destroying bradykinin and for converting angiotensin I to angiotensin II. This observation led to the synthesis of angiotensin-converting enzyme (**ACE**) inhibitors. Bradykinin-potentiating and ACE-inhibiting peptides have also been found in a number of other crotaline venoms (genera *Bothrops* and *Agkistrodon*). To date, four sarafotoxins have been isolated from the venom of the Israeli burrowing asp (*Atractaspis engaddensis*) (Fig. 2). They show 60 per cent sequence homology with the endothelins, which are also 21-amino acid polypeptides. Sarafotoxins and endothelins are potent vasoconstrictors (including coronary arteries), delay atrioventricular conduction, and are positively inotropic.

Fig. 10 Venom apparatus of viperine and crotaline snakes. (a) Venom gland of Palestine viper (*Vipera palaestinae*). (b) Venom gland of Western rattlesnake (*Crotalus viridis*). C, compressor glandulae muscle; VG, venom gland; AG, accessory gland; F, fang. (Dissection by Professor E. Kochva, reproduced from Gans, C. and Gans, K.A. (eds), 1978, *Biology of the reptilia*, vol 8. Academic Press, London, by permission.)

Fig. 11 Gross bilateral conjunctival oedema (chemosis) in a Burmese rice farmer 48 h after being bitten by a Russell's viper. (Copyright D.A. Warrell.)

Fig. 12 Haemorrhagin activity. An erythrocyte (E) spurting through an open endothelial junction (J) between endothelial cells (En) from the lumen (L) of a rat mesenteric blood vessel, 5 min after exposure to habu (*Trimeresurus flavoviridis*) venom. Note extensive destruction of the basement membrane (Bm), and failure of the platelet (P) to undergo viscous metamorphosis. (By courtesy of Dr A. Ohsaka and Academic Press, reproduced from Ohsaka A, Suzuki K, Ohashi M (1975). *Microvascular Research* **10**, 208).

Snake venoms can cause haemostatic defects in a number of different ways: venom procoagulant enzymes, many of them serine proteases, activate the blood clotting cascade at various sites. Some Viperidae venoms contain thrombin-like fibrinogenases which remove fibrinopeptides from fibrinogen directly. Others activate endogenous plasminogen. Venoms may induce or inhibit platelet aggregation. Spontaneous systemic bleeding is caused by haemorrhagins, metalloendopeptidases, some with disintegrin-like and other domains, which damage vascular endothelium (Fig. 12). The combination of consumption coagulopathy, thrombocytopenia, and vessel wall damage can result in massively incontinent bleeding, a common cause of death after bites by Viperidae, Australasian Elapidae, and the few medically important Colubridae. Many venoms are haemolytic *in vitro*, but clinically significant intravascular haemolysis, apart from the microangiopathic haemolysis associated with disseminated intravascular coagulation, is seen only after bites by *D. russelii* (Sri Lanka and India), and some *Bothrops* and colubrid species. Acute renal tubular necrosis may be caused by severe hypotension, disseminated intravascular coagulation (*D. russelii*), a direct nephrotoxic effect of the venom (*D. russelii*), and myoglobinuria secondary to generalized rhabdomyolysis (sea snakes, *D. russelii* in Sri Lanka and India, and tropical rattlesnakes). Neurotoxic polypeptides and phospholipases block neuromuscular transmission causing death through bulbar or respiratory paralysis.

Clinical features

Fear and treatment effects as well as the venom contribute to the symptoms and signs of snake bite. Even patients who are not envenomed may feel flushed, dizzy, and breathless and may notice constriction of the chest, palpitations, sweating, and acroparaesthesiae. Tight tourniquets may produce congested and ischaemic limbs; local incisions at the site of the bite may cause bleeding, and sensory loss and herbal medicines often induce vomiting. The earliest symptoms directly attributable to the bite are local pain and bleeding from the fang punctures, followed by pain, tenderness, swelling and bruising extending up the limb, lymphangitis, and tender enlargement of regional lymph nodes. Early syncope, vomiting, colic, diarrhoea, angio-oedema, and wheezing may follow bites by some snakes (e.g. European Vipera, *D. russelii*, *Bothrops* spp., Australian elapids, and *Atractaspis engaddensis*). Nausea and vomiting is a common early symptom of systemic envenoming.

Bites by Colubridae (back-fanged snakes)

Severe envenoming causes repeated vomiting, colicky abdominal pain, headache, widespread systemic bleeding with extensive ecchymoses, incoagulable blood, intravascular haemolysis, and renal failure. Local swelling and bruising may be the only results of envenoming. The first symptoms of envenoming may be delayed for 24 to 72 h after the bite.

Bites by Atractaspididae (burrowing asps or stiletto snakes)

Local effects are pain, swelling, blistering, necrosis, and tender enlargement of local lymph nodes. Violent gastrointestinal symptoms (nausea, vomiting, and diarrhoea), anaphylaxis (dyspnoea, respiratory failure), and electrocardiogram (**ECG**) changes (atrioventricular block, ST, T-wave changes) have been described in patients envenomed by *A. engaddensis*.

Bites by Elapidae (cobras, kraits, mambas, African garter snakes, coral snakes, and Australasian snakes)

Bites by kraits, mambas, coral snakes, and some cobras (e.g. *N. haje*, *N. nivea* and *N. philippinensis*) produce minimal local effects, but the venoms of African spitting cobras (*N. nigricollis*, *N. mossambica*, etc.) and Asian cobras (*N. naja*, *N. kaouthia*, *N. sumatrana*, etc.) cause tender local swelling, blistering, and superficial necrosis which may be extensive (Fig. 13). 'Skip' lesions, separated by apparently normal areas of skin, are a typical finding (Fig. 14). However, elapid venoms are best known for their neurotoxic effects. Early symptoms, before there are objective neurological signs, include vomiting, 'heaviness' of the eyelids, blurred vision, paraesthesias around the mouth, hyperacusis, headache, dizziness, vertigo, hypersalivation, congested conjunctivas, and 'gooseflesh'. Paralysis is first detectable as ptosis and external ophthalmoplegia appearing as early as 15 min after the bite, but sometimes it is delayed for 10 h or even more than 24 h following death-adder (Acanthophis) bites. Later the face, palate, jaws, tongue, vocal cords, neck muscles, and muscles of deglutition may become paralysed (Fig. 15). The pupils are dilated. Respiratory failure may be precipitated by airway obstruction at this stage, or later after paralysis of intercostal muscles and the diaphragm. Neurotoxic effects are completely reversible, either acutely in response to antivenom or anticholinesterases (for example, following bites by Asian cobras, some Latin American coral snakes—*Micrurus* spp., and Australasian death adders—Acanthophis) or they may wear off spontaneously in 1 to 7 days.

Envenoming by terrestrial Australasian elapids produces four main groups of symptoms: neurotoxicity (Fig. 16), haemostatic disturbances and, rarely, generalized rhabdomyolysis and renal failure. Painful regional lymph nodes are a useful sign of impending systemic envenoming, but local

Fig. 13 Extensive necrosis of skin and subcutaneous tissues in a Nigerian girl bitten 9 days previously on the elbow by a black-necked or spitting cobra (*Naja nigricollis*). (Copyright D.A. Warrell.)

Fig. 14 Sierra Leonian woman showing 'skip lesion' separated by an area of unaffected skin after envenoming by a black-necked spitting cobra. (Copyright D.A. Warrell.)

signs are usually mild, except after bites by the king brown or Mulga snake (*Pseudechis australis*). Early symptoms include vomiting, headache and syncopal attacks.

Patients 'spat' at by spitting elapids may develop venom ophthalmia. There is intense pain in the eye, blepharospasm, palpebral oedema, and leucorrhoea (Fig. 17(a)). Corneal erosions can be seen by slit-lamp or fluorescein examination in more than half of patients spat at by *N. nigricollis*. Rarely, venom is absorbed into the anterior chamber causing hypopyon and anterior uveitis. Secondary infection of corneal abrasions may lead to permanent blinding opacities or panophthalmitis (Fig. 17(b)).

Bites by sea snakes and sea kraits
Patients envenomed by sea snakes notice headache, a thick feeling of the tongue, thirst, sweating, and vomiting. Between 30 min and 3.5 h after the

Fig. 15 Neurotoxic envenoming. Ptosis, ophthalmoplegia, and inability to open the mouth and protrude the tongue in a Sri Lankan patient envenomed by the common krait (*Bungarus caeruleus*). (Copyright D.A. Warrell.)

Fig. 16 Generalized paralysis, including ptosis, external ophthalmoplegia, inability to open the mouth, protrude the tongue, swallow or speak, and respiratory paralysis requiring mechanical ventilation in a Papua New Guinean man bitten 24 h previously by a taipan (*Oxyuranus scutellatus canni*). (Copyright D.A. Warrell.)

bite there is generalized aching, stiffness, and tenderness of the muscles. Trismus is common. Later there is generalized flaccid paralysis. Myoglobinuria appears 3 to 8 h after the bite. Myoglobin and potassium released from damaged skeletal muscles can cause renal failure, while hyperkalaemia may precipitate cardiac arrest.

Bites by Viperidae (vipers, adders, rattlesnakes, lance-headed vipers, moccasins, and pit vipers)
Viper venoms usually produce more severe local effects than do those of other snakes. Swelling may become detectable within 15 min but is sometimes delayed for several hours. It spreads rapidly, sometimes involving the whole limb and adjacent trunk. There is associated pain and tenderness in regional lymph nodes, with bruising of overlying tissues and lymphangitic lines. Bruising, blistering, and necrosis may appear during the next few days (Fig. 18). Necrosis can be severe following bites by some rattlesnakes, lance-headed vipers (genus *Bothrops*), Asian pit vipers, and the large African *Bitis* species (puff adder, Gabon, and rhinoceros-horned vipers, etc.). When the envenomed tissue is contained in a tight fascial compartment such as the pulp space of digits or the anterior tibial compartment, ischaemia may result (Fig. 19). Absence of swelling 2 h after a viper bite suggests that there has been no envenoming. However, fatal envenoming by a few species can occur in the absence of local signs (for example, *C. d. terrificus*, *C. scutulatus*, and Burmese Russell's viper). Haemostatic abnormalities are characteristic of envenoming by Viperidae. Persistent bleeding from fang puncture wounds, venepuncture or injection sites, other new and partially healed wounds, and postpartum, indicates that the blood is incoagulable. Spontaneous systemic haemorrhage is most often detected in the gingival sulci (Plate 4). Epistaxis, haematemesis, cutaneous ecchymoses, haemoptysis, and subconjunctival, retroperitoneal, and intracranial haemorrhages (Fig. 20) are also reported. Patients envenomed by Burmese Russell's vipers may suffer haemorrhagic infarction of the anterior pituitary (Sheehan's syndrome) (Fig. 21). Hypotension and shock are common in patients bitten by North American rattlesnakes (e.g. *C. adamanteus*, *C. atrox*, and *C. scutulatus*), *Bothrops*, *Daboia*, and *Vipera* species (e.g. *V. palaestinae* and *V. berus*). The central venous pressure is usually low and the pulse rate rapid, suggesting hypovolaemia resulting from extravasation of fluid into the bitten limb. Patients envenomed by Burmese Russell's vipers and children

envenomed by *Vipera berus* show evidence of generally increased vascular permeability. Direct myocardial involvement is suggested by an abnormal ECG or cardiac arrhythmia. Patients envenomed by some species of the genera *Vipera* and *Bothrops* and Australasian elapids may experience early transient and recurrent syncopal attacks associated with features of an autopharmacological or anaphylactic reaction, such as vomiting, sweating, colic, diarrhoea, shock, and angio-oedema. These symptoms may appear as early as 5 min or as late as many hours after the bite. Early collapse after bites by Australian brown snakes (genus *Pseudonaja*) and tiger snakes (genus *Notechis*) has been attributed to coronary and pulmonary thromboembolism. Renal failure is a common mode of death in patients envenomed by Viperidae. Victims of Russell's viper may become oliguric within a few hours of the bite and complain of loin pain suggesting renal ischaemia. Neurotoxicity, resembling that seen in patients bitten by Elapidae, is a feature of envenoming by a few species of Viperidae (e.g. *C. d. terrificus,* berg adder—*Bitis atropos* and other small *Bitis* species, and the Sri Lankan *D. russelii*). There is evidence of generalized rhabdomyolysis (Fig. 22), but progression to respiratory or generalized paralysis is unusual.

Fig. 18 Severe blistering in a Thai boy bitten on the leg by a Malayan pit viper (*Calloselasma rhodostoma*). (Copyright D.A. Warrell.)

Envenoming by European vipers

The common viper or adder (*V. berus*) (Fig. 9), the only venomous snake found in Britain, occurs in England, Wales, Scotland, and northern Europe, extending into the Arctic Circle and through Asia as far east as Sakhalin Island and south to northern Korea. There are four other vipers that are widely distributed in mainland Europe: the nose-horned or sand viper (*V. ammodytes*) in the Balkans, Italy, Austria, and Romania; the asp viper (*V. aspis*) in France (south of Paris), Spain, Germany, Switzerland, and Italy; Lataste's viper (*V. latasti*) in Spain and Portugal, and Orsini's viper (*V. ursinii*) in south-eastern France, central Italy, and Eastern Europe. The Montpellier snake (*Malpolon monspessulanus*) is a large back-fanged colubrid snake whose bite can cause transient mild symptoms.

Clinical features of European viper bite Pain usually develops quickly at the site of the bite and local swelling is evident within a few minutes, but is sometimes delayed for 30 min or longer. Local blisters containing blood are uncommon. Swelling and bruising may advance to involve the whole limb within 24 h, extend on to the trunk, and in children become generalized. A few cases of intracompartmental syndromes and necrosis have been described. Pain, tenderness, and enlargement of local lymph nodes is sometimes noticeable within hours. Marked lymphangitis and bruising of the affected limb appears within a day or two. Dramatic, early systemic symptoms may appear within 5 min of the bite or be delayed for many hours. They include retching, vomiting, abdominal colic, diarrhoea, incontinence of urine and faeces, sweating, vasoconstriction, tachycardia, shock, and

(a)

(b)

Fig. 17 Venom ophthalmia caused by the black-necked spitting cobra (*Naja nigricollis*). (a) Acute venom ophthalmia showing intense painful inflammation and discharge. (b) In this case, the corneal injury was neglected and so secondary infection developed, necessitating enucleation of the eye. (Copyright D.A. Warrell.)

Fig. 19 Extensive necrosis of skin and muscle including the contents of the anterior tibial compartment in a patient bitten by a common lancehead (*Bothrops atrox*) in Brazil. (Copyright D.A. Warrell.)

Fig. 20 CT scan showing intracranial haemorrhage in a child bitten by a common lancehead (*Bothrops atrox*) in Ecuador. The fluid level in the larger collection of blood indicates that the blood was incoagulable. (Copyright Hospital Vozandes Quito.)

Fig. 22 Brazilian girl bitten 24 h previously by a tropical rattlesnake (*Crotalus durissus terrificus*). She has bilateral ptosis, paralysis of the facial muscles, and gross myoglobinuria resulting from generalized rhabdomyolysis. (Copyright D.A. Warrell.)

angio-oedema of the face, lips, gums, tongue, throat, as well as epiglottis, urticaria, and bronchospasm. These symptoms may persist for as long as 48 h. Hypotension is the most important sign. It usually develops within 2 h, and may be transient (resolving spontaneously within 2 h), or persistent, recurrent, or progressive, and fatal. ECG changes include flattening or inversion of T waves, ST elevation, second-degree heart block, and cardiac brady- and tachyarrhythmias, atrial fibrillation, and myocardial infarction. Defibrinogenation (incoagulable blood) or milder degrees of coagulopathy and spontaneous bleeding into the gastrointestinal tract, lungs (Fig. 23), or urinary tract are uncommon. Other clinical features include fever, drowsi-

ness, and, rarely, coma and seizures secondary to hypotension or cerebral oedema, respiratory distress/pulmonary oedema (in children), acute renal failure, cardiac arrest, intrauterine death, acute gastric dilatation, and paralytic ileus. Laboratory findings include a neutrophil leucocytosis (more than 20 000/μl in severe cases), thrombocytopenia, initial haemoconcentration and later anaemia resulting from extravasation into the bitten limb, and, rarely, haemolysis, elevation of serum creatine kinase, and metabolic acidosis. Deaths usually occur between 6 and 60 (average 34) h after the bite. Most adder bites cause only trivial symptoms, but patients must be assessed individually. Children may be severely envenomed: in a French series there were three deaths in a group of seven children aged between 2½

Fig. 21 Haemorrhagic infarction of the anterior pituitary in a Burmese patient who died after being bitten by a Russell's viper (*Daboia russelii siamensis*). (By courtesy of Dr U Hla Mon, Yangon, Myanmar.)

Fig. 23 Chest radiograph of a 9-year-old girl, 3 days after being bitten by *Vipera berus*, showing interstitial pulmonary bleeding. (By courtesy of Dr R. Pugh, Hull, and *The Practitioner*.)

and 10 years. The dangers of adder bite should not be underestimated. The antivenom treatment of adder bite is discussed below.

Laboratory investigations

The peripheral neutrophil count is raised to 20 000 cells/μl or more in severely envenomed patients. Initial haemoconcentration, resulting from extravasation of plasma (*Crotalus* species and Burmese *D. russelii*), is followed by anaemia caused by bleeding or, more rarely, haemolysis. Thrombocytopenia is common following bites by pit vipers (e.g. *C. rhodostoma, Crotalus viridis helleri*) and some Viperidae (e.g. *Bitis arietans* and *D. russelii*), but is unusual after bites by *Echis* species. A useful test for venom-induced defibrinogenation is the 20-min whole-blood clotting test. A few millilitres of venous blood is placed in a new, clean, dry, glass test tube, left undisturbed for 20 min, and then tipped once to see if it has clotted or not. Incoagulable blood indicates systemic envenoming (consumption coagulopathy or anticoagulant) and may be diagnostic of a particular species (for example, *Echis* species in the northern third of Africa). Patients with generalized rhabdomyolysis show a steep rise in serum creatine kinase, myoglobin, and potassium levels. Black or brown urine suggests generalized rhabdomyolysis or intravascular haemolysis. Concentrations of serum enzymes, such as creatine kinase and aspartate aminotransferase, are moderately raised in patients with severe local envenoming, probably because of local muscle damage at the site of the bite. High concentrations suggest generalized rhabdomyolysis. Urine should be examined for blood/haemoglobin, myoglobin and protein, and for microscopic haematuria and red cell casts. Electrocardiographic abnormalities such as sinus bradycardia, ST–T changes, various degrees of atrioventricular block, and hyperkalaemic changes may be seen.

Immunodiagnosis

Specific snake venom antigens have been detected in wound swabs, aspirates or biopsies, serum, urine, cerebrospinal fluid, and other body fluids. Of the various techniques for their detection, radioimmunoassay is probably the most sensitive and specific, but enzyme immunoassay (**EIA**) has been the most widely used. Under ideal conditions, relatively high venom antigen concentrations (wound swabs or aspirates) may be detected quickly enough (15–30 min) to allow the selection of the appropriate monospecific antivenom. A commercial test kit for Australian elapids is produced by CSL, Melbourne. For retrospective diagnosis, including forensic cases, tissue around the fang punctures, wound and blister aspirate, serum, and urine should be stored for EIA immunodiagnosis.

Management of snake bite

First aid

The patient should be reassured and moved to the nearest hospital or dispensary as quickly, as comfortably and passively as possible. The bitten limb should be immobilized with a splint or sling and all unnecessary movement discouraged.

Most traditional first aid methods are potentially harmful and should not be used. Local incisions and suction do not remove venom effectively and may introduce infection, damage tissues, and cause persistent bleeding. Vacuum extractors, potassium permanganate, and ice packs may potentiate local necrosis. Electric shocks may act as counterirritants but are dangerous and have not been proved beneficial. Tourniquets and compression bands are potentially dangerous as they can cause gangrene (Fig. 24), increased fibrinolysis, and bleeding in the occluded limb, peripheral nerve palsies, compartmental ischaemia, and intensification of local signs of envenoming.

The pressure immobilization method developed by the late Struan Sutherland and his colleagues in Australia involves bandaging the entire bitten limb as tightly as for a sprained ankle, using a long crêpe bandage, starting at the toes or fingers, and incorporating a splint (Fig. 25). In animals, this method exerted a pressure of about 55 mmHg and was effective in prevent-

Fig. 24 Gangrene of forearm in a Thai patient who applied a tight tourniquet above the elbow for several hours after being bitten by a Malayan pit viper. (Copyright D.A. Warrell.)

ing the systemic uptake of Australian elapid and some other venoms. Anecdotal experience supports the use of the method. Several reported patients have deteriorated after release of the pressure bandage. Prospective clinical studies are needed to assess the risks and benefits of this interesting technique. In the meantime, it is recommended for the first-aid of bites by Australasian elapids, sea snakes, and other elapid snakes whose venoms can have a rapid neurotoxic effect (e.g. kraits, coral snakes, and some cobras). The method is not recommended for bites by snakes whose venoms cause massive local swelling and necrosis as these effects may be accentuated by the bandage, which will increase pressure in fascial compartments, risking ischaemic necrosis.

Pursuing and killing the snake is not recommended, but if the snake has been killed it should be taken with the patient to hospital, but it must not be handled as even a severed head can inject venom.

Patients being transported to hospital should lie on their left side to prevent aspiration of vomit. Persistent vomiting can be treated with chlorpromazine by intravenous injection (25–50 mg for adults, 1 mg/kg for

Fig. 25 Sutherland's pressure immobilization method for envenoming by neurotoxic species, such as Australasian elapids. (By courtesy of Australian Venom Research Unit, University of Melbourne.)

children). Syncope, shock, angio-oedema, and other autonomic symptoms can be treated with 0.1 per cent adrenaline (epinephrine) by subcutaneous injection (0.5 ml for adults, 0.01 ml/kg for children) and an antihistamine such as chlorphenamine (chlorpheniramine) maleate by intravenous injection (10 mg for adults, 0.2 mg/kg for children). Patients with incoagulable blood will develop haematomas after intramuscular and subcutaneous injections, and so the intravenous route should be used whenever possible. Respiratory distress and cyanosis should be treated by clearing the airway, giving oxygen, and, if necessary, assisted ventilation. If the patient is unconscious and no femoral or carotid pulses can be detected, cardiopulmonary resuscitation must be started immediately.

Hospital treatment

Clinical assessment

In most cases of snake bite there are uncertainties about the species and the quantity and composition of venom injected, which can be resolved only by admitting the patient for at least 24 hours of observation. Local swelling is usually detectable within 15 min of pit viper envenoming and within 2 h of envenoming by most other vipers, but may not develop in patients bitten by some neurotoxic species such as kraits, coral snakes, and sea snakes. Fang marks are sometimes invisible. Tender enlargement of regional lymph nodes draining the bitten area is an early sign of envenoming by Viperidae, some Elapidae, and Australasian elapids. All the tooth sockets should be examined meticulously as this is usually the first site of spontaneous bleeding (Plate 4): other common sites are the nose, conjunctivas, skin, and gastrointestinal tract. Persistent bleeding from venepuncture sites and other wounds implies incoagulable blood. Hypotension and shock are important signs of hypovolaemia or cardiotoxicity, seen particularly in patients bitten by North American rattlesnakes and some Viperinae (e.g. *V. berus*, *D. russelii*, *V. palaestinae*). Ptosis is the earliest sign of neurotoxic envenoming (Fig. 15). Respiratory muscle power should be assessed objectively and repeatedly, for example by measuring vital capacity. Trismus and generalized muscle tenderness suggest rhabdomyolysis (sea snakes). If a procoagulant venom is suspected, the coagulability of whole blood should be checked at the bedside using the 20-min, whole-blood clotting test.

Antivenom treatment

The most important decision is whether or not to give antivenom, the only specific treatment for envenoming. There is now abundant evidence that in patients with severe envenoming the benefits of this treatment far outweigh the risks of antivenom reactions (see below). Antivenom has reduced the mortality of systemic envenoming by *Echis ocellatus* in Nigeria from 20 to 3 per cent and by *C. d. terrificus* in Brazil from 74 to 12 per cent. Antivenoms are effective in reversing hypotension caused by *V. berus* envenoming and coagulopathies caused by *Bothrops* species, *D. russelii*, *C. rhodostoma*, *T. albolabris*, and *Oxyuranus scutellatus*. Antivenom, also known as antivenin, antivenene, and antisnakebite serum, is the partially purified immunoglobulin (whole IgG, F(ab′)$_2$, or Fab fragments) of horses or sheep which have been immunized with venom.

General indications for antivenom

Antivenom is indicated if there are signs of systemic envenoming such as:

(1) haemostatic abnormalities, for example spontaneous systemic bleeding, incoagulable blood, or thrombocytopenia;

(2) neurotoxicity;

(3) hypotension and shock, abnormal ECG, or other evidence of cardiovascular dysfunction;

(4) generalized rhabdomyolysis.

Supporting evidence of severe envenoming is a neutrophil leucocytosis, elevated serum enzymes such as creatine kinase and aminotransferases,

haemoconcentration, severe anaemia, myoglobinuria, haemoglobinuria, methaemoglobinuria, hypoxaemia, and acidosis.

In the absence of systemic envenoming, local swelling involving more than half the bitten limb, extensive blistering or bruising, bites on digits, and rapid progression of swelling are indications for antivenom, especially in patients bitten by species whose venoms are known to cause local necrosis (e.g. Viperidae, Asian cobras, and African spitting cobras).

Special indications for antivenom

Some developed countries can afford a wider range of indications.

United States and Canada

After bites by the most dangerous rattlesnakes (*C. atrox, C. adamanteus, C. viridis, C. horridus*, and *C. scutulatus*) antivenom therapy should be given early, even before systemic envenoming has become obvious. Rapid spread of a local swelling is considered an indication for antivenom, as is immediate pain or any other symptom or sign of envenoming after bites by coral snakes (*Micruroides euryxanthus, Micrurus fulvius*, and *M. tener*).

Australia

Antivenom should be given to any patient with proved or suspected snake bite if there are tender regional lymph nodes or any other evidence of systemic spread of venom, and in anyone effectively bitten by an identified highly venomous species.

Europe

(Adder—*Vipera berus*—and other European Vipera). Zagreb antivenom, or Protherics ViperaTAb (Table 1), is indicated to prevent morbidity and reduce the length of convalescence in patients with moderately severe envenoming, as well as to save the lives of severely envenomed patients. Indications are:

(1) a fall in blood pressure (systolic to <80 mmHg, or by more than 50 mmHg from the normal or admission value) with or without signs of shock;

(2) other signs of systemic envenoming (see above) including spontaneous bleeding, coagulopathy, pulmonary oedema or haemorrhage (shown by chest radiograph), ECG abnormalities, and a definite peripheral leucocytosis (more than 15 000/µl) and elevated serum creatine kinase;

(3) severe local envenoming—swelling of more than half the bitten limb developing within 48 h of the bite—even in the absence of systemic envenoming;

(4) in adults, swelling extending within 4 h beyond the wrist after bites on the hand or beyond the ankle after bites on the foot within 4 h of the bite.

Patients bitten by European Vipera who show any evidence of envenoming should be admitted to hospital for observation for at least 24 h. Antivenom should be given whenever there is evidence of systemic envenoming ((1) or (2) above), even if its appearance is delayed for several days after the bite.

Prediction of antivenom reactions

Skin and conjunctival tests do not predict early (anaphylactic) or late (serum sickness type) antivenom reactions and should not be used.

Contraindications to antivenom

Atopic patients and those who have reacted previously to equine antiserum are at increased risk of developing severe antivenom reactions. In such cases, antivenom should be given only if there is severe envenoming. Reactions may be prevented or ameliorated by pretreatment with subcutaneous adrenaline (epinephrine), antihistamine, and hydrocortisone, or a continuous intravenous infusion of 1:1 000 000 adrenaline while antivenom is being given. However, this prophylaxis is not safe enough to be recommended for routine use. Rapid desensitization is not recommended.

Selection and administration of antivenom

Antivenom should be given only if its stated range of specificity includes the species responsible for the bite. Opaque solutions should be discarded, as precipitation of protein indicates loss of activity and an increased risk of reactions. Expiry dates quoted on ampoules are often very conservative for commercial reasons. Liquid and lyophilized antivenoms stored below 8 °C usually retain most of their activity for 5 years or more. Monospecific (monovalent) antivenom is ideal if the biting species is known. Polyspecific (polyvalent) antivenoms are used in many countries because of the difficulty in identifying the species responsible for bites. Polyspecific antivenoms may be effective but a higher dose is required because they contain less of the specific neutralizing antibody per unit of immunoglobulin than monospecific antivenoms. Antivenoms may exhibit a range of paraspecific neutralizing activity. For example, the South African Institute for Medical Research's 'polyvalent antivenom', which is raised against the venoms of 10 species, has paraspecific activity against a further five species.

It is almost never too late to give antivenom while signs of systemic envenoming persist, but, ideally, it should be given as soon as it is indicated.

Antivenom has proved effective up to 2 days after sea snake bites and, in patients still defibrinated, weeks after bites by Viperidae. In contrast, local envenoming is probably not reversible unless antivenom is given within a few hours of the bite. The intravenous route is the most effective. An infusion of antivenom diluted in approximately 5 ml of isotonic fluid/kg body weight is easier to control than an intravenous 'push' injection of undiluted antivenom given at the rate of about 4 ml/min, but there is no difference in the incidence or severity of antivenom reactions in patients treated by these two methods.

Dose of antivenom

Manufacturers' recommendations are based on mouse protection tests and may be very misleading. Few clinical trials have been performed to establish appropriate starting doses, and in most countries antivenom is used empirically. Many hospitals in the rural tropics give a standard dose of 1 to 2 ampoules to every patient who claims to have been bitten, irrespective of clinical severity. This practice squanders scarce, expensive antivenom and exposes non-envenomed patients to the risk of reactions. Some suggested initial doses are given in Table 1. *Children must be given the same dose as adults.*

Table 1 Guide to initial dosage of some important antivenoms

Species		Manufacturer, antivenom	Approximate
Latin name	English name		initial dose
Acanthophis spp.	Death adder	CSL,* monospecific	3000–6000 units
Bitis arietans	Puff adder	Aventis-Pasteur Fav Afrique and Favi Rept; SAIMR;[+] polyspecific	80 ml
Bothrops jararaca	Jararaca	Brazilian manufacturers, Bothrops polyspecific	20 ml
Bungarus caeruleus	Common krait	Indian manufacturers, polyspecific	100 ml
Calloselasma (Agkistrodon) rhodostoma	Malayan pit viper	Thai Red Cross, Bangkok, monospecific Thai Government Pharmaceutical Organization, monospecific	100 ml 50 ml
Crotalus adamanteus	Eastern diamondback rattlesnakes	Protherics 'CroFab'	7–15 vials
C. atrox	Western diamondback rattlesnakes	Protherics 'CroFab'	7–15 vials
C. viridis subspp.	Western rattlesnakes	Protherics 'CroFab'	7–15 vials
Daboia (Vipera)	Russell's vipers	Myanmar Pharmaceutical Industry, monospecific	40 ml
russelii		Indian manufacturers, polyspecific Thai manufacturers, monospecific	100 ml 50 ml
Echis spp.	Saw-scaled or carpet vipers	SAIMR[+], Echis, monospecific; Aventis-Pasteur 'Fav Afrique'	20 ml
Elapidae (Hydrophiinae)	Sea snakes	*CSL, sea snake/tiger snake	1000 units
Naja kaouthia	Monocellate Thai cobra	Thai Red Cross, monospecific	100 ml
N. naja	Indian cobra	Indian manufacturers, polyspecific	100 ml
Notechis scutatus	Tiger snake	CSL*, monospecific	3000–6000 units
Pseudechis textilis	Eastern brown snake	CSL*, monospecific	3000–6000 units
Oxyuranus scutellatus	Taipan	CSL*, monospecific	12 000 units
Trimeresurus albolabris	Green pit viper	Thai Red Cross, monospecific	100 ml
Vipera berus	European adder	Immunoloski Zavod-Zagreb Vipera, polyspecific Protherics Fab. monospecific 'Vipera TAb'	10 ml 100–200 mg
V. palaestinae	Palestine viper	Rogoff Medical Research Institute, Tel Aviv, Palestine, viper-monospecific	50–80 ml

* Commonwealth Serum Laboratories, Australia.

[+] South African Institute for Medical Research.

Response to antivenom

Often, there is marked symptomatic improvement soon after antivenom has been injected. In shocked patients, the blood pressure may rise and consciousness return (*C. rhodostoma*, *V. berus*, *Bitis arietans*). Neurotoxic signs may improve within 30 min (*Acanthophis* spp, *N. kaouthia*), but the response usually take several hours. Spontaneous systemic bleeding usually stops within 15 to 30 min and blood coagulability is restored within 6 h of antivenom treatment, provided a neutralizing dose has been given. More antivenom should be given if severe signs of envenoming persist after 1 to 2 h, or if blood coagulability is not restored within about 6 h. Systemic envenoming may recur hours or days after an initially good response to antivenom. This is explained by the continuing absorption of venom from the injection site after clearance of antivenom from the bloodstream. The apparent serum half-lives of antivenoms in envenomed patients range from 26 to 95 h. Envenomed patients should therefore be assessed daily for at least 3 or 4 days.

Antivenom reactions

Early (anaphylactic) reactions

These develop within 10 to 180 min of starting antivenom in between 3 and 84 per cent of patients. The incidence increases with dose and decreases when more highly refined antivenom is used, and when administration is by intramuscular rather than intravenous injection. The symptoms are itching, urticaria, cough, nausea, vomiting, other autonomic manifestations, fever, and tachycardia. Up to 40 per cent of patients with early reactions develop systemic anaphylaxis: hypotension, bronchospasm, and angio-oedema. Deaths are rare, but individual cases, such as the asthmatic boy who died from anaphylactic shock after receiving Pasteur antivenom in England in 1957, have been widely publicized and have led to an unreasonable rejection of antivenom treatment. Early antivenom reactions are unlikely to be type-I, IgE-mediated hypersensitivity reactions to equine serum protein. They result from complement activation by immune complexes or aggregates of IgG.

Pyrogenic reactions

Pyrogenic reactions result from contamination of the antivenom with endotoxin-like compounds. Fever, rigors, vasodilatation, and a fall in blood pressure develop 1 to 2 h after treatment. In children, febrile convulsions may be precipitated.

Late reactions

Late reactions of serum sickness type may develop between 5 and 24 (mean 7) days after antivenom therapy. The incidence of these reactions and the speed of their development increases with the dose of antivenom. Clinical features include fever, itching, urticaria, arthralgia (sometimes involving the temporomandibular joint), lymphadenopathy, periarticular swellings, mononeuritis multiplex, albuminuria, and, rarely, encephalopathy. This is a classical immune complex disease.

Treatment of antivenom reactions

Adrenaline (epinephrine) is the effective treatment for early reactions; 0.5 to 1.0 ml of 0.1 per cent (1 in 1000, 1 mg/ml) is given by intramuscular injection to adults (children 0.01 ml/kg) at the first signs of a reaction. The dose may be repeated if the reaction is not controlled. Patients with profound hypotension, severe bronchospasm, or laryngeal oedema may be given adrenaline by slow intravenous injection (0.5 mg diluted in 20 ml of isotonic saline over 10–15 min). A histamine anti-H$_1$ blocker, such as chlorphenamine (chlorpheniramine) maleate (10 mg for adults; 0.2 mg/kg for children) should be given by intravenous injection to combat the effects of histamine release during the reaction. Pyrogenic reactions are treated by cooling the patient and giving antipyretics. Late reactions respond to an oral antihistamine such as chlorphenamine (2 mg every 6 hours for adults; 0.25 mg/kg per day in divided doses for children) or to oral prednisolone (5 mg every 6 hours for 5 to 7 days for adults; 0.7 mg/kg per day in divided doses for children).

Supportive treatment

Neurotoxic envenoming

Bulbar and respiratory paralysis may lead to death from aspiration, airway obstruction, or respiratory failure. A clear airway must be maintained and, if respiratory distress develops, a cuffed endotracheal tube should be inserted or a tracheostomy performed. Provided they are adequately ventilated, patients with neurotoxic envenoming remain fully conscious with intact sensation. Patients have been effectively ventilated manually (by Ambu bag or anaesthetic bag), as in the 1952 poliomyelitis epidemic in Copenhagen, for 30 days and have recovered after 10 weeks of mechanical ventilation. Although artificial ventilation was first suggested for neurotoxic envenoming more than 100 years ago, patients continue to die because they are denied this simple procedure. Anticholinesterases have a variable but potentially useful effect in patients with neurotoxic envenoming, especially when postsynaptic neurotoxins are involved. The 'Tensilon test' should be performed in all cases of severe neurotoxic envenoming, as with suspected myasthenia gravis. Atropine sulphate (0.6 mg for adults; 50 μg/kg for children) or glycopyrronium is given by intravenous injection followed by an intravenous injection of edrophonium chloride (10 mg for adults; 0.25 mg/kg for children). Patients who respond convincingly can be maintained on neostigmine methyl sulphate (50–100 μg/kg) and atropine, every 4 hours by continuous infusion.

Hypotension and shock

If the central venous pressure is low or there is other clinical evidence of hypovolaemia, a plasma expander, preferably fresh whole blood or fresh-frozen plasma, should be infused. If there is evidence of increased capillary permeability (e.g. facial and conjunctival oedema, serous effusions, haemoconcentration, hypoalbuminaemia, etc.) it may be safer in the long term to rely on a selective vasoconstrictor such as dopamine (starting dose 2.5–5 μg/kg per min by intravenous infusion). Delayed hypotension developing about one week after bites by Burmese *D. russelii* may respond to intravenous hydrocortisone.

Oliguria and renal failure

Urine output, serum creatinine, urea, and electrolytes should be measured each day in patients with severe envenoming and in those bitten by species known to cause renal failure (e.g. *D. russelii*, *C.d. terrificus*, *Bothrops* spp., sea snakes). If urine output drops below 400 ml in 24 h, urethral and central venous catheters should be inserted. If urine flow fails to increase after cautious rehydration, diuretics should be tried (e.g. furosemide (frusemide)) by slow intravenous injection, 100 mg followed by 200 mg, and then mannitol. Dopamine (2.5 μg/kg per min by intravenous infusion) has proved effective in some patients bitten by Russell's vipers. If these measures are ineffective, the patient should be placed on strict fluid balance. Peritoneal or haemodialysis will usually be required. In Rangoon, the mortality of established renal failure following *D. russelii* envenoming has been reduced to less than 30 per cent by using peritoneal dialysis, usually for only 72 h.

Local infection at the site of the bite

Bites by some species (e.g. *Bothrops* spp., *C. rhodostoma*) are likely to be complicated by local infections caused by bacteria in the snake's venom or on its fangs. This should be prevented with penicillin, chloramphenicol, or erythromycin and a booster dose of tetanus toxoid, especially if the wound has been incised or tampered with in any way. An aminoglycoside such as gentamicin should be given for 48 h if there is evidence of local necrosis.

Management of local envenoming

Bullae are best left intact. The bitten limb should not be elevated as this increases the risk of intracompartmental ischaemia. Once definite signs of necrosis have appeared (blackened anaesthetic area with putrid odour or signs of sloughing), surgical debridement, immediate split-skin grafting, and broad-spectrum antibiotic cover are indicated.

Intracompartmental syndrome and fasciotomy

Increased pressure within tight fascial compartments such as the digital pulp spaces and anterior tibial compartment may cause ischaemia. This complication is most likely after bites by North American rattlesnakes, *Calloselasma rhodostoma*, *Trimeresurus flavoviridis*, *Bothrops* spp., and *Bitis arietans*. The signs are excessive pain, weakness of the compartmental muscles and pain when they are passively stretched, hypoaesthesia of skin supplied by nerves running through the compartment, and obvious tenseness of the compartment. Detection of arterial pulses by palpation or Doppler does not exclude intracompartmental ischaemia. Intracompartmental pressures exceeding 45 mmHg carry a high risk of ischaemic necrosis. In these circumstances, fasciotomy may be justified, but it did not prove effective in saving envenomed muscle in experimental animals. Fasciotomy is contraindicated until blood coagulability has been restored. Early adequate antivenom treatment will prevent the development of intracompartmental syndromes in most cases. Necrosis of digits is especially common.

Haemostatic disturbances

Once specific antivenom has been given to neutralize venom procoagulants, restoration of coagulability and platelet function may be accelerated by giving fresh whole blood, fresh-frozen plasma, cryoprecipitates (containing fibrinogen, factor VIII, fibronectin, and some factors V and XIII) or platelet concentrates. Heparin has been used to treat a variety of snake bites, usually with disastrous results. Heparin did not prove beneficial in patients envenomed by *Echis ocellatus*.

Other drugs

Corticosteroids, antifibrinolytic agents (aprotinin–Trasylol and ε-aminocaproic acid), antihistamines, trypsin, and a variety of traditional herbal remedies have all been used, but none has proved effective and many are potentially harmful.

Treatment of snake venom ophthalmia

When cobra venom is 'spat' into the eyes, first aid consists of irrigation with generous volumes of water or any other bland liquid which is available. Unless a corneal abrasion can be excluded by fluorescein staining or slit-lamp examination, treatment should be the same as for any corneal injury: a topical antimicrobial such as tetracycline or chloramphenicol should be applied. Instillation of antivenom is not recommended. A 0.1 per cent adrenaline eyedrop preparation relieves the pain.

Interval between bite and death

Exceptionally, patients may die 'within a few minutes' (reputedly after a bite by the king cobra, *Ophiophagus hannah*) or as long as 41 days (*E. carinatus*) after snake bite. However, most deaths occur about 8 h after cobra bites (*N. naja*), 18 h after krait bites (*Bungarus caeruleus*), 16 h after North American rattlesnake bites (*Crotalus* spp.), 3 days after *D. russelii* bites, and 5 days after *Echis* bites.

Prevention of snake bite

To reduce the risk of bites, snakes should never be disturbed, attacked, cornered, or handled, even if they are thought to be a harmless species or appear to be dead. Venomous species should never be kept as pets or as performing animals. In snake-infested areas, boots, socks, and long trousers should be worn for walks in undergrowth or deep sand, and a light should always be carried at night. Collecting firewood, dislodging logs and boulders with bare hands, pushing sticks or digits into burrows, holes, and crevices, climbing rocks and trees covered with dense foliage, and swimming in overgrown lakes and rivers are particularly hazardous activities. Unlit paths and gutters are especially dangerous after heavy rains. To prevent sea-snake bites, fishermen should not touch these animals when they are caught in nets or on lines, swimmers and divers should not aggravate them and should avoid wading in the sea, especially in muddy estuaries, in

sand, or near coral reefs. It is futile and ecologically undesirable to attempt to exterminate venomous snakes. Various substances toxic to snakes, such as insecticides and methylbromide, have been used to keep human dwellings free of these animals. However, no effective but harmless snake repellent has been discovered.

Immunization against envenoming

The idea of inducing protective levels of antibodies against lethal venom components in high-risk populations by pre-exposure immunization has been tried, with inconclusive results, in Japan (*T. flavoviridis*) and considered in Burma (*D. russelii*). To be effective, high titres of a neutralizing antibody would have to be present at the time of the bite. The accelerated secondary response stimulated by envenoming would be too late to be useful.

Venomous lizards

Of the lizards, two species—the gila monster (*Heloderma suspectum*) and Mexican beaded lizard (*H. horridum*), up to 60 to 80 cm long—are venomous (Plate 5). They occur in the south-western United States, western Mexico, and Central America as far south as Guatemala. Venom from mandibular glands is conducted along grooved lower teeth. It contains lethal gila and horridum glycoprotein toxins, phospholipase A$_2$, and several fascinating bioactive peptides: helospectins I and II and helodermin (vasoactive intestinal peptide analogues) and extendins-3 and -4 (glucagon-like peptide-1 analogues). Humans are rarely bitten. The lizard clings on with a bulldog-like grip and may leave radiolucent teeth in the wound. There is immediate severe local pain and regional lymphadenopathy. Systemic symptoms include weakness, dizziness, hypotension, syncope, sweating, rigors, tinnitus, nausea, vomiting, leucocytosis, and ECG changes. There are no reliable reports of fatalities, but a patient envenomed by *H. suspectum* developed refractory hypotension resulting in myocardial infarction and renal failure and associated with coagulopathy. Specific antivenom is not available. Strong analgesia may be required. Hypotension should be treated with plasma expanders and, if persistent, with a pressor agent such as dopamine.

Poisonous amphibians

The moist skin of amphibians such as frogs, toads, newts, and salamanders is an accessory respiratory organ, which is protected from micro-organisms by highly toxic secretions containing amines, peptides, proteins, steroids, and alkaloids. Some compounds are synthesized *de novo*, while others are sequestered from prey such as ants, beetles, and millipedes. The bitter flavour and lethal effects of these secretions and the vivid warning coloration of many species defend them against predators. The skin of poison frogs (Dendrobatidae) of Central and South America secrete lipophilic alkaloids such as batrachotoxins (*Phyllobates* spp.), which activate sodium channels; histrionico toxins (*Dendrobates histrionicus*) (Plate 6), which block nicotinic receptors; pumiliotoxins (*D. pumilio*), which affect sodium channels; and epibatidine (*Epipedobates tricolor*), a powerful analgesic and nicotinic receptor agonist. Two Colombian tribes, the Embará and Noanamá Chocó, use the skin poisons of three species of Phyllobates to coat the tips of their blow-gun darts (Plate 7). Some toads can squirt venom from their parotid glands, this contains bufadienolides which affect membrane Na$^+$/K$^+$-ATPase. When licked or put in the mouth by dogs or children or when ingested as Chinese traditional medicines such as *Kyushin*, *Yixin Wan*, or the topical aphrodisiac *Ch'an-Su*, the poisons can cause fatal digoxin-like poisoning. Symptoms include hypersalivation, cyanosis, cardiac arrhythmias, and generalized convulsions. Antidigoxin antibodies ('Digibind') have some therapeutic effect.

The skin of three species of newts, genus *Taricha*, from the western United States, contains tarichatoxins identical to tetrodotoxin, which also occurs in some toads, frogs, fish, crustaceans, and octopuses (see below). Tetrodotoxin can be absorbed through the gastric mucosa, explaining the death of a man who swallowed a 20-cm long Oregon rough-skinned newt (*Taricha granulosa*). He developed paraesthesia of the lips, progressing to more generalized numbness and weakness, and had a cardiopulmonary arrest about 2 h after swallowing the newt.

Poisonous birds

The feathers, skin, and breast muscles of three species of pitohui or thickhead, passerine birds from New Guinea (genus *Pitohui*, Pachycephalidae) contain homobatrachotoxin, a potent steroidal alkaloid that activates sodium channels and was originally isolated from the skin of South American poison-dart frogs (*Phyllobates*, Dendrobatidae—see above). Poisonous pitohuis have an unpleasant peppery odour and their skin has a bitter flavour. Contact with their feathers causes numbness and burning of the tongue, lip or skin wounds, and sneezing. This may be a protective mechanism, and the striking 'warning' coloration of the hooded pitohui (*P. dichrous*) (Plate 8) may be the subject of Müllerian mimicry by less poisonous species. Judging by their reputation in Papua New Guinea, other species, including birds of paradise and the blue-capped Ifrita (*Ifrita kowaldi*), may also prove to have poisonous tissues.

Venomous fish

More than 100 species of fish can inflict dangerous stings on humans. Venom is injected through spines in front of the fins and tail and in the gill covers. The Indo-Pacific region and other tropical waters have the richest venomous fish fauna, but dangerous species such as sharks, chimaeras, and weevers also occur in temperate northern waters and a number of large rivers in South American, West Africa, and Southeast Asia are inhabited by freshwater stingrays (*Potamotrygon* spp.). The following groups are capable of fatal envenoming: Squaliformes (sharks and dogfish), Rajiformes (stingrays and mantas), Siluroidei (catfish), Trachinidae (weevers), Scorpaenidae (scorpionfish and stonefish), and Uranoscopidae (stargazers and stonelifters). Venom glands are embedded in grooves in the spines or, in the case of stingrays, lie beneath a membrane covering the long barbed precaudal spine.

Incidence and epidemiology

Weeverfish are common around the British coast especially in Cornwall. Hundreds of stings occur in some years, with a peak incidence in August and September. A total of 58 cases were seen at one hospital at Pula on the Adriatic coast over a period of 13 years. It has been estimated that there are 1500 stings by rays and 300 stings by scorpionfish in the United States each year. Stings by venomous freshwater rays (*Potamotrygon hystrix*, *P. motoro*) are common in the Amazon region of Brazil and especially in Acré. In 4 years, 81 cases of stonefish (*Synanceja* spp.) sting were seen in Pulau Bukom Hospital near Singapore. Ornate, but aggressive and venomous members of the genera *Pterois* and *Dendrochirus* (lion, zebra, tiger, turkey, or red fire fish) (Plate 9), which are popular aquarium pets, often sting their owners on the fingers. Most fish stings are inflicted on the soles of the feet of people wading near the shore or in the vicinity of coral reefs. Venomous fish are effectively camouflaged (*Synanceja* spp.) or lie partly covered by sand. Stingrays lash their tails at the intruding limb and usually impale the ankle (Plate 9). Fatal fish stings are very rarely reported.

Venom composition

The instability of most fish venoms at normal ambient temperatures has made them difficult to study. Stingray and weeverfish venoms contain peptides, enzymes, and a variety of vasoactive compounds such as kinins, 5-hydroxytryptamine, histamine, and catecholamines. Pharmacological effects include local necrosis, direct actions on cardiac skeletal and smooth muscle resulting in ECG changes, hypotension, paralysis, and central nervous system depression.

Clinical features

Immediate sharp, agonizing pain is the dominant symptom. Hot, erythematous swelling extends up the stung limb and may persist with pain for several days and be complicated by necrosis (Plate 10) and secondary infection by marine *Vibrio* spp. (such as *V. vulnificus*) and other unusual bacteria, particularly if the spine remains embedded in the wound. Stingray spines, which are up to 30 cm long, can cause severe lacerating injuries especially to the lower legs, but if the victim inadvertently lies on the ray or falls onto it, the spine may penetrate the thoracic or abdominal cavities with fatal results.

Systemic effects are uncommon after weever stings (Trachinidae), but people stung by rays or Scorpaenidae (scorpion- and stone-fish) may develop nausea, vomiting, signs of autonomic nervous system stimulation; such as diarrhoea, sweating and hypersalivation; cardiac arrhythmias, hypotension, respiratory distress, neurological signs, and generalized convulsions. Patients have died within 1 h of being stung by *Synanceja verrucosa*.

Treatment

Pain is alleviated by immersing the stung limb in water which is uncomfortably hot (but less than 45 °C) yet not scalding. The 50 °C recommended by some authorities will cause a full thickness scald! Temperature can be assessed with the unstung limb. Addition of magnesium sulphate is unnecessary. Injection of a local anaesthetic is less effective even when applied as a ring block in the case of stung digits, but a local nerve block with 0.5 per cent of plain bupivacaine does seem to work. The venomous spine (which may be barbed), fragments of membrane, and other foreign material should be removed as soon as possible. Systemic effects must be treated symptomatically. An adequate airway should be established and cardiopulmonary resuscitation may be needed. Severe hypotension may respond to adrenaline (epinephrine), bradycardia to atropine. The Commonwealth Serum Laboratories (**CSL**) in Australia manufacture an antivenom specific for *Synanceja trachynis*, *S. verrucosa*, and *S horridus*. This has paraspecific activity against the venoms of the North American scorpionfish (*Scorpaena guttata*) and some other members of the Scorpaenidae. One ampoule (2 ml or 2000 units) is given intravenously for each two puncture marks found at the site of the sting. The dose is increased for patients with severe symptoms. Antibiotic treatment for secondary infections should take into account the range of possible marine pathogens. Ciprofloxacin covers *Vibrio* and *Aeromonas* spp.

Prevention

Fish stings can be prevented by employing a shuffling gait when wading, by avoiding handling living or dead fish, and by keeping clear of fish in the water, especially in the vicinity of tropical reefs. Footwear protects against most species except stingrays.

Poisoning by ingestion of aquatic animals

Acute gastrointestinal symptoms ('food poisoning') after eating seafood are usually caused by bacterial or viral infections such as *Vibrio parahaemolyticus* (crustaceans, especially shrimps), *V. cholerae* (crabs and molluscs), non-O group 1 *V. cholerae* (oysters), *V. vulnificus* (oysters), *Aeromonas hydrophila* (frozen oysters), *Plesiomonas shigelloides* (oysters, mussels, mackerel, cuttlefish), *Shigella* spp. (molluscs), *Campylobacter jejuni* (clams), *Salmonella typhi* (molluscs), hepatitis A virus (molluscs, especially clams and oysters), Norwalk virus (clams and oysters), and astro- and caliciviruses (cockles and other molluscs). Botulism has been caused by eating smoked fish and canned salmon; and in Japan and elsewhere, fish and molluscs became contaminated with methyl mercury from industrial waste, causing severe neurological damage and fetal abnormalities ('Minamata disease').

Toxins in seafood may also give rise to gastrointestinal neurotoxic and histamine-like symptoms. Two main syndromes are described.

Gastrointestinal and neurotoxic syndromes

Nausea, vomiting, abdominal colic, tenesmus, and watery diarrhoea may precede neurotoxic symptoms of paraesthesia of the lips, buccal cavity, and extremities, distorted temperature perception (so that cold objects impart a burning sensation like dry ice), myalgia, progressive flaccid paralysis, dizziness, ataxia, cardiovascular disturbances, bradycardia, and rashes. Important causes of this syndrome are:

1. *Ciguatera fish poisonings*—Symptoms develop between 1 and 6 h (extreme range, minutes to 30 h) after eating fish such as groupers, snappers, parrot fish, mackerel, moray eels, barracudas, and jacks. These are warm-water shore or reef fish. The global incidence is thought to exceed 50 000 cases per year. Up to 1 per cent of the population may be affected each year (e.g. in Kiribati, Tokelau, and Tuvalu in the Pacific region) with a case fatality of 0.1 per cent. The toxins responsible are polyethers—such as ciguatoxin (activates Na$^+$ channels), maitotoxin (activates Ca^{2+} channels), and scaritoxin, ultimately derived along the food chain from benthic dinoflagellates such as *Gambierdiscus toxicus*. They are concentrated in the liver, viscera, and gonads, especially of large carnivorous fish. The increasing market for exotic fish from the Caribbean and elsewhere has led to cases of ciguatera in Britain. Gastrointestinal symptoms resolve within a few hours, but paraesthesiae and myalgia may persist for a week or even months. Similar symptoms (chelonitoxication) may follow ingestion of marine turtles in the Indo-Pacific area, but the case fatality is much higher.

2. *Tetrodotoxin poisoning*—Scaleless porcupine, sun, puffer, and toad fish (order: Tetraodonitiformes) may become highly poisonous at certain seasons, such as May to June, the spawning season in Japan. Tetrodotoxin, an aminoperhydroquinazoline, is one of the most potent non-protein toxins known. It produces neurotoxic and cardiotoxic effects by blocking voltage-gated sodium ion channels. It is found: concentrated in the ovaries, viscera, and skin of tetraodontiform fish; in the skin of newts (genus *Taricha*), frogs and toads (genera *Colostethus, Atelopus, Bracycephalus*), and salamanders; in the saliva of octopuses; from the digestive glands of several species of gastropod molluscs; in a starfish, flat worm (*Planorbis* spp.), and Nemertine worms in Japan; and is produced by some bacteria (*Pseudomonas* spp.).

   Puffer fish ('fugu') is particularly popular in Japan where, despite stringent regulations, there are still cases of tetrodotoxin poisoning, with about four deaths each year. Neurotoxic symptoms develop within 10 to 45 min and death from respiratory paralysis usually occurs between 2 and 6 h after eating the fish. There may be no gastrointestinal symptoms. Erythema, petechiae, blistering, and desquamation may appear.

3. *Paralytic shellfish poisoning*—Bivalve molluscs, such as mussels, clams, oysters, cockles, and scallops (and also xanthid, coconut, and horseshoe crabs) may acquire tetrahydropurine neurotoxins such as saxitoxin from dinoflagellates (*Alexandrium* spp.). These may be sufficiently abundant between latitudes 30 °N and 30 °S during the warmer months of May to October to produce a 'red tide'. The dangerous season is signalled by the deaths of large numbers of fish and sea birds. Symptoms develop within 30 min of ingestion and may progress to fatal respiratory paralysis within 12 h in 8 per cent of cases. Milder gastrointestinal and neurotoxic symptoms (neurotoxic shellfish poisoning) without paralysis can follow the ingestion of molluscs contaminated by brevitoxins from *Gymnodinium breve*. These microalgae can also cause a 'red tide'. In the United Kingdom there have been several outbreaks of neurotoxic red-whelk (*Neptunea antiqua*) poisoning attributable to tetramine.

4. *Amnesic shellfish poisoning*—develops after ingestion of mussels and other molluscs contaminated with domoic acid from diatoms (*Pseudonitzschia* spp.). Gastroenteritis starts within 24 h of exposure and, in severe cases, within 48 h there is headache and coma followed by short-term memory loss.

Histamine-like syndrome (scombrotoxic poisoning)

The red flesh of scrombroid fish (tuna, mackerel, bonito, and skipjack) and of canned non-scrombroid fish, such as sardines and pilchards, may be decomposed by the action of bacteria such as *Proteus morgani* and *Klebsiella pneumoniae*, which decarboxylate muscle histidine into saurine, histamine, cadaverine, and other unidentified toxins: 100 g of spoiled fish may contain almost 1 g of histamine. Histamine absorbed from the gut is normally broken down by N-methyl-transferase and diamine oxidase (histaminase), but if the histamine concentration is very high, or the patient is taking a diamine oxidase inhibitor such as isoniazid (as antituberculosis chemotherapy), scombrotoxic poisoning may result. Toxic fish may produce a tingling or smarting sensation in the mouth when eaten. Within minutes or up to a few hours after ingestion, flushing, burning, sweating, urticaria, and pruritis may develop with headache, abdominal colic, nausea, vomiting, diarrhoea, bronchial asthma, giddiness, and hypotension.

Diagnosis and treatment

The differential diagnosis includes bacterial and viral food poisoning and allergic reactions.

No specific treatments or antidotes are available, but gastrointestinal contents should speedily be eliminated by emetics and purges. Activated charcoal adsorbs saxitoxin and other shellfish toxins. Mannitol has been advocated for ciguatera poisoning. Atropine is said to improve gastrointestinal symptoms and sinus bradycardia in patients with gastrointestinal and neurotoxic poisoning. Calcium gluconate may relieve mild neuromuscular symptoms. Oximes and anticholinesterases appear ineffective in ciguatera and tetrodotoxin poisoning, respectively. Patients who develop respiratory paralysis should be intubated and ventilated. The symptoms of scombrotoxic poisoning can be alleviated with antihistamines and bronchodilators.

Prevention

Ciguatera toxin, tetrodotoxin, scombrotoxins and some other marine toxins are heat-stable so cooking does not prevent poisoning. Some toxins are fairly water-soluble and may be leached out by soaking, so water in which fish are cooked should not be drunk. In tropical areas, the flesh of fish should be separated as soon as possible from the head, skin, intestines, gonads, and other viscera which may contain high concentrations of toxin. All scaleless fish should be regarded as potentially tetrodotoxic and very large fish carry an increased risk of being ciguatera-toxic. Moray eels should never be eaten because of the high risk of unusually rapid and severe ciguatera fish poisoning. Scombroid poisoning can be prevented by eating fresh fish or by freezing them as soon as possible after they are caught. Shellfish should not be eaten during the dangerous seasons and when there are red tides.

Poisoning by ingesting carp's gallbladder

In parts of the Far East, the raw bile and gallbladder of various species of freshwater carp (e.g. the grass carp *Ctenopharyngodon idellus*, 'plaa yeesok' *Probarbus jullienii*) are believed to have medicinal properties. Patients in China, Taiwan, Hong Kong, Japan, Thailand, and elsewhere have developed acute abdominal pain, vomiting, and watery diarrhoea 2 to 18 h after drinking the raw bile or eating the raw gallbladder of these fish. One patient developed flushing and dizziness. Hepatic and renal damage may develop, progressing to oliguric or non-oliguric acute renal failure (acute tubular necrosis). The hepatonephrotoxin has not been identified, but is heat-stable and may be derived from the carp's diet.

Venomous marine invertebrates (Cnidarians (coelenterates): jellyfish, cubomedusoids, sea wasps, Portuguese-men-o'-war or bluebottles, hydroids, stinging corals, sea anemones, etc.)

The tentacles of cnidarians are armed with millions of nematocysts (stinging capsules). When triggered by contact or chemicals, stinging hairs are everted at enormous acceleration and force, penetrating the skin. These produce lines of painful irritant weals. Cnidarian venoms contain peptides and other vasoactive substances such as 5-hydroxyhistamine, histamine, prostaglandins, and kinins which cause immediate excruciating pain, inflammation, and urticaria.

Epidemiology

The most dangerous species, the box jellyfish, cubomedusoid, sea wasp, or indringa (*Chironex fleckeri*) of northern Australia, has caused more than 70 deaths since 1883. Most stings occur in December and January. Fatal jellyfish stings in the Indo-Pacific region—from India, north to the Philippines, and east to Bougainville Island—are attributable to *Chiropsalmus quadrumanus* and *C. quadrigatus*. Fatal stings have also been inflicted by the Portuguese man-o'-war (*Physalia* spp.) and the Chinese jellyfish *Stomolophus nomurai*. Many stings in northern Queensland are caused by *Carukia barnesi* and other tiny cubomedusoids (Irukandji stings). Hundreds of thousands of swimmers off the northern Adriatic coast were stung by a plague of *Pelagia noctiluca* during the summers of 1977 to 1979. Stings by the sea anemone, *Anemonia sulcata*, are also reported from the coasts of Slovenia and Croatia.

Clinical features

Nematocyst stings may leave a diagnostic pattern on the skin: *C. fleckeri* produces wide, striated brownish-purple weals (Plate 11), whereas *C. barnesi* causes a transient erythematous macule and the Portuguese man-o'-war (genus *Physalia*) produces chains of oval weals surrounded by erythema. Immediate severe pain is the commonest symptom. Chirodropids (genera *Chironex* and *Chiropsalmus*) cause the most severe systemic symptoms such as respiratory arrest, generalized convulsions, pulmonary oedema, and cardiac arrest within minutes of the accident. Other systemic effects include cough, nausea, vomiting, abdominal colic, diarrhoea, rigors, severe musculoskeletal pains, and profuse sweating. 'Irukandji' syndrome consists of severe musculoskeletal pain, anxiety, trembling, headache, piloerection, sweating, tachycardia, hypertension, and pulmonary oedema starting about 30 min after a sting by *C. barnesi* (and at least seven other species of tiny cubomedusoids) and persisting for hours. *Physalia* species can also cause severe systemic envenoming, including intravascular haemolysis, peripheral gangrene, and renal failure.

Treatment

Patients stung by jellyfish must be removed from the water as soon as possible to prevent drowning. The aim is to prevent a further discharge of nematocysts on fragments of tentacles stuck to the skin. Alcoholic solutions such as methylated spirits and suntan lotion, the traditional remedy, cause massive discharge of nematocysts. Commercial vinegar or a 3 to 10 per cent aqueous acetic acid solution are, however, effective against stings by *Chironex* spp. and other cubozoans, including Irukandji. Baking soda and water (50 per cent (w/v)) is effective for the widely distributed Atlantic genus, *Chrysaora*. Vinegar is not recommended for stings by *Chrysaora*, *Physalia*, or *Stomalophus* spp. Ice packs relieve the intense pain. Pressure immobilization may increase the amount of venom injected and is not recommended. Cardiopulmonary resuscitation has proved life-saving in several Australian

patients who became cyanosed, comatose, and pulseless. A specific 'sea wasp' antivenom for *C. fleckeri* is manufactured in Australia. Treatment with verapamil is not recommended.

Prevention

Bathers, especially children, should keep out of the sea at times of the year when dangerous cnidarians are prevalent, especially when warning notices have been put up; or they should bathe in 'stinger-resistant' enclosures, but these do not exclude Irukandji. Wet or 'Lycra' suits, nylon stockings, and other clothing will protect against nematocyst stings.

Echinodermata (starfish and sea urchins)

These animals are protected by hard exoskeletons with numerous long, sharp projecting spines and grapples (globiferous pedicellariae) which can release venom when embedded in the skin. Severe pain and local swelling may result, and sometimes systemic effects such as syncope, numbness, generalized paralysis, aphonia, respiratory distress, cardiac arrhythmias, and even death. Embedded fragments of spines may lead to secondary infection and chronic granulomas or damage to bones and joints.

Treatment

Hot water (see above) may relieve the pain. Skin penetrated by the spines, usually the soles of the feet, should be softened with 2 per cent salicylic acid ointment or acetone. The spines can then be squeezed out or removed surgically. No antivenoms are available.

Mollusca (cone shells and octopuses)

The 500 species of cone shells (genus *Conus*) are carnivorous marine snails that harpoon their prey (fish, polychaete worms, and other molluscs), implanting a radular tooth charged with venom containing a mixture of small (10–30 amino acid) peptide toxins. These include: conotoxins which block acetylcholine receptors and voltage-sensitive Ca^{2+} and Na^+ channels; conantokins which are *N*-methyl-D-aspartate receptor antagonists with anticonvulsant activity; and conopressins which target vasopressin receptors. Cone shells are attractive and valuable collectors' items. People who pick them up may be stung. Symptoms of envenoming are nausea, vomiting, paraesthesia and numbness of the lips and site of sting, numbness, dizziness, ptosis, diplopia, dysarthria, dyspnoea, and loss of consciousness. In a series of 35 cases mostly stung by *Conus geographus* reported in Japan (1896–1996), 10 died within 2 to 5 h of the sting (Plate 12).

Several species of small octopus found in the Australian and West Pacific region (blue ringed octopuses—genus *Hapalochlaena*—Plate 13) can inject salivary tetrodotoxin when they bite swimmers with their powerful beaks. These bites are painful and cause local bleeding, swelling, and inflammation. Severe neurotoxic symptoms, and even fatal generalized paralysis, may develop within 15 min of the bite.

Treatment

No antivenoms are available. Cardiopulmonary resuscitation and mechanical ventilation may be required.

Venomous arthropods (Hymenoptera (bees, wasps, yellowjackets, hornets, and ants))

The commonest and most severe stings from *Hymenoptera* spp. are caused by members of the families Apidae (e.g. honey bees, *Apis mellifera*, *A.. cerania*, bumble bees, etc.), Vespidae (e.g. wasps, genera *Polistes* and *Paravespula*), American yellowjackets and 'hornets' (genera *Vespula* and

Dolichovespula) and European and Asian true hornets (genus *Vespa*), and Formicidae (e.g. fire ants, genus *Solenopsis*). Allergic reactions to single stings from *Hymenoptera* spp. are common, whereas toxic reactions resulting from many stings are rare, except in the Americas. Venom allergens include phospholipases A, hyaluronidase, acid phosphomonoesterases, and melittin (*A. mellifera*). Non-allergenic compounds include vasoactive amines such as histamine, 5-hydroxytryptamine, catecholamines and kinins, cholinesterase (in the venom of the common European wasp (*Paravespula germanica*), pheromones, and 2-methylpiperidine alkaloids in venoms from *Solenopsis* (fire ant) spp.

Epidemiology

Fewer than 10 people die from hymenopteran sting anaphylaxis in England and Wales each year, 2 or 3 per year in Australia, and in the United States there are between 40 and 50 deaths per year. The incidence of systemic reactions to stings by *Hymenoptera* spp. has been reported as 0.4 to 0.8 per cent in children. In an adult population in the United States, the prevalence of systemic allergic sting reactions was found to be 4 per cent; 20 per cent of this population showed evidence of venom hypersensitivity (skin tests or radioallergosorbent test, **RAST**). In Britain, most patients allergic to bee venom are beekeepers or their relatives. Since the escape of swarms of African honey bees (*A. m. scutellata*) in Brazil, in 1957, this aggressive strain has spread throughout Latin America and north as far as Las Vegas in the United States. About 30 deaths from mass attacks by these bees have been reported each year. Two species of fire ants, *Solenopsis richteri* and *S. invicta*, were imported into the United States from South America in 1918 and have now spread to 13 southern states where an estimated 2.5 million individuals are stung each month. The incidence of systemic allergic reactions is about 4 per 100 000 population per year, and there have been fatalities.

Clinical features

Toxic effects

In non-sensitized individuals, a sting, which, in the case of Vespidae and Apidae, introduces about 50 μg of venom, will rapidly produce a hot, red, painful swelling and weal a few centimetres in diameter, which persists for a few hours. These effects are dangerous only if the airway is obstructed, for example following stings on the tongue. As few as 30 stings can cause fatal systemic envenoming in children, but children and adults have survived more than 1000 stings by *A. mellifera*. In some patients, symptoms have suggested histamine toxicity: vasodilatation, hypotension, vomiting, diarrhoea, throbbing headache, coma, and bronchoconstriction. In Latin America, victims of attacks by *A. m. scutellata* have shown evidence of generalized rhabdomyolysis (grossly elevated serum creatine kinase, aminopeptidases, and myoglobin), intravascular haemolysis, hypercatecholaminaemia (hypertension, pulmonary oedema, myocardial damage), bleeding, hepatic dysfunction, and acute renal failure (Plate 14). In non-sensitized people, stings form *Solenopsis* spp. produces pain, itching, swelling, and erythema around a central weal which last a few hours, and later vesicles or pustules. In an unsensitized patient an estimated 10 000 *S. invicta* stings caused no systemic envenoming.

Allergic effects

Clinical suspicion of dangerous venom hypersensitivity arises when systemic symptoms follow a sting. Patients may die within minutes of the sting. Systemic symptoms include: a tingling scalp; itching of the palms, soles, axillas, and perineum, becoming generalized; flushing; dizziness; syncope; wheezing; abdominal colic (uterine colic in women), diarrhoea, incontinence of urine and faeces; tachycardia and visual disturbances; all developing within a few minutes of the sting. Over the next 15 to 20 min, urticaria, angio-oedema of the lips, gums, and tongue, a generalized redness of the skin with swelling, oedema of the glottis, profound hypotension, and coma may develop. A few patients develop serum sickness a week or more after the sting. Some patients with sting allergy have other evidence of an atopic disposition. Reactions are enhanced by β-blockers.

Diagnosis of anaphylaxis and venom hypersensitivity

Serum concentrations of mast-cell tryptase may be raised for up to 6 h after an anaphylactic attack, distinguishing this diagnosis from panic attacks and other causes of collapse. Type I hypersensitivity is confirmed by detecting venom-specific IgE in the serum using RAST or by prick skin tests. Patients who have suffered a systemic reaction, have a 50 to 60 per cent risk of a reaction to their next sting. Local reactions, even massive ones involving persistent swelling of the whole stung limb, in the absence of systemic symptoms do not predict a systemic reaction when stung again. Children who have generalized urticaria after a sting have only a 10 per cent chance of a systemic reaction when restung. Hypersensitivity to venom may be lost spontaneously, especially by children and young adults. The RAST test can be used for a postmortem diagnosis of Hymenoptera sting anaphylaxis.

Treatment

The barbed stings of Apidae remain embedded at the site of the sting and continue to inject venom, so they should be removed immediately by any means possible. Vespids can withdraw their stings and sting repeatedly. Wasp stings may become infected because these insects feed on rotting meat. Domestic meat tenderizer (papain) diluted roughly 1:5 with tap water is said to produce immediate relief of pain. Ice packs and aspirin are also effective. Systemic but not topical antihistamines can be used for more severe local reactions. Massive local reactions may require aspirin, nonsteroidal anti-inflammatory agents, or even corticosteroids. **Systemic anaphylaxis** must be treated with 0.1 per cent (1:1000) adrenaline (epinephrine) (0.5–1 ml for adults; 0.01 mg/kg for children) given by intramuscular injection, or, if the patient is unconscious or pulseless, diluted 1:100 000, by intravenous injection. In rare cases, blood pressure fails to respond even to large doses of adrenaline and plasma expanders. These patients should be given cardiopulmonary resuscitation, selective bronchodilators such as salbutamol, pressor agents such as dopamine, and intravenous histamine H_1 and H_2 blockers such as chlorphenamine (chlorpheniramine) maleate (10 mg for adults; 0.2 mg/kg for children) and cimetidine. Corticosteroids probably have no effect in acute anaphylaxis but may prevent relapses a few hours later. Patients who know they are hypersensitive should wear an identifying tag (such as provided by Medic-Alert in Britain) as they may be discovered unconscious after being stung. They should be trained to give themselves adrenaline using an 'EpiPen' or similar apparatus. Adrenaline delivered by a pressurized inhaler ('Medihaler-Epi') or squirted down the endotracheal tube produces transient blood levels insufficient to combat anaphylaxis. Respiratory tract obstruction and shock are the main causes of death.

Severe envenoming from multiple stings by *Hymenoptera* spp. should be treated with adrenaline, intravenous antihistamines (doses as above), and corticosteroids. Intensive care is essential. Intravenous mannitol and bicarbonate may protect the kidneys from the damaging effects of myoglobinuria and haemoglobinaemia ('pigment nephropathy'), as in patients with the crush syndrome. Experimental antivenoms have been produced but are not yet commercially available. Exchange transfusion or plasmapheresis might be considered to remove venom in severe cases. Renal dialysis is often needed.

Prevention

Patients over the age of 25 years who have a history of systemic anaphylaxis following a sting and who have evidence of hypersensitivity (venom-specific IgE detectable in the serum or a positive skin test) should be considered for desensitization with purified venoms. This treatment proved significantly more effective than placebo or the previously used whole body extracts of *Hymenoptera* spp. in preventing anaphylactic reactions to sting challenge. Desensitization usually involves weekly visits to the hospital for at least 8 weeks for the administration of gradually increasing doses of venom. When protection has been demonstrated by the patient's ability to tolerate 100 µg of venom (equivalent to two stings) they are ready for maintenance therapy, usually 100 µg of venom every 4 to 8 weeks. A period of 2 to 5 years of maintenance desensitization is recommended, after which more than 90 per cent of subjects will remain protected against systemic reactions after stopping treatment. Desensitization is complicated by systemic reactions in 5 to 15 per cent of patients and by local reactions in 50 per cent.

Wasps are attracted by sweet things and meat in kitchens, greengrocers, orchards, and vineyards. Vespidae are attracted by brightly coloured floral patterns and perfumes. Hornets are attracted by light. Some species are so aggressive that their nests must be eradicated before their territory can be used for farming.

Venomous lepidoptera

The stinging hairs of some species of adult moths can cause contact dermatitis and urticaria ('lepidopterism'), while caterpillars can produce local or even systemic effects ('erucism'). Venomous lepidoptera are found in all parts of the world, but most cases of lepidopterism are reported from Middle and Southern America. Severe cutaneous urticating eruptions (Plate 15) can be caused by caterpillars of the genus *Megalopyge* (called 'puss-moths' in the southern United States) and by adult female moths of the genus *Hylesia* which have barbed setae ('flechettes') on their abdomens. Epidemics of stings by these moths have been described, especially from coastal areas of Brazil, Peru, Venezuela, and Mexico. Caterpillars of the genus *Lonomia* (*L. obliqua*, *L. achelous*) can inject through their bristles venom containing a plasminogen activator, plasmin-like enzyme, protease-activating factors V and XIII, and prothrombin, resulting in defibrinogenation, spontaneous bleeding into the skin, urinary tract, and even fatal intracranial haemorrhage (Plate 16). Laboratory findings in envenomed patients are decreased plasma fibrinogen, factor V, factor XIII, and plasminogen concentrations, as well as increased fibrin(ogen) degradation products and fibrinolytic activity but a normal platelet count.

In Pará State, Brazil, rubber tappers are frequently in contact with caterpillars (*Premolis semirufa*) whose stinging hairs can cause a disabling arthritis of the hands ('pararama').

Venomous coleoptera (beetles)

The most famous vesicating beetle is 'Spanish fly'—*Lytta vesicatoria* (Meloidae—blister beetles). Its venom contains cantharidin, which causes blistering when applied to the skin and priapism (hence its reputation as an aphrodisiac) and renal failure when given systemically or absorbed after eating the legs of frogs which have fed on meloid beetles.

'Nairobi eye' and similar blistering conditions in Australia and South-East Asia are caused by species of the genus *Paederus* (Staphylinidae) (Plate 17). A typical skin lesion (dermatitis linearis) consists of erythema, itching, and blistering caused by inadvertently crushing and smearing the beetle. Systemic symptoms such as fever, arthralgia, and vomiting may arise in severe cases. The active principle pederin is the most complex non-proteinaceous insect toxin known. Treatment is palliative. The toxin is easily spread to other sites such as the eye by fingers.

Scorpions (Scorpiones: Buthidae, Scorpionidae)

Species capable of inflicting fatal stings occur in North Africa and the Middle East (genus *Androctonus*, *Buthus*, and *Leiurus*); South Africa (*Parabuthus* spp.); India (*Mesobuthus tamulus*); North, Central and Southern America, Trinidad, and Tobago (genera *Tityus* (Plate 18) and *Centruroides*). Scorpion toxins target Na⁺, K⁺, Ca²⁺, and Cl⁻ channels causing direct effects and the release of neurotransmitters such as acetylcholine and catecholamines.

Epidemiology

There have been no deaths from scorpion sting in the United States since 1968. However, between 1000 and 2000 deaths were reported each year in Mexico, but recently this number has declined dramatically. Case fatality is highest (formerly about 50 per cent) in children less than 4 years old. In Trinidad, stings by *Tityus trinitatis* are an occupational hazard of sugar cane and cocoa plantation workers. In the 1960s, there were 33 deaths in a group of 698 cases. Mortality was 25 per cent in children under 5 years compared to 0.25 per cent in adults. In Brazil, mortality was about 1 per cent in adults and 15 to 25 per cent in children less than 6 years old. In India, many people are stung by the red scorpion (*Mesobuthus tamulus*) with fatalities in adults and children.

Clinical features

Intense local pain is the commonest symptom. There may be slight local oedema and tender enlargement of regional lymph nodes, but stings by *Hemiscorpius lepturus* (Iran, Iraq, Pakistan, and Yemen) cause a local macular lesion which may blister and become necrotic resulting in sloughing of a large area of skin (Plate 19). Systemic symptoms may develop within minutes or be delayed for as much as 24 h. Symptoms vary depending on the species and geographical area. Scorpion venoms stimulate the release of acetylcholine and catecholamines, often resulting in initial cholinergic and later adrenergic symptoms. Early symptoms include vomiting, profuse sweating, piloerection, alternating brady- and tachycardia, abdominal colic, diarrhoea, loss of sphincter control, and priapism. Later, severe life-threatening cardiorespiratory effects may appear: hypertension, shock, tachy- and bradyarrhythmias, ECG changes (Fig. 26), and pulmonary oedema (Fig. 27) with or without evidence of myocardial dysfunction. Severe cardiovascular complications are particularly associated with stings by *Leiurus quinquestriatus*, *Mesobuthus tamulus*, and *Tityus* species. Stings by the North American *Centruroides sculpturatus* produce neurotoxic effects such as fasciculation, spasms, respiratory paralysis, and convulsions. Victims of the Trinidad black scorpion (*Tityus trinitatis*) develop severe abdominal pain with nausea, vomiting and haematemesis, hyperglycaemia, and biochemical evidence of acute pancreatitis.

Treatment

Pain responds temporarily to local infiltration or ring block with local anaesthetic. Local injection of emetine or dehydroemetine is said to relieve the pain but may cause necrosis. Parenteral opiate analgesics, such as pethidine or morphine, may be required, but are said to be dangerous in victims of *C. sculpturatus*.

Antivenom is manufactured in a number of countries. Its use is strongly advocated in Africa and the Americas, but ancillary pharmacological treatment is regarded as being much more important in the Middle East and India. However, if specific antivenom is available it should be administered intravenously as soon as possible in patients with systemic envenoming and in young children stung by dangerous species, even before the development of these symptoms. Patients with cardiovascular symptoms benefit from vasodilator treatment with α-blockers (e.g. prazosin), calcium-channel blockers (e.g. nifedipine), or ACE inhibitors (e.g. captopril). Atropine should not be used except in cases of life-threatening sinus bradycardia. The use of cardiac glycosides and β-blockers is controversial. Anticonvulsants such as phenobarbital (phenobarbitone) are recommended for neurotoxic symptoms.

Prevention

Scorpions can be kept out of houses by including a row of ceramic tiles in the outside wall, making the doorsteps at least 20 cm high, and using residual insecticides, such as 1 per cent lindane or dieldrin powders.

Spiders (Araneae)

All but one family of this enormous order are venomous, but few species have proved dangerous to humans. Spiders bite with a pair of small fangs,

(a)

(b)

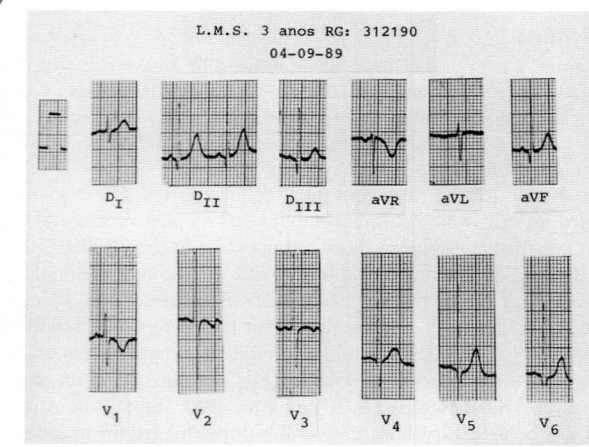

(c)

Fig. 26 Electrocardiographic changes caused by envenoming by the Brazilian scorpion (*Tityus serrulatus*). (By courtesy of Dr Carlos Amaral, Belo Horizonte, Brazil.) (a) ECG of 3-year-old girl 2 h after sting, showing sinus tachycardia and mild T-wave and ST-segment changes in the inferior and anterior leads. (b) Same patient 24 h after the sting, showing sinus tachycardia with marked ST downsloping and ST displacement in the inferior and anterolateral leads. (c) ECG of the same patient 3 days after the sting, showing return to normal sinus rhythm and ST pattern.

the chelicerae, to which the venom glands are connected (Plate 20). There are four medically important genera of venomous spiders: *Loxosceles* cause necrotic araneism and *Latrodectus*, *Phoneutria*, and *Atrax* cause neurotoxic araneism.

Epidemiology

Loxosceles laeta (Plate 21) is widely distributed and causes many bites in people in Central and Southern America, especially in Chile, where the mortality ranges from 1 to 17 per cent. *L. reclusa*, the brown recluse spider, caused at least 200 bites and six deaths in the United States during the last century. More than 60 cases were reported from Texas between 1959 and 1962. Bites by *L. rufescens* have been reported from the Mediterranean region, North Africa, and Israel. Most bites from *Loxosceles* spp. occur in bedrooms while people are asleep or dressing, and in the United States a number of men were bitten on the genitalia while they sat on outdoor lavatories in which the spiders had spun their webs. *Latrodectus tredecimguttatus* (sometimes referred to, loosely, as 'tarantula') lives in fields in Mediterranean countries and has been responsible for a series of epidemics of bites. In Italy, 946 cases were reported between 1946 and 1951. *L. hasseltii*, the Australian redback spider (Plate 22), causes up to 340 bites each year in Australia and 20 deaths have been reported. The black widow spider (*L. mactans*) was responsible for 63 deaths in the United States between 1950 and 1959. Other species of *Latrodectus* are found in Latin America.

Phoneutria nigriventer (Plates 20 and 23), the banana spider, causes bites and deaths in South American countries. These spiders have been imported to temperate countries on bunches of bananas, causing a few bites and

(a)

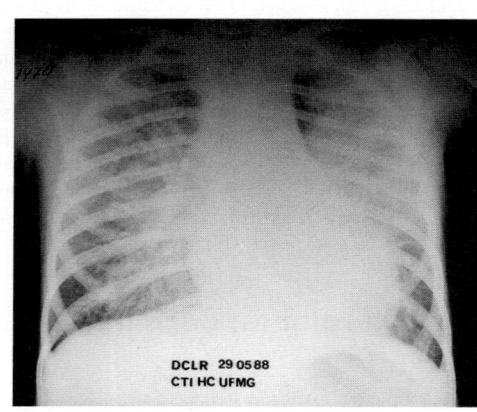

(b)

Fig. 27 Pulmonary oedema caused by *Tityus serrulatus* envenoming. (By courtesy of Dr Carlos Amaral, Belo Horizonte, Brazil.) (a) Chest radiograph of a 9-year-old girl 24 h after sting, showing alveolar infiltrates in both lungs with air bronchograms. The heart size is increased. (b) Chest radiograph of 7-year-old girl 10 h after sting, showing bilateral pulmonary oedema with enlarged heart.

deaths. The funnel web spiders (genus *Atrax*) are restricted to south-eastern Australia and Tasmania. The Sydney funnel web spider (*A. robustus*) occurs only within a 160-mile (256 km) radius of Sydney. The aggressive males of this species caused at least 13 deaths between 1927 and 1980. Members of the related genera *Hadronyche* and *Missulina* may be equally dangerous. In England, mild neurotoxic araneism has been described after bites by *Steatoda nobilis* (Theridiidae) and the woodlouse spider (*Dysdera crocata*).

Necrotic araneism

The bite itself is usually painless and unnoticed. Burning develops over several hours at the site of the bite, with swelling and development of a characteristic macular lesion (Plate 24(a)) which shows areas of red (vasodilatation), white (vasoconstriction), and blue (prenecrotic cyanosis). Eventually the lesion forms a blackened eschar (Plates 24(b) and (c)) which sloughs in a few weeks, sometimes leaving a necrotic ulcer. The necrotic area may, rarely, cover an entire limb. Facial lesions may cause much oedema. Some 13 per cent of cases have systemic symptoms such as fever, headaches, scarlatiniform rash, jaundice, methaemoglobinaemia, and haemoglobinuria resulting from intravascular haemolysis. Renal failure may ensue. The average case fatality is about 5 per cent.

Neurotoxic araneism

The bite is very painful but local signs are minimal (*L. mactans*) or moderate (*L. hasselti*). After about 30 min there is painful regional lymphadenopathy, then headache and nausea and vomiting, with local sweating and piloerection ('gooseflesh') (Plate 25) and painful muscle spasms and tremors that may be severe enough to embarrass respiration. Local sweating and piloerection at the site of the bite is very suggestive of neurotoxic araneism. Other features include tachycardia, hypertension, restlessness, irritability, psychosis, priapism, and rhabdomyolysis. The 'facies latrodectismica' is a painful grimace caused by facial spasm and trismus associated with swollen eyelids, congested conjunctivas, flushing, and sweating (*L. tredecemguttatus*). Similar effects are seen in patients bitten by *Phoneutria* and *Atrax* spp.

First-aid treatment

In the case of bites by spiders with rapidly acting and potent venoms, such as *A. robustus* and *Hadronyche* species, firm crêpe bandaging and splinting of the bitten limb may delay venom spread until the patient reaches hospital.

Specific treatment

Antivenoms for a bite from *Latrodectus* spp. are made in Australia, the United States, Russia, Italy, Croatia, South, Africa and South America; for *Atrax* spp. bites in Australia; for *Loxosceles* spp. in Peru, Brazil, and Argentina; and for *Phoneutria* spp. in Brazil. Neurotoxic araneism seems more responsive to antivenom than does the necrotic type.

Supportive treatment

Oral dapsone (100 mg twice daily) is said to reduce the extent of necrotic lesions by inhibiting neutrophil degranulation. Calcium gluconate (10 ml of a 10 per cent solution, given by slow intravenous injection) relieves the pain of muscle spasms caused by the venom of *Latrodectus* spp. rapidly and more effectively than muscle relaxants such as diazepam or methocarbamol. Antihistamines, corticosteroids, α-blockers, and atropine have also been advocated. For necrotic araneism cause by *Loxosceles* spp. surgical debridement, corticosteroids, antihistamines, and hyperbaric oxygen all have their advocates, but there is no basis for recommending their use.

Ticks (Acari)

Taxonomy and epidemiology

Ticks, with mites, form the order Acari of the class *Arachnida*. Adult females of about 34 species of hard tick (family *Ixodidae*) and immature specimens of nine species of soft ticks (family *Argasidae*) have been implicated in human tick paralysis. The tick's saliva contains a neurotoxin which causes presynaptic neuromuscular block and decreased nerve-conduction velocity. The tick embeds itself in the skin with its barbed hypostome introducing the salivary toxin while it engorges with blood.

Although tick paralysis has been reported from all continents, most cases occur in western North America (*Dermacentor andersoni*), eastern United States (*D. variabilis*), and eastern Australia from north Queensland to Victoria (*Ixodes holocyclus* known as the bush, scrub, paralysis-, or dog tick). In British Columbia there were 305 cases with a 10 per cent mortality between 1900 and 1968. About 120 cases have been reported in the United States, and in New South Wales there were at least 20 deaths between 1900 and 1945.

Clinical features

Ticks are picked up in the countryside or from domestic animals, particularly dogs, in the home. The majority of patients and almost all fatal cases are children. After the tick has been attached for about 5 or 6 days a progressive ascending, lower motor neurone paralysis develops with paraesthesiae. Often a child, who may have been irritable for the previous 24 h, falls on getting out of bed first thing in the morning and is found to be weak or ataxic. Paralysis increases over the next few days: death results from bulbar and respiratory paralysis and aspiration of stomach contents. Vomiting is a feature of the more acute course of *Ixodes holocyclus* envenoming.

This clinical picture is often misinterpreted as poliomyelitis. Other neurological conditions, including Guillain–Barré syndrome, paralytic rabies, Eaton–Lambert syndrome, myasthenia gravis, or botulism, may also be suspected. Diagnosis depends on finding the tick, which is likely to be concealed in a crevice, orifice, or hairy area of the body. The scalp is the commonest place. Fatal tick paralysis has been caused by a tick attached to the tympanic membrane.

Treatment

The tick must be detached without being squeezed. It can be painted with ether, chloroform, paraffin, petrol, or turpentine, or prised out between the partially separated tips of a pair of small, curved forceps. Following removal of the tick there is usually a rapid and complete recovery; but in Australia, patients have died after the tick has been detached. An antivenom, raised in dogs, is available in Australia, and, recently, rabbits have been used to produce an antitoxin against *I. holocyclus* saliva. This is recommended for severely affected or very young patients; 20 to 30 ml are given intravenously.

Centipedes (Chilopoda)

Many species of centipedes can inflict painful bites (Fig. 28), producing swelling, inflammation, and lymphangitis. Systemic effects such as vomiting, headache, cardiac arrhythmias, and convulsions are extremely rare and the risk of mortality was probably greatly exaggerated in the older literature. The most important genus is *Scolopendra* which is distributed throughout tropical countries. Local treatment is the same as for scorpion stings. No antivenom is available.

Millipedes (Diplopida)

Most species possess glands in each of their body segments which secrete, and in some cases squirt out, irritant liquids for defensive purposes. These

Fig. 28 Venom 'jaws' (modified limbs) of a Thai centipede (*Scolopendra* species). (Copyright DA Warrell.)

contain hydrogen cyanide and a variety of aldehydes, esters, phenols, and quinonoids. Members of at least eight genera of millipedes have proved injurious to humans. Important genera are *Rhinocricus* (Caribbean), *Spirobolus* (Tanzania), *Spirostreptus* and *Iulus* (Indonesia), and *Polyceroconas* (Papua New Guinea). Children are particularly at risk when they handle or try to eat these large arthropods. When venom is squirted into the eye, intense conjunctivitis results and there may be corneal ulceration and even blindness. Skin lesions initially stain brown or purple, blister after a few days, and then peel. First aid is generous irrigation with water. Eye injuries should be treated as for snake venom ophthalmia (see above).

Leeches (Phylum Annelida, Class Hirudinea)

Leeches are blood-sucking, hermaphroditic, egg-laying annelids which have elongated annulated bodies. They attach themselves to leaves, rocks. or the host by a posterior sucker. To feed, the leech applies its anterior sucker containing the mouth armed with three radially arranged jaws which make a Y-shaped incision. Blood is sucked out by the action of the muscular pharynx. To prevent blood clotting, the saliva contains a histamine-like vasodilator and anticoagulants, such as: hirudin from the medicinal leech (*Hirudo medicinalis*), which inhibits thrombin and factor IXa; hementin from *Haementeria ghilianii*, which is directly fibrinolytic; and hementerin from *H. depressa* (= *H. lutzi*), a plasminogen activator. Other enzymes include esterases, antitrypsin, antiplasmin, and antielastase. Recombinant hirudin is now produced as a therapeutic anticoagulant. The medicinal leech is still used by plastic surgeons to reduce haematomas under skin grafts; the wound may become infected with *Aeromonas hydrophila* which lives symbiotically in the leech's gut.

Two groups of leeches cause human morbidity and even mortality in tropical countries.

Land leeches

Species of the genera *Haemadipsa* and *Phyrobdella* are 1 to 8 cm long. They infest, often in enormous numbers, the damp, leafy floor and low vegetation of rainforests, choosing game trails and watering places. By standing on the posterior sucker and waving the anterior sucker, they can sense their prey with amazing efficiency. They drop on to the prey or pursue it with a looping or lashing motion. These leeches usually attach themselves to the lower legs or ankles and are adept at penetrating clothing, even long trousers tucked into socks and lace-up boots. The bite is usually painless and infested persons may not realize what has happened until they hear a squelching sound, notice that their feet are warm and wet, and see blood welling over the tops of their boots. Land leeches ingest about 1 ml of blood

in one hour and then drop off, but the wound continues to bleed for some time and forms a fragile clot.

Aquatic leeches

These species may be swallowed by those who drink stagnant water or even mountain stream water, or they may attack bathers, entering the mouth, nostrils, eyes, vulva, vagina, urethra, or anus. The enormous brightly coloured buffalo leech (*Hirudinaria manillensis*) of South-East Asia, is up to 16 cm long and can ingest 1 ml of blood in 10 min. *Limnatis nilotica* occurs around the Mediterranean, Middle East, and North Africa. *Myxobdella africana* occurs in East Africa. *Dinobdella ferox* (5 cm long) is found in Asia. Some aquatic leeches are very slow feeders and may remain attached for days or even weeks.

Clinical features

The main effect is blood loss, but other symptoms include pain caused by the bite, secondary infection, a residual itching, and phobia. Ingested aquatic leeches usually attach to the pharynx but may penetrate the bronchi or oesophagus. *H. manillensis* entering via the anus can reach the rectosigmoid junction of the bowel causing perforation and peritonitis. Patients with a leech in the pharynx often have a feeling of movement at the back of the throat with cough, hoarseness, stridor, breathlessness, epistaxis, haemoptysis, and haematemesis. Fatal upper airway obstruction may result. Bleeding may persist for up to a week after the leech has dropped off. In rural Thailand, vaginal bleeding in girls who have swum in ponds or canals is often attributable to infestation by aquatic leeches. Sexual abuse may be wrongly inferred if this diagnosis is not considered. Transmission of rinderpest and other viruses, leptospirosis, and *Trypanosoma cruzi* has been suggested but not proved. Secondary infection of medicinal leech bites by *Aeromonas hydrophila* has been described.

Treatment

Leeches will detach if a grain of salt, a lighted match or a cigarette, alcohol, turpentine, or vinegar are applied. Local bleeding can be stopped by applying a styptic, such as silver nitrate or a firm dressing. Aquatic leeches that have penetrated the respiratory, upper gastrointestinal, genitourinary tracts, or rectum must be removed by endoscope. Spraying with 30 per cent cocaine, 10 per cent tartaric acid, or dilute (1:10 000) adrenaline (epinephrine) makes the leech detach from the nasopharynx, larynx, trachea, or oesophagus, while irrigation with a concentrated salt solution may be effective in the genitourinary tract and rectum. Leeches should not be pulled off so roughly that the mouth parts are left in the wound as this will lead to a chronic infection. Antimicrobial treatment of secondary bacterial infections (e.g. of *Aeromonas hydrophila* with cefuroxime or a quinolone) may be required.

Prevention

This can be achieved by impregnating clothing, especially the bottoms of trousers and socks, with repellents such as dibutyl phthalate and diethyl toluamide. They may also be applied to the skin and the inside and outside of footwear. If these compounds are not available, invasion of footwear during jungle walks can be prevented, rather messily, by rolling a rope of tobacco in the tops of the socks and keeping the feet well soaked with water. Children should be discouraged from bathing in leech-infested waters and all drinking water should be boiled or filtered.

Further reading

Mechanical injuries caused by animals

Barss PG (1982). Injuries caused by garfish in Papua New Guinea. *British Medical Journal* **284**, 77–9.

Barss P, Ennis S (1988). Injuries caused by pigs in Papua New Guinea. *Medical Journal of Australia* **149**, 649–56.

Baxter DN, *et al.* (1984). The deleterious effects of dogs on human health. *Community Medicine* **6**, 29–36, 185–97, 198–203.

Middaugh JP (1987). Human injury from bear attacks in Alaska, 1900–1985. *Alaska Medicine* **29**, 121–6.

Wallet T (1978). *Shark attack and treatment of victims in South African waters.* Purnell, Cape Town.

Venomous mammals

Fenner PJ, Williamson JA, Myers D (1992). Platypus envenomation: a painful learning experience. *Medical Journal of Australia* **157**, 829–32.

Venomous snakes

Gopalakrishnakone P, ed (1994). *Sea snake toxinology*, pp 1–36. Singapore University Press,

Harvey AL, ed (1991). *Snake toxins. International encyclopedia of pharmacology and therapeutics*, Section 134. Pergamon Press, New York.

Meier J, White J, eds (1995). *Handbook of clinical toxicology of animal venoms and poisons.* CRC Press, Boca Raton, FL.

Reid HA (1976). Adder bites in Britain. *British Medical Journal* **2**, 153–6.

Reid HA, *et al.* (1963). Clinical effects of bites by Malayan viper (*Ancistrodon rhodostoma*). *Lancet* **i**, 617–21.

Russell FE (1980). *Snake venom poisoning.* Lippincott, Philadelphia, PA.

Sutherland SK, Tibballs J (2001). *Australian animal toxins. The creatures, their toxins and care of the poisoned patient*, 2nd edn. Oxford University Press, Melbourne.

Theakston RDG, Warrell DA (1991). Antivenoms: a list of hyperimmune sera currently available for the treatment of envenoming by bites and stings. *Toxicon* **29**, 1419–70.

Warrell DA (1990). Treatment of snake bite in the Asia-Pacific region: a personal view. In: Gopalakrishnakone P, Chou LM, eds. *Snakes of medical importance (Asia-Pacific region).* Singapore University Press.

Warrell DA (2003). Epidemiology, clinical features and management of snakebites in Central and South America. In Campbell J, Lamar WW, Greene H, eds. *Venomous reptiles of the Americas.* Cornell University Press, Ithaca NY (in press).

Warrell DA, ed (1999). WHO/SEARO Guidelines for the clinical management of snake bites in the South East Asian region. *South East Asian Journal of Tropical Medicine and Public Health* **30**(Suppl 1), 1–85.

Venomous lizards

Bogert CM, Martin del Campo R (1956). The Gila monster and its allies. *Bulletin of the American Museum of Natural History* **109**, 1–238.

Preston CA (1989). Hypotension, myocardial infarction and coagulopathy following Gila monster bite. *Journal of Emergency Medicine* **7**, 37–40.

Russell FE, Bogert CM (1981). Gila monster, venom and bite—a review. *Toxicon* **19**, 341–59.

Poisonous amphibians

Brubacher JK, *et al.* (1996). Treatment of toad venom poisoning with digoxin-specific Fab fragments. *Chest* **110**, 1282–8.

Daly JW (1998). Thirty years of discovering arthropod alkaloids in amphibian skin. *Journal of Natural Products* **61**, 162–72.

Hitt M, Ettinger DD (1986). Toad toxicity. *New England Journal of Medicine* **314**, 1517–18.

Kwan T, Dino Paiusco A, Kohl L (1992). Digitalis toxicity caused by toad venom. *Chest* **102**, 949–50.

Myers CW, Daly JW, Malkin B (1978). A dangerously toxic new frog (Phyllobates) used by the Emberá Indians of Western Colombia with discussion of blowgun fabrication and dart poisons. *Bulletin of the American Museum of Natural History* **161**(Art 2), 307–66.

Poisonous birds

Dumbacher JP, *et al.* (1992). Homobatracho-toxin in the genus *Pitohui*: chemical defense in birds? *Science* **258**, 799–800.

Venomous fish

Castex MN (1967). Fresh water venomous rays. In: Russell FE, Saunders PR, eds. *Animal toxins*, pp 167–76. Pergamon Press, Oxford.

Halstead BW (1988). *Poisonous and venomous marine animals of the world*, 2nd revised edition. Darwin Press, Princeton.

Lehane L, Rawlin GT (2000). Topically acquired bacterial zoonoses from fish: a review. *Medical Journal of Australia* **173**, 256–9.

Maretić, Z. (1973). Some epidemiological, clinical and therapeutic aspects of envenomation by weever fish sting. In: De Vries A, Kochva E, eds. *Toxins of animal and plant origin*, pp 1055–65. Gordon and Breach, New York.

Sutherland SK, Tibballs J (2001). *Australian animal toxins. The creatures, their toxins and care of the poisoned patient*, 2nd edn. Oxford University Press, Melbourne.

Williamson JA, *et al.*, eds (1996). *Venomous and poisonous marine animals: a medical and biological handbook.* University of New South Wales Press, Sydney.

Poisoning by ingestion of aquatic animals

Bagnis RA, *et al.* (1979). Clinical observations on 3009 cases of Ciguatera (fish poisoning) in the Southern Pacific. *American Journal of Tropical Medicine and Hygiene* **28**, 1067–73.

Daranas AH, Norte M, Fernández JJ (2001). Toxic marine micro-algae. *Toxicon* **39**, 1101–32.

Halstead BW (1988). *Poisonous and venomous marine animals of the world*, 2nd revised edition. Darwin Press, Princeton.

Trishnananda M, *et al.* (1966). Poisoning following the ingestion of the horseshoe crab (*Carcinoscorpius rotundicauda*): report of four cases in Thailand. *Journal of Tropical Medicine and Hygiene* **69**, 194–6.

Uragoda CG, Kottegoda SR (1977). Adverse reactions to isoniazid on ingestion of fish with a high histamine content. *Tubercle* **58**, 83–9.

Williamson JA, *et al.*, eds. (1996). *Venomous and poisonous marine animals: a medical and biological handbook.* University of New South Wales Press, Sydney.

World Health Organization (1984). *Aquatic (marine and fresh water) biotoxins.* Environmental Health Criteria, 37. WHO, Geneva.

Poisoning by ingestion of carp's gallbladder

Lin YF, Lin SH (1999). Simultaneous acute renal and hepatic failure after ingesting raw carp gall bladder. *Nephrology, Dialysis and Transplantation* **14**, 2011–12.

Venomous marine invertebrates

Beadnell CE, *et al.* (1992). Management of a major box jellyfish (*Chironex fleckeri*) sting. *Medical Journal of Australia* **156**, 655–8.

Halstead BW (1988). *Poisonous and venomous marine animals of the world*, 2nd revised edn. Darwin Press, Princeton.

Hartwick R, *et al.* (1980). Disarming the box-jellyfish. Nematocyst inhibition in *Chironex fleckeri*. *Medical Journal of Australia* **1**, 15–20.

Martin JC, Audley I (1990). Cardiac failure following Irukandji envenomation. *Medical Journal of Australia* **153**, 164–6.

Olivera BM, Cruz LJ (2001). Conotoxins, in retrospect. *Toxicon* **39**, 7–14.

Pereira PL, *et al.* (2000). Pressure immobilisation bandages in first-aid treatment of jelly fish envenomation: current recommendation reconsidered. *Medical Journal of Australia* **173**, 650–2.

Sutherland SK, Tibballs J (2001). *Australian animal toxins. The creatures, their toxins and care of the poisoned patient*, 2nd edn. Oxford University Press, Melbourne.

Williamson JA, *et al.*, eds. (1996). *Venomous and poisonous marine animals: a medical and biological handbook.* University of New South Wales Press, Sydney.

Venomous arthropods

British Society for Allergy and Clinical Immunology Working Party (1993). Position paper on allergen immunotherapy. *Clinical and Experimental Allergy* 23(Suppl 3), 19–22.

de Shazo RD, Butcher BT, Banks WA (1990). Reactions to the stings of the imported fire ant. *New England Journal of Medicine* 323, 462–6.

França FOS, et al. (1994). Severe and fatal mass attacks by 'killer' bees (Africanised honey bees—*Apis mellifera scutellata* in Brazil: clinicopathological studies with measurement of serum venom concentrations. *Quarterly Journal of Medicine* 87, 269–82.

Hunt J Jr, et al. (1978). A controlled trial of immunotherapy in insect hypersensitivity. *New England Journal of Medicine* 2991, 157–61.

McHugh SM, et al. (1995). Bee venom immunotherapy induces a shift in cytokine responses from a TH-2 to a TH-1 dominant pattern: comparison of rush and conventional immunotherapy. *Clinical and Experimental Allergy* 25, 828–38.

Mueller UR (1990). *Insect sting allergy. Clinical picture, diagnosis and treatment.* Gustav Fischer, Stuttgart.

Piek T (1986). *Venoms of the* Hymenoptera. *Biochemical, pharmacological and behavioural aspects.* Academic Press, London.

Winston ML (1992). *Killer bees. The Africanized Honey Bee in the Americas.* Harvard University Press, Cambridge, Mass.

Venomous lepidoptera

Kelen EMA, Picarelli ZP, Duarte AC (1995). Hemorrhagic syndrome induced by contact with caterpillars of the genus *Lonomia* (Saturniidae, Hamileucinae). *Journal of Toxicology. Toxin Reviews* 14, 283–308.

Venomous coleoptera (beetles)

Eisner T, et al. (1990). Systemic retention of ingested cantharidin by frogs. *Chemoecology* 1, 57–62.

Frank JH, Kanamitsu K (1987). *Paederus sensulato* (Coleoptera: Staphylinidae): natural history and medical importance. *Journal of Medical Entomology* 24, 1555–91.

Roberts JI, Tonking HD (1935). Notes on an East African vesicant beetle, *Pederus crebripunctatus* Epp. *Annals of Tropical Medicine and Parasitology* 29, 415–20.

Southcott RV (1989). Injuries from Coleoptera. *Medical Journal of Australia* 151, 654–9.

Scorpions

Amaral CFS, et al. (1991). Electrocardiographic, enzymatic and echocardiographic evidence of myocardial damage after *Tityus serrulatus* scorpion poisoning. *American Journal of Cardiology* 67, 655–7.

Amaral CFS, De Rezende NA, Freire-Maia L (1993). Acute pulmonary edema after *Tityus serrulatus* scorpion sting in children. *American Journal of Cardiology* 71, 242–5.

Bawaskar HS, Bawaskar PH (1992). Management of the cardiovascular manifestations of poisoning by the Indian red scorpion (*Mesobuthus tamulus*). *British Heart Journal* 68, 478–80.

Bettini S, ed (1978). *Athropod venoms. Handbook of experimental pharmacology,* Vol 48, p 977. Springer-Verlag, Berlin.

Brownell P, Polis G, eds (2001). *Scorpion biology and research.* Oxford University Press, New York.

Fet V, et al., eds (2000). *Catalog of the scorpions of the world. (1758–1998).* New York Entomological Society, New York.

Freire-Maia L, Campos JA, Amaral CFS (1996). Treatment of scorpion envenoming in Brazil. In: Bon C, Goyffon M, eds. *Envenomings and their treatments,* pp 301–10. Edition Fondation Marcel Mérieux, Lyon.

Gueron M, Ilia R, Sofer S (1992). The cardiovascular system after scorpion envenomation. A review. *Clinical Toxicology* 30, 245–8.

Keegan HL (1980). *Scorpions of medical importance.* University Press of Mississippi, Jackson.

Polis GA, ed (1990). *The biology of scorpions.* Stanford University Press, Stanford, CA.

Radmanesh M (1990). Clinical study of *Hemiscorpion lepturus* in Iran. *Journal of Tropical Medicine and Hygiene* 93, 327–32.

Waterman JA (1938). Some notes on scorpion poisoning in Trinidad. *Transactions of the Society of Tropical Medicine and Hygiene* 31, 607–24.

Spiders

Clark RF, et al. (1992). Clinical presentation and treatment of black widow spider envenomation: a review of 163 cases. *Annals of Emergency Medicine* 21, 782–7.

Maretić Z, Lebez D (1979). *Araneism with special reference to Europe.* Novit, Pula-Ljubjan, Yugoslavia.

Southcott RV (1976). Arachnidism and allied syndromes in the Australian region. *Records of the Adelaide Children's Hospital* 1, 97–186.

Sutherland SK, Tibballs J (2001). *Australian animal toxins. The creatures, their toxins and care of the poisoned patient,* 2nd edn. Oxford University Press, Melbourne.

Warrell DA, et al. (1991). Neurotoxic envenoming by an immigrant spider (*Steatoda nobilis*) in southern England. *Toxicon* 29, 1263–5.

Ticks

Gothe R, Kunze K, Hoogstraal H (1979). The mechanism of pathogenicity in the tick paralyses. *Journal of Medical Entomology* 16, 357–69.

Murnaghan MF, O'Rourke FJ (1978). Tick paralysis. In: Bettini S, ed. *Arthropod venoms. Handbook of experimental pharmacology,* Vol 48, p 419. Springer-Verlag, Berlin.

Pearn J (1977). The clinical features of tick bite. *Medical Journal of Australia* 2, 313.

Stone BF (1987). Toxicoses induced by ticks and reptiles in domestic animals. In: Harris JB, ed. *Natural toxins: animal, plant and microbial,* pp 56–71. Oxford University Press, Oxford.

Millipedes

Bettini S, ed (1978). *Arthropod venoms. Handbook of experimental pharmacology,* Vol 48, p 977. Springer-Verlag, Berlin.

Radford AJ (1975). Millipede burns in man. *Tropical and Geographical Medicine* 27, 279–87.

Leeches

Adams SL (1988). The medicinal leech. A page from the Annelids of Internal Medicine. *Annals of Internal Medicine* 109, 399–405.

Cundall DB (1986). Severe anaemia and death due to the pharyngeal leech *Myxobdella africana. Transactions of the Royal Society of Tropical Medicine and Hygiene* 80, 940–4.

Editorial (1992). Hirudins: return of the leech? *Lancet* 340, 579–80.

Keegan HL (1963). Leeches as pests of man in the Pacific region. In: Keegan HL, McFarlane WR, eds. *Venomous and poisonous animals and noxious plants of the Pacific region,* pp 99–104. Pergamon Press, Oxford.

Sawyer RT (1986). *Leech biology and behaviour.* Oxford University Press, Oxford.

Snower DP, et al., eds (1989). *Aeromonas hydrophila* infection associated with the use of medicinal leeches. *Journal of Clinical Microbiology* 27, 1421–2.

Websites

WCH Clinical Toxinology Resource (covers venomous animals world-wide).
    www.toxinology.com.
Venomous Snake Systematics.
    sbsweb.bangor.ac.uk/˜bss166/update.htm.
Australian Venom Unit.
    www.pharmacology.unimelb.edn.au/avruweb/index.htm.
Shark attacks.
    www.flmnh.ufl.edu/fish/Sharks/ISAF/ISAF.htm.
Arachnids.
    www.ufsia.ac.be/Arachnology.

8.3 Poisonous plants and fungi

M. R. Cooper, A. W. Johnson, and H. Persson

There are relatively few plants and fungi that cause serious poisoning, but some have a very wide geographical distribution: in this group are oleanders (*Nerium* and *Thevetia* spp.), monkshood (*Aconitum napellus*), thorn apple (*Datura* spp.), angels' trumpets (*Brugmansia* spp.), *Euphorbia* spp. and the death cap fungus (*Amanita phalloides*).

Most incidents with plants occur in small children and are entirely accidental. Adults may sometimes confuse edible and toxic plants, but are more often poisoned by deliberate ingestion of those with psychoactive properties; ingestion of toxic plants as a means of suicide occurs sporadically in most parts of the world but in Sri Lanka and South India yellow oleander (*Thevetia peruviana*) is a common agent of suicide. In many countries poisoning by fungi is a more prominent medical problem than poisoning by plants, and is mostly the result of misidentification.

The general principles for treatment of poisoning outlined elsewhere (see Chapter 8.1) also apply to plant and fungal poisoning. In most cases only simple measures (applied at home) are necessary, such as rinsing of the mouth and giving peroral fluids for dilution. However, if a highly toxic plant or fungus has been ingested in significant amounts, energetic gut decontamination is required, including gastric emptying and administration of activated charcoal, to which most of the toxins bind well. Symptomatic and supportive care should be given as necessary, and specific antidotes are available for a few types of poisoning.

Plant poisoning

Clinical effects can be used to classify plant poisoning. However, poisoning by some plants causes symptoms of more than one type, and the severity may vary according to the sensitivity of the individual.

Digestive tract irritation

Some plants have very irritant sap: that of cuckoo pint (*Arum maculatum*), dumb cane (*Dieffenbachia* spp.) (Plate 1), elephant's ear (*Philodendron* spp.), and black bryony (*Tamus communis*) contains calcium oxalate, and that of *Euphorbia* spp., mezereon, and spurge laurel (*Daphne* spp.) diterpene esters. These cause immediate soreness, reddening, and even blistering of the lips and mouth, salivation, and dysphagia.

With most plants, however, the first signs of poisoning are nausea, abdominal cramps, and vomiting. In many cases the vomiting may eliminate the poisonous substances and partly prevent the development of further toxic effects; elimination is also promoted by the associated diarrhoea. Toxic agents causing irritation of the stomach and intestines include anthraquinones found in *Aloe* spp. and purging buckthorn (*Rhamnus cathartica*), cytisine in *Laburnum* spp. (Plate 2), lectins in *Jatropha*, protoanemonin in *Anemone* spp. and *Helleborus* spp., saponins in horse chestnut (*Aesculus hippocastanum*) and ivy (*Hedera* spp.), and viscotoxins in mistletoe (*Viscum album*). Unidentified irritants are present in white bryony (*Bryonia dioica*), holly (*Ilex* spp.), *Lantana camara*, privet (*Ligustrum vulgare*), pokeweed (*Phytolacca americana*), and snowberry (*Symphoricarpos alba*). With other plants, some of which are much more toxic than those mentioned so far, the start of gastrointestinal symptoms is delayed for several hours (up to 2 days). The toxins responsible include colchicine in autumn crocus (*Colchicum autumnale*) and glory lily (*Gloriosa superba*), the very highly toxic lectins in jequirity beans (*Abrus precatorius*) (Plate 3), castor beans (*Ricinus communis*) (Plate 4), and false acacia (*Robinia pseudoacacia*), oxalic acid in some members of the Polygonaceae family, solanine in *Solanum* spp. (Plate 5), and unidentified agents, such as that in spindle (*Euonymus europaeus*).

After ingestion of plants containing irritant sap, rational procedures to follow are rinsing of the mouth and dilution by drinking fluids; the addition of activated charcoal may be beneficial. Gastric emptying is rarely indicated, unless large amounts or highly toxic plants have been ingested. Symptomatic care is given as required.

Cardiovascular disturbances

In addition to the well-known effects of the cardiac glycosides of foxglove (*Digitalis purpurea*) (Plate 6), there are various other plants that produce the digitalis-like effects seen in digoxin overdosage (see Chapter 15.5.1): lily of the valley (*Convallaria majalis*), bluebell (*Hyacinthoides non-scripta*), oleander (*Nerium oleander*) (Plate 7), and yellow oleander (*Thevetia peruviana*). Cardiovascular effects are also induced by aconitine in *Aconitum* spp. (Plate 8) and larkspurs (*Delphinium* spp.). Aconitine causes a burning sensation in the mouth and pharynx, gastrointestinal symptoms, paraesthesia, and, in particular, cardiac arrhythmias (mainly ventricular) that may prove fatal. Other examples of cardiovascular toxins are: andromedotoxins (grayanotoxins) in mountain laurel (*Kalmia latifolia*), *Menziesia* spp., *Pieris* spp., and *Rhododendron* spp., phoratoxin in American mistletoes (*Phoradendron* spp.), proveratrines in *Veratrum* spp., taxines in yews (*Taxus* spp.) (Plate 9), and veratrine in death camas (*Zigadenus* spp.). These cardiac glycosides also irritate the digestive tract.

Gastric emptying (avoid ipecacuanha) is performed and activated charcoal administered if the ingested dose and time since ingestion indicate its usefulness. In addition to symptomatic and supportive care, digoxin-specific antibodies (ovine Fab fragments such as 'Digibind' and 'DigiTab') have been used successfully in reversing life-threatening digitalis effects in plant poisoning, notably poisoning by *Thevetia peruviana* (Apocynaceae), a common agent of suicide in South Asia, and anecdotally in poisoning by other Apocynaceae and even toad skin toxins. In experimental animals, fructose-1,6-diphosphate has also proved effective. Ingestion of aconitine alkaloids also requires vigorous gastrointestinal decontamination, careful cardiac monitoring, and treatment of arrhythmias.

Central nervous effects

Some plants contain hallucinogenic compounds, for which they are smoked, chewed, eaten, or infused in water to make teas. Among the plant hallucinogens are tetrahydrocannabinols in cannabis (*Cannabis sativa*), alkaloids in khat (*Catha edulis*) (Plate 10), D-lysergic acid amide in morning glory (*Ipomoea* spp.), mescaline in peyote (*Lophophora williamsii*), myristicin in nutmeg (*Myristica fragrans*), and vincristine and vinblastine in periwinkle (*Vinca* spp.); others contain hyoscine (see atropine-like effects below).

Patients who have taken hallucinogens require reassurance and supportive treatment.

A number of plants contain convulsants, although actual clinical cases mainly involve Umbelliferae, such as cowbane (*Cicuta virosa*) and hemlock water dropwort (*Oenanthe crocata*) that contain cicutoxin and oenanthotoxin respectively. Other convulsants include hypoglycin A in ackee (*Blighia sapida*), coriamyrtin in *Coriaria myrtifolia*, anthracenones in *Karwinskia humboldtiana*, tetranortriterpenes in chinaberry (*Melia azedarach*), alkaloids in moonseed (*Menispermum canadense*), podophylloresin in May apple (*Podophyllum peltatum*), and strychnine and brucine in nux vomica (*Strychnos nux-vomica*). Cicutoxin, one of the most potent convulsants known, may cause an extremely dramatic syndrome with gastroenteritis, increased secretions, and long-lasting intense episodes of generalized tonic-clonic convulsions, resulting in severe metabolic acidosis and multiple organ failure. Consumption of unripe ackee fruit (*Blighia sapida*) causes epidemic vomiting (Jamaican vomiting sickness) and a toxic hypoglycaemic syndrome which can result in fatal encephalopathy.

Treatment is symptomatic and supportive, aiming at control of convulsions and secondary effects.

Atropine-like effects

The tropane alkaloids atropine, hyoscine (scopolamine), and hyoscyamine present in some plants of the Solanaceae competitively inhibit the muscarinic effects of acetylcholine and block the parasympathetic nervous system. This will cause a classic anticholinergic syndrome. *Datura stramonium* is used as a hallucinogen in parts of Africa (for example in Niger where it is known as 'sobi-lobi') (Plate 18). The symptoms may vary depending on the proportion of the alkaloids in the different plants. Typical is a warm, dry-skinned and dry-mouthed, thirsty, anxious, excited, and hallucinating patient. Facial flushing, tachycardia, and mydriasis are also common. In serious cases, arrhythmias, urinary retention, psychosis, convulsions, coma, and respiratory failure may ensue; fatal outcome has been reported. The plants in this group include angels' trumpets (*Brugmansia* spp.) (Plate 17) and thorn apple (*Datura stramonium*), which are among the most common plants involved in poisoning cases worldwide, deadly nightshade (*Atropa belladonna*) (Plate 16) and henbane (*Hyoscyamus niger*). Unilateral dilatation of the pupil (gardener's mydriasis), usually without systemic effects, may be seen in gardeners who rub their eyes after handling members of the Solanaceae such as angels' trumpets (*Brugmansia* spp.).

Gastrointestinal decontamination is performed, if appropriate, considering ingested dose and time since ingestion. A quiet environment, with reassurance and good symptomatic and supportive care, is basic. In cases where typical central and peripheral anticholinergic effects are present, specific treatment with physostigmine, 1 to 2 mg intravenously in adults (children 0.02 to 0.04 mg/kg), may be useful in reversing hallucinations, delirium, and psychotic behaviour. Physostigmine should be withheld if cardiotoxic agents have been ingested or there is widening of the QRS complexes.

Nicotine-like effects

Nicotine in tobacco plants (*Nicotiana tabacum*) and other alkaloids with similar actions, such as coniine from hemlock (*Conium maculatum*) (Plate 15), used for judicial executions in ancient Athens, first stimulate and then paralyse all autonomic ganglia. Centrally, small doses cause respiratory stimulation, while large doses can lead to convulsions and arrest of respiration. Many other symptoms may occur but they are complex and unpredictable. Nicotine-like effects occur with gelsemine and related alkaloids in yellow jessamine (*Gelsemium sempervirens*), cytisine in *Laburnum* spp., and lobeline in *Lobelia* spp.

Gastrointestinal decontamination by gastric lavage (not ipecacuanha-induced emesis because of rapid onset of symptoms) and administration of activated charcoal are indicated at an early stage. In severe cases, extensive symptomatic and supportive care may be necessary.

Liver damage

Various plants in the Compositae (*Senecio* spp.), Leguminosae (*Crotalaria* spp.), and Boraginaceae (*Heliotropium* and *Symphytum* spp.) (Plate 11) as well as some in other families contain pyrrolizidine alkaloids, which principally affect the liver. Poisoning has occurred from contamination of cereal crops by these plants and their subsequent incorporation into bread, and from their use in herbal medicines and bush teas. These alkaloids can cause acute damage to the liver (veno-occlusive disease), which has occurred mainly in Jamaica, India, and Afghanistan. Symptoms, including nausea, abdominal pain and distension, hepatomegaly, and sometimes fever and vomiting, first appear a few days after ingestion. A chronic cirrhosis of the liver can occur in people ingesting small quantities of pyrrolizidine alkaloids over a long period.

Treatment can only be supportive as, once absorbed, there is no specific method of preventing the toxic effects of these alkaloids.

Kidney damage

This can occur after ingestion of plants rich in oxalates, for example the leaves of rhubarb (*Rheum rhabarbarum*) and docks and sorrels (*Rumex* spp.). Nephrotoxicity may also occur after ingestion of terpene-containing plants, such as *Daphne mezereum* and *Juniperus sabina*.

Fluid replacement is essential and generous hydration advisable to promote renal excretion of oxalates.

Hydrocyanic acid toxicity

Parts of some plants contain relatively high concentrations of cyanogenic glycosides. The most likely sources are the kernels of fruits of *Prunus* species (almonds, apricots, cherries, peaches, etc.) or of loquat (*Eriobotrya japonica*), a large number of apple pips (*Malus* spp.), the berries or leaves of the cherry laurel (*Prunus laurocerasus*), or inadequately prepared cassava (*Manihot esculenta*) (see below). The glycosides will release cyanide only when the kernels or other plant material are being chewed. This takes some time, so the onset of symptoms is not so rapid as after ingestion of inorganic cynanide compounds. In practice, cyanide poisoning from plants (with the exception of cassava) is a rare phenomenon.

When it is suspected that large amounts of cyanogenic glycosides have been ingested, gastrointestinal decontamination is indicated. If typical symptoms ensue, treatment is the same as for hydrocyanic acid poisoning from any other source (see Chapter 8.1).

Skin damage

The most common form of skin damage by plants is a non-allergic dermatitis that results from direct contact with various plants that contain irritants, for example the stinging hairs of the stinging nettle (*Urtica dioica*), the diterpene-containing latex of *Euphorbia* spp., or the calcium oxalate crystals of *Dieffenbachia* spp. and other members of the Araceae family. There are also allergic forms of dermatitis that result from hypersensitivity to plant allergens. The most common and severe forms of allergic contact dermatitis in the United States are caused by poison ivy (*Rhus radicans*) (Plate 12) and western poison oak (*Toxicodendron diversilobum*), and in the United Kingdom by a primula (*Primula obconica*), but such cutaneous hypersensitivity can occur to a very large number of vascular plants.

Contact with the sap of some plants followed by exposure to sunlight (ultraviolet radiation) can give rise to a characteristic skin reaction. Phototoxic psoralens (furanocoumarins) are present in various members of the Umbelliferae, including giant hogweed (*Heracleum mantegazzianum*) (Plate 13), other *Heracleum* spp., and parsnips (*Pastinaca sativa*), and also celery (*Apium graveolens*), especially when infected with the pink rot fungus (*Sclerotinia sclerotiorum*). Other psoralen-containing plants are rue (*Ruta graveolens*) (Plate 14) and the gas plant (*Dictamnus albus*). Typical lesions in dermatitis caused by psoralens are erythema, papules, vesicles, and enormous bullae localized to exposed areas of skin.

Treatment is as for a chemical burn. Psoralens can also induce hyper-pigmentation that can last for several months.

Food plant toxicity

The following toxins are present in plants used regularly for food:

1. Lectins. These phytohaemagglutinins are glycoproteins, and beans (Leguminosae) are the main food source. The lectins are not readily digested by pepsin and have a strong affinity for the intestinal mucosa, where they prevent absorption of carbohydrates. Adequate cooking destroys the lectins, but eating raw or incompletely cooked beans can cause diarrhoea, while long-term exposure can lead to retarded growth and may even be fatal.

2. Cyanogens. Cyanogenic glycosides are present in some staple foods, such as cassava, sweet potato, and yam, all of which can be made safe to eat by adequate soaking, drying, or fermentation. Chronic poisoning may cause tropical ataxic neuropathy and spastic paraparesis ('konzo').

3. Alkaloids. Dangerously high quantities of these may develop in some plant foods, for example potato tubers that have sprouted or been stored in the light and become green. The green colour is chlorophyll and is harmless, but under conditions where greening occurs the gly-coalkaloid solanine and its derivatives will also have been produced; these exhibit anticholinesterase activity.

4. Oxalates. These accumulate in some members of the Polygonaceae, notably rhubarb, of which only the red leaf stalks should be eaten, and then only after cooking.

5. Polyphenols. These are a possible cause of upper digestive tract cancers that may develop after eating sorghum, or taking teas or alcoholic drinks containing high concentrations of tannins.

Some specific diseases attributable to plants are: lathyrism, a paralytic disease caused by a neurotoxic amino acid in chick peas (*Lathyrus sativus*); favism that occurs among natives of some Mediterranean and Middle Eastern countries who have a genetic deficiency of glucose-6-phosphate dehydrogenase and cannot digest broad (fava) beans (*Vicia faba*); and Jamaican vomiting sickness that results from eating the unripe fruits of the ackee (*Blighia sapida*). Other foods that cause poisoning are the seeds of *Mucuna pruriens*, flour ground from the cones of cycads (for example *Zamia* spp.) (Plate 19), and young fronds of bracken fern (*Pteridium aquilinum*).

Herbal medicines

It should not be assumed that herbal preparations are safe because they are 'natural', and some may have harmful effects that are not immediately obvious, for example carcinogenicity, hepatotoxicity, or teratogenicity. For example, plants of the genus *Aristolochia* are constituents or contaminants of some Chinese herbal medicines (such as 'Mu Tong' and 'Fang Ji') and can cause genotoxic carcinogenesis and interstitial nephritis. Adulteration of herbal medicines with cheaper ingredients, heavy metals, and orthodox drugs is not uncommon.

Fungal poisoning

Fungal poisoning (mycetismus) is a sporadic problem in many parts of the world. It is usually accidental, occasionally homicidal or suicidal, and may become epidemic when conventional food is scarce in times of war or famine. In 2000, outbreaks of mushroom poisoning involving 212 people with 17 deaths were reported from Voronezh and Volgograd in Russia.

The toxicity of fungi may vary with location, season, and in different years; for some mushroom toxins there may also be a variation in the susceptibility of individuals. Cases of fungal poisoning can be classified into those that develop signs of toxicity within a few hours of ingestion, or after a delay of 10 (occasionally 6) to 24 h or several days.

Symptoms that develop within a few hours

Gastroenteritis

Few of the chemical agents responsible for this type of poisoning have been identified. The fungi in this group include flat-capped psalliota (*Agaricus placomyces* or *A. praeclavesquamosus*), yellow-staining mushroom (*Agaricus xanthodermus*), honey fungus (*Armillaria mellea*), the devil's mushroom (*Boletus satanas*), *Chlorophyllum molybdites* (*Lepiota morgani*), *Entoloma* spp., *Hebeloma* spp., wax caps (*Hygrocybe* spp.), sulphur tuft (*Hypholoma fasciculare*), milk caps (*Lactarius* spp.), shaggy parasol (*Macrolepiota rhacodes*), broad-gilled agaric (*Megacollybia platyphylla*), Jack-o'lantern or copper trumpet (*Omphalotus olearius*), pink coral fungus (*Ramaria formosa*), brittle gills (*Russula* spp.), earthballs (*Scleroderma* spp.), and spotted tricholoma (*Tricholoma pardinum*).

Gastrointestinal symptoms usually start within a few hours and resolve fairly quickly, but are sometimes more intense and result in fluid and electrolyte imbalance.

Treatment is symptomatic and admission to hospital is seldom necessary, but may occasionally be required, especially in children and the elderly.

Cholinergic symptoms

The parasympathomimetic effects of muscarine, which is the toxic ingredient of certain *Inocybe* and *Clitocybe* species, include abdominal pain and diarrhoea, sweating, lacrimation, salivation, myosis, bronchorrhoea, and sometimes bronchospasm, bradycardia, and hypotension. Only trace amounts of muscarine occur in fly agaric (*Amanita muscaria*) (Plate 20) after which the toxin was named.

Treatment is specific and includes 1 to 2 mg of atropine in adults (children 0.02 mg/kg) that effectively antagonizes muscarinic overstimulation. The dose is repeated as required.

Mental confusion

This may result from poisoning by panther cap (*Amanita pantherina*), fly agaric (*Amanita muscaria*), and *Amanita strobiliformis*, whose active ingredients are isoxazoles (ibotenic acid and muscimol) that act as γ-aminobutyric acid agonists. Anxiety, euphoria, visual disturbances, erratic behaviour, hallucinations, and gastrointestinal symptoms may occur, and peripheral anticholinergic symptoms are also frequently observed; the occasional appearance of muscarine symptoms in *Amanita muscaria* poisoning is a rare phenomenon.

Treatment is symptomatic and supportive. Diazepam, 5 to 10 mg in adults (children 0.1 to 0.2 mg/kg), repeated as required, can be given for sedation. In severe cases with evident psychotic behaviour, chlorpromazine or haloperidol may be useful.

Hallucinations

These are mainly visual and are the predominant feature in poisoning by psilocybin, a tryptamine derivative. Psilocybin and related substances are found in *Psilocybe* species and several other genera of (usually small) fungi, often collectively called 'magic mushrooms'; among these are some *Conocybe* spp., *Gymnopilus* spp., *Panaeolina foenisecii*, *Panaeolus* spp., *Pluteus* spp., and *Stropharia* spp. These fungi are eaten because of their psychoactive properties. The effects of the toxin are similar to those of LSD (stimulation of central and blockade of peripheral serotonin receptors). Other early symptoms are relaxation, euphoria, depersonalization, and altered sense of time and space. Less pleasurable, but equally typical symptoms, are vertigo, bizarre and terrifying hallucinations, anxiety, agitation, tachycardia, mydriasis, and flushing. Gastrointestinal symptoms, apart from nausea, are uncommon. Occasionally fever and seizures are observed in children. Sometimes frightening flashbacks occur after days or weeks.

Treatment is symptomatic, with reassurance and rest in a quiet environment. In cases of severe anxiety and agitation, diazepam may be given; in addition haloperidol or chlorpromazine is often necessary.

Alcohol-associated effects

When alcohol is taken at the same time as some fungi, notably an ink cap (*Coprinus atramentarius*) but also club foot (*Clitocybe clavipes*), or up to 5 days after they are eaten, a reaction similar to that induced by disulfiram (Antabuse) used for treating alcoholics (see Chapter 26.7.1) is produced. The skin becomes flushed, and sweating, mydriasis, nausea, anxiety, dyspnoea, and hypotension can occur as a result of the accumulation of acetaldehyde, because the toxin (named coprine in *C. atramentarius*) blocks the liver enzyme aldehyde dehydrogenase.

Treatment is symptomatic and supportive.

Symptoms with delayed onset

Severe gastroenteritis

Gastrointestinal symptoms that appear after a long latent period followed by liver damage, and sometimes also by kidney damage, are typical of poisoning by amatoxins, a group of cyclic octapeptides occurring in the death cap (*Amanita phalloides*) (Plate 21), which is by far the most common cause of death from the ingestion of fungi. Amatoxins also occur in the destroying angel (*Amanita virosa*), the fool's mushroom (*Amanita verna*) and some *Galerina* and *Lepiota* spp. (in particular *Galerina marginata* and *Lepiota cristata*). These toxins inhibit transcription from DNA to mRNA by blocking RNA polymerase II (B). This results in deficient protein synthesis and subsequent cell death. The main target organs are the intestinal mucosa, liver, and kidneys.

Abdominal pain and vomiting, but in particular a severe, watery diarrhoea, start 10 to 24 h (more rarely at 6 h but normally around 12 h) after ingestion. Dehydration and exhaustion will ensue. Sometimes there is a transient recovery, after which the signs and symptoms of liver damage gradually appear from the second day. Hepatic failure may ensue, and this is the cause of death in fatal cases. Impaired kidney function is common initially because of dehydration; kidney dysfunction at a later stage is normally an indication of toxic renal damage and is a poor prognostic sign.

The mainstay of treatment is early admission to hospital, with rapid correction of fluid, electrolyte, and metabolic disturbances, adequate and preferably slightly increased diuresis for the first few days, and multiple oral doses of activated charcoal until 3 days after ingestion. Silibinin (also called silybin or silymarin), the main active constituent of milk thistle (*Silybum marianum*), reduces hepatic amatoxin uptake and, although its value in the clinical setting is controversial, it should be considered in patients who present after significant ingestion, as judged from their history and clinical findings. The dose of silibinin is 5 mg/kg intravenously over 1 h, followed by 20 mg/kg/24 h as a continuous infusion for 3 days after ingestion. Benzylpenicillin in large doses may be an alternative, if silibinin is not available. Haemodialysis or haemoperfusion is not indicated, unless the patient is admitted very early and before the onset of symptoms (very unusual) or in cases where there is pre-existing renal dysfunction. Liver transplantation may be the only therapeutic option.

Gastrointestinal and central nervous effects

The toxin gyromitrin, found in the false morel (*Gyromitra esculenta*), decomposes in the stomach to form hydrazines (in particular monomethylhydrazine). Hydrazines block pyridoxine synthesis, cause glutathione depletion in erythrocytes, and form free oxygen radicals that may bind to macromolecules in the liver. Gastrointestinal symptoms, associated with headache, vertigo, sweating, diplopia, nystagmus, ataxia, cramps, delirium, and sometimes coma, appear 6 to 24 h after ingestion or inhalation of cooking vapour. Severe poisoning may also cause hypoglycaemia, hepatic damage, and haemolysis; renal damage has also been reported.

Apart from symptomatic and supportive care, treatment includes administration of pyridoxine at 25 mg/kg over 30 min to prevent and control neurological symptoms; repeat doses may be required. It is advisable to administer a glucose infusion and to maintain adequate diuresis.

Kidney failure

Poisoning characterized by kidney dysfunction after a latent period of 2 to 4 days, in milder cases even up to 2 weeks, is typical of the group of brownish-orange *Cortinarius* spp. (*C. orellanus*, *C. speciosissimus*, and *C. splendens*) that contain orellanine, a highly nephrotoxic tetrahydroxylated di-*N*-oxidized bipyridine, and some less toxic derivatives such as orelline. During the latent period some patients may have diffuse gastrointestinal symptoms (often a day or more after the mushroom meal), but this is not the rule. This lack of early warning signs makes *Cortinarius* poisoning especially insidious, and patients are almost invariably admitted to hospital when the renal damage is already established and treatment procedures to prevent the toxic effects are no longer relevant. Typically, symptoms appear days after the meal, with fatigue, intense thirst, headache, chills, and abdominal, lumbar, and flank pain. After a transient polyuric phase, oliguria and anuria may follow. Renal function will recover in some cases, whereas in others kidney failure is permanent.

As these patients are normally admitted very late, management possibilities are restricted to monitoring of renal function and symptomatic care, including haemodialysis. In cases of persistent renal failure, kidney transplantation may be an alternative to chronic dialysis. If admitted during the first day, vigorous gut decontamination and haemoperfusion for poison elimination may be considered on theoretical grounds.

Allergic reactions

The roll-rim cap (*Paxillus involutus*) (Plate 22), previously eaten with impunity, may suddenly give rise to an immunohaemolytic anaemia in which decreased haemoglobin levels result in shock and even renal insufficiency. A respiratory allergy, called farmer's lung, results from inhaling spores of the mould *Faenia rectivergula* that is sometimes present on grain or hay. Spores of oyster mushrooms (*Pleurotus ostreatus*) or puffballs (*Lycoperdon* spp.) can also cause respiratory allergies. Skin allergies have been reported with the shiitake mushroom (*Lentinus elodes*).

Ergotism and mycotoxicoses

The ascomycete fungus *Claviceps purpurea* infects (Plate 23) cereal crops, in which its hard, purplish-black fruiting bodies or sclerotia (ergots) develop in the seed heads. Ergots contain several alkaloids that can cause disease when flour made from contaminated grain is eaten. There are two forms of ergotism ('St Anthony's fire'): vasoconstriction, sometimes leading to loss of extremities through gangrene (occurring after small quantities of contaminated food have been eaten over a long period) and a less common, acute form characterized by muscular tremors, convulsions, and hallucinations.

Other potent toxins (mycotoxins) are produced by some moulds (*Acremonium*, *Alternaria*, *Aspergillus*, *Fusarium*, *Penicillium*) that develop on growing crops, particularly if wet and harvested late, but occur mainly in cereal grains, rice, or nuts stored under damp, inadequately ventilated conditions. Intoxication may result from ingestion or inhalation. Aflatoxins (from *Aspergillus* spp.), ochratoxins (from *Aspergillus ochraceus* and *Penicillium verrucosum*), and trichothecenes and zearalenone (from *Fusarium* spp.) have been detected in foods and are suspected of causing immunosuppression, myelosuppression, hepatotoxicity, nephrotoxicity, neurotoxicity, dermatotoxicity, oestrogenicity, mutagenicity, teratogenicity, and carcinogenicity (liver, colon, alveolar cells). Ochratoxin A, which inhibits mitochondrial oxidative phosphorylation in the proximal tubule of the nephron, has been implicated as a possible cofactor in Balkan nephropathy.

Specific mycotoxins can be detected at 0.1 ng/ml by radioimmunoassay and enzyme immunoassay.

Sources of information

A directory of poison information centres worldwide is kept by the International Programme on Chemical Safety (IPCS), WHO, Geneva. A computerized, image-based, identification system for poisonous plants and fungi has been developed by the Royal Botanic Gardens, Kew, in collaboration with the Medical Toxicology Unit of Guy's and St Thomas' Hospital Trust, London. The system, called *Poisonous Plants and Fungi in Britain and Ireland* is available on CD-ROM from the Royal Botanic Gardens, Kew. Similar systems are being developed for other countries.

Further reading

Bresinsky A, Besl H (1990). *A colour atlas of poisonous fungi. A handbook for pharmacists, doctors, and biologists*, transl. N.G. Bisset. Wolfe, London.

Cooper MR, Johnson AW (1998). *Poisonous plants and fungi in Britain. Animal and human poisoning*, 2nd edn. The Stationery Office, London.

Eddleston M *et al.* (2000). Anti-digoxin Fab fragments in cardiotoxicity induced by ingestion of yellow oleander: a randomised controlled trial. *The Lancet* **355**, 967–72.

Everist SL (1981). *Poisonous plants of Australia*, 2nd edn. Angus and Robertson, Sydney.

Frohne D, Pfänder HJ (1997). *Giftpflanzen: ein Handbuch für Apotheker, Ärzte, Toxikologen und Biologen*, 4th edn. Wissenschaftliche Verlagsgesellschaft, Stuttgart. (An English translation of the first edition, by N.G. Bisset was published as *A colour atlas of poisonous plants* by Wolfe, London, 1984.)

Lovell CR (1993). *Plants and the skin*. Blackwell Scientific, Oxford.

Malloy CD, Marr JS (1997). Mycotoxins and public health. *Journal of Public Health Management Practice* (3) 61–9.

Meda HA *et al.* (1999) Epidemic of fatal encephalopathy in preschool children in Burkina Faso and consumption of unripe ackee (*Blighia sapida*) fruit. *The Lancet* **353**, 536–40.

Parish RC, Doering PL (1986). Treatment of *Amanita* mushroom poisoning. A review. *Veterinary and Human Toxicology* **28**, 318–22.

Turner NJ, Szczawinski AF (1991). *Common poisonous plants and mushrooms of North America*. Timber Press, Portland, OR. (Reprinted 1995.)

Watt JM, Breyer-Brandwijk MG (1962). *The medicinal and poisonous plants of southern and eastern Africa*, 2nd edn. Livingstone, Edinburgh.

8.4 Occupational and environmental health and safety

8.4.1 Occupational and environmental health and safety

J. M. Harrington with contributions from K. Gardiner, I. S. Foulds, T. C. Aw, E. L. Baker, and A. Spurgeon

General introduction

J. M. Harrington

Definition and scope

Occupational health is that area of public health concerned with managing the health of working people. Occupational health professionals include physicians, nurses, hygienists (scientists with experience in monitoring and more importantly controlling the exposure of working people to chemical, physical, and biological agents in their place of work), toxicologists, and—increasingly these days—psychologists to the assess the psychosocial aspects of work. Safety engineers are responsible for prevention and investigation of accidents at work (see under Occupational safety).

Occupational health issues can be promoted by these professionals, but for long-term success it is crucial that both managers and the workforce consider it an integral part of their working practices and philosophy. It is in everyone's interest that the workforce is 'happy, healthy, and here'!

History of occupational disease

Stone Age flint knappers were probably exposed to airborne silica dust during their work. However, life expectancy then was probably shorter than the pathogenesis of silicosis. Some industries like mining have always been hazardous. The ancient Egyptians recognized this by restricting such work to slaves and criminals. By the Middle Ages, the plight of the free miner had been recognized by Georgius Agricola (1494–1555) and Paracelsus (1493–1541). Agricola not only described the 'galloping consumption' of Carpathian silver miners but also proposed ways of reducing the dust in mines by improved ventilation.

The first authoritative treatise on occupational disease was written by Ramazzini (1633–1764). His book *De Morbis Artificium* is unsurpassed in its classic descriptions of many occupational diseases ranging from mercurialism in mirror workers to repetitive strain injury in clerical workers. The Industrial Revolution in Britain brought occupational diseases to the attention of Parliament, largely through the work of philanthropists like Robert Owen, Robert Peel, and Lord Shaftesbury. Early legislation to control the worst vicissitudes of factory labour was emasculated by Parliament but the process had begun. The First Act of 1802 (which, interestingly, introduced the concept of limiting the hours of work) was followed by others leading to the 1833 Act which saw the start of His/Her Majesty's Factory Inspectorate (HMFI)—an enforcing authority.

By the early twentieth century the toxic effects of arsenic, mercury, phosphorus, and lead were so common that notification of these diseases became required by law and compensation for ill health was granted. Clearly, working conditions in the Western world have improved greatly since then but the recent revelations about factory life in Eastern Europe as well as the working conditions for many in Third World countries demonstrate an important tenet of occupational health practice: that is, while occupational disease may be preventable, the continued—often necessary—use of hazardous materials and processes ensures that many such diseases cannot be eliminated, only controlled.

Occupational health services

The notion that employers should provide health care for workers is hardly new. During the fourteenth century, the Pope — not an employer in this connection! — decreed that prostitutes should be examined regularly for evidence of sexually transmitted disease. Whether the results were significant epidemiologically is not recorded. The first recognizable occupational health service in England began in the mid eighteenth century when the London (Quaker) Lead Company recognized the adverse effect of mining on workers and provided health and welfare services in northwest England. Since then, occupational health provision has expanded along different lines in different countries.

The International Labour Organization (Convention 161, 1985) urged members 'to develop progressively occupational health services for all workers …. The provision made should be adequate and appropriate to the specific needs of the undertaking.' Services are not universally available and interpretation of the requirements varies greatly between countries and employment sectors. Initially, most services arose from a mixture of philanthropy and self-interest; the theory being that the healthy worker was likely to be more productive. Present-day services range from total health care including primary care and hospital medicine (as in the states of Eastern Europe), to industry-specific systems concerned almost solely with the adverse health effects of a single industrial environment (as with the extractive, offshore, and chemical industries). Services in the United States and much of Europe may include general health promotion and education, but much inequity in health care exists between enterprises within the same country.

Recent increase in the provision of occupational health services has followed the enactment of effective health and safety legislation. The Health and Safety at Work etc. Act (1974) in the United Kingdom is an example. Some countries such as the Nordic countries, The Netherlands, and Australia, require the provision of occupational health services by law. Statutory provision of such services in the United Kingdom and the United States is limited to particular industrial sectors and specific occupational exposures such as ionizing radiation, heavy metals, fibrogenic materials, and carcinogens. In general, major Health and Safety Acts will 'enable' a variety of government departments to create legislation in the form of 'regulations' requiring action from employers in particular occupational and environmental circumstances. The increasing attention paid in the United Kingdom to public health issues has enhanced the chances of improving occupational health services, although, counterintuitively, many of the larger industrial enterprises are divesting themselves of an 'in-house' service.

The European Community, through 'directives', increasingly drives the occupational health and safety agenda in member states requiring them to modify or create legislation in response.

The latest moves from Brussels have been to encourage the delivery of occupational health to all by 'competent' persons, although the mode of delivery—even the definition of competent—has been left to member states for interpretation.

An ideal 'menu' of such services depends on many variables including the industrial sector, existing legislation, management/employee collaboration, the availability of employment, and compensation for damage. Most importantly, the level of service provided should be based on a thorough risk assessment of the work processes in that organization and a clear and logical procedure of risk management.

To deliver even such a basic service will require multidisciplinary teams including trained physicians, hygienists, and nurses. Few companies have such services and many are too small even to contemplate such provision.

Developments will be tempered primarily by the economic climate, perceptions of what constitutes occupationally mediated disease, and political will. However, an exponential rise in legal action, insurance costs, and compensation will play a significant part in persuading management that competent occupational health services are an absolute requirement of profitable organizations. If this is to encompass the small and medium-sized enterprises then provision must come either from larger employers (such as the National Health Service) or from private providers. It is important to remember that in the United Kingdom, for example, companies employing fewer than 250 people account for 99 per cent of all businesses and 40 per cent of the working population.

Prevention

The prevention of occupational disease depends upon recognition of the condition as occupational, assessment of the level and duration of exposure and hence its possible effects, control of the problem at source, audit of the risk management procedures, and perhaps health surveillance of those exposed using suitable techniques. These procedures are dealt with later in the chapter.

Recognition of diseases as occupational may vary from country to country. The EC has proposed a harmonization of national lists of occupational disease for the purpose of compensation of workers.

Compensation for occupational diseases

In the early years of Western industrialized society, the chances of a worker winning compensation for an occupationally related disease or injury were slim, resting as they did on a successful common law suit against the employer for negligence. Such cases are still notoriously difficult to win. However, by the end of the nineteenth century, many countries in Europe as well as the United States had passed workman's compensation laws of one sort or another. Such schemes were usually restricted to specified diseases or occupations. For example, the 1897 Act in Britain was for accidents only, with six diseases added in the 1906 Act. Today the Industrial Injuries Scheme extends to 67 diseases.

The principles underlying such schemes are that they should be 'no fault', that the disease should be, with reasonable certainty, caused by work, and that the benefit claimed should offset job loss, wage earning deficit, disability, or provide death benefit to the next of kin. While the scheme in Britain has suffered considerable erosion over the last 10 years, similar schemes exist in one form or another in all EC member states with the exception of The Netherlands where compensation for ill health is of a more general nature. Advice on proposed additions to the list of compensatable diseases is made in the member states by government appointed advisory groups. In Britain, this group is the Industrial Injuries Advisory Council which reports to the Secretary of State for Work and Pensions.

New EC recommendations propose that national schemes be made uniform. In addition, the EC wishes to see the introduction of a concept to aid those who can prove they have an occupationally related disease which is not on the standard list—the so-called 'individual proof' system. In Britain such a dual system of specified agents and individual claim opportunities exists only for asthma. No specific agents are listed for dermatitis.

It is important that the clinician is aware of such schemes. If the disease and work exposure seem related, and are listed, the patient should be advised to claim for compensation.

Further reading

Adams RM (1999). *Occupational skin disease*, 3rd edn. WB Saunders, Philadelphia.

Cox RAF, ed (2000). *Fitness to work; the medical aspects*, 3rd edn. Oxford Medical Publications, Oxford.

Harrington JM *et al.* (1998). *Occupational health*, 4th edn. Blackwell Scientific, Oxford.

International Labour Office (1998). *Encylopaedia of occupational health and safety*, 4th edn. International Labour Office, Geneva.

Levy BS, Wegman DH (2000). *Occupational health*, 4th edn. Little, Brown, Boston.

Parkes WR, ed (1994). *Occupational lung disorders*, 3rd edn. Butterworth, London. (4th edn in preparation.)

Baxter P *et al.*, eds (2000). *Hunters' diseases of occupation*, 9th edn. Hodder and Stoughton, London

Health and Safety Executive (1998). *Help on work-related stress. A short guide*, INDG 281. Health and Safety Executive, London.

Assessment of the workforce and their environment

K. Gardiner and J. M. Harrington

Introduction

Occupational health comprises recognition, evaluation, and control. Control (including prevention) is the paramount element; there is no point in knowing what may happen or diagnosing what has happened if no remedial action is taken. For too long, society/industry has relied on occupational physicians to identify the failures in control by means of diagnosing occupationally related disease without giving sufficient weight to the need for control and therefore prevention.

As a result of this realization, current health and safety legislation is driven by risk assessment, i.e. those who generate the risk(s) are responsible for undertaking an assessment, the detail of which must be commensurate with the complexity of the situation and the ultimate risk. It follows from this that the quantified risk must be managed, and hence employers must now add risk management to their portfolio of activities.

Before embarking on any evaluation, especially where there is suspicion of occupational aetiology, great care needs to be exercised beforehand to determine what the legislation requires, what the known toxicological/health effects are, previous evidence from similar circumstances/environments, etc. This is the 'recognition' aspect, and highlights the necessity not only to be well informed but also competent (i.e. to be able to interpret and act upon the information appropriately).

Evaluation

One aspect of occupational medicine, distinct from most others, is that commonly one is dealing with groups rather than individual patients. In the main, this acts to complicate the evaluation as interindividual variance is added to the intrinsic intraindividual variance (for example, two people exposed to exactly the same quantity of toluene over the same time period will not excrete the same amount of urinary hippuric acid or excrete it at the same rate). In order to minimize any erroneous decisions and to maximize the usefulness of any information, evaluation of the workforce (and workplace) must be conducted in a systematic manner. This is often achieved by posing a number of simple questions.

The most fundamental of these questions is why? It is essential that the rationale for evaluating an individual or group is clear and justifiable. However, as occupational health professionals exist to eliminate ill health at work their priority must always be to eliminate problems in the workplace immediately rather than to delay while quantifying them. The law is prescriptive for only for a limited number of hazards (ionizing radiation, lead, asbestos).

Where large groups are involved, it may be necessary to evaluate a subset—this is the 'who' question. When there is no other over-riding need for selection (such as those working for extended periods (more than 8 h per day), those working at an elevated metabolic/breathing rate, those already unwell, or those likely to undertake unusual or unscheduled tasks (maintenance)), individuals should be chosen randomly.

The timing of measurements (i.e. 'when') is often critical. Should health outcome measures be taken before, during, or after the putative exposure or is there some legislative requirement that dictates the timing? For example, urinary mandelic acid (for styrene exposure) is best collected at the end of a working shift whereas urinary trichloroacetic acid (for trichloroethylene exposure) is best measured at the end of the working week, this being determined, in part, by the differing half-lives of the substances concerned.

Usually, the issue of what to assess is self-evident, but, as with all other aspects of this systematic approach, answers to the questions are interlinked, certainly with the 'why' question. For example, is biological monitoring or biological effect monitoring required? The former is the detection of a chemical or its metabolite in a biological sample as a measure of exposure. The latter is measurement of a change in some biochemical or physiological variable to indicate the effect of the contaminant on the body.

Choice of an appropriate technique for making these measurements should be based where possible on sensitivity and specificity.

The technique should be both suitable and sufficient for its purpose. For example, in the diagnosis of occupational asthma suitable techniques include peak flow meters, simple spirometry (time–volume curves), and whole-body plethysmography, but the simplest of these may be adequate.

Remedial action

The law is clear: the employer must adapt the workplace to be a safe environment for the employees. The employees should not have to adapt themselves to the stresses and strains of their work. Despite this philosophy, it is common for the chain of control to start with ineffective pre-employment medicals whose aim is only to avoid exposing people to contaminants likely to exacerbate allergies or other diseases.

Control is often viewed as a physical alteration of the workplace (engineering) or alteration of the behaviour of the workforce (administrative). It is preferable to have designed the workplace appropriately in the first place. Unfortunately, most control is required remedially, after an unacceptable level of risk has been identified as a result of a formal risk assessment. Remedial action may involve:

- elimination—removal of the process;
- contaminant substitution—replacemnt of the contaminant with one carrying a lower risk;
- process modification (temperature, agitation, enclosure, etc.);
- substance modification (wavelength, form, size, etc.);
- isolation/segregation (time, distance, shielding);
- local extract ventilation;
- minimization of the duration and frequency of exposure;
- education and training and the use of personal protective equipment.

Occupational dermatology

I. S. Foulds

An occupational dermatosis is a pathological condition of the skin for which occupational exposure can be shown to be a major contributory factor. Legal definitions vary between countries. In the United Kingdom the majority are defined by Prescribed Disease D5 of the Department of Health and Social Security as 'non-infective dermatitis of external origin (including chrome ulceration of the skin but excluding dermatitis due to ionizing particles or electromagnetic radiation other than radiant heat)'. However, this definition may exclude newly described dermatoses, and in the case of occupationally acquired hypomelanosis a new category (Prescribed Disease C25) was necessary.

Incidence

The true incidence of occupational dermatoses is difficult to obtain, as in some countries occupational accidents and illnesses are not differentiated, and others fail to separate dermatitis from other skin diseases. Few statistics are derived from short absences from work or disease without disability, and most information is based on compensation paid.

Dermatitis, mostly due to irritant contact factors, accounts for 95 per cent of all occupational dermatoses. In the United Kingdom a million working days a year may be lost from such conditions. The diagnosis and management is discussed elsewhere (see Chapter 23.1).

Some managers and even some doctors believe that people with dermatitis are out to obtain whatever they can in the way of compensation. However, in times of high unemployment, many people are reluctant to seek help in case they are labelled as suffering from industrial dermatitis and are then transferred to less skilled work with the loss of bonuses or even their jobs. Once labelled in this way, they are unlikely to find alternative employment.

Many employers believe that they do not have a problem with dermatitis, but careful inspection of employees' skin shows that the condition may be present in up to a third of the workforce. Considerable time is lost due to dermatitis and suffering due to discomfort, depression, and social ostracism is impossible to quantify.

Employees' and employers' attitudes to dermatitis

As with many skin diseases there are many myths attached to dermatitis. The 'leper approach' still exists. Many people believe that dermatitis is infectious and can be passed on by towels and touching; this results in the affected individual becoming socially isolated. Under no circumstances should dermatitis ever be regarded as infectious. It can only be acquired by wear and tear occurring to the skin or by the development of an allergy to a substance that has been in contact with the skin. Affected individuals therefore should not have unnecessary restrictions placed on them.

When someone develops severe occupational dermatitis this is often apparent to their colleagues who, after discussion, may think that their own skin problems are also occupationally related. However, since skin diseases are common, individual problems may be falsely attributed to a work-related cause. With outbreaks of apparent dermatitis, great care is needed in handling the situation to identify the causes and differentiate those with occupationally related problems from those with other skin diseases. It may be necessary to ask for the help of a dermatologist with specialist knowledge if the confidence of the workforce is to be maintained.

Barrier creams

No cream provides a barrier to penetration of substances into the skin. In fact, in some situations they may actually enhance penetration. Although there are numerous formulations available, they can be divided into those suitable for dry or for wet work.

The main benefit they offer is from their bases such as lanolin which may help to improve the hydration (suppleness) of the skin, with the result that, when cleansers are used, less degreasing of the skin occurs. In theory, this may help to reduce irritant contact dermatitis from repeated hand washing. There is no evidence that barrier creams protect against sensitizers, and occasionally sensitization may occur to some of the constituents of the cream. The use of a barrier cream may give an employee a false sense of security and lead to increased skin abuse.

Skin cleaning

When substances remain on the skin after the working day, the risk of irritation or sensitization is increased. The most efficient skin cleaners, however, are often the most irritant of substances due to their solvent or detergent content. If cleaners are too mild for the task, workers will often use degreasing agents in the manufacturing process, for example solvents or paraffins, to obtain adequate cleaning. Although these substances will 'clean' they are potentially very irritant with repeated use. It is often not appropriate to provide one type for different jobs. Agents should be chosen that clean adequately in a short period of time without having too strong a degreasing effect.

After-work creams

There are many such creams, essentially moisturizers, which have the benefit of increasing the hydration of the skin following cleaning at the end of the day. They are of particular benefit in occupations where excessive drying of the skin may occur. Their use should be encouraged where hot air driers are used as these tend to dry the skin unduly.

Skin protection

In industrial situations the hands and forearms are most at risk. The use of proper gloves (along with gauntlets or arm bands to prevent powders entering under the cuff) coupled with a high standard of hygiene, can minimize contact and provide adequate protection. Where moving machinery is present, wearing gloves may pose a potential danger. Even when gloves are used, they may be taken off to undertake tasks requiring manual dexterity, resulting in contaminated hands being placed back inside the gloves.

A wide range of materials have been used to manufacture gloves including cotton, leather, nylon, glass fibre, acrylonitrile, rubber, neoprene, butyl rubber, viton, polyurethane, PVC, PVA, and Teflon. These confer individual benefits in specific occupational applications.

Non-dermatitic occupational dermatoses

These form a minority of occupational dermatoses and awareness of their existence is important for those involved in managing skin patients. The more important are briefly mentioned below:

1. Psoriasis (see Chapter 23.1) may erupt at sites of injury or as a response to friction in manual workers. When this occurs on the hands, it may be confused with dermatitis although vesicles (blisters) are not found in psoriatic skin.

2. Infections include anthrax (albeit rare in the United Kingdom), human papilloma virus warts, orf (a poxvirus), and fungal infections such as tinea pedis and cattle ringworm (*Trichophyton mentagrophytes*).

3. Chronic paronychia due to candida occurs in those exposed to wet work.

4. Acne may be caused by a variety of chemicals including oils, coal tar chlorphenols, and petroleum products. Chloracne is a particularly refractory form of acne caused by halogenated aromatic chemicals, which may also cause systemic toxicity. Mild cases may be difficult to differentiate from conventional acne but multiple comedones (blackheads) are found over the malar regions. Industrial accidents can result in exposure and subsequent symptoms: for example in 1976 an explosion in a chemical plant near Seveso, Italy resulted in the exposure of the local population to 2,3,7,8-tetrachlorodibenzo-*p*-dioxin which caused severe systemic and cutaneous symptoms.

5. Vitiligo may be occupationally acquired. Several substituted phenols including *p*-tertiary-butyl phenol and monobenzyl ether of hydroquinone may cause hypomelanosis indistinguishable from vitiligo.

6. Scleroderma may be caused by exposure to vinyl chloride, and has been reported with trichlorethylene and organic solvents. Scleroderma-like lesions have also been reported in people exposed to epoxy resin fumes, and silicosis associated with scleroderma has been reported in miners.

7. A variety of chemicals may cause alteration of skin pigment; for example mercury and silver, which causes argyria.

8. Occupationally induced itching may occur in atopic individuals who exhibit dermographism due to histamine release from mast cells caused by fibres typically around 3 μm in size which can penetrate the skin. This occurs with exposure to glass fibres, ceramic fibres, and fibreglass.

Occupational cancer (see also Chapter 6.1)

J. M. Harrington

Background

Georgius Agricola's account in 1555 of the illnesses of Carpathian silver miners includes evidence of a rapidly progressive and fatal lung disorder. The fact that these mines are now known to contain uranium ore suggests that exposure to radon gas may well have been high enough to cause lung cancer in the miners. Nevertheless, it is Percival Pott's description in 1775 of an excess risk of scrotal cancer in postpubertal chimney sweeps that first raised the possibility of chemicals—particularly polynuclear aromatic hydrocarbons (PAH)—causing cancer. Confirmatory evidence from animal experiments did not arrive until 1915 and the first carcinogenic hydrocarbon was identified by Kennaway in 1924 as 1,2,5,6-dibenzanthracene.

While the polynuclear aromatic hydrocarbons were generating interest as skin carcinogens, clinical observations of dyestuff workers were suggesting a link between bladder cancer and aromatic amines. In 1895, Rehn described three cases in a group of 45 workers in Germany involved in the preparation of fuchsin. Further reports followed from other countries and the classic studies of Case and his colleagues in the 1950s showed that 2-naphthylamine and benzidine were human carcinogens in manufacturing and user industries. 2-napthylamine was a contaminant of the antioxidant used in tyre manufacture. Rehn discovered that an organ distant from the point of first contact could bear the main force of the carcinogenic effect if its exposure was most prolonged and most intense.

In the same year that Rehn made his discovery, Röntgen discovered X-rays and 3 years later, the Curies isolated radium. Unfortunately, knowledge of the carcinogenic properties of ionizing radiation came from the skin and bone marrow cancers suffered by these early pioneers with confirmatory animal data following soon after. The bone sarcomas noted in laboratory animals were followed by human evidence in the 1930s among the painters of luminous dials who used radium-235 and mesothorium. The inventor of the luminous paint, Dr von Sochocky, died of aplastic anaemia in 1928. Again in the 1930s, case reports were appearing of lung cancer (an unusual tumour in those days) in workers exposed to asbestos fibre. In asbestosis cases the incidence was reported as 18 per cent and reports of pleural mesothelioma followed a decade or so later.

Thus, within a century of Rehn's discovery, chemical carcinogenesis had become a well-recognized phenomenon with much of the evidence coming from occupational studies.

Diagnosis

Clinical acumen remains of paramount importance. It is clinicians who have played the major role in discovering new causes of cancer with confirmatory evidence coming from laboratory studies and epidemiological investigations (see Fig. 1).

Such information is collated and interpreted by various national and international agencies. The most reliable source is the monograph series of the International Agency for Research on Cancer (**IARC**) based in Lyon. To date they have published over 70 such monographs with several updating supplements. When a patient is diagnosed as having cancer, it is important that the clinician should review the occupational history to consider an occupational cause. If this seems probable, enquiries should be made to see if state compensation is available for that cancer and that workplace exposure.

Attribution of cancer to occupational causes

The most widely accepted estimates of the proportion of all cancers attributable to occupational exposures is 4 per cent with a range of 2 to 8 per cent for a developed country like the United States. For the 20 per cent or so of the population in which occupationally related cancers are almost exclusively concentrated (manual workers aged 20 or over, in mining, agriculture, and industry broadly defined), perhaps as much as one lung or bladder cancer in every five may be attributed to workplace exposure.

In addition, it is necessary to consider other exposures which may interact with workplace exposures. These are particularly relevant when considering the relative effectiveness of removing or reducing exposure to one or more jointly acting agents. Few good studies have been completed on interaction, but there is good evidence for the multiplicative effects of cigarette smoking and asbestos exposure in the genesis of lung cancer. Besides asbestos, interactions have been demonstrated to be at least additive for tobacco consumption and exposure to arsenic and nickel compounds as well as ionizing radiation.

Tables 1 and 2 show some important examples of occupational exposures causing cancer.

Polynuclear aromatic hydrocarbons

Polynuclear aromatic hydrocarbons are a large and complex group of compounds mainly generated during the incomplete combustion of carbonaceous products, of which coal and oil result in the most important occupational exposures. Cigarette smoke contains a number of these compounds and so it is often difficult to distinguish lifestyle from occupational factors. The site of action of these compounds is mainly the lung, skin, and bladder. The industries most prominently linked to such exposures are coke ovens, gas production, steel industries, aluminium refineries, iron and steel foundries as well as workers exposed to exhaust fumes from soot, pitch, tar, and petroleum products.

Aromatic amines

Aromatic amines are a group of chemically similar compounds which have particular importance as dyestuffs or antioxidants or as intermediates in dye production. Some are known human bladder carcinogens, a larger number are known animal carcinogens but for which human data are limited or lacking. The more potent carcinogens are now banned.

Metals and metalloids

The most important carcinogenic metals are compounds of arsenic, chromium, and nickel. Arsenic and its compounds cause lung and skin cancer,

Table 1 Industrial processes causally associated with human cancer. The suspected target organs are in parentheses. (Based on *IARC Monographs* vols. 1–71 1972–99)

Industry	Human target organs
Aluminium production	Lung, bladder (haemopoietic/lymphatic system, oesophagus, stomach)
Auramine, manufacture of	Bladder
Boot and shoe manufacture and repair	Haemopoietic/lymphatic system, nasal sinus (bladder, digestive tract)
Coal gasification	Skin, lung, bladder
Coke production	Skin, lung, kidney
Furniture and cabinet making	Nasal sinus
Haematite mining, underground, with exposure to radon	Lung
Iron and steel founding	Lung (digestive tract, genitourinary tract, haemopoietic/lymphatic system)
Isopropyl alcohol manufacture, strong acid process	Nasal sinus (larynx)
Magenta, manufacture of	Bladder
Painters (occupational exposure as)	Lung (oesophagus, stomach, bladder)
Rubber industry	Bladder, (haemopoietic/lymphatic system, lung, renal tract, digestive tract, skin, liver, larynx, brain, stomach)

and these risks occur in the extraction of metalliferous ores (which are frequently contaminated by arsenic compounds) and in the now limited use of arsenic in pesticides and other industrial usages. Hexavalent chromium compounds used in the pigment and plating industries have been shown to cause lung cancer. Lung and nasal cancer are associated with the refining of nickel and the most likely causative agents are the oxidic and sulphidic nickel compounds. Other metals for which there is evidence of carcinogenicity include beryllium and cadmium.

Other organic compounds

Benzene is widely used in industry both as the base compound and as an important building block in the organic chemical industry. It causes leukaemia and aplastic anaemia. Vinyl chloride monomer, which is the starting point for synthesis of polyvinyl chloride, causes angiosarcoma of the liver. The most potent lung carcinogens are apparently the chloromethyl ethers which are used in ion exchange resins. Other suspect organics include acrylonitrile, acrylamide, butadiene, diethyl sulphate, epichlorhydrin, ethylene dibromide, formaldehyde, styrene oxide, tetrachloroethylene, and trichlorothylene.

Industrial processes

Some processes listed in Table 1 are linked to specific exposures, such as polynuclear aromatic hydrocarbons in aluminium production and radon in underground mining. For others such as boot and shoe manufacture, furniture making, and painting, the specific relevant exposures have not been identified.

Musculoskeletal disorders

T. C. Aw

Musculoskeletal disorders rank alongside stress as a major cause of workplace ill health. As musculoskeletal disorders are common in the general population, their suspected relationship to specific occupations or activities can often be difficult to confirm. A combination of occupational, psychological, personal, social, and home factors may be involved. The epidemic

Fig. 1 The scientific basis for establishing occupational causality.

of repetitive strain injury in Australia during the 1980s highlighted the complex interaction of symptoms, group perceptions, and employment.

Repetitive strain injury

This term was coined to describe pain and discomfort in the wrist and forearm associated with the performance of repeated tasks, mainly at work. Other terms used synonymously are cumulative trauma disorder, occupational overuse syndrome, and work-related upper limb disorder, with some terms restricting the definition to conditions in upper limbs caused by work. Unfortunately, there is no widely accepted case definition, and several disorders such as carpal tunnel syndrome, de Quervain's disease, epicondylitis, and tenosynovitis are often included in the entity. Clusters of cases have been recognized in occupational groups such as typists, telephonists, computer keyboard operators, musicians, cleaners, hairdressers, butchers, and assembly line workers. While the wrist and forearm are the anatomical regions most frequently affected, the symptoms are often very diffuse and the shoulder and neck may also be involved. Risk factors common to many cases are:

(1) repeated movements at certain joints, often through the full range of movements, for example flexion and extension at the wrists;

(2) constrained postures, sometimes at the extremes of the range of movements, and often against pressure or force.

Table 2 Chemicals and groups of chemicals causally associated with human cancer for which exposure has been mostly occupational. The suspected target organs are in parentheses. (Based on *IARC Monographs* vols. 1–71, 1972–99)

Chemical	Human target organ
4-Aminobiphenyl	Bladder
Arsenic and arsenic compounds*	Skin, lung (liver, haematopoietic system, gastrointestinal tract, kidney)
Asbestos	Lung, pleura, peritoneum, gastrointestinal tract, larynx
Benzene	Haemopoietic system
Benzidine	Bladder
Bis (chloromethyl) ether and chloromethyl methyl ether (technical grade)	Lung
Chromium compounds, hexavalent*	Lung (gastrointestinal tract)
Coal tars	Skin, lung (bladder)
Coal tar pitches	Skin, lung, bladder (gastrointestinal tract, haemopoietic/lymphatic system)
Ethylene oxide	Lymphatic and haemopoeitic systems
Inorganic acid mists (strong) containing sulphuric acid	Larynx
Ionizing radiation	Haemopoietic/lymphatic system, bone, skin, and other organs depending on exposure and type of radiation
Mineral oils, untreated and mildly treated	Skin (respiratory tract, bladder, gastrointestinal tract)
Mustard gas (sulphur mustard)	Lung, larynx, pharynx
2-Naphthylamine (and other aromatic amines)	Bladder (liver)
Nickel and nickel compounds*	Nasal sinus, lung (larynx)
Radon (and its decay products)	Lung
Shale oils	Skin (colon)
Soots	Skin, lung
Talc containing asbestiform fibre	Lung (pleura)
Vinyl chloride	Liver, lung, brain, lymphatic and haematopoietic systems (gastrointestinal tract)

*The evaluation of carcinogenicity in humans applies to the group of chemicals as a whole and not necessarily all individual chemicals within the group.

Low back pain

This is possibly the commonest musculoskeletal condition experienced by people at work. Poor lifting and manual handling techniques and sitting for prolonged periods in the course of work activities (for example professional drivers) are contributory factors. Nurses, porters, and brick-layers are groups with a high prevalence of low back pain. The total cost of sickness absence, early retirement, and treatment for low back pain in many countries is considerable.

Occupations associated with musculoskeletal disorders

Several occupations are associated with a high risk of sustaining an occupationally related musculoskeletal injury. These include fractures and joint damage in construction workers, miners, and deep sea fishermen, avascular bone necrosis from decompression sickness in tunnellers and divers, acroosteolysis in workers exposed to vinyl chloride monomer, and septic bone and joint lesions from brucellosis in meat process workers. The joints of coal-face workers, farmers, and professional dancers are subjected to frequent heavy impact loading leading to a high incidence of degenerative changes of the hip and knee.

Clinical investigations and management

Several investigations such as erythrocyte sedimentation rate, C-reactive protein, rheumatoid factor, and imaging may help to exclude an underlying medical condition.

The management of a case of occupational musculoskeletal disorder requires alleviation of symptoms and the consideration of modifications to the system of work or the layout of the workstation. Non-steroidal anti-inflammatory medication and physiotherapy can reduce pain, discomfort, and limitation of function. Localized areas of inflammation will respond to local injections of corticosteroids. Physical therapy procedures and occasionally surgery may be considered. There should be an evaluation of ergonomic factors in the design of equipment at the individual's workplace. This requires attention to the adequacy of the workstation, ease of access of the worker to tools, components, and other equipment, and the suitability of the general work environment—its lighting, temperature, humidity, and noise. Training in proper methods of lifting and manual handling is essential.

Musculoskeletal disorders affecting occupation

Patients with known arthritic disease, such as rheumatoid arthritis and systemic lupus erythematosis, need to be assessed for the effect that the condition may have on the performance of their work duties. The fluctuating nature of most forms of chronic arthritis makes precise predictions difficult. Physical disability can improve despite persistence of the disease. This is due both to the beneficial effects of treatment and to the patient's adaptation to the consequences of the disease.

Cardiovascular system

J. M. Harrington

Cardiovascular disease is the major cause of mortality and morbidity in industrialized countries (see Section 15). The association between personal risk factors and cardiovascular disease is well known, but less attention has been paid to occupational and environmental influences.

There is good evidence from the classical studies of London bus drivers and conductors that sedentary workers have a higher risk of ischaemic heart disease than those who are more active. There is some evidence linking job stress and heart disease. The Whitehall II studies suggest that control over one's job is an important factor in determining subsequent risk of myocardial infarction.

Exposure to chemicals such as carbon disulphide, chlorinated organic solvents, nitroglycerine, and vinylchloride monomer may contribute to cardiovascular disease. The cardiovascular effects of exposure to heavy metals are largely secondary to their nephrotoxic effects. Toxic industrial gases produce their effect secondary to anoxia. Among physical agents, vibration is known to cause peripheral vascular disease and acute high exposure to noise is known to raise blood pressure. Workers on rotating shifts have an increased risk of ischaemic heart disease.

Genitourinary system

J. M. Harrington

The kidney plays a crucial role in the excretory and detoxification mechanisms of the body. Perhaps the most effective detoxification manoeuvre of the liver is to increase the polarity or acidity of the absorbed substance. This, in turn, increases the water solubility of the chemical and hence its renal excretion. The kidney, therefore, bears the brunt of many exposures to toxic chemicals. Some toxic substances do reach the kidney unchanged but most are metabolized to some extent or other. Some, such as cadmium, become sequestered in the renal cortex while others, such as the aromatic amines, are present in the bladder long enough and at a high enough concentration to induce malignant change in the transitional cell epithelium.

Sudden, severe exposures to some chemicals can cause acute nephropathy. Such compounds may damage the kidney directly due to their intrinsic nephrotoxicity or may induce secondary damage due to prerenal effects, such as the haemolysis following arsine exposure. Hypovolaemic shock can follow acute fluid loss or extreme heat, while post-traumatic renal failure can follow crush injuries or high-voltage electric shock, both of which cause muscle necrosis. Chronic lower-dose exposure leading to nephropathy is more commonly associated with metals or organic solvents.

The metals most commonly implicated in renal disease are mercury, cadmium, lead, and, perhaps, uranium (see Chapter 8.1). Mercury exposure resulting in acute tubular necrosis or the nephrotic syndrome is most unusual these days. Under present-day workplace exposures, the effects of inhaled mercury vapour or absorption of mercury salts are more likely to cause mild proteinuria and limited tubular dysfunction. Biological monitoring of mercury-exposed workers has had to become more sophisticated. Sensitive tests of urinary enzymes, such as N-acetyl-β-D-glucosamidase, are necessary to detect those subtle effects. Similarly, modern industrial exposures to cadmium rarely result in the proximal or distal tubular dysfunction or renal cortical damage that was more prevalent in the past. However, cadmium is only slowly leached from the renal cortex and remains a potentially serious long-term cumulative poison. The environmental cadmium contamination which caused widespread tubular dysfunction with hypercalciuria and osteomalacia in multiparous postmenopausal Japanese women (Itai-Itai disease) has not been described in the West. Lead nephropathy is also a rarity nowadays, but was not uncommon in the early part of this century. Lead is capable of causing damage to all parts of the nephron. More subtle tests of renal enzymes are now needed to assess the effects of lead exposure on the kidney. Soluble uranium compounds such as uranium hexafluoride have been shown to be potent nephrotoxins after acute accidental exposure but this problem is virtually unknown in a well-controlled modern facility.

Chlorinated aliphatic solvents such as carbon tetrachloride and chloroform can cause the hepatorenal syndrome. The renal damage is largely an effect on the proximal tubular epithelium which can lead to tubular necrosis and acute oliguric renal failure. The weight of evidence from case–control studies of workers exposed to solvent suggests an excess risk of glomerulonephritis. The mechanism is unclear, but a link with Goodpasture's syndrome suggests possible autoimmune damage to the glomerular basement membrane.

Although the prostate possesses the curious ability to concentrate (and excrete) heavy metals, little evidence exists of occupationally related prostatic disease. Earlier reports of a link between cadmium exposure and prostatic cancer have not been confirmed. Cancers of the urinary tract associated with occupational exposure to aromatic amines and polynuclear aromatic hydrocarbons were described earlier.

Gastrointestinal tract

T. C. Aw

The gastrointestinal tract acts as a semipermeable membrane through which ingested pollutants are absorbed. There are defence mechanisms that limit the damage to the gastrointestinal tract from such pollutants, and minimize their absorption. The mucous lining of the gut and diarrhoea and vomiting form part of these defence mechanisms. Hence, systemic absorption via the gastrointestinal tract plays a relatively minor role in causing occupational disease.

Acute gastroenteritis may follow the ingestion of chemicals such as soluble salts of heavy metals.

The liver is frequently at risk from occupational exposures, as it is the target organ for detoxification and metabolism of absorbed compounds. A wide variety of infectious and chemical agents cause different types of hepatocellular injury which may eventually lead to cirrhosis and liver failure (Table 3).

The haemopoietic system

T. C. Aw

The metal most frequently associated with bone marrow damage is inorganic lead. Lead causes anaemia by inhibiting the enzymes involved in haem synthesis and also by haemolysis. Determination of blood lead levels

Table 3 Effects of occupationally related hepatotoxins. (From Harrington JM, Gill FS, Aw TC *et al.* (1998). *Occupational health*, 4th edn. Blackwell Scientific, Oxford)

| Effect | Substance | |
	Organic	Inorganic
Centrilobular necrosis	Acrylonitrile	Antimony
	Carbon tetrachloride	Arsenic
	Chlorinated hydrocarbon insecticides	Boranes
	Chlorinated naphthalenes	Phosphorus (yellow)
	Dimethyl hydrazine	Selenium
	Dimethyl nitrosamine	Thallium
	Dinitrophenol	
	Ethyl alcohol	
	Halothane	
	Methyl chloride	
	Nitrobenzene	
	Phenol	
	Polychlorinated biphenyls	
	Tetrachloroethylene	
	1,1,1-Trichloroethane	
	Trichloroethylene	
	Trinitrotoluene	
	Toluene	
	Vinyl chloride	
	Halothane	
Hepatic infections	Viral hepatitis (A,B,C)	
	Leptospirosis	
	Q fever	
	Schistosomiasis	
	Amoebiasis	
Cholestatic cholangiolytic	Methylene dianiline	
	Organic arsenicals	
	Toluene diamine	

is used in the monitoring of lead-exposed workers. A diagnosis of lead poisoning is supported by symptoms of malaise, colic, and constipation, signs of anaemia and peripheral motor neuropathy (rare, usually only in severe cases), and laboratory evidence of basophilic stippling of erythrocytes, elevated blood lead, low haemoglobin, raised free erythrocyte protoporphyrin, and raised urinary δ-aminolaevulinic acid. Indications of excessive lead absorption should lead to removal of the affected worker from further occupational exposure, with full investigation into the circumstances of exposure to lead at work and possibly elsewhere.

Massive intravascular haemolysis is caused by acute exposure to arsine, phosphine, and stibine. These are gases encountered in the smelting and refining of metals, galvanizing processes, and in certain soldering procedures. They are formed from the reaction between nascent hydrogen and arsenic, phosphorus, and antimony respectively.

Occupational exposure to ionizing radiation can occur following the industrial use of radioactive sources to test the integrity of welds, in the health-care industry, and in nuclear power stations (see Chapter 8.5.9).

Benzene is encountered in the petroleum industry, and is used as a starter chemical for the production of other aromatic organic compounds. Its effects on the haemopoietic system include early platelet deficiency, mild haemolysis, and pancytopenia. Major effects are aplastic anaemia and lymphoid and myeloid leukaemia.

Methaemoglobinaemia can result from exposure to occupational and environmental agents such as nitrates, and nitro and amino derivatives of aromatic compounds. Specific examples are aniline, aminobenzene, nitrobenzene, and nitrates in the soil.

Infections

T. C. Aw

Certain industries are associated with an increased risk of occupational infections, and the health-care industry is possibly the best example of this. Working in tropical environments also exposes workers to the risk of tropical diseases. Occupational and environmental infections involve a range of organisms from viruses, rickettsiae, bacteria, and fungi to larger organisms such as parasites and insects. Occupations involved include farming, forestry, and sewage work.

In the health-care industry, blood-borne infections such as hepatitis B and human immunodeficiency virus (**HIV**) pose practical problems for the safety of staff during contact with infected patients, and the safety of patients during contact with infected staff. Worldwide, several dozen cases of HIV have been documented to have occurred in health-care workers following contact with infected blood or body fluids from patients. These have involved needlestick injuries, mainly from contaminated hollow-bore needles, or substantial blood contamination of damaged skin. Only two cases of HIV transmission from health-care workers to patients have been noted. One involved a dentist and the other an orthopaedic surgeon. With hepatitis B, the incidence of outbreaks from doctor to patient and vice versa is much more common. Until recently, transmission of hepatitis B from doctor to patient was thought to involve only those who were e-antigen positive carriers. There have been several cases to date involving surface-antigen positive but e-antigen negative carriers. This has led to a review of occupational procedures that may pose a risk to patients from such carriers. Protection of health-care staff from hepatitis B infection involves the intramuscular administration of yeast-derived genetically engineered vaccines (plasma-derived vaccines were previously used) to staff at risk. The vaccine does not protect against other hepatitis infections (hepatitis C, D, and G) which are similar to hepatitis B in their transmission and sequelae. Other occupational infections affecting staff in microbiological laboratories and other health-care workers include tuberculosis, salmonellosis, syphilis, and malaria.

The reproductive system

T. C. Aw

Occupational and environmental exposures may affect female and male reproductive systems and influence different stages in the outcome of pregnancy. Children can be affected by parental exposure to physical and chemical hazards.

The male reproductive system

Exposure to the pesticides 1,2-dibromo-3-chloropropane (**DBCP**) and chlordecone (Kepone), are among the best documented cases. Liquid DBCP was used as a nematocide for crops. Chlordecone was used as an insecticide. Gynaecomastia has been reported in male workers following prolonged contact with oestrogenic agents such as diethylstilbestrol, and in those involved in the preparation of oral contraceptive products.

Effects on the male reproductive system may also occur following exposure to heat (potentially a problem in workplaces such as foundries), microwave and ionizing radiation, cytotoxic drugs, animal growth promoters, fumigants such as ethylene dibromide, and heavy metals, for example lead, manganese, and mercury compounds.

The female reproductive system

Effects on the female reproductive system range from alterations in the menstrual cycle—both the amount of menstrual flow as well as the regularity of cycles—spontaneous abortions, and infertility. Rubella can be a problem for female health-care workers and those working in microbiological laboratories, especially if adequate procedures are not in place for occupational health vetting and immunization of this occupational group. Concerns about an increase in spontaneous abortions amongst female anaesthetists exposed to anaesthetic gases were investigated, and recent reviews of the findings suggest that the evidence is weak. Nevertheless, occupational exposure standards were set in the United Kingdom in 1996 for limiting workplace exposure to nitrous oxide, halothane, enflurane, and isoflurane. Similar concerns about working with visual display units (such as computer monitors) and spontaneous abortions led to several large-scale epidemiological studies. These studies indicated that the association could well have occurred by chance, given that spontaneous abortions are relatively common events and that there has been a rapid increase in use of visual display unitss in recent years.

Other occupational and environmental exposures that can affect the female reproductive system are ionizing radiation, cytotoxic drugs, lead, and ethylene oxide.

Other environmental effects

Environmental contamination with 'endocrine-disruptors' such as plasticizers has been thought to be responsible for an alteration to the sex ratio of fish populations. Pollution from similar organic compounds has been suggested to be contributing to the decline in mean sperm counts for male populations in several parts of Europe. These observations have led to proposals for testing chemicals for endocrine disrupting properties.

Neurological disorders

E. L. Baker

Neurological disorders caused by exposure to chemicals

Central nervous system effects

Exposure to chemicals, primarily encountered by workers in manufacturing, construction, and agricultural jobs, can cause transient and persistent effects on the central nervous system (Table 4). Transient central nervous system dysfunction is most commonly caused by exposure to volatile organic solvents, to organophosphate insecticides, or to carbon monoxide. In each instance, these substances, acting through different mechanisms,

Table 4 Central nervous system syndromes caused by workplace toxins

Disorders	Manifestations	Causal agent
Acute intoxication	Light-headedness	Carbon monoxide
	Loss of consciousness	Organic solvents
	Death (rare)	Organophosphates
Organic affective syndrome	Fatigue	Organic solvents
	Irritability	Lead
	Depression	Mercury
		Styrene
Chronic toxic encephalopathy	Impaired neurobehavioural function (symptoms as above)	Organic solvents
		Lead
Psychosis	Marked emotional instability	Carbon disulphide
		Manganese (rare)
		Toluene (rare)

may cause central nervous system dysfunction ranging from acute intoxication manifested by light-headedness and dizziness to loss of consciousness and even death. Persistent central nervous system sequelae may occur following one exposure episode if exposure levels are high and the time of exposure is prolonged.

Persistent central nervous system dysfunction, manifesting as neurobehavioural performance deficits, has been reported following chronic exposure to moderate concentrations of various agents encountered in the workplace and occasionally in the environment. This syndrome, chronic toxic encephalopathy, consisting primarily of memory impairment, impaired psychomotor function, and mood disorders, has been seen following chronic exposure to lead, styrene, and certain organic solvents. In more severe cases the deficits persist, but do not progress, following cessation of exposure. If behavioural symptoms are present without evidence of abnormal neurobehavioural test performances (i.e. organic affective syndrome) reversal of these manifestations usually occurs following cessation of exposure.

Peripheral nervous system effects
Exposure to certain agents (Table 5) may cause either motor or sensorimotor polyneuropathy. Rarely, exposure to lead at high levels for long periods may cause upper extremity motor neuropathy, consisting of wrist extension weakness or wrist drop. Certain substances (for example acrylamide, hexacarbon solvents, and certain organophosphorus compounds) may act as axonal toxins causing a mixed sensorimotor polyneuropathy manifesting as symmetrical, distal sensory loss. Upon removal from exposure, the symptoms usually recede over a period of months with modest or no residual damage.

Table 5 Peripheral nervous system syndromes caused by workplace toxins

Disorders	Manifestation	Causal agent
Motor neuropathy	Wrist weakness	Lead
Mixed sensori-motor neuropathy	Symmetrical distal sensory loss, mild motor dysfunction	Acrylamide
		Arsenic
		Carbon disulphide
		Carbon monoxide (rare)
		DDT (rare)
		n-Hexane
		Methyl n-butyl ketone
		Mercury
		Organophosphorus compounds (selected agents)

Other nervous system effects
A variety of other neurological effects have been reported following exposure to toxic agents in the environment (Table 6). In most cases, symptoms recede once exposure has ceased.

Neurological disorders caused by physical factors

Repetitive trauma disorders
See under Musculoskeletal disorders and Section 18.

Entrapment neuropathies
In certain occupations, sustained postures such as working overhead may cause muscular hypertrophy or other changes resulting in entrapment of nerve roots or individual nerves. Such conditions are diagnosed by obtaining a careful work history and are managed by modification of the work environment.

Vibration-induced neuropathy (see also Section 24)
Certain jobs involving the use of vibrating hand tools or pneumatic drills may be responsible for the occurrence of peripheral neuropathy. These disorders may originate from a combination of physical trauma to the nerve itself as well as damage to blood vessels which supply the nerves.

The role of psychology in occupational health

A. Spurgeon

There is growing recognition of the importance of psychological factors in a range of occupational health concerns. The following represents the main

Table 6 Other neurological manifestations following exposure to toxic agents in the workplace

Manifestation	Causal agent
Ataxic gait	Acrylamide
	Chlordane
	Chlordecone (Kepone)
	DDT
	Manganese
	Methyl mercury
Bladder neuropathy	Dimethylaminopropionitrile
Constricted visual fields	Organic mercury
Cranial neuropathy	Carbon disulphide
	Trichlorethylene
Headache	Lead
	Nickel
Impaired visual acuity	n-Hexane
	Methanol
	Organic mercury
Increased intracranial pressure	Organotin compounds
Opsoclonus	Chlordecone (Kepone)
Paraplegia	Organotin compounds
Parkinsonism	Carbon disulphide
	Carbon monoxide
	Manganese
Seizures	Lead
	Organic mercury
	Organochlorine insecticides
	Organotin compounds
Tremor	Carbon disulphide
	Chlordecone (Kepone)
	DDT
	Manganese
	Mercury

Table 7 Factors in the working environment that have been identified as potential psychosocial hazards

Stressor type	Example
Job content	Work overload
Working hours	Shiftwork, overtime
Organizational culture	Lack of communication, participation
Work role	Ambiguity, conflict
Interpersonal relationships	Harassment
Career structure	Job insecurity
Physical environment	Noise, poor ergonomic design

areas where psychology is now considered to have a significant contributory role.

Occupational stress

Reports of work-related stress have increased dramatically in recent years. A number of factors in the working environment have been identified as potential psychosocial hazards. These are usually categorized as in Table 7.

Prolonged exposure to one or more of these conditions may result in a range of symptoms of psychological distress such as feelings of anxiety, irritable or aggressive behaviour, lack of concentration, lack of confidence and an inability to make decisions, sleep disturbance, and fatigue. There may also be associated physical symptoms such as frequent headaches and nausea. Occupational stress is often identified as a result of the individual's inappropriate (maladaptive) coping strategies such as frequent short-term absences, alcohol and other substance abuse, poor time-keeping, and by uncharacteristically poor work performance. Effective management of occupational stress usually requires an integrated approach which includes attention to both the workplace and the individual and consists of intervention at three levels:

1. Primary intervention focuses on the identification of particular sources of stress in the working environment and the institution of measures to eliminate or reduce these.

2. Secondary intervention focuses on improving the coping skills of employees by the use of specific forms of stress management training (for example relaxation, conflict management, assertiveness, time management) and health promotional activities. These are particularly appropriate where workplace stressors are intrinsic to the particular occupation and therefore non-removable, for example the potential for aggressive confrontation with members of the public.

3. Tertiary intervention is concerned with counselling and rehabilitation of psychologically distressed individuals. The source of stress may often be multifactorial, and not therefore solely work-related, but it has an impact upon work performance and may be exacerbated by the demands of work

Neurobehavioural effects (see Sections 24 and 26)

The response to hazard exposure

A growing number of occupational health complaints are characterized by a lack of a firm diagnosis or clear occupational causation. These include, in particular, complaints which consist of a range of non-specific symptoms, typically headache, fatigue, nausea, depressed mood, cognitive confusion, and sometimes eye and nasal irritation. They are reported in diverse situations such as in air-conditioned offices (sick-building syndrome), proximity to low-frequency electromagnetic fields and perceived exposure to very low (often undetectable) levels of chemicals. In addition the prevalence of musculoskeletal complaints in many workplaces has been shown to be related to the presence of psychosocial hazards. At an individual level the reporting of such complaints, the decision to be absent from work, and the subsequent response to treatment and the duration of absence from work also appear to be strongly related to psychological factors. An important element is the structure of health beliefs and attitudes which the individual

brings to the situation. This influences their response to real or perceived exposure to hazards by determining their selection of which information to attend to and their subsequent interpretation of that information. Specific examples of syndromes with these features which occur in both an occupational and wider community setting may be multiple chemical sensitivity and chronic fatigue syndrome. Current approaches to effective management of these and other similar conditions favour a 'biopsychosocial' approach which rejects the artificial distinction between a physically and a psychologically based complaint and treats both physical and psychological symptoms simultaneously.

Risk perception

Individual response to exposure to hazards is one aspect of the wider subject of risk perception. Public and individual perceptions of risk are invariably at odds with quantitative risk assessment based on real data. Risk perception and associated safety behaviour are known to depend on a range of attitudinal factors, notably whether exposure to the hazard is perceived to be voluntary or involuntary, whether the consequences are perceived to be short or long term, who is perceived to be responsible or to benefit, the perceived importance or vulnerability of those at risk, and the level of concern generated by the media and the activity of pressure groups. Modern approaches to risk assessment accept that subjective and objective evaluations of risk should both be taken into account when defining the tolerability of any risk to individuals or groups, either in the workplace or in the wider environment. In addition, communication about risk is unlikely to be effective if it does not take account of the existing attitudes and beliefs of the audience and the reasoning behind these. The application of this to the development of a positive safety culture is discussed elsewhere.

8.4.2 Occupational safety

Richard T. Booth

Introduction

Accidents at work occur under a variety of circumstances. A few serious accidents involve fires and explosions in chemical process plants, and transportation disasters. But the vast majority of accidents involve everyday events such as contact with moving machinery, falls, cuts from handling materials, slipping on or striking against objects, and injuries from hand tools. Road accidents at work are the main cause of occupational fatalities. Despite the diversity of accidents, it is now agreed that the causes of all these accidents and principles of safety management are common to all, and to the control of health hazards at work.

The regulation of occupational safety in the United Kingdom evolved along two largely independent pathways. The first was the development of legislative controls of safety, gradually embracing an increasing range of hazards and of industries and employers. The second pathway was the development of safety management.

The distinctive feature of industry- and hazard-based safety legislation from 1844 was that the regulators identified the hazards, implicitly assessed the risks (largely as a reaction to events), and prescribed 'blanket' rule-based control standards. Safety was driven by legislation, and a knowledge of the law was the foundation of workplace controls, as described in 1972 by the Robens' Report for the Committee on Safety and Health at Work.

In contrast, safety management began (in Great Britain at least) after World War I, promoted by the British Industrial Safety First Movement, later the Royal Society for the Prevention of Accidents. Industrial accident prevention was seen as being achieved by committees, workers' participation, the employment of safety officers, joint accident investigations, and the promotion of a positive safety culture.

Limitations of this approach were the tendency to distance safety management from operational management generally, the adoption of a reactive approach to prevention, seeing accident causation in very simple terms, and a predilection for panaceas, such as 'accident proneness'.

The first determined attempt to amalgamate these two pathways or 'traditions' of safety within a framework of law was proposed by the Robens' Report. The Committee recognized that much safety law was outdated, too detailed, prescriptive, and legalistic. Robens proposed the wholesale repeal of the then existing law and its replacement with 'goal-setting' legislation. The Robens' philosophy was partly realized by the Health and Safety at Work, etc. Act of 1974, but arguably only fully implemented in the early 1990s as a result the European Union (**EU**) Framework and other directives (heavily influenced in most cases by experience in Great Britain), together with the government's deregulation initiatives. Whereas traditional law drove the safety system, the contemporary doctrine is that the law should underpin good, and promote best, practice. To a large extent, the Health and Safety Commission and the Health and Safety Executive (**HSC, HSE**) together became not just the custodian of the law, but also the custodian of good practice (as evidenced by standards) and the prime mover of the safety system. The duty of employers was no longer slavishly to adhere to a set of statutory rules, but to develop their own safety organization and arrangements that could be shown to follow good practice, which employers' and employees' organizations had been involved in framing.

The last 30 years have therefore seen the recognition of safety as an integral part of company management. Risk assessment is accepted as the essential basis for prevention.

The size of the problem

During 1998 to 1999, 188 employees were killed at work in Great Britain. In addition, 65 self- employed people and 369 members of the public (including trespassers and suicides on the railways) received fatal injuries at work. The numbers of non-fatal accidents are less certain. Accidents at work in Great Britain should be reported to the relevant enforcing authority under the terms of the Reporting of Injuries, Diseases and Dangerous Occur-

rences Regulations 1995 (**RIDDOR**). However, the Department of Employment in its in 1992 Labour Force Survey suggested that only about 30 per cent of reportable accidents to employees were reported. Reporting levels vary sharply in different employment sectors; from 80 per cent in the energy sector to 17 per cent in agriculture. Only about 5 per cent of reportable accidents to the self-employed are reported.

In 1991, the HSE argued, from the evidence of reported accidents, that accident rates in Great Britain were lower than in other industrialized countries. But the findings of the Labour Force Survey suggest that the lower accident rates in Great Britain may be partly a consequence of serious under-reporting and also a result of differences in reporting criteria. Notably, the published Great Britain data do not include fatal and serious injury from occupational road accidents. These data are included in reports from many EU countries. Some further reservations about accident data as a measure of safety performance are mentioned later.

Table 1 shows the frequency, causes, and results of different kinds of accident. Accidents leading to fatal injuries can be markedly different from those leading to major injuries. Falls on the level cause most major injuries, but few fatalities. Falls from heights and injuries from moving/falling objects contribute substantially to both severity categories.

Table 2 shows the kinds of injuries associated with fatal and serious nonfatal accidents. Fractures (15 per cent), concussion and internal injuries (14 per cent), and injuries of more than one type (26 per cent) were the injuries most often associated with fatality. Nearly three-quarters of all major injuries are attributable to fractures. The nature of injury was unknown in 9.3 per cent of cases, presumably because these details were not given on the standard pro-forma but were included in supplementary documents that did not find their way into the statistics.

The evolution of safety management

Accident prevention requires the creation, and maintenance, of a safe working environment, and the promotion of safe behaviour—the avoidance of error—by those doing hazardous work. However, safety management has emphasized the prevention of repetitions of accidents that have

Table 1 Kinds of accident: fatal and non-fatal major[1] injuries to employees for Great Britain. Numbers averaged for the 4 years 1996/97–1999/2000[2]

Kind of accident	Fatal injuries		Non-fatal major injuries	
	No.	%	No.	%
Contact with moving machinery	16	8.3	1762	6.2
Struck by moving object, including flying/falling item	35	18.1	4460	15.8
Struck by moving vehicle	36	18.7	920	3.3
Struck against something fixed or stationary	2	1.0	1404	5.0
Injured while handling, lifting, or carrying	1	0.5	2857	10.1
Slip, trip, or fall on same level	2	1.0	8730	30.9
Falls from heights	52	26.9	5277	18.7
Trapped by something collapsing or overturning	12	6.2	186	0.7
Drowning or asphyxiation	6	3.1	53	0.2
Exposure to, or contact with, a harmful substance	4	2.1	862	3.0
Exposure to fire	4	2.1	82	0.3
Exposure to explosion	4	2.1	57	0.2
Contact with electricity or electrical discharge	14	7.3	230	0.8
Injured by an animal	1	0.5	169	0.6
Acts of violence	1	0.5	666	2.4
Other kinds of accident	2	1.0	503	1.8
Injuries not classified by kind	1	0.5	55	0.2
Totals	**193**	**100.0**	**28273**	**100.0**

Note that the numbers of accidents have been rounded to whole numbers. Percentages are based on the unrounded numbers.

[1] Major injuries are defined under RIDDOR, and include fractures, amputations, losses of consciousness due to lack of oxygen, and any injury that results in the person injured being admitted immediately into hospital for more than 24 hours.

[2] The data in Table 1 and Table 2 below for 1999/00 are provisional.

Derived from Table A1.9 of HSC (2000).

Table 2 Nature of injury: fatal and non-fatal major injuries to employees for Great Britain. Numbers averaged for the four years 1996/97–1999/00

Nature of injury	Fatal injuries		Non-fatal major injuries	
	No.	%	No.	%
Amputation	0	0.0	1184	4.2
Loss of sight of eye	0	0.0	128	0.5
Fracture	29	15.0	20661	73.1
Dislocation	0	0.0	1179	4.2
Concussion and internal injuries	27	14.0	521	1.8
Lacerations and open wounds	4	2.1	1358	4.8
Contusions	11	5.7	506	1.8
Burns	8	4.2	790	2.8
Poisonings and gassings	11	5.7	213	0.8
Sprains and strains	0	0.0	405	1.4
Superficial injuries	0	0.1	341	1.2
Natural causes	1	0.5	10	0.0
Other injuries caused by contact with electricity	12	6.2	165	0.6
Injuries of more than one type	50	25.9	432	1.5
Injuries not elsewhere specified	22	11.4	241	0.9
Injuries not known	18	9.3	141	0.5
Totals	**193**	**100.0**	**28275**	**100.0**

Note that the numbers of injuries have been rounded to whole numbers. Percentages are based on the unrounded numbers.
Derived from Table A1.9 of HSC (2000).

already occurred, using information derived from detailed accident investigations. Accidents meriting investigation usually involve a casualty, and it is not surprising that the behaviour of those injured may dominate the minds of the investigators. Reactive prevention tends to be easier than proactive prevention. Assessing risks and devising preventive plans without the help of accident data is difficult: it involves weighing the probabilities of a wide range of unwanted outcomes, and preparing an integrated control plan to cope with all the detected hazards.

Key features of the traditional approach were the search for a primary accident cause, and the debate about whether the primary cause was an unsafe act or an unsafe condition.

Most practical accident prevention involved the preparation of a safety rule designed to prevent a recurrence of the unsafe act, or a physical safeguard to obviate the unsafe condition existing immediately before the accident.

The causation debate, with its political overtones and desire to apportion blame, often missed three crucial inter-related, issues:

- The concept of a single primary cause for an accident is a bizarre simplification of a complex multicausal process. The term 'unsafe act' embraces a wide range of unintentional errors and intentionally risky behaviour 'violations'.

- The distinction between the contribution of unsafe conditions and unsafe acts in causation has masked the more important distinction between the relative contribution of conditions and behaviour in prevention, and the need for prevention plans to promote both safe conditions and safe behaviour.

- The argument has focused almost exclusively on the errors made by those people involved in the accidents, not the managers and engineers whose errors (remote in time and place from the accident) may have created a physical environment conducive to the risk of serious accidents.

The safety management approach proved inadequate to cope with major hazards created by rapidly developing technology. Preventive measures may be rendered obsolete by each technical advance. Rules and safeguards devised in the aftermath of accidents may later be perceived as overzealous and may conflict with the needs of both employers and employees to get the job done. Both parties may tacitly conspire to evade the safety rules or to defeat the physical safeguards. Measures taken to prevent one specific accident may conflict with the measures adopted to prevent a different accident, and with production-oriented rules. Rule books and legislation drawn may become incomprehensible and contradictory. At least two company rules may exist for any situation: the rule to get the job done in time, and a more demanding rule that may be invoked when things go wrong.

Proactive safety management

Accident investigations and prevention programmes must address the distinctive elements of the accident causation process described below.

Multicausality

Few accidents are associated with a single cause. Rather, they happen as a result of a chance concatenation of many distinct causative factors, each one necessary but not sufficient to cause a final breakdown. The coverage of prevention plans should therefore seek to permeate all aspects of the organization's activities. Accident investigators should continue to seek out causative factors even when 'a familiar, abnormal event is found which is therefore accepted as explanation, and a cure is known'.

Active and latent failures

Active failures are errors that have an immediate adverse effect, while latent failures lie dormant in an organization becoming evident only when combined with local triggers. The triggers are the active failures: unsafe acts, and unsafe conditions such as mechanical failure.

Skill-, rule-, and knowledge-based errors, and violations

The standard framework for classifying error is the skill—rule—knowledge-based model.

Skill-based errors involve 'slips' or 'lapses' in highly practised and routine tasks. Knowledge-based errors are failures to create an adequate new rule to cope with a situation. Violations, or risk taking, are another category of error. Someone deliberately does something contrary to a rule, such as an approved operating procedure.

Hazard identification, risk assessment, and preventive action

These are the essential foundation of safety management—the avoidance of latent failures and of safe personal behaviour in the face of danger—the avoidance of active failures.

To create and maintain a safe working environment, and to work safely in a dangerous environment, people must have the knowledge and skills and must know the rules, and be motivated, to:

(1) identify hazards;

(2) assess accurately the priority and importance of the hazards (risk assessment);

(3) recognize and accept personal responsibility for dealing with the hazards in an appropriate way;

(4) have appropriate knowledge about what should be done (including specified rules);

(5) have the skills to carry out the appropriate necessary sequence of preventive actions, including monitoring the adequacy of the actions, and taking further corrective action.

The organization should be aware of circumstances where managers, supervisors, and other personnel may:

- underestimate the magnitude of risks;
- overestimate their ability to assess and control risks;
- have an impaired ability to cope with risks.

The aims of safety management

The aim of safety management is not limited to hazard identification, control, and monitoring. Employers must plan for safety. Decisions have to be made about priorities for resource allocation, training needs, the appropriate risk-assessment methods to be adopted, the need to assess human reliability, and the choice of tolerable-risk criteria. Safety criteria should underpin every decision made by the enterprise and must be considered as an integral part of day-to-day decision-making. The employer must establish an organization and communications systems that helps to integrate safety within the management process, and which ensures that everyone is fully informed about safety issues, and ideally has had an opportunity to discuss them.

Key functions of safety management

1. *Policy and planning*: relies on the determination of safety goals, objectives, and priorities, and a programme of work designed to achieve the objectives, which is subject to measurement and review.

2. *Organization and communication*: involves establishing clear lines of responsibility and two-way communications at all levels.

3. *Hazard management*: depends on ensuring that hazards are identified, risks assessed, and control measures determined, implemented, and subject to measurement and review.

4. *Monitoring and review*: requires the establishment of whether the above steps are in place, in use, and work in practice.

The four key elements of safety management are underpinned by the requirements of the Management of Health and Safety at Work Regulations 1999.

Safety management and safety culture

These procedures and systems are necessary elements of an effective safety programme, but are not the whole story. There is a danger that an organization's safety policies, plans, and monitoring arrangements, although appearing well considered and comprehensive, may create an aura of respectability which disguises sullen scepticism or false perceptions among influential people at management and shop-floor levels.

The concept of safety culture

The Health and Safety Commission has defined safety culture as follows:

> The safety culture of an organization is the product of individual and group values, attitudes, competencies, and patterns of behaviour that determine the commitment to, and the style and proficiency of, an organization's health and safety programmes.

> Organizations with a positive safety culture are characterized by communications founded on mutual trust, by shared perceptions of the importance of safety, and by confidence in the efficacy of preventive measures.

The Confederation of British Industry has reported the results of a survey of 'how companies manage health and safety'. The idea of the culture of an organization was incorporated in the report's title 'Developing a safety culture'. The dominant themes to emerge were:

(1) the crucial importance of leadership and the commitment of the chief executive;

(2) the executive safety role of line management;

(3) involvement of all employees;

(4) openness of communication; and

(5) demonstration of care and concern for all those affected by the business.

The Health and Safety at Work Act requires all companies employing five or more people to prepare a health and safety policy. A written corporate statement on the safety policy and organization is a crucial element in the promotion and maintenance of a positive safety culture within the organization, and of high standards of safety awareness in the minds of both management and workforce.

The policy should embody a positive approach to the management of safety. It must be more than a one-off event written to fulfil the letter of the Act; its objective should be to establish the corporate attitude to safety and the necessary organization through which the safety objectives can be assured. This must be subject to regular, systematic review.

Monitoring safety performance

Many companies measure safety performance merely by counting the number of accidents, a belated and potentially misleading statistic. In many organizations there are not enough accidents to determine whether differences between sites or over time are due to real differences, or to chance. Company and national accident statistics are influenced by variations in the time that individuals choose to take off for a given injury severity.

The design of a health and safety monitoring system for an enterprise must address two crucial issues:

1. There is no single unambiguous measure of safety performance that is resistant to abuse. Accident data must be combined with other measures.

2. Monitoring should be designed to both check and promote compliance.

Performance measures should be designed to permeate every activity within the organization. A battery of distinctive tests should be incorporated into the safety programme, so that the limitations of one are balanced by the strengths of another.

Safety auditing

Proprietary safety auditing systems are often used to measure safety performance, and to identify aspects of safety management requiring improvement. Audits typically comprise a checklist with about 400 questions and a scoring system. These audits allow companies to compare their safety management procedures against objective criteria, but some companies may try to improve their audit score in ways that do not lead to real improvements in safety.

Safety training

In the past, too much training was of poor quality and of doubtful effectiveness, but training is an essential part of the company's safety arrangements. The Institution of Occupational Safety and Health have published a safety training policy that emphasizes the need for:

(1) explicit training in organizations to promote and maintain a positive safety culture;

(2) training of senior managers to be competent in strategic safety management;

(3) training of managers and workers to be competent in hazard identification, risk assessment, and control;

(4) training of trainers to be competent in safety training;

(v) in-company evaluation of training effectiveness.

Further reading

Booth RT (2000). Challenges and opportunities facing the Institution of Occupational Safety and Health. *Journal of The Institution of Occupational Safety and Health* **4**, 7–21.

Committee on Safety and Health at Work (Robens Committee) (1972). *Safety and health at work*. HMSO, London.

Confederation of British Industry (1990). *Developing a safety culture*. CBI, London.

Department of Employment (1992). Health and safety statistics 1990–1991. *Employment Gazette* (*Occasional Supplement 3*) **100**, September.

Hale AR, Glendon AI (1987). *Individual behaviour in the control of danger*. Elsevier, Amsterdam.

Health and Safety Commission (1991). *Second report: human reliability assessment—a critical overview. ACSNI Study Group on human factors*. HMSO, London.

Health and Safety Commission (1993). *Third report: organising for safety— ACSNI study group on human factors*. HMSO, London.

Health and Safety Commission (2000). *Health and safety statistics 1999/2000*. HSE Books, Sudbury, Suffolk, UK.

Health and Safety Executive (1991). *Workplace health and safety in Europe*. HMSO, London.

Health and Safety Executive (1997). *Successful health and safety management*, Health and Safety Series booklet HS G 65. HSE Books, Sudbury, Suffolk, UK.

Heinrich HW (1969). *Industrial accident prevention*, 4th edn. McGraw Hill, New York.

Institution of Occupational Safety and Health (1992). *Institution policy statement on safety training*. IOSH, Leicester.

International Nuclear Safety Advisory Group (1988). *Basic safety principles for nuclear power plants*, Safety Series No 75-INSAG-3. International Atomic Energy Authority, Vienna.

International Nuclear Safety Advisory Group (1991). *Safety culture*, Safety Series No 75-INSAG-4. International Atomic Energy Authority, Vienna.

Rasmussen J (1987). Reasons, causes and human error. In: Rasmussen J, Duncan K, Leplat J, eds. *New technology and human error*, pp. 293–301. Wiley, Chichester, UK.

Reason JT (1990). *Human error*. Cambridge University Press.

Zohar D (1980). Safety climate in industrial organisations: theoretical and applied implications *Journal of Applied Psychology* **65**, 96–102.

8.5 Environmental diseases

8.5.1 Environmental extremes—heat

M. A. Stroud

Thermoregulation in the heat

Most of human evolution took place in Africa and hence all races are heat tolerant. Indeed, we try to maintain a near tropical microclimate against our skin, by using clothing to reduce heat loss to our surroundings. Our thermal balance is regulated by the hypothalamus which integrates information from skin temperature sensors with core temperature data from receptors in the walls of large blood vessels and in the brain. Rising temperatures trigger both behavioural and physiological responses.

Behavioural changes include reducing physical activity, altering clothing, and seeking shade or cool shelter. Cold drinks are also helpful. Although these responses seem simplistic, decisions may not be straightforward. If physical activity is low and water is in short supply, it is better to increase clothing cover and protect yourself from high radiant heat inputs. If activity must be continued and water is freely available, minimal clothing to permit maximal sweat evaporation is preferable. Immediate physiological responses involve vasodilatation of skin and subcutaneous blood vessels to enhance surface heat loss from radiation, conduction, and convection. The vasodilatation is triggered by a sympathetic cholinergic reflex in response to skin warming with additional direct effects of heat on arteriolar tone. In a resting individual, skin vasodilatation can maintain thermal equilibrium in environmental temperatures up to 32°C, but with higher temperatures or heat production from activity, core temperatures will rise. This will trigger sweating to promote evaporative cooling.

Heat acclimatization

Repeated heat exposure can increase our capacity to lose heat by about 20-fold. This is partly due to greater skin blood flow from increases in circulating volume and improved vasodilatory responses, but changes in sweating responses are more important. In the non-acclimatized, sweating is triggered by a rise in core temperature of about 1°C and maximum rates are limited to about 0.5 l/h. Following acclimatization, a 0.5°C core rise will trigger the response and rates may exceed 2.0 l/h. Acclimatization also leads to aldosterone-mediated reductions in sodium loss in both sweat and urine. The acclimatized individual therefore requires no sodium supplementation and giving supplements can delay the acclimatative process. Avoiding them altogether, however, does risk salt depletion in non-acclimatized persons during prolonged heat stress. Acclimatization develops swiftly and around 90 per cent of maximum heat tolerance is present after 7 to 10 days on which core temperature has risen by more than 1°C for more than 1 h. Physical exertion combined with heat makes changes even more rapid. After returning to cool environments, adaptation is lost in 20 to 40 days.

Susceptibility to heat-related illness

Although we are generally heat tolerant, heat-related illness is relatively common and a number of factors increase vulnerability. Above an environmental temperature of about 35°C, we tend to gain heat from our surroundings and this, along with metabolic heat production, can only be lost via evaporation of sweat. High humidity, hot environments are therefore the greatest threat. Acclimatization status has a marked influence on heat-related risks with the unacclimatized prone to hyperthermia and salt depletion. The fully acclimatized are vulnerable to dehydration from high sweat rates. Dehydration in itself limits sweating capacity and skin blood flow and hence increases risks. It can occur easily since thirst is a poor trigger for adequate drinking. Sweat rates can also exceed gut capacity for water absorption.

Prolonged physical activity can cause heat illness under quite modest environmental conditions. This is particularly common when individuals are obliged to wear insulative or non-vapour-permeable clothing. Military heat casualties are sometimes due to these factors but there have also been fatalities in soldiers who have been heat susceptible for no obvious cause. Such genetic or constitutional vulnerability should be suspected whenever a heat-related problem occurs following relatively modest heat stress. These individuals should be strongly advised to avoid similar circumstances in future. Obesity and poor physical fitness are further risk factors in the heat, as is diabetic autonomic dysfunction. The elderly are generally heat sensitive and, in addition, are prone to problems from the increased circulatory demands of vasodilatation. Drugs can also induce heat illness (see below).

Heat exhaustion

Most casualties in hot environments suffer from heat exhaustion. There is usually a history of prolonged heat stress followed by nausea, weakness, headache, thirst, and sometimes collapse. Patients appear dehydrated with a tachycardia and low blood pressure. If hyperthermic, the casualty should be complaining of feeling hot and should appear flushed and sweaty. The absence of these symptoms and signs, especially with a very high core temperature, suggests heat stroke. Heat exhaustion is ascribable to sodium and/or water depletion but discriminating between the predominant loss can be difficult. Sodium depletion tends to be greater if the casualty was poorly acclimatized and hence sweated relatively more sodium than water. Conversely, water depletion is more common in acclimatized individuals. Muscle cramps or whole body dehydration without marked changes in haematocrit or serum proteins are suggestive of excessive sodium loss, but serum sodium tends to be normal in such cases unless enthusiastic fluid replacement without salt has led to hyponatraemia. This sometimes occurs in runners following marathons in hot environments. In predominantly water-depleted heat exhaustion, haematocrit, serum proteins, and serum sodium tend to be high. Renal impairment occurs in either form of heat exhaustion and the treatment of both types often requires 5 to 10 l of oral or intravenous fluids in the first 24 h. Sodium supplementation is given as appropriate but if unsure about sodium status it is usually safer to provide some than to precipitate acute hyponatraemia.

Heat stroke

Mild heat stroke has occurred when a hot environment or high activity levels have led to pyrexia with cerebral disturbance. Core temperature is usually 38 to 41°C. The condition frequently follows heat exhaustion but temperature rise may have occurred rapidly with no time for salt or water depletion. Sufferers have headaches and may be either drowsy or irritable. They often hyperventilate. The great danger is progression to more severe heat stroke, in which core temperature reaches levels that cause irreversible denaturing of proteins. This usually occurs at above 41.5°C. Damage is widespread and particularly effects brain, liver, kidney, and muscle. Furthermore, the hypothalamic thermoregulatory centre may fail, switching off vasodilatation and sweating, and switching on cold defences inappropriately. Patients may therefore claim to feel cold and on examination may be shivering with a dry, vasoconstricted skin. A disastrous vicious cycle of increasing temperatures can then ensue.

Treatment for all heat stroke requires early recognition and rapid cooling. Tepid water and fan-assisted evaporation may be more effective than cold water immersion which can limit heat loss through intense peripheral vasoconstriction. Intraperitoneal fluids, paralysis, and ventilation may be needed and, in extremis, cooling by cardiac by-pass should be considered. Hyperkalaemia, hypocalcaemia, acidosis, rhabdomyolysis, disseminated intravascular coagulation, and hepatic or renal failure are all common complications. Ventricular fibrillation is a frequent terminal event. Even if apparently resuscitated and cooled successfully, a 12 to 24-h 'lucid interval' may precede major deterioration. Permanent neurological damage is common.

Drug-induced heat illness

Many drugs can cause mild degrees of pyrexia by inducing local or systemic inflammation or hypersensitivity. Some also increase susceptibility to environmental heat by inhibiting central thermoregulation (e.g. barbiturates and phenothiazines) or reducing sweating capacity (e.g. anticholinergics). Salicylate overdose can generate heat stroke by increasing metabolic heat production while impairing hypothalamic regulation. There are two types of heat-related drug reaction, however, which are particularly dangerous.

Malignant hyperpyrexia

This is usually a dominantly inherited condition although different gene defects may effect families. Administration of a variety of anaesthetic agents, including halothane and suxamethonium, leads to rapid, massive heat production from generalized increases in skeletal muscle tone. Contraction is triggered at the muscle cell membrane and hence neuromuscular blocking agents are ineffective. Intravenous dantrolene, an inhibitor of muscle calcium flux, is helpful and can be used along with ventilation and cooling/supportive measures. Fatalities are common and it is therefore important to avoid risks whenever possible. In patients with a relevant personal or family history, in whom an anaesthetic is unavoidable, oral dantrolene should be given prior to the use of low-risk agents.

Neuroleptic malignant syndrome

This condition has similarities to malignant hyperpyrexia but is induced by idiosyncratic reactions to normal doses of antidopaminergic drugs including phenothiazines and butyrophenones. The onset is less rapid than malignant hyperpyrexia, occurring over a few days. The increased muscle tone is also induced presynaptically and hence neuromuscular blocking agents help. Some recreational drugs such as ecstasy may induce this type of response, although most cases of ecstasy-induced hyperthermia are probably cases of heat stroke induced by enthusiastic dancing with limited fluid intake in hot, humid environments.

Further reading

Hodgson P (1991). Malignant hyperthermia and the neuroleptic malignant syndrome. In: Swash M, Oxbury J, eds. *Clinical neurology*, pp. 1344–5. Churchill Livingstone, Edinburgh.

Hubbard RW, Armstrong LE (1988). The heat illnesses: biochemical, ultrastructural, and fluid-electrolyte considerations. In: Pandolf KB, Sawka MN, Gonzalez R, eds. *Human performance physiology and environmental medicine at terrestrial extremes*, pp. 305–59. Benchmark, Indianapolis.

Stroud MA (1993). Environmental temperature and physiological function. In: Ulijaszek SJ, Strickland SS, eds. *Seasonality and human ecology*, pp 38–53. Cambridge University Press.

8.5.2 Environmental extremes—cold

M. A. Stroud

It has only been 10 000 to 15 000 years since ancestral humans dwelt exclusively in warm or hot climates. Humans are therefore poorly cold adapted and hypothermia occurs quite frequently even in temperate regions. With water immersion it may occur in the tropics. In truly cold areas, there is also the risk of non-freezing cold injury and frostbite. Nevertheless, behavioural changes allow us to operate safely in the coldest environments.

Thermoregulation in the cold

Core temperatures in the cold are usually maintained by adjustments in clothing and physical activity. The latter can increase heat production from a resting 100 watts to 1 to 2 kilowatts. This is very effective. While it takes highly specialized, multilayered clothing to keep warm while inactive in an environment of +5°C, clothing insulation equivalent to normal office dress (1 clo) will maintain core temperature at −20°C when working moderately hard.

Our limited physiological cold protection is under hypothalamic control. Falling surface and, to a lesser extent, core temperatures lead to decreased blood flow in the skin due to increased sympathetic adrenergic tone and direct cooling effects of cold on skin arterioles. This minimize surface heat loss. Unfortunately, vasoconstriction also leads to severe cooling of the hands and feet with problems of temporary skin numbness and muscle weakness, and risks of more permanent peripheral cold injury. It is often this peripheral cooling that limits our capacity to work in the cold.

Falling skin temperatures will also lead to higher resting muscle tone and shivering, especially when declining core temperature releases hypothalamic inhibition of shivering. These mechanisms can only increase resting heat production to around 500 watts and, unlike newborn infants and some other mammals, adult humans cannot add significant non-shivering heat production to this figure.

Effects of falling core temperature

Falling core temperature leads to progressive decline in function. At 34 to 36°C, hypothermic individuals are conscious of feeling cold and try to move around, add clothing, or seek shelter. Simultaneously, physiological defences are activated. With further falls, mental and physical problems increase with some individuals becoming withdrawn while others exhibit aggression or disinhibition. Once core temperatures reach 33 to 34°C, victims often stagger and become confused or drowsy. It is also around this point that 'paradoxical undressing' may occur. This phenomenon is well described and appears to be due to hypothalamic dysfunction with alteration of set-point temperature. Victims therefore think that they are hot and appropriate behavioural and physiological responses disappear. At core temperatures varying between 26°C and 32°C, coma will ensue and between 17 to 26°C cardiac output becomes inadequate to sustain life for prolonged periods. The risk of ventricular fibrillation is also high. Nevertheless, successful resuscitations of victims with core temperatures below 15°C have been reported.

Causes of hypothermia

A number of factors increase hypothermic risk. Wetting of skin or clothing extracts enormous amounts of heat and reduces insulation of garments. Complete immersion is particularly hazardous and globally, more than 100 000 people per year die of cold shock or inexorable hypothermia in the water. This far exceeds deaths from drowning without cold. Winds also increase environmental cooling and a still air temperature of +5°C equates to −50°C if wind speed is 40 km/h. Coupled with rain, these effects often contribute to hypothermic accidents amongst hill walkers and mountaineers, although in these cases fatigue may contribute. Prolonged exertion depletes muscle glycogen which reduces heat production capacity from both exercise and shivering. A low blood glucose also impairs hypothalamic temperature control.

Small, thin individuals cool easily due to increased surface-to-volume ratios. They also have reduced subcutaneous insulation and low heat producing mass. A fat individual can maintain core temperature at rest, even if mean skin temperature is 12°C, whereas a thin individual struggles to maintain thermal equilibrium with a skin temperature of 25°C. Sometimes, however, rapid cooling can have benefits. A small child in cold water may cool so rapidly that vagally triggered bradycardia and lowered brain metabolic demands may permit successful resuscitation after very prolonged immersion.

The elderly may also be small and thin and are at risk of so-called 'urban hypothermia'. Poverty, illness, immobility, malnutrition, and a less sensitive regulatory system may contribute but, in many cases, hypothermia on admission to hospital is secondary to other pathology, for example a stroke may have led to prolonged immobility in a cool environment. Drugs that impair consciousness or induce vasodilatation are risk factors, and alcohol is particularly hazardous. Alcoholics with no fixed abode and tendency for hypoglycaemia are frequent urban cold casualties.

Hypothermic illness

General management of the hypothermic casualty is similar to that for any comatose or semicomatose individual. Abnormalities in blood gases, pH, electrolytes, and glucose are common, and pancreatitis or rhabdomyolysis are recognized complications. Accurate measurement of core temperature is surprisingly difficult and axillary, tympanic, and oral temperatures can all be misleading. A low reading rectal thermometer is best. Hypothermia has one, very specific risk. Pronouncement of death is fraught with difficulty since profound bradycardia, minimal stroke volume, and marked respiratory depression occur. The old adage that you are 'never dead unless warm and dead' must be taken seriously.

A variety of rewarming methods are available. Warm blankets and hot drinks will suffice in many cases but, although used widely, metallized 'space blankets' are of no proven benefit. Warmed intravenous fluids are helpful and, in extreme cases, peritoneal warmed fluids or cardiac bypass can be used. Specialized equipment providing heated, humidified air also permits core rewarming. Hot baths are effective but difficult to utilize safely since a paradoxical fall in core temperature can occur as blood flow is rapidly restored to cold limbs. In general, if cooling was prolonged in onset or duration, rewarming must be undertaken with extreme caution. In critical cases, where rapid rewarming is needed, full resuscitation facilities must be available, although safe defibrillation in the presence of water is impossible.

Careful monitoring during rewarming is vital. Blood volumes are often low due to early cold-induced diuresis followed by the inability of hypothermic kidneys to retain salt and water. In immersion casualties, hydrostatic effects on the limbs may have promoted additional fluid loss and, if possible, these individuals must be kept recumbent throughout rescue and rewarming to minimize risks from extreme postural hypotension. Warming cell membranes are extremely unstable and uncontrollable fluxes in potassium and other electrolytes may occur although care must be taken in interpreting biochemical results from cold peripheral blood sampling.

Non-freezing cold injury

Local temperatures of less than12°C prevent normal membrane pumping and paralyse nerve and muscle conduction. If such cooling is prolonged, permanent damage may ensue. Immersion in cold water is particularly likely to cause this type of damage and soldiers in military campaigns are frequent victims of 'trench foot'. Long-term damage is likely whenever an anaesthetic, paralysed, cold region becomes hot, red, painful, and swollen after rewarming, although this change may take several days. Degeneration of nerve and muscle can then follow leading to prolonged anaesthesia, muscle contractures, or inappropriate peripheral vascular control with intolerance to local heat or cold. There may be slow improvement over months or years.

Frostbite

Human tissues freeze at around −2°C. Ice forms outside cells but the remaining extracellular fluid becomes hyperosmolar and hence severe intracellular dehydration occurs. This denatures proteins. Vascular endothelial cells are particularly vulnerable and following rewarming small blood vessels may leak plasma and then become blocked by red cell sludge and clot. Additional ischaemic necrosis is then superimposed on the frost damage.

Frozen tissues appear hard and white and are anaesthetic. Rewarming leads to pain and swelling often accompanied by blistering. Deep freezing results in irreversible necrosis but appearances can be misleading and early amputation of digits should be avoided. If still frozen, rewarming is best achieved rapidly by using immersion in water at 40 to 42°C, although any thawing should be avoided if refreezing is likely. Once thawed, treatment is similar to that used for burns with prevention of infection paramount. Generous analgesia is required.

Further reading

Granberg PO (1997). Cold injury. In: Chant ADB, Barros D'Sa AAB, eds. *Emergency vascular practice*, pp. 119–34. Arnold, London.

Hamlet MP (1988). Human cold injuries. In: Pandolf KB, Sawka MN, Gonzalez R, eds. *Human performance physiology and environmental medicine at terrestrial extremes*, pp. 435–66. Benchmark, Indianapolis.

Stroud MA (1993). Environmental temperature and physiological function. In: Ulijaszek SJ, Strickland SS, eds. *Seasonality and human ecology*, pp. 38–53. Cambridge University Press.

8.5.3 Drowning

Peter J. Fenner

Introduction

Drowning is an important cause of accidental death and neurological damage, particularly in children, and is usually preventable. Drowning is listed in the Global Burden of Disease Study as the fourth most common injury worldwide (behind road-traffic accidents, self-inflicted injuries, and violence but ahead of war deaths), and is the twentieth most common cause of death worldwide, with numbers estimated at 504 000 each year.

Drowning is defined as death from suffocation by submersion in a liquid, usually freshwater or seawater. Near-drowning is survival, at least temporarily, from suffocation by submersion.

Mortality and morbidity

Acute hypoxia is the cause of the haemodynamic effects and death. Neurological morbidity in survivors of near-drowning includes difficulty with learning, memory, attention, and planning and cerebral palsy. A major study of childhood immersions has shown that approximately 68 per cent of survivors have no neurological defect, 29 per cent have some deficit, and 3 per cent will live in a permanent vegetative state. Economic costs to the community are immense.

Epidemiology

Bathtub and bucket drownings may involve infants and toddlers under the age of 12 months. Ten per cent of fatal bucket or tub immersions are the result of child abuse. Drowning rates in young children worldwide, many of whom are unsupervised, have decreased little despite preventive strategies such as fencing swimming pools. However, despite the lack of preventive strategies aimed at older children, drowning rates in older children have declined dramatically in the last decade. Ocean drownings are less common than freshwater drownings. Fewer children swim unsupervised in the ocean, and the preventive and rescue efforts of lifesaving and lifeguard associations guarding the beaches have proved effective, especially in Australia and the United States. Reasons for variations in rates of drowning include climate, the availability of beaches, lakes, and other natural and artificial water sources, employment of lifeguards at water parks, use of different kinds of vessels suitable for recreation (kayaks, personal watercraft, etc.), provision and use of lifejackets, and popularity of hobbies, pastimes, and professions associated with a risk of drowning (for example fishing). Recently a study provided proof of the principle that an unexplained drowning or near drowning may have a genetic basis.

Ethnicity

White American children aged 1 to 4 years have twice the drowning rate of African-American children of a similar age, these occurring mainly in residential swimming pools. Conversely, among children and young people aged 5 to 19 years, the rate of drowning in African-Americans is greater than for white Americans. In Australia deaths from drowning in Aboriginal children are more frequent than in whites.

Alcohol

Alcohol affects vision, balance, and movement and is a risk factor in drowning for both adolescent and adult swimmers, as well as for boat operators and passengers, who may fall overboard while intoxicated. Some 25 to 50 per cent of adult drowning victims may have had some exposure to alcohol at the time of rescue, resuscitation, or death.

Pathophysiology

Early animal studies in unanaesthetized dogs suggested that spontaneous respiratory efforts continue for around 60 s after immersion. Complete cardiac arrest supervenes after 4.5 min (mean 262 s). Aspiration is usual in drowning and near-drowning. It has been suggested that approximately 10 to 15 per cent of drowning victims do not aspirate water ('dry' drowning, possibly occurring from laryngeal spasm). However, further studies of these data by Modell suggest the conclusion may be without foundation and the effect may be due to cardiac standstill or other causes of sudden death; careful postmortem examination is required.

The haemodynamic effects following inspiration of liquid are the same irrespective of whether hypotonic, isotonic, or hypertonic solutions are involved, and are similar to anoxic controls. Both groups show a rapid fall in cardiac output, an increase in pulmonary capillary wedge pressure, central venous pressure, and pulmonary vascular resistance. Reduction in the dynamic compliance of the lungs is similar following inspiration of all types of solutions. However, aspiration of large volumes of hypertonic seawater draws fluid by osmosis from the circulation into the lung, resulting in fluid-filled, non-ventilated but perfused alveoli, incapable of normal gas exchange. Aspiration of large amounts of hypotonic fresh water may cause sufficient absorption of fluid into the circulation from the alveoli to cause both acute hypervolaemia and haemolysis, although within an hour redistribution of fluid and pulmonary oedema occurs, causing a decreased circulating blood volume. Although Modell suggested that 85 per cent of human drowning victims aspirate only 22 ml/kg of water or less, Conn estimated that water equivalent to about 10 per cent of body weight may be absorbed from the lungs during freshwater drowning.

The brain has a limited ability to maintain ATP anaerobically when cerebral blood flow is reduced. Without cerebral blood flow, the brain suffers irreparable damage within 4 to 6 min. There is some potential, however, for the restoration of activity for up to 60 min of total anoxia in hypothermia. Death or severe neurological impairment occurs after sumbersion of more than 5 to 10 min. Bystanders' estimates of sumbersion time are usually inaccurate.

Hypothermia

Submersion (not immersion) in ice-water with associated hypothermia is an important cause of near-drowning. Continuous aspiration of cold water results in rapid reduction in the core temperature while the circulation is intact. Such victims may survive, protected by hypothermia, with little or no neurological deficit after long submersion with extreme anoxia. In water at 16 °C with maximum submersion for 10 min or less, a good outcome could often be predicted.

Intact neurological survival occurred in a 6-year-old boy with a rectal temperature of 16.4 °C. after submersion for 65 min when the blood was rewarmed over 96 min in steps of 3 °C. In adults, success is less common. A notable exception was a 31-year-old man with a core temperature of 23 °C who had been asystolic for 80 min and was warmed by cardiopulmonary bypass and recovered. In warm-water drownings, Frates was unable to show any statistically significant correlation between duration of submersion and survival.

Causes of drowning

Drowning occurs in many different situations including accidental immersion of people with poor or no swimming ability, with head and neck injuries, following cardiac and neurological emergencies (including epilepsy), as a result of impaired ability (including the effects of alcohol and drugs), metabolic disease (including hypoglycaemia), and even child abuse and murder. In countries with large coastlines or bathing beaches, drowning is common and is often caused by swimmers being caught in rip currents (large volumes of water returning back out to sea after onshore wave action): there is no such entity as the frequently suggested 'undertow'.

Swimmers in difficulty may be able to shout for help but, contrary to public opinion, those drowning do not. Most drowning victims adopt a characteristic vertical position in the water—legs hang vertically, head tilted back for quick exhalation and inhalation before bobbing under water, with no time nor sufficient breath to call for help. After only 20 to 60 s, victims may submerge permanently.

Clinical features

Prognostic indicators

Success or failure of the resuscitation of the near-drowned depends on the promptness and adequacy of emergency resuscitation and subsequent respiratory intensive care. Up to 25 per cent of drowning victims presenting to the emergency department will die and a further 6 per cent have neurological sequelae.

Those with a normal chest radiograph on admission survive. Pao_2 may not relate to radiographic appearances. Although the cause and pathophysiological changes of pulmonary insufficiency vary depending on the type and volume of fluid aspirated, serum electrolytic and haemoglobin concentrations (or haematocrit) are unhelpful in predicting survival.

Cardiovascular status

This is a better guide to outcome than the neurological status. Mortality is high in victims with circulatory arrest on admission but victims with sinus rhythm, reactive pupils, and neurological responsiveness at the scene of immersion have good outcomes. Victims who are asystolic on arrival at hospital and remain comatose for more than 3 h have a poor outcome unless they are hypothermic. Rapid hypothermia from sudden submersion in cold water (see Chapter 8.5.2) carries a relatively good prognosis, compared with hypothermia after prolonged submersion and cardiac arrest.

Neurological status

Victims who are alert when medical help arrives have a survival rate approaching 100 per cent, whereas the prognosis in those who are comatose with fixed dilated pupils is poor. Victims with blunted consciousness have a survival rate of 87 per cent with no neurological defects, 2 per cent with minor defects, and 11 per cent die. Approximately 40 to 50 per cent of victims who are comatose on arrival have incapacitating brain damage. Those with no spontaneous limb movements and abnormal brainstem function 24 h after the accident have a poor neurological outcome.

A modified Glasgow coma score is helpful in evaluating neurological injury. A score of 5 or less predicts a mortality risk of over 80 per cent. Pupil reactions at the time of arrival differentiate survivors from fatalities but could not differentiate between those with minor or incapacitating neurological deficits. Fixed dilated pupils or total flaccidity are associated with a high mortality. Victims with any motor activity, even posturing or seizures in the immediate postresuscitation period, had a higher incidence of intact survival, but posturing movements persisting or recurring after 12 to 24 h, indicate a high probability of severe brain damage.

An abnormal computed tomography scan in the initial 36 h following an immersion incident is associated with a dismal prognosis. Magnetic resonance imaging with qualitative and quantitative magnetic resonance spectroscopy data may allow a more accurate prognosis.

The gravity of the early clinical state, the estimated duration of cardiorespiratory arrest, the severity of the hypothermia, seizures, and paroxysmal motion activity do not determine the severity of near-drowning encephalopathy. Early EEG patterns with moderate background activity, sleep patterns, response to auditory and painful stimulations, and numerous beta rhythms suggest a good outcome whereas bad outcomes are suggested by high-voltage, rhythmic delta waves, biphasic sharp waves, monotonous EEG, 'burst-suppression' pattern, and the absence of beta rhythms. Chil-

dren without spontaneous movements and normal brainstem function 24 h after near-drowning suffer severe neurological deficits or death.

Treatment

The near-drowning victim must be treated immediately for ventilatory insufficiency, hypoxia, and the resulting acidosis. A successful outcome depends on early effective resuscitation at the scene and on competent intensive life support. Australian surf lifesaving teaching has shown that respiratory resuscitation in deep water can be effective.

Immediate

Lying the victim on his or her side for assessment of the airway and breathing will assist drainage of any excess water from the lungs. On-site cardiopulmonary resuscitation is necessary, with all victims having supplemental oxygen as soon as possible, preferably at the scene using positive airway pressure (bag, valve, mask). An oropharyngeal airway or endotracheal tube should be inserted in comatose victims if suitably qualified personnel are present. Pulse oximetry is helpful. Vomiting and regurgitation are a significant risk during early resuscitation. Respiratory and cardiopulmonary arrest may occur after an apparently successful rescue, mandating close, uninterrupted monitoring and the early administration of oxygen to all immersion victims.

On hospital arrival

On arrival at the hospital, after initial establishment of a clear airway and cardiocirculatory support, arterial blood gas tensions and pH should be measured. The pH of the blood will indicate whether a metabolic acidosis remains secondary to a significant period of hypoxia.

Mechanical ventilation may be necessary with positive end-expiratory pressure or continuous positive airway pressure. A central venous catheter, or pulmonary artery catheter in selected cases, helps to assess the effective circulating blood volume to guide fluid therapy.

In both freshwater and seawater aspiration, large volumes of intravenous colloid are usually needed while circulating blood volume and cardiac output are estimated. Failure of response to intravascular replacement with 20 ml/kg of colloid is an indication for starting inotropes. Steroid and prophylactic antibiotic therapy do not appear to increase the chance of survival.

Inpatient treatment

Extracorporeal membrane oxygenation has been used successfully for the treatment of adult respiratory distress syndrome secondary to near-drowning, although this addresses only the pulmonary not the cerebral injury. Patients with severe hypoxaemia may also have irreversible cerebral ischaemia.

If adult respiratory distress syndrome occurs, it is usually within 6 h of admission. There is evidence that alveolar epithelial barrier function is well preserved even after aspiration of large quantities of hypertonic salt water. Surfactant has been used with some success in refractory respiratory failure in near-drowning, but it is expensive.

The risk of secondary pneumonia is high, especially when mechanical ventilation has been used. Although prophylactic antibiotics are not recommended broad-spectrum antibiotics may be required. Mild reversible renal impairment (serum creatinine <0.30 mmol/l (3.4 mg/dl)) is usual but severe acute renal failure (ARF) requiring dialysis can occur. It is recommended that any patient who presents after near-drowning or immersion should be assessed for potential ARF by serial estimations of serum creatinine, particularly when there is an increase in the initial serum creatinine, marked metabolic acidosis, an abnormal urinalysis, or marked lymphocytosis.

Prevention of drowning

Swimming pools and natural bodies of water present the greatest risk to young children. Preventive measures include public educational campaigns in the media, education and supervision by the parents, training in cardiopulmonary resuscitation, and better safety standards and safety devices, including pool fencing. The number of pool drownings in Brisbane (Australia) decreased after legislation made pool fencing compulsory. Strategies for the prevention of drowning should also consider hazards in rural areas.

The swimming and safety skills of young children may be improved by training. Education of the public is essential—in Australia only 17 per cent of surf rescues and resuscitations occurred within patrolled areas (up to 95 per cent successful resuscitation), while 55 per cent were saved and resuscitated outside patrolled areas (62 per cent successful); resuscitation success rates fell with increasing distance from patrolled areas. Some 5 per cent of all non-boating drownings in Australia were overseas tourists; 89 per cent of these were drowned in the ocean.

Eighty-nine per cent of children aged 35 to 59 months and 6 per cent of those younger than 3 years of age are sometimes bathed without adult supervision. An adult should supervise infants aged under 3 and all epileptic children in the bath.

Deaths from drowning in accidents involving boating and personalized water craft can be prevented by using lifejackets (personal flotation devices), but as many as 50 per cent of boaters do not use them. Efforts to increase their use should target adolescents, adults, and boating enthusiasts, especially those using motor boats. Specific measures tailored to prevent drowning associated with vessels capsizing and sinking in Alaska's commercial fishing industry have been successful.

More men than women drown in most age groups, probably reflecting an overestimation of their abilities, and more alcohol consumption. Middle-aged men dominate the group who die of cardiac events (mostly on the surface). Those who die of breath-holding hypoxia tend to be young males. Hyperventilation to increase breath-hold time is a dangerous practice that should be discouraged. Drownings are rare at supervised water parks, probably because of the large number of lifeguards on duty.

Further reading

Cummins P, Quan L. (1999). Trends in unintentional drowning. The role of alcohol and medical care. *Journal of the American Medical Association*, **281**: 2198–202.

DeNicola LK, Falk JL, Swanson ME, Gayle MO, Kissoon N. (1997). Submersion injuries in children and adults. *Critical Care Clinics*, **13**: 477–502.

Manolios N, Mackie I. (1988). Drowning and near-drowning on Australian beaches patrolled by lifesavers: a 10-year study, 1973–1983. *Medical Journal of Australia*, **148**:165–171.

Modell JH, Layon AJ. (1999). Drowning and near-drowning. In: Lungdren CEG, Miller JN, eds. *The lung at depth*. New York: Marcel Dekker Inc., 395–417.

Orlowski JP. (1987). Drowning, near-drowning, and ice-water submersion. *Pediatric Clinics of North America*, **34**: 75–92.

Pearn J. (1987). Drowning and near drowning. Paediatric emergencies. In: Black JA, ed. *Medical aspects of drowning in children*, 2nd edn. London: Butterworths.

Spicer ST, Quinn D, Nyi NN, Nankivell BJ, Hayes JM, Savdie E. (1999). Acute renal impairment after immersion and near-drowning. *Journal of the American Society of Nephrology*, **10**: 382–6.

8.5.4 Diseases of high terrestrial altitudes

D. Rennie

High altitude terrain and populations

Until the late nineteenth century, mountains were viewed by Europeans as dangerous, mysterious, hostile, and remote. Yet there is evidence that mountainous regions have, for many thousands of years, been the home of large and elaborate civilizations such as that of the Incas, which in the fifteenth century included Ecuador to the north and much of northern Chile and Argentina some 5000 km to the south, an empire of at least 12 million people. The Altiplano or high plateau of the Andes is still home to millions of descendants of these Incas, many of whom have never been below altitudes around 4000 m above sea level.

Temperature tends to determine the fauna and flora. Since, other things being equal, temperature falls with increasing altitude, the high altitude climate tends to be an arctic one. The snow line and tree line become lower with increasing distance from the equator and to live, work, hunt, and cultivate at altitudes above 3000 m is possible only within about 40° of the equator. This includes the Andes of Ecuador, Bolivia, Peru, and northern Chile, the Rocky Mountains in the United States, the high lands of east Africa, the Caucasus, the Pamirs, and the Himalayas, but does not include, for example, the European Alps.

The fall in temperature of some 1°C for every 150 m rise in altitude, irrespective of latitude, and the high winds increase the danger of cold injury. The low humidity contributes greatly to fluid loss and dehydration, as does the increased solar radiation, which may be very much exaggerated by reflection from the snow. These factors are, however, common to most arctic environments and are discussed elsewhere.

The fact that so many people of diverse races have been born and have lived at such altitudes, and the fact that, excluding Antarctica, about 2.5 per cent of the land lies above 3000 m, gives high altitude physiology and medicine an economic, political, and cultural relevance. As modern transport brings the highest mountains within range of the meanest purse, tourists, hikers, mountaineers, and downhill and cross-country skiers, as well as mining engineers, geologists, and surveyors, are flocking up into the hills. Every day in July and August about 3600 people visit the summit of Pike's Peak in Colorado (4300 m) and there is now even a 42-km marathon race up and down that mountain. In 1950, three expert Western climbers first reached the base of the ice fall below Mount Everest's Western Cwm, at 5300 m. Twenty-five years later, in a mere 4 weeks, well over 500 inexpert tourists did so.

The vast majority of mankind lives below 1000 m altitude and, though there is an exponential rise in the numbers of lowlanders going to high altitude, they cannot assume that the ascent can be made with impunity.

Hypoxia

Though the proportion of oxygen in the air (20.93 per cent) is the same at every altitude, the atmospheric pressure decreases with increasing altitude. The total atmospheric pressure at sea level (barometric pressure, PB varies but is usually around 760 torr (mmHg) (101 kPa) and that due to oxygen (the partial pressure of oxygen) is 20.93 per cent of this, that is 159 torr (21.2 kPa). In the lung, the air is rapidly saturated with water vapour at body temperature. At any altitude this is 47 torr (6.25 kPa) at 37°C. The actual combined pressures of gas taken into the lungs is therefore PB–47 torr and the inspired oxygen tension (PIo_2) is 20.93 per cent of this: $0.2093 \times (PB–47)$. At sea level this is $0.2093 \times (760–47) = 149$ torr (19.8 kPa). At about 5500 m the atmospheric pressure is about half that at sea level and at the summit of Everest (8848 m) the atmospheric pressure is about 250 torr (33 kPa; one-third that at sea level) and the partial pressure of oxygen is $0.2093 \times 250 = 52.3$ torr (7 kPa). The partial pressure of water, however, reduces the PIo_2 from 52.5 torr to $0.2093 \times (250-47) = 42.5$ torr (5.7 kPa). It is clear that the fraction of total inspired gas pressure due to water vapour, which at sea level is 6 per cent, increases with altitude. At the summit of Everest it will be nearly 19 per cent and at 19 200 m (63 000 feet), the total pressure of inspired gases would be a fatal 47 torr—fatal because all of it would be water vapour. Conversely, the proportion of inspired gas due to oxygen, which is 19.6 per cent at sea level, is reduced to 17 per cent at the summit of Everest.

Following a plane's sudden decompression or a rapid balloon ascent, for example, a resting man, just up from sea level, would lose consciousness in a matter of minutes at altitudes between 6400 and 7300 m ($PAo_2 = 24$–15 torr; 3.2–2 kPa) and in seconds above 7300 m (PAo_2 below 15 torr; 2 kPa), yet during 1 year (1978–9) a total of 14 men, on the three highest peaks in the world (Everest, K2, and Kanchenjunga) were not only fully conscious at rest more than 1000 m higher than this but were able to climb over difficult terrain in bad weather to their respective summits (8848 m, 8611 m, and 8598 m) all without the benefit of supplemental oxygen.

Acclimatization

The difference between the ineffectual newcomer on arrival at high altitudes and the resident is the sum of a myriad of physiological adjustments called 'acclimatization'. This seems to depend solely upon the length of exposure and the age when first exposed and has little to do with genetic factors. The time of greatest adjustment is in the hours and days after arrival at a higher altitude, but changes may continue for years.

The alterations in response to hypoxia affect every tissue. They may be summarized as a series of adjustments which boost oxygen supply to the mitochondria by keeping the partial pressure of oxygen in the tissue capillaries as high as possible, by decreasing the distance oxygen has to diffuse in the tissues, and by increasing the concentrations of respiratory enzymes. A few of the principal steps involved may be summarized as follows.

Ventilation

When PAo_2 has fallen to 55 to 60 torr (7.3–7.9 kPa) at an altitude of about 2000 to 3000 m, the peripheral chemoreceptors are stimulated by hypoxia and ventilation is increased. This initial reaction is amplified over the next 3 or 4 days so that PAo_2 levels which are only very slightly lower than normal (as one would find at, say, 1000 m altitude) now begin to stimulate ventilation. After a few weeks of sojourn, however, ventilation slowly decreases and this process continues for years, though ventilation is always higher in sojourners than in people who were born and have lived all their lives at altitude. With exercise, ventilation increases more at high altitude than at sea level and more in sojourners than in natives.

Driving respiration by hypoxia implies, from the point of view of carbon dioxide (CO_2), 'hyperventilation', since CO_2 is blown off and a respiratory alkalosis develops. The Pco_2 falls in a linear manner with altitude, and the alkalosis is only partly compensated by a rise in urinary excretion of bicarbonate. The effect of the increased ventilation is rapidly to increase the alveolar oxygen pressure by reducing the oxygen gradient between ambient and alveolar air and by reducing $PAco_2$.

Pulmonary diffusion

Though no increase in pulmonary diffusing capacity occurs in sojourners at high altitude, natives have increased pulmonary diffusing capacity with a lowered alveolar–arterial oxygen gradient, associated with an increased capillary surface for diffusion. This is due to an opening up of pulmonary capillaries, and to polycythaemia which decreases the distance necessary for gaseous diffusion. In the newcomer to high altitude, exercise is accompanied by a marked fall in arterial oxygen saturation, in contrast to the unchanged values on exercise at sea level, and this may be partly due to a limitation in diffusion.

Circulation

Though there is an abrupt increase in cardiac output on ascent to high altitude, there follows a progressive decrease in stroke volume and maximal cardiac output is reduced at all levels of exercise including maximal exercise. There is no evidence for insufficient myocardial oxygenation and there is argument about whether or not the myocardium is actually depressed by the hypoxia. There is an immediate alteration in the distribution of blood flow. For example coronary and cutaneous flow both fall, cerebral and retinal flow increase, renal flow temporarily decreases, and then, with acclimatization, returns to normal.

The oxygen-carrying ability of the blood is considerably increased by the massive increase in red cell production, in total red cell mass, and, more importantly, in tissue capillarity. It is somewhat offset by the higher haematocrit which increases the blood viscosity and decreases the rate of flow. The shift in the oxy–haemoglobin dissociation curve to the right, which occurs on ascent and is due to an increase in red cell 2,3-diphosphoglycerate, favours unloading of oxygen to the tissues, but this particular adjustment is offset by the shift to the left caused by alkalosis.

Tissue adaptations

Apart from the very major role of increased tissue capillarity which reduces the average capillary–mitochondrial distance and so dramatically reduces the distance for diffusion, increased myoglobin facilitates oxygen diffusion and there is an increase both in mitochondrial density and in many enzymes of the respiratory pathway (e.g. in cytochrome oxidase).

Oxygen uptake

Though the oxygen uptake at rest is not diminished even at very high altitudes, above an altitude of 1500 m the maximal oxygen uptake, $\dot{V}o_{2max}$, falls about 10 per cent for each gain in altitude of 1000 m between 1500 and 6700 m and though it is improved by administration of pure oxygen, it does not return to normal until several days after descent. The cause of this drop in $\dot{V}o_{2max}$ has been debated. If, at any one altitude, the work load is increased, $\dot{V}o_2$ may reach a maximum but ventilation, already increased at high altitude, is still able to increase further and so does not seem to be the factor limiting $\dot{V}o_{2max}$.

At altitude, as opposed to at sea level, arterial oxygen saturation falls with increasing exertion, but at moderate altitudes rises again near maximal exertion. There is probably no increase in alveolar–arterial oxygen gradient and, because of the rise in haemoglobin, the amount of oxygen carried is kept up. Diffusion may be a little limited but diffusion and the blood's oxygen carrying capacity are probably not factors limiting $\dot{V}o_{2max}$. After a few days at high altitude, however, maximal heart rate and, particularly, maximal cardiac stroke volume are reduced, the cause being unclear, and so the inability of the heart to go on increasing cardiac output seems to be the reason for the fact that $\dot{V}o_{2max}$ declines progressively with increases in altitude.

Extreme altitudes

At extreme values, where every increment in height results in a precipitous fall in $\dot{V}o_{2max}$, the oxygen cost of the work of ventilation rises considerably and it assumes an even greater proportion of total oxygen cost when $\dot{V}o_{2max}$ is reduced to really low levels. Moreover, the maximal ventilation itself is reduced at such altitudes and, in addition, there is a diffusion defect within the lungs which becomes very marked on exercise. This, together with the steady decline in maximal cardiac output, causes maximal oxygen uptake to fall very precipitously at 8848 m where PB is around 250 torr almost to resting or basal levels of oxygen uptake, a figure of about 5 m/kg per min. The state of a climber at 8000 m who is comfortable resting in his tent but whose $\dot{V}_{O_2max}$ is reached when he puts on his boots, for example, is perilous.

Alveolar gas samples taken on the summit of Everest (8848 m; barometric pressure 253 torr, 33.4 kPa) show an inspired P_{O_2} = 43 torr (5.68 kPa), and alveolar P_{O_2} = 35 torr (4.62 kPa). Estimated arterial gas values are: P_{O_2} = 28 torr (3.7 kPa); P_{CO_2} = 7.5 (0.99 kPa); pH = greater than 7.7; oxygen saturation = 70 per cent. A number of reports have suggested mild, possibly permanent, defects in cognition in climbers who have ascended to extreme high altitudes.

Illness due to altitude

Acute mountain sickness

For centuries it has been known that when lowland dwellers climb mountains some of them become ill. The illness, usually called acute mountain sickness, generally begins after a few hours, and is characterized by non-specific symptoms such as headache and vomiting. In the vast majority of people it is transient and trivial but in a few becomes progressive, severe, and may be fatal. It is to some extent relieved by breathing oxygen and it is cured by descent to sea level. Its cause is unknown.

Acute mountain sickness may be more than a temporary annoyance. It is of concern because it is probably a manifestation of mild, transitory cerebral oedema, and in a small proportion of cases this oedema may worsen and become clinically overt (high altitude cerebral oedema). Acute mountain sickness is also associated with, and made much worse by, the increased hypoxia consequent upon high altitude pulmonary oedema.

Symptoms and signs

Symptoms come on between 8 and 96 h after ascent and include, after an initial euphoria, lethargy, headache, fitful sleep with arousals, an increasingly severe headache, often occipital, nausea, vomiting, dizziness, and loss of balance. The sufferer lies groaning in his sleeping bag, refusing food, and dozing. After a day or two of rest, the symptoms disappear and are soon forgotten, yet they may recur on further ascent to a greater altitude.

The signs are few: an irritable, depressed, but usually fit person, often, because he is starved, smelling of ketones and vomit, and holding his aching head. The most useful diagnostic sign is ataxia. Occasionally the patient, especially if vomiting and taking diuretics, may be too dehydrated and hypotensive to stand up. At this stage crackles may be heard in more than a quarter of people examined.

In a few, the symptoms rapidly worsen with the onset of pulmonary oedema. Soon the breathlessness, even at rest, is extreme and may be accompanied by a dry cough. The patient, anxious and sometimes incoherent, becomes progressively more dyspnoeic and sometimes orthopnoeic. He is very cyanosed, with a mild pyrexia (38.3°C), a pronounced tachycardia, and sometimes mild hypotension. There are no signs of cardiac failure, but loud crackles can easily be heard all over the chest and frothy sputum, sometimes tinged with blood, wells out of the mouth and nose.

Pulmonary oedema, if very severe, decreases oxygenation and so tends to be accompanied by high altitude cerebral oedema but each syndrome may occur independently as features of acute mountain sickness. In cerebral oedema without pulmonary manifestations, the patient, having had progressively worsening symptoms of acute mountain sickness for several days, becomes incoherent, hallucinated, and too ataxic and drowsy to stand up or look after himself. He may be unable to get out of his tent, or he may do so and then fall into a snow drift and lie there. Soon he is stuporose and snoring stertorously. His sleeping bag may be wet with urine and in a few hours he is in deepening coma. There are rarely any localizing signs; mild bilateral papilloedema is characteristic.

Predisposing factors

Males and females are equally likely to develop the acute mountain sickness syndrome, and the incidence is inversely related to age. There is no good evidence that the incidence of acute mountain sickness relates to prior physical fitness as expressed by, say, maximal oxygen consumption, and much anecdotal evidence from many experienced observers is that there is no such relationship. We now know, however, that statistically-speaking, the higher the vital capacity, the less the chance of acute mountain sickness and there is increasing evidence that susceptibility to acute mountain sickness is correlated with a poor ventilatory response to hypoxia, measured at sea level. Many other physiological functions have been measured at sea level but none usefully predict whether any one individual will develop acute mountain sickness. Factors related statistically to the occurrence of acute mountain sickness are severe exertion, pre-existing respiratory infection, starting an ascent at a higher altitude; previous acute mountain sickness, especially pulmonary oedema; and having a low vital capacity and a poor ventilatory response to hypoxia. Healthy, high-altitude dwellers seem to be at unusually high risk of pulmonary oedema after brief descent to lower altitudes followed by reascent.

Pathophysiology

On ascent to high altitudes, a great many factors affect cerebral oxygenation: an increase in the rate and depth of breathing; a fall in plasma volume and increase in haemoglobin; an increase in cerebral blood flow due to hypoxic cerebral vasodilatation (to some extent off set by hypocapnic cerebral vasoconstriction); and increases in brain oxygen extraction. The net result is that cerebral oxygen delivery and metabolism are both normal at the sort of altitudes most climbers are likely to experience. But this is not to say that all brain function is normal. There is now good evidence, for example, that at levels of hypoxia frequently met by climbers the synthesis of neurotransmitters such as serotonin is diminished, and this may explain the changes in mood and reversible defects in cognition that have been reported.

Patients with acute mountain sickness, whether this is due to failed or exaggerated physiological adjustments to hypoxia, tend to have ventilation that is inappropriately low for the altitude. They thus have lower blood oxygen and higher P_{CO_2} levels. Pulmonary oedema causes a vicious cycle of deepening hypoxia.

People with acute mountain sickness also have an antidiuresis and retain fluid. The skull is a rigid box, so small increases in volume lead to large increases in pressure, and recent work suggests that those people who have relatively large ratios of cerebrospinal fluid to brain volume may be able to displace the cerebrospinal fluid more easily and so be protected. There is movement of fluid into the cells, and considerable hypoxic cerebral vasodilatation. As Hackett has argued, neither is sufficient to cause high altitude cerebral oedema. The finding, using MRI, of oedema of the white matter in cerebral oedema of high altitude lends support to the concept that in acute mountain sickness there is vasogenic cerebral oedema. This is an oedema due to movement of fluid and proteins from inside the blood vessels across the blood–brain barrier, perhaps due to a failure of vascular autoregulation and transmittal of increased pressures to the capillaries. This fits with the observation that steroids, which are useful in high altitude cerebral oedema and in prevention of acute mountain sickness, are effective only in the vasogenic sort of cerebral oedema. Hypoxia stimulates the formation of inducible nitric oxide synthase (iNOS) which increases the permeability of the blood–brain barrier, and iNOS may be the cause of the oedema where cerebral capillary pressure is already raised. Autopsies in people who have died from cerebral oedema have shown, besides oedema, numerous tiny haemorrhages from the capillaries.

Moderate acute mountain sickness is associated with oedema of the brain, but exposure to high altitude causes increased brain volume (increased brain water, or blood volume, or both) in men whether they have acute mountain sickness or not. The reason why some individuals are susceptible to developing symptoms is not known, but there is increasing interest in the idea that susceptibility might depend on the ability of an individual's craniospinal anatomy to accommodate volume increases. Since the mean volume needed to raise intracranial pressure 10-fold is 26 ml for an adult, small individual differences in compliance on the part of the intraspinal space might explain differences in susceptibility. Evidence that mild acute mountain sickness is due to cerebral oedema is as yet lacking, though this is likely.

It is known that on ascent to high altitude there is a shift in blood from the systemic 'capacitance vessels' (veins) to the pulmonary circuit. Exercise and cold increase this shift, while phentolamine, an α-adrenergic blocker, decreases pulmonary vascular resistance and improves gas exchange in high altitude pulmonary oedema. In addition, there is a greater than normal hypoxic pulmonary arterial vasoconstriction with a rise in pulmonary artery pressure. Nifedipine, which reduces pulmonary arterial pressure, has been shown to be effective in both the prevention and treatment of high altitude pulmonary oedema. Neither of these processes causes the pulmonary oedema but both contribute to it. Cardiac function is not impaired. Pulmonary wedge pressures, reflecting average pulmonary venous pressures, are normal, as are atrial pressures.

The oedema fluid of people suffering from high altitude pulmonary oedema has been shown, using bronchopulmonary lavage, to be high in protein content, which is characteristic of a breakdown in vascular permeability, and not like that of 'high-pressure' cardiogenic pulmonary oedema. Recent work, however, suggests a more complex picture. Albumin escape rates into the alveolae may not be sufficiently increased in high altitude pulmonary oedema, and the increased alveolar protein might be due to water reabsorption from the alveolae. The oedema fluid also contains large numbers of cells, the vast majority of them macrophages as well as markers of chemotactic activity and inflammation. Various mediators of inflammation, such as E-selectin, are raised early in high altitude pulmonary oedema. This accords with the observation that upper respiratory infections seem to predispose to high altitude pulmonary oedema, but recent studies suggest that the high permeability leak is non-inflammatory.

Cases of high altitude pulmonary oedema after minimal exertion at modest altitudes, in people with congenital absence of the right pulmonary artery, suggest that pulmonary hypertension and shearing forces due to a massively increased circulation (in these cases through one lung) might together contribute to high altitude pulmonary oedema. It seems that in high altitude pulmonary oedema some lung capillary beds are closed off, whether by hypoxic vasoconstriction or by capillary wall oedema and thrombosis. The ventilation/perfusion mismatch increases hypoxia and there is diversion of the whole circulation through the remaining, widely patent capillaries, which are damaged both by the increased pressure and the shear stress of the large flow. As a consequence, they leak in a patchy fashion, causing the typical patchy appearance on radiographs of high altitude pulmonary oedema. Nitric oxide improves high altitude pulmonary oedema by reducing this ventilation/perfusion mismatch.

Incidence

Lacking rigorous, large-scale studies, we can say that acute mountain sickness has been reported below 1550 m, is uncommon below 3000 m, and that the higher the altitude, the faster the ascent, and the greater the exertion the higher the incidence (from fewer than 10 per cent to 60 per cent), and the worse the illness.

Most large studies suggest that some symptoms, for example a bad headache that is not relieved by 600 mg of aspirin, occur in over half of lowlanders going to above 4000 m and that over 10 per cent of climbers have more than one severe symptom at that altitude. High altitude pulmonary oedema occurs in about 5 per cent of people at that altitude, but symptomless crackles in the lung in almost a quarter. Cerebral oedema, which takes a few days to develop, is less common, occurring in perhaps 0.5 to 2 per cent.

Diagnosis

The differential diagnosis is small. For mild acute mountain sickness the non-specific symptoms mean that hypothermia, exhaustion, and dehydration should be considered. The effects of alcohol and marijuana may duplicate those of acute mountain sickness. For pulmonary and cerebral oedema, only infectious diseases (pneumonia or meningoencephalitis) are likely possibilities, though carbon monoxide poisoning due to poorly venti-

lated tents occurs. Periodic breathing with apnoeic phases is normal at high altitude and not by itself a cause for alarm, though it may be very marked in cerebral oedema. Fever is moderate in high altitude pulmonary oedema, which is accompanied by extreme tachycardia and cyanosis, without purulent sputum. In cerebral oedema there is no meningism and little if any pyrexia, nor evidence of ear infection or of localizing signs. There is a striking absence of any signs of cardiac decompensation (cardiac enlargement, raised neck veins). Giving oxygen—which is expensive, often not available, and has to be given in 4 to 5 l/min amounts—frequently produces equivocal results as everyone at high altitude, with almost any illness or none at all, feels temporarily better on oxygen.

All illnesses improve on descent, but the very dramatic recovery on descent in acute mountain sickness, and particularly in pulmonary and cerebral oedema, is so striking as to be diagnostic in itself. Numerous cases have been described of people unconscious and worsening at 4000 m who were fully conscious at 3000 m.

The physician who sees the patient on descent is, however, usually obliged to perform a battery of tests on the patient who, except in the case of very prolonged cerebral oedema, is recovering fast. The chest radiograph will show scattered fluffy patches of oedema; the electrocardiogram shows simple right ventricular hypertrophy and 'strain', and the cerebrospinal fluid will be normal.

Prophylaxis

Acute mountain sickness and its complications are the consequence of ascent that for any one individual is too high or too fast and are therefore easily and completely preventable by going up slowly. Everyone going to high altitudes has the responsibility to set a schedule for themselves that includes frequent rests, and that allows them to descend at will. Acute mountain sickness affects the capacity to reason, so everyone must also take responsibility for their fellows, realizing that pulmonary or cerebral oedema can be rapidly fatal and that it is often simple to walk a sufferer down 1000 m, whereas a few hours delay can endanger the patient's life and that of scores of rescuers. Even now, communications are frequently faulty, planes and helicopters may not exist or may crash, or be unable to get near. Energetic propaganda advising slow ascent and rest days and nights has been shown to lower the incidence of acute mountain sickness.

Since insensible water loss is increased due to the increased exertion, the extra ventilation and the dry air, every effort must be made to avoid dehydration, by drinking enough to urinate clear, dilute urine. The climber should also eat plenty, especially carbohydrates. There is evidence that sleeping tablets, which further lower the already lowered oxygen saturation during sleep should be avoided.

Acetazolamide, 5 mg/kg per day, reduces the incidence and severity of acute mountain sickness when taken before and during ascent. It probably works by decreasing cerebrospinal fluid formation and, more importantly, stimulating nocturnal respiration by causing an intracellular acidosis in the respiratory centre so that periodic episodes of apnoea, which are very common at altitude, are abolished and blood oxygen saturation is never allowed to fall. Its principal side-effect is tingling in the hands, feet, and around the mouth.

Dexamethasone, (2 mg every 6 h or 4 mg every 12 h) a glucocorticoid effective in the management of cerebral oedema, has been shown to prevent acute mountain sickness, while reducing the retinal arterial dilation that follows exposure to hypoxia.

Treatment

Rest, aspirin for headache, and a descent of 500 m or so for a couple of nights usually suffice, though ataxia may require the patient be assisted down further. Acetazolamide (250 mg, 8-hourly), started 12h before ascent, increases oxygenation during sleep and relieves symptoms. Dexamethasone (4 mg 6-hourly) is highly effective. Diuretics are logical, given the water retention. The presence of pulmonary oedema or coma necessitates urgent removal down at least 1000 m, and careful observation. In addition to descent, oxygen, should be administered (if necessary through an endotracheal tube at a rate of 5–6 l/min). Immediate descent by even a small amount may save the lives of such critically ill patients, and reliance on air evacuation is dangerous.

In pulmonary oedema, sit the patient up if this makes him comfortable and give frusemide (20–40 mg orally) and morphine (15 mg intravenously). Both these drugs divert blood from the pulmonary to the systemic circuit. Frusemide causes a diuresis and morphine decreases anxiety and respiration rate.

The calcium blocker, nifedipine, prevents high altitude pulmonary oedema in susceptible subjects, improves oxygenation, and reduces the excessive rise in pulmonary artery pressure in pulmonary oedema. It works by improving the matching of perfusion to ventilation, by lessening the formation of oedema fluid, and by decreasing the inflammatory response. Its side-effects (hypotension and tachycardia) suggest that its use should be limited to established oedema. Further studies may confirm that inhaled nitric oxide is useful.

A portable, light-weight hyperbaric bag, made of impermeable nylon, has been developed. The victim lies inside while the air pressure is increased using a foot pump, by 104 torr. For example at 4200 m, where ambient barometric pressure is 449 torr, the pressure in the bag, 553 torr, would be equivalent to an altitude of 2544 m. This is therefore equivalent to taking the patient down 1656 m. Controlled clinical trials have shown the bag to be effective in acute mountain sickness and mild pulmonary oedema, and expeditions should consider taking such bags with them, though descent is still the best, quickest, and usually the safest therapy.

In cerebral oedema, intravenous dexamethasone in large doses (e.g. 8 mg) should be given to reduce the oedema. A cuffed endotracheal tube should be passed, the lungs kept inflated and the bladder kept empty with a Foley catheter (all these devices should form part of the kit of a responsible physician travelling at high altitudes).

Prognosis

This depends not merely on the altitude and terrain but on the speed with which early signs are noticed by the patient's colleagues and their determination and skill in evacuating him to lower altitudes immediately. Once pulmonary oedema and to the rarer but more dangerous cerebral oedema have developed, the patient probably has about a one-third chance of dying. If he lives, full recovery is the rule.

Retinal haemorrhage of high altitude

On ascent, there a considerable increase in cerebral and retinal blood flow. Ophthalmoscopy around 5000 to 6000 m has shown a 20 to 25 per cent increase in diameter of both arteries and veins, and striking increase in the tortuosity of these vessels (Fig. 1). Suffusion of the optic disc with blood due to capillary dilatation may delude the examiner into diagnosing papilloedema.

Studies have shown that one-third to one-half of symptomless climbers descending from between 7000 and 8000 m down to 5000 m altitude develop flame-shaped retinal haemorrhages (Fig. 2). The haemorrhages are usually near the optic disc, may be of any size, and are usually unnoticed and resolve on descent, unless they are at the fovea, where they may leave a permanent blind spot.

They may be caused by transmission of high thoracic pressures developed during straining or prolonged coughing, and transmitted through a vasculature dilated because of hypoxia. It is probable that the finding of retinal haemorrhages in someone at high altitude is not by itself a reason to counsel descent.

Peripheral oedema

Swelling of hands, face, and ankles may occur in climbers on ascent to high altitude, just as on long-continued hiking at sea-level, and rarely there may be gross anasarca. The oedema is more common in women than in men though no association with menses has been found. It is associated with acute mountain sickness and pulmonary oedema but may occur by itself, and it is relieved by the diuresis that accompanies descent.

Fig. 1 The left optic fundus of a 26-year-old male climber photographed at 5900 m altitude. Both the veins and arteries are dilated and tortuous and there is hyperaemia of the optic disc as well as mild papilloedema. The climber had severe headache, nausea, and vomiting.

Other illnesses of high altitudes

People frequently ask their physicians whether their hearts will be all right at high altitude. The physiological facts are that the normal heart is not limited by heights up to the top of Everest. Unhappily, the doctor has no tests that are sensitive or specific enough to give an accurate prediction, unless the patient has symptoms. The doctor has to remind the prospective trekker that he or she is going on an adventure, and getting away from, among other things, good emergency medical treatment. The physician should be very hesitant to forbid any activity which may have great meaning to the patient, in the absence of actual, as opposed to theoretical, evidence that it is harmful.

On theoretical grounds, people with diseases which limit ventilation, diffusion of oxygen, circulation, and tissue adaptation, will fare badly at high altitudes. Often, however, there is little evidence and doctors should be cautious about the constraints they place on a patient's activities and frank about our ignorance.

Chronic mountain sickness (Monge's disease)

This is a clinical syndrome affecting a few very long-term residents at altitudes, and equivalent to the alveolar hypoventilation syndrome seen at sea level. It is to be distinguished from the persistent failure of a newcomer to

Fig. 2 The left optic fundus of a fit and symptomless 28-year-old male climber photographed at 5900 m altitude. The vessels are dilated, as in Fig. 1, but are less tortuous. Retinal haemorrhages are shown.

adjust to the altitude which results in weeks or even months of acute mountain sickness. It usually occurs in men between the ages of 20 and 50, and the symptoms are of headache, dizziness, depression, irritability, and, most strikingly, drowsiness and even episodes of coma. The signs are those of polycythaemia that is excessive for the altitude (in the high 70s) and cyanosis with suffused, congested conjunctiva, ear lobes, cheeks, and lips, as well as clubbed finger nails. Signs of congestive heart failure may be present. Poor ventilation is reflected by a low oxygen saturation and arterial $P\text{CO}_2$. The right heart may be enlarged on chest radiograph and there is evidence of right ventricular hypertrophy on ECG, itself a reflection of marked pulmonary hypertension. All the symptoms, signs, and physiological abnormalities are cured by descent to sea level, and sufferers should move there permanently.

Myocardial infarction

All idigenous populations studied at high altitudes have, compared with people in the West, low rates of coronary disease, perhaps because they exercise more, eat less (especially less salt), have lower serum lipids and have less hypertension. In the United States, the decline in mortality from arteriosclerotic disease with increasing altitude may be due to migration down to lower altitudes of people liable to coronary disease.

The physician at sea level is often asked by people whether it is safe for them to go up to 3000 or 4000 m altitude to ski or to climb. Logic dictates that as the myocardium has no oxygen reserves, as myocardial oxygen extraction even at sea level leaves no room for improvement, and as coronary flow is decreased, people who have poor coronary circulation will be at great risk when they ascend from sea level and start hard exercise. There are, however, no credible studies, with useful denominators, to guide the physician. A prudent physician might tell the patient not to ascend until he is fit to take exercise at sea level, but unless the patient has had a previous myocardial infarction, we have no evidence that an electrocardiogram, with or without exertion or breathing low oxygen mixtures simultaneously, has any predictive value at all, and the patients' previous history of fitness and of illness is likely to be far more useful.

Pulmonary emboli

Deep vein thrombosis tends to occur in climbers at very high altitudes partly because the erythropoietic stimulus never shuts off above an altitude of about 5500 m so that the blood is very viscous and partly because of dehydration and enforced inactivity due to storms. Pulmonary emboli, sometimes fatal, occur. Evacuation to lower altitudes and the administration of aspirin as an anticoagulant should be tried.

Sickle-cell anaemia

Since cells containing HbS sickle, when hypoxic, become sticky and rigid, it is not surprising that homozygous cases of HbS (sickle-cell anaemia) are at great danger from high altitude. In Denver, at 1609 m, people who are heterozygotes (sickle-cell trait) apparently lead normal lives, but cases of splenic infarction in people with sickle-cell trait have been described in men at between 3500 and 4500 m. One should be cautious in advising anyone with sickle-cell trait to exercise at altitudes above about 2000 m.

Further reading

Grissom CK, Elstad MR (1999). The pathophysiology of high altitude pulmonary edema. *Wilderness and Environmental Medicine* 10, 88–92.

Hackett PH (1999). The cerebral etiology of high-altitude cerebral edema and acute mountain sickness. *Wilderness and Environmental Medicine* 10, 97–109.

Hackett PH, Roach RC (1994). High altitude medicine and physiology. In: Auerbach PS, ed. *Management of wilderness and environmental emergencies*, 4th edn. C.V. Mosby, St Louis.

Hackett PH, Roach RC (2001). High altitude illness. *New England Journal of Medicine* 345, 107–14.

8.5.5 Aerospace medicine

D. M. Denison and M. Bagshaw

Introduction

Aviation medicine concerns the welfare of humans in flight through the Earth's atmosphere, an oxygen-rich gas that shields the ground below from solar radiation above. Held to the Earth by gravity, compressed under its own weight, the atmosphere is denser close to the ground than further away. Long waves of infrared light penetrate it easily but heat the ground below. Hot ground reradiates some of this heat at shorter wavelengths which are absorbed by carbon dioxide and water vapour, making the air close to the ground much warmer than that higher up. Short waves of ultraviolet sunlight, absorbed by oxygen molecules early in their journey, create a belt of warm ozone at high altitudes. Some rays intercepted in the same region generate secondary rays that extend lower down. Very few reach the ground. At sea level the atmosphere exerts a pressure of about 760 mmHg (101 kPa); it is variably moist, has a temperature that ranges from –60 °C to +60 °C, and moves at wind speeds from 0 to 160 km/h. With increasing altitude, the temperature, pressure, and water content of the atmosphere fall and wind speeds increase. Some of these features are summarized in Fig. 1. On ascent conditions generally become more severe and more uniform, so turbulence decreases. Most flights through the atmosphere last for a day or less, but some balloon flights persist for longer. The main medical problems of flight through the atmosphere are hypoxia, confining people to small spaces, exposing them to high accelerations, and getting them back to the ground safely should something go wrong.

Space medicine concerns the welfare of humans in flight through vacuums remote from the Earth, the protection of its atmosphere, and the pull of its gravity. Here the problems are those of very prolonged flight times, preserving the pressure and composition of a self-contained gaseous environment, much greater radiation hazards, coping with weightlessness, and engineering the safety of extravehicular excursions that may last several hours.

Atmospheric pressure

Total gas pressure falls with altitude in a regular, almost exponential way, halving every 18 000 ft (5500 m), as in Fig. 2. The oxygen content of the atmosphere (20.93 per cent) is constant to very high altitudes, so the same curve can be used to obtain the ambient oxygen pressure by rescaling the ordinate (also shown in Fig. 2). The oxygen pressure of physiological importance is that which exists in ambient air when it is warmed and wetted on entering the bronchial tree. This process necessarily raises water vapour pressure to about 47 mm Hg, regardless of the total gas pressure outside. The oxygen pressure in moist inspired gas ($P\text{IO}_2$) fully saturated with water vapour at 37 °C is given by the relationship:

$$P\text{IO}_2 = F\text{IO}_2\,(PB - 47)$$

where $F\text{IO}_2$, the fractional concentration of oxygen in the inspirate, is 0.2093 when air is inspired.

Atmospheric temperature

Atmospheric temperature drops more or less linearly with altitude, at about 2 °C/1000 ft (300 m), to the tropopause (40 000 ft (12 200 m)), is stable at –56 °C up to about 80 000 ft (24 400 m)and then rises to almost body temperature at about 150 000 ft (46 000 m), but by then air density is so low that its temperature is unimportant (cf. the dense cold air below).

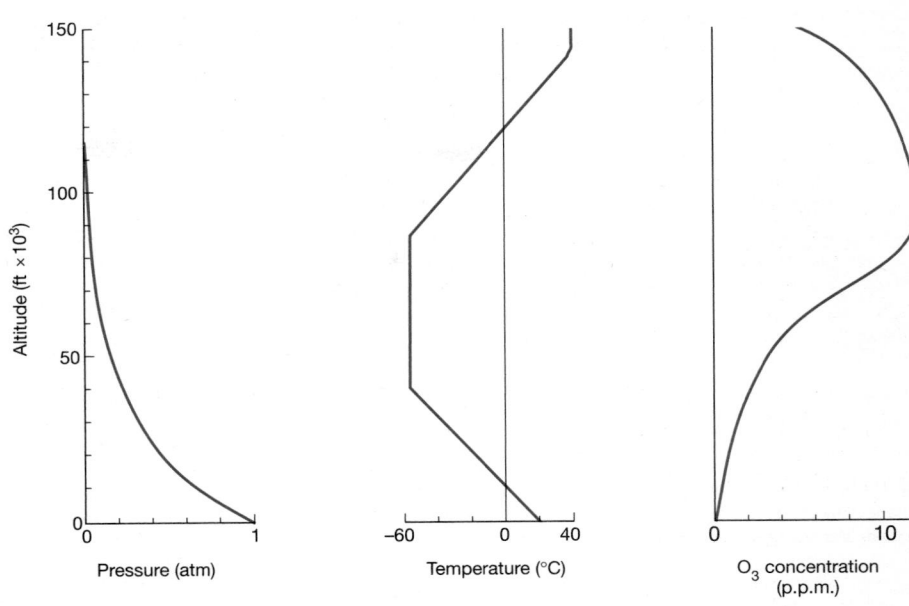

Fig. 1 Some physical features of the Earth's atmosphere, showing the variations in barometric pressure, air temperature, and ozone concentration with altitude. (NB: There is an international aviation safety convention that all altitudes are given in feet.) The shaded diagram on the left illustrates how the Earth's atmosphere is compressed under its own weight. The atmosphere absorbs much solar radiation.

Atmospheric ozone

Atmospheric ozone is formed by irradiation of diatomic oxygen molecules which dissociate into atoms. At very high altitudes the ultraviolet irradiation is so intense that all oxygen exists in the monatomic form. Lower down, some of the monatomic oxygen produced higher up combines with oxygen molecules to form the triatomic gas O_3 (ozone), at concentrations from 1 to 10 parts per million (**ppm**). The ozonosphere normally exists between 40 000 and 140 000 ft (12 200 and 42 700 m), i.e. from one-fifth to one-thirtieth of an atmosphere. Below 40 000 ft (12 200 m) the irradiation is normally too weak for significant amounts of ozone to form. Concentrations of 1 ppm at sea-level cause lung irritation. Ten times that concentration can cause fatal lung oedema. Although the ozonosphere is at much lower pressure, the ventilation systems of aircraft flying at very high altitudes can take in the ozone and compress it to partial pressures at which pulmonary irritation is a credible hazard.

Mechanical aspects

Propeller-driven aircraft need sufficient air to bite on but not enough to slow them down. They fly best at altitudes below 30 000 ft (9150 m), but if cruising above 10 000 ft (3000 m) they need pressurization to prevent cabin

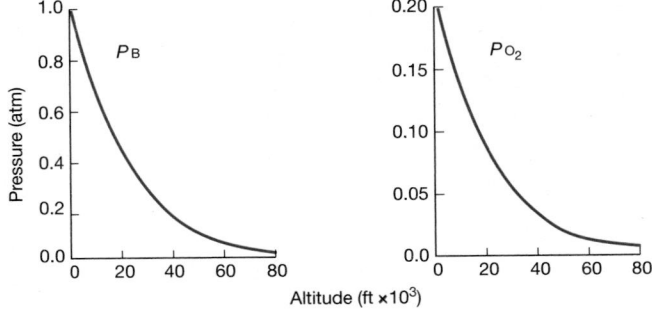

Fig. 2 The variations of barometric pressure (PB) and ambient oxygen pressure (Po_2) with altitude.

altitudes rising above about 8000 ft (2440 m). They use control surfaces and the resistance of the atmosphere to force changes in direction and ambient air to ventilate the pressurized cabins. Aircraft cabins are usually pressurized and ventilated with sufficient air from outside to dilute the carbon dioxide excreted by the occupants' lungs to an ambient partial pressure of 3 mmHg (0.4 kPa) or less. Many studies have shown that exposure to carbon dioxide at such levels increases lung ventilation slightly and appropriately, but has no other ill effects. Submariners have accepted for many years, with good evidence, a carbon dioxide partial pressure of 7 mmHg (0.9 kPa) as a safe upper limit for continuous exposure of healthy adults for 3 months. Because the ventilating air is dry, humidity in the cabin is low. This dries out the mouth and nose, which is marginally uncomfortable but has no other ill effects. Total water loss from this cause per person over a 10 h flight would be about 100 g.

Jet aircraft propel themselves by throwing a stream of hot gas behind them, but they need atmospheric oxygen to ignite the fuel that does this. They fly best at altitudes above 30 000 ft (9150 m) but below 65 000 ft (19 800 m). Generally, they use control surfaces and the resistance of the atmosphere to change direction and use ambient air to ventilate their pressurized cabins. However, some aircraft, such as 'jump jets', can also manoeuvre by changing their direction of thrust.

Rockets take an oxygen supply with them, and fly best in a vacuum. Space flights are commonly of long duration. There is no atmosphere for control surfaces to work against, or to be compressed to ventilate. Thus all navigation has to be achieved by directional motors and the pressure and composition of cabin atmospheres has to be maintained by on-board systems.

The atmosphere permits vehicles to travel through it at very high speeds. Usually these are achieved and lost so gradually that the changes of pace pass unnoticed, but so-called 'agile' aircraft can make continuous high-speed turns, sustained for a minute or more. The accelerations that such turns produce are proportional to the square of the vehicle's speed and inversely proportional to the radius of its turning circle (as shown in Fig. 3). Because the aircraft turns by applying its broad wing surface to the air, these accelerations are almost perpendicular to that surface and roughly parallel to the long axes of the people within. Most often, aircraft make 'head to the middle' turns, and blood and loosely tethered organs like the

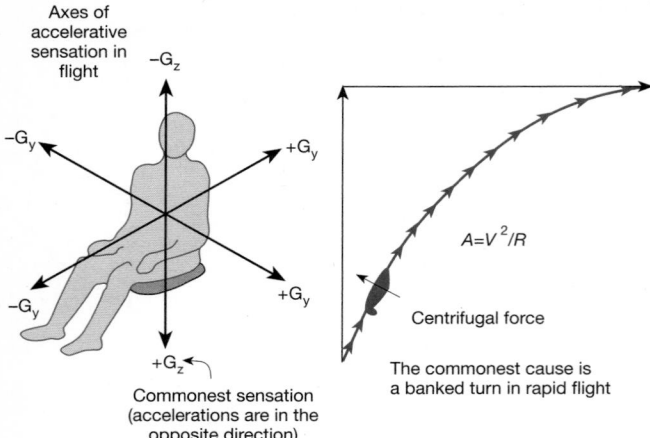

Fig. 3 The axes of acceleration in flight are labelled according to the sensations experienced by the aviator. Thus, when the pilot is accelerated upwards ($+G_z$) the body fluids and tissues sare felt to sink towards the feet.

liver and heart fall towards the feet (positive '*g*' or $+G_z$ accelerations). Healthy unprotected adults, sitting erect in 'head to the middle' turns will 'black out' at about $+3G$. Protective devices that raise intrathoracic pressure and apply counterpressure to the abdomen and legs during 'head to the middle' turns can maintain consciousness up to about $+10G$. When aircraft make 'head-out' turns, (negative '*g*' or $-G_z$ accelerations), mobile organs and blood are forced towards the head, eventually leading to 'red-out'.

In brief, the important features of the atmosphere are that its temperature and pressure fall and radiation intensities rise with altitude. In addition there is a poisonous belt of ozone at high altitude. The atmosphere also permits vehicles to travel at high speeds and make sustained severe accelerations. The biochemical and mechanical hazards posed by these stresses are extremely challenging but on the whole they only affect professional aircrew. The main biochemical risk, shared by many patients at sea-level and all who fly, is hypoxia.

Biochemical hazards

Hypoxia

Oxygen has a dual role in most animal cells, as it is life-giving and extremely poisonous at the same time. In air, or dissolved in simple solution, it is benign and only ionized with difficulty. However, once an electron is successfully attached to an oxygen molecule it becomes a highly corrosive superoxide ion, forming a cascade of other very destructive oxygen radicals. This is an essential feature of oxygen toxicity, which is discussed in Chapter 8.5.6. Superoxide dismutase and various peroxidases have evolved to protect most cells from the effects of spontaneous formation of oxygen radicals by quenching the ions as rapidly as they appear.

More recently in evolution, other enzymes developed which harness this property of oxygen molecules in a controlled way. There are three sorts: oxidases, oxygenases, and hydroxylases. Quantitatively, cytochrome a_3 oxidase is the most important because, using oxygen as the ultimate electron sink, it allows many metabolic processes to proceed and at the same time unlocks and traps most of the energy the body needs (oxidative phosphorylation). However, several other oxidases that release this energy are unable to trap it. They are used to denature various unwanted products of metabolism.

Oxygenases introduce an oxygen molecule into organic molecules creating new compounds. Although these enzymes, of which there are many, only consume a small fraction of the body's total oxygen requirement, they are particularly important because they are responsible for production and

dismemberment of many critical compounds such as the amine transmitters of the brain.

Hydroxylases insert one atom of oxygen and another of hydrogen into organic molecules. They too are responsible for many critical metabolic processes and for the denaturation of many drugs in the liver, kidney, and elsewhere.

These enzymes handle virtually all the oxygen uptake measured at the lips but differ in their affinity for oxygen, described by the Michaelis constant (for oxygen). This constant (K_{mO_2}) is that partial pressure of oxygen which, when all other factors are equal, just allows an oxygen-consuming reaction to proceed at half its maximum velocity. The major oxidase (cytochrome a_3), which is the cocatalyst of oxidative phosphorylation, has a very high oxygen affinity and thus a very low K_{mO_2}, of 1 mmHg or less. That means this particular type of oxygen consumption, representing 80 to 90 per cent of the whole, can proceed full tilt down to very low levels of oxygen supply indeed. By contrast (Fig. 4), the other enzymes, which are quantitatively less important but qualitatively critical, have Michaelis constants for oxygen that vary from 5 to 250 mmHg. A fall in oxygen supply will influence these processes long before oxidative phosphorylation is affected and at times when overall oxygen consumption is diminished little if at all.

Although Fig. 2 describes how ambient oxygen pressure is related to altitude, it does not convey the measure of oxygen supply critical to humans, namely the pressure of oxygen to be found in the lungs. That pressure is determined by two equations (Fig. 5). The alveolar ventilation equation states that alveolar CO_2 pressure (P_ACO_2) depends only on CO_2 excretion ($\dot{M}CO_2$) and alveolar ventilation ($\dot{V}a$), so:

$$P_ACO_2 = k(\dot{M}CO_2/\dot{V}a).$$

The alveolar air equation states that since at any one time there is a fixed trading ratio between oxygen uptake and CO_2 excretion ($R = \dot{M}CO_2/\dot{M}O_2$), alveolar oxygen pressure (P_AO_2) can be calculated from the moist inspired oxygen pressure ($P_IO_2{}^*$) and alveolar P_CO_2, so:

$$P_AO_2 = P_IO_2{}^* - (P_ACO_2/R).$$

Progressive hypoxia leads to a mild hyperventilation (i.e. a rise in $\dot{V}a$ and fall in P_ACO_2). Knowing this it is possible to sketch a graph of alveolar oxygen pressure against altitude as in Fig. 6(a).

When arterialized blood leaves a healthy lung it has an oxygen pressure some 10 mmHg less than that in the alveoli, due to uneven matching of ventilation to perfusion, some anatomical shunting, and an almost nominal obstacle to diffusion. In resting people, the alveolar–arterial oxygen

Fig. 4 Curves of oxygen uptake ($\dot{M}O_2$) as a fraction of the theoretical maximum ($\dot{M}O_2$max) against the partial pressure of oxygen (P_O_2) for a family of oxygen-handling enzymes with Michaelis constants for oxygen (K_{mO_2}) from 1 to 250 mmHg.

The **Alveolar ventilation equation** ignores dead-space, and supposes there is a stream of oxygen-rich CO_2 free gas, V_A and says, for practical purposes:

$$P_{ACO_2} \propto \dot{M}_{CO_2}/V_A$$

$\dot{V}_A$

Minus the almost equal O_2 uptake, $\dot{M}_{O_2}$

Plus the CO_2 output, $\dot{M}_{CO_2}$

The **Alveolar air equation** pictures V_A trapped in a bag, and notes there must be a link between the rise in P_{CO_2} and the fall in P_{O_2}, so that, for most practical purposes:

$$P_{AO_2} = P_{IO_2} - P_{ACO_2}/R$$

$\dot{V}_A$

Rise $\propto \dot{M}_{CO_2}$

Fall $\propto \dot{M}_{O_2}$

Partial pressure

Time

$\dot{M}_{CO_2}$ $\dot{M}_{O_2}$

Fig. 5 Graphical representations of the alveolar ventilation and alveolar air equations.

gradient does not change much with altitude, although the relative importance of the factors contributing to it alter considerably; so subtracting a further 10 to 15 mmHg describes the relation between arterial oxygen pressure and altitude (also shown in Fig. 6).

The most important change is the loss of the head of pressure driving oxygen from the alveoli to blood, as the fall in alveolar P_{O_2} is much greater than that in mixed venous P_{O_2} (because of the shape of the oxygen dissociation curve). As a result the alveolar–venous gradient for oxygen diffusion is smaller and equilibration slower than at ground level.

People ascending to altitude in a matter of minutes, rather than over several days, make two adaptive responses to hypoxia: an increase in blood flow and the modest hyperventilation mentioned previously. These limit but do not abolish the effects of lack of oxygen. The consequences (Fig. 7) include loss of night vision, impairment of the ability to learn complex and then simple tasks, a deterioration in the performance of already learnt skills, a progressive loss of muscular power (aerobic capacity), and eventually loss of consciousness, convulsions, and death.

As Fig. 7 shows, people abruptly exposed to altitudes of 10 000 ft (3000 m) and above are mentally unreliable and physically weak. This altitude is taken as the ceiling above which it is mandatory to provide aviators with oxygen. To be safe, the ceiling that is actually used is almost always 8000 ft (2440 m), at which barometric pressure is 565 mmHg, arterial oxy-

gen pressure is around 55 mmHg (i.e. sitting just at the top of the sloping part of the oxyhaemoglobin dissociation curve), and venous oxygen pressures have only fallen by 1 to 2 mmHg. It is the maximum cabin altitude that is generally permitted in civilian passenger aircraft. There is some evidence that, even at this altitude, people tire more quickly and learn more slowly than at ground level. Some aircraft have a lower maximum cabin altitude, but this requires a stronger and thus heavier cabin to contain the higher pressure, or engines producing a higher mass flow (such as the Concorde supersonic transport aircraft) which makes the aircraft less economical to run.

Two physiological features of altitude hypoxia are especially important in aviation. The first is a total lack of awareness that the mind is breaking down. This means that an affected individual cannot be relied upon to take corrective action, however well trained. It follows that protective equipment has to be designed to sense the hypoxia and come into operation automatically. The second feature, known as the time of useful consciousness, describes how rapidly consciousness is lost and thus dictates how quickly this equipment must respond.

The time of useful consciousness is the interval after the onset of hypoxia during which an aviator can be relied upon to act sensibly. This is a difficult characteristic to test, as sophisticated abilities need to be sampled in an adequate and time-consuming way at moments when the level of consciousness may be changing rapidly. Many studies have confirmed the general relation between this time interval and the altitude of sudden exposure, which is shown in Fig. 8(a). The time of useful consciousness diminishes from about 4 min at 25 000 ft (7620 m) to a minimum of roughly 15 s, which is reached at 35 000 (10 700 m) to 40 000 ft (12 200 m). This asymptote represents the sum of the 7 s or so required for blood to travel from the

Fig. 6 (a) Variations in moist inspired, alveolar, and arterial oxygen pressure (P_{O_2}) with altitude in normal men. (b) The conventional oxygen–haemoglobin dissociation curve of whole blood plotted to the same pressure scale as the left-hand graph, so that arterial O_2 content can be read directly (at the same horizontal level as the P_{O_2} curve. It also emphasizes that the arteriovenous oxygen content difference (a–vΔ) is proportional to the ratio of oxygen uptake ($\dot{M}_{O_2}$) to local blood flow (Q).

Fig. 7 A summary of the functional consequences of altitude hypoxia.

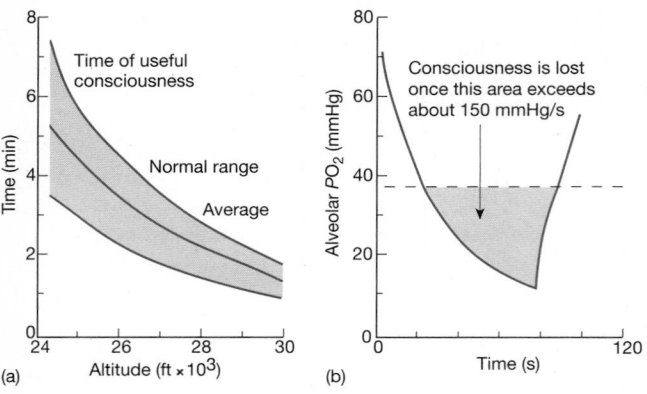

Fig. 8 (a) Variations in the time of useful consciousness with altitude. (b) One way of expressing the dose of hypoxia needed to bring about the loss of consciousness.

lungs to the brain and the equal time needed for the brain to consume the oxygen that is already dissolved in its substance.

Some recent studies have defined the dose of hypoxia that can be suffered before useful consciousness is lost. In trained and healthy men breathing normally (i.e. with an alveolar P_{CO_2} of 35 to 40 mmHg), it is equivalent on a curve of alveolar P_{O_2} against time, to an area of 150 mmHg s, where P_{O_2} is less than 38 mmHg (Fig. 8(b)). However, this is sensitive to many other factors, of which the most important are the degree of hyperventilation and the acceleration that the person is exposed to at the time. Hyperventilation causes cerebral vasoconstriction, and a 'positive g' opposes the upward flow of blood to the brain (see below). Sometimes deterioration in consciousness is quickened by vasovagal syncope, but more often the heart is beating quite rapidly as consciousness is lost. Exertion also quickens loss of consciousness, as mentioned previously, because it forces blood to rush through the lungs, leaving insufficient time for oxygen equilibration.

The minimum cabin pressure of 565 mmHg (75.1 kPA) (8000 ft (2440 m)) in commercial passenger aircraft, is sufficiently low to bring a normal person's arterial P_{O_2} along the plateau of the oxyhaemoglobin dissociation curve until it is sitting just at the top of the steep part (Fig. 6). Because their blood is still fully saturated with oxygen they will not be cyanosed at this altitude. At ground level, many people with chest diseases have arterial oxygen pressures that are as low as 55 to 60 mmHg (or even lower, in which case they become cyanosed). As they ascend to 8000 ft (2440 m) their arterial P_{O_2} will fall further. If their hypoxaemia at ground level is due to a mismatch of ventilation to perfusion, as is usually the case, the drop in arterial P_{O_2} will not be as extensive as in normal people (about 40 mmHg), but if it is due to diffusion defect associated with desaturation on exertion, as in some fibrotic conditions, it may be greater. However, in either event, it can be reversed completely by the administration of oxygen, because 30 per cent oxygen at 8000 ft (2440 m) is equivalent to breathing air at ground level. The medical services of all the major airlines can provide a personal oxygen supply for any passenger if they are given notice beforehand. (It is worth checking the altitudes of the patient's destination and of any stopping point *en route* at the same time.)

Oxygen equipment and pressure cabins

Aircraft that fly below 10 000 ft (3000 m) do not need any oxygen equipment at all. Most of those that fly higher have reinforced cabins capable of holding a higher pressure inside them than out. These are of two sorts, the high-differential type, seen in passenger and transport aircraft generally, and the low-differential variety found in military high-performance aircraft. The former, holding a high transmural pressure, usually prevent pressure falling below 565 mmHg (8000 ft (2440 m)). They provide an environment in which oxygen equipment is not needed routinely and the

occupants breathe cabin air. However, it is always possible that the pressure-cabin system can fail, allowing the pressure within to fall to the level of that outside. This fall can be limited by descent to a lower altitude, but it is not always practical to put the aircraft into a very steep dive, for reasons of structure or air traffic control. Similarly, it is not always practical to descend below 10 000 ft (3000 m) because, in mid-Atlantic for example, there may not be sufficient fuel for the vehicle to reach the nearest land through the dense air at the lower altitudes. For these reasons, if there is a cabin-pressure failure, an emergency oxygen supply is available for passengers and crew.

A high-differential cabin limits the vehicle's range and manoeuvrability. It also increases the risk of catastrophic damage if the fuselage is punctured. So, military high-performance aircraft are fitted with low-differential cabins. These usually prevent cabin pressure falling below 280 mmHg (37.2 kPA) (equivalent to a pressure altitude of 25 000 ft (7620 m)). That is the level at which decompression sickness becomes a serious hazard (see below). In such aircraft, oxygen equipment is needed routinely.

Sometimes military air crew have to escape in flight. The faster the aircraft is travelling the more difficult this is to do. All modern fighters are equipped with ejection seats to launch the crew into the air stream and get them clear of the tail. Usually, the ejected crew free-fall in their seats until below 10 000 ft (3000 m). This gets them through the cold hypoxic upper air as quickly as possible. A small seat- or suit-mounted emergency oxygen supply sees them safely through this stage. Then their parachutes deploy automatically as they are released from their seats to get them safely to ground.

Mechanical effects of pressure change

In civilian passenger and transport aircraft the climb to cruise altitude takes about 30 min and involves a fall of about 200 mmHg (26.6 kPA) in cabin pressure (to the equivalent of 8000 ft (2440 m)). Descent to the ground takes much the same time. Body fluids and tissues generally are virtually incompressible and do not alter shape to any important extent when such pressures changes are applied. The same is true of cavities such as the lungs, gut, middle ear, and facial sinuses that contain air, provided that they can vent easily. Gas-containing spaces that cannot vent easily behave differently.

The thoracoabdominal wall can develop transmural pressures of +100 mmHg or so briefly, but is normally flaccid and has a transmural pressure of a few millimetres of mercury. Gas within will usually be at a pressure very close to that outside, and must follow Boyle's law. Ascent from ground level (760 mmHg) to 8000 ft (2440 m) (565 mmHg) will expand a given volume of trapped gas in a completely pliable container by about 35 per cent, which is equivalent to a radial increase of 10 per cent if it were in a sphere or 18 per cent in a cylinder of fixed length. In the abdomen this may cause slightly uncomfortable gut distension in healthy people but it is not an important problem.

The time constant of emptying of a lung that is kept full by continued decompression is less than 1 s in healthy people (peak expiratory flow is normally 1.5 lungfuls/s). Evidence from very rapid decompressions in fighter aircraft shows that healthy people at functional residual capacity can tolerate decompressions of about 200 mm Hg, from about 280 mm Hg to 80 to 120 mm Hg, which are complete in as little as 0.1 s. Even very diseased lungs can vent themselves over a minute or so. In consequence, the risk of lung rupture in normal flight is extremely rare (Fig. 9).

The cavity of the middle ear poses a separate problem since it vents easily but sometimes fails to fill because the lower part of the Eustachian tube behaves as a non-return valve, especially when it is inflamed. As a result, the cavity equilibrates quite easily on ascent but does not refill on descent, and the ear-drum bows inwards, causing pain that can be severe.

Altitude-induced decompression sickness

If ambient pressure falls quickly to less than half its original value, the gas dissolved in blood and tissue fluids may come out of solution precipitously,

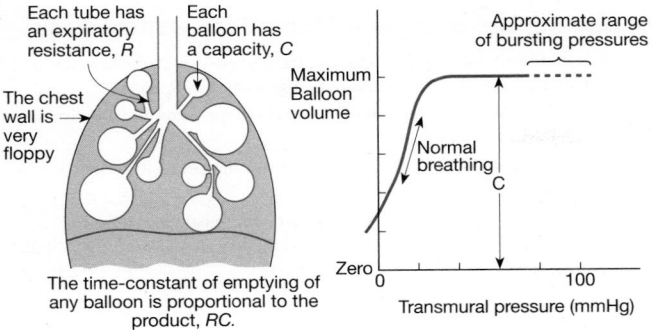

Fig. 9 A graphical summary of the factors determining lung rupture.

forming bubbles and obstructing flow in small blood vessels. The time symptoms take to develop varies widely between individuals and shortens markedly as the altitude of exposure rises. A guide to these times and variability is given in Fig. 10. Symptoms usually resolve quickly after a descent of a few thousand feet and rarely persist after descent to ground level, on oxygen. Should they persist, treatment should be along the lines detailed in Chapter 8.5.6. The risk continues to be significant in some military flights but, with the exception of passengers who have been scuba-diving very recently, it is not a hazard in commercial flights (see below).

Medical problems

Most doctors at times have to consider whether their patients are fit to fly as passengers. No aircraft flight is without risk. These risks include mechanical failure of the aircraft, adverse weather conditions, pilot error, and medical incapacitation of aircrew. Commercial flying, however, is very safe. Worldwide, the accident rate is 1 in 2 million flying hours with some countries achieving 1 in 5 million flying hours. Medical conditions causing temporary or incomplete incapacitation of passengers are not uncommon in flight. The stress of modern of travel should not be underestimated. Passengers on international flights are required to check in at least 2 h before departure, airports often have very long walkways and it may be difficult to obtain help. Many passengers are elderly with heavy luggage, and flight legs may often take 12 h or more.

No significant mental or physical ill effects in healthy people can be attributed to the pressure or composition of cabin atmospheres in normal commercial passenger flight. Flights generate other concerns, namely those of jet-lag, ear and sinus problems, deep vein thrombosis, cross-infections, the safe transport of passengers who are unwell, and the medical fitness of aircrew.

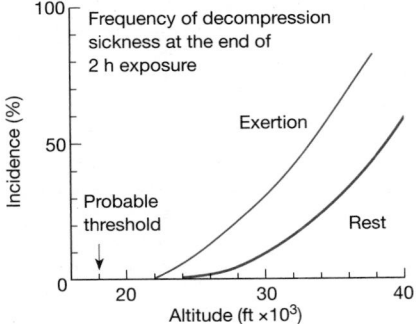

Fig. 10 The incidence of decompression sickness (percentage) at the end of 2 h of exposure to various altitudes in men at rest, or exerting themselves.

Jet-lag or circadian dysrhythmia

When people are transported across two time zones or more, bodily rhythms, especially sleep/wake cycles,are disturbed and take several days to readjust, at the rate of 1 day per time zone crossed. As a result people feel sleepy when they need to be awake and vice versa. These effects are compounded by interrupted sleep and physical inactivity on prolonged flights. The combined effects may increase people's vulnerability to infections but at present there is no good evidence that this is so. What is clear is that jet-lag affects the ability to think straight for a while and may well interfere with the ability to drive. A number of studies are in progress.

Ear and sinus problems

As the pressure in the cabin changes, gases trapped in the body expand and contract. This can lead to a little abdominal discomfort on ascent and relief on descent, but matters little in healthy passengers. However, air trapped in the nasal sinuses and the cavity of the middle ear can cause pain, commonly more marked on descent than ascent. Swallowing, jaw-wriggling, and nose-blowing manoeuvres usually sort things out, but passengers who know they have active ear or sinus problems should take decongestants with them and, if the problems are more than trivial, seek medical advice beforehand.

Cross-infection

Transmissible respiratory infections, such as tuberculosis, can be passed to fellow passengers in flight via person to person droplet spread The major obstacle to study is that passengers disperse widely and rapidly soon after landing and may not associate or report infections subsequent to flight. The risk of cross-infection in aircraft is reduced by passing recirculated cabin air through high-efficiency particulate filters which have an efficiency in excess of 96 per cent.

Deep vein thrombosis

There is a evidence that people obliged to sit in cramped positions for a long time, whether in underground bomb shelters, cars, trains, planes, or at home, may be more to liable to develop deep vein thrombosis. Ironically, this was first recognized explicitly during the airborne bombardment of London in 1940. The condition is notoriously difficult to diagnose. Again, because passengers disperse far and wide and may not link thromboembolic phenomena with recent journeys, the evidence relating the condition to flight is unsatisfactory. The mild hypoxia of commercial flight produces complex changes in clotting mechanisms. The topic is highly controversial. Good epidemiological studies are required. Passengers who have recently given birth or suffered abdominal or pelvic surgery, or are taking hormonal medication, are at increased risk and should take medical advice before travelling. The advice is usually simple: 'walk around as much as you can during the flight'.

Passengers who are unwell

Although the reduced total and oxygen pressures of the cabin atmosphere have little effect on healthy people, they can adversely affect passengers who are already unwell. Those at risk are people with definite heart or lung disease or recent chest or abdominal surgery. Almost all can be transported safely provided that the carrier knows beforehand. Usually the provision of 2 to 4 litres of oxygen per minute is sufficient for those with heart and lung problems. Passengers in late pregnancy or with a recent pneumothorax or very recent surgery need particular care.

Amongst the apparently well, those with recent fractures should note that air trapped beneath their plaster casts may expand so new casts should be split before travel. Patients who have recently undergone clinical procedures that introduce gas into the body (for example arthroscopies, air encephalograms, pulmonary needle biopsies) should not fly until it is known that the gas has been resorbed. Passengers should not scuba-dive in the 12 h before flight because otherwise they may suffer decompression illness *en route*. This should be increased to 24 h if the dive depth exceeded 30 ft (9 m). If an apparently fit passenger develops progressive limb pain in flight, oxygen should be given immediately and the passenger advised to stay at ground level for at least 12 h at the next landing point.

Methods of safe transport are well understood. The essence of the problem is passenger education. Passengers should be given accurate and easily understood information about the very slight risks of flying and about when they should seek medical advice or inform the carrier before flying. A number of carriers provide helpful information on their web sites (for example: http://www.britishairways.com/heath).

Medical fitness of aircrew

Commercial aircrew are responsible for very expensive vehicles and for many lives. In battle, military aircrew may be responsible for much more expensive vehicles and weapons and for very many more lives. Because of this and the great costs of training, military forces and airlines demand the highest physical and psychological standards of aircrew. The medical criteria set for entry to training are usually higher than those for aircrew who are already trained and experienced. Commercial and private aircrew need a current certificate that they are 'fit to fly', which can only be provided by authorized medical examiners. In Europe medical standards for commercial aircrew are imposed by the Joint Aviation Authorities in line with the standards set by the International Civil Aviation Authority.

Summary

Aerospace medicine is a subject that is largely understood. The major peer-review journal in the field is *Aviation, Space and Environmental Medicine*, published by the Aerospace Medical Association. 'Fitness to fly' certificates for commercial and military aircrew can only be provided by authorized medical examiners. Further epidemiological studies are needed on deep vein thrombosis, the effects of jet-lag, and the transmission of respiratory infections resulting from commercial flights. For the care of individual patients, airline medical services are a valuable source of advice and will provide in-flight supplies of oxygen if needed. Specialist organizations can supply medical and nursing support for patients who are too ill to travel alone. Surprisingly few patients are truly too unfit to fly.

Further reading

General

Campbell RD, Bagshaw M (1999). *Human performance and limitations in aviation*. Blackwell Science, Oxford.

Coker RK, ed (2001). Managing passengers with lung disease planning air travel: British Thoracic Society recommendations. *Thorax* (in press).

DeHart RL, Millet KC, Murphy J, eds (1996). *Fundamentals of aerospace medicine*. Williams and Wilkins, Philadelphia.

Ernsting J, Nicholson AN, Rainford DJ (1999). *Aviation medicine*, 3rd edn. Butterworth Heinemann, London.

House of Lords Inquiry (2000). *Air travel and health*. Her Majesty's Stationery Office, London.

Jagoda A, Pietrzak M (1997). Medical emergencies in commercial air travel. *Emergency Medicine Clinics of North America* 1, 251–60.

Joint Aviation Authorities (1996). *Joint aviation requirements: flight crew medical requirements* (JAR/FCL/Part 3-Medical). Westwood Digital, Cheltenham.

Rosenberg CA, Pak F (1997). Emergencies in the air: problems, management and prevention. *Journal of Emergency Medicine* 15, 159–64.

Thibault C (1997). Special Committee report: cabin air quality. *Aviation, Space and Environmental Medicine* 68, 80–2.

Concerning the deep vein thrombosis controversy

Bendz B *et al.* (2000). Association between acute hypobaric hypoxia and activation of coagulation in human beings. *Lancet* 356, 1657–8.

Ferrari E *et al.* (1999). Travel as a risk factor for venous thromboembolic disease. *Chest* 15, 40–444.

Kraaijenhagen RA *et al.* (2000). Travel and the risk of venous thrombosis. *Lancet* 356, 1492–3.

Miller A, ed (1997). Suspected acute pulmonary embolism: a practical approach; British Thoracic Society recommendations. *Thorax* 52 (Suppl. 4), 1–24.

8.5.6 Diving medicine

D. M. Denison and T. J. R. Francis

Introduction

Divers are exposed to many hazards. Frequently it is too late or impractical to give specific help once trouble occurs, so diving medicine is largely concerned with prevention. It depends upon a thorough understanding of the jobs that divers do and the risks that they run completing them. Almost every diving accident is due to a failure of education or equipment design.

Leaving a typical shore (Fig. 1), the sea bed falls with a slope of about 1 in 50 until it is 200 to 300 m deep. This shallow stretch is the continental shelf. The bed then angles more steeply (roughly 1 in 15), as the continental slope, to descend to vast flat expanses of soft mud, the abyssal plains, at depths of 3 to 6 km, interrupted by occasional mountains and chasms. The deepest point is just over 11 km below the surface. Water is almost incompressible. Ambient pressure rises linearly with depth by 1 atmosphere for every 10 m descent. Diving is confined largely to the continental shelves, i.e. to pressures of 1 to 30 atmospheres.

Currents, arising from differences in water temperature and salinity, course across the abyssal plains and well up the continental slopes as mineral-rich streams to supply vegetable life in sunlit upper zones. Animals that feed on these plants or each other are concentrated so that 80 per cent of the biomass lies in the top 200 m, mainly close to the shore. Together, these sites form an area equal to that of Africa, infinitely more fertile and, as yet, virtually unfarmed.

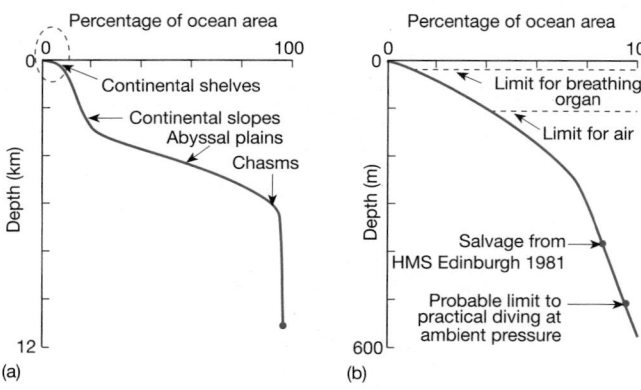

Fig. 1 (a) A cumulative depth versus area plot of the oceans. (b) A similar plot of the top 600 m, including the continental shelves.

Limitations to diving

At the surface, tidal currents are accelerated or slowed down by features of the shore but often exceed the speed at which people can swim (Fig. 2(a)). It may only be practical to dive in slack water, i.e. for an hour or two each day. Waves are often sufficiently high to prevent divers being launched or recovered safely (Fig. 2(b)). Tidal currents tunnelled along marine canyons, and springs of fresh water or falls of cold ocean water can carry divers in unexpected directions without them being aware.

Dawn arrives late and dusk comes early to the sea. Light that is not reflected at the surface is absorbed and scattered, halving its intensity with every 1 or 2 m of descent. It is effectively 'night' below 80 m. Most sports diving takes place in clear shallow waters at placid times of the year. Professional diving, for example harbour work, hull inspections and repairs, pipeline surveys, oil-rig work, and wreck salvage, occurs throughout the year, alongside or beneath large obstructions, in turbid waters where finding the task, let alone completing it, may be very demanding. Artificial illumination is often ineffective because of backscattering.

Underwater, binaural localization of sound is poor. Noises are transmitted almost five times as fast and many times more efficiently through water than air. Loss of air conduction raises auditory thresholds by 30 to 60 dB. Neoprene foam hoods that keep the head warm raise thresholds by a further 30 dB or so. Superior transmission of sound also increases susceptibility to blast injury.

All of the oceans except for the surface waters of tropical seas are too cold for individuals to remain in for long without insulation (Fig. 3). In air, people maintain body temperature at 37 °C with minimal effort when the air temperature is 18 to 24 °C, the zone of thermal neutrality. In water, this zone is high and narrow (35.0 to 35.5 °C). Loss of tactile discrimination and manual dexterity are major problems when working in cold water.

Problems of simple immersion

On immersion blood is displaced upwards from the abdomen and legs, some 500 ml entering the chest, distending the large veins and the right atrium. Local stretch receptors signal an excess circulating volume and promote diuresis. On emmersion the displaced blood drops down from the chest revealing hypovolaemia.

Effort in water is lost in moving, making most tasks more tiring and less efficient than on land (Fig. 4). The maximum sustained thrust that swimmers can develop is about 5 kg, which is just enough for propulsion at 1 to 2 knots. On full inspiration an adult swimmer is about 2.5 kg positively buoyant and needs half of their maximum swim power to descend. A swimmer breathing out to residual volume will be about 2.5 kg negatively buoyant and will need half of their maximum swim power to ascend. The swimmer's almost weightless body can be displaced with ease. The body can be poised at will but body weight can no longer be used to apply leverage or torque, or to stay in place when a current is running.

Considerations before diving—fitness to dive

Divers have a physically demanding job and often work in sites remote from medical aid. They must be strong and free of any active or latent condition that could erupt while they are away. Military and commercial divers must have annual medical examinations for 'fitness to dive', and sports divers are urged strongly to do likewise. The medical checks have three aims: to determine whether candidates are fit to swim in swift currents and rough waters at remote sites, to discover whether they are fit enough to rescue a fellow diver in trouble, and to find out if they have any specific problems that would make them a liability to themselves or others under water.

Divers are expected to be bodily fit and mentally stable and free of conditions such as epilepsy and ill-controlled diabetes or asthma. They should not be addicted to alcohol or any other drug and they should not have a history, or other evidence, of obstructive lung disease, ruptured eardrums, or aural surgery. Divers who are generally fit to dive should not be allowed to do so when they have chest, upper airway, or ear infections, or if they become obese. They should not dive while taking any medication that could impair their ability to think clearly or orientate themselves in space correctly.

Three unresolved issues in 'fitness to dive' assessments cause concern: the role of lung function tests, the significance of a probe-patent foramen ovale, and how to deal with a history of asthma.

The role of lung function tests

If a candidate runs several kilometres a day, is a good swimmer, was always good at games at school, and has no history of recent respiratory disease it is very likely that they will be fit enough to dive. The forced expired volume

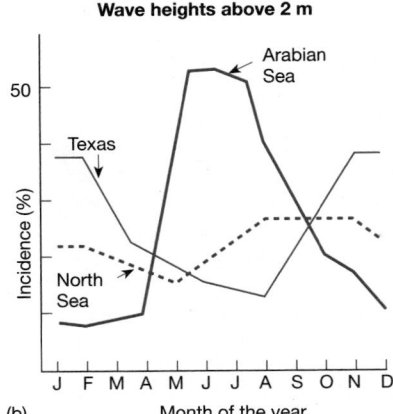

Fig. 2 (a) A plot of the usual and the not uncommonly seen tidal currents in eight diving sites around the world. (b) A plot of the percentage incidence of waves exceeding a height of 2 m at different times of the year in three of the diving sites.

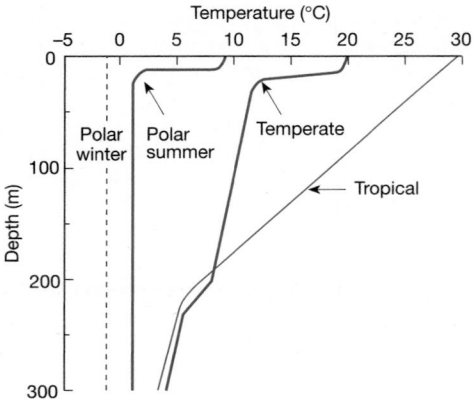

Fig. 3 Variations in sea temperature with site and depth. Note that water temperatures of less than 20 °C are too cold for unclothed individuals to stay in for very long.

in 1 s (**FEV1**), which should be more than 75 per cent predicted, if multiplied by 35, measures the most air that the subject can process in 1 min. The forced vital capacity (**FVC**), which is a guide to the volume of useable lung, should also be more than 75 per cent predicted because there is good evidence that subjects with a low FVC and, by inference, lungs that are too small for their bodies, are more liable to lung rupture on rapid ascents. The FEV1/FVC ratio is not especially helpful. The expiratory flow rate that matters in diving is the peak expiratory flow (**PEF**)/FVC ratio which is a reasonable measure of the time constant of emptying when the lung is full. The peak expiratory flow rate should be at least one and a half predicted FVC per second.

Patent foramina ovale

On most ascents many bubbles can be detected in systemic venous blood. The bubbles are normally trapped unnoticed in pulmonary capillaries. One in four healthy people has a slightly patent foramen ovale that may allow bubbles to pass into the left heart causing cerebrospinal or coronary gas

Fig. 4 A comparison of oxygen consumption ($\dot{M}O_2$) when pedalling a cycle ergometer in air and under water, (a) at a constant speed (60 rev/min) and (b) at a constant light load. Note the high cost of moving the limbs through water. Most people's aerobic capacity is about 2.5 litres O_2/min.

embolism. Four out of five of the victims of cerebrospinal gas embolism in diving have patent foramina, but it is unclear whether that is cause or effect. Systemic venous bubbles are common but arterial gas embolisms are rare. Bubbles have complicated inflammatory interactions with vessel walls, and any significant load arriving in the lung could trigger pulmonary vasoconstriction, raising right heart pressures and opening a previously 'closed' foramen. Present evidence does not justify excluding one-quarter of the population from diving, as gas embolism is rare.

A history of asthma

It has been the custom to bar candidates with a history of asthma from diving, because of the fear that they were more likely to rupture their lungs on fast ascents. However, childhood asthma often disappears and very many people with current mild asthma are known to have completed very many dives without ill effect. It seems there is a case for relaxing this requirement slightly, but three questions prevail: is the candidate fit enough to cope with a diving emergency, liable to exercise-induced asthma, or likely to bronchoconstrict on the inhalation of salt water? Perhaps the most reasonable view at present is to allow a candidate with very mild asthma to dive, provided that they can demonstrate a stable and essentially normal spirometry over a 2-month period, that they do not have exercise-induced asthma, and that they do not constrict abnormally to a saline aerosol challenge.

Problems of descent

On leaving the surface, gas in the chest, abdomen, and clothing is subject to Boyle's law. Vertical movements may quickly become uncontrolled because of the positive feedback between depth and buoyancy. The deeper divers go, the denser they become and the more rapidly they fall. The higher they rise, the less dense they become and the faster they ascend. The chest wall can only maintain a pressure difference equivalent to 1 or 2 m of water, so the gas within the respiratory tract (lungs, upper airways, sinuses, the middle ear, and the Eustachian tubes) is virtually at the same pressure as the surrounding sea. The lung of a person breath-hold diving to 30 m (4 atmospheres absolute) is compressed from total lung capacity to residual volume, so they will need half of their aerobic capacity to ascend. Gas in clothing exaggerates these changes, leaving little margin for controlling unexpected ascent or descent.

Descent may lead to several mechanical problems that become obvious early in a dive (suit/facemask squeeze, lung squeeze, sinus squeeze, middle-ear squeeze, inner-ear squeeze, reversed ear syndrome, alternobaric vertigo, and caloric vertigo). These occur commonly, even on breath-hold dives.

The squeezes

On descent, rising ambient pressure may force the diver's face into the air-filled mask, uless the mask is vented, leading to facial oedema and subconjunctival haemmorhages. These will resolve spontaneously and need no treatment. Similarly a dry suit, particularly if poorly tailored, can pinch the skin resulting in linear wheals that are commonly distributed around the neck, axillae, and groins. Again, these require no active intervention but should not be confused with the cutaneous signs of decompression illness. Occasionally suit squeeze can be severe enough to limit a diver's movements in a deep-water emergency. Increasing ambient pressure compresses the lung according to Boyle's law but more blood is drawn into the chest to replace the vanishing lung so lung sqeeze is only serious at great depths in breath-hold dives. When gas in obstructed sinuses is compressed, sinus walls become oedematous and may bleed. The blood or clot is usually expelled by trapped gas expanding on ascent.

When gas trapped in the middle ear contracts it draws the ear drum inwards and the round and oval windows of the inner ear outwards. Difficulty in clearing the ears is the commonest problem in diving. Attempts to clear them by over-vigorous Valsalva manoeuvres have the opposite effects. If one ear clears much before the other disorientation may occur due to uneven stimulation (alternobaric vertigo). If the external auditory canals are unequally blocked at the start of a dive, cool water will enter one canal before the other leading to caloric vertigo. Drum ruptures in any of these conditions normally heal spontaneously. Diving should not be permitted until the drums have healed. Persistent ruptures require surgery.

Problems at the bottom of a dive

For more sustained dives, gas must be delivered to the diver at the same pressure as the surrounding water. It can be sent via an umbilical pipe from the surface, in which case it can flush through the helmet or face mask continuously—which is wasteful of gas but easily engineered—or it can supply a regulating valve that provides gas on demand only. Alternatively, the diver can take self-contained underwater breathing apparatus (scuba). This feeds a demand regulator and rarely lasts for more than 1 h. Professional divers often use a combination of all three systems, i.e. a surface-demand supply for routine use, with a helmet-flushing capability for occasional comfort or emergency use, and a small, back-mounted gas supply ready in case the surface supply fails. Sustained dives can cause biochemical problems (nitrogen narcosis, oxygen toxicity, and the high-pressure nervous syndrome). These influence the choice of the breathing mixture to be used.

Nitrogen narcosis

Air can be breathed safely down to depths of 50 m, although tests of sophisticated cerebral function show that there is already some impairment at 20 m. Below 50 m, mental deterioration becomes obvious, manifested by actions such as divers offering their mouthpiece to neighbouring fish. This occurs as further nitrogen dissolves in some parts of nerve membranes, making them thicker. Replacing the nitrogen with smaller helium molecules allows divers to go deeper. Changes in function develop within minutes and are rapidly reversible, because they depend purely on passive chemical solution. If divers breathe an oxygen–helium mix rather than air they can descend to the lowermost parts of the continental shelves (730 m) without narcosis. Nitrogen narcosis is a wholly preventable hazard of diving, which can be completely reversed within minutes by ascent and needs no treatment.

Oxygen toxicity

Oxygen becomes toxic to the lungs when alveolar oxygen pressure exceeds half an atmosphere, and it becomes toxic to the nervous system when the alveolar, and so arterial, oxygen pressure exceeds 2 atmospheres. Effects are due to complex chemical interactions, rather than physical solution, and so take time to develop and reverse. Oxygen damages the lung by irritating its endothelial and epithelial surfaces. The time taken for symptoms to appear depends upon the dose. It varies from several hours at half an atmosphere Po_2 to a few hours at 2 atmospheres. Above that pressure, the neurological sequelae overshadow the pulmonary damage that still occurs (Fig. 5).

High-pressure nervous syndrome

At great depths, people breathing oxygen–helium mixtures show neurological disturbances due to direct compression of nerve tissues, making parts of the membranes thinner. Nerve impulses travel more easily and

Fig. 5 Commonly observed pulmonary and central nervous O_2 toxicity versus time curves related to inspired Po_2 (Po_2) (constructed from the data of many workers).

convulsions result. Thickening the tissues with some nitrogen prevents this and allows divers to go deeper.

Problems of ascent

Return to the surface poses three hazards: expansion of gases trapped in sinuses, lung rupture, and decompression sickness.

Expansion of gas in sinuses

If gases trapped in sinuses cannot escape on ascent they will press on the walls and eventually burst them. Rupture of the ethmoid sinus is rare but feared because of the risk of cerebral infection.

Lung rupture

In a sustained dive the lungs contain enough gas to burst them on ascent unless they are adequately vented. The full lung has a bursting pressure of about 75 mmHg (1 m of seawater) and time constants of emptying that are close to 0.3 s. Divers are taught to exhale continuously whenever they ascend, and to ascend no faster than the bubbles they exhale. In such ascents the lungs have time to empty sufficiently and the risk of rupture is low.

Lung rupture often occurs in divers breath-holding on ascent or ascending too fast. Central tears lead to mediastinal emphysema. Peripheral tears cause pneumothorax. Gas may also enter the circulation as air emboli. Escaped gas expands as the ascent continues, making matters worse. The victim may lose consciousness immediately but otherwise notes dyspnoea, cough, or haemoptysis a few minutes later. Voice change and discomfort in the throat or behind the sternum may also be noticed. There may be surgical emphysema of the neck and upper chest, increased cardiac dullness or crepitus, and/or evidence of a pneumothorax. If air embolism has occurred there will be additional neurological signs. Uncomplicated pneumomediastinums, superficial emphysema, or non-tension pneumothorax are treated by oxygen alone. They should not be positive-pressure ventilated. Tension pneumothorax needs an immediate chest drain. Patients with neurological signs should be recompressed as soon as possible.

Decompression sickness occurs because during any dive extra inert gas, usually nitrogen or helium, goes into passive solution in tissues. On ascent this gas can come out of solution in an uncontrolled way, forming bubbles in the circulation and within tissues. As the ascent continues, these bubbles increase in size and number, blocking blood vessels and distorting or rupturing cells. On redescent the bubbles contract and are eventually resorbed. If the first or the subsequent ascent is slow enough, few if any bubbles are

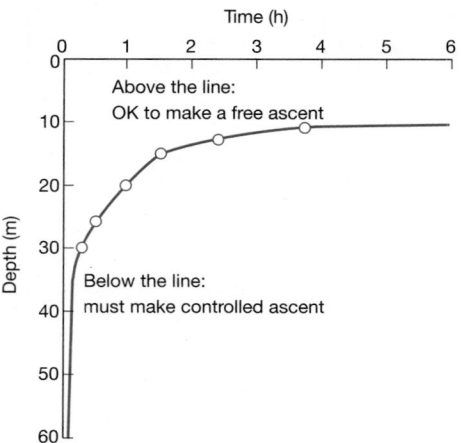

Fig. 6 The 'no-stop' diving curve that determines whether a dive has been shallow and brief enough for the diver to make a free ascent to the surface.

formed, the extra gas diffuses into the bloodstream and out of the lungs easily, and the diver reaches the surface unharmed.

A vast amount of experimental work has been done to determine the safe limits to 'no-stop' diving (Fig. 6) and the depth–time profiles that have to be followed on returning to the surface after any longer dive. Knowledge of safe practice is tabulated in a series of lengthy decompression schedules, which can be obtained from diving clubs or the helplines given below. After very long dives the ascent is very slow and can take several days.

About 1 per cent of dives conducted to recommended schedules, and many badly conducted dives, lead to decompression sickness. The most common presentation in military and commercial diving is limb pain, commonly of the shoulders or elbows in divers and of the knees and hips in tunnel workers. Pain may present a few minutes after a dive or as much as 24 h after the diver has left the water, often as a dull and poorly localized ache of gradual onset. It is not usually made worse by movement of the joint, although weight bearing may make knee pain worse. Physical signs of inflammation are uncommon. Left untreated, the pain will regress and disappear over 2 or 3 days. Recompression commonly improves the pain quickly.

Although sports divers also experience limb pain, neurological symptoms are more prevalent. Sensory disturbance is common, with numbness and paraesthesiae being frequent manifestations, often patchily distributed with no clear dermatomal or peripheral nerve distribution. A particularly fulminant form commences with girdle pain accompanied by loss of sensation and power in the lower limbs. Involvement of the brain is common and may be subtle. Denial is a frequent feature. Any of the higher functions can be involved, including loss of short-term memory, altered affect, visual disturbance, and loss of consciousness. Involvement of the inner ear can present in an identical manner to inner ear squeeze.

Divers who display any manifestation of decompression illness within 24 h of a dive should be managed as if they have the condition. This involves instigating first aid measures and obtaining an informed opinion. The two mainstays of the first aid management are the provision of oxygen (as close to 100 per cent as possible) and rehydration. Within the United Kingdom, informed opinions can be obtained from the British Hyperbaric Association or the Institute of Naval Medicine via their 24-h helplines (0831 151523 and 02392 768026 respectively).

All but trivial cases of decompression illness should be recompressed as soon as possible. It is an effective treatment. The object is to reduce the size of existing bubbles and prevent the formation of new ones, before irreversible infarction and oedema occur.

Problems after the dive

Most ascents are associated with the appearance of many bubbles in systemic venous streams, but these do not usually cause symptoms and so such dives are considered to be 'safe'. Decompression tables that have been established experimentally define the boundaries beyond which more than 2 or 3 per cent of divers will experience symptoms of decompression illness. Such dives are 'unsafe'. There is no doubt that the neurological or other sequelae to unsafe dives may fail to resolve completely, but these are regarded as the consequences of unsafe practices. More recently, diving physicians have been asking whether 'safe' dives lead to insidious, cumulative damage. Although the damage is slight or subclinical, there is definite evidence now that they do. Autopsies on asymptomatic divers with no history of acute decompression illness have revealed that their brains and spinal cords contain considerably more microinfarcts than those of non-diving controls. More importantly, radiographs of the long bones of divers and caisson workers show increasing numbers of aseptic infarcts in a sizeable minority (up to 11 per cent). The incidence is higher in those with a history of overt decompression illness but also occurs in those without. Infarcts can occur after a single decompression, but their incidence rises with age, depth, and diving intensity. Those in the shafts of bone are asymptomatic, but those at juxta-articular surfaces can be severely disabling (dysbaric osteonecrosis). They are more common in caisson workers than divers, but are even seen in professional breath-hold divers, such as the Ama of Japan, in whom the dissolved gas burden must be light. The aetiology is unknown, but gas embolism is the favoured explanation.

Commercial diving, especially saturation diving, causes the lung's total and vital capacities to expand, its FEV1:FVC ratio to fall, and its pulmonary capillary blood volume, as judged by carbon monoxide transfer, to fall. The effects are slight but definite and may be cumulative. The expansions in lung volumes are attributed to the training effects of breathing compressed gases for long times. The fall in the FEV1:FVC ratio is mainly due to the rise in FVC but there are hints of additional small-airway damage. The fall in pulmonary capillary blood volume appears to be due to transient episodes of hyperoxia during saturation diving procedures, but may also be associated with the influx of bubbles from systemic veins on 'safe' decompressions.

It is also known that commercial divers develop a mild degree of high-tone deafness, currently attributed to the noise of gas flows within their helmets.

Codes of safe diving practice given in the Health and Safety Executive's Diving Operations at Work Regulations 1998 and the Compressed Air Regulations 1996 have been accepted nationally and internationally.

Conclusion

Diving is a sometimes very vigorous activity that demands a high degree of mental and physical fitness. It exposes people to several physical and chemical challenges that are reasonably well understood. Because it takes place remote from medical help, there is a strong emphasis on prevention of illness by following safe practices. The practices have been developed empirically on the non-appearance of symptoms in brief trains of dives. There are now indications that these practices may not be quite as safe as first thought, but the cumulative effects are generally slight.

Further reading

Bennett PB, Elliott DH, eds (1993). *The physiology and medicine of diving*, 4th edn. Saunders, London.

Bove AA, ed (1997). *Diving medicine*, 3rd edn. WB Saunders, Philadelphia.

Edmonds C, Lowry C, Pennefather J, eds (1993) *Diving and sub-aquatic medicine*, 3rd edn. Butterworth-Heinemann, London.

Lundgren C, ed (1999). *The lung at depth*. Marcel Dekker, Basle.

8.5.7 Lightning and electrical injuries

Chris Andrews

Introduction

Lightning is a powerful force; it provides spectacular displays and has evoked an extensive mythology. The comparatively recent discovery and distribution of electricity have had an equally profound effect, and provide truth to the adage that 'electricity is a good servant and a bad master'.

Epidemiology

Lightning injury

The accepted case fatality of lightning shock is around 30 per cent. Estimated mortality is around 0.3 per million population in the United States each year, compared with 1.5 per million in Singapore, 0.3 per million in Australia, and fewer than 0.1 per million in the United Kingdom.

In the early part of the twentieth century, most individuals struck were outdoor workers (67 per cent) and outdoor recreationalists (28 per cent). The present corresponding figures are 45 per cent and 50 per cent, which may be explained by changes in social and work habits. Indoor strikes (for example by current conducted through communication or power apparatus) continue to account for about 5 per cent of these accidents.

Males are more often injured than females (1.67 males to 0.33 females); the age group most at risk are those aged 20–29 years. Risky situations include sheltering under trees, on open water, on tractors and in open fields, and playing golf. Regional differences correlate well with storm activity and population density in that area.

Electrical injury

Industrial and domestic situations are the two main areas in which electrical injury occurs.

Electrocution ranks fifth in the causes of workplace death, accounting for the death of 10 000 workers each year in the United Sates, with a further 10 million being injured. Most of the victims work for utility companies, followed by mining and construction workers. Contact with power lines causes 53 per cent of fatal shocks, and contact with power tools account for a further 22 per cent. The most dangerous times of day seem to be between 10 a.m. and 3 p.m. on Mondays, Tuesdays, and Thursdays. Most of the victims are trade and labouring staff; sales, clerical, and professional categories are at least risk. Metal ladders and antennas are particularly dangerous and can be hoisted easily into overhead power lines. Codes of safe practice are written accordingly.

In domestic situations, contact with overhead lines is again important. Faulty repair of equipment and faulty apparatus, wiring, and especially power and extension cords account for large numbers of deaths and injuries. Children are at particular risk. Death from domestic electric shock has shown a marked decrease with the introduction of residual current devices (known as RCDs). These detect a large proportion of potentially dangerous situations—they sense if current is diverted from the supply main to earth and interrupt it in a matter of milliseconds.

Mechanisms of injury

Lightning injury

Lightning injury may be sustained in four separate ways. First, a person may be struck directly. Secondly, a nearby object, such as a tree or a building, may be struck, and someone in direct contact with it may receive a shock. Thirdly, without direct contact an arc may 'jump' to a nearby person from the struck object, thereby generating a 'side flash'. Finally, as current disperses away from the base of a strike to ground, an individual may divert current flowing in the ground to themselves. This is termed shock due to increase in earth potential. Recently a fifth mechanism has been proposed — the transient flow of current due to corona and streamer formation.

Both cardiac and respiratory function cease instantaneously under lightning strike, the cardiac arrest being asystolic. Cardiac function restarts under local pacemaker control, but respiratory function does not recommence and secondary hypoxic cardiac arrest supervenes.

The major cranial orifices are portals of entry for lightning current, and from there pathways to the brainstem are short. Respiratory function is thought to be affected there, and thence conduction through the cerebrospinal fluid and then blood to the myocardium.

The QT prolongation resulting from lightning injury may predispose to episodic arrythmias. There is no evidence to that lightning inhibits body metabolism. Resuscitation is as urgent as with any other injury.

Electrical injury

With electric shock it is important to assess the points of entry and exit and the pathway of current through the body. Once the pathway has been determined, a locus for expected injury can be established and the flow of current can be estimated from the applied voltage divided by the impedance of the proposed pathway. Most impedance is in the skin barriers, and the impedance demonstrated is non-linear. There is an initial (contact) impedance which decreases as current flow continues. Impedance also varies with time since application, contact surface area, and frequency.

For currents with a frequency of 15 to 100 Hz, externally applied from hand to hand or hand to foot, relevant parameters include 0.5 mA as the threshold of perception and 10 mA for 'let go' current. A 50 per cent chance of fibrillation exists at 2000 mA conducted for 10 ms, or at the other extreme 100 mA conducted for 10 s. Direct internal application of less than 200 μA to the heart muscle may induce fibrillation.

Joule heating may account for tissue damage in the path of the current. It may be calculated from the power dissipation in the tissue—the square of the tissue current times its impedance, the former often being hard to estimate. The complex phenomenon of electroporation, where cell membranes are breached by the electrical induction of unstable pores in the membrane, may alternatively lead to cell death.

Presentation of the injured person

Lightning injury

A witnessed strike offers the best chance of resuscitation. The victim is not dangerous to touch, and does not constitute a risk to the rescuer. Immediate cardiopulmonary resuscitation is paramount. It has been stated that:

> Any person found with linear burns and clothing exploded off should be treated as the victim of a lightning strike. Feathering burns are pathognomic of lightning injury and occur in no other type of injury. …Another complex diagnostic of lightning injury includes linear or punctate burns, tympanic membrane rupture, confusion, and outdoor location…
>
> Cooper *et al.* (2000)

In assessing a lightning victim, the following features must be sought.

Cardiovascular and pulmonary consequences

Asystolic arrest is the main cardiac event in lightning injury. ECG signs may take many forms, with ischaemic and infarct forms. They almost invariably resolve completely over time. Alterations in QT interval and arrythmias of many kinds are seen. ECG changes may not occur until late in the course, and so are a poor diagnostic tool. Respiratory arrest is common. A person not suffering cardiopulmonary arrest is highly unlikely to die from lightning strike ($p < 0.0001$).

Neurological consequences

Direct neural injury may occur both centrally and peripherally. All forms of intracranial bleeding have been reported. Direct cerebral damage particularly affects the basal ganglia, cerebellum, and brainstem. Dural tears, scalp haematomata, and fractures are also seen. Seizures occur as a result of anoxia and injury.

Peripheral nerve injury, including autonomic injury, can give prolonged and long-lasting disability which often develops late. Other late features include spinal cord atrophic paralysis, cerebellar ataxia, inco-ordination, paraesthesiae, and aphasiae. Ongoing complex regional pain syndromes may be seen.

Keraunoparalysis and burns

Over 70 per cent of victims demonstrate keraunoparalysis. This is a syndrome of cold, pulseless, mottled, and asensory extremities. The syndrome resembles a compartment syndrome and occurs in the line of passage of the strike current. It resolves spontaneously within 24 h with no sequelae, and requires no surgical intervention.

Burns are of minor consequence in lightning injury, and again require little intervention. Entry and exit burns may be full thickness though small. Arborescent (feathering) burns resemble fern-like patterns on the skin. Their aetiology is unknown, but they fade within 24 h. Linear burns are due to the passage of hot plasma tongues over the skin. Eschar is simply allowed to separate without further treatment. Flash may be seen, like sunburn or welder's flash, from the profound radiation of the strike. Sheet burns resulting from efflux of hot plasma may be a variant of linear burning, since both seem to follow moisture and sweat lines. There may be contact burns from heated metal such as buckles and coins.

Eye, ear, and explosive injuries

The explosive force of the lightning insult blasts clothing apart, and may cause percussive injury to the lungs and abdominal viscera. Tympanic membranes are usually ruptured, perhaps from the explosive force of the strike. Percussive eye injury, particularly retinal, has been reported. Cataracts may develop much later.

Other injuries

Renal and haematological damage have occasionally been reported. In pregnant women the fetus is unlikely to survive. Menstrual and sexual difficulties have been reported.

Electrical injury

In contrast to lightning injury, victims may suffer prolonged attachment to the source of electrical current, making them dangerous to touch. Before resuscitation they must be removed from the current source, and this usually means interrupting the current flow at the supply point.

Burns are far more serious, and may merit intense surgical treatment. The likelihood of internal burning (remembering the possibility of electroporation) may require further surgical intervention. Cardiac and respiratory burns may also exist.

Cardiovascular consequences

Fibrillation is the most common cardiac abnormality following electrical injury. Cardiopulmonary resuscitation is urgently required. Electricity suppliers have standard first aid/resuscitation procedures. Cardiac dysfunction may persist for long periods, and ECG signs may not resolve.

Neurological and muscular consequences

Neural injury may be categorized into early and late syndromes, at cerebral, cord, and peripheral level.

Early tetanic muscular contraction locks the victim onto the electrical conductors. This tetany may compromise respiratory function. Neurological injury may be hard to distinguish from hypoxic and vasospastic injury. Similarly, neural injury is often hard to separate from ischaemic injury due to vessel spasm. Early and late generalized convulsions may occur. Pareses and paraesthesiae may develop, both early and late.

In the long term complex regional pain syndromes and other chronic pain syndromes must be considered.

Burns

Burns are often severe in electrical injury and merit much treatment effort. Arc and flame burns and contact burns from current entry and exit are seen. For example, tetanic gripping of the electrical conductor causes grasp burns to the hand.

Severe internal thermal or electroporation damage may occur. The management is largely surgical. Joints, ligaments, and tendons may be severely damaged by the heat generated, and osteonecrosis may be seen.

Other aspects

Widespread muscle damage generates myoglobin that must be cleared by the kidney with a severe risk of renal damage. Other metabolic and biochemical disturbances secondary to hypoxia may develop. Massive hyperkalaemia has implications for the use of depolarizing muscle relaxants.

Eye damage includes retinal damage, with punctation and detachment, and thermal damage to other media. During follow-up the possibility of ocular pareses and cataracts must be recognized.

After shock during pregnancy the prognosis for the fetus is poor. Non-focal injury is more likely in survivors.

Psychological consequences of electrical and lightning injuries

Although electrical and lightning injuries are fundamentally different in nature and management, their psychological sequelae are similar. Sequelae may be disabling. To a large extent psychological consequences of persisting pain and dysfunction cannot be separated from organic psychological consequences.

Emotional sequelae include depression, often with organic features. It is hard to separate this from the emotional reaction to injury and continuing disability. Aggression, anxiety, and phobic features are common. Marital disharmony commonly follows social withdrawal, disinterest, and a fatigue state. Loss of interest in sex and in relationships, together with a feeling of fault or guilt, may be associated. Sleep disturbance is common.

There is loss of short-term memory with impaired concentration, higher mental functions, and loss of identity and ability.

Treatment of the injuries

First, urgent and life-saving treatment must be administered. Secondly, there must be surveillance for delayed sequelae, and thirdly long-term monitoring for morbidity, including cataract formation and psychological problems.

Lightning injury

First the casualty is resuscitated and evacuated. Cardiopulmonary resuscitation is continued until medical emergency help is obtained. Ventilation and cardiac support may be required.

ECG monitoring must be used to detect subtle effects like QT prolongation. Associated trauma is treated.

In the long term, patients are observed for development of pain syndromes. Ocular and auditory function are monitored. Sensitivity to the psychological sequelae is required, and preventive interviewing may be useful.

Carbemazepine, gabapentin, clonazepam, flecainide, and mexilitine are useful to control neurally derived pain and resulting weakness. An antidepressant (see below) is a useful adjunct to this.

Electrical injury

Urgent life support is indicated. Ventilatory and inotropic support and correction of arrhythmias may be required.

For burns, progressive debridement and/or amputation may be needed. Renal damage should be prevented.

Associated trauma is treated. Ocular and auditory function are monitored and psychological disturbances are reviewed. In the long term surveillance is similar to lightning injury.

Psychological elements

In all cases the management of the psychological syndrome is paramount and may be the greatest determinant of long-term functional capability. Awareness of the impact of the injury on employment and relationships and social networks is fundamental. Cognitive and computer aids are being developed.

An antidepressant such as a selective serotonin reuptake inhibitor, possibly citalopram, paroxetine, venlafaxine, or a tricyclic such as clomipramine, may be useful.

Early and continuing neuropsychological assessment is desirable.

Controversy

The place of polaxamers in discovering the extent of electroporation and in delineating debridement levels is of great interest.

The mechanisms of the psychological disability remain to be elucidated. Victims are frequently 'written off' as malingering or simply depressed, when a more extensive syndrome exists. The useful duration of monitoring of otherwise asymptomatic people has not been determined.

Further reading

Andrews CJ (1996). Electric shock and lightning strike. In: Pearn J, ed *The science of first aid*. St John's Ambulance Press, Canberra.

Andrews CJ *et al.* (1992) *Lightning injuries: electrical, medical and legal aspects*, chapter 17, pp. 148–70. CRC Press, Boca Raton, FL.

Bridges J *et al.* (1985). *Electric shock safety criteria*. Pergamon, Oxford.

Cooper MA (1980). Lightning injuries: prognostic signs for death. *Annals of Emergency Medicine* 9, 134.

Cooper MA, ed. (1995). *Seminars in Neurology* 15 (3, 4). Special issues on lightning and electrical injuries.

Cooper MA *et al.* (2000). Lightning injuries. In: Auerbach P, ed *Wilderness medicine*, 4th edn, chapter 3, pp. 73–111. Mosby, St Louis, MO.

Lee RC, Capelli-Schellpfeffer M, Kelley K (1994). Electrical injury. *Annals of the New York Academy of Science* 720.

Lee RC, Cravalho EG, Burke JF (1992). *Electric trauma*. Cambridge University Press, Cambridge.

8.5.8 Podoconiosis

S. M. Evans, J. J. Powell,
and R. P. H. Thompson

Introduction

Podoconiosis (from the Greek *podos* 'of the foot' and *konia* 'dust'), named and characterized by the late Dr Ernest W. Price, is a non-filarial form of elephantiasis affecting the feet and legs of barefoot agrarian communities. It is endemic in parts of Africa, Central and South America, northwest India, and Indonesia. The disease is an obstructive lymphopathy, caused by the penetration of fine particles of silica and aluminosilicates into the tissues of the foot.

Aetiology

Areas of high prevalence are typified by a reddish brown volcanic soil that has a high clay content and is extremely slippery after rain. A large proportion of the soil comprises particles of less than 2 µm in diameter, in which the aluminosilicate kaolinite predominates. Other environmental features of areas in which podoconiosis occurs include high altitude (1250 to 2500 m), average daytime temperatures of 20 °C, and a high hot-seasonal rainfall in excess of 1000 mm annually. In these conditions, weathering of the volcanic alkali basalt rock favours formation of a fertile clay soil, which attracts subsistence farming and a largely barefooted population. In adjacent, tropical, non-endemic, lowland areas, more complete chemical degradation of the parent rock reduces soil fertility and also the biological activity of the soil particles.

The greater exposure of men to soil particles during farming is probably responsible for their higher incidence of podoconiosis compared with that of women. In areas of high prevalence, for example in highland areas of East Africa, up to 70 adults in every 1000 are affected. There appears to be a familial tendency to develop the disease, and this may reflect an inherited inability of the immune system to process and detoxify ultrafine particles. The socio-economic consequences of belonging to such a family, in terms of marriage opportunity and employment, are considerable.

Microparticles

Using polarized light microscopy, birefringent particles are frequently seen in lymph node macrophages, but in tissue sections from the foot electron microscopy is needed. Price's X-ray microanalytical studies of the tissues of the foot and femoral nodes in areas with podoconiosis demonstrated the presence of ultrafine particles, consisting mainly of silicon and aluminium with smaller amounts of titanium and iron. Particles were found both within macrophage phagolysosomes (Fig. 1) and free within the tissue, and their elemental compositions matched those of the fine particles of the local soil. Morphological analysis identified kaolinite (an aluminosilicate), amorphous silica, titanium and iron oxides, with some quartz, exactly as in the local soil. Such mineral particles are also found in many areas of the world without podoconiosis so the exact reason for their pathogenicity can only be hypothesized. However, fine particles have been shown to be important aetiological agents in a number of human diseases, in particular chronic inflammatory lung conditions such as silicosis and asbestosis, and asthma.

In podoconiosis, the small size of the particles is likely to play an important role in dictating toxicity. Evidence for this comes from data showing that a significantly higher proportion of the soil in endemic areas consists of particles less than 5 µm in diameter than in neighbouring non-endemic areas. Indeed, particles released after digestion of diseased femoral lymph nodes were found to range in size from 0.3 to 6.0 µm. Transcutaneous entry of macromolecules and micron-sized particles is well recognized, but it may be facilitated in podoconiosis by the presence of larger, abrasive crystals of quartz in the silt fraction of the soil.

The volcanic origin of the rock is clearly important. Using thermoluminescence, specific defects in the crystal lattice, which are fixed in the rock as the hot volcanic lava undergoes rapid cooling, have been identified in microparticles from affected areas. Furthermore, newly fractured mineral crystals exhibit much higher reactivity than those that have been weathered. The microtopography of particle surfaces has been analysed by thermostimulated exoelectronic emission, which also identified a characteristic peak in soil fractions from endemic areas.

Another factor is persistence, since the particles are not easily dissolved or degraded in the tissues. In experiments with cultured murine macrophages, soil particles from endemic areas were toxic at a lower concentration than the corresponding soil fraction from non-endemic areas. Thus, the particles have a direct toxicity to immunocytes but this could be modified by interactions with other ions (such as iron) or biomolecules.

Once internalized, toxic mineral microparticles exert a range of effects, from mild irritation to extensive fibrosis and obstructive lymphopathy.

Pathology

The earliest histological feature of podoconiosis is seen in the dermis where collections of lymphocytes accumulate around channels of the superficial lymphatic plexus, sweat ducts, and sweat glands. A chronic inflammatory infiltrate is evident in the adventitia of the deeper lymphatic vessels, with subendothelial oedema gradually replaced by fibrosis. Similarly, lymph node capsules are thickened by fibrosis and the interfollicular sinuses become dilated and packed with lymphocytes. Macrophages are evident in the cortex of the node and frequently contain aggregations of particles, which often exhibit birefringence. With increasing severity of disease, fibrosis becomes more advanced, especially at the corticomedullary boundary.

Clinical appearances

The clinical manifestations of podoconiosis depend upon the degree to which fibrosis occurs in the dermis. Two main types are described, although most cases show features of both types, between the two extremes.

In the soft or 'water-bag' type, there is little dermal fibrosis and minimal hyperkeratotic change. The skin is smooth and can be grasped between the fingers. Lymphoedema is marked and extends gradually from the dorsum of the foot to involve the whole lower leg. The swollen limb pits on pressure (Fig. 2(a)).

By contrast, the hard or 'leathery' type is characterized by extensive dermal fibrosis, which may be more than 3 cm thick. The skin is fixed to

Fig. 2 Clinical types of elephantiasis. (a) The soft or 'water-bag' type. Swelling is readily reduced by compression or elevation. The skin is soft and can be pinched off the bones. (b) The hard or 'leathery' type. The skin is rough and fixed to deeper tissues. Nodulation is seen on the toes and dorsum of the foot.

Fig. 1 Electron micrograph of a femoral lymph node of an elephantiasic person. Note the two macrophages on the left, the upper of which contains a number of clumps of microparticles. X-ray analysis showed that most of these were silica with varying amounts of aluminium, iron, and titanium (×7200).

deeper tissues, does not pit, and hyperkeratosis and hyperpigmentation are marked. In front of the ankle and behind the toes, there may be many folds of firm, rough skin, which are easily traumatized, and multiple nodules often develop (Fig. 2(b)).

A subgroup of the hard or 'leathery' type is the 'slipper' type, in which hyperkeratosis is distributed around the back of the heel, the borders of the sole, over the toes and on to the dorsum of the foot. Lymphatic obstruction is confined to the deep lymphatics of the plantar region so that the dermal fibrotic reaction occurs in the distribution of a slipper.

Natural history

Podoconiosis usually starts between the ages of 10 and 20 and progresses at a variable rate over months or years. The first symptoms are a burning sensation of the soles of the feet and itching of the lower legs, usually intermittent and unilateral at first, especially in bed at night or after exertion. Uncovering or raising the leg usually alleviates symptoms, but alcohol consumption, exercise, or menstruation may exacerbate them. The first swelling is usually evident just proximal to the first toe cleft, and spreads after a time to involve the rest of the dorsum of the foot, and later the whole lower leg. The chronic progression of the disease is marked by intensification of the burning discomfort and itching, and it may be punctuated by acute episodes of lymphangitis. Infected ulcers and cellulitis may complicate the clinical picture. Both legs are always involved, although there may be considerable asymmetry. Once established, the femoral lymph nodes are often enlarged and tender but they rarely suppurate.

Management

Price has emphasized the importance of obtaining the co-operation and understanding of patients in order to maximize the benefits of intervention.

The mineral load in the tissues cannot be reduced once it has been absorbed. Therefore, the main strategy is aimed at prevention. Provision of footwear is the most obvious protection, and it is highly effective, but matting to cover the bare ground of residential huts is also used. Occasionally, it is possible to arrange a change of employment or residence.

Anti-inflammatory analgesics, such as aspirin, are effective for burning discomfort. Reduction of oedema will improve itching, more easily accomplished in the early phases of the disease and in the soft or 'water-bag' type. Elevation of the foot of the bed and elasticated stockings may be sufficient initially, but a programme of treatment using compressive methods (compressive bandaging or intermittent compression machines) is needed in more advanced cases.

Finally, a variety of traditional drugs in tropical Africa, derived from plants, has been used in podoconiosis with the aim of reducing fibrosis and progression of the disease. Some of these contain benzopyrones, coumarin, and toxerutin, which may have antifibrogenic properties, but none has yet been convincing in the long-term control of limb swelling in this unpleasant and disfiguring disease.

Further reading

Blanke JH *et al.* (1983). Correlations between elephantiasis and thermoluminescence of volcanic soil. *Radiation Effects* **73**, 103–13.

Blundell G, Henderson WJ, Price EW (1989). Soil particles in the tissues of the foot in endemic elephantiasis of the lower legs. *Annals of Tropical Medicine and Parasitology* **83**, 381–5.

Davies JE, Townsend PD (1990). Exoemission of Ethiopian soils and the endemicity of non-filarial elephantiasis. *Radiation Protection Dosimetry* **4**, 185–8.

Harvey RJ, Powell JJ, Thompson RPH (1996). A review of the geochemical factors linked to podoconiosis. In: Appleton JD, Fuge R, McCall GJH, eds *Environmental geochemistry and health*, Geological Society special publication 113, pp 255–60. Geological Society, Bath.

Price EW (1990). *Podoconiosis: non-filarial elephantiasis*. Oxford University Press, Oxford.

Price EW, Plant DA (1990). The significance of particle size of soils as a risk factor in the etiology of podoconiosis. *Transactions of the Royal Society of Tropical Medicine and Hygiene* **84**, 885–6.

Spooner NT, Davies JE (1986). The possible role of soil particles in the aetiology of non-filarial endemic elephantiasis: a macrophage cytotoxicity assay. *Transactions of the Royal Society of Tropical Medicine and Hygiene* **80**, 222–5.

8.5.9 Radiation

J. R. Harrison

There are two types of radiation: ionizing and non-ionizing. The former includes radiation from naturally occurring sources, such as radon gas or cosmic rays, and man-made sources, such as X-rays. The latter includes radiation from natural ultraviolet light and radiowaves and man-made emissions from radio transmitters and mobile phones. In all cases the electromagnetic radiation may cause biological damage by the deposition of energy in the body. They have the capacity to produce early acute effects and some have the ability to produce late effects, such as cancer. High doses can cause early death.

Ionizing radiation

Physicians are likely to become involved with radiation issues if people are over-exposed. For example, the theft of a caesium-137 radiotherapy source in Goiânia, Brazil led to 50 people being over-exposed, resulting in four deaths. In that incident large areas of land and property were contaminated. In the accident at the Chernobyl nuclear power plant 28 members of the workforce died of radiation-related injuries. The release of radioactivity also led to widespread contamination of houses, land, and foodstuffs. Experience shows that in these situations both individual and public health concerns dominate the agenda and place a burden on health professionals.

In the early twentieth century, due to a lack of knowledge about the harmful biological effects of ionizing radiation, many radiologists received high doses to their hands (often calibrating their machines by an erythema dose). Subsequently many died of radiation-induced cancers.

Atoms, radioactivity, and radiation

Some isotopes of elements are unstable and undergo radioactive decay. The time necessary to reach a stable form depends on the element and ranges from a few fractions of a second to several thousand years. The unit for radioactivity is the becquerel (Bq): 1 Bq equals one atomic disintegration per second. The average amount of natural potassium-40 (^{40}K) in every kilogram of the average person is 60 Bq. This means that about 15 million ^{40}K atoms disintegrate inside a person each hour.

Electromagnetic radiation (X-rays and gamma rays) or subatomic particles such as alpha and beta particles and neutrons can all interact with matter and tissues and cells. The different types of radiation penetrate matter, the extent of the penetration being determined by the size, charge, and energy of the particle/wave. Alpha particles are stopped by a thin piece of paper or the dead layer of the skin, while beta particles can penetrate the hand but will be stopped by a thin sheet of aluminium. X- and gamma rays penetrate the body and an aluminium sheet but are stopped by lead. Neutrons penetrate most materials but may be stopped by thick polythene or concrete (hydrogenous materials). These overall properties of radiation affect the degree of cellular damage following exposure and the methods needed for protection.

Ionizing radiation has sufficient energy to break chemical bonds and ionize atoms and molecules, producing ion pairs. These ions are charged and are capable of causing further ionization and energy deposition leading to physicochemical changes in cellular constituents. Some of these changes may be of no biological consequence and others may be repaired, but there is a finite probability that damage may cause cell death or irreparable damage to vital cell constituents such as the DNA.

Dose quantities

The absorbed dose is a measure of the mean energy absorbed by unit mass of tissue, and the absorbed dose in gray (Gy) is equal to the deposition of one joule (J) of energy in one kilogram (kg) of tissue. Overall, the greater the dose, the greater the likelihood of a biological effect being seen.

Various radiation and tissue weighting factors are used to convert the absorbed dose in gray to an effective dose in sievert (Sv). This system allows external and internal exposures to be combined into one dose—on the basis of equality of risk. Once a radionuclide is incorporated it will continue to expose surrounding tissues until it finally decays or is excreted.

Submultiples of the gray and sievert are commonly used, such as the milligray (mGy) and millisievert (mSv), which is one-thousandth of a sievert. For example, the world average individual dose received due to exposure to natural background radiation is about 2 mSv per year compared with the occupational dose limit of 20 mSv per year.

Acute radiation sickness

An acute exposure (measured in seconds, minutes, or hours) causes cell damage, the severity of which depends on the tissue type, or even death. It is characterized by a sudden sensation of anorexia or nausea and is soon followed by vomiting and sometimes diarrhoea. In the sensitive mucosal stem cells of the gastrointestinal tract, in particular in the stomach and small intestine, 5-hydroxytryptamine (**5-HT₃**) is released into the bloodstream which stimulates the nausea/vomiting centres in the brain and other 5-HT₃ receptors. There is a concomitant increase in bowel motility, which may be caused by bile salts acting on the damaged mucosa. The total spectrum of effects is dependent upon the dose but may be anorexia, nausea and vomiting, and diarrhoea. Radiation sickness extends beyond the early symptoms, as damage to other tissues, such as the bone marrow, causes lowering of blood cell counts leaving the body vulnerable to infection. High radiation doses can also lead to permanent sterility, serious damage to other organs, and to death (with or without medical treatment).

Many other symptoms may arise which depend on the dose, the dose rate, and the area of the body affected. These might include loss of hair, skin burns, or haemorrhages in the short term and increased incidence of cancer in the long term. These symptoms may vary due to individual susceptibility and because in most uncontrolled situations the nature of the exposure is non-uniform. In radiotherapy, where exposures are controlled and fractionated to enable normal sensitive tissues to recover between treatments, nausea and/or vomiting usually only occur where there is a high-dose total-body irradiation, for example in the ablation of bone marrow for subsequent bone marrow transplantation. It is normal to give antiemetics such as ondansetron (a 5-HT₃ antagonist) to reduce such side-effects.

At doses greater than 1 Gy significant reductions in blood cell counts follow depletion of the bone marrow, and can lead to reduced resistance to infections, haemorrhages, and anaemia. If there is significant direct exposure or surface contamination with radioactive materials skin burns may occur leading to further fluid loss and the danger of infection. The acute symptoms are sometimes grouped together and called the acute radiation syndrome. Combined injuries have a worse prognosis, and this is important in medical management. Without medical treatment an acute dose of approximately 4 Gy is likely to lead to death within 60 days in 50 per cent of those exposed. Doses in excess of 10 Gy are likely to result in earlier death, even with treatment. Similar doses over longer periods (days, weeks) may cause a variety of symptoms, but death is unlikely as the cells and tissues have time to repair the damage.

The following figures are given as guidelines for adults: anorexia may be seen in 5 per cent of those at 0.4 Gy and 95 per cent at 3 Gy, nausea in 5 per cent at 0.5 Gy and 95 per cent at 4.5 Gy, vomiting in 5 per cent at 0.6 Gy and 100 per cent at 7 Gy, and diarrhoea in 5 per cent at 1 Gy and over 20 per cent at 8 Gy. If the time from exposure to onset of any of the above symptoms is less than 1 h the dose is likely to be more than 3 Gy, if more than 3 h the dose is likely to be more than 1 Gy, and if they last for more than 24 h the dose is likely to be more than 6 Gy. These general spectra can be helpful to physicians as an aid to medical triage before more refined estimates can be made.

Clinical treatment of radiation injuries

General

Experience from many radiation accidents has shown that the heterogeneous nature of the exposures tends to confound both the clinical and pathological picture so that estimating the scale of the radiation damage and exposure is difficult. The early treatment of conventional injuries is the main factor that determines survival in patients who have been accidentally irradiated.

Casualties on admission can be classified into four treatment categories: mild, moderate, severe, and lethal. Stating specific dose ranges for these categories is not possible, primarily because of the difficulty in converting an exposure to a meaningful tissue dose; however, equivalent whole-body dose ranges would be less than 2 Gy, 2 to 5 Gy, 5 to 10 Gy, and more than 10 Gy respectively. The most reliable prognostic guides for treatment in the early stage are the change in levels of blood cells, which relates to dose, and cytogenetics, which will give a good estimate of dose.

The degree of radiation-induced marrow aplasia (reversible or irreversible) may not be known for days because of the uncontrolled nature of the exposure and the likelihood that it was non-uniform and heterogeneous. However, assessment of the dose, while important, is secondary to the treatment.

Reliable triage and good clinical care based on comprehensive biological data will ensure the best chance of recovery provided that some critical stem cells survive the radiation exposure. There is a need for biological monitoring, such as absolute lymphocyte counts and cytogenetics, to assess the effective dose and the probability of survival.

Sepsis

The suppression of bone marrow activity will reduce the resistance to bacterial and viral infections. For febrile neutropenic casualties, blood, urine, and faecal samples for cultures need to be taken on admission. Patients must be started on broad-spectrum antimicrobials and these should be given until the patient is afebrile. Experience has shown that fungal lung infections can be the cause of late deaths when all the other radiation effects have been stabilized. Early use of antifungal agents and gammaglobulin for viral infections is essential.

Marrow aplasia

Following a suspected high radiation exposure, initial patient assessment should be based on dosimetric testing (biological, physical), daily full blood counts, viral titres (for cytomegalovirus and HIV for example), HLA subtyping for possible bone marrow transplantation, and the administration of haematopoietic growth factors (colony stimulating factors such as granulocyte or granulocyte/macrophage colony stimulating factors). Particular care is needed if the patient has other injuries, such as pulmonary infections, burns, or smoke inhalation.

Subsequent supportive therapy might include platelet transfusions, particularly if surgery is indicated for other injuries. Other treatments might include the use of thrombopoietic drugs. However, bone marrow transplants should only be given if an autologous donor is available.

Gastrointestinal

Vomiting should be controlled by use of effective antiemetics such as ondansetron. This relaxes the gut and reduces mechanical damage to the lining of the small intestine. Antiemetics also help to reduce fluid loss. Diarrhoea should be treated with fluids and electrolytes and efforts should be made to improve host defences by elemental diets, vitamins, and glutamine parenterally or intravenously.

Cutaneous

Remove all clothing as soon as possible, bathe very gently in lukewarm baths, use acetic acid or ion exchangers if surface contamination is thought to be soluble caesium, and only remove contamination mechanically from the soles of the feet or the palms of the hands.

Later treatments might include the use of topical creams, systemic aci-tretin, and gamma interferon. These have been found to be helpful in treating the chronic skin damage seen in the Chernobyl firefighters.

Combined injury

Radiation injury is not immediately life threatening; initial care should address the associated conventional injuries, for example thermal burns and wounds. After stabilization, radio-isotope decontamination should be performed before emergency surgery, definitive care, and treatment of radiation injuries. Collection of biological samples during the resuscitation stages will supplement the initial data collected during triage. Ideally, definitive care should immediately follow resuscitation.

Management of soft tissue wounds requires alternative ways to close wounds, for example biological wound coverings and skin grafts. Surgical correction of life-threatening and other major injuries should be carried out as soon as possible (within 36 to 48 h); elective procedures should be postponed until late in the convalescent period (45 to 60 days) following haematopoietic recovery. Treatment of thermal burns should include early excision of potentially septic tissue and closure of the wounds, preferably by skin grafting.

Counselling

Overexposure to ionizing radiations increases the risk of subsequent radiation-induced cancers. So it is important that over-exposed patients are counselled on the radiation risks in comparison with other risks in life. Experience from the Chernobyl accident has shown that many people have unwarranted fears from their radiation exposures due to poor communications and a lack of trust.

Non-ionizing radiation

Ultraviolet radiation

The main organs affected by ultraviolet radiation are the skin and the eye. There is evidence that ultraviolet radiation can also induce changes in the immune system but the significance of this to humans is not yet clear. The most serious health effects are the cutaneous malignancies.

The skin

Short-term effects
Short-term skin effects are sunburn, principally consisting of erythema and oedema, both of which may be very severe. In some people this sunburn is followed by increased production of melanin (a suntan). A suntan is not an indication of good health and only offers minimal protection against further exposure. It is a sign that damaged skin is attempting to protect itself from further harm.

Long-term effects
The most serious long-term effect is the induction of cancer. The non-melanoma skin cancers are mainly basal cell carcinomas and squamous cell carcinomas. They are relatively common in white populations, although they are rarely fatal. The overall incidence is difficult to assess because of under-reporting. Malignant melanoma is the main cause of death from skin cancer, particularly in young people, although its incidence is lower than that of non-melanoma skin cancers. The risk of developing malignant melanoma has increased substantially in white populations for several decades, and the annual incidence in the United Kingdom is now approaching 10 new cases per 100 000. Chronic exposure to solar radiation causes photoageing of the skin, which is characterized by a leathery, wrinkled appearance and loss of elasticity. A small quantity of ultraviolet radiation is beneficial in terms of vitamin D synthesis in the skin.

The eye

Responses of the human eye to acute exposure to ultraviolet radiation include photokeratitis and photoconjunctivitis. Repeated exposure is also a major factor in the causation of non-malignant clinical lesions of the cornea and conjunctiva such as climatic droplet keratopathy, pterygium, and, probably, pinguecula. Epidemiological data on cataract formation in highly exposed people suggest that cumulative exposure to ultraviolet radiation is a principal causative factor in the development of, at least, cortical cataracts, although the extent to which this is an important risk factor for cataracts in the general population is unclear.

Immune responses

Biological studies have shown that exposure to ultraviolet radiation can suppress the normal antigen-specific immune response to some skin tumours and to various skin pathogens, although immunity acquired from prior infection is not affected. The significance for human health of ultraviolet radiation-induced immune suppression is not clearly established at present.

Radiofrequency electromagnetic waves

The possible hazards to humans of exposure to high-intensity radiofrequency electromagnetic waves are more controversial, but individuals chronically exposed to such radiation at high intensity have been reported as developing such conditions as anaemia, alopecia, or psychological disorders. In animal studies, changes in the high spontaneous rate of cancer in particular strains have been reported. The widespread use of radiofrequency microwaves (in mobile phones and ovens for home and restaurant cookery) has made their safety a more important question. With the exception of the danger from induction heating, with consequent damage due to thermal burns, there is no evidence that there is significant risk of danger to the general public from the use of such appliances. The National Radiological Protection Board has given advice that acceptable exposures should not result in a rise in body temperature of more than 0.5 °C as shown by skin and rectal temperature. Local tissue temperatures should not exceed 38 °C for the head, 39 °C for the trunk, or 40 °C for the limbs.

Magnetic fields

With the increasing use of magnetic resonance imaging interest has developed in the possible hazards to humans of exposure to strong and varying magnetic fields. Once again, the biological evidence is largely anecdotal and in part contradictory, and mainly involves transient psychological changes. The National Radiological Protection Board has recommended that for static magnetic fields the individual being imaged should not be exposed to a field greater than 2.5 tesla (T) to the whole or a substantial portion of the body. There is no evidence so far to suggest that the embryo is sensitive to magnetic fields and radiofrequency at the intensities encountered in clinical magnetic resonance imaging, but it is felt to be prudent to exclude pregnant women during the first trimester.

Summary

The man-made use of ionizing radiation in medicine and industry and for nuclear power has shown that high doses are lethal and early (deterministic) effects are visible and can be shorten life. Latent (stochastic) effects, particularly cancers, are well documented and risk estimates based on the study of occupationally and medically exposed cohorts are reasonably robust. Legislative dose limits will prevent deterministic effects and reduce the risk of stochastic effects to an acceptable level, although all doses should be kept as low as reasonably practicable. Information on the possible health effects of radiofrequencies and electromagnetic fields is less robust. However, the degree of risk acceptable to the public and workforce is likely to change.

Further reading

Berry RJ (1986). The radiologist as a guinea pig: radiation hazards to man as demonstrated in early radiologists, and their patients. *Journal of the Royal Society of Medicine* **79**, 506–9.

IAEA (International Atomic Energy Agency) (1988). *The radiological accident in Goiânia.* IAEA, Vienna.

ICRP (International Commission on Radiological Protection) (1991). *1990 Recommendations of the International Commission on Radiological Protection,* ICRP Publication 60.

International Atomic Energy Agency and World Health Organization (1998). *Diagnosis and treatment of radiation injuries,* Safety Report series no 2. IAEA, Vienna.

International Atomic Energy Agency and World Health Organization (1998). *Planning the medical response to radiological accidents,* Safety Report series no 4. IAEA, Vienna.

MacVittie TJ, Weiss JF, Browne D, eds (1996). *Advances in the treatment of radiation injuries,* Advances in the Biosciences vol. 94. Pergamon, Oxford.

Mettler FA, Upton AC (1995). *Medical effects of ionizing radiation,* 2nd edn. WB Saunders, Philadelphia.

NRPB (National Radiological Protection Board) (1999). Board atatement: advice on the 1998 ICNIRP guidelines for limiting exposure to time-varying electric, magnetic and electromagnetic fields (up to 300 Ghz). *Documents of the National Radiological Protection Board* **10**, no 2.

WHO (World Health Organization) (1996). *Health consequences of the Chernobyl accident,* WHO Scientific Report. WHO, Geneva.

8.5.10 Noise

R. McCaig and T. C. Aw

Introduction

Noise is one of the most prevalent hazards in the workplace, particularly where there is a large manufacturing sector. In developed countries exposure to noise remains a significant occupational health problem with well-established sources of exposure in engineering, printing, textiles, and other production processes being supplemented by those in entertainment and broadcasting, and, more recently, by the growth of telephone customer service centres, where workers are potentially exposed to noise from head sets. Although it has been known for over a century that excessive exposure to noise results in hearing loss, it is only within the last 20 to 30 years that comprehensive hearing conservation programmes have been adopted in industry. Noise-induced hearing loss, which is entirely preventable, remains a common occupational injury.

The vibration of objects in air propagates acoustic energy which impinges on the tympanic membrane. The subjective effect of this energy may be pleasant, as in speech or music, yet it retains the potential to be harmful at sufficient intensities. The term 'noise' generally refers to loud or harsh sound of any kind. The ear is sensitive to a very wide range of pressure change and, to accommodate this, a logarithmic scale is required. A reference pressure of 0.000 02 pascal (Pa), the threshold of hearing, is used and a rating in decibels is obtained from the formula:

$$\text{sound pressure} = 20 \log_{10} \frac{\text{measured pressure}}{\text{reference pressure}} \text{ decibel (dB)}.$$

Thus a sound pressure of 0.2 Pa is equivalent to 80 dB, and one of 2.0 Pa to 100 dB.

A sound pressure level of 60 dB may be found in an office environment and levels between 90 dB and 100 dB in factories. Simple instruments are available to measure sound levels. However, the full characterization of a noise source requires more complex analysis, including the frequency spectrum. Most noise sources operate continuously but some produce intermittent peaks of exposure (impulse noise) arising from sources such as drop forging or the detonation of explosives. Separate criteria for the risk of damage apply to these two types of exposure.

In a normal young adult the ear is sensitive to a range of frequencies from about 20 Hz up to 20 kHz . The ear and brain together are not equally sensitive to all frequencies of sound, being markedly less sensitive at frequencies below 500 Hz and above 4 kHz. The more sensitive frequencies which lie in between 500 Hz and 4 kHz are those required for the perception of speech. Sound level meters contain filtering circuits which allow them to mimic the response of the human ear to sound. Different weightings are available, related to the subjective loudness of sounds. The one most commonly used is the A scale, reported as dB(A).

The effects of noise

Exposure to noise results in both physiological and pathological changes. An early response to acute noise exposure is an increase in blood pressure. More prolonged exposure to a sufficient intensity of noise causes a temporary shift in the threshold of hearing (temporary threshold shift). This may be experienced as a transient dullness of hearing and can be measured objectively. If exposure to noise is prolonged over months and years, a permanent threshold shift can result. Along with a reduction in the sensitivity of hearing, the person also experiences difficulty in differentiating similar sounds, particularly those of the consonants which are heard over a frequency range of 700 Hz to 4 kHz. With severe hearing loss there may be loudness recruitment; when sound intensity is increased beyond the now elevated threshold of hearing, a rapid and uncomfortable increase is experienced in the sound perceived. Noise-induced hearing loss may also be accompanied by tinnitus.

Excessive noise exposure causes damage to the outer hair cells of the cochlea, with breakage and disruption of the pattern of cilia on these cells which operate as local electromechanical amplifiers within the cochlea. When stimulated by oscillations of the basilar membrane at the appropriate frequency these cells contract and, by means of the cilia, pull down the overlying tectorial membrane. In doing so the inner end of the tectorial membrane is brought more closely into contact with the cilia of the inner hair cells, increasing their stimulation and that of the nerve fibres leaving the cells. Thus the outer hair cells assist frequency selectivity and amplification within the cochlea. Noise damage physically disrupts this amplification mechanism.

The 'non-auditory' effects attributed to noise include changes in both performance and health. Exposure to unwanted background noise, in particular speech, can disturb the performance of mental tasks. However, it has not been clearly established that environmental noise, for example around airports, results in an increase in psychiatric morbidity within the surrounding community. There is better evidence that environmental noise from road traffic is associated with an increase in cardiovascular morbidity but such an association has not been established in occupational settings.

Hearing loss

Permanent hearing loss is first detected as a reduction in hearing thresholds at the higher frequencies on the audiogram. Typically, this begins at 4 kHz and, with time, affects the adjacent frequencies creating a 'notch' pattern in the audiogram, described as the 4 kHz dip (Fig. 1). This sensitivity arises from the structure and configuration of the outer ear and the cochlea. With continuing exposure this hearing loss will extend to the lower frequencies and the thresholds will worsen (Fig. 2). Much of the damage is incurred during the initial years of exposure. Younger people may not be aware of hearing loss. It is in early middle age when the difference in hearing thresholds between those exposed to noise and the non-exposed becomes more

Fig. 1 Hearing loss after continuing noise exposure. Initially the lower frequencies are largely unaffected and there is recovery in the higher frequencies, appearing as a characteristic notching of the audiogram.

obvious. Thereafter this difference is reduced, as presbyacusis (the reduction in hearing threshold with age) affects both groups.

The management of workers regularly exposed to noise should centre on the reduction of noise at source. A programme of screening audiometry should be introduced where daily personal exposure to noise (a time-weighted measure) is of the order of 85 to 90 dB(A), and in conformity with relevant national legislation and guidance. The technical requirements for industrial hearing conservation audiometry are specified in ISO 6189. Measures are normally taken to avoid temporary threshold shifts at the time of testing, with examinations repeated every 2 to 3 years.

Where abnormalities are detected, it is important to establish the history of occupational and leisure noise exposure, the use of hearing protection, exposure to ototoxic drugs and chemicals, and relevant past diseases and injuries, and tinnitus. Otoscopic examination, bone conduction audiometry, tympanometry to determine middle ear function, and evoked response audiometry may have a role in clinical assessment. Referral for a specialist opinion is relevant where pathology other than noise-induced hearing loss is suspected (such as the rare acoustic neuroma) and where it is thought that a hearing aid or tinnitus masker may be of help to the individual. In some countries noise-induced hearing loss results in the payment of compensation to workers and, where appropriate, individuals should be advised of their eligibility. Redress may also be available through the civil courts.

Hearing conservation

All workers exposed to noise should be included in a hearing conservation programme. This will include measures to control noise at source, the marking of remaining noisy areas, the use of hearing protectors, and the training of workers. In many countries this is required by national legislation. Where this is not the case, published damage risk criteria, for example ISO 1999, can be used to determine risk and the need for intervention. Control at source can be achieved, for example, by redesigning parts and machinery or by providing soundproof enclosures. This is always preferable to reliance on the use of hearing protectors, which must be fitted correctly and used continuously during the period of exposure to noise. This can be difficult to achieve in practice, particularly in the absence of good supervision. Hearing loss found on the audiogram can, however, be persuasive evidence to the worker of the need for improved hearing protection. Health professionals have a role in education in support of hearing conservation.

Further reading

Axelson A *et al.* (1996) *Scientific basis of noise-induced hearing loss.* Thieme, New York.

Fig. 2 With continuing noise exposure the extent of loss increases and extends into the lower frequencies.

International Organization for Standardization (1983). *Acoustics—pure tone air conduction threshold audiometry for hearing conservation purposes*, ISO 6189. International Organization for Standardization, Geneva.

International Organization for Standardization (1990). *Acoustics— determination of occupational noise exposure and estimation of noise-induced hearing impairment*, ISO 1999. International Organization for Standardization, Geneva.

8.5.11 Vibration

Tar-Ching Aw and R. McCaig

Definition

Vibration is 'the mechanical oscillation of a surface around its reference point'. Workplace exposure to vibration results in local effects, mainly on the hands when the vibration is transmitted to the upper limbs, and as general systemic effects (mainly low back pain) when vibration is transmitted to the whole body. The clinical syndrome in the former has been termed 'vibration white finger' or 'hand–arm vibration syndrome'.

Exposure

Occupational exposure to whole-body vibration occurs in drivers of tractors, forklift trucks, mobile cranes, buses, lorries, and in helicopter pilots. The nature of the surface over which the vehicle is driven may be as important as the characteristics of the vehicle. Hand–arm vibration exposure occurs in factory workers involved in fettling, chipping, grinding, riveting, swaging, and using handheld pneumatic hammers, drills, chisels, and polishing and rotary tools. It also affects forestry, agricultural, and woodworkers using chain saws, miners drilling rock surfaces, and construction and road workers using drills and compactors. It has been estimated that around 3 per cent of the working population are occupationally exposed to sources of vibration.

Clinical effects

Whole-body vibration

Exposure to whole-body vibration causes physiological changes to the cardiovascular, respiratory, and musculoskeletal system. Clinical effects attributed to whole-body vibration include headache, motion sickness, sleep and visual disturbances, and urinary and abdominal complaints. The only effect with reasonable evidence of association with whole-body vibration is low back pain. In drivers, low back pain may occur as a result of vibration, poor posture within the vehicle cab, and/or other work duties such as loading and lifting.

Hand–arm transmitted vibration

This causes secondary Raynaud's phenomenon which manifests as frequent prominent episodic pallor of the digits, usually on exposure to cold. Patients frequently describe digital pallor in the morning, or following an outdoor activity such as fishing or gardening, especially in cold weather. The vascular changes may be accompanied by neurological and musculoskeletal effects which contribute to the disability experienced. Vascular and sensorineural effects may appear and progress independently. The latent period between initial exposure and development of symptoms is usually 5 to 10 years, although periods as short as 6 months or as long as 20 years have been noted depending on the intensity and duration of exposure. The sequence of colour change in the affected digits include pallor, a bluish hue due to cyanosis, and redness with spontaneous reversal of the vascular spasm.

Neurological effects include paraesthesia, reduced temperature perception, loss of manual dexterity, and pain. Severe tingling and discomfort often follow rapid warming of the hands. Loss of proprioception causing the inability to distinguish and hold small objects such as coins or to button up clothes contributes to physical and social disability. Musculoskeletal effects are not as well established, but muscle weakness, exostoses and cysts in the carpal bones, carpal tunnel syndrome, osteoarthritis, and Dupuytren's contracture have been associated with exposure to vibration.

Diagnosis

For a diagnosis of hand–arm vibration syndrome, the following criteria should be met:

(a) there must be evidence of sufficient exposure to vibration;

(b) episodic pallor of the digits and/or sensorineural effects should be confirmed;

(c) other causes of Raynaud's phenomenon or sensory changes must be considered.

The presence of associated musculoskeletal features would add support to the diagnosis. Physical examination may show callosities on the hands, loss of sensation in the affected digits, and muscle weakness, although there may be no obvious abnormalities, especially in the early stages of the disease.

Various clinical and special tests have been used in the evaluation of patients with hand–arm vibration syndrome. These include digital blood pressure measurements, vibrotactile thresholds, sensory aesthesiometry, and cold provocation tests. The clinical and occupational history is of greater importance than the results of any of the various tests in the diagnosis of hand–arm vibration syndrome.

The differential diagnosis should include other causes for Raynaud's phenomenon (constitutional or secondary to rheumatoid arthritis, systemic lupus erythematosus, scleroderma, and other autoimmune disorders, cryoglobulinaemia, frostbite, and the thoracic outlet syndrome). Use of ergot, clonidine, and β-blockers, occupational exposure to vinyl chloride monomer, and heavy cigarette smoking may be contributory factors.

Management, treatment, and prevention

The severity of hand–arm vibration syndrome can be staged using the Stockholm Workshop Scale (Table 1). The grade of the disorder is indicated by the stage and the number of affected fingers on each hand; for example, '2L(2)/1R(3)' refers to two digits at stage 2 in the left hand; and three digits at stage 1 in the right hand.

Engineering controls can minimize the transmission of vibration from machinery to the body or hands. The patient may be able to continue in their job following such action. Where the condition is severe and the source of vibration cannot be eliminated, redeployment should be considered. In early cases redeployment may arrest or reverse the progression of symptoms. In severe cases the disease can progress regardless of removal from further exposure to vibration.

Advice to the patient includes avoidance or reduction of further exposure to vibration, use of appropriate gloves, keeping the body and hands warm, especially in cold weather, and cessation of cigarette smoking. Vasodilatory drugs such as tolazoline, inositol, and cyclandelate, and calcium antagonists such as verapamil and nifedipine, angiotensin-converting enzyme inhibitors, prostaglandins, and stanazolol have been tried with varying success.

A diagnosis of Raynaud's phenomenon should always include detailed inquiry into occupational exposure to vibration. The diagnosis of a case of

Table 1 Stockholm Workshop Scale: classification of the hand–arm vibration syndrome

Stage	Grade	Description
Vascular component		
0		No attacks
1	Mild	Occasional attacks affecting only the tips of one or more fingers
2	Moderate	Occasional attacks affecting distal and middle (rarely also proximal) phalanges of one or more fingers
3	Severe	Frequent attacks affecting all phalanges of most fingers
4	Very severe	As in stage 3, with trophic changes in the finger tips
Sensorineural component		
0_{SN}		Vibration-exposed but no symptoms
1_{SN}		Intermittent numbness with or without tingling
2_{SN}		Intermittent or persistent numbness, reduced sensory perception
3_{SN}		Intermittent or persistent numbness, reduced sensory tactile discrimination and/or manipulative dexterity

hand–arm vibration syndrome should be viewed as a sentinel event warranting further investigation of the workplace to assess whether improvements in work practices can be implemented to prevent other cases from occurring.

Further reading

Griffin MJ (1997). Measurement, evaluation, and assessment of occupational exposures to hand-transmitted vibration. *Occupational and Environmental Medicine* **54**, 73–89.

Pelmear PL, Wasserman DE (1998). *Hand–arm vibration: a comprehensive guide for occupational health professionals*, 2nd edn. OEM Press, Beverly Farms, MA .

8.5.12 Disasters: earthquakes, volcanic eruptions, hurricanes, and floods

Peter J. Baxter

Deaths from natural disasters present a rising global trend. In the last half of the twentieth century, about 250 great natural disasters hit the planet, killing at least 1.4 million people and disrupting the lives of many millions more. At least 130 million people are affected each year by disasters and this number is rapidly increasing. Between 500 and 700 natural catastrophes are recorded every year and in the late 80s and 90s individual events entailed extremely large economic losses. Most human and economic losses have been from earthquakes, windstorms, and floods (Fig. 1). Global changes responsible for the worsening impact of disasters include the continuing, usually unplanned, expansion of populations into more and more exposed areas and the environmental degradation that is increasing the vulnerability of settlements, especially in heavily urbanized areas. This reckless development is going on throughout the world, even in areas of well-known risk.

Climate forecasts of an increase in the world's average temperature of 1.0 to 3.5°C and warming of the oceans could increase the potential for more intense hurricanes over wider areas and, in temperate regions, more severe wind storms and fluctuations in rainfall (floods and drought) and rising sea levels, increasing the frequency of severe coastal floods.

Predisaster measures

Disaster is the result of a vast ecological breakdown in the relation between humans and their environment, a serious and sudden (or slow, as in drought) event on such a scale that the stricken community needs extraordinary efforts to cope with it, often with outside help or international aid. Accurately forecasting the timing and size of natural disasters is rarely possible. This places major constraints on preventing loss of life by timely evacuation of people from the areas at risk. Disasters are quite different from major incidents in that normal lifelines and infrastructure usually break down. But despite their chaotic elements, disasters are amenable to scientific study and communities can develop planning and preparedness measures to reduce their impacts. Health workers have a key role in hazard management in risk assessment, predisaster planning and preparedness, as well as the emergency response.

Earthquakes

Many parts of the world are known to be at risk from devastating earthquakes, but it remains impossible to predict where and when a quake will strike. Most deaths and injuries are caused by collapsing buildings. Secondary causes such as fires can be important. Timber, masonry, reinforced concrete, and other types of buildings inflict injuries in different ways and to different degrees of severity when they collapse. In masonry buildings, an important cause of death is often suffocation from the weight and dust from the wall or roof material which buries the victims. The impacts of falling masonry cause crush injuries to the head and chest, external or internal haemorrhage, and chest compression (traumatic asphyxia). Little is know about the survival time of people trapped in collapsed buildings, but most victims die immediately or within 24 h, depending upon such factors as the severity of aftershocks, fire outbreaks, and rainfall. Rapid extrication of survivors and application of first aid by the uninjured immediately after the event could save up to 25 to 50 per cent of injured victims. The greatest demand for emergency medical services is within the first 24 h and the need for emergency treatment fades after 3 to 5 days. Causes of delayed death include dehydration, hypothermia, crush syndrome, and postoperative sepsis. Most of those requiring medical assistance suffer minor injuries such as lacerations and contusions.

A great earthquake struck Kobe City in Japan on 17 January 1995. It exposed serious flaws in the Japanese emergency services, as well as showing the need for comprehensive planning for medical care and welfare in earthquake-prone countries. The scale of disaster was beyond all expectations. The immediate victims included 5520 dead (10 per cent killed in fires) and 41 527 wounded. Four days later, 342 000 people (10 per cent of the total population of the region) were staying in shelters at a time of

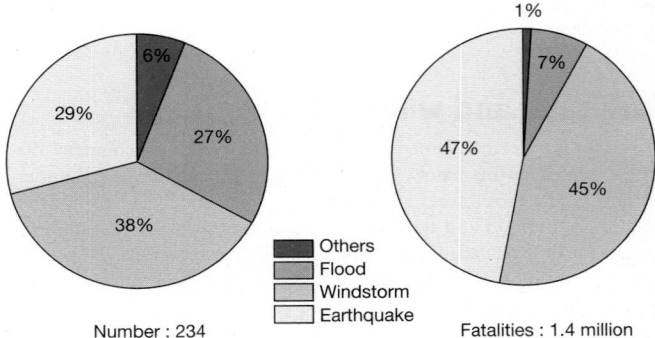

Fig. 1 Great natural catastrophes 1950 to 1999

subzero temperatures. The plight of the elderly was not appreciated, as many of their carers were either dead or surviving as victims themselves. About 80 per cent of hospitals in the area were damaged, 7 per cent completely destroyed. Undamaged hospitals lacked the structural means to adapt rapidly to deal with overwhelming numbers of casualties requiring emergency care; the breakdown of supplies and water, electricity, and gas and failure of communications badly hampered other hospitals that were still functioning. The transfer of pharmaceuticals and medical equipment took longer than expected. The economic losses exceeded 100 billion US dollars, making it the costliest natural disaster in the world to date.

Volcanic eruptions

About 500 to 600 volcanoes around the world are known to be capable of eruptive activity and several major eruptions occur every year. The vast majority of volcanoes are explosive and unpredictable in behaviour, providing little opportunity for people to escape unless full evacuation measures are taken as soon as premonitory signs develop. This is in contrast to the less common lava flow eruptions, where people can normally escape by the time the lava flow heads towards them. Most deaths and injuries in explosive eruptions (such as engulfed ancient Pompeii) are caused by pyroclastic flows and surges, which are clouds of hot ash and gas that can travel at hurricane speeds. Survival is uncommon but victims will have extensive and severe skin burns, as well as inhalation injuries. The worst volcanic disaster in the twentieth century was at St Pierre, Martinique, in 1902, when 28 000 people were killed in a laterally directed pyroclastic surge. One of the most dangerous volcanoes in the world is Vesuvius, Italy, where uncontrolled building has resulted in over one million people living in an area which could be devastated by pyroclastic flows in a new eruption. Another major cause of death is lahars or wet flows of debris, either ash that has built up on the slopes of the volcano or unstable masses that are mobilized during the eruption or by rain, or rarely by release of water from a crater lake. The eruption of Ruiz del Nevada volcano in Colombia in 1984 triggered a lahar (mud flow) by rapid melting of the glacier at the summit, the melt waters rushing down valleys and mixing with debris as they went. Although adequate warning could have been given to the people below, lack of preparedness meant that the lahar engulfed towns including Armero, killing around 24 000 people. In one of the largest eruptions of the century, at Mount Pinatubo in the Philippines in 1991, 50 000 people were successfully evacuated from the threat of pyroclastic flows, but over 300 people died while sheltering in their homes from the collapse of roofs due to the accumulated weight of rain and ash.

The eruption of the Soufriere Hills volcano on the tiny Caribbean island of Montserrat began in July 1995 and gradually escalated, forcing the evacuation of thousands of people from their homes because of the threat of pyroclastic flows. By 1997, these flows had devastated the southern part of the island, evicting three-quarters of the population of 12 000 people. Air pollution from volcanic gases and ash has been a major consideration because of the close proximity of the population to the volcano and the frequent eruption of fine, respirable ash containing hazardous amounts of the crystalline silica mineral, cristobalite, which can cause silicosis.

Hurricane and windstorm

Hurricanes are one of a broad class of extreme weather phenomena that include winter storms (snow, sleet, freezing rain, and freezes), thunderstorms (e.g. tornadoes, heavy rains, lightning, wind, and hail), extreme precipitation (e.g. flood and flash floods), and windstorms. Hurricanes (or typhoons as they are called in the Western Pacific) are tropical cyclones that form over warm oceans with ocean surface temperatures over 26°C. Once over land they soon run out of energy and rapidly abate, but can still cause flooding from heavy rain. Very high wind speeds, up to 250 km/h, are restricted to a relatively narrow track, usually no more than 150 km wide, within which localized gusts may even achieve tornado speeds and be

extremely destructive. However, most deaths and injuries are not from the effect of wind on people (who normally remain inside for protection) or from building damage (building collapse or being struck by flying debris). Instead, deaths and injuries are very commonly the result of flooding from the sea surge as the hurricane strikes land, concurrent heavy rainfall (typically up to 60 cm, over a larger area and extending further inland than wind speed) and resulting landslides. Hurricanes lift the sea, forming a sea surge that typically rises 3 to 4 m above existing tides, with the wind generating waves on top of these.

Hurricane Andrew, which struck Florida in August 1992, was the most destructive natural disaster in the history of the United States and the third most intense storm to strike the United States in the twentieth century. Andrew developed sustained wind speeds above 250 km/h, even greater in localized tornado-like gusts. Mitigation measures (evacuation of three-quarters of a million people) held the death toll at 43. The most destructive effects of storm surge are on beaches and offshore islands, but in low-lying regions these can extend as far as 40 km inland. A dome of water lifted by the hurricane may be up to 100 km wide on open coasts. Such a surge drowned at least 200 000 people in Bangladesh in 1970. During a 2-week period in October/November 1998, Hurricane Mitch battered Central America. It unexpectedly slowed to a tropical storm and years of rainfall fell on Central America within a few hours. The result was about 13 000 slope failures and landslides, adding to the destruction of extensive flooding. Over 20 000 people were killed and over two million people left homeless.

Over 90 per cent of fatalities in hurricanes are drownings associated with storm surges or floods. Other causes of death include burial beneath houses collapsed by wind, penetrating trauma from broken glass or wood, blunt trauma from floating objects or debris, or entrapment in mudslides. The number of severe trauma patients among survivors is usually small; the greatest need in the postimpact phase is the provision of adequate shelter, water, food, and clothing, and sanitation. Most suffer from lacerations caused by flying glass or other debris, or minor trauma such as closed fractures and puncture wounds. After Hurricane Mitch the incidence of cholera and other water-borne diseases (leptospirosis, dengue, and malaria) increased, particularly in the urban areas.

Floods

In addition to the major losses of life that can be caused by hurricanes and their associated sea surges, floods mostly result from moderate to large events (rainfall, snow melt, high tides) occurring within the expected range of stream flow or tidal conditions. In Britain, as in many countries with low-lying coastal land, the hazard of coastal flooding from sea surges and high tides dominates over river flooding, although the latter is more frequent. Floods have been particularly devastating in China, with such notable historic disasters as the flooding of the Hung Ho in 1887 and 1931 claiming 900 000 and 3.7 million lives respectively. Over 40 million people are estimated to be affected yearly by flood. Flood warning and forecasting, combined with effective land management, community preparedness, and evacuation planning, are as essential as engineered river and coastal defences.

The primary cause of death from floods is drowning, but trauma from impacts with floating debris and hypothermia due to cold exposure is also important. The portion of survivors requiring emergency medical care is small, most injuries being minor, such as lacerations. This absence of victims with severe or multiple trauma is likely to reflect the long delay in reaching survivors, so they die from their injuries or from exposure before search and rescue teams can arrive. Increased morbidity and mortality in survivors who experience flooding was reported in the year after the East Coast Flood in 1953 and a river flood in Bristol in 1968; an increase in suicides and mental health problems were found in the aftermath of severe flooding caused by heavy rains in central Europe in July 1997.

Postdisaster relief

Myths surrounding postdisaster relief include:

- any kind of international assistance is needed;
- the affected population is too shocked and helpless to take responsibility for their own survival;
- natural disasters trigger secondary disasters through outbreaks of communicable diseases;
- life gets back to normal after a few weeks.

Most deaths in sudden-onset disasters happen long before outside aid arrives. However, relief teams have an important role in restoring roads and bridges, bringing in potable water, ensuring solid waste management, food protection, vector control, and sanitation. Attendances at medical facilities may return to normal within a few days of a disaster, and restoration of primary care then becomes a top priority rather than emergency treatment.

Epidemiology has an important role in postdisaster assessment and health surveillance, particularly where relocation of large populations has occurred, as well as investigating the causes of mortality and morbidity in disasters, including mental ill health and long-term health sequelae.

Further reading

Coburn A, Spence R (1992). *Earthquake protection*. Wiley, Chichester.

Lumley JSP, Ryan JM, Baxter PJ, eds (1996). *Handbook of the medical care of catastrophes*. Royal Society of Medicine, London.

Noji EK, ed. (1997). *The public health consequences of disasters*. Oxford University Press, New York.

Pielke RA Jr, Pielke RA Sr (1997). *Hurricanes: their nature and impacts on society*. Wiley, Chichester.

Smith K, Ward R (1998). *Floods: physical processes and human impacts*. Wiley, Chichester.

9

Principles of clinical pharmacology and drug therapy

9 Principles of clinical pharmacology and drug therapy

Andrew Herxheimer*

Clinical pharmacology is the application of scientific principles to understanding the ways in which drugs behave and work in humans. Such understanding underlies rational drug therapy. Every decision to prescribe or use a drug comprises a series of separate decisions that are usually taken at great speed and often without enough thought. The main questions that must be decided are:

1. Does this patient's problem require a drug? What is likely to happen if no drug is used?

2. If a drug is needed, what type of drug action would be most appropriate?

3. Which class of drug will best provide the desired action?

4. Which particular drug in that class should be chosen, and in what pharmaceutical form?

5. What dose is to be used, how often, and at what times of the day or in what circumstances?

6. For how long is the drug to be used, initially and in the long term?

7. Will the cost of the drug matter to the patient?

8. How will the drug treatment fit into the overall treatment plan?

9. Will it be necessary to review the treatment? If so, when, how, and by whom?

10. What will the patient need to understand about treatment? Who will communicate this, and how?

11. What other help may the patient need to use the treatment optimally?

In a consultation all these questions cannot be considered from scratch. The physician must therefore answer as many of them beforehand as possible. This can be done with the help of appropriate therapeutic guidelines and a good formulary (which is really a specialized collection of guidelines concerning mainly one aspect of treatment, the choice of drug). Guidelines exist to provide thoroughly prepared decision paths for the common problems. The time and effort saved by using them enables physicians to focus on those aspects of an individual patient and problem that require individual adaptation of or departure from the relevant guideline. A guideline is like the trunk and large branches of an easily climbed tree—a decision tree. Once in the crown one is free to decide which small branch or leaf is the best. Many of the questions listed can only be answered satisfactorily after discussion between patient and doctor. For example, the patient's attitude to and feelings about taking medicines often determines whether or not to use a drug; the formulation chosen is influenced by the patient's needs or preference, for example difficulty in swallowing tablets or aversion to suppositories; the dosage regimen must be practicable for the patient. The best treatment decisions build on the patient's as well as the clinician's knowledge and experience. The clinician therefore has to find out about patients' experience of treatments—this should always be part of taking the history, but it is often forgotten.

The treatment history gives a necessary background for prescribing decisions because it can indicate how effective or ineffective previous treatment has been, and whether previous treatment has caused problems that should be avoided in the future. It can warn of possible interactions. It will show what the patient knows and believes about drugs and other treatments, as well as what he or she does not know about his/her treatment, and would like to know. Areas to ask about include:

- medicines currently being used, including dosage

- previous hospital treatment

- previous treatment from the family doctor

- 'alternative' treatments such as herbal or homeopathic medicines, acupuncture

- self-prescribed medicines

- past bad experiences with medicines, fears or worries about medicines.

Benefit and harm in prescribing

A doctor who prescribes a drug does so expecting that it will help the patient, and believing that any disbenefits, which may range from minor inconvenience or discomfort to a chance of serious harm, are acceptable. Such judgements are often referred to as assessments of the 'benefit/risk ratio', but this is a meaningless and confusing term. Risk means 'probability of harm', whereas benefit usually means 'amount of benefit'. Both benefit and harm have two dimensions, magnitude and probability, which must be clearly separated. Unfortunately we have no word for 'probability of benefit'.

The data that we have on benefits differ greatly from those used to estimate harm. Knowledge of the benefits to be obtained from a drug is almost always greater than knowledge of the harm that it may do. This is because the initial clinical research on a drug is done explicitly to assess the hoped-for benefits, which must occur in a high proportion of patients if the drug is to be useful, whereas harmful effects, especially unexpected ones, cannot be looked for in clinical trials—which are anyway too small to detect uncommon ones. Serious harm tends to affect relatively few patients and often is not suspected or discovered until a drug has been widely used for at least several years. As a result much less is known about the adverse effects of new drugs than about their benefits, and knowledge about harm accrues remarkably slowly in the first few years of a drug's life. If the drug is widely used, more of the iceberg gradually becomes visible. Because of the unknown risks of new drugs, it is better to choose older established drugs unless there is a clear reason for preferring a particular new drug.

Another dimension that must be considered is time: benefits are typically seen quickly, many adverse effects may not occur for years. That makes

* Much has been taken from Aronson and White's excellent text in the third edition of the *Oxford Textbook of Medicine*.

it even harder to weigh benefits against harm. Often they just cannot be compared. Two examples illustrate the problem.

First, in the case of pneumococcal pneumonia treated with penicillin, a cure is known to be likely and adverse effects are usually few and minor. However, if the patient is known to be allergic to penicillin, the risk of a serious adverse effect becomes too great and the benefit no longer outweighs the risk; in such a case another antibiotic would be used. In this example the balance of benefit and harm is easily determined.

In contrast, consider the treatment with warfarin of a patient with atrial fibrillation and a history of bleeding peptic ulcer. Which outweighs the other: the potential benefit of preventing an embolic stroke by using the anticoagulant, or the risk of causing serious gastrointestinal bleeding? These two are not readily comparable, but a decision has to be made. It may be decided to use warfarin and hope to prevent serious bleeding with a proton pump inhibitor such as omeprazole, arguing that the degree of morbidity from an embolic stroke is likely to be more serious than that from an acute gastrointestinal bleed, with an approximately equal risk of mortality. But the patient may strongly dislike having to attend for regular monitoring of the anticoagulant effect (international normalized ratio, INR). There is no right answer.

The balance of benefit and harm from a particular treatment depends on four major factors:

(1) the seriousness of the illness;
(2) the effectiveness of the treatment;
(3) the seriousness of possible adverse effects;
(4) the risk of possible adverse effects.

If a disease is life threatening, if the drug to be used is highly effective and the only one available, and if the risk of serious adverse effects is negligible, the balance clearly favours the treatment. At the other end of the spectrum, if the disease is trivial, if the treatment is not very effective and more effective and safer alternatives exist, and if the risk of serious adverse effects is high, the likely harm outweighs the benefit. Table 1 illustrates this spectrum. Most cases lie somewhere between these two extremes.

The example of phenylbutazone, a highly effective non-steroidal anti-inflammatory drug, illustrates the principles involved. Use of the drug has a risk of marrow aplasia of between 1 in 30 000 and 1 in 100 000. While no other equally effective drugs existed, the benefit from phenylbutazone was considered great enough to outweigh the relatively high risk of marrow aplasia. However, once other equally effective and safer drugs became available, the risk of its adverse effects was seen to outweigh whatever benefit it gave, and its use was restricted.

Note that in making this decision to restrict the use of phenylbutazone the benefit was considered not in absolute terms but in relation to the severity of the disease and the benefit obtainable from other drugs. While phenylbutazone was more potent therapeutically than other available drugs it was considered highly beneficial, but when equally effective drugs arrived its net benefit was perceived to be less, although the therapeutic effect of the drug itself had not changed during that time. Phenylbutazone is still used today in some cases of severe ankylosing spondylitis that have responded poorly to other anti-inflammatory drugs. In those cases doctors and patients seem to believe that the benefit outweighs the risk of marrow aplasia.

Efficacy, effectiveness, efficiency of drugs

These terms need to be distinguished. Efficacy refers to any arbitrarily chosen effect, which may or may not be clinically relevant. It is best avoided in clinical contexts. Effectiveness means clinical effectiveness, and is defined as the likelihood and extent of the desired effects on the patient.

Efficiency is the ratio of effectiveness to cost: it is clearly more efficient to use the cheaper of two equally effective, equally safe, and equally reliable drugs.

The therapeutic index of a drug

The therapeutic index of a drug is the ratio of the dose at which adverse effects become important to that at which a therapeutic benefit is expected. This index does not have a numerical value, as precise estimates of these doses are not available and vary from person to person. Instead, drugs are divided into two categories, those with high and low therapeutic indices. For example, in the absence of hypersensitivity, penicillins have a high therapeutic index; very large doses can be given without fear of adverse effects. In contrast, digoxin has a low therapeutic index; it takes very little more to cause toxicity than to produce therapeutic benefit. Drugs with a low therapeutic index include the aminoglycoside antibiotics, anticoagulants, anticonvulsants, antihypertensives, some antiparasitic and antiviral drugs, cardiac glycosides, cytotoxic and immunosuppressant drugs, oral contraceptives, sympathomimetics, and drugs that act on the brain.

The benefit for a particular drug is more likely to outweigh the risk of harm if the drug has a high therapeutic index. In choosing between two equally effective drugs, one would choose the one with the higher therapeutic index.

Formularies

Formularies are lists of medicines for prescribers and pharmacists, intended to guide the choice and facilitate the dispensing of medicines. Many give details of the formulation and doses of drugs. Each formulary is produced primarily for a particular group, usually the prescribers in one country or region or institution, or even one practice. Most formularies are restrictive, that is they make a more or less narrow choice of medicines from all those available that could be used. This is typical for the formulary of a hospital, or of a health maintenance organization. A hospital formulary lists only the preparations that are stocked in the hospital pharmacy; a health maintenance organization formulary only those that the organization will pay for. The British National Formulary, probably the best known and most widely used formulary of all, differs in this respect, for it includes all medicines available for prescription in Britain, whether they are good choices and recommended or not. However, in every section concise and critical 'notes to facilitate the selection of suitable treatment' precede the list. These notes help prescribers everywhere (not only in Britain) to think, and add greatly to the value of the book, especially since it is updated twice a year and accessible electronically (http://bnf.org).

The WHO 'Model list of essential drugs'

In many poor countries large sections of the population have no access to drugs or health care, and governments cannot afford to provide necessary drugs. To help them to use their limited funds in the best ways, the World Health Organization has since 1978 published a regularly updated 'Model list of essential drugs'. Essential drugs are defined as 'those that satisfy the health care needs of the majority of the population; they should therefore be available in adequate amounts and in the appropriate dosage forms'. The WHO list is called a model list because it cannot be used as it stands but must be adapted to the needs and priorities of individual countries. That is

Table 1 The factors that affect the benefit to risk ratio

Seriousness of the indication	Efficacy of drug	Adverse reactions severity	Risk of adverse reactions	Alternative treatment efficacy	Alternative treatment safety	Benefit/harm relationship
Threatens life	High	Trivial	Rare	Poor	Poor	Excellent
Trivial	Poor	Serious	Frequent	Good	Good	Not acceptable

Table 2 The four processes of clinical pharmacology and the questions with which they are associated in relation to drug therapy

Process	Question
Pharmaceutical	Is the drug getting into the patient from the appropriate formulation?
Pharmacokinetic	Is the drug getting to its site of action?
Pharmacodynamic	Is the drug producing the required pharmacological effect?
Therapeutic	Is the pharmacological effect being translated into an appropriate therapeutic effect?

not easy, and WHO offers governments help with it and related work. Many developing countries now have an essential drugs programme.

The principles of clinical pharmacology

Drug therapy can be considered under four headings—pharmaceutical, pharmacokinetic, pharmacodynamic, and therapeutic—the four major processes of clinical pharmacology, each of which is associated with a question about drug therapy (Table 2, Fig. 1).

The pharmaceutical process

The pharmaceutical process concerns the question 'Is the drug getting into the patient from the appropriate formulation?'

Usually there is no need to worry about the formulation of a drug, beyond deciding whether to use the oral or parenteral route. For example, oral frusemide (furosemide) or bumetanide are prescribed as tablets. But sometimes the decision is harder. For example, in Britain six different oral lithium formulations exist, differing in strength and absorption characteristics. Glyceryl trinitrate is formulated for use orally, sublingually, buccally, transdermally, and as a spray. To understand the differences it is necessary to understand the concept of systemic availability.

Systemic availability

Systemic availability (commonly called bioavailability) is the proportion of administered drug that reaches the systemic circulation and is available for distribution to the site of action. The term usually refers to formulations given orally, but it can also refer to other routes of administration, such as intramuscular or transdermal.

When a drug is given intravenously it all enters the systemic circulation (systemic availability = 100 per cent).

When a drug is given orally in solution all the drug is immediately available for absorption. How much of it enters the systemic circulation will depend on the extent of absorption and the metabolic effect of the liver as it passes through for the first time (the so-called first-pass effect).

When a drug is given orally as a tablet or capsule the amount that enters the systemic circulation also depends on the properties of the formulation, including how fast the tablet disintegrates and how fast the drug particles dissolve in the intestinal fluid—the 'pharmaceutical availability'.

Fig. 1 The four processesses of clinical pharmacology in relation to drug therapy.

Prescribers rely on the pharmacist and pharmaceutical chemist to provide formulations of high stability and predictable pharmaceutical availability. When different formulations of the same drug are available the doctor may have to decide which to prescribe. This may be particularly important for drugs with a low therapeutic index, for which differences in pharmaceutical availability will matter. For example, if a patient is taking a formulation of low pharmaceutical availability that is producing a good therapeutic effect, switching to one of high availability can cause adverse effects.

Special drug formulations

Most drugs are given orally; oral formulations include elixirs, ordinary (quick-release) tablets and capsules, and modified-release formulations. However, drugs may be given by other routes, including sublingually, buccally, rectally, transdermally, by inhalation, and by injection intravenously, subcutaneously, intramuscularly, or locally.

Modified-release formulations

'Modified-release' formulations are oral formulations with some special release mechanism. Most are intended to prolong the duration of action of a drug and to smooth its effects by gradual release during the dosage interval. Examples include formulations of theophylline, nifedipine, diltiazem, and lithium. Prescriptions of these drugs should specify the exact formulation, as formulations differ in systemic availability.

Sublingual, buccal, rectal formulations

Drugs that are absorbed through the oral or rectal mucosa enter veins and pass into the systemic circulation intact, avoiding first-pass metabolism in the liver. For example, sublingual glyceryl trinitrate is effective in doses about 10 times less than those required by mouth and the effect is rapid. Rectal administration achieves a direct effect on the large bowel (for example corticosteroids in ulcerative colitis).

Transdermal formulations

Some drugs are well absorbed through the skin, and their transdermal administration via 'patches' allows controlled release of small amounts over many hours. Examples are glyceryl trinitrate in the long-term treatment of angina pectoris, transdermal hyoscine for travel sickness, estradiol as hormone replacement therapy, and nicotine for stopping smoking.

Inhalations

Inhaled formulations come in several forms, with different intentions. Sodium cromoglicate is in a powder for inhalation, designed to act locally on the bronchioles in the management of asthma. Salbutamol aerosol, on the other hand, is designed to produce bronchodilatation by a metered dose ($100\ \mu g$) of droplets, small enough ($2–5\ \mu m$) to reach the bronchioles. About 10 per cent of any inhaled drug reaches the bronchial tree, the rest being lost in the air, absorbed from the oropharynx, or swallowed. Nebulizers provide continuous administration of aerosolized drugs for short periods.

Subcutaneous, intramuscular, and local injections

The rate of absorption of insulin from the site of subcutaneous injection is controlled by its physical state (for example crystalline or non-crystalline), its zinc or protein content, and the nature and pH of the buffer in which it is suspended. Thus, soluble insulin has a rapid onset and short duration of action (about 6 h), while ultralente insulin, which has large crystals and a high zinc content, begins to act at about 7 h and acts for about 36 h.

Drugs are sometimes absorbed erratically from intramuscular injection sites; for phenytoin and diazepam the intramuscular route should be avoided if possible. Absorption may be retarded by the use of thick oils, which slow down diffusion of the drug from the site of injection and retard intramuscular absorption—for example vasopressin tannate in oil used in diabetes insipidus, and fluphenazine decanoate in oil in schizophrenia.

Some local anaesthetic injections contain adrenaline, which by vasoconstriction prevents rapid removal of the drug from the injection site.

Combination formulations in oral therapy

Combination products are seductive, but should be used only when at least two criteria are met:

- the frequency of administration of the two drugs is the same;
- the fixed doses in the combination product are therapeutically and optimally effective in most cases (i.e. when it is not necessary to alter the dose of one drug independently of the other).

Acceptable combination products include:

- Aspirin plus codeine (cocodaprin) or paracetamol plus dihydrocodeine (codydramol), pairs of drugs that have different analgesic actions (which summate) and different adverse effects (which do not).
- Levodopa plus a peripherally-acting dopa decarboxylase inhibitor (benserazide or carbidopa); the peripheral action of the decarboxylase inhibitor blocks peripheral metabolism of levodopa, which is free to enter the brain, where it is converted to the pharmacologically active product dopamine, producing the therapeutic effect in Parkinson's disease.
- Combined oral contraceptives, which contain an oestrogen and a progestogen.
- Ferrous sulphate plus folic acid, used to prevent anaemia in pregnancy.
- Coamoxiclav (amoxicillin plus clavulanic acid); the β-lactamase inhibitor, clavulanic acid, prevents the breakdown of amoxicillin by bacterial penicillinase, so broadening its spectrum.

The patient's use of the medicine: compliance and concordance

Compliance is used as a technical term for the extent to which the patient follows a prescribed regimen. However, the word has unwelcome overtones, implying orders that the patient is expected to obey. The word 'concordance' has been introduced to supplant it, to make it clear that therapeutic decisions are best arrived at jointly by prescriber and patient agreeing on what to do. If both understand and accept the reasons for a particular choice, then the patient will be more committed to it than if a choice is imposed without explanation or discussion. This partly accounts for the wide variation in 'non-compliance', which in different studies has been found to be as low as 10 per cent and as high as 90 per cent. Compliance is affected not only by the behaviour of patient and doctor, but also by the nature of the treatment and the type of illness.

The nature of the treatment

Apart from the cost to the patient (which matters greatly in some countries), two main aspects of the treatment itself determine compliance, the complexity of the regimen and adverse effects. The complexity of the prescribed regimen involves two factors: the frequency of administration (the more often during the day patients have to take a drug the less likely they are to take it) and the number of drugs prescribed (the more drugs prescribed the less likely is overall compliance). It is difficult to take several medications at different dosages that involve different numbers of tablets at different times of the day.

If patients experience symptoms that they attribute to adverse drug effects (for example diarrhoea due to antibiotics or sedation due to anticonvulsants), then, unless they can be persuaded that the likely benefits of treatment outweigh the disadvantages, they will stop taking the medicine. Some patients, notably children and the elderly, have problems with certain formulations, for example sickly elixirs or large, dry, bitter tablets.

The type of illness

People who are severely mentally disturbed, for example patients with schizophrenia or manic-depressive psychosis, often take medicines unreliably.

Physical disability may cause difficulty even in patients who want to take their medicine. For example patients with rheumatoid arthritis who cannot reach the tablets or cannot remove the top of a child-proof container, cannot take them without help.

Sometimes a good response to treatment leads patients to stop. For example, patients with tuberculosis need long courses of several drugs to eradicate the infection; motivation may wane once the symptoms have resolved, risking reactivation and the emergence of resistant bacilli.

Some diseases may promote compliance. Patients with insulin-dependent diabetes easily become very ill quite quickly if they forget to take their insulin, and that is likely to make them comply, although they may not use it precisely as advised. Patients in whom a β-blocker or vasodilator has largely prevented anginal attacks will be conditioned to good compliance.

The patient's behaviour

People tend to forget to take medicines, or can't be bothered; they may feel no need for treatment (for example in asymptomatic hypertension); they may be unclear about the prescribing instructions; they may not want to feel dependent or be thought to be dependent on 'drugs'. There may be social or physical reasons why they cannot reach a pharmacist, financial difficulties, or everyday inconveniences in carrying and taking the medication. (See www.dipex.org/hypertension, for interviews in which patients talk about their tablets.)

The doctor's behaviour

The enthusiasm and confidence with which a treatment is prescribed, and the extent to which these attitudes are transmitted to the patient, may influence not only compliance but also the response to therapy. This is partly related to the placebo effect.

Methods of assessing compliance

It is important to assess compliance both in everyday practice and in clinical trials. The most obvious and usually the easiest approach is to ask the patient whether he or she has been taking the drugs, and whether there have been any problems. If the doctor is non-judgmental and indicates that difficulties are common, the patient is encouraged to be open.

Less directly one can ask to see the patient's tablets: this confirms that the prescription has been cashed. Counting the tablets left in the bottle is a guide to how many have been taken, but some may have been thrown away. Recording devices fitted in the caps of medication containers can record the frequency and exact timing of the opening of the container, and are useful in research.

When a patient is vague or untrustworthy, measurement of some compounds in the plasma or urine may give a good indication of compliance, but this does not allow for patients who take their treatment only on the day they visit the doctor. The compound measured may be the drug itself (for example phenytoin or lithium in the plasma, or salicylate in the urine) or a marker (for example riboflavin, which is easily detected in the urine).

Detecting the pharmacological effect of a drug can also give evidence of compliance; for example, the response of the heart rate for β-blockers, the prothrombin time for oral anticoagulants, and the reticulocyte count for haematinics. Failure to detect the pharmacological effect of a drug implies non-compliance or inadequate dosage. During long-term antibiotic therapy for urinary tract infection, antibacterial activity in the urine can be measured.

Obviously, if the desired therapeutic effect occurs the question of compliance is unimportant. However, a good therapeutic outcome may occur irrespective of the treatment used. It would be wrong to attribute a good outcome to the effect of a drug that the patient may not have taken; this is an important principle in clinical trials.

Methods of improving compliance

Compliance can be improved by supervised administration of the drug, by removing barriers to compliance, by simplifying the therapeutic regimen, and by educating the patient on the need to take the medicine, with reminders when possible.

Supervised administration Administration of a drug by the doctor or nurse ensures compliance. This is possible in hospital or when only occasional administration is required (for example intramuscular injections of vitamin B_{12}, long-acting depot injections of neuroleptics in the treatment of schizophrenia, and supervised twice-weekly antituberculosis therapy). Sometimes a single dose of a drug can be given at the time of consultation, rather than a short course of tablets (for example an intramuscular antibiotic in the treatment of gonorrhoea). In some cases, a relative or other carer can give the drug at home.

Removing barriers to compliance Compliance may be encouraged by prescribing pleasant-tasting elixirs rather than tablets for children and the elderly, and by using a drug or formulation that minimizes adverse effects.

Simplification of the therapeutic regimen The therapeutic regimen can be simplified by reducing both the number of drugs a patient has to take and the frequency of administration. This can sometimes be done with the help of modified-release or combination formulations.

Education and reminders Educating the patient about why treatment is necessary (for example, treating hypertension or diabetes reduces the risk of serious complications) is time consuming but undoubtedly improves compliance. In the treatment of certain infections (as in patients with AIDS or tuberculosis and in typhoid carriers) the importance to the community should also be explained.

Even when patients are well motivated, reminders to take the treatment may improve compliance as it is easy to forget to take medication. Many medicines for long-term use are dispensed in a 'calendar pack', for example oral contraceptives.

Patients can be helped by a clearly written list of their current drugs, explaining the names, and labelling medicine bottles clearly. Information leaflets may also help to educate and remind them about their treatment.

The pharmacokinetic process

Pharmacokinetics concerns the question 'Is the drug getting to its site of action?' It comprises absorption and systemic availability, distribution, metabolism, and excretion.

Absorption and systemic availability

After an oral dose the amount of drug that reaches the systemic circulation depends on its absorption and how far it escapes metabolism in the gut, the liver, and the lungs. This is called its systemic availability (or bioavailability).

Systemic availability is defined in terms of the amount of administered drug that reaches the systemic circulation intact and the rate at which that happens. The rate of availability depends on pharmaceutical factors (see above) and gastrointestinal absorption, presystemic metabolism being relatively unimportant. But the extent of availability depends on both the extent of absorption and the extent of presystemic metabolism.

Figure 2 illustrates what is meant by the rate and extent of systemic availability. It shows three curves representing the theoretical plasma concentrations resulting over time after the same oral dose of three different formulations of the same drug. Each curve has three important attributes: the peak concentration (C_{max}), the time taken to reach the peak (t_{max}), and the total area under the curve (**AUC**). C_{max} and t_{max} are measures of the rate of availability, and the total AUC is a measure of its extent. In the three hypothetical cases the rates of availability clearly differ. For formulation I the systemic availability is rapid, perhaps too rapid, leading to potentially toxic plasma concentrations. Formulation II is less quickly available and plasma concentrations never reach the potentially toxic range. Formulation III is slowly available and plasma concentrations after a single dose are always subtherapeutic. However, in contrast to the rate of availability, the extent of availability of these three formulations, as assessed by the AUC, is the same in each case.

For drugs whose action may depend on the threshold plasma concentration achieved after a single dose (for example analgesics), such differences

Fig. 2 The theoretical plasma concentrations resulting over time after the oral administration of three different formulations of the same dose of the same drug. The profile in each case depends on both the rate and the extent of systemic availability.

may be important. Thus, for the rapid relief of pain a soluble aspirin formulation, giving a curve like formulation II, would be preferable to an enteric-coated formulation, giving a curve like that of formulation III.

A curve of type I can be therapeutically useful if a very fast rate of absorption is needed to produce a quick therapeutic effect, for example sublingual glyceryl trinitrate to relieve an acute attack of angina pectoris, although it is also more likely to cause headache by dilating extracranial blood vessels.

For drugs whose action is related to a steady-state concentration during multiple dosing, the differences in rate of availability become less important and the chief consideration is the extent.

The rate of absorption

Gastrointestinal motility

Drugs are absorbed mainly in the upper small intestine, and altered gastric emptying therefore alters the rate. For example, in migraine the rate of absorption of analgesics is reduced because of reduced gastric motility, delaying the response to an oral analgesic. This delay can be reduced by giving metoclopramide, which hastens gastric emptying.

When a drug dissolves more slowly than the stomach empties, increased gastrointestinal motility may reduce both the rate and extent of absorption. Thus, in severe diarrhoea enteric-coated formulations may pass through the gut intact.

Malabsorption

Drug absorption is often impaired in patients with malabsorption, but not always. For example, the absorption of propranolol, cotrimoxazole, and cefalexin is increased in patients with coeliac disease. Digoxin, however, is less well absorbed from tablets in patients with coeliac disease, radiation-induced enteritis, and other gastrointestinal disease, and thyroxine absorption is impaired in coeliac disease.

Food

Food may alter the rate and extent of absorption of drugs. For example, eggs impair iron absorption, and milk (and any calcium, aluminium, magnesium, or ferrous salt) impairs tetracycline absorption by the formation of an insoluble chelate. But such effects are rarely important clinically.

First-pass metabolism

First-pass metabolism is metabolism that occurs before the drug enters the systemic circulation. This may happen in the gut lumen (for example with benzylpenicillin or insulin), the gut wall (tyramine, chlorpromazine), the liver (the most important), and the lungs (various amines).

Many drugs undergo first-pass metabolism in the liver. For instance, propranolol is metabolized to 4-hydroxypropranolol, which is pharmacologically inactive.

When first-pass metabolism results in the formation of compounds with less pharmacological activity than the parent compound, the drug's efficacy

is lower after oral than intravenous administration. In some cases (for example insulin) metabolism is so extensive that oral therapy is impossible. However, such a drug given sublingually, rectally, or transdermally, can bypass the liver (see above).

Distribution

Protein binding

Many drugs are bound to circulating proteins, usually albumin (acidic drugs), but also globulins (hormones), lipoproteins, and acid glycoproteins (basic drugs). Only non-protein-bound drug can bind to cellular receptors, pass across tissue membranes, and reach cellular enzymes, thus being distributed to other body tissues, metabolized, and excreted (for example by the kidney). Thus, changes in protein binding may sometimes cause changes in drug distribution. However, such changes matter only if the drug is more than 90 per cent bound in the plasma and is not widely distributed to body tissues. This is important mainly with phenytoin and warfarin.

The albumin binding of drugs may be changed in renal impairment (the explanation for this is unknown), hypoalbuminaemia (drug binding is reduced when the plasma albumin concentration falls below 25 g/l), the last trimester of pregnancy (during which protein binding is reduced partly because of hypoalbuminaemia), and displacement by other drugs.

The binding of drugs to α_1-acid glycoprotein is increased after trauma and surgery, and in inflammatory diseases and infections. For example, the binding of quinine is increased in malaria.

Tissue distribution

The extent of drug distribution to the tissues of the body varies widely. Some drugs enter only the body fluids, while others are bound extensively in tissues. The distribution of drugs to different tissues is influenced by plasma-protein binding, specific receptor sites in tissues (for example the binding of cardiac glycosides to Na^+,K^+-ATPase in cell membranes throughout the body), regional blood flow (well-perfused organs, such as the heart, kidneys, and liver, accumulate drugs more than poorly perfused organs, such as fat and bone), lipid solubility (non-polar relatively lipid-soluble drugs enter tissues more readily than polar compounds), active transport across cell membranes (for example the adrenergic neurone-blocking drugs), and the effects of other drugs (tricyclic antidepressants inhibit the active transport of the adrenergic neurone blockers, reducing their access to the site of action in the brain, and thus their efficacy).

In some diseases drug distribution is altered for unknown reasons. In renal failure, apart from its effect on protein binding, the distribution of some drugs (for example insulin and digoxin) may also be decreased. In cardiac failure the distribution of some antiarrhythmic drugs, such as disopyramide, is reduced. Obesity and malnutrition influence the distribution of drugs that are highly fat soluble (anaesthetics for example).

Metabolism

Most drugs are metabolized in the liver. Examples of other sites are: suxamethonium in the plasma; insulin and vitamin D in the kidneys; cytosine arabinoside, cyclophosphamide, and other cytotoxic drugs in many cells; and acetylcholine and other neurotransmitters at synapses and within nerves.

Drug metabolism occurs in two phases:

1. Phase I metabolism involves chemical alteration of the basic structure of the drug, for example by oxidation, reduction, or hydrolysis. Oxidation reactions are further subdivided according to whether or not they are effected by the cytochrome-linked mixed function oxidases. Examples of phase I reactions include the N-demethylation of diazepam to desmethyldiazepam, an active metabolite with a long duration of action, and the oxidation of ethanol to acetaldehyde.

2. Phase II metabolism involves conjugation, for example by sulphation, glucuronidation, methylation, or acetylation. Some drugs are conjugated without prior phase I transformation, while others undergo

phase I metabolism before conjugation can occur. The end products of conjugation are compounds that are more water soluble and therefore more rapidly excreted by the kidneys. They are usually, though not always, pharmacologically inactive. Examples of phase II reactions are the glucuronidation of paracetamol, the *N*-acetylation of hydralazine and procainamide, and the methylation of desipramine to its active metabolite imipramine. A conjugated product may sometimes be further metabolized. For example, oestrogens are excreted via the bile, deconjugated in the gut by bacteria, and then reabsorbed.

The end-result of drug metabolism is inactivation, but during the process compounds with pharmacological activity may be formed. An inactive compound may be metabolized to an active one; inactive drugs administered for the effects of their active metabolites are called 'prodrugs'. Levodopa, for Parkinson's disease, can be regarded as a prodrug because it enters the brain and is there metabolized to dopamine. Usually a pharmacologically active compound is transformed to inactive compounds, but sometimes other active compounds are formed first. Examples of parent drugs with active metabolites include diamorphine (which is rapidly metabolized to morphine) and some benzodiazepines (such as diazepam, metabolized to desmethyldiazepam).

Some active compounds are metabolized to toxic compounds. Examples include pethidine (meperidine), the accumulation of whose toxic metabolite norpethidine limits the duration of therapy, and phenytoin, whose main metabolite may inhibit the further metabolism of phenytoin. The normally minor metabolic pathway by which paracetamol is metabolized to a toxic metabolite is enhanced in overdose because the usual detoxifying pathways are saturated (see Chapter 8.2.1).

The factors that affect hepatic drug metabolism are genetic (see pharmacogenetics below), other drugs (see drug interactions below), hepatic blood flow (for drugs that are rapidly cleared), liver disease (only important in extensive liver disease or when there is arteriovenous shunting), and age. The metabolism of some drugs is impaired in old people and in babies younger than about 6 months, particularly premature babies. In both cases this is due to reduced activity of the hepatic microsomal drug metabolizing enzymes. For example, in neonates uridine 5-diphosphate glucuronyl transferase, which conjugates chloramphenicol, is relatively inactive; neonates eliminate chloramphenicol slowly, and may suffer peripheral circulatory collapse (the 'grey syndrome') when given it in weight-related doses that do not harm adults.

Excretion

The kidney is the main route of drug excretion. Other, usually minor, routes include the lungs (important for paraldehyde), breast milk, sweat, tears, and genital secretions (alarming if the patient is not expecting the orange-red discoloration caused by rifampicin), saliva, and bile. Excretion in bile can lead to the reabsorption of some compounds in the gut, for example chloramphenicol (whose inactive metabolites are reactivated by hydrolysis in the gut), oestrogens (which bacteria in the gut deconjugate), morphine, rifampicin, and tetracyclines.

Renal excretion of drugs involves three main processes (Fig. 3): glomerular filtration, passive tubular reabsorption, and active tubular secretion. Thus:

Total renal clearance = Clearance by filtration + Clearance by secretion − Retention by reabsorption.

If a drug is mainly metabolized to inactive compounds, renal function will not greatly affect elimination of the active compound. However, if the drug or an active metabolite is excreted unchanged via the kidneys, changes in renal function will influence its elimination.

Glomerular filtration

All drugs are filtered at the renal glomerulus. The extent of filtration is directly proportional to the glomerular filtration rate (**GFR** = 120 ml/min) and to the fraction of unbound drug in the plasma (*fu*). Thus:

Rate of clearance by filtration = $fu \times$ GFR.

Fig. 3 A diagrammatic representation of a nephron, showing the sites of the three major processes of drug excretion via the kidney.

If the total renal clearance of a drug is equal to $fu \times$ GFR then it is cleared principally by filtration. It may, of course, also be affected by the other two mechanisms, secretion and reabsorption, but in that case those effects must balance each other. Examples of drugs whose clearance is similar to the GFR (after correction for protein binding) are digoxin, gentamicin, procainamide, methotrexate, and ethambutol. As creatinine is cleared mainly by filtration, the creatinine clearance is useful in estimating the clearance rates of these drugs.

Passive tubular reabsorption

Drugs are passively reabsorbed by the renal tubules. The elimination of drugs with very low rates of renal clearance (i.e. approaching urine flow rate, or about 1–2 ml/min) will be significantly affected by changes in urine flow rate (because a doubling of flow rate will increase their rate of clearance by 1–2 ml/min, i.e. twofold). However, for weak acids and weak bases the main factor affecting passive reabsorption is the pH of the renal tubular fluid, because the extent of their ionization (and therefore of their passive reabsorption) depends on the pH when seen in relation to the pK_a of the drug. For example, in an alkaline urine weak acids with a pK_a below 7.5, such as aspirin, are more highly ionized, and therefore less well reabsorbed. The reverse is true for weak bases with a pK_a greater than 7.5, such as amphetamine, whose reabsorption is reduced, and whose clearance is therefore enhanced, by an acid urine. These principles are sometimes put to use in the treatment of overdose (see Section 8). Renal failure alters passive reabsorption indirectly, by changing urine flow rate and pH.

Active tubular secretion

If the renal clearance of a drug is greater than expected by filtration, it is also secreted actively by the proximal tubule. Penicillin is an example. Some drugs inhibit active tubular secretion, and this explains some drug interactions (see below).

Plasma half-life ($t_{1/2}$)

The half-life of a drug is the time it takes for the plasma concentration or amount of drug in the body to halve. In most cases it is constant, no matter what the starting concentration or amount. After one half-life, 50 per cent of the drug will be eliminated, after two half-lives 75 per cent (50 + 25 per cent), and so on. Thus, it takes between four and five half-lives for about 95 per cent of the drug to be eliminated. If the half-life of the drug is prolonged (as for digoxin in renal failure), elimination will take proportionately longer. The rate at which drug accumulates in the body during regular multiple dosing is determined by the half-life. Just as it takes four half-lives for 95 per cent of the drug to be eliminated after withdrawal, it takes four half-lives for about 95 per cent of steady state to be reached during regular administration (Fig. 4(a) and Fig. 5, bottom and middle curves).

The delay in reaching a steady state can be overcome by giving a loading dose. When a drug has a half-life greater than 24 h (for example digoxin, 40 h; digitoxin 7 days; *S*-warfarin, 32 h), it takes several days or weeks of regular administration of the same daily dose before the steady-state plasma concentration or amount of drug in the body is reached. Such a delay may be unacceptable if the eventual steady-state plasma concentration is needed for a therapeutic effect. In such cases a loading dose can be given in order to boost the amount of drug in the body to the required level. Thereafter the regular maintenance dose is given to maintain the steady state (Fig. 4(b) and Fig. 5, top curve).

Non-linear kinetics

Although the pharmacokinetics of most drugs are linear, some are not. This means that some aspect of their kinetics becomes saturated in the therapeutic dosage range, so that a linear increase in dosage does not produce a proportionate increase in plasma concentration or effect. The prime example is phenytoin, whose enzymatic metabolism in the liver becomes saturated at dosages in the therapeutic range; plasma phenytoin concentrations therefore increase non-linearly with dosage.

The pharmacodynamic process

The pharmacodynamic process describes all those matters concerned with the pharmacological actions of a drug, whether they lead to therapeutic effects or adverse effects. The associated question is 'Is the drug producing the required pharmacological effect?'

Drugs produce their pharmacological effects in many different ways, often by stimulating or blocking a receptor (Table 3).

Fig. 5 Plasma quinine concentrations in cerebral malaria during repeated administration of 5 mg/kg every 8 h (bottom curve), repeated administration of 10 mg/kg every 8 h (middle curve), and repeated administration of 10 mg/kg every 8 h after a loading dose of 20 mg/kg (top curve). (From White NJ et al. (1983). Quinine loading dose in cerebral malaria. *American Journal of Tropical Medicine and Hygiene* **32**, 1–5, with permission.)

Actions via direct effects on receptors

Receptors are proteins situated either in cell membranes or within the cellular cytoplasm. For each type a specific group of ligands, drugs or endogenous substances exists that bind to the receptor and produce pharmacological effects. Ligands are of three types: agonists, antagonists, and partial agonists.

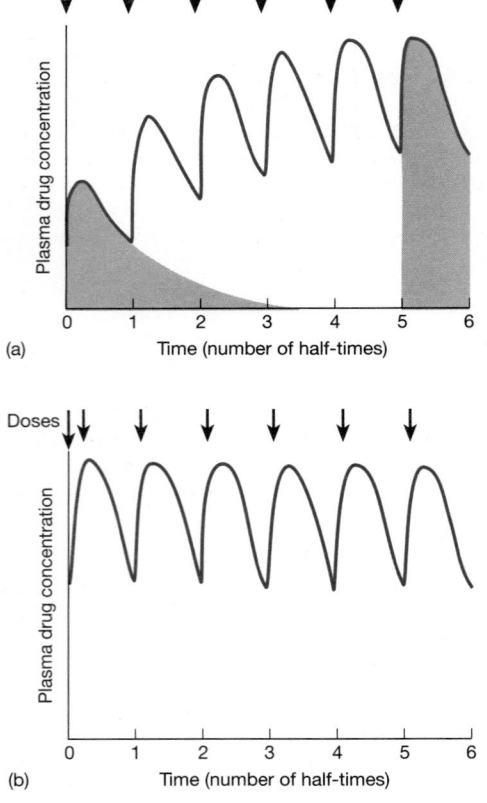

Fig. 4 (a) The theoretical plasma concentrations of a drug over time during its repeated oral administration. With repeated doses the drug accumulates to an eventual steady state. (b) If the correct loading dose is given a steady state can be achieved rapidly and then maintained by giving a smaller maintenance dose. In this example, because the drug is being given once every half-life the maintenance dose is half the loading dose.

Table 3 The types of pharmacological actions of drugs

Actions	Examples
Actions via receptors	
Agonist at a receptor	Morphine
Antagonist at a receptor	Naloxone
Partial agonist at a receptor	Pentazocine
Actions via second messengers	Lithium
Indirect alterations of the effects of endogenous agonists	
Physiological antagonism (insulin)	Glucagon
Increase in endogenous release (monoamines)	Amphetamine
Inhibition of endogenous reuptake (monoamines)	Antidepressants
Inhibition of endogenous metabolism (GABA)	Vigabatrin
Prevention of endogenous release (aldosterone)	ACE inhibitors
Inhibition of transport processes	Diuretics
Actions on enzymes	
Enzyme inhibition	Warfarin
Enzyme activation	Thrombolytic drugs
Enzymatic action	Factor VIII
Other miscellaneous effects	
Chelating agents	Penicillamine
Osmotic diuretics	Mannitol
Volatile general anaesthetics	Halothane
Replacement drugs	Iron salts

GABA, γ-aminobutyrate; ACE, angiotensin-converting enzyme.

Agonists bind to a receptor and produce a response. For example, morphine is an agonist at μ opioid receptors, which mediate its analgesic action.

Antagonists (or blockers) prevent an agonist from binding to a receptor and thus prevent its effects. However, pure antagonists do not themselves have any pharmacological actions mediated by receptors. For example, naloxone is an opioid-receptor antagonist; when it binds to opioid receptors it prevents or reverses the effects of morphine and other opiates.

Unlike a full agonist, which is capable of producing a maximal response when it binds to enough receptors, a partial agonist cannot produce the maximal response of which the tissue is capable, even when it binds to the maximum number of available receptors. Thus, above a certain level of binding a partial agonist may bind to receptors without producing any further increase in effect. However, in so doing it may prevent the action of other agonists, and may thus behave as an antagonist. This mixture of actions is called partial agonism. For example, buprenorphine is a mixed opioid agonist/antagonist at μ receptors. If used in combination with a high dose of a pure agonist it will tend to oppose its action rather than supplement it.

Receptor subtypes

In some cases a receptor may have subtypes, for which certain ligands may have some selectivity. For example, of at least three subtypes of opioid receptors, μ and δ are both involved in analgesia, gastrointestinal motility, and respiratory depression, and κ is involved in analgesia, sedation, and miosis. These receptors are variably distributed in the nervous system. Most opiates act at μ receptors, but none is completely selective and they may act at other subtypes.

Long-term effects of drugs at receptors

During long-term therapy the effects of a drug may be altered by adaptive responses, usually accompanied by either increases ('upregulation') or decreases ('downregulation') in receptor numbers. Such changes may explain both beneficial and adverse effects of drugs. Examples include:

- The therapeutic response to antidepressants, perhaps related to changes in receptors in the brain secondary to the actions of these drugs on neurotransmitter uptake. This could explain why the therapeutic response to antidepressants takes a few weeks.

- The way in which the response to levodopa in Parkinson's disease changes during long-term administration (producing, for example, the 'on–off' effect).

- Withdrawal syndromes that may occur because long-term changes become unopposed when the drug is withdrawn, for example after the long-term abuse of opiates, or the use of benzodiazepines in chronic anxiety.

Actions via direct effects on second messengers

When an agonist stimulates a membrane-bound receptor its effect is produced in one of two ways: either through a so-called second messenger (see Fig. 6) or by changing the activity of an ion channel linked to the receptor. Some drugs may act by affecting second messengers directly. For example, lithium may work by inhibiting phosphatidylinositol turnover at different sites. Theophylline and caffeine work by inhibiting the breakdown of cyclic AMP.

Actions via indirect alterations of the effects of endogenous agonists

Some drugs indirectly alter the effect of an endogenous agonist rather than acting via a receptor. Some oppose the physiological effects of others. For example, glucagon is a physiological antagonist of the actions of insulin and can be used to treat hypoglycaemia.

Increase in endogenous release

Some drugs enhance the action of endogenous agonists by increasing their release. For example, amphetamines increase the release of dopamine from

Fig. 6 A schematic representation of the second-messenger systems that mediate the effects of drugs acting at receptors. PIP_2, phosphatidylinositol bisphosphate; DG, diacyl glycerol; IP_3, inositol triphosphate.

nerve endings. Because amphetamines can cause a syndrome resembling schizophrenia, this action has led to the idea that schizophrenia may be related to excess dopamine action in the brain.

Prevention of endogenous release

If a drug prevents the release of an endogenous agonist it will reduce its effects. For example, angiotensin-converting enzyme inhibitors prevent the formation of angiotensin II; this prevents the release of endogenous aldosterone, resulting in potassium retention.

Inhibition of endogenous reuptake

Some drugs inhibit the reuptake of endogenous agonists, enhancing their effects. For example, many antidepressants inhibit the reuptake by neurones of certain neurotransmitters, such as noradrenaline and 5-hydroxytryptamine.

Inhibition of endogenous metabolism

Some drugs potentiate endogenous agonists by inhibiting their metabolism. For example, vigabatrin inhibits the metabolism of γ-aminobutyrate in the brain, enhancing its actions and suppressing seizures.

Actions via the inhibition of transport processes

Because cations (such as sodium, potassium, and calcium) and other substances (such as organic acids in the kidneys) have so many important roles in the maintenance of normal cellular function, inhibition of their transport is an important type of mechanism of drug action.

Diuretics

Most diuretics act by inhibiting sodium reabsorption in the renal tubules. The loop diuretics frusemide (furosemide) and bumetanide inhibit Na/K/Cl cotransport in the ascending limb of Henle's loop. The thiazide diuretics inhibit Na/Cl cotransport in the proximal segment of the distal convoluted tubule. The potassium-sparing diuretic amiloride inhibits sodium channels in the distal segment of the distal convoluted tubule.

Calcium antagonists

The calcium antagonists, such as verapamil, diltiazem, and the dihydropyridines (for example nifedipine), inhibit the transport of calcium via potential-operated calcium channels. The different calcium antagonists have different selectivities for calcium channels in different tissues, and have various actions. For example, verapamil has an antiarrhythmic action in the heart, and nifedipine a vasodilator action on peripheral arterioles.

Drugs acting on potassium channels

Potassium channels in cell membranes control the rate of efflux of potassium from the cells. Cellular activity is reduced by drugs that open K^+ channels and increased by drugs that close them.

Drugs that open potassium channels include vascular smooth muscle relaxants, such as minoxidil and hydralazine. Drugs that close them include the sulphonylureas, which increase the release of insulin from pancreatic β cells, and 3,4-diaminopyridine, which increases the release of acetylcholine at the neuromuscular junction.

Actions via enzyme inhibition

Some drugs act by directly inhibiting enzymes.

Neostigmine is a reversible cholinesterase inhibitor. It increases the concentration of acetylcholine at the muscle motor endplate, improving neuromuscular transmission. Xanthine and hypoxanthine are oxidized to uric acid by xanthine oxidase; this is inhibited by allopurinol, which therefore reduces the synthesis of uric acid in gout.

The monoamine oxidase inhibitors inhibit the metabolism of the monoamines 5-hydroxytryptamine, noradrenaline, and dopamine in the brain, and they presumably produce their antidepressant effect by this action. Just as drugs that act via receptors may be selective for a subtype of receptor, so monoamine oxidase inhibitors may be selective for one subtype of monoamine oxidase. For example, selegiline selectively inhibits monoamine oxidase type B: it inhibits the metabolism of dopamine in the brain and enhances the action of levodopa in parkinsonism. However, because gut monoamine oxidase is of type A, selegiline does not produce the 'cheese reaction' (due to tyramine and other amines, see below) that non-selective monoamine oxidase inhibitors do. In contrast, the antidepressant moclobemide selectively inhibits monoamine oxidase A; although it inhibits the metabolism of tyramine in the gut it does not inhibit its metabolism by monoamine oxidase B after absorption.

The cardiac glycosides act by inhibiting the Na/K pump, changing the disposition of sodium, which secondarily changes calcium disposition within cells.

Other drugs that act via enzyme inhibition include warfarin (vitamin K epoxide reductase), aspirin and other non-steroidal anti-inflammatory drugs (the enzymes involved in prostaglandin synthesis), angiotensin-converting enzyme inhibitors, disulfiram (alcohol dehydrogenase), some anticancer drugs such as cytarabine (DNA polymerase), and some anti-infective drugs (bacterial or viral enzymes; for example, trimethoprim inhibits bacterial dihydrofolate reductase, the quinolones inhibit bacterial DNA gyrase, and zidovudine and didanosine inhibit the reverse transcriptase of HIV).

Danazol and stanozolol are examples of drugs that inhibit an enzyme indirectly—they stimulate the production of an inhibitor of C1 esterase and are used to treat hereditary angio-oedema, in which there is reduced plasma activity of the inhibitor.

Actions via enzyme activation or direct enzymatic activity

Some drugs activate enzymes or are themselves enzymes.

The clotting and fibrinolytic factors are enzymes, and certain drugs that act on clotting and fibrinolysis do so by increasing their activity. Heparin acts by activating antithrombin III. The thrombolytic drugs streptokinase, alteplase, and anistreplase activate plasminogen.

Clotting factor deficiencies can be treated by replacing deficient enzymes of the clotting pathway, for example factor VIII in patients with haemophilia, and fresh frozen plasma in warfarin toxicity. Pancreatic enzymes are used in treating malabsorption in patients with chronic pancreatic insufficiency.

L-Asparaginase is an enzyme that hydrolyses asparagine, an essential amino acid in neoplastic cells. Some patients with acute lymphoblastic leukaemia may be helped by depriving their leukaemic cells of asparagine.

Actions via other miscellaneous effects

Chelating agents

Drugs that chelate metals can be used to hasten their removal from the body. Calcium sodium edetate chelates many divalent and trivalent metals and is used to treat poisoning, particularly with lead. Dimercaprol chelates some heavy metals and is used to treat mercury and gold poisoning. Desfer-

rioxamine chelates iron and is used in treating iron poisoning and the iron overload that occurs with repeated blood transfusion (as in thalassaemia). Penicillamine chelates copper and is used in treating hepatolenticular degeneration (Wilson's disease); it is also used to complex cystine and thus prevent renal damage in cystinuria.

Osmotic diuretics

Mannitol is freely filtered at the glomerulus but the renal tubules reabsorb only a little. It therefore increases the concentration of osmotically active particles in the tubular fluid and takes water with it.

Volatile general anaesthetics

General anaesthetics form a diverse group of agents, such as the halogenated hydrocarbons (halothane, trichloroethylene), and non-halogenated agents (nitrous oxide, ether, cyclopropane), which produce similar effects on the brain. Their main action is probably on the lipid matrix of the biological membrane, changing its biophysical properties, and so altering ion fluxes or other functions that influence neuronal excitability.

Replacement of vitamins and minerals

Some drugs are used simply to replace deficiencies, for example ferrous salts in iron deficiency anaemia and hydroxocobalamin (vitamin B_{12}) in vitamin B_{12} deficiency.

Stereoisomerism and drug action

Stereoisomerism (chirality) of organic compounds is due to asymmetry in one or more of their atoms (usually carbon), resulting in two structures (enantiomers) that cannot be superimposed on each other.

The terminology used to describe chiral compounds is complex, but in summary some are called R and S (from the Latin rectus = right and sinister = left), others D and L (from the Latin dexter = right and laevus = left), and yet others d and l. Examples of drug enantiomers are R-warfarin and S-warfarin, D-glucose (dextrose) and L-glucose (laevulose), and d-propranolol and l-propranolol.

Of all synthetic drugs used in clinical practice about 40 per cent are chiral and about 90 per cent of those are marketed in the racemic form (i.e. as an equal mixture of the two enantiomers). Examples include d,l-propranolol and R,S-warfarin. Naproxen is one of the few examples of a synthetic compound that is marketed as a single enantiomer. In contrast, naturally occurring and semisynthetic compounds are almost all chiral and almost all are marketed as a single isomer. Examples include D-glucose (dextrose) and the naturally occurring amino acids (for example L-dopa).

Enantiomers often have differing actions. For example, l-propranolol is a β-blocker, while d-propranolol has membrane stabilizing activity like that of local anaesthetics; l-sotalol is a β-blocker, while d-sotalol has antiarrhythmic effects like those of amiodarone.

Sometimes the difference between enantiomers is a difference between therapeutic and adverse effects, as dramatically demonstrated by the example of thalidomide whose R enantiomer is hypnotic but whose adverse effects seem to be due to the S enantiomer.

In some cases, differences between enantiomers are limited to differences in potency. For example, S-warfarin and R-warfarin have the same anticoagulant actions, but the former is about five times more potent.

Sometimes enantiomeric differences tell us something about the mechanism of action of a drug. For example, S-timolol is a more potent β-blocker than R-timolol, but both are equally effective in reducing intraocular pressure in patients with glaucoma. This suggests that timolol lowers the intraocular pressure by a mechanism unrelated to β-blockade.

One enantiomer may be eliminated differently from the body than the other. For example, the half-lives of S-warfarin and R-warfarin are 32 h and 54 h, and the routes of metabolism are to 7-hydroxywarfarin for S-warfarin and to warfarin alcohols for R-warfarin. This is important in some drug interactions with warfarin, because some drugs (such as metronidazole) that inhibit the metabolism of warfarin, primarily affect the more potent enantiomer, S-warfarin.

Pure enantiomers of synthetic drugs are expensive to make, but new techniques may reduce the costs and lead to the emergence of more formulations of pure enantiomers for clinical use.

The therapeutic process

The question associated with the therapeutic process is 'Is the pharmacological effect being translated into a therapeutic effect?'

Translation of pharmacological effect into therapeutic effect during short-term therapy

The short-term therapeutic and toxic effects of drugs occur as a result of the pharmacological actions discussed above. However, the translation of molecular and cellular pharmacological effects into the therapeutic or toxic effect is not a simple process, but one that involves several translational stages at different pharmacological and physiological levels.

Take, for example, the action of salbutamol, a β_2-adrenoceptor agonist, in the treatment of asthma. Salbutamol stimulates bronchial β_2-adrenoceptors, and so increases the activity of adenylate cyclase; this is its pharmacological effect at the molecular level. The increase in adenylate cyclase activity leads to an increase in the intracellular concentration of cyclic AMP, a pharmacological effect at the cellular level. The increase in cyclic AMP in some way alters the function of bronchial smooth muscle cells, and results in an inhibition of the release of inflammatory mediators from bronchial mast cells, with effects on cell physiology. All this in turn results in bronchodilatation, an effect on tissue physiology. Bronchodilatation improves lung function, an effect on organ physiology. Finally, the patient can breathe more easily, the desired clinical effect.

This analysis of the short-term effects of drugs teaches us several things about drug action: how drug action may be modified; how therapeutic and adverse effects may be mediated via different pharmacological effects; the relation between the pharmacological effects of a drug and the rate of onset or duration of its action; and drug/disease interactions.

How drug action may be modified

It is often possible to modify the action of a drug beneficially or adversely. For example, one would expect a xanthine derivative, such as theophylline, which increases cellular cyclic AMP concentrations by the inhibition of phosphodiesterase, to potentiate the action of salbutamol at the stage at which it alters adenyl cyclase activity. This turns out to be both a beneficial and an adverse clinical interaction—beneficial because theophylline enhances the therapeutic action of salbutamol, adverse because it also enhances the hypokalaemia that salbutamol may cause by stimulating Na^+/K^+-ATPase.

Different pharmacological actions may mediate therapeutic and adverse or other effects

Some drugs have more than one molecular mechanism of action, and two different therapeutic effects of a drug may result from different actions. For example, tetracycline acts against bacteria by interfering with their protein synthesis, but in acne it helps by interfering with sebum production in sebaceous glands.

Similarly, a therapeutic effect may be brought about by one pharmacological action and an adverse effect by another. For example, the therapeutic effect of salbutamol results from its action on β_2-adrenoceptors, but it causes the unwanted effect of tachycardia by stimulating β_1-adrenoceptors.

Different therapeutic or adverse effects may be produced by the actions of a single drug on the same or a similar molecular mechanism in different tissues. For example, the inhibition of β_2-adrenoceptors causes bronchoconstriction in the lungs of susceptible people and impairs glycogenolysis in the liver.

Peripheral or non-therapeutic effects of drugs can be clinically important in several ways. For example, aminoglycoside antibiotics can all damage the inner ear, leading to impaired hearing or loss of balance; these effects are quite separate from the antibiotic activity of these drugs but must be

Fig. 7 The effect of metoclopramide on the absorption of paracetamol. When metoclopramide (10 mg intravenously) was given with paracetamol (1.5 g orally) the rate of paracetamol absorption was increased, as evidenced by a higher and earlier peak paracetamol plasma concentration. (Adapted from Nimmo J *et al.* (1973). Pharmacological modification of gastric emptying: effects of propantheline and metoclopramide on paracetamol absorption. *British Medical Journal* i, 587–9, with permission.)

considered when choosing dosage regimens and mean that plasma concentration must be monitored.

The relation between the pharmacological actions of a drug and the rate of onset and duration of its effects

The rate of onset of action of a drug depends not only on its pharmacokinetics (i.e. the time it takes for the appropriate amount of drug to build up at the site of action; Fig. 4), but also on how long it takes for the full pharmacodynamic sequence of events to unroll. In the case of salbutamol the time between β_2-adrenoceptor stimulation and bronchodilatation (Fig. 7) is of the order of a few minutes. However, for other drugs the sequence of events takes much longer. For example, corticosteroids react with a receptor protein in cellular cytoplasm to form a steroid–receptor complex. This complex enters the cell nucleus, where it binds to chromatin and directs the genetic apparatus to transcribe RNA. This leads, for instance in liver cells, to the production of enzymes involved in gluconeogenesis and amino acid metabolism. Once the steroid has bound to its intracellular receptor it sets off a sequence of reactions that then has its own timescale, independent of the quantity of steroid, either in the blood or combined with the receptor. The induction of protein synthesis by RNA transcription takes several hours and each new protein has its own biological lifespan. This is why the effect takes hours or days to occur.

Similarly, the duration of action of a drug is related not only to the time it takes for the drug to be cleared from the body, but also to the duration of its pharmacological effects. For example, aspirin inhibits cyclo-oxygenase by acetylating a serine moiety at the active site of the enzyme. In platelets prostaglandin synthesis is thus inhibited for the lifetime of the platelet. So, although aspirin leaves the body within a few hours, its effect on platelets lasts for days.

Drug/disease interactions

Because of the complex links between the pharmacological effects of a drug and its therapeutic or adverse effects, the pathophysiology of the disease being treated, or of other incidental diseases, can variously alter the way in which the pharmacological effect is translated into a therapeutic effect.

The use of digoxin in cardiac failure is an example of the ways in which drug/disease interactions may influence therapy. Digoxin inhibits the activity of the membrane-bound Na/K pump. This is its pharmacological effect at the molecular level, which increases the intracellular concentration of sodium, and thereby alters the intracellular disposition of calcium (a pharmacological effect at the cellular level). This in turn leads to an alteration in the action potential of cardiac muscle (a physiological effect at the cellular level), which then causes an increase in the rate of contractility of the myocardial fibres (a physiological effect at the tissue level). Consequently cardiac output increases (a physiological effect at the level of the whole organ).

If this chain of events occurs without interruption the clinical result will be relief of the signs and symptoms of heart failure. However, drug/disease interactions can alter the therapeutic outcome at various stages in the chain. Thus, potassium depletion enhances the binding of digoxin to the Na/K pump and this increases the extent of inhibition of sodium transport, which can in turn cause digoxin toxicity. In hyperthyroidism the nature of the interaction between digoxin and the Na/K pump is altered, resulting in resistance to the inhibitory effects of digoxin. Increasing the dose may merely cause digoxin toxicity without ever producing a therapeutic effect. In patients with chronic cor pulmonale, digoxin may inhibit the Na/K pump and may even cause cardiac arrhythmias without ever increasing the rate of myocardial contractility. This may be because of tissue hypoxia and acidosis in cor pulmonale, which may also contribute to an increased risk of digoxin-induced cardiac arrhythmias without benefiting patients with acute myocardial infarction. In patients with hypertrophic obstructive cardiomyopathy, although digoxin increases the rate of myocardial contractility, this is not translated into an increase in cardiac output, as left ventricular outflow remains obstructed.

Thus even when it can be shown that a drug is having its expected action at a particular pharmacological or physiological level, it cannot automatically be assumed that it will have a consequent therapeutic effect.

Interactions with circadian phase

Most bodily functions vary in a circadian rhythm - for example sleep and wakefulness, urinary excretion, secretion of hormones—and drug effects are liable to differ at different phases of the rhythm. In some instances the difference is dramatic. For example melatonin taken late in the afternoon evening advances the circadian phase, and sleepiness comes earlier, whereas taken in the morning the same dose retards circadian phase. Bright light switches off the body's own melatonin release, darkness switches it on. So in the morning exogenous melatonin prolongs the effect of darkness, late in the day it switches on the response to darkness early. Another example is related to the secretion of cortisol by the adrenal cortex. A high plasma cortisol concentration inhibits corticotrophin release from the pituitary. Corticotrophin is secreted at night, and plasma cortisol peaks around 8 a.m., and about then the corticotrophin concentration is zero. Exogenous cortisol given at this time cannot inhibit corticotrophin release because none is occurring. But given in the evening it will completely inhibit corticotrophin release during the night. For this reason cortisol given once daily in the morning causes much less pituitary inhibition than the same dose given in the evening, or than doses spread over the 24 hours. Circadian therapeutics are complicated to study, and so far few practical examples are known. An important principle that is likely to find increasing application is that the 'hour of greatest therapeutic effect' will differ from the 'hour of greatest toxicity', since therapeutic and toxic effects are mediated by widely differing mechanisms. This could be exploited to increase the safety margin or tolerability of treatment, for example in cancer chemotherapy.

Translation of pharmacological effect into therapeutic effect during long-term therapy

During prolonged therapy adaptation may develop to the short-term pharmacological effects of the drug (Table 4), with several consequences.

Therapeutic effects through adaptation

In immunization, by adapting to an initial immunological challenge the immune system develops the ability to respond to a subsequent similar challenge, tetanus immunization for example.

Although tricyclic antidepressants rapidly inhibit reuptake of noradrenaline and 5-hydroxytryptamine in the brain, the therapeutic effect of these drugs takes 1 to 2 weeks to become evident. The brain adapts to the increased concentrations of noradrenaline and 5-hydroxytryptamine in the synaptic cleft in certain areas, where the sensitivity of responses to neuro-

Table 4 The different ways in which adaptation to drug effects may become apparent clinically

Effect	Example
Therapeutic effects through adaptation	Immunization and vaccination. Tricyclic antidepressants
Tolerance (increasing ineffectiveness of therapy):	
Target cell tolerance	Depletion of noradrenaline by ephedrine. Change in sulphydryl function by nitrates
Opioid tolerance	
Physiological homoeostatic mechanisms	Hydralazine (reflex tachycardia). Acetazolamide (acidosis reversing hypokalaemia)
Metabolic autoinduction	Barbiturates, carbamazepine
Withdrawal syndromes:	
Through receptor changes	Opioids, alcohol, benzodiazepines, β-blockers
Through physiological adaptation	Corticosteroids
Adverse effects directly due to adaptation	Tardive dyskinesia due to dopamine antagonists

transmitters is decreased by 'downregulation'; part of this adaptive effect could be the pharmacological action through which these drugs produce their therapeutic effects.

Tolerance: increasing ineffectiveness of therapy

Tolerance is a state of decreased responsiveness to a drug, resulting from previous exposure, either to the same drug or to one with similar short-term effects.

For example, it can develop to the vasoconstricting effects of ephedrine nosedrops, used to treat vasomotor rhinitis: as ephedrine acts by releasing noradrenaline from sympathetic nerve endings, when the noradrenaline is depleted the ephedrine can no longer be effective.

Patients who take long-term glyceryl trinitrate, particularly from transdermal patches, become tolerant and may not respond to its acute effects. To avoid this, a patch should be applied for no longer than 18 h. This effect probably reflects depletion of tissue sulphydryl groups by oxidation to disulphide groups.

Physiological tolerance by homoeostatic mechanisms

Secondary hyperaldosteronism is a physiological response to sodium loss produced by loop or thiazide diuretics. The enhanced potassium excretion that it causes may be obviated by using a potassium-sparing diuretic (for example amiloride) or the aldosterone antagonist spironolactone.

Another type of physiological tolerance occurs in patients given the diuretic acetazolamide. This is a powerful kaliuretic and can cause severe potassium depletion when it is first given. However, because it inhibits carbonic anhydrase activity in the kidney it causes bicarbonate depletion, and the resulting acidosis causes retention of potassium. Thus, potassium depletion due to acetazolamide lasts for only a few days or weeks.

Metabolic tolerance Metabolic tolerance results from faster metabolism of the drug. The commonest cause is induction of hepatic microsomal drug metabolizing enzymes by drugs such as barbiturates, phenytoin, or carbamazepine. In a particular case, the hepatic inactivation of the carbamazepine is increased after long-term exposure to carbamazepine itself (the phenomenon known as 'autoinduction'), and tolerance occurs spontaneously. Induction of drug metabolism can lead to adverse drug reactions (see below).

Withdrawal syndromes

A common, though not inevitable, outcome of an adaptive response to long-term drug use is the occurrence of a withdrawal response, which occurs either when the drug is withdrawn or when an antagonist is given, and which usually takes the form of some sort of adverse reaction.

A withdrawal syndrome occurs in opiate addicts when the opiate is withdrawn or when an antagonist, such as naloxone, is given. The symptoms consist of yawning, rhinorrhoea, and sweating, followed by shivering and goose flesh ('cold turkey'); later, nausea, vomiting, diarrhoea, and hypertension may occur. The acute syndrome subsides within a week, but the addict may be anxious and sleep badly for several weeks or months after. This syndrome can be avoided by introducing increasing doses of methadone as the opiate is withdrawn, as the later withdrawal of methadone, which has a much longer duration of action than morphine, may not result in this syndrome.

Delirium tremens may occur on withdrawal of alcohol from chronic alcoholics. This syndrome consists of disorientation and visual hallucinations. Withdrawal of benzodiazepines after long-term therapy may result in a disturbance of sleep pattern (rebound insomnia associated with abnormal sleep patterns), agitation, restlessness, and occasionally epileptic convulsions.

The risk of angina pectoris, myocardial infarction, and arrhythmias is increased in patients with ischaemic heart disease when β-adrenoceptor antagonists are withdrawn after long-term use. This may be due to an increase in the numbers of cardiac β-adrenoceptors, with increased sensitivity to the β-adrenergic effects of sympathetic stimulation.

Angina and even myocardial infarction have been reported in munitions workers who have become tolerant of the effects of nitroglycerine (glyceryl trinitrate) and have taken a break from work.

Long-term therapy with corticosteroids suppresses pituitary secretion of adrenocorticotrophic hormone, leading to adrenal cortical atrophy. When treatment is suddenly withdrawn, secretion of adrenocorticotrophic hormone by the pituitary may take several weeks or months to recover. Because the adrenal cortex has to increase in size again in order to become normally responsive to adrenocorticotrophic hormone the patient is at great risk of an addisonian crisis if stressed.

Adverse effects directly due to adaptation

Patients taking a neuroleptic drug (for example chlorpromazine, fluphenazine, or haloperidol) continuously for a long time commonly develop abnormal movements (known collectively as tardive dyskinesia). The face, mouth, and tongue are often affected, with stereotyped sucking and smacking of the lips, lateral jaw movements, and darting movements of the tongue. Occasionally more widespread dyskinesia may resemble choreoathetosis. The long-term blockade of brain dopamine function with neuroleptics is thought to lead to increased sensitivity to the effects of dopamine in certain areas of the brain, perhaps by increasing the number of dopamine receptors. Tardive dyskinesia may result from such increased sensitivity in extrapyramidal areas of the brain.

Adverse drug reactions

Adverse effects are unwanted effects of drugs, and they may be either toxic effects or side-effects. A toxic effect is an adverse effect that arises through an exaggeration of the pharmacological action that is responsible for the therapeutic effect of the drug (for example arrhythmias due to digoxin), and is therefore dose related. A side-effect is an adverse effect that arises through some pharmacological action other than that which produces the therapeutic effect (for example the anticholinergic effects of tricyclic antidepressants); such effects may or may not be dose related. The term 'adverse effects' covers all types of unwanted effects.

Incidence

The risks of adverse drug reactions have been variously estimated as follows:

- 10 to 20 per cent of hospital inpatients suffer an adverse reaction;

- 0.24 to 2.9 per cent of deaths in hospital inpatients are due to adverse reactions;

- 0.3 to 5.0 per cent of hospital admissions are due to adverse reactions.

Classification (see Table 5)

Dose-related adverse reactions

Dose-related adverse drug reactions are usually due to a pharmacokinetic or pharmacodynamic abnormality producing an exaggeration of a known pharmacological effect of the drug. The pharmacological effect that proves adverse may be the same as that which achieves the therapeutic effect (for example hypoglycaemia due to insulin), or due to another effect occurring in parallel (the anticholinergic action of tricyclic antidepressants, producing a dry mouth or urinary retention).

Dose-related adverse reactions may occur because of variations in the pharmaceutical, pharmacokinetic, or pharmacodynamic properties of a drug, often due to some disease or pharmacogenetic characteristic of the patient. These mechanisms are illustrated below.

Pharmaceutical defect

Adverse reactions can be caused by a contaminant, for example pyrogens or even bacteria in intravenous formulations, if quality control breaks down. If a febrile reaction occurs in a patient being given an infusion, the drip should be taken down and all its components sent for bacteriological investigation. The manufacturer should be urgently notified.

Out-of-date formulations may sometimes cause adverse reactions because of degradation products. For example, outdated tetracycline may cause Fanconi's syndrome, because it is degraded to anhydrotetracycline and epiandrotetracycline. The omission of the preservative citric acid from tetracycline formulations has reduced the risk of this effect, but has not removed it completely.

Table 5 Classification of adverse drug reactions

Dose-related effects
Pharmaceutical variation
Pharmacokinetic variation
    Pharmacogenetic variation:
    Hepatic disease
    Renal disease
    Cardiac disease
    Thyroid disease
    Drug interactions
Pharmacodynamic variation:
    Hepatic disease
    Altered fluid and electrolyte balance
    Drug interactions
Non-dose-related effects
Immunological reactions
Pseudoallergic reactions
Pharmacogenetic variation
Long-term effects
Adaptive changes
Rebound phenomena
Other long-term effects
Delayed effects
Carcinogenesis
Effects concerned with reproduction:
    Impaired fertility
    Teratogenesis: adverse effects on the fetus during the early
      stages of pregnancy
    Adverse effects on the fetus during the later stages of
      pregnancy
    Drugs in breast milk

Pharmacokinetic variation

Normal individuals vary greatly in their rate of elimination of drugs. This variation is greatest for drugs cleared by hepatic metabolism and is determined by several factors, which may be genetic, environmental (diet, smoking, alcohol), or hepatic (blood flow and intrinsic drug-metabolizing capacity). On top of this normal variation specific pharmacogenetic or hepatic abnormalities may be associated with adverse reactions. In addition, renal and cardiac disease can change drug pharmacokinetics. Pharmacogenetics is discussed below.

The reserve of the liver parenchyma is large, and adverse reactions due to impaired hepatic metabolism are uncommon. Nevertheless, in patients with severe liver disease care must be taken, particularly with drugs with a low therapeutic index and those subject to extensive first-pass elimination. For example, hepatocellular dysfunction, as in severe hepatitis or advanced cirrhosis, may reduce the clearance of drugs for which the capacity of the liver is limited, phenytoin, theophylline, and warfarin for example. Porto-systemic shunting in portal hypertension, associated with cirrhosis, reduces the clearance of drugs normally cleared rapidly by the liver, for example morphine and other narcotic analgesics, propranolol, labetalol, and chlor-promazine.

Drugs that the kidneys excrete unchanged, or whose active metabolites are excreted, will accumulate in renal failure. Important examples include digoxin, lithium, tetracyclines, aminoglycoside antibiotics, and vancomycin.

Pharmacodynamic variation

People vary greatly in their pharmacodynamic responses, and that variability may be compounded by the effects of disease, as the following examples show.

Liver disease may influence pharmacodynamic responses to certain drugs by several mechanisms. Blood clotting may be impaired in cirrhosis and acute hepatitis because of reduced production of clotting factors; patients with oesophageal and gastric varices caused by portal hypertension in cirrhosis are also at risk of bleeding. Drugs that may impair haemostasis, or that may predispose to bleeding by causing gastric ulceration, should be avoided; these include anticoagulants and non-steroidal anti-inflammatory drugs (for example aspirin, indometacin, ibuprofen).

In patients with hepatic encephalopathy (hepatic coma or precoma), the brain is more sensitive to the effects of sedating drugs. It is therefore wise to avoid opioid and other narcotic analgesics and barbiturates; chlorpromazine dosage should be reduced. Chlormethiazole or a short-acting benzodiazepine may be used cautiously as a tranquillizer.

Diuretics used to treat ascites and peripheral oedema may precipitate hepatic encephalopathy, particularly if diuresis is too rapid.

In hepatic cirrhosis, certain drugs may exacerbate sodium and water retention; they include indometacin, corticosteroids, and carbamazepine.

The pharmacodynamic effects of some drugs may be altered by changes in fluid and electrolyte balance. For example, both hypokalaemia and hypercalcaemia potentiate the toxic effects of digoxin. The class I antiarrhythmic drugs, such as quinidine, procainamide, and disopyramide, may be more arrhythmogenic in hypokalaemic patients, and this combination particularly increases the risk of polymorphous ventricular tachycardia. Hypocalcaemia prolongs the action of muscle relaxants such as tubocurarine. Fluid depletion enhances the hypotensive effects of antihypertensive drugs.

Non-dose-related adverse reactions

Non-dose-related adverse drug reactions are caused by immunological and pharmacogenetic mechanisms. Allergic drug reactions are:

- Unrelated to the usual pharmacological effects of the drug.
- A delay often occurs between the first exposure to the drug and the subsequent adverse reaction.
- Very small doses of the drug may elicit the reaction once allergy is established.

- The reaction disappears on withdrawal; and the illness is often recognizable as a form of immunological reaction, for example rash, serum sickness, anaphylaxis, asthma, urticaria, angio-oedema.

Factors associated with an increased risk of allergic drug reactions include a history of allergic disorders (patients with a history of atopic disease and those with hereditary angio-oedema) and HLA status (the risk of nephrotoxicity from penicillamine is increased in patients with the HLA types B8 and DR3, and reduced in patients with HLA DR7; the risk of skin reactions with penicillamine is associated with HLA DRw6, and that of thrombocytopenia is associated with HLA DR4; patients with HLA DR4 also have a greater risk of the lupus-like syndrome (see below) when it is associated with hydralazine).

Drug allergy and its manifestations are classifiable according to the classification of hypersensitivity reactions, i.e. into four types, I to IV (see Section 5).

Type I reactions (anaphylaxis; immediate hypersensitivity)

In type I reactions the drug or metabolite interacts with IgE molecules fixed to cells, particularly tissue mast cells and basophil leucocytes. This triggers a process that leads to the release of pharmacological mediators (histamine, 5-hydroxytryptamine, kinins, and arachidonic acid derivatives), which cause the allergic response.

Clinically, type I reactions manifest as urticaria, rhinitis, bronchial asthma, angio-oedema, and anaphylactic shock. Drugs likely to cause anaphylactic shock include penicillins, streptomycin, local anaesthetics, and iodide-containing radiographic contrast media.

Type II reactions (cytotoxic reactions)

In type II reactions a circulating antibody of the IgG, IgM, or IgA class interacts with a hapten (drug) combined with a cell membrane constituent (protein), to form a hapten–protein/antigen–antibody complex. Complement is then activated and cell lysis occurs. Most examples are haematological: thrombocytopenia from quinidine or quinine ('gin and tonic purpura'), and occasionally rifampicin; 'immune' neutropenia, which can be difficult to distinguish from neutropenia occurring as a direct toxic effect on the bone marrow—phenylbutazone, carbimazole, tolbutamide, anticonvulsants, chlorpropamide, and metronidazole have all been incriminated; and the haemolytic anaemias that penicillins, cephalosporins, rifampicin, and quinidine can also produce by this mechanism.

Type III reactions (immune complex reactions)

In type III reactions, antibody (IgG) combines with antigen, that is the hapten–protein complex, in the circulation. The complex so formed is deposited in the tissues, complement is activated, and damage to capillary endothelium results.

Serum sickness, with fever, arthritis, enlarged lymph nodes, urticaria, and maculopapular rashes, is the typical drug reaction of this type. Penicillins, streptomycin, sulphonamides, and antithyroid drugs may cause it. Another type III reaction is the acute interstitial nephritis that may be caused by penicillins, some non-steroidal anti-inflammatory drugs, and some diuretics.

Type IV reactions (cell-mediated or delayed hypersensitivity reactions)

In type IV reactions, T lymphocytes are sensitized by a hapten–protein antigenic complex. When the lymphocytes meet the antigen an inflammatory response ensues. Examples are the contact dermatitis caused by local anaesthetic creams, antihistamine creams, and topical antibiotics and antifungal drugs. Rashes in response to sulphonamides and thiacetazone are more common in people infected with HIV.

Pseudoallergic reactions

'Pseudoallergy' (included here for convenience) is a term applied to reactions that resemble allergic reactions clinically but for which no immunological basis can be found. For example, asthma and rashes caused by aspirin are pseudoallergic reactions. In some asthmatics aspirin may trigger an attack of asthma. Aspirin-sensitive asthmatics are often sensitive to other salicylates and to other non-steroidal anti-inflammatory drugs, such as indometacin and ibuprofen. In addition, about half of aspirin-sensitive asthmatics are also sensitive to tartrazine (E102), a yellow dye used to colour some medicines and foodstuffs.

In some patients the administration of ampicillin or amoxicillin causes a maculopapular erythematous rash resembling the toxic erythema which can occur in penicillin hypersensitivity. However, the so-called ampicillin rash seems not to have an immunological origin. It can be distinguished from true penicillin hypersensitivity by its later onset after the first dose (typically 10–14 days compared with 7–10 days in penicillin hypersensitivity, though they overlap) and non-recurrence after re-exposure. Unlike penicillin hypersensitivity it carries no increased risk of a serious allergic response to other penicillins. An ampicillin rash occurs in about 1 per cent of the normal population, but in a much higher proportion of some groups of patients: it occurs almost invariably in patients with some viral infections (for example infectious mononucleosis, cytomegalovirus infection, measles), lymphomas, and leukaemias, and the risk is increased in patients taking allopurinol.

Clinical manifestations of allergic reactions

The immunological mechanistic approach does not always fit the clinical presentation, in which one is generally faced with some allergic syndrome.

Drug fever as an isolated phenomenon can occur with penicillins, phenytoin, hydralazine, and quinidine. Such fevers are usually of low grade and the patient is generally not very ill. The fever subsides within a few days of stopping the drug. With the penicillins it can sometimes be difficult to distinguish drug fever from a fever that persists because of resistant infection. Fever is also a manifestation of the neuroleptic malignant syndrome, a rare serious idiosyncratic adverse reaction of unknown cause, usually manifested by a sudden onset of fever, akinesia, rigidity, reduced consciousness, and autonomic disturbances including tachycardia and hypertension; it can kill, and demands emergency treatment by active cooling and intravenous dantrolene.

Rashes of several types may occur, including toxic erythema (due for example to antibiotics, sulphonamides, thiazide diuretics, frusemide (furosemide), sulphonylureas, phenylbutazone), urticaria (penicillins, codeine, dextrans, radiographic contrast media), erythema multiforme (penicillins, sulphonamides, barbiturates, phenylbutazone), erythema nodosum (sulphonamides, oral contraceptives), cutaneous vasculitis (sulphonamides, thiazide diuretics, allopurinol, indometacin, phenytoin), exfoliative dermatitis and erythroderma (gold salts, phenylbutazone, isoniazid, carbamazepine), photosensitivity (amiodarone, sulphonamides, thiazide diuretics, sulphonylureas, tetracyclines, phenothiazines, nalidixic acid), fixed eruptions (barbiturates, sulphonamides, tetracyclines), and toxic epidermal necrolysis (Lyell's syndrome) (phenytoin, sulphonamides, gold salts, tetracyclines, allopurinol).

Drugs may produce thrombocytopenic purpura (for example quinine, digitoxin, rifampicin) or purpura from capillary damage or fragility without thrombocytopenia (corticosteroids, thiazide diuretics).

A syndrome mimicking systemic lupus erythematosus, often involving joints and generally without renal involvement, may follow treatment with hydralazine, procainamide, phenytoin, or ethosuximide. Although this reaction is conveniently discussed here it is to some extent dose dependent, as the risk is increased at higher drug doses, and with hydralazine and procainamide it is more common among slow acetylators.

Asthma occurring as a pseudoallergic reaction to non-steroidal anti-inflammatory drugs and tartrazine has been noted above. Other adverse reactions in the lung include pneumonitis associated with the lupus-like syndrome (see above), pulmonary eosinophilia, and fibrosing alveolitis.

Jaundice may occur as an allergic response to some drugs through either cholestasis (for example with phenothiazines, erythromycin, and chlorpropamide) or generalized liver damage (for example with halothane, isoniazid and monoamine oxidase inhibitors).

Long-term effects causing adverse reactions

Some adverse effects during long-term therapy are related to both the duration of treatment and the dose.

Adaptive changes

These are the basis of some adverse reactions. Examples include the development of tolerance to and physical dependence on narcotic analgesics, and tardive dyskinesia in some patients receiving long-term neuroleptic therapy for schizophrenia.

Rebound phenomena

When adaptive changes occur during long-term therapy, sudden withdrawal of the drug may result in rebound reactions. Examples include the typical syndromes that occur after the sudden withdrawal of narcotic analgesics or of alcohol (delirium tremens). Sudden withdrawal of barbiturates may result in restlessness, mental confusion, and convulsions, and a similar syndrome in which anxiety features prominently may occur after the sudden withdrawal of benzodiazepines. Sleeplessness may also be a feature of the sudden withdrawal of these and a variety of other hypnotic drugs. Sudden withdrawal of some antihypertensive drugs may result in rebound hypertension; this was common with clonidine. Sudden withdrawal of β-adrenoceptor antagonists may result in rebound tachycardia and arrhythmia, sometimes precipitating myocardial ischaemia.

Sudden withdrawal of corticosteroids can cause acute adrenal insufficiency; after long-term administration withdrawal should be very slow.

Reversal of the effects of heparin with protamine sulphate may be associated with rebound hypercoagulability and an increased risk of thromboembolism. However, this risk may have to be taken when heparin overdosage has caused life-threatening bleeding. But the withdrawal of oral anticoagulants, such as warfarin, does not lead to rebound hypercoagulability.

Other long-term effects

Chloroquine may accumulate in the corneal epithelium (causing a keratopathy) and in the retina (causing a pigmentary retinopathy and blindness). The former occurs in over 90 per cent of patients on long-term therapy; the latter is less common but it is more serious. The risk increases with daily doses of over 4 mg/kg and in patients also taking probenecid.

Some of the long-term adverse effects of amiodarone are caused by the deposition in the tissues of lipofuchsin, including a neuropathy, pulmonary alveolitis, liver damage, microdeposits in the cornea, and skin phototoxicity.

Delayed effects causing adverse reactions

Carcinogenesis

The incidence of vaginal adenocarcinoma is increased in the daughters of women who took diethylstilbestrol during pregnancy (hoping to prevent threatened abortion). The incidence of uterine endometrial carcinoma is probably increased in women taking oestrogen replacement therapy for menopausal symptoms, and oral contraceptives increase the incidence of benign liver tumours. Anabolic steroids carry an increased risk of liver tumours.

Various anticancer drugs increase the risk of tumours. Examples include the increased risk of bladder cancer with long-term cyclophosphamide, and of non-lymphocytic leukaemias with alkylating agents such as melphalan, cyclophosphamide, and chlorambucil. Similarly, patients on immunosuppressive drug regimens, such as azathioprine with corticosteroids, have a greatly increased risk of developing lymphomas. This has mainly been noted after renal transplantation, but also in other patients.

Adverse reactions associated with reproduction

Some drugs impair fertility. For example, cytotoxic drugs can cause ovarian failure with amenorrhoea. Sperm production may be reversibly impaired by sulphasalazine, nitrofurantoin, monoamine oxidase inhibitors, and anti-malarials, and irreversibly by cytotoxic drugs.

Teratogenesis

Teratogenesis occurs when a drug taken early in pregnancy causes a developmental abnormality in a fetus. The first trimester of pregnancy, and particularly the period from the second to the eighth weeks of gestation, the period of organogenesis, is the most critical, and during this time drugs may cause structural abnormalities. The brain is vulnerable throughout pregnancy.

For a drug to be teratogenic it must first pass across the placenta. The drugs that do this are those that have a low molecular weight, are poorly ionized at physiological pH, and are very fat soluble. The few drugs that do not pass across the placenta illustrate these principles. For example, heparin is ionized and of high molecular weight and tubocurarine is ionized and relatively lipid insoluble; neither crosses the placenta. However, most drugs in the maternal circulation do reach the fetus to some extent.

If a drug is a known teratogen in humans or animals then the data sheet will say so. However, if a drug is not known to be teratogenic in humans, lack of evidence of teratogenicity in animals cannot be taken as evidence that the drug is not teratogenic in humans. Many new drugs are introduced with the advice that they should not be taken during pregnancy, simply for lack of evidence. Table 6 gives important examples of drugs to avoid during pregnancy.

Adverse effects on the fetus during the later stages of pregnancy

Some drugs that are not teratogenic may have adverse effects on the fetus if given later in pregnancy. Table 7 lists some important drugs that should be avoided or used with care during later pregnancy (some throughout the whole duration of pregnancy).

What should be done if a woman of childbearing potential is given a drug, and then finds out days or weeks later that she is pregnant? First, it is important to identify the drug and the exact time of exposure to it. If it is a known or a likely teratogen, the relation between the time of exposure and the likely time of conception should be determined. It is sometimes possible to identify the precise date of conception, but if it is not, one should try to estimate the gestational age by carefully documenting the recent menstrual history and, if necessary, date the pregnancy by ultrasound. If exposure to a known teratogen has occurred during the first 8 weeks of pregnancy, further investigation may be necessary to identify precise fetal abnormalities. For example, ultrasound can detect many structural abnormalities, and neural tube defects may be diagnosed by measuring serum

Table 6 Some important drugs that may be harmful during early pregnancy

Drug	Effect
Alcohol	Fetal alcohol syndrome
Androgens	Virilization and multiple congenital defects
Antineoplastic agents	Multiple congenital defects
Carbimazole	Aplasia cutis
Corticosteroids (high dosages)	Cleft palate
Cyproterone	Feminization of male fetus
Diethylstilbestrol	Vaginal adenosis and adenocarcinoma in daughters
Distigmine	Increased uterine tone
Ergotamine	Increased uterine tone
Fibrinolytic drugs	Placental separation
Lithium	Cardiovascular and other malformations
Misoprostol	Increased uterine tone
Phenytoin	Fetal hydantoin syndrome
Tetracyclines	Yellow discoloration of teeth, inhibition of bone growth
Valproate	Neural tube defects
Vitamin A analogues	Congenital defects
Warfarin	Multiple congenital defects

Table 7 Drugs to be avoided or used with care during later pregnancy

Drug(s)	Risk to fetus or neonate
Aminoglycoside antibiotics	Eighth nerve damage
Antithyroid drugs	Goitre and hypothyroidism
Aspirin	Kernicterus, haemorrhage (also maternal)
Benzodiazepines	'Floppy infant' syndrome
Chloramphenicol	Peripheral vascular collapse
Disopyramide	May induce labour
Fibrinolytic drugs	Fetal/maternal haemorrhage
Misoprostol	May induce labour
Narcotic analgesics	Respiratory depression. Opiate withdrawal syndrome if mother dependent
Nitrofurantoin	Haemolysis
Non-steroidal anti-inflammatory drugs	Closure of the ductus arteriosus. Delayed and prolonged labour
Pethidine	Respiratory depression
Sulphonamides	Kernicterus
Sulphonylureas	Hypoglycaemia
Tetracyclines	See Table 6
Thiazide diuretics	Thrombocytopenia
Warfarin	Fetal or retroplacental haemorrhage

and amniotic α-fetoprotein concentrations. In such circumstances any advice on termination of a pregnancy should be based on a consideration of the risk of fetal abnormality from both published information and investigation of the individual case.

Adverse reactions to drugs in breast milk

Some drugs can cause adverse effects in babies after ingestion in breast milk. These include drugs that are so extensively excreted in the milk as to cause dose-related adverse effects in the infant, and drugs that do not necessarily enter the milk in large amounts, but whose adverse effects are not dose related. The latter include drugs that may cause hypersensitivity reactions (for example penicillins and sulphonamides), and drugs that are hazardous to babies with glucose 6-phosphate dehydrogenase deficiency (for example nitrofurantoin and primaquine). Drugs to be avoided are listed, for example, in the British National Formulary and the Physician's Desk Reference. If the safety of a drug is in doubt it is best either to choose another drug or, if the drug must be used, to advise the mother to suspend breast feeding.

Methods used in detecting adverse reactions

During the period of clinical trial that a drug undergoes before its general release only the most frequent of adverse reactions will be detected, because so few patients are studied. We need methods for detecting adverse reactions as quickly as possible after marketing, for confirming that the events detected are truly adverse reactions, and for assessing their overall incidence, so that we can try to judge the balance of benefit and harm. Table 8 summarizes some methods of doing this.

Prevention of adverse effects: the role of consumers†

Ordinary people taking a medicine do not usually expect unwanted effects, even if they have received information about them from their doctor, the pharmacist, or most often in the leaflet with the medicine. Most people are optimists, and believe that a medicine prescribed by a doctor or sold in a pharmacy will not cause them any problem—though others might suffer some unpleasant effects.

The aim of information that patients get about adverse effects is to warn that such effects may occur, so that they can:

† Text previously published in *Thérapie*.

Table 8 Some postmarketing surveillance schemes and their advantages and disadvantages

Scheme	Advantages	Disadvantages
Anecdotal reports	Simple, cheap	Rely on individual vigilance and astuteness. Only detect relatively common effects
Voluntary organized reporting	Simple	Under-reporting. Reporting bias by 'bandwagon' effect
Intensive event monitoring	Easily organized	Selected population studied for a short time
Cohort studies	Can be prospective; good at detecting effects	Very large numbers required. Very expensive
Case–control studies	Excellent for validation and assessment	Will not detect new effects. Expensive
Population statistics	Large numbers can be studied	Difficult to coordinate. Quality of information may be poor. Too coarse
Record linkage	Excellent if comprehensive	Time consuming. Expensive. Retrospective. Relies on accurate records

(1) assess the potential disadvantages of the medicine, before deciding whether to take it ;

(2) connect an adverse event with the taking of the medicine and take appropriate action.

What the information rarely, if ever, does is to explain in what specific ways adverse effects may be prevented or at least minimized. There are even many doctors who do not understand this very clearly. The necessary strategy has several components, each related to a particular category of adverse effects.

First come the dose-dependent effects known to occur in everybody if the dose is high enough. They can be prevented or minimized by keeping the dosage as low as possible. If harm is more likely with long continued use of the drug, then the duration of use should be limited, as for example with the neuroleptic antipsychotic drugs.

Second, the effects of drug interactions, which can be prevented by avoiding concurrent use of interacting drugs, or minimized by very careful monitoring if the drugs are essential.

Third are new adverse effects that have not yet been reported, and are a puzzling and unpleasant surprise for everyone concerned. These generally affect such a small proportion of patients that they have remained undetected in premarketing clinical trials. Such surprises are rarer after a drug has been widely used for several years. They can therefore be partially prevented by avoiding the use of new drugs whenever possible, at least during the first few years of their life. If there is a compelling reason for using a new drug, this should be explained to the patient and documented in the records. Furthermore, use of the new drug should be monitored more closely than would be necessary with an older and familiar drug. It is thus important that patients should know whenever the drug prescribed for them is new.

Fourth, adverse effects may result when a prescriber uses a drug with which he or she is insufficiently familiar. So when a doctor is not sure what to prescribe, and at last finds something to try in one of his or her compendia, the patient can reasonably ask how familiar the doctor is with that drug. If it is new to the doctor, then hesitation is appropriate and it may be reasonable to seek a second opinion from someone more experienced.

Fifth, some individuals are especially liable to suffer adverse effects. They may have a genetic abnormality—for example they may be poor metabolizers of a wide range of drugs, or they may lack normal plasma cholinesterase, leading them to suffer suxamethonium apnoea. The development of genetic testing in the coming years will greatly help to identify these people and so enable us to protect them from many kinds of drug-related harm. Meanwhile the best that can be done is always to take a careful medication history, asking about any previous bad experience with medicines, and where a genetic problem is suspected, also a family history. When a genetic abnormality has led to an adverse effect, the patient must be given detailed information about it so that he or she can warn any treating doctor in order to avoid future dangerous exposures.

It can be concluded from all this that all of us, as consumers who are liable to become patients at some time, need to understand a few fundamental principles:

1. All drugs have not only the intended beneficial effects, but can and often do cause harmful or unpleasant effects as well. This knowledge should influence the decision whether or not to accept medication that the doctor or pharmacist or anyone else proposes.

2. Harmful or unpleasant effects are more likely and are often worse with higher than lower doses. It is therefore important to use the lowest dosage that works, and to do so with the doctor's help.

3. Well known and established drugs are safer than new or relatively untried drugs. It is therefore best to avoid new drugs unless there is a convincing reason for using one.

4. If it is necessary to use more than one medicine at the same time, it is important to check that they are safe to use together, and to monitor their use with special care.

5. People can differ greatly in how drugs affect them. We should each learn from our own personal experiences with medicines, and make sure our doctors learn from them too in what they prescribe for us individually.

It will take much effort to educate consumers to the point where they can apply these principles in consultations with health professionals and in their use of medicines. We as professionals must take the lead and teach them, at least by example.

Finding the lowest effective dose: two examples†

A retired economist's hypertension was well controlled by atenolol 25 mg/day, but she was bothered by her slow pulse rate, often below 60 beats/min, and asked her doctor if she could take a smaller dose. He said yes, why not.

The 25 mg tablets are not scored, but the patient succeeded in cutting them more or less in half, rejecting any fragments that looked too small. The blood pressure remained well controlled on half the previous dose, and the pulse rate rose modestly.

Another patient, a biologist with ischaemic heart disease, had a raised serum cholesterol, which a low-fat diet had reduced only slightly to 6.1 mmol/l. On simvastatin 10 mg/day this fell to 5.3 mmol/l, which was still above the target level of 4.5. Simvastatin is made only in 10, 20 and 40 mg tablets, so the doctor wanted to prescribe 20 mg/day. The patient felt that doubling the dose might be unnecessary, so the doctor suggested taking 15 mg/day or one and a half tablets. (That is easier to remember than taking one tablet (10 mg) and two (20 mg) on alternate days.) Although the tablets are not scored they have an oval shape and are easy to break in two. The dose of approximately 15 mg/day lowered the serum cholesterol to 4.4 mmol/l.

Biological variation is often neglected in clinical trials and in the dosage recommendations that are derived from them. New drugs are commonly marketed at higher doses than some patients need, because the company wants to be sure of achieving a therapeutic effect in the majority. The result is that the most sensitive patients get more than they need or than is good

† We are indebted to *Health Which?* (October, 2000), p.15. Consumers Association, London for permission to reproduce these examples.

for them. It is worth asking patients about their experience of drugs—whether they have found small doses effective in the past, or whether they have been ineffective. Dose titration with the patient's help can on occasion improve treatment. And to facilitate this, all tablets should be scored—manufacturers please note.

Drug interactions

A drug interaction occurs when the effects of one drug (the object drug) are altered by the effects of another drug (the precipitant drug). Usually this results in an adverse drug reaction, but in a few cases a drug interaction may prove beneficial. Interactions form about 7 per cent of all adverse drug reactions; among the few patients who die from adverse drug reactions (about 4 per cent of all deaths) about a third are due to interactions.

Drugs likely to precipitate interactions include the following: drugs that are highly protein bound (aspirin, phenylbutazone, sulphonamides, and trichloracetic acid, a metabolite of chloral hydrate), as they are likely to displace object drugs from protein-binding sites; those that stimulate the metabolism of other drugs, including various anticonvulsants (phenytoin, carbamazepine, phenobarbital), rifampicin, griseofulvin. Those that inhibit the metabolism of other drugs, including allopurinol, chloramphenicol, cimetidine, metronidazole and other imidazoles (for example ketoconazole), monoamine oxidase inhibitors, azapropazone and related drugs, and quinolone antibiotics (for example ciprofloxacin); those that affect renal function and alter the renal clearance of object drugs (for example diuretics, probenecid).

The most likely object drugs in interactions are those that have a steep dose–response curve (i.e. drugs for which a small change in dose results in a relatively large change in therapeutic effect, important in interactions causing decreased efficacy of the object drug), and those that have a low therapeutic index (i.e. drugs for which the dose at which toxic effects start to occur is little more than the therapeutic dose, important in interactions causing toxic effects of the object drug). Drugs that fulfil these criteria include the aminoglycoside antibiotics, anticoagulants, anticonvulsants, antihypertensive drugs, cardiac glycosides, cytotoxic and immunosuppressant drugs, oral contraceptives, and drugs that act on the central nervous system.

Drug interactions can be classified by mechanism; Table 9 lists some important examples.

Pharmaceutical interactions

Pharmaceutical interactions are physicochemical, either of a drug with an intravenous infusion solution or of two drugs in the same solution. Such interactions result in the loss of activity of the object drug. Pharmaceutical interactions are too numerous to remember in detail, but they can be avoided by adhering to some simple principles. These include giving intravenous drugs by bolus injection if possible or via an infusion burette, by not adding drugs to infusion solutions other than dextrose or saline, and by avoiding mixing drugs in the same infusion solution, unless the mixture is known to be safe (for example potassium chloride with insulin).

Pharmacokinetic interactions

Pharmacokinetic interactions occur when the precipitant drug alters the absorption, distribution, or elimination (metabolism or excretion) of the object drug.

Absorption interactions

One drug can alter the absorption of another, but such effects are rarely important. Exceptions include the interactions of cholestyramine with warfarin and digitoxin, whose initial absorption and reabsorption after biliary excretion are reduced resulting in increased dosage requirements. Oestrogens are metabolized in the liver and some of their metabolites are excreted in the bile, deconjugated by bowel organisms, and reabsorbed. The effect of the combined oral contraceptive can therefore be reduced and pregnancy can result if a poorly absorbed antibiotic such as ampicillin prevents the bacterial deconjugation of the oestrogen.

Table 9 Mechanisms of drug interactions and some important examples

Mechanism	Example	Outcome
Physicochemical	Calcium gluconate plus sodium bicarbonate	Precipitation of calcium carbonate in infusion solution
Altered absorption	Reabsorption of oestrogens reduced by antibiotics	Unwanted pregnancy
	Gastric emptying increased by metoclopramide	Increased rate of absorption of simple analgesics
Altered protein binding	Displacement of phenytoin by aspirin	Phenytoin toxicity (transient)
Increased metabolism	Oestrogen metabolism increased by carbamazepine, griseofulvin, phenytoin, rifampicin	Unwanted pregnancy
Reduced metabolism	Warfarin metabolism inhibited by amiodarone, azapropazone, chloramphenicol, cimetidine	Warfarin toxicity
	Theophylline metabolism inhibited by erythromycin	Theophylline toxicity
	Phenytoin metabolism inhibited by isoniazid	Phenytoin toxicity
	Azathioprine metabolism inhibited by allopurinol	Azathioprine toxicity
	Amine metabolism inhibited by monoamine oxidase inhibitors (includes tyramine in foods and phenyl-propanolamine in cold cures)	Acute severe hypertension
Reduced renal elimination	Penicillin/cephalosporin excretion reduced by probenecid	Prolonged duration of antibiotic action
	Lithium excretion reduced by diuretics	Lithium toxicity
	Digoxin excretion reduced by amiodarone, quinidine, verapamil	Digoxin toxicity
Drug effects altered at the same site	Naloxone displaces opioids from opioid receptors	Reversal of opioid toxicity
	Vitamin K competes with warfarin for epoxide reductase	Reversal of the effect of warfarin
	β-blockers and verapamil	Risk of heart failure or arrhythmias
	Effects of warfarin enhanced by tetracyclines	Warfarin toxicity
	Fibrates and statins	Increased risk of rhabdomyolysis/renal failure
Drug effects altered at different sites	Effects of psychoactive drugs enhanced by alcohol	Increased sedation
	Cytotoxic drugs act at different stages of the cell cycle	Therapeutic potentiation in cancer chemotherapy
Drug effects altered indirectly	Aspirin causes gastric bleeding and reduces platelet aggregation	Increased risk of bleeding with warfarin and impaired haemostasis
	Diuretics cause potassium loss; enhanced effects of antiarrhythmic drugs	Enhanced effects of digoxin (risk of toxicity, risk of ventricular tachycardia)

There are two good examples of beneficial absorption interactions. Metoclopramide hastens gastric emptying and so hastens the absorption of analgesics used to treat an acute attack of migraine (Fig. 7). Charcoal binds certain drugs in the gut and thus prevents their initial absorption or their reabsorption after biliary excretion or intestinal secretion. This is valuable in the treatment of self-poisoning with drugs such as phenobarbital and tricyclic antidepressants.

Protein-binding displacement interactions

Displacement of one drug by another from its sites of binding to plasma proteins will cause an increase in the circulating concentration of unbound drug, and thus the potential for an increased effect of the displaced drug. Such interactions are important if the object drug is highly protein bound (greater than 90 per cent) and has a low apparent volume of distribution. The important drugs concerned are warfarin, phenytoin, and tolbutamide.

The most common precipitant drugs in protein-binding displacement interactions are sulphonamides, salicylates, and chloral hydrate and some of its congeners (because of their metabolite, trichloracetic acid). In addition, valproate specifically displaces phenytoin.

However, the importance of protein-binding displacement interactions has been exaggerated, and they are often clinically unimportant. The reason is that when drugs such as warfarin, phenytoin, and tolbutamide are displaced their rates of clearance increase in proportion to the degree of displacement. This means that the total concentration of drug in the plasma will fall after displacement, negating the initial effect. Thus, if the patient weathers the initial increase in unbound concentration of the object drug, the interaction will not matter.

Interactions through induction of metabolism

Certain drugs increase ('induce') drug metabolism by increasing the amount of endoplasmic reticulum in hepatocytes and by increasing the content of cytochrome P450 enzymes and cytochrome c reductase, which catalyse mainly oxidative reactions. Induction of the metabolism of an object drug in this way causes a reduction in its effects (resulting, for example, in epileptic fits while on phenytoin, or pregnancy while on an oral contraceptive). Drugs that induce drug metabolism include barbiturates, carbamazepine, griseofulvin, phenytoin, and rifampicin.

Interactions through inhibition of metabolism

Certain drugs inhibit drug metabolism. Interactions of this type fall into two categories: those in which the precipitant drug inhibits one or more particular cytochrome P450 enzymes and those involving other specific metabolic pathways.

Important examples of inhibition of drug metabolism by inhibition of oxidative reactions are: inhibition of warfarin metabolism by cimetidine (Fig. 8), metronidazole, and other imidazoles, chloramphenicol, norfloxacin, and other quinolones, phenylbutazone, azapropazone, sulfinpyrazone; inhibition of phenytoin metabolism by isoniazid; inhibition of theophylline metabolism by quinolone and macrolide antibiotics.

The interaction of allopurinol with azathioprine and 6-mercaptopurine results from the effect of inhibition of a specific metabolic pathway. Both 6-mercaptopurine and azathioprine (which is metabolized to 6-mercaptopurine) are metabolized by xanthine oxidase, which allopurinol inhibits.

The interaction of monoamine oxidase inhibitors with dietary tyramine results in severe hypertension, which can kill. Inhibition of monoamine oxidase results in an increase in the noradrenaline content of sympathetic nerve endings. When tyramine is ingested monoamine oxidase normally inactivates it in the gut wall; however, when monoamine oxidase is inhibited tyramine passes through the gut wall and liver and reaches the systemic circulation. Tyramine releases noradrenaline from its increased stores in nerve endings and a hypertensive crisis results.

Excretion interactions

Most interactions involving drug excretion occur in the kidneys.

Fig. 8 An example of an interaction involving inhibition of drug oxidation. Plasma warfarin concentrations and the prothrombin time both rose after cimetidine (200 mg three times daily) was introduced in volunteers taking daily maintenance doses of warfarin. (Adapted from Serlin MJ et al. (1979). Cimetidine: interaction with oral coagulants in man. The Lancet **ii**, 317–19, with permission. ©The Lancet.)

Inhibition of renal tubular secretion

Probenecid inhibits the tubular secretion of penicillins and cephalosporins, prolonging their therapeutic effects. Quinidine, verapamil, and amiodarone inhibit the tubular secretion of digoxin and salicylates inhibit the active secretion of methotrexate; in both cases toxic effects can occur.

Increased renal tubular reabsorption

Diuretics that inhibit renal tubular sodium reabsorption cause compensatory reabsorption of lithium with consequent toxicity.

Reduced renal tubular reabsorption

Changing the pH of the urine will alter the reabsorption of drugs that are subject to passive reabsorption. This is put to use in the treatment of overdose with salicylates and amphetamines (by alkalinizing or acidifying the urine respectively).

Pharmacodynamic interactions

Pharmacodynamic interactions occur when the precipitant drug alters the effect of the object drug at its site of action.

Interactions at the same site

Direct pharmacodynamic interactions occur when two drugs either act on the same site (antagonism or synergism) or act on two different sites with a similar end result. Many antagonistic interactions are therapeutically beneficial, including the reversal of the effects of opiates with naloxone and the reversal of the actions of warfarin by vitamin K. In contrast, synergistic interactions are often adverse. The effects of warfarin may be increased or decreased by changes in the affinity of warfarin for vitamin K epoxide reductase (clofibrate, D-thyroxine, anabolic steroids), alterations in the synthesis rate of clotting factors (anabolic steroids), changes in the activity of clotting factors (tetracyclines), or decreased availability of vitamin K secondary to decreased plasma lipids (D-thyroxine, anabolic steroids).

The effects of depolarizing skeletal muscle relaxants are potentiated by some antibiotics (for example aminoglycosides, polymixin B, and colistin) and by quinidine and quinine. These interactions are due to the curare-like effects of the precipitant drugs on the motor endplate of skeletal muscle.

Concurrent use of verapamil and a β-adrenoceptor antagonist increases the risks of cardiac arrhythmias and heart failure.

Interactions at different sites

Drugs that depress central nervous function may potentiate each other, whether or not they have effects on the same receptors. The most common example is that of alcohol with any centrally acting drug (Fig. 9).

Fig. 9 A pharmacodynamic interaction. Neither doxepin (20 mg three times daily) nor amitriptyline (20 mg three times daily) alone altered the reaction time. Alcohol alone prolonged the reaction time slightly at all times of testing after drug administration (30, 90, and 150 min). However, the combination of alcohol with either doxepin or amitriptyline prolonged the reaction time by much more than one would expect from the separate effects of each component of the combination. (Adapted from Seppala T, *et al.* (1975). Effect of tricyclic antidepressants and alcohol in psychomotor skills related to driving. *Clinical Pharmacology and Therapeutics* **17**, 515–22, with permission.)

Other examples include the many combinations of cytotoxic drugs used to treat lymphomas and leukaemias, and the use of combinations of antibiotics in the treatment of some infections, even when only one organism is implicated (for example in infective endocarditis and tuberculosis). These are beneficial interactions.

Indirect pharmacodynamic interactions

In indirect pharmacodynamic interactions a pharmacological, therapeutic, or toxic effect of the precipitant drug in some way alters the therapeutic or toxic effect of the object drug, but the two effects are not themselves related and do not themselves interact.

Warfarin and other anticoagulants may be involved in indirect interactions if platelet aggregation is reduced (for example by salicylates, dipyridamole, sulfinpyrazone, mefenamic acid, and other non-steroidal anti-inflammatory drugs), when there is drug-induced thrombocytopenia, if a drug causes gastrointestinal ulceration (for example aspirin and other non-steroidal anti-inflammatory drugs), or if a drug causes enhanced fibrinolysis (for example the biguanides).

Alterations in fluid and electrolyte balance may secondarily alter the effects of some drugs. The effects of cardiac glycosides and the arrhythmogenic effects of some antiarrhythmic drugs (such as quinidine, procainamide, and phenytoin) are increased by potassium depletion (due to potassium-wasting diuretics, corticosteroids, and purgatives for example).

Pharmacogenetics

Pharmacogenetics is the study of the influence of heredity on the pharmacokinetics of drugs and pharmacodynamic responses to them.

Pharmacokinetic defects

The extent to which an individual metabolizes a drug is, at least in part, genetically determined. For example, monozygotic twins metabolize drugs similarly, while dizygotic twins often do not. For most drugs the variability in metabolism is unimodally distributed. However, for some the distribution is bimodal or trimodal, indicating that separate populations of people metabolize those drugs at different rates. The important pathways of drug metabolism subject to pharmacokinetic variability are acetylation, hydroxylation, and suxamethonium hydrolysis.

Acetylation

Some drugs are acetylated by the hepatic enzyme *N*-acetyltransferase, which is distributed bimodally. Fast acetylators have more *N*-acetyltransferase in the liver than slow acetylators; this is inherited as an autosomal dominant trait. The ratio of fast:slow acetylators varies among races, being for example 40:60 in Europe, 85:15 in Japan, and 95:5 in the Inuit. Drugs affected are isoniazid, hydralazine, procainamide, phenelzine, dapsone, and some sulphonamides. Slow acetylators require lower doses of isoniazid and hydralazine than fast acetylators in the treatment of tuberculosis and hypertension respectively. They are also more likely to develop the lupus erythematosus-like syndrome caused by isoniazid, hydralazine, and procainamide, and the peripheral neuropathy caused by isoniazid (which can be prevented or treated with pyridoxine). The interaction between isoniazid and phenytoin, in which isoniazid inhibits phenytoin metabolism, resulting in phenytoin toxicity, occurs more frequently among slow acetylators.

The acetylator status of an individual is easily assessed by giving a sulphonamide, such as sulphadimidine or sulphapyridine, orally and measuring the relative proportions of acetylated and total sulphonamide in a sample of urine passed 5 to 6 h later.

Oxidation

Certain varieties of oxidation are bimodally distributed, but in contrast to acetylation this is a heterogeneous group of defects and they are not all uniformly due to decreased amounts of enzyme. Individuals with impaired and normal oxidation are classified as poor and extensive metabolizers respectively. The main type of defect is the debrisoquine type, an autosomal recessive defect of cytochrome P450 of the type CYP2D6. It occurs in about 9 per cent of Caucasians, and has a lower prevalence in other racial types.

Other drugs that are affected include captopril, codeine, flecainide, metoprolol, nortriptyline, propafenone, and timolol. The dose-related adverse effects of these drugs (for example central nervous system toxicity with nortriptyline) are more likely in poor hydroxylators. Quinidine inhibits some oxidative reactions and may turn an extensive metabolizer of the debrisoquine type into a poor metabolizer.

The metabolism of mephenytoin is mediated by cytochrome CYP2C, whose activity is bimodally distributed. Poor metabolizers of proguanil (used to prevent malaria) do not convert it to the active form cycloguanil, and may fail to respond to treatment.

Sulphoxidation of penicillamine is polymorphic. Poor sulphoxidation is associated with a fourfold increase in the risk of adverse effects in rheumatoid arthritis. Adverse reactions to gold salts containing a thiol group may also be linked to poor sulphoxidation.

Disease associations with polymorphic metabolism

As some diseases may be related to the effects of environmental chemicals, it is of interest that polymorphic acetylation, hydroxylation, and sulphoxidation have other clinical associations. For example, the risks of bladder cancer may be increased in slow acetylators, of parkinsonism in poor debrisoquine hydroxylators, of bronchogenic carcinoma in extensive debrisoquine hydroxylators, and of primary biliary cirrhosis in poor sulphoxidizers.

Suxamethonium hydrolysis

Suxamethonium (succinylcholine) is metabolized in the plasma by the non-specific esterase pseudocholinesterase. Normally this happens quickly and neuromuscular blockade lasts only a few minutes. However, in some people the pseudocholinesterase is of abnormal affinity and amount, and metabolizes the suxamethonium only slowly, resulting in prolonged neuromuscular blockade. Three types of abnormalities of pseudocholinesterase occur, each inherited in autosomal recessive fashion, the dibucaine-resistant, fluoride-resistant, and 'silent' gene types.

Some individuals, perhaps 1 in 1000, have a two- or threefold higher concentration of pseudocholinesterase in the plasma and resist the effects of suxamethonium.

Pharmacodynamic defects

Some biochemical abnormalities make individuals peculiarly sensitive or resistant to the effects of certain drugs.

Red cell enzyme defects (see Section 22)

Unusual drug reactions may affect people whose erythrocytes are deficient in any one of three different but functionally related enzymes, glucose-6-phosphate dehydrogenase, glutathione reductase, and methaemoglobin reductase, which help to prevent the oxidation of various cell proteins. If such an erythrocyte is exposed to an oxidizing agent, haemolysis occurs, probably because of unopposed oxidation of sulphydryl groups in the cell membrane.

Porphyria (see Section 11)

The hepatic porphyrias, acute intermittent porphyria and porphyria cutanea tarda, are characterized by abnormalities of haem biosynthesis. Certain drugs may precipitate an attack of porphyria.

Malignant hyperthermia

This is a serious, potentially fatal, complication of general anaesthesia with halothane, methoxyflurane, and suxamethonium. It affects about 1 in 20 000 anaesthetized patients and is inherited in autosomal dominant fashion. The body temperature rises acutely to 40 to 41 °C, with muscle stiffness, tachycardia, sweating, cyanosis, and tachypnoea. Dantrolene, which decreases the amount of calcium released from sarcoplasmic reticulum, is effective.

Corticosteroid glaucoma

Intraocular pressure rises during daily use of corticosteroid eyedrops, and the rise is trimodally distributed, 65 per cent, 30 per cent, and 5 per cent of individuals having small, medium, and large increases in pressure. Those who have a large increase in pressure are at increased risk of glaucoma. Inheritance is autosomal recessive.

Vitamin D-resistant rickets

Three varieties of rickets are resistant to the effects of vitamin D (cholecalciferol): familial hypophosphataemic rickets, vitamin D dependency, and Fanconi's syndrome (see Section 12).

Coumarin resistance

Coumarin resistance is a rare defect in which 20 times the usual dose may be required to produce satisfactory anticoagulation. It has autosomal dominant inheritance; the mechanism may be resistance of the vitamin K epoxide reductase to inhibition by warfarin.

Monitoring drug therapy

Monitoring drug therapy usually involves trying to measure the clinical response directly. If this is difficult, or is not related directly in time to a dose of the drug, another measure of the pharmacological effect may be required. In some cases it may be necessary to resort to measurement of the plasma concentration of the drug.

Monitoring the therapeutic effects of drugs

Some events can be directly monitored in the individual patient, while some are monitored in a population. The latter can be applied to the individual only in terms of a statistical probability derived from the observed population variability. Examples of therapeutic events that can be monitored in the individual include frequency of seizures during anticonvulsant drug therapy, muscle power during treatment of myasthenia gravis, the frequency of attacks of angina pectoris, and body weight during diuretic therapy.

Preventive measures in medicine cannot be monitored in the individual and their effects must be gauged by population studies. Examples include the frequency of infections after immunization, the reduction of the risks of hypertension by diuretics, and the prevention of the complications of myocardial infarction by streptokinase and aspirin.

Monitoring the pharmacodynamic effects of drugs

In some circumstances the pharmacological effect of a drug can be carefully measured, followed sequentially, and used as a guide to drug therapy even though it may not be correlated precisely with the therapeutic effect. Examples include the effect of insulin on the blood glucose concentration in diabetes mellitus, anticoagulants on the prothrombin time, bronchodilators on FEV_1 and peak flow rate in bronchial asthma, and cancer chemotherapy on tumour markers.

Monitoring drug pharmacokinetics (plasma concentration measurement)

This is useful for a few drugs, namely those for which:

- there is difficulty in measuring or interpreting the clinical evidence of therapeutic or toxic effects.
- the relation between dose and plasma concentration is unpredictable.
- there is a good relation between plasma concentration and effect, which have a low therapeutic index, and which are not metabolized to active metabolites.

The drugs for which plasma concentrations are commonly and usefully measured are listed in Table 10.

Measurement may be useful when individualizing therapy (for example at the start of therapy when the relation between dose and plasma concentration in the individual is uncertain, when rapid changes in renal function alter the relation between dose and plasma concentration, or when another drug alters the relation between dose and plasma concentration), in the diagnosis of suspected toxicity, and in assessing compliance (see above).

Phenytoin

Plasma concentrations of phenytoin in the toxic range are quite well related to its acute toxic effects, but not to its long-term adverse effects, such as gingival hyperplasia, hirsutism and acne, and folate and vitamin D deficiencies. At low dosages it takes about 2 weeks of maintenance therapy to reach steady state after a change in dose, and the higher the plasma concentration the longer it takes (up to 3 weeks or longer in some patients). For this reason the dosage should not be changed too frequently. Provided the sample is not taken too soon after a dose (i.e. within 1 to 2 h), the time of sampling hardly matters for phenytoin, as plasma concentrations fluctuate little between doses.

Table 10 Usual therapeutic and toxic plasma concentrations of commonly measured drugs

Drug	Concentration below which a therapeutic effect is unlikely	Concentration above which a toxic effect is more likely
Gentamicin*	5 µg/ml (peak)	12 µg/ml (peak), 2 µg/ml (trough)
Digoxin	1.0 nmol/1	3.8 nmol/1
Cyclosporin†	80–200 nmol/1	170–300 nmol/1
Lithium	0.4 mmol/1	1.0 mmol/1
Phenytoin	40 µµmol/l	80 µmol/l
Theophylline	55 µmol/1	100 µmol/1

* Conventional dosage regimens.
† Measured in whole blood by specific radioimmunoassay or high-performance liquid chromatography; the actual results depend on the laboratory in which the measurement is made.

Digoxin

Plasma digoxin concentrations correlate well with toxic effects but not with the therapeutic effect within the therapeutic dosage range. The time of blood sampling should be at least 6 h after the previous dose, and 12 h is the best time in patients taking once daily treatment. During regular maintenance dosage without a loading dose, steady state is reached after about 7 days (normal renal function) to 18 days (functionally anephric). The relation between dose and plasma digoxin concentrations is altered by renal impairment (which reduces the clearance of digoxin), for example in older people, and drug interactions (see above). Factors that alter the link between the concentrations and effects of digoxin, and which make it difficult to interpret the plasma concentration, include potassium depletion (which increases the effect of a given concentration of digitalis on the heart) and thyroid disease (hyperthyroidism decreases responsiveness and hypothyroidism increases it). Children younger than 6 months have lower plasma digoxin concentrations at a given dose than older children and adults, and they are also more resistant to the pharmacodynamic actions of digitalis; in them plasma digoxin concentrations cannot be clearly interpreted.

Lithium

Serum lithium concentrations correlate quite well with the therapeutic effect in the range 0.4 to 0.8 mmol/l. At 1.0 to 1.5 mmol/l the incidence of both acute toxicity and long-term adverse effects is increased. Concentrations above 1.5 mmol/l should be avoided. Blood samples should be taken at exactly 12 h after the previous dose, or as near to that as possible. It takes about 3 days for steady state to be reached during regular maintenance therapy, but patients vary widely, and in some it may take a week.

Monitoring of plasma lithium concentration is necessary for several reasons. Lithium is nephrotoxic and is excreted by the kidneys; toxicity is thus self-perpetuating because it causes renal damage, further retention of lithium, and further toxicity. Systemic availability varies from person to person, is altered by diarrhoea, and varies for different formulations. Changes in sodium balance alter the renal excretion of lithium; for example, renal sodium loss induced by diuretics leads to lithium retention.

Aminoglycoside antibiotics

The same principles apply to all the aminoglycoside antibiotics and we shall take gentamicin as an example. The relation between the plasma concentration of gentamicin and its therapeutic efficacy is complicated by the fact that different organisms have different sensitivities to the antibiotic. The toxic effects of gentamicin on the ears and kidneys are related to the 'peak' concentration (the highest concentration measured after a dose, usually occurring about 1 h after an intramuscular injection or the start of an intravenous infusion) and the 'trough' concentration (the concentration measured just before the next dose is due).

With standard regimens a peak plasma concentration of 5 to 9 mg/l is generally considered necessary, although when gentamicin is used together with benzylpenicillin to treat bacterial endocarditis, lower plasma gentamicin concentrations may be effective. Bacteriological measurement of *in vitro* inhibitory concentrations will help to guide therapy. Expert advice on dosage and target plasma concentrations should be obtained.

Theophylline

Plasma theophylline concentrations correlate well with therapeutic and toxic effects. Measurement is essential in any patient who has been taking oral theophylline and is to be given it intravenously.

Ciclosporin

Ciclosporin is generally measured in whole blood and the result of the assay may depend on whether the measurement technique is by immunoassay or high-performance liquid chromatography. The time to steady state is about 2 days and samples should be taken just before the next dose is due. Factors that alter the whole blood concentration of ciclosporin without a change in dose include reduced absorption (due to diarrhoea or reduced bile-salt production), reduced metabolism (due to liver disease or inhibition by drugs such as ketoconazole and cimetidine or grapefruit juice), and increased metabolism (due to enzyme-inducing drugs).

Further reading

Clinical pharmacology

Laurence DR, Bennett PN, Brown MJ (1997). *Clinical pharmacology*, 8th edn. Churchill Livingstone, Edinburgh. [Lively and readable, with interesting and stimulating quotations and references.]

Ritter JM, Lewis LD, Mant TGK (1999). *A textbook of clinical pharmacology*, 4th edn. Arnold, London. [Well organized, illustrated with many clinical case vignettes.]

Pharmacological effects of drugs

Rang HP, Dale MM, Ritter JM (1999). *Pharmacology* 4th edn. Churchill Livingstone, Edinburgh.

Pharmacokinetics

Rowland M, Tozer TN (1994). *Clinical pharmacokinetics. Concepts and applications*, 3rd edn. Lea and Febiger, Philadelphia. [An excellent text that needs to be worked through systematically. Covers basic concepts, principles of kinetics as applied to drugs, therapeutic regimens, and individualization of therapy. Well illustrated with practical problems.]

Adverse effects of drugs

Dukes MNG, Aronson JK, eds (2000). *Meyler's side effects of drugs*, 14th edn. Elsevier, Amsterdam. [Adverse reactions to drugs discussed under the headings of the individual drugs or groups of drugs, arranged in chapters according to class of drug. Good indexes with separate listings for drugs and diseases. Supplemented by *Side effects of drugs Annuals*. Elsevier, Amsterdam, published annually since 1977. A special feature is minireviews of specific topics, distinguished from the main text typographically.]

Herxheimer A (1991). How much drug in the tablet? *Lancet* **337**, 346–8.

Inman WHW, ed (1986). *Monitoring for drug safety*, 2nd edn. MTP, Lancaster.

Monitoring drug therapy

Aronson JK, Hardman M, Reynolds DJM (1993). *ABC of monitoring drug therapy*. BMJ Publications, London. [Introduction to the principles of monitoring drug therapy by plasma drug concentration measurement, with separate monographs for each important drug.]

Useful website

The British National Formulary http://bnf.org.

10

Nutrition

10.1 Diseases of overnourished societies and the need for dietary change

J. I. Mann and A. S. Truswell

Introduction

Nutrition issues at different stages of technical and economic development

Inappropriate nutrition contributes to illness and premature death in populations throughout the world. The nutritional problems of a country depend more upon the stage of technical and economic development than geographical location (Table 1). Until about 10 000 years ago our ancestors were hunter–gatherers. There are few contemporary hunter–gatherers left, but some of these have been studied, for example !Kung bushmen. Hunter–gatherers collected a wide range of plant foods, but also ate meat and fish. They ate little salt, alcohol, or milk (other than breast milk as infants), little cereal, and no refined sugar apart from honey. Studies of contemporary hunter–gatherers indicate that they do not become obese but may experience seasonal hunger. We infer also that malnutrition was uncommon unless illness or injury supervened. High blood pressure or coronary heart disease would have been rare and plasma cholesterol was probably low. Teeth were worn down by hard food and caries was rare. With prolonged lactation, births were spaced fairly widely. The weaning period of childhood was precarious but general nutritional health was good. *Homo sapiens* evolved as hunter–gatherers and it is unlikely there has been sufficient time to adapt physiologically to many modern foods.

Many contemporary people in the Third World are peasant agriculturists living a way of life similar to that of the rural population of Western Europe and North America until the industrial revolution. They tend to rely on the one crop with the best yield and are vulnerable to crop diseases or crop toxins and droughts. Milling and refining cereals increases the risk

Table 1 Nutrition issues at different stages of technical and economic development

Hunter–gatherers
Occasional seasonal hunger
Malnutrition uncommon
General nutritional health good
Peasant agriculturists
Single crop staple
Clinical disorders may result from single or multiple nutrient deficiencies
Hypertension may occur
Urban slum and periurban shanties
Inadequate breast feeding
Inadequate food
Diarrhoea and other infective disorders, especially in young children
Marasmus
Obesity and alcoholism may occur
Affluent societies
High fat energy dense diets
Physical inactivity
Obesity, coronary heart disease, and hypertension common
Malnutrition may occur in frail elderly and sick

of malnutrition. Though some foods are stored, diet is seasonal. Malnutrition can occur from lack of essential nutrients in the staple food, for example vitamin A deficiency, pellagra, kwashiorkor, and iodine deficiency disorders. Hypertension occurs (salt is available) but coronary heart disease is rare.

Urban slum and periurban shanties are homes for an increasing proportion of the growing populations of Third World countries who are pouring into overcrowded, unsanitary accommodation in vast, polluted cities. Conditions are reminiscent of the slums of London, Manchester, and New York in the nineteenth century. These people have lost their contact with the land and food traditions and for them food is expensive. Mothers of young children have to go out to work. Breast feeding is impossible and it is very difficult to keep bottle feeds hygienic. Young children are most susceptible to diarrhoeal and other infectious diseases; these, with the mothers' absence and inadequate food, can lead to marasmus. Among adults, however, some become obese, others may be alcoholics.

In affluent societies, the prosperous people in the First World do not have to worry about the problems of getting food and keeping it uninfected. Food is cheap for them and they can eat their favourite food all year round. There is a multiplicity of nutrition advice and concerns with breakthroughs and scares, science, and pseudoscience about all food. The diet is high in fat and dense in energy. Obesity and its related disorders, coronary heart disease and hypertension (with its complications), are the principal causes of death. While sports are watched on television by millions, many ordinary citizens do not undertake any physical activity that promotes health. Obesity is unfashionable but difficult to avoid and increasing. Malnutrition occurs in the frail elderly and the sick but this malnutrition is usually subclinical and identified mainly by biochemical tests.

As mortality due to infectious disease is reduced by antibiotics and immunization in most Third World countries, and as their people are living longer and increasingly adopting Western foods and labour-saving techniques, non-communicable diseases are the major causes of death. These non-communicable diseases formerly affected only the ruling and merchant elite of developing countries but there is now a growing epidemic of obesity, diabetes, hypertension, and coronary heart disease. Health authorities in all but the least developed countries have the formidable task of providing education and food policies both to prevent malnutrition and at the same time to prevent overnutrition.

Epidemiological methods used to study nutrition-related diseases

The nutritional component of non-communicable diseases is more difficult to study than classical nutrition deficiency diseases because they develop slowly and are multifactorial. The dietary factor may be a 'risk factor' rather than a direct cause. However, there is now convincing evidence that dietary change can appreciably reduce the risk of some important non-communicable diseases. Very often the first clue to the association between a food or nutrient and a disease comes from observing striking differences in disease incidence between countries (or groups within a country) which correlate with differences in nutritional intake. Sometimes, dietary changes over time in a single country have been found to coincide with changes in disease rates. Such observations give rise to hypotheses about possible diet–disease links, rather than proof of causation because many potential causative factors may be confounded by parallel dietary changes.

Retrospective or case–control studies have sometimes been used as a rapid and inexpensive way of testing hypotheses. A series of people who have been diagnosed with, for example, cancer of the large bowel, are asked what they usually eat, or what they ate before they became ill. These 'cases' are compared with at least an equal number of 'controls', people without bowel cancer, matched for age, gender, and, if possible, social condition. Weaknesses of the method include the possibility that the disease may affect food habits, that cases cannot recall their diet accurately before the cancer was diagnosed, that controls may have some condition that affects dietary habits, or that food intakes are recorded from cases and controls in a different way ('bias'). Furthermore, it is conceivable (and for coronary heart disease and cancer, likely) that dietary factors may operate many years before the condition comes to light.

Prospective or cohort studies avoid the biases involved in asking people to recall past eating habits. Information about food intake and other characteristics are collected well before onset of the disease. Large numbers of people must therefore be interviewed and examined; they must be of an age at which bowel cancer (say) starts to be fairly common (i.e. middle aged) and in a population which has a fairly high rate of this disease. The healthy cohort thus examined and recorded is then followed up for five or more years. Eventually, a proportion will be diagnosed with bowel cancer and the original dietary details of those who develop cancer can be compared with the diets of the majority who have not developed the disease. Usually, a number of dietary and other environmental factors are found to be more, or less, frequent in those who develop the disease. These, then, are apparent risk factors, or protective factors. However, they are not necessarily the operative factor. Fruit consumption may appear to be protective but perhaps, in this cohort, smokers eat less fruit and smoking may be more directly related. This confounding has to be quantified by analysing the data to see the relationship of fruit to the disease at different levels of smoking.

Definitive proof that a dietary characteristic is a direct causative or protective factor may come from one or more randomized, controlled, prevention trials. These involve either the addition of a nutrient or other food component as a supplement to those in the experimental group and a placebo taken by the control group, or the prescription of a dietary regime to the experimental group while the controls continue to follow their usual diet. Disease (and death) outcomes in the two groups are compared. Such trials have the advantage of being able to prove causality as well as potential cost/benefit of the dietary change. However, they are costly to carry out because it is usually necessary to study large numbers of people over a prolonged period. Quite often a single trial does not, in itself, produce a definitive answer but by combining the results of all completed trials in a meta-analysis more meaningful answers are obtained.

Much research involving the role of diet in chronic, degenerative disease has centred around the effects of diet on modifying risk factors rather than the disease itself. For many chronic diseases there are biochemical markers of risk. High plasma cholesterol, for example, is an important risk factor for coronary heart disease. Innumerable studies have examined the role of different nutrients and foods on plasma cholesterol or other risk factors. Such studies are cheaper and easier to undertake than population-based studies since far fewer people are studied over a relatively short period of time. They have helped to find which foods lower cholesterol and so should help protect against coronary heart disease. It is this information that has formed the basis of the public health messages which may have contributed to the decline in the incidence of coronary disease in most affluent societies over the last 20 years.

In this age of evidence-based medicine one would ideally like to see the results of randomized, controlled trials before offering dietary advice. However, this may be impossible to achieve. For example a clinical trial to demonstrate that a particular dietary manipulation will reduce the risk of

cancer may require a trial of such magnitude and duration that it is impractical and a decision as to whether or not to recommend dietary change will need to be based on a lesser degree of evidence. Such evidence might include consistent, strong associations in longitudinal studies, biological plausibility, and corroborative experimental evidence. A dose–response relationship between the putative causal factor and the disease provides particularly strong evidence that the association is causal and that modification may reduce risk.

Tools of the trade for nutritionists

The methods for measuring food and drink intake are important tools for those who study diet–chronic disease relationships. Many studies have examined the association between changing patterns of food consumption at a national level and disease rates in various countries. Such studies do no more than provide clues for further research since the dietary data do not accurately reflect the consumption by individuals. Dietary intake of individuals is assessed by means of food frequency questionnaires, diet records, and recalls which all have different strengths and weaknesses. A weakness of most methods of assessing dietary intake is that some people, especially those who are overweight or obese, tend to underestimate their intake. Food composition tables are required to convert information gathered regarding food intake to consumption of energy and essential nutrients. Sometimes it is more reliable to assess the intake of a nutrient by measuring the level in the blood or urine or activity in the body than attempting to calculate intake from a diet record or food frequency questionnaire. Urinary sodium and iodine are examples of such biomarkers. Glutathione peroxidase activity provides a measure of assessing selenium status in those with a relatively low intake.

Coronary heart disease

Experimental, epidemiological, and clinical trial data provide strong evidence for the role of nutritional factors in the aetiology of coronary heart disease and the potential for dietary modification to reduce cardiovascular morbidity and mortality in the population as a whole, in individuals at high risk, and in those who have already experienced a cardiovascular event. Prospective studies suggest a wide range of foods and nutrients which may be involved (Table 2). Foods which increase the risk of coronary heart disease, when consumed in large amounts, probably do so because they are rich in saturated or *trans*-unsaturated fatty acids, and dietary cholesterol. 'Protective' foods contain several different nutrients which may reduce cardiovascular risk. Oily fish is rich in very long chain polyunsaturated fatty acids (eicosapentaenoic and docosahexaenoic acids; C20:5,*n*-3, C22:6,*n*-3). Fruit and vegetables are good sources of antioxidant nutrients, folate, and other biologically active substances. Nuts contain several potentially 'protective' fatty acids (oleic and linoleic acids; C18:1, C18:2) as well as vitamin E. Whole grain cereals are good sources of dietary fibre as well as some unsaturated oils. An example of the findings in one epidemiological study are given in Table 3. Each of the nutrients mentioned has an appropriately favourable or adverse effect on one or more of the cardiovascular risk factors (Table 4). The fact that some prospective studies suggest a protective effect of antioxidants derived from foods, whereas others have found particular benefit from antioxidant nutrient supplements, represents the single inconsistency in a very large body of data.

Clinical trials have shown that when diet is modified to facilitate appropriate changes in the nutrients mentioned above, levels of risk factors are altered in a favourable direction and cardiovascular events are reduced, even when the intervention is started in middle age with cardiovascular disease already present. The various trials have involved different dietary interventions so that formal meta-analysis is inappropriate, nevertheless it is possible to draw certain general conclusions regarding likely benefit from various dietary changes. Most have aimed for a reduction in plasma cholesterol by manipulation of dietary fat intake. For every 1 per cent reduction in plasma cholesterol a 2 to 3 per cent reduction in cardiovascular events

Table 2 Foods and nutrients which may promote or protect against coronary heart disease

Promoting Foods	Nutrients	Protective Foods	Nutrients
High fat dairy products	Saturated fatty acids	Fruits	Dietary fibre (non-starch polysaccharide)
Fatty meats	*Trans* unsaturated fatty acids	Vegetables	Linoleic acid (C18:2, *n*-6), α-linolenic acid (C18:3, *n*-3)
Eggs	Dietary cholesterol	Whole-grain cereals	Antioxidant nutrients, especially vitamin E and flavonoids
Margarine[a]		Oily fish Nuts Alcohol	Folate

[a] Margarines containing appreciable quantities of *trans* unsaturated fatty acids

occurs. Thus an 8 to 10 per cent reduction in cholesterol, which can be achieved by modifying the nature of dietary fat (replacing saturated fatty acids with mono- and *cis*-polyunsaturated fatty acids and cereals, vegetables, and fruit) will result in appreciable benefit. Trials which have examined potential benefits of dietary manipulations other than those designed to lower plasma cholesterol suggest that further clinical benefit might accrue from favourable changes in other risk factors. Consumption of oily fish two or more times per week, or a small amount of fish oil taken as a supplement, have been shown to reduce cardiovascular death in those with pre-existing coronary artery disease. While increased intakes of vegetables and fruit may confer a cardioprotective effect, there is at present no convincing evidence from clinical trials of benefit associated with the use of antioxidant nutrient supplements. The role of margarines rich in plant sterols and stanols, which may further lower dietary cholesterol by preventing absorption and reabsorption of dietary cholesterol, is yet to be established.

Community programmes, aiming to achieve dietary change along the lines indicated here, have been shown to reduce cardiovascular risk factors and one—the North Karelia Project in Finland—has shown that, in the intervention county, cardiovascular disease mortality decreased to a greater extent than might have been expected on the basis of experience in other Finnish provinces. The availability of appropriate food choices at reasonable cost is an essential component of any programme aimed at reducing cardiovascular risk, since rates are highest in those of the lowest socioeconomic status. While those at the highest personal risk are likely to show the greatest individual benefit from dietary and lifestyle changes, national coronary heart disease rates will only be reduced if changes are made by the population at large. The main purpose of such recommendations is to reduce the risk of morbidity and mortality from coronary heart disease in those who are in the prime of life. Even greater reduction in morbidity and mortality and an improvement in life expectancy may occur in succeeding generations who will have reduced lifetime exposure to risk factors related to lifestyle.

Hypertension

Over 30 years ago, Dahl drew attention to the correlation between salt intake and prevalence of hypertension in populations. This and other similar studies were flawed by methodological difficulties associated with measuring salt intake and blood pressure. The more recent Intersalt Study used standardized blood pressure measurements and 24-h urinary sodium excretion, the best available method of assessing intake. The study, which involved 52 centres in 32 countries, suggested that a difference in sodium intake of around 100 mmol/day over a 30-year period might be expected to result in differences of approximately 10 mmHg in systolic blood pressure and 6 mmHg in diastolic blood pressure. Meta-analyses of observational data and intervention trials show broadly comparable results. In one such meta-analysis, of 68 crossover trials and 10 randomized controlled trials of dietary salt reduction, it appears that a reduction of daily sodium intake of about 50 mmol (about 3 g salt) would, after a few weeks, lower systolic blood pressure by an average of 5 mmHg and by 7 mmHg in those with high blood pressure; diastolic blood pressure would be lowered by half as much. It is estimated that such a reduction in salt intake by a whole Western population would reduce the incidence of stroke by 26 per cent and of coronary heart disease by 15 per cent. Reduction also in the amount of salt added to processed foods would lower blood pressure by twice as much and could prevent as many as 70 000 deaths per year in Britain. The heterogeneity in the response of individuals to sodium restriction suggests the possible existence of a group of hyper-responders but there is as yet no clear indication as to how such individuals might be defined.

Table 3 Relative risk and 95 per cent confidence intervals (CI) of coronary heart disease according to specified intake of wholegrain foods in the Nurses Health Study (75 521 women aged 38–63 years at baseline); multivariate relative risk adjusted for other cardiovascular risk factors

Whole-grain food	Relative risk					P for trend
	Almost never	<1 serving/week	2–4 servings/week	5–6 servings/week	>1 serving/day	
Whole-grain breakfast cereal Relative risk (95 per cent CI)	1.00	0.89 (0.72,1.10)	0.72 (0.56, 0.92)	0.82 (0.66, 1.02)	0.76 (0.57, 1.00)	0.007
Cooked oatmeal (servings/d) Relative risk (95 per cent CI)	1.00	0.92 (0.79,1.08)	0.70 (0.49, 0.98)	1.41 (0.75, 2.66)	1.10 (0.45, 2.68)	0.68
Brown rice (servings/d) Relative risk (95 per cent CI)	1.00	0.86 (0.72,1.02)	0.77 (0.45, 1.32)	0.45 (0.06, 3.20)	–	0.04
Wheat germ (servings/d) Relative risk (95 per cent CI)	1.00	0.55 (0.37, 0.81)	1.11 (0.64, 1.93)	0.41 (0.15, 1.10)	–	0.01
Bran (servings/d) Relative risk (95 per cent CI)	1.00	0.76 (0.59, 0.98)	0.68 (0.44, 1.03)	0.63 (0.42, 0.95)	–	0.001

Reproduced from Liu S *et al.* (1999). Whole-grain consumption and risk of coronary heart disease: results from the Nurses' Health Study. *American Journal of Clinical Nutrition* **70**, 412–19, with permission.

Table 4 Some effects of nutrients which promote or protect against coronary heart disease on cardiovascular risk factors

Nutrient	Effect
Promoting	
Saturated fatty acids	↑ total and LDL cholesterol
	↑ thrombogenesis
	↓ insulin sensitivity
Trans unsaturated fatty acids	↑ total and LDL cholesterol and Lp(a)
Dietary cholesterol (when taken in large amounts)	↑ total and LDL cholesterol
Protective	
Dietary fibre	↓ total and LDL cholesterol
	↑ insulin sensitivity
Folic acid	↓ homocysteine
Antioxidant nutrients	↓ oxidation of LDL
Unsaturated fatty acids (C18:2,*n*-6); C18:3,*n*-3; C20:5,*n*-3; C22:6,*n*-3)	↓ thrombogenesis

↑ increase; ↓ decrease

Several mechanisms have been suggested to explain the association between salt intake and blood pressure, including reduced urinary sodium excretion and fluid retention by some individuals, increased sympathetic nervous system activity and impaired baroreflex function, and alterations of ion transport in vascular smooth muscle.

Obese people have higher blood pressures than non-obese people and if they lose weight blood pressure falls even if the usual salt intake is maintained on the restricted diet. An Australian trial showed, in a clinical trial setting, that weight reduction (maximum loss of 7.4 kg) compared favourably with metoprolol in the treatment of mild hypertension, and diet was associated with an improved plasma lipid profile not seen on the drug.

In epidemiological studies, blood pressure increases progressively when reported alcohol intake increases above three drinks per day. Several intervention studies have shown that reduction of alcohol intake can produce an appreciable reduction in blood pressure amongst hypertensive heavy drinkers. For example one study showed that replacing standard beer (5 per cent alcohol) with a reduced alcohol beer (0.9 per cent alcohol) produced a reduction in alcohol intake from 450 to 64 ml/week and a significant fall in blood pressure.

High intakes of potassium and calcium and a vegetarian diet have also been shown to be associated with reduced levels of blood pressure. However, it was previously believed that these were relatively unimportant compared with dietary sodium and overweight. The recent DASH (Dietary Approaches to Stop Hypertension) trial has shown a remarkably powerful blood pressure-lowering effect in association with a diet rich in fruit, vegetables, and low-fat dairy products. In hypertensive individuals, systolic and diastolic blood pressures were lowered by 11 and 6 mmHg respectively, compared with the control group. Smaller changes were seen in the normotensive group, 3 and 9 mmHg for systolic and diastolic pressures respectively. These findings require confirmation.

Diabetes mellitus

Diet undoubtedly plays an important aetiological role in type 2 diabetes mellitus. As early as 1920, Himsworth suggested that excessive intake of energy, deficiency of dietary carbohydrate, and possibly an excessive intake of fat might increase the risk of diabetes. His conclusions were largely based on the improved glucose tolerance observed in non-diabetic individuals eating a high carbohydrate compared with a high fat/low carbohydrate diet. He also noted the association between high carbohydrate intakes and reduced mortality from diabetes and the fact that newly diagnosed diabetic patients were found to have a high intake of total energy (especially energy derived from fatty foods) before the onset of symptoms than non-diabetic controls. Although Himsworth's findings are based on studies which may

not fulfil the criteria required of modern nutritional epidemiology, the conclusions have largely been confirmed by subsequent epidemiological and clinical studies.

Epidemiological surveys and longitudinal studies in many countries confirm the striking association between increasing degrees of obesity and the risk of developing type 2 diabetes mellitus. The association is strongest in those with central (android) obesity and those with a family history of the condition, reflecting the importance of genetic determinants (see also Chapter 10.5). While energy intake in excess of requirements is now universally accepted as an important risk determinant, controversy has raged with regard to the extent to which macronutrient distribution and some micronutrients might be involved in the aetiology of type 2 diabetes. Epidemiological evidence suggests that the condition is uncommon in people eating a range of 'traditional diets' high in fresh fruit, vegetables, and cereals, and therefore high in starches and non-starch polysaccharides and low in fat. Diabetes prevalence seems to increase rapidly when traditional lifestyles are exchanged for the Western way of life, particularly when such transitions occur over a short time span. Such changes have been clearly demonstrated in Micronesians, Polynesians, American Indians, and Aboriginal Australians, as well as Chinese and Asian immigrants to Mauritius. A sharp rise in the frequency of type 2 diabetes mellitus also emerges from studies of Asian Indian immigrants to Fiji, South Africa, and Britain, and of Chinese in Singapore, Taiwan, and Hong Kong. The change from traditional to a Western diet is usually accompanied by a reduction in physical activity. As lifestyle change starts to occur in China and India, by far the most populous countries, type 2 diabetes mellitus may create an enormous public health problem. Indeed, it seems reasonable to claim that the disease has already reached epidemic proportions in many indigenous populations amongst whom it is difficult to disentangle the relative importance of genetic and environmental factors. By contrast, North Western Europeans and Anglo-Celts have a relatively low susceptibility to diabetes.

It is not yet clear whether any single attribute of the Western way of life is particularly important in increasing the risk of diabetes. Excess sucrose has been largely exonerated as an important dietary factor in the aetiology of type 2 diabetes, except perhaps when, alongside a high intake of fat, it contributes towards an excessive energy intake. A high intake of saturated fatty acids undoubtedly further decreases insulin sensitivity, an underlying abnormality in type 2 diabetes. One large prospective study of health professionals in the United States has found that a high intake of low glycaemic index foods (i.e. predominantly carbohydrate-containing foods producing a relatively low glycaemic excursion after ingestion when compared with a comparable amount of glucose) tends to protect against type 2 diabetes and that the effect is independent of other individual dietary attributes. A low level of physical activity appears to be an important predisposing factor for obesity and hence type 2 diabetes. Thus, it seems most likely that a combination of factors is responsible.

Australian Aboriginals who have adopted a Western diet have high rates of diabetes. A study in Australia showed that reverting to their traditional lifestyle is associated with a marked improvement in several indices of carbohydrate metabolism. Many studies in affluent societies have shown that weight reduction in overweight people, those with impaired glucose tolerance, and people with diabetes can often result in normal, or near normal, blood glucose levels without the need for oral hypoglycaemic therapy. Furthermore, diets high in soluble forms of non-starch polysaccharides and in which low glycaemic index carbohydrate-containing foods predominate can improve glycaemic control in those with diagnosed diabetes, independent of an effect on body mass. However, in people who are not overweight, sufficient improvement to reduce the need for drug therapy and achieve even near normal blood glucose concentrations is seen only with extreme dietary change (i.e. diets consisting largely of raw and unprocessed foods and exceptionally low in fat). Intervention studies in people with impaired glucose tolerance suggest that risk of progression to diabetes can be reduced and that this results chiefly from weight loss rather than modification of individual nutrients. However, the largest intervention study involving advice to modify diet and increase physical activity carried out so far has been in progress for 6 years, and there is a suggestion that the condition may relapse with time, possibly as a consequence of reverting to previous lifestyle habits. Thus, while it appears that reducing the level of obesity in the population at large is the single measure most likely to reduce overall rates of type 2 diabetes mellitus in high-risk groups, the extent to which risk reduction can be achieved in practice remains to be established.

Although diet is important in the management of type 1 diabetes, nutritional factors do not appear to have contributed to the aetiology of the disease to the same extent as for type 2 diabetes mellitus. Genetic and other environmental factors are believed to be more important. Recent studies have suggested, however, that infants who have been breastfed may have a reduced risk of type 1 diabetes mellitus in later life and this observation could be linked with immune mechanisms known to be associated with this condition.

Cancers

The development of cancer involves several stages and occurs over a long period of time. Nutritional factors may operate at one or more of these stages. During the first stage of initiation, the DNA of the healthy cell is damaged by chance mutation or a carcinogen. During the promotion (second) stage, the 'initiated' cells may be exposed to promoters, environmental factors, which create conditions which favour their growth over that of normal cells. This phase tends to be prolonged and may be delayed or accelerated by environmental factors. Genetic factors also operate. Ultimately, preneoplastic cells are formed which differ in appearance and function from normal cells. During the final stage of progression, additional mutations tend to occur leading to the transformation of preneoplastic to neoplastic cells. Nutritional factors may act as carcinogens or promoters. Given this long natural history of the disease process, it is hardly surprising that few data from intervention trials are available and data relating dietary factors to various cancers are derived from epidemiological associations and animal experiments. Nevertheless Doll and Peto have estimated that about one-third of all cancers in Western countries may be attributed to diet. The dietary and nutritional factors which may play a role in human cancer are listed in Table 5.

Breast cancer is a common cancer amongst women in the Western world. There is a strong, positive correlation between fat intake and breast cancer rates in different countries and a pooled analysis of case–control studies suggest an increase in relative risk of breast cancer associated with a high fat intake in postmenopausal but not premenopausal women. Animals given chemical carcinogens develop fewer tumours if they are given a low fat diet. However, prospective studies have not confirmed higher rates of breast cancer in women with high fat intakes. Thus, it is not absolutely clear whether fat intake is a risk factor *per se* or simply a marker for some other important environmental factor operating in countries with high rates of breast cancer. Furthermore, high fat intakes may be associated with obesity, high circulating endogenous oestrogens, and early menarche, all of which have been clearly established as risk factors. Plant oestrogens (isoflavones from soy products, lignans in wholegrain cereals and vegetables) may also be protective by increasing the length of the menstrual cycle, thus reducing the number of menstrual cycles and reducing exposure to peak hormone levels.

Cigarette smoking is unquestionably the most important cause of lung cancer, one of the most common cancers. However, vegetables and fruit have consistently been shown to have a protective effect in more than 30 case–control and prospective studies. A large clinical trial in which heavy smokers were given supplements of α-tocopherol, β-carotene (presumed to be the protective factors in vegetables and fruit), or placebo, showed no clinical benefit but with hindsight the results were not surprising. It seems most unlikely that the carcinogenic effects of prolonged, heavy cigarette smoking can be reversed by vitamin supplements given over a short period of time.

Colorectal cancer is the second most common cause of cancer amongst males. A low intake of vegetables and non-starch polysaccharide appear to be the most consistent dietary factors associated with increased risk. Non-starch polysaccharide escapes digestion in the small intestine and is fermented in the large bowel by the colonic microbial flora. Short chain fatty acids are produced, one of which, butyrate, is an antiproliferative agent. Non-starch polysaccharide may further reduce the risk of large bowel cancer by stimulating bacterial growth and increasing the biomass as well as the unfermented non-starch polysaccharide binding with water, so leading to an increase in stool weight, dilution of colonic contents, and faster transit time through the large bowel. High fat diets are associated with increased concentration of bile acids in the colon. These are converted to secondary bile acids, of which deoxycholic acid is a known promoter of

Table 5 Nutritional determinants of various cancers

Factor	Cause + Prevent –	Cancers
Dietary fat	+	Colorectal, breast, prostate, pancreas
ω3-PUFA	–	Colorectal, breast
ω3-PUFA	+	Prostate, breast, ovary (endocrine-related)
Fish oils	–	Colorectal, breast
Obesity	+	Colorectal, oesophagus, breast, endometrium, gallbladder
Exercise, lack of	+	Colorectal
Meat	+	Colorectal, breast
Protein	+	Colorectal, pancreas, breast, prostate
Soy	–	Breast
Grilled, fried meat	+	Colon
Salt	+	Stomach
Salted foods	+	Stomach, colorectal
Pickled, 'processed' foods	+	Stomach, nasopharyngeal
Mouldy foods (e.g. aflatoxin)	+	Oesophagus, stomach, liver
Sugar	+	Breast, pancreas
Iron	+	Colorectal
Calcium	–	Colorectal
Milk	–	Oesophagus, stomach
Folic acid	–	Cervix, colorectal
Nitrates	+	Stomach
Alcohol	+	Liver, pancreas, oesophagus, colorectal, head and neck, mouth, stomach, breast
Fruits, vegetables		
Antioxidants: selenium, vitamins C, E, retinoids (vitamin A), β-carotene, carotenoids (lyopene, lutein)	–	Epithelial cancers, especially respiratory and alimentary tracts: lung, nasopharynx, oesophagus, stomach, colorectal, mouth, pancreas, breast, bladder, cervix, prostate
Non-nutritive plant chemicals: glucosinolates, indoles, flavanoids, sulphur compounds	+/–	Digestive tract
Dietary fibre, non-starch polysaccharides	–	Colorectal
Resistant starch	–	Colorectal
Plant sterols	–	Breast, prostate, hormone-dependent

The evidence for many of the relationships is not yet conclusive; this list is not exhaustive.
PUFA = polyunsaturated fatty acids.

large bowel cancer. A 4-year intervention trial has shown that a low fat diet (fat providing less than 25 per cent total energy) plus 25 g wheat bran daily can reduce the frequency of large adenomas in the large bowel but this has not been confirmed in two other comparable studies. There is insufficient evidence to reliably incriminate another potentially deleterious factor: high intake of red meat. However, it is possible that the method used for cooking meat may be important. Increased intakes of heterocyclic amines may form on the surface of cooked meat, especially during grilling, frying, or cooking on a barbecue. It has also been suggested that n-3 polyunsaturated fatty acids may be protective because they slow down the rate of cell division of mucosal colonic cells.

Cancer of the prostate is the third most common cancer in males, with a seventy-fold variation in incidence, the highest rates (in the United States, Europe, and Australasia) being associated with the highest intakes of fat. In contrast with most other sites, there appears to be no protective effect of vegetables and fruit.

Cancer at all other sites is less frequent, but nutritional causes appear to be involved for some. Alcohol appears to play an important role in cancers of the mouth, pharynx, oesophagus, and liver. Obesity is an important factor in endometrial cancer and may have some role in postmenopausal breast cancer in women and bowel cancer in men. A high intake of salted foods may be involved in cancer of the stomach and vegetables and fruit appear to be protective against cancers at most sites.

Obesity (see also Chapter 10.5)

Obesity is the most obvious and important nutritional disease in affluent societies, its comorbidities including type 2 diabetes, coronary heart disease, hypertension, stroke, gallstones, osteoarthritis, some cancers, and obstructive sleep apnoea. Obese people may also be disadvantaged in terms of social, economic, and psychological effects. The psychological well being of children may be particularly affected. Most of the adverse consequences of obesity are appreciably reduced by weight loss, though gallstone formation may not be reduced. While the genetic component of obesity is acknowledged, the dramatic increase in prevalence in virtually all westernized countries in recent years provides ample evidence of the overwhelming importance of environmental factors. Inactivity is unquestionably an important cause but increased consumption of readily available 'convenience' and other energy-dense foods contribute to an energy intake in excess of expenditure. It seems unlikely that the epidemic of obesity will be reversed unless the nutritional environment in which we live is altered by creating more opportunities for physical activity and improving availability of food choices, and providing appropriate health education.

Diverticular disease of the colon

The first suggestion that deficiency of non-starch polysaccharides in the diet may be implicated in the aetiology of diverticular disease of the colon came from striking geographical variations in its prevalence and the documented increase in disease rates in several European countries since the 1920s. These variations and trends in rates are certainly compatible with a causative link with low non-starch polysaccharide diets but could also be explained by several alternative dietary and other environmental influences. The best-documented evidence comes from comparisons of asymptomatic groups of vegetarians and meat eaters who volunteered to have a barium meal. Radiological diverticular disease was found more frequently amongst non-vegetarians (33 per cent) than vegetarians (12 per cent) who had appreciably higher intakes of non-starch polysaccharide. Furthermore, when comparing individuals with and without diverticular disease in both the vegetarian and non-vegetarian groups, those with diverticular disease had appreciably lower intakes of non-starch polysaccharide than those with no evidence of diverticulae following barium meals. Animal experiments provide support (for example rats given a diet low in non-starch polysaccharide have been shown to develop diverticulae, as do rabbits fed with

white bread, sugar, and vitamins, and given prostigmine). An increase in non-starch polysaccharide intake is widely recommended to patients with symptomatic diverticular disease, a treatment justified by the findings of some (but not all) controlled clinical trials.

Plausible theories concerning pathogenesis have been suggested; small, hard faeces, undoubtedly seen with a diet deficient in non-starch polysaccharide, are associated with narrowing of the colon and the formation of closed segments in which pressure increases. Additional work is needed by colonic muscles to provide the pressure to move the more solid faeces, producing muscular hypertrophy in addition to the diverticula at sites of weakness where blood vessels penetrate the muscular coat.

Dental caries

Dental caries was exceptionally rare among young people in ancient Britain. Surveys over the past 15 years have suggested that as many as 80 per cent of 5-year-olds require treatment for dental caries and about 10 per cent of all children enter school with more than half their teeth seriously decayed. Some 5 per cent of the adult population in England and Wales and 15 per cent of that in Scotland are edentulous by the age of 30 years. Several strands of evidence suggest a nutritional cause. Amongst the indigenous population of many countries where unrefined foods form the bulk of the diet (e.g. China, Uganda) dental caries once had a very low prevalence. Within a few years of the addition of sugar and other refined foods the frequency showed a rapid increase. A similar change has been shown experimentally in monkeys. In a classical experiment carried out in a Swedish mental hospital, volunteers given toffee apples, chocolate, and caramel in addition to their controlled diet had a thirteen-fold greater number of tooth surfaces becoming carious each year, compared with those eating the controlled diet alone. While frequency, timing, and amount of extrinsic sugars may be important in the aetiology there is no doubt that fluoride in the water or in tooth paste can profoundly reduce the risk of dental caries.

Constipation and the irritable bowel syndrome

Nine-nine per cent of a large population sample studied in Britain reported that they defecated at least three times per week but perceived constipation is a frequent complaint. Approximately 3 per cent of all prescriptions written in the National Health Survey (in the United Kingdom) were for purgatives and laxatives, at a cost of around £4 000 000, and many times this amount must have been spent in buying these preparations over the counter. In another survey, 6 per cent of people aged between 18 and 80 years described straining when passing stools. No data are available concerning the frequency of passing small stools. There seems little doubt that constipation is uncommon in populations with a high intake of non-starch polysaccharide. In rural Africa, stool weights are frequently around 500 g daily, and bowel transit times around 40 h. In Britain, stool weights in non-vegetarians are more usually around 100 g (with a very wide range), whereas in vegetarians the average stool weight is over 200 g. Factors other than non-starch polysaccharide might be involved but British vegetarians and non-vegetarians with high average daily intakes of non-starch polysaccharide have transit times of less than 75 h and rarely report constipation, whereas those with lower intakes have transit times ranging from 20 to 124 h and frequently complain of constipation. There is no doubt that increasing the non-starch polysaccharide content of the diet (especially that derived from cereals) relieves the symptoms of constipation, an observation now confirmed by controlled clinical trials. There is no direct evidence of a causal link between a diet low in non-starch polysaccharide and the irritable bowel syndrome, but diets rich in non-starch polysaccharide are widely recommended in its treatment and are believed to be of value, even in the absence of formal clinical trials.

Osteoporosis

Osteoporosis is an important cause of morbidity amongst the elderly, especially in women, and the incidence of osteoporotic fractures is increasing steadily as people are living longer. In 1990, there were an estimated 1.66 million hip fractures world-wide. By the year 2025, it is projected that there will be 1.16 million hip fractures in men and 2.78 million in women due to osteoporosis. The aetiology of osteoporosis is complex; women have a lower peak bone mass than men and then lose bone rapidly after the menopause in association with a decline in oestrogens. Women lose approximately half their trabecular bone and a third of their cortical bone, while men lose a third of their trabecular bone and a fifth of their cortical bone. Genetic factors influence peak bone mass and bone loss and these may operate by some of the well-known risk factors: strong family history of osteoporosis, short stature, early menopause, and white or Asian race. However, there are also clearly established environmental factors, including leanness (genetic factors probably operate in addition), multiparity, cigarette smoking, and excessive alcohol intake. The role of dietary calcium has been uncertain but there is now convincing evidence that the best way of avoiding osteoporotic fractures in later life is to achieve optimal skeletal mass for one's genetic potential and to retain this as long as possible. The best means of doing so is by ensuring lifelong adequate consumption and maximum absorption and retention of calcium. The need for substantial amounts of dietary calcium, taken in conjunction with physiological amounts of vitamin D, is particularly important during the periods of growth, pregnancy, lactation, and in the postmenopausal years.

Other diseases

Gallstones, appendicitis, haemorrhoids, varicose veins, and hiatus hernia all occur frequently in developed countries and rarely in developing countries but the evidence linking these diseases to a nutritional cause in tenuous. Gallstones are undoubtedly associated with obesity. Both gallstones and appendicitis are more common in non-vegetarians than vegetarians and there are some rather indirect data suggesting an association with diets high in sugars and deficient in non-starch polysaccharides. The addition of bran to the diet can make bile less saturated and experimentally induced gallstones in animals tend to be reduced if foods rich in non-starch polysaccharides are given. Data from the United Kingdom and South Africa taken together provide interesting information concerning appendicitis; appendicitis rates were compared in two matched South African Caucasian groups, the privileged group living in university halls of residence and the other living in the establishments for the indigent where the diets contained more fibre. Annual rates were 7.8 and 1.8 per thousand, respectively. Of course, factors other than diets might explain this but the rates were strikingly similar to those found in an almost identical study in Bristol (7.6 per thousand in a public school and 0.8 per thousand in an orphanage).

The case for dietary change

Nutrition research often generates results which may be translated by researchers, self-styled 'experts', or the media into potentially confusing and conflicting messages. It is therefore critically important for governments, who develop food and nutrition policies, for doctors, others involved in health and nutrition education, and for consumers to have authoritative recommendations which represent consensus opinions of nutrition scientists. Terminology regarding such recommendations has been confusing, but the most recent British Government publication suggests a new approach. Dietary reference values are intended for policy makers and health professionals who recommend diets for individuals. These include population averages (sometimes also recommended individual minimum and maximum intakes) for the macronutrients, average requirements for total energy, and reference nutrient intakes (previously referred to as recommended dietary intakes or allowances) for vitamins and minerals.

The latter values are defined as levels of intake which will satisfy the requirements of the great majority in any given population. Thus, the reference nutrient intake is set at two (estimated) standard deviations above the average of all individual requirements for each nutrient. While this approach helps to ensure nutritional adequacy, the situation has become more complex with the suggestion that some nutrients might confer protection against certain chronic diseases when intakes exceed the reference nutrient intake. Thus, it is now considered necessary to set an upper safe level beyond which toxic effects may occur. These dietary reference values will be largely meaningless to the population at large. For the general public, dietary guidelines have been developed to translate dietary reference values into practical advice.

The dietary reference values for macronutrients (Table 6) are based to a considerable extent on the evidence-based data which suggest that alteration of dietary fat intake from that typical of most Western countries is likely to reduce population and individual risk of coronary heart disease. The emphasis is on reduction of saturated and *trans* unsaturated fatty acids and the recommendation represents a substantial reduction from present levels of intake. The recommended intake of *cis*-monounsaturated acids is similar to that at present but adherence to the recommendation for saturated fat will inevitably lead to an alteration in source, from animal to vegetable, since at present much of both mono- and saturated fatty acids are derived from the same animal sources. The total intake of *cis*-polyunsaturated fatty acids has been set at a level slightly higher than at present but the proportions of *n*-3 and *n*-6 are not specified. However, a recent European consensus group has suggested that those not eating fish at least once a week should consider obtaining 200 mg of very long chain *n*-3 polyunsaturated fatty acid daily from other sources. In view of the growing evidence that plant *n*-3 polyunsaturated fatty acid might independently reduce coronary heart disease risk, an intake of 2 g/day or 1 per cent total energy from α-linolenic acid is also recommended. The group advised against the use of *n*-3 to *n*-6 ratios but favoured separate recommendations for α-linolenic acid, marine *n*-3 polyunsaturated fatty acid, and linoleic acid.

Only about 50 g of carbohydrate daily is required to avoid ketosis and at the other end of the range of intake many populations maintain an adequate nutritional status when carbohydrate provides up to 80 per cent total energy. However, most Western societies are unaccustomed to a high carbohydrate intake and are reluctant to accept substantial increases. Therefore, a modest increase in total carbohydrate is advised with a limitation on the use of non-milk extrinsic sugars because of their role in dental caries, especially when consumed frequently. Furthermore, foods high in

Table 6 Dietary reference values for fat and carbohydrate for adults as a percentage of daily total energy intake (percentage of food energy)

Nutrient	Individual minimum	Population average	Individual maximum
Saturated fatty acids		10 (11)	
cis-Polyunsaturated fatty acids		6 (6.5)	10
n-3	0.2		
n-6	1.0		
cis-Monounsaturated acids		12 (13)	
trans Fatty acids		2(2)	
Total fatty acids		30 (32.5)	
Total fat		33 (35)	
Non-milk extrinsic sugars	0	10 (11)	
Intrinsic and milk sugars and starch		37 (39)	
Total carbohydrate		47 (50)	
Non-starch polysaccharides (g/day)	12	18	24

extrinsic sugars are energy-dense and contain relatively few essential nutrients. On the other hand, it is considered appropriate (Table 6) that intrinsic sugars (that is those incorporated into the cellular structure of foods), milk sugars, and starches should provide the balance of dietary energy not provided by protein, fat, and non-milk extrinsic sugars, that is, an average of 37 per cent total dietary energy. Foods containing these macronutrients are usually good sources of essential micronutrients as well as dietary fibre (non-starch polysaccharide), an increase in which is also recommended because of the convincing evidence for benefit in terms of bowel function and possible benefits regarding a range of diseases of the large intestine, diabetes, and cardiovascular disease.

It seems conceivable that these recommendations regarding carbohydrate may be modified in the future. It is becoming increasingly clear that the health benefits associated with carbohydrate-containing foods are principally derived from carbohydrates which are not digested and absorbed in the small intestine but which enter the large bowel where they undergo fermentation or act as stool-bulkers. The process of fermentation leads to the production of fatty acids which are useful not only as fuel sources but by their antiproliferative effect may also reduce the risk of colon cancer. Carbohydrates which undergo fermentation include oligosaccharides, resistant starch, and certain non-starch polysaccharides such as gum, pectins, and mucilages. Those which remain intact and act as stool bulkers include cellulose, hemicellulose, and lignin. The suggestion that complex carbohydrates may confer health benefits is becoming outmoded since many forms of starch are rapidly digested and absorbed as sugars. Thus the extent and speed with which carbohydrates are digested and absorbed in the small intestine provide the best indicator for health-promoting, carbohydrate-rich foods. The most useful, simple indicator of this is the glycaemic index (Fig. 1). A recent World Health Organization Expert Consultation has suggested that this index might guide the choice of carbohydrate-containing foods, the lower glycaemic index foods being the preferred food choices (see Table 7).

The glycaemic index concept does have limitations. It is important to emphasise that it should not be used for carbohydrate-containing foods which are also high in fat. These will usually have a low glycaemic index but

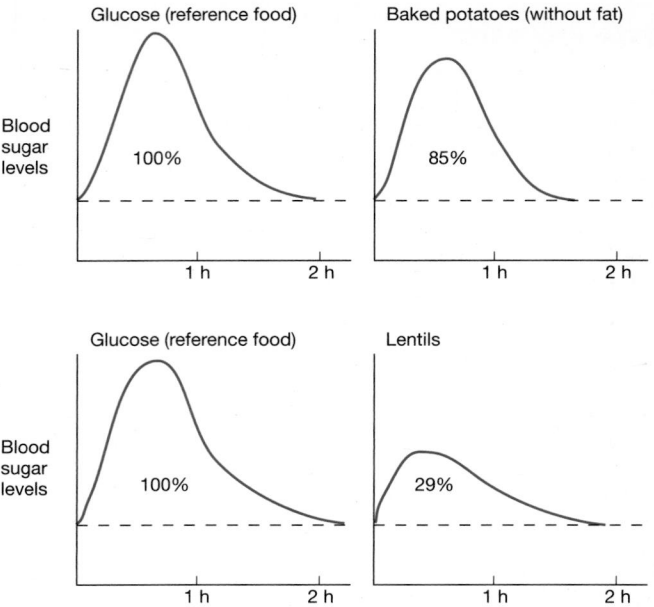

Fig. 1 Calculation of the glycaemic index of a food. The area under the blood glucose curve is calculated geometrically using the fasting level as baseline and expressed as a percentage of that seen after consumption of 50 g pure glucose. In practice, 8 to 12 people are tested and the mean of the group is the glycaemic index of the test food.

are obviously not regarded as the best choices. Sucrose and sucrose-rich foods will also have a relatively low glycaemic index because of their fructose content. While the detrimental effects of sucrose have been overstated in the past, sucrose confers no health benefits other than acting as an

Table 7 Glycaemic index (GI) of selected foods (glucose = 100)

High GI foods					
Cocopops	77	Wholemeal bread	77	French fries[a]	75
Cornflakes	77	Rye, blackbread	76	Watermelon	72
Rice Bubbles	89	Puffed crispbread	81	Corn chips	72
Weetabix	75	Water crackers	78	Jelly beans	80
Rice, calrose	83	Potato, baked	85	Glucose	100
Moderate GI foods					
Muesli, untoasted	56	Beetroot	64	Orange juice	57
Rice, basmati	59	Potato, new	62	Soft drink, carbonated	68
White bread	70	Banana	60	Popcorn	55
Ryvita	69	Pineapple	66	Potato crisps[a]	57
Biscuits, Arrowroot	69	Raisins	64	Honey	58
Shortbread	64	Rockmelon	65	Sucrose	59
Ice cream	61	Sultanas	56		
Low GI foods					
All Bran	30	Carrots	49	Apple	36
Porridge	50	Sweet corn	48	Apricot (dried)	43
Muesli, toasted[a]	43	Peas (green)	48	Grapes	43
Rice, white long grain	50	Sweet potato	48	Orange	43
Instant noodles	47	Yams	35	Peach, canned in juice	30
Pasta, spaghetti	41	Baked beans	48	Peach, fresh	28
Bread, heavy grain	45	Haricot beans	38	Pear	36
Rye bread, pumpernickel	50	Butter beans	31	Whole milk	27
Biscuits, oatmeal	55	Chickpeas	33	Yoghurt, low fat	33
Banana cake[a]	47	Kidney beans	27	Apple juice	41
Sponge cake	46	Soya beans	18	Chocolate[a]	49
Apple muffin[a]	44	Lentils	28	Fructose	20

[a] Food with a high fat content

energy source. Given the need to reduce energy dense foods in many countries sucrose-rich foods are not generally encouraged.

While appropriate distribution of macronutrients might be expected to reduce cardiovascular risk, improve bowel function, and probably also reduce the risk of certain cancers and other diseases of the large bowel, it is imperative to consider the extent to which diet can influence obesity and its comorbidities, especially type 2 diabetes which accounts for a public health problem of enormous magnitude. Increasing carbohydrate-containing foods rich in non-starch polysaccharide at the expense of saturated fat is likely to enhance satiety and so help to reduce excessive energy intake. However, increasing energy output by increasing physical activity is an equally essential component of public health measures designed to stem the tide of the obesity epidemic occurring in most affluent societies and many developing countries.

Reference nutrient intakes (adequate for most individuals) are provided for vitamins and minerals; selected examples are shown in Table 8. Clinical vitamin deficiencies, discussed in detail in Chapter 10.3 are uncommon in affluent societies except in at-risk subgroups within populations. For example immigrants who have migrated from sunny, tropical to high latitude, cloudy countries may be at risk of vitamin D deficiency; strict vegetarians (who consume no animal or dairy products) may become deficient in vitamin B_{12}, and disadvantaged groups (especially the very young, pregnant and lactating women, and the elderly) may have generally inadequate intakes.

On the other hand, inappropriate intakes of certain minerals are fairly common. Many groups are particularly vulnerable to iron deficiency, due to high physiological requirements (infants and toddlers, adolescents, pregnant women), high losses (menstruating women), or poor absorption (the elderly and people consuming foods high in inhibitors of absorption, such as fibre and tannin in tea). Vegetarians are also at increased risk of iron deficiency even when total intake of iron appears to be adequate since non-haem iron from plant foods is less bioavailable than haem iron from animal sources. Bioavailability is enhanced by the consumption, at the same time, of vitamin C. Iodine and selenium are deficient in soils in various parts of the world. Clinical selenium deficiency has only been reported from China

though the consequences of lesser degrees of selenium deficiency have yet to be established with certainty, especially in regions where soils are known to be deficient (e.g. the South Island of New Zealand). Endemic iodine deficiency is widespread, especially in the Himalayas and the Andes, and clinical deficiency states are largely avoided by the use of iodized salt and sanitizers containing iodine used by the dairy industry. Interestingly, in New Zealand where goitre due to iodine deficiency had virtually been eliminated, mild iodine deficiency appears to be reoccurring possibly as a result of reduced use of iodized salt and the introduction by the dairy industry of alternative sanitizers. Young women often have insufficient calcium to help achieve peak bone mass, and older women may have an inadequate intake to help reduce an age-related bone loss.

Excessive intakes of sodium, to such an extent that it probably contributes to hypertension and its consequences, are common throughout the Western world. Targets for reduction may be more important than reference nutrient intakes for sodium. An intake of 100 mmol/day (2.3 g/day), a level currently exceeded in most countries, might be an appropriate maximum.

Folate is probably the best example of a nutrient for which intakes greater than those recommended have been shown to confer benefit. Intakes of 400 µg or more per day (reference nutrient intake 200 µg/day) can appreciably reduce the risk of neural tube defects. Furthermore, the potential for folate to reduce cardiovascular risk by a reduction in plasma homocysteine concentrations may provide further justification for higher recommended intakes if the trials underway at present demonstrate reduced cardiovascular risk. There is evidence that higher than recommended intakes of several antioxidant nutrients reduces subsequent cardiovascular risk and possibly also the risk of certain cancers. However, there are insufficient data regarding optimum intakes to contemplate firm recommendations at present.

Dietary assessment methods are not sufficiently sensitive to determine accurately intake of several important nutrients so that in order to assess either adequacy or excess in an individual or group of individuals for clinical or research purposes it is necessary to use biomarkers. Intakes of iodine and sodium are assessed by measuring amounts in 24-h urine collections.

Table 8 Reference nutrient intakes for selected vitamins and minerals

Age	Vitamin B_{12} µg/day	Folate µg/day	Vitamin A µg/day	Vitamin D µg/day	Calcium mmol/day	Sodium[a] mmol/day	Iron µmol/day	Zinc µmol/day	Iodine µmol/day
0–3 months	0.3	50	350	8.5	13.1	9	30	60	0.4
4–6 months	0.3	50	350	8.5	13.1	12	80	60	0.5
7–9 months	0.4	50	350	7	13.1	14	140	75	0.5
10–12 months	0.4	50	350	7	13.1	15	140	75	0.5
1–3 years	0.5	70	400	7	8.8	22	120	75	0.6
4–6 years	0.8	100	500	–	11.3	30	110	100	0.8
7–10 years	1.0	150	500	–	13.8	50	160	110	0.9
Males									
11–14 years	1.2	200	600	–	25.0	70	200	140	1.0
15–18 years	1.5	200	700	–	25.0	70	200	145	1.0
19–50 years	1.5	200	700	–	17.5	70	160	145	1.0
50+ years	1.5	200	700	[d]	17.5	70	160	145	1.0
Females									
11–14 years	1.2	200	600	–	20.0	70	260[b]	140	1.0
15–18 years	1.5	200	600	–	20.0	70	260[b]	110	1.1
19–50 years	1.5	200	600	–	17.5	70	260[b]	110	1.1
50+ years	1.5	200	600	[d]	17.5	70	160	110	1.1
Pregnancy	[c]	+100	+100	10	[c]	[c]	[c]	[c]	[c]
Lactation									
0–4 months	+0.5	+60	+350	10	+14.3	[c]	[c]	+90	[c]
4+ months	+0.5	+60	+350	10	+14.3	[c]	[c]	+40	[c]

[a] mmol sodium = 23 mg.

[b] Insufficient for women with high menstrual losses where the most practical way of meeting iron requirements is to take iron supplements.

[c] No increment.

[d] After 65 years of age the reference nutrient intake is 10 µg/day for men and women.

Measurement of folate concentration in the serum or red blood cells provide a good estimate of intake since the amounts in fruit and vegetables vary enormously and are also dependent upon shelf-life and method of preparation. Fatty acid composition of serum or red cell membrane provides an indication of the nature of dietary fat intake. For some nutrients which are not always readily bioavailable adequacy of intake must be assessed by alternative means. In the case of iron, measurement of ferritin in the blood (indicating iron stores) is a more useful indicator of iron status than dietary intake (see also Chapter 22.4.4).

Substantial changes in what have become traditional eating habits of many affluent societies are required in order to achieve the advised changes in distribution of macronutrients and recommended intake of all essential micronutrients. A multifocal approach is necessary if there is to be a real chance of achieving dietary change. At the policy making and government level, there needs to be a serious commitment to enabling the population as a whole to make appropriate food choices. Fatty cuts of meat, high-fat products (e.g. meat pies), and convenience foods (e.g. fish and chips, burgers) are relatively inexpensive and therefore frequently eaten by those of lower socio-economic status who have the highest rates of coronary heart disease. Policies are required which ensure that more appropriate food choices are available at reasonable cost. This is not easy to achieve in many Western countries where farmers may have considerable political influence and subsidies may be available for some high-fat dairy products such as butter and cheese. Governments and intergovernmental agencies also have the responsibility for ensuring that food labels and health claims are accurate, interpretable, and likely to facilitate health-promoting food choices, a particularly important issue given the increased consumption of packaged food.

Dietary guidelines are necessary to provide clear directions to individuals and families who wish to aim for a healthy diet pattern. These guidelines vary slightly from country to country though some are almost universal (see Box 1). Others are less consistent (see Box 2). The public also need education regarding food groups and the nutrients they contain, the interpretation of food labels, the meaning of health claims, and the methods of food preparation. The increased use of convenience and packaged food has meant that many people no longer possess basic cooking skills. They also need (and want) to know the merits and demerits of obtaining certain essential micronutrients by taking supplements or fortified food products rather than conventional foods.

Doctors are frequently asked to give nutritional advice but may lack the necessary expertise. Dietitians, nutritionists, and appropriately trained practice nurses, play an invaluable role in providing the public with practical advice to facilitate changes from the typical Western diet as well as providing instruction regarding therapeutic diets for those with diseases requiring specific diet therapy. The enormous potential for dietary change to reduce the effects of a wide range of diseases should encourage physicians to approach the nutritional management of their patients with enthusiasm.

Box 1　Dietary guidelines for which there is almost complete agreement

1. Eat a nutritionally adequate diet composed of a variety of foods.
2. Eat less fat, particularly saturated fat.
3. Adjust energy balance for body weight control—less energy intake, more exercise.
4. Eat more wholegrain cereals, vegetables and fruits.
5. Reduce salt intake.
6. Drink alcohol in moderation, if you do drink.

Box 2　Additional dietary guidelines in some countries

1. Recommendation regarding sugar and sugary foods may vary from 'no increase' to 'decrease'.
2. Drink plenty of fluids each day.
3. Make sure you get enough calcium or milk.
4. Eat foods containing iron.
5. Do not eat too much protein.
6. Limit caffeine intake.
7. Drink fluoridated water.
8. Preserve the nutritive value of food (by good food preparation).
9. Eat three good meals a day.

Further reading

COMA–CHD Panel on Dietary Reference Values of the Committee on Medical Aspects of Food Policy (1991). *Report on Health and Social Subjects: 41. Dietary Reference Values for Food Energy and Nutrients for the United Kingdom.* HMSO, London.

de Deckere EAM, Korver O, Verschuren PM, Katan MB (1998). Health aspects of fish and n-3 polyunsaturated fatty acids from plant and marine origin. *European Journal Clinical Nutrition* **52**, 749–53.

Department of Health (1994). *Report on Health and Social Subjects: 46. Nutritional aspects of cardiovascular disease. Report of the Cardiovascular Review Group Committee on Medical Aspects of Food Policy.* HMSO, London.

Mann J, Truswell AS, eds. (2002). *Essentials of Human Nutrition*, 2nd edn. Oxford University Press.

Truswell AS (1999). *ABC of Nutrition*, 3rd edn. BMJ Books, London.

World Heath Organization/Food and Agriculture Organization (1998). *Carbohydrates in Human Nutrition.* FAO Food and Nutrition Paper 66. Report of a Joint FAO/WHO Expert Consultation. Rome.

10.2 Nutrition: biochemical background

Keith N. Frayn

Introduction: flux of 'energy substrates'

Food intake is sporadic: for most people it occurs in three major boluses each day. Energy expenditure, however, is continuous, with variations during the day that bear no resemblance to the pattern of energy intake, except that over some reasonable period of time (a week or more) the two will, in most people, match almost exactly. Therefore the body has developed complex systems that direct nutrients into storage pools when they are in excess, and that regulate the 'mobilization' of nutrients from these pools as they are needed. The situation is analogous to the petrol (gas) tank of a motor car and the throttle that regulates fuel oxidation, except that in the motor car there is just one fuel and just one engine: in humans there are three major nutrients and a variety of tissues and organs, each of which may have its own preferences for fuels, that vary with time. The fact that we can carry on our daily lives without thinking about whether to store or mobilize fuels, and which to use, attests to the remarkable efficiency of these control systems.

The body's principal macronutrient stores are listed in Table 1 and are related to daily fluxes in the body.

The regulation of macronutrient flux

The need for the co-ordinated control of nutrient storage and mobilization, to flux between tissues and along the many metabolic pathways, is met by a complex series of control mechanisms. These may be viewed on several levels.

The simplest involves the effects of substrate concentration, and is dependent upon the kinetic properties of enzymes and transport proteins. An illustration is the uptake of glucose by the liver. The facilitated carrier responsible for entry of glucose into the hepatocyte, GLUT2, has a high Michaelis constant, K_m (around 10–20 mmol/l), for glucose and a high capacity. The first enzyme of glucose metabolism in the hepatocyte, hexokinase IV (glucokinase), has similar properties. Therefore, flux of glucose into the hepatocyte is dependent upon the extracellular to intracellular concentration gradient. When glucose is absorbed from the small intestine and transported to the liver in the portal vein the hepatocyte is subject to an external glucose concentration of perhaps 10 mmol/l, and acts as a 'sink' to remove glucose and buffer fluctuations in delivery of glucose to the systemic circulation. In contrast, the glucose transporter in the brain, GLUT3, has a low K_m (around 1–3 mmol/l), and glucose utilization is therefore almost constant while the plasma glucose concentration varies within the normal physiological range. Within tissues the same may be true. The aminotransferases (transaminases) that catalyse the removal of amino groups from amino acids, the first step in their catabolism, have a high K_m and high capacity, and again flux is driven by concentration. Hans Krebs showed that this was one explanation for the old observation that an increase in protein intake is followed by rapid oxidation of the excess amino acids.

The next level involves more specific interaction of nutrients, or pathway intermediates, with enzymes, usually through allosteric effects (binding of the effector alters the conformation of the enzyme and hence its catalytic properties). There are many examples in the metabolism of carbohydrate, fat, and protein. The enzyme 6-phosphofructo-1-kinase (which converts fructose-6-phosphate to fructose-1,6-bisphosphate in the pathway of glycolysis) is a good example, subject to allosteric regulation by many compounds that relate to the 'energy status' of the cell. For instance, it is activated by AMP (indicating energy shortage) and inhibited by ATP. Such mechanisms undoubtedly provide important 'fine tuning' of flux along various pathways entirely in accord with the modern view that regulation of flux does not reside in certain 'rate-limiting steps' but is distributed amongst many steps along a pathway.

These mechanisms operate essentially within one tissue. However, the co-ordination of nutrient metabolism requires considerable interaction between tissues and organs. This co-ordination is largely brought about by

Table 1 Macronutrient stores in relation to daily intake

Macronutrient	Total amount in body	Energy equivalent (MJ)	Days' supply if the only energy source	Daily intake (g)	Daily intake as percentage of store
Carbohydrate:	0.6 kg	8.5	< 1	300	60
free glucose	12 g				
liver glycogen	100 g				
muscle glycogen	500 g				
Fat (triacylglycerol):	12–18 kg	550	56	100	0.7
circulating in plasma	5 g				
stored in adipocytes	12–18 kg				
Protein and amino acids:	12 kg	200	(20)	100	0.8
free amino acids	100 g				
protein	12 kg				

These are very much typical rounded figures. Days' supply is the length of time for which this store would last if it were the only fuel for oxidation at an energy expenditure of 10 MJ/day: the figure for protein is given in parentheses since protein does not fulfil the role of an energy store in this way.

the hormonal and nervous systems. Certain hormones play a particularly important role in regulation of macronutrient flux (Table 2). The role of the nervous system in metabolic regulation is often difficult to assess. For instance, whilst the effects of adrenaline are properly regarded as hormonal, liberation of noradrenaline from sympathetic nerve endings in tissues may bring about identical effects and can be difficult to distinguish. The somatic nervous system (motor neurones innervating skeletal muscle) has clear effects, for example stimulation of breakdown of muscle glycogen linked to muscle contraction. The autonomic nervous system probably plays multiple roles, but some are indirect: for example regulation of blood flow and cardiac output, thus affecting delivery of substrate to tissues, and regulation of the secretion of pancreatic hormones.

The effects of hormones are mediated in many ways, but may be divided into acute effects (usually acting within seconds or minutes), often brought about through reversible (de)phosphorylation of enzymes, and longer-term effects (hours or days), brought about by regulation of gene expression. The former are usually exerted through binding to cell surface receptors linked to a variety of second messenger systems, the latter through nuclear receptors (for example for glucocorticoids and thyroid hormones). However, the distinction is not absolute: insulin, for example, brings about both acute and longer-term effects through binding to the same cell surface receptor.

A further level of co-ordination is through the effects of nutrients themselves, or important cellular components such as cholesterol, upon gene expression. This can be seen as a longer-term mechanism to ensure that metabolism is appropriate to the diet being ingested and the lifestyle followed. A variety of nutrient response elements are being discovered in the promoter regions of genes for enzymes concerned with substrate metabolism. Particular examples are the carbohydrate response element (upregulating expression of genes for glucose metabolism such as pyruvate kinase in the glycolysis pathway), the sterol response element (cellular sterols downregulate expression of the low-density lipoprotein receptor and the enzymes of cholesterol biosynthesis) and response elements for fatty acid derivatives. Fatty acids affect gene expression through a family of transcription factors known as the peroxisome proliferator activated receptors which act in turn upon the peroxisome proliferator response elements. These were discovered through the effects of a diverse group of compounds that promote proliferation of peroxisomes in the rodent liver. Now they are recognized as factors that mediate the response to dietary fatty acids. They are summarized in Table 3.

Table 2 Major hormonal effects on intermediary metabolism

Hormone	Origin	Target tissue	Major metabolic effects	Comments
Insulin	Pancreatic islets (β-cells)	Liver	Stimulation of glycogen synthesis/suppression of glycogen breakdown	Regulates glucose storage in liver
			Stimulation of glycolysis/suppression of gluconeogenesis	Regulates hepatic glucose output
			Suppression of fatty acid oxidation/ketogenesis	Via malonyl CoA
			Stimulation of triacylglycerol synthesis	
			Stimulation of cholesterol synthesis	
		Skeletal muscle	Stimulation of glucose uptake	Regulates glucose uptake by muscle
			Stimulation of glycogen synthesis	
			Net protein anabolic effect	Insulin may suppress protein breakdown more than stimulation of protein synthesis
		Adipose tissue	Activation of triacylglycerol removal from plasma	Via lipoprotein lipase
			Suppression of fat mobilization	Via hormone-sensitive lipase
Glucagon	Pancreatic islets (α-cells)	Liver	Stimulation of glycogen breakdown/suppression of glycogen synthesis	In effect the regulation is via the insulin/glucagon ratio
			Stimulation of gluconeogenesis/suppression of glycolysis	
			Stimulation of fatty acid oxidation/ketogenesis	
Adrenaline	Adrenal medulla	Adipose tissue	Stimulation of fat mobilization	Via hormone-sensitive lipase
		Skeletal muscle	Stimulation of glycogen breakdown	Acts in concert with muscle contraction
Tri-iodothyronine	Thyroid	All oxidative tissues	Increase in basal metabolism	
Cortisol	Adrenal cortex	Liver	Stimulation of gluconeogenesis	
		Skeletal muscle	Generally catabolic effect	
		Adipose tissue	Promotes site-specific fat deposition (central depots) and fat mobilization (peripheral depots)	
Growth hormone	Anterior pituitary	Liver	Stimulation of gluconeogenesis	Direct effect – other effects are mediated indirectly via insulin-like growth factors
		Adipose tissue	Stimulation of fat mobilization	This is an acute effect: chronically, growth hormone promotes mobilization from central fat depots
Insulin-like growth factors (IGF) I and II	Liver (IGF-I) and other tissues (both)	Several	Generally insulin-like acute effects on metabolism	Physiological role is probably longer-term effects on growth
Leptin	Adipose tissue	Hypothalamus	Suppression of appetite; possibly stimulation of energy expenditure	Latter effect prominent in rodents, may not occur in humans
		Reproductive system	Signals sufficient fat stores for reproduction to be possible	As with effects on hypothalamus, leptin (or absence thereof) may be a signal of starvation rather than of plenty

Table 3 Peroxisomal proliferator activated receptors (PPARs): tissue distribution and effects of activation.

Receptor	Main tissue distribution	Genes whose expression is increased by PPAR activation	Genes whose expression is suppressed by PPAR activation
PPAR-α	Liver (main site) Kidney, heart, muscle, brown adipose tissue	Apolipoprotein AI Apolipoprotein AII Enzymes of peroxisomal fatty acid oxidation Liver FABP CPT-1 Enzymes of mitochondrial fatty acid oxidation	Apolipoprotein CIII
PPAR-δ*	Widespread	Not known, although HDL concentrations increase with activation	Not known
PPAR-γ1	Widespread at low levels		
PPAR-γ2	Adipose tissue	Factors involved in adipocyte differentiation Adipose tissue FABP (also known as aP2) Lipoprotein lipase Fatty acid transport protein Acyl CoA synthase GLUT4 Phosphoenolpyruvate carboxykinase	Leptin

*Also known as PPAR-β, NUC 1, FAAR (fatty-acid activated receptor).

Abbreviations: CPT-1, carnitine palmitoyltransferase-1; FABP, fatty acid binding protein; GLUT4, insulin-regulated glucose transporter; HDL, high-density lipoprotein.

(Reproduced from Gurr MI, Harwood JL, Frayn KN (2001). *Lipid biochemistry*, 5th edn. Blackwell Scientific, Oxford, with permission)

Carbohydrate metabolism in the postabsorptive and postprandial states

The postabsorptive state

In the overnight-fasted (postabsorptive) state, no glucose enters the plasma from the small intestine. Glucose in the plasma turns over at about 2 mg/kg body weight/min (200 g/24 h). About one-half of this will be consumed by the brain. Of the remainder, a considerable proportion will be utilized by blood cells and peripheral tissues by anaerobic glycolysis, thus returning lactate to the liver for reconversion to glucose (Fig. 1). This is the Cori cycle.

Glucose is produced by hepatocytes from glycogen breakdown and from gluconeogenesis. Net glycogen breakdown is stimulated by the relatively low insulin/glucagon ratio after overnight fasting. The major substrates for gluconeogenesis are lactate and pyruvate, released from blood cells and peripheral tissues, together with alanine and glycerol. The pathway of gluconeogenesis predominates over that of glycolysis, again because of the relatively low insulin/glucagon ratio.

Glucose metabolism following a meal

When a meal enters the system, this pattern of metabolism changes rapidly. About 12 g of free glucose are present in the circulation and extravascular space. Typically, a single meal will provide about 100 g of glucose, entering the circulation over perhaps 60 min. In order to minimize variations in plasma glucose concentration, co-ordinated mechanisms come into play to suppress the production of endogenous glucose and to increase the rate of removal of glucose from the circulation.

Much of the incoming glucose may be taken up by hepatocytes as described earlier, but some enters the systemic circulation, from where it can stimulate pancreatic insulin secretion (and somewhat suppress glucagon secretion, although this is not so marked an effect). Insulin is liberated into the portal vein. Thus, the liver is exposed at this time to high concentrations of glucose (from the small intestine) and insulin. The net effect is to reverse net glycogenolysis, so that net glycogen synthesis begins. In addition gluconeogenesis is suppressed and glycolysis favoured (Fig. 1). Hepatocyte glucose output is therefore rapidly suppressed and converted to a net uptake of glucose. At the same time, utilization of glucose by insulin-sensitive peripheral tissues such as skeletal muscle and adipose tissue is increased. The main mechanism of this short-term change is the recruitment of the insulin-regulated glucose transporter GLUT4 to the cell membrane from an intracellular pool. However, the reduction in concentration of plasma non-esterified fatty acids (see below) will also remove inhibition of glucose uptake caused by fatty acid oxidation. Within muscle, glycolysis and glycogen synthesis will be stimulated by insulin. In adipose tissue, increased glucose uptake provides glycerol-3-phosphate (formed from glycolysis) for esterification of fatty acids (see below). Thus, insulin is the key

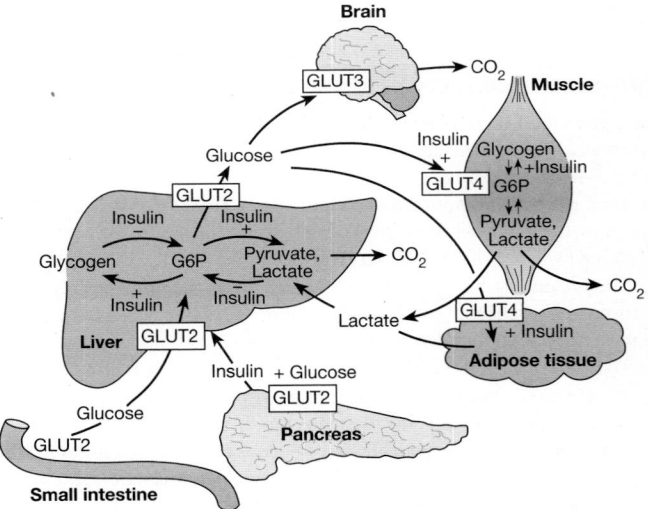

Fig. 1 Overview of carbohydrate metabolism. Pathways in the liver shown as regulated by insulin are probably controlled by the insulin/glucagon ratio (high in the fed state, low in fasting). In muscle, contraction is an important stimulus for glycogen breakdown and glycolysis. Adrenaline also contributes. Not shown is the significant glucose uptake by red blood cells and other glycolytic tissues, returning lactate to the liver. GLUT2 is the high-K_m non-insulin regulated glucose transporter (i.e. the glucose flux is determined by concentration), GLUT3 is the low-K_m brain glucose transporter (the glucose flux is relatively independent of concentration within the normal range), and GLUT4 the insulin-regulated glucose transporter. G6P is glucose 6-phosphate.

regulator of the rapid changes that occur in glucose metabolism in the post-prandial state: it brings about glucose storage as glycogen, and promotes the utilization of glucose at the expense of fatty acids.

Fat metabolism in the postabsorptive and postprandial states

Forms of fat in the circulation (see Chapter 11. 6)

Fatty acids circulate in various forms: as non-esterified fatty acids, as tria-cylglycerol (triglyceride) fatty acids, esterified to glycerol in phospholipids, and esterified to cholesterol as cholesteryl esters. The first two are involved in 'energy metabolism'. The main carriers of triacylglycerol in the circu-lation are the triacylglycerol-rich lipoproproteins, chylomicrons secreted from the small intestine and transporting dietary fat, and very low-density lipoprotein particles secreted from the liver, transporting endogenous tria-cylglycerol. In the postabsorptive state, chylomicron triacylglycerol secre-tion will be virtually zero. Secretion of very low-density lipoprotein is a means of exporting fat from the liver to peripheral tissues. In these tissues it is hydrolysed by the enzyme lipoprotein lipase situated in the capillaries of skeletal muscle, adipose tissue, mammary glands, and other tissues that use fatty acids. Lipoprotein lipase acts on the circulating triacylglycerol-rich particles to liberate fatty acids which may diffuse into the parenchymal cells (muscle fibres, adipocytes, etc.). Lipoprotein lipase in skeletal muscle is downregulated by insulin, whereas that in adipose tissue is upregulated by insulin. In the postabsorptive state muscle lipoprotein lipase is likely to predominate as the site of removal of triacylglycerol from the very low-density lipoprotein particles. The fatty acids can then be used as an oxida-tive fuel by the muscle. In this process very low-density lipoprotein particles lose their triacylglycerol core and become relatively enriched with cholesterol and phospholipids. After several cycles through such capillary beds, they are reduced to simple particles with a core of cholesteryl ester and an outer phospholipid shell: in fact, low-density lipoprotein particles, the main carrier of cholesterol in the circulation.

Non-esterified fatty acids and 'energy transport'

Fat is mobilized from adipose tissue stores in the form of non-esterified fatty acids (Fig. 2). The adipocyte has a central droplet of triacylglycerol, which is hydrolysed by the intracellular enzyme hormone-sensitive lipase, releasing glycerol and non-esterified fatty acids. These fatty acids are liber-ated into the plasma bound to albumin for transport to other tissues, including liver and skeletal muscle. Hormone-sensitive lipase is stimulated by catecholamines but powerfully suppressed by insulin, each exerting control over reversible (de)phosphorylation (see Fig. 2) (insulin leads to dephosphorylation and deactivation). Thus, it is active in the postabsorp-tive state when there is a call upon the body's fat stores. It is also activated during exercise, mainly by catecholamine stimulation. The turnover of non-esterified fatty acids in the plasma is rapid. They are the major oxida-tive fuel in muscle after overnight fast (glucose only supplies around 5 to 10 per cent of the oxidative fuel for skeletal muscle in this state), and in the liver they are both a fuel for oxidation and a substrate for synthesis of tria-cylglycerol that will be exported as very low-density lipoprotein. A typical concentration of non-esterified fatty acids in the plasma after overnight fast is 500 μmol/l, one-tenth that of glucose, but because of their rapid turnover and their larger molecular mass fatty acids account for about twice the 'energy turnover' of glucose in the circulation.

Disposition of dietary fat

Dietary fat is almost entirely (typically 95 per cent or more) in the form of triacylglycerol. A typical meal might contain 30 to 40 g of fat. The typical

Fig. 2 Overview of fat metabolism. Triacylglycerol (TAG) enters the circulation from the diet in the form of chylomicrons. Fatty acids are taken up by tissues through the action of the enzyme lipoprotein lipase (LPL). Adipose tissue TAG is the major store. It is mobilized in times of energy demand by the enzyme hormone-sensitive lipase (HSL), liberating non-esterified fatty acids (NEFA) into the circulation, from where they may be taken up by a number of tissues and used for synthesis of new TAG and for oxidation. Major points of hormonal regulation are shown (italic).

plasma triacylglycerol concentration in a healthy subject is 1 mmol/l, con-fined to the vascular space; this means that about 3 g of triacylglycerol is present in the circulation. Therefore, as in the case of glucose, the amount in a meal could overwhelm the system unless co-ordinated mechanisms come into play to ensure its rapid dispersion.

Dietary triacylglycerol is digested in the stomach and small intestine and packaged by the enterocytes of the duodenum and proximal ileum into chylomicrons, which enter the circulation via the lymphatics (Fig. 2). Therefore, unlike other nutrients absorbed from the small intestine, they bypass the liver on first passage. The chylomicrons also carry other lipid constituents of food, including cholesterol and fat-soluble vitamins. In the circulation their fate is similar to that of very low-density lipoprotein par-ticles, although the tissue-specific regulation of lipoprotein lipase ensures that adipose tissue (where lipoprotein lipase is upregulated by insulin) is a major site of clearance of their triacylglycerol. The pathway of triacylgly-cerol synthesis in adipocytes, as in the liver, is stimulated by insulin. There-fore, there is a short and energy efficient pathway for storage of dietary fatty acids in adipose tissue (Fig. 2). The half-life of chylomicron triacylglycerol in the circulation is about 5 min. After hydrolysis of most of the triacylgly-cerol, the remnant particles are removed by receptors in the liver and other tissues. Thus dietary cholesterol which remains in the remnant particles along with most fat-soluble vitamins is transported mainly to the liver.

Provided that a meal contains carbohydrate or protein, stimulation of insulin secretion will rapidly suppress the mobilization of adipose tissue fat stores, and concentrations of non-esterified fatty acids in the plasma will fall after a meal. Therefore utilization of fatty acids by tissues such as skel-etal muscle and liver will be reduced simply by lack of availability. As noted above, this reduces competition for oxidation in muscle, further increasing glucose utilization. In liver, the lack of non-esterified fatty acids is likely to decrease the secretion of very low-density lipoprotein triacylglycerol. Insulin appears also to suppress very low-density lipoprotein triacylglycerol secretion directly. This is somewhat controversial, and the effects of insulin may be different in the acute, postprandial situation from the situation of prolonged hyperinsulinaemia (as in insulin resistance). Within the liver, insulin powerfully stimulates esterification of fatty acids (for triacylglycerol synthesis) at the expense of oxidation of fatty acids (see below), so the suppressive effect of insulin on very low-density lipoprotein triacylglycerol secretion can only be short-term. Nevertheless, it seems an exact parallel with the suppression of hepatic glucose output by insulin.

Inter-relationships between carbohydrate and fat metabolism

Links between carbohydrate and fat

In mammals, fat cannot be converted to glucose in a net sense (for each molecule of acetyl CoA entering the tricarboxylic acid cycle, two molecules of CO_2 are produced). Glucose can, however, be converted to fat: acetyl CoA produced by pyruvate dehydrogenase leaves the mitochondrion (being transported across the mitochondrial membrane as citrate, then 'liberated' by the cytosolic enzyme ATP-citrate lyase), and is then a substrate for the pathway of *de novo* lipogenesis, which begins with the enzyme acetyl CoA carboxylase (forming malonyl CoA). At one time it was believed that *de novo* lipogenesis was a major route for laying down storage fat. Although this may be true in small rodents under some conditions, many measurements made in recent years have confirmed that this pathway makes a quantitatively small contribution to triacylglycerol synthesis in humans. Instead, it seems that almost all the triacylglycerol that we deposit in adipose tissue arises from dietary fatty acids, taken up from circulating triacylglycerol-rich lipoproteins by the lipoprotein lipase pathway (see Chapter 4.3).

The lack of quantitatively significant interconversion of carbohydrate and fat has led to the suggestion that we may view carbohydrate and fat balance as independent. This view is entirely erroneous. Despite the lack of interconversion, carbohydrate balance strongly influences fat balance, and vice versa. These influences occur at a number of levels.

At a chronic level, ingestion of a high-carbohydrate diet will induce enzymes of fat synthesis and downregulate enzymes of fatty acid oxidation, through insulin- and carbohydrate-response elements in the promoter regions of the genes in question. On a whole-body but more acute level there are clear hormonal effects. Principal amongst these is carbohydrate-induced insulin secretion. Insulin, as outlined above (see Chapter 4.3), powerfully suppresses the release of non-esterified fatty acids from adipose tissue. Therefore, when carbohydrate is readily available, fat stores are conserved.

The glucose–fatty acid cycle

Beyond this, there are specific cellular mechanisms that regulate the relative oxidation of carbohydrate and fat. These probably operate in a number of tissues although they have been most studied in skeletal and heart muscle and in liver. In 1963 Philip Randle and colleagues described the glucose–fatty acid cycle, which encompasses one aspect of this mutual relationship between carbohydrate and fat oxidation. It is summarized in Fig. 3. The concept was based upon observations that availability of fatty acids reduced the oxidation of glucose in skeletal and cardiac muscle. The mechanism involves generation of acetyl CoA from β-oxidation of fatty acids. A high ratio of acetyl CoA to free CoA within the mitochondrion inhibits pyruvate dehydrogenase. In addition, export of citrate to the cytoplasm would inhibit phosphofructokinase, and consequent accumulation of glucose-6-phosphate would inhibit uptake of hexokinase and glucose. The precise

Fig. 3 The glucose–fatty acid cycle. When glucose and insulin concentrations are high, release of non-esterified fatty acid (NEFA) from adipose tissue is suppressed, and glucose utlization predominates in insulin-sensitive tissues such as skeletal muscle. In the fasting state (glucose and insulin concentrations are low) NEFA utilization predominates, reinforced by inhibitory effects of the products of β-oxidation of fatty acids on glucose uptake and oxidation. This may have pathological significance in that states in which NEFA concentrations tend to be high (e.g. type 2 diabetes) will be associated with resistance of glucose utilization to insulin.

mechanism has since been disputed, but the basic observation has been confirmed many times. The glucose–fatty acid cycle describes the normal interplay between fat and carbohydrate oxidation, but has also been invoked (following a suggestion made in the original paper in 1963) to explain pathological situations involving excess availability of fat and insulin resistance of glucose uptake (for example type 2 diabetes and obesity).

Glucose and the regulation of fatty acid oxidation

An additional mechanism was first described in 1977 by Denis McGarry and Daniel Foster. They were following up a longstanding observation that the generation of ketone bodies by the liver (a reflection of β-oxidation of fatty acids) was suppressed by insulin or in livers from carbohydrate-replete animals. They showed that malonyl CoA, the first committed intermediate in the pathway of *de novo* lipogenesis (produced by acetyl CoA carboxylase; see above), strongly inhibited fatty acid oxidation. This inhibition is mediated via the enzyme carnitine palmitoyltransferase-1 (also called carnitine acyltransferase-1) in the mitochondrial membrane. Carnitine palmitoyltransferase-1 is responsible for the transport of fatty acids from the cytoplasm to the mitochondrion for β-oxidation. Acetyl CoA carboxylase is activated by insulin (both by increased gene transcription and by reversible dephosphorylation). Hence in a carbohydrate-replete state malonyl CoA will be formed and fatty acid oxidation inhibited (Fig. 4).

This is now recognized as a widespread regulatory mechanism. There are two isoforms of acetyl CoA carboxylase. Acetyl CoA carboxylase 1, expressed in lipogenic tissues such as liver and adipose tissue, appears to be involved in *de novo* fatty acid synthesis. Acetyl CoA carboxylase 2 is expressed more in tissues oxidizing fatty acids such as heart and skeletal muscle and is thought to produce malonyl CoA for regulatory rather than synthetic purposes. In fact, in muscle the pathway of fatty acid synthesis does not occur (fatty acid synthase is not expressed). Muscle carnitine palmitoyltransferase-1 is more sensitive to inhibition by malonyl CoA than is the liver enzyme. The ability of glucose to inhibit the oxidation of fatty acids in muscle has recently been clearly demonstrated *in vivo*, and has been termed the 'reverse glucose–fatty acid cycle'.

Fig. 4 The inhibition of fatty acid oxidation when glucose and insulin concentrations are high. Pathways are: 1, fatty acid 'activation' (fatty acyl CoA synthase); 2, transfer of acyl CoA into the mitochondrion via carnitine palmitoyltransferase-1 (CPT-1); 3, β-oxidation; 4, glycolysis (cytosolic) followed by pyruvate dehydrogenase (mitochondrial); 5, transfer of acetyl CoA to the cytosol via the citrate shuttle (details not shown); 6, acetyl CoA carboxylase (ACC) to form malonyl CoA, which is a powerful inhibitor of CPT-1; 7, fatty acid synthesis (not present in all tissues in which this mechanism operates, for example skeletal muscle).

Protein and amino acid metabolism and their regulation

Since there are 20 different amino acids incorporated into protein, and a variety of other amino acids that have important biological rules, it is essential for this purpose to generalize somewhat about amino acid and protein metabolism.

The body pools of protein and amino acids, and their turnover, are summarized in Fig. 5. Insulin exerts a net anabolic role on body protein, mainly in skeletal muscle, whereas thyroid hormones and cortisol are generally 'catabolic'. Anabolism is also stimulated by anabolic steroids, by physical training, and during growth by the insulin-like growth factors.

Dietary protein, digested in the small intestine and absorbed as free amino acids and short peptides, enters the portal vein. In the enterocytes of the small intestine some amino acids, especially glutamine, are removed for use as an oxidative fuel. The remaining products of digestion next meet the liver where further preferential extraction takes place. Amino acid oxidation is, under most circumstances, the major oxidative pathway in the liver. About 60 per cent of incoming amino acids may be directed into immediate oxidation. The rate of hepatic protein synthesis is also high, and since much of the protein is secreted (for example albumin), this represents a net loss of

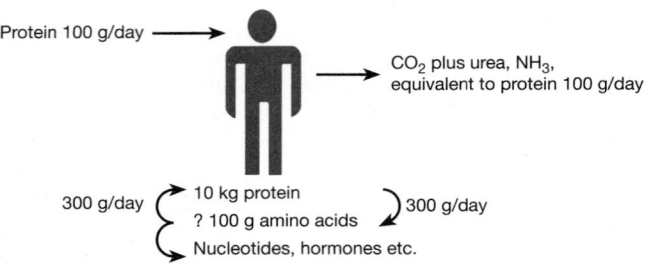

Fig. 5 The body pools of protein and amino acids, and their turnover. Figures are approximate.

amino acids from the liver (perhaps a further 20 per cent of the incoming amino acids). The remaining mixture of amino acids, around 20 per cent of those absorbed, enters the systemic circulation. This mixture is enriched in the branched chain amino acids leucine, isoleucine, and valine, which have a special role in muscle.

Urea synthesis takes place only in the liver. (The pathway is present in the brain but this is not a significant site of blood urea production.) Therefore, amino acids released from proteolysis in peripheral tissues must be transported, or must transfer their amino nitrogen, to the liver. This results in considerable interaction between the pathways of amino acid, carbohydrate, and fat metabolism. Measurements of arteriovenous differences across muscle and adipose tissue show that the release of the two amino acids alanine and glutamine predominates. Since glutamine carries two nitrogens it is, under most circumstances, the predominant carrier of nitrogen. Arteriovenous difference measurements across the splanchnic bed (by catheterization of the hepatic vein) show an almost identical pattern for uptake: removal of alanine and glutamine far exceeds that of other amino acids. Therefore amino acids in tissues including muscle and adipose tissue must transfer their amino nitrogen to alanine (by transamination with pyruvate) and glutamine (formed from glutamate, itself arising by transamination with 2-oxoglutarate). The aminotransferases (transaminases) bring about this transfer. It is important that the 2-oxoacid acceptors, pyruvate and 2-oxoglutarate, are common metabolic intermediates and thus readily available.

Much of the alanine released from skeletal muscle comes from transamination of pyruvate formed in glycolysis. Within the liver the amino group can be transferred further, for example to oxaloacetate, forming aspartate which is one of the immediate donors of nitrogen to the urea cycle. The pyruvate thus formed may be a substrate for gluconeogenesis, producing glucose that can be recycled to peripheral tissues. This metabolic cycle has been called the glucose–alanine cycle. It closely parallels the Cori cycle (see above).

The other route of entry of nitrogen into the urea cycle is ammonia. In peripheral tissues ammonia may be formed by the oxidative deamination of glutamate, catalysed by glutamate dehydrogenase. This reaction, in combination with the aminotransferases, can be seen to capture amino nitrogen from a number of amino acids. However, blood ammonia concentrations are very low (it is highly toxic) and instead it seems to be 'fixed' in the amido group of glutamine by the enzyme glutamine synthetase. In the liver the ammonia required for the urea cycle may be formed from the amido nitrogen of glutamine, removed by the enzyme glutaminase, or by the oxidative deamination of glutamate. There is also a supply of ammonia from the small intestine.

An important aspect of the large store of muscle protein is that it represents a potential source of synthesis of new glucose during fasting. In that situation, while the brain continues to require glucose for oxidation, and as glycogen reserves are depleted, new glucose can only be formed from glycerol, released in adipose tissue lipolysis, and from amino acids. The pathways described above are for the transfer of nitrogen, but not necessarily of carbon, to the liver. To explain the latter, we have to invoke pathways whereby amino acid carbon can also be exported. Amino acids whose 2-oxoacid can enter the tricarboxylic acid cycle may generate pyruvate (which can also accept amino nitrogen to become alanine). Pairs of amino acids can provide all the carbons necessary for glutamine synthesis.

Further reading

Frayn KN (1996). *Metabolic regulation: a human perspective*. Portland Press, London.

Friedman JM, Halaas JL (1998). Leptin and the regulation of body weight in mammals. *Nature* **395**, 763–70.

Havel RJ (1997). Postprandial lipid metabolism: an overview. *Proceedings of the Nutrition Society* **56**, 659–66.

McGarry JD (1979). Lilly Lecture 1978. New perspectives in the regulation of ketogenesis. *Diabetes* **28**, 517–23.

Nonogaki K (2000). New insights into sympathetic regulation of glucose and fat metabolism. *Diabetologia* **43**, 533–49.

Nordlie RC, Foster JD, Lange AJ (1999). Regulation of glucose production by the liver. *Annual Review of Nutrition* **19**, 379–406.

O'Brien RM, Granner DK (1996). Regulation of gene expression by insulin. *Physiological Reviews* **76**, 1109–61.

Randle PJ *et al.* (1963). The glucose-fatty acid cycle. Its role in insulin sensitivity and the metabolic disturbances of diabetes mellitus. *The Lancet* **1**, 785–9.

Sidossis LS, Wolfe RR (1996). Glucose and insulin-induced inhibition of fatty acid oxidation: the glucose-fatty acid cycle reversed. *American Journal of Physiology* **33**, E733–E738.

Zammit VA (1999). The malonyl-CoA-long-chain acyl-CoA axis in the maintenance of mammalian cell function. *Biochemical Journal* **343**, 505–15.

Zierler K (1999). Whole body glucose metabolism. *American Journal of Physiology* **276**, E409–E426.

10.3 Vitamins and trace elements

M. Eastwood

Vitamins are diverse organic compounds that the body cannot synthesize; they are required in small amounts to contribute to health.

Historical background

Our understanding of the role of vitamins comes from clinical observations, nutritional experiments in animals, and studies using purified preparations of the active principle used to treat deficiency states. Early pioneers differentiated dietary deficiency from infection and other causes of disease. Scurvy was once the scourge of mariners and explorers, but the clinical trials of Lind (1753), confirmed by Captain Cook on his voyages, showed the benefits of citrus fruits. Many years later, Holst and Froelich (1907) produced scurvy in guinea-pigs by dietary deprivation.

Rickets arose in sun-starved urban slums, and Trousseau noted the beneficial effects of cod liver oil (1860). Ejikmann and Grijns fed chickens the same diet as their patients who had beriberi (1897); neuropathy in the chickens resolved when the diet contained whole-grain, rather than polished, rice. In the 1900s Gowland Hopkins, the discoverer of vitamins, described a fat-soluble, essential growth accessory food factor A in milk. This was differentiated from water-soluble accessory food factor B by McCollum and Davis. Mellanby treated rickets in puppies with a fat-soluble food factor D. Lucy Wills described the megaloblastic anaemia of pregnancy in 1931, which is now known to be caused by a deficiency of folic acid.

In 1894 Atwater published a table of food composition and dietary standards for the United States. The first *USA Recommended Daily Allowances* was published in 1941. Food rationing in Britain during the Second World War was a triumph for the science of applied nutrition. The natural development of this work was the emergence of recommended daily intakes that recognized the differing requirements of the young and growing, pregnant and lactating, middle-aged and old, and ill; with this, developed the concept of the optimal intake for optimal nutritional status. The isolation and chemical synthesis of the vitamins and their active principles provided formidable challenges to scientists, rewarded by eight Nobel prizes in Medicine and Physiology and four in Chemistry. In 1976, Linus Pauling advocated gram intakes of ascorbic acid as a prevention against the common cold. Pauling thus founded 'orthomolecular medicine'.

The traditional classification of vitamins into water and lipid soluble and by their associated deficiency conditions becomes less useful as their biochemical roles are better understood. An inadequate dietary vitamin intake will result in specific cellular failure and even death. There is a dose–response relationship with vitamin intake from the physiological through the pharmacological to the toxic. Recommendations for vitamin intake for different ages, needs, and communities are based on dietary intake, bioavailability, steady-state concentrations in plasma and tissue at defined intakes, urine excretion, adverse effects, biochemical and molecular function, and freedom from deficiency. With increasing intake, either orally or as an infusion, a vitamin is distributed through the body fluids and tissues until the saturation point is exceeded. The prescription of vitamins parenterally, bypassing the absorptive processes, also has dosage implications.

The carotenoids illustrate the complexity of vitamins in physiology, pharmacology, and as toxins. Carotenoids are used by archaebacteria to reinforce cell membranes, their long, rigid carbon backbone acting as a rivet across the membrane. The polyene chain of between 9 and 11 double bonds serves to harvest light energy in plants, and, as the pigment retinal, is a visual pigment in animals. The linear system of conjugated C=C bonds make for a high reducing and antioxidant potential. Carotenoids act as the coloration in plants and to protect egg proteins against the enzymatic activity of proteases. Retinoic acid in animals and abscisic acid in plants act as hormones. When retinoids and carotenoids were used in lung cancer chemoprevention trials, the incidence of cancer increased, ascribed possibly to the increase in the oxidized products of β-carotene. A mix of vitamins and antioxidants might prevent such oxidation. Such a mix can be found in fruit and vegetables, which emphasizes the benefit of a good diet containing five portions (60 to 150 g) of fruit and vegetables a day.

Vitamin C (ascorbic acid)

Ascorbic acid is a simple sugar that reversibly oxidizes to dehydroascorbate. Dietary sources are fresh fruit and fruit juices, especially blackcurrants, guavas, green leafy vegetables, and fresh milk. Ascorbic acid is readily oxidized during cooking—a process accelerated by traces of copper in alkaline solution. Since humans, guinea-pigs, the Indian fruit-eating bat, the red vented bulbul, and some birds are unable to synthesize ascorbic acid, it thus represents a vitamin in these species. Ascorbic acid

- is a water-soluble, non-specific radical-trapping antioxidant and reducing agent which is present in all tissues;

- acts synergistically with vitamin E;

- is involved in copper-containing hydroxylase enzymes (e.g. proline and lysine hydroxylase), and is important in collagen metabolism and 2-oxoglutarate-linked iron hydroxylases;

- is involved in carnitine biosynthesis, which is necessary for fatty acid transport from the cytosol into mitochondria; and

- is involved in the synthesis of hormones (e.g. epinephrine (adrenaline)).

Ascorbic acid is rapidly absorbed from the small intestine. The plasma concentration (5 per cent as dehydroascorbate) and dietary intake are in a sigmoidal relationship (80 μmol/l on 100 mg/day) which plateaus at 1000 mg/day intake. The body pool size is 900 mg (5 mmole in the normal adult): approximately 3 per cent, irrespective of pool size, is degraded each day and excreted in the urine as free ascorbic acid, dehydroascorbate, or diketogulonate. High tissue concentrations at birth steadily decline with increasing age.

A shortfall in vitamin C intake without clinical scurvy may be associated with a reduction in the body's water-soluble antioxidant capacity, the consequences of which are still being debated. The young and elderly are particularly at risk of scurvy, which results from an inadequate intake of ascorbic acid. Clinical scurvy appears after 4 weeks on an ascorbic acid-deficient diet when the body pool is less than 300 mg (1.7 mmole). There is a failure of connective tissue collagen synthesis, and cartilage, bone, and dentine growth are all compromised. Tissues bleed readily, and heal poorly due to defective intracellular linkages between the endothelial cells and capillary basement tissue. Individuals are initially lethargic and irritable. Characteristic livid-coloured, spongy, bleeding gingivitis of the gums develops, and scurvy buds appear in the papillae between the teeth. Large or microscopic haemorrhages occur in the gums, as well as in the eyes (especially bulbar conjunctiva), subcutaneous tissues, synovia of joints, and beneath the periosteum of bones. Perifollicular bleeding occurs in the dependent parts of the body, later becoming more generalized. Fatal haemorrhages may also occur in the brain or heart muscle. Keratin-like material heaps on the surface of hair follicles, through which a deformed corkscrew hair projects. Other signs include dependent oedema, oliguria, depression, megaloblastic or normoblastic anaemia, and superinfection. Infants present with irritability, tender legs, and pseudoparalysis. Scurvy buds, but not gingivitis, occur in edentulous infants. Large subperiosteal haemorrhages develop over the long bones, especially the femur.

Diagnosis requires an awareness of the condition, a careful dietary history, and a clinical examination. The patient can improve on hospital diet alone. Ascorbic acid is measured in plasma or whole blood. While leucocyte or buffy-coat vitamin C concentrations reflect tissue concentrations, this is complicated in disease by different leucocytes types which vary in number and ascorbic acid content.

Requirements

The optimum dietary intake of ascorbic acid has yet to be defined. The body can be saturated with 1 g/day for 5 days. Recommendations for dietary intake range from 40 to 200 mg per day. An upper limit of intake is recommended at 1 to 2 g/day, based upon body saturation figures rather than toxicity. During pregnancy and lactation, intake should be between 100 and 200 mg daily. The ascorbic acid content of breast milk varies between 30 and 80 mg/l which provides 25 mg per day, clinical scurvy has not been observed in fully breast-fed infants. The ascorbic acid intake of the elderly is generally adequate but should be monitored. The pharmacological use of ascorbic acid is extensive and imaginative.

Biotin

Biotin contains a ureido group in a five-membered ring fused with a tetrahydrothiophene ring with a five-carbon side chain terminating in a carboxyl group. Dietary biotin is found in yeast, bacteria, liver, kidney, egg yolks, cooked cereals, pulses, nuts, chocolates, and some vegetables. Biotin is a cofactor for the acetyl-coenzyme A (**CoA**), propionyl CoA, and pyruvate carboxylase systems involved in the incorporation of bicarbonate as a carboxyl group into substrates in fatty acid synthesis and gluconeogenesis. Biotin is absorbed from the upper gastrointestinal tract. Raw egg white contains the glycoprotein avidin (molecular weight, 68 000) which binds biotin with a high affinity and prevents biotin absorption. Biotin is transported in plasma to the liver for storage. It is metabolized before excretion in the urine as biotin, bisnorbiotin, and biotin sulphoxide.

Biotin deficiency results in fatigue, depression, sleepiness, nausea, loss of appetite, muscle pain, hyperaesthesia and paraesthesia, alopecia, dermatitis, conjunctivitis, smooth tongue, and dry skin. Individuals receiving treatment for epilepsy are at risk of biotin deficiency. There are no indications that excess biotin is toxic. Body stores are measured by plasma biotin concentrations, and lymphocyte propionyl CoA carboxylase and its activation index (ratio of enzyme activity incubated with and without biotin) or urinary 3-hydroxy isovalerate.

Requirements

The dietary requirement of biotin is not known with certainty. The average intake of a British adult ranges from 10 to 70 µg/day, which is seen to be adequate. In infants, preterm to 5 years, an intake between 5 and 25 µg/day is suggested.

Niacin: nicotinic acid and nicotinamide

Niacin is a B vitamin. It occurs in food as nicotinic acid, as a pyridine nucleotide coenzyme derivative (NAD and NADP), as an amide, nicotinamide (niacinamide), or as a nicotinoyl ester, niacytin in maize. Nicotinic acid is found in meat, poultry, fish, wholemeal cereals, pulses, and coffee. Nicotinic acid is synthesized from tryptophan, catalysed by kynureninase and kynurenine hydroxylase which are vitamin B_6 and riboflavin dependent. A deficiency of either vitamin B_6 or riboflavin may aggravate niacin deficiency. Some 60 mg of dietary tryptophan generates 1 mg of nicotinic acid. The nicotinic acid equivalent is the dietary nicotinic acid content plus 1/60th of the dietary tryptophan.

Nicotinamide is a component of the coenzymes nicotinamide adenine dinucleotide (**NAD+**) and nicotinamide adenine dinucleotide phosphate (**NADP+**, also known as triphosphopyridine nucleotide (**TPN+**)). NAD coenzymes are biological carriers of reducing equivalents, that is to say electrons, during metabolic oxidation to NADH+. NADH+ acts as a true coenzyme in enzymes involved in epimerization, aldolization, and elimination.

The various conjugated forms of niacin are hydrolysed and absorbed in the upper gastrointestinal mucosa as the free acid. Niacytin from maize is neither hydrolysed nor absorbed. In Central America, maize is eaten as tortillas, in which lime water hydrolyses the nicotinoyl ester component. Niacin and tryptophan deficiencies occur in poor populations dependent upon maize for their protein intake. Zein, the principal maize protein, is deficient in tryptophan. Protein energy malnutrition, dietary amino acid imbalances (for example, an excess leucine intake), anaemia, and other vitamin deficiencies worsen the problem. Dietary fortification with other proteins is necessary.

An inadequate dietary intake of 1- to 2-months' duration leads to significant tissue depletion and pellagra, which if untreated progresses to death. There is no apparent tissue storage of this vitamin. The vitamin is excreted in the urine as nicotinuric acid, nicotinamide-*N*-oxide and 5'-methylnicotinamide. Pellagra is characterized by dermatitis, diarrhoea, and dementia; the disease is chronic with a seasonal periodicity. Individuals suffer weight and stamina loss, which is worsened by secondary bacterial and parasitic infections. Erythematous dermatitis is symmetrically distributed on skin exposed to sunlight and mechanical irritation. In chronic pellagra the skin looks sunburnt. In severe cases, gastrointestinal disturbances occur with diarrhoea. There can be glossitis, angular stomatitis, cheilosis, and an inflamed tongue, and secondary infection of the mouth. Mild mental changes include anxiety and irritability progressing to manic depressive illness. There may be paraesthesia in the lower limbs, with loss of vibration sense and proprioception leading to ataxia and spasticity.

Pellagra can occur in alcoholism, malabsorption syndromes, and Hartnup disease. Mild cases rapidly improve on treatment with niacin or a suitable dietary protein supplementation. Oral nicotinamide (100 mg every 4 h) results in symptom resolution within 24 h, although mental symptoms, especially dementia, may be unresponsive to treatment. Nicotinic acid may cause unpleasant flushing and burning sensations. A supplementary diet containing good-quality protein and all of the vitamins is important. Nicotinic acid, but not nicotinamide, is used therapeutically for hyperlipidaemias at a dose of 2 to 6 g/day, but it can be hepatotoxic.

Microbiological methods provide the most sensitive means of measuring niacin and nicotinamide in serum, urine, and food. Alternatively, urinary nicotinamide, *n*-methyl nicotinamide (**NMN**), is measured over a defined time or as a ratio of creatine in urine. Urinary *N*-methyl-2-piridone-5-carboxamide (2-pyridone) excretion is a more sensitive measurement in borderline cases of nicotinamide deficiency, and is expressed in relation to urinary creatinine excretion.

Requirements

These are related to dietary tryptophan intake. A protein intake of between 60 and 85 g/day contains approximately 13 mg tryptophan/g, equivalent to between 13 and 17 mg/day of niacin. The recommended intake as niacin equivalents is 6.6 mg (54 μmole)/4185 J (4.185 J = 1 kCal). Hormonal changes during pregnancy affect tryptophan metabolism, so that 30 mg of tryptophan is equivalent to 1 mg of dietary niacin. Breast milk should provide not less than 3.5 mg preformed niacin/4185 J. Mature human milk provides preformed niacin (2.7 mg/l), therefore an increment of 2 mg/day niacin for the nursing mother is suggested.

Pantothenic acid

Pantothenic acid is the dimethyl derivative of butyric acid joined by a peptide linkage to α-alanine. The active form, 4'-phosphopantetheine, is present in all tissues. Pantothenic acid is thermo- and acid-labile. It is widely available in animal-based foods, especially liver, although cereals and legumes are also sources. 4'-Phosphopantetheine is a constituent of CoA and acyl carrier protein. CoA plays a central role in intermediary metabolism, fatty-acid β-oxidation, sterol synthesis, and other acetylation processes. Acyl carrier protein is an acyl carrier in the synthesis of lipids. Pantothenic acid is found in food as the coenzyme CoA or acyl carrier protein form and is hydrolysed by a pancreatic enzyme before absorption. Urinary excretion is in the free acid form.

Pantothenic acid is not stored in the body. Although no specific deficiency syndrome has been recorded, pantothenic acid deficiency may occur as part of the overall problem in people who are severely malnourished. No toxic intakes have been recorded. There is no biochemical method for measuring pantothenic acid status in humans.

Requirements

Most human diets provide 3 to 10 mg of pantothenic acid per day. A safe and adequate intake is between 3 and 7 mg per day, including during pregnancy and lactation. Infants require 1.7 mg/day; human milk provides 2.6 mg/day. Infant formula milk should contain at least 2 mg/litre.

Riboflavin

Riboflavin is a substituted alloxazine ring linked to ribotol, an alcohol derived from the pentose sugar ribose. It is light sensitive. Dietary sources are liver, milk, cheese, eggs, some green vegetables, and beer. Other sources are yeast extracts (for example, Marmite) and meat extracts (for example, Bovril). Riboflavin in the diet exists in either the free form or the phosphorylated coenzyme form.

Riboflavin links with phosphoric acid as flavin mononucleotide (or riboflavin–5'-phosphate) (FMN), which with adenosine monophosphate (AMP) forms flavin adenine dinucleotide (FAD): the prosthetic groups of the flavoprotein enzymes. Flavoproteins are involved in redox processes involving the hydrogen-transfer chain in the mitochondria and the production of ATP. FAD/FMN acts as a coenzyme in oxidation/reduction reactions, electron transport, oxidative phosphorylation (for example, succinic dehydrogenases), and fatty-acid β-oxidation.

Riboflavin is absorbed from the upper gastrointestinal tract, there is no specific storage tissue, and it is excreted in the urine either free or in small amounts of hydroxylated products. Chronic infection can affect urinary riboflavin excretion. A deficiency of riboflavin causes cheilosis, angular stomatitis, superficial interstitial keratosis of the cornea, and nasolabial seborrhoea. Riboflavin deficiency may impair iron absorption. No toxic effects have been shown for riboflavin.

Riboflavin status can be estimated from the urinary riboflavin:creatinine ratio, which is insensitive at low intakes. The erythrocyte glutathione reductase activation coefficient (EGRAC) measures tissue saturation and long-term riboflavin status.

Requirements

Adults, including the elderly, need between 1 and 1.5 mg of riboflavin per day. The average riboflavin content of breast milk in Britain is approximately 0.3 mg/l, which is dependent upon maternal intake. Intakes should increase by 0.3 mg/day during pregnancy, and 0.5 mg/day during lactation. Recommended intakes for children range from 0.4 mg/day for infants up to 3 months of age and 1.0 mg/day thereafter.

Thiamin

Thiamin hydrochloride consists of a substituted pyrimidine ring linked by a methylene group to a sulphur-containing thiazole ring. All animal and plant tissues contain thiamin, usually in the phosphorylated form. The important sources are plant seeds and cereal germ, nuts, peas, beans, pulses, and yeast. Losses occur with cooking and alkaline pH. Thiamin diphosphate is the coenzyme in α-ketoacids and decarboxylation reactions involved in the oxidative decarboxylation of pyruvic acid to acetyl-CoA, and the transketolase reaction in the hexose monophosphate shunt. Thiamin may also play a role in neural excitation mechanisms.

Absorption is from the upper gastrointestinal tract, followed by phosphorylation to the active diphosphate form. There is no body store and the only reserve is the vitamin functionally bound to enzymes. Multiple end-products are excreted in the urine. Beriberi is caused by dietary thiamin deficiency, a disease that was endemic in the East as a result of the ingestion of polished rice which is deficient in the vitamin. Carbohydrate metabolism is impaired by a deficiency of thiamin pyrophosphate, a coenzyme necessary for the decarboxylation of pyruvate to acetyl-CoA. Pyruvic and lactic acid accumulate in the body. The clinical presentations of thiamin deficiency are:

- wet beriberi (high-output cardiac failure);
- dry beriberi (polyneuropathy);
- infantile beriberi;
- neuropathy and cardiomyopathy in chronic alcoholism; and the
- Wernicke–Korsakoff syndrome.

Initially the symptoms are of non-specific malaise and evidence of early cardiac failure and neuropathy. Wet beriberi is characterized by left- and right-sided high-output cardiac failure, cardiomegaly, hypotension, rapid deterioration, and death. Dry beriberi is a polyneuropathy affecting motor and sensory nerves. Initially there is paraesthesia progressing to painful muscle wasting and polyneuritis. Total sensory loss occurs and patients become immobile and emaciated; they are at a high risk for the development of Wernicke–Korsakoff's encephalopathy. Infantile beriberi occurs in breast-fed infants of thiamin-deficient mothers, usually when they are between 2- and 5-months old. In the acute form, the child is restless, distressed with evidence of high output cardiac failure; convulsions may develop and the child becomes comatose. In the chronic form, the child is fretful, sleeps poorly, and the muscles may be flaccid. Cardiac failure, gastrointestinal symptoms, and sudden death are common. Alcoholic neuropathy presents with a sensory and motor neuropathy sometimes complicated by cardiomyopathy. Sensory nerve dysfunction includes paraesthesia and severe nerve pain. Motor nerve lesions are of both upper and lower motor neurone type. A patient with Wernicke–Korsakoff syndrome is disorientated and apathetic. Nystagmus, ataxia, and confabulation are not infrequent consequences of lesions in the brainstem, diencephalon, and cerebellum.

Treatment is with intramuscular thiamin 25 mg twice daily for 3 days, and thereafter 10 mg two or three times daily. The reversal of the wet type of beriberi is rapid. Improvement is slow for dry beriberi, especially for the neurological abnormalities. In infantile beriberi, both mother (10 mg thiamin twice daily) and the infant (thiamin intramuscularly 10 to 20 mg/day for 3 days, and thereafter 5 to 10 mg twice daily) are treated. Beriberi can be prevented by eating thiamin-containing foods, unmilled or thiamin-fortified rice, or thiamin supplements.

Long-term intakes in excess of 50 mg per kg body weight/day are toxic, leading to headaches, irritability, insomnia, rapid pulse, weakness, contact dermatitis, pruritus, and even death. Thiamin status can be measured by urinary thiamin and the thiamin:creatinine ratio with or without a loading dose, or by the reactivation of the cofactor-depleted red-cell enzyme transketolase *in vitro*.

Requirements

Thiamin requirements are related to energy and carbohydrate metabolism. The average requirement for adults, normal pregnancy or lactation, and children is 0.4 mg/4185 J and not less than 0.8 mg/day for adults with a supplement of 0.6 mg/4185 J during pregnancy and lactation. Human breast milk contains the equivalent of 0.3 mg/4185 J. The elderly may require 1 mg/day.

Vitamin B₆ (pyridoxine)

Pyridoxine is to be found in several forms: pyridoxal, pyridoxamine, and pyridoxine. This family of vitamin B₆ compounds is found in many foods: cereals, meat (particularly liver), fruits, and leafy and other vegetables. The free form is common in plants, the phosphorylated form, pyridoxamine phosphate, in animal tissues. Pyridoxal-5'-phosphate is a coenzyme and plays a major role in the intermediary metabolism of amino acids, in α-decarboxylation, aldolization, and transamination reactions. Pyridoxal-5'-phosphate acts as a coenzyme with glycogen phosphorylase in muscle, and has a role in the actions on hormones which modulate gene expression. Vitamin B₆ is absorbed in the free form and phosphorylated for use in enzymes. There is no specific storage in tissues and it is excreted in urine largely as 4-pyridoxic acid.

Primary dietary deficiency has not been reported in adults, largely because of the wide availability of the vitamin. A biochemical deficiency occurs in alcoholics. Patients taking isoniazid may develop a pyridoxine deficiency and neuropathy. Women taking massive supplements of between 2 and 7 g/day, a dose which has been recommended for alleviating premenstrual symptoms, may develop a sensory neuropathy.

There is no single marker sensitive at all levels of dietary intake. Biochemical markers include plasma pyridoxal phosphate concentrations, red-cell transaminase activation, and the urinary excretion of vitamin B₆ degradation products. Metabolic loading tests also measure vitamin B₆ status, including the tryptophan- and methionine-load tests.

Requirements

The total body pool of vitamin B₆ is 15 μmole (4 mg)/kg, 80 per cent of which is in muscle, with a half-life of 33 days. Adults, pregnant and lactating women, and the elderly require a daily intake of 13 μg/g of protein (approximately 4 mg/day). The vitamin B₆ content of human breast milk is low at between 40 and 100 μg/l (or 3–8 μg vitamin B₆/g protein). Infants under 3 months of age require 6 μg/g protein, increasing to up to 13 μg/g protein at 7 to 10 years.

Folate (folic acid, folacin)

Sources of folate include liver, yeast extract, and green leafy vegetables. Folates are derivatives of folic acid (pteroylglutamic acid) including the folylpolyglutamate found in foods. Folic acid is a pterin ring (2-amino, 4-hydroxypteridine) attached to *p*-aminobenzoic acid conjugated to L-glutamic acid (**PteGlu**). Variants include:

- di-(7,8-tetrahydrofolic acid) (**DHF**) and tetra-(5,6,7,8-tetrahydrofolic acid) (**THF**) reduced forms of the pteridine ring;
- one-carbon substitution (methyl, formyl, methenyl, methylene, or formimino) at positions N5 or 10: 5-formyl-THF, 10-formyl-THF, 5-formimino-THF, 5,10-methenyl-THF, 5,10-methylene-THF, and 5-methyl-THF;
- a chain of 4–6 glutamates attached to the L-glutamate.

Folic acid gives and receives 1-carbon groups on the N5 or N10 position in nucleic acid and amino acid biosynthetic reactions. Most dietary folate is in the polyglutamyl form, which is hydrolysed to monoglutamate before being absorbed from the duodenum. A brush-border glutamyl carboxypeptidase is inhibited by alcohol, which is of relevance in alcoholic folic deficiencies. Folate bound to a milk protein is absorbed from the ileum. Folic acid is stored in the liver. Plasma folates are mainly 5-methyl-THF monoglutamate. Within cells, 5-methyl–THF is converted to THF polyglutamates, the main cellular forms of folic acid.

Folate polyglutamates do not readily cross cell membranes. The polyglutamate form has two functions: storage; and as a coenzyme for normal 1-carbon metabolism (for which it is the most efficient coenzyme). The 5-methyl group is transferred to homocysteine (creating methionine and THF); the enzyme is the vitamin B₁₂-dependent methionine synthase, wherein methionine, folic acid, and vitamin B₁₂ interlink.

Reactions in which folate is involved include:

- methylation of amino acids;
- serine reversibly interconverting with glycine;
- methionine interconverting with homocysteine (methionine is the precursor of *S*-adenosyl-L-methionine (**SAM**), a methyl donor in the methylation of lipids, hormones, DNA, cell division, and proteins); and
- thymidine and purine synthesis.

Folic acid deficiency may arise:

- as a dietary deficiency;
- in malabsorption syndromes;
- where there are excessive demands, as with increased cell proliferation (for example, in leukaemias and haemolytic anaemias);
- where drugs interfere with folic acid metabolism; and
- in the rare inborn errors of folic metabolism.

Folic acid deficiency is an important cause of megaloblastic anaemia, never to be confused with vitamin B₁₂ deficiency.

Neural tube defects (**NTDs**) are congenital deformities of the spinal cord and brain: spina bifida, anencephaly, encephalocele, and iniencephaly. Folic acid is involved in the aetiology of NTDs. The precise mechanism is unclear, but there may be an underlying genetic predisposition involving a variant of 5,10-methyl-THF reductase. Closure of the neural tube occurs early in pregnancy thereby making aetiological studies difficult. The results of recommendations to take folic acid supplements prophylactically are encouraging.

Epidemiological studies suggest an increased risk of vascular disease associated with hyperhomocysteinaemia. Homocysteine is reversibly methylated to methionine, a step which involves folate, vitamin B₁₂, and vitamin B6. Supplementation of these vitamins has been proposed to reduce the putative dangers of hyperhomocysteinaemia.

Folate status is measured by the folate concentration in serum and red cells. Red-cell folate levels reflect body stores. A coincidental measurement of serum vitamin B₁₂ is important.

Requirements

Children and adults, including the elderly, need a folate intake of 200 μg/day. Women planning a pregnancy should increase their intake of folic acid to 0.4 mg/day by capsule supplement. If there has been a previous

NTD-affected pregnancy then 5 mg of folic acid/day preconception is suggested. A problem is that some pregnancies are unplanned. Dietary supplementation is impractical. Total folic acid excretion in breast milk averages 40 µg/day, and an additional maternal intake of 60 µg per day is required.

Vitamin B₁₂

Vitamin B_{12} is a cobalt-containing corrinoid, four linked pyrrole rings (corrin) co-ordinating with a central cobalt atom. The cobinamides necessary for human well being are methylcobalamin, adenosylcobalamin, hydroxycobalamin, and cyanocobalamin. Micro-organisms, including colonic flora, synthesize cobalamin. Yeast is a source of cobalamin, primarily as adenosyl- and hydroxocobalamin. Methyl cobalamin is found in egg yolk, cheese, and cow's milk. A vegan diet carries a risk of vitamin B_{12} deficiency.

The reactions requiring vitamin B_{12} include:

- isomerization of methylmalonyl-CoA to succinyl-CoA (methyl malonic acid concentrations increase in cases of vitamin B_{12} deficiency);
- methyltransferase reactions: for example, homocysteine to methionine, i.e. the transfer of a methyl group from 5-methyl-TFH to homocysteine which converts homocysteine to methionine.

Vitamin B_{12} has an important role in the maintenance of myelin. Deoxyadenosyl B_{12} is essential for propionyl-CoA reactions by transmutation of methylmalonyl-CoA to succinyl-CoA.

Vitamin B_{12} binds to food proteins and is released by saliva, acid pH, and pepsin, depending upon the mode of cooking and type of food protein. Vitamin B_{12} at stomach pH forms complexes with glycoproteins, transcobalamin, haptocorrin, and intrinsic factor. In the duodenum, cobalamin is released by pancreatic enzymes and alkaline pH and binds solely to intrinsic factor. The vitamin B_{12}/intrinsic factor complex is absorbed from the ileum through a specific receptor. Cobalamin is released from intrinsic factor, converted (80 per cent to methyl and also adenosyl and hydroxy forms) and carried in the blood by transcobalamins I, II, and III. Of these, transcobalamin II releases vitamin B_{12} to the tissues to be stored in the adenosyl form. The total body cobalamin content in adults is between 2 and 5 mg, most of which is stored in the liver. Turnover is 0.1 per cent of the body pool each day. There is efficient conservation by the kidneys and the enterohepatic circulation. Most vitamin B_{12} is excreted in urine and small amounts in faeces, including unabsorbed bacterially synthesized vitamin B_{12}. The relationship between dietary intake and serum concentrations is not linear because the body stores of vitamin B_{12} are largely in the liver.

Vitamin B_{12} deficiency results in megaloblastic anaemia and neurological disorders, especially in the posterolateral columns of the spinal cord. Causes of deficiency are dietary (vegans), lack of intrinsic factor (Addison's pernicious anaemia, gastric resection), intestinal colonization by bacteria and parasites (for example, tapeworms), and ileal resection. The megaloblastic anaemia is due to a lack of vitamin B_{12} for methionine synthase, insufficient methionine regeneration, and 5,10-methylene-THF and deficient thymidylate synthesis. In vitamin B_{12} deficiency, odd number 15- and 17-carbon fatty acids and branch-chain fatty acids are synthesized and incorporated into an unstable myelin nerve sheath. An inability to regenerate methionine from homocysteine, for the S-adenosylmethionine generation necessary for myelin proteins, leads to demyelination.

The efficiency of vitamin B_{12} absorption is measured by the Schilling test or by a whole-body scanner.

Requirements

A dietary intake of between 1 and 2 µg/day for adults of all ages is protective. In pregnancy there is a compensatory increased absorption so that 1.5 µg/day is sufficient. During lactation an increment of 0.5 µg/day should ensure an adequate supply in breast milk (0.2 to 1.0 µg/l). The requirement for infants is of the order of 0.1 µg/day and for children aged 3 to 10 years,

0.5 to 1.0 µg/day. Vitamin B_{12} has extremely low toxicity and as much as 3 mg/day may be taken.

Vitamin A

The vitamin A family (retinoids) are related to the plant pigment carotene. Dietary vitamin A comes in two forms: from animal sources, preformed, vitamin A fatty-acid esters; or from plant, provitamin A carotenoids. β-Carotene, a provitamin A carotenoid, consists of two retinol molecules. Retinol is vitamin A alcohol, a hydrocarbon chain with a betaionone ring at one end and an alcohol group at the other, usually esterified with a fatty acid (retinyl esters) as the *all-trans* stereoisomer. The *cis* configuration isomer (11 or 13 position) is less potent. Retinol can be oxidized to an aldehyde (retinal) or acid (retinoic acid). Retinol and carotene are readily oxidized and are protected by vitamin E.

Retinol is present in dairy products, liver, and fatty fish liver oils. Carotenes are found predominantly in green vegetables as well as in yellow and red fruits and vegetables. Vitamin A is essential for the maintenance of epithelial tissue, visual function, and the immune system. Most actions of vitamin A in development, differentiation, and metabolism are mediated through retinoid receptors of the nuclear steroid receptor family of proteins that bind retinoic acid and regulate gene expression.

The photopigment rhodopsin is formed by the protein opsin and 11-*cis* retinal. A photon of light converts the *cis* retinal to the *trans* form, which reversibly dissociates from the opsin and is seen as light. Retinyl esters are hydrolysed by pancreatic hydrolases and the enteric mucosa. β-Carotene is cleaved to two retinols by β-carotene 15,15'-deoxygenase, and carotenoids oxidatively cleave to retinal and apocarotenoids. Retinal is reduced to retinol, esterified with long-chain fatty acids, and transported to the liver as retinyl long-chain fatty esters in chylomicrons through the lymph. Retinol is a major liver storage form and circulates to tissues, bound to retinol binding protein. There is an enterohepatic circulation of retinoids.

Vitamin A deficiency is a major worldwide cause of blindness, due to a poor dietary intake of green vegetables, fruit, and dairy produce. Malabsorption is a less common cause. Vitamin A deficiency results in reduced rhodopsin in the retinal rods resulting in loss of vision. Xerophthalmia causes blindness in 500 000 young children each year, especially amongst bottle-fed infants and breast-fed infants with vitamin A-deficient mothers. Protein calorie malnutrition compounds the problem during weaning. Vitamin A deficiency aggravates damage from other causes of keratoconjunctivitis, for example measles. Epithelial surfaces undergo squamous metaplasia, followed by corneal ulceration and irreversible visual damage. Clinical forms are:

- conjunctival xerosis (Bitots's spots are white plaques of thickened conjunctival epithelium indicative of vitamin deficiency in the young);
- corneal xerosis;
- keratomalacia, leading to blindness;
- night blindness, an early symptom with or without xerophthalmia;
- xerophthalmia fundi; and
- corneal scars.

Vitamin A is important in epithelial metabolism. Deficiency leads to epithelial metaplasia and inappropriately keratinized epithelium in the mucous membranes of the respiratory, gastrointestinal, and genitourinary tract. Sebaceous glands become blocked thereby causing follicular keratosis.

Prophylaxis demands education in the eating of dark-green vegetables. Where xerophthalmia is endemic, vitamin A is given prophylactically in capsule form or by food fortification. Frank deficiency is treated by high-potency Vitamin A: 200 000 IU for 2 days, and a third dosage at least 2 weeks later. Thereafter, improved diet and supplementation is obligatory. Corneal ulceration is treated by antibiotics, and the response is rapid. Vitamin A deficiency is a putative risk factor for childhood morbidity and death, especially for the underweight and premature infant.

β-Carotene is not toxic, but high intakes lead to a yellow appearance sparing the eyes (hypercarotenaemia). Polar bear's liver, rich in retinol, is toxic and ingestion can cause drowsiness, headache, vomiting, and excess peeling of the skin. Large intakes of retinol are teratogenic. Pregnant women should be careful not to exceed the recommended intake of vitamin A in the first trimester.

Plasma retinol is an insensitive indicator of vitamin A status. The relative-dose-response (**RDR** test), which measures retinol transport by the retinol binding protein, is used as a functional test for calculating retinol stores. The concentration of plasma carotenoids reflects short- to medium-term intakes. The following are equipotent to 1 μg of *all-trans*-retinol equivalents/day: 3.33 IU vitamin A, 3.5 nmol retinol or retinyl ester, or 6 μg *all-trans*-β-carotene.

Requirements

Adults require 500 μg retinol equivalents/day; infants, 250 to 350 μg retinol equivalents/day; children, 350 μg retinol equivalents/day; pregnancy, an increment of 100 μg retinol equivalents/day, particularly during the third trimester. Lactation requires an increment of 300 μg retinol equivalents/day. Breast milk vitamin A concentration should exceed 1.5 mmol/l.

Vitamin D

The vitamin D family of sterols includes vitamin D_3 (cholecalciferol) and vitamin D_2 (ergocalciferol). Cholecalciferol is to be regarded as a hormone rather than a vitamin, and is produced by the ultraviolet irradiation of dietary 7-dehydrocholesterol (provitamin D_3) in the skin. The extent of exposure to sunlight determines production. Cholecalciferol is also available in fatty fish (for example, cod), eggs, and chicken liver. Ergocalciferol is also the result of the exposure of ergosterol (provitamin D_2) to ultraviolet light. Ergocalciferol differs from cholecalciferol in having an extra methyl group at C-24 and a double bond at C-22,23. 1,25-dihydroxycholecalciferol vitamin D (**1,25(OH)2D**) regulates calcium and phosphate absorption, metabolism, and export into the bloodstream. Such regulation is through steroid:thyroid hormone nuclear receptors. $1,25(OH)_2D$ is also a developmental hormone inhibiting proliferation and promoting differentiated function in cells.

Dietary vitamin D is absorbed in the small intestine, as a lipid, transported to the liver bound to α-globulin (*trans*-calciferol) in chylomicrons. Both vitamin D_2 and vitamin D_3 are inactive. They are converted in the liver by a P-450 inducable microsomal enzyme into 25-hydroxy vitamin D (**25(OH)D**), which has modest biological activity, before plasma transport on a specific globulin. The active form of vitamin D is $1,25(OH)2D$ formed in the kidney by a mitochondrial hydroxylase acting on 25(OH)D. The half-life of $1,25(OH)_2D$ is less than 24 h. All forms of vitamin D are stored in fat. Vitamin D is 24-hydroxylated and, as the glucuronide, is excreted in bile into an enterohepatic circulation.

The prime consequence of vitamin D deficiency is rickets, caused by a failure to mineralize the bony skeleton. The epiphyseal cartilage replacement is defective, leading to an overgrowth of subperiosteal osteoid tissue and poor mineralization of the bone matrix resulting in soft bones. The type of bony abnormalities depends on the age of onset and the weight-bearing bones involved. The appearance of the rachitic child is deceptive, the child may appear quite well or be restless with hypotonic muscles and twisted limbs' postures. The abdomen is swollen and the child suffers from diarrhoea, respiratory infection, and delayed tooth development. In the infant, the commonest abnormality is enlargement of the end of the radius and the costochondral junction—termed the ricketic rosary. Later there is bossing of the frontal and parietal bones and delayed closure of the anterior fontanel; so-called 'pigeon chest' can result, which is an undue prominence of the sternum and a transverse depression from the costal margins towards the axillae. All are due to pressure on the soft bones when the child is supine. In the walking child, the weight-bearing bones bend, kyphosis of the spine and bowing of the lower ends of the femur, tibia, and fibula result.

Pelvic deformity can make delivery difficult in subsequent pregnancies. Tetanic spasm can occur, whereby spasm of the hands, feet, and vocal chord result in high-pitched cries and breathing problems.

Diagnosis is based on the clinical appearance and measurements of plasma alkaline phosphatase (although interpretation of the results is difficult in the growing child) and plasma 25(OH)D levels. There are several risk factors:

- inadequate exposure to sunlight (dependent on latitude, in the United Kingdom 30- to 90-min exposure of the face and legs per day will restore 25(OH)D concentrations;
- strict vegetarianism;
- a vitamin D-deficient mother breast feeding her baby;
- high melanin content in the skin, which screens the metabolically active skin sites; and
- malabsorption.

Prevention of vitamin D deficiency requires a supplement of 10 μg of vitamin D daily or regular exposure to sunlight in well-nourished individuals.

Osteomalacia, may present with muscular weakness and a waddling gait. Bone pain, tetany, and spontaneous fractures may develop. Radiographic features include bone rarification, pseudofractures, and Looser's zones at points of compression stress. Renal disease, from many causes, may be associated with impaired renal synthesis of $1,25(OH)_2D$. A failure of 25-hydroxylation of vitamin D can occur in hepatic disease. Dietary vitamin D intake may be important in immunity to tuberculosis, and 25-OH vitamin D deficiency may contribute to the occurrence of tuberculosis. Hypervitaminosis occurs during infant supplementation and replacement therapy. Plasma calcium concentrations increase with tetany, ECG changes with resultant convulsions, and occasionally death. Vitamin D in milligram amounts is poisonous, and is used as a rodenticide.

The best measure of the vitamin status in humans is the plasma 25(OH)D concentration.

Requirements

No minimum dietary intake has been identified for adults exposed to ample sunlight. However, 10 μg/day vitamin D is recommended for those with poor sun exposure. Breast-milk vitamin D concentrations are low (0.25–1.25 μg/litre) and are reduced in the winter. Vitamin D intakes are a problem for the 6- to 12-month-old baby dependent upon modestly fortified weaning foods. The diet thereafter expands and the plasma 25(OH)D concentrations are usually satisfactory. Pregnant and lactating women should receive supplementary vitamin D at 10 μg/day. Where the elderly are insufficiently exposed to the summer sun, their stores may be reduced and a supplement of 10 μg/day vitamin D is recommended.

Vitamin K

Vitamin K, a naphthoquinone, occurs in two forms in human nutrition: vitamins K_1 and K_2. Vitamin K_1 of plant origin is a phytylmenaquinone (also known as phylloquinone or phytylmenadione) and consists of 2-methyl-1,4-naphthoquinone (menadione or menaquinone) attached to a 20-carbon phytyl side chain. Vitamin K_2 is one of several homologues produced by bacteria with 4 to 13 isoprenyl units in the side chain (menaquinone-4 to -13). Vitamin K_1 is present in fresh green vegetables (for example, broccoli, lettuce, cabbage, and spinach) and beef. Vitamin K is involved in the synthesis of proteins central to blood coagulation, namely prothrombin and factors VII, IX, and X. Vitamin K is necessary for the post-translational carboxylation of glutamic acid in the coagulation proteins. γ-Carboxyglutamate allows the binding of calcium and phospholipids in the formation of thrombin.

Vitamin K is absorbed as a lipid, and is transported from the intestine in the blood in chylomicrons as β-lipoproteins. Vitamin K_2 of bacterial origin is absorbed from the colon. When there is vitamin K deficiency, the blood clotting time is prolonged and factor VII, IX, and X activities are reduced. Deficiency is uncommon in adults. However, in infants deficiency results from a sterile intestinal tract and the inadequate vitamin K content of human and cow's milk. The problem is compounded by the immature liver of the infant being slow to synthesize prothrombin. Acquired deficiencies occur as a result of any cause of lipid malabsorption and after bowel sterilization with broad-spectrum antimicrobial agents. Vitamin K deficiency may also result from the regular ingestion of liquid paraffin, since the vitamin partitions preferentially into this non-absorbed, non-polar hydrocarbon oil and is excreted rather than absorbed. Liquid paraffin is still used in many parts of the world as a regular aperient, principally by the elderly.

Natural vitamin K preparations are free from toxic effects. There are naturally occurring vitamin K antagonists—for instance, spoilt sweet clover produces a dicoumarol that prolongs the prothrombin time of the cow, thereby causing a bleeding condition. Drugs designed to prolong prothrombin time were developed as a result of this observation. Vitamin K deficiency can be detected by the 'prothrombin time' test which measures prolongation of clotting time.

Requirements

The children and adult dietary requirements of phylloquinone are between 0.5 and 1.0 μg/kg body weight per day. Vitamin K in human breast milk is as the phylloquinone and the concentration varies between 1 and 10 μg/l. An adequate intake for breast-fed infants is 8.5 μg phylloquinone/day. Vitamin K is given as supplements in malabsorption syndromes and prophylactically for haemorrhagic disease of the newborn.

Vitamin E

The vitamin E family consists of fat-soluble biologically active tocopherols and tocotrienols. The tocopherols are the most potent, their activity depending upon the position and number of methyl substitutions. α-Tocopherol, is the most potent; γ-tocopherol and γ-tocotrienol have activity of 48 and 20 per cent, respectively, when compared to α-tocopherol.

Vegetable oils—wheat germ, sunflower seed, cottonseed, safflower, palm, rape seed, and other oils are abundant sources of vitamin E. The free-radical scavenging properties of vitamin E are a function of the fused chroman ring system, the phytyl side chain facilitates entry into the hydrophobic environment of the membrane. Ascorbic acid may reduce tocopheroxyl radicals formed by the scavenging of free radicals during metabolism. This enables a molecule of tocopherol to scavenge many radicals. The absorption of the vitamin is incomplete and varies between 20 per cent and 80 per cent. Vitamin E enters the systemic circulation in chylomicrons and very low-density lipoproteins (**VLDL**) and coincidentally protect the polyunsaturated fatty acids (**PUFA**) which are also transported. Lipoprotein lipase controls uptake by the liver or transfer to other lipoproteins. The normal lipoprotein concentrations of vitamin E as α-tocopherol range from 11 to 37 μmol/l. α-Tocopherol forms 90 per cent of the vitamin E found in tissues, including all cell membranes where it inhibits the non-enzymatic oxidation of PUFA by molecular oxygen. Biochemical deficiency may occur as a result of gastrointestinal malabsorption and in premature infants. Vitamin E deficiency has been implicated in peripheral neuropathy associated with malabsorption syndromes and often accounts for the acanthocytosis, retinitis pigmentosa, and neurological features in Bassen-Kornzweig disease (abetalipoproteinaemia). Patients with fat malabsorption due to cystic fibrosis, coeliac disease, prolonged cholestasis, and after massive small intestinal resections are particularly at risk from vitamin E deficiency; supplements prevent and may slowly ameliorate the neurological deficit. Homozygosity for inactivating mutations in the α-tocopherol transfer protein is a cause of isolated vitamin E deficiency and ataxia which closely resembles the spinocerebellar ataxia of Friedreich's disease. Patients with

Friedreich's ataxia in the absence of frataxin mutations should be investigated for vitamin E deficiency and defects in the tocopherol transfer protein; vitamin E supplements may slowly improve this condition. Longstanding profound deficiency of vitamin E is associated with progressive spinocerebellar ataxia, visual loss due to retinitis pigmentosa, haemolysis (with red cell acanthocytosis), upward visual gaze palsies, dementia, and muscle weakness. If detected, vigorous long-term vitamin E supplementation is indicated as well as attention to the primary cause of the deficiency. There appears to be no adverse effects from large doses of vitamin E up to 3200 mg/day.

Vitamin E status can be measured from the plasma tocopherol concentration, or expressed as a ratio of total blood lipids or vitamin E:cholesterol. A functional test of vitamin E status is the hydrogen peroxide haemolysis test (erythrocyte stress test).

Requirements

The average intake in Britain is 6 mg/day, most of which is derived from fats, oils, and cereals. The dietary requirement is determined by the PUFA content of membranes and tissues and the PUFA content of the diet. The relationship between PUFA intake and vitamin E requirements is not a simple linear relationship. Intakes of 4 mg and 3 mg of α-tocopherol equivalents per day, respectively, for men and women have been regarded as adequate, but may be too low. Alternatively, and better, would be 0.4 mg α-tocopherol equivalents per gram of dietary PUFA/day, thereby increasing the recommendation to 7 mg. This formula might also be used for infants. Human breast milk contains 10 mg of α-tocopherol equivalents/l in colostrum, reducing to 3.2 mg/l at 12 days and thereafter.

Trace elements

Trace elements are important, since they:

- act as cofactors in enzyme oxidation–reduction reactions;
- maintain the specific configuration of proteins;
- are incorporated into the structure of hormones; and
- play a structural and catalytic role in gene expression and transcriptional regulation of genes.

Trace elements are required in small amounts. The trace elements contained in soil and drinking water vary from area to area, which determines the variation in intake seen in different communities. The amount and chemistry of dietary constituents eaten with the trace elements affects the absorption efficiency of the essential elements. The absorption of calcium and trace metals (for example, zinc) can be inhibited by dietary phytate. Copper absorption is reduced by competitive interactions affecting its solubility. A mild degree of iron depletion increases not only iron absorption but also lead, zinc, cadmium, cobalt, and manganese.

Individual trace elements

[The following abbreviations are used below: At wt, atomic weight; val, valency; iso, natural isotope; Abund, natural abundance in earth's crust as a per cent of the total.]

Cobalt

At wt: 59; val: 2, 3; iso: 59; abund: 0.0018 per cent

Sources are wholemeal flour and seafoods. Cobalt's role is as a component of vitamin B12. Uncomplexed cobalt can be absorbed and subsequently excreted in urine. Intakes of cobalt are approximately 5 μmole/day and the total body content is 1.5 mg (7.5 μmole). In Quebec, a cobalt-containing beer improver (15 μmol of cobalt/l) proved to be toxic; its best customers developed severe cardiomyopathy.

Chromium

At wt: 52; val: 2, 3; iso: 50, 52, 53, 54; abund 0.033 per cent.

Chromium is present in most foods especially wheat germ, molasses, green beans, and broccoli. Dietary intakes vary between 5 and 100 μg/day, but absorption is meagre at 1 per cent. The plasma concentration of chromium is 0.3 μg/ml bound to transferrin, and it is excreted in urine. Deficiency increases the risk of type II diabetes mellitus and cardiovascular disease. The recommended adult intake is 0.5 μmole/day and between 2 and 19 nmole/kg per day for children and adolescents. The adult body contains 100 to 200 μmole. The chromium content of human milk is 0.06 to 1.56 ng/ml. Chromium in high dosage is well tolerated.

Copper

At wt: 64; val: 1, 2; iso: 63, 65; abund: 0.010 per cent.

Good sources of copper include green vegetables, fish, oysters, and liver. Copper is required by the immune, nervous, and cardiovascular systems for skeletal development, iron metabolism, red-cell formation, and enzymes including cytochrome oxidase and superoxide dismutase. Between 35 and 70 per cent of ingested copper is actively absorbed, but this is affected by age and the chemistry of accompanying food. Copper is concentrated in the liver, excreted in bile, and lost in faeces. In plasma, copper is bound to caeruloplasmin and albumin. The total amount of copper in an adult is approximately 2 mmole (50 to 120 mg). Copper accumulates in the fetal liver for early extrauterine life, premature birth results in depleted copper stores. Copper deficiency in adults has not been reported, but patients taking large doses of the chelator penicillamine for cystinuria and as a second-line agent in rheumatoid arthritis, are at risk. Poisoning with copper presents with haemolysis and brain and hepatocellular damage. The requirement for adults (including during pregnancy) is 1.5 to 3 mg/day, children range 0.6 to 1.5 mg/day. An infant requires 0.4 to 0.6 mg/day.

Iodine

At wt: 127; val: 1; iso: 127; abund: 6×10^{-6} per cent.

Iodine is present in modest amounts in most food and drinking water. Seafood, milk, and meat are good sources. Iodine is required for thyroxine 3,5,3',5'-tetraiodothyronine (T4) and 3,5,3'-tri-iodothyronine (T3). Selenium and zinc are important in the conversion of T4 to the active T3, catalysed by selenium-dependent iodothyronine deiodinase. Dietary iodine from food and water is absorbed as inorganic iodide and transported to the thyroid gland. The body content of iodine is between 20 and 50 mg (160 to 400 μmole).

Goitre results from iodine deficiency and is endemic in mountainous areas. Some 800 million people are at risk of iodine deficiency, of whom 190 million may develop goitres and more than 3 million are cretinous. These populations have an iodine intake less than 25 μg/day—the required intake being 80 to 150 μg/day. Iodine replacement is essential for these populations and may be added to food, salt, or water or by the direct administration of iodine. Goitre may also arise through eating plants containing goitrogens (for example, thiocyanate in cassava, maize, bamboo shoots, etc.) Maternal iodine deficiency is associated with perinatal death, stillbirths, spontaneous abortions, endemic cretinism, and congenital abnormalities. Thyroxine is essential for brain development during the first 2 years of life. A modest increase in the incidence of hyperthyroidism occurs following the ingestion of iodized salt preparations in individuals over 40 years of age.

Thyroid hormone and urinary iodine measurements reflect iodine status. Adults require 140 μg/day, babies 40 μg/day, infants 50 μg/day, and children 50 to 140 μg/day. Intake should increase to 175 μg/day during pregnancy and 200 μg/day with lactation. Breast milk contains 44 to 93 μg/litre, an adequate iodine intake.

Magnesium

At wt: 24; val: 2; iso: 24, 25, 26; abund: 1.94 per cent.

Magnesium is present in most foods, particularly chlorophyll-containing vegetables. Magnesium is absorbed from the distal intestine and excretion is through the kidneys. Magnesium homeostasis includes reabsorption of endogenous magnesium from enteric secretions. The plasma concentration varies between 0.6 and 1.0 mmol/l, and adult whole-body magnesium is 1 mole or 25 g—two-thirds in bone with phosphate and bicarbonate, the remainder being complexed with ATP. Magnesium is a cofactor for cocarboxylase and is involved in the replication and transcription of DNA and translation of RNA. Magnesium deficiency is manifested by progressive muscle weakness, failure to thrive, neuromuscular dysfunction, arrhythmias, hallucinations, positive Trousseau's sign, coma, and death. Malabsorption, alcohol abuse, and diuretics are causes of a low serum magnesium levels.

Urinary magnesium is an approximate measure of dietary intake. Typically, a diet in the United Kingdom contains between 8 and 17 mmole of magnesium/day (200 to 400 mg). Adults (including during pregnancy), require between 8 and 10.3 mmole/day (200 to 250 mg). Human breast milk contains 0.12 mmole (2.8 mg)/litre. The lactating mother should increase her magnesium intake by 2.0 mmole/day (50 mg). Babies require 30 mg/day, infants 75 mg/day, and children 80 to 200 mg/day

Manganese

At wt: 55; val: 2, 4; iso: 55; abund: 0.085 per cent.

Tea, cereals, legumes, and leafy vegetables are good sources of manganese. Manganese is a cofactor and enzyme activator. Manganese absorption is only 3 to 4 per cent efficient. Calcium, phosphorous, fibre, and phytate interact with and reduce manganese absorption. The plasma concentration is between 1 and 2 μg/g bound to transferrin, the body pool contains 0.3 mmole, and excretion is in bile. Manganese deficiency in man has not been reported. The average intake in Britain is 2 to 5 mg/day, half from tea. Safe intakes for adults are more than 1.5 mg (25 μmole)/day and for children and infants more than 16 μg (0.3 μmole)/kg per day. Breast milk contains 15 μg/litre.

Molybdenum

At wt: 96; val: 2, 3, 4; iso: 92, 94, 95, 96, 97, 98, 100; abund: 7×10^{-4} per cent

Important dietary sources are wheat flour and its germ, legumes, and meat. Molybdenum is a cofactor for oxidases important in the metabolism of DNA and sulphites. Intestinal absorption efficiency is high at 40 to 100 per cent. Plasma concentration is 1 μg/100 ml, and molybdenum is bound to protein. Storage is in the liver and excretion in urine. There are no reports of molybdenum deficiency in man. Gout has been attributed to high molybdenum intakes of 10 to 15 mg/day. Adults require between 75 and 200 μg of molybdenum/day (0.75 to 4 μmole/day). Breast-fed infants require 1.0 μg/kg per day. Babies require 15 to 30 μg/day, infants 20 to 40 μg/day, and children 40 to 100 μg/day.

Nickel

At wt: 59; val: 2, 3; iso: 58, 60, 61, 62, 64; abund: 0.018 per cent

It has not been established whether nickel is essential in humans. Absorption is 3 to 6 per cent of the dietary intake. Plasma concentrations are between 2 and 4 μg/100 ml, some of which is bound to albumin. Nickel is excreted in urine. Nickel deficiency might result in depressed growth and haemopoesis. Requirements are unknown, but intakes in the United Kingdom are about 140 μg/day (2.4 μmole/day).

Phosphorus

At wt: 31; val: 3, 5; iso: 31; abund: 0.12 per cent.

Phosphorus is present in all natural foods, the usual diet in Britain providing 1.5 g of phosphorus daily. Phosphorus is an important physiological component: with calcium, of the bony skeleton; of adenosine triphosphate

(ATP) in oxidative phosphorylation; in nucleic acids through phosphorylation of nucleotides; and in enzyme control through phosphorylation by protein kinases. Phosphorus is absorbed as free inorganic phosphorus from the diet (controlled by 1,25(OH)$_2$ vitamin D) at both the brush-border and basolateral membranes. The plasma concentration of phosphorus is between 0.8 and 1.4 mmol/l and it is excreted in both urine and faeces. The bony skeleton contains 80 per cent of the body content of phosphorus as the calcium salt, 19 to 29 mmole (600 to 900 g). Recommended phosphorus requirements are equimolar to calcium.

Selenium

At wt: 79; val: 2, 4; iso: 74, 76, 77, 78, 80, 82; abund: 8×10^{-5} per cent

Selenium is found in food as selenoamino acids, selenoproteins, and as selenide, selenite, or selenate. The main sources of selenium are cereals, meat, and fish. Selenium is a cofactor of certain enzymes (for example, iodothyronine deiodinase and glutathione peroxidases). Both selenium and vitamin E are important in stabilizing lipid membranes by inhibiting oxidative damage. Absorption is efficient at 35 to 85 per cent. The plasma concentration of selenium is between 7 and 30 µg/100 ml protein bound. Excretion is in urine and possibly bile. In New Zealand, Venezuela, and China both the soil and population can be deficient in selenium. In China, selenium deficiency is associated with the childhood cardiomyopathy, Keshan's disease.

In certain areas of Tibet and Nepal, Kashin-Beck disease, a degenerative arthropathy associated with selenium deficiency, is endemic. Iodine deficiency, resulting in hypothyroidism and goitre, is an associated risk factor for Kashin-Beck disease even in individuals with normal serum selenium concentrations. The precise relationship between iodine deficiency and selenium status in areas where selenium deficiency is endemic remains to be established—especially in patients with Kashin-Beck disease.

Urinary selenium output, red-cell selenium levels, or glutathione peroxidase activity are markers of recent and medium-term dietary intake. Adults require 75 µg/day (0.9 µmole/day). Fertility requires an adequate selenium intake, but the pregnant woman has no additional dietary selenium requirements. Lactation requires an increase in dietary intake of 15 µg/day (0.2 µmole/day). Breast-fed infants should receive approximately 10 µg/day (0.1 µmole/day) and children 15 to 30 µg/day (0.2 to 0.4 µmole/day). Breast milk contains 20 to 60 µg/litre of selenium.

Silicon

At wt: 28; val: 4; iso: 28, 29, 30; abund: 25.8 per cent

Cereal grains and other sources of dietary fibre are important sources of silicon. The role of silicon in human nutrition may be important in cartilage and connective tissue as the human aorta, trachea, lungs, and tendons are rich in silicon. Silicic acid is readily absorbed. The body storage pool is approximately 3 g (1 mole) in a 60-kg man; the plasma monosilicic acid concentration is 500 µg/100 ml. The dietary requirements of silicon are unknown.

Sulphur

At wt: 32; val: 2, 4; iso: 32, 33, 34, 36; abund: 0.048 per cent

Sulphur occurs in: proteoglycans; dermatan, chondroitin and keratin sulphate; glutathione; and coenzymes including coenzyme A. Cysteine, methionine, and disulphide crosslinkage are important in proteins, and sulphate is involved in detoxification processes. Sulphur is absorbed as amino acids, which are subsequently desulphated, and excreted in urine as sulphates. Dietary intake is of the order of 0.7 mg (22 µmole)/day. The dietary requirements of sulphur are unknown.

Zinc

At wt: 65; val: 2; iso: 64, 66, 67, 68, 70; abund: 0.02 per cent

Dietary sources are meats, whole grains, legumes, and oysters. Zinc is required as a cofactor in DNA synthesis, cell division, and protein synthesis. Zinc-finger 'proteins' are important as gene transcriptional regulators. It has long been believed that zinc is important for wound healing. Approximately 20 per cent of dietary zinc is absorbed complexed with amino acids, phosphates, and organic acids. Phytates and oxalates form insoluble complexes which inhibit absorption. The normal plasma concentration of zinc is between 80 and 110 µg/100 ml, complexed with albumin. The adult body content of zinc is over 2 g (30 mmole). Bone, the prostate, semen, and the choroid of the eye all contain high concentrations of zinc. Loss of zinc from the body is in faeces.

Zinc is widely available in foods so dietary deficiency is rare, and only reported in malabsorption and in male dwarfs in Iran. The clinical signs are growth retardation, hypogonadism, bullous-pustular dermatitis, paronychia, lethargy, hepatosplenomegaly, and iron deficiency anaemia which responds to zinc supplements (15 mg three times/day). Zinc deficiency has been reported as a feature in a number of diseases, including the florid deficiency state and skin condition acrodermatitis enteropathica, an autosomal recessive trait leading to selective impairment of zinc uptake by the upper small intestinal mucosa. Similar signs may be observed in patients with severe malabsorption due to Crohn's disease and other intestinal disorders, especially those associated with a loss of inflammatory cells in the gut lumen. Excessive zinc can lead to nausea, vomiting, and fever.

The plasma concentration of unhaemolysed zinc is a measure of a person's current zinc status. Zinc in the red-blood cells and hair gives a long-term assessment of zinc status. Adults of all ages (and during pregnancy and lactation) require between 12 and 15 mg of zinc (110 to 145 µmole)/day. Infants need between 4 and 5 mg/day; however, human milk is not a rich source of zinc (2–3 mg/litre) and the infant depends very much on the stores obtained during its last 3 months of interuterine life. Children require 10 to 15 mg/day

Further reading

General

Eastwood M (1997). *Principles of human nutrition.* Aspen, Gaithersburg, MD.

Panel on Dietary Reference Values of the Committee on Medical Aspects of Food Policy (1991). *Report on Health and Social Subjects 41. Dietary reference values for food energy and nutrients for the United Kingdom.* HMSO, London.

Powers HJ (1997). Vitamin requirements for term infants: considerations for infant formulae. *Nutrition Research Reviews* 10, 1–33.

Sadler MJ, Strain JJ, Caballero B, eds. (1999). *Encylopedia of human nutrition.* Academic Press, San Diego, CA.

Ziegler EE, Filer LJ Jr, eds. (1996). *Present knowledge in nutrition*, 7th edn. ILSI Press, Washington DC.

Carotenoids as background examples

Cox DN *et al.* (1998). Take five, a nutrition education intervention to increase fruit and vegetables intakes. *British Journal of Nutrition* 80, 123–31.

Vershinin A (1999). Biological functions of carotenoids—diversity and evolution. *Biofactors* 10, 99–104.

Wang XD, Russell RM (1999). Procarcinogenic and anticarcinogenic effect of β-carotene. *Nutritional Reviews* 57, 263–72.

Vitamin C

Benzie IFF (1999). Vitamin C: prospective functional markers for defining optimal nutritional status. *Proceedings of the Nutrition Society* 58, 469–76.

Sauberlich HE (1994). Pharmacology of vitamin C. *Annual Review of Nutrition* 14, 371–91.

Thiamin, biotin, and pantothenic acid

Bender DA (1999). Optimum nutrition: thiamin, biotin and pantothenate. *Proceedings of the Nutrition Society* 58, 427–33.

Folate

Butterworth CE Jr, Bendich A (1996). Folic acid and the prevention of birth defects. *Annual Review of Nutrition* **16**, 73–97.

McNulty H (1997). Folate requirements for women *Proceedings of the Nutrition Society* **56**, 291–303.

Scott JM (1999). Folate and vitamin B12. *Proceedings of the Nutrition Society* **58**, 441–8.

Selhub J (1999). Homocysteine metabolism. *Annual Review of Nutrition* **19**, 217–46.

Vitamin B₁₂

Scott JM (1999). Folate and vitamin B12. *Proceedings of the Nutrition Society* **58**, 441–8.

Vitamin A

McClaren DS (1980). *Nutritional ophthalmology*. Academic Press, London.

Semba RD (1997). Vitamin A and human immunodeficiency virus disease. *Proceedings of the Nutrition Society* **56**, 459–69.

Thurnham DI, Northrop-Clewes CA (1999). Optimal nutrition: vitamins and the carotenoids. *Proceedings of the Nutrition Society* **58**, 449–57.

Vitamin D

Nutritional aspects of bone; a symposium (1997). *Proceedings of the Nutrition Society* **56**, 903–87.

Wilkinson RJ et al. (2000). Influence of vitamin D deficiency and vitamin D receptor polymorphisms on tuberculosis among Gujarati Asians in west London: a case control study. *Lancet* **355**, 618–21.

Vitamin E

Gabsi S, et al. (2001). Effect of vitamin E supplementation in patients with ataxia with vitamin E deficiency. *European Journal of Neurology* **8**, 477–81.

Halliwell B (1996). Antioxidants in human health and disease. *Annual Review of Nutrition* **16**, 33–50.

Moreno-Reyes R, et al. (1998). Kashin-Beck osteoarthropathy in rural Tibet in relation to selenium status. *New England Journal of Medicine* **339**, 1112–20.

Morrisey PA, Sheehy PJA (1999). Optimal nutrition: vitamin E. *Proceedings of the Nutrition Society* **58**, 459–68.

Stevenson VL, Hardie RJ (2001). Acanthocytosis and neurological disorders. *Journal of Neurology* **248**, 87–94.

Traber MG, Sies H (1996). Vitamin E in humans: demand and delivery. *Annual Review of Nutrition* **16**, 321–47.

Trace elements

Arthur JR, Beckett GJ, Mitchell JH (1999). The interactions between selenium and iodine deficiencies in man and animals. *Nutrition Research Reviews* **12**, 55–73.

Cousins RJ (1994). Metal elements and gene expression. *Annual Review of Nutrition* **14**, 449–69.

Failla ML (1999). Considerations for determining 'optimal nutrition' for copper, zinc, manganese and molybdenum. *Proceedings of the Nutrition Society* **58**, 497–505.

Goyer RA (1997). Toxic and essential metal interactions. *Annual Review of Nutrition* **17**, 37–50.

Lukaski HC (1999). Chromium as a supplement. *Annual Review of Nutrition* **19**, 279–302.

10.4 Severe malnutrition

Alan A. Jackson

Introduction

Severe malnutrition reflects a society which is not able to meet its basic needs for health care and survival. It is the consequence of a range of factors which together characterize underdevelopment, poverty and deprivation, an insanitary environment, frequent infections, and food which is poor in quality or limited in availability. A series of vicious cycles operate within individuals and across generations, limiting the ability of vulnerable groups, families, and individuals to cope with the harsh realities of a hostile environment, either through the exigencies of nature or a human unwillingness to share the available resources with greater equity. Across the globe, severe malnutrition is a common condition during childhood and is most prevalent amongst the poorest in developing countries, but it is also found with uncomfortable frequency amongst the most deprived of every society, including those in Europe and North America. It is a frequent aspect of clinical medicine in patients who, for any reason, have a loss of appetite or a reduction in food intake. The same principles of management and care apply wherever the problem is found.

Malnutrition at any age impairs the ability to perform and function. Children with severe malnutrition are at risk of serious, life-threatening problems which require urgent attention. More insidiously, malnutrition during childhood stunts development and leaves a scar which remains for the rest of that person's life. This lost potential can express itself as an increased risk of ill health, as impaired intellectual development leading to poor school performance, or in limited physical development leading to poorer work performance. Once part of an individual's potential for development has been lost, the clinical and social implications tend to be cumulative. On a global scale, the sum total of the loss of individual capability represents a fundamental brake on aspirations for social and economic development. Throughout the world, 54 per cent of childhood deaths can be attributed directly or indirectly to malnutrition, amounting to 11.6 million 1995. This burden is not spread evenly between different parts of the world. For the worst affected countries, as many as 50 per cent of children under 5 have malnutrition which is severe enough to threaten life, most frequently in sub-Saharan Africa and Southeast Asia. This is representative of the day-to-day situation, and is not a peculiarity of special emergencies.

Notwithstanding the large number of children with severe malnutrition, over the past 20 years there has been a shift to the right of the curve for the distribution of the height and weight of children, indicating a general improvement and marked success for specific interventions. Thus, change is possible and when suitable measures are put in place sustained improvement can be achieved. However, there is absolutely no basis for complacency, as recent figures suggest a slowing down, or even a reversal, of this improvement. This may relate to an inability to control infections effectively, with tuberculosis, malaria, and diarrhoea continuing to play a major role and the HIV epidemic making a significant contribution. The world's population continues to increase, so an improvement in percentage terms

Table 1 The case mortality for severe malnutrition has failed to improve because of four major errors of management (from Scholfield C and Ashworth A (1996). Why have mortality rates for severe malnutrition remained so high? *Bulletin of the World Health Organization* **74**, 223–9)

1.	The assumption that a low plasma albumin concentration is the basis of oedema and can be effectively treated with a high-protein diet
2.	The use of diuretics for the treatment of oedema
3.	Early use of iron supplements to treat anaemia
4.	Failing to differentiate that the acute illness should be managed before any attempts to correct weight loss

does not necessarily mean a decrease in the absolute numbers of malnourished people across the globe.

Severe malnutrition is a late stage in a process where an individual has had inadequate access to sufficient energy and nutrients for a period of time. During this time the function of the body changes and there are important ways in which severely malnourished children are different from normal children. They do not respond to medical treatment in the way that would be expected, and if they are treated in the same way as normal children they will very likely die. Based upon best practice mortality would be expected to be around 5 per cent, but in many centres case mortality has remained unchanged for 50 years, around 50 per cent, with four major errors in care occurring in about 80 per cent of centres (Table 1).

The World Health Organization (**WHO**) has produced guidelines on effective treatment in 10 steps (Fig. 1). During the early period of care the order in which different aspects of treatment are carried out is critical for a successful outcome. A central feature is that as a first step the body's cellular machinery has to be repaired if function is to be restored. Silent infections are common. There have been unusual losses of nutrients from the body which cannot be corrected adequately on a standard diet. The damaged systems of the body are not able to cope with excess energy or further stress. Effective treatment requires the ordered correction of the underlying problems before any attempts are made to correct the tissue deficits.

Clinical syndromes

Severe malnutrition can present with an array of clinical symptoms and signs, which depend upon the duration of the illness, the extent of coinfection, the particular pattern of nutrient deficiencies and metabolic disturbances, and other associated complications such as diarrhoea and vomiting with attendant disturbances in fluid and electrolytes (Table 2). All descriptions of the condition emphasize one or other feature of the presentation. The archetypal descriptive terms for childhood malnutrition, kwashiorkor, marasmus, or marasmic kwashiorkor, were originally used to characterize clinical syndromes.

The first description of the kwashiorkor syndrome emphasized the development, location, and timing of the skin lesion, with progression from friable hyperpigmented skin, which stripped to reveal hypopigmented

Activity	Initial treatment		Rehabilitation	Follow-up
	days 1–2	days 3–7	weeks 2–6	weeks 7–26
Treat or prevent: hypoglycaemia hypothermia dehydration				
Treat Infection				
Correct electrolyte imbalance				
Correct micronutrient deficiencies	←— without iron —→	←— with iron —→		
Begin feeding				
Increase feeding to recover lost weight ('catch-up growth')				
Stimulate emotional and sensorial development				
Prepare for discharge				

Fig. 1 WHO recommendations for the 10-step approach to the management of severe malnutrition.

skin which ulcerated easily to provide a ready portal for infection—lesions distinct from pellagra. Other features such as abnormal affect and hepatomegaly were noted, but were less remarkable. Placing emphasis upon variability in clinical presentation has made comparison difficult and encouraged the idea that the underlying pathophysiology, and hence its treatment, differs in important ways between locations. This has diverted attention from similarities in the fundamental changes which take place across the range of clinical presentations. Identifying differences in clinical presentation for this complex disorder are less important than thought previously for successful management.

The function of the body is controlled through the integration of many systems. A fault in any one has implications for the function of all the others. Thus, there is the need for adequate amounts of energy, energy-generating nutrients (carbohydrate, lipid, and protein), minerals, and a range of micronutrients for the body to function effectively in a harmonized way. Lack of any component, or an imbalance, leads to deranged handling of others. By adopting an agreed classification relevant comparisons have been drawn and it is clear that the range of clinical features represent varying manifestations of a clinical disorder with the interaction of qualitative and quantitative factors. The quantitative change results from an inadequate intake of food and leads to a wasting syndrome, classically marasmus, with the progressive loss of tissue, especially marked for subcutaneous fat and muscle. The result is a thin appearance, with pinched

Table 2 Important clinical features to enable immediate clinical decisions for emergency management of severe malnutrition

Feature	Details/relevance
Anthropometry	Stunting, wasting, presence of pitting oedema
Gastrointestinal	History of anorexia, poor appetite, vomiting, diarrhoea. Appearance of mouth. Distended or scaphoid abdomen, with succussion splash
Liver	Degree of enlargement, jaundice, petechiae
Cardiovascular	Circulatory collapse, anaemia, shock (depleted intravascular volume, cold hands and feet, weak radial pulse, diminished consciousness) ± signs of 'dehydration' (sunken eyes, sunken fontanelle, decreased skin turgor)
Infection	Hypothermia, fever, localizing signs (respiratory distress, broken skin, mouth, ears)
Specific deficiencies	Eye signs of xerophthalmia, vitamin A

features, thin arms and legs, and a scaphoid abdomen. Qualitative changes are usually associated with unusual losses of nutrients from the body, for example through diarrhoea or infection, reordered metabolism to deal with metabolic stress, or the toxic effects of a range of noxious exposures. The end result of this process is likely to be the loss of cellular integrity and control, leading to oedema.

Classification

Severe malnutrition is defined as severe wasting (less than 70 per cent, or a score of less than –3 standard deviations, weight for height, compared with the National Centre for Health Statistics/World Health Organization (NCHS/WHO) reference), or the presence of oedema of both feet, or clinical signs of severe malnutrition, reflecting that there are quantitative and qualitative changes taking place (Table 3). The more severely malnourished an individual, the greater the risk of complications and the risk of an adverse outcome is related to the severity of the weight deficit or the extent to which normal function is deranged. An effective classification differentiates those at greatest risk, guides suitable interventions, and helps determine the extent to which interventions have successfully corrected the problem. These changes can all be marked either quantitatively or qualitatively.

Quantitative measures indicate the extent to which the expected pattern of growth in height and weight has not been achieved: low height for age, low weight for height, and low weight for age. Low height for age (shortness or stunting) is indicative of longer-term malnutrition or poor health. Low weight for height (thinness or wasting) implies recent or continuing current severe weight loss. Low weight for age (insufficient weight relative to age) implies stunting and/or wasting. Weight is more easily measured than height and assessing weight for age is the simplest way of excluding severe malnutrition in the absence of oedema. This has been the basis of a widely used system of classification—the Gomez classification. Weight for age is influenced by both height for age and weight for height. Where deprivation is common there is a high prevalence of low height for age, and weight for age is more strongly influenced by stunting than by wasting, and requires broader public health approaches for its alleviation being unlikely to respond in the short term to aggressive clinical intervention. The prevalence of stunting starts to increase at around 3 months of age, and the process of stunting slows down at around 3 years of age, after which mean heights run parallel to the reference. Weight for height has the advantage that it can be used when age is not known reliably and suggests recent severe weight loss, indicating those children who are most likely to benefit

Table 3 Classification of malnutrition. The diagnoses are not mutually exclusive

Moderate malnutrition	Severe malnutrition
Symmetrical oedema	
No	Yes (oedematous malnutrition)*
Weight for height	
SD score between –3 and –2† (70 to 79%)‡	SD score below –3 (< 70%) (severe wasting)§
Height for age	
SD score between –3 and –2 (85 to 89%)	SD score below –3 (< 85%) (severe stunting)

*This includes kwashiorkor and marasmic kwashiorkor in older classifications. To avoid confusion with the clinical syndrome of kwashiorkor, which includes other features, the term 'oedematous malnutrition' is preferred.

†Below the NCHS/WHO reference; the SD score is defined as the deviation of the value for the individual from the median value for the reference population, divided by the standard deviation of the reference population.

‡Percentage of the median NCHS/WHO reference.

§This corresponds to marasmus (without oedema) in the Wellcome clinical classification, and to grade III malnutrition in the Gomez system. To avoid confusion the term severe wasting is preferred.

from immediate aggressive nutritional intervention and support. The rate at which weight improves is used to assess progress during recovery, and success of care is indicated by the achievement of a weight which is appropriate for the individual's height. The Waterlow classification usefully identified the relationship between height and weight and suitable cut-off points for intervention.

Qualitative criteria are more difficult, because of their variability and uncertainty about whether they mark any particular pathophysiological process. It has been agreed that the presence of pitting oedema is the archetype of qualitative change, identified as kwashiorkor in the Wellcome classification and now called oedematous malnutrition. In milder forms oedema might be restricted to the limbs, but embraces the entire body in more severe forms. Obtaining a reliable measure of body weight is difficult in the presence of oedema, because of the uncertain contribution of oedematous fluid. The overall appearance might be of a child who superficially appears full, but has evident wasting below the oedema when examined carefully with the clothes removed. Poor appetite or anorexia might be very common, but is not used as a diagnostic criterion. Multiple infection is common and often silent, so that specific sites of infection may be difficult to identify or localize. A high index of suspicion is required for the presence of silent infections, which should be presumed to be present. Infection is not part of the diagnostic criteria.

Natural history and clinical presentation

Inadequate nutrition slows the pace of growth and development and the greater the severity of the limitation or insult, or the longer its duration, the greater the difference between the achieved development and that expected. The stress of an insult of greater severity evokes a metabolic response which is associated with a loss of body weight and a reordering of function, so that resources and effort devoted to growth and development are diverted to maintain the integrity of the individual. The nutritional health of the infant is critically determined by how well prepared the mother was to carry the pregnancy, and the effectiveness with which breast feeding is established and maintained. During pregnancy and for the first months of life the infant is totally dependent upon the mother for its nutrient supply. During early pregnancy there is the elaboration and maturation of function in the fetus. The last trimester is of critical importance as it is when the fetus accumulates effective reserves of nutrients, helping survival and facilitating development during the first year of life. The fetus accumulates reserves of energy, as subcutaneous lipid, and of minerals and vitamins, such as iron, zinc, copper, vitamin A, riboflavin, or pyridoxine, in liver and muscle. At birth the relative protection of the intrauterine environment is replaced by the many hazards of the external world. Gastrointestinal and respiratory infection are amongst the serious dangers to survival and breast feeding provides effective protection from both. Even in affluent societies breast feeding provides the infant with a level of protection against ill health that identifies effective breast feeding as a singularly important feature in any rational policy in public health nutrition. There is a massive increase in the risk of ill health for infants who are not breast fed during the early months of life. This risk is magnified enormously for infants exposed to unsanitary environments with limited access to health care. Anything which limits the growth of the fetus, impairs its development, or causes it to be delivered early will limit its ability to cope with extrauterine life, and increase the risk of problems, infections, and malnutrition. There is enhanced mother–infant bonding and emotional development with breast feeding, and other special benefits include the remarkable bioavailability of energy and nutrients, the presence of non-nutritional factors, protective factors, and growth factors.

Screening: identification and prevention

Malnutrition is a preventable condition and the early identification of those at risk and the implementation of interventions which correct underlying problems and prevent further deterioration is central to strategies for effective care. Early growth failure can be detected by regular weighing, as an integral part of immunization and other health programmes. A series of plotted weights is most valuable and intervention is required for those whose weight crosses two growth centiles on successive measurements. If measurements are only available for a single time point, then height for age and weight for height provide an indication of any past or ongoing growth failure. Advice and demonstration of best practice in child care and feeding may be sufficient to correct a mild degree of growth failure, but persistent or more severe growth failure require closer investigation to exclude underlying problems. Poor anthropometry, with a history of poor appetite and weight loss, should always be taken very seriously and pursued until a cause has been identified and corrected. Severe malnutrition is a medical emergency.

Childhood malnutrition is a clinical problem for the individual, but is also a symptom of ineffective public health policy. Targeted interventions should address the immediate needs of the child, but should also embrace broader considerations. For the child, there is the need to effectively immunize against infection, recognize and treat infection in a timely way, and ensure an effective period of nutritional support following infection. For the family, there is the need to enhance the child rearing skills of the parents, create a stimulating environment, acquire and practice simple skills in hygiene and food preparation, and strengthen family dynamics and coping strategies. For the community, there is the need to improve the economic base of households, increase food purchasing power, increase food security or household food availability, and to treat specific nutrient deficiencies. Sound hygienic practices have to be strengthened at the group or household level, and where necessary the amount and quality of water and the safe and effective removal of solid waste improved. Each activity can exert a beneficial effect on growth and development. Any one might be relatively easy to introduce, but the real difficulty is to ensure that all are sustained. The need is for a fundamental change in the health culture and the creation of a framework of behaviour in which development activities become rooted and take place as a matter of course. A failure to establish and maintain an effective system of health care leads to a progressive deterioration in the clinical state of the most vulnerable infants leading eventually to severe malnutrition.

Aetiology and pathophysiology

Children may become malnourished simply because there is not enough food available, but sick malnourished individuals have no appetite for food. It seems paradoxical that a child who has obviously lost weight and needs to eat may refuse food even when it is readily available. If food is forced there is the possibility that the child will become worse, or even die. In managing severe malnutrition appetite is one of the most important symptoms. A loss of appetite is an important protective mechanism against consuming food which is likely to stress the systems of the body. In experimental studies there are two major biological reasons why appetite is lost: a deficiency of a specific nutrient and infection. Severe malnutrition is a disorder which results from the interaction of three distinct but related processes, each of which appears to be related directly to the food consumed, but none of which can be easily understood simply by a consideration of food:

- reductive adaptation
- inflammatory and immune responses
- specific nutrient deficiencies.

Food helps meet the many needs for normal function, growth, and development in childhood, but also the ability to cope with environmental challenge. A diet which is adequate but marginal under normal circumstances is inadequate for the increased demands during recovery from frequent intercurrent illness with the double burden of the need for catch-up growth and to make good the unusual losses of nutrients during the infective episode itself. The time available for successful convalescence, before the next bout of infection, is too short to adequately make up the deficit.

Reductive adaptation: failure to meet the usual demands of the body for macronutrients

Reductive adaptation takes place when the demands of the body for energy and nutrients are not adequately met by the dietary intake. The general features are similar regardless of the basis for the inadequate intake. It is a general response to preserve essential function, but carries a cost. Normal metabolism takes place within a highly regulated environment, through the control and integration of exchange and turnover amongst cells and tissues. For the cellular machinery of the body to remain functionally intact and operationally effective requires a constant supply of energy and other nutrients. An estimated one-third of resting energy expenditure may be consumed through the synthesis and degradation of macromolecules such as protein, and a further third is associated with the movement of material across membranes, for example through the pumping activity of the sodium/potassium pump, Na^+/K^+-ATPase. These processes represent the internal work of the body at cellular level and underlie the functioning of all the organs and tissues. They take place continuously and the total activity can be measured as energy expenditure. As food consumption is intermittent the processes are independent of the immediate food intake. However, a sustained lack of food leads to progressive impairment of the cellular machinery as damage due to the wear and tear of normal use can no longer be replaced effectively.

Structure

When food consumption is significantly reduced, metabolic processes continue to enable the body to function, and the energy to support these processes is derived from reserves within the body. The body is in negative energy balance, and tissue mass cannot be maintained, leading to loss in weight. The losses are uneven between tissues, with major losses in subcutaneous fat and muscle and relative preservation of the metabolically more active visceral tissues. One important consequence is that heat generated by muscle is reduced and at the same time insulation in the skin is impaired leading to greater heat loss. The altered body composition underlies all anthropometric methods which are used to assess nutritional status. In addition to the changes in mass, efficiencies in the utilization of energy have to be found.

Function

Efficiencies are achieved by reducing the amount of work carried out by the body. External work is reduced by decreasing physical activity. Internal work is reduced by decreasing cellular metabolic activity, with subsequent effects upon tissue function. Significant efficiencies might be achieved for the major energy-consuming processes such as membrane pumping, protein turnover, and cellular replication. Fundamental to maintaining the chemical environment of cells is the relative distribution of potassium in the intracellular space and sodium in the extracellular space. As potassium tends to leak out of the cell and sodium tends to leak into the cell, for the cell membrane to maintain the effective partitioning of electrolytes requires that sodium is pumped out of the cell in exchange for potassium, consuming ATP. The cell membrane tends to become more 'leaky' in malnutrition as its lipid composition changes, and the Na^+/K^+-ATPase is downregulated as one way in which to reduce energy expenditure. Therefore compared with normal, all people with malnutrition have reduced intracellular potassium and increased intracellular sodium, hence decreased total body potassium and increased total body sodium, which is not identified necessarily on standard biochemical tests. The ability to maintain protein synthesis is fundamental but energetically expensive; energetic efficiency requires a reduction in protein synthesis, which is not divided equally amongst tissues. Liver normally accounts for about 25 per cent of protein synthesis, with the synthesis of nutrient transport proteins

playing a critical role in the delivery of lipid, minerals, and vitamins to the other tissues. Reduced synthesis of nutrient transport proteins may save energy, but at the cost of reduced delivery to peripheral tissues; thus for example limited synthesis of apolipoproteins limits the delivery of lipid to peripheral tissues and enhances the accumulation of lipid in liver. Cellular replication is energetically demanding, requiring the ready availability of all nutrients. A reduction in cellular replication provides efficiencies in energy and nutrient use but impairs the function of systems critically dependent upon cellular replication: the skin, gastrointestinal tract, respiratory tract, and the immune system.

Functional and metabolic cost of reductive adaptation

The function of the cells in all tissues is affected by reductive adaptation. With relative protection of more vital functions, the cost is a reduction in those functions which are not immediately vital but which provide the functional reserve capability which enables the metabolic flexibility to respond to a changed internal environment or a challenge from the external environment. As a consequence, changes which would be readily managed in the normal state present a metabolic stress in the reductively adapted state. What would normally be a modest challenge can induce a major metabolic perturbation. Reductive adaptation represents the loss of reserve capacity, which leads to increased metabolic brittleness and vulnerability. The cellular machinery is no longer capable of responding effectively to the usual challenges. There is a change in the function of all systems.

Gastrointestinal tract

There is loss of mucosa and submucosal tissues, loss of gastric acidity, and a reduced capacity for digestion and absorption. This leads to impaired bioavailability of nutrients from food, decreased transit time, and predisposition to small bacterial overgrowth. An impaired ability to repair and maintain the integrity of the endothelium predisposes to bacterial translocation and overexposure to endotoxins.

Skin

The skin wastes, loses its ability to maintain heat, and readily becomes breached and infected.

Immune system

There is increased exposure to pathogens and a decreased capacity to respond (inflammation and immune response see below).

Liver

There is downregulation of synthetic and excretory processes. The reduced functional reserve makes it more difficult to maintain glucose homeostasis in the face of increased bacterial exposure. Intermediary metabolism is impaired and transport proteins for the delivery of lipid, vitamins, and minerals to other parts of the body are reduced. The formation of clotting factors is impaired. Reduced bile and bile salt formation affect digestion. Metabolism and clearance of drugs, toxins, and xenobiotics is also reduced.

Cardiovascular system

A reduction in the functional reserve of the heart, slower pulse, and increased circulation time make heart failure more likely if excess fluid is given intravenously. There is poor circulatory control with a tendency to reduced intravascular volume with an expanded interstitial fluid space.

Iron is an integral part of haemoglobin in red cells, involved in the transport of oxygen from the lungs to the tissues. The mass of red cells is related to the amount of oxygen which has to be transported, which in turn relates to the mass of active lean tissue. As part of reductive adaptation there is a decrease in the lean tissue of the body with an associated decrease in the red cell mass. The iron which is released from haemoglobin is not required immediately for the formation of more red cells. The level of iron in the body is controlled by the rate at which it is absorbed from the gastrointestinal tract, as once in the body there are no recognized mechanisms through which iron can be lost. Therefore, the iron released from red cells cannot be excreted and is placed into storage. Free iron is highly reactive and acts as a focus for uncontrolled excess generation of free radicals, thereby damaging other cellular components. Excess iron is stored in the liver, bound to ferritin. A demand for ferritin synthesis is energetically expensive and diverts amino acids from the formation of other proteins. As part of reductive adaptation, the ability to effectively sequester iron in a chemically quiescent state is impaired.

Renal
There is decreased functional capacity of the kidney, with an impaired ability to concentrate, dilute, or acidify urine.

Muscle
Muscle mass is reduced and muscle function impaired by reduced potassium, which together lead to reduced generation of heat.

Brain
Brain function is relatively well preserved. Nevertheless there is blunting of higher functions with decreased mentation, apathy and depression, and impaired control of hormonal and integrative responses. There is a decrease in activity, poor work performance, and a decrease in discretionary activities, which together contribute to a slowing of learning.

Infection: the inflammatory and immune responses

Survival in a potentially hostile world requires effective non-specific and specific defence mechanisms. Non-specific physical barriers (skin and mucous membranes) and chemical protection (gastric acidity, secretions such as tears, mucins, etc.) depend upon cellular replication, which is less well maintained during reductive adaptation and even minor damage leads to a breach which is not repaired. Local damage with bacterial invasion usually elicits local inflammation, a systemic or acute phase response, and a specific immune response. The mounting, co-ordination and regulation of an effective response requires energy, increased cellular replication, and protein synthesis. The changes in hormones and cytokines associated with reductive adaptation impair the establishment and control of normal inflammatory and immune responses. The localized signs of tissue damage or infection—enlarged lymph nodes, enlargement of the spleen or liver, and the normal features of the acute phase response (fever, rapid pulse, and respiration)—are blunted or lost in malnutrition, making diagnosis more difficult.

Loss of appetite is a central feature of a more severe acute phase response, as the body raids its own tissues for the nutrients it requires to satisfy this unusual demand. There is a shift from the usual pattern of protein synthesis with less emphasis on growth. As muscle wastes the amino acids are made available for the synthesis of proteins for the immune system and the liver shifts from synthesizing large amounts of nutrient transport proteins to the formation of acute phase response proteins which limit cell damage and help repair. Albumin synthesis is inhibited, and it is redistributed to the third space leading to a reduced plasma albumin concentration. The low albumin which is frequently seen in malnourished people reflects the presence of an ongoing infection rather a dietary deficiency of protein. Correcting the problem requires that the underlying infection be effectively treated, not that dietary protein be increased. The cells of the inflammatory and immune systems increase their utilization of glucose, with increased gluconeogenesis from amino acids. A feature of the acute phase response is a profound change in the handling of micronutrients. There is a block in the absorption of iron. Net tissue breakdown releases components for which there is no immediate use. The circulating concentrations may be reduced (iron and zinc which are sequestered in the liver), or increased (copper), and there may be increased losses from the body in urine or stools (zinc and vitamin A). In childhood, diarrhoea is a frequent accompaniment of infection, which adds an excessive loss of nutrients from the body, especially potassium, magnesium, zinc, and vitamin A.

Specific nutrient deficiencies

Deficiency of specific nutrients is the most difficult aspect of severe malnutrition to manage effectively. Whereas in classical deficiency states, inadequate dietary intake is usually the major underlying cause, in severe malnutrition it is the failure to correct excessive losses of nutrients which leads to major imbalances. Major losses of intracellular nutrients can be difficult to identify with reliability for three reasons:

(1) Losses of intracellular content may not be readily identified using standard biochemical tests on blood, for example potassium.

(2) Bone acts as a very effective buffer for many nutrients and therefore severe total body depletion can develop without obvious biochemical change or loss of function, for example magnesium.

(3) During an inflammatory response, redistribution of nutrients within the body makes standard tests for nutrient deficiency very difficult to interpret, for example vitamin A, zinc, or iron.

Infection causes an unbalanced loss of nutrients, which may be obvious in association with diarrhoea and vomiting, but may be more subtle as in the increased urinary losses of vitamin A and zinc which are an integral feature of the acute phase response. For an individual consuming a diet which is marginal in one or other nutrient, increased losses may make the critical difference to achieving balance, which cannot be restored unless additional nutrients are provided during the convalescent period. All cellular functions are likely to be affected to a greater or lesser degree by specific deficiencies, but one process which is of special importance is the ability to cope with 'free radicals' or oxidative induced cell damage.

Antioxidant protection

In severe malnutrition there is a major imbalance between the potential for damage induced by free radicals and protective antioxidant systems. Infection, oxidative burst, and free iron all contribute to an increased potential for damage. Mortality is greatest in those with an obvious impairment of the antioxidant defences. Children with oedematous malnutrition have severely reduced concentrations of glutathione in blood and mortality is highest in those with impaired activity of glutathione peroxidase. Although the pattern varies with location, deficiencies of micronutrients are common and result in impaired cell function and membrane damage. The many layers of antioxidant protection which are specific for each compartment of the cell provide a measure of safety. However, the system is potentially vulnerable to deficiencies or limitations in multiple micornutrients, for example niacin, folate, thiamine, riboflavin, cobalamin, ascorbic acid, carotenoids, tocopherol, selenium, zinc, copper, magnesium. A deficiency might not be readily identifiable, either clinically or biochemically, and a high index of suspicion is required.

Oedema

Oedema reflects an inability to maintain the correct distribution of fluid in the intracellular space, the vascular space, and the interstitial space, and is a final common pathway representing a loss of metabolic control. Incorrect approaches to the management of oedema—the use of diuretics or the use of high protein diets—are amongst the commonest reasons for increased mortality. The rationale behind the incorrect approach to management presumes that oedema is simply the consequence of hypoalbuminaemia, itself the result of inadequate dietary protein. There are profound perturbations of protein metabolism in kwashiorkor, but these are due to concurrent infection, loss of appetite, and increased losses of nitrogen in stools rather than a diet deficient in protein. A low plasma albumin usually indicates an acute phase response to an unrecognized infection. Treatment with a high-protein diet or infusions of albumin does not correct the oedema, but does increase mortality. A low plasma concentration of albumin might contribute to formation of oedema, but is seldom the sole or primary cause. Although diuretics exert a direct effect on cell membranes, giving a diuretic is less likely to be effective if the intravascular space is reduced.

Table 4 Major factors which contribute to the development of pitting oedema in severe malnutrition

Hypoalbuminaemia	Associated with impaired protein metabolism, infection or stress, impaired hepatic function, toxic damage
Salt and water retention	Potassium deficiency, phosphate deficiency, acid–base imbalance, impaired renal function
Impaired membrane function	Altered composition (phospholipid composition and fatty acid profile). Impaired or downregulation of Na^+K^+-ATPase. Free radical induced damage

Diuretics which lead to increased urinary losses of potassium make the underlying problem of a deficiency of body potassium even worse.

The normal distribution of water between the different body compartments is tightly controlled through a number of interlinked factors. Disruption of one or more of these factors may lead to the development of oedema, and will need to be corrected for the oedema to be effectively cleared (Table 4).

Potassium deficiency leads to retention of sodium. Altered membrane structure and reduced activity of Na^+/K^+-ATPase allows intracellular potassium to fall and intracellular sodium to rise. All malnourished individuals should be presumed to be deficient in potassium and to have excess intracellular sodium, regardless of the composition of the plasma measured on routine biochemistry. Indeed plasma sodium concentrations might be low and it is tempting to give extra sodium, which is absolutely the wrong thing to do. There is more than enough sodium in the body, but it is in the wrong place. A direct approach which seeks to correct the disordered biochemistry is less likely to succeed than an approach which recognizes that the fundamental problem is that of disordered cellular function. Similar factors lead to cellular damage in any severely undernourished person, and by treating the malnutrition and repairing the metabolic machinery of the cells of the body, oedema will be effectively treated. What is required is generous supplements of potassium and correction of the underlying membrane dysfunction, which enables fluid and electrolyte balance to be restored. There is a close metabolic interdependence of potassium and magnesium, both of which are readily lost from the body in diarrhoea. It is extremely difficult to correct potassium deficiency in the presence of an associated magnesium deficiency, or to correct a magnesium deficiency in the face of a potassium deficiency. They have to be corrected together.

Principles of care

Phases of treatment: the 10 steps (Fig. 1, Table 5)

One of the important reasons why mortality from malnutrition has not been reduced in many centres is because the primary objective of treatment has been to try and correct the obvious weight deficit. In attempting to replace the lost tissue as soon as possible, generous intakes of food have been provided, encouraged and even forced. If appetite is poor, or anorexia is a feature, then generous forcefeeding by nasogastric tube has been used. This can be very dangerous. The 10-step approach to treating malnutrition clearly identifies that treatment must be divided into different phases: the cellular machinery has to be repaired before it can be used to enable tissue growth.

Two clinical features which are directly related to specific nutrient deficiencies and are particularly difficult to manage are oedema and persistent diarrhoea. Any specific nutrient deficiency impairs cellular function and increases the risk of infection. Infection increases nutrient losses through tissue wasting as an intrinsic feature of the acute phase reaction and as vomitus or diarrhoea. Increased generation of free radicals is part of the body's attempts to deal with infecting organisms, and deficiencies of specific micronutrients directly impair the ability to cope with free radical gen-

eration. Even if an individual recovers from an infection, nutrients which have been depleted from the body are not easily replaced. This has two important effects. Firstly, the individual is deficient in a specific nutrient and carries the specific and general features of the deficiency, importantly loss of appetite. Secondly, if the deficiency is severe it may be very difficult for it to be corrected by consuming a normal diet without the addition of specific nutrient supplements. Under this circumstance, poor appetite, persistent reductive adaptation, and continued risk of further infection is maintained.

If energy is provided in excess of the requirements for maintenance, there are few ways in which it can be excreted or handled metabolically. Any significant excess is deposited as new tissue, either as cells or as cells filled with fat. There is a considerable underlying drive to form new cells, but in addition to energy this requires the availability of all the nutrients contained within the cell structure. When specific deficiencies have not been corrected individual nutrients are limiting for cell formation and it is not possible to handle the excess energy through the formation of new tissue. The excess energy creates a very serious metabolic upset (see recovery syndrome below). Therefore, during the period when nutrient deficiencies are being corrected and infections treated it is important to give sufficient energy to cover the needs of the body, but not so much that the body is forced to make new tissue. This is the basis for identifying the different phases of treatment: first to repair the machinery and gain control of metabolism by providing only enough energy to satisfy the needs for maintenance, but not enough to drive growth. Managing reductive adaptation, specific nutrient deficiencies, infection, and free radical-induced membrane and cellular damage lie at the heart of the problems associated with immediate care during the resuscitation period.

A loss of appetite is an important protective mechanism limiting food consumption which is likely to stress the systems of the body. In experimental studies there are two major biological reasons why appetite is lost: a deficiency of a specific nutrient and infection. Hence, the loss of appetite is a cardinal sign of an underlying metabolic problem which is ongoing. If the problem is identified and corrected, then appetite is restored very quickly. Most malnourished children have a profound loss of appetite due to a combination of infection and deficiencies of specific nutrients which interact to

Table 5 Outline clinical management of severe malnutrition.

1. Resuscitate

Manage infection, fluid and electrolyte imbalance and shock: oxygen, glucose, reduce heat loss, give antibiotics, maintain circulation, treat vitamin A deficiency

2. Stabilize

Control energy and protein intake at maintenance: 400 kJ/kg/day (100 kcal/kg/day), 1 to 1.5 g protein/kg/day

Small frequent meals: eight meals every 3 h, or six meals every 4 h, throughout 24 h

Correct deficiencies of specific nutrients by addition to food: potassium (4 mmol/kg/day), magnesium (0.4 mmol/kg/day), folic acid (1 mg/day), zinc (2 mg/kg/day), copper (0.3 mg/kg/day), multivitamin supplement

Treat bacterial infection: broad spectrum antibiotics, cotrimoxazole or ampicillin with gentamycin

Treat small bowel overgrowth with metronidazole

Treat helminth infections with mebendazole

Transfuse for severe anaemia

Topical treatment and care for skin lesions

Exclude tuberculosis

Give sensory stimulation and emotional support

3. Weight gain (rapid catch-up growth)

Ad libitum intake to achieve at least 600 kJ/kg/day (150 kcal/kg/day), 4 g protein/kg/day

Continue with micronutrient supplements

Add supplemental iron

Give sensory stimulation and emotional support

make the problem worse. Correcting the loss of appetite is central to effective care. The restoration of appetite marks the restoration of metabolic control and is a key component of therapy and a marker of progress. Once the emergency treatment required to resuscitate the child has been completed, the emphasis of care is to treat the underlying problems which are associated with a loss of appetite.

Resuscitation

Severely malnourished children present a medical emergency because of two sets of problems: the deadly triad of infection, hypothermia, and hypoglycaemia, and marked fluid and electrolyte disturbances (Table 5).

The deadly triad: hypoglycaemia, hypothermia, and infection

Brain cells are absolutely dependent upon a regular supply of glucose and oxygen to maintain the availability of ATP. Death occurs within 5 min if the supply of either is impaired, through poor circulation, reduced respiration, or a low blood glucose. The glucose required is either made in the liver or taken in the diet. Reductive adaptation limits the capacity for glucose formation and delivery and a regular dietary supply is required if blood concentrations are to be maintained. The availability of glucose for the brain can be impaired if there is competition from other tissues or functions, for example in order to maintain body temperature or to deal with infection. Malnourished individuals generate less heat and have reduced thermal insulation and therefore cool rapidly when exposed. Any attempt to generate more heat consumes glucose and other energy-providing fuels. A normal effective response to infection is a burst of activity in white blood cells which place heavy demands on available glucose, competing with the brain and leading to hypoglycaemia, and increasing the rate of heat loss leading to hypothermia. Therefore, the triad of hypoglycaemia, hypothermia, and infection indicate a very serious situation in which the body is no longer able to adequately maintain the supply of glucose to support essential functions. The treatment is to increase the supply by giving oral or intravenous glucose, reducing competing demands through decreasing the amount of heat lost, and by effectively treating infections. To deliver glucose and oxygen to the brain effectively requires an adequate circulation, which is compromised with intravascular dehydration. The correction of dehydration is closely associated with the correction of electrolyte imbalances, with energy homeostasis, and with normal cellular function. Care has to be taken to ensure that each is corrected in concert with the other to ensure that imbalances do not arise. All malnourished individuals are deficient in potassium and carry excess sodium.

Specific micronutrients: vitamin A, zinc, and iron

Iron is highly reactive chemically, and fulfils many important functions related to the generation of energy for normal cellular function. High reactivity, if not adequately controlled, carries the potential for cell damage. Red cell mass reduces in malnutrition as the lean body mass decreases. The iron is not used for further haemoglobin formation and cannot be excreted so has to be stored innocuously, as any which is unbound is liable to increase oxidative cell damage. In severe malnutrition there is increased stored iron and free iron. The available iron is not used for haemoglobin formation and giving iron supplements to treat anaemia simply adds to the load, stresses the system further, and increases mortality, especially in the presence of infection such as malaria. Initially, it is more important to repair and restore the capacity to cope with free radicals by improving vitamin and trace element status. Later, when the acute problems have been resolved, the iron will be removed from storage and used to form new tissue. As stored iron is used up, supplemental iron will have to be provided to keep pace with the rate of tissue demand.

Blindness and other eye signs of overt vitamin A deficiency are common in many parts of the world. Less obvious changes lead to impaired integrity of mucosal surfaces in the gastrointestinal and respiratory tract, lowering resistance to gastroenteritis and respiratory infections. During infection vitamin A is lost from the body, severe deficiency may develop rapidly, and the eye signs often deteriorate during early treatment. In areas where vitamin A deficiency is common, a large dose of vitamin A given very early in the treatment is an urgent necessity.

Zinc is required for the function of a wide range of enzymes, and a deficiency has widespread effects. A shortage of zinc impairs the replication of cells such as the gut mucosa, leading to further mucosal damage and increased diarrhoea. Zinc deficiency leads to diarrhoea and diarrhoea leads to zinc deficiency. Similar changes take place in damaged skin leading to ulcerated skin which is readily damaged with mild trauma.

Persistent diarrhoea

Many malnourished children have diarrhoea which can take time to settle. The diarrhoea may be infective in origin or have an infective component, due to viruses, bacteria, fungi, or helminths. However, diarrhoea which has persisted for any time will also have an element due to specific nutrient deficiencies (zinc and vitamin A) or chemical injury (bile salt deconjugation). With continued diarrhoea there are ongoing losses of nutrients. Few bacteria exist in the healthy small intestine, but small bowel overgrowth develops readily in malnutrition, due to a combination of gastric achlorhydria, reduced motility (potassium and magnesium deficiency), leading to bile salt deconjugation, damaged mucosa, and bacterial translocation. For the bowel to repair and re-establish its resistance requires adequate nutrients, most especially zinc, vitamin A, and folates. Thus the effective treatment of chronic diarrhoea requires a three-pronged approach: correction of potassium deficiency, treatment of bacterial overgrowth (with metronidazole), and effective repletion of specific nutrient deficiencies (such as zinc, vitamin A, and folate).

Management

The objectives of the resuscitation phase are to stabilize vital functions, by giving oxygen, supporting respiratory and cardiac function, and correcting fluid imbalance, to ensure that adequate amounts of glucose are delivered to the brain. Body temperature must be maintained by maintaining glucose supply to the system, limiting heat loss through the skin, and starting to control infection. As the capacity for the body to carry out metabolic functions is impaired, external support has to be supplied regularly on a 24-h cycle. The regular intake of small amounts over 24 h (especially at night) is a very effective way of achieving this (Table 5). All infections must be treated. Specific nutrient deficiencies must be corrected, but no iron or extra sodium should be provided. The metabolic state must be controlled by limiting the intake of energy and protein to that required to maintain body weight, and ensuring that there is no excess (see below). These steps will enable the repair of the metabolic machinery and allow cellular function to move towards normal. The response to a successful intervention will be a return of appetite; the patient will feel better and smile.

Recovery syndrome

Limited availability of one or more nutrients leads to competition between all cells for the little available. Some nutrients become relatively more deficient, upsetting the balanced function between tissues and the clinical signs of a deficiency become more obvious. There is a similar explanation for why the clinical signs of a deficiency are not always apparent, even though the body might be particularly deficient. During reductive adaptation, the demand for nutrients is decreased, and the signs of a deficiency are masked. Signs of deficiency become exposed in rapidly dividing tissues, when the demand for nutrients is greatest. Vitamin A and zinc are examples, but the same principles apply to many other nutrients, especially the B vitamins. The recovery or refeeding syndrome develops when individuals who have undergone reductive adaptation are suddenly provided with a relative excess of food. Excess energy drives metabolism while specific nutrient deficiencies are inadequately corrected and the metabolic machinery is still compromised. The syndrome may vary in its details, but consists of left- and right-sided heart failure associated with an overloaded circulation. This may progress to vascular collapse with abdominal distension as the circulating vascular volume is poured into the bowel as a profound secretory diarrhoea. The first sign of the onset of the recovery syndrome is an increase in pulse and respiratory rate. If food continues to be consumed at the same rate the load on the heart will progress to heart failure. This is a medical emergency, and it is vitally important that the food intake is reduced or stopped. If the changes are identified early and are relatively mild, then food intake should be reduced. If the condition has advanced and is severe then it may be necessary to stop all food for 12 to 24 h. The problem will then resolve.

Replacing lost weight

The ultimate objective of treatment is to replace the lost tissue. Cellular hypertrophy and hyperplasia are critically dependent upon and limited by the available energy and nutrients. For tissue of average composition the formation of 1 g tissue requires 20 kJ of energy. A normal 1-year-old infant gains 1 g/kg body weight/day, but for catch-up weight gain during recovery from malnutrition weight it is possible to form tissue at up to 20 g/kg/day, by consuming an additional 400 kJ/kg/day. Achieving this requires an energy-dense diet which is consumed throughout the 24 h of the day. Energy is necessary but not sufficient for new tissue formation. The nutrients needed for the formation of cell membranes and protoplasm are required in adequate amounts and suitable proportions. As the lean body mass grows it has an increased need for oxygen, and the red blood cell mass increases. Iron is taken out of storage to form new red cells, and eventually these stores are depleted with the need to add supplemental iron to the diet. There is an increased demand for amino acids to meet the needs of new tissue formation. It is safe to allow quite large intakes of protein. As the amino acids are deposited in tissue and do not accumulate in the free form there is no risk of toxicity. However, to meet the pattern of amino acids required by the body will require the endogenous biosynthesis of relatively large amounts of the 'non-essential' amino acids in the body, which in itself will require the generous availability of minerals and vitamins.

Important general aspects of care

The physical care which is provided to correct the biochemical, metabolic, and infective problems is critical for success. However, there is also the need to address the broader needs of the child for healthy development. In part this is provided by creating a warm, caring environment, in part by suitably structured activities which provide an appropriate level of stimulation to encourage brain function to recover and develop.

All aspects of care need skill and sympathy. The severely malnourished child is desperately sick and must be nursed as a critically ill child with minimum physical disturbance. With correct treatment, progress can be very rapid, and it is desirable to involve the parents and siblings, to encourage and demonstrate preferred childcare practices. This will facilitate the transfer between hospital and home, and make it more likely that the practices become embedded. Less seriously ill children can be effectively managed as outpatients, using the same principles and approach to the management decisions.

Further reading

Calder PC, Jackson AA (2000). Undernutrition, infection and immune function. *Nutrition Research Review* **13**, 3–29.

De Onis M, Blossner M (1997). *WHO global database on child growth and malnutrition.* WHO, Geneva.

Khanum S, Ashworth A, Huttly SRA (1994). Controlled trial of three approaches to the treatment of severe malnutrition. *The Lancet* **344**, 1728–32.

Scholfield C, Ashworth A (1996). Why have mortality rates for severe malnutrition remained so high? *Bulletin of the World Health Organization* **74**, 223–9.

Waterlow JC (1992). *Protein-energy malnutrition.* Edward Arnold, London.

WHO (1995). Physical status: the use and interpretation of anthropometry. *Report of a WHO Expert Committee*, WHO Technical Report Series no.854. WHO, Geneva.

WHO (1999). *Management of severe malnutrition: a manual for physicians and senior health workers.* WHO, Geneva.

WHO/UNICEF (2000). *Management of the child with a serious infection or severe malnutrition: guidelines for care at the first-referral level in developing countries.* WHO, Geneva.

10.5 Obesity

Peter G. Kopelman and Stephen O'Rahilly

Historical introduction

Obesity is now so common that it may replace undernutrition and infectious disease as one of the most significant contributors to global ill health. Modern research shows that obesity represents an important and defined medical disorder. Investigations into the genetic contribution to weight gain and the intra-abdominal distribution of fat (central obesity) have identified certain ethnic groups and susceptible families who are specifically at risk. There is, moreover, increasing awareness that overweight and obesity are key factors in the development of other chronic diseases, in particular type 2 diabetes and coronary heart disease, to which they contribute to the high mortality. Obesity can no longer be dismissed as a cosmetic problem affecting certain individuals: it is, in effect, an epidemic that requires effective measures for its prevention and management.

Definition of overweight and obesity

In clinical practice body fat is most commonly and simply estimated by using a formula that combines weight and height. The underlying assumption is that most variation in weight for persons of the same height is due to fat mass. The formula most frequently used in epidemiological studies is the body mass index (**BMI**), which is the weight in kilograms divided by the square of the height in metres. BMI is strongly correlated with densitometric measurements of fat mass adjusted for height in middle-aged adults. The main limitation of the BMI is that it does not distinguish fat mass from lean mass.

Measurements of body circumference are important because excess visceral (intra-abdominal) fat is itself a potential risk factor for chronic diseases, independent of total adiposity. Waist circumference and the ratio of waist circumference to hip circumference are practical measures for assessing upper body fat distribution, although neither provides a precise estimate of visceral fat. Measurement of skinfold thickness with callipers provides a more precise assessment of body fat, especially if taken at multiple sites. Skinfolds are useful in the estimation of fatness in children, for whom standards have been published. However, these measurements are more difficult to make in adults (particularly in the very obese), are subject to considerable variation between observers, require accurate callipers, and do not provide any information on abdominal and intramuscular fat. In general they are not superior to simpler measures of height and weight.

Measurement of bioimpedance is based on the principle that lean mass conducts current better than fat mass because it is primarily an electrolyte solution. A measurement of the resistance to a weak current (impedance) applied across the extremities provides an estimate of body fat when combined with height and weight and an empirically derived equation. Although impedance devices are simple and practical to use, they neither measure fat nor predict biological outcomes more accurately than the simpler anthropometric measurements. Table 1 lists the methods used to characterize obesity.

Defining a 'healthy weight' for a particular society is not straightforward. There are methodological difficulties that derive from a definition based on total mortality rates. People frequently lose weight as a consequence of illness, unrecognized at the time of survey, that is ultimately fatal. This gives an appearance of a higher mortality among those with lower weights (reverse causation). The effect can be minimized by either excluding persons with diagnoses that might affect weight and/or those who report recent weight loss, or excluding those who die during the first years of follow-up. A second concern is the confounding factors that may distort the association between body weight and mortality: cigarette smoking is of particular importance. The Nurses Health Study, which prospectively studied 116 000 women in the United States during a 17-year period, shows a U-shaped relationship between mortality and BMI in an overall age-adjusted analysis. However, the relationship becomes a simple positive association when reverse causation is accounted for and the analysis is limited to those who have never smoked.

There is a close relationship between BMI and the incidence of several chronic conditions caused by excess fat (Fig. 1)—type 2 diabetes, hypertension, coronary heart disease, and cholelithiasis. This relationship is approximately linear for a range of BMIs less than 30: American women with a BMI of 26 have a twofold increased risk of coronary heart disease compared with women with a BMI of less than 21, and an eightfold increased risk of developing type 2 diabetes. The equivalent figures for American men are a 1.5-fold increase and a fourfold increase. The risk of hypertension is doubled in both men and women with a BMI of 26. All

Table 1 Practical clinical methods for assessment of an obese subject

Characteristic of obesity measured	Methods
Body composition	BMI
	Underwater weighing
	Dual-energy X-ray absorptiometry
	Isotope dilution
	Bioelectrical impedance
	Skinfold thickness
Regional distribution of fat	Waist circumference; waist to hip ratio
	Computed axial tomography
	Ultrasound
	Magnetic resonance imaging
Energy intake	Dietary recall or record
	Macronutrient composition' by prospective dietary record or dietary 'questionnaire
Energy expenditure	Doubly labelled water
	Indirect calorimetry (resting)
	Physical activity level by questionnaire
	Motion detector
	Heart rate monitor

Fig. 1 Relation between body mass index (BMI) up to 30 and the relative risk of type 2 diabetes, hypertension, coronary heart disease, and cholelithiasis. Panel A shows these relations for women, initially 30 to 55 years of age, who were followed up for 18 years. Panel B shows the same relations for men, initially 40 to 65 years of age, who were followed up for 10 years. (From Willett WC, Dietz WH, Colditz GA (1999) *New England Journal of Medicine* **341**, 427–33, with permission of the authors and the Editor.)

risks are greatly increased for those subjects with a BMI greater than 29, independent of gender.

Body mass index can be used to estimate the prevalence of obesity within a population and the associated risks. It does not, however, account for the wide variation in the nature of obesity between different individuals and populations. A World Health Organization Expert Committee has proposed a classification of overweight and obesity that applies to both men and women and to all adult age groups (Table 2).

Waist circumference correlates with measures of risk for coronary heart disease such as hypertension or blood lipid concentrations. The choice of cut-off points on the waist circumference continuum involves a reciprocity between sensitivity and specificity similar to that for BMI. An expert panel has suggested increased risks if the waist circumference is more than 102 cm for men and more than 89 cm in women. However, lower cut-off points are associated with a two- to threefold increase in the relative risk of type 2 diabetes. Gender-specific cut-off points for waist circumference may guide the interpretation of values for adults: proposed cut-off levels are shown in Table 3. Level 1 is designed to alert clinicians to potential risk while level 2 should initiate therapeutic action. It must be emphasized that

Table 2 Cut-off points proposed by a World Health Organization (WHO) Expert Committee for the classification of overweight. Body mass index (BMI) is the weight in kilograms divided by the height in metres^2

BMI	WHO classification	Popular description
< 18.5	Underweight	Thin
18.5–24.9	–	'Healthy', 'normal', 'acceptable'
25–29.9	Grade 1 overweight	Overweight
30.0–39.9	Grade 2 overweight	Obese
40.0 or greater	Grade 3 overweight	Morbid obesity

these figures reflect knowledge acquired largely from epidemiological studies in developed countries. Preliminary information from developing nations indicates that lower cut-off levels for both BMI and waist circumference are appropriate for certain populations, who are at particular risk from comparatively modest degrees of overweight.

Epidemiology of overweight and obesity

The value of estimating prevalence and secular trends in overweight and obesity for identifying those at risk cannot be overemphasized. Conservative estimates of the economic costs of obesity in developed countries are between 2 and 7 per cent of the total health costs: this confirms that obesity represents a significant portion of expenditure in national health care budgets.

The range of BMI varies significantly according to the stage of economic transition and associated industrialization of a country: the shift from dietary deficit to one of dietary excess. As the proportion of the population with a low BMI decreases, there is an almost reciprocal increase in the proportion of the population with a BMI above 25. This indicates the tendency for a population-wide shift as socio-economic conditions improve so that overweight replaces thinness. Importantly, changes in adult prevalence of overweight and obesity are reflected by an even more striking changes in childhood and adolescence in both industrialized and developing countries. The early onset of obesity leads to an increased likelihood of obesity in later life, as well as an increased prevalence of obesity-related disorders.

Obesity, defined as a BMI of more than 30, is a common condition in Europe and the United States. The most comprehensive information in Europe comes from the data collected between 1983 and 1986 for the MONICA study. On average 15 per cent of men and 22 per cent of women were found to be obese, with overweight being much more common among women than men. More than half the adult population between 35 and 65 years of age in Europe were either overweight or obese. In England and Wales the most recent health survey has confirmed an increase in the prevalence of obesity in adults from 6 per cent of men and 8 per cent of women in 1980 to 17 per cent of men and 21 per cent of women in 1998. National surveys in the United States have shown a marked increase in the prevalence of obesity over time. The striking increase in prevalence between 1980 and 1994 confirms that population-wide increases in overweight and obesity may occur over short periods. The most recent data from the United States, derived from the third NHANES (1988 to 1994),

Table 3 Gender- specific waist circumferences that denote 'increased risk' (level 1) and 'substantially increased risk' (level 2) of metabolic complications associated with obesity in Caucasians. Level 1 is intended to alert clinicians to potential risk for coronary heart disease while level 2 should initiate therapeutic action

	Increased risk of complications	Substantially increased risk of complications
Men	94 cm or greater	102 cm or greater
Women	88 cm or greater	88 cm or greater

shows about 20 per cent of American men and about 25 per cent of American women to be obese. Subanalysis shows African-American women and other minority populations to have particularly high rates of obesity. Obesity is likewise prevalent in Latin America and is a particular problem in the Caribbean.

The increasing prevalence of obesity is not confined to Europe and the Americas. In Southeast Asia a dramatic rise is being seen in all populations. Obesity is now more prevalent in Malaysia than undernutrition in both urban and rural communities, but the most striking figures come from the Pacific region. In urban Samoa the prevalence of obesity is estimated as greater than 75 per cent of adult women and 60 per cent of adult men. High prevalence rates are also observed in the Middle East.

Aetiology of human obesity

At its simplest level the 'cause' of obesity is already known. By definition it results from an imbalance between energy intake and energy expenditure. In any individual, excessive caloric intake or low energy expenditure, or both, may explain the development of obesity. A third factor, so-called 'nutrient partitioning', a term reflecting an individual's propensity to store excess energy as fat rather than lean tissue, may contribute but will not be discussed further here. Multiple studies over several decades have attempted to clarify the relative roles of energy intake, energy expenditure, and nutrient partitioning in human obesity. The lack of consensus, despite intensive efforts, reflects a number of problems inherent in the study of the obese state. These include the heterogeneity of human obesity and errors in measurements of energy intake and expenditure, combined with the minor degrees of energy imbalance required to accumulate fat tissue over time, and the confounding effect of obesity *per se* on the measurement of physiological parameters.

Role of altered energy intake in the pathogenesis of obesity

It is surprising that no direct correlation has been reported between increasing prevalence of obesity and increased energy intake in developed nations given the ready availability of highly palatable foods. Underreporting of food intake confounds the understanding of the role of energy intake in the aetiology of obesity. Underreporting is an almost invariant feature of obesity, with comparisons of energy intake and expenditure in obese subject showing a consistent shortfall in self-reported food intake of approximately 30 per cent of the energy requirements. It is thus extremely difficult to obtain reliable data on the energy intake of free-living obese subjects.

Role of altered energy expenditure in the development and maintenance of obesity

The principal components of energy expenditure are resting metabolic rate, which represents the energy cost of maintaining physiological homeostasis, and physical activity, being the most variable component and representing 20 to 50 per cent of total energy expenditure. Resting energy expenditure is readily measured by indirect calorimetry, and the use of water labelled with two stable isotopes allows accurate measurements of total energy expenditure over a 10- to 20-day period. Studies of age- and sex-matched pairs of lean and obese women following an imposed activity schedule clearly demonstrate consistently higher energy expenditure in obese subjects compared with their lean pairs. The measurement of energy expenditure within the home, using doubly labelled water, shows comparable values between obese and lean subjects when corrected for different body sizes. Thus, a defect in metabolic mechanisms controlling energy expenditure has not been identified in human obesity. However, studying subjects when they are already obese is always confounded by the energy cost of the increased fat and associated lean mass, and corrections made for these may be insufficiently precise.

Prospective studies of energy expenditure in groups of individuals are more informative. Longitudinal studies of Pima Indians in Arizona suggest that the risk of a weight gain of 10 kg during a 4-year follow up is sevenfold higher in those in the lowest tertile of relative resting metabolic rate compared with those in the highest tertile. Nevertheless, even in a population which is predisposed to obesity, resting metabolic rate only predicts 40 per cent of the weight gain. No association has been observed between resting metabolic rate and 10-year weight gain in a Dutch population, and results from other studies have also questioned the validity of such an association.

In developed countries there is a relationship between low levels of physical activity and obesity. A longitudinal Finnish study found that those reporting physical exercise three or more times each week had on average lost weight since a preceding survey. By contrast, those who undertook little physical activity gained weight and had twice the risk of gaining 5 kg or more. Among children in the United States, the relative risk of obesity is 5.3 times greater for children who watch television for five hours or more each day compared with those children who watch for less than two hours, even after correcting for a wide range of socio-economic variables.

In the United Kingdom, a study combining data on energy intake and physical activity in relation to the secular increase in adult obesity showed no relationship between total energy intake or fat consumption and the prevalence of obesity, but a close relationship between proxy measures of physical activity (television viewing and car ownership).

Environmental and cultural factors in obesity

The evidence for the critical role of environmental factors in the development of obesity comes from migrant studies and the 'Westernization' of diet and lifestyles in developing countries. The dramatic increase in age-standardized prevalence of obesity (> 60 per cent in men and women) in the Naurians in Micronesia and Polynesians in Western Samoa is closely paralleled by alterations in diet and lifestyle. A marked change in BMI is frequently witnessed in migrant studies, where populations with a common genetic heritage live under new and different environmental circumstances. Pima Indians living in the United States are on average 25 kg heavier than Pima Indians living in Mexico.

In men and women the prevalence of overweight and obesity increases with age until 50 to 60 years; it is particularly apparent between the ages of 20 and 40 years. There are large, usually unexplained, variations between ethnic groups—this is particularly apparent in women in the United States with the rapidity of change occurring with increasing affluence of particular groups (22 per cent of Causian women are obese, 30 per cent of African-American women, and 34 per cent of Mexican-American women). In industrialized countries, a higher prevalence of overweight and obesity is observed in those with lower educational attainments and low income, although the reverse may be seen in developing countries. There is a tendency for overweight to increase after marriage and with increasing parity. Dietary intake and physical activity are crucially important factors in increasingly affluent societies.

The analysis of the prevalence of obesity by socio-economic status in England and Wales demonstrates a strong social class gradient, especially in women, ranging from 10.7 per cent in social class 1 (high) to 25 per cent in social class V (low). Interestingly, this is accompanied by marked differences in measures of physical activity, with social classes IV and V spending significantly more time watching television and being more likely to define themselves as inactive than those in social class 1.

Genetic factors in obesity

Evidence from twin, adoption, and family studies shows unequivocally that inherited factors contribute importantly to interindividual differences in fat mass. Studies of identical twins raised separately are particularly striking; they demonstrate a much closer correlation of BMI with biological rather than adoptive family members. The identification of genetic variants influencing human fat mass is a cherished goal of obesity research; it is only recently that the first mutations causing human obesity have been found. In general, mutations have been found in those rare children with extreme obesity and clear evidence for monogenic inheritance. The discovery of these defects has been dependent on rapid advances in mouse genetics. The seminal murine discovery is that of the novel adipocyte hormone leptin, which is deficient in the obese ob/ob mouse. Administration of recombinant leptin by injection restores ob/ob mice to normal body weight and corrects the associated metabolic and reproductive malfunction.

The discovery of leptin and the identification of its receptor, which is highly expressed in the hypothalamus, has advanced the understanding of molecular mechanisms within the hypothalamus that regulate appetite and energy expenditure. A particularly important element of this system is the group of neurones in the arcuate nucleus expressing pro-opiomelanocortin and the melanocortin 4 receptor, to which peptides derived from pro-opiomelanocortin bind. Thus far, five different genetic defects causing monogenic human obesity have been identified. These include mutations in leptin and the leptin receptor and two defects involving the pro-opiomelanocortin system, mutant pro-opiomelanocortin and mutant melanocortin 4 receptor. A single obese subject with mutations in a prohormone convertase enzyme shows major defects in pro-opiomelanocortin processing that may account for the obese phenotype (Table 4). These discoveries have shown for the first time that rare forms of severe human obesity may occur as a result of unitary molecular lesions within the appetite control pathway making such cases largely resistant to voluntary or imposed dietary restrictions.

Genetic studies in the more common forms of obesity have yet to have the same tangible success that has been seen with monogenic subtypes. Nevertheless, rapid progress has been made in the identification of chromosomal loci containing genes conferring susceptibilty to obesity. In particular, a region of chromosome 2 has been reported in independent studies of different racial groups to influence obesity-related phenotypes. It is of note that this region contains the pro-opiomelanocortin gene. Given the speed of progress of the Human Genome Project, it may not be long before this locus and other variants responsible for obesity syndromes are identified.

Gene/environment interaction

Obesity represents a heterogeneous group of conditions with multiple causes. Body weight is determined by an interaction between genetic, environmental, and psychosocial factors acting through the physiological mediators of energy intake and expenditure. Fatness runs in families, but the influence of the genotype on the aetiology of obesity may be attenuated or exacerbated by non-genetic factors. The genetic influences appear to operate through susceptibility genes. Such genes increase the risk of developing a characteristic but are not essential for its expression or, by themselves, sufficient to explain the development of a disease The susceptible gene hypothesis is supported by findings from twin studies in which pairs of twins were exposed to periods of positive and negative energy balance. The differences in the rate of weight gain, the proportion of weight gained, and the site of fat deposition showed greater similarity within pairs than between pairs. This suggests that differences in genetic susceptibility within a population determine those who are most likely to become obese in any given set of environmental circumstances. Implicit to the susceptible gene hypothesis is the role of environmental factors that unmask latent tendencies to develop obesity.

Pathophysiology of obesity

Obesity causes or exacerbates many disorders, both independently and in association with other diseases. In particular, it is associated with the development of diabetes mellitus, coronary heart disease, an increased incidence of certain forms of cancer, obstructive sleep apnoea, and osteoarthritis of large and small joints. The Build and Blood Pressure Study has shown that the adverse effects of excess weight tend to be delayed, sometimes for

Table 4 Genetic and clinical characteristics associated with monogenic causes of human obesity

Syndrome	Locus/mode of Inheritance	Obesity characteristics	Other features
Prader–Willi	15q11: imprinted gene	Feeding difficulties at birth, followed by extreme hyperphagia and weight gain with generalized obesity from age 2–3 years. Short stature	Hypogonadism, hypotonia, small hands and feet, scoliosis, learning difficulties, behaviour problems
Bardet–Biedl	16q21, 11q13, 15q22, 3p12: all recessive	Overlap with Lawrence–Moon–Bardet–Biedl (which is characterized by progressive spastic paraparesis and without polydactyly); onset of generalized obesity in first 2 years. Short stature	Retinitis pigmentosa, hypogonadism, learning difficulties, polydactyly
Cohen	8q22–23: recessive	Truncal obesity from mid-childhood	Hypogonadism, delayed puberty with or without hypogonadism
Alstrom	2p12–13: autosomal recessive	Normal height, truncal obesity from mid-childhood	Hypogonadism, blindness in infancy from retinal degeneration, deafness, insulin resistance, diabetes mellitus, progressive nephropathy
Edwards			Similar to Alstrom but with pigmented retinopathy
Klinefelter's	XXY	Adult onset with peripheral distribution. Tall with eunuchoid proportions	Hypogonadal, moderate learning difficulties, gynaecomastia
Albright hereditary osteodystrophy (Gs Alpha mutations)	Autosomal recessive	Childhood onset	Round face, variable hormone resistance including TSH, PTH, short fourth metacarpal
Congenital leptin deficiency	Autosomal recessive	Childhood onset, generalised obesity, normal stature, marked hyperphagia	Hypogonadism, insulin resistance
Prohormone convertase 1	Autosomal recessive	Childhood onset—one subject described to date	Hypogonadism, hyperproinsulinaemia, reactive hypoglycaemia, hypoadrenalism
Leptin receptor	Autosomal recessive	Childhood onset—three subjects described to date	Hypogonadism, short stature, hypothyroidism
POMC	Autosomal recessive	Childhood onset—two subjects described to date	Hypoadrenalism, red hair, pale skin
MC4R	Autosomal dominant	~10 subjects described to date	None

Abbreviations: TSH, thyroid-stimulating hormone; PTH, parathyroid hormone; POMC, pro-opiomelanocortin; MC4R, melanocortin 4 receptor.

10 years or longer. Life insurance data and epidemiological studies confirm that increasing degrees of overweight and obesity are important predictors of decreased longevity. In the Framingham Heart Study, the risk of death within 26 years increased by 1 per cent for each extra pound (0.45 kg) increase in weight between the ages of 30 and 42 years, and by 2 per cent between the ages of 50 and 62 years. Despite this evidence many clinicians consider obesity to be a self-inflicted condition of little medical significance.

Obesity and type 2 diabetes mellitus

Obesity is accompanied by an elevated fasting level of plasma insulin and an exaggerated insulin response to an oral glucose load. Overall fatness and the distribution of body fat influence the metabolism of glucose through independent but additive mechanisms. Increasing upper body obesity is accompanied by a progressive increase in the response of glucose and insulin to an oral glucose challenge, and there is a positive correlation between increasing upper body obesity and resistance to the effects of insulin. Posthepatic insulin delivery is increased in upper body obesity, leading to more marked peripheral insulin concentrations which, in turn, lead to peripheral resistance to insulin.

Differences in the ability of insulin to suppress lipolysis, and of catecholamines to stimulate lipolysis, also vary according to fat distribution. These factors contribute to an exaggerated release of free fatty acids from abdominal adipocytes into the portal system. Free fatty acids have a deleterious effect on uptake of insulin by the liver and contribute to the increased hepatic gluconeogenesis and hepatic glucose release observed in upper body obesity. Insensitivity to insulin is not confined to adipocytes, and is accentuated by the resistance of skeletal muscle to insulin.

The elevation in plasma free fatty acids, particularly postprandially when their concentration is usually suppressed by insulin, leads to an inappropriate maintenance of glucose production and an impairment in the use of glucose by the liver (impaired glucose tolerance). Reduced hepatic clearance of insulin leads to increased peripheral (systemic) insulin concentrations and to a further downregulation of insulin receptors.

In the initial phases of this process, the pancreas can respond by maintaining a state of compensatory hyperinsulinaemia. With ever increasing plasma concentrations of free fatty acids, the insulin-resistant individual cannot maintain this state of compensatory hyperinsulinaemia, and hyperglycaemia prevails. Hyperinsulinaemia and insulin resistance contribute to the characteristic alterations in the profile of plasma lipids which are associated with obesity: elevated fasting concentration of triglycerides in the plasma, reduced high-density lipoprotein (**HDL**) cholesterol, marginal elevations in the concentration of cholesterol and low-density lipoprotein (**LDL**) cholesterol, and an increase in the number of ApoB-carrying lipoproteins.

Prospective population studies confirm a close association between increasing body fatness and type 2 diabetes. In the Nurses Cohort Study, BMI was the dominant predictor of the risk of diabetes after adjustment for age. In this study the risk of diabetes was increased fivefold for those with a BMI of 25, 28-fold for those with a BMI of 30 and 93-fold for those with a BMI of 35 or greater. Women who gained 8 to 10.9 kg in weight during the period of study had a 2.7-fold increased risk of diabetes compared with women of stable weight. Similarly, the risk of diabetes in men increases for all BMI levels of 24 or above. The distribution of fat tissue is also independently associated with diabetes: a waist circumference of more than 102 cm (40 in) increases the risk of diabetes 3.5-fold even after controlling for the BMI.

Fetal nutrition

Recent evidence suggests that undernutrition of the fetus during intrauterine development determines the later onset of obesity, hypertension, and type 2 diabetes, independent of genetic factors. Such a phenomenon sug-

gests the possibility of long-term programming of genetic expression as a consequence of altered intrauterine growth: Barker has proposed that an adverse nutritional environment *in utero* causes defects in the development of body organs, leading to a 'programmed' susceptibility that interacts with later diet and environmental stresses to cause overt disease many decades later. In support of this hypothesis is the finding of an inverse relationship between birthweight and systolic blood pressure and type 2 diabetes in both men and women in later life, with the highest mean systolic blood pressures and blood glucose concentrations being observed in those with the lowest birthweight and highest current weight.

Cardiovascular function in obesity

The effects of increased body fatness on cardiovascular function are predictable. Total body oxygen consumption is increased due to an increase in lean tissue mass as well as the oxidative demands of metabolically active adipose tissue, and this is accompanied by an absolute increase in cardiac output. However, the values are within the normal range when they are normalized to body surface area. The total blood volume in obesity is increased in proportion to body weight, such that obesity can be regarded as a state of expanded volume. This increase in blood volume contributes to an increase in the left ventricular preload and an increase in resting cardiac output. The increased demand for cardiac output is achieved by an increase in stroke volume while the heart rate remains comparatively unchanged. The obesity-related increase in stroke volume results from an increase in diastolic filling of the left ventricle. The volume expansion and increase in cardiac output lead to structural changes in the heart. The increase in left ventricular filling results in an increase in the size of the left ventricular cavity and an increase in wall stress. As left ventricular dilatation is accompanied by myocardial hypertrophy, the ratio between the radius of the ventricular cavity and wall thickness is preserved. This thickening of the wall with dilatation results in eccentric hypertrophy. The mass of the left ventricle increases directly in proportion to BMI or the degree of overweight. The blood pressure is a function of cardiac output and the vascular resistance against which the blood is pumped—systemic vascular resistance. An elevated cardiac output is common with moderate obesity, but not all obese patients are hypertensive. However, in those subjects where systemic resistance is increased, the combination of hypertension and obesity results in an increase in the dimensions of the ventricular wall disproportionate to the chamber radius, which eventually leads to concentric hypertrophy.

The cardiovascular adaptation to the increased intravascular volume of obesity may not completely restore normal haemodynamic function. Marked systolic dysfunction occurs when the ventricle can no longer adapt to volume overload. Dilatation of the left ventricular cavity radius reduces ventricular contractility. Despite an elevation in cardiac output, obese individuals have been shown to have depressed myocardial contractility proportional to excess weight. With left ventricular hypertrophy, reduced ventricular compliance alters the ability of the chamber to accommodate an increased volume during diastole and this results in diastolic dysfunction. A combination of systolic and diastolic dysfunction progresses to clinically significant heart failure. Body weight, independent of several traditional risk factors, was directly related to the development of congestive cardiac failure in the Framingham Heart Study.

In addition to congestive cardiac failure, the presence of hypertrophy of the left ventricle has been associated with a greater risk of morbidity and mortality from coronary heart disease and sudden death as well as arrhythmia. In the Framingham Heart Study, the 26-year incidence of coronary heart disease in women and men was related proportionately to excess weight. The incidence of coronary heart disease increased by a factor of 2.4 in obese women and a factor of two in obese men under the age of 50 years. The independent risk of coronary heart disease attributed to obesity in multivariate analysis may reflect other important mediators such as upper body fat, altered blood flow and haemostasis, hyperinsulinaemia, or sleep apnoea.

Sleep-breathing abnormalities in obesity

An increased amount of fat in the chest wall and abdomen has a predictable effect on the mechanical properties of the chest and the diaphragm and leads to an alteration in respiratory excursions during inspiration and expiration, reduced lung volume, and mismatched regional ventilation. The increased mass of fat additionally decreases compliance of the respiratory system as a whole. All of these changes are significantly exaggerated when an obese person lies flat. The mass loading effect of fat requires the respiratory muscles to exert increased force to overcome the excessive elastic recoil and there is an associated increase in the elastic work of breathing. The changes in respiratory function related to obesity are most important during sleep.

During rapid eye movement sleep, there are decreases in voluntary muscle tone with reduced arterial oxygen saturation and a rise in carbon dioxide in all individuals, but these changes are especially marked in obese subjects. Irregular respiration and occasional apnoeic episodes often occur in lean people during rapid eye movement sleep but obesity, with its influence on respiratory mechanics, increases their frequency and may result in severe hypoxia and cardiac arrhythmias. Studies of obese men and women have demonstrated that the obstruction occurs in the larynx and is associated with loss of tone of the pharyngeal and glossal muscles, in particular the genioglossus muscle. Relaxation of the genioglossus allows the base of the tongue to fall back against the posterior pharyngeal wall, occluding the pharynx. This results in a temporary cessation of breathing (apnoea) and transient hypoxia. It is not uncommon to observe saturation values as low as 6.5 kPa during rapid eye movement sleep in some obese subjects while their awake arterial blood gases are normal.

A few obese patients suffer a marked depression in both hypercapnic and hypoxic respiratory drives accompanied by abnormal and irregular patterns of breathing during sleep and (eventually) in the waking state. Characteristically, such individuals show frequent and prolonged episodes of sleep apnoea—sleep is disturbed with frequent awakening related to the resumption of breathing following an apnoeic episode. Daytime somnolence soon intervenes accompanied by persistent hypoxia/hypercapnia, pulmonary hypertension (superimposed upon an increased circulatory volume), and right-sided cardiac failure. Such changes constitute the clinical manifestation of the obesity-hypoventilation syndrome (formerly known as the Pickwickian syndrome).

In the Swedish Obese Subjects study (SOS), which examined 3034 subjects with a BMI over 35, over half of men and one-third of women reported snoring and apnoea. In contrast, 15.5 per cent of Swedish men of comparable age were self-reported habitual snorers.

An increased risk of myocardial infarction and stroke has been reported in sleep apnoea. Snoring is a strong risk factor for sleep-related strokes, while symptoms of sleep apnoea increase the risk for cerebral infarction.

Other complications associated with obesity

Gallbladder disease is the most common digestive disease in obese individuals; it has a progressive and linear risk from a BMI of 20 upwards. Liver abnormalities are described in obesity mainly due to fatty infiltration but, on occasions, associated with fibrosis and/or cirrhosis. Certain forms of cancer are more common in obese subjects: colorectal and prostate in obese men, carcinoma of the gallbladder, breast, and endometrium in obese women. Osteoarthritis frequently accompanies obesity, while bone density tends to be increased in obese subjects. Obesity in women is also associated with menstrual irregularity and infertility; obesity may be, but is not always, associated with the polycystic ovary syndrome. Table 5 lists the morbidity associated with increasing body weight.

Table 5 Systemic comorbidities associated with obesity

Cardiovascular	Hypertension
	Coronary heart disease
	Cerebrovascular disease
	Varicose veins
	Deep vein thrombosis
Respiratory	Breathlessness
	Sleep-related hypoventilation
	Sleep apnoea
	Obesity hypoventilation syndrome
Gastrointestinal	Hiatus hernia
	Gallstones
	Fatty liver and cirrhosis
	Colorectal cancer
Metabolic	Dyslipidaemia
	Insulin resistance
	Type 2 diabetes mellitus
	Hyperuricaemia
Endocrine	Increased adrenocortical activity
	Altered circulating and binding of sex steroids
	Breast cancer
	Polycystic ovary syndrome
	Hirsutism
Locomotor	Osteoarthritis
	Nerve entrapment
Renal	Proteinuria
Genitourinary	Endometrial cancer
	Prostate cancer
	Stress incontinence
Skin	Acanthosis nigricans
	Lymphoedema
	Sweat rashes

Clinical assessment

Clinical setting

The usual principles for a medical consultation are applicable to the assessment of an overweight patient. The consultation room should preferably be properly equipped with larger than average chairs, access for wheelchairs for patients with mobility problems and medical equipment of appropriate size (examination couch, blood pressure cuff, weighing scales, stadiometer, and tape measure).

Historical background

Table 6 outlines the areas of medical history that should be investigated. The history of weight gain should be described in detail to identify possible causes and to assess the patient's insight and understanding of the factors causing weight gain. It is also useful to distinguish obesity which began in childhood from that occurring later in life either in relation to specific physiological 'critical periods' or illness. A number of syndromes are associated with the onset of obesity in childhood, but the longevity of the history and the associated clinical features generally make such cases obvious (Table 4). Disease involving the hypothalamus can often be distinguished from 'spontaneous' or 'simple' obesity by a shorter duration of weight gain and specific symptoms related to associated endocrine disturbances. The identification of the single gene disorders involving leptin and its signalling pathways are somewhat more difficult to distinguish from simple obesity, but extreme weight gain from early childhood, a positive family history, and the associated clinical features described in Table 4 are all characteristic. The most common single gene disorder causing obesity, melanocortin 4 receptor deficiency, is problematic as there are no pathognomonic features, but the diagnosis should be considered in cases of early onset familial obesity, usually with a clear dominant inheritance.

Table 6 Key points to cover when taking a history from an obese patient

- Medical history, risk factors and established complications from obesity—enquire about snoring and daytime somnolence
- Body weight history (landmarks for weight gain: puberty, employment, marriage, pregnancies, age at menopause, injuries resulting in periods of immobility etc.)
- History of previous treatment(s) for obesity (including successes and failures)
- Family history of obesity, related diseases, and risk factors (i.e. type 2 diabetes, hypertension, premature coronary heart disease and gallstones)
- Dietary history including usual eating pattern, alcohol intake
- Activity and lifestyle
- Relevant social history including cigarette smoking
- Drug history—drugs associated with weight gain, e.g. phenothiazines, tricyclics, anticonvulsants, lithium, anabolic and glucocorticoid steroids
- In women, menstrual history (irregular menses associated with polycystic ovary syndrome)

The measurement of serum leptin is not recommended as a routine examination, but in cases of severe early onset obesity this should be undertaken, since, although it is rare, congenital leptin deficiency is a potentially treatable disorder.

Clinical examination

An outline of a scheme for clinical examination is given in Table 7. Height should be measured accurately using a stadiometer and weight measured by accurate scales calibrated against known weights. Fat distribution is assessed by measurement of the waist circumference and is used to refine an assessment of risk for patients with a BMI of 25 to 34.9. Waist circumference is taken as the midpoint between the lower rib margin and the iliac crest. An examination of the skin is important: thin, atrophic skin is a feature of excess corticosteroids; acanthosis nigricans (pigmented 'velvety' skin creases, especially in the axillae) suggests insulin resistance; severe hirsutism in women may indicate polycystic ovary syndrome. A neck circumference of more than 43 cm (17 in) indicates a likelihood of obstructive sleep apnoea, while abnormal external gonadal status accompanied by intellectual impairment may suggest a rare genetic syndrome.

Assessment of risk

An assessment of an obese patient's absolute risk status requires an assessment of associated disease conditions (established coronary heart disease, other atherosclerotic diseases, type 2 diabetes, and sleep apnoea), other

Table 7 Checklist of key points in the examination and investigation of an obese patient

Examination
  Height, weight—calculate BMI
  Blood pressure
  Waist circumference
  Neck circumference
  Any evidence of cardiac valvular disease
  Any evidence of pulmonary hypertension, cor pulmonale, or congestive cardiac failure
  Signs of hyperlipidaemia
  Signs of thyroid disease
  Ophthalmic evidence of diabetes or sustained hypertension
Investigations
  Fasting blood glucose
  Fasting lipid profile
  Strip test for urine glucose and protein
  Free thyroxine and thyroid-stimulating hormone

obesity-associated diseases such as gynaecological abnormalities, osteo-arthritis, gallstones, and stress incontinence, and cardiovascular risk factors. These will include cigarette smoking, hypertension, high-risk LDL cholesterol (> 4 mmol/litre), low HDL cholesterol (< 1 mmol/litre), impaired fasting blood glucose levels, and a family history of premature coronary heart disease. Patients can be classified as being of high absolute risk if they have three of these risk factors and will usually require therapeutic intervention.

In the obese patient who smokes, cessation of smoking is a major goal of risk management. An obstacle to cessation of smoking is the attendant weight gain. The weight gained on stopping smoking is less likely to impair health than is continued smoking. For this reason, cessation of smoking should be advocated at the same time as measures to prevent weight gain.

Assessment of motivation to lose weight

Not all patients are prepared for weight reduction despite a referral to a medical practitioner. It is often useful to confirm that a patient understands the need for weight loss and is prepared to follow medical advice to achieve and maintain an agreed weight goal.

Treatment

The recommendation to treat overweight and obesity is based on evidence that relates obesity to increased mortality and the results from randomized controlled trials which demonstrate that weight loss reduces the risk of disease. Professional, governmental, and other bodies have drawn up guidelines for obesity management. These strategies for providing care to the obese patient provide useful and evidence-based guidance for clinical management.

Aims for a weight loss programme

Any treatment programme for overweight and obese patients should place equal importance on the problem of weight reduction and the maintenance of the lowered weight. Obesity may not respond to conventional methods of treatment such as a low-calorie diet: its management frequently requires an individually tailored approach.

Goals of weight loss

The success or failure of a treatment programme may be judged by an arbitrarily chosen target weight or percentage weight loss. After an initial period of relatively rapid reduction of weight, an average continuing loss of anything up to 1 kg per week should be considered acceptable. Assessment of success must take account of the age of the patient, the initial degree of obesity, the presence of indicators of associated risk or complications, and previous attempts at weight control. Weight loss goals for overweight and obese patients should be tailored to the individual. A weight loss of 5 per cent of the initial body weight will result in some improvement, while a loss of 10 per cent is of major benefit with clinically useful changes such as a lowered blood pressure, reduction in levels of plasma total cholesterol and triglycerides, an increase in HDL cholesterol, and a significant improvement in diabetic control (Table 8). The primary goal of treatment is a 10 per cent reduction from the initial weight; successful weight loss should be regarded as a loss of more than 5 per cent of the initial weight with the consequent amelioration of risk factors; very successful weight loss would be a loss of more than 20 per cent in obese patients. Weight loss should be approached incrementally with new goals for weight loss negotiated with the patient once the original target has been achieved. Goals for older patients (more than 65 years) will be different from those for younger patients—data suggest that a population becomes heavier with age whereas the risk from obesity does not increase proportionally. In some patients, particularly older patients, prevention of further weight gain may be more appropriate than actual weight loss.

Table 8 Potential health benefits that may accrue from the loss of 10 kg from the initial body weight in those patients with comorbidities.

Mortality	20–25% fall in total mortality
	30–40% fall in diabetes-related deaths
	40–50% fall in obesity-related cancer deaths
Blood pressure	Fall of about 10 mmHg in both systolic and diastolic values
Diabetes	Reduces risk of developing diabetes by > 50%
	Fall of 30–50% in fasting glucose
	Fall of 15% in haemoglobin A1c
Lipids	Fall of 10% in total cholesterol
	Fall of 15% in LDL cholesterol
	Fall of 30% in triglycerides
	Increase of 8% in HDL cholesterol

Adapted from Jung RT. *British Medical Bulletin*, 1977; **53**: 311, with permission

Dietary treatment of obesity

Control of diet is the focus of management of overweight and obese patients, and its primary importance must be emphasized. Long-term changes in food choices, eating behaviour, and lifestyle are needed, rather than a temporary restriction of specific foods. The treatment should be nutritionally sound and aim to promote a healthier diet while moderating energy intake and increasing physical activity. Such a treatment may require a period of supervision for at least 6 months. A review of 48 randomized control trials shows that an average weight loss of 8 per cent of the initial body weight can be obtained over 3 to 12 months with a low-calorie diet, and that this weight loss effects a decrease in abdominal fat.

The weight-reducing dietary regimen tailored to an individual's need should initially provide a 600 kcal/day (2.5 MJ/day) energy deficit, based on estimated initial maintenance energy. The diet may best be achieved by a reduction in overall fat intake and will mean, for example, an energy prescription of approximately 1500 kcal/day (6.27 MJ/day) for a moderately active woman of average height aged between 31 and 60 years, and approximately 1800 to 2000 kcal/day (7.52 to 8.36 MJ) for a man of similar age and activity. For overweight patients with a BMI in the range of 27 to 35, a decrease of 300 to 500 kcal/day (1.25 to 2.1 MJ/day) will result in weight loss of about 0.25 to 0.5 kg/week. For more severely obese patients, with a BMI greater than 35, deficits of 500 to 1000 kcal/day (2.1 to 4.2 MJ/day) will lead to weight loss of 0.5 to 1 kg/week. After 6 months, the rate of weight loss usually declines and the weight remains constant because of less expenditure of energy at the lower weight. A further adjustment of calorie intake will be indicated at this stage.

Very low calorie diets

The use of very low calorie diets should only be considered after the failure of determined attempts to lose weight with conventional restriction of normal diets. Their use should follow all of the recommendations from the Committee on Medical Aspects of Food Policy, in particular that such preparations must provide a minimum of 400 kcal (1.7 MJ) per day for women and 500 kcal (2.1 MJ) per day for men. It must be recognized that these diets do not alter eating habits or weight loss beneficially in the longer term. Very low calorie diets may occasionally be useful in the hospital setting for rapid weight loss before surgery. Evidence from randomized trials confirms that over the longer term (more than a year) weight loss following very low calorie diets is no different from that obtained with a low-calorie diet.

Behaviour management

Behavioural interventions seek to alter an individual's lifestyle. Behavioural weight control programmes encourage patients to become more aware of their eating and physical activity and focus on changing the lifestyle and environmental factors that influence their behaviour. All dietary regimens should ideally be linked to behavioural therapy: such therapy may be used by self-help groups. The key difference between behavioural methods and other forms of treatment for obesity is that they lay particular emphasis on personal responsibility for initiating and maintaining treatment rather than the imposition of external authority.

In most trials, behavioural intervention has produced consistent short-term weight loss. Recent studies suggest that a focus on calorie restriction and reduced fat intake, as part of the behavioural approach, is more successful than calorie restriction alone. Studies of methods that seek to avoid circumstances that induce excessive eating are inconclusive, whereas behavioural programmes which provide appropriate foods may be of value. Evidence from randomized controlled trials confirms that behavioural strategies reinforce changes in diet and physical activity in obese adults to produce weight loss in the range of 10 per cent over 4 months to 1 year. Longer-term follow-up shows a return to baseline weight in the absence of continuing behavioural intervention. Trial evidence suggests that behavioural therapy, when used in combination with other weight loss methods, induces further short-term (up to a year) weight loss and that extended treatment programmes improve long-term maintenance of weight.

Exercise and physical activity

When physical activity or exercise alone is used in the treatment of obesity, weight losses are modest and average 2 to 3 kg. This weight loss, although small, exceeds that predicted if direct energy expenditure calculations are performed. For any given weight loss, the loss of fat-free mass is less in exercising versus non-exercising subjects: this is important because fat-free mass is the best predictor of resting metabolic rate which is the largest contributor to total daily energy expenditure. A review of randomized controlled trials provides strong evidence that physical activity alone in obese adults results in modest weight loss and increased cardiovascular fitness.

Regular exercise results in reduction in blood pressure, both in association with or independently of weight loss, and an improvement in atherogenic lipid profiles. A reduction in plasma triglycerides and low-density lipoprotein cholesterol and elevation of high-density lipoprotein cholesterol has been reported with exercise and physical training in obese patients. Exercise also has beneficial effects on glucose metabolism and the sensitivity of skeletal muscle to insulin. However, persuading an obese person to participate in long-term exercise programmes, and to maintain exercise as part of daily routine, is not easy. It is not necessary for the obese patient to increase maximal oxygen uptake by strenuous exercise to derive benefit from exercise: metabolic evidence of improvement in fitness is achieved with less vigorous exercise such as walking increased distances and swimming. The risks from exercise are small, provided it is introduced gradually and pre-existing conditions such as osteoarthritis and ischaemic heart disease are taken into account. The results from randomized controlled trials suggest that a combination of diet and exercise generally produces more weight loss than diet alone, including decreased abdominal fat. More importantly, subjects who exercise adhere to the prescribed diet better than those who do not exercise. One of the most consistent findings in randomized controlled trials of the effect of exercise is the maintenance of weight loss for 2 years.

Drug treatment

The criteria applied to the use of an antiobesity drug should be similar to those applied to the treatment of other relapsing disorders. Many drugs have been advocated over the years as treatment for obesity. Some of these compounds are effective, but many are ineffective. The use of drugs in the management of obesity is bedevilled by the limitations of the available published scientific evidence. It is therefore important that doctors who use these drugs make themselves fully familiar with either the primary literature for any drug, or an authoritative summary document.

Indications for antiobesity drug treatment

It may be appropriate to consider drug treatment if after at least 3 months of supervised diet, exercise, and behavioural management, or at a subsequent review, a patient's BMI is equal to or greater than 30 and weight loss is less than 10 per cent of the presenting weight. In certain clinical circumstances it may also be appropriate to consider antiobesity drug treatment for those patients with established comorbidities whose BMI is 27 or greater, if this is permitted by the drug's licence.

The initiation of drug treatment will depend on the clinician's judgement about the risks to an individual from continuing obesity: drug treatment may be particularly appropriate for patients with comorbid risk factors or complications from their obesity. A drug should not be considered ineffective because weight loss has stopped, provided that the lowered weight is maintained. However, continuation of the drug should depend on the balance between the health benefits of maintained weight and the potential adverse effects of the drug.

Types of drug treatment for obesity

There are currently two categories of antiobesity drugs—those which act on the gastrointestinal system (pancreatic lipase inhibitors) and those which act on the central nervous system to suppress appetite.

Drugs acting on the gastrointestinal system (pancreatic lipase inhibitors)

Orlistat inhibits pancreatic and gastric lipases thereby decreasing the hydrolyisis of ingested triglycerides. It produces a dose-dependent reduction in absorption of dietary fat that is near maximum at a dose of 120 mg three times daily. These actions lead to weight loss in obese subjects. Adverse effects of Orlistat are predominantly related to malabsorption of fat. These include loose or liquid stools, faecal urgency, and oily discharge; they can be associated with malabsorption of fat-soluble vitamins. As the consumption of a high-fat meal will inevitably lead to severe gastrointestinal symptoms, it is possible that some of the weight loss with Orlistat treatment results from an 'antabuse effect', enforcing behavioural change; Orlistat is not itself systemically absorbed.

Centrally acting antiobesity drugs

Drugs which act on the central nervous system can be divided into three groups: those acting via serotoninergic (5-hydroxytryptamine) pathways, for example fenfluramines, those acting via noradrenergic pathways, for example phentermine, and those acting via serotoninergic and noradrenergic pathways, for example sibutramine.

- Drugs acting on serotoninergic pathways: The two drugs from this category, fenfluramine and dexfenfluramine, principally act by releasing serotonin from synapses in the central nervous system; they have only a modest action on inhibiting the reuptake of serotonin into nerve terminals. Because the fenfluramines have been withdrawn they will not be considered further.

- Drugs acting on catecholamine pathways: Phentermine is a phenylethylamine derivative with minor sympathomimetic and stimulant properties whose antiobesity action is due to suppression of appetite. Phentermine has also been withdrawn and will not be considered.

- Drugs acting on noradrenergic and serotoninergic pathways: Sibutramine promotes a sense of satiety through its central action as an inhibitor of serotonin and noradrenaline reuptake. It may also have an enhancing effect on thermogenesis through stimulation of peripheral noradrenergic receptors. Sibutramine is well absorbed following oral ingestion and undergoes first-pass metabolism in the liver to produce two active metabolites that have long elimination half-lives. This enables sibutramine to be given on a single daily basis at a starting dose of 10 mg. Adverse effects include nausea, dry mouth, rhinitis, and constipation. The noradrenergic actions of the drug may cause an increase in blood pressure and heart rate in some patients, or prevent the

expected fall in these parameters with weight loss. The drug should be used with caution in hypertensive patients.

Drugs not appropriate for the treatment of obesity

There is no published evidence to suggest that bulk forming agents (e.g. methyl cellulose) have any beneficial long-term action for weight reduction. Diuretics, human chorionic gonadotrophin, amphetamines, dexamphetamines, and thyroxine are not treatments for obesity and should never be used to achieve weight loss. Under no circumstance should thyroxine be prescribed for obesity in the absence of biochemically proven hypothyroidism. Metformin and acarbose may be useful in the management of the obese non-insulin-dependent diabetic patient: they have no proven efficacy for obesity alone and are not licensed for such use.

Prescribing antiobesity drug treatment

A review of randomized controlled trials provides good evidence that pharmacological therapy combined with diet, lifestyle modification, and physical activity results in weight loss in obese adults that is significantly greater than placebo when the drugs are used for 6 months to 2 years. Experience of the use of antiobesity drugs gained during 12- to 24-month randomized controlled trials indicates that approximately 30 to 40 per cent of the actively treated patients respond as judged by a 5 to 10 per cent reduction in body weight maintained over 12 months. The weight loss occurs in the 'responder' group within 12 weeks. This indicates a suitable time period when 'responders' to drug treatment can be identified and a decision taken to continue the medication. Continual assessment of drug therapy for efficacy and safety is essential. If the drug is effective in helping a patient to lose and/or maintain weight loss, and there are no serious side-effects, it may be continued. If not, it should be discontinued. Once a weight loss target has been achieved, there should be an opportunity for renegotiation of a new target, if indicated, and/or long-term monitoring with reinforcement. Combination therapy of two drugs is contraindicated because of lack of evidence of safety.

Figure 2 summarizes recommendations for the appropriate use of an antiobesity drug.

A system of regular medical audits should be a prerequisite of a weight management programme with a record of results and audit action.

Surgical treatment of obesity

There are two operative procedures currently used for the surgical treatment of obesity: gastric restriction and gastric bypass operations.

Gastric restriction involves the creation of a small capacity compartment (less than 20 ml) by either a combination of vertical stapling and a constrictive band opening or a circumgastric band pinching off a small proximal pouch. A modification of the latter procedure is an inflatable circumgastric band attached to a subcutaneous reservoir which allows access by a hypodermic syringe to inject or withdraw fluid thereby tightening or enlarging the band width.

Gastric bypass is performed by stapling shut a vertically oriented pouch of less than 20 ml and connecting this pouch to the jejunum transected 50 cm from the ligament of Treitz (Roux-en-Y gastric bypass). Published evidence confirms that this procedure produces greater weight loss but is accompanied by more frequent adverse effects including 'dumping'.

Most surgical procedures used in the treatment of obesity have been performed laparoscopically which reduces the requirement for sedating pain medication and facilitates prompt postoperative mobilization.

The initial findings from the Swedish Obese Subjects study of severely obese subjects (those with a BMI of more than 40) indicate that weight loss of approximately 30 kg over 2 years is associated with a 60 per cent reduction in plasma insulin, a 25 per cent decrease in plasma glucose and triglycerides, and a 10 per cent reduction in blood pressure. Furthermore, this degree of weight loss resulted in a 14-fold reduction in the risk of developing diabetes and a three- to fourfold risk reduction for the development of hypertension, hypertriglyceridaemia, and low HDL cholesterol levels. Poor

Fig. 2 Suggestions for the practical management of antiobesity drug treatment.

health-related quality of life was dramatically improved after gastric restriction surgery, while only minor fluctuations in health-related quality of life were observed in subjects treated by conventional dietary methods. The positive changes in health-related quality of life at 2 years were related to the magnitude of weight loss: the greater the weight loss, the greater the improvement in health-related quality of life.

Randomized controlled trials confirm that surgery for obesity is an option for carefully selected patients with clinically severe obesity (BMI ≥ 40 or BMI ≥ 35 with comorbid conditions) when less invasive methods of weight loss have failed, and the patient is at high risk for obesity-associated morbidity and mortality. The nature of the surgical procedures necessitates long-term hospital follow-up for such patients.

Weight maintenance

In most patients obesity results not from an inability to lose weight but a profound difficulty in maintaining a lowered weight. A programme to enable the individual to maintain their lowered weight must follow any successful weight loss. A combination of appropriate eating, physical activity, and reinforcement of behavioural methods is the most successful in the long term. Physicians and others can reinforce the importance of this approach but the ultimate responsibility for following such advice must lie with the patient.

Management of obesity during pregnancy

In pregnancy, a weight gain of 12 kg in women of normal weight is associated with the best outcome. By contrast, in women who start pregnancy with a BMI of more than 28, the lowest perinatal mortality is seen with a weight gain of only 4 kg. In pregnancy the aim is thus to limit total weight gain in obese women to 4 kg: the mother-to-be can achieve this by following a nutritionally balanced eating programme prescribed by a registered dietitian, throughout pregnancy.

Management of obesity in childhood

The management of overweight and obesity in children follows the same principles as for adults except that the use of medication is not recommended. Dietary intervention to reduce calorie intake needs to be tempered by a necessity to provide adequate micronutrients such as iron and calcium. Early treatment of childhood obesity has the advantage that it provides the opportunity for the child to 'grow' into their weight. In other words, height may continue to increase for many years and the child main-

taining his/her weight will achieve a more favourable body habitus. Any form of dietary restriction must be combined with a regular exercise programme—the design of the activity programme needs to be tailored to the skills of the child and may include walking, swimming, and jogging.

Prevention

The two priority areas for public health strategies aimed at preventing obesity are increasing physical activity and improving the quality of the available diet within a community. However, such strategies must address the need to improve the population's understanding of the nature of obesity and its management and reduce exposure to an environment which promotes obesity. Achievement of these aims requires the involvement of individuals, their families, health professionals, health services, and a commitment from all sectors of the community.

Further reading

Barsh GS, Farooqi IS, O'Rahilly S (2000). Genetics of body weight regulation: applications and opportunities. *Nature* **404**, 644–51.

Chan JM *et al.*(1994). Obesity, fat distribution and weight gain as risk factors for clinical diabetes in men. *Diabetes Care* **17**, 961–9.

Clinical Guidelines, National Heart, Lung and Blood Institute Web site: http://www.nhlbi.nih.gov/nhbli/cardio/obes/prof/guidelns/ob_gdlns.htm

Royal College of Physicians of London (1998). *Clinical management of overweight and obese patients with particular reference to the use of drugs.* Royal College of Physicians, London.

Farooqi IS *et al.* (1999). Effects of recombinant leptin therapy in a child with congenital leptin deficiency. *New England Journal of Medicine* **341**, 879–84.

Flegal KM, Carroll MD, Kuczmarski RJ, Johnson CL (1998). Overweight and obesity in the United States: prevalence and trends, 1960–1994. *International Journal of Obesity* **22**, 39–47.

Glenny A-M *et al.* (1997). The treatment and prevention of obesity: a systematic review of the literature. *International Journal of Obesity* **21**, 715–37.

Grunstein RR (1998). Pulmonary function, sleep apnoea and obesity. In: Kopelman PG, Stock MJ, eds. *Clinical obesity*, pp 248–89. Blackwell Science, Oxford.

Hubert HB *et al.* (1983). Obesity as an independent risk factor for cardiovascular disease: a 26-year follow-up of participants in the Framingham heart study. *Circulation* **67**, 968–77.

Kopelman PG (2000). Obesity as a medical problem. *Nature* **404**, 635–643.

Kral J (1998). Surgical treatment of obesity. In: Kopelman PG, Stock MJ, eds. *Clinical obesity*, pp 545–63 Blackwell Science, Oxford.

Lew EA (1985). Mortality and weight: insured lives and the American Cancer Study. *Annals of Internal Medicine*, **103,** 1024–9.

Manson JE *et al.* (1995). Body weight and mortality among women. *New England Journal of Medicine* **333**, 677–85.

Prentice AM, Jebb SA (1995). Obesity in Britain: gluttony or sloth? *British Medical Journal* **311**, 437–9.

Ravussin E *et al.* (1988). Reduced rate of expenditure as a risk factor for body weight. *New England Journal of Medicine* **318**, 467–72.

Willett WC, Dietz WH, Colditz GA (1999). Guidelines for healthy weight. *New England Journal of Medicine* **341,** 427–33.

World Health Organization (1997). *Obesity: preventing and managing the global epidemic.* WHO, Geneva.

World Health Organization Expert Committee (1995). *Physical status: the use and interpretation of anthropometry.* WHO Technical Report Series no. 854. WHO, Geneva.

World Health Organization MONICA Project (1988). Geographical variation in the major risk factors of coronary heart disease in men and women aged 35–64 years. *World Health Statistics Quarterly* **41**, 115–40.

Zhang Y *et al.* (1994). Positional cloning of the mouse obese gene and its human homologue. *Nature* **372**, 425–32.

10.6 Special nutritional problems and the use of enteral and parenteral nutrition

M. Elia

Anorexia is a common consequence of disease. Undernutrition may increase morbidity after elective surgery and accidental injury, produce non-specific symptoms such as lethargy, depression, and fatigue, reduce tolerance to cytotoxic drugs or radiotherapy, and prolong the hospital stay.

It is possible to administer sufficient nutrients to individuals at risk of malnutrition, including those with gastrointestinal failure and severe burns, and those who are unconscious. Artificial nutritional support may be given in nursing homes and even at home so that it has become an important aspect of treatment.

The benefits of nutritional support depend on the severity of the disease and on nutritional status; this assessment of clinical and nutritional status is the first important step in rationalizing its use.

Nutritional screening and assessment

A well-structured history may provide useful information about possible undernutrition and the likelihood of specific nutrient deficiencies. Detecting malnutrition in routine clinical practice should be simple, reliable, and reproducible. Criteria for detecting malnutrition include the following: a body mass index of less than 18.5 kg/m² (chronic protein–energy undernutrition) or less than 20 kg/m² with a history of weight loss; unintentional weight loss of more than 10 per cent of body weight during the preceeding 6 months; and associated reduction in food intake/reduced appetite. The history may also reveal underlying psychosocial problems (loneliness, bereavement, isolation, alcoholism) and physical disabilities (active disease; for example painful mouth conditions, difficulties with eating and swallowing, inability to self-care) that are likely to have contributed to the weight loss. It is obvious that these underlying problems will also have to be addressed as part of the management.

The clinical history may indicate specific nutrient deficiencies: blood loss leads to iron deficiency; previous gastric surgery to vitamin B₁₂ or iron deficiency; coeliac disease may lead to folic acid and iron deficiency; and intestinal resections or fistulae associated with large amounts of intestinal effluents lead to deficiency of many nutrients including sodium, magnesium, and zinc. However, it is often difficult to establish the diagnosis of specific nutrient deficiencies from the history alone.

A dietary history may alert the clinician to major reductions in dietary intake and may indicate the likelihood of specific nutrient deficiencies. For example: anaemia in a vegan may be due to an inadequate intake of vitamin B₁₂; a diet poor in fruit and vegetables may predispose to vitamin C deficiency; a diet poor in fish and margarine (which is normally supplemented with vitamin D) may predispose to rickets or osteomalacia, especially in housebound individuals not exposed to sunlight.

Clinical examination

The relationship of height to weight provides a useful indication of nutritional status. In children an inadequate intake frequently results in growth

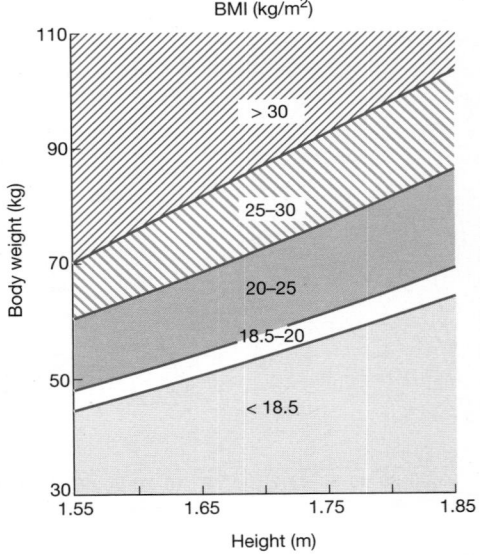

Fig. 1 Ranges of body mass index (weight (in kg)/height²(in m²)): less than 17, moderate to severe chronic protein–energy malnutrition (severe if less than 15); 17 to 20, chronic protein–energy malnutrition but some normal subjects; 20 to 25, desirable (some authorities 19 to 25); 25 to 30, mildly overweight (grade 1 obesity); 30 to 40, grade II obesity; over 40, grade III obesity.

retardation. Centile charts are useful for this assessment, particularly if sequential measurements are made. In adults an inadequate intake leads to wasting. The body mass index (weight (in kg)/height² (in m²)) can give some indication of the extent of depletion (Fig. 1), as can skinfold thickness (measured with a caliper), arm circumference, and arm muscle area (calculated from the arm circumference and skinfold thickness at the level at which the circumference was measured) (Fig. 2). However, the range of normality is large, and it is possible for subjects to lose a substantial amount of body weight, adipose tissue, or muscle mass and still exhibit normal indices (Figs. 1 and 2), or even above the normal range (for example obese individuals). It is therefore more useful to undertake sequential rather than single measurements.

An overall impression of nutritional status (subjective global assessment) may emerge from a combination of history and clinical examination. The examination should assess muscle wasting, the amount of subcutaneous fat, and the presence of oedema. Many other signs may be useful, especially on examining the limbs and integument (Table 1): chelosis or stomatitis may be the result of deficiency of vitamin B complex (but angular stomatitis is common in elderly subjects and may also result from badly fitting dentures); atrophic glossitis may result from folate or vitamin B₁₂ deficiency (this may also result from antibiotic therapy); koilonychia may

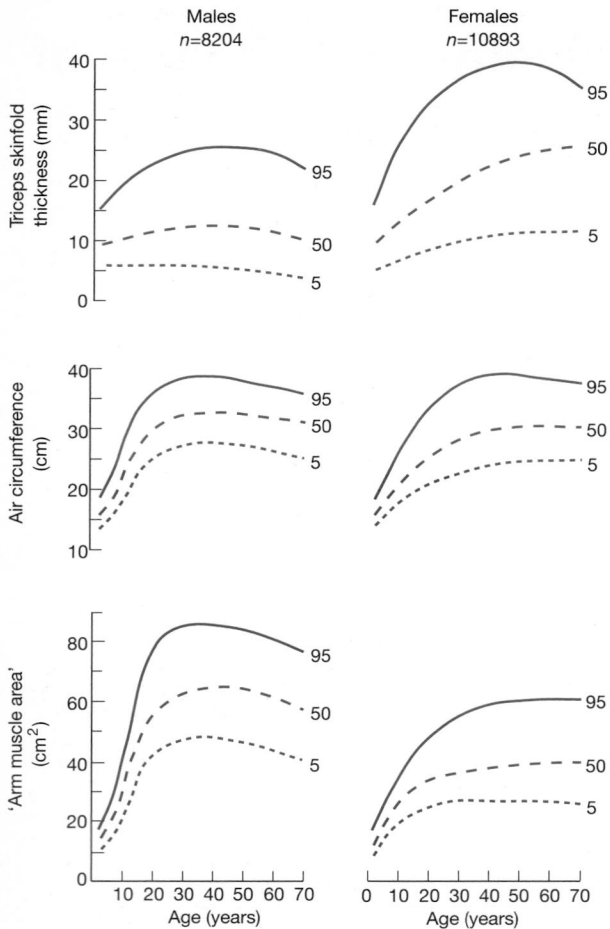

Males
n=8204

Females
n=10893

Fig. 2 Percentile curves of triceps skinfold thickness and the estimated mid-upper arm cross-sectional muscle are of American citizens. Based on the United States Health and Nutrition Survey (Frisancho 1981, 1984).

Table 1 Signs of specific nutrient deficiencies on examining the limbs and integument

Nutrient	Sign
Vitamin B₁₂	Anaemia (megaloblastic), atrophic tongue, peripheral neuropathy and subacute combined degeneration of the cord (e.g. absent ankle jerks and upgoing toes)
Folic acid	Anaemia (megaloblastic), atrophic tongue
Vitamin A	Xerophthalmia, hyperkeratosis of the skin
Vitamin C	Easy bruising (positive Hess test)
Vitamin K	Easy bruising (negative Hess test)
Vitamin D	Rickets (swollen wrists, rickety rosary, knock knees), tetany and positive Trousseau's sign (hypocalcaemia), proximal myopathy
Thiamin	Peripheral neuropathy (dry beriberi), oedema (wet beriberi)
Iron	Anaemia (microcytic hypochromic), koilonychia, angular stomatitis, atrophic tongue
Zinc	Bulbous pustular peristomal and acral dermatitis, loss of hair
Magnesium	Tetany, positive Trousseau's sign
Essential fatty acids	Diffuse scaly dermatitis

result from severe iron deficiency; tetany may occur in patients with vitamin D deficiency, or hypomagnesaemia; and a rash (acrodermatitis enteropathica) may occur in zinc deficiency. In alcoholics the presence of Wernicke's encephalopathy, Korsakoff's psychosis, and peripheral neuropathy point to the likelihood of thiamin deficiency. Easy bruising may be a sign of scurvy or vitamin K deficiency.

Since the signs and symptoms of many nutrient deficiencies are non-specific, they are often present in a severe form before they can be detected clinically. Deficiencies are usually present in combinations rather than in isolation. The key is to remember to include nutritional causes in the differential diagnosis.

Preventing and treating malnutrition and the indications for artificial nutritional support

Malnutrition in a variety of clinical conditions has been linked to poor outcome. This, together with the high prevalence of malnutrition reported in hospitals, has contributed to enthusiasm for artificial nutritional support. However, there are many simple things that the clinician can do to improve nutritional state. Nausea may be helped by an antiemetic. A person with dysphagia due to an oesophageal stricture may be helped by the provision of sloppy or liquid meals rather than solid foods. In contrast, patients with neurological disorders of swallowing may benefit from more viscous liquids. Pain causes anorexia, and its relief may improve appetite. Dedicating time to feeding weak and elderly patients may do much to improve their nutrition or at least prevent malnutrition. This task may be undertaken by nurses, health care assistants, or relatives.

When intake is inadequate, oral supplements may be tried. If these fail, enteral or parenteral nutrition may have to be used (see below for indications). In some patients it is immediately obvious that artificial nutritional support is necessary. This applies to patients who are unconscious (and likely to remain unconscious for a long period), and those who are unable to swallow or have intestinal failure. It also may apply to patients subjected to major surgery, for example oesophagogastrectomy, who are routinely prevented from eating for a week or more until the anastomosis has adequately healed, and patients receiving aggressive chemotherapy for haematological malignancies (bone marrow transplantation). These latter patients typically develop severe inflammation of the mouth and other parts of the gastrointestinal tract, so that artificial nutritional support (enteral or parenteral nutrition) may be required.

Oral or enteral nutrition should be used where possible because it is simpler, cheaper, and more physiologically acceptable than parenteral nutrition. In addition, enteral nutrition appears to be better than parenteral nutrition in maintaining the integrity of the 'gut barrier', which prevents bacteria and associated endotoxins from entering the systemic circulation. General and specific recommendations about the use of enteral tube feeding are given in Table 2. Some of these guidelines also apply to parenteral nutrition but only when the gut is not available for feeding. Well-recognized indications are prolonged gastrointestinal failure in the form of ileus, peritonitis, severe and recurrent pancreatitis, high intestinal fistulae, short bowel syndrome, or severe inflammatory disease of the intestine, for example severe mucositis following cytotoxic therapy, or Crohn's disease complicated by fistulae. The use of parenteral nutrition in the postoperative period is discussed separately.

Infusion of nutrients into peripheral veins has often been associated with rapid development of phlebitis and venous occlusion. These complications may be reduced by infusing solutions of lower osmolarity (a larger volume, less glucose, and more fat—since fat emulsions have an osmolarity close to that of blood), through suitable fine-bore cannulae. Small doses of heparin and/or corticosteroids and vasodilatory glycerin trinitrate skin patches may prevent venous occlusion. However, peripheral parenteral venous feeding has obvious limitations for patients with poor peripheral venous access and for those requiring prolonged infusions of hypertonic solutions.

Nutritional requirements

Protein and energy

Recommendations about nutrient intake depend on disease activity and nutritional state. Figure 3 shows the effects of increasing nitrogen intake on the nitrogen balance in subjects who are close to energy equilibrium. Normal individuals in energy balance achieve nitrogen balance at a mean intake of 0.1 g N/kg. The World Health Organization recommends a minimum of 0.12 g N/kg, to take into account the variability between individuals (+2 standard deviations). A greater intake produces little improvement in nitrogen balance in normal subjects. In contrast, depleted individuals, particularly those without associated inflammatory or infective disease, achieve a progressively greater positive balance as more nitrogen is taken in (Fig. 3).

Negative nitrogen balance in catabolic states is due to a combination of the disease itself, which enhances both net muscle proteolysis and liver gluconeogenesis, immobility, and the effect of drugs such as steroids. The catabolism is usually greatest within the first few days of injury but in patients suffering from burns it may continue for weeks. In well-nourished patients (such as those with sepsis, trauma, or burns) who are close to energy balance, an increase in nutritional intake results in improved nutri-

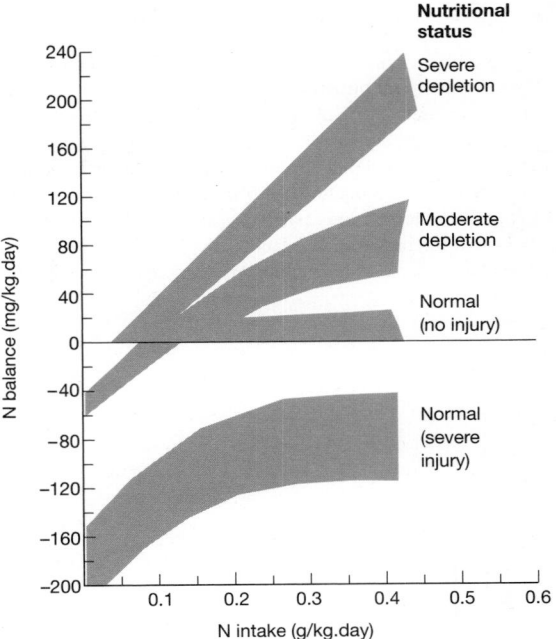

Fig. 3 Relationship between nitrogen intake (1 g N = 6.25 g protein) and nitrogen balance in subjects who are receiving sufficient energy to be close to energy balance (see text).

Table 2 Guidelines for the use of enteral nutrition in the adult patient (based on the American Society of Parenteral and Enteral Nutrition Board of Directors 1987)

1. Clinical settings where artificial enteral nutrition should be a part of routine care

    (a) Protein energy malnutrition (greater than 10 per cent weight loss) with little or no oral intake for the previous 5 days

    (b) Less than 50 per cent of the required oral nutrient intake for the previous 7–10 days

    (c) Severe dysphasia or swallowing-related difficulties, e.g. head injury, strokes, motor neurone disease

    (d) Major, full-thickness burns

    (e) Massive small bowel resection in combination with parenteral nutrition (in patients with 50–90 per cent small bowel resection, enteral nutrition is given to hasten gut regeneration and return to oral intake)

    (f) Low-output enterocutaneous fistulae (< 500 ml/day)* (elemental diets may hasten closure of fistula)

2. Clinical conditions where enteral nutrition would normally be helpful

    (a) Major trauma (see 1(a) and 1(b))

    (b) Radiation therapy (see 1(a) and 1(b))

    (c) Mild chemotherapy (see 1(a) and 1(b))

3. Clinical settings where enteral nutrition is of limited or undetermined value

    (a) Intensive chemotherapy (parenteral nutrition is often indicated)

    (b) Immediate postoperative period or poststress period (especially if an adequate oral intake will be resumed within 5 to 7 days)

    (c) Acute enteritis

    (d) Less than 10 per cent remaining small intestine (parenteral nutrition is usually indicated)

4. Clinical settings in which enteral nutrition should not be used

    (a) Complete mechanical intestinal obstruction

    (b) Ileus or intestinal hypomotility

    (c) Severe uncontrollable diarrhoea

    (d) High-output fistulae

    (e) Severe acute pancreatitis

    (f) Shock

    (g) Aggressive nutritional support not desired by the patient or legal guardian, and such action being in accordance with hospital policy and existing law

    (h) Prognosis not warranting aggressive nutritional support

*If the fistula is proximal, the feeding should be distal. If the fistula is distal, sufficient proximal length must be present to allow sufficient absorption. Fistulae due to malignancy, radiation, and distal obstruction are unlikely to close spontaneously.

tional balance. However, as Fig. 3 indicates, the relationship between intake and nitrogen balance is disturbed so that the more severe the injury, the greater the catabolism. In practice, many patients become malnourished following a severe catabolic injury, so that the response to nutrient intake is intermediate between malnutrition uncomplicated by disease and severe injury uncomplicated by malnutrition.

From these different responses (Fig. 3) some general recommendations emerge for nitrogen intake. (Fig. 4). The recommended energy intake also varies with the clinical state. In well-nourished individuals who are likely to receive nutritional support for long periods, it is wise to aim for energy balance. In the depleted patient, it is desirable to achieve a positive energy balance (as well as a positive nitrogen balance), whereas in obese individuals, loss of adiposity (while limiting the loss of lean tissue) is desirable.

In calculating energy requirements it is also important to remember that reduced physical activity often offsets any increase in basal metabolic rate due to disease. Even in ambulatory patients receiving parenteral nutrition in hospital and at home, total 24-h energy expenditure has often been found to be 1700 to 2300 kcal/day (7140 to 9660 kJ/day).

Energy requirement varies substantially with body size, nutritional status, and disease activity. Approximate estimates for requirements are given in Fig. 4. Most hospitalized adult patients generally require 1500 to 2500 kcal (6300 to 10 500 kJ)and between 10 and 15 g N/day. In prescribing artificial feeding it is often possible to approximate the requirements to the contents of three or four standard regimens, to monitor the patient's progress, and to adjust accordingly. The intake of energy can sometimes be reduced in the acute phase of disease, when there is metabolic instability and substantial intolerance to nutrients such as glucose, or in obese individuals. The intake of protein may be reduced in hepatic encephalopathy, and in renal failure if the aim is to reduce the uraemia and either to avoid dialysis or to increase the interval between dialyses. However, protein requirements are frequently administered and the patient is dialysed according to needs. Fluid restriction may limit the administration of nutrients and a compromise between the general clinical and nutrient needs may be necessary.

Fluid

Usually 1.5 to 3.0 litres of fluid are given to adults receiving enteral (around 1.5–2.0 litres) or parenteral nutrition (around 1.5–3.0 litres), but different intakes may be required. Particularly high fluid and electrocyte requirements are necessary in patients with large-output intestinal fistulae. Usually the fluid allocated to nutritional support is restricted, partly because the patient may already be receiving fluid for other purposes (for example infusions of drugs and blood), and partly because the clinical conditions demand it. Low fluid intake may be necessary in oedematous patients, those with renal hepatic or cardiac failure, and patients who have suffered a recent head injury. After head injury fluid restriction is frequently recommended to limit brain oedema, which can adversely affect clinical outcome; however, some head-injured subjects may develop diabetes insipidus, when extra fluid is required. Patients with burns also have high fluid requirements. On the other hand, many acute diseases (such as various forms of trauma or injury) are associated with impaired renal excretion of water and salt loads, and therefore fluid balance has to be monitored carefully. In the intensive care unit, fluid intake is often modified according to measurements of central venous pressure. Major changes in body weight from one day to the next can also help in the assessment of fluid requirement since these predominantly reflect changes in fluid balance.

Minerals and trace elements

For many adult patients receiving artificial nutritional support, the recommended intake of sodium and potassium is 50 to 100 mmol/day. Chloride intake is usually similar to that of sodium, and phosphate is usually prescribed at a dose of 20 to 40 mmol/day. However, since artificial nutrition is used in a wide range of patients with different disorders it is not surprising that mineral requirements vary considerably. For example, sodium restriction may be necessary in patients with renal, hepatic, and cardiac failure who are prone to fluid retention. Additional sodium is required in patients with increased gastrointestinal effluents. The additional requirements of sodium and potassium can be predicted from effluent composition as indicated in Table 3. Note that the loss of 1 litre of gastrointestinal fluid may more than double the sodium requirements while affecting potassium requirements to a much smaller extent. However, more potassium may be required in patients with excessive renal losses. Potassium requirements may double in patients receiving amphotericin B, which is often given to recipients of a bone marrow transplant. Adequate amounts of potassium and phosphate, which are predominantly intracellular ions, are also necessary during repletion of lean tissue. Indeed, deficiencies of these substances can exacerbate negative nitrogen balance.

The recommended intakes of calcium, magnesium, and many trace elements are quite different for oral/enteral nutrition compared with intravenous nutrition (Table 4). This is because the gut only absorbs a proportion of these nutrients, sometimes less than 10 per cent (for example in the case of chromium). Prolonged intravenous administration of trace elements at the dose recommended orally may prove to be toxic. One of the functions of the gut is to limit the uptake of potentially toxic substances that may be present in excess in the diet or in the gut. The gut is the most important organ regulating the availability to the body of some trace elements, as in the case of iron and manganese for which there is little capacity for disposal by other organs such as the kidney or liver. However, the gut does not appear to be so important in the regulation of fluorine, iodine, or selenium status.

The requirements of trace elements in various diseases are not clearly established, although patients with intestinal fluid losses may have substantially greater requirements for zinc (see footnote to Table 4).

Vitamins

In contrast to the intravenous recommendations for trace elements, which are generally lower (sometimes by severalfold) than those given orally, the reverse is true for vitamins (Table 5). This is partly because the vitamins are

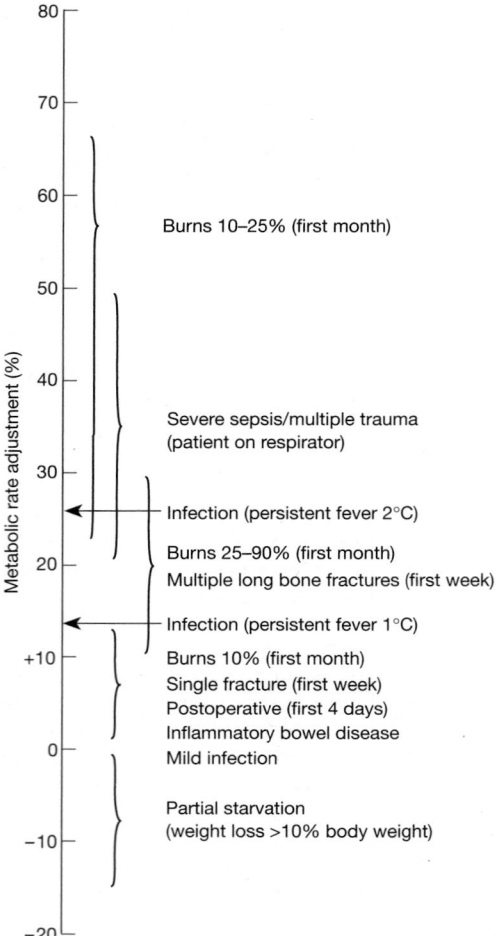

Fig. 4 Guidelines for estimating the approximate energy and nitrogen (N) requirements (1 g N = 6.25 g protein) for an adult patient receiving artificial nutritional support (based on Elia 1994). Energy: 1, Estimate the approximate basal metabolic rate of a normal adult with the same weight as the patient from standard reference tables. 2, Adjust the basal metabolic rate for disease according to the accompanying nonogram. 3, Add a combined factor for activity and thermogenesis (mainly diet induced)—bed-bound plus10 per cent; bed-bound, mobile/sitting, plus 15 to 20 per cent; mobile on ward, plus 25 per cent. 4, If an increase in energy stores is required add 400 to 800 kcal/day (1680 to 3360 kJ/day). If a decrease in energy stores is required energy intake can be reduced. Protein: 1, Consult the nonogram to determine the degree of hypermetabolism—0 per cent, 0.17 g N/kg/day ('normal' protein requirement); 5 to 25 per cent, 0.2 g N/kg/day; more than 25 per cent, 0.20 to 0.25 g N/kg/day. 2, If patient is depleted can increase to 0.25 (0.2 to 0.3) g N/kg/day For obese individuals with a body mass index of 30 to 40 kg/m² use about 75 per cent of the value estimated from body weight and for those with a body mass index over 40 kg/m² use about 60 to 65 per cent of the value estimated from body weight

Table 3 Approximate electrolyte content of intestinal effluents (mmol/l)

	Na	K	HCO₃	Cl
Gastric	60	15	–	90
Pancreatic	140	5	90	75
Biliary	140	5	35	100
Small intestinal	100	10	25	100
Diarrhoea	60	30	45	45

Table 4 Recommended daily oral and parenteral intakes of calcium, magnesium, and trace elements in adults

Mineral or trace element	Oral (mg)*		Intravenous (mg)†
	Men	Women	
Calcium	800	800	240–400
Magnesium	350	280	140–290
Iron	10	15	1–2
Zinc	15	12	2.5–4.0‡
Copper	1.5–3.0	1.5–3.0	0.5–1.5
Iodine	0.15	0.15	0.1–0.2
Manganese	2–5	2–5	0.15–0.8§
Fluorine	1.5–4.0	1.5–4.0	1–3
Chromium	0.05–0.20	0.05–0.20	0.007–0.013§
Selenium	0.070	0.055	0.03–0.06
Molybdenum	0.075–0.25	0.075–0.25	0.015–0.030

*Recommended dietary allowances (National Research Council 1989). The values are for adult males (79 kg) and non-pregnant, non-lactating women (63 kg) aged 25 to 50 years. Values for those aged over 50 years are generally identical. Some values are indicated as ranges because there is less information on which to base precise recommendations.
†Based on American Medical Association (1989) and Elia (1994).
‡Add 2 mg in the acute catabolic state and 12 to 17 mg per litre of intestinal effluent lost.
§These doses, especially those at the upper end of the range, are probably overestimates since they have been reported to result consistently in supraphysiological concentrations.

generally absorbed to a much greater extent than most trace elements, and partly because their requirement probably increases in many diseases. Although the vitamin requirements in particular diseases, especially infective and active inflammatory ones, are not well established, the requirements for some vitamins may be considerably greater than in health. In addition, some vitamins may degrade during the preparation and storage of parenteral nutrition solutions. For example vitamin A, riboflavin, and vitamin K are photosensitive, and vitamin C may degrade in the presence of trace elements and oxygen. Thiamin can degrade in the presence of sulphite, which is used as a preservative, and vitamin A palmitate may be adsorbed on some plastic storage bags or administration sets. It should be

Table 5 Recommended oral and parenteral intake of vitamins in adults

Vitamin	Oral (mg)*		Parenteral (mg)†
	Men	Women	
Water soluble			
Thiamin (B$_1$)	1.5	1.1	3.0
Riboflavin (B$_2$)	1.7	1.3	3.6
Niacin (B$_5$)	19	15	40
Pyridoxine (B$_6$)	2.0	1.6	4.0
Folate (B$_9$)	0.2	0.18	0.4
B$_{12}$	0.002	0.002	0.005
Pantothenic acid (B$_3$)	4–7	4–7	15
Biotin (B$_7$)	0.03–0.1	0.03–0.1	0.1
Ascorbic acid (C)	60	60	100
Fat soluble			
Vitamin A‡	1	0.8	1.0
Vitamin D§	0.005	0.005	0.005
Vitamin E¶	10	8	10
Vitamin K	0.08	0.65	–

*Recommended dietary allowances (National Research Council 1989). The values relate to adult males (79 kg) and non-pregnant, non-lactating females (63 kg) aged 25–50 years. Values for those aged >50 years are similar to those indicated. Some values are indicated as ranges because there is less information on which to base allowances.
†Based on American Medical Association (1979).
‡Retinol equivalents: 1 retinol equivalent = 6 μg β-carotene.
§As cholecalciferol: 10 μg cholecalciferol=400 IU vitamin D.
¶α-tocopherol equivalents: 1 mg D-α-tocopherol = 1 α-tocopherol equivalent.

also be remembered that some patients are depleted of vitamins prior to the initiation of therapy, and therefore extra intake is necessary to replete the stores.

Manufactured enteral feeds have a long shelf-life and contain trace elements and vitamins. Parenteral feeds have a shorter shelf-life and vitamins and trace elements are often added shortly before use because of the concern about stability (see above). Vitamin K need not be added routinely in parenteral feeds and particular care must be taken in patients who are on anticoagulants. Sufficient quantities of this vitamin are normally synthesized in the gut but a weekly intramuscular dose is often recommended, especially in those receiving antibiotics that affect the metabolism of intestinal bacteria. More frequent doses may be given to patients with liver disease who have a coagulation problem and are at risk of gastrointestinal bleeding.

Although deficiencies are not likely to develop for months or possibly years (vitamin A, vitamin D, vitamin B$_{12}$), it is usual practice to administer a mixture of trace elements and vitamins from the outset even if nutritional support is only likely to be required for a few weeks. This is because the stores of some (mainly water-soluble vitamins such as thiamin and riboflavin) are very small. Furthermore, some patients are malnourished at presentation so that the stores of other trace elements or vitamins may already be depleted.

Complications of artificial nutritional support: prevention, treatment, and monitoring

A summary of the complications that may be encountered during parenteral and enteral nutrition is given in Table 6.

Parenteral nutrition

Mechanical

Complications related to the insertion of a central venous catheter, usually into the subclavian vein, are not common, although pneumothorax may occur in 2 to 3 per cent of cases (the frequency depends on the expertise of the person involved in the procedure). The insertion of the catheter is carried out under aseptic conditions and the position of the catheter tip is confirmed radiologically after insertion. Radiography also helps exclude other complications such as pneumothorax.

Many of the risks associated with parenteral nutrition can be reduced by following appropriate protocols. For example, laying the patient head down while changing feeds and checking the position of locks prevents air embolism. The use of strict aseptic techniques is essential to prevent catheter-related sepsis (see below).

Occlusion of the catheter may result from reflux of blood into the catheter, but it may also result from coagulation of the feed, especially when all-in-one solutions which include lipid are infused. The incidence of catheter blockage depends on how long the catheter is used for, the diameter of the catheter, the type of catheter (soft polyurethane and Teflon catheters are said to have a lower risk of thrombosis than rigid polyethylene catheters), and the type of feed administered (all-in-one mixtures tend to cause line blockage more readily). In patients receiving cyclic nocturnal feeding, flushing the catheter with heparin (50 IU/ml) at the end of feeding reduces the risk of thrombosis. Some recommend routine inclusion of heparin (2–3 IU/ml) in the parenteral nutrition solution to prevent both catheter blockage and local venous thrombosis. Several methods may be tried to unblock an occluded catheter. Gentle suction may remove the clot. The clot may be lysed by inserting a solution of urokinase (5000 U/ml) for about 1 h. Alcohol (50 per cent) may be used in a similar way to dissolve lipid-associated occlusions. Insertion of hydrochloric acid (1 M) into the catheter is another potentially effective method.

Infections

Catheter-related infection is an important complication. The infecting organisms are typically derived from the skin (for example *Staphylococcus*

Table 6 Some complications associated with enteral and parenteral nutrition

Parenteral	Enteral
Mechanical	
Catheter malposition	Tube malposition (e.g. placement in trachea)
Insertion trauma: pneumothorax, arterial/venous damage (bleeding), branchial plexus injury, chylothorax, cardiac injury, cardiac arrhythmia, fistula	Insertion trauma: nasogastric damage to nasal septum, oesophagus, stomach; perforation (rare); tracheobroncheal fistula (rare)
	Gastrostomy/enterostomy: damage to stomach, small bowel, bleeding; peritonitis; leakage, irritation, and infection around the ostomy
Catheter blockage, kinking, or occlusion	Tube blockage, kinking, or occlusion
Catheter embolus	Loss of tube into gastrointestinal tract
Air embolus	
Thrombosis and embolism from catheter tip or vein surrounding catheter	
Feed/flow related	
Substrate overload	Diarrhoea or constipation
Glucose: hyperglycaemia and hyperosmolarity (flow related)	Bloated abdomen and/or cramps
Fat: infusional hyperlipidaemia	Regurgitation/aspiration pneumonia
Amino acids: hyperammonaemia (infants); uraemia (renal disease)	Hyperglycaemia
Infections	
Catheter-related sepsis	Infection of feed or administration set
Infected feed/administration set	Infection around ostomy
Infection around catheter entry site	
Metabolic	
Fluid and electrolyte disturbances	Fluid and electrolyte disturbances
Deficiency syndromes, e.g. trace elements, vitamins, essential fatty acids	Deficiency syndromes (rare with standard feeds in typical patients)
Hyper/hypoglycaemia	Hyper/hypoglycaemia
Substrate overload (see text)	
Organ tissue dysfunction	
Abnormal liver function	Mainly disease related
Intestinal atrophy (source of bacterial sepsis)	Aspiration pneumonia may precipitate respiratory distress
Respiratory distress (excess nutrient administration)	
Metabolic bone disease	
Allergic reactions	
For example to lipid (rare)	Occasionally with some feed constituents (avoided with elemental diets)
Psychological	
Anxiety	As for parenteral
Depression	
Abnormal self-image	
Social isolation (home nutrition)	

aureus, *Staphylococcus epidermidis*), although a variety of other organisms from the systemic circulation including Gram-negative organisms and fungi may seed on to the catheter tip, especially when it is associated with a fibrin clot. Catheter-related sepsis can largely be avoided by the use of aseptic techniques during insertion of the catheter and during the change of feeds, and by avoiding the use of the central venous catheter for purposes other than feeding, such as blood sampling or the administration of drugs and blood.

When catheter-related sepsis is strongly suspected and the patient is unwell and deteriorating, the catheter should be removed. However, it should be remembered that most episodes of pyrexia are not due to catheter-related sepsis, and the skill of the physician/surgeon in diagnosing alternative causes (such as wound infection, pyrexia of trauma, urinary tract infection in patients with urinary catheters, pulmonary embolism) can prevent unnecessary removal of central venous catheters and the hazards that accompany recannulation. Blood cultures taken both from the central venous line and a peripheral vein and a swab from the catheter enteral site may help to identify the type of organism causing sepsis, and the likelihood that it is related to the catheter.

The procedure of tunnelling the line under the skin from its site of insertion (typically the subclavian vein) to the anterior chest wall makes dressing and care of the catheter easier, and the location is often more comfortable for the patient. However, there is little evidence that the use of a tunnelling procedure reduces the incidence of catheter-related sepsis.

Multilumen catheters are sometimes required for multiple uses (sampling and administration of blood, and use for infusion of parenteral solutions including drug therapy). They have the advantage of convenience, especially in patients with limited peripheral venous access. Reports suggest that such catheters become infected more frequently than single-lumen catheters used solely for parenteral nutrition but this is not surprising because multilumen catheters are used in patients who have more severe disease.

Metabolic complications

Fluid and electrolyte abnormalities are common during parenteral nutrition. This is largely because the underlying condition may result in excess fluid and electrolyte losses (postoperative nasogastric losses, intestinal fistula, etc.) or retention (renal, cardiac, and hepatic failure). Drug therapy may also affect acid–base fluid and electrolyte status. Clinicians involved with the nutritional support of the patient must liaise closely with those involved with other aspects of management. The nutrition team has an important role, partly because it can make the necessary daily adjustments of fluid and electrolytes in the parenteral nutrition solution and partly because it can make adjustments to other minerals or micronutrients that are not administered routinely to ill patients, for example additions of zinc and magnesium in patients with persistent loss of intestinal effluent. Magnesium deficiency may lead to neuromuscular excitability and tetany. It may also produce hypocalcaemia which is not corrected by calcium administration. Zinc deficiency may impair wound healing and produce severe dermatitis.

Hyperglycaemia is common in patients receiving parenteral nutrition in hospital. This is largely because glucose intolerance is frequently associated with severe disease. It can be managed by reducing the intake of glucose (with or without an increase in lipid intake) or by administering insulin, either as a constant infusion or by intermittent subcutaneous or intramuscular injections, at a dose determined by blood glucose concentrations. Particularly high glucose concentrations may occur if the rate of infusion of nutrients is not adequately regulated. Without the use of an infusion pump the rate of infusion may increase severalfold to cause severe hyperglycaemia, hyperosmolarity, headaches, vomiting, and an impaired level of consciousness.

Abnormal liver-related tests are frequently observed in patients receiving parenteral nutrition in hospital, for example increased activities of glutamate oxaloacetate transaminase, serum glutamic pyruvic transaminase, and alkaline phosphatase. These frequently reflect the underlying disease (such as sepsis, malignancy, inflammatory bowel disease, pre-existing liver disease) but other factors may be involved: infusion of lipid or excess glucose (leading to hepatic steatosis); bacterial overgrowth in the intestine; and biliary sludge and even gallstones. The prolonged absence of oral intake during parenteral nutrition fails to stimulate normal gallbladder contraction and this is probably responsible for the development of biliary sludge. Detailed investigation of abnormal liver function (biochemical tests, ultrasound scans, and sometimes liver biopsy) may, on occasion, be necessary to discover the underlying pathology.

Deficiencies of phosphate and essential fatty acids have both been reported during parenteral nutrition, arising from their lack of inclusion in parenteral nutrition solutions. Phosphate deficiency can cause muscle weakness and impair the utilization of protein. It also causes hypercalcaemia and, in the long term, bone disease. Deficiency of essential fatty acids produces alopecia, thrombocytopenia, anaemia, and a skin rash as early as 6 weeks after starting intravenous nutritional support without fat. Biochemically, it is diagnosed by an increase in the triene to tetraene ratio (> 0.4) since, in the absence of linoleic acid, oleic acid is metabolized to eicosatrienoic acid. The condition is more likely to develop in patients receiving continuous rather than intermittent parenteral nutrition, because essential fatty acids from the endogenous lipid stores are continually prevented from being released by hyperinsulinaemia. The deficiency syndrome is rapidly reversed by administering an intravenous lipid. Regular application to the skin of oils containing essential fatty acids allows sufficient absorption of fatty acids to treat or prevent this syndrome.

In patients intolerant of lipid (for example patients with hyperlipidaemia and some patients with renal or hepatic disease or diabetes) hypertriglyceridaemia results. This may affect the assays of a number of standard biochemical tests and dilute other plasma constituents (thereby causing pseudohyponatraemia). Visual inspection of plasma for lipid several hours after cessation of the lipid infusion can alert the clinician to this problem. Measurement of plasma triglycerides provides a more accurate assessment.

Lipid infusion has been implicated in affecting the function of some organs. For example, hepatic steatosis may cause abnormal liver function tests, and lung deposition in patients with respiratory distress can impair pulmonary function by reducing the permeability of the lung to gases.

Excessive administration of glucose may also have adverse respiratory effects. This is because glucose produces 30 per cent more CO_2 per MJ than fat, and an even greater amount of CO_2 per MJ when there is net lipogenesis from carbohydrate. Furthermore, excessive administration of glucose increases energy expenditure (dietary-induced thermogenesis) to a greater extent than fat. In patients with impaired pulmonary function this may precipitate respiratory failure, or impair weaning of a patient with respiratory failure from a respirator. However, with the typical amount of glucose infused in most patients this is a theoretical rather than a practical occurrence and the use of high-fat regimens is generally not indicated.

Metabolic bone disease (mainly osteoporosis) is associated with long-term parenteral nutrition (usually home parenteral nutrition). Several factors may contribute, including corticosteroid therapy, the underlying disease, and immobility. Excess amino acid intake and heparin have also been implicated. Aluminium toxicity has been implicated as a cause of a painful metabolic bone disorder.

Trace element and vitamin deficiencies may occur in patients on long-term parenteral nutrition. Usually this is due to the prescription of insufficient amounts, but excessive losses of intestinal effluents may also be responsible. Deficiencies of several trace elements have been described, for example copper, zinc, iron, selenium, as well as case reports of chromium and molybdenum deficiencies. Several vitamin deficiencies have also been described, including biotin deficiency (eczematous dermatitis, hair loss, depression, anorexia) which is rare under normal circumstances, and night blindness due to vitamin A deficiency. These should be uncommon if appropriate protocols are followed.

Enteral nutrition

The complications most associated with enteral feeding in hospitalized patients include nausea or vomiting (10–20 per cent), abnormal bloating and cramps, diarrhoea (5–30 per cent), and constipation (but mainly in long-term feeders at home). Delayed gastric emptying is a feature of many conditions including postoperative abdominal surgery, head injury, and severe sepsis. Gastric stasis may lead to accumulation of feed in the stomach, so that eventually the patient develops nausea and vomiting.

In unconscious patients and those with an impaired swallowing reflex, vomiting may lead to aspiration pneumonia, which is one of the most serious complications of enteral nutrition. Gastro-oesophageal regurgitation may also predispose to aspiration pneumonia. Some of the effects of poor gastric emptying can be prevented by administering the feed directly into the small intestine. A nasogastric tube may be placed in the small intestine under radiographic control, endoscopically, or during surgery. In those at risk of gastric stasis/regurgitation, gastric pooling can be checked by intermittent aspiration through tubes with a sufficiently wide bore. Continuous infusion of feed into the stomach can prevent the sudden gastric disturbance associated with bolus feeding. The use of an infusion pump to control delivery of feed into the stomach can prevent gastric flooding associated with inadequate manual flow control systems. The use of metoclopramide or erythromycin, which stimulate gastric emptying, may be beneficial. Erythromycin acts as a motilin receptor agonist.

Despite the frequency of diarrhoea in patients receiving enteral tube feeding in hospital, the mechanism is not entirely understood. However, it is often associated with antibiotic therapy. Lactose intolerance has also been implicated but most enteral feeds are free of lactose. Rapid delivery of nutrients into the gastrointestinal tract may lead to diarrhoea, especially if the delivery is postpyloric. Here the protective effect of the pylorus in regulating delivery of nutrients into the small intestine is bypassed. Other factors have been implicated, including bacterial contamination of enteral diets, an underlying gastrointestinal disease, the use of laxatives, lack of dietary fibre, and neuroendocrine reflexes whereby the administration of feed in the stomach or upper small intestine cause secretion of fluid in the small and large bowel. Diarrhoea may be prevented by taking care not to contaminate the feed with bacteria, controlling the rate of feed infusion, and/or treating the underlying condition. Drugs such as codeine phosphate or loperamide may help to control the symptoms.

Constipation may also complicate long-term enteral nutrition, particularly in elderly, inactive subjects. Lack of fibre has been implicated, but the constipation remains despite fibre supplements.

Another potential problem is regurgitation of feed in patients with impaired gastro-oesophageal function, such as elderly people with a hiatus hernia who have an impaired swallowing reflex. This may lead to aspiration pneumonia which can be avoided by administering the feed with the upper part of the body elevated to an angle of about 30°; in those with a high risk of aspiration, it is best to administer the feed directly into the small intestine (jejunostomy feeding).

Several metabolic disturbances have been described during enteral feeding: hyperglycaemia in glucose-intolerant subjects; rebound hypoglycaemia after sudden withdrawal of feed; disturbances in plasma potassium, depending on the patient's renal and gastrointestinal function and the potassium content of the feed; hypophosphataemia during refeeding. Refeeding malnourished subjects may produce hypophosphataemia and hypokalaemia as lean tissues containing these electrolytes are accreted. New legislative regulations implemented in the European Community in 1999, which demand that the micronutrient to energy ratio is within a specific range, should reduce the incidence of trace element, mineral and vitamin deficiencies.

The complications of enteral nutrition at home are similar to those in hospital. However, lack of enteral access (due to tube blockage or dislodgement) can be an important problem, because it may lead to dehydration, especially in those with swallowing-related problems who are prevented from drinking. Flushing of the tubes with water at the end of each feeding period can prevent tube blockage. A blocked tube may be unblocked by flushing it with water in the first instance, followed by a warm solution of sodium bicarbonate or by digesting the coagulated feed with pancreatic enzymes. Fizzy cola drinks may also be effective in unblocking tubes. If a gastrostomy or enterostomy tube has been dislodged, it is important to replace it quickly because the stoma may rapidly close up and make further access difficult.

General monitoring of patients on artificial nutritional support

Careful observations should be made of the patient shortly after the start of enteral or parenteral nutrition to assess feed tolerance. In patients receiving parenteral nutrition, urine should be analysed every 4 h to check for glycosuria, and blood glucose should be measured in these patients and others with suspected glucose intolerance. The development of glycosuria in previously stable patients without glycosuria may indicate the development of a complication such as infection before it has been diagnosed clinically in hospital. Routine measurements of temperature, pulse, blood pressure, and fluid balance are also essential. Changes in daily weight are the best indices of day-to-day changes in fluid balance. In the longer term, changes in weight usually indicate changes in lean and adipose tissue in response to the support provided.

The frequency with which other investigations are carried out depends on the patient and the underlying condition (see also above). In patients with large losses of gastrointestinal fluids or those on long-term parenteral nutrition (especially when there is little or no enteral or oral intake) an assessment of trace element and/or vitamin status is often necessary. The catheter site should be inspected regularly as a possible source of infection, and fresh dressings applied according to standard protocols.

In patients receiving enteral tube feeding, it is important to assess feed tolerance by ensuring that gastric pooling does not occur, especially in those at risk of gastric stasis and those with an impaired swallowing reflex. The development of diarrhoea should be investigated promptly so that appropriate action (such as adjustment of infusion rate or eradication of specific gastrointestinal pathogens) can be taken.

Nutritional aspects of specific conditions

The reader is referred to other sections for information on nutritional and fluid and electrolyte aspects of various clinical conditions, for example acute and chronic renal failure, malabsorption syndrome, hyperlipidaemia, diabetes mellitus, cystic fibrosis, short bowel syndrome, and enterocutaneous fistulae. Nutritional aspects of other conditions that have recently gained prominence are discussed here.

Acquired immune deficiency syndrome (AIDS)

AIDS has important nutritional consequences. Early studies suggested that weight loss at death was commonly over 20 per cent of body weight, and sometimes more than 40 per cent of body weight. Severe weight loss occurs in low-income countries but in more developed countries where protease inhibitors have been extensively used, survival has been prolonged and the frequency of severe undernutrition has been reduced. These changes have been associated with the development of a syndrome that includes abnormal central fat distribution, hyperlipidaemia, and a tendency to lactic acidosis. In the long term, the risks of malnutrition may be replaced by an increased risk of cardiovascular disease. Important clinical problems evident in the era before antiprotease therapy remain relevant to patients in high-income countries, especially at presentation, as well as those in countries where protease inhibitors are not widely used.

Acute weight loss is usually a consequence of acute infections, whereas more chronic loss is usually associated with an enteropathy. There are many direct causes of weight loss. Food intake is usually decreased during acute infections, but during recovery it may be normal or even greater than nor-

mal. In advanced AIDS decreased food intake is often associated with opportunistic infections in the mouth, pharynx, and oesophagus, which may cause pain and dysphagia. Associated malignancy (Kaposi's sarcoma and non-Hodgkin's lymphoma) may also lead to anorexia. Furthermore, antifungal and antiviral drugs can cause nausea, vomiting, and anorexia, and the use of chemotherapeutic agents for malignancy can produce stomatitis, pharyngitis, and oesophagitis, which can make swallowing painful and distressing. The enteropathy can be caused by many pathogens and can lead to steatorrhoea, fluid and electrolyte disturbances, and trace element and vitamin deficiencies. Neurological disease is also often associated with malnutrition. Dysphagia and coma obviously lead to reduced nutrient intake and malnutrition, and 'dementia', which may affect half the patients with advanced AIDS, may make dietary assessment and management particularly difficult.

Treatment of the underlying condition, such as mouth, throat, and other systemic infections which cause dysphagia, or systemic infections which cause anorexia, can do much to improve nutritional status. There is substantial anabolic potential between acute infective episodes, and the rapid diagnosis and treatment of such infections produce better nutritional results than delayed treatment.

Nutritional assessment should begin at the outset and changes in body weight in relation to the disease process should be closely monitored. Psychological evaluation and social counselling should not be neglected. Anxiety, apathy, and depression are common and may lead to self-neglect, irregular food intake, and deterioration of nutritional status. Support should begin with general nutritional advice about diet, but it may need to progress to the use of supplements and, occasionally, enteral tube feeding or parenteral nutrition.

Surveys have shown that many patients with AIDS take supplements of vitamins and trace elements. In some cases, ingestion of a large excess of micronutrients leads to toxicity.

Burns

Severe burns provide one of the most powerful catabolic stimuli. The injury response may persist for weeks or months during the period of wound healing. It is not surprising that the nutritional requirements of such patients are greater than for most other catabolic states (see Fig. 4). Inappropriate nutritional support to metabolically unstable patients (burned or non-burned subjects) may cause severe metabolic disturbances: thus before aggressive nutritional support is started, shock and acid–base disturbances should be at least stabilized.

With minor burns a normal oral intake, with or without supplements, is all that is required. However, with severe burns, anorexia is frequently severe and prolonged, and artificial nutritional support is usually required.

Feeding through a nasogastric tube is often well tolerated. However, the use of enteral tube feeding may be restricted early after burns because of gastric stasis or ileus. In most patients gastrointestinal motility improves within 2 to 4 days, so that more nutrients can be administered. Nevertheless, it is important to aspirate the gastric contents intermittently, especially in the early phase after burns, to ensure that there is no gastric pooling. The fluid and electrolyte requirements are often considered in association with nutritional needs, and frequently extra fluid is drunk or given through the enteral feeding tube or an intravenous line, to match the increased fluid losses from the skin surface. Some units routinely provide extra micronutrients, but the extent to which vitamin and trace element requirements are increased after burns is poorly defined.

In patients with severe burns, and those with other associated problems such as intra-abdominal injuries and sepsis, smoke inhalation, and multiorgan failure resulting in artificial ventilation, ileus often persists. In others, the gastrointestinal tract may not tolerate sufficient enteral nutrition to meet the increased requirements of the patient. Some patients, particularly those with severe burns, may thus need both enteral and parenteral nutrition. The enteral feeding is to be encouraged because it may maintain gut integrity, prevent bacterial translocation from the gut into the systemic circulation, and speed up the transition from parenteral nutrition to normal oral intake.

Head injury

Head injury provides another important indication for artificial nutritional support, especially since many patients have an impaired level of consciousness for prolonged periods.

Head injury frequently coexists with other major injuries, with the result that there is a severe hypermetabolic and catabolic response (for example, the negative nitrogen balance may be greater than 20 g N/day in the first week after injury even when a limited intake of nutrients is provided).

Immobility contributes to the loss of muscle bulk and weight loss can occur very rapidly. One of the main constraints to the use of enteral tube feeding is delayed gastric emptying, which frequently lasts for more than 10 days after severe head injury. This may be due to the injury alone but it may also be due to associated abdominal trauma. The use of traditional nasogastric feeding techniques in such patients often makes it difficult to provide the full nutritional requirements within 1 to 2 weeks. The impaired level of consciousness and poor or absent swallowing reflex also means that gastric pooling and aspiration are not uncommon. Parenteral nutrition has been used routinely in some centres but more recently increasing emphasis has been placed on enteral feeding, partly because it may prevent mucosal atrophy and bacterial translocation from the gut, and partly because parenteral nutrition is associated with a number of potentially serious complications, such as catheter-related sepsis (see above). Therefore, attempts have been made to improve methods of delivering nutrients enterally. This includes the use of pump-assisted delivery and the use of metoclopramide and erythromycin to stimulate gastric emptying. Attempts have also been made to introduce feeds directly into the small intestine, either endoscopically or under radiological control. Bypassing the stomach can allow sufficient delivery of feed to be achieved, but displacement of the tube back into the stomach may occur. Another way of dealing with the problem of gastric stasis is to place jejunostomy tubes, using a laparoscopic percutaneous procedure. Preliminary results of feed tolerance in non-randomized studies of injury are encouraging but further work is needed, particularly since the tubes may be regurgitated back into the stomach.

In patients in whom enteral feeding is not successful, for example when there is poor gastric emptying, difficulties in placing a nasojejunal tube, or severe feed-induced diarrhoea, parenteral nutrition is indicated.

Acute pancreatitis

In patients with acute pancreatitis, malnutrition may arise because of anorexia, prolonged ileus, and catabolic complications such as necrotizing pancreatitis (in around 15 per cent of patients) and pancreatitic infection (in around 4 per cent of patients). There is also concern that enteral feeding will stimulate pancreatic exocrine function and precipitate further attacks of pancreatitis or delay recovery from the initial attack. Therefore, parenteral nutrition was routinely advocated for severe and complicated cases of acute pancreatitis. Parenteral nutrition continues to have an important role in the management of acute pancreatitis, especially when it is complicated by enteric fistulae or when enteral nutrition cannot be used to administer sufficient nutrients to meet needs. However, the recent trend is to use less parenteral nutrition and more delivery of nutrients directly into the jejunum. This trend has come about because there is no evidence that parenteral nutrition improves clinical outcome compared with no nutritional support in patients with mild to moderate pancreatitis. There is also no evidence that jejunal feeding adversely affects outcome by stimulating exocrine pancreatic secretions. Indeed, three recent randomized controlled trials suggest that early nasojejunal feeding (2 days after the onset of pancreatitis) has advantages over parenteral nutrition with respect to the severity of subsequent disease (Ranson criteria, in a study of predominantly mild acute pancreatitis, and other indices of the inflammatory response in a study of more severe pancreatitis), and septic complications (in studies of

severe pancreatitis). Enteral tube feeding is more physiological and cheaper. Although clinical attitudes are changing, it is necessary to confirm by large randomized controlled studies that jejunal feeding attenuates the inflammatory response and improves clinical outcome to a greater extent than parenteral nutrition. In practice it is also necessary to ensure that there are adequate facilities for placing nasogastric tubes (for example radiologically or endoscopically), and for dealing with tubes that coil back into the stomach.

Transplantation

Artificial nutritional support is variably required for patients requiring a transplanted organ. With renal transplantation, where the gastrointestinal tract is not affected unless surgical complications occur, it is usual to eat normally shortly after the surgery.

Patients with liver or heart plus lung transplants are usually artificially ventilated in the intensive care unit after transplantation. Artificial nutritional support is often given during this period, especially in those with pre-existing malnutrition or postoperative complications. In those with substantial malnutrition, attempts should be made to improve nutritional status before the procedure.

Artificial nutritional support may also be required following treatment with cytotoxic drugs or radiotherapy. In bone marrow transplantation the use of aggressive cytotoxic therapy or radiotherapy may result in inflammation of the mucous membranes of the gastrointestinal tract from mouth to rectum beginning a few days after cytotoxic therapy. Swallowing then becomes painful and diarrhoea a problem. The severity of this mucositis may limit the dose of cytotoxic drugs used. A nasogastric tube is often uncomfortable to such patients, and bleeding may occur from friction with the inflamed mucosa, especially in those with thrombocytopenia, and parenteral nutrition is often required.

There is much research interest in the use of specific nutrients or bioactive substances to protect the mucosa of the gut from damage by cytotoxic drugs or radiotherapy but these have not found their place in routine clinical practice. Graft-versus-host reactions may also be accompanied by gastrointestinal symptoms. Severe, prolonged, watery diarrhoea, amounting to several litres a day, presents a serious problem. Parenteral nutrition is usually necessary after intestinal transplantation, partly because the pre-existing bowel disease produces malnutrition (many patients receiving bowel transplants are on long-term parenteral nutrition prior to the transplant), and partly because it is necessary to ensure that sufficient time has been allowed after transplant surgery to ensure that anastomoses have adequately healed and that mucosal integrity has recovered. Fluid electrolyte and trace elements may need to be given in increased amounts to balance the increased loss associated with gastrointestinal effluents. The protein and energy requirements of patients receiving transplants can be calculated according to the scheme indicated in Fig. 4.

Perioperative nutrition

Although malnutrition may be present before to elective surgery, it is more likely to occur postoperatively, especially in those with complications. Many studies have been undertaken to assess whether perioperative artificial nutritional support reduces the complication rate after surgery. They have produced conflicting results, with some suggesting improvements, others no significant effect, and in yet others an increase in infective complications (such as catheter-related sepsis) when parenteral nutrition is used. These conflicting results have occurred at least partly because of the multiple other factors that affect the outcome of surgery (age, sex, severity of disease, skill of the surgeon, nursing care, presence or absence of a nutrition team, and preoperative nutritional status). The results are also affected by the type of nutritional support provided. Preoperative enteral tube feeding has been reported to improve clinical outcome, but few studies of this exist. Postoperative oral supplements and supplementary enteral tube feeding have been have been reported to improve clinical outcome in malnourished patients with a fractured hip or femur. Postoperative supplements and enteral tube feeding in more well-nourished individuals has produced clinical benefit in only some studies. Perioperative parenteral nutrition has been more controversial.

The largest multicentre trial of perioperative parenteral nutrition (The Veteran Affairs Total Parenteral Nutrition Co-operative Study Group) involved several hundred patients undergoing elective abdominal and thoracic surgery. The routine administration of parenteral nutrition (from up to 2 weeks before surgery and at least 3 days after surgery) provided no overall benefit. However, in the subgroup of patients who were severely malnourished, perioperative nutritional support decreased the non-infective complications from 42 per cent to between 5 and 23 per cent (depending on the method used to define malnutrition). This and other studies emphasize the importance of patient selection for nutritional support. It is obvious, for instance, that other patient groups, such as those with prolonged ileus, massive bowel resection, fistulae, or recurrent severe pancreatitis, are likely to benefit from parenteral nutrition. Meticulous fluid and electrolyte balance is of major importance (see Table 3) in those with fistulae, nasogastric aspirates, or multiorgan failure.

Patients with prolonged anorexia and intra-abdominal sepsis are also likely to benefit from nutritional support. Parenteral nutrition may be required for long periods, for instance in the patient in whom the fluid output from a fistula gradually decreases in the absence of oral food intake, or after massive intestinal resection (short bowel syndrome) when intestinal adaptation may take weeks or months. In some patients with the short bowel syndrome (less than 25 cm of the small intestine remaining) such support will be required indefinitely.

Home nutritional support

One of the most important recent developments in clinical nutrition is the use of artificial nutrition in the community. In many developed countries there is now more tube feeding taking place in the community than in hospital. Furthermore, the increasing emphasis on home enteral tube feeding is likely to continue. Home parenteral nutrition is also increasing, but it is used there much less than in hospitals. In low-income countries the trend towards home care has been limited by the lack of an adequate infrastructure and organization, which are necessary to train, discharge, and monitor patients, and to ensure that the feeds and accessories are delivered to the home regularly and reliably.

Artificial nutritional support at home has a number of advantages over treatment in hospital. Patients frequently feel more comfortable in the familiar home environment, where many of them not only care for themselves but also for other family members. Affected adults may frequently go to work and children attend school. The treatment of patients at home is cheaper and frees beds for the use of other patients. Treatment at home does involve a major commitment on the part of the patient or carer and serious complications may arise.

Indications

Since most malnutrition occurs in the community, it is necessary to identify patients who are likely to benefit from simple dietary measures, the use of mixed macronutrient supplements, and home parenteral nutrition or home enteral tube feeding. The type of treatment depends on whether the gastrointestinal tract is available for the digestion and absorption of nutrients. In the case of artificial nutritional support, it is necessary to ensure that the patients or carers are able to perform the necessary tasks to a sufficiently high standard.

Food and oral supplements

When malnourished patients do not respond adequately to simple dietary advice (for example frequent ingestion of appetizing high energy density meals or snacks), mixed solid or liquid macronutrients can be given. A

systematic review of 84 trials of oral nutritional supplements in the community concluded that the supplements were much more likely to produce benefit in patients with a body mass index of less than 20.0 kg/m² than in those with a body mass index of more than 20 kg/m². Furthermore, in patients with a body mass index of less than 20 kg/m² the supplements largely added to oral intake, whereas in those with a body mass index of more than 20 kg/m² they largely replaced oral food intake. The benefits varied according to the disease. In patients with chronic obstructive airways disease the supplements increased muscle strength, walking distance, and well being. In children with cystic fibrosis they improved growth, and in elderly subjects they reduced the number of falls and increased activities of daily living. In patients with HIV infection they improved immune function tests. In general improvements were not noted unless body weight increased by more than 5 per cent. Supplements were found to be of little or no value in patients who had a body mass index of more than 20 kg/m².

Home parenteral nutrition

Intestinal failure due to Crohn's disease (with or without fistulae) is the most common indication in the United Kingdom. The short bowel syndrome, motility disorders (such as scleroderma, and pseudo-obstruction), congenital bowel disease, and radiation enteritis are also important indications. Home parenteral nutrition has also been used in patients with malignancy (usually those with intestinal obstruction) and in patients with AIDS who are unable to tolerate enteral nutrition.

Home enteral tube feeding

The principal indications are those associated with swallowing difficulties. These may be obstructive (such as malignancy of the upper gastrointestinal tract) or non-obstructive and due to neurological disorders (for example strokes, Parkinson's disease, motor neurone disease, multiple sclerosis, and primary muscle diseases that affect swallowing). In children, although a neurological disorder of swallowing is an important indication, chronic anorexia leading to failure to thrive is perhaps more common (due to, for example, congenital malformations, severe cystic fibrosis, inborn errors of metabolism, and some gastrointestinal disorders such as Crohn's disease).

Age distribution

Many patients receiving enteral nutrition at home are elderly: this is not surprising since conditions such as stroke, motor neurone disease, and oesophageal malignancy typically occur in the elderly. Home tube feeding is also relatively common in children, mainly in those aged less than 10 years. This age distribution has particular implications for home care. Many elderly people are unable to care for themselves because of weakness, immobility, arthritis, poor eyesight or hearing, etc., and therefore a carer, usually a family member, has to be identified. Similarly, carers are frequently required for children on home enteral nutrition.

The age distribution of patients on home parenteral nutrition is different, partly because the indication is often Crohn's disease, which occurs predominantly in subjects aged 20 to 50 years.

Management

The principles of artificial nutritional support at home are similar to those in hospital. Management begins with nutritional screening, so that patients with malnutrition or at high risk of malnutrition are identified, as well as the underlying risk factors (see section on nutritional screening and assessment). Nutritional goals are set, the underlying psychosocial and physical problems (active disease) are addressed, and nutritional counselling and support are provided. Normal food is encouraged whenever possible, but when this is inadequate supplements may be used. This type of nutritional support is normally initiated in the community, whereas home enteral and parenteral nutrition is usually initiated in specialist centres. Special considerations apply to patients receiving home enteral and parenteral nutrition.

Psychological evaluation

The thought that artificial nutritional support may have to be given at home for months or years may surprise some patients and they may find it difficult to accept the concept. Nevertheless, given appropriate support, as the patient or carer gains confidence their fears and anxieties frequently subside. It is always essential to involve family members (or the carer) as well as the patient. Contact with patients who are already on home treatment may do much to reassure. School-age children may also have particular difficulties in coming to terms with this form of therapy, but careful counselling and the use of nocturnal feeding alone frequently allows them to adjust, attend school, and lead a reasonably normal life.

Training

The training should be supervised only by those experienced in the field. Despite pressure for hospital beds, discharge should not take place until it is clear that the patient is adequately skilled and appropriate arrangements have been made at home.

Patients (or carers of the patients) requiring artificial nutrition at home should learn the basic principles of nutritional support and of asepsis. They should know how to program the infusion pump that delivers the nutrients, how to add solutions to the feed (if required), how to connect and disconnect the feeds to the catheter/tube, how to change dressings, how to recognize problems associated with feeding, such as a blocked catheter and infection, and how to recognize hyper/hypoglycaemia, measure blood glucose, and screen for glycosuria. Training is often helped by audiovisual aids and written instruction, and reinforced by repeated practice. A trial of home nutritional support over a weekend may be a useful way of assessing the patient's ability to adjust and cope.

Evaluation of the home environment

An assessment of the home environment is essential before discharge. There must be space available for the storage of feeds and accessories. A refrigerator is usually necessary for storage of parenteral nutrition solutions and drugs. Modifications to the home can be made to allow routine activities to be carried out more efficiently. A wheelchair or other extra equipment may be very useful for some patients, such as a bed harness for very disabled patients and adjustable V-shaped boards for children with cystic fibrosis who require physiotherapy and postural drainage of lung secretions.

Financial arrangements

Financial arrangements for home artificial nutrition clearly vary from country to country and in different parts of the same country. A clear statement about finances should be made prior to discharge. In many countries patients and/or carers are entitled to some sort of financial or other support. These should be made known to those entitled to receive them.

Written instructions and follow-up arrangements

Prior to discharge all patients should have written instructions for the routine procedures for home nutritional support and how to recognize and act when complications arise. Patients/carers should also have the telephone number of the appropriate health professional to contact in an emergency, on a 24-h basis.

Outcome

The outcome of home nutritional support varies considerably, depending on the underlying condition and the initial selection criteria.

Home parenteral nutrition

The most extensive analysis of outcome of patients on home parenteral nutrition has come from North America (Fig. 5). For a variety of con-

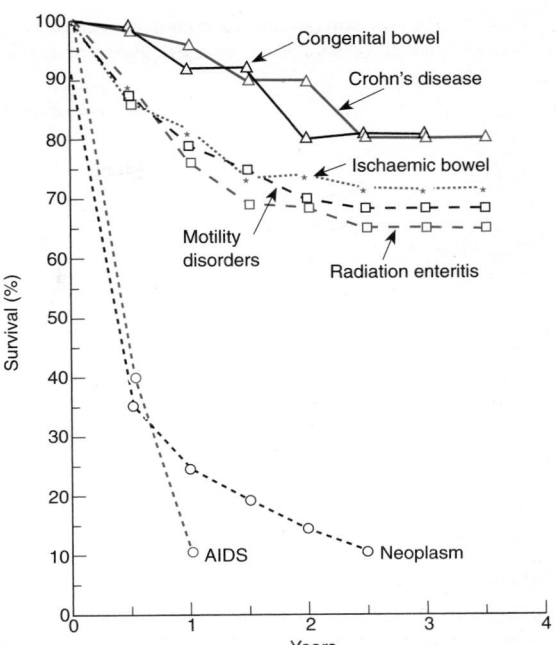

Fig. 5 Survival of different groups of patients receiving home parenteral nutrition (from Howard et al. 1991).

ditions (congenital bowel disease, Crohn's disease, motility disorders of the gut, and radiation enteritis), there is a substantial mortality in the first 2 years (10–30 per cent), but few deaths occur after this period. The mortality is usually due to the underlying condition, although a few deaths arise from complications of parenteral nutrition. Mortality in patients receiving home parenteral nutrition for AIDS and malignancy has been reported to be high (Fig. 5). For example, in one survey the mortality of AIDS patients receiving parenteral nutrition in the pre-antiprotease era was as high as 93 per cent in a year. This mortality in AIDS and malignancy clearly depends on when nutritional support is started in relation to the stage and severity of the disease. Such a high mortality dictates that such treatment should only be offered to those in whom there is good reason to expect a substantial consequent improvement in the quality of life.

In that context in general, the British Artificial Nutrition Survey has revealed that 71 per cent of patients on home parenteral nutrition undertook full normal activity, 13 per cent limited activity, and the remaining 16 per cent were housebound. Seventy-one per cent were independent, 19 per cent required some help or total help, and only 10 per cent of patients were severely disabled and heavily dependent on others.

Home enteral tube feeding

The British Artificial Nutrition Survey has provided outcome data on patients receiving home enteral and parenteral nutrition (Table 7). Only 62 per cent of patients on home enteral tube feeding were continuing at 1 year. Twenty-two per cent died whilst receiving tube feeding, but the total mortality is likely to have been greater because some patients almost certainly died after stopping tube feeding. However, there was great variability in the outcome, which was related to age, and both type and stage of disease.

Despite the high mortality, many family members feel that the quality of life of affected individuals frequently improves, or does not deteriorate. They appreciate and enjoy being with the affected family member, even in the face of a poor prognosis. In a survey of children receiving home tube feeding, predominantly for failure to thrive, parents reported greater freedom because they did not have to spend so much time trying to feed their

Table 7 One-year outcome of adult patients receiving home enteral tube feeding (HETF) and home parenteral nutrition (HPN) in Great Britain (all values are percentages),. Based on the British Artificial Nutrition Survey (Elia *et al*. 2001)

	Died whilst on HETF/HPN	Withdrew/ refused or in hospital	Returned to full oral feeding	Continuing
HETF				
All diagnoses (*n* = 16 247)	33.8	2.1*	14.3	45.7
Cerebrovascular accident (*n* = 6044)	33.1	1.5	12.9	52.7
Oesophageal cancer (*n* = 1812)	46.6	3.0	23.3	27.1
Motor neurone disease (*n* = 925)	62.9	0.9	1.3	34.8
Multiple sclerosis (*n* = 911)	14.2	1.6	3.6	80.6
Cerebral palsy (*n* = 270)	10.0	0.4	5.6	84.1
HPN				
All diagnoses (*n* = 467)	8.1	2.6*	13.1	74.2
Crohn's disease (*n* = 188)	3.7	3.7	16.5	76.1

*Time spent in hospital less 1 per cent for HETF and less 2 per cent for HPN.

children as previously. They also reported that their children were happier and more active than before tube feeding.

Monitoring

Patients on home nutritional support should be seen at regular intervals, at a frequency determined by the needs of the patient or carer and the stability of the clinical condition. It is necessary to assess whether the initial goals have been met, and if not a decision has to be made whether new goals should be set or the management changed in an attempt to meet the initial goals. Functional outcome measures, such as walking distance in patients with respiratory or motor disabilities, or eating capabilities, are particularly important. For example, patients with swallowing problems may improve and return to normal oral feeding. If swallowing function is not assessed intermittently in certain patient groups (for example those with strokes) home enteral tube feeding may continue unnecessarily. Nutritional assessment is often based on changes in growth or body weight (taking into consideration the presence or absence of oedema), but changes in skinfold thicknesses and arm muscle circumference and a variety of biochemical parameters may also be used (for example urinary creatinine in accurately collected 24-h urine specimens is a reasonable index of muscle mass).

The need for blood counts, urea and electrolytes, and liver function tests varies, depending on the clinical situation. They are more often required for those taking parenteral nutrition. Measurements of trace elements and vitamins are sensible for patients receiving long-term artificial nutrition, particularly those receiving parenteral nutrition.

Ethical considerations

Legal and ethical considerations about indications and when to start and terminate home nutritional support vary from country to country. Furthermore, the law prohibits discontinuation of nutritional support in some states in America but not in others. Particularly difficult ethical issues concern patients with dementia who stop eating for unknown reasons, and those who are unconscious or have very severe disabilities that are likely to deteriorate.

The role of nutrition teams in the management of patients in hospital and at home

Nutritional support is required for a wide range of patients distributed in different wards. A nutrition team, consisting of a clinician, a specialist nurse, dietitian, pharmacist, and possibly others such as a chemical pathologist and bacteriologist, can advise, supervise, and co-ordinate the management of patients, and maintain high standards of care. It has been shown repeatedly that such teams minimize the incidence of complications associated with nutritional support, avoid unnecessary nutritional support, and reduce wastage of feeds. The reduction in the incidence of catheter-related sepsis alone, from a rate of 25 per cent to 3 per cent has substantial economic implications, since one episode of catheter-related sepsis in a British hospital is currently estimated to cost between £1500 and £5000. Nutrition teams also have an important role to play in training patients for home support, providing advice, co-ordinating the supply of feeds and other equipment to the home, and supervising follow-up.

Further reading

American Medical Association (1979). Guidelines for essential trace element preparations for parenteral use. A statement by the nutrition advisory group. *Journal of the American Medical Association* **241**, 2051–4.

American Medical Association Department of Foods and Nutrition (1979). Multivitamin preparations for parenteral use. *Journal of Enteral and Parenteral Nutrition* **3**, 258–62.

American Society of Parenteral and Enteral Nutrition Board of Directors (1987). Guidelines for the use of enteral nutrition in the adult patient. *Journal of Parenteral and Enteral Nutrition* **11**, 435–9.

Elia M (1993). Artificial nutritional support in clinical practice in Britain. *Journal of the Royal College of Physicians* **27**, 1–15.

Elia M (1994). Home enteral nutrition: general aspect and a comparison between the United States and Britain. *Nutrition* **10**, 1–9.

Elia M, Jebb SA (1994). Nutrition. *Medicine International* **22**, 381–420.

Elia M *et al.* (2001). *Trends in artificial nutrition in the UK during 1996-2000*. British Association for Parenteral and Enteral Nutrition (BAPEN), Maidenhead, UK.

Frisancho AR (1981). New norms of upper limb fat and muscle areas for assessment of nutritional status. *American Journal of Clinical Nutrition* **34**, 2540–5.

Frisancho AR (1984). New standards of weight and body composition by frame size and height for the assessment of nutritional status of adults and the elderly. *American Journal of Clinical Nutrition* **40**, 808–19.

Green CJ (1999). Existence, causes and consequences of disease-related malnutrition in the hospital and the community, and clinical and financial benefits of nutritional intervention. *Clinical Nutrition* **18** (Suppl. 2), 3–28.

Howard L *et al.* (1991). Four years of North American Registry home parenteral nutrition outcome data and their implications for patient management. *Journal of Parenteral and Enteral Nutrition* **15**, 384–91.

Matarese LE, Gottlschlich MM (1998). *Contemporary nutrition support practice: a clinical guide*. WB Saunders, Philadelphia.

National Research Council (1989). *Recommended dietary allowances*, 10th edn. National Academy Press, Washington, DC.

Rombeau JL and Rolandelli RH (1997). *Enteral and tube feeding*. WB Saunders, Philadelphia.

Shenkin A, Wretlind A (1977). Complete intravenous nutrition including amino acids, glucose and lipids. In: Richards JJ, Kinney JM, eds. *Nutritional aspects of care in the critically ill*, pp 345–65. Churchill Livingstone, Edinburgh.

Stratton R, Elia M (1999). A critical systematic analysis of the use of oral nutritional supplements in the community. *Clinical Nutrition* **18** (Suppl. 2), 29–84.

Taylor S, Goodinson-McLaren S (1992). *Nutritional support: a team approach.* Wolfe Publishing, London.

The Veteran Affairs Total Parenteral Nutrition Co-operative Study Group (1991). Peri-operative total parenteral nutrition in surgical patients. *New England Journal of Medicine* **325**, 525–32.

Wilcock H, Armstrong J, Cottee S (1992). Artificial nutrition in a health district with particular reference to tube feeding. *Health Trends* **23**, 93–100.

Index

Note: Numbers 1., 2. and 3. preceding the page numbers denote the volume. Numbers in italic refer to tables and/or illustrations separate from the text.